Spinal Anatomy and Surgical Approaches

Degenerative Disorders of the Cervical Spine

Degenerative Disorders of the Thoracic and Lumbar Spine

CAMPBELL'S OPERATIVE ORTHOPAEDICS

CAMPBELL'S OPERATIVE ORTHOPAEDICS

THIRTEENTH EDITION

Frederick M. Azar, MD
Professor
Department of Orthopaedic Surgery and Biomedical Engineering
University of Tennessee–Campbell Clinic
Chief of Staff, Campbell Clinic
Memphis, Tennessee

James H. Beaty, MD
Harold B. Boyd Professor and Chair
Department of Orthopaedic Surgery and Biomedical Engineering
University of Tennessee–Campbell Clinic
Memphis, Tennessee

S. Terry Canale, MD
Harold B. Boyd Professor and Chair Emeritus
Department of Orthopaedic Surgery and Biomedical Engineering
University of Tennessee–Campbell Clinic
Memphis, Tennessee

EDITORIAL ASSISTANCE
Kay Daugherty and **Linda Jones**

GRAPHIC ASSISTANCE
Shawn Maxey

ELSEVIER

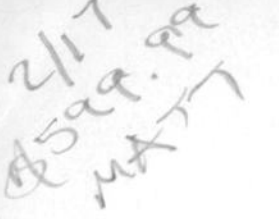

ELSEVIER

1600 John F. Kennedy Blvd.
Ste. 1800
Philadelphia, PA 19103-2899

CAMPBELL'S OPERATIVE ORTHOPAEDICS, THIRTEENTH EDITION **ISBN: 978-0-323-37462-0**
INTERNATIONAL EDITION **ISBN: 978-0-323-43380-8**

Notices

Knowledge and best practice in this field are constantly changing. As new research and experience broaden our understanding, changes in research methods, professional practices, or medical treatment may become necessary.

Practitioners and researchers must always rely on their own experience and knowledge in evaluating and using any information, methods, compounds, or experiments described herein. In using such information or methods they should be mindful of their own safety and the safety of others, including parties for whom they have a professional responsibility.

With respect to any drug or pharmaceutical products identified, readers are advised to check the most current information provided (i) on procedures featured or (ii) by the manufacturer of each product to be administered, to verify the recommended dose or formula, the method and duration of administration, and contraindications. It is the responsibility of practitioners, relying on their own experience and knowledge of their patients, to make diagnoses, to determine dosages and the best treatment for each individual patient, and to take all appropriate safety precautions.

To the fullest extent of the law, neither the Publisher nor the authors, contributors, or editors, assume any liability for any injury and/or damage to persons or property as a matter of products liability, negligence or otherwise, or from any use or operation of any methods, products, instructions, or ideas contained in the material herein.

International Standard Book Number: 978-0-323-37462-0

Executive Content Strategist: Dolores Meloni
Senior Content Development Manager: Taylor Ball
Publishing Services Manager: Patricia Tannian
Senior Project Manager: John Casey
Design Direction: Renee Duenow

Printed in Canada

9 8 7 6 5 4 3 2 1

IN MEMORY

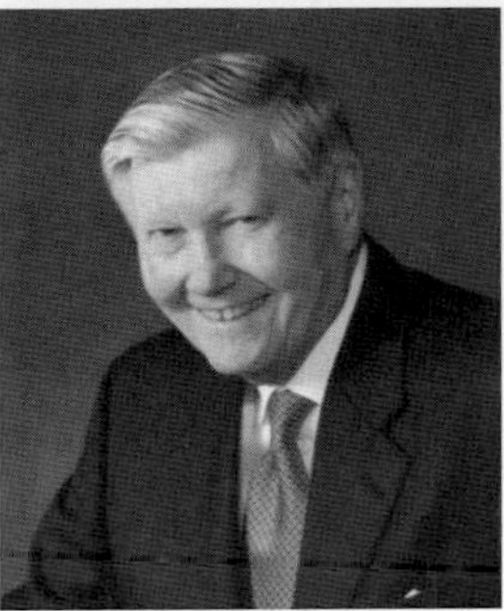

Lee W. Milford, MD
1922–2013

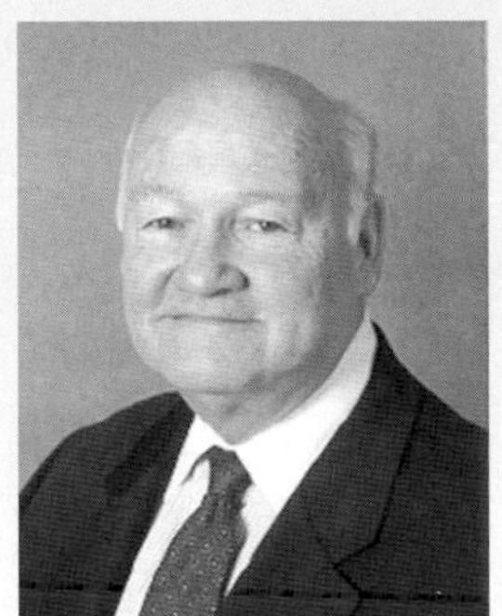

Robert E. Tooms, MD
1933–2013

Since the last edition of this text, we have lost two of our friends and mentors, Dr. Lee Milford and Dr. Robert Tooms, both of whom made important contributions to several editions of *Campbell's Operative Orthopaedics*. Dr. Milford was responsible for the first chapter in the book to focus on surgery of the hand. In the 7th edition of *Campbell's Operative Orthopaedics* (1987), he established the format for the hand section of the text by dividing the enormous amount of information from one chapter into 18 more focused chapters. His hand surgery chapters formed the basis of three monographs (*The Hand*). Dr. Tooms also expanded his area of expertise, taking amputation from a single chapter to multiple, anatomy-based chapters. His compassion for and dedication to amputees, especially children, are evident in his work. He was an early adopter of total joint arthroplasty and contributed some of the first chapters on total knee and total ankle arthroplasty. The experience and expertise of these two staff members added immensely to the value of our book, and we hope subsequent editions have remained true to their example.

DEDICATION

This 13th edition of *Campbell's Operative Orthopaedics* is dedicated to all of the contributors, present and past, without whose knowledge and dedication this text would be impossible. Over the years, nearly 100 authors have freely shared their time and knowledge with their colleagues, residents, fellows, and medical students. Their varied areas of expertise have allowed our text to cover a wide array of orthopaedic conditions and procedures and to keep information current. The willingness of these experts in their respective fields to take the time and make the effort to contribute well thought out and well-written chapters is a large part of the ability of *Campbell's Operative Orthopaedics* to remain relevant and useful for almost 80 years.

CONTRIBUTORS

FREDERICK M. AZAR, MD
Professor
Director, Sports Medicine Fellowship
University of Tennessee–Campbell Clinic
Department of Orthopaedic Surgery and Biomedical Engineering
Chief-of-Staff, Campbell Clinic
Memphis, Tennessee

JAMES H. BEATY, MD
Harold B. Boyd Professor and Chair
University of Tennessee–Campbell Clinic
Department of Orthopaedic Surgery and Biomedical Engineering
Memphis, Tennessee

CLAYTON C. BETTIN, MD
Instructor
University of Tennessee–Campbell Clinic
Department of Orthopaedic Surgery and Biomedical Engineering
Memphis, Tennessee

JAMES H. CALANDRUCCIO, MD
Associate Professor
Director, Hand Fellowship
University of Tennessee–Campbell Clinic
Department of Orthopaedic Surgery and Biomedical Engineering
Memphis, Tennessee

FRANCIS X. CAMILLO, MD
Associate Professor
University of Tennessee–Campbell Clinic
Department of Orthopaedic Surgery and Biomedical Engineering
Memphis, Tennessee

S. TERRY CANALE, MD
Harold B. Boyd Professor and Chair Emeritus
University of Tennessee–Campbell Clinic
Department of Orthopaedic Surgery and Biomedical Engineering
Memphis, Tennessee

DAVID L. CANNON, MD
Associate Professor
University of Tennessee–Campbell Clinic
Department of Orthopaedic Surgery and Biomedical Engineering
Memphis, Tennessee

KEVIN B. CLEVELAND, MD
Instructor
University of Tennessee–Campbell Clinic
Department of Orthopaedic Surgery and Biomedical Engineering
Memphis, Tennessee

ANDREW H. CRENSHAW JR, MD
Associate Professor
University of Tennessee–Campbell Clinic
Department of Orthopaedic Surgery and Biomedical Engineering
Memphis, Tennessee

JOHN R. CROCKARELL JR, MD
Professor
University of Tennessee–Campbell Clinic
Department of Orthopaedic Surgery and Biomedical Engineering
Memphis, Tennessee

GREGORY D. DABOV, MD
Assistant Professor
University of Tennessee–Campbell Clinic
Department of Orthopaedic Surgery and Biomedical Engineering
Memphis, Tennessee

RAYMOND J. GARDOCKI, MD
Assistant Professor
University of Tennessee–Campbell Clinic
Department of Orthopaedic Surgery and Biomedical Engineering
Memphis, Tennessee

BENJAMIN J. GREAR, MD
Instructor
University of Tennessee–Campbell Clinic
Department of Orthopaedic Surgery and Biomedical Engineering
Memphis, Tennessee

JAMES L. GUYTON, MD
Associate Professor
University of Tennessee–Campbell Clinic
Department of Orthopaedic Surgery and Biomedical Engineering
Memphis, Tennessee

JAMES W. HARKESS, MD
Associate Professor
University of Tennessee–Campbell Clinic
Department of Orthopaedic Surgery and Biomedical Engineering
Memphis, Tennessee

ROBERT K. HECK JR, MD
Associate Professor
University of Tennessee–Campbell Clinic
Department of Orthopaedic Surgery and Biomedical Engineering
Memphis, Tennessee

SUSAN N. ISHIKAWA, MD
Assistant Professor
Co-Director, Foot and Ankle Fellowship
University of Tennessee–Campbell Clinic
Department of Orthopaedic Surgery and Biomedical Engineering
Memphis, Tennessee

MARK T. JOBE, MD
Associate Professor
University of Tennessee–Campbell Clinic
Department of Orthopaedic Surgery and Biomedical Engineering
Memphis, Tennessee

DEREK M. KELLY, MD
Associate Professor
University of Tennessee–Campbell Clinic
Department of Orthopaedic Surgery and Biomedical Engineering
Memphis, Tennessee

DAVID G. LAVELLE, MD
Associate Professor
University of Tennessee–Campbell Clinic
Department of Orthopaedic Surgery and Biomedical Engineering
Memphis, Tennessee

SANTOS F. MARTINEZ, MD
Assistant Professor
University of Tennessee–Campbell Clinic
Department of Orthopaedic Surgery and Biomedical Engineering
Memphis, Tennessee

ANTHONY A. MASCIOLI, MD
Assistant Professor
University of Tennessee–Campbell Clinic
Department of Orthopaedic Surgery and Biomedical Engineering
Memphis, Tennessee

BENJAMIN M. MAUCK, MD
Instructor
University of Tennessee–Campbell Clinic
Department of Orthopaedic Surgery and Biomedical Engineering
Memphis, Tennessee

MARC J. MIHALKO, MD
Assistant Professor
University of Tennessee–Campbell Clinic
Department of Orthopaedic Surgery and Biomedical Engineering
Memphis, Tennessee

WILLIAM M. MIHALKO, MD
Professor, H.R. Hyde Chair of Excellence in Rehabilitation Engineering
Director, Biomedical Engineering
University of Tennessee–Campbell Clinic
Department of Orthopaedic Surgery and Biomedical Engineering
Memphis, Tennessee

ROBERT H. MILLER III, MD
Associate Professor
University of Tennessee–Campbell Clinic
Department of Orthopaedic Surgery and Biomedical Engineering
Memphis, Tennessee

G. ANDREW MURPHY, MD
Associate Professor
Co-Director, Foot and Ankle Fellowship
University of Tennessee–Campbell Clinic
Department of Orthopaedic Surgery and Biomedical Engineering
Memphis, Tennessee

ASHLEY L. PARK, MD
Clinical Assistant Professor
University of Tennessee–Campbell Clinic
Department of Orthopaedic Surgery and Biomedical Engineering
Memphis, Tennessee

EDWARD A. PEREZ, MD
Associate Professor
Director, Trauma Fellowship
University of Tennessee–Campbell Clinic
Department of Orthopaedic Surgery and Biomedical Engineering
Memphis, Tennessee

BARRY B. PHILLIPS, MD
Associate Professor
University of Tennessee–Campbell Clinic
Department of Orthopaedic Surgery and Biomedical Engineering
Memphis, Tennessee

DAVID R. RICHARDSON, MD
Associate Professor
Co-Director, Foot and Ankle Fellowship
University of Tennessee–Campbell Clinic
Department of Orthopaedic Surgery and Biomedical Engineering
Memphis, Tennessee

MATTHEW I. RUDLOFF, MD
Assistant Professor
University of Tennessee–Campbell Clinic
Department of Orthopaedic Surgery and Biomedical Engineering
Memphis, Tennessee

JEFFREY R. SAWYER, MD
Professor
Director, Pediatric Orthopaedic Fellowship
University of Tennessee–Campbell Clinic
Department of Orthopaedic Surgery and Biomedical Engineering
Memphis, Tennessee

DAVID D. SPENCE, MD
Assistant Professor
University of Tennessee–Campbell Clinic
Department of Orthopaedic Surgery and Biomedical Engineering
Memphis, Tennessee

THOMAS W. THROCKMORTON, MD
Professor
Director, Resident Education
University of Tennessee–Campbell Clinic
Department of Orthopaedic Surgery and Biomedical Engineering
Memphis, Tennessee

PATRICK C. TOY, MD
Assistant Professor
University of Tennessee–Campbell Clinic
Department of Orthopaedic Surgery and Biomedical Engineering
Memphis, Tennessee

WILLIAM C. WARNER JR, MD
Professor
University of Tennessee–Campbell Clinic
Department of Orthopaedic Surgery and Biomedical Engineering
Memphis, Tennessee

JOHN C. WEINLEIN, MD
Assistant Professor
University of Tennessee–Campbell Clinic
Department of Orthopaedic Surgery and Biomedical Engineering
Memphis, Tennessee

A. PAIGE WHITTLE, MD
Associate Professor
University of Tennessee–Campbell Clinic
Department of Orthopaedic Surgery and Biomedical Engineering
Memphis, Tennessee

KEITH D. WILLIAMS, MD
Associate Professor
Director, Spine Fellowship
University of Tennessee–Campbell Clinic
Department of Orthopaedic Surgery and Biomedical Engineering
Memphis, Tennessee

DEXTER H. WITTE, MD
Clinical Assistant Professor of Radiology
University of Tennessee–Campbell Clinic
Department of Orthopaedic Surgery and Biomedical Engineering
Memphis, Tennessee

PREFACE

Over the past four years, our authors have exhaustively reviewed a multitude of new techniques, new equipment, and new information in the world literature to produce a comprehensive update of our textbook. This edition reflects the growing numbers of less-invasive surgical techniques and devices that are being described, with promising results reported, and many arthroscopic and endoscopic techniques that continue to expand their indications. Over the last several years, ambulatory surgery centers have become an important part of orthopaedic surgery—from ligament repair to total joint arthroplasty—and outpatient orthopaedic surgery is now more frequently performed than standard hospital-based surgery in many centers. With knowledge and technology expanding and evolving at an ever-increasing speed, we have attempted to include the latest orthopaedic procedures while retaining as a foundation many of the classic techniques.

As always, the Campbell Foundation staff—Kay Daugherty and Linda Jones, editors; Shawn Maxey, graphics; and Tonya Priggel, librarian—were essential in the production of this edition. Thanks to Kay and Linda for taking sometimes illegible notes on a napkin and translating them into eloquent English, to Shawn for keeping track of the hundreds of illustrations, and to Tonya for always locating the latest information on any topic. As many of our orthopaedic colleagues who have visited our institution can affirm, the piles of references, rough drafts, and jammed-full file folders that occupy the office floor are a testament to this monstrous undertaking. Our thanks, too, to Taylor Ball, Content Development Editor; Dolores Meloni, Executive Content Strategist; and John Casey, Senior Project Manager, at Elsevier publishing, who provided much guidance, encouragement, and assistance and who, while they may have doubted that we would get material in on time, never expressed anxiety. We also are most appreciative of the worldwide community of orthopaedic surgeons for their expertise and innovation without which our book would not be possible. Without their zeal to learn, teach, and contribute to the body of orthopaedic knowledge, our purpose would be compromised.

We are most grateful to our families, especially our wives, Sissie Canale, Terry Beaty, and Julie Azar, who patiently endured our total immersion in the publication process.

Technology has made the exchange of information easier and faster, but, as noted by one pundit, we can "drown in technology" and the "fog of information can drive out knowledge." We have attempted to take advantage of current technology while presenting information in a consistent and concise manner that clears the "fog" and adds to knowledge. Dr. Campbell noted many years ago, "The purpose of this book is to present to the student, the general practitioner, and the surgeon the subject of orthopedic surgery in a simple and comprehensive manner." We hope that this edition continues to live up to his standards.

Frederick M. Azar, MD
James H. Beaty, MD
S. Terry Canale, MD

CONTENTS

VOLUME I

PART I GENERAL PRINCIPLES

PART II RECONSTRUCTIVE PROCEDURES OF THE HIP IN ADULTS

PART III RECONSTRUCTIVE PROCEDURES OF THE KNEE IN ADULTS

PART IV RECONSTRUCTIVE PROCEDURES OF THE ANKLE IN ADULTS

PART V RECONSTRUCTIVE PROCEDURES OF THE SHOULDER AND ELBOW IN ADULTS

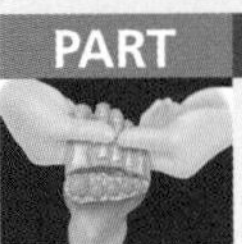

PART VI AMPUTATIONS

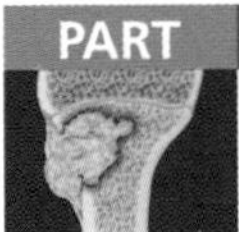

PART VII INFECTIONS

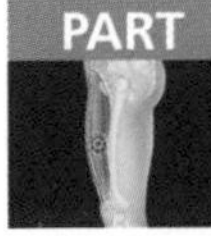

PART VIII TUMORS

PART XIX THE FOOT AND ANKLE

VIDEO CONTENTS

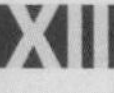

PART XIII SPORTS MEDICINE

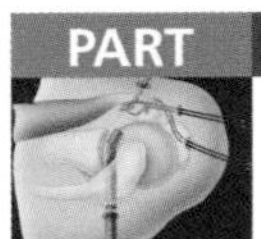

PART XIV ARTHROSCOPY

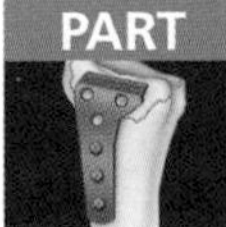

PART XV FRACTURES AND DISLOCATIONS IN ADULTS

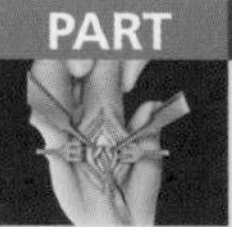

PART XVIII THE HAND

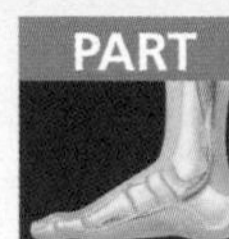

PART XIX THE FOOT AND ANKLE

PART IX

CONGENITAL AND DEVELOPMENTAL DISORDERS

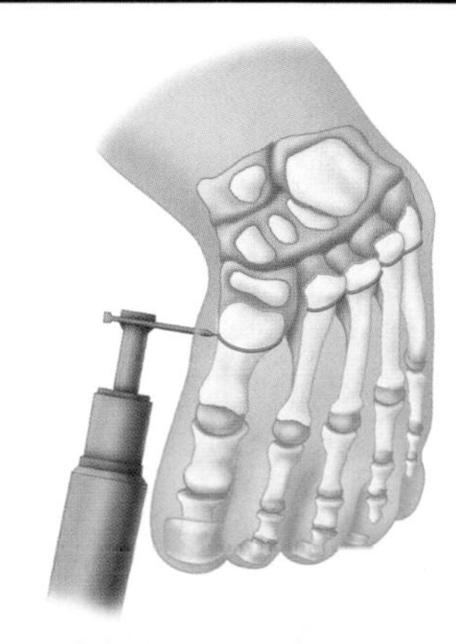

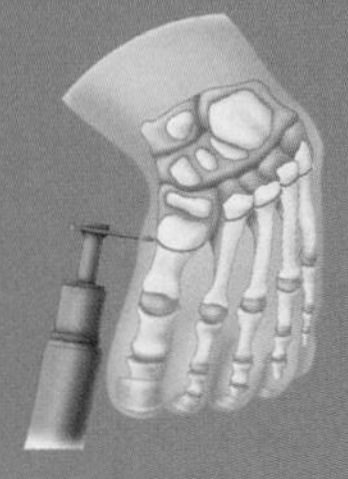

CHAPTER 29

CONGENITAL ANOMALIES OF THE LOWER EXTREMITY

Derek M. Kelly

This chapter describes congenital anomalies of the foot and lower extremity. Congenital anomalies of the hip and pelvis are described in Chapter 30, and congenital anomalies of the trunk and upper extremities are described in Chapter 31. Congenital anomalies of the spine are discussed in Chapters 43 and 44, and congenital anomalies of the hand are discussed in Chapter 79. Many of the operative techniques described here are useful for other conditions and are found in the references in other chapters.

ANOMALIES OF THE TOES

The most common anomaly of the toes is polydactyly, the presence of supernumerary digits. Others are syndactyly (webbed toes), macrodactyly (enlarged toes), and congenital contracture or angulation. Any of these conditions may require surgery. When surgery is contemplated for anomalies of the toes, several factors must be considered, including cosmesis, pain, and difficulty in fitting shoes, but overall long-term function of the foot is the primary concern. A satisfactory clinical result should correct all of these problems.

POLYDACTYLY

Polydactyly of the toes may occur in established genetic syndromes but occurs most commonly as an isolated trait with an autosomal dominant inheritance pattern and variable expression. The overall incidence of polydactyly is approximately two cases per 1000 live births. Surgical treatment of polydactyly is amputation of the accessory digit. Preoperative radiographs should be obtained to detect any extra metatarsal articulating with the digit, which should be amputated with its associated digit (Fig. 29-1). Occasionally, a combined polydactyly-syndactyly deformity requires more complex surgical correction (Fig. 29-2), such as resection of the more peripheral digit using residual skin for coverage.

Venn-Watson classified polydactyly and directed attention to the difference between preaxial and postaxial types (Fig. 29-3). In preaxial polydactyly, the most medial great toe usually is excised. The remaining great toe should have a careful repair of the capsule if necessary to prevent a progressive hallux varus; Kirschner wire fixation is used for 4 to 6 weeks. A more recent classification system by Seok et al. focuses on the importance of associated syndactylism, axis deviation, and metatarsal extension, with each of these factors resulting in a higher rate of unsatisfactory results after surgical correction.

AMPUTATION OF AN EXTRA TOE (SIMPLE POSTAXIAL POLYDACTYLY)

TECHNIQUE 29-1

- At the base of the toe to be amputated, make an oval or racquet-shaped incision through the skin and fascia, preserving extra skin to ensure tension-free closure after amputation of the extra digit (Fig. 29-4).
- Draw the tendons distally as far as possible and divide them.
- Incise the capsule of the metatarsophalangeal joint transversely, dissect it from the metatarsal, and disarticulate the joint.

- With an osteotome or bone-cutting forceps, sharply resect any bone that may have protruded from the metatarsal head.
- If the radiograph has revealed an extra metatarsal, resect it after continuing the incision proximally on the dorsolateral aspect of the foot. A complete extra ray amputation may require transfer of the peroneus brevis tendon insertion with partial resection of the lateral border of the cartilaginous cuboid.

See also Video 29-1

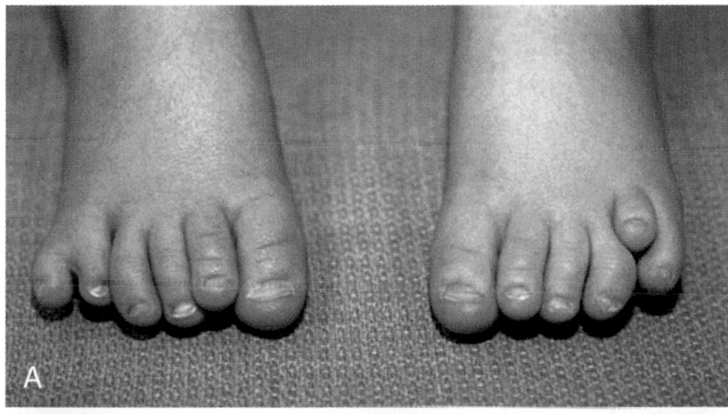

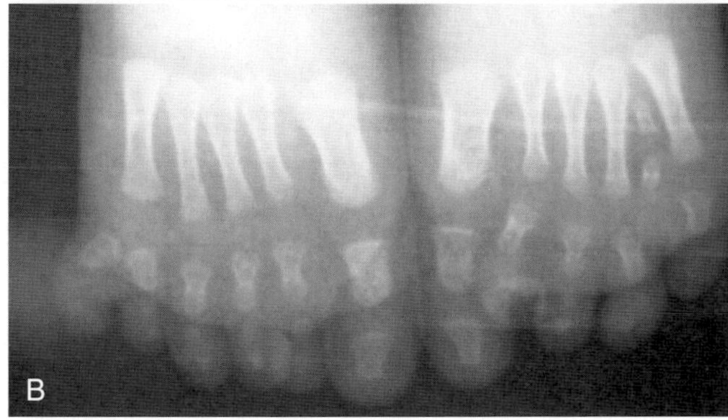

FIGURE 29-1 **A,** Bilateral polydactyly in 6-month-old infant. **B,** Accessory metatarsal of left foot can be seen on radiograph.

SYNDACTYLY

Syndactyly of the toes rarely interferes with function, and surgery is indicated primarily for cosmetic reasons; the same technique is used as for the fingers (see Chapter 79). Syndactyly is commonly associated with polydactyly in the foot, and removal of the more medial or lateral digit is typically preferred.

MACRODACTYLY

Macrodactyly occurs when one or more toes or fingers have hypertrophied and are significantly larger than the surrounding toes or fingers. The most common associated conditions are neurofibromatosis, hemangiomatosis, and congenital lipofibromatosis. Surgery is indicated to relieve functional symptoms, primarily pain or difficulty in fitting shoes. The cosmetic goal is to alter the abnormal appearance of the toes

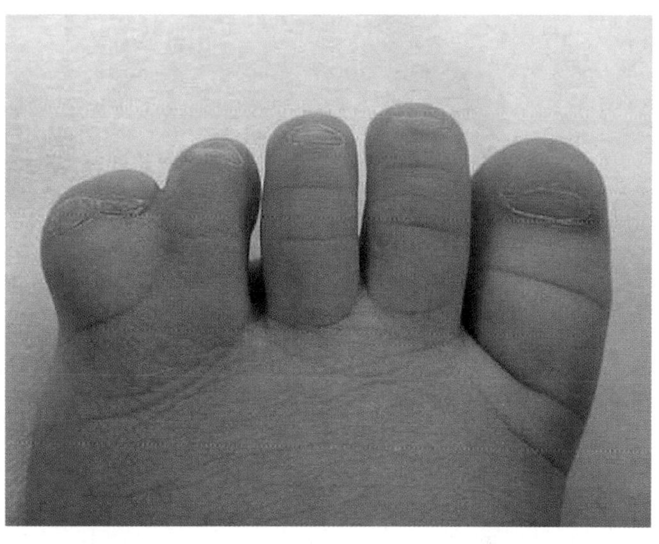

FIGURE 29-2 Complex polydactyly-syndactyly of left fifth toe with bony and soft-tissue syndactyly. (From Lee HS, Park SS, Yoon JO, et al: Classification of postaxial polydactyly of the foot, Foot Ankle Int 27:356, 2006.)

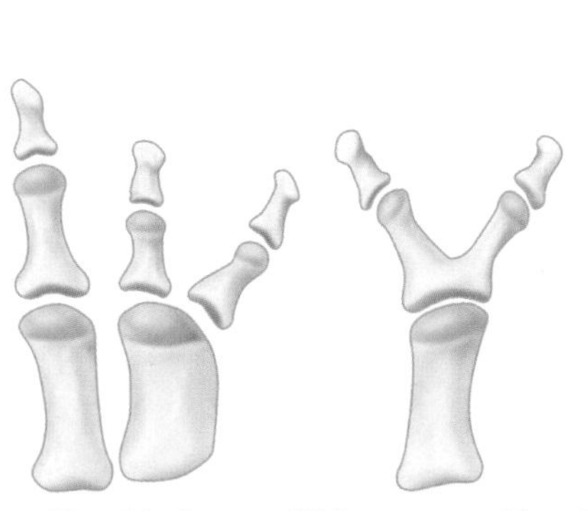

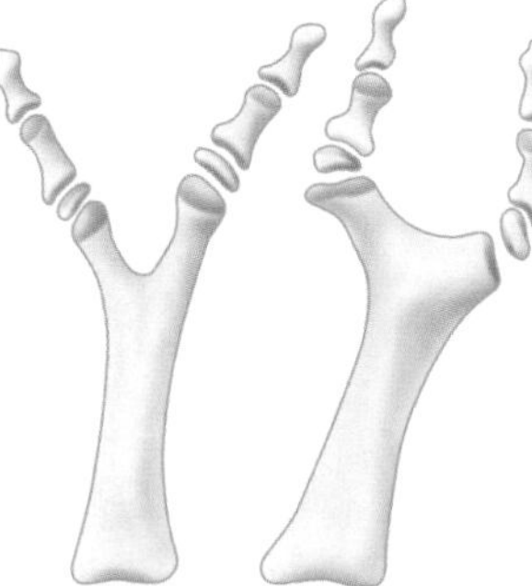

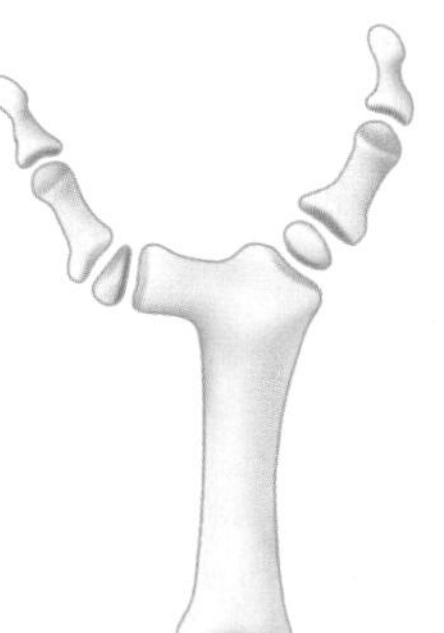

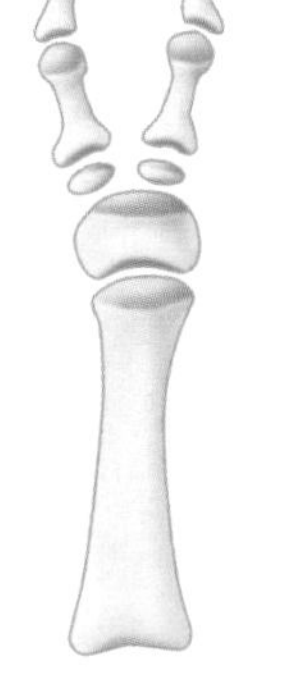

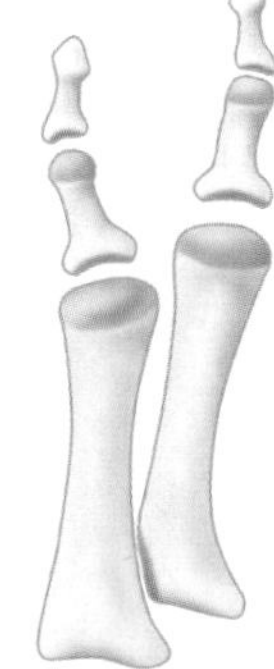

FIGURE 29-3 Venn-Watson classification of polydactyly. **A,** Preaxial polydactyly. **B,** Postaxial polydactyly.

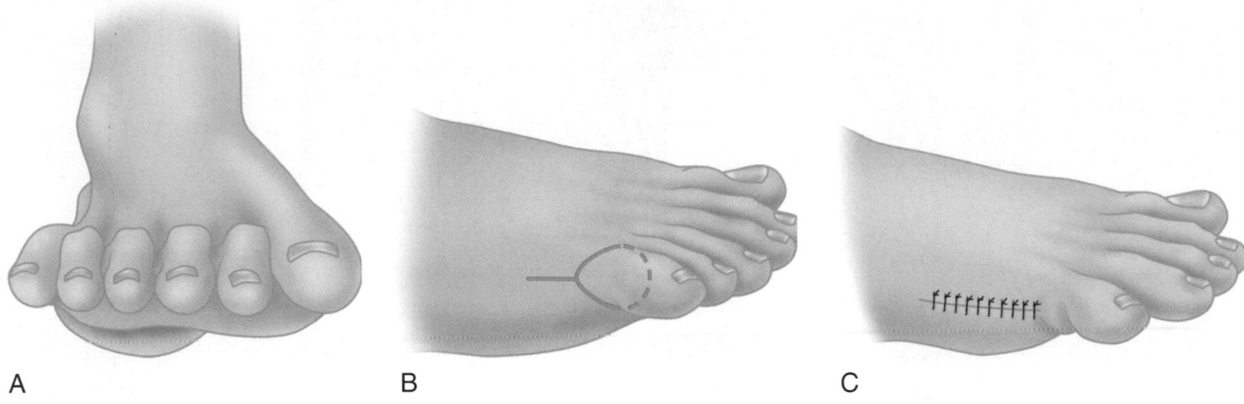

FIGURE 29-4 Polydactyly. **A,** Front view of foot. **B,** Outline of incision passing through web space between fifth and sixth toes and extending in racquet-shaped incision along lateral border of foot. **C,** Surgical excision of supernumerary digit. **SEE TECHNIQUE 29-1.**

and foot and to achieve a foot similar in size to the opposite foot (Fig. 29-5).

Many operative procedures have been described for the treatment of macrodactyly, including reduction syndactyly, soft-tissue debulking combined with ostectomy or epiphysiodesis, toe amputation, and ray amputation. Soft-tissue debulking combined with ostectomy or epiphysiodesis can be used in the initial treatment of a single digit with macrodactyly; the recurrence rate with this technique is virtually 100%. Ray resection, combined with debulking repeated as necessary has been recommended; however, when the great toe is involved, the result often is only fair, and repeated soft-tissue debulking may be necessary. When enlargement of the toe or forefoot is less severe, epiphysiodesis of the phalangeal physes is recommended when the toe reaches adult size; debulking is repeated as necessary. Ray amputation is indicated in patients with massive enlargement of the bone and soft tissues, and is also the procedure of choice for severe recurrence after reduction syndactyly or soft-tissue debulking. Hallux valgus may occur after resection of the second ray and occasionally requires surgical correction during adolescence.

TSUGE RAY REDUCTION

The Tsuge procedure is an additional option for pedal macrodactyly treatment. It is a rare procedure for a rare condition; however, according to the authors, the benefit of this procedure is that it debulks and shortens the toe but maintains good cosmesis by preserving the toenail.

TECHNIQUE 29-2

(TSUGE)

- After administering general anesthesia and placing a tourniquet, make a midaxial fish-mouth incision (Fig. 29-6A).
- Dissect sharply down the plantar aspect of the distal and middle phalanges.
- Disarticulate the distal interphalangeal joint.
- Identify and protect the neurovascular bundles within the dorsal flap. Do not excise or debulk.
- Release the flexor digitorum longus and extensor digitorum longus tendon insertions from the distal phalanx and tag these (maintain and protect the extensor digitorum longus attachment to the middle phalanx).
- Using a microsagittal saw, make a coronal cut along the distal phalanx, excising the plantar portion and leaving approximately a third of the phalanx beneath the nail plate and matrix (Fig. 29-6B).
- Make a transverse cut across the distal phalanx, excising the physis (Fig. 29-6C).
- Skeletonize the middle phalanx dorsally, protecting the extensor attachment.
- Make a similar size-matched coronal cut in the middle phalanx at the one-third dorsal to two-thirds plantar level.
- Create a transverse osteotomy across the dorsal aspect of the middle phalanx, leaving the physis still attached to the plantar aspect of the residual bone.
- Excise the distal aspect of the dorsal middle phalanx (Fig. 29-6D).
- Shorten the remaining plantar aspect of the middle phalanx if needed to the desired length of the toe.
- Bring the dorsal sliver of the distal phalanx, which contains the nail, proximally and fit it to the plantar portion of the middle phalanx (Fig. 29-6E) and secure the transferred bone with a small Kirschner wire or suture lasso.
- Reattach the flexor digitorum longus tendon to the remaining middle phalanx using Vicryl suture (Ethicon, Somerville, New Jersey, USA). Reattach the extensor digitorum longus tendon to the middle phalanx.
- Deflate the tourniquet and obtain hemostasis using bipolar electrocautery.
- After the bony work, debulk any redundant plantar flap of tissue and fat (Fig. 29-6F) to allow wound closure (Fig. 29-6G).
- Copiously irrigate the wound and close with absorbable suture. As a result of the digital shortening, a dorsal bump just proximal to the nail is created.
- Apply a sterile dressing and a well-padded short leg walking cast.

POSTOPERATIVE CARE. The patient is allowed weight bearing as tolerated.

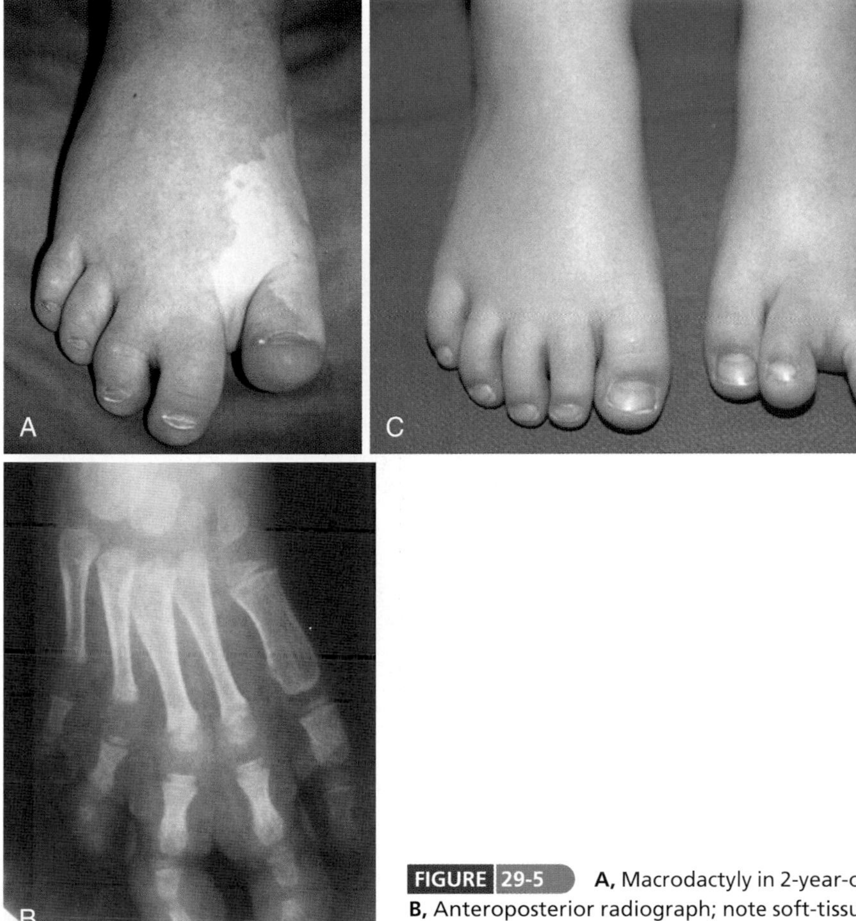

FIGURE 29-5 **A,** Macrodactyly in 2-year-old child with Klippel-Trenaunay-Weber syndrome. **B,** Anteroposterior radiograph; note soft-tissue hypertrophy of second and third ray phalanges. **C,** Clinical appearance of macrodactyly in another child.

RAY REDUCTION

TECHNIQUE 29-3

- Outline dorsal skin incisions along the ray to be reduced, with a single long incision or multiple small incisions along the metatarsal and phalanges.
- Debulk any fibrofatty tissue, protecting the digital neurovascular bundles.
- Osteotomize the metatarsal neck and shorten the metatarsal by removing a segment of sufficient length to match this metatarsal to the others.
- Fuse the physis at the level of the metatarsal head. If necessary, repeat this process for any phalanges until the ray has been shortened to normal length.
- Insert a smooth, longitudinal Kirschner wire from the tip of the toe to the base of the metatarsal to align the ray.
- Secure hemostasis, close the wound with interrupted sutures, and apply a short leg cast.

POSTOPERATIVE CARE. The Kirschner wire is removed at 6 weeks, and a short leg walking cast is worn until any bony procedures have healed.

RAY AMPUTATION

TECHNIQUE 29-4

- Outline the ray to be amputated with skin flaps to include amputation from the tip of the toe to the base of the metatarsal.
- Make dorsal and plantar incisions starting over the metatarsophalangeal joint, with connecting incisions in the web space of adjacent toes. Continue the incisions proximally, dorsally and plantarward, to the base of the metatarsal to be resected (Fig. 29-7).
- Amputate the metatarsal and its associated phalanges and any surrounding hypertrophied soft tissue. Protect the neurovascular bundles that supply adjacent toes.
- After adequate resection of tissue, close the wound with interrupted sutures in the usual manner.

POSTOPERATIVE CARE. A short leg cast is applied to protect the wound until healing occurs at 4 to 6 weeks.

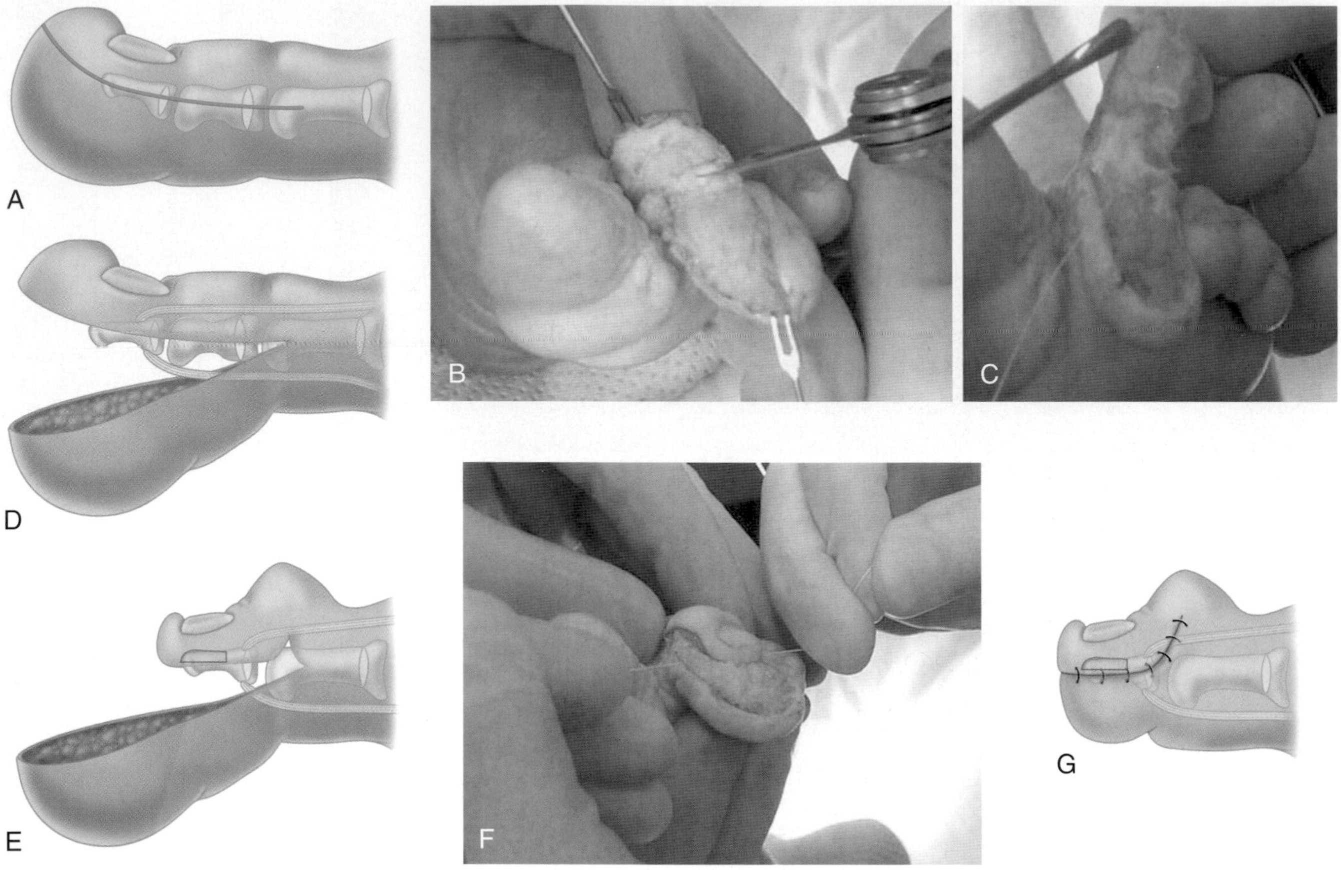

FIGURE 29-6 Tsuge ray reduction procedure. **A,** Fish-mouth incision made to the level of the proximal phalanx. **B,** Coronal osteotomy of the distal phalanx. **C,** Physis is removed by transverse osteotomy from remaining dorsal bone. Plantar portion is removed. **D,** Osteotomy and removal of dorsal middle phalanx. **E,** Dorsal third of distal phalanx is fixed to plantar two-thirds of middle phalanx and tendons reattached. **F,** Fibrofatty issue remains when digit is shortened, creating a dorsal bump. **G,** Excess tissue is debulked. (From Morrell NT, Fitzpatrick J, Szalay EA: The use of the Tsuge procedure for pedal macrodactyly: relevance in pediatric orthopaedics, J Pediatr Orthop B 23:260, 2014.) **SEE TECHNIQUE 29-2.**

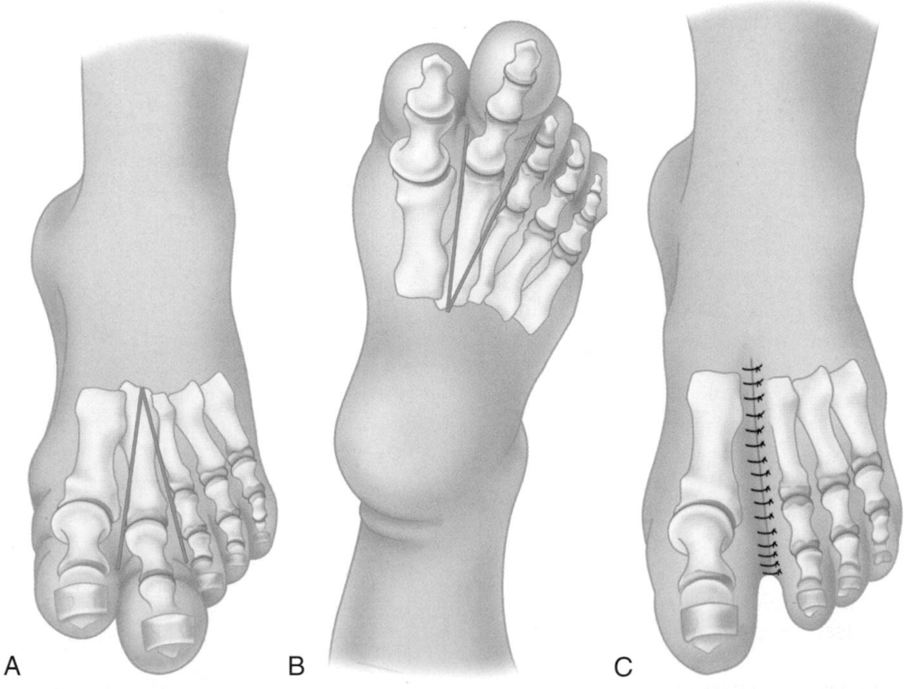

FIGURE 29-7 Ray amputation for macrodactyly. **A,** Incision on dorsal surface of foot. **B,** Plantar incision. **C,** Closed incision after amputation. **SEE TECHNIQUE 29-4.**

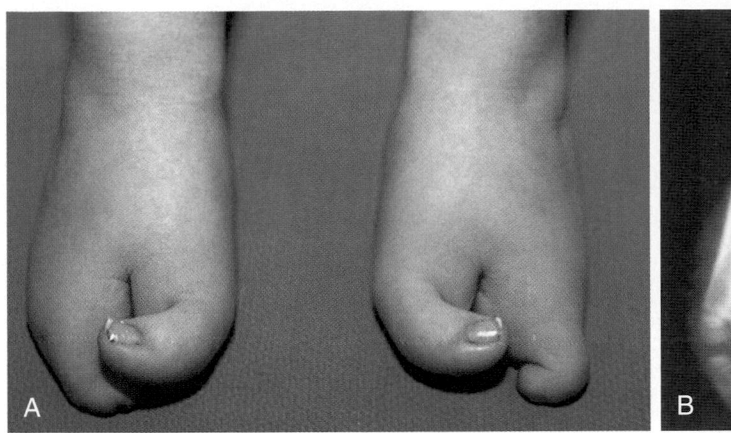

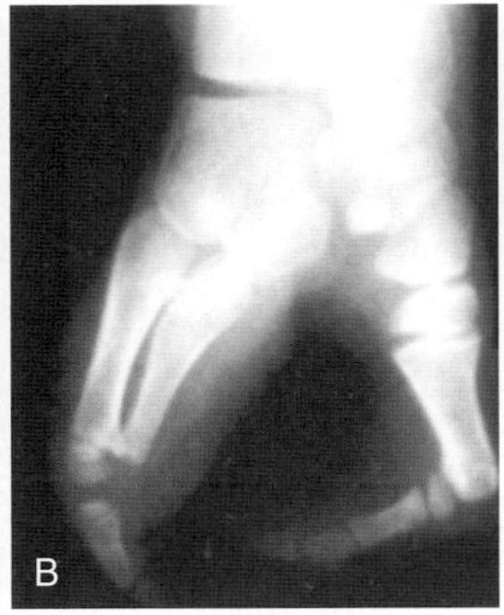

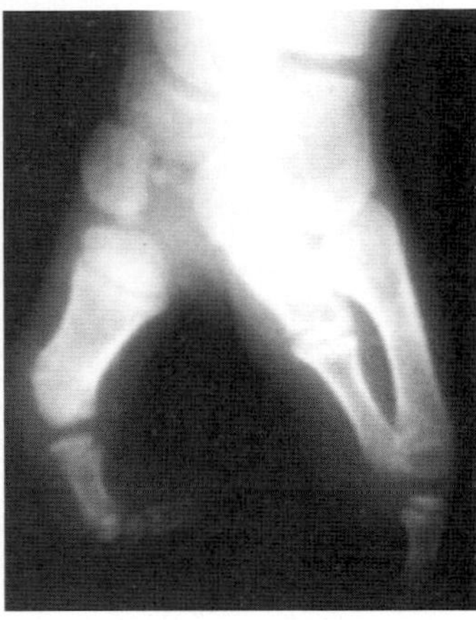

FIGURE 29-8 **A,** Bilateral cleft foot in 4-year-old boy. **B,** Anteroposterior view; note angular deformity of metatarsophalangeal joints of great toe and fifth toe.

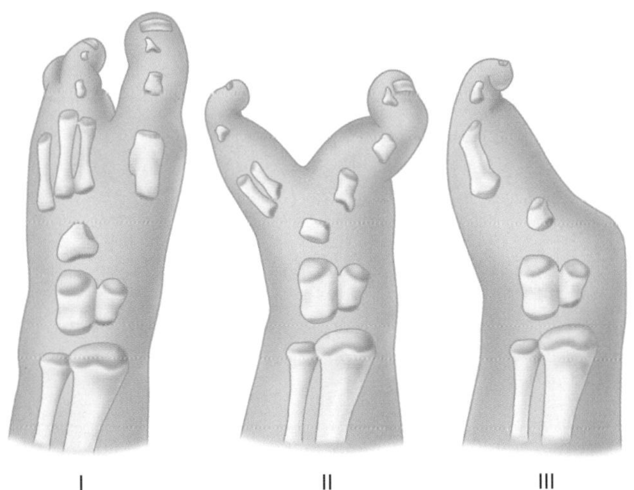

FIGURE 29-9 Clinical classification of cleft foot deformity (see text).

CLEFT FOOT (PARTIAL ADACTYLY)

Cleft foot (lobster foot) is an anomaly in which a single cleft extends proximally into the foot, sometimes as far as the midfoot. Generally, one or more toes and parts of their metatarsals are absent, and often the tarsals are abnormal. Although the deformity varies in degree and type, the first and fifth rays are usually present (Fig. 29-8). If a metatarsal is partially or completely absent, its respective toe is always absent. Blauth and Borisch classified the deformities into six types based on the number of metatarsal bones present. Type I and type II are cleft feet with minor deficiencies, both having five metatarsals. The metatarsals are normal in type I and partially hypoplastic in type II. The number of identifiable metatarsals decreases progressively: type III, four metatarsals; type IV, three metatarsals; type V, two metatarsals; and type VI, one metatarsal.

Abraham et al. described a simplified clinical classification on which they based treatment recommendations (Fig. 29-9). Type I has a central ray cleft or deficiency (usually second or third rays or both) extending up to the midmetatarsal level without splaying of medial or lateral rays. For this type of cleft foot, they recommended soft-tissue syndactylism with partial hallux valgus correction if needed; however, this type of deformity typically results in little functional limitation and is primarily a cosmetic concern. Type II has a deep cleft up to the tarsal bones with forefoot splaying, for which they recommended soft-tissue syndactylism, with first-ray osteotomy if needed, before age 5 years. Type III is a complete absence of the first through third or fourth rays, for which they did not recommend surgery; Abraham et al. recommended syndactylism for all type II cleft feet in the first 3 years of life while the forefoot is still supple. All of their patients older than 5 years with type II deformities had first ray amputation.

Any surgery for cleft foot should improve function and appearance. When surgical correction is performed, dorsal and plantar flaps are raised from the skin of the apposing surfaces, which are then sutured together (Fig. 29-10). Any bony or joint deformity of the first or fifth ray should be corrected at the time of surgery (Fig. 29-11). This may require capsulotomies and osteotomies of any retained rays. If pin fixation is used for fixation of osteotomies of the phalanges or metatarsals, the pins and short leg cast are removed 6 weeks after surgery, and a short leg walking cast or cast boot may be worn for an additional few weeks.

Wood, Peppers, and Shook described a simplified cleft closure using rectangular flaps. According to these authors, this technique is easier than techniques using multiple triangular flaps and produces superior cosmetic results. They recommended correction of the cleft foot at 6 months old because of fewer anesthesia risks, minimal growth deformities, and malleability of the soft tissues.

SIMPLIFIED CLEFT CLOSURE

TECHNIQUE 29-5

(WOOD, PEPPERS, AND SHOOK)

- At least two metatarsals must be present for good cleft closure.

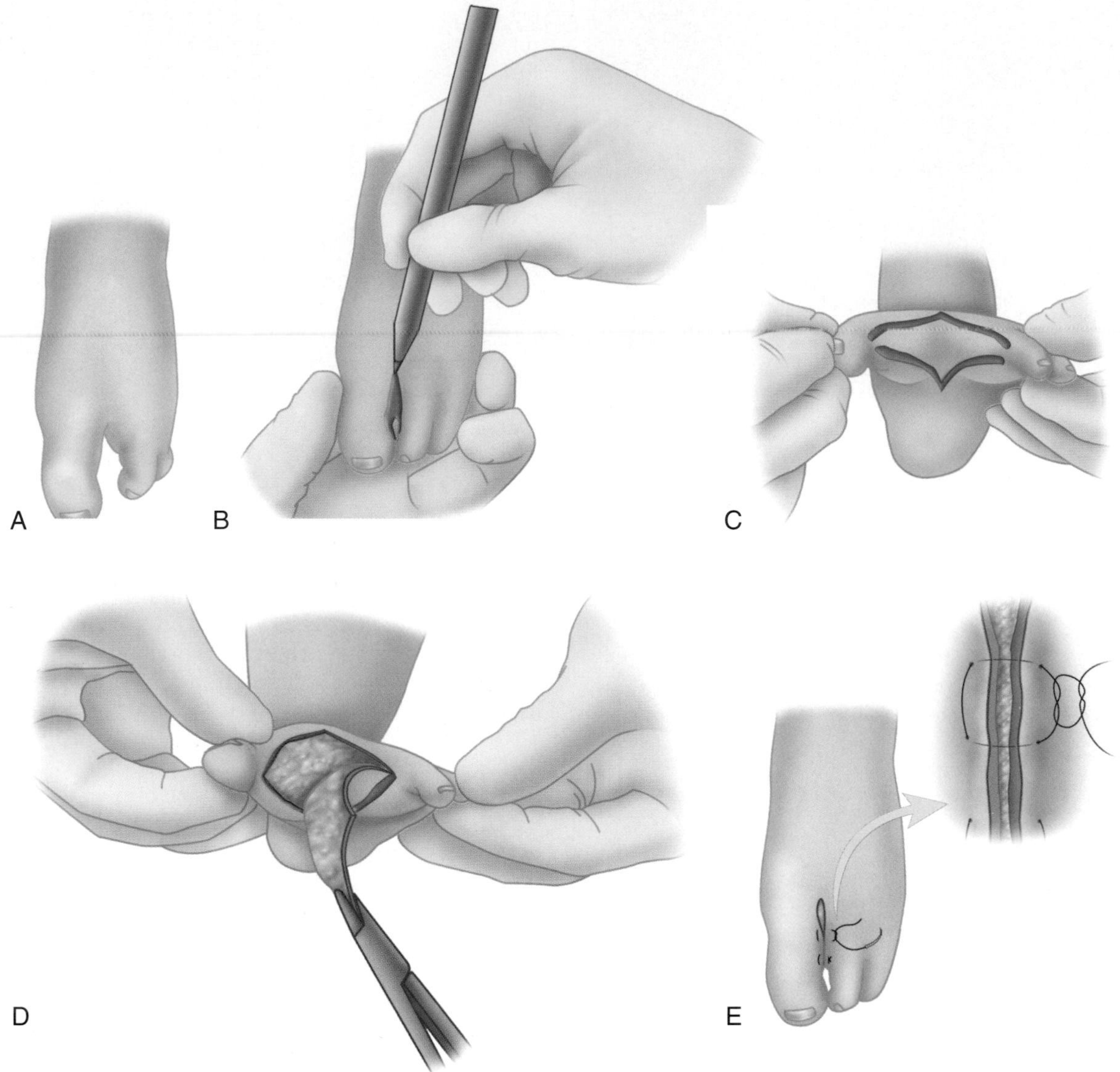

FIGURE 29-10 Syndactylism of cleft. **A-C,** Cleft is manually closed, and cleavage area is marked with sterile ink pen on dorsum and sole of foot. **D,** Skin and some subcutaneous tissue is removed as outlined by ink lines. **E,** Undermined skin edges are approximated with horizontal mattress sutures.

- On the lateral side, or fifth ray, raise a rectangular flap, starting from the plantar surface of the foot to the dorsum (Fig. 29-12A). This does not include fascia but includes a fairly thick flap with fat.
- Exactly opposite this flap on the medial side, or first ray, raise a rectangular flap starting on the dorsum of the foot to the plantar aspect. Repeat this two or three times until the skin of the entire cleft is removed (Fig. 29-12B).
- At the longest toe, raise a distally based flap for suturing to the adjacent toe to make a wide web.
- If the toes spring apart, make a closing wedge osteotomy at the base of each metatarsal to centralize the toes (Fig. 29-12C) and stabilize the osteotomies with Kirschner wires (Fig. 29-12D).
- To stabilize the intermetacarpal distance further and unload tension on the surgical flaps, reconstruct the intermetacarpal ligament with local ligamentous tissue, joint capsule, or tendon obtained from the cleft foot or with autograft plantaris tendon or fascia lata.
- Close the wound in routine fashion, and apply a cast.

POSTOPERATIVE CARE. At 3 weeks, weight bearing in a walking cast is allowed. At 6 weeks, the cast is discontinued, and the Kirschner wires are removed.

CONTRACTURE OR ANGULATION OF THE TOES

Congenital contracture, angulation, or subluxation of the fifth toe is a fairly common familial deformity, but rarely causes symptoms. The anomaly is rarely disabling, and surgery

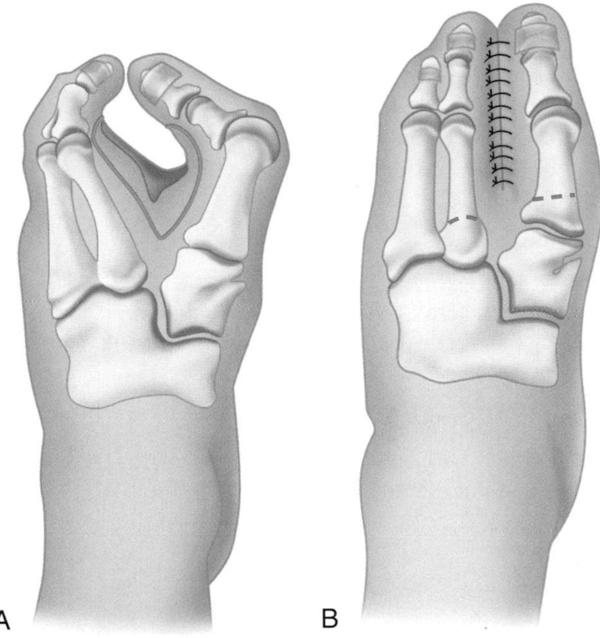

FIGURE 29-11 Correction of cleft foot. **A,** Skin incisions along cleft between abnormal rays of foot. **B,** Artificial syndactyly created after excision of skin cleft, apposition of rays, and osteotomies of metatarsals.

usually is indicated only to improve function of the foot or make shoe fitting easier. The direction of angulation of the fifth toe determines the operative procedure. Surgical procedures for the correction of an angulated toe include soft-tissue correction alone, soft-tissue correction with proximal phalangectomy, and amputation.

CORRECTION OF ANGULATED TOE

TECHNIQUE 29-6

- Administer an ankle block anesthetic (see Chapter 80), and inflate a sterile ankle tourniquet.
- Approach the fifth metatarsophalangeal joint through a Z-plasty incision. With the toe held in the corrected position, draw the central limb of the Z-plasty along the band of contracted skin to the fourth web space. Create the proximal and distal limbs of the Z-plasty of equal lengths (Fig. 29-13). Make the angle of the Z-plasty 60 degrees, which allows maximal elongation along the longitudinal axis of the Z-plasty when the limbs are transposed.
- Release the extensor digitorum longus tendon of the fifth toe in a long, oblique fashion.
- Release the dorsal and medial capsule and place the toe in the corrected position.
- Transpose the two limbs of the Z-plasty and suture them with interrupted absorbable sutures.

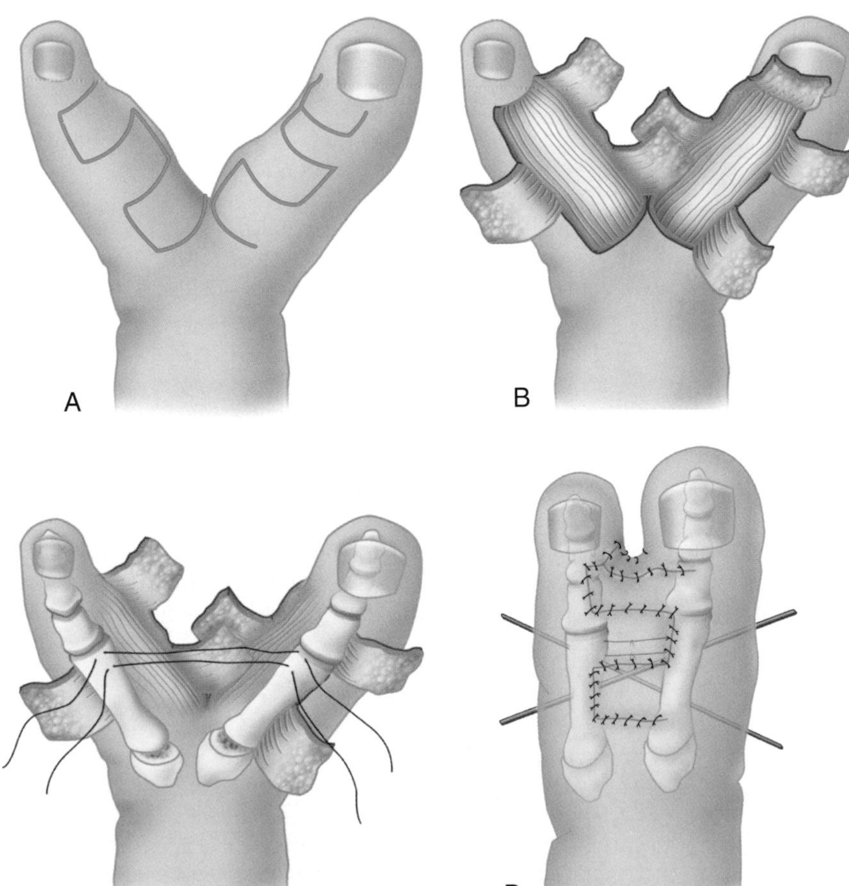

FIGURE 29-12 Cleft foot closure (see text). **A,** Rectangular flaps are raised on both rays. **B,** Flaps are raised until skin of entire cleft is removed. At distal tip of longer toe, flap is raised to suture to adjacent toe to make wide toe web. **C,** If toes spring apart, closing wedge osteotomy is made at base of each metatarsal to centralize bones. **D,** Kirschner wires are inserted to maintain position. **SEE TECHNIQUE 29-5.**

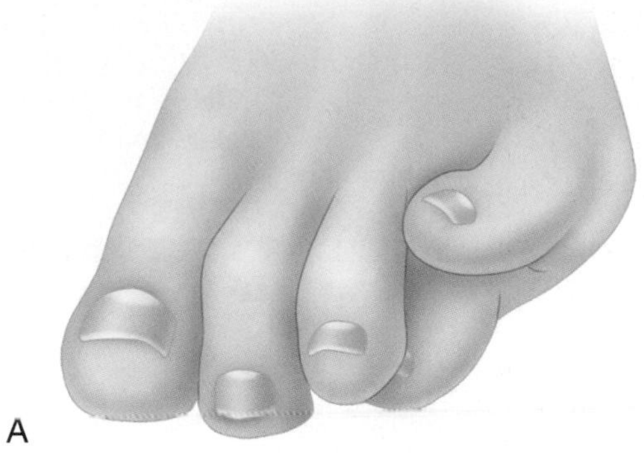

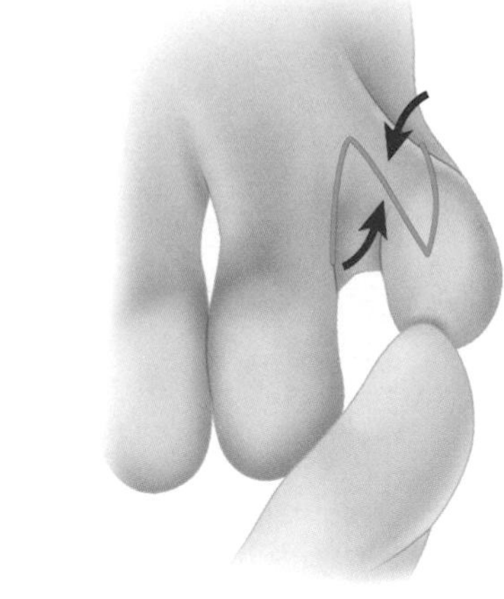

FIGURE 29-13 Correction of congenital crossover fifth toe. **A,** Preoperative appearance. **B,** Z-incision with 60-degree angles. Arrows indicate direction flaps are transposed to allow lengthening along longitudinal axis of Z-plasty. (From Thordarson DB: Congenital crossover fifth toe correction with soft-tissue release and cutaneous Z-plasty, Foot Ankle Int 22:511, 2001.) **SEE TECHNIQUE 29-6.**

Butler arthroplasty can be done for correction of a dorsally overriding fifth toe. One complication of Butler arthroplasty is the potential for vascular damage caused by excessive tension on the neurovascular bundle. This complication can be prevented by (1) avoiding any tension on the neurovascular bundle, (2) taking care not to manipulate or exert traction on the toe, and (3) avoiding the use of circumferential taping or rigid splinting.

ARTHROPLASTY OF THE FIFTH METATARSOPHALANGEAL JOINT

TECHNIQUE 29-7

(BUTLER)

- After preparing and draping the foot and applying a tourniquet, make a double racquet incision, with the dorsal handle following the extensor longus tendon and the plantar handle inclined laterally to provide a circumferential incision (Fig. 29-14A).
- To expose the contracted extensor tendon, elevate skin flaps by blunt dissection, protecting the neurovascular bundle (Fig. 29-14B).
- Transect the extensor tendon to the fifth toe and divide the dorsal aspect of the metatarsophalangeal joint capsule (Fig. 29-14C).
- The toe should now partially rotate downward and laterally into the correct position. In long-standing deformities, the plantar aspect of the capsule is adherent and prevents full reduction of the proximal phalanx on the metatarsal during derotation of the toe.
- If necessary, separate the adherent plantar capsule by blunt dissection and divide it transversely to allow the toe to lie freely in a fully corrected position (Fig. 29-14D and E).
- Close the skin with multiple interrupted sutures and apply a light dressing to the suture line (Fig. 29-14F and G).

POSTOPERATIVE CARE. A short leg cast or postoperative surgical shoe may be worn, with a light dressing only over the fifth toe. Protected activity is allowed as tolerated.

CONGENITAL HALLUX VARUS

Congenital hallux varus is a deformity in which the great toe is angled medially. The varus deformity of the toe varies in severity from only a few degrees to 90 degrees. The hallux varus can occur at the metatarsophalangeal joint with a normal metatarsal or it can occur in association with other deformities of the medial foot such as bracket epiphysis or preaxial polydactyly.

Typically, congenital hallux varus is unilateral and is associated with one or more of the following: (1) a short, thick first metatarsal; (2) accessory bones or toes; (3) varus deformity of one or more of the four lateral metatarsals; and (4) a firm fibrous band that extends from the medial side of the great toe to the base of the first metatarsal (Fig. 29-15). The explanation for this anomaly is that two great toes originate in utero, but the medial or accessory one fails to develop. Later, the rudimentary medial toe, together with the band of fibrous tissue, acts like a taut bowstring and gradually pulls the more fully developed great toe into a varus position.

The proper treatment for congenital hallux varus depends on the severity of the deformity and the rigidity of the contracted soft structures. A metatarsal epiphyseal bracket can be treated with physiolysis if performed very early or physiolysis combined with corrective osteotomy if performed later for milder hallux varus (Fig. 29-16). An osteotomy without physiolysis has an increased risk of recurrence, and the use of a bone graft increases the risk of fusing the epiphyseal bracket. A fat graft can be used as interposition material; however, Choo and Mubarak noted that fat attaches poorly to the diaphysis. Several of their patients developed a peripheral bar at the proximal metaphyseal-epiphyseal junction causing recurrent deformity. They recommended using polymethyl methacrylate as interposition material.

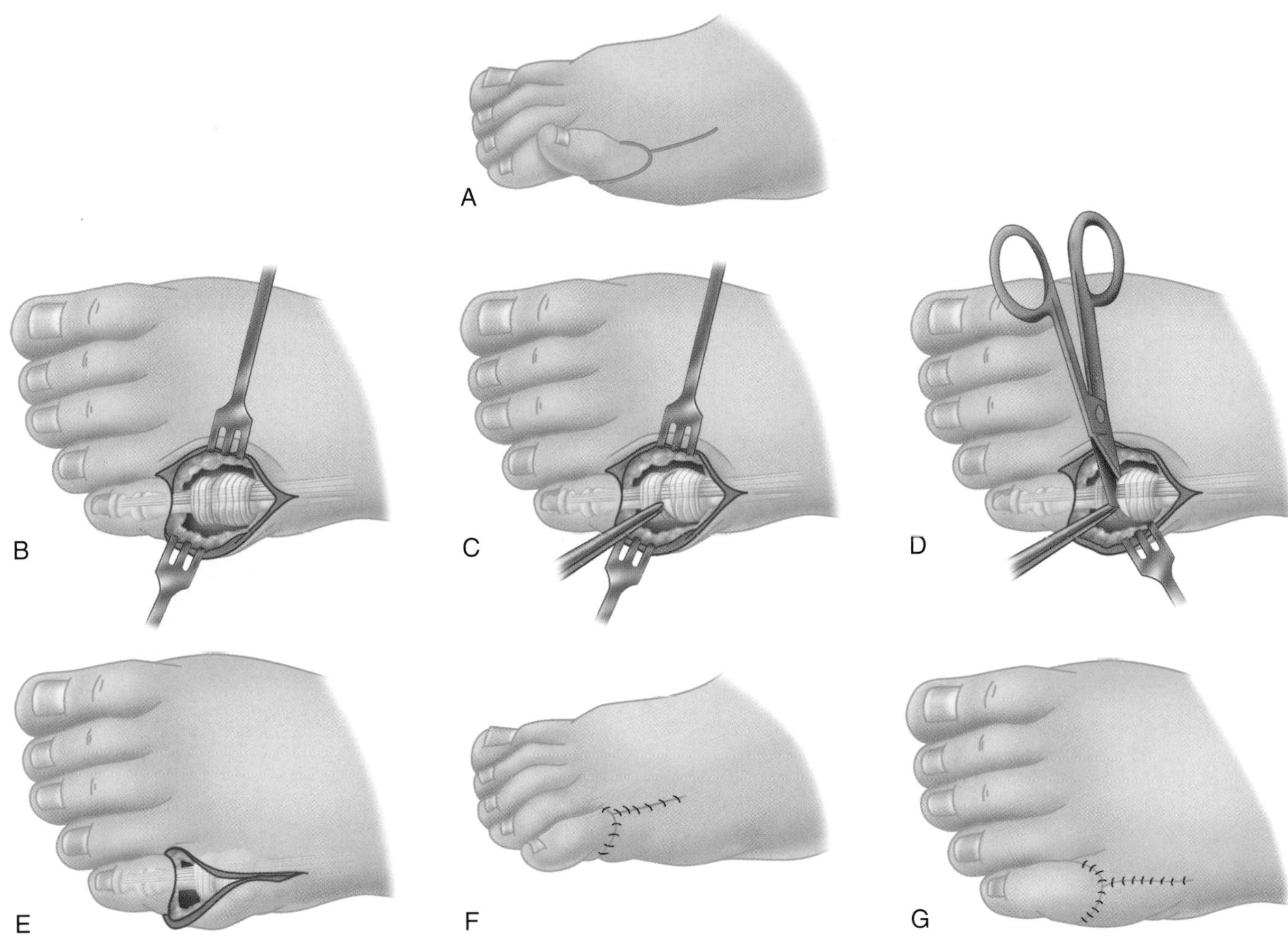

FIGURE 29-14 Butler arthroplasty. **A,** Double racquet incision. **B,** Exposure of extensor tendon. **C,** Transection of extensor tendon. **D,** Separation of adherent capsule. **E,** Corrected position of toe. **F** and **G,** Skin closure. **SEE TECHNIQUE 29-7.**

The Farmer technique is effective in correcting moderate deformity. The operation of Kelikian et al. is also satisfactory for severe deformity with an excessively short first metatarsal (Fig. 29-17). Each of these procedures is designed to create a syndactyly between the second toe and the hallux to maintain deformity correction. If the deformity is complicated by traumatic arthritis of the metatarsophalangeal joint, arthrodesis of this joint (see Chapter 81) is indicated. In rare cases, if the deformity is too severe either to be corrected or to undergo arthrodesis, amputation is indicated.

CREATION OF SYNDACTYLY OF THE GREAT TOE AND SECOND TOE FOR HALLUX VARUS

TECHNIQUE 29-8

(FARMER)

- Raise a broad Y-shaped flap of skin and subcutaneous tissue from the dorsal surface of the web between the first and second toes (Fig. 29-18); base the flap dorsally in the space between the first and second metatarsals, and include in it the skin contiguous with the web distally along the two toes for one third of their length.
- From the medial edge of the base of the flap, curve the incision medially and slightly distally across the medial aspect of the first metatarsophalangeal joint. Deepen this incision transversely through the medial part of the capsule of the first metatarsophalangeal joint.
- Move the great toe laterally against the second toe and create a syndactyly between these two toes by suturing the apposing skin edges together.
- A smooth longitudinal Kirschner wire can be inserted from the tip of the great toe into the first metatarsal to align the great toe in a neutral position.
- Excise any accessory phalanx or hypertrophic soft tissue from the great toe through a separate dorsomedial incision.
- Swing the Y-shaped flap of skin and subcutaneous tissue medially and suture it in place to cover the defect in the skin on the dorsal and medial aspects of the first metatarsophalangeal joint.

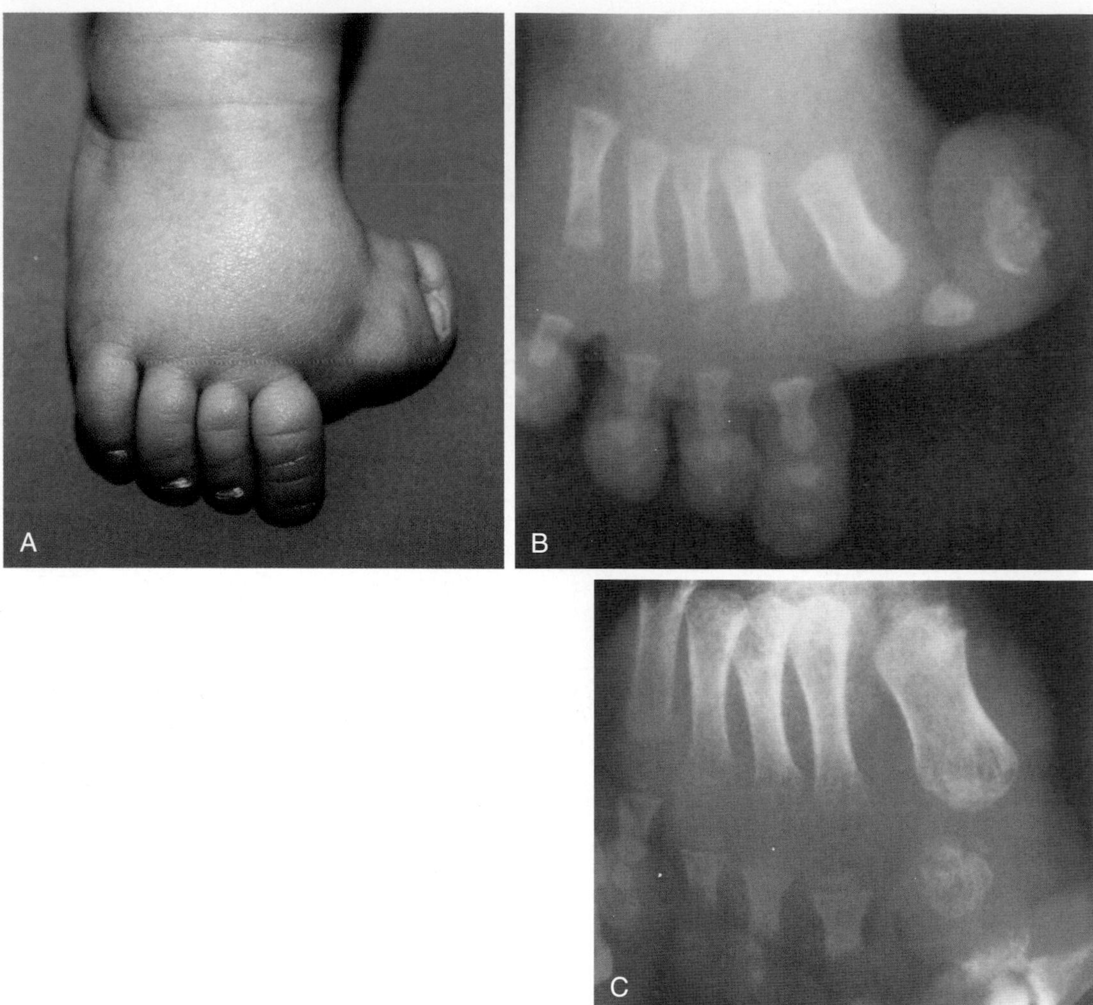

FIGURE 29-15 **A,** Congenital hallux varus of right foot. **B,** Anteroposterior radiograph; note short first metatarsal and accessory distal phalanx. **C,** Appearance after surgical correction.

- In an alternative technique described by Farmer, the Y-shaped flap of skin and subcutaneous tissue is raised from the plantar surface of the foot (Fig. 29-19); the rest of the procedure is the same as already described, with the flap swung medially to cover the defect in the skin at the first metatarsophalangeal joint. Any defect that cannot be closed by the flap either is left open to heal secondarily or is covered by a full-thickness skin graft.

POSTOPERATIVE CARE. The foot is immobilized in a cast. At 6 weeks, the cast and pins are removed, and full activities are allowed.

CONGENITAL METATARSUS ADDUCTUS

Metatarsus adductus, which consists of adduction of the forefoot in relation to the midfoot and hindfoot, is a common anomaly, often causing intoeing in children. It can occur as an isolated anomaly or in association with clubfoot. Among children with metatarsus adductus, 1% to 5% also have developmental dysplasia of the hip or acetabular dysplasia.

Clinically, metatarsus adductus can be classified as mild, moderate, or severe (Fig. 29-20). In the mild form, the forefoot can be clinically abducted to the midline of the foot and beyond (Fig. 29-21A). The moderate form has enough flexibility to allow abduction of the forefoot to the midline, but usually not beyond (Fig. 29-21B). In rigid metatarsus adductus, the forefoot cannot be abducted at all. There also may be a transverse crease on the medial border of the foot or an enlargement of the web space between the great and second toes. In general, mild metatarsus adductus resolves without treatment. Moderate or severe metatarsus adductus is best treated initially by serial stretching and casting for 6 to 12 weeks, or until the foot is clinically flexible.

Metatarsus adductus may be seen as a residual deformity in patients previously treated surgically or nonsurgically for congenital clubfoot. This residual metatarsus adductus can be rigid, indicating fixed positioning of the forefoot on the midfoot and hindfoot, or it can be dynamic, caused by imbalance of the anterior tibial tendon during gait. The rigidity or flexibility of the forefoot should be determined before undertaking any surgical correction in an older child. Metatarsus adductus, particularly in its milder forms, is often only a

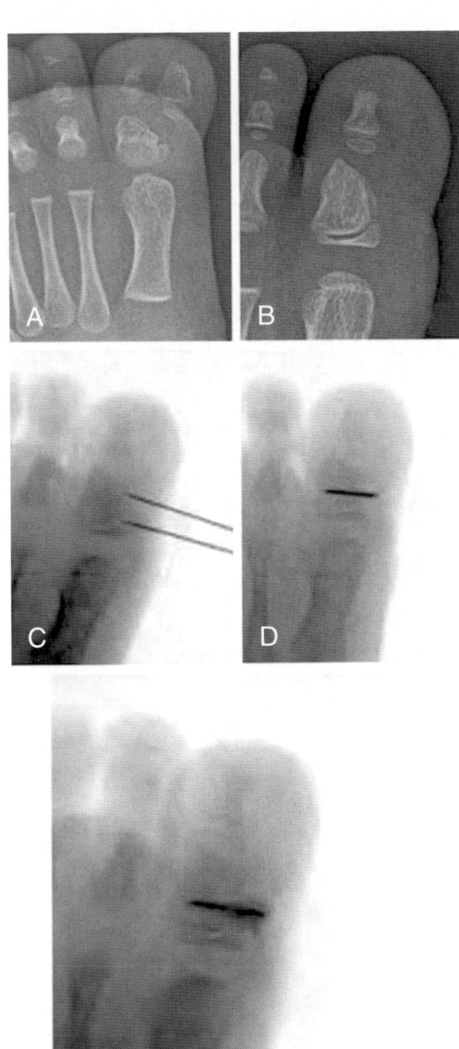

FIGURE 29-16 Epiphyseal bracket. **A,** Foot with preaxial polydactyly had reconstruction. **B,** Several months later an epiphyseal bracket of the proximal phalanx was noted with early ossification. **C,** The patient had excision of the hallux bracket. Intraoperative imaging demonstrating two needles at edges of bracket. **D,** Kirschner wire placed transversely through proximal phalanx. **E,** Polymethyl methacrylate cement was placed around wire. (From Choo AD, Mubarak SJ: Longitudinal epiphyseal bracket, J Child Orthop 7:449, 2013.)

cosmetic concern. However, shoewear may also become an issue as the child ages.

TREATMENT

In a young child, surgery is not indicated until conservative treatment has failed. When a child passes the appropriate age for serial stretching and casting, surgery becomes a reasonable option. Indications for surgery include pain, objectionable appearance, and difficulty in fitting shoes because of residual forefoot adduction. Numerous soft-tissue and bony procedures have been described for correction of metatarsus adductus. We prefer to tailor the surgery to the age and deformity of the particular child (Box 29-1).

DOME-SHAPED OSTEOTOMIES OF METATARSAL BASES

Berman and Gartland recommended dome-shaped osteotomies for all five metatarsal bases for resistant forefoot adduction in children 4 years old and older (Fig. 29-22). For a mature foot with uncorrected metatarsus adductus, or if all of the medial soft-tissue structures are contracted, they recommended a laterally based closing wedge osteotomy through the bases of the metatarsals. Correcting the alignment without shortening the lateral border of the foot can

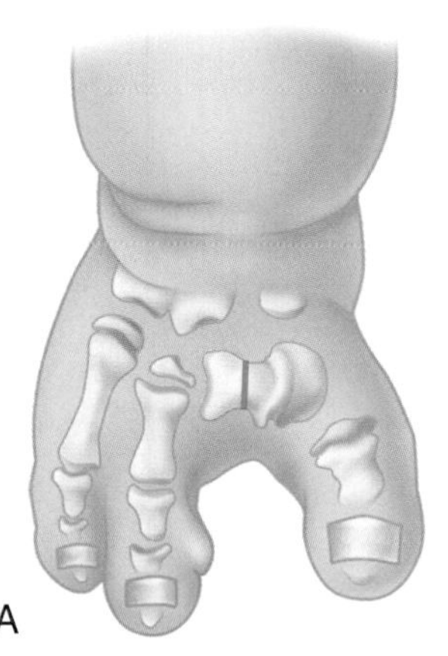

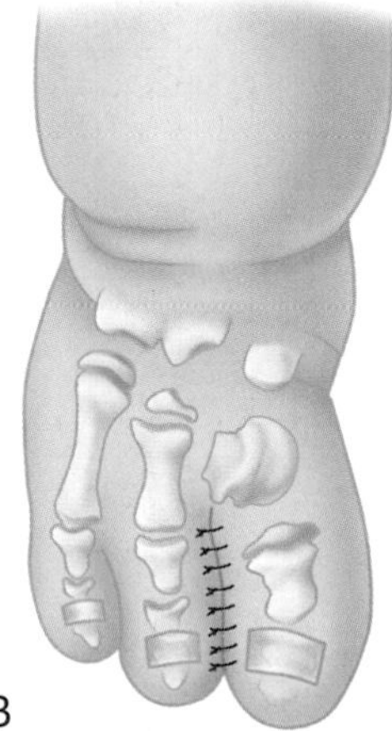

FIGURE 29-17 Kelikian procedure for congenital hallux varus. **A,** Preoperative appearance of foot. **B,** After artificial syndactyly.

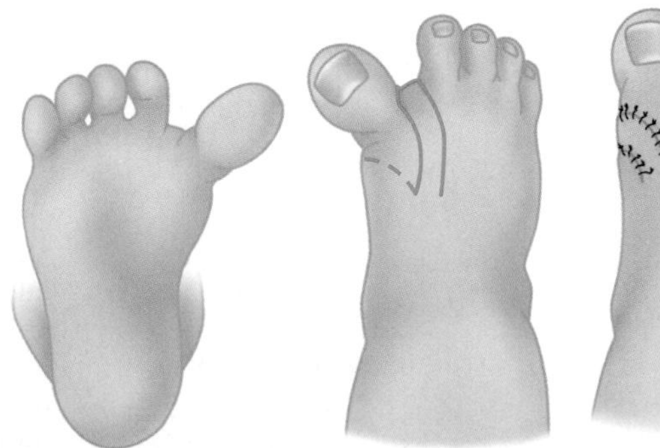

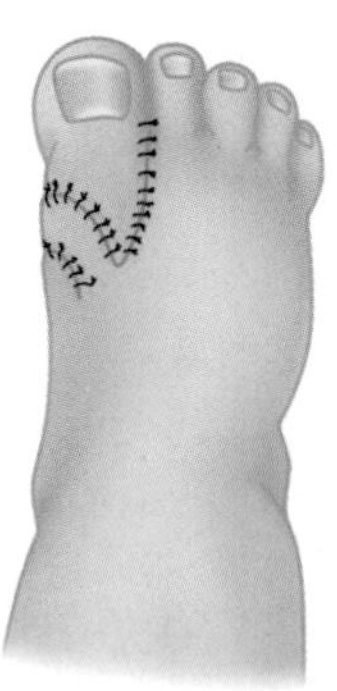

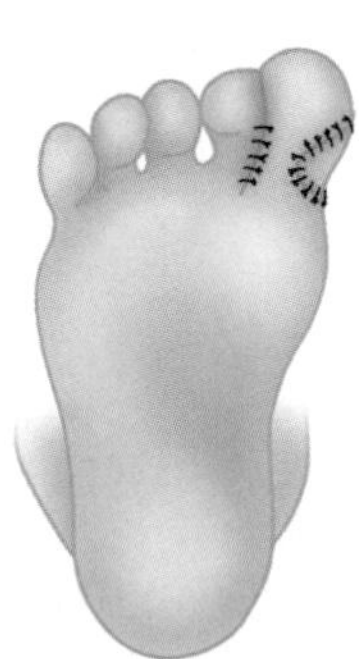

FIGURE 29-18 Farmer procedure for congenital hallux varus (see text). **SEE TECHNIQUE 29-8.**

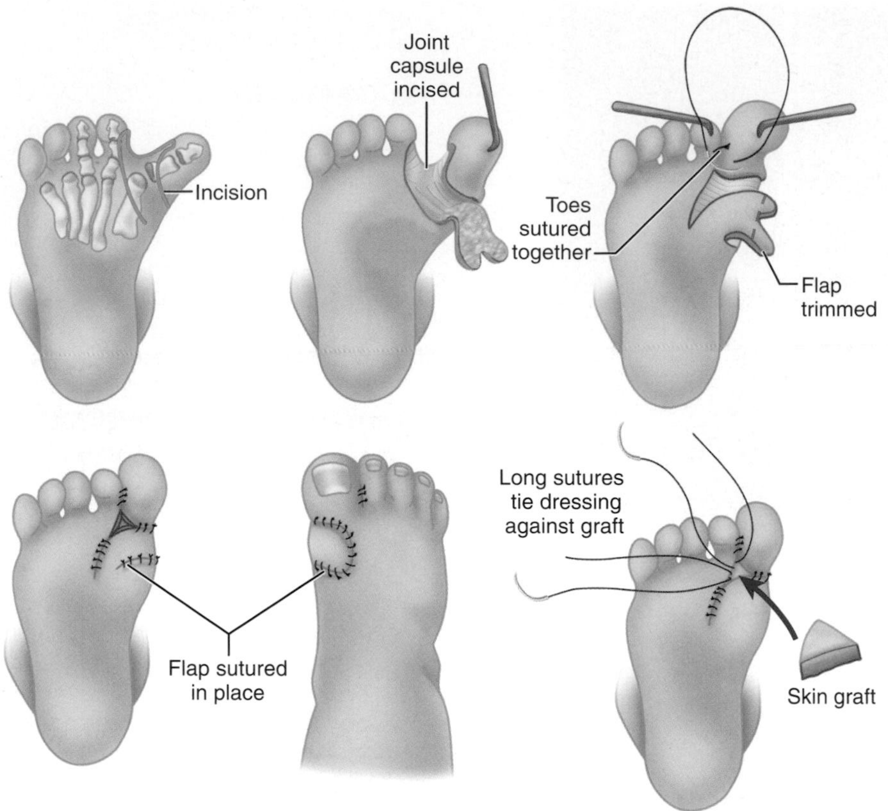

FIGURE 29-19 Alternative Farmer procedure for congenital hallux varus (see text). **SEE TECHNIQUE 29-8.**

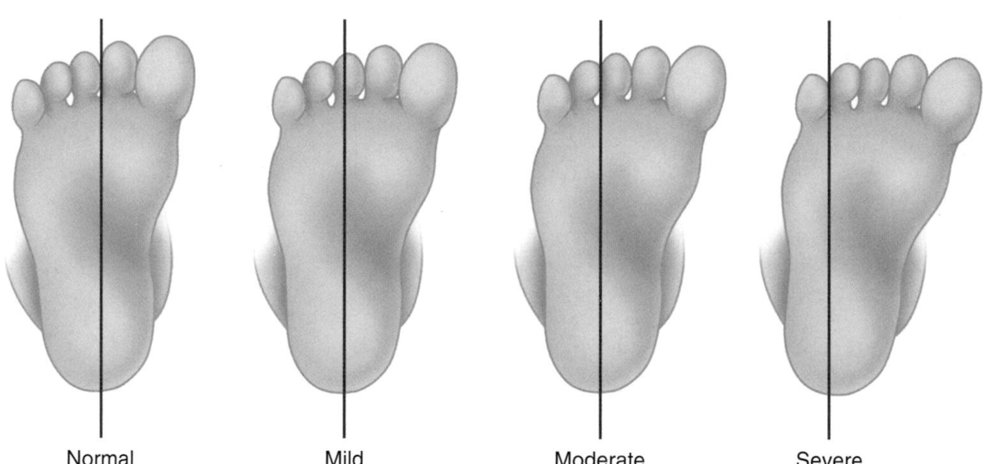

FIGURE 29-20 Heel bisector defines relationship of heel to forefoot from left to right: normal (bisecting second and third toes), mild metatarsus adductus (bisecting third toe), moderate metatarsus adductus (bisecting third and fourth toes), and severe metatarsus adductus (bisecting fourth and fifth toes).

cause excessive tension on the skin on the medial border or on the neurovascular bundle posterior to the medial malleolus. Steinmann pins inserted parallel to the medial and lateral borders of the foot are usually necessary to hold the foot in the corrected position until the osteotomies have healed. Without internal fixation, the soft tissue on the medial side may cause recurrence of deformity.

TECHNIQUE 29-9

(BERMAN AND GARTLAND)

- Approach all five metatarsal bases dorsally. Make two longitudinal dorsal incisions, one between the first and second metatarsals and the other overlying the fourth.

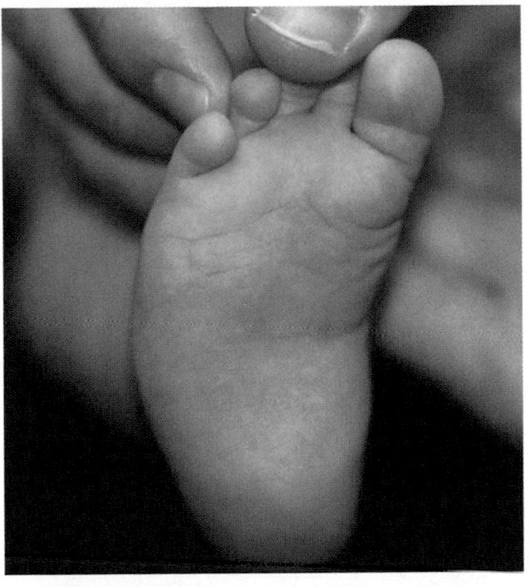

FIGURE 29-21 Congenital metatarsus adductus. Moderate deformity.

BOX 29-1

Treatment of Metatarsus Adductus

None: mild deformities resolve
Serial stretching and casting: rarely for moderate and severe deformities
Surgery: deformity uncorrected by conservative treatment
- Pain
- Objectionable appearance
- Difficulty in fitting shoes

2-4 years: Tarsometatarsal capsulotomies (Heyman, Herndon, and Strong)
≥4 years: Multiple metatarsal osteotomies (Berman and Gartland); medial cuneiform, lateral cuboid double osteotomy

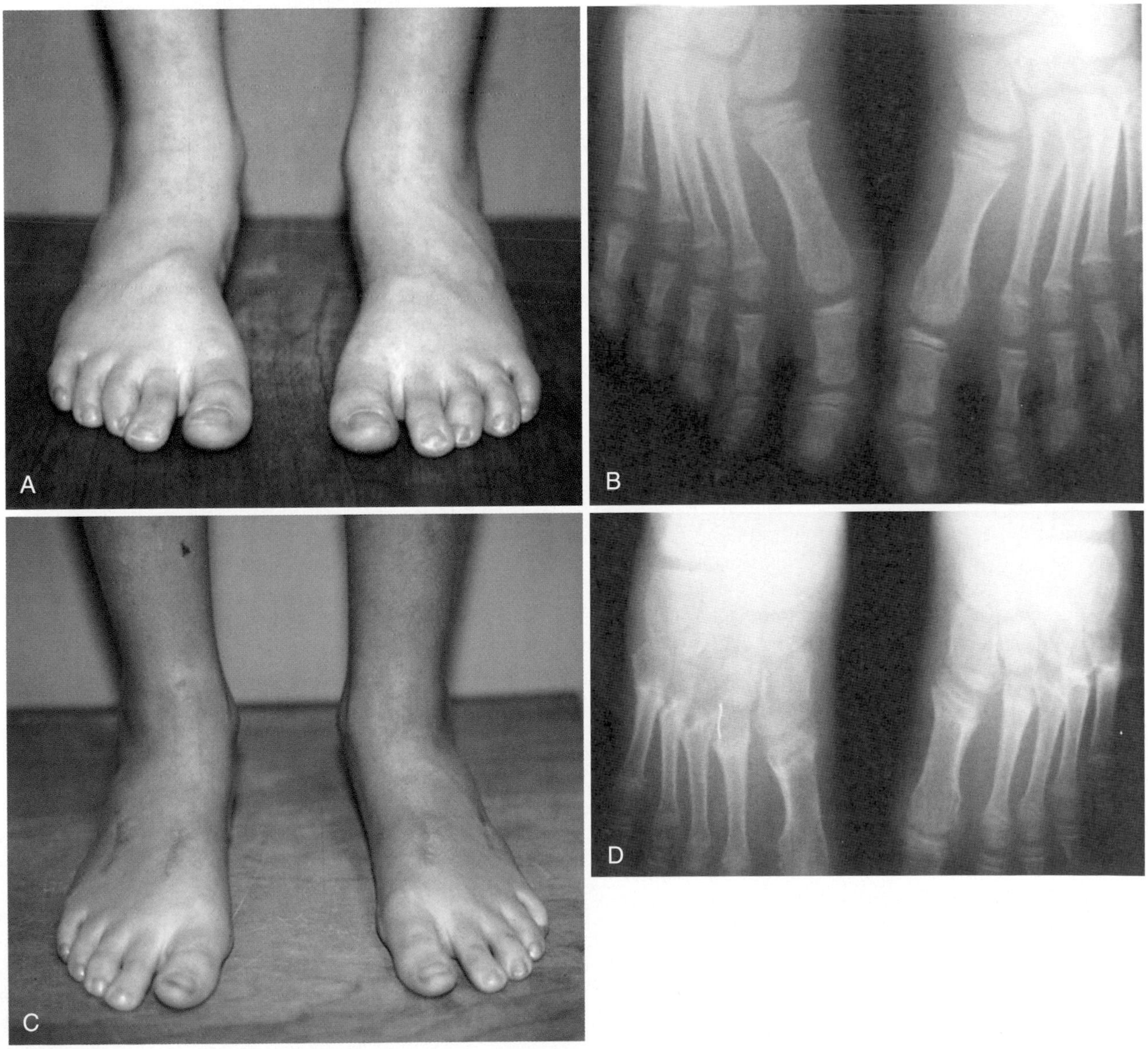

FIGURE 29-22 **A** and **B,** Rigid metatarsus adductus in 8-year-old child. **C** and **D,** After multiple metatarsal osteotomies. **SEE TECHNIQUE 29-9.**

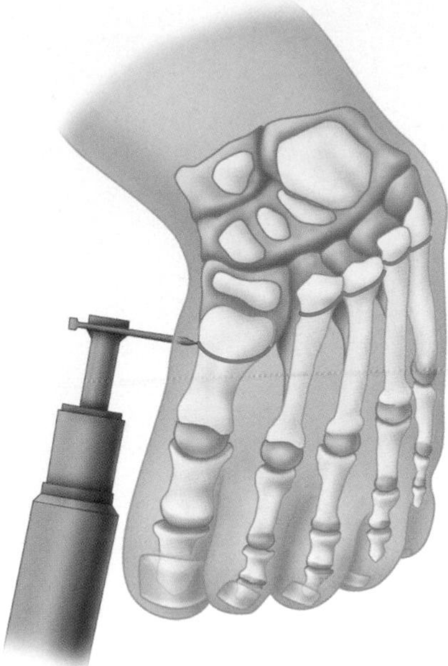

FIGURE 29-23 Berman and Gartland technique for metatarsal osteotomies. Dome-shaped osteotomy is completed at base of each metatarsal. **SEE TECHNIQUE 29-9.**

Protect the extensor tendons and superficial nerves and preserve the superficial veins as much as possible.

- Expose subperiosteally the proximal metaphysis of each metatarsal, and with a small power drill make a dome-shaped osteotomy in each with the apex of the dome proximally (Fig. 29-23). Avoid the physis at the base of the first metatarsal.
- If adequate correction cannot be obtained by these osteotomies, resect small wedges of bone based laterally at the osteotomies as needed.
- Align the metatarsals and transfix the foot in the corrected position with small, smooth Steinmann pins inserted proximally through the shafts of the first and fifth metatarsals and across the osteotomies in these bones and, if needed, in all five metatarsals. Prevent dorsal or volar angulation and overriding of the fragments.
- Before closing the wound, check the placement of the pins, position of the osteotomies, and forefoot alignment by radiographs (Fig. 29-24). The anteroposterior talus–first metatarsal angle should be corrected to 0 to 10 degrees.

POSTOPERATIVE CARE. A short leg cast is applied with the foot in the corrected position. At 6 weeks, the cast and pins are removed, and weight bearing is begun, commonly in a walking cast or cast boot for 2 to 4 weeks.

For the osteotomy portion of the above technique, Knorr et al. described using the Cahuzac technique of percutaneous osteotomies of the metatarsals in children with metatarsus adductus. The approach uses a beaver blade to create two small incisions over the base of the second metatarsal and the third intermetatarsal space. A high-speed surgical burr is

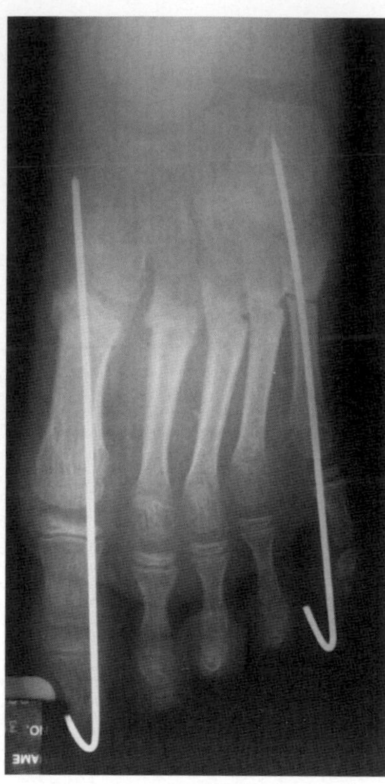

FIGURE 29-24 Completed osteotomies with Steinmann pins inserted to hold corrected position. **SEE TECHNIQUE 29-9.**

used to create a percutaneous osteotomy of the second through fourth metatarsal bases. Percutaneous cuneometatarsal capsulotomy is performed with a 19-gauge needle. The forefoot is manipulated and stabilized with an obliquely oriented, percutaneous 2-mm Kirschner wire from the first metatarsal into the tarsal bones.

CUNEIFORM AND CUBOID OSTEOTOMIES

McHale and Lenhart recommended opening wedge osteotomy of the medial cuneiform and closing wedge osteotomy of the cuboid for correction of deformities in the midfoot with severe shortening of the medial column ("bean-shaped" foot).

TECHNIQUE 29-10

(MCHALE AND LENHART)

- With the anesthetized patient supine, make a small longitudinal incision over the cuboid (Fig. 29-25A).
- Remove a 7- to 10-mm wedge with its base in a dorsolateral position (Fig. 29-25B).
- Approach the medial cuneiform by using part of the distal extension of the medial incision (Fig. 29-25A) or a 2-cm incision medially over the medial cuneiform.
- Make the osteotomy in the cuneiform, leaving the anterior tibial tendon attached to the distal piece of bone.

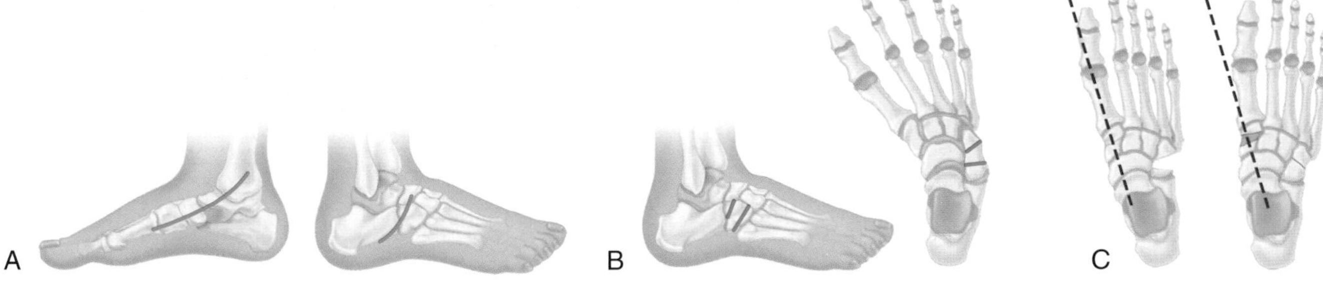

FIGURE 29-25 Osteotomies of medial cuneiform and cuboid for correction of residual deformity. **A,** Lateral and medial incisions. **B,** Removal of dorsolateral wedge from cuboid. **C,** Placement of wedge in osteotomy in medial cuneiform. **SEE TECHNIQUE 29-10.**

- Spread the medial cuneiform osteotomy with a smooth spreader and insert the wedge of bone removed from the cuboid, with the base of the wedge straight medially (Fig. 29-25C).
- Check clinical correction of the deformity. If the lateral border of the foot still appears prominent (midfoot supination has not been corrected), remove a larger wedge of bone from the cuboid.
- Use two smooth Kirschner wires to fix the foot in the corrected position. Insert one pin through the cuboid, starting in the calcaneus and exiting through the base of the fifth metatarsal. Place the other pin through the first web space, through the medial cuneiform and tarsal navicular, and into the talus.
- Confirm the position of the pins and the correction of the bony deformity with radiographs.
- After correct positioning of the foot, the lateral three toes may remain in passively uncorrectable flexion. If so, perform simple flexor tenotomy.
- Close the wounds and apply a short leg cast with thick padding to allow for swelling.

POSTOPERATIVE CARE. At 2 weeks, the wounds are checked, and a more form-fitting, non–weight-bearing cast is applied. The pins are removed at 6 weeks, and a weight bearing cast is applied. A cast or cast boot is worn until bony union is evident on radiographs, usually at 8 to 12 weeks.

ANOMALIES OF THE FOOT

CONGENITAL CLUBFOOT (TALIPES EQUINOVARUS)

The incidence of congenital clubfoot is approximately one in every 1000 live births. Although most cases are sporadic occurrences, families have been reported with clubfoot as an autosomal dominant trait with incomplete penetrance. Bilateral deformities occur in 50% of patients. In patients with bilateral deformity, the severity and response to treatment is highly correlated between the two feet.

Several theories have been proposed regarding the cause of clubfoot, but the underlying cause of clubfoot is still mostly unknown. One theory is that a primary germplasm defect in the talus causes continued plantarflexion and inversion of this bone, with subsequent soft-tissue changes in the joints and musculotendinous complexes. Another theory is that primary soft-tissue abnormalities within the neuromuscular units cause secondary bony changes. There may be a vascular cause because many children with clubfoot have a hypertrophic anterior tibial artery or other vascular anomalies.

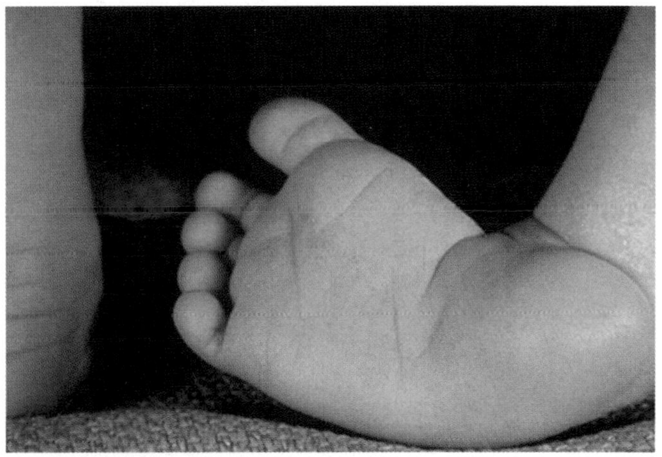

FIGURE 29-26 Congenital clubfoot in newborn. Posterior view—inversion, plantarflexion, and internal rotation of calcaneus and cavus deformity with transverse plantar crease.

Several authors have documented abnormal distribution of type I and type II muscle fibers in clubfeet. The abnormal foot may be one half to one size smaller in length and width.

Multiple studies have demonstrated no correlation between clubfoot and developmental dysplasia of the hip. It is thought that a routine clinical examination screening is all that is needed for the evaluation of hip pathology in children born with a clubfoot deformity.

The pathologic changes caused by congenital clubfoot must be understood if the anomaly is to be treated effectively. The four basic components of clubfoot are cavus, adduction, varus, and equinus. The deformity varies in severity, from a mild positional clubfoot that is passively correctable to near the neutral position to a much more severe clubfoot with extreme, rigid hindfoot equinus and forefoot adduction. The typical deformity is shown in Fig. 29-26. Clubfoot often is accompanied by internal tibial torsion. The ankle, midtarsal, and subtalar joints all are involved in the pathologic process.

Turco attributed the deformity to medial displacement of the navicular and calcaneus around the talus. The talus is forced into equinus by the underlying calcaneus and navicular, whereas the head and neck of the talus are deviated medially. From a three-dimensional perspective, the relationship of the calcaneus to the talus is characterized by abnormal rotation in the sagittal, coronal, and horizontal planes. As the calcaneus rotates horizontally while pivoting on the interosseous ligament, it slips beneath the head and neck of the talus anterior to the ankle joint, and the calcaneal tuberosity moves toward the fibular malleolus posteriorly. The proximity of the calcaneus to the fibula is primarily caused by horizontal rotation of the talocalcaneal joint, rather than by equinus alone. The heel appears to be in varus because the calcaneus rotates through the talocalcaneal joint in a coronal plane and horizontally. The talonavicular joint is in an extreme position of inversion as the navicular moves around the head of the talus. The cuboid is displaced medially on the calcaneus.

In a three-dimensional clubfoot computer model, the talar neck has been shown to be internally rotated relative to the ankle mortise, but the talar body is externally rotated in the mortise. The calcaneus is significantly internally rotated with the sloped articular facet of the calcaneocuboid joint causing additional internal rotation of the midfoot.

Contractures or anomalies of the soft tissues exert further deforming forces and resist correction of bony deformity and realignment of the joints. Talocalcaneal joint realignment is opposed by the calcaneofibular ligament, the superior peroneal retinaculum (calcaneal fibular retinaculum), the peroneal tendon sheaths, and the posterior talocalcaneal ligament. Resisting realignment of the talonavicular joint are the posterior tibial tendon, the deltoid ligament (tibial navicular), the calcaneonavicular ligament (spring ligament), the entire talonavicular capsule, the dorsal talonavicular ligament, the bifurcated (Y) ligament, the inferior extensor retinaculum, and occasionally the cubonavicular oblique ligament. Internal rotation of the calcaneocuboid joint causes contracture of the bifurcated (Y) ligament, the long plantar ligament, the plantar calcaneocuboid ligament, the navicular cuboid ligament, the inferior extensor retinaculum (cruciate ligament), the dorsal calcaneocuboid ligament, and occasionally the cubonavicular ligament.

The metatarsals also are often deformed. They may deviate at the tarsometatarsal joints, or these joints may be normal, and the shafts of the metatarsals themselves may be adducted.

If the clubfoot is allowed to remain deformed, many other late adaptive changes occur in the bones. These changes depend on the severity of the soft-tissue contractures and the effects of walking. In untreated adults, some joints may spontaneously fuse, or they may develop degenerative changes secondary to the contractures.

The initial examination of the foot and the progress of treatment should depend on clinical judgment and occasionally radiographic examination.

RADIOGRAPHIC EVALUATION

If the clubfoot deformity is somewhat atypical, is associated with a global genetic or neurologic condition, or appears resistant to initial nonoperative treatment, imaging evaluation should be included. In a nonambulatory child, standard radiographs include simulated weight-bearing anteroposterior and stress dorsiflexion lateral radiographs of both feet. Standing anteroposterior and lateral standing radiographs may be obtained for an older child. Alternatively, ultrasonography has been proposed as a radiation-free imaging modality and could be used in locations familiar with the technique.

TABLE 29-1

Progression of Foot Angles in Normal Feet Over Average 6-Year Follow-Up

ANGLE	AVERAGE FIRST VISIT (DEGREES)	AVERAGE LAST VISIT (DEGREES)
ANTEROPOSTERIOR VIEW		
Talocalcaneal	36.3	27.4
Calcaneal–second metatarsal	14.4	12.3
Talus–first metatarsal	16.9	8.1
LATERAL VIEW		
Talocalcaneal	46	44.2
Calcaneal–first metatarsal	150	148
Tibiocalcaneal	61.5	73.2
Talus–first metatarsal	16.3	12.1
Talocalcaneal index	83	71.6

Important angles to consider in the evaluation of clubfoot are the talocalcaneal angle on the anteroposterior radiograph, the talocalcaneal angle on the lateral radiograph, the tibiocalcaneal angle, and the talus–first metatarsal angle (Fig. 29-27). The anteroposterior talocalcaneal angle in normal children ranges from 30 to 55 degrees (Table 29-1). In clubfoot, this angle progressively decreases with increasing heel varus. On the dorsiflexion lateral radiograph, the talocalcaneal angle in a normal foot varies from 25 to 50 degrees; in clubfoot, this angle progressively decreases with the severity of the deformity to an angle of 0 degrees, or parallelism. The tibiocalcaneal angle in a normal foot is 10 to 40 degrees on the stress lateral radiograph. In clubfoot, this angle generally is negative, indicating equinus of the calcaneus in relation to the tibia. Finally, the talus–first metatarsal angle is a radiographic measurement of forefoot adduction. This is useful in the treatment of metatarsus adductus alone but is equally important in the treatment of clubfoot to evaluate the position of the forefoot. In a normal foot, this angle is 5 to 15 degrees on the anteroposterior view; in clubfoot, it usually is negative, indicating adduction of the forefoot.

CLASSIFICATION

Two of the more commonly used classifications by Pirani et al. and Diméglio et al. are based solely on physical examination requiring no radiographic measurements or other special studies. Pirani's system is composed of six different physical examination findings and includes a hindfoot contracture score and a midfoot contracture score (Table 29-2), each scored 0 for no abnormality, 0.5 for moderate abnormality, or 1 for severe abnormality. Each foot is assigned a total score, the maximum being 6 points, with a higher score indicating a more severe deformity. In the system of Diméglio

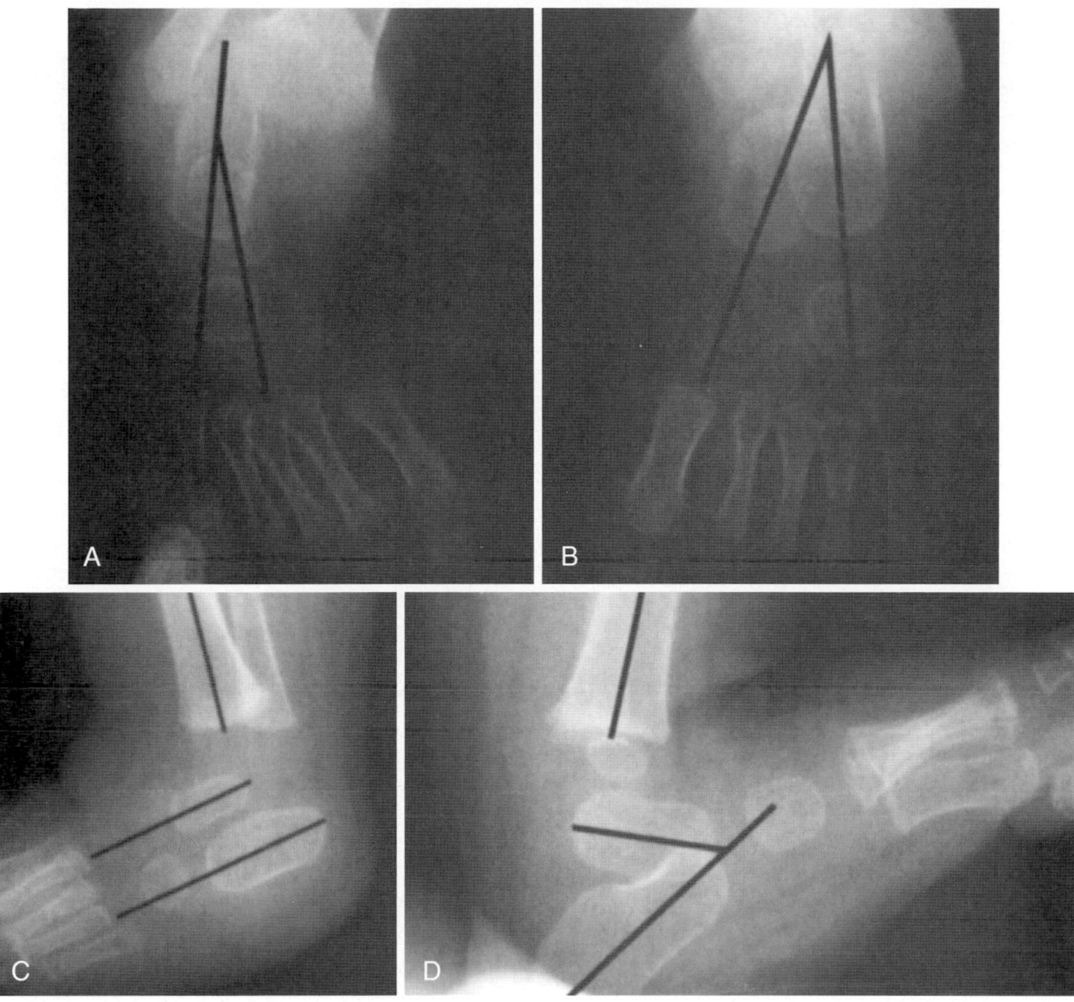

FIGURE 29-27 Radiographic evaluation of clubfoot. **A,** Anteroposterior view of right clubfoot with decrease in talocalcaneal angle and negative talus–first metatarsal angle. **B,** Talocalcaneal angle on anteroposterior view of normal left foot. **C,** Talocalcaneal angle of 0 degrees and negative tibiocalcaneal angle on dorsiflexion lateral view of right clubfoot. **D,** Talocalcaneal and tibiocalcaneal angles on dorsiflexion lateral view of normal left foot.

et al, four parameters are assessed on the basis of their reducibility with gentle manipulation as measured with a handheld goniometer: (1) equinus deviation in the sagittal plane, (2) varus deviation in the frontal plane, (3) derotation of the calcaneopedal block in the horizontal plane, and (4) adduction of the forefoot relative to the hindfoot in the horizontal plane (Fig. 29-28). In a comparison of the two systems both were shown to have good interobserver reliability after the initial learning phase. Routine clinical use of one or both of these classification systems can be helpful in determining prognosis and documenting maintenance of correction or recurrence over time.

NONOPERATIVE TREATMENT

The initial treatment of clubfoot is nonoperative. Various treatment regimens have been proposed, including the use of corrective splinting, taping, and casting. Although a number of various casting techniques are used, the most widely accepted technique is that described by Ignacio Ponseti and consists of weekly serial manipulation and casting during the first weeks of life.

PONSETI CASTING TECHNIQUE FOR CORRECTION OF CLUBFOOT DEFORMITY

Successful correction of clubfoot deformity generally is reported in more than 90% of children 2 years and younger treated with Ponseti casting even after previous unsuccessful nonoperative treatment. Multiple studies have highlighted the success and reproducibility of the Ponseti method even in developing nations. Achilles tenotomy generally is required, and anterior tibial tendon transfer may be added to the casting routine when necessary. Bleeding complications have been reported after percutaneous tenotomy from injury to the peroneal artery or the lesser saphenous vein; making a small open incision directly over the tendon before severing it, making the tenotomy from medial to lateral (Fig. 29-29), and using a more rounded beaver-eye blade can help avoid vascular injury.

Reported recurrence rates after Ponseti casting range from 10% to 30%; however, many recurrent deformities can be treated successfully with repeat casting, with or without the addition of Achilles tenotomy or anterior tibial tendon transfer. Numerous authors have noted that the most

TABLE 29-2

Pirani Classification of Clubfoot Deformity

PHYSICAL EXAMINATION FINDINGS	SCORE OF 0 NO ABNORMALITY	SCORE OF 0.5 MODERATE ABNORMALITY	SCORE OF 1 SEVERE ABNORMALITY
Severity of posterior crease (foot held in maximal correction) (HCFS 1)	Multiple fine creases	One or two deep creases	Deep creases of arch change contour
Emptiness of heel (foot and ankle in maximal correction) (HCFS 2)	Tuberosity of calcaneus easily palpable	Tuberosity of calcaneus more difficult to palpate	Tuberosity of calcaneus not palpable
Rigidity of equinus (knee extended, ankle to ankle maximally corrected) (HCFS 3).	Normal ankle dorsiflexion	Ankle neutral, but not fully dorsiflexes beyond	Cannot dorsiflex neutral
Severity of medial crease (foot held in maximal correction) (MFCS 1)	Multiple fine creases	One or two deep creases	Deep creases change contour of arch
Curvature of lateral border of foot (MFCS 2)	Straight	Mild distal curve	Curve at calcaneocuboid joint
Palpation of lateral part of head of talus (forefoot fully abducted) (MCFS 3)	Navicular completely "reduces"; lateral talar head cannot be felt	Navicular partially "reduces"; lateral head less palpable	Navicular does not "reduce"; lateral talar head easily felt
Medial malleolar–navicular interval (foot held in maximal correction)	Definite depression felt	Interval reduced	Interval not palpable
Fibula-Achilles interval (hip flexed, knee extended, foot and ankle maximally corrected)	Definite depression felt	Interval reduced	Interval not palpable
Rigidity of adductus (forefoot is fully abducted)	Forefoot can be overcorrected into abduction	Forefoot can be corrected beyond neutral, but not fully	Forefoot cannot be corrected to neutral
Long flexor contracture (foot and ankle held in maximal correction)	MTP joints can be dorsiflexed to 90 degrees	MTP joints can be dorsiflexed beyond neutral but not fully	MTP joints cannot be dorsiflexed to neutral

Modified from Flynn JM, Donohoe M, Mackenzie WG: An independent assessment of two clubfoot-classification systems, J Pediatr Orthop 18:323, 1998.
HCFS, Hindfoot contracture score; *MFCS*, midfoot contracture score; *MTP*, metatarsophalangeal.

important factor in avoiding recurrent deformity is patient compliance with the postoperative brace wear regimen. Although the Ponseti method is ideally used in newborns, many studies have demonstrated successful use of the Ponseti method in older children or children with recurrent deformities after initial casting treatment. Although the success rates are lower in older children, nonoperative treatment should be considered the first line of treatment even in a toddler.

Strict adherence to the principles described by Ponseti is important to achieve optimal results. Only a few modifications to his original technique have demonstrated equivalent results. An accelerated casting program biweekly can result in more rapid correction of the deformity without compromising outcome. Fiberglass casting material has been shown to provide similar results to plaster casts. Bracing up to the age of 4 years may be superior to discontinuing brace treatment at the age of 3 years as originally described.

Application of Ponseti Casts. The Ponseti method consists of two phases: treatment and maintenance. The treatment phase should begin as early as possible, optimally within the first two weeks of life; however, older children also can be treated nonoperatively using Ponseti's principles. Gentle manipulation and casting are done weekly, although more frequent cast changes over a shorter period of time have been advocated by some authors. The order of correction by serial manipulation and casting should be as follows: first, correction of forefoot cavus and adduction; next, correction of heel varus; and finally, correction of hindfoot equinus. Correction should be pursued in this order so that a rocker-bottom deformity is prevented by dorsiflexing the foot through the ankle joint rather than the midfoot. Each cast holds the foot in the corrected position, allowing it to reshape gradually. Generally five to six casts are required to correct the alignment of the foot and ankle fully. Before application of the final cast, most infants require percutaneous Achilles tenotomy (Fig. 29-29) to gain adequate lengthening of the Achilles tendon and prevent a rocker bottom deformity.

The first cast application corrects the cavus deformity by aligning the forefoot with the hindfoot, supinating the forefoot to bring it in line with the heel, and elevating (dorsiflexing) the first metatarsal (Fig. 29-30A). The casts should be applied in two stages: first, a short leg cast to just below the knee, then extension above the knee when the plaster sets. Long leg casts are essential to maintain a strong external rotation force of the foot beneath the talus, to allow adequate stretching of the medial structures, and to prevent cast slippage.

One week after application, the first cast is removed, and after about 1 minute of manipulation, the next toe-to-groin cast is applied (Fig. 29-30B). Manipulation and casting at this

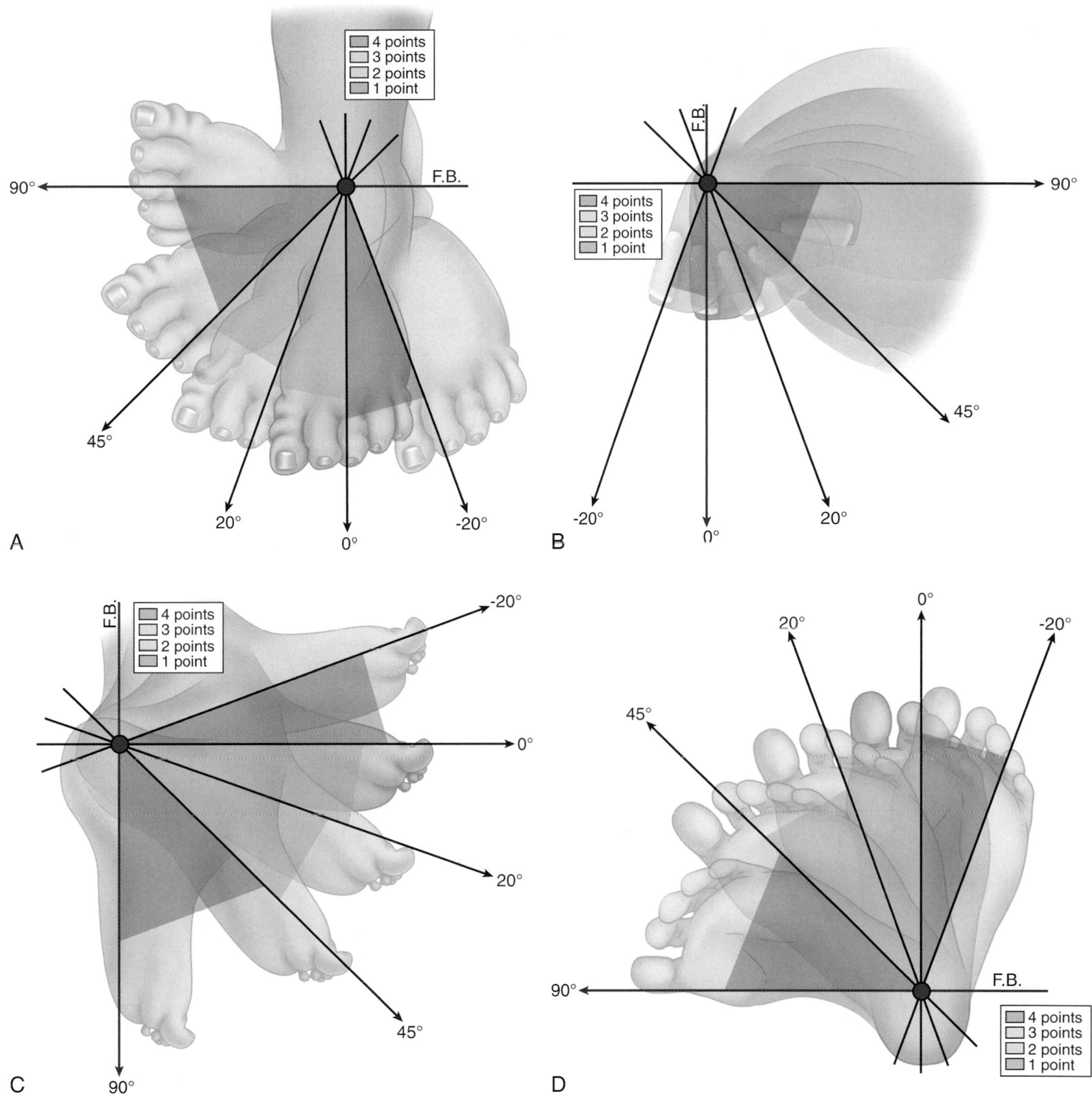

FIGURE 29-28 Classification of clubfoot severity by Diméglio (see text and Table 29-3). **A,** Equinus deviation. **B,** Varus deviation. **C,** Derotation. **D,** Adduction. (From Diméglio A, Bensahel H, Souchet P, et al: Classification of clubfoot, J Pediatr Orthop B 4:129, 1995.)

stage are focused on abducting the foot around the head of the talus, with care to maintain the supinated position of the forefoot and avoid any pronation. During these manipulations, the navicular can be felt reducing over the talar head by a thumb placed on the head of the talus. It is crucial that forefoot derotation occur about the talus rather than the calcaneocuboid joint and the heel should not be directly manipulated. Maintaining forefoot supination throughout the process and correcting the talonavicular subluxation without producing a rocker-bottom deformity will cause the calcaneus to abduct and evert. Final correction of residual calcaneus deformity can then be achieved with a percutaneous Achilles tenotomy.

Manipulation and casting are continued weekly for the next 2 to 3 weeks to abduct the foot gradually around the head of the talus. The foot should never be actively pronated; however, the amount of supination is gradually decreased over these several casts until the forefoot is in neutral position

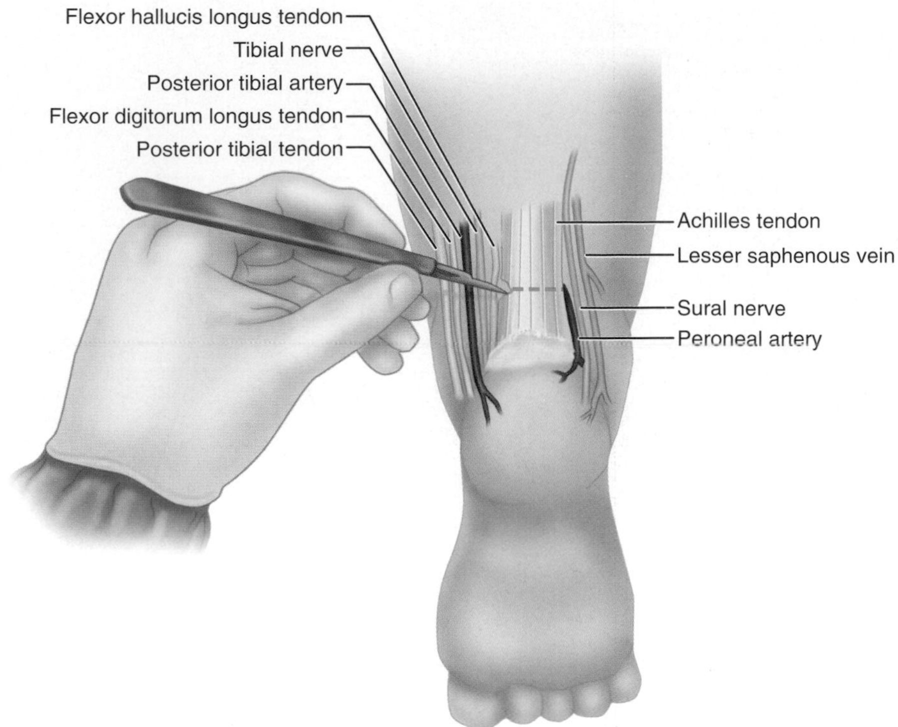

FIGURE 29-29 Technique of percutaneous Achilles tenotomy from medial to lateral; note proximity of peroneal artery, lesser saphenous vein, and sural nerve to lateral edge of tendon.

relative to the longitudinal axis of the foot (Fig. 29-30C). Ideally each cast should be removed just before repeat manipulation and casting, and a variety of casting materials can be used with similar success.

The final cast is applied with the foot in the same maximally abducted position and dorsiflexed 15 degrees. In most children, a percutaneous Achilles tenotomy is done to prevent development of a rocker-bottom deformity. This procedure can either be performed in the clinic with local skin anesthesia, or in the operating room under sedation or general anesthesia. The benefit of tenotomy in the clinic setting is a reduced need for anesthesia and prolonged fasting; however, the operating room offers the ability to more easily control any excess bleeding that may occur. The foot is cast in the final position of approximately 70 degrees of abduction and 15 degrees of dorsiflexion for 3 weeks (Fig. 29-30D). Five or six casts usually are necessary to correct the clubfoot deformity.

Maintenance Phase. When the final cast is removed, the infant is placed in a brace that maintains the foot in its corrected position (abducted and dorsiflexed). The brace (foot abduction orthosis) consists of shoes mounted to a bar in a position of 70 degrees of external rotation and 15 degrees of dorsiflexion. The distance between the shoes is set at about 1 inch wider than the width of the infant's shoulders (Fig. 29-31).

Multiple different types of shoes and bars have been designed and proposed. In some cases, it may be necessary to experiment with different combinations to find a brace that will lead to maximal compliance. The brace is worn 23 hours each day for the first 3 months after casting and then while sleeping for 3 to 4 years. Brace wear compliance is of upmost importance in maintaining correction and preventing recurrence. Frequent follow-up during the bracing period is essential to encourage continued compliance and to detect early recurrence.

MANAGEMENT OF RECURRENCE

Recurrence of the deformity is infrequent if the bracing protocol is followed closely. Early recurrences (usually mild equinus and heel varus) are best treated with repeat manipulation and casting. The first cast may require some dorsiflexion of the first ray if cavus deformity is present. Subsequent casts abduct the foot around the talar head, correcting the varus and ultimately allowing ankle dorsiflexion. Achilles tendon lengthening (Fig. 29-29) may be necessary if dorsiflexion is insufficient; transfer of the anterior tibial tendon (see Chapter 34) may be necessary to help maintain correction, particularly in children with persistent dynamic inversion.

OPERATIVE TREATMENT

Surgery in clubfoot is indicated for deformities that do not respond to conservative treatment by serial manipulation and casting. Often in children with a significant rigid clubfoot deformity, the forefoot has been corrected by conservative treatment, but the hindfoot remains fixed in varus and equinus, or the deformity has recurred. Surgery in the treatment of clubfoot must be tailored to the age of the child and to the deformity to be corrected.

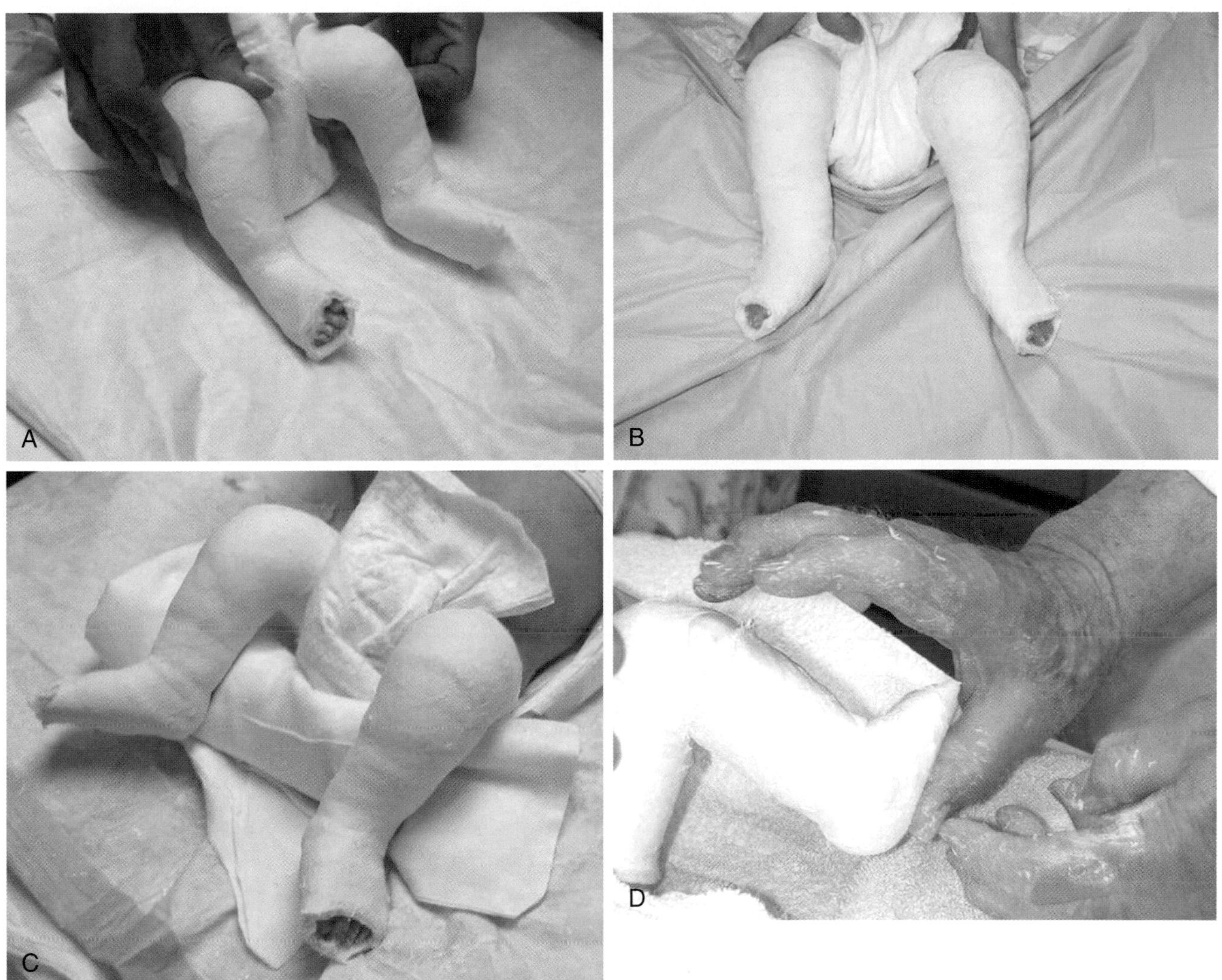

FIGURE 29-30 Technique of Ponseti casting for clubfoot correction (see text). **A,** First cast; note positioning of forefoot to align with heel, with outer edge of foot tilted even farther downward because of Achilles tendon tightness. **B,** Second cast is applied with outer edge of foot still tilted downward and forefoot moved slightly outward. **C,** Third cast; Achilles tendon is stretched bringing outer edge of foot into more normal position as forefoot is turned farther outward. **D,** Final cast; Achilles tendon is stretched more with foot pointed upward. (From Scher DM: The Ponseti method for clubfoot correction, Oper Tech Orthop 15:345, 2005.)

Extensive release that includes the posterolateral ligament complex most often is required for severe deformity. The procedure described by McKay takes into consideration the three-dimensional deformity of the subtalar joint and allows correction of the internal rotational deformity of the calcaneus and release of the contractures of the posterolateral and posteromedial foot. A modified McKay procedure through a transverse circumferential (Cincinnati) incision is our preferred technique for the initial surgical management of most clubfeet.

General principles for any one-stage extensile clubfoot release include (1) release of the tourniquet at the completion of the procedure, obtaining hemostasis by electrocautery, and (2) careful subcutaneous and skin closure, with the foot in plantarflexion, if necessary, to prevent tension on the skin. The foot can be placed in a fully corrected position 2 weeks after surgery at the first postoperative cast change. Surgery can be done with the child supine or prone, at the discretion of the surgeon.

TRANSVERSE CIRCUMFERENTIAL (CINCINNATI) INCISION

One option for comprehensive release is the use of the transverse circumferential incision, also known as the Cincinnati incision. This incision provides excellent exposure of the subtalar joint and is useful in patients with a severe internal rotational deformity of the calcaneus. One potential problem with this incision is tension on the suture line when attempting to place the foot in dorsiflexion to apply the postoperative cast. To avoid this, the foot can be placed in plantarflexion in the immediate postoperative cast and then in dorsiflexion to the corrected position at the first cast change when the wound has healed at 2 weeks. This cast change frequently requires sedation or outpatient general anesthesia.

If primary skin closure is difficult in a foot in a fully corrected position, a fasciocutaneous flap closure can be

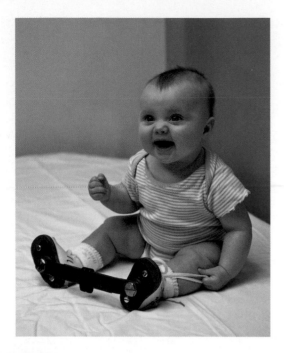

FIGURE 29-31 Foot abduction orthosis consists of shoes mounted to bar in 70 degrees external rotation and 15 degrees dorsiflexion.

used. The rotation of V-Y flaps allow complete wound closure without any skin tension.

TECHNIQUE 29-11

(CRAWFORD, MARXEN, AND OSTERFELD)

- Begin the incision on the medial aspect of the foot in the region of the naviculocuneiform joint (Fig. 29-32A).
- Carry the incision posteriorly, gently curving beneath the distal end of the medial malleolus and ascending slightly to pass transversely over the Achilles tendon approximately at the level of the tibiotalar joint (Fig. 29-32B).
- Continue the incision in a gentle curve over the lateral malleolus and end it just distal and slightly medial to the sinus tarsi (Fig. 29-32C).
- Extend the incision distally medially or laterally, depending on the requirements of the operation.

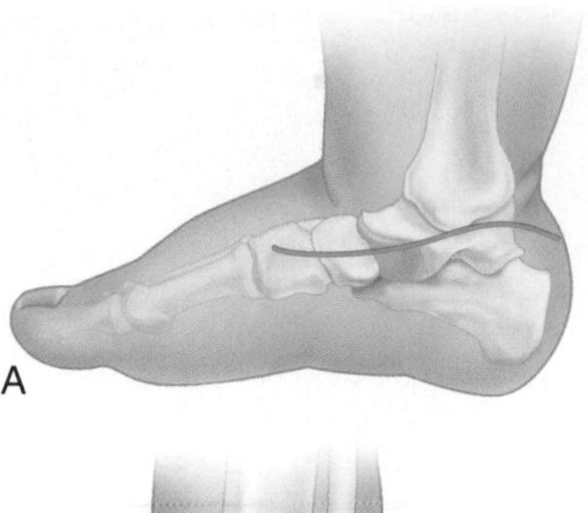

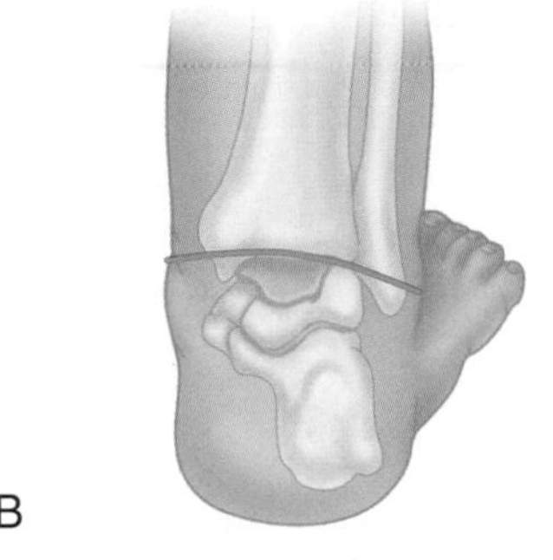

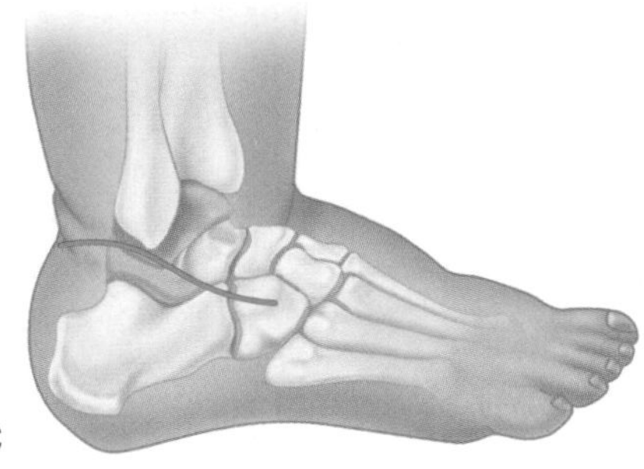

FIGURE 29-32 Transverse circumferential (Cincinnati) incision as described by Crawford et al. **A,** Medial view. **B,** Posterior view. **C,** Lateral view. **SEE TECHNIQUES 29-11 AND 29-20.**

EXTENSILE POSTEROMEDIAL AND POSTEROLATERAL RELEASE

TECHNIQUE 29-12

(MCKAY, MODIFIED)

- Incise the skin through a transverse circumferential (Cincinnati) incision, preserving if possible the veins on the lateral side and protecting the sural nerve.
- Dissect the subcutaneous tissue up and down the Achilles tendon to lengthen the tendon at least 2.5 cm in the coronal plane. If sagittal plane lengthening is done, the lateral attachment of the Achilles tendon to the calcaneus should be preserved to aid in correction of hindfoot varus.
- Incise the superior peroneal retinaculum off the calcaneus at the point where it blends with the sheath of the Achilles tendon.
- Dissecting carefully, release the peroneal tendons from their sheaths and protect them with a vessel loop, then separate the calcaneofibular and posterior calcaneotalar ligaments, the thickened superior peroneal retinaculum, and the peroneal tendon sheath.
- Incise the calcaneofibular ligament close to the calcaneus (this ligament is short and thick and attached very close to the apophysis).
- Incise the lateral talocalcaneal ligament and the lateral capsule of the talocalcaneal joint from their attachments to the calcaneocuboid joint to the point where they enter the sheath of the flexor hallucis longus tendon posteriorly. In more resistant clubfeet, the origin of the extensor digitorum brevis, cruciate crural ligament (inferior extensor retinaculum), dorsal calcaneocuboid ligament, and, occasionally, cubonavicular oblique ligament must be dissected off the calcaneus to allow the anterior portion of the calcaneus to move laterally.

- On the medial side, dissect free the neurovascular bundle (medial and lateral plantar nerves and associated vascular components) into the arch of the foot, preserving the medial calcaneal branch of the lateral plantar nerve. Protect and retract the neurovascular bundle with a small Penrose drain or vessel loop. Complete dissection of the medial and lateral neurovascular bundle throughout the arch of the foot.
- Enter the compartment of the medial plantar neurovascular bundle and follow it into the arch of the foot well beyond the cuneiforms; elevate the abductor hallucis muscle to enter the plantar aspect of the foot.
- Enter the sheaths of the posterior tibial tendon, the flexor hallucis longus and flexor digitorum longus tendons, and protect each of these structures.
- Section the narrow strip of fascia between the medial and lateral branches of the plantar nerve to allow the abductor hallucis to slide distally.
- Enter the sheath of the posterior tibial tendon just posterior to and above the medial malleolus. Split the sheath and superficial deltoid ligament up the tibia until the muscle can be identified.
- Lengthen the tendon by Z-plasty at least 2.5 cm proximal from the medial malleolus to the maximal distance allowed by the incision. Starting from the point at which the flexor digitorum longus and the flexor hallucis longus tendons cross, sharply dissect both sheaths from the sustentaculum tali, moving in a proximal direction until the talocalcaneal joint is entered.
- Continue the dissection down and around the navicular, holding the distal segment of the lengthened posterior tibial tendon attached to the bone.
- Open the talonavicular joint by pulling on the remaining posterior tibial tendon attachment and carefully cut the deltoid ligament (medial tibial navicular ligament), talonavicular capsule, dorsal talonavicular ligament, and plantar calcaneonavicular (spring) ligament close to the navicular.
- Enter and carefully expose by blunt dissection and retraction the interval between the dorsal aspect of the talonavicular joint and the extensor tendons and neurovascular bundle on the dorsum of the foot. Do not dissect or disturb the blood supply to the dorsal aspect of the talus.
- Follow through with the dissection, incising the capsule of the talonavicular joint all the way around medially, inferiorly, superiorly, and laterally. Inferior and lateral to the joint is the bifurcated (Y) ligament; incise both ends of this ligament to correct the horizontal rotation of the calcaneus.
- Complete the release of the talocalcaneal joint ligaments and capsule by incising the remaining medial and posteromedial capsule and superficial deltoid ligament attached to the sustentaculum tali. Do not incise the talocalcaneal ligaments (interosseous ligaments) at this time.
- Retract the lateral plantar nerve, detach the origin of the quadratus plantae muscle using a periosteal elevator on the medial inferior surface of the calcaneus, and expose the long plantar ligament over the plantar calcaneocuboid ligament and the peroneus longus tendon.
- At this point, the talus should roll back into the ankle joint, exposing at least 1.5 cm of hyaline cartilage on its body. If this does not happen, incise the posterior talofibular ligament. If the talus still does not roll back into the ankle joint, cut the posterior portion only of the deep deltoid ligament.
- The decision must be made as to the necessity of dividing the interosseous talocalcaneal ligament to correct the horizontal rotational abnormality through the talocalcaneal joint. This decision depends on the completeness of the correction and the mobility of the subtalar complex, as determined by the position of the foot.
- Line up the medial side of the head and neck of the talus with the medial side of the cuneiforms and medially push the calcaneus posterior to the ankle joint while pushing the foot as a whole in a posterior direction. Examine the angle made by the intersection of the bimalleolar ankle plane with the horizontal plane of the foot; if the angle is 85 to 90 degrees, the ligament need not be cut. In children older than 1 year of age, such an incision generally is necessary, however, because the ligament usually has become broad and thick, preventing derotation of the talocalcaneal joint.
- After the foot has been satisfactorily corrected, pass a small Kirschner wire through the talus from the posterior aspect into the middle of the head. Positioning the pin in a slightly lateral direction in the head of the talus is beneficial in older children with more pronounced medial deviation of the talar head and neck because it allows lateral displacement of the navicular and cuneiforms on the head of the talus to eliminate forefoot adduction.
- Pass the pin through the talonavicular joint and cuneiforms and out the forefoot on either the medial or the lateral side of the first metatarsal. While an assistant inserts the pin, mold the forefoot out of adduction. Cut off the end of the pin close to the body of the talus. The pin can be left out of the skin on the dorsum of the forefoot or just under the skin requiring a small incision later for removal in the operating room.
- Check for proper positioning of the foot: The longitudinal plane of the foot is 85 to 90 degrees to the bimalleolar ankle plane, and the heel under the tibia is in slight valgus.
- If the talocalcaneal ligament has been divided, insert a pin through the calcaneus, burying it deep in the talus from the plantar surface. Do not penetrate the ankle joint.
- Suture the posterior tibial and Achilles tendons snugly with the foot in slight dorsiflexion. Lengthening of the flexor digitorum longus is rarely required, but the flexor hallucis longus is typically tight with the foot in the corrected position. The flexor hallucis longus tightness can be corrected by a fractional lengthening at the musculotendinous junction, a Z-lengthening of the tendon, transection of the tendon after formal tenodesis to the flexor digitorum longus at the master knot of Henry (preferred technique), or by flexor tenotomy at the level of proximal phalanx of the great toe.
- Reposition the lengthened posterior tibial tendon in its sheath and repair the sheath beneath the medial malleolus. With the fibrofatty tissue left attached to the

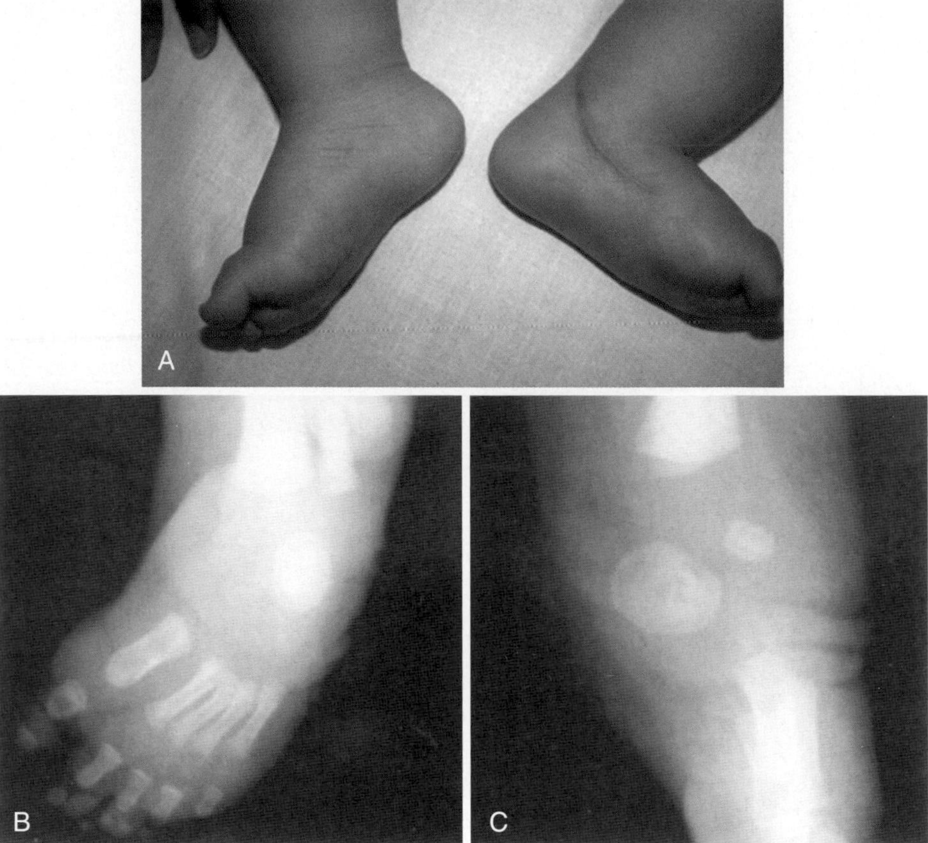

FIGURE 29-33 Modified McKay procedure using Cincinnati incision. **A,** Clinical appearance after correction. **B** and **C,** Preoperative anteroposterior and lateral radiographs. **SEE TECHNIQUE 29-12.**

calcaneus anterior to the Achilles tendon, cover the lateral aspect of the ankle joint. Keep the peroneal tendons and sheaths from subluxating around the fibula by suturing the sheaths of the peroneal tendons to the fibrofatty flap. Close the subcutaneous tissue and skin with interrupted sutures.

- Apply nonadherent dressing and, very loosely, apply a padded long leg cast with the foot in plantarflexion and the flexed to 90 degrees (Fig. 29-33).

POSTOPERATIVE CARE. A long leg cast is applied with the foot in plantarflexion. At 2 weeks, the cast is changed, and the foot is placed in the corrected position. This can be done with sedation or general anesthesia as an outpatient procedure. At 6 weeks, the cast and pins are removed in the operating room (Fig. 29-34). Correction is maintained in an ankle/foot orthosis.

Special attention should be given to two specific problems in clubfoot. The first is residual hindfoot equinus in children 6 to 12 months old who have obtained adequate correction of forefoot adduction and hindfoot varus. This equinus can be corrected adequately by Achilles tendon lengthening and posterior capsulotomy of the ankle and subtalar joints without an extensive one-stage posteromedial release. Careful intraoperative assessment is necessary to determine if a more extensive release is required instead of a limited procedure that corrects only hindfoot equinus. The heel varus and internal rotation must have been corrected adequately if Achilles tendon lengthening and posterior capsulotomy are to be used alone.

The second specific problem is dynamic metatarsus adductus caused by overpull of the anterior tibial tendon in older children who have had correction of clubfoot. In the rare child with symptoms, the treatment of choice is transfer of the anterior tibial tendon to the lateral cuneiform. The forefoot must be flexible for a tendon transfer to succeed (see Technique 34-9).

ACHILLES TENDON LENGTHENING AND POSTERIOR CAPSULOTOMY

TECHNIQUE 29-13

- Make a straight longitudinal incision over the medial aspect of the Achilles tendon, beginning at its most distal point and extending proximally to 3 cm above the level of the ankle joint. Carry sharp dissection through the subcutaneous tissue.

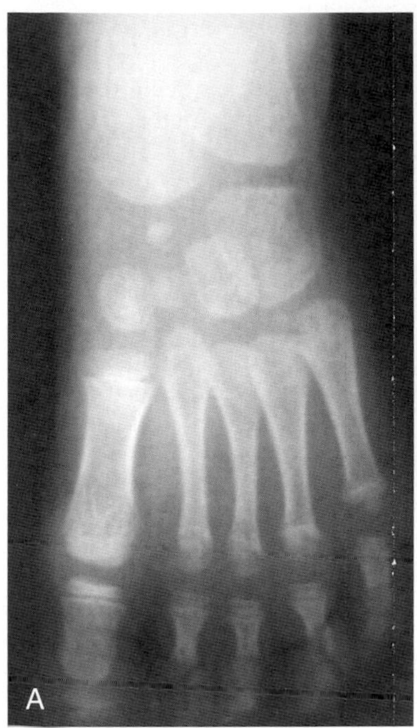

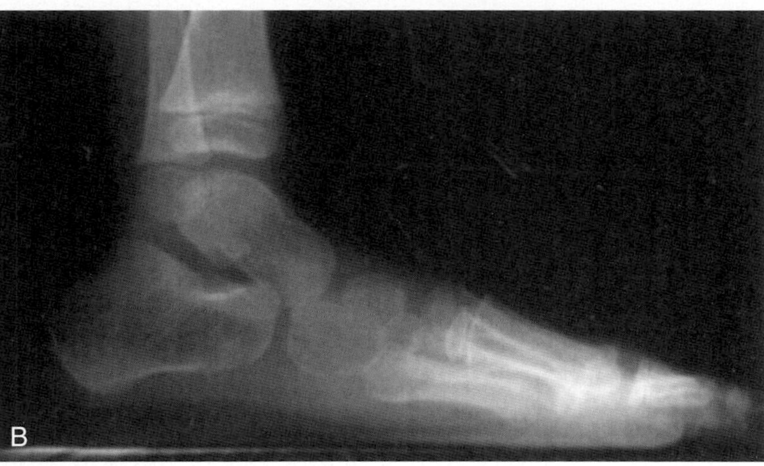

FIGURE 29-34 **A** and **B**, Radiographic appearance of left foot in 6-year-old child who had modified McKay procedures at 6 months of age. **SEE TECHNIQUE 29-12.**

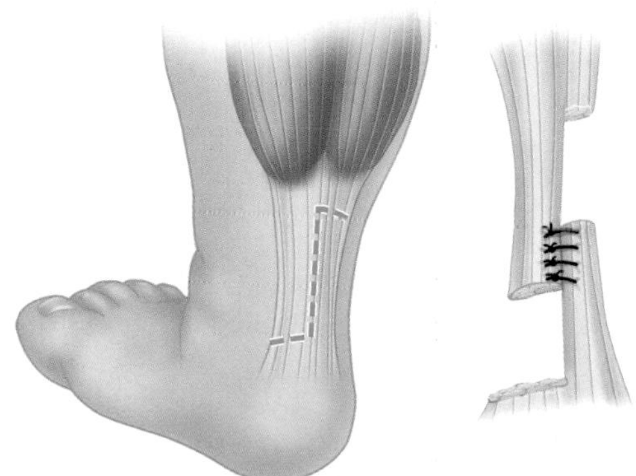

FIGURE 29-35 Achilles tendon lengthening (see text). **SEE TECHNIQUE 29-13.**

- Identify the Achilles tendon and make an incision through the peritenon medially. Dissect the Achilles tendon circumferentially to expose it for a length of 3 to 4 cm.
- Perform a tenotomy of the plantaris tendon if it is present.
- Identify medially the flexor hallucis longus, flexor digitorum communis, and posterior tibial tendons and the neurovascular bundle; protect these with Penrose drains.
- Perform a Z-plasty to lengthen the Achilles tendon by releasing the medial half distally and the lateral half proximally for a distance of 2.5 to 4 cm (Fig. 29-35).
- Gently debride pericapsular fat at the level of the subtalar joint.
- Identify the posterior aspect of the ankle joint by gentle plantar flexion and dorsiflexion of the foot. If the ankle joint cannot be easily identified, make a small vertical incision in the midline until synovial fluid exudes from the joint.
- Perform a transverse capsulotomy at the most medial aspect, stopping at the sheath of the posterior tibial tendon and the most lateral articulation of the tibiofibular joint. Do not divide the posterior tibial tendon sheath and its underlying deep deltoid ligament.
- If posterior subtalar capsulotomy is required, enter the subtalar joint at the most proximal aspect of the sheath of the flexor hallucis longus tendon, and extend the capsulotomy medially and laterally as necessary.
- Place the foot in 10 degrees of dorsiflexion and approximate the Achilles tendon to assess tension. Place the foot in plantarflexion and repair the Achilles tendon at the appropriate length.
- Deflate the tourniquet, obtain hemostasis with electrocautery, and close the wound in layers.
- Apply a long leg, bent-knee cast with the foot in 5 degrees of dorsiflexion.

POSTOPERATIVE CARE. The cast is removed 6 weeks after surgery. Postoperative bracing with an ankle-foot orthosis can be used for 6 to 9 months longer.

Several long-term evaluations of surgically treated clubfeet have demonstrated good results. The feet typically are plantigrade, functional, and relatively painless; however, persistent stiffness and mild discomfort with prolonged standing or activity are common.

RESISTANT CLUBFOOT

Treatment of residual or resistant clubfoot in an older child is one of the most difficult problems in pediatric orthopaedics. The deformity may take many forms, and there are no clear-cut guidelines for treatment. Each child must be evaluated carefully to determine which treatment would best correct his or her particular functional impairment. Thorough physical examination should include careful assessment of the forefoot and hindfoot. Residual forefoot deformity should be determined to be either dynamic (with a flexible forefoot) or rigid. The amount of inversion and eversion of the calcaneus and dorsiflexion and plantarflexion of the ankle should be determined. Any prior surgical procedures causing significant scarring around the foot or loss of motion should be noted. Standing anteroposterior and lateral radiographs should be obtained to assess anatomic measurements; if the clubfoot deformity is unilateral, the opposite foot can be used as a control for measurements. All possible causes of the persistent deformity, including underlying neuropathy, abnormal growth of the bones, or muscle imbalance, should be investigated. Most deformities have been reported to result from undercorrection at the time of the primary operation caused by failure to release the calcaneocuboid joint and plantar fascia and failure to recognize residual forefoot adduction on intraoperative radiographs; however, over-correction with hindfoot valgus or dorsal subluxation of the navicular is not uncommon.

Incomplete correction may not be obvious at the time of surgery, but it becomes apparent with growth as the persistent deformities become more evident (Fig. 29-36). Clubfoot that appears by clinical and radiographic evaluation to be uncorrected may not always require surgery. The functional ability of the child, the severity of symptoms associated with the deformity, and the likelihood of progression if the deformity is left untreated must be considered when treatment decisions are being made. Repeat manipulation and casting should always be considered as an option for the recurrent clubfoot. Many difficult foot deformities can be improved or corrected with a series of repeat manipulations and castings.

Even if the repeat casting does not completely correct the residual or recurrent deformity; parts of the deformity often can be improved, lessening the degree of surgery required for full correction.

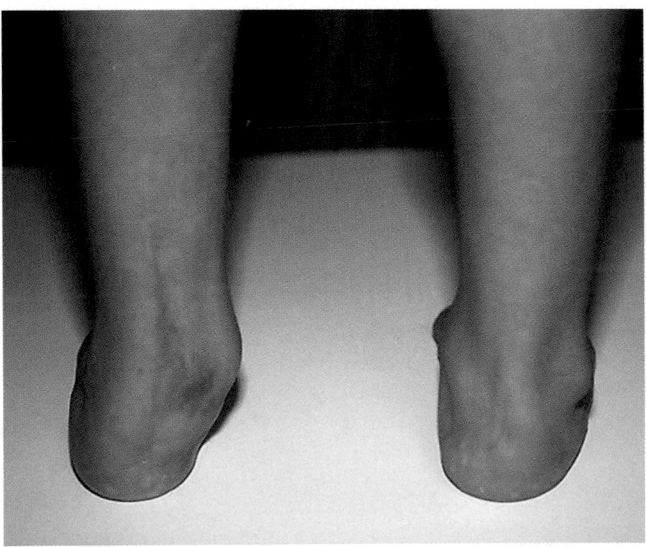

FIGURE 29-36 Overcorrection of left clubfoot deformity apparent in 6-year-old girl.

The basic surgical correction of resistant clubfoot includes soft-tissue release and bony osteotomies. The appropriate procedures and combination of procedures depend on the age of the child, the severity of the deformity, and the pathologic processes involved. In general, the older the child, the more likely it is that combined procedures will be required. Children 2 to 3 years old may be candidates for the modified McKay procedure (see Technique 29-12), but if previous soft-tissue release has caused stiffness of the subtalar joint, osteonecrosis of the talus, or severe skin contractures, osteotomies are a better choice. Children older than 5 years almost always require osteotomies for correction of resistant deformity; children 1 to 5 years old constitute a gray area in which treatment guidelines are unclear and careful judgment is required. The separate components of the residual deformity must be assessed accurately and treatment directed appropriately. Common components of resistant clubfoot deformity are adduction or supination, or both, of the forefoot, a short medial column or long lateral column of the foot, internal rotation and varus of the calcaneus, and equinus.

Correction of the forefoot with residual adduction or supination or both is similar to correction of isolated metatarsus adductus by multiple metatarsal osteotomies or by combined medial cuneiform and lateral cuboid osteotomies, when the deformity is in the forefoot. Because dynamic supination and adduction often are caused by overactivity of the anterior tibial tendon and underactivity of the peroneal tendon, a tendon-balancing procedure may be the most reasonable solution in the flexible foot.

Evaluation of the hindfoot should determine whether the deformity is caused by isolated heel varus, a long lateral column of the foot, or a short medial column. In children younger than 2 or 3 years who have had no previous surgery, residual heel varus may be corrected by extensive subtalar release, but children 3 to 10 years old who have residual soft-tissue and bony deformities usually require combined procedures.

Ankle valgus must be differentiated from hindfoot valgus because the methods and timing of surgical correction are different. For symptomatic ankle valgus, percutaneous medial malleolar epiphysiodesis using a 4.5-mm cortical screw has been recommended.

For isolated heel varus with mild supination of the forefoot, a Dwyer osteotomy with a lateral closing wedge osteotomy of the calcaneus can be performed. Opening wedge osteotomy of the calcaneus occasionally is followed by sloughing of tight skin along the incision over the calcaneus. Consequently, although some height of the calcaneus is lost after a lateral closing wedge osteotomy, most authors now prefer lateral closing wedge osteotomy with Kirschner wire fixation, if necessary. The ideal age for the operation is 3 to 4 years, but there is no upper age limit.

If the hindfoot deformity includes heel varus and residual internal rotation of the calcaneus with a long lateral column of the foot, the Lichtblau procedure may be appropriate. This procedure corrects the long lateral column of the foot by a closing wedge osteotomy of the lateral aspect of the calcaneus or by cuboid enucleation. The best results with this procedure are obtained in children 3 years old or older in whom the calcaneus and lateral column are long relative to the talus. Potential complications include the development of a "Z"-foot, or "skew"-foot, deformity.

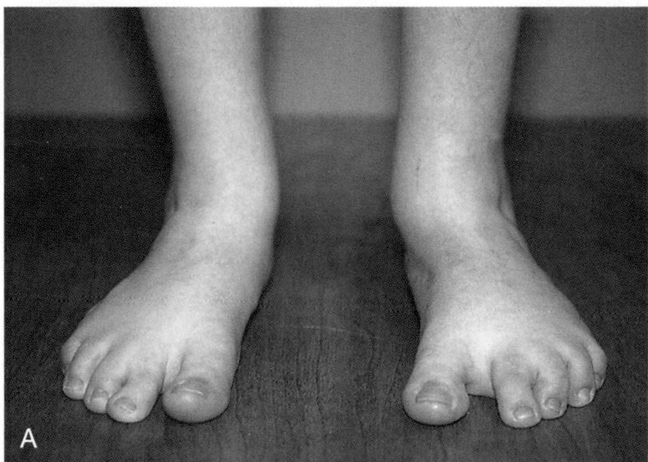

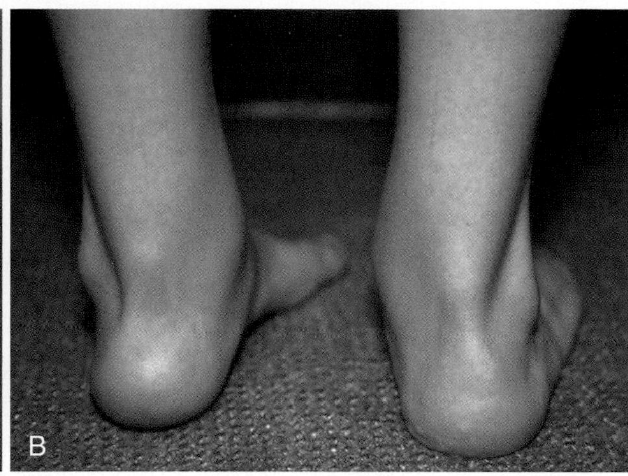

FIGURE 29-37 A and B, Deformities in 12-year-old boy after undercorrection of left clubfoot. Note metatarsus adductus, heel varus, and internal tibial torsion.

Adductus of the forefoot, as measured by the calcaneal–second metatarsal angle has been reported to improve after combined cuboid-cuneiform osteotomy, with no further surgery required.

Residual heel equinus can be corrected by Achilles tendon lengthening and posterior ankle and subtalar capsulotomies in a younger child with a mild deformity. In rare cases, an isolated, fixed equinus deformity in an older child requires a Lambrinudi arthrodesis. Anterior distal tibial hemiepiphysiodesis as a method to correct ankle equinus has been shown to be ineffective in achieving the desired clinical result.

Good long-term results have been reported with complete soft-tissue release and calcaneocuboid fusion for recurrent clubfoot, possibly avoiding the needed for later triple arthrodesis.

Talonavicular arthrodesis also has been described for residual midfoot deformities with or without lateral column shortening and a calcaneal wedge osteotomy with improvement in symptoms. This should be carefully considered if much of the foot motion is occurring at this joint.

If all three deformities are present in a child older than 10 years (Fig. 29-37), triple arthrodesis may be appropriate. Internal tibial torsion occasionally occurs with resistant clubfoot deformity but rarely requires derotational osteotomy. Before tibial osteotomy is considered, it must be determined absolutely that the pathologic condition is confined to the tibia and is not a resistant deformity in the foot.

Correction using the Ilizarov device, with or without bony procedures, has been described for correction in children with severe soft-tissue and bony deformities.

The principles of Ilizarov correction of severe resistant clubfoot include stable bone fixation to the tibia as well as pin fixation to the talus, calcaneus, and forefoot. Some advocate partial soft-tissue release before gradual correction, but the risk of wound complications is greatly increased by this approach. After correction, soft-tissue release with or without arthrodesis also may be required to maintain correction and prevent recurrence. This approach offers the ability to maintain foot length while achieving a plantigrade position and three-dimensional deformity correction. However, the psychologic impact of Ilizarov treatment must be carefully considered, and rehabilitation can be quite challenging.

OSTEOTOMY OF THE CALCANEUS FOR PERSISTENT VARUS DEFORMITY OF THE HEEL

Dwyer reported osteotomy of the calcaneus for relapsed clubfoot using an opening wedge osteotomy medially to increase the length and height of the calcaneus. The osteotomy is held open by a wedge of bone taken from the tibia. A modification of this technique is a laterally based closing wedge osteotomy of the calcaneus.

TECHNIQUE 29-14

(DWYER, MODIFIED)

- Expose the calcaneus through a lateral incision over the calcaneus, cuboid, and base of the fifth metatarsal.
- Expose the lateral surface of the bone subperiosteally and with a wide osteotome resect a wedge of bone based laterally large enough, when removed, to permit correction of the heel varus. Do not injure the peroneal tendons.
- Remove the wedge of bone, place the heel into the corrected position and close the incision with interrupted sutures.
- If necessary, fix the osteotomy with a Kirschner wire.
- Apply a short leg cast with the foot in the corrected position.

POSTOPERATIVE CARE. The Kirschner wire is removed at 6 weeks, and casting is discontinued at 8 to 12 weeks.

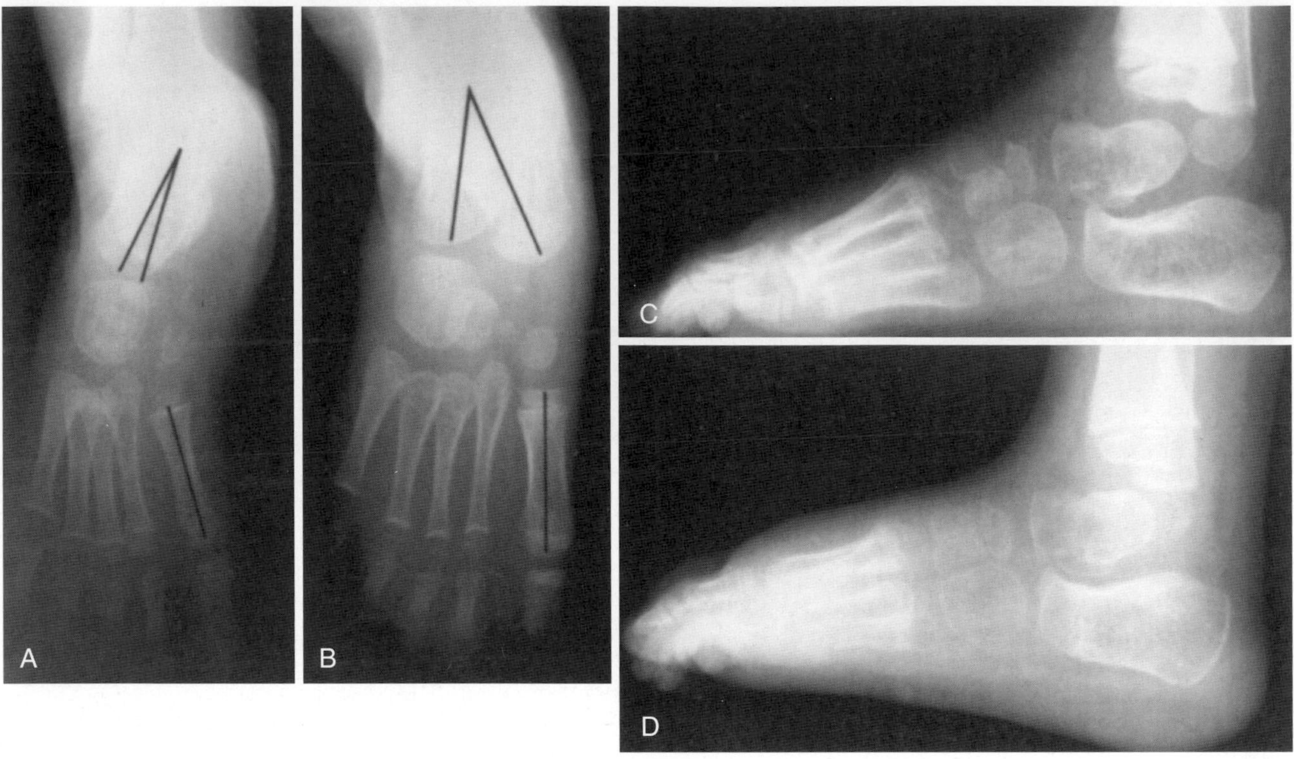

FIGURE 29-38 **A-D,** Severe residual clubfoot deformity in 5-year-old child on anteroposterior (**A**) and lateral (**C**) radiographs. **B** and **D,** After Lichtblau procedure. **SEE TECHNIQUE 29-15.**

MEDIAL RELEASE WITH OSTEOTOMY OF THE DISTAL CALCANEUS

An alternative to calcaneocuboid arthrodesis is lateral closing wedge osteotomy of the calcaneus, as described by Lichtblau (Fig. 29-38). This procedure may prevent the long-term stiffness of the hindfoot seen with the Dillwyn-Evans procedure.

TECHNIQUE 29-15 *Fig. 29-39*

(LICHTBLAU)

- If soft-tissue release medially is required, make an incision on the medial aspect of the foot beginning about 1 cm below the medial malleolus, crossing the tuberosity of the navicular, and sloping downward to the base of the first metatarsal. Identify and free the superior border of the abductor hallucis muscle, and reflect it plantarward.
- Isolate the posterior tibial tendon at its insertion on the beak of the navicular, dissect it from its sheath, and perform a Z-plasty about 1 cm from its insertion. Allow the proximal end of the tendon to retract, using the distal end as a guide to the talonavicular joint.
- Resect the tendon sheath overlying the joint and open it generously on its medial, dorsal, and plantar aspects.
- Open the flexor tendon sheaths and lengthen them by Z-plasty technique.
- Make a lateral incision 4 cm long centered over the calcaneocuboid joint.

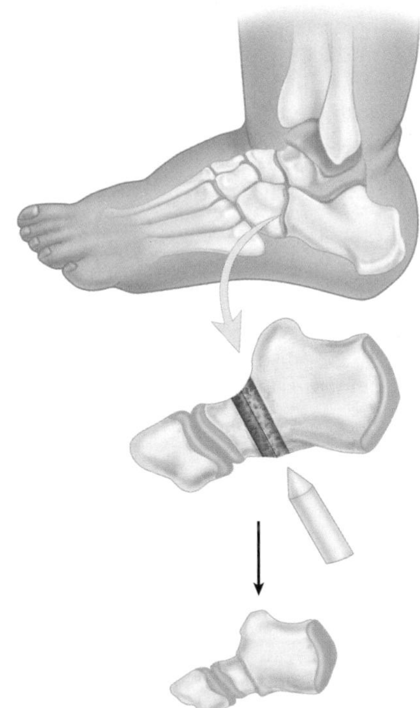

FIGURE 29-39 Lichtblau procedure (see text). **SEE TECHNIQUE 29-15.**

- Dissect the origin of the extensor digitorum brevis muscle from the calcaneus and reflect it distally to permit exposure and opening of the calcaneocuboid joint.
- Identify the distal end of the calcaneus and perform a wedge-shaped osteotomy, removing about 1 cm of the distal and lateral border of the calcaneus and 2 mm of the distal and medial border. Leave the articular surface of the calcaneus intact.
- Bring the cuboid into contact with the distal end of the calcaneus at the osteotomy site and evaluate the amount of correction of the varus deformity. If the cuboid cannot be closely approximated to the calcaneus, resect more of the calcaneus.
- A smooth Kirschner wire can be inserted across the calcaneocuboid joint to fix the osteotomy.
- Repair all soft tissues and close the subcutaneous tissue and skin. Apply a long leg cast with the foot in the corrected position.

POSTOPERATIVE CARE. The long leg cast is changed to a short leg cast 3 weeks after surgery. The short leg cast is worn for 6 more weeks. The pin is removed at 8 to 12 weeks.

SELECTIVE JOINT-SPARING OSTEOTOMIES FOR RESIDUAL CAVOVARUS DEFORMITY

Described by Mubarak and Van Valin, selective joint-sparing osteotomies of the foot can be used for multiple etiologies that result in rigid cavus and cavovarus foot deformities, including hereditary motor sensory neuropathies, traumatic brain injury, spinal cord lipoma, and residual or recurrent clubfoot. The technique involves stepwise correction of each aspect of the deformity with a closing wedge osteotomy of the first metatarsal, opening plantar wedge osteotomy of the medial cuneiform, closing wedge osteotomy of the cuboid, osteotomies of the second and third metatarsals, sliding osteotomy of the calcaneus, plantar fasciotomy, and peroneus-to-brevis transfer. Indications for this procedure are rigid cavus or cavovarus deformity, ankle or foot instability symptoms including pain, painful metatarsal heads and callosities, and ankle or foot sprains or fractures.

TECHNIQUE 29-16

(MUBRAK AND VAN VALIN)

- To correct rigid cavus, make an incision along the medial foot over the first metatarsal and medial cuneiform.
- Partially free the anterior tibial tendon to expose the cuneiform.
- Under fluoroscopic guidance, place intraosseous needles or small Kirschner wires in the mid-portion of the medial cuneiform and 1 cm distal to the first metatarsal physis. Take care not to disturb the physis.
- Perform a dorsal, closing-wedge osteotomy of the first metatarsal by removing a large 20- to 30-degree wedge (Fig. 29-40A). Then create a plantar-based, opening wedge osteotomy of the medial cuneiform and insert the bone wedge (Fig. 29-40B). Stabilize both osteotomies with Kirshner wires.
- To correct forefoot varus, make a longitudinal lateral incision overlying the cuboid. Identify the calcaneocuboid and cuboid-fifth metatarsal joints with fluoroscopy and protect these joints. Create a laterally based, closing-wedge osteotomy of the cuboid by removing a triangular wedge of bone with a base size of 5 to 10 mm (Fig. 29-40C). Stabilize the osteotomy with a Kirshner wire.
- If second and third metatarsal head prominence remains after the osteotomies have been completed, dorsal closing wedge osteotomies of the second and third metatarsals are required (Fig. 29-40C). Make a single incision overlying the bases of the second and third metatarsals. Create dorsally a slightly lateral based closing wedge osteotomy of the base of each metatarsal and stabilize them with intramedullary Kirshner wires.

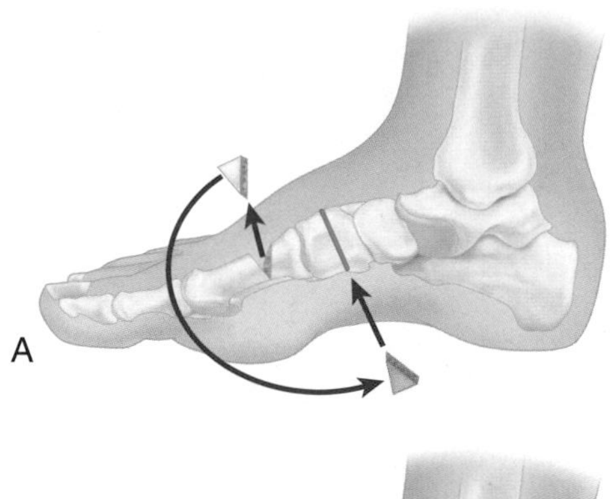

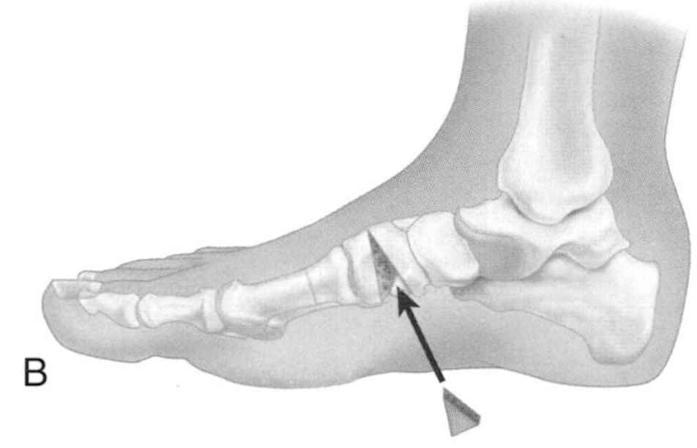

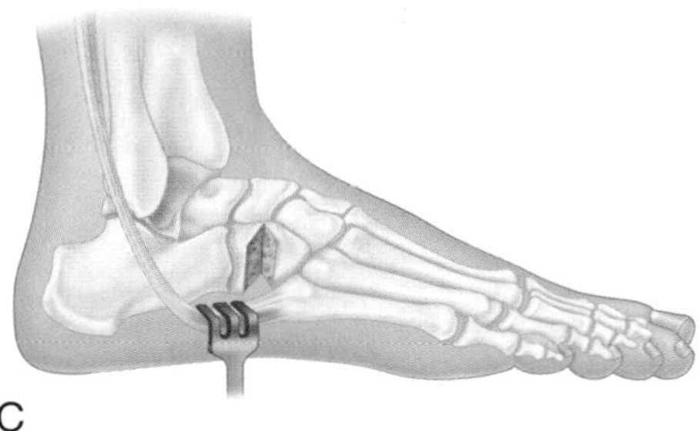

FIGURE 29-40 Selective joint sparing osteotomies (Mubarak and Van Valin). **A,** Dorsal closing-wedge osteotomy of the first metatarsal. **B,** Plantar-based opening-wedge osteotomy of the medial cuneiform. **C,** Laterally-based closing-wedge osteotomy of the cuboid. **SEE TECHNIQUE 29-16.**

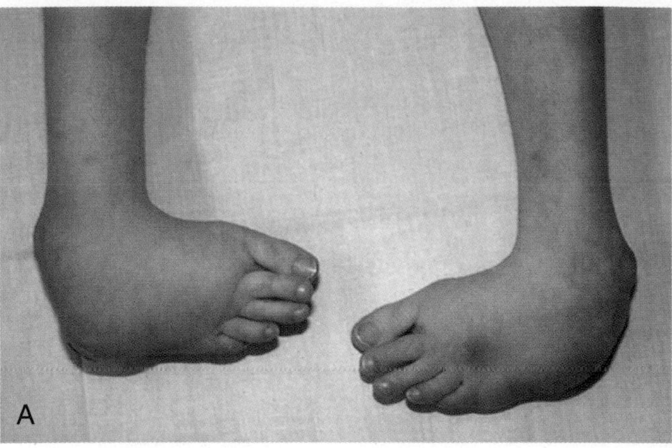

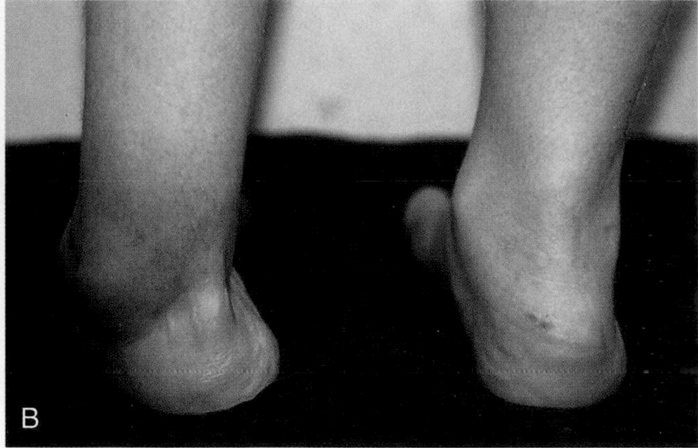

FIGURE 29-41 **A,** Untreated clubfoot in 14-year-old girl. **B,** Recurrent left hindfoot varus in 8-year-old girl.

- For rigid hindfoot varus, perform a Dywer osteotomy of the calcaneus (Technique 29-14).
- Next, evaluate the plantar fascia. If this structure is tight, perform a plantar fasciotomy (Technique 83-6 in Tenth Edition).
- For deformities caused by neurologic conditions, consider a peroneus longus-to-brevis transfer. Through the same incision used for the cuboid osteotomy, release the peroneus longus just under the cuboid and reattach it to the brevis.
- Close the incision. Apply a bivalved, short leg cast.

POSTOPERATIVE CARE. The bivalved cast is closed at 1 week. Non–weight bearing is continued for 4 weeks. Then the pins are removed under sedation anesthesia and a short leg cast is applied. Weight bearing is allowed in the second cast for 4 more weeks.

TRIPLE ARTHRODESIS AND TALECTOMY FOR UNCORRECTED CLUBFOOT

Triple arthrodesis and talectomy generally are salvage operations for uncorrected clubfoot in older children and adolescents (Figs. 29-41 and 29-42). Triple arthrodesis corrects the severely deformed foot by a lateral closing wedge osteotomy through the subtalar and midtarsal joints. Functional results generally are improved despite postoperative joint stiffness. Talectomy should be reserved for severe, untreated clubfoot; for previously treated clubfoot that is uncorrectable by any other surgical procedures; and for neuromuscular clubfoot.

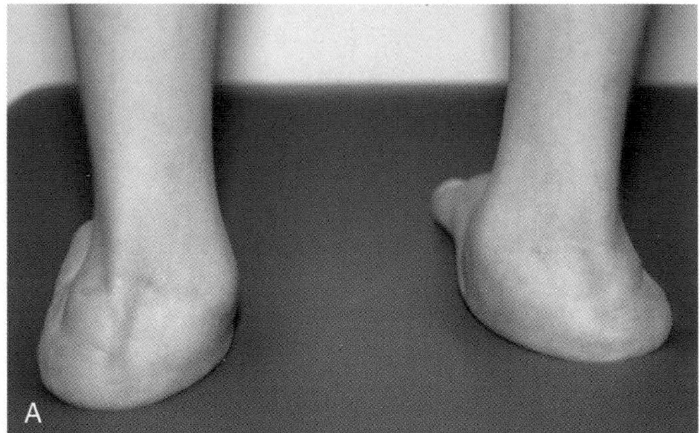

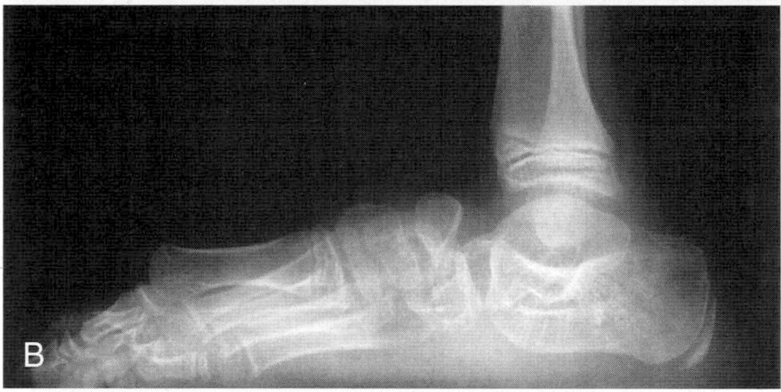

FIGURE 29-42 **A,** Overcorrected clubfoot in 12-year-old boy showing hindfoot valgus, dorsal dislocation of navicular on talus, and dorsal bunion deformity. **B,** Standing lateral radiograph.

TRIPLE ARTHRODESIS

TECHNIQUE 29-17

- Make an incision along the medial side of the foot parallel to the inferior border of the calcaneus.
- Free the attachments of the plantar fascia and of the short flexors of the toes from the plantar aspect of the calcaneus.
- By manipulation, correct the cavus deformity as much as possible.
- Through an oblique anterolateral approach, expose the midtarsal and subtalar joints (Fig. 29-43).
- Resect a laterally based wedge of bone that includes the midtarsal joints. Resect enough bone to correct the varus and adduction deformities of the forefoot.
- Through the same incision, resect a wedge of bone, again laterally based, which includes the subtalar joint. Resect enough bone to correct the varus deformity of the calcaneus. If necessary, include in the wedge the navicular and most of the cuboid and lateral cuneiform and the anterior

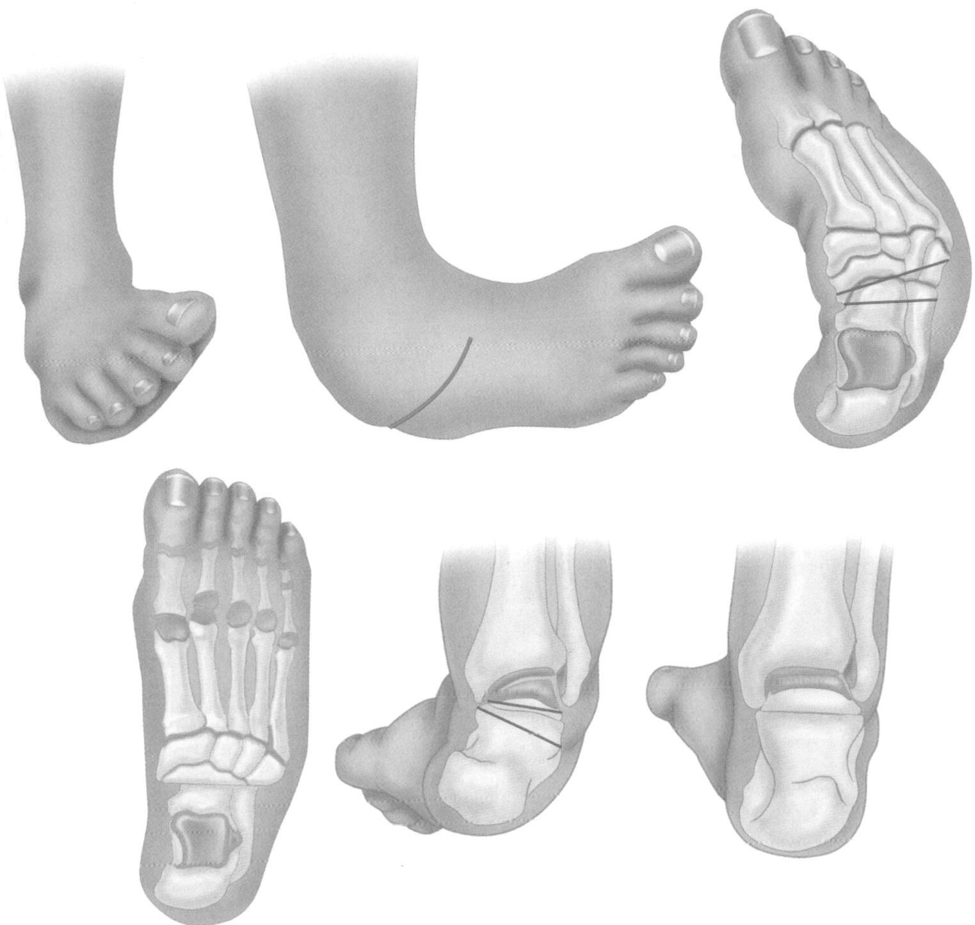

FIGURE 29-43 Arthrodesis for persistent or untreated clubfoot. Area between blue lines represents amount of bone removed from midtarsal region and subtalar joint in moderate fixed deformity. In severe deformity, wedge may include large part of talus and calcaneus and part of cuneiforms. **SEE TECHNIQUE 29-17.**

part of the talus and calcaneus, and in the second wedge include much of the superior part of the calcaneus and the inferior part of the talus.

- Lengthen the Achilles tendon by Z-plasty and perform a posterior capsulotomy of the ankle joint. By manipulating the ankle, correct the equinus deformity.
- Hold the correct position with a Kirschner wire inserted through the calcaneocuboid and talonavicular joints or with staple fixation.

POSTOPERATIVE CARE. With the foot in the corrected position and the knee flexed 30 degrees, a long leg cast is applied from the base of the toes to the groin. The Kirschner wire and cast are removed at 6 weeks. A short leg walking cast is worn for 4 more weeks.

TALECTOMY

Trumble et al. described a talectomy for clubfoot deformity in patients with myelomeningocele, but the technique can be modified for treatment of a severe, resistant, idiopathic clubfoot deformity.

TECHNIQUE 29-18

(TRUMBLE ET AL.)

- Expose the talus through an incision parallel to the inferior border of the calcaneus (Fig. 29-44A). If additional soft-tissue release is required, talectomy can be done after circumferential release (see Technique 29-11).
- Carry the dissection to the prominent lateral articular margin of the navicular in the interval between the extensor digitorum longus and peroneus tertius tendons. Invert and plantar flex the forefoot.
- Place a towel clip around the neck of the talus and deliver it into the wound; dissect all of its ligaments (Fig. 29-44B). Excise the talus intact because retained remnants of cartilage may interfere with proper positioning of the foot; these remnants also may grow and cause later deformity and loss of correction.
- Derotate the forefoot and displace the calcaneus posteriorly into the ankle mortise until the navicular abuts the anterior edge of the tibial plafond. The exposed articular surface of the tibial plafond should be opposite the middle articular facet of the calcaneus. If necessary to obtain adequate posterior displacement, excise the tarsal navicular.

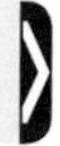

- Section the deltoid and the lateral collateral ligaments of the ankle.
- Correct equinus deformity of the hindfoot by sectioning the Achilles tendon and allowing its proximal end to retract.
- In feet with uncorrected, severe equinovarus deformity, the dome of the talus may be extruded anterior to its normal relationship in the ankle mortise. Adaptive narrowing of the mortise may require release of the anterior and posterior tibiofibular ligaments of the syndesmosis to allow proper posterior positioning of the calcaneus.
- In the proper plantigrade position, the long axis of the foot should be aligned at a right angle to the bimalleolar axis of the ankle, not to the axis of the knee joint. This usually requires 20 to 30 degrees of external rotation of the foot.
- When the proper position has been achieved, insert one or two Steinmann pins from the heel through the calcaneus and into the distal tibia.
- Apply a long leg cast with the knee flexed to 60 degrees.

POSTOPERATIVE CARE. The Steinmann pins are removed at 6 weeks and a below-knee, weight-bearing cast is applied. The cast is worn for 12 more weeks.

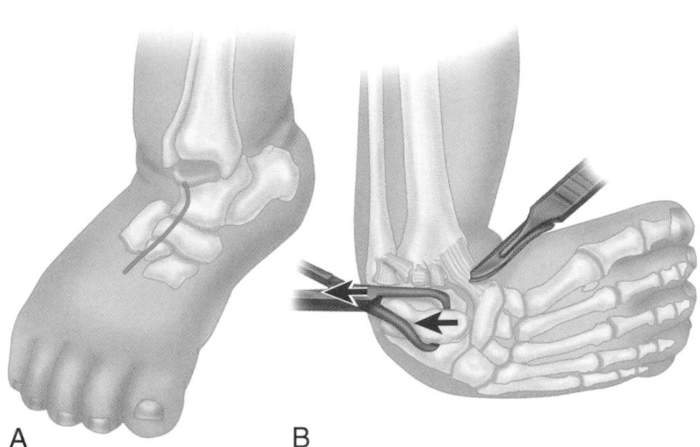

FIGURE 29-44 Talectomy. **A,** Anterolateral skin incision. **B,** Total talectomy. **SEE TECHNIQUE 29-18.**

DORSAL BUNION

Dorsal bunions that develop after clubfoot surgery have been attributed to muscle weakness, particularly of the triceps surae, wherein a bunion develops as the patient tries to push off with the toe flexors to compensate for the weakness of the triceps, or imbalance between the anterior tibial muscle and an impaired peroneus longus muscle. Most authors recommend transfer of the flexor hallucis longus to the neck of the first metatarsal, combined with bony correction by plantar closing wedge osteotomy of the first metatarsal (Fig. 29-45).

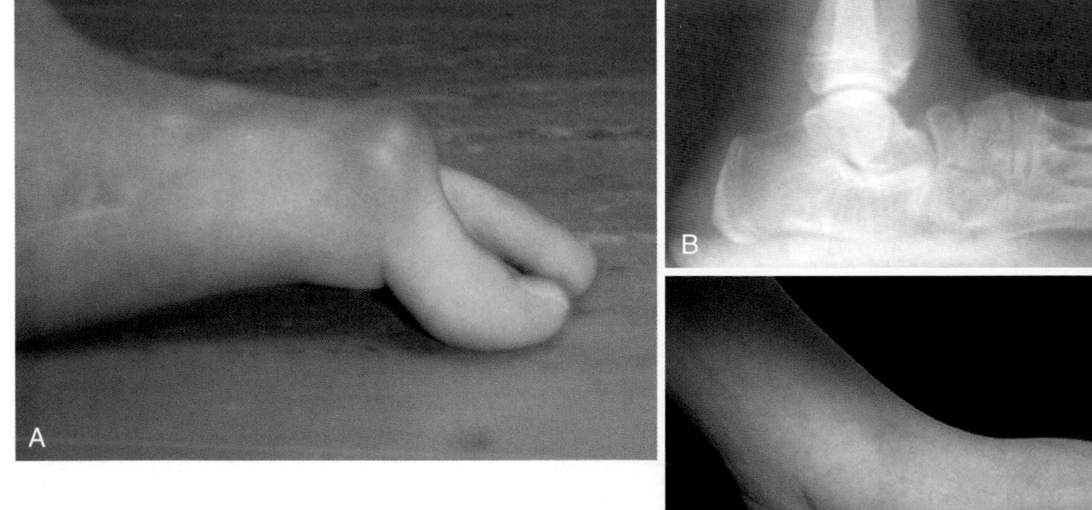

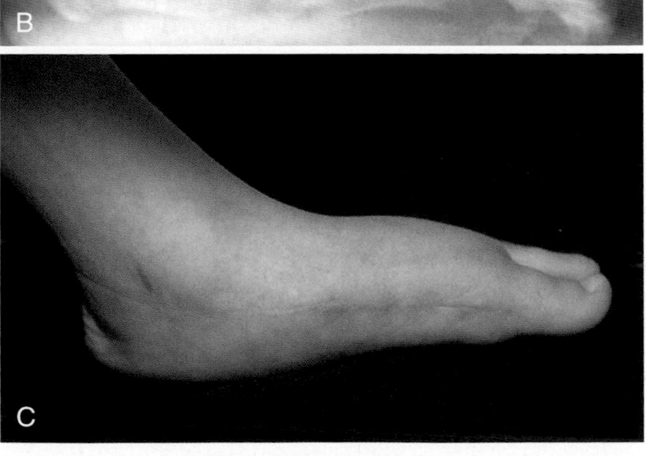

FIGURE 29-45 **A,** Dorsal bunion in 9-year-old boy after clubfoot release at 9 months of age. **B,** Lateral view of dorsal bunion at metatarsophalangeal joint of left great toe. **C,** Postoperative appearance of left foot after plantar closing wedge osteotomy of first metatarsal with transfer of flexor hallucis longus to first metatarsal neck. **SEE TECHNIQUE 29-18.**

FIRST METATARSAL OSTEOTOMY AND TENDON TRANSFER FOR DORSAL BUNION

TECHNIQUE 29-19

(SMITH AND KUO)

- Through a medial incision, expose the first metatarsal and perform a proximal plantar closing wedge osteotomy.
- Bring the metatarsal into alignment with the forefoot by plantarflexion and insert a Kirschner wire for fixation.
- Carry the incision distally, or make a second incision at the metatarsophalangeal joint to allow identification and transection of the flexor hallucis longus tendon.
- Drill a hole in the distal first metatarsal neck in a dorsal-to-plantar direction.
- Pass the flexor hallucis tendon through the hole and suture it back on itself.
- Close the wounds and apply a short leg, non–weight-bearing cast.

POSTOPERATIVE CARE. Non–weight bearing is continued in the cast for 6 weeks, after which the Kirschner wire is removed. A walking cast is worn for 4 weeks. Full activity usually can be resumed at 3 to 4 months.

CONGENITAL VERTICAL TALUS

Congenital vertical talus, rocker-bottom flatfoot, or congenital rigid flatfoot must be distinguished from flexible pes planus commonly seen in infants and children. Congenital vertical talus may be associated with numerous neuromuscular disorders, such as arthrogryposis and myelomeningocele, but it also may occur as an isolated congenital anomaly.

CLINICAL AND RADIOGRAPHIC FINDINGS

Congenital vertical talus usually can be detected at birth by the presence of a rounded prominence of the medial and plantar surfaces of the foot produced by the abnormal location of the head of the talus (Fig. 29-46). The talus is so distorted plantarward and medially as to be almost vertical. The calcaneus also is in an equinus position, but to a lesser degree. The forefoot is dorsiflexed at the midtarsal joints, and the navicular lies on the dorsal aspect of the head of the talus. The sole is convex, and there are deep creases on the dorsolateral aspect of the foot anterior and inferior to the lateral malleolus.

As the foot develops and weight bearing is begun, adaptive changes occur in the tarsals. The talus becomes shaped like an hourglass but remains in so marked an equinus position that its longitudinal axis is almost the same as that of the tibia, and only the posterior third of its superior articular surface articulates with the tibia. The calcaneus remains in an equinus position also and becomes displaced posteriorly, and the anterior part of its plantar surface becomes rounded. Callosities develop beneath the anterior end of the calcaneus and along the medial border of the foot superficial to the head of the talus. When full weight is borne, the forefoot becomes severely abducted, and the heel does not touch the floor. Adaptive changes occur in the soft structures. All the capsules, ligaments, and tendons on the dorsum of the foot become contracted. The posterior tibial and peroneus longus and brevis tendons may come to lie anterior to the malleoli and act as dorsiflexors rather than plantar flexors.

Congenital vertical talus can be difficult to distinguish from severe pes planus, although the two can be differentiated by the use of appropriate radiographs or ultrasound. The plantarflexion lateral radiograph is most helpful to confirm the diagnosis of congenital vertical talus (Fig. 29-47).

TREATMENT

Congenital vertical talus is difficult to correct and tends to recur. Dobbs described the use of outpatient serial casting to achieve relaxation of the dorsolateral structures of the foot and partial or complete reduction of the talonavicular joint followed by percutaneous retrograde pinning or open reduction and retrograde pinning of the talonavicular joint in the operating room. Once the talonavicular joint is stabilized by pin fixation, percutaneous Achilles tenotomy is done to achieve ankle dorsiflexion without persistent rocker-bottom deformity. Excellent results in terms of clinical appearance, function, and deformity correction have been reported by a number of authors, and this technique has emerged as a

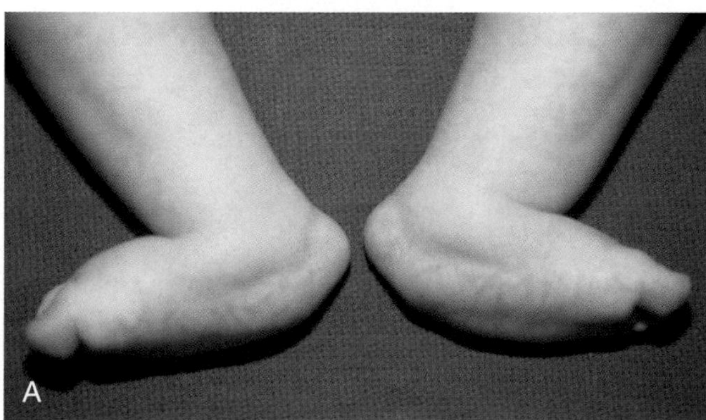

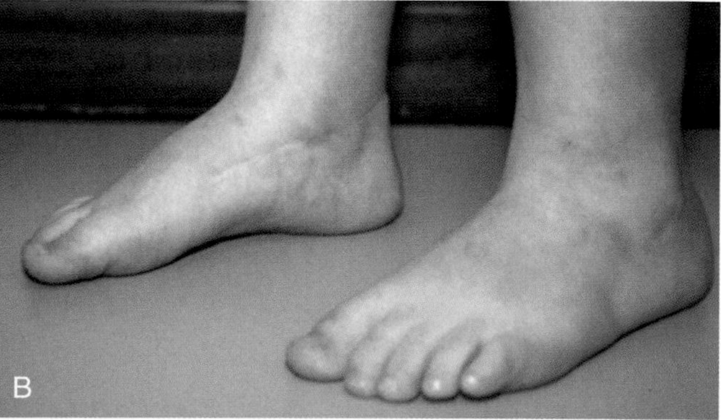

FIGURE 29-46 **A,** Bilateral congenital vertical talus in 14-month-old child. **B,** At 6 years of age, after bilateral operative correction at age 14 months in which transverse circumferential approach was used.

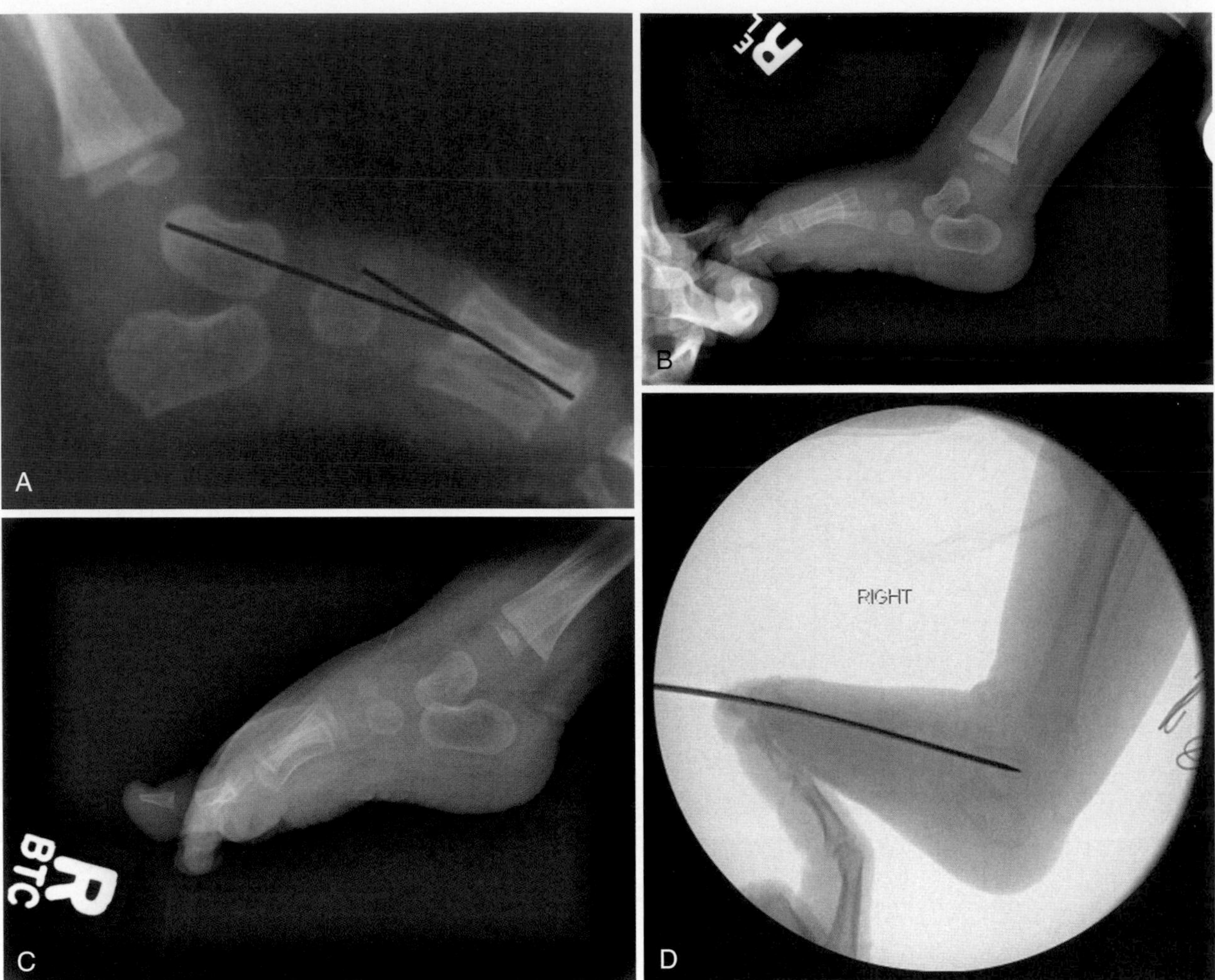

FIGURE 29-47 Plantarflexion lateral stress radiographs in diagnosis of congenital vertical talus. **A,** In normal foot, long axis of first metatarsal passes plantarward to long axis of talus. **B,** Forced plantarflexion lateral demonstrates inability of first metatarsal to line up with the talus. **C,** After 5 weeks of casting the plantarflexion lateral demonstrates good alignment of the first metatarsal and talus. **D,** After percutaneous pinning of talonavicular joint and percutaneous Achilles tenotomy.

viable initial option for many patients with congenital vertical talus.

Persistent or recurrent deformity after a trial of casting may necessitate more extensive operative intervention, particularly in children with more severe or rigid deformities.

The exact surgery indicated is determined by the age of the child and the severity of the deformity. Children 1 to 4 years old generally are best treated by open reduction and realignment of the talonavicular and subtalar joints. Occasionally, in children 3 years old or older who have a severe deformity, navicular excision is required at the time of open reduction. Children 4 to 8 years old can be treated by open reduction and soft-tissue procedures combined with extraarticular subtalar arthrodesis. Children 12 years old or older are best treated by triple arthrodesis for permanent correction of the deformity.

Kodros and Dias reported a single-stage procedure in which a threaded Kirschner wire is used as a "joystick" to manipulate the talus into correct position. The corrected position is held with threaded Kirschner wires across the talonavicular and subtalar joints (Fig. 29-48).

For a young child with a mild or moderate deformity, the technique of Kumar, Cowell, and Ramsey is recommended.

OPEN REDUCTION AND REALIGNMENT OF TALONAVICULAR AND SUBTALAR JOINTS

TECHNIQUE 29-20

(KUMAR, COWELL, AND RAMSEY)

- Make the first of three incisions on the lateral side of the foot, centered over the sinus tarsi, or use the transverse circumferential (Cincinnati) approach (Fig. 29-32), which we prefer. Avoid entering the sinus tarsi laterally.
- Expose the extensor digitorum brevis and reflect it distally to expose the anterior part of the talocalcaneal joint.
- Identify the calcaneocuboid joint and release all tight structures around it, including the calcaneocuboid ligament.

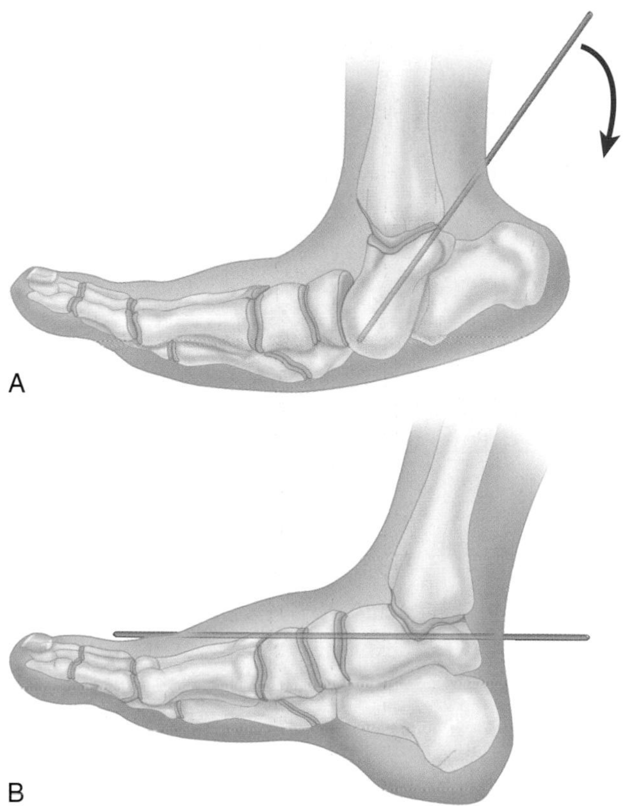

FIGURE 29-48 Single-stage correction of congenital vertical talus. **A,** After soft-tissue release, a threaded Kirschner wire is placed axially in the vertical talus from posterior and is used as "joystick" to manipulate talus into reduced position. **B,** Wire is advanced across talonavicular joint.

- Make the second incision on the medial side of the foot, centered over the prominent head of the talus. This exposes the head of the talus and medial part of the navicular.
- The anterior tibial tendon also is exposed; if the tendon is contracted, lengthen it by Z-plasty. Alternatively, release the anterior tibial tendon from its attachment to the medial cuneiform and first ray and transpose it into the planter aspect of the repaired talonavicular capsule.
- Release all tight structures on the medial and dorsal aspects of the head of the talus and the navicular. Free also the anterior part of the talus from its ligamentous attachments to the navicular and calcaneus. This includes releasing the dorsal talonavicular ligament, the plantar calcaneonavicular ligament, and the anterior part of the superficial deltoid ligament. If necessary, divide part of the talocalcaneal interosseous ligament so that the talus can be easily maneuvered into position by a blunt instrument. If the peroneal, extensor hallucis longus, and extensor digitorum longus tendons remain contracted, expose and lengthen them by Z-plasty. Alternatively, perform a fractional lengthening of these tendons through an anterior incision at the musculotendinous junction.
- Make a third incision 2 inches long on the medial side of the Achilles tendon. Lengthen this tendon by Z-plasty, and, if necessary, perform a capsulotomy of the posterior ankle and subtalar joints.
- The talus and calcaneus can now be placed in the corrected position, and the forefoot can be reduced on the hindfoot.
- Pass a Kirschner wire through the navicular and into the neck of the talus to maintain the reduction. Obtain anteroposterior and lateral radiographs to confirm reduction of the vertical talus (Fig. 29-49).
- Reconstruct the talonavicular ligament, repair any lengthened tendons, transfer the anterior tibial tendon to the plantar aspect of the talonavicular joint capsule, and close the wound in layers.
- Apply a long leg cast with the knee flexed and the foot in proper position.

POSTOPERATIVE CARE. At 8 weeks, the cast and Kirschner wire are removed. A new long leg cast is applied, and this type of cast is worn for 1 month. A short leg cast is worn for an additional month. The foot is supported in an ankle-foot orthosis for another 3 to 6 months.

OPEN REDUCTION AND EXTRAARTICULAR SUBTALAR FUSION

Coleman et al. described open reduction and extraarticular subtalar fusion in older children with severe or recurrent deformities. This technique combines the procedure of Kumar et al. with a Grice-Green fusion performed 6 to 8 weeks later. Dennyson and Fulford modified this technique by using screw fixation across the talocalcaneal joint.

TECHNIQUE 29-21

(GRICE-GREEN)

- Make a short curvilinear incision on the lateral aspect of the foot directly over the subtalar joint.
- Carry the incision down through the soft tissues to expose the cruciate ligament overlying the joint. Split this ligament in the direction of its fibers and dissect the fatty and ligamentous tissues from the sinus tarsi.
- Dissect the short toe extensors from the calcaneus and reflect them distally. The relationship of the calcaneus to the talus now can be determined, and the mechanism of the deformity can be shown.
- Place the foot in equinus and invert it to position the calcaneus beneath the talus.
- A severe, long-standing deformity may require division of the posterior capsule of the subtalar joint or removal of a small piece of bone laterally from beneath the anterosuperior articular surface of the calcaneus.
- Insert an osteotome or broad periosteal elevator into the sinus tarsi and block the subtalar joint to evaluate the stability of the graft and its proper size and position.
- Prepare the graft beds by removing a thin layer of cortical bone from the inferior surface of the talus and superior surface of the calcaneus (Fig. 29-50).

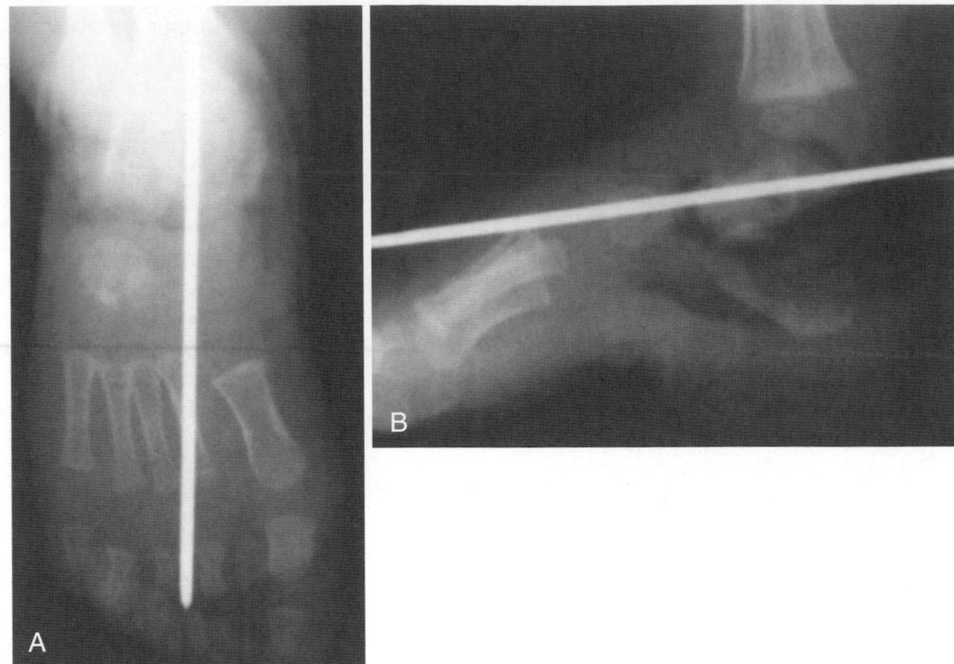

FIGURE 29-49 Intraoperative radiographs after correction of congenital vertical talus through transverse circumferential approach. **A,** Anteroposterior view shows correction of talocalcaneal and talus–first metatarsal angles. **B,** Lateral view shows corrected position of talus and reduction of navicular and forefoot after fixation with single Steinmann pin. **SEE TECHNIQUE 29-20.**

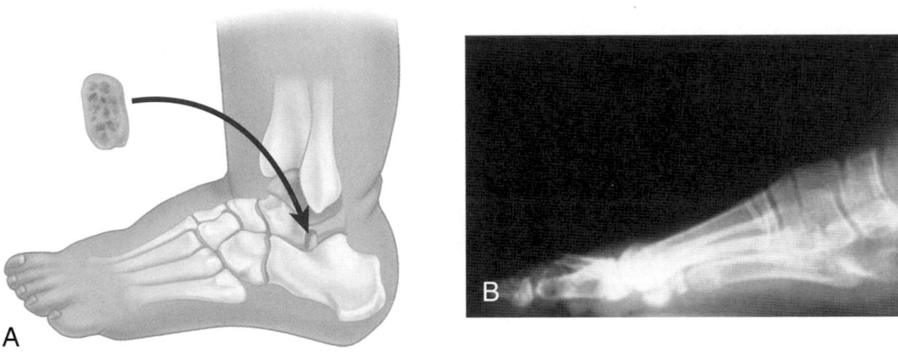

FIGURE 29-50 Grice-Green subtalar fusion. **A,** Preparation of graft bed and placement of graft in lateral aspect of subtalar joint. **B,** Lateral view of 10-year-old patient who had open reduction and Grice-Green fusion for congenital vertical talus at 3 years of age. **SEE TECHNIQUE 29-21.**

- Make a linear incision over the anteromedial surface of the proximal tibial metaphysis, incise the periosteum, and take a block of bone large enough for two grafts (usually 3.5 to 4.5 cm long and 1.5 cm wide). As an alternative to tibial bone, a short segment of the distal fibula or a circular segment of the iliac crest can be used.
- Cut the grafts to fit the prepared beds. Use a rongeur to shape the grafts so that they can be countersunk into cancellous bone to prevent lateral displacement.
- With the foot held in a slightly overcorrected position, place the grafts in the sinus tarsi. Evert the foot to lock the grafts in place.
- If a segment of the fibula or iliac crest is used, a smooth Kirschner wire can be used to hold the graft in place for 12 weeks, or a screw can be inserted anteriorly from the talar neck into the calcaneus for rigid fixation (Fig. 29-51).
- The foot should be stable enough to allow correction of equinus deformity by Achilles tendon lengthening if necessary.
- Apply a long leg cast with the knee flexed, the ankle in maximal dorsiflexion, and the foot in the corrected position.

POSTOPERATIVE CARE. The long leg cast is worn for 12 weeks, and weight bearing is not allowed. The Kirschner wire is removed, and a short leg walking cast is worn for 4 more weeks.

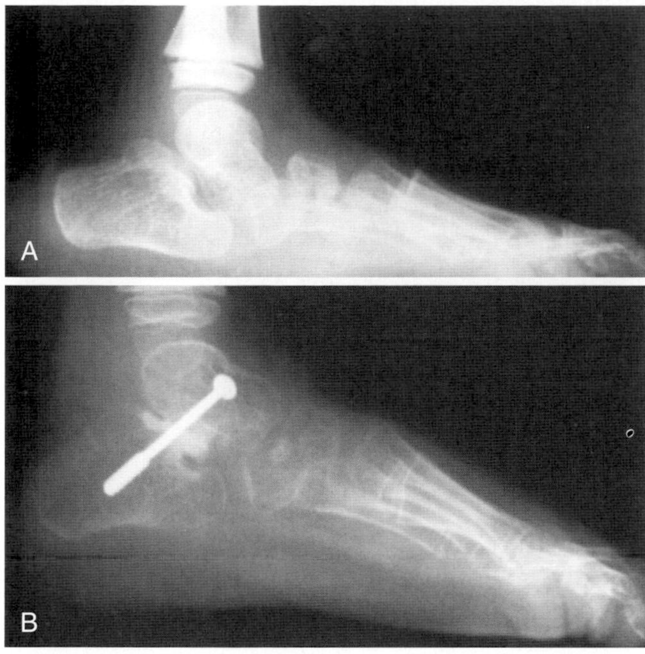

FIGURE 29-51 A, Congenital vertical talus in 6-year-old child. B, Corrected position of talus fixed with screw through neck of talus into calcaneus, as described by Dennyson and Fulford. Bone graft in middle and posterior aspects of subtalar joint. **SEE TECHNIQUE 29-21.**

TRIPLE ARTHRODESIS

Older children (>12 years) with uncorrected vertical talus who have pain or difficulty with shoe wear can be treated with triple arthrodesis. The procedure generally requires medial and lateral incisions and adequate osteotomies to place the foot in a plantigrade position, a technique similar to that used for correction of a severe tarsal coalition deformity (see Chapter 82).

ANOMALIES OF THE LEG

CONGENITAL ANGULAR DEFORMITIES OF THE LEG

Congenital angular deformities of the leg are primarily of two kinds: deformities in which the apex of the angulation is anterior and deformities in which it is posterior. In both, the tibia often is bowed not only anteriorly or posteriorly, but also medially or laterally. Anterior bowing of the tibia is commonly associated with neurofibromatosis.

Posterior angular deformities of the tibia tend to improve with growth (Fig. 29-52). A limb-length discrepancy also may be present, ranging from several millimeters to several centimeters. Children with these deformities should be examined yearly for any potential limb-length discrepancy that may require limb equalization, usually by an appropriately timed epiphysiodesis or limb lengthening in severe deformities.

Anterior angular deformities of the tibia are more worrisome because of their potential association with congenital pseudarthrosis of the tibia. Occasionally, these tibias maintain a normal medullary canal and show no evidence of narrowing or of the sclerotic "high-risk tibia." If any indication

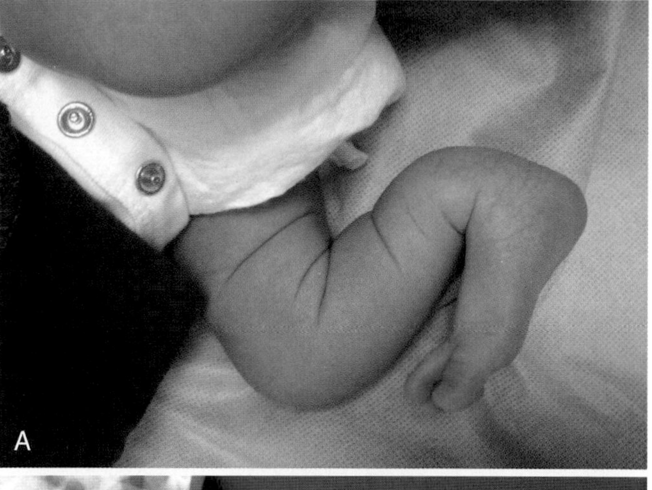

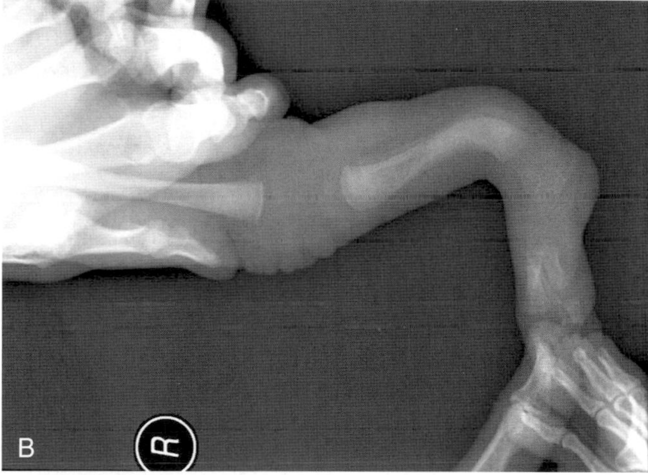

FIGURE 29-52 Congenital posteromedial bowing of right tibia. A, Clinical appearance. B, Radiographic appearance.

of narrowing of the medullary canal is present or develops in an anteriorly bowed tibia, the limb should be braced until skeletal maturity is reached.

Unilateral anterior bowing of the tibia with duplication of the great toe has been described as a distinct syndrome, which should be considered in the differential diagnosis of anterolateral tibial bowing and should not be mistaken for congenital pseudarthrosis. Associated conditions, in addition to duplication of the great toe, include shortening of the tibia that results in significant leg-length discrepancy, clinodactyly, and anomalous maturation of the carpal bones and metacarpals.

CONGENITAL PSEUDARTHROSIS OF THE FIBULA AND TIBIA

Congenital pseudarthrosis is a specific type of nonunion that at birth is either present or incipient. Its cause is unknown, but it occurs often enough in patients with either neurofibromatosis or related stigmata to suggest that neurofibromatosis, if not the cause of congenital pseudarthrosis, is closely related to it. Congenital pseudarthrosis most commonly involves the distal half of the tibia and often that of the fibula in the same limb. The true cause of the poor healing potential of the bone at the pseudarthrosis site is unknown; however, hamartomatous thickened fibrous tissue with limited vascular

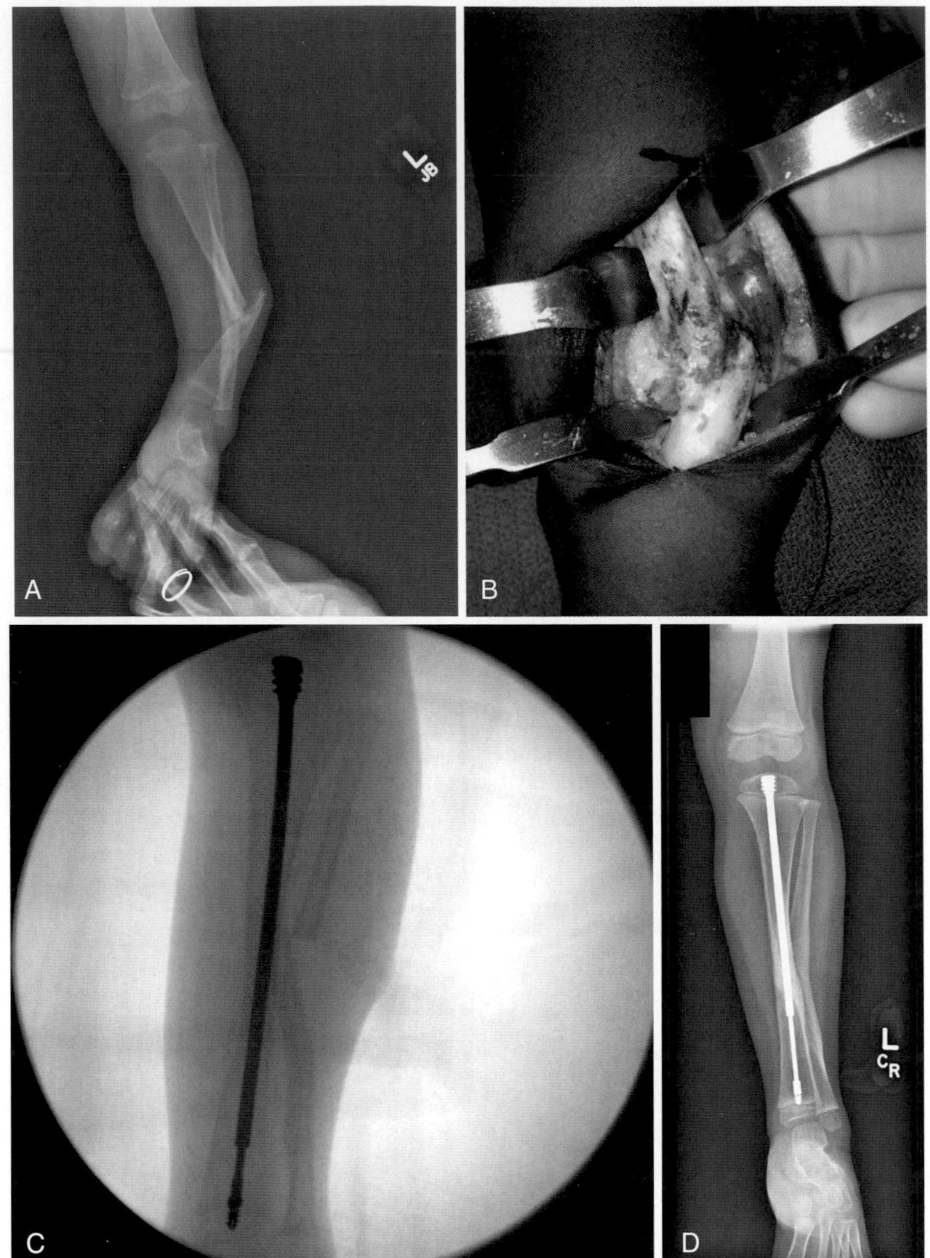

FIGURE 29-53 Congenital pseudarthrosis. **A,** Radiograph of 3-year-old with established nonunion present since birth. **B,** Intraoperative photo of hamartomatous tissue. **C,** Postoperative radiograph demonstrating stabilization of tibia using telescoping intramedullary rod following surgical debridement, iliac crest bone graft, and bone morphogenetic protein placement. **D,** Healed nonunion 10 months postoperatively.

ingrowth is seen universally at the site of the pseudarthrosis (Fig. 29-53).

■ FIBULA

Congenital pseudarthrosis of the fibula often precedes or accompanies the same condition in the ipsilateral tibia. Several grades of severity of this pseudarthrosis are seen: bowing of the fibula without pseudarthrosis, fibular pseudarthrosis without ankle deformity, fibular pseudarthrosis with ankle deformity, and fibular pseudarthrosis with latent pseudarthrosis of the tibia. Sometimes it even develops between the time of successful bone grafting of a pseudarthrosis of the tibia and skeletal maturity; because the lateral malleolus becomes displaced proximally, a progressive valgus deformity of the ankle develops.

Until skeletal maturity is reached, the ankle can be stabilized by an ankle-foot orthosis. At maturity, any significant deformity can be treated by supramalleolar osteotomy made through essentially normal bone, and union of the osteotomy can be expected. Langenskiöld devised an operation for children, however, to prevent this valgus deformity or halt its progression. He created a synostosis between the distal tibial and fibular metaphyses. Because in congenital pseudarthrosis securing union by bone grafting may be as difficult in the

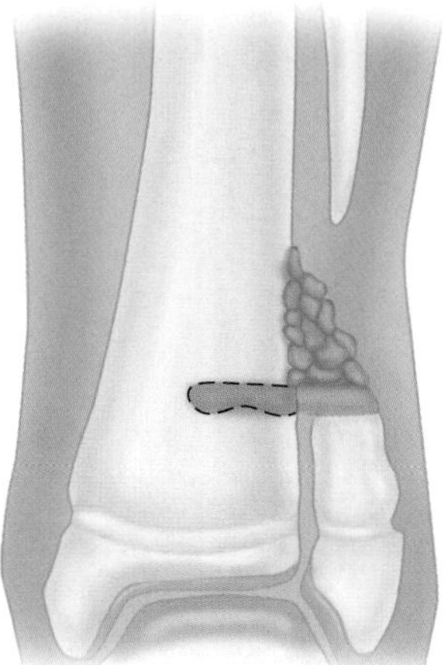

FIGURE 29-54 Langenskiöld technique for creating synostosis between distal tibial and fibular metaphyses to prevent valgus deformity of ankle in congenital pseudarthrosis of fibula (see text). **SEE TECHNIQUE 29-22.**

fibula as in the tibia, an operation that prevents the ankle deformity without grafting in fibular pseudarthrosis is useful (Fig. 29-54).

TIBIOFIBULAR SYNOSTOSIS

TECHNIQUE 29-22

(LANGENSKIÖLD)

- Make a longitudinal incision anteriorly over the distal fibula.
- Divide the fibula 1 to 2 cm proximal to the level of the distal tibial physis and excise the cone-shaped part of the distal fibular shaft.
- In the lateral surface of the tibia, at the level of the cut surface of the fibula, and at the attachment of the interosseous membrane, make a hole as wide as the diameter of the fibula. Proximal to the hole, remove the periosteum and interosseous membrane from the tibia over an area of several square centimeters.
- From the ilium, obtain a bone graft the same width as that of the hole in the tibia and long enough to extend from the lateral surface of the fibula into the spongy bone of the tibial metaphysis.
- Insert the graft perpendicular to the long axis of the limb so that it rests on the cut surface of the fibula and extends into the slot in the tibial cortex.
- Pack spongy iliac bone in the angle between the proximal surface of the graft and the lateral surface of the tibia.
- Apply a cast from below the knee to the base of the toes.

POSTOPERATIVE CARE. At 2 months, full weight bearing in the cast is allowed, and at 4 months the cast is discontinued.

TIBIA

Congenital pseudarthrosis of the tibia is rare, with an incidence of approximately one in 250,000 live births. Most large series report 50% to 90% association of this disorder with the stigmata of neurofibromatosis, including skin and osseous lesions.

CLASSIFICATION

Multiple classification systems have been created to describe congenital pseudarthrosis of the tibia. These classification systems tend to be more descriptive of the radiographic appearance of the lesion at a particular course in the disease and often provide little insight into the correct type of treatment or prognosis. Nevertheless, a descriptive classification can be helpful for communication between treating physicians and is important from a historical standpoint. We prefer the Boyd classification of congenital pseudarthrosis of the tibia:

Type I pseudarthrosis occurs with anterior bowing and a defect in the tibia present at birth. Other congenital deformities also may be present.

Type II pseudarthrosis occurs with anterior bowing and an hourglass constriction of the tibia present at birth. Spontaneous fracture, or fracture after minor trauma, commonly occurs before 2 years of age. This is the so-called high-risk tibia. The tibia is tapered, rounded, and sclerotic, and the medullary canal is obliterated. This type is the most common, is often associated with neurofibromatosis, and has the poorest prognosis. Recurrence of the fracture is common during the growth period but decreases in frequency with age and generally ceases to occur after skeletal maturation (Fig. 29-55).

Type III pseudarthrosis develops in a congenital cyst, usually near the junction of the middle and distal thirds of the tibia. Anterior bowing may precede or follow the development of a fracture. Recurrence of the fracture after treatment is less common than in type II, and excellent results after only one operation have been reported to last well into adulthood (Fig. 29-56).

Type IV pseudarthrosis originates in a sclerotic segment of bone in the classic location without narrowing of the tibia. The medullary canal is partially or completely obliterated. An “insufficiency” or “stress” fracture develops in the cortex of the tibia and gradually extends through the sclerotic bone. With completion of the fracture, healing fails to occur, and the fracture widens and becomes a pseudarthrosis. The prognosis for this type generally is good, especially when it is treated before the insufficiency fracture becomes complete (Fig. 29-57).

Type V pseudarthrosis of the tibia occurs with a dysplastic fibula. A pseudarthrosis of the fibula or tibia or both may develop. The prognosis is good if the lesion is confined to the fibula. If the lesion progresses to a tibial pseudarthrosis, the natural history usually resembles that of type II pseudarthrosis.

Type VI pseudarthrosis occurs as an intraosseous neurofibroma or schwannoma that results in a pseudarthrosis. This is extremely rare. The prognosis depends on the aggressiveness and treatment of the intraosseous lesion.

A more recent and simplified classification system proposed by Johnston et al. could guide treatment and prognosis. This classification scheme includes (1) the presence or absence of

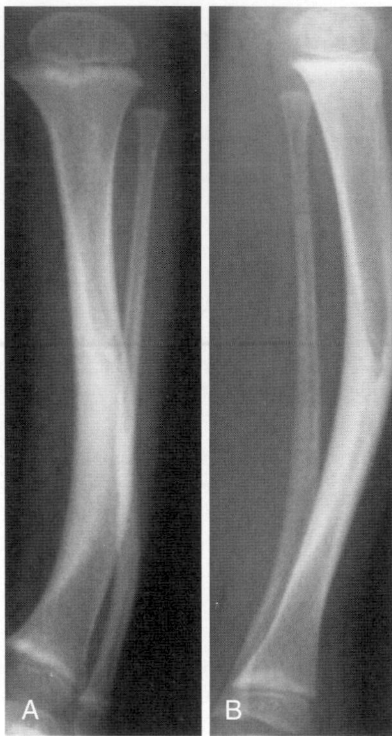

FIGURE 29-55 Type II congenital pseudarthrosis of tibia. **A,** Anteroposterior view of left tibia. **B,** Lateral view. Note anterior bowing and narrow, sclerotic medullary canal.

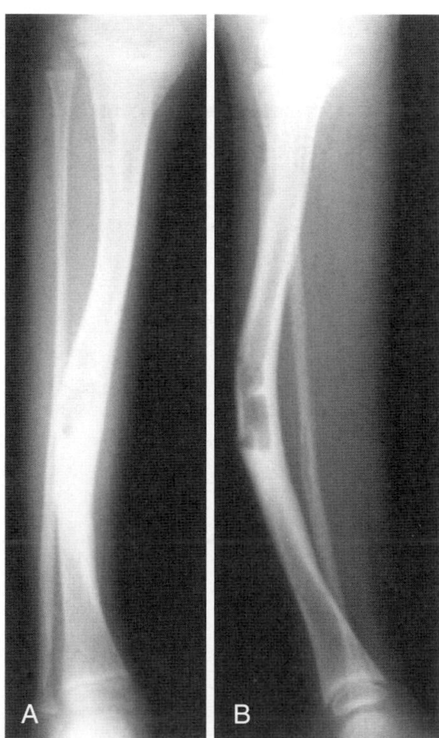

FIGURE 29-56 Type III congenital pseudarthrosis of tibia. **A,** Anteroposterior view of right tibia. **B,** Lateral view. Note cyst formation in middle third of tibia with anterior bowing and narrow medullary canal distal to cyst.

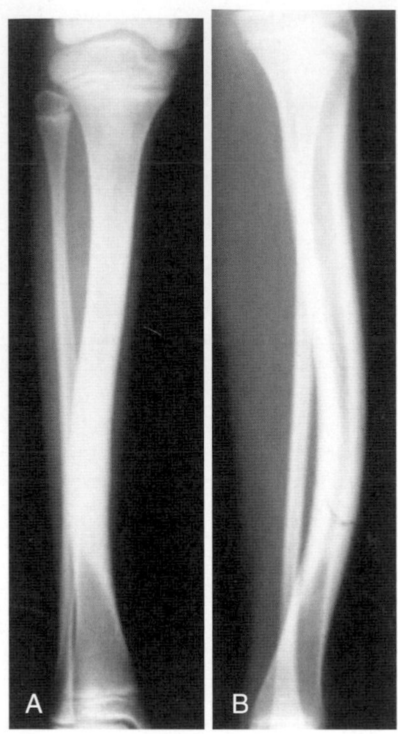

FIGURE 29-57 Type IV congenital pseudarthrosis of tibia. **A,** Anteroposterior view of right tibia. **B,** Lateral view. Note fracture in anterior cortex in distal third of tibia.

a fracture and (2) age of first fracture, before or after age 4 years. Under this classification scheme, fractured tibias require surgical treatment while intact tibias can be treated with observation and splinting.

For those tibias that require surgery, the treatment involves first resecting the entire pseudarthrosis, leaving a bone gap and soft-tissue defect that must be treated regardless of the descriptive radiographic classification before surgical resection.

TREATMENT

Treatment of congenital pseudarthrosis of the tibia depends on the age of the patient and the presence or absence of a fracture. Before walking age, little treatment is required for a pseudarthrosis, but once the child begins to ambulate, the leg should be immobilized in a clamshell orthosis and protected. If no fracture is present, the child can be treated in a brace until skeletal maturity with close follow-up. Once a true pseudarthrosis of the tibia develops, it cannot be expected to heal when treated by casting or bracing alone.

Initial surgical management of tibial pseudarthrosis involves resection of the entire pseudarthrosis and surrounding hamartomatous tissue, restoration of mechanical alignment and intramedullary fixation. These three basic principles often are augmented by a combination of primary shortening, bone transport, supplemental bone grafting, and bone morphogenetic protein. Osseous union probably is more difficult to obtain in this condition than in any other (31% to 56% reported successful treatment). Even when union is obtained, it often is transient, and refracture, leg-length discrepancy, and malalignment may require further surgical management and possibly amputation.

Amputation is rarely, if ever, considered in the initial management of congenital pseudarthrosis of the tibia; however, amputation is frequently required and should be discussed early as a possible outcome of attempted treatment. Factors favoring amputation include anticipated shortening of more than 2 or 3 inches (5 to 7.5 cm), a history of multiple failed surgical procedures, and stiffness and decreased function of a limb that would be more useful after an amputation and prosthetic fitting.

INTRAMEDULLARY FIXATION

Although many techniques have been described, the most commonly used is the intramedullary rodding technique described by Anderson et al. The pseudarthrosis is often quite distal in the tibia, making intramedullary fixation alone inadequate and unstable. Therefore, the ankle joint often must be crossed by the rod to provide additional stability in these very distal pseudarthroses. The rod can migrate with growth, resulting in restoration of some ankle motion over time or can be surgically advanced to a position above the ankle once solid union has been achieved. For those lesions that appear more proximal in the tibia, it might be possible to avoid crossing the ankle joint. In these cases, larger rod diameter or an interlocking option could aid in stability.

VASCULARIZED GRAFT

Resection of the pseudarthrosis with reconstruction using a free vascularized bone graft with either fibular or iliac crest grafts (Fig. 29-58) also has been described with good results.

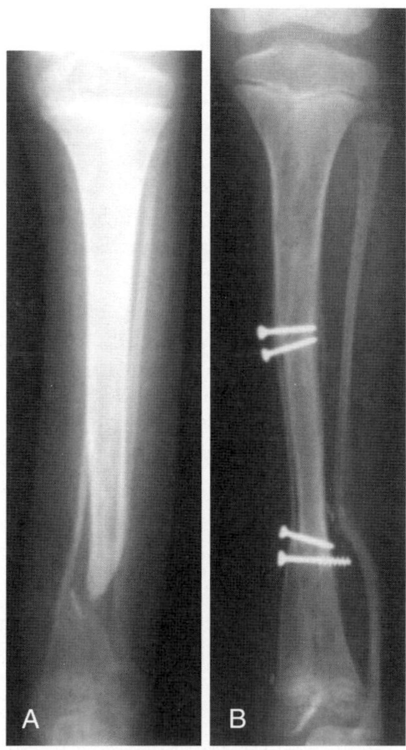

FIGURE 29-58 Congenital pseudarthrosis of tibia treated with vascularized fibular bone graft. **A,** Preoperative radiograph of tibia with established distal pseudarthrosis after multiple failed surgical procedures. **B,** Three years after repair with vascularized fibular graft.

The procedure requires experience with microvascular techniques, however, and two surgical teams are advantageous, one to harvest the graft while the second prepares the pseudarthrosis site to receive the graft. Vascularized fibular grafts may be indicated for pseudarthroses with gaps of more than 3 cm and for pseudarthroses in which multiple surgical procedures have failed.

ILIZAROV

In addition, good preliminary results were reported with the Ilizarov technique, but problems have included difficulty transporting the proximal tibia, "docking" malalignment, and poor quality of regenerated bone, leading to refracture. For most established pseudarthroses, initial treatment should be intramedullary rodding and bone grafting. The Ilizarov approach with bone transport does offer the advantage of maintaining or gaining tibial length.

BONE MORPHOGENETIC PROTEIN

Multiple reports have documented the successful use of recombinant human bone morphogenetic protein (rhBMP) in the treatment of congenital pseudarthrosis of the tibia. Both currently available forms (rhBMP-2 and rhBMP-7) of this protein have been used. In each series, BMP was used in conjunction with other accepted forms of bony stabilization such as intramedullary fixation. Early union rates have been favorable, but long-term follow-up and prospective comparative studies are needed to better understand the long-term efficacy and safety of these treatments. Because the treatment of congenital pseudarthrosis of the tibia is challenging, BMPs should be considered as an adjunct to treatment.

INSERTION OF WILLIAMS INTRAMEDULLARY ROD AND BONE GRAFTING

TECHNIQUE 29-23 *Fig. 29-59*

(ANDERSON ET AL.)

- Position the patient supine on a radiolucent operating table and apply a tourniquet to the thigh.
- Expose the ipsilateral iliac crest and harvest as much cancellous bone and bone from the outer table as can be obtained safely.
- Approach the tibia through an anterior incision that is centered over the pseudarthrosis and just lateral to the tibial crest. Divide the deep fascia of the anterior compartment at this level.
- Subperiosteally, expose the normal bone of the tibial shaft just proximal and distal to the pseudarthrosis.
- Completely excise the bone and fibrous tissue at the pseudarthrosis until normal medullary bone of both tibial fragments is exposed. Resection generally results in tibial shortening of 1 to 3 cm.
- Tibial union may be difficult to achieve in patients with a normal fibula; therefore a fibular osteotomy should be considered to allow adequate approximation of the two ends of the tibia.

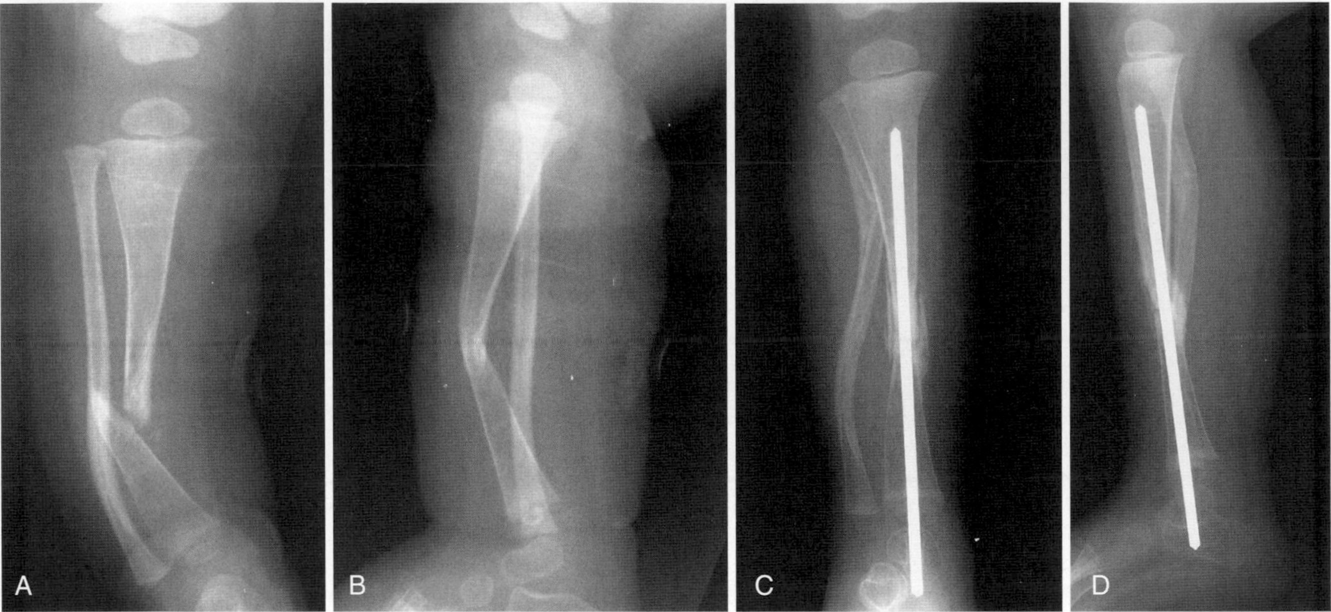

FIGURE 29-59 Insertion of Peter Williams rod for congenital pseudarthrosis of tibia, as described by Anderson et al. **A,** Anteroposterior view of type II congenital pseudarthrosis of tibia in 16-month-old child. **B,** Lateral view. **C,** Postoperative anteroposterior view. **D,** Postoperative lateral view. **SEE TECHNIQUE 29-23.**

- Ream the medullary canals of both tibial fragments with a drill or small curet or both.
- The Williams device consists of an indwelling rod and an insertion rod. The indwelling rod is smooth and cylindrical and varies in diameter. The proximal end is machined to a diamond tip, and the distal blunt end is threaded internally for approximately 15 mm so that a second (insertion) rod of equal outside diameter can be attached to it temporarily. The insertion rod is machined proximally so that its external threads screw into the distal end of the indwelling rod, and it is machined distally to a diamond tip.
- To determine the rod length needed, make a lateral radiograph to determine the expected length of the leg after the affected bone and fibrous tissues have been removed, and the angular deformity has been corrected.
- Drive the coupled rods into the distal part of the tibia at the site of the osteotomy, across the ankle and subtalar joints, and out the sole through the heel pad. When the rod is placed across the ankle joint, it is important to correct valgus deformity of the ankle and dorsiflexion deformity of the foot, which are the inevitable consequences of weight bearing on an anterolaterally bowed tibia. Fluoroscopy is helpful during this part of the procedure.
- Approximate the tibial fragments and drive the rod retrograde into the region of the proximal tibial metaphysis, nearly to the tibial physis, but not encroaching on it. Unscrew the insertion rod a single full turn and verify the junction of the rod on a lateral radiograph.
- Fully disassemble (unscrew) the insertion rod and remove it, leaving the distal end of the implanted rod in the calcaneus.
- Pack the autologous corticocancellous bone strips from the iliac crest around the osteotomy and secure them with circumferential sutures of fine stainless steel or, as have been used more recently, absorbable sutures.
- Prophylactic fasciotomies often are required before wound closure.
- Close the subcutaneous tissue and skin and apply a long-leg cast.

POSTOPERATIVE CARE. The duration of immobilization and the type of cast are determined by the amount of healing noted on clinical and radiographic examinations. When healing is sufficient, the cast is discontinued. Removal of the cast and institution of progressive weight bearing usually are possible several months after surgery. A knee-ankle-foot orthosis or patellar tendon–bearing brace is worn until skeletal maturity is reached.

COMPLICATIONS

STIFFNESS OF THE ANKLE AND HINDFOOT

A stiff ankle should be expected until the distal tip of the rod is proximal to the ankle joint after longitudinal growth of the distal end of the tibia. Even if stiffness persists, it rarely hampers functional results.

REFRACTURE

Refracture is common in patients with pseudarthroses, despite apparently solid clinical and radiographic union. Refracture can be managed with casting or removal and replacement of the intramedullary rod with additional bone grafting. Because of the likelihood of refracture, removal of the rod after union is not recommended until skeletal maturity has been reached.

VALGUS ANKLE DEFORMITY

The distal tibial fragment must be fixed so that valgus deformity of the ankle is corrected at the time of placement of the intramedullary rod. Intraoperative fluoroscopy is useful for monitoring this procedure. Long-term bracing is mandatory during the growth years to minimize progressive valgus ankle deformity, or surgical treatment with the Langenskiöld procedure may be indicated.

Valgus deformity has been found to be significantly more frequent when the fibula is left intact than when fibular osteotomy is done (with or without fibular fixation). In addition, the presence of fibular insufficiency (fracture or prepseudarthrotic lesion) appears to be highly prognostic for subsequent valgus deformity, whether or not the fibula eventually healed.

TIBIAL SHORTENING

Tibial shortening should be anticipated in almost all these children. The maximal projected shortening in the patients of Anderson et al. was 4 cm. In selected patients, tibial shortening can be treated by a well timed contralateral epiphysiodesis or limb lengthening of the proximal tibia. The Ilizarov technique may be useful initially in severe cases with significant shortening and a wide nonunion or in patients in whom medullary nailing and standard bone grafting procedures fail.

CONSTRICTIONS OF THE LEG

A congenital circumferential constriction, or "Streeter" band of the soft tissues of the leg (Fig. 29-60) is rare, occurring in 1 per 10,000. These lower extremity bands often are associated with other anomalies, such as absent digits, foot deformities, constriction bands on the upper extremity, cleft palate, and heart defects.

The deep fascia may be affected, and usually the lymphatic vessels and superficial circulation are partially obstructed. Distal to the constriction there may be persistent pitting edema that may or may not be cured by excising the constriction. Fractures of the tibia and fibula at the level of the constriction have been reported. In marked contrast to congenital pseudarthrosis, after successful treatment of the constriction, the fractures heal promptly without surgery.

Traditionally, constriction bands have been released in two or three stages to prevent vascular compromise of the distal part of the extremity. More recently, however, several authors have reported good results with one-stage release. The advantages of a one-stage release include easier postoperative care, especially in infants, and avoidance of a second or third operation with additional periods of anesthesia.

Hennigan and Kuo divided 135 constriction bands in 73 patients into four zones (Fig. 29-61). Most (50%) were in zone 2, between the knee and ankle. They also classified the bands according to severity: grade 1 bands involved subcutaneous tissue, grade 2 bands extended to the fascia, grade 3 bands extended to the fascia and required release, and grade 4 bands were congenital amputations.

Amputation may be the only treatment option for severe type 3 bands (Fig. 29-62). The prevalence of clubfoot in patients with congenital constricting bands ranges from 12% to 56%.

All neurologic deficits were in children with grade 3 bands in zone 2, and clubfoot in these children required numerous and more extensive surgeries, with poorer results than those in children with no neurologic deficits. These authors suggested early complete soft-tissue release, along with consideration of tendon transfers, and noted that bony surgery eventually becomes necessary, and prolonged bracing will be needed to prevent recurrence.

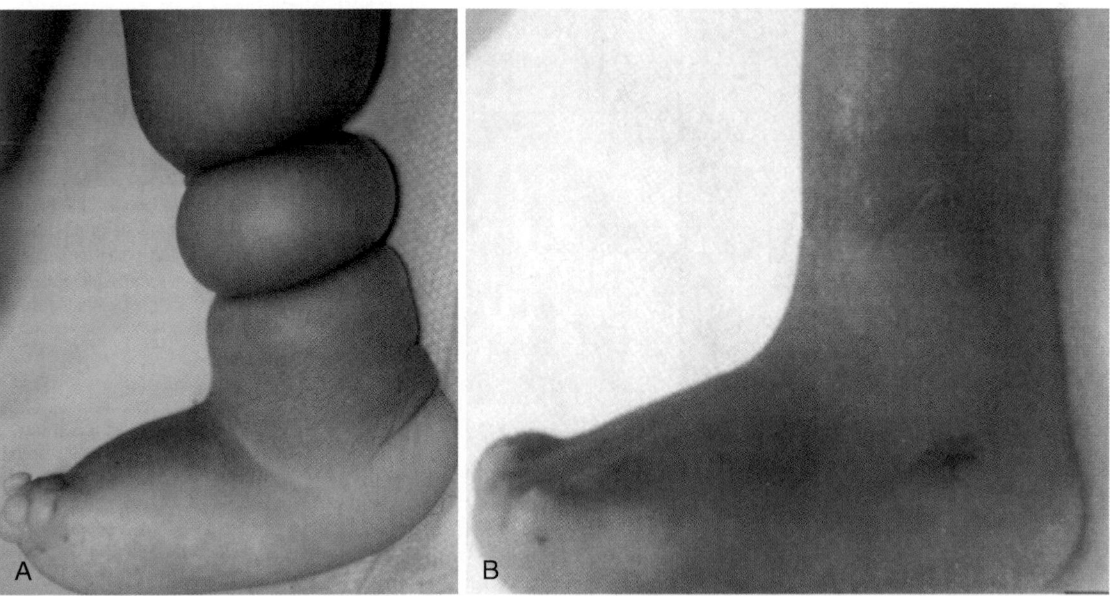

FIGURE 29-60 **A,** Congenital constriction of leg and congenital vertical talus. **B,** Appearance after excision of constricting bands. (From Gabos PG: Modified technique for the surgical treatment of congenital constriction bands of the arms and legs of infants and children, Orthopedics 29:401, 2006.)

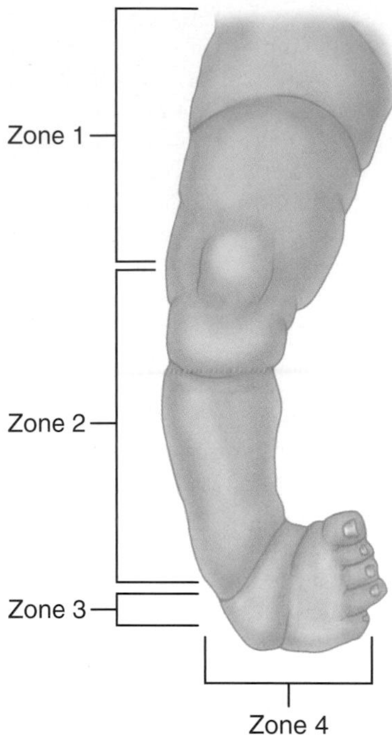

FIGURE 29-61 Zones of constricting bands described by Hennigan and Kuo (see text).

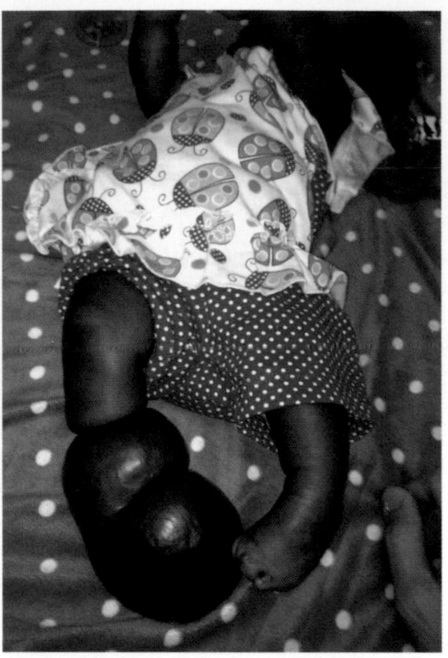

FIGURE 29-62 Amputation may be the only treatment option for severe type 3 bands.

ONE-STAGE OR TWO-STAGE RELEASE OF CIRCUMFERENTIAL CONSTRICTING BAND

TECHNIQUE 29-24

(GREENE)

- Excise a 1- to 2-mm margin of normal skin and subcutaneous tissue to minimize the risk of recurrence. For a two-stage procedure only excise 180 degrees.
- Resect all constricted fascia and muscle that have been converted to dense fibrous connective tissue.
- After resection of the dermal layers within the constriction band, identify the vascular and neurologic structures proximal and distal to the band by careful dissection as the skin and subcutaneous tissue are undermined.
- If subcutaneous tissue is excessive, especially on the dorsum of the fingers, debulking should be done.
- Close the skin with multiple Z-plasties, fashioning fairly large flaps at an angle of 60 degrees (Fig. 29-63).

POSTOPERATIVE CARE. A pressure bandage is applied from proximal to the area of surgery to the distal end of the limb. With young children, a cast or plaster splint is applied and worn for 2 to 3 weeks until the incision has healed.

CONGENITAL HYPEREXTENSION AND DISLOCATION OF THE KNEE

Congenital hyperextension of the knee is only the lowest grade of an abnormality that is divided into three grades according to severity: grade 1, congenital hyperextension; grade 2, congenital hyperextension with anterior subluxation of the tibia on the femur; and grade 3, congenital hyperextension with anterior dislocation of the tibia on the femur (Fig. 29-64). Congenital hyperextension or dislocation of the knee usually is associated with skeletal abnormalities elsewhere in the extremity such as hip dysplasia (Fig. 29-65).

It has been postulated that the basic defect in congenital dislocation of the knee is absence or hypoplasia of the cruciate ligaments, although others consider these findings a result of the dislocation.

The pathologic condition usually varies with the severity of the deformity, but always the anterior capsule of the knee and the quadriceps mechanism are contracted. As the severity of the anterior displacement of the tibia increases, other findings include intraarticular adhesions and other abnormalities within the joint and hypoplasia or absence of the patella. Fibrosis and loss of bulk of the vastus lateralis muscle have been noted, as well as, obliteration of the suprapatellar pouch from the adherent quadriceps tendon and lateral displacement of the patella. In severe anterior dislocation, the collateral ligaments have been shown to course anteriorly from their femoral attachments, and anterior subluxation of the hamstring muscles in some patients to function as extensors of the knee in this deformed position.

The treatment of congenital hyperextension of the knee depends on the severity of the subluxation or dislocation and the age of the patient. In a newborn with mild-to-moderate

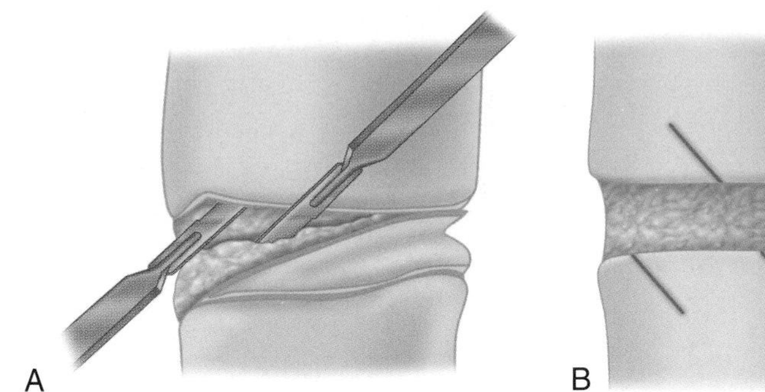

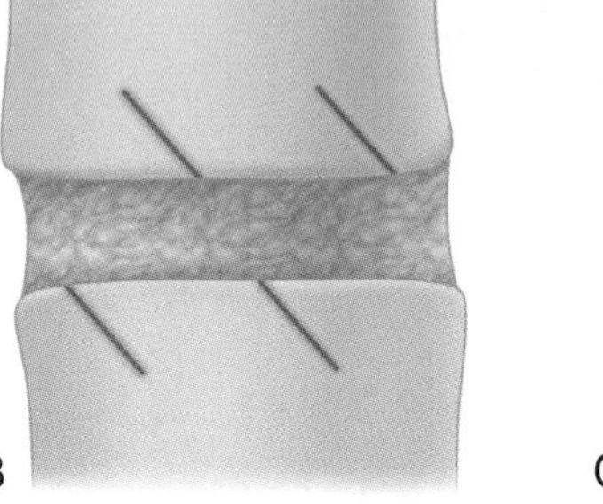

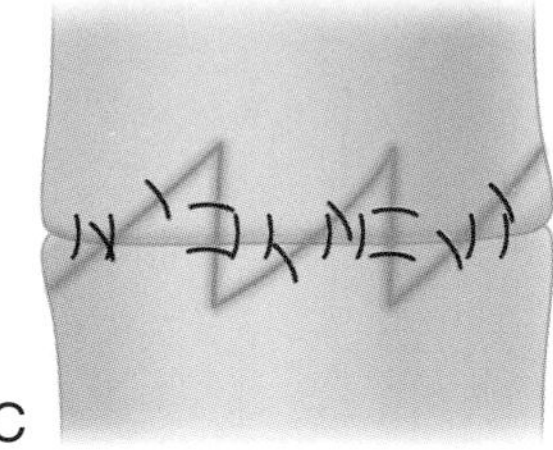

FIGURE 29-63 Congenital constriction release and Z-plasty. **A,** Excision of constriction band and undermining of skin edges. **B,** Z-plasty incisions at 60 degrees. **C,** Repair of Z-plasties with simple or mattress sutures. **SEE TECHNIQUE 29-24.**

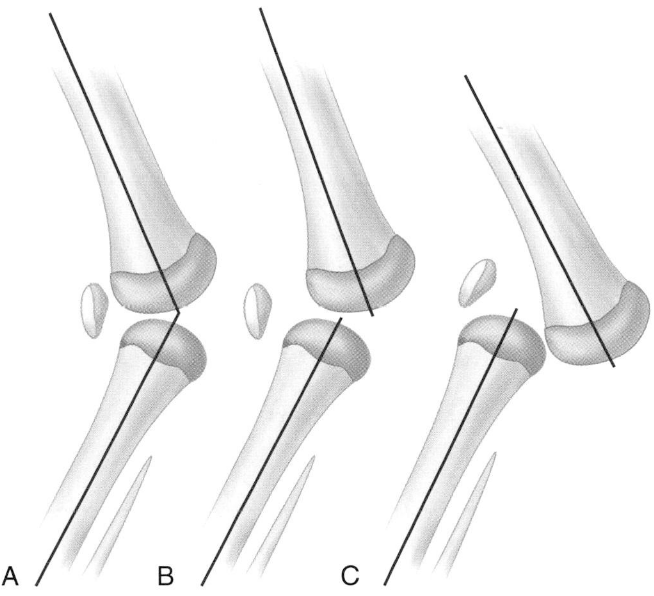

FIGURE 29-64 **A,** Congenital hyperextension of the knee. **B,** Subluxation of knee. **C,** Dislocation of knee.

hyperextension or subluxation, conservative treatment methods, such as the use of the and serial casting to increase knee flexion followed by a Pavlik harness for a few weeks to prevent early recurrence are likely to succeed. Roach and Richards proposed two criteria for successful nonoperative treatment of congenital knee dislocation: radiographic evidence of reduction and knee flexion to 90 degrees or more. According to most authors, nonoperative treatment can be continued for 3 months. In children who do not respond to conservative measures, the use of skeletal traction for correction is an option, but the deformity is difficult to correct with this method. In older children with moderate or severe subluxation or dislocation, surgery is indicated. In a child with congenital dislocation of the knee and congenital dislocation of the hip, surgical correction of the knee first is advisable. However, Johnston et al. described a single-stage correction for both deformities with similar outcomes to staged reconstructions.

Curtis and Fisher described a procedure for correction of congenital dislocation of the knee that is recommended for children 6 to 18 months old. The technique combines anterior capsular release, lengthening of the quadriceps mechanism, and release of intraarticular adhesions. Occasionally, the articular surfaces of the knee remain abnormal if the deformity recurs. Ideally, a functional range of motion can be obtained. In rare cases osteotomy of the femur or tibia may be required in an older child. When needed, femoral shortening can be a good adjunct to quadricepsplasty with good mid-term to long-term function.

Joseph et al. proposed some modifications to the Curtis and Fisher procedure that includes a laterally based incision, a more extensive, tongue-type release of the quadriceps tendons, and avoidance of dissection up to and including the collateral ligaments. These modifications were designed to correct specific problems such as anterior wound dehiscence, inadequate quadriceps tendons length, and postoperative knee instability caused by a collateral transection, respectively.

Dobbs proposed a less invasive treatment of congenital dislocation of the knee that involves serial casting and mini-open tenotomy of the quadriceps with additional anterior capsulotomy if required. This protocol resulted in successful deformity correction in 14 of 16 knees, with two knees requiring additional surgery. Longer follow-up is needed to determine the lasting effects of this treatment.

CAPSULAR RELEASE AND QUADRICEPS LENGTHENING FOR CORRECTION OF CONGENITAL KNEE DISLOCATION

TECHNIQUE 29-25

(CURTIS AND FISHER)

- Make a long anterior midline incision starting superomedially at the level of the middle third of the femur and extending inferolaterally to the tibial tuberosity. Alternatively, Joseph described exposure through a lateral incision with fewer wound complications.
- Expose the anterior thigh muscles and divide the quadriceps mechanism superior to the patella by either an

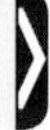

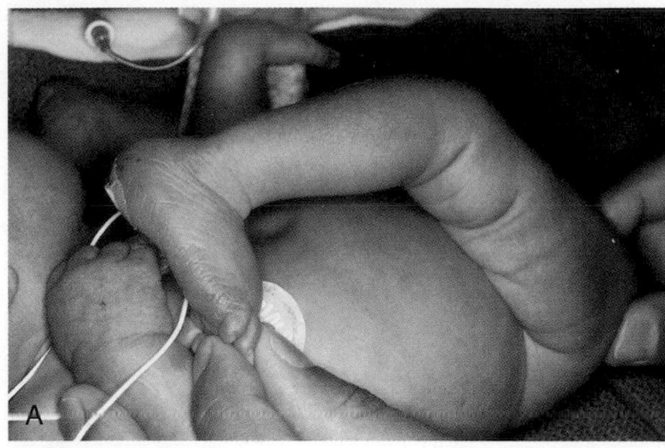

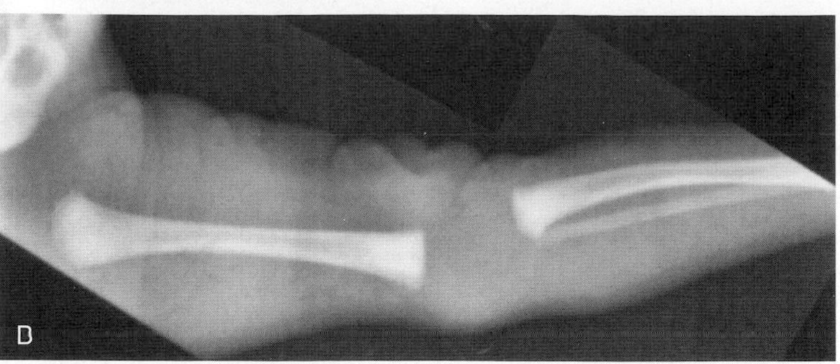

FIGURE 29-65 Congenital dislocation of knee. **A,** Clinical photograph of a child with congenital hyperextension deformity of the knee. **B,** Lateral radiograph after partial correction of the deformity demonstrates persistent anterior subluxation of the tibia. (Courtesy of Jay Cummings, MD.)

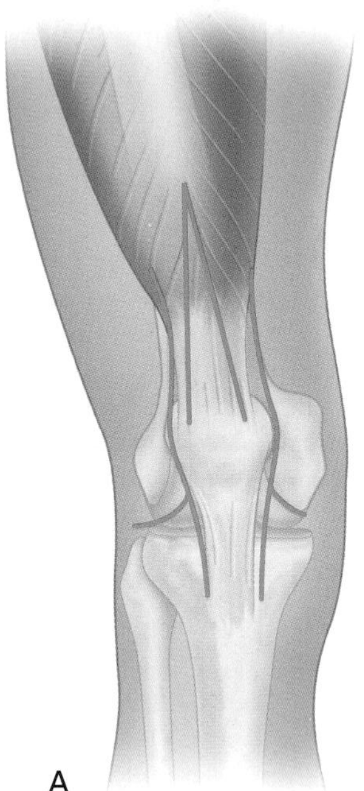

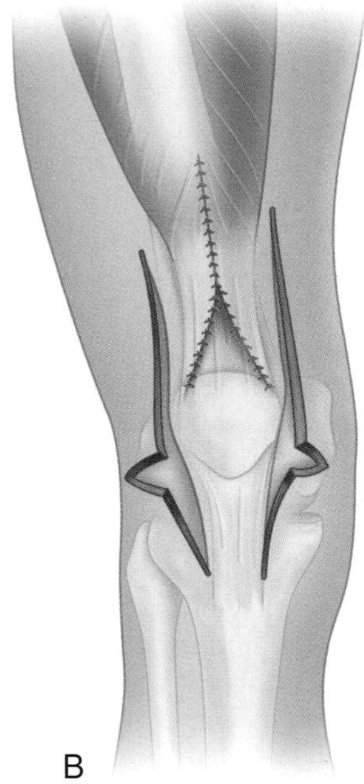

FIGURE 29-66 Curtis and Fisher technique for congenital dislocation of knee. **A,** Lines of incision to release anterior capsule medially and laterally and medial and lateral retinaculum of quadriceps mechanism. **B,** Correction after soft-tissue release and lengthening of rectus femoris muscle. **SEE TECHNIQUE 29-25.**

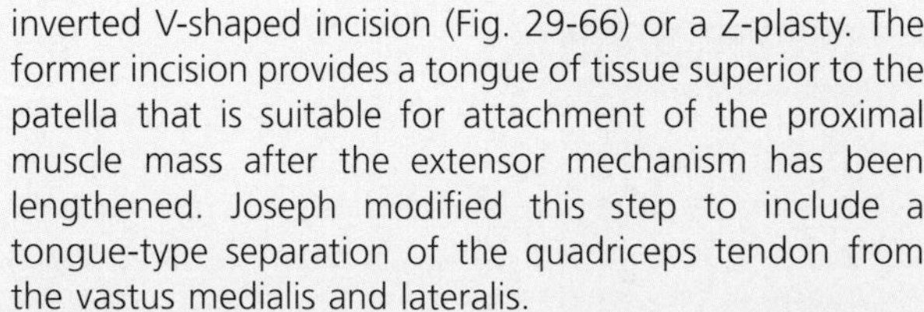
inverted V-shaped incision (Fig. 29-66) or a Z-plasty. The former incision provides a tongue of tissue superior to the patella that is suitable for attachment of the proximal muscle mass after the extensor mechanism has been lengthened. Joseph modified this step to include a tongue-type separation of the quadriceps tendon from the vastus medialis and lateralis.

- Divide the anterior capsule transversely and extend the incision posteriorly to the tibial and fibular collateral ligaments. Mobilize and displace these ligaments posteriorly as the knee is flexed. In some, dissection to the level of the collateral ligaments can be avoided as long as they can be displaced posteriorly.
- If the patella is displaced laterally, release the lateral part of the patellar tendon and the vastus lateralis so that the patella can be moved to its proper location on the femoral condyles.
- Release any tight iliotibial band and lengthen the fibular collateral ligament if needed.
- Mobilize all normal-appearing quadriceps muscle and align it in the long axis of the femur to exert a direct pull on the patella.
- Suture the lengthened quadriceps mechanism with repair of the vastus medialis muscle to the lengthened rectus femoris.
- Evaluate tracking of the patella from extension to 90 degrees of flexion.
- Close the wound and apply a long leg cast with the knee flexed 30 degrees.

POSTOPERATIVE CARE. If the anterior skin is under excessive tension, the cast can be changed at 2 weeks with the use of outpatient anesthesia. At 4 to 6 weeks, the cast is removed, and active and passive exercises are begun. In older patients, continuous passive motion can be used to regain motion during the first 3 to 6 weeks after surgery, and a long leg brace is worn for 6 to 12 months to prevent hyperextension of the knee.

CONGENITAL DISLOCATION OF THE PATELLA

Congenital dislocation of the patella often is familial and bilateral. Occasionally, it is accompanied by other abnormalities, especially arthrogryposis multiplex congenita and Down syndrome. It is persistent and irreducible and usually accompanied by abnormalities of the quadriceps mechanism. The vastus lateralis may be absent or severely contracted, and the patella may be dislocated laterally and attached to the anterior aspect of the iliotibial band. Often the patella is small and misshapen and in an abnormal location in the quadriceps mechanism. Genu valgum and external rotation of the tibia

TABLE 29-3

Two Types of Congenital Dislocation of the Patella

PERSISTENT DISLOCATION	OBLIGATORY DISLOCATION
Patella is dislocated lateral and persistent in that location	Patella dislocates and reduces spontaneously with flexion and extension of knee joint
Often obvious in infancy	Usually present at 5-10 years old
Frequently associated with generalized syndrome	Usually isolated anomaly
Knee flexion contracture is present	Range of knee motion usually normal
Nearly always produces little functional disability	May be well tolerated with little functional disability
Early surgical correction	Surgical correction can be delayed until patient is symptomatic

Adapted from Eilert RE: Congenital dislocation of the patella, Clin Orthop Relat Res 389:22, 2001.

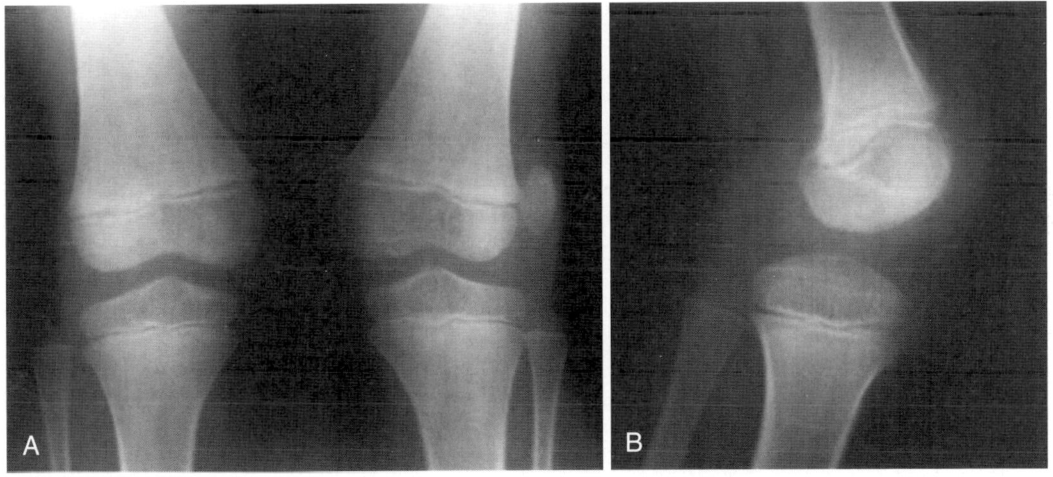

FIGURE 29-67 Untreated congenital dislocation of left patella in 5-year-old boy. **A,** Anteroposterior view shows fixed lateral dislocation. **B,** On lateral view, patella appears absent because of superimposed femoral condyles.

on the femur commonly develop. The capsule on the medial side of the knee is stretched, the lateral femoral condyle is flattened, or the insertion of the patellar tendon is located more laterally than normally.

Eilert noted that two clinical syndromes have been described in the literature: congenital dislocation of the patella or fixed lateral dislocation of the patella and habitual dislocation of the patella, which he suggested should be more accurately termed "obligatory dislocation" of the patella. These two syndromes have different clinical presentations (Table 29-3), and the timing of surgical correction is different.

The diagnosis of congenital dislocation of the patella often is difficult to make before the patient is 3 to 4 years old because of lack of ossification of the patella; however, more severe cases, with associated knee flexion contractures, can be diagnosed soon after birth. Magnetic resonance imaging (MRI) can show the cartilaginous patella lying lateral to the femur and can confirm the diagnosis when congenital lateral patellar dislocation is suspected. Several authors have described the use of ultrasound to define the position of the cartilaginous patella. Because the severity of the deformity is directly related to the length of time that the deformity is allowed to remain uncorrected, surgery can be done as soon as the diagnosis is made to try to prevent a valgus, flexion, or external rotation deformity of the knee (Fig. 29-67).

The underlying pathologic condition of congenital or habitual dislocation of the patella is contracture of the quadriceps mechanism, which is more severe in patients with congenital dislocations. Operative techniques vary according to the extent and degree of these operative findings. The primary objective is release of the contracted structures on the lateral side of the patella (the lateral capsule, iliotibial band, and lateral portion of the quadriceps) to allow reduction of the patella. Medial plication of the lax capsule is necessary to stabilize the reduced patella. In most patients, especially younger children, extensive lateral release and capsular plication are sufficient to obtain patellofemoral congruency. In older children, advancement of the vastus medialis often is necessary to tighten the muscle and improve muscle action.

LATERAL RELEASE AND MEDIAL PLICATION

TECHNIQUE 29-26

(BEATY; MODIFIED FROM GAO ET AL. AND LANGENSKIÖLD)

- Make a midline incision from the distal aspect of the femur to the tibial tuberosity. Perform a full-thickness skin dissection over the patella to expose the medial and lateral aspects of the knee joint and the quadratus femoris muscle.
- Release the vastus lateralis from its most proximal muscle origin in the quadratus femoris to the level of the joint. This may require release of the iliotibial band laterally to the intermuscular septum.
- Because a midline surgical incision over the patella tends to heal with more proliferative scarring in children than in adults, Eilert suggested making the surgical incision over the anterolateral knee so that the scar is not under direct pressure against the patella. The incision must be long enough to expose a sufficient portion of the quadriceps muscle so that it can be realigned, and in an infant with congenital patellar dislocation, the incision may extend halfway up the thigh.
- Occasionally, the rectus femoris must be dissected and lengthened by a Z-plasty.
- Incise the vastus medialis obliquus from its origin proximally and distally from the patella, the medial capsule, and the patellar tendon.
- Reduce the patella into the femoral groove.
- Reattach laterally and distally the vastus medialis obliquus to the patellar tendon and medial retinaculum to secure the patella in the femoral groove.
- When the initial suture has been placed distally, move the knee through a gentle range of motion to assess reduction and tracking of the patella in the femoral groove. If the tension is too tight on the vastus medialis obliquus, remove the suture and transfer the muscle slightly proximally. If the tension is too lax, attach the vastus medialis obliquus farther distally and laterally.
- Occasionally, the patella is so unstable that the gracilis or semitendinous tendon must be divided at the musculotendinous junction and transferred into the patella as a checkrein for added stability. The vastus medialis obliquus is sutured to the remaining retinaculum of the patella and the quadratus femoris.
- Continue the repair of the vastus medialis obliquus proximally and distally.
- Move the knee again through a range of motion to ensure reduction of the patella in the femoral groove and normal tracking during flexion and extension.
- Deflate the tourniquet and obtain hemostasis with electrocautery. Insert a drain deep into the wound and close the subcutaneous tissue and skin.
- Apply a long leg cast with the knee in 30 degrees of flexion.

POSTOPERATIVE CARE. The cast is removed approximately 6 weeks after surgery, and active and passive range-of-motion exercises are begun.

CONGENITAL DEFICIENCIES OF THE LONG BONES

The first scientific approach to the problem of congenital long bone deficiencies was devised by Frantz and O'Rahilly in 1961. Their widely-used classification system described deficiencies as terminal or intercalary. In terminal deficiencies, there is an amputation with no body parts distal to the site (Fig. 29-68A). In intercalary deficits, a middle segment is missing, but the distal segments are present (Fig. 29-68B). Terminal and intercalary deficiencies are defined further as transverse or longitudinal. The complete absence of a hand at the wrist is a terminal transverse deficiency. A complete hand without a radius or ulna is an intercalary transverse deficiency. An example of a terminal longitudinal deficiency is fibular hemimelia, in which the lateral two rays also are missing. Fibular hemimelia in which the foot is normal is an intercalary longitudinal deficiency.

TIBIAL HEMIMELIA

Since the disorder was first described by Otto in 1941, tibial hemimelia has been known by a variety of names, including congenital longitudinal deficiency of the tibia, congenital dysplasia of the tibia, paraxial tibial hemimelia, tibial dysplasia, and congenital deficiency or absence of the tibia. This condition actually represents a spectrum of deformities, ranging from total absence of the tibia (the most severe form) to mild hypoplasia of the tibia (the least severe form). The incidence has been estimated at one in 1 million live births, and the condition may be bilateral in 30% of patients. It usually occurs sporadically, although familial cases with either autosomal dominant or recessive transmission patterns have been reported. There are multiple distinct syndromes that have tibial hemimelia as a component including polydactyly–triphalangeal thumb syndrome (Werner syndrome), tibial hemimelia diplopodia, tibial hemimelia–split hand/foot syndrome, tibial hemimelia–micromelia–trigonal brachycephaly syndrome, and femoral bifurcation-tibial hemimelia-hand ectrodactyly (Gollop-Wolfgang Complex). The exact cause is multifactorial, and a variety of gene defects have been discovered. However, it does not appear that one particular gene mutation or one inheritance pattern can be used to explain all cases.

The involved leg is short, and the fibular head is palpable if it is proximally displaced. The foot is held in severe equinovarus, and the hindfoot is stiff (Fig. 29-69). In older children, the proximal tibial anlage may be palpable, even if it is not radiographically visible. The knee is generally flexed, and in more severe deformities, quadriceps insufficiency causes a lack of knee extension. Careful clinical evaluation of the quadriceps extensor mechanism is important because this has significant prognostic value regarding the potential for reconstruction of the knee. Femoral hypoplasia may be seen.

CLASSIFICATION

The most widely used classification scheme for tibial hemimelia is that of Jones, Barnes, and Lloyd-Roberts (Fig. 29-70), which is based on the early radiographic presentation. Treatment recommendations are given for each type.

In type 1A deformity, there is a complete radiographic absence of the tibia and a hypoplastic distal femoral epiphysis (compared with the normal side) (Fig. 29-71A). In type 1B

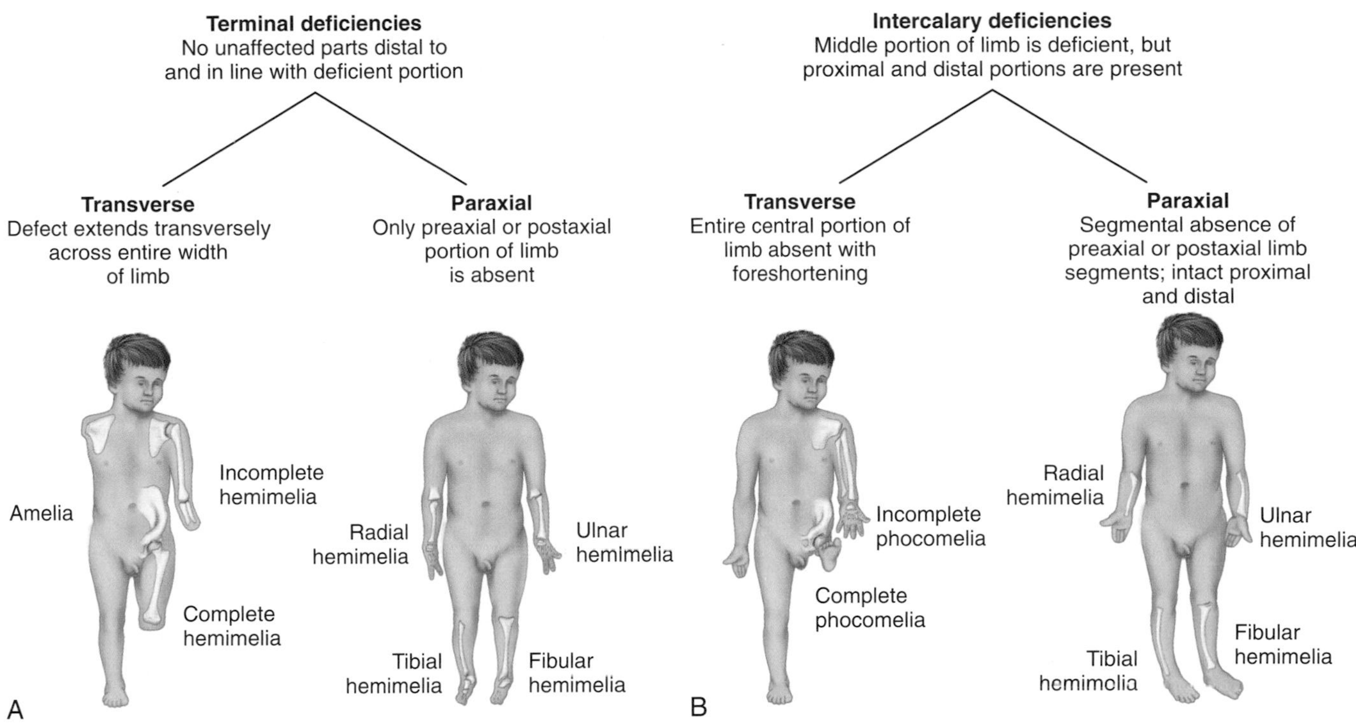

FIGURE 29-68 Frantz-O'Rahilly classification of congenital limb deficiencies. **A,** Terminal deficiencies. **B,** Intercalary deficiencies.

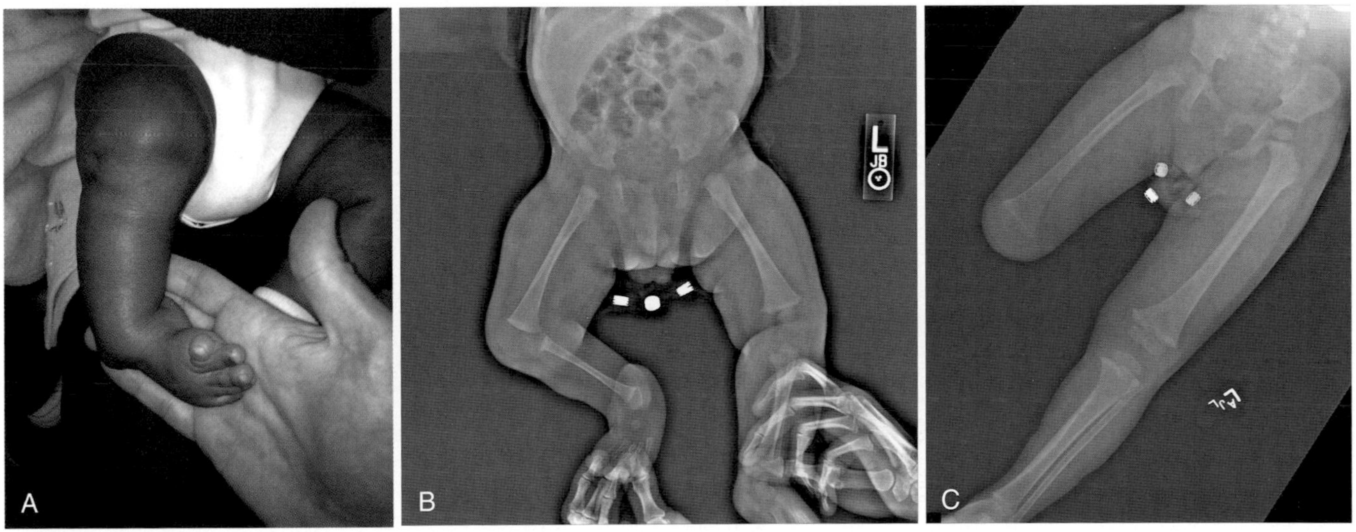

FIGURE 29-69 **A,** Jones type I deformity with rigid foot deformity and absent quadriceps function. **B,** Complete radiographic absence of the tibia. **C,** Radiograph after knee disarticulation.

deformity, there also is no radiographic evidence of a tibia, but the distal femoral epiphysis appears more normal in size and shape. This difference is crucial because the type 1B deformity has a proximal tibial cartilaginous anlage that can be expected to ossify with time. Arthrography, ultrasound, and MRI have shown this cartilaginous anlage in type 1B deformities (Fig. 29-71B, right). In time, the proximal tibial anlage of a type 1B deformity may ossify to become a type 2 lesion.

In type 2 deformity, a proximal tibia of varying size is present at birth. The fibula usually is normal in size, but the head is proximally dislocated (Fig. 29-71B, left).

Type 3 deformity, in which the proximal tibia is not radiographically visible, is rare. The distal tibial epiphysis sometimes is visible, along with a mature distal metaphysis; however, there may be only a diffuse calcified density within the distal tibial anlage. The distal femoral epiphysis usually is well formed, but the upper end of the fibula is proximally

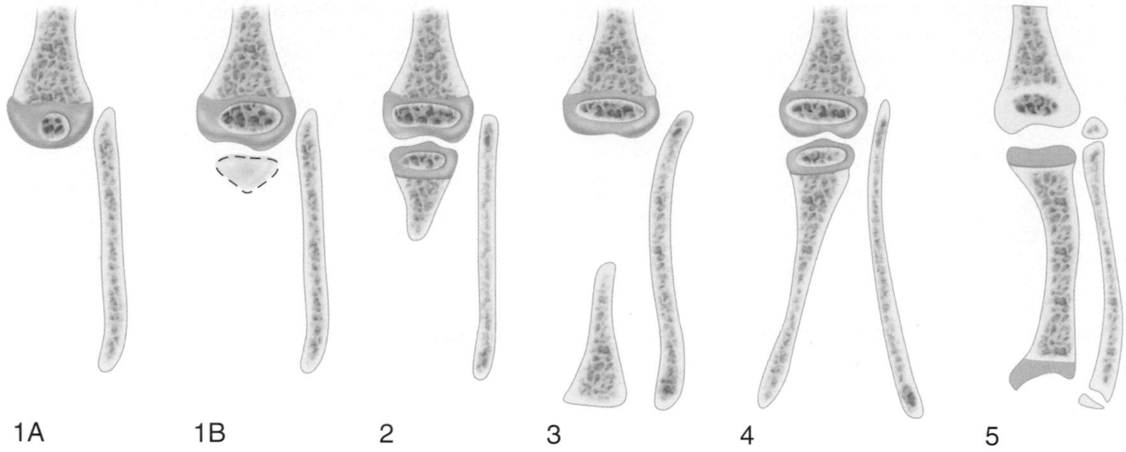

FIGURE 29-70 Classification of tibial hemimelia. In type 1A, fibula is dislocated proximally, tibia is not radiographically evident, and distal femoral epiphysis is smaller than on normal side. In type 1B, fibula is dislocated proximally, and proximal tibial anlage may be visible at birth on ultrasound or magnetic resonance imaging, but not on plain radiographs. Type 2 deformity has proximal dislocation of fibula and radiographically visible proximal tibia with normal-appearing knee joint. In type 3 deformity, fibula is dislocated proximally, distal tibia is radiographically visible, but proximal tibia is not seen. In rare type 4 deformity, fibula has migrated proximally, with diastasis of distal tibiofibular joint. Type 5 Birch modification of Jones classification to include global shortening of the tibia relative to the fibula.

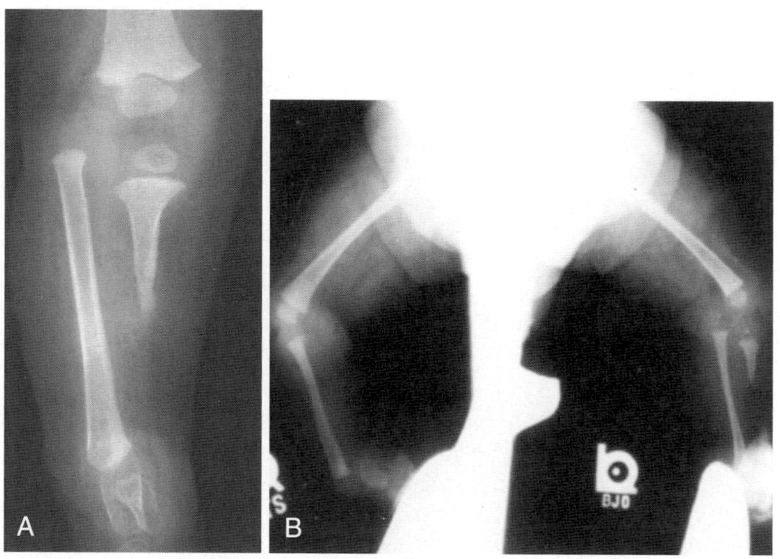

FIGURE 29-71 **A,** Congenital tibial hemimelia type 1A. **B,** Bilateral tibial hemimelia (right type 1B and left type 2).

dislocated. Although the distal femoral epiphysis usually is of normal size, the knee generally is unstable.

In type 4 deformity, which is rare, the tibia is shortened, and there is a proximal migration of the fibula with distal tibial fibular diastasis (Fig. 29-72). This deformity also has been called congenital diastasis of the ankle joint and congenital tibiofibular diastasis. Clinton and Birch, in their 37-year review of 125 limbs with tibial hemimelia, noted no true type 3 deformities. They also proposed the addition of a Jones type 5, which involves global tibial shortening relative to the fibula of varying severity.

A more recent classification takes into account the MRI, ultrasonographic, and intraoperative findings of the cartilaginous anlage both proximally and distally. This classification includes seven types, with "a" and "b" subtypes depending on the presence or absence of cartilaginous portions (Fig. 29-73). This classification includes global shortening of the tibia, which was previously not classified in the Jones system. Although not currently widely used, this system may become more mainstream in the years to come.

In tibial hemimelia, the superficial peroneal nerve may terminate at the level of the ankle. Leg muscles that normally insert on the plantar surface of the foot tend to blend into a common tendon sheet. The talus and calcaneus frequently are congenitally fused. The anterior tibial artery is absent, and the plantar arterial arch is incomplete. Similar vascular findings in clubfoot and tibial hemimelia suggest reduced vascular flow as a cause. Associated anomalies generally are most

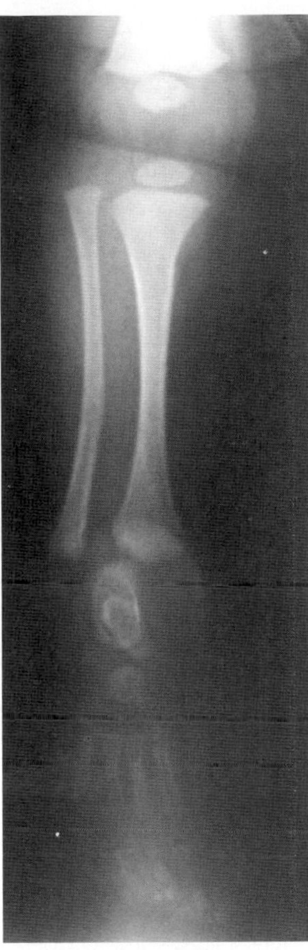

FIGURE 29-72 Newborn with congenital diastasis of ankle representing type 4 tibial hemimelia; note absence of first ray.

severe when the tibia is least developed. In type 4 deformities, the distal tibial epiphysis may be absent.

TREATMENT

As with all congenital lower limb deficiencies, the goal of treatment is a functional limb equal in length to the normal limb. The type of surgical treatment depends on the radiographic classification and clinical appearance. For severe deficiencies, amputation and prosthetic rehabilitation are the most practical means of treatment.

Jones Type 1A Tibial Hemimelia. The two options for treatment of type 1A deformities are knee disarticulation and knee reconstruction (with or without foot amputation). The easiest and frequently most effective option is knee disarticulation followed by fitting with an above-knee prosthesis. This option provides a definitive solution with one operation and is indicated when there is no intact quadriceps-patellar tendon complex (Figure 29-69). Knee disarticulation is preferred over above-knee amputation because above-knee amputation for type 1A deformity may result in skin problems from bony stump overgrowth. Because the ultimate femoral growth often is diminished, the end result of a knee disarticulation may be a functional above-knee amputation level. Children treated in this manner are almost uniformly active, functional prosthetic users. Attempts to correct the equinovarus and absent knee joint frequently result in repeated operations and eventual failure. The Brown procedure, transfer of the proximal fibula under the distal femur in type 1A deformities, has not produced stable long-term results. It may be reasonable to preserve the foot in bilateral deformities because limb-length discrepancy is not a consideration, but attempts to reconstruct the knee in conjunction with foot amputation have produced mixed results.

Jones Type 1B and 2 Tibial Hemimelia. In type 1B and type 2 deformities, a functional knee joint exists, and knee disarticulation is not required if the quadriceps mechanism is present and functional. A proximal tibiofibular synostosis combined with a Syme amputation or distal reconstruction is the treatment of choice (Fig. 29-74).

Putti used a side-to-side configuration (Fig. 29-75C), but most authors now prefer end-to-end alignment between the tibial remnant and the fibula. Although it would seem preferable to wait until the proximal tibial anlage ossifies, stability can be achieved even when the proximal tibia is purely cartilaginous. At a second stage, the foot is amputated to make prosthetic rehabilitation easier. Retention of the foot during the proximal tibial reconstruction is helpful because it serves as a fixation point for a long leg cast. Making a synostosis between the fibula and tibia creates a more uniform, in-line, weight bearing mechanical axis. When the fibula is not transferred to the tibia, a peculiar, curved, hypertrophied fibula develops, causing a secondary deformity. Fusing the fibula underneath the tibia encourages its transformation into a more tibia-like bone. The Syme amputation is preferred to a through-bone amputation to prevent transdiaphyseal problems of bony stump overgrowth and to preserve maximal length of the stump. Another option, if the tibial segment is long enough, involves the creation of a synostosis between the distal tibia and fibula (Fig. 29-76). The Ertl amputation results in a functional transtibial amputation with a proposed decreased risk of bone overgrowth.

Authors have attempted to treat types 1B and 2 tibial hemimelia with surgical equalization of leg length, production of a plantigrade foot, and creation of a stable knee. Traditional leg-lengthening procedures, soft-tissue reconstruction, and casting have not reliably achieved these goals in patients with tibial hemimelia; however, the Ilizarov method offers a viable option for reconstruction in selected cases. These decisions can be quite difficult. Amputation is an undesirable option for many families who hope for a normal limb. Therefore, the expected function of the reconstructed limb, the multiple surgical procedures required, and the prolonged time in an external fixator frame must be weighed carefully against the function that can be obtained with timely amputation and prosthetic management. Other ingenious procedures have been used for reconstruction in children with tibial hemimelia.

In patients with tibial hemimelia and ipsilateral femoral deficiency, arthrodesis of the fibula to the distal femur can be performed or, in younger children, chondrodesis, aligning the fibula directly with the femur and the intercondylar notch. Combining this with a Syme amputation significantly lengthens the effective lever arm of the femur.

Although Syme and Boyd amputations have been the accepted treatments to make prosthetic rehabilitation easier, other alternatives have been described. If a family is absolutely opposed to amputation of the foot, an acceptable alternative is reconstruction of the foot and ankle complex by

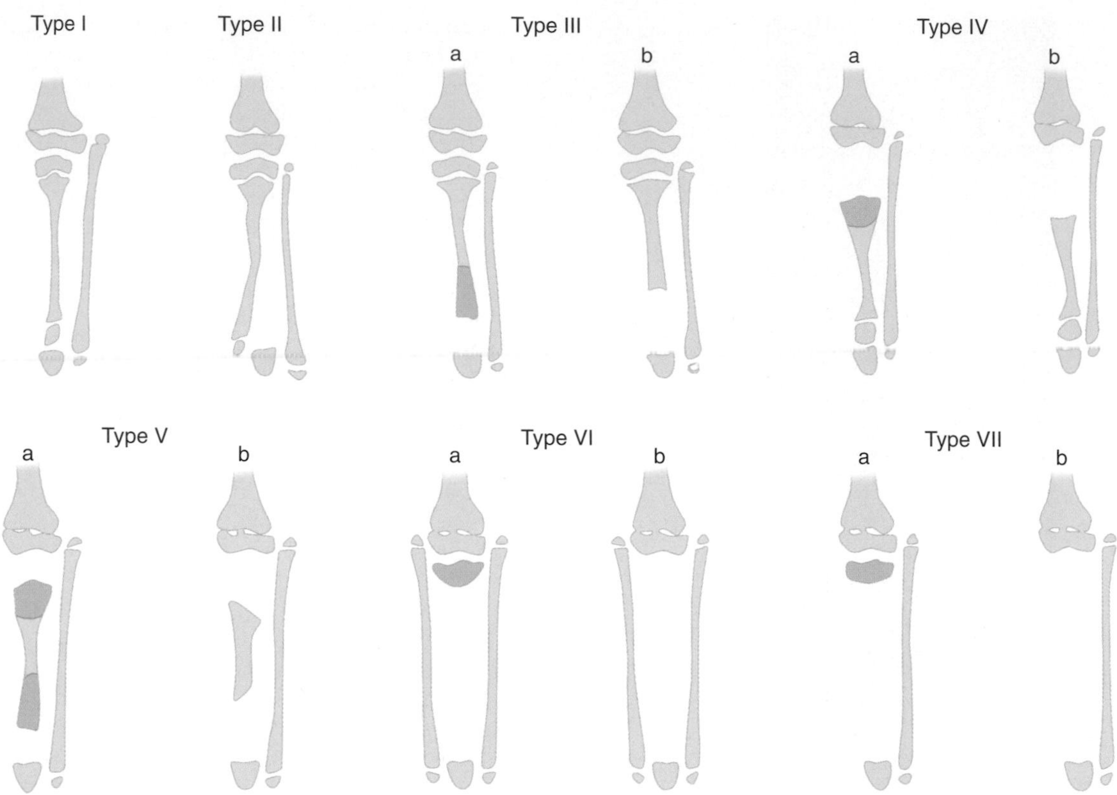

FIGURE 29-73 Weber classification of tibial hemimelia based on severity in a higher maturation level. Type I, hypoplasia; type II, diastasis; type III, distal aplasia; type IV, proximal aplasia; type V, bifocal aplasia; type VI, agenesia with double fibula; type VII, agenesia with single fibula. (Type [a] is with cartilaginous anlage and [b] is without cartilaginous anlage; tan represents bone, and blue represents cartilage). (From Weber M: New classification and score for tibial hemimelia, J Child Orthop 2:169, 2008.)

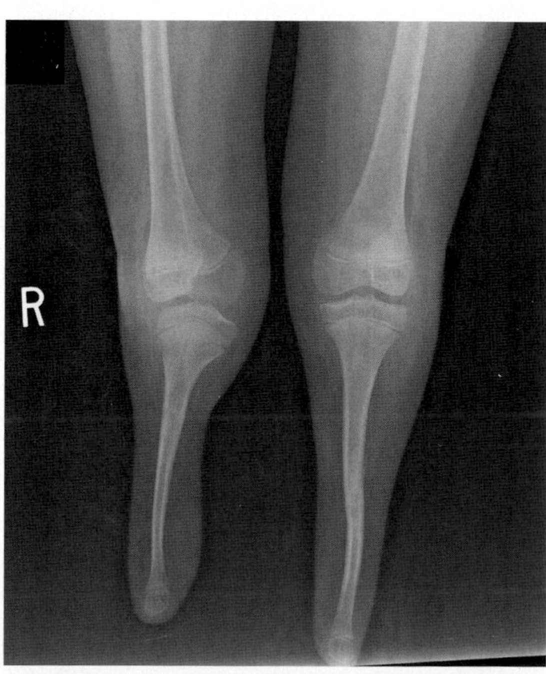

FIGURE 29-74 Follow-up after fibula to tibia transfer and Syme amputation. **SEE TECHNIQUE 29-28.**

implanting the distal fibula into the talus in an extreme equinus position to increase the length of the limb (Fig. 29-75A). Prostheses can be constructed to take advantage of this extra length while accommodating the foot.

Some authors recommend knee disarticulation even in type 2 deficiencies if severe knee flexion contractures are present before surgery. Finally, proximal tibiofibular synostosis is not absolutely indicated for all type 2 deformities; the literature contains reports of satisfactory prosthetic rehabilitation after Syme amputation alone; however, if the fibula is transferred under the tibial remnant, it can be expected to remodel reliably and form into a large, tibia-like bone eventually.

Jones Type 3 Tibial Hemimelia. Type 3 deficiencies are extremely rare and in the limited reports available have been treated with a variety of amputations. In some patients, tibiofibular synostosis may be possible.

Jones Type 4 Tibial Hemimelia. For patients with type 4 deficiencies, treatment must be individualized. Syme amputation provides excellent function. Customized reconstruction of the ankle joint to retain the foot and ankle also has been described. Most patients can be treated with combinations of distal tibiofibular synostosis and distal fibular epiphysiodesis. Equinovarus deformities of the foot, if present, require soft-tissue releases.

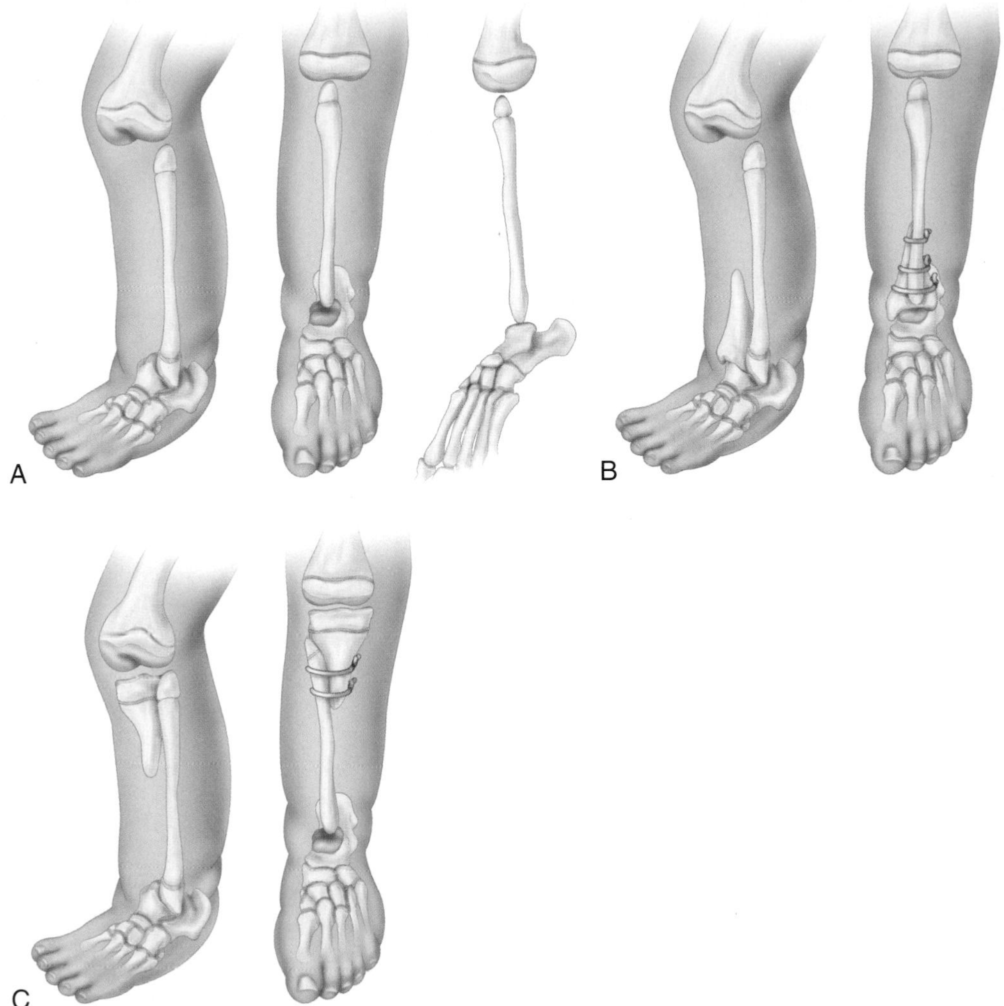

FIGURE 29-75 Variations of Putti procedure for reconstruction of congenital absence of tibia. **A,** Fibula is inserted into hindfoot with foot in severe equinus to lengthen limb. Fibula also has been transferred to intercondylar notch. **B,** Fibula has been transferred to intercondylar notch, and distal tibiofibular synostosis has been created. **C,** Type 2 deficiency. Fibula has been synostosed to proximal tibia and inserted into hindfoot with foot positioned in equinus to obtain additional length. End-to-end synostosis is preferred; if side-to-side synostosis is performed, transverse screw can be used for fixation.

DISTAL FIBULOTALAR ARTHRODESIS

TECHNIQUE 29-27

- Place the patient supine on the operating table.
- Approach the distal fibulotalar articulation anterolaterally to expose both bones.
- Dissect soft tissue to allow central placement of the body of the talus onto the distal end of the fibula.
- Create a trough through the dome of the talus into which the distal fibula is placed plantigrade and in neutral alignment with the foot.
- If necessary, fix the fibulotalar articulation with longitudinal and crossed Kirschner wires.
- Remove the cartilage from the distal fibular epiphysis and from the dome of the talus to allow bone-to-bone contact.
- Close the wound and apply a long leg, bent-knee cast.

POSTOPERATIVE CARE. The cast is worn until the arthrodesis has united, usually at 12 to 16 weeks.

PROXIMAL TIBIOFIBULAR SYNOSTOSIS

TECHNIQUE 29-28 *Fig. 29-74*

- Make an anterolateral incision beginning at the proximal tibia and extending distally and anteriorly to the middle third of the tibia. Identify and protect the peroneal nerve.
- Dissect a sufficient portion of the anterior compartment musculature from the proximal medial tibia to expose the proximal tibial cartilaginous anlage (in type 1B deficiency) or the bony proximal tibia (in type 2 deficiency).

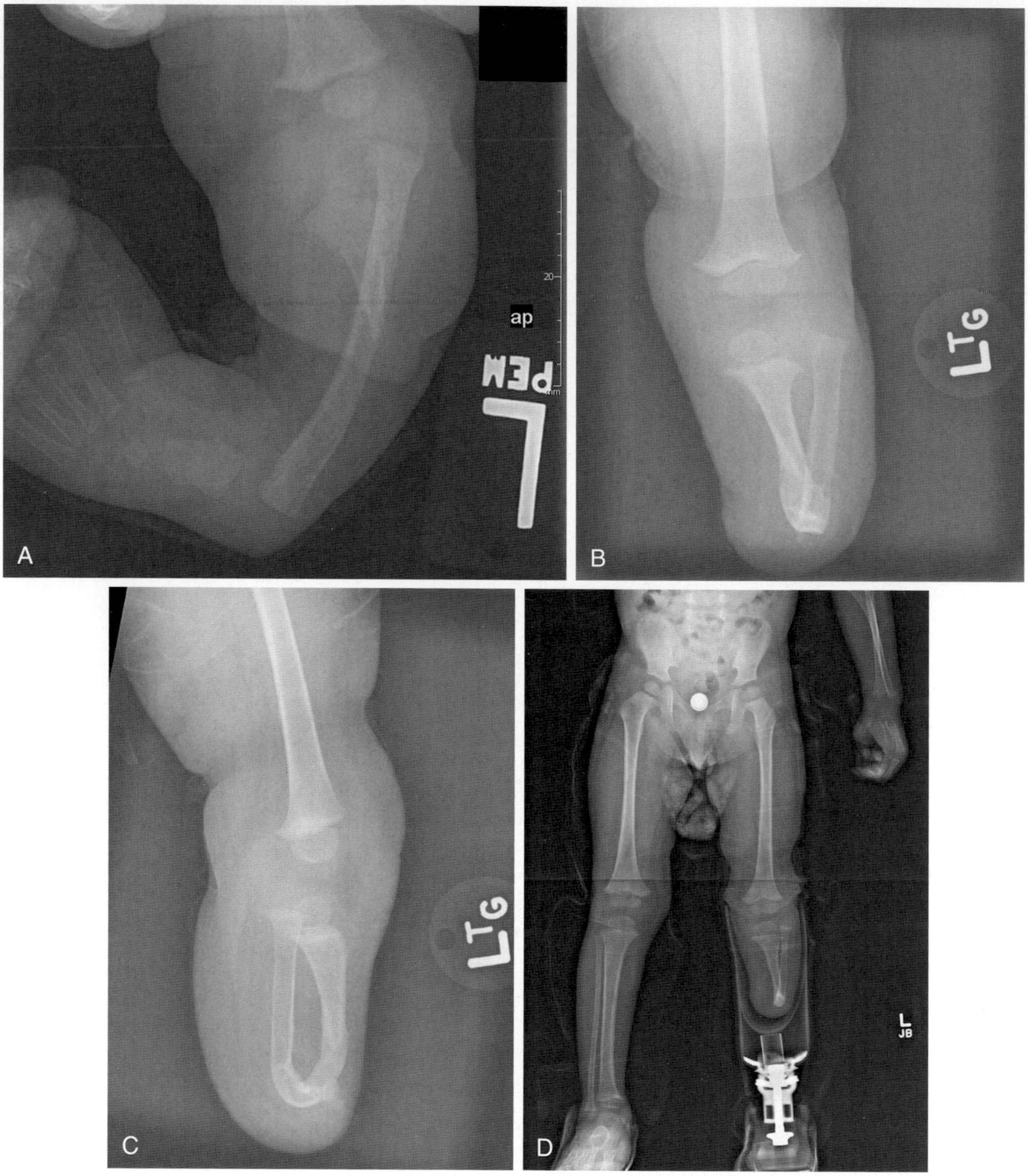

FIGURE 29-76 **A,** Jones type II hemimelia with significant tibial shortening and rigid foot deformity. **B,** Posterior Ertl amputation (anteroposterior view). **C,** Lateral view. **D,** Prosthetic fitting.

- Leave the proximal attachments of the fibula intact, but perform a subperiosteal dissection of the fibula.
- At an appropriate point opposite the distal end of the proximal tibial anlage, perform an osteotomy of the fibula.
- Drill a Steinmann pin of appropriate size distally through the medullary canal of the fibula out the plantar aspect of the foot.
- Reduce the fibula on the proximal tibia and drive the medullary pin retrograde into the proximal tibial remnant.
- If necessary, pass the pin into the distal femur for stability.
- Distally, bend the pin 90 degrees and cut it off below the level of the skin to be removed 6 to 8 weeks later. Immobilize the leg in a cast. Alternative fixation techniques can include screws, cross pins, and cerclage wires.

At a later date, the foot may be amputated. In some patients, the foot may be salvaged with a combination of soft-tissue release, Ilizarov technique, and talectomy or arthrodesis as needed. The tip of the proximal tibial remnant should be sectioned sufficiently to create a wide surface for either chondrodesis or synostosis with the fibula. The periosteum of the fibula should be sutured to the proximal tibial remnant, if possible, to prevent reformation of the fibula to its proximal remnant.

FIBULAR HEMIMELIA

Fibular hemimelia, also known as congenital absence of the fibula, congenital deficiency of the fibula, paraxial fibular hemimelia, and aplasia or hypoplasia of the fibula, is the most common long bone deficiency (followed by aplasia of the radius, femur, tibia, ulna, and humerus). Whether or not dysgenesis and relative ischemia affect the developing mesenchyme and cause the skeletal dysplasia seen in fibular hemimelia is still conjectural. There are no clear genetic or toxic pathogenetic mechanisms. Fibular hemimelia consists of a spectrum of anomalies, the least severe being mild fibular shortening and the most severe being total absence of the fibula associated with defects in the foot, tibia, and femur. Because of the myriad anomalies associated with even mild fibular deficiency, postaxial hypoplasia may be a more descriptive designation for this condition.

The clinical presentation depends on the specific classification and associated anomalies. Generally, there is leg-length discrepancy with equinovalgus deformity of the foot, flexion contracture of the knee, femoral shortening, instability of the knee and ankle, and a stiff hindfoot with absent lateral rays (Fig. 29-77). Although equinovalgus is the most common foot deformity, equinovarus and calcaneovalgus also have been reported. Clinical problems are leg-length inequality and foot and ankle instability. In bilateral involvement, the leg-length discrepancy generally is manifested as disproportionate dwarfism because both sides usually are affected to a similar degree.

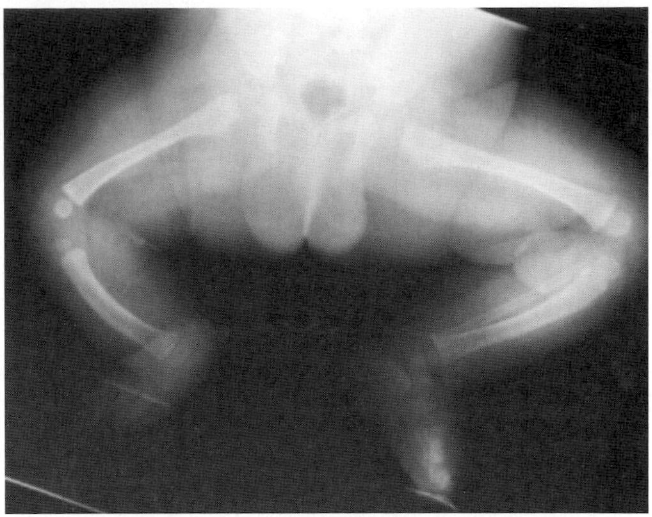

FIGURE 29-77 Radiograph of infant with classic fibular hemimelia. Femur and tibia are both short, and foot is in valgus with absent lateral rays.

CLASSIFICATION

A useful classification scheme proposed by Achterman and Kalamchi (Fig. 29-78) distinguishes a type 1 deformity (hypoplasia of the fibula) from a type 2 deformity (complete absence of the fibula). Type 1 deformities are subdivided further into type 1A and type 1B. In type 1A, the proximal fibular epiphysis is distal to the proximal tibial epiphysis, and the distal fibular epiphysis is proximal to the talar dome. In type 1B, the deficiency of the fibula is more severe, with 30% to 50% of the length missing, and no distal support for the ankle joint (Fig. 29-79). Abnormalities of the femur are common, as is hypoplasia of the patella and lateral femoral condyle. The cruciate ligaments also are clinically unstable. Angulation of the tibia is found most often in patients with type 2 deficiencies. Ball-and-socket ankle joints are present in most patients with type 1A deficiencies, and more severe foot and ankle problems are found in patients with type 2 deformities. Some patients with type 2 deformities have relatively stable ankle joints, however, despite the absence of a fibula, and others have complete instability of the tibiotalar articulation. Tarsal coalitions and absence of the lateral rays are common.

Another classification by Birch et al. takes overall limb-length inequality and foot function into account when determining treatment (Table 29-4).

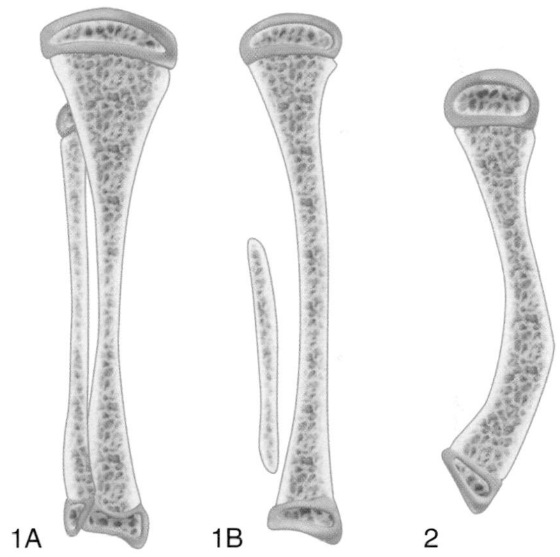

FIGURE 29-78 Achterman and Kalamchi classification of fibular hemimelia. Type 1A: proximal fibular epiphysis is more distal, and distal fibular epiphysis is more proximal than normal. Type 1B: more severe deficiency of fibula with at least 30% to 50% of fibula missing and no distal support to ankle joint. Type 2: complete absence of fibula with bowing and shortening of tibia.

The foot is considered functional if it can be made plantigrade and has three or more rays. Limb-length inequality is determined by a full-length radiograph or scanogram. The percentage of shortening remains constant in 85% of fibular deficiency patients. If both limbs are involved, the longer limb is considered “normal” and the percentage of shortening is measured relative to the “normal” limb.

TREATMENT

At the initial evaluation, the physician should attempt to predict the ultimate limb-length discrepancy, based on the

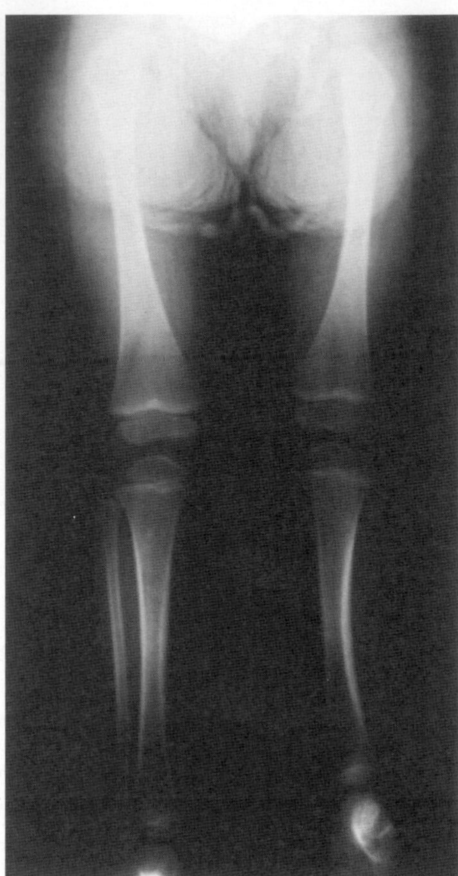

FIGURE 29-79 Achterman and Kalamchi type 1B fibular hemimelia with very hypotrophic, faintly visible fibula; mild shortening of femur; and moderate shortening of tibia.

TABLE 29-4

Fibular Deficiency: Functional Classification and Treatment Guidelines (Birch)

CLASSIFICATION	TREATMENT
TYPE I: FUNCTIONAL FOOT	
IA: 0%-5% inequality	Orthosis, epiphysiodesis
IB: 6%-10% inequality	Epiphysiodesis ± limb lengthening
IC: 11%-30% inequality	1 or 2 limb-lengthening procedures or amputation
ID: >30% inequality	>2 limb-lengthening procedures or amputation
TYPE II: NONFUNCTIONAL FOOT	
IIA: Functional upper limb	Early amputation
IIB: Nonfunctional upper limb	Consider limb salvage procedure

current percentage of shortening. Generally, because the percentage of shortening in an infant remains relatively constant throughout childhood, reasonable predictions of final leg-length discrepancy can be made based on very early radiographs. The function of the foot also is assessed as described.

For a patient with a functional foot and minimal limb-length inequality (≤5%), the goals of treatment are equalization of limb length and correction of the foot deformity. Shoe lifts are prescribed during the growth period, and epiphysiodesis of the normal leg is performed at the appropriate time so that leg lengths are equal at the end of skeletal growth. If contralateral epiphysiodesis or shortening would result in unacceptable overall diminution of height, the physician is faced with a difficult decision: either the short leg is lengthened, or the foot is amputated, and length is equalized with a prosthesis.

For inequality of 6% to 10%, appropriately timed epiphysiodesis can be used with or without limb lengthening in patients with a functional foot. Stevens and Arms recommended combining limb lengthening with hemiepiphysiodesis of the distal femur or ankle or both to correct valgus alignment. They also suggested that adjunctive contralateral epiphysiodesis might be preferable to repeated limb lengthening, emphasizing the multiple procedures that may be required for associated deformities. For patients with 11% or more limb-length inequality and a functional foot, a difficult decision must be made whether to undertake limb salvage with multiple lengthening or amputation. McCarthy et al. found that patients who had amputations were able to perform more activities, had less pain, were more satisfied, had a lower complication rate, and had undergone fewer surgical procedures than patients with tibial lengthenings; however, the decision to proceed with amputation is often a difficult one for families to make.

For more severe deformities of the foot, those with less than three rays or rigid equinovalgus, early amputation and prosthetic reconstruction usually are considered the best options for these nonfunctional feet; however, if the upper limbs also are severely affected, salvage of the deformed foot may be beneficial to maintain global function.

Choi et al. (2000) noted that the distal tibial epiphysis in patients with fibular hemimelia often is wedge-shaped, and they found that the severity of the wedging was predictive of the severity of foot deformity after tibial lengthening. In patients with mildly wedged epiphyses (type I), varying degrees of mild growth retardation and minimal foot deformity should be anticipated; in patients with moderately wedged epiphyses (type II), worsened asymmetric growth retardation and progressive foot deformity should be expected; and in patients with severely wedged epiphyses (type III), severe growth retardation and severe foot deformities should be expected.

When the foot is to be salvaged, various reconstructive procedures have been described. For equinovalgus deformity, posterior and lateral releases are required. The Achilles tendon and the fibrocartilaginous anlage of the absent fibula must be released. In older children, ankle valgus can be corrected with a dome or varus supramalleolar osteotomy. Varus osteotomy shortens the limb but also eliminates the medial prominence associated with a simple closing wedge osteotomy (Fig. 29-80). A Wiltse osteotomy corrects the translational deformity (Fig. 29-81).

When the foot is amputated, Syme amputation is typically performed. At the time of amputation any residual bowing of the tibia can be corrected with an osteotomy, or this angular correction can be postponed to an older age. Although a Boyd amputation offers greater length than a Syme procedure, it should be used cautiously in very young children because the

Boyd amputation leaves a remnant of calcaneus that can migrate posteriorly (Fig. 29-82). Prophylactic sectioning of the Achilles tendon should be considered when amputation is performed for congenital limb deficiencies. Cruciate deficiency is common in patients with fibular hemimelia. However, the treatment of anterior cruciate ligament deficient knees remains controversial. Some authors have found good function and health status relative to age-matched controls over long-term follow-up in patients with anterior cruciate ligament deficient knees and a wide variety of fibular hemimelia severity and treatments.

Others have suggested that anterior cruciate ligament reconstruction should be consider for athletes with fibular hemimelia and anterior cruciate ligament insufficiency, with expectation of good results and function after reconstruction.

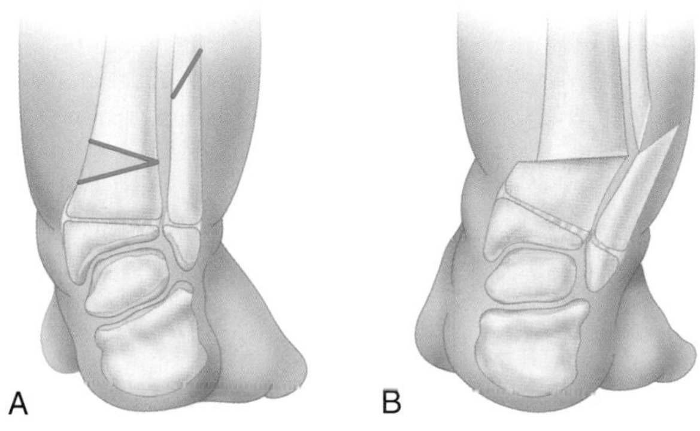

FIGURE 29-80 **A** and **B,** Closing wedge technique can result in translation deformity with prominent medial malleolus (**B**).

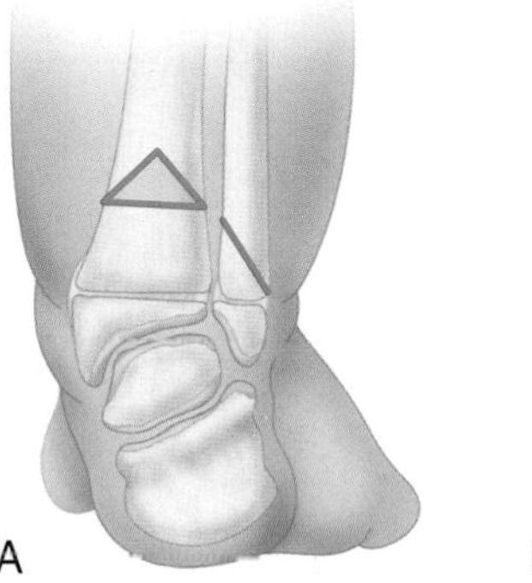

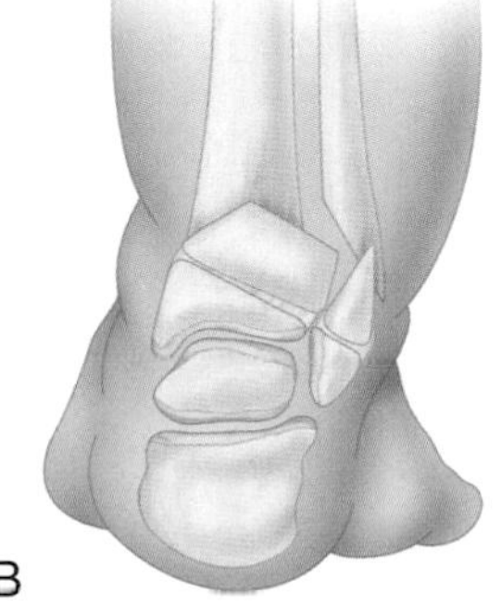

FIGURE 29-81 Wiltse varus osteotomy for valgus ankle deformity. This osteotomy corrects translation that occurs during closing wedge osteotomy. **A,** Translatory shift occurs because deformity is present in ankle joint, and osteotomy is done more proximally in metaphysis. **B,** Translating distal fragment laterally results in more natural contour of ankle. **SEE TECHNIQUE 29-29.**

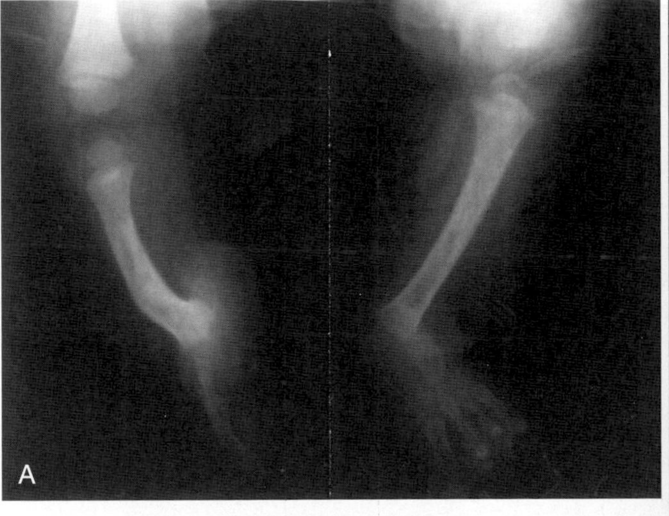

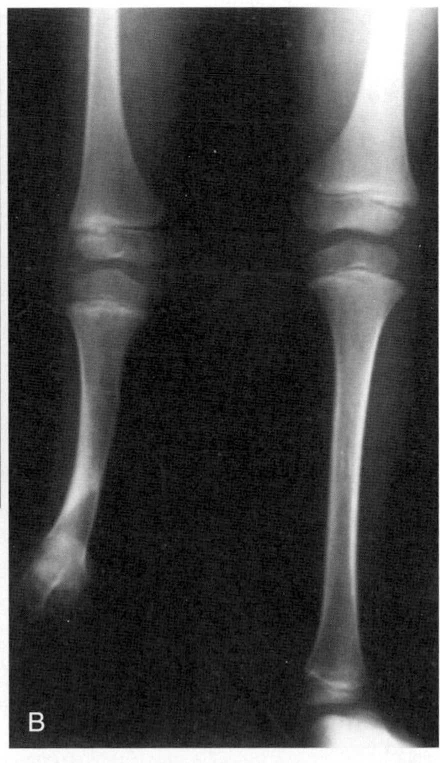

FIGURE 29-82 **A,** Bilateral type 2 deficiencies affecting right side more severely than left side—four rays on left foot and only three on right. **B,** After Boyd amputation on right and foot centralization on left. (Courtesy of Robert N. Hensinger, MD.)

VARUS SUPRAMALLEOLAR OSTEOTOMY OF THE ANKLE

TECHNIQUE 29-29

(WILTSE)

- Make an anterior approach to the distal tibia and a lateral approach to the distal fibula.
- Create a triangular osteotomy, removing a segment of bone that can be used for bone grafting (Fig. 29-81A). Make the base of the triangle parallel to the floor, but not parallel to the ankle joint.
- Make an oblique osteotomy of the distal fibula.
- Displace the distal segments proximally and laterally to avoid excessive prominence of the medial malleolus (Fig. 29-81B).
- Fix the osteotomy with Steinmann pins and apply a long leg cast.

POSTOPERATIVE CARE. Weight bearing is not allowed until the osteotomies have healed adequately.

PROXIMAL FEMORAL FOCAL DEFICIENCY

Similar to many other congenital longitudinal and transverse deficiencies, proximal femoral focal deficiency (PFFD) includes a broad spectrum of defects. Mild forms result in minor hypoplasia of the femur, whereas severe involvement may result in near complete agenesis of the femur (Fig. 29-83). Most commonly, PFFD consists of a partial skeletal defect in the proximal femur with a variably unstable hip joint, shortening, and associated other anomalies. Most patients with PFFD, especially patients with bilateral involvement, have associated anomalies, the most common of which are fibular hemimelia and agenesis of the cruciate ligaments of the knee. A variety of other congenital anomalies have been reported in association with PFFD, including clubfoot, talocalcaneal coalitions, congenital heart anomalies, spinal dysplasia, and facial dysplasias.

The incidence of PFFD has been reported to be one per 50,000 live births. Maternal diabetes has been implicated in femoral hypoplasia.

CLASSIFICATION

Aitken's four-part classification scheme (classes A, B, C, and D) is one of the earliest attempts to provide a systematic taxonomy of this condition (Table 29-5).

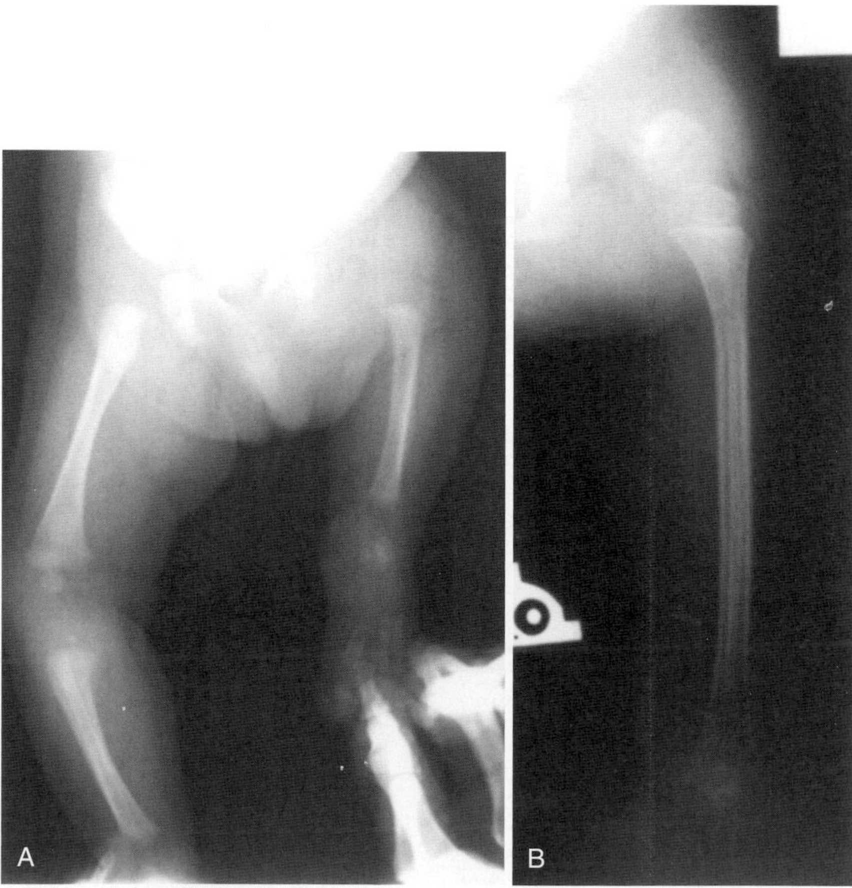

FIGURE 29-83 **A,** Infant with severe proximal femoral focal deficiency. In addition to absent femur, tibia is short and lateral ray is absent. **B,** At 5 years of age, after Boyd amputation. Distal femoral epiphysis is seen, but there is no femoral shaft or head. Acetabulum shows no sign of development. Cartilaginous anlage of distal femoral epiphysis was present at birth but not yet radiographically evident.

TABLE 29-5

Proximal Focal Femoral Deficiency (Aitken Classification)

TYPE	FEMORAL HEAD	ACETABULUM	FEMORAL SEGMENT	RELATIONSHIP AMONG COMPONENTS OF FEMUR AND ACETABULUM AT SKELETAL MATURITY
A	Present	Normal	Short	Bony connection between components of femur Femoral head in acetabulum Subtrochanteric varus angulation, often with pseudarthrosis
B	Present	Adequate or moderately dysplastic	Short, usually proximal bony tuft	No osseous connection between head and shaft Femoral head in acetabulum
C	Absent or represented by ossicle	Severely dysplastic	Short, usually proximally tapered	May be osseous connection between shaft and proximal ossicle No articular relation between femur and acetabulum
D	Absent	Absent Obturator foramen enlarged Pelvis squared in bilateral cases	Short, deformed	None

Modified from Herring JA: Tachdjian's Pediatric Orthopaedics, Fourth Edition, Philadelphia, Elsevier, 2014.

In class A, there is a normal acetabulum and femoral head with shortening of the femur and absence of the femoral neck on early radiographs. With age, the cartilaginous neck ossifies, although this frequently is associated with a pseudarthrosis. This may heal, but the usual radiographic picture shows severe coxa vara with significant shortening of the limb. Class B is similar to class A in that an acetabulum and femoral head are present; however, there is no bony connection between the proximal femur and the femoral head, and a pseudarthrosis is present. In class C, there is further degradation in the formation of the hip, characterized by a dysplastic acetabulum, absent femoral head, and short femur. A small, separate ossific tuft can be seen at the proximal end of the femur. In class D, the acetabulum, femoral head, and proximal femur are totally absent, and, in contrast to class C, there is no ossified tuft capping the proximal femur. Class D patients often have bilateral anomalies.

Other authors have expanded the definition of PFFD to include lesser expressions of femoral malformation. In his evaluation of 125 patients with PFFD, Pappas described nine classes that ranged in severity from complete absence of the proximal femur (class I) to mild femoral aplasia (class IX).

TABLE 29-6

Nine Pappas Classes of Congenital Abnormalities of the Femur

	CLASS I	CLASS II (AITKEN D)	CLASS III (AITKEN B)	CLASS IV (AITKEN A)
	Tibia			
Femoral Shortening (%)		70-90	45-80	40-67
Femoropelvic abnormalities	Femur absent Ischiopubic bone structures underdeveloped and deficient Lack of acetabular development	Femoral head absent Ischiopubic bone structures delayed in ossification	No osseous connection between femoral shaft and head Femoral head ossification delayed Acetabulum may be absent Femoral condyles maldeveloped Irregular tuft on proximal end of femur (rare)	Femoral head and shaft joined by irregular calcification in fibrocartilaginous matrix
Associated abnormalities	Fibula absent	Tibia shortened Fibula, foot, knee joint, and ankle joint abnormal	Tibial shortened 0-40% Fibula shortened 5-100% Patella absent or small and high riding Knee joint instability common Foot malformed	Tibia shortened 0-20% Fibula shortened 4-60% Knee joint instability frequent Foot small with infrequent malformations
Treatment objectives	Prosthetic management	Pelvic-femoral stability through prosthetic management	Union between femoral shaft and hip for stability Prosthetic management	Union between femoral head, neck, and shaft Prosthetic management

From Pappas AM: Congenital abnormalities of the femur and related lower-extremity malformations: classifications and treatment, J Pediatr Orthop 3:45, 1983.

The Pappas class II corresponds to the Aitken class D, the Pappas class III corresponds to the Aitken class B, and the Pappas class IV and class V may be correlated with the Aitken class A (Table 29-6). Kalamchi et al. developed a simplified classification scheme for congenital deficiency of the femur that included five groups: group I, short femur and intact hip joint; group II, short femur and coxa vara of the hip; group III, short femur, but well-developed acetabulum and femoral head; group IV, absent hip joint and dysplastic femoral segment; and group V, total absence of the femur. Group III is further subdivided into type A (bony defect of the femoral neck eventually ossifies) and type B (bony defect does not ossify and results in a persistent pseudarthrosis).

Gillespie and Torode identified two major groups for treatment purposes. Group I patients had a hypoplastic femur in which the hip and the knee were reconstructible, and leg equalization was sometimes possible. Group II patients exhibited a "true" PFFD in which the hip joint was markedly abnormal. Although some of these patients had tenuous connections between the femoral head and the proximal femur, the alignment and surrounding musculature were markedly abnormal. Also, these legs were too shortened, rotated, and marred by flexion contractures of the hip and knee to be reconstructible. These patients required only reconstructive procedures that make prosthetic fitting easier.

TREATMENT

The major problems with PFFD are limb-length inequality and variable inadequacy of the proximal femoral musculature and hip joint. Treatment is highly individualized and ranges

CLASS V (AITKEN A)	CLASS VI	CLASS VII	CLASS VIII	CLASS IX
48-85	30-60	10-50	10-41	6-20
Femur incompletely ossified, hypoplastic, and irregular Midshaft of femur abnormal	Distal femur short, irregular, and hypoplastic Irregular distal femoral diaphysis	Coxa vara Hypoplastic femur Proximal femoral diaphysis irregular with thickened cortex Lateral femoral condyle deficiency common Valgus distal femur	Coxa valga Hypoplastic femur Femoral head and neck smaller Proximal femoral physis horizontal Abnormality of femoral condyles common, with associated bowing of shaft and valgus of distal femur	Hypoplastic femur
Tibia shortened 4-27% Fibula shortened 10-100% Knee-joint instability common Severe malformations of foot common	Single-bone lower leg Patella absent Foot malformed	Tibia shortened <10-24% Fibula shortened <10-100% Lateral and high-riding patella common	Tibia shortened 0-36% Fibula shortened 0-100% Lateral and high-riding patella common Foot malformed	Tibia shortened 0-15% Fibula shortened 3-30% Additional ipsilateral and contralateral malformations common
Prosthetic management	Prosthetic management	Extremity length equality Improved alignment of (a) proximal and (b) distal femur	Extremity length equality Improved alignment of (a) proximal and (b) distal femur	Extremity length equality

from amputation and prosthetic rehabilitation to limb salvage, lengthening, and hip reconstruction. The natural history of the particular variant and the limitations of surgical reconstruction must be considered.

Often no surgical reconstruction of any kind is indicated. Bilateral PFFD is best treated nonoperatively (Fig. 29-84). These patients can walk well without prostheses, but for social or cosmetic reasons extension prostheses may be provided. The patients learn to accept their short stature and are quite functional. Foot surgery may be required to correct other anomalies. Limb lengthening is not indicated in these patients because extreme lengthening would be necessary, and the hips are unstable. Knee fusion is not indicated because the knee functions in conjunction with the hip pseudarthrosis to provide useful motion.

Most children with PFFD can learn to walk without a prosthesis, but a prosthesis helps equalize leg lengths. For selected patients, prosthetic management that incorporates the patient's foot without surgical treatment can be used for PFFD, but, more commonly, this type of prosthetic management is used a temporary solution in a younger patient until definitive surgery is performed (Figure 29-85). An alternative approach is to use the prosthesis to mold the foot into equinus so that it fits into an above-knee amputation prosthetic socket. The socket is fashioned to include the entire femur. Later an arthrodesis can be done, if necessary, to make prosthetic fitting easier. It is possible, however, that some knee motion within the stump of the prosthesis may serve as a protective mechanism for the abnormal proximal hip. If a knee arthrodesis is performed, the potential benefits in gait and prosthetic

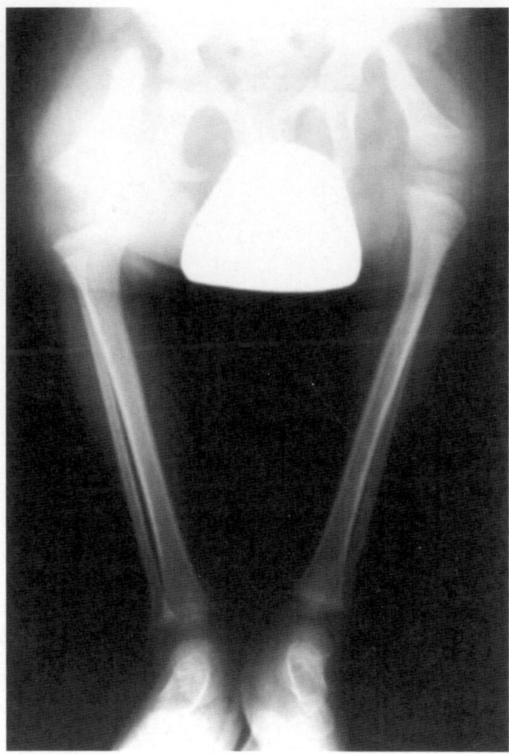

FIGURE 29-84 Severe (Aitken class D) bilateral proximal femoral focal deficiency in 3-year-old boy; note total lack of formation of acetabulum.

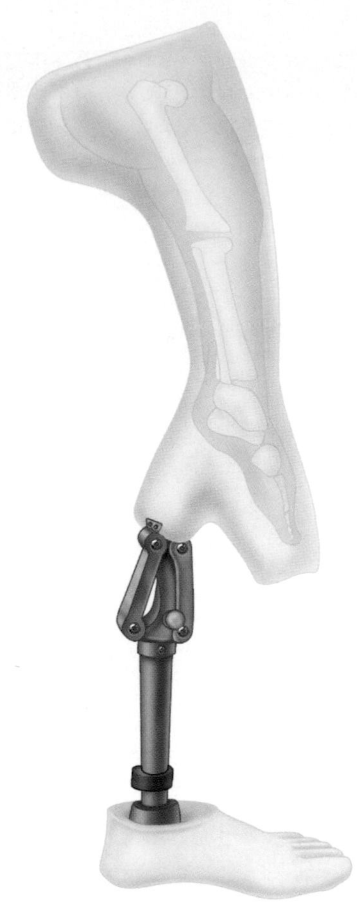

FIGURE 29-85 Prosthesis incorporating foot.

fitting may be outweighed by the increased stress placed on the proximal femur and proximal hip articulation and pseudarthrosis, if present.

Once it is determined that surgical treatment is necessary, two key factors must be assessed: stability of the hip joint and percentage of limb-length inequality. For patients with a stable hip and predicted length of more than 50% of the contralateral limb, limb lengthening (as described later in this chapter) should be considered. Knee fusion and Syme amputation or knee fusion and rotationplasty are indicated for patients with a stable hip and limb length less than 50% of the contralateral extremity. Finally, if the hip is unstable, stability can be achieved with a Steel or Brown fusion of the femur to the pelvis followed by Syme amputation or rotationplasty.

Stable Hip and Minimal Shortening. When there is a stable hip and relatively little shortening (<50% predicted length), salvage of the limb often is preferred. For patients with a femoral head and an acetabulum (Aitken class A and class B), many authors have recommended surgery to establish continuity between the femoral head and the femur. Because of poor bone stock, surgery is best delayed until ossification of the femoral head and proximal metaphysis is adequate, even then supplemental autogenous bone grafting may be needed at the pseudarthrosis site. Although the radiographic picture may be improved with correction of the proximal pseudarthrosis, it remains to be shown that function is improved. Many patients treated nonoperatively have good motion and reasonably good function. For less severe PFFD (Pappas class VII, class VIII, and class IX), hip reconstruction is limited to osteotomies that improve biomechanical alignment. Care must be taken not to damage the proximal femoral physis in these children who already have problems with diminished growth of the femur.

Surgical limb lengthening, with or without contralateral shortening, should be considered only if the femur is intact. Ten to 12 cm has been recommended as the maximal amount of lengthening possible in a single long bone with congenital deficiency and, combined with contralateral shortening, 17 to 20 cm as the maximal amount of inequality that can be corrected. Limb lengthening should be done only in a femur with more than 50% of predicted femoral length or less than 20 cm of projected shortening; other prerequisites for lengthening include hip stability and a stable, plantigrade foot. Regardless of technique, limb lengthening in patients with PFFD is difficult, with the ever-present danger of knee and hip subluxation. For large discrepancies, lengthening can be done in stages: one at 4 or 5 years of age, a second at 8 or 9 years, and a third during adolescence. Depending on the predictions of the patient's overall height based on the normal leg, a contralateral epiphysiodesis may be indicated.

Limb lengthening procedures place stress on the hip and knee. Bowen et al. emphasized the importance of avoiding hip subluxation and dislocation during femoral lengthening in patients with unilateral femoral shortening. They identified several factors that predict progressive subluxation or dislocation of the hip during femoral lengthening: (1) type of

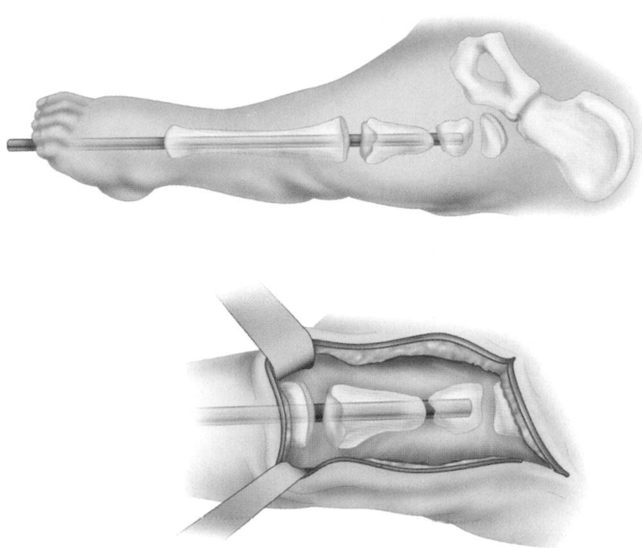

FIGURE 29-86 When proximal femur is small, with pseudarthrosis between femoral neck and shaft, it can be stabilized to create better lever arm. Simultaneous knee arthrodesis can be performed to create one-bone leg. If possible, medullary fixation should stop just short of proximal femoral epiphysis.

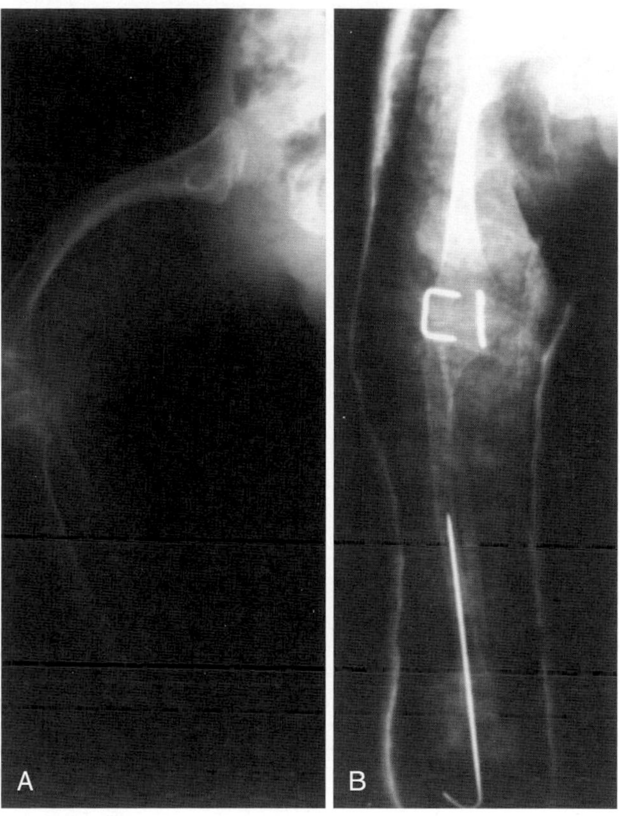

FIGURE 29-87 **A,** Proximal femoral focal deficiency in 7-year-old child; femur is severely shortened, and tibia is relatively hypoplastic. **B,** After Boyd ankle amputation, stabilization with medullary Steinmann pin, and staple arthrodesis of knee joint, patient can be rehabilitated as after knee disarticulation.

deformity (Kalamchi classification), (2) the combined abnormality of coxa vara plus the varus bow of the femoral shaft, and (3) acetabular dysplasia present before lengthening. No hip abnormalities occurred after lengthening in patients with Kalamchi type I or II deficiencies, but progressive subluxation or dislocation of the hip occurred in patients with type IIIA femurs with a combined coxa vara plus varus bow of the femoral shaft of less than 115 degrees and an acetabular index of more than 25 degrees. They recommended correction of the varus bow of the femur and the neck-shaft angle to 120 degrees and the acetabular index to less than 25 degrees before lengthening of type IIIA femurs.

Stable Hip and Severe Shortening. Knee arthrodesis (Fig. 29-86) with foot amputation, rather than limb lengthening, often is the preferred treatment for patients with severe shortening and stable hips (Fig. 29-87). Knee arthrodesis as described by King serves to create a single bony segment from the tibia and shortened femur to function as an above-knee amputation after foot amputation.

Unstable Hip. For more severe deformities in which the hip is unstable and there is no femoral head or acetabulum (Aitken class C and class D or Pappas class II and class III), many authors recommend that no attempt be made at hip reconstruction, although there are notable exceptions. Steel iliofemoral fusion (Fig. 29-88), which requires a simultaneous Chiari osteotomy (reference Chiari osteotomy in the hip anomalies chapter) to create a suitable bony bed to receive the small femoral remnant, allows the knee joint to assume the function of the hip joint. The femoral fragment is fused in a 90 degree flexed position relative to pelvis so than knee extension now serves as hip flexion. Additional bone graft to ensure fusion has been recommended for Steel fusions. Closing wedge osteotomies can be used to eliminate the anterior bowing of the femur and allow additional hip flexion for sitting. The Brown modification (Fig. 29-89) of the Steel fusion partially addresses this concern by rotating the femoral fragment 180 degrees. With this technique, the femoral segment is fused to the pelvis in the extended position. In this position, former knee flexion now functions as hip flexion and former ankle dorsiflexion now functions as knee flexion. Iliofemoral fusion may limit mobility of the limb. Even with a certain amount of instability, the knee generally functions as a hinge, providing flexion and extension only. Rotation and abduction are lost after iliofemoral arthrodesis.

KNEE FUSION FOR PROXIMAL FEMORAL FOCAL DEFICIENCY

TECHNIQUE 29-30

(KING)

- Make an S-shaped incision to expose the distal femur and proximal tibia anteriorly.
- With an oscillating saw remove the proximal aspect of the proximal tibial epiphysis until the ossific nucleus is seen. Then remove the entire distal femoral epiphysis. The remaining tibial epiphysis and distal femoral metaphysis will be approximated and stabilized to achieve fusion.

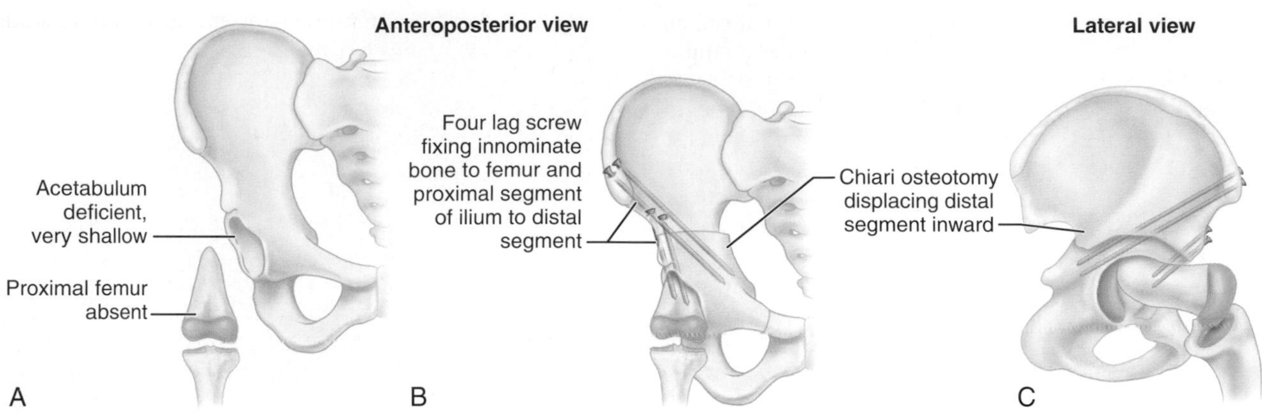

FIGURE 29-88 Steel iliofemoral fusion. **A,** Proximal femur is absent. **B,** The femur has been shortened to just above the distal physis and rotated 180 degrees so that popliteal fossa now faces anteriorly. A Chiari pelvic osteotomy has been fixed with two screws; this is optional depending on bony contact of the femur to the pelvis. The femur is fixed to the pelvis with several screws. **C,** Lateral view of the final position of the femur. It is important that the femur be shortened as much as possible and that the femoral epiphysis be ablated.

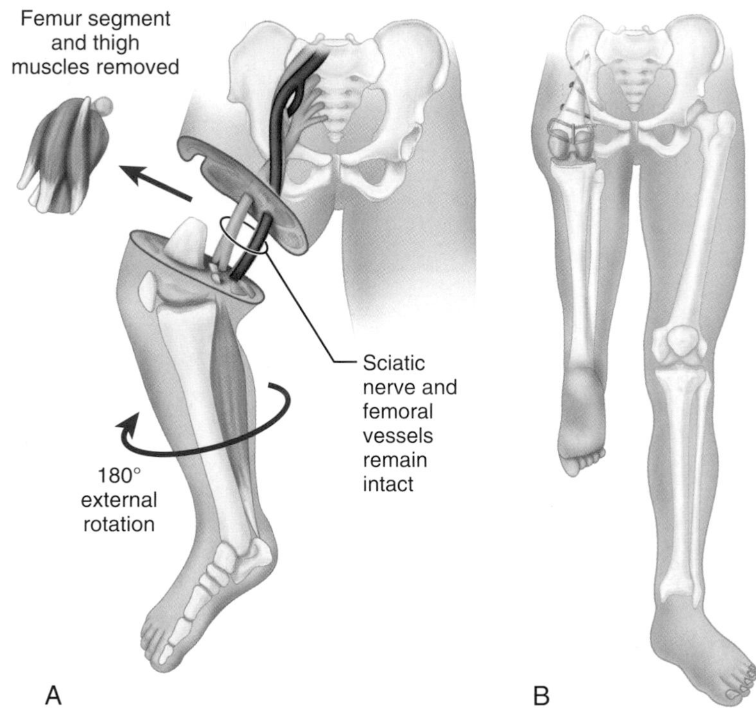

FIGURE 29-89 Rotationplasty and femoropelvic arthrodesis (see text). **A,** Proximal part of femur (with hypoplastic head) and surrounding thigh muscles are removed, and leg is rotated 180 degrees. **B,** Limb is rotated, and residual femur is attached to pelvis.

- Insert an intramedullary rod into the proximal tibia in an antegrade fashion until it exits the plantar surface of the foot.
- Completely excise the patella to prevent patellofemoral symptoms later in life.
- Next, approximate the two bony surfaces, taking care to ensure proper rotational alignment while maintaining a straight segment.
- Advance the rod retrograde into the intramedullary canal of the femoral segment.
- Close the wound in routine manner and apply a hip spica cast.

POSTOPERATIVE CARE. The spica cast and rod are removed in the operating room when bony union at the arthrodesis site is achieved, usually at 6 weeks. Amputation of the foot often is done at the time of rod removal.

For removal of the foot, ankle disarticulation, Syme amputation, or Boyd amputation can all be used. The heel pad is stabilized by either the Syme or the Boyd amputation, an advantage over simple ankle disarticulation. The Boyd amputation saves the entire calcaneus and provides a slightly more bulbous stump and additional length. If the combined length of the tibia, femoral remnant, and foot is greater than the femur on the opposite side, however, taking into account potential growth, there is no advantage in the small increase and additional length provided by the Boyd amputation.

Prosthetic reconstruction can be made easier in severe cases by a Syme amputation. The child is observed with serial scanograms until sufficient data have been collected to construct a working Moseley straight-line graph; then further surgery can be planned. If knee arthrodesis is selected to improve fitting of a prosthesis and gait, the physes around the knee can be epiphysiodesed if necessary to ensure that the prosthetic knee is at the same level as the contralateral normal knee when the child reaches skeletal maturity. Precise predictions are unnecessary because small amounts of additional shortening in the involved leg can be readily accommodated by the prosthesis. If the involved femorotibial unit is longer than the contralateral normal femur, however, the prosthetic knee must be placed in either a very proximal or a very distal position, which is less cosmetically desirable (Fig. 29-90). Although this can be treated with a leg-shortening procedure at skeletal maturity, a simpler preventive procedure, such as a well-timed epiphysiodesis during the growing years, is preferable.

Rotationplasty. Rotationplasty (Van Nes procedure) can be used as an alternative to knee arthrodesis and amputation. This reconstruction should be considered in patients who, because of significant femoral shortening, are not candidates for femoral lengthening. The procedure combines arthrodesis of the knee with rotation of the distal tibia 180 degrees externally so that the ankle joint becomes a functional knee joint: ankle plantarflexion becomes "knee" extension, and ankle dorsiflexion becomes "knee" flexion. A reasonably stable hip joint and a well-functioning ankle are required for this technique. Many patients with PFFD also have fibular hemimelia, with a poorly functioning ankle joint. An arc or ankle motion of at least 90 degrees is required for rotationplasty reconstruction to be beneficial. The femur, knee, and tibia should equal the length of the opposite femur, but this usually is not the case, so ipsilateral knee epiphysiodesis is done to equalize the reconstructed femoral unit and the contralateral normal femur.

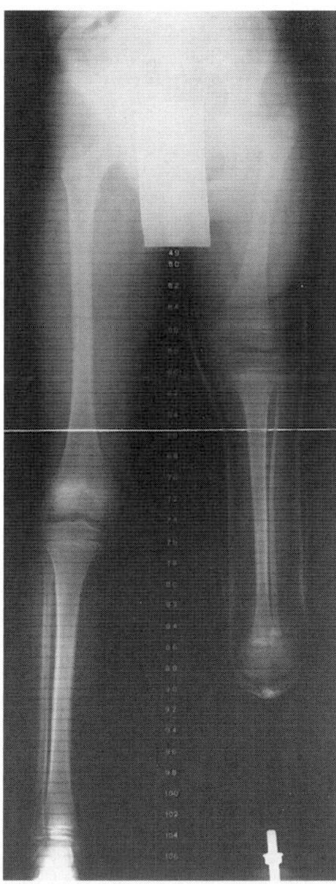

FIGURE 29-90 Twelve-year-old child with previous Boyd amputation but no knee arthrodesis. Prosthetic management is that of below-knee amputation, but result is cosmetically poor because of extremely long "tibia."

Brown described a modification of the Van Nes procedure in which the limb is completely detached except for the sciatic nerve and the femoral vessels, the proximal part of the dysplastic femur and some muscles are resected, the residual limb is externally rotated 180 degrees, and the rotated distal part of the femur is fused to the pelvis (Fig. 29-89). With this procedure, the rotated knee functions as a hip with flexion and extension, and the rotated ankle acts as a knee, allowing patients to function as below-knee amputees. Brown noted that because the muscles distal to the knee are not disturbed, the problem of derotation of the limb, a frequent problem after Van Nes rotationplasty, does not occur.

Some significant problems must be discussed with the patient and parents before undertaking this type of reconstruction. First, the appearance of the leg, with the foot rotated backward (Fig. 29-91), can be psychologically disturbing; great care should be taken in the preoperative consultation to make this clear. It is helpful to have another patient who has already undergone the procedure demonstrate how the prosthesis functions. If such a patient is unavailable, the family should be shown photographs and drawings of a rotationplasty. Another problem, especially in young children, is derotation of the surgically rotated foot, which has been reported to occur in as many as 50% of patients. Compared with a Syme amputation, rotationplasty has been shown to result in a slightly more (10%) energy-efficient gait, although an electromyographic and gait analysis study showed that older patients generally had lower functional scores, shorter walking distances, and worse gait patterns. Younger patients were better able to adapt to the altered anatomic and functional situation and to develop good function.

ROTATIONPLASTY

TECHNIQUE 29-31

Fig. 29-92

(VAN NES)

- Position the patient supine and drape the entire limb free so that the skin is exposed from the toes to the iliac crest. Place a small towel under the sacrum.
- Begin the incision proximal and lateral to the knee and extend it across the knee distally along the subcutaneous crest of the tibia.

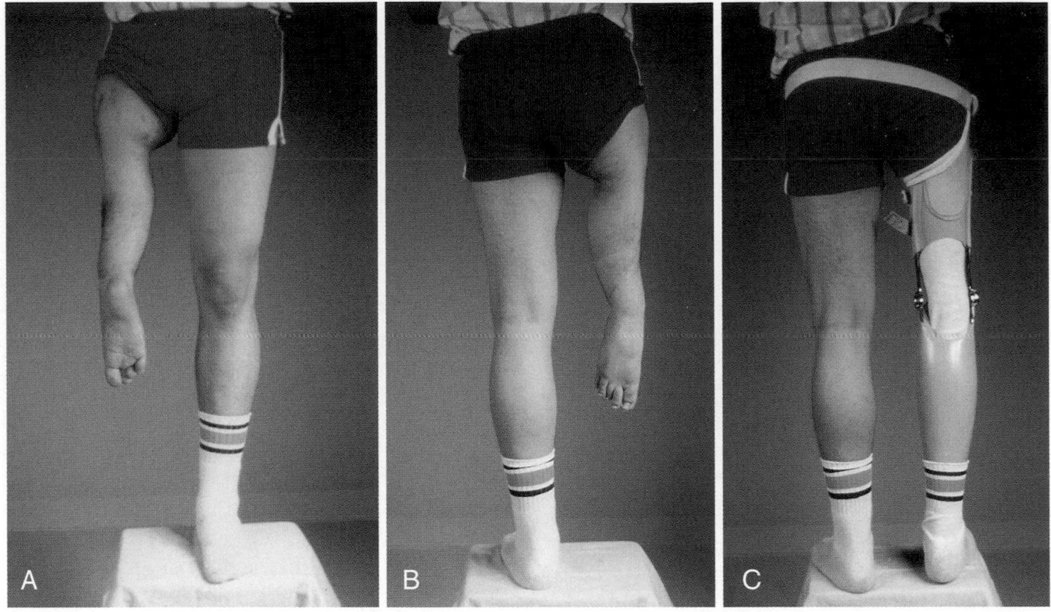

FIGURE 29-91 Appearance of limb after Van Nes rotationplasty: front view (**A**), back view (**B**), and with prosthesis (**C**).

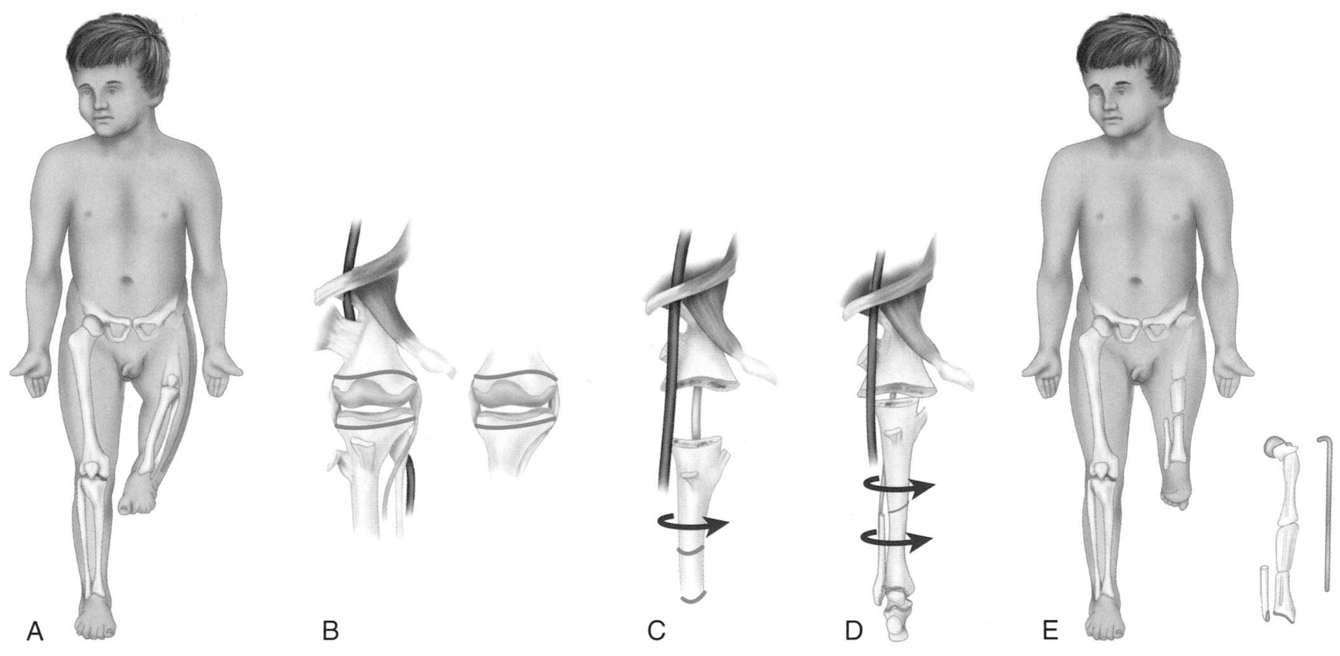

FIGURE 29-92 Van Nes rotationplasty. Preoperatively, ankle joint of shortened extremity is approximately at level of opposite knee joint. **A,** Long incision on lateral aspect of leg extends from hip to midshaft of tibia. **B,** Quadriceps and sartorius tendons are taken down distally to expose adductor hiatus and femoral artery; peroneal nerve is dissected free. **C,** After resection of knee joint and freeing of femoropopliteal artery, tibia is externally rotated 140 degrees. **D,** Further rotation of 40 degrees more is possible after tibial osteotomy, allowing stretch on soft tissues to spread over greater distance. External rotation is preferred to internal rotation to prevent stretching of peroneal nerve. **E,** Fixation with medullary Rush rod. **SEE TECHNIQUE 29-31.**

- Elevate the flaps medially and laterally to expose the knee capsule and patellar tendon.
- Divide the patellar tendon and open the knee capsule transversely.
- Apply traction on the capsule proximally and distally to expose the knee joint fully by dividing the collateral ligaments and the anterior, medial, and lateral capsule.
- On the medial side, carefully dissect out the insertion of the adductor magnus up to the level of the femoral artery.
- Divide the adductor magnus to enable the artery to derotate anteriorly and to limit postoperative derotation.
- Trace the femoral artery distally and posteriorly as it becomes the popliteal artery.
- Divide the medial hamstring muscles at their insertion.

- On the lateral side, carefully dissect out the peroneal nerve. If the fibula is deficient, the anatomic relationship between the peroneal nerve and the proximal fibular head may be abnormal. To prevent damage to the peroneal nerve, trace the nerve proximally to its point of origin on the sciatic nerve. Release any fascial attachments distally over the peroneal nerve.
- After the major neurovascular structures have been completely identified and protected, divide the posterior knee capsule, and section the origins of the gastrocnemius heads.
- The only remaining attachments from the femur to the tibia are the skin, subcutaneous tissues, and neurovascular structures. Release the lateral hamstrings.
- With an osteotome or oscillating saw, remove the articular cartilage of the proximal tibia down to the level of the proximal tibial epiphysis. Do not damage the proximal tibial physis.
- If the leg needs to be shortened, shorten the femur by removing the distal femoral epiphysis and physis.
- Insert an intramedullary Rush rod through the distal femur proximally, exiting through the piriformis fossa into the buttock. If necessary, ream the femur with a drill to prevent comminution during nail insertion.
- Make a small incision in the buttock where the nail exits.
- Remove the nail and reinsert it from proximal to distal through the femur and into the tibia, stopping short of the distal tibial physis. While the nail is being inserted, rotate the tibia externally to relax the peroneal nerve.
- Gently transfer the femoral popliteal artery anteriorly through the adductor hiatus.
- If the leg cannot be comfortably rotated through the knee resection, obtain additional rotation through a separate osteotomy in the midshaft of the tibia, which also is stabilized by the intramedullary nail.
- Additional shortening can be performed through the tibia if necessary. In such instances, a fibular osteotomy also is performed.
- Attempt to rotate the extremity 180 degrees. If the rotation places too much torque on the vascular structures, and the distal pulses are lost, derotate the leg through the knee until the pressure on the vessels is relieved.
- Close the wounds and apply a spica cast that maintains rotation.

POSTOPERATIVE CARE. If derotation of the foot was required to relieve vascular pressure, the foot is rotated serially using successive hip spica casts to turn the foot on the axis of the intramedullary nail. When the osteotomies have healed, the child is fitted with a modified below-knee prosthesis. Although it is possible to amputate the toes to make the foot look more like a below-knee stump and less like a "backward" foot, most patients decline this option.

Amputations. Although most of the basic surgical principles of amputation in adults apply to children, there are important differences. Most amputations in children are performed for congenital conditions. Either the child is born without a portion of the limb, or an amputation is performed to make reconstruction and prosthetic rehabilitation easier in a deficient limb. Trauma accounts for most acquired amputations in children. In contrast to typical adult dysvascular patients, children may tolerate skin grafts over stumps and, to a certain extent, tension at the suture line. Most revision surgeries in children with congenital amputations involve the lower extremity. Revision amputation surgery in upper extremity limb deficiencies rarely is required.

Prosthetic fitting after amputation in children should begin after complete wound healing and standard stump preparation. A rigid postoperative plaster dressing that is bivalved to allow for swelling is preferred. When the wounds are sufficiently healed, stump wrapping with elastic bandages is begun to prepare the stump for a prosthesis. Phantom pain and phantom sensations are problems in child amputees, especially after tumor surgery. Neuroma formation is rare, but gentle handling of the nerves and sectioning with a sharp knife without applying excessive traction on the nerves should be routine in all amputation surgery in children.

In planning amputation surgery, maximal length should be preserved to provide maximal lever arm strength for powering a prosthesis. Physes should be preserved whenever possible to ensure continued growth of the limb. This is especially true for the physes around the knee, which provide most of the growth in the lower extremity, and the physes around the shoulder and wrist, which provide most of the longitudinal growth of the upper extremity. Although amputation through a long bone in a growing child can result in appositional terminal overgrowth, this is not an adequate reason for sacrificing length. In below-knee amputations in young children, it is highly likely that the fibula, and to a lesser extent the tibia, will overgrow, but this can be satisfactorily remedied by revision surgery. Although knee disarticulation would prevent overgrowth, it is far more important to preserve the knee joint to power a below-knee prosthesis than to prevent overgrowth of the stump. Even short below-knee segments should be preserved if possible in growing children. Because the proximal tibial physis contributes most of the growth of the tibia, an initially short stump has the potential to become a longer, more functional stump. In older children, it is possible to lengthen a short below-knee stump using the Ilizarov technique to provide a more functional stump in selected patients.

Terminal overgrowth has been reported most frequently in the humerus, followed by the fibula, tibia, and femur. Because it seems to be caused by appositional periosteal bone formation distally and not by epiphyseal growth proximally (Fig. 29-93), epiphysiodesis does not prevent stump overgrowth. A variety of techniques have been devised to prevent stump overgrowth, but none has been completely successful. Small bone spurs that form at the edge of the transected bone do not constitute true overgrowth and rarely require surgical removal. Stump overgrowth occurs in congenital and traumatic amputations.

Patellar dislocations and patella alta are common problems in adolescents with below-knee amputations, presumably caused by the force of the patellar tendon-bearing prosthesis against the lower surface of the patella. Elongation of the patellar tendon might be prevented by earlier modification of the prosthesis to distribute the force around a greater area rather than concentrating it on the patellar tendon.

Ankle Disarticulation. Although standard amputation techniques are described in Chapter 15), important variations

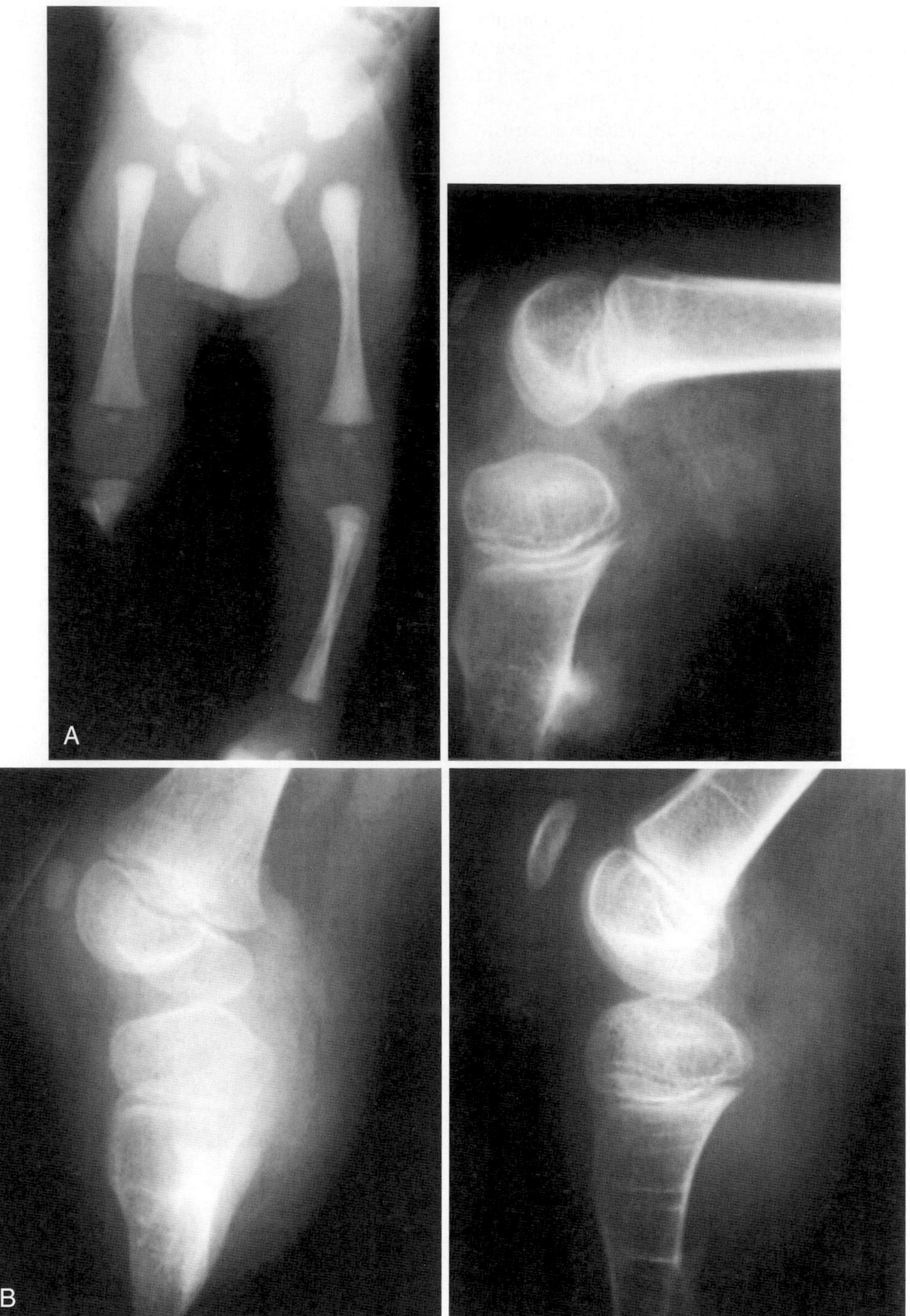

FIGURE 29-93 **A,** Newborn with congenital amputation through proximal tibia. **B,** At 5 years of age, continued growth of distal stump and penciling resulted in protrusion of bone from skin. (Courtesy of Robert N. Hensinger, MD.)

of amputations around the ankle exist for reconstruction in children with congenital limb deficiencies. The two most common reconstructive amputations performed for these children are the Syme and Boyd procedures. The Syme amputation is a modified ankle disarticulation. The Boyd procedure amputates all of the foot bones except the calcaneus and fuses the calcaneus to the distal tibia.

Many studies have documented excellent results with both procedures, and there are pros and cons to each. There is no clear consensus in the literature regarding the preferred technique. The problems encountered in Syme amputations in children have been overgrowth of retained portions of calcaneus apophyses, heel pad migration, and formation of exostoses. The advantages of the Boyd operation are the additional length gained and the prevention of the posterior displacement of the heel pad, which occurs in many patients with Syme amputations. In the Boyd amputation, it is important to align the calcaneus properly. If the calcaneus is not aligned correctly, it angulates into equinus and interferes with weight bearing.

A problem common to the Syme and the Boyd amputations is the flare of the distal tibial metaphysis, which gives a bulbous shape to the distal stump and necessitates a special prosthesis with a removable medial window. In children with congenital limb deficiencies, such as tibial or fibular hemimelia, the distal ankle is relatively hypoplastic, however, so a bulbous stump usually is not a problem.

SYME AMPUTATION

TECHNIQUE 29-32

- Make a fish-mouth incision beginning at the lateral malleolus, extending over the dorsum of the foot, and ending 1 cm distal to the medial malleolus (Fig. 29-94A). The plantar portion should extend distally enough to allow adequate skin closure anteriorly.
- Place the foot in as much equinus as possible to expose the anterior ankle capsule and divide it.
- Divide the deltoid ligament between the talus and the medial malleolus, but do not damage the nearby posterior tibial vessels.
- Section the lateral ligament between the calcaneus and the tibula.
- Grasp the talus with a large clamp and force it further into equinus to permit dissection of the posterior ankle capsule.
- Make a subperiosteal dissection of the posterior aspect of the calcaneus through the ankle joint.
- Cut the Achilles tendon at its point of insertion into the calcaneus, but do not "button hole" it through the skin.
- Place further traction on the hindfoot and further hyperflexion into equinus and dissect the soft tissues with a periosteal elevator and a knife, staying in the subperiosteal plane to avoid damaging the heel pad.
- Continue the dissection until the entire calcaneus has been excised (Fig. 29-94B).
- To anchor the heel pad, drill holes in the anterior aspect of the distal tibia and use stout sutures from the distal aspect of the heel pad, anchoring it in the aponeurosis of the distal tibia (Fig. 29-94C).
- In children, it is unnecessary to remove the cartilage of the distal tibia, but if desired the flare of the medial malleolus and distal fibula can be trimmed to create a more even weight-bearing surface.
- Pull the flexor tendons distally, transect them, and allow them to retract.
- Ligate the posterior and anterior tibial arteries as far distally as possible to prevent ischemic necrosis of the flaps.
- Insert suction drains in the wound and close the skin in layers (Fig. 29-94D).
- Apply a rigid plaster dressing to diminish pain after surgery; bivalve the cast to allow for swelling.

POSTOPERATIVE CARE. Weight bearing on the stump in a cast is delayed until the wound has healed adequately.

BOYD AMPUTATION

TECHNIQUE 29-33

- Make a fish-mouth incision as described for the Syme amputation.
- Elevate the skin flaps proximally and amputate the forefoot through the midtarsal joints.
- Excise the entire talus, using sharp dissection.
- With an oscillating saw or osteotome, transect the distal end of the calcaneus (Fig. 29-95A).

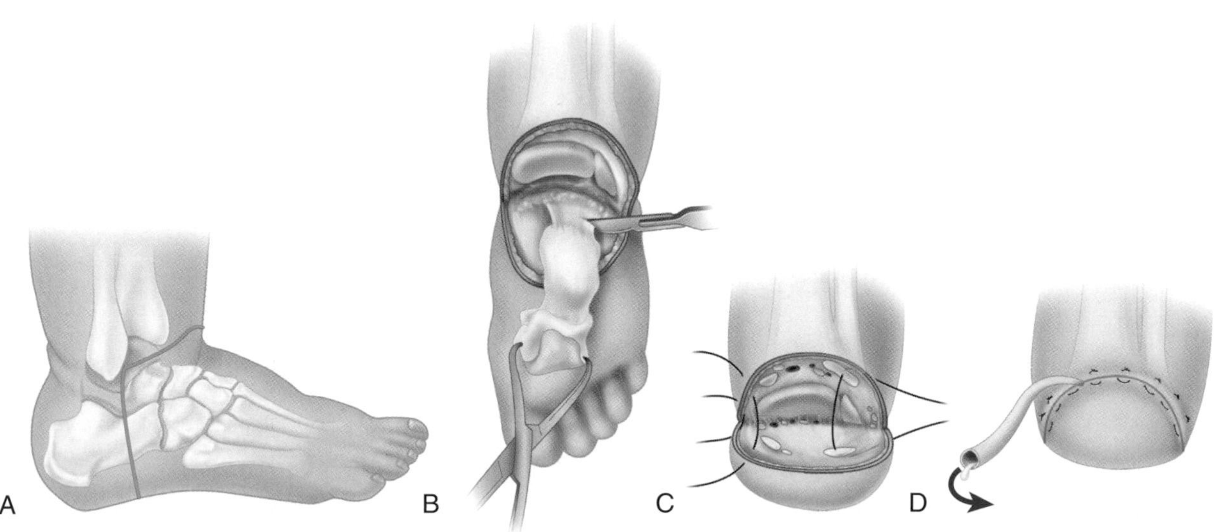

FIGURE 29-94 Syme amputation. **A,** Fish-mouth incision. **B,** Enucleation of talus and calcaneus. **C,** Plantar flap sutured to distal tibia. **D,** Completed closure with drain in place. **SEE TECHNIQUE 29-32.**

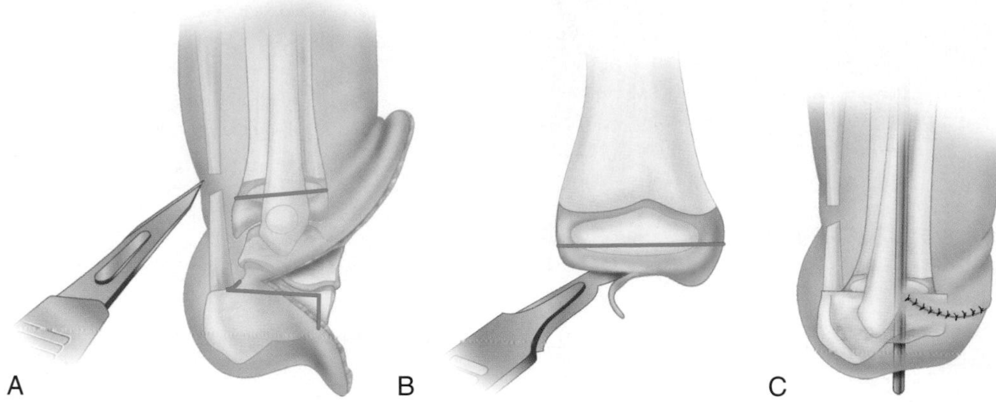

FIGURE 29-95 Boyd amputation. **A,** Fish-mouth incision; shaded areas represent resected bone. **B,** Cartilage of distal tibia is removed by shaving gradually until bony epiphysis is reached; calcaneus is shifted anteriorly, and Achilles tendon is sectioned to prevent it from migrating proximally. **C,** Fixation with smooth medullary pin aids fusion of calcaneus to distal tibial epiphysis. **SEE TECHNIQUE 29-33.**

- In a similar manner, remove the articular surface of the subtalar joint on the calcaneus perpendicular to the long axis of the tibia.
- Resect an adequate amount of the distal tibial articular cartilage so that the bony epiphysis of the distal tibia is exposed (Fig. 29-95B).
- Shape the calcaneus to fit accurately against the surface of the distal tibial epiphysis. Stabilize this with a smooth Steinmann pin that enters the heel pad and provides fixation to the tibia by crossing the distal tibial physis into the metaphysis.
- Occasionally, the Achilles tendon must be severed to allow accurate positioning of the calcaneus.
- Shift the calcaneus anteriorly before fixing it with the Steinmann pin (Fig. 29-95C).
- Section the medial and lateral plantar nerves and allow them to retract.
- Section the posterior and anterior tibial arteries as far distally as possible to prevent wound necrosis.
- Close the wound over drains and apply a plaster cast. A hip spica cast may be necessary for young children.

POSTOPERATIVE CARE. The pin usually can be removed at 6 weeks, and a new cast is applied and worn for an additional 6 weeks. After this, the stump usually has healed sufficiently for prosthetic rehabilitation.

LIMB-LENGTH DISCREPANCY

Limb-length equality in the lower extremity is not only a cosmetic concern, but also a functional concern. The short leg gait is awkward, increases energy expenditure because of the excessive vertical rise and fall of the pelvis or compensatory ankle movements and may result in back pain from long-standing significant discrepancies. Compensatory scoliosis and decreased spinal mobility also have been reported with discrepancies of 1.2 to 5.2 cm; however, it should be noted that limb length inequalities of 0.5 to 2 cm are common in the normal, asymptomatic population.

Limb length inequality of more than 2.5 cm has traditionally been considered significant, with an increased likelihood of knee, hip, and lumbar spine pain; however, support for this exact value is lacking in the literature. The management of a patient with limb-length inequality is quite complex, and multiple factors including cause of the discrepancy, associated conditions, pain, and patient/family expectations must be taken into account along with the measured difference before treatment is undertaken.

Limb-length inequality may be acquired and result from trauma or infection that damages the physis, from asymmetric paralytic conditions (e.g., poliomyelitis or cerebral palsy), or from tumors or tumor-like conditions that affect bone growth by stimulating asymmetric growth, such as occurs with juvenile rheumatoid arthritis or postfracture hypervascularity. Idiopathic unilateral hypoplasia and hyperplasia are other common causes of limb-length discrepancy. Finally, congenital conditions such as femoral or fibular deficiency or tibial hemimelia can cause the inequality.

The treatment of limb-length discrepancy must be tailored to the specific conditions and needs of the individual patient. Treatment plans can be formulated only after a careful evaluation that includes assessment of the chronologic and skeletal ages of the patient, the current and predicted discrepancy in the limb lengths, the predicted adult height, the cause of the discrepancy, the functional status of the joints, and the social and psychologic background of the patient and family.

CLINICAL ASSESSMENT

Clinical evaluation should include assessment for any rotational and angular deformities, foot height differences, scoliosis, pelvic obliquity, and joint mobility and function. In certain paralytic conditions, particularly spastic diplegia, flexion contractures of the knee and hip make the limb appear shorter than it really is on clinical and radiographic examinations; however, mild shortness of the paralytic side can improve gait by allowing the paralytic foot to clear the floor more easily during the swing phase of gait.

The simplest means of measuring limb-length discrepancy is to place wooden blocks of known heights under the

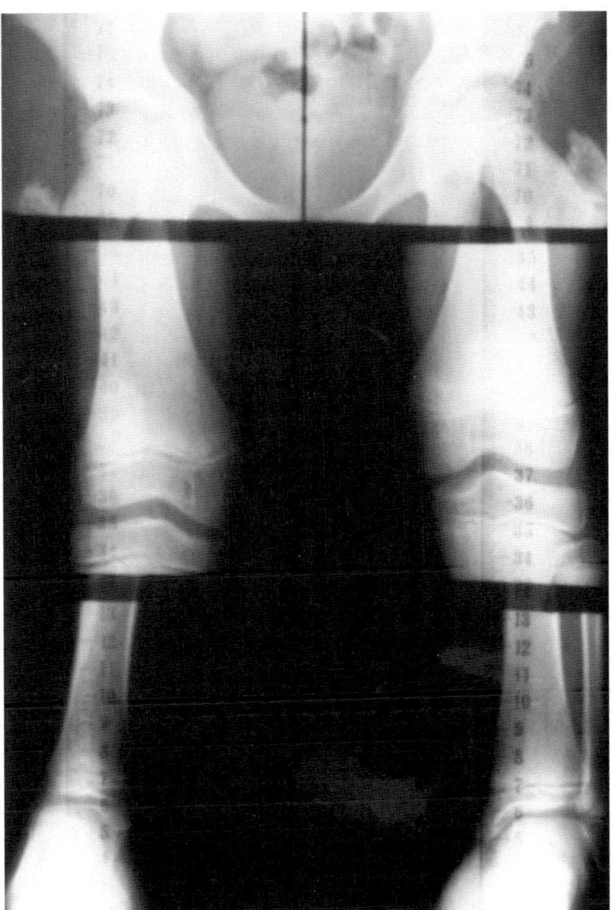

FIGURE 29-96 Scanogram obtained for evaluation of limb-length discrepancy in 12-year-old boy with fibular hemimelia on right.

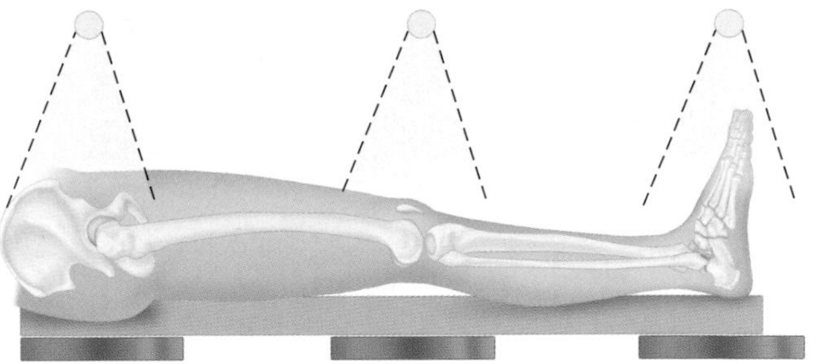

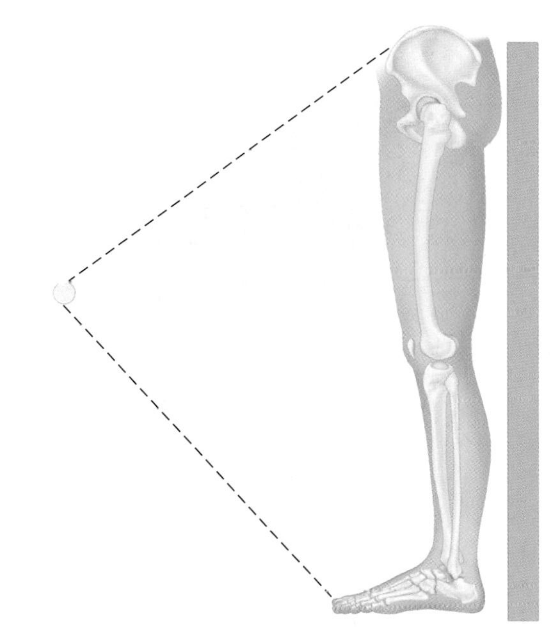

FIGURE 29-97 Scanogram compared with standing orthoradiograph.

short leg until the pelvis is level; however, asymmetric pelvic development or pelvic obliquity can cause miscalculation. Measurement also can be made from the anterior superior iliac spine to the medial malleolus, but this measurement may not be accurate because of patient positioning. Supine and prone Galeazzi measurements can help to localize the discrepancy to the femoral or tibial segment respectively.

RADIOGRAPHIC ASSESSMENT

Radiographic measurements are an essential part of the evaluation of limb length inequality, and they are important for accuracy because clinically palpable landmarks may be inaccurate. Two commonly used radiographic techniques for measuring lower limb-length discrepancy are the standing orthoradiograph and the scanogram. The orthoradiograph is made on a long cassette that includes the hip, knee, and ankle on a single exposure. A magnification marker placed on the leg at the level of the bone minimizes magnification error. The scanogram uses separate exposures of the hip, knee, and ankle, so there is little parallax error (Figs. 29-96 and 29-97).

It does require that the child remain still for all three exposures, however. Although the parallax error is greater with standing orthoradiographs; they do offer the additional benefit of showing limb alignment, as well as reducing the exposure to ionizing radiation. With either study, it is imperative that the legs be positioned with the patellae facing forward.

Skeletal age is an important factor to include when making treatment decisions. A view of the left wrist is obtained to estimate skeletal age from the Greulich and Pyle atlas; however, this is unnecessary for children younger than 5 years old because the skeletal and chronologic ages are not significantly different in these children. Although the use of the Greulich and Pyle atlas is an important part of the overall assessment of skeletal age, it should be noted that the standard deviation for this atlas is one page either way.

CT scanograms have been proposed as an improvement over standard scanograms because the radiation exposure is less, and accuracy is not compromised. On lateral CT scanograms, accurate measurement can be made of even a limb with a flexion deformity. On biplanar CT scanograms, foot height also can be measured. EOS®, slot scanning technology (EOS Imaging, Paris, France), offers an alternative in some centers (Fig. 29-98). Benefits include simultaneously obtained biplanar, upright images of the entire length of both lower extremities with little to no magnification error, and lower

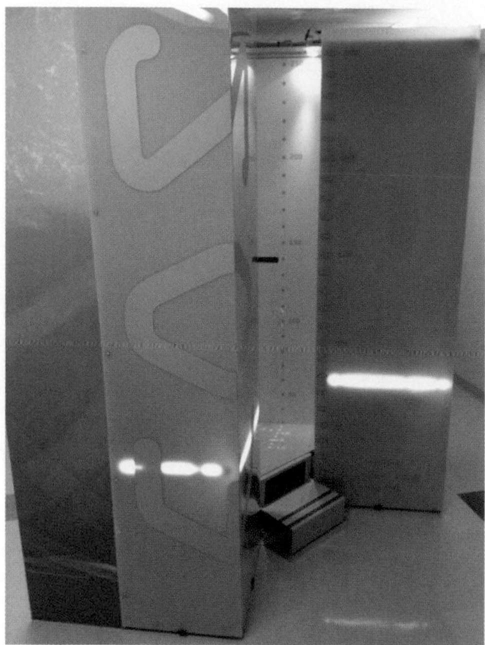

FIGURE 29-98 EOS machine.

radiation exposure. To avoid motion artifact, the child must remain still throughout the short scan time. This technology has been shown to provide greater accuracy and reliability over more traditional imaging modalities.

TECHNIQUES FOR PREDICTING GROWTH REMAINING

Multiple techniques are used to predict growth and to help the surgeon determine the timing of limb equalization procedures. One is the Green-Anderson growth-remaining chart. Proper use of this chart requires the clinician to estimate the percentage of growth inhibition for the patient by taking two interval measurements separated by at least 3 months. The growth difference between the involved limb and the normal limb is multiplied by 100, and that result is divided by the growth of the normal limb. Moseley simplified the Green-Anderson chart by mathematically manipulating the original data to allow it to fit on a straight-line graph that is visually graphic and easier to apply (Fig. 29-99). It avoids the need for mathematical calculations of growth inhibition and provides a ready prediction of the results of epiphysiodesis, lengthening, and shortening (Box 29-2). Reference slopes are provided for predicting future limb growth after epiphysiodesis of the distal femur, the proximal tibia, or both. The difference between the slopes of the normal leg and the short leg is the growth inhibition. Lengthening of the short leg in a growing child can be depicted by a sharp vertical rise, followed by a continued gradual slope equivalent to the slope of growth before lengthening (Fig. 29-100).

One criticism of the Green-Anderson tables and the Moseley straight-line graph for limb-length discrepancy is that they do not include an estimation for foot height. A discrepancy of 4 cm by radiographic scanograms may be 5 cm by the clinical block technique if the short leg also has a small foot and ankle unit.

There are some fundamental problems with the Green-Anderson and the Moseley methods. The original data for growth and height may not be applicable to modern children. The skeletal age according to Greulich and Pyle's atlas is at best an approximation. Human growth is not always mathematically predictable because it is influenced by nutritional, metabolic, hormonal, and socioeconomic factors as well as the cause of the leg-length discrepancy. Limb-length discrepancy in some children with juvenile rheumatoid arthritis and Perthes disease may follow an upward slope/downward slope pattern in which the discrepancy corrects itself. In overgrowth after a femoral fracture, the pattern of growth may level off, and after a short period the discrepancy remains constant. Despite these atypical patterns, most leg-length discrepancies follow the traditional growth prediction curves.

Simpler methods of predicting growth are available. The Menelaus method is convenient because it requires no special charts or graphs and relies on chronologic age rather than skeletal age. Menelaus assumes that in adolescents older than 9 years of age, the distal femur grows ⅜ inch (9 mm) per year, the proximal tibia grows ¼ inch (6 mm) per year, and growth ceases at age 14 years in girls and at age 16 years in boys. Using his technique, Menelaus achieved a final limb-length discrepancy of less than ¾ inch in 94 patients who underwent epiphysiodesis.

Paley, Bhave, Herzenberg, and Bowen developed a "multiplier" method for predicting limb-length discrepancy at skeletal maturity. Using available databases, they divided femoral and tibial lengths at skeletal maturity (L_m) by femoral and tibial lengths (L) at each age for each percentile group. The resultant number was called the multiplier (M). This multiplier is used in formulas to predict limb-length discrepancy and the amount of growth remaining and to calculate the timing of epiphysiodesis. According to these authors, the multiplier method allows for a quick calculation of predicted limb-length discrepancy at skeletal maturity, without the need to plot graphs, and is based on one or two measurements. A simple chart of multipliers and several formulas are all that is required (Table 29-7).

The multiplier method can be applied to total limb-length discrepancy, including femoral, tibial, and foot-height differences. Clinical data in their study confirmed that the multiplier method correlated closely with the Moseley method.

In a group of patients with limb lengthenings, there was no difference in the accuracy of the two methods; in a group with epiphysiodeses, the multiplier method was more accurate. In two later clinical validation studies, Aguilar et al. showed the multiplier method to be more accurate than the Moseley and Anderson methods; the multiplier method also was quicker and simpler to use, requiring only one data point for predicting limb length at maturity. No matter the method used; all are, at best, approximations. A final clinical discrepancy of 1 to 1.5 cm after treatment should be considered an excellent outcome.

TREATMENT

The goals of treatment are a balanced spine and pelvis, equal limb lengths, and a correct mechanical weight-bearing axis. In patients with rigid scoliosis and an oblique lumbosacral takeoff, some degree of limb-length discrepancy may be desirable to preserve a balanced spine. By convention, the term epiphysiodesis is used to describe the arrest of growth

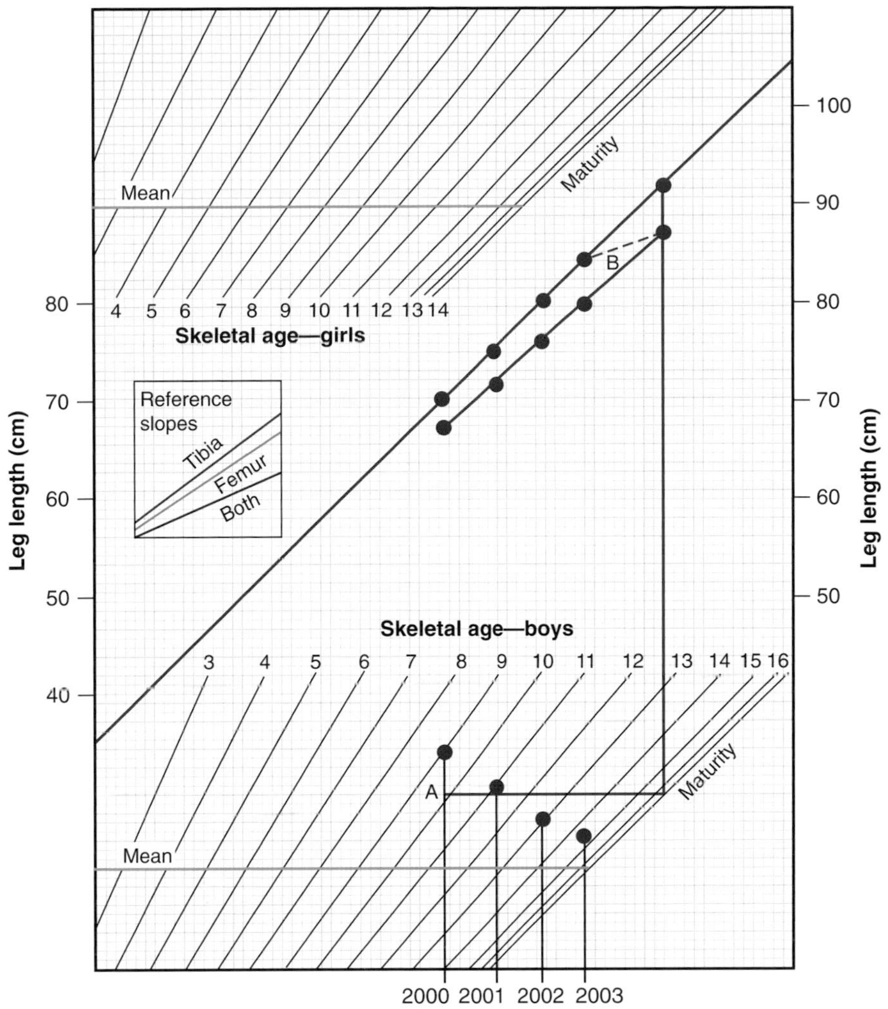

FIGURE 29-99 Moseley straight-line graph. Example shown is boy with idiopathic hemiatrophy observed clinically for 4 consecutive years. In 2000, longer leg measured 70 cm, shorter leg was 67 cm, and bone age was 9 years. Additional scanograms and bone age radiographs are plotted as shown. Horizontal straight line (*A*) extends to maturity line with equal number of skeletal ages above and below line. At skeletal maturity, longer leg is projected to measure 92 cm, and shorter leg is projected to measure 87 cm. Broken line (*B*) represents projected growth of longer leg if epiphysiodeses of distal femur and proximal tibia are performed when longer leg reaches 84 cm in length, obtaining limb equalization by skeletal maturity.

of a particular physis. It should be noted that physeal, rather than epiphyseal, growth is halted through this process, and the term physiodesis might be a more accurate term. Nevertheless, epiphysiodesis is used through the remainder of the chapter when discussing cessation of physeal growth.

Four types of treatment are available for limb-length equalization: shoe lift or prosthetic conversion, epiphysiodesis of the long leg, shortening of the long leg (in patients too old for epiphysiodesis), and lengthening of the short leg. Judicious combinations of ipsilateral lengthening and contralateral epiphysiodesis can be used for significant discrepancies to reduce the amount of lengthening required.

For small discrepancies of 1.5 cm or less, no treatment is necessary. If a patient desires, a 1-cm shoe lift can be provided to wear inside the shoe. The lift need not compensate for the entire discrepancy because people rarely stand erect with both knees and hips straight, and many people have small (1 cm) differences that are functionally insignificant. The degree of discrepancy that can be compensated for with an internal shoe lift is limited; however, and for differences of 2 to 4 cm, a lift on the outside of the shoe is necessary. For small discrepancies, a heel lift can be used, and for larger differences, a full-sole lift is needed. A shoe lift can be used for large discrepancies if the patient declines shortening or lengthening. Lifts of 5 to 10 cm are unsightly and unstable, however, and may require additional uprights or an ankle-foot orthosis to help support the ankle.

Many children reject shoe lifts on reaching adolescence, preferring instead to walk with compensatory mechanisms, including ankle equinus, pelvic tilt, and contralateral knee flexion. Nevertheless, shoe lifts often are beneficial in this age group as a trial to allow the patient to assess the potential benefits of a proposed surgical option. Extension prostheses are “modified shoe lifts” in that the foot is not amputated.

BOX 29-2

Instructions for Using Moseley Straight-Line Graph for Leg-Length Inequality

Depiction of Past Growth

- At each office visit, obtain three values:
  - Length of the normal leg measured by orthoradiograph from the most superior part of the femoral head to the middle of the articular surface of the tibia at the ankle
  - Length of the short leg
  - Radiographic estimate of skeletal age
- Place the point for the normal leg on the normal leg line of the appropriate length.
- Draw a vertical line through that point the entire height of the graph and through the skeletal age "scalar" area of either boys or girls; this line represents the current skeletal age.
- Place the point for the short leg on the current skeletal age line of the correct length.
- Mark the point where the current skeletal age line intersects that sloping "scalar" in the skeletal age area that corresponds to the radiographic estimate of skeletal age.
- Plot successive sets of three points in the same fashion.
- Draw the straight line that best fit the points plotted previously for successive lengths of the short leg.
- *Discrepancy* is represented by the vertical distance between two growth lines.
- *Inhibition* is represented by the difference in the slope between the two growth lines, taking the slope of the normal leg as 100.

Prediction of Future Growth

- Extend to the right growth line of the short leg.
- Draw the horizontal straight line that best fits the points plotted previously in the skeletal age area.
- *Growth percentile* is represented by the position of that horizontal line and indicates whether the child is taller or shorter than the mean.
- *Skeletal age scale* is represented by the intersections of this horizontal line with the scalars in the skeletal age area. The maturity point is the intersection of the line with the maturity scale.
- Draw a vertical line through the maturity point. This line represents maturity and the cessation of growth. Its intersection with the growth lines of the two legs represents their anticipated lengths at maturity.
- In keeping a child's graph up to date, it is recommended that these lines be drawn in pencil. The addition of further data makes this method more accurate and may require slight changes in the positions of these lines.

Effects of Surgery

Epiphysiodesis

- Ascertain the length of the normal leg just before surgery, and mark that point on the normal leg line.
- From that point draw a line parallel to the reference point for the particular physis fused. This is the new growth line for the normal leg (contribution of physes to total growth of leg: distal femur, 37%; proximal tibia, 28%; both, 65%).
- The percentage decrease in slope of the new growth line (taking the previous slope as 100%) exactly represents the loss of the contribution of the fused physis or physes.

Lengthening

- Draw the growth line for the lengthened leg exactly parallel to the previous growth line but displaced upward by a distance exactly equal to the length increase achieved. Because the physes are not affected, the growth rate is not affected and thus the slope of the line is unchanged.

Timing of Surgery

Epiphysiodesis

- Project the growth line of the short leg to intersect the maturity line, taking into account the effect of a lengthening procedure if necessary.
- From the intersection with the maturity line, draw a line whose slope is equal to the reference slope for the proposed surgery.
- The point at which this line meets the growth line of the normal leg indicates the point at which surgery should be done. This point is defined not in terms of the calendar but in terms of the length of the normal leg.

Lengthening

- Because lengthening procedures do not affect the rate of growth, the timing of this procedure is not critical and is governed by clinical considerations.

Postoperative Follow-Up

- Draw the new growth line of the normal leg as explained under Effects of Surgery.
- Data are plotted exactly as before except that the length of the short leg is plotted first and is placed on the growth line previously established for the short leg.

Instead, the foot is forced into an equinus position and is fitted into a custom prosthesis that has a prosthetic foot distal to the natural foot. Conversion with a Syme or Boyd amputation is preferred, however, to make prosthetic fitting easier.

OPERATIVE TREATMENT

Theoretically, lengthening of the short limb is the optimal treatment, but technical difficulty and frequent complications of lengthening procedures have made epiphysiodesis a more attractive option for small discrepancies. For growing children, epiphysiodesis is a relatively simple procedure with reasonably low morbidity and fast recovery. In adolescents too old for effective epiphysiodesis, limb shortening is accurate, safe, and simple, with a complication rate only slightly higher than epiphysiodesis. Joint stiffness after shortening is rare because the muscles are made slack by shortening of the limb, in contrast to lengthening, which frequently results in permanent joint stiffness and subluxation.

Shortening and epiphysiodesis have several disadvantages: (1) the normal limb is operated on rather than the pathologic limb, and if there is a deformity in the short limb, a second operation may be necessary to correct that

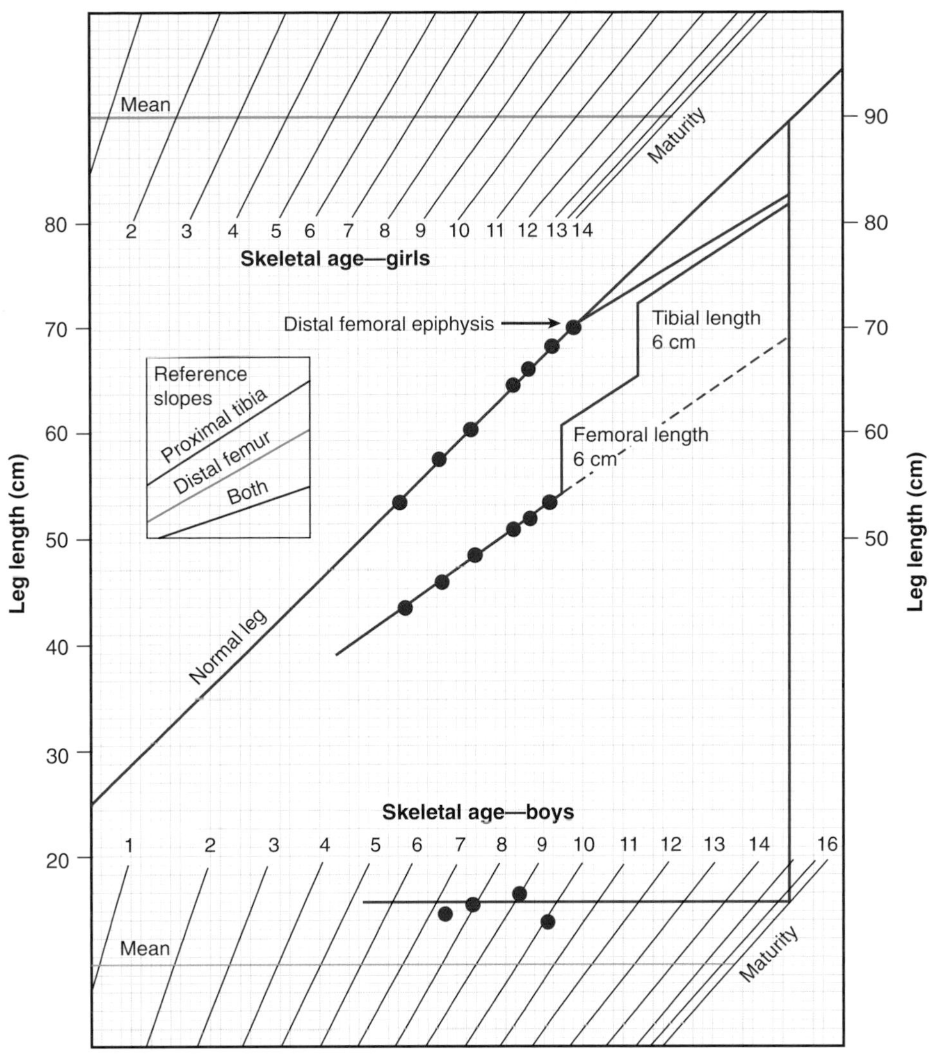

FIGURE 29-100 Moseley graph of patient with congenitally short femur and fibular hemimelia shows plan of femoral lengthening, tibial lengthening, and distal femoral epiphysiodesis.

deformity; (2), the resulting body proportions may be cosmetically displeasing after shortening; (3) the degree of shortening possible is limited because of the inability of the muscles to adapt to shortening of more than 5 cm; and (4) the final height after shortening or epiphysiodesis may be unacceptably low.

EPIPHYSIODESIS

Phemister described epiphysiodesis in 1933, and his original technique, with minor modifications, has been widely used for limb-length equalization. Most authors recommend epiphysiodesis when 2 to 5 cm of shortening is required; however, Menelaus and others recommended epiphysiodesis for discrepancies of 8 to 10 cm to avoid the complications of limb lengthening. Currently, epiphysiodesis is not recommended for shortening of more than 5 cm.

A newer technique of epiphysiodesis involves the use of percutaneous instrumentation, to obliterate the physis through small, cosmetically pleasing incisions (Technique 29-35).

Angled curets can be used instead of high-speed burrs to scrape the epiphyseal cartilage. It should be noted that normal physeal anatomy often contains multiple undulations or peaks and valleys. Care should be taken to obliterate as much of the physis as possible so that growth arrest is complete and predictable.

Métaizeau et al. described a technique for percutaneous epiphysiodesis using transphyseal screws (PETS) (Technique 29-36).

In 32 patients with leg-length discrepancies, PETS reduced the final discrepancy to less than 1 cm in 82% and to 5 mm or less in 56%. PETS has also shown success in the correction of angular deformities of the lower extremity. Multiple authors have cited as advantages of PETS simplicity of the technique, short operating time, rapid postoperative rehabilitation, and potential reversibility. However, there seems to be a lag time before the PETS technique produces the desired effect; therefore, the epiphysiodesis should be performed up to 1 year before the time predicted for a formal open procedure.

TABLE 29-7

Lower Limb Multipliers for Boys and Girls

AGE	MULTIPLIER	
(year + month)	*Boys*	*Girls*
Birth	5.080	4.630
0 + 3	4.550	4.155
0 + 6	4.050	3.725
0 + 9	3.600	3.300
1 + 0	3.240	2.970
1 + 3	2.975	2.750
1 + 6	2.825	2.600
1 + 9	2.700	2.490
2 + 0	2.590	2.390
2 + 3	2.480	2.295
2 + 6	2.385	2.200
2 + 9	2.300	2.125
3 + 0	2.230	2.050
3 + 6	2.110	1.925
4 + 0	2.000	1.830
4 + 6	1.890	1.740
5 + 0	1.820	1.660
5 + 6	1.740	1.580
6 + 0	1.670	1.510
6 + 6	1.620	1.460
7 + 0	1.570	1.430
7 + 6	1.520	1.370
8 + 0	1.470	1.330
8 + 6	1.420	1.290
9 + 0	1.380	1.260
9 + 6	1.340	1.220
10 + 0	1.310	1.190
10 + 6	1.280	1.160
11 + 0	1.240	1.130
11 + 6	1.220	1.100
12 + 0	1.180	1.070
12 + 6	1.160	1.050
13 + 0	1.130	1.030
13 + 6	1.100	1.010
14 + 0	1.080	1.000
14 + 6	1.060	NA
15 + 0	1.040	NA
15 + 6	1.020	NA
16 + 0	1.010	NA
16 + 6	1.010	NA
17 + 0	1.000	NA

MULTIPLIER METHOD FOR PREDICTING LOWER LIMB–LENGTH DISCREPANCIES

Length at Skeletal Maturity

$Lm = L \times M$

This formula can be used to determine the length of the femur, tibia, femur and tibia, or entire lower limb, including the foot height. It applies equally to the short and long limbs.

Congenital Limb-Length Discrepancy

$\Delta m = \Delta \times M$

This formula can be used to determine limb-length discrepancy in patients with congenital short femur, fibular hemimelia, hemihypertrophy, or hemiatrophy.

TABLE 29-7

Lower Limb Multipliers for Boys and Girls—cont'd

AGE	MULTIPLIER	
(year + month)	*Boys*	*Girls*

Developmental Limb-Length Discrepancy

$\Delta m = \Delta + (I \times G)$

where $I = 1 - (S - S)/(L - L)$ and $G = L(M - 1)$. This formula can be used to determine limb-length discrepancy in patients with Ollier disease, poliomyelitis, or growth arrest. It also can be used to determine discrepancy in patients with a congenital discrepancy. It also is useful in predicting the growth-remaining discrepancy in patients who have already undergone one or more limb-lengthening procedures.

Timing of Epiphysiodesis

$L\varepsilon = Lm - G\varepsilon$

and

$M\varepsilon = Lm/L\varepsilon$

Look in the multiplier table for the value of $M\varepsilon$ and determine which age corresponds to this multiplier value. This is the age of the patient at the time of epiphysiodesis.

G, Amount of growth remaining; I, amount of growth inhibition; L, current length of long limb; L, length of long limb as measured on previous radiographs (preferably made at least 6 or 12 months before current radiographs); Lm, length of femur or tibia at skeletal maturity; M, multiplier; S, current length of short limb; S, length of short limb as measured on previous radiographs (preferably made at least 6 or 12 months before current radiographs); Δ, current limb-length discrepancy; Δm, limb-length discrepancy at skeletal maturity; ε, desired correction following epiphysiodesis; Gε, amount of femoral or tibial growth remaining at age of epiphysiodesis ($G\varepsilon = \varepsilon/0.71$ for femur and $\varepsilon/0.57$ for tibia); Lε, desired length of bone to undergo epiphysiodesis at time of epiphysiodesis; Mε, multiplier at age of epiphysiodesis.

From Paley D, Bhave A, Herzenberg JE, et al: Multiplier method for predicting limb-length discrepancy, J Bone Joint Surg 82A:1432, 2000.
NA, Not applicable.

PHYSEAL EXPOSURE AROUND THE KNEE

TECHNIQUE 29-34

(ABBOTT AND GILL, MODIFIED)

- Flex the knee 30 degrees to relax the hamstring muscles and make a lateral incision 6.5 cm proximal to the lateral femoral condyle, continuing distally between the biceps tendon and iliotibial band to the fibular head and extending anteriorly over the lateral aspect of the tibia.
- Enter the interval between the lateral intermuscular septum and the vastus lateralis.
- Cauterize the superior geniculate arteries.
- Make a vertical incision in the periosteum over the physis and identify the thin "white line" of cartilage.
- Protect the peroneal nerve behind the fibular head and incise the periosteum over the anterior aspect of the fibular head.
- Reflect the anterior compartment muscles off the tibia distally to expose the proximal tibial physis.
- On the medial side, make a curved incision starting at the adductor tubercle and continuing first posteriorly and then anteriorly along the sartorius tendon. Ligate the geniculate arteries.
- Open the periosteum of the distal femur between the vastus medialis and intermedius muscles. Keep the dissection subperiosteal to avoid entering the knee joint.
- Over the proximal tibia, retract the pes anserinus tendon posteriorly, ligate the geniculate arteries, and make a vertical incision to aid in subperiosteal exposure to locate the physis.

Four short (2.5 cm) incisions can be used rather than two long ones to improve cosmesis. Dissection of the peroneal nerve is not mandatory. Fluoroscopy or image intensification, using needles to locate the physes, is helpful in placing the incisions. Preoperative radiographs showing the relation of the distal femoral physis to the patella also aid placement of the incision.

EPIPHYSIODESIS

TECHNIQUE 29-35 *Fig. 29-101*

(PHEMISTER)

- Expose the epiphyseal plate as described in Technique 29-33.
- At a point equidistant from the anterior and posterior surfaces of the bone excise a rectangular section of cortex 3 cm long and 1 to 1.5 cm wide that crosses the physeal plate.
- Both anterior and posterior to the defect thus created chisel out the epiphyseal plate for a distance of 3 to 5 cm in each direction and to a depth of about 1 cm.

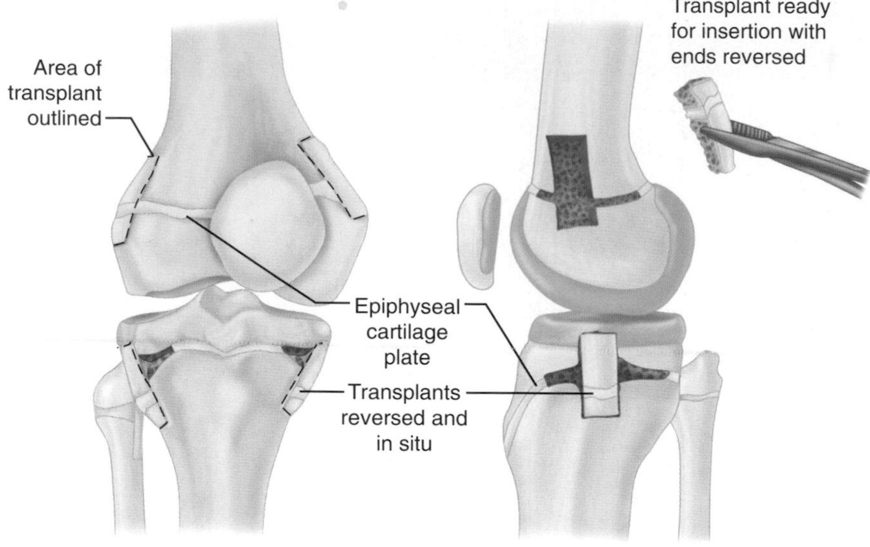

FIGURE 29-101 Phemister epiphyseodiaphyseal fusion. **SEE TECHNIQUE 29-35.**

- Reinsert the section of cortex into its original bed but with its ends reversed. Repeat the procedure on the opposite condyle.
- To arrest the proximal fibular epiphysis completely, excise the plate in an anteroposterior plane with an osteotome and a small curet and fill its space with small bone chips.

POSTOPERATIVE CARE. The extremity is immobilized for 3 weeks. Full weight bearing may usually be allowed at 1 month.

PERCUTANEOUS EPIPHYSIODESIS

TECHNIQUE 29-36

(CANALE ET AL.)

- After administration of general anesthesia, place the patient supine on the operating table. Prepare the limb in the standard fashion and drape it free. A tourniquet can be used if desired.
- Place a hemostat on the lateral aspect of the leg to locate the lateral portion of the distal femoral physis. After it has been located with image intensification, make small medial and lateral stab wounds approximately 1.5 cm long.
- Place a smooth Steinmann pin or Kirschner wire into the physis and drill it into the side of the distal femoral physis. Confirm correct positioning of the pin on anteroposterior and lateral image intensification views. Rotate the image intensifier rather than the leg because rotation of the leg causes the iliotibial band and medial musculature to tighten and interfere with placement of instruments.
- Place a cannulated reamer over the guide pin (Fig. 29-102A and B) and drill into the physis approximately halfway across; verify this with image intensification.
- After removal of the reamer, introduce a high-speed pneumatic drill with a dental burr. Protect the skin during drilling to prevent heat necrosis of the skin; using a guard for the dental burr is helpful.
- As an alternative, use angled and straight curets to remove the physis (Fig. 29-102C). Ream the physis proximally and distally, anteriorly and posteriorly, especially at the periphery, to create a "bull's eye" effect in the center of the physis at the lateral periphery.
- It is unnecessary to remove the entire physis. A lucent area or blackout effect is noted on image intensification where the physis and surrounding bone have been removed. If the "bull's eye" effect is not achieved, use a curet or larger reamer (e.g., from an adult compression hip screw set), and repeat the procedure on the medial side with frequent image intensification evaluation. Often the medial and lateral defects can be connected.
- Thoroughly irrigate to remove all loose pieces of cartilage and cancellous bone.
- Close the wounds with subcutaneous sutures and apply a sterile dressing.
- The same technique is used in the proximal tibial physis except that the tibial physis is more undulating than the femoral and requires more careful drilling. Epiphysiodesis of the proximal fibular physis may be unnecessary, especially if the desired growth arrest in the proximal tibia is less than 2.5 cm. Perform proximal fibular epiphysiodesis with a small Steinmann pin, a small cannulated reamer, and a hand drill or curet under direct vision through a

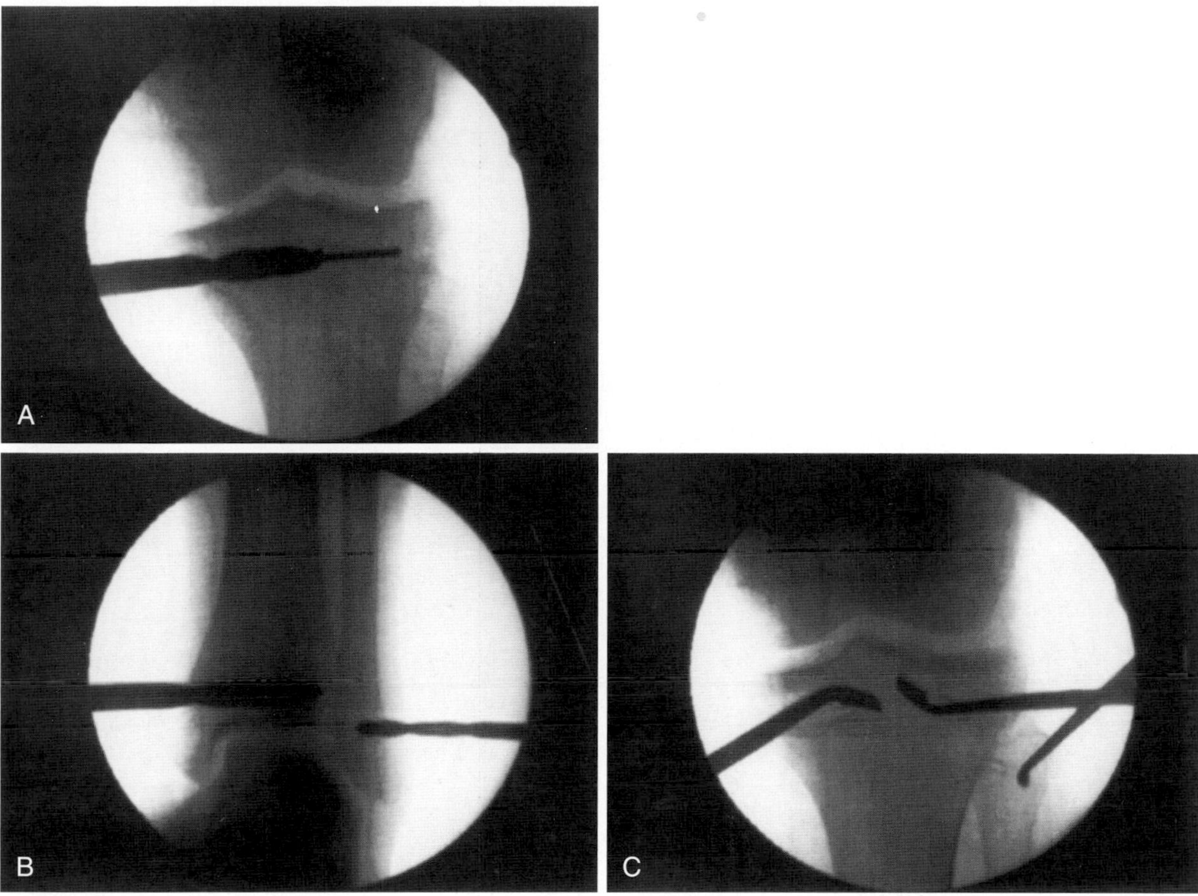

FIGURE 29-102 **A,** Insertion of cannulated reamer over guide pin in proximal tibia. **B,** Percutaneous drilling of distal tibial and fibular physes. **C,** Alternative method of using curets inserted through drill holes in cortex. **SEE TECHNIQUE 29-36.**

small separate incision. Because of the possibility of mechanical or thermal damage to the peroneal nerve, take great care in this area.

- As a modification of this technique, a radiolucent imaging table can be used instead of a fracture table. Use a tourniquet and make the stab wound large enough to insert a ¼-inch drill bit to broach the cortex. Curet the physis with angled and straight curets, using the image intensifier as needed (Fig. 29-102C).
- In the proximal tibia, it is important to palpate the fibular head, make the incision over the physis under image control, and stay anterior. A drill is not required to broach the proximal fibular cortex; a small, straight curet works well and does not risk injury to the peroneal nerve.

POSTOPERATIVE CARE. Immediate weight bearing in a soft knee immobilizer is allowed. The immobilizer is worn for approximately 2 to 3 weeks. If femoral and tibial epiphysiodeses have been done, a knee immobilizer is worn for 10 to 14 days, and then active range-of-motion exercises are begun. Crutches are used for guarded weight bearing for the first 4 weeks.

PERCUTANEOUS TRANSEPIPHYSEAL SCREW EPIPHYSEIODESIS

TECHNIQUE 29-37

(MÉTAIZEAU ET AL.)

- Prepare and drape the entire lower limb from groin to foot.
- Through a small stab incision over the lateral aspect of the distal femoral metaphysis, drill a hole directed obliquely downward and medially.
- Aiming slightly posterior to the midcoronal plane of the femur, advance the drill past the anatomic axis to cross the physis at the junction of its middle and inner thirds, and stop just short of the articular surface of the medial femoral condyle.
- Insert a cancellous screw with long threads; a cancellous screw with short threads and a washer can be used.
- Insert the second screw from the medial aspect, symmetrically to the first screw in relation to the anatomic axis of the distal femur, but slightly anterior to the midcoronal plane to avoid the first screw (Fig. 29-103).

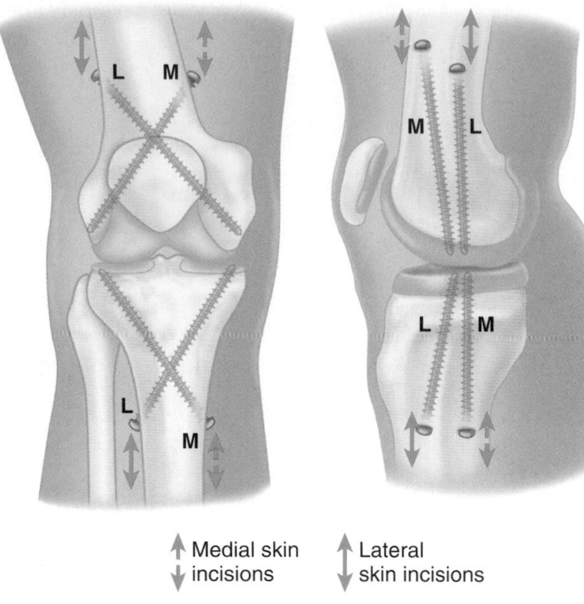

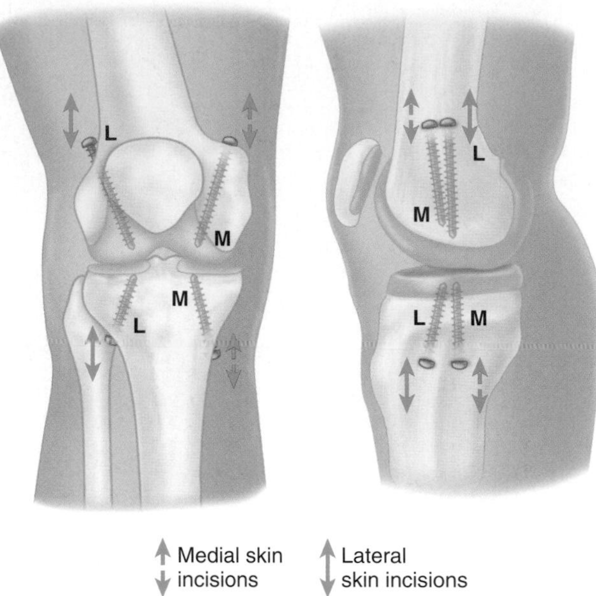

FIGURE 29-103 Percutaneous epiphysiodesis using transphyseal screws. Paired crossed transphyseal screws across distal femoral and proximal tibial physes. L, lateral screws; M, medial screws. **SEE TECHNIQUE 29-37.**

FIGURE 29-104 Percutaneous epiphysiodesis using transphyseal screws. Nonintersecting transphyseal screws. Each pair crosses physis, one screw at either end of its middle third. L, lateral screws; M, medial screws. **SEE TECHNIQUE 29-37.**

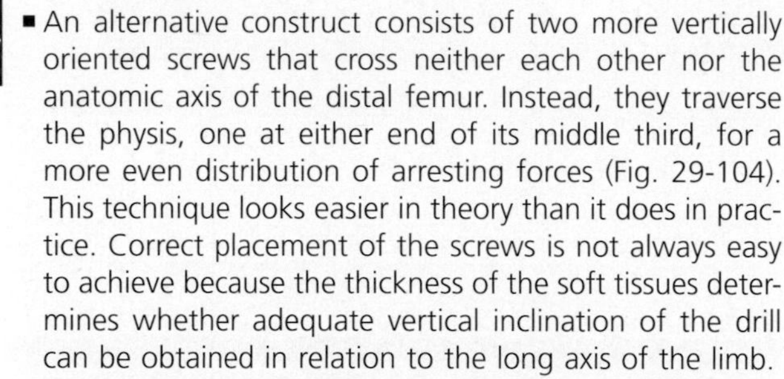

- An alternative construct consists of two more vertically oriented screws that cross neither each other nor the anatomic axis of the distal femur. Instead, they traverse the physis, one at either end of its middle third, for a more even distribution of arresting forces (Fig. 29-104). This technique looks easier in theory than it does in practice. Correct placement of the screws is not always easy to achieve because the thickness of the soft tissues determines whether adequate vertical inclination of the drill can be obtained in relation to the long axis of the limb.
- Begin insertion of the lateral tibial screw just posterior to the tibial crest to avoid the muscles of the anterior compartment of the leg. Direct it medially, upward and slightly posteriorly, to cross the physis at the junction of its middle and medial thirds (Fig. 29-103). An alternative construct can be used in which screws do not cross each other or the anatomic axis of the tibia (Fig. 29-104).
- After insertion of all screws, fully flex the knee to free any adhesions between screws and the quadriceps apparatus.

Proximal fibular epiphysiodesis is done only if more than 2 cm of tibial correction is needed. Percutaneous insertion of a screw across the proximal fibular epiphysis is dangerous. A short incision is required to identify and protect the peroneal nerve. Open curettage also can be done through a small anterior approach.

An alternative method of epiphysiodesis is physeal stapling or tension plating (Fig. 29-105). Although this technique is largely reserved for hemiepiphysiodesis in angular corrections, it can be used for complete epiphysiodesis if implants are used on both sides of the physis. However, this technique for complete epiphysiodesis has been shown to be inferior to physeal ablation. Dual plating technique also has the advantage of potential growth resumption with implant removal; however, restoration of normal growth often is unpredictable after implant removal, and careful timing of epiphysiodesis is still important. Recently, implant failures

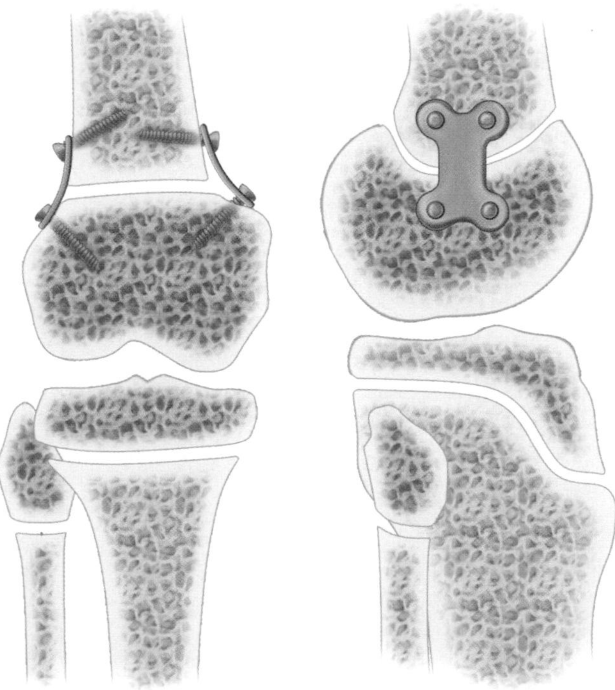

FIGURE 29-105 Tension plate epiphysiodesis. **SEE TECHNIQUE 29-38.**

have been described with the use of a single two-hole plate, and the use of additional plates or larger, four-hole plates should be considered. Most of these plating system are non-locking, which allows some degree of screw divergence within the plate as the physis continues to grow. It is likely that growth arrest does not occur until maximal screw divergence is reached. Therefore, it is advisable to place the screws in a divergent fashion at the time of implantation to allow growth arrest to occur as quickly as possible.

Regardless of the technique used, careful timing and consideration of the final height of the knee are important. For discrepancies involving the femur and tibia, epiphysiodesis of both may be required to ensure that the knees and pelvis are level. Operative complications are uncommon; reported complications include cutaneous nerve entrapment, infection, asymmetric growth arrest, undercorrection, and overcorrection, and implant failures.

TENSION PLATE EPIPHYSIODESIS

TECHNIQUE 29-38 *Fig. 29-105*

- Expose the physis as described in Technique 29-33, taking care to avoid significant disruption the periosteum or perichondral ring.
- Using fluoroscopy, place a reference wire in the center of the physis. To avoid asymmetric growth arrest, the pin should be in the center of the physis on the lateral fluoroscopic projection. Alternatively, the reference pin can be placed more anteriorly or posteriorly to achieve some degree of extension or flexion, respectively, at the physis.
- Next place the appropriate size plate over the reference wire using the centering hole.
- Place guide pins in the metaphyseal and epiphyseal holes for cannulated systems and drill over the guide pins. For noncannulated systems, simply drill the metaphyseal and epiphyseal holes.
- Place screws in the metaphyseal and epiphyseal holes to secure the tension plate to the bone surface. These screws should be placed in a divergent fashion because growth arrest does not begin until the screws reach the angular divergence allowed by the screw-plate interface.
- Close the wounds with subcutaneous sutures and apply a sterile dressing.

POSTOPERATIVE CARE. Immediate weight bearing with crutches is allowed; a soft knee immobilizer is worn for 2-3 weeks.

LIMB SHORTENING

Shortening usually is reserved for skeletally mature patients with a discrepancy greater than 2 cm, who can accept the loss of stature necessary to equalize limb lengths. When planning surgery, ultimate length and alignment should be considered. Wagner outlined the standard approach to limb shortening, but improvements have been made in femoral shortening techniques, such as a closed technique for diaphyseal shortening described by Winquist. In the femur, 5 to 6 cm is the maximal length that can be removed without seriously affecting muscle function; in the tibia, the maximum probably is 2 to 3 cm; however, removal of up to 5 cm of the tibia has been reported.

In general, femoral shortening is tolerated better than tibial shortening because the soft-tissue muscular envelope is much larger, making skin closure easier, offering a better cosmetic result, and ensuring prompt union of the osteotomy. If the discrepancy is largely confined to the tibia, however, tibial shortening is preferred to make the knee heights level.

Wagner recommended metaphyseal osteotomy if angular or rotational correction is required, and diaphyseal osteotomy if shortening alone is necessary. Proximal metaphyseal osteotomy of the femur has fewer complications than distal osteotomy, which may compromise knee motion. Additionally, proximal femoral shortening has less negative effect on the strength of the quadriceps. Distal femoral metaphyseal osteotomy should be avoided unless necessary for correction of angular deformity. The development of interlocking intramedullary fixation has made diaphyseal shortening preferable to metaphyseal osteotomy in the femur, even if rotational correction is needed. Shortening over an intramedullary rod should be delayed until complete skeletal maturity has been reached, or the entry portal of the nail should be the greater trochanter instead of the piriformis fossa to decrease the risk of femoral head osteonecrosis.

PROXIMAL FEMORAL METAPHYSEAL SHORTENING

TECHNIQUE 29-39 *Fig. 29-106*

(WAGNER)

- Before surgery, plan the osteotomy to provide the needed angular correction
- Through a proximal lateral incision, split the fascia lata and elevate the vastus lateralis and the periosteum.
- Fashion an insertion site for the right-angle blade plate or hip screw according to the preoperative plan.
- Mark the bone to control rotation, and remove the proscribed segment with an oscillating saw. Leave a spike of medial cortex and lesser trochanter intact to act as a buttress.
- Remove the segment, and bring the distal fragment into direct apposition with the proximal segment.
- Apply the osteosynthesis plate and insert the screws to create compression across the osteotomy.

DISTAL FEMORAL METAPHYSEAL SHORTENING

TECHNIQUE 29-40 *Fig. 29-107*

(WAGNER)

- Before surgery, make a careful plan for the resection and angular correction.

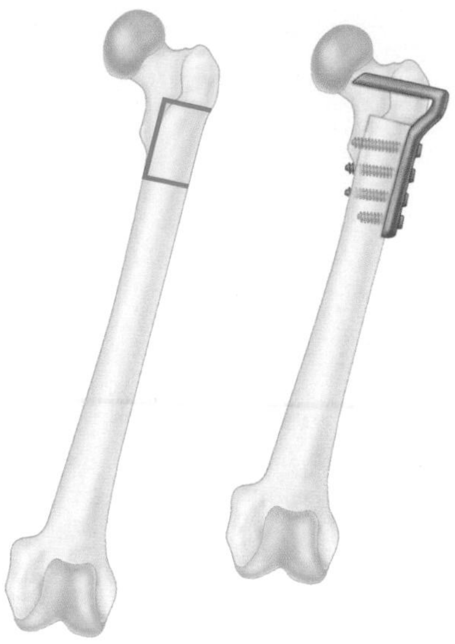

FIGURE 29-106 Wagner technique for proximal femoral metaphyseal shortening. **SEE TECHNIQUE 29-39.**

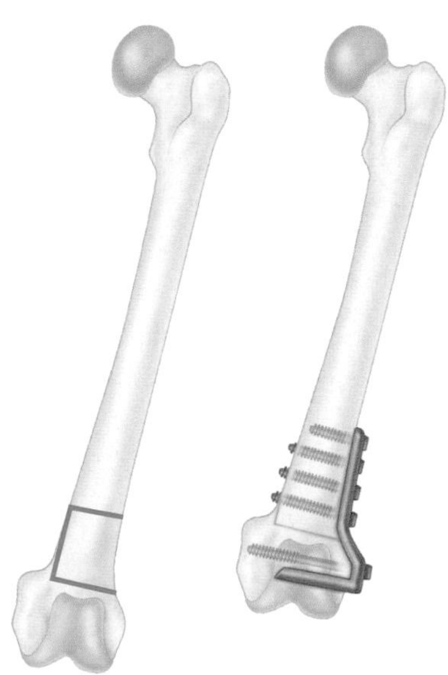

FIGURE 29-107 Wagner technique for distal femoral metaphyseal shortening. **SEE TECHNIQUE 29-40**

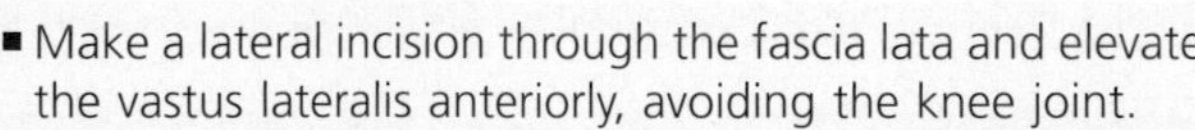

- Make a lateral incision through the fascia lata and elevate the vastus lateralis anteriorly, avoiding the knee joint.
- Use the blade plate seating device to prepare the entrance for the blade plate.
- With an oscillating saw, make the proximal osteotomy and then the distal osteotomy. For added stability, try to preserve a medial spike of bone with the distal fragment.
- Impact the two fragments and apply the blade under compression, or insert a distal femoral sliding screw and fixation plate device.

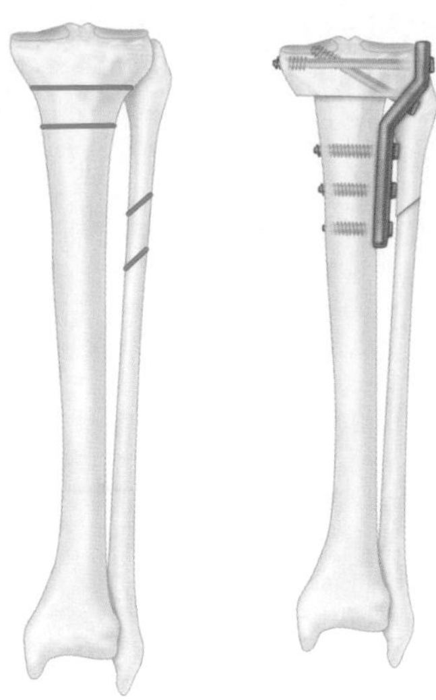

FIGURE 29-108 Wagner technique for proximal tibial metaphyseal shortening. **SEE TECHNIQUE 29-41.**

PROXIMAL TIBIAL METAPHYSEAL SHORTENING

TECHNIQUE 29-41 *Fig. 29-108*

(WAGNER)
- Through a lateral incision, resect a portion of the fibula at the junction of the proximal and middle thirds.
- Make a separate anterior incision to expose the proximal tibia subperiosteally.
- Resect the desired amount of bone (no more than 4 cm except in unusual circumstances) below the tibial tuberosity with an oscillating saw.
- Hold the two bone ends under compression with a T-plate.
- Perform a prophylactic fasciotomy.
- Wound closure may be difficult because of the nature of the skin around the proximal tibia.

TIBIAL DIAPHYSEAL SHORTENING

TECHNIQUE 29-42

(BROUGHTON, OLNEY, AND MENELAUS)
- Make a longitudinal incision over the anteromedial surface of the tibia.
- Perform a subperiosteal dissection and make a step-cut osteotomy, removing the desired amount of bone and allowing for 5 to 7.5 cm of overlap after shortening.
- Through a separate incision, remove an equivalent amount of bone from the midshaft of the fibula (Fig. 29-109A).

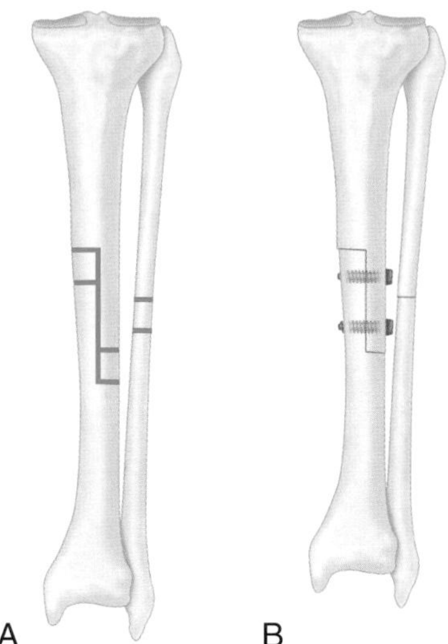

FIGURE 29-109 **A** and **B,** Technique for tibial diaphyseal shortening in skeletally immature patients. **SEE TECHNIQUE 29-42.**

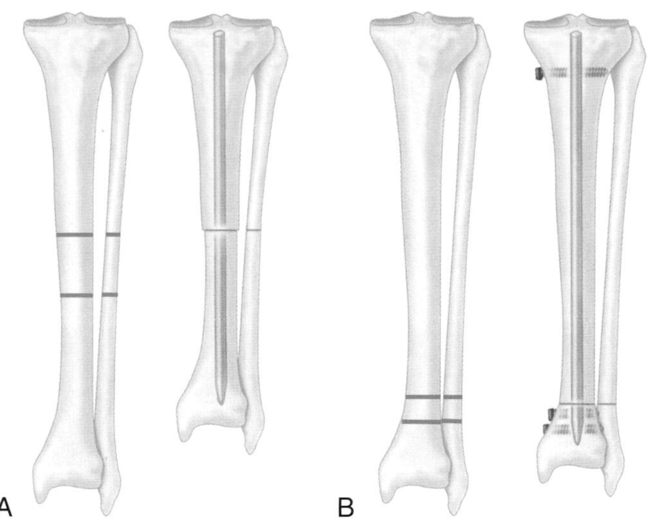

FIGURE 29-110 **A,** Diaphyseal shortening with medullary fixation. **B,** Distal tibial shortening with locked intramedullary nail. **SEE TECHNIQUE 29-42.**

- Shorten the leg and fix the step-cut osteotomy with two lag screws (Fig. 29-109B) or, in mature patients, with an intramedullary nail (Fig. 29-110). This is the only technique indicated in skeletally immature patients.

CLOSED FEMORAL DIAPHYSEAL SHORTENING

TECHNIQUE 29-43

(WINQUIST, HANSEN, AND PEARSON)

- Position the patient on a fracture table in the supine "scissor" position.
- Use the standard techniques for closed medullary nailing (see Chapter 53) and ream to the desired width in 0.5-mm increments. Consider venting the distal metaphyseal-diaphyseal junction with a 4.8-mm cannulated drill bit to prevent fat embolism.
- Adjust the saw for the appropriate depth according to the preoperative plan and insert the saw until, with the blade fully retracted, the measuring device is seated firmly against the greater trochanter.
- While an assistant applies pressure to hold the measuring device in place for the proximal and the distal cuts, deploy the saw blade in increments, making complete revolutions (Fig. 29-111A). If necessary, back up one index notch to repeat the cuts if the blade is getting stuck.
- Slowly continue cutting until the final index mark is reached, at which point the blade is fully deployed. The most difficult area to cut is posteriorly in the linea aspera. If necessary, complete the cut percutaneously with a thin osteotome. The next larger size blade and cam can be inserted to get a larger cutting diameter, but this can be difficult if the canal is not reamed widely enough.
- After completing the first cut, retract the blade fully.
- Remove the foot from the fracture table and angulate the distal femur 60 to 70 degrees in all directions to complete the osteotomy; replace the traction.
- Advance the measuring device handle distally while holding the locking nut in place. The distance that develops between these two components should equal the amount of femur to be resected.
- Spin the locking nut distally to lock the measuring device handle.
- With an assistant holding the measuring device firmly against the greater trochanter, make the second (proximal) osteotomy in the same fashion as the first.
- After completing the second osteotomy, retract the blade fully and remove the saw. The resected bone should be subtrochanteric rather than diaphyseal to lessen the effect on the quadriceps mechanism.
- Insert an internal chisel of appropriate size, hook the medial aspect of the intercalary segment, and pound on the handle backward with a tuning-fork hammer to split the bone (Fig. 29-111B).
- Repeat this maneuver at least one more time on the lateral segment.
- Use the hook of the chisel to push the fragments away from the canal.
- Have the unscrubbed assistant again remove the foot from the fracture table and impact the osteotomy, displacing the segmental fragments to either side, using the chisel to manipulate the fragments if necessary.
- In some cases, splitting of the "napkin ring" resected bone piece is unsuccessful. Should this occur, make a small lateral incision to remove the intercalary segment.
- Pass a nail-driving guidewire across the osteotomy and insert an appropriate-size nail for fixation while the unscrubbed assistant maintains rotational alignment.

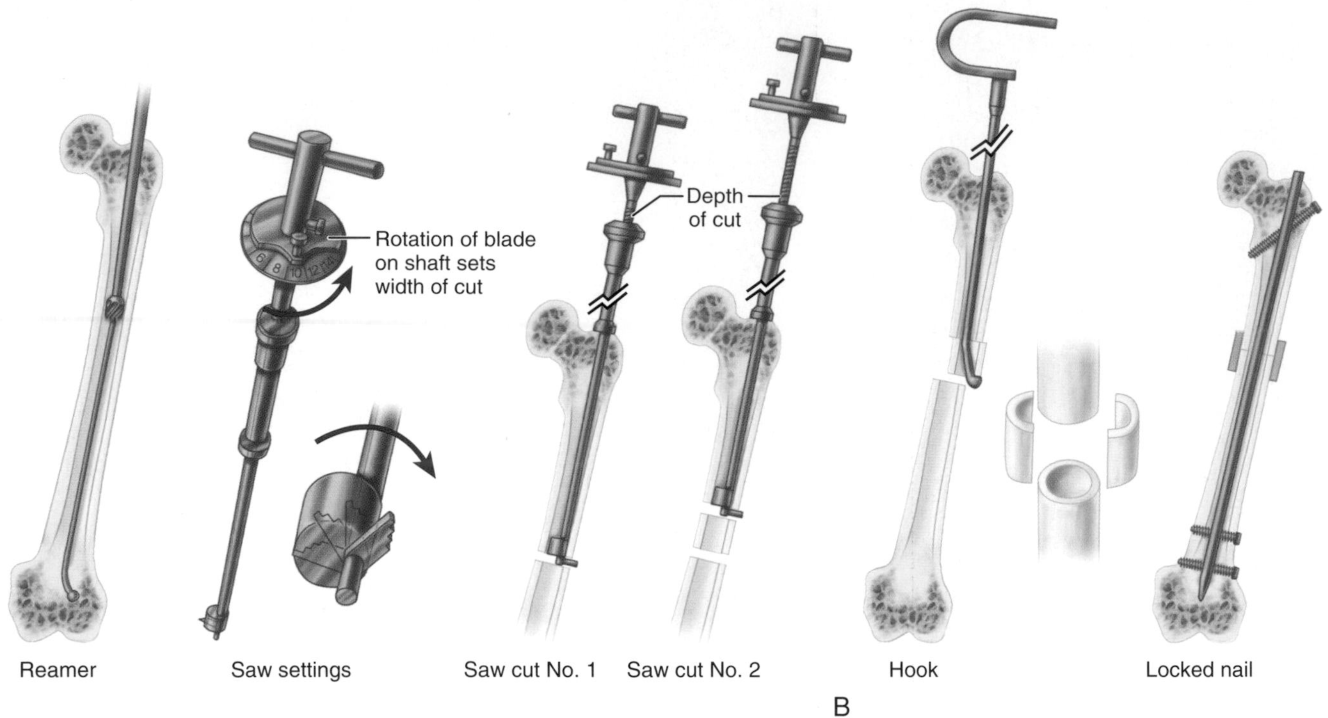

FIGURE 29-111 Closed femoral diaphyseal shortening, as described by Winquist et al. (see text). **A,** Medullary canal is reamed with standard cannulated reamer. Special medullary saw is inserted into reamed canal. One or two rotations are made with saw at each setting, and saw is progressively opened until blade is completely exposed. **B,** After both saw cuts have been made, intercalary segment is split using back-cutting chisel. Rotational alignment and distraction can be controlled with locked medullary nail. **SEE TECHNIQUE 29-43.**

- Lock the nail proximally and distally for rotational control and to prevent inadvertent lengthening postoperatively (Fig. 29-112).
- Steinmann pins can be inserted into the lateral aspect of the femoral condyle and the greater trochanter just before the first osteotomy to serve as references for rotational alignment control.
- Check rotational alignment before leaving the operating room.

POSTOPERATIVE CARE. A knee splint is used to stabilize the shortened quadriceps mechanism, and a vigorous strengthening program is begun. Rehabilitation is faster if the patient has participated in a quadriceps-strengthening and hamstring-strengthening program before surgery. Rotation or distraction at the osteotomy site may occur if a locked nail is not used.

LIMB LENGTHENING

A limb-lengthening program requires a patient and family fully committed to maximal participation in an extended project. The success of limb lengthening depends largely on the patient's efforts in physical therapy and the care of the external fixator. Although technical improvements have reduced the frequency with which major complications associated with limb lengthening occur, the process remains difficult and should be performed by surgeons with appropriate experience.

Shortening procedures are preferable for many patients who are candidates for limb lengthening. Patients who are unable to participate in frequent follow-up or who do not have the support to care for the fixator properly and to undergo vigorous physical therapy are best treated by means other than lengthening. Candidates for limb lengthening and their parents benefit from meeting other patients in various stages of the lengthening process.

Acute long bone lengthening seldom is indicated; however, Salter described acute distraction and interposition grafting through the innominate bone. Millis and Hall reported a modification of this technique; they achieved an average lengthening of 2.3 cm in 20 patients with acetabular dysplasia with femoral shortening, pure limb-length inequality, decompensated scoliosis, and primary intrapelvic asymmetry. This technique may be useful in patients who also require acetabular reconstruction, but epiphysiodesis or gradual distraction lengthening techniques are more reliable alternatives for isolated limb-length discrepancy.

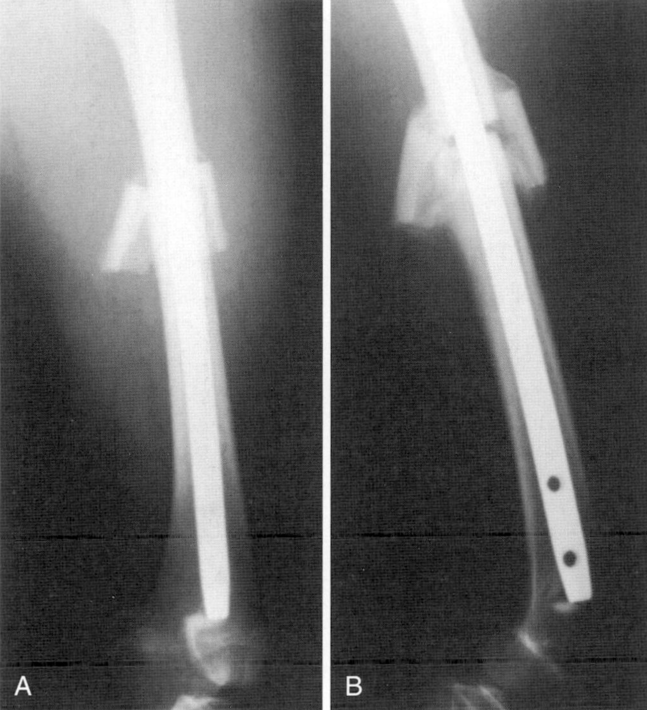

FIGURE 29-112 **A,** Sixteen-year-old girl underwent 4-cm closed femoral shortening. Shortly after surgery, intercalary fragment is seen around site of osteotomy, acting as bone graft. **B,** Osteotomy has healed 8 weeks later. At least 4 mm of distraction occurred after osteotomy. Locking of nail is recommended to preserve alignment and length, if necessary. **SEE TECHNIQUE 29-43.**

TRANSILIAC LENGTHENING

TECHNIQUE 29-44

(MILLIS AND HALL)

- Use the anterior ilioinguinal approach to the pelvis described for the Salter innominate osteotomy (see Chapter 30).
- Use a Gigli saw to make the osteotomy from the sciatic notch to the anterior inferior iliac spine (Fig. 29-113A).
- Insert a lamina spreader into the anterior aspect of the osteotomy.
- Have an assistant apply caudally directed pressure on the iliac crest to prevent displacement of the proximal fragment by shear force through the sacroiliac joint, while another assistant applies traction to the femur, keeping the knee flexed to relax the sciatic nerve.
- Fashion a full-thickness block of iliac crest into a trapezoid. The height of the graft directly superior to the acetabulum determines the amount of lengthening.
- Wedge the iliac graft into the distraction site (Fig. 29-113B) and hold it with two large, threaded Steinmann pins that transfix the proximal fragment, the graft, and the distal supraacetabular fragment (Fig. 29-113C).

POSTOPERATIVE CARE. Traction is applied for 5 days. Range-of-motion exercises are begun at 3 days, and touch-down weight bearing is allowed at 7 days. Full weight bearing is delayed until graft incorporation is evident on radiographs, usually at 3 to 6 months.

Lengthening by callotasis (or low energy corticotomy followed by gradual distraction of the bone fragments with a mechanical apparatus) has been the basic procedure for limb lengthening since Putti's report of the technique in 1921. Osteotomy and fixation techniques have been modified by several authors, but the principles remain the same. The corticotomy should be made by low-energy methods, usual multiple percutaneous drill holes connected by an osteotome, with care taken to avoid significant disruption of the surrounding soft tissues. Distraction should begin after a brief latent period of 1 to 3 weeks to allow for early callous formation. The rate of distraction should be approximately 1 mm per day divided over four 0.25-mm increments. The formation of the distraction regenerate should be closely monitored with frequent radiographic assessment, and the rate of distraction should be altered accordingly to avoid premature consolidation or poor regenerate formation. No matter what type of external apparatus is used, the device should remain in place for 1 month for every 1 cm of length achieved. Despite careful technique and excellent patient cooperation, high complication rates are reported with all methods, including deep infection, nonunion, fracture after device removal, malunion, joint stiffness, and nerve palsy.

Several fixators were developed, including Wagner's low-profile, monolateral fixator, DeBastiani's Orthofix, the Ilizarov device, and the Taylor Spatial Frame, all of which have undergone numerous modifications. The original Wagner device is adjustable in only two planes, and the Hoffman modification is adjustable in one additional plane. DeBastiani's device (Orthofix) has modular components that allow certain simple angular corrections. The Ilizarov device is extremely modular and can be adapted with extensions and hinges to lengthen and correct angular and translational deformities simultaneously. Rotational deformities can be corrected either at the time of fixator application or later by applying outriggers to the rings.

The Taylor Spatial Frame also has been used for deformity correction and lengthening. This frame uses the slow correction principles of the Ilizarov system but adds a six-axis deformity analysis incorporated in a computer program. The Taylor Spatial Frame has been shown to have a steep learning curve and has a high cost. In addition, no differences between the Taylor and Ilizarov frames have been noted in terms of lengthening index and complication rate, although rotational, translational, and residual deformity correction may be easier with the Taylor frame.

The circular devices are more difficult to apply than the monolateral fixators, and extensive training and experience are recommended before using them. For detailed descriptions of the components of these fixators, preoperative planning, and frame construction and application, see Chapter 53.

Internal lengthening devices were developed to eliminate the problems associated with pin track infection and

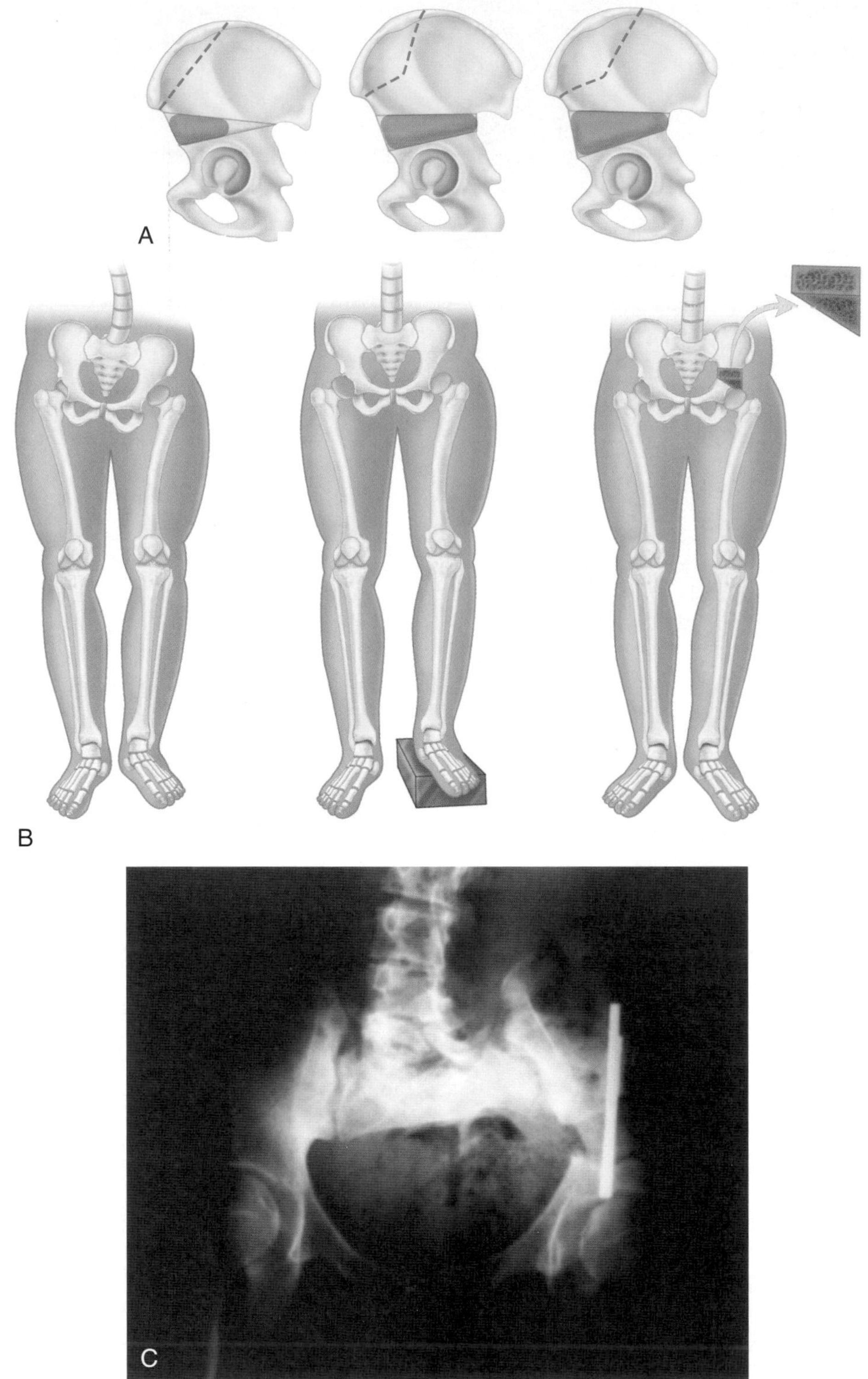

FIGURE 29-113 **A,** Acute transiliac lengthening accomplished by modification of Salter technique. Instead of triangular graft, square or trapezoidal graft is used. Lengthening is greater with larger grafts. **B,** Acetabular dysplasia and mild limb-length inequality. Pelvic obliquity results in compensatory scoliosis. In middle figure, block has been placed beneath shorter leg. Although this balances pelvis and straightens spine, it causes acetabulum to be even more vertical. On right, transiliac lengthening has been performed to improve femoral acetabular coverage and regain length. **C,** Transiliac lengthening with trapezoidal graft. **SEE TECHNIQUE 29-44.**

soft-tissue transfixation, to maintain mechanical alignment and stability during lengthening and consolidation, and to improve patient comfort and tolerance. Lengthening of these devices may be initiated by rotation of the involved limb (Albizzia nail; DePuy Australia Pty Ltd, Mount Waverly, Australia); controlled rotation, ambulation, and weight bearing (Intramedullary Skeletal Kinetic Device; Orthofix, McKinney, Tex); an implanted electrically activated motorized drive (Fitbone; Wittenstein Igersheim, Germany), or an externally applied magnetic field (PRECICE Nail, Ellipse Technologies, Inc., Irvine CA, USA or the PHENIX M2 Lengthening nail; Phenix Medical, France).

These intramedullary devices do not allow for gradual correction of angular deformities because they can only lengthen in one plane; therefore, any angular deformities must be corrected at the time of nail insertion or by other means after lengthening. There are a number of studies demonstrating difficulty in controlling rate of growth using the Intramedullary Skeletal Kinetic Device (ISKD) nail, and many authors are suggesting alternative devices.

Finally, some authors have reported the use of an intramedullary nail or submuscular plate in addition to an external fixator for distraction osteogenesis.

With most of these techniques, distraction osteogenesis is done with the use of an external device as described above, and the submuscular plate or intramedullary nail is then used to stabilize the regenerate as it consolidates, allowing earlier removal of the external device.

TIBIAL LENGTHENING

TECHNIQUE 29-45

(DEBASTIANI ET AL.)

- Place the patient supine on a radiolucent table.
- Resect 2 cm of the distal fibula through a lateral approach.
- Use the mated Orthofix drills, drill guides, and screw guides to insert the conical, self-tapping cortical and cancellous screws.
- Insert a cancellous screw 2 cm distal to the medial aspect of the knee, parallel to the knee joint.
- Place the appropriate rigid template parallel to the diaphysis of the tibia and insert the distalmost screw.
- Go to the proximal part of the template and insert the next screw in the fourth template hole distal to the upper screw. The last screw to be placed is in the distal template, in the hole farthest away from the distalmost screw.
- Remove the template and perform a corticotomy just distal to the tibial tuberosity.
- Incise the anterior skin and periosteum longitudinally.
- Under direct vision, drill a series of unicortical holes in the tibia. Set the drill stop at 1 cm to prevent penetration of the marrow.
- Use a thin osteotome to connect the drill holes and to divide along the posteromedial and posterolateral cortices as much as can be done safely.
- Flex the tibia at the corticotomy to crack the posterior aspect of the tibia.
- Apply the Orthofix lengthener. If the fracture fixation device is used, fix the ball joint rigidly with a small amount of methylmethacrylate.
- Suture the periosteum and close the skin over drains.

POSTOPERATIVE CARE. Partial weight bearing and physical therapy are begun immediately. Distraction is delayed until callus is visible on radiographs, usually by 10 to 15 days. Distraction is begun at 0.25 mm every 6 hours but can be reduced if pain or muscle contraction occurs. Radiographs are made 1 week after distraction begins to ensure a complete corticotomy and are made at 4-week intervals thereafter. If the regenerated callus is of poor quality, distraction is stopped for 7 days. Recompression is indicated for gaps in the callus and for evidence of excessive neurovascular distraction. When the desired length is obtained, the body-locking screw mechanism is tightened, and the distraction mechanism is removed from the fixator. Full weight bearing is allowed until good callus consolidation is seen, then the body-locking screw is unlocked to allow dynamic axial compression. The fixator is removed when corticalization is complete. If stability is confirmed, the screws are removed. If there is any doubt as to stability of the bone, the fixator is replaced for an additional period.

TIBIAL LENGTHENING

TECHNIQUE 29-46 *Fig. 29-114*

(ILIZAROV, MODIFIED)

- Frame preconstruction involves assembling a frame consisting of four equal Ilizarov rings sized to the patient; use the smallest diameter rings that leave sufficient space for swelling after surgery. There should be one fingerbreadth of space between the proximal ring and the tibial tuberosity and two fingerbreadths posteriorly at the largest diameter of the posterior calf muscles (Fig. 29-115A). The most proximal ring can be a ⅝-inch ring to allow more knee flexion after surgery, especially if the ipsilateral femur is to be lengthened at the same time, because full rings would touch each other with relatively little knee flexion.
- Connect the upper two rings with 20-mm threaded, hexagonal sockets for better stability. In small patients, there may be room proximally for only one ring and a drop wire (Fig. 29-115B). The distal two rings can be spaced farther apart than the top two rings for better stability, but for significant lengthening it is better to have the distal two-ring construct relatively farther away from the intended proximal metaphyseal corticotomy site; such an arrangement maximizes the amount of soft tissue available for stretching, contributing to the overall lengthening.
- For initial preconstruction, use only two connections between each pair of rings, one anteriorly and one directly posteriorly. Plan the frame so that the central connection

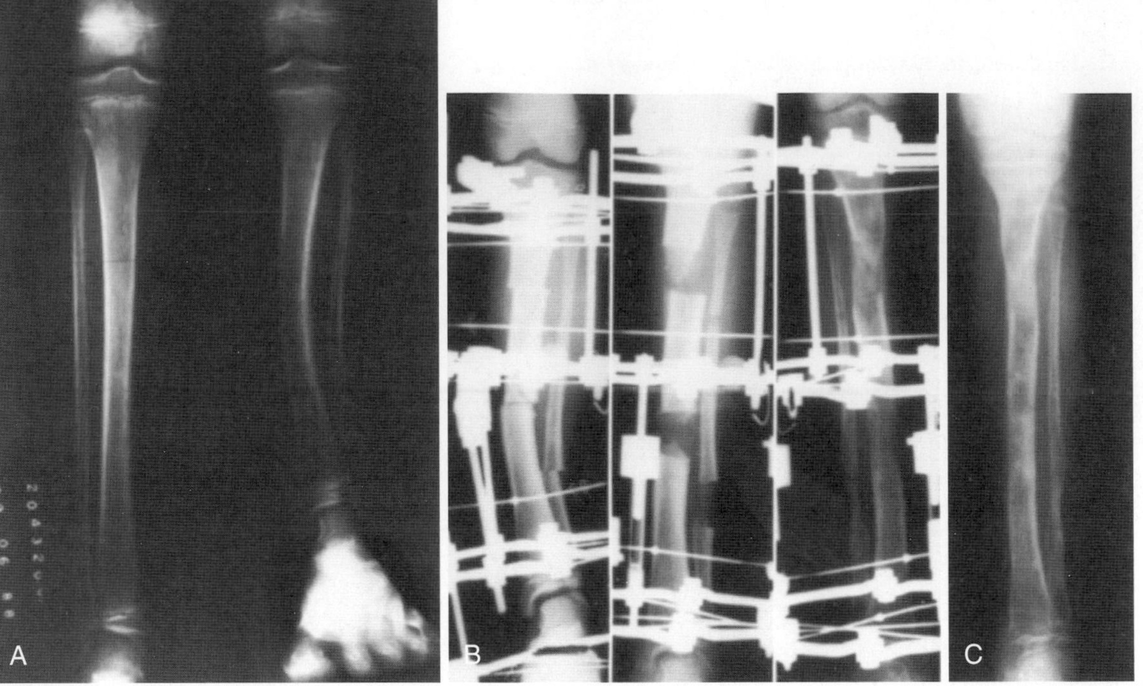

FIGURE 29-114 **A,** Congenital posteromedial bowing of tibia in 11-year-old girl. Although deformity largely corrected spontaneously, child is left with 6 cm of shortening and valgus angulation in midshaft of tibia. **B,** Double-level tibial lengthening. Lower corticotomy is made at apex of angular deformity in midshaft, and upper corticotomy could have been made more proximally in metaphyseal region. After distraction with appropriately placed hinge, more distal corticotomy not only opens up for elongation but also corrects valgus deformity. **C,** Final result after removal of fixator shows excellent regenerated bone in gaps. This 6-cm lengthening required 41/2 months in fixator. Premature consolidation of proximal fibular osteotomy resulted in spontaneous proximal fibular epiphysiolysis. **SEE TECHNIQUE 29-46.**

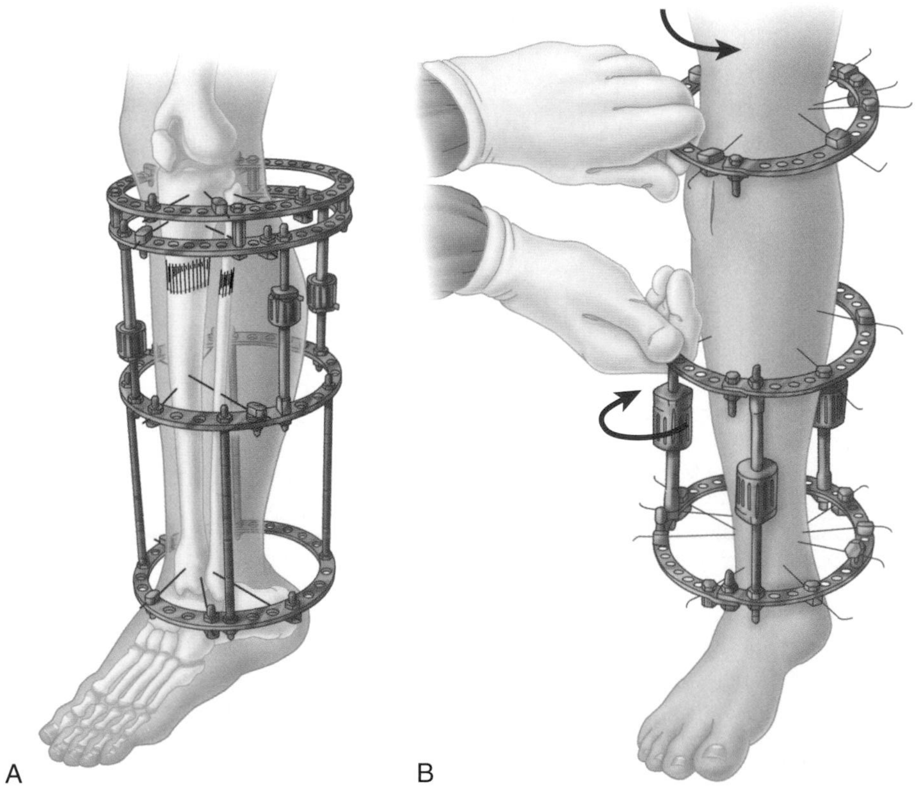

FIGURE 29-115 Typical Ilizarov frame for moderate tibial lengthening. **A,** In skeletally immature child with intact physes, proximal segment would not have enough room for two rings. Single ring distal to proximal tibial epiphysis is used with drop wire for additional segmental stabilization of proximal segment. For significant amount of lengthening, third ring can be placed more distally to allow greater mass of soft tissue for recruitment into lengthening process. **B,** If necessary, Ilizarov rings can be used to complete the posterior aspect of the corticotomy by externally rotating the distal segment. **SEE TECHNIQUE 29-46.**

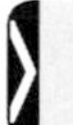

bolts are centered directly over the tibial tuberosity and the anterior crest of the tibia.

- Assemble all rings symmetrically.
- To compensate for the anterior and valgus angulation that often occurs during tibial lengthening, some surgeons connect the upper two-ring set to the lower set with anterior and posterior threaded rods attached to the lower of the proximal two rings with conical washer couples. These allow a tilt of 7 degrees to be built into the system.
- Adjust the frame so that the proximal rings are higher anteriorly and medially. The frame is applied in this "cock-eyed" position, but after the corticotomy is made, the conical washer bolts are removed and all four rings are brought into parallel alignment, placing the tibia in about 5 degrees of prophylactic recurvatum and varus.
- More often, a symmetrically aligned frame is used without any prophylactic positioning. Instead, careful attention is paid to the follow-up radiographs during lengthening. If axial deviations are found at the end of lengthening, corrective hinges are placed onto the ring to obtain proper alignment.
- For frame application, position the patient on a radiolucent table and apply a tourniquet to the upper thigh.
- Through a lateral incision, expose the midfibula by subperiosteal dissection and transect it with an oscillating saw.
- Release the tourniquet and close the fibular wound in layers.
- Under fluoroscopic control, insert a reference wire from medial to lateral, perpendicular to the long axis of the tibia (for a normally aligned leg), just below the proximal tibial physis. Use 1.8-mm wires in large children and adolescents and 1.5-mm wires in smaller children.
- Attach the preassembled frame to this reference wire.
- Place another wire from the fibula to the tibia just proximal to the distal tibial physis. Use the standard Ilizarov principles of wire insertion and fixation at all times (see Chapter 53).
- Wires should be pushed or gently tapped through the soft tissues rather than drilled, especially when exiting close to neurovascular structures.
- When passing wires through the anterior compartment muscles, hold the foot dorsiflexed for the same reason.
- Incise the skin to allow passage of olive wires.
- Never pull or bend a wire to the ring. Instead, build up to the wire with washers or posts as necessary to avoid undue torque and undesirable moments on the tibia.
- Tension the wires to 130 kg, unless the wire is suspended off a ring, in which case 50 to 60 kg of tension is used to prevent warping of the ring. It is best to use two wire tensioners to tighten two wires simultaneously on the same ring, if possible, to prevent warping of the ring.
- After tensioning and securing the wires, cut the ends long (about 4 cm) and curl the ends of the wire directly over the wire-fixation bolt to allow later retensioning, if necessary. Bend the cut wire points into available ring holes so that they do not injure the patient or staff members.
- After the first two wires have been attached to the frame and tensioned, the frame can act as a drill guide for placement of the remaining wires. The wires in the first ring are the initial transverse reference wire and a medial face wire that is parallel to the medial surface of the tibia.
- Place a third wire from the fibular head into the tibia to prevent dissociation of the proximal tibiofibular joint during lengthening. This wire does not risk damage to the peroneal nerve if the fibular head is readily palpable. Do not use an olive wire because it would compress the proximal tibiofibular joint. Ideally, this wire should be proximal to the proximal fibular physis.
- In the second ring, place a transverse wire and another medial face wire, avoiding the pes anserinus tendons, if possible.
- Because there is a strong tendency to valgus during proximal tibial lengthening, place olive wires on the top and bottom rings laterally and on the middle two rings medially to function as fulcrums for bending the tibia into varus. Half-pins (5 mm or 6 mm) are now used more frequently, especially in the diaphysis.
- For corticotomy, remove the two threaded rods connecting the proximal fixation block with the distal fixation block.
- Make a 2-cm incision over the crest of the tibia just below the tibial tuberosity.
- Incise the periosteum longitudinally and insert a small periosteal elevator.
- Elevate a narrow portion of periosteum the width of the small periosteal elevator along the medial and lateral surfaces of the tibia.
- Insert a 1.2-cm (½ inch) osteotome transversely into the thick anterior cortex.
- Use a 5-mm (¼ inch) osteotome to score the medial side and then the lateral side. The periosteal elevator can be placed flush along the bone to act as a directional guide for the osteotome.
- The corticotomy is guided by feel and by hearing the sound change when the osteotome exits the back cortex. On the medial side, no important structures are at risk; on the lateral cortex, the posterior tibial muscle belly is between the tibia and the deep neurovascular structures.
- After cutting the medial and lateral cortices, withdraw the osteotome and reinsert it along the medial cortex.
- Turn the osteotome 90 degrees to spread the cortices and crack the posterior cortex. Repeat this maneuver at the lateral cortex, if needed.
- Although Ilizarov recommended not violating the medullary canal, most Western surgeons have adopted DeBastiani's method of making several front-to-back drill holes to weaken the posterior cortex. The corticotomy also can be completed by externally rotating the distal tibia, but do not internally rotate the tibia for fear of stretching the peroneal nerve.
- For proximal or distal tibial metaphyseal "corticotomies," a Gigli saw makes a smooth osteotomy without risk of fracture into adjacent pin sites. The Gigli saw method requires two transverse incisions, one anteriorly and one posteromedially. Subperiosteal dissection with a small elevator is done on all three sides of the tibia. Right-angle and curved clamps are used to pass a heavy suture, which is tied to the Gigli saw. The suture can be passed before frame application and the Gigli saw after completion of

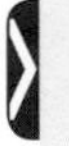

the fixation. When activating the saw, assistants must retract the skin edges. Care is taken to protect the medial face periosteum at the final part of the osteotomy.

- For frame assembly, reduce the fracture, and insert four distraction rods or graduated telescopic rods, approximately 90 degrees apart, between the middle two rings.
- Close the corticotomy site, over a drain if necessary, and apply compressive dressings.
- Dress the wire sites with foam sponges held in place by plastic clips or rubber stoppers. If rubber stoppers are used, put them on before fixing the wires to the rings.

POSTOPERATIVE CARE. Physical therapy and crutch walking with partial weight bearing are begun immediately. Distraction is delayed for 5 to 7 days. In children, the distraction rate is 0.25 mm four times per day. The patient and family are taught to care for the pins before discharge from the hospital, usually 5 to 7 days after surgery. Radiographs are made 7 to 10 days after distraction is begun to document separation at the corticotomy site. Regenerated bone should be seen in the gap by 4 to 6 weeks, although linear streaks of regenerated bone usually are visible before then, especially in younger children. If the regenerated bone formation is insufficient, the rate of distraction should be slowed, stopped, or in some instances temporarily reversed. Weight bearing and functional activity of the limb aid in maturation of the regenerated bone. During distraction, knee flexion contractures and ankle equinus contractures can be prevented with prophylactic splints and orthoses. The fixator is removed when there is evidence of corticalization of the regenerated bone, and the patient is able to walk without aids.

For significant lengthening, especially when ankle mobility is abnormal before surgery, the foot can be fixed into the lengthening device by inserting an olive wire from each side of the calcaneus at divergent angles to one another. These are attached to an appropriate-size half-ring. This half-ring must be within 2 cm of the back of the heel to capture the obliquely placed wires anteriorly. The heel ring is connected to the lowest ring of the lengthening frame with short plates and threaded rods. The heel ring and wires can be removed after lengthening is complete to prevent subtalar stiffness. A custom orthosis can be constructed to accommodate the foot construct.

For lengthening of more than 6 cm, double-level lengthening speeds the process and reduces the time in fixation by about 40%. In this modification, three rings are used, with a drop wire off each ring to give "bilevel" fixation at each segment (Fig. 29-115). The fibula should have one wire transfixing it at each of the three rings. Two fibular osteotomies and two corticotomies are required, one of each just below the proximal ring and one of each just above the distal ring. A heel ring and wires are added to prevent equinus of the ankle. The bottom two rings can be connected to provide a stable handle on the distal segments to complete the proximal corticotomy, and the top two rings can be connected to complete the distal corticotomy.

If a fixed knee contracture develops during lengthening, the physical therapy treatments should be done more often. If the knee contracture does not respond to physical therapy and splinting, the frame can be extended proximally to the thigh with a cuff cast incorporating a ring and a hinge incorporated at the approximate axis of rotation of the knee. The device can be used to distract and correct the knee contracture slowly.

To correct other deformities of the tibia while lengthening, the Ilizarov frame can be modified with hinges to effect angular and translational correction simultaneously. Internal rotation can be corrected distally by osteotomy at the time of fixator application. Proximally, internal rotation should be corrected gradually after lengthening is complete but before the regenerated bone is solid. Use of the Ilizarov device for multiplane corrections should be attempted only by surgeons with experience in these techniques.

TIBIAL LENGTHENING OVER INTRAMEDULLARY NAIL (PRECICE INTRAMEDULLARY LENGTHENING SYSTEM, ELLIPSE TECHNOLOGIES, IRVINE, CA, USA)

TECHNIQUE 29-47

(HERZENBERG, STANDARD, GREEN)

- Preoperative planning is essential to determine the amount of lengthening required, the correct nail length, and correct location for the tibial corticotomy.
- Place the patient supine, with the hip and knee flexed and the affected leg hanging vertically down over a padded bar or sterile triangle, avoiding any pressure on the fibular head (common peroneal nerve). Patient positioning for the PRECICE procedure is the same as that for other intramedullary nailing procedures.
- Create an osteotomy of the fibula through a separate incision to allow distraction of the tibial osteotomy. Consider prophylactic fasciotomies as well as a gastrocsoleus recession if indicated (Chapter 33).

VENTING OF INTRAMEDULLARY CANAL

- Drill two or three 4-mm or 5-mm diameter holes in the tibia, across both cortices and into the intramedullary canal. Position the vent at the level of the planned corticotomy. Venting reduces intramedullary pressure during reaming.
- Reamings from the vent holes will serve as additional bone graft.

SYNDESMOSIS SCREW

- A cannulated screw should be placed across the tibia and fibula distal to the tip off the nail (see syndesmotic screw placement, Chapter 54).
- Syndesmotic screw fixation ensures that the fibula lengthens with the tibia.
- Place a proximal syndesmotic screw (if needed) after final nail insertion.

NAIL INSERTION

- Make a 5-cm vertical skin incision in the midline, centered at the level of the tibial plateau. Ensure that the entry portal is no more than 1 cm distal to the anterior edge of the tibial plateau; a more distal entry point may result in damage to the posterior cortex.
- Reflect the skin and subcutaneous tissues medially until the medial border of the patellar tendon is visible, make an incision medial to the tendon and proximal to the tibial tuberosity, and retract the tendon laterally to allow identification of the midpoint of the anterior margin of the tibial plateau.
- Use an awl or cannulated opening reamer over a guidewire to open the medullary canal in the midline. Use image intensification in the sagittal and frontal planes to confirm that the tip of the reamer and guide pin are in the line of the tibial canal.
- Insert the ball tipped guidewire until its tip sits 3 to 4 cm beyond the planned distal end of the nail.
- Reaming begins with an 8-mm flexible reamer and increases in 0.5-mm increments. Ream 2.0 mm beyond the planned implant diameter.
- Connect the appropriate diameter and length PRECICE nail to the proximal guide arm. Verify correct alignment of the proximal interlocking screws by passing a drill bit through the guide and screw hole in the implant.
- Advance the nail to just above the level of the planned osteotomy.
- Remove the guide rod to complete the corticotomy.

OSTEOTOMY

- Complete the osteotomy at the level of the vent holes. The appropriate osteotomy level is commonly at the junction of the upper and middle thirds of the tibia (Fig. 29-116).
- To make the osteotomy, create additional drill holes at the level of the previously placed vent holes. Preserve the periosteum to protect the blood supply to the regenerated bone. Complete the osteotomy with multiple passes with a small osteotome. The posterior cortex may be difficult to cut and can be broken through osteoclasis by rotating the limb.
- Test that the two bone segments rotate freely and independently of each other.

NAIL INSERTION (CONT'D)

- Advance the nail beyond the osteotomy to the desired level.
- Using the proximal screw guide, place two bicortical locking screws.
- With a freehand technique (see Chapter 53), insert two distal locking screws.

CLOSURE

- After careful irrigation to remove any remaining bone fragments from the proximal wound, insert closed suction drainage, close the incisions in layers in the usual fashion, and apply firm dressings to prevent hematoma formation.

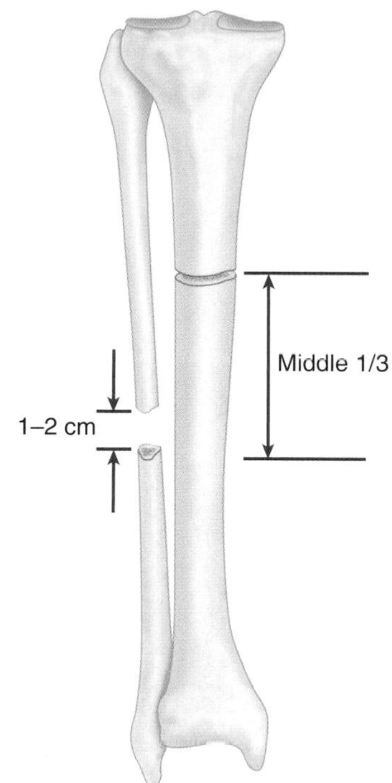

FIGURE 29-116 **Location of osteotomies for tibial lengthening with intramedullary skeletal kinetic distractor (see text).** (From Cole JD: Intramedullary skeletal kinetic distractor: tibial surgical technique: technique manual, Orthofix, McKinney, Tex.) **SEE TECHNIQUE 29-47.**

INTRAOPERATIVE EXTERNAL REMOTE CONTROL (ERC) DISTRACTION

- Locate the center of the magnet with image intensification and mark the skin. The mark should be frequently refreshed postoperatively.
- Place the ERC in a sterile bag and place over the skin mark.
- Activate the ERC to distract the PRECICE nail 1.0-2.0 mm to verify correct functioning of the system. It takes 7 minutes for 1.0 mm of lengthening. It is not necessary to retract the device.

POSTOPERATIVE CARE. The drains are removed at 24 to 48 hours after surgery. Partial weight bearing with crutches is allowed at 1 week and is continued throughout the lengthening and consolidation phases. Full weight bearing is not allowed until cortication of the regenerated bone is evident in three of four cortices during the end of the consolidation phase. Isometric exercises for the whole limb are encouraged early. Gentle knee mobilization can be started after about 4 days within the limits of comfort. Lengthening should be initiated 7 to 8 days after surgery. Daily lengthenings are typically 0.5-1.0 mm divided into two to four sessions. The physician and his staff should properly train the patient on use of the ERC. Weekly radiographic evaluation is important to monitor progress. Removal of the PRECICE is recommended 12-18 months after radiographic evidence of full bony consolidation.

FEMORAL LENGTHENING

TECHNIQUE 29-48

(DEBASTIANI ET AL.)

- Place the patient supine on a radiolucent table.
- Use the mated drills, drill guides, and screw guides to insert the conical self-tapping cortical and cancellous screws.
- Insert a cortical screw at the level of the lesser trochanter, perpendicular to the shaft of the femur.
- Attach the rigid template and insert the distalmost screw, lining the template up parallel to the shaft of the femur.
- Return to the proximal end of the template and insert the next screw in the fourth template hole distal to the upper screw. The last screw to be placed is in the distal template, in the hole farthest away from the distalmost screw.
- Remove the template and perform a corticotomy 1 cm distal to the proximal two screws (just distal to the iliopsoas insertion).
- Incise the anterior thigh skin longitudinally and dissect bluntly between the sartorius muscle and the tensor fasciae latae muscle and through the substance of the vastus intermedius and rectus femoris muscles. Incise the periosteum longitudinally and elevate it laterally and medially.
- Under direct vision, drill a series of 4.8-mm unicortical holes in the visible aspect of the anterior two thirds of the circumference of the femur (Fig. 29-117A). Set the drill stop at 1 cm to prevent penetration of the marrow.
- Use a thin osteotome to connect the drill holes without violating the marrow. Flex the femur at the corticotomy to crack the posterior cortex, completing the corticotomy. Do not use the Orthofix pins as handles to complete the corticotomy, or they may loosen.
- Reduce the fracture and apply the Orthofix lengthener. If the Orthofix fracture-fixation device is used, fix the ball joint rigidly with a small amount of methylmethacrylate. The Orthofix slide-lengthening device can be used with or without swivel clamps.
- If swivel clamps are used, blocking them with methylmethacrylate should be considered. The slide lengthener is especially useful for double-level lengthening.

Price recommended acute valgus of a few degrees for subtrochanteric lengthening to help prevent the common problem of varus at this level. Adductor tenotomy also is advised. Suture the periosteum and close the skin over drains. The use of six pins has been recommended for femoral lengthening to gain stability and to resist a tendency for varus deviation (Fig. 29-117B).

POSTOPERATIVE CARE. Postoperative care is the same as that for tibial lengthening (Technique 29-46).

FEMORAL LENGTHENING

TECHNIQUE 29-49

(ILIZAROV, MODIFIED)

- Frame preconstruction includes the following considerations. The standard femoral lengthening frame consists of a proximal fixation block made of two arcs, a distal fixation block made of two identically sized rings, and an

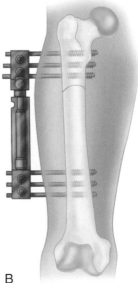

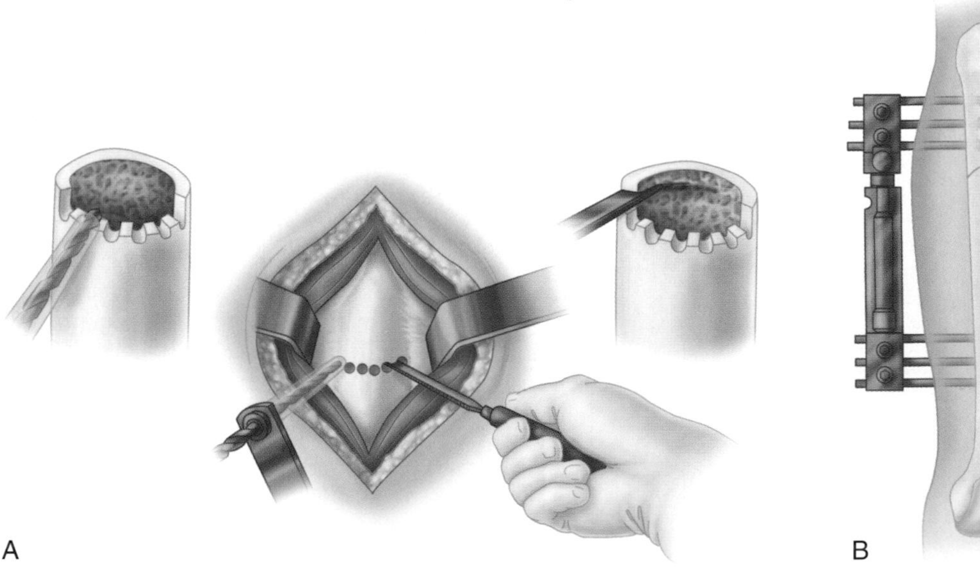

FIGURE 29-117 **A,** DeBastiani technique for corticotomy. Using limited open exposure and a 4 or 5 mm drill, multiple holes are drilled in anterior half of bone. These are connected with 5-mm osteotome, which also is used to complete corticotomy posteriorly. **B,** Orthofix device for femoral lengthening. To control varus deviation, three screws are used proximally and three distally, or frame can be applied with prophylactic valgus built into construct. **SEE TECHNIQUES 29-48 AND 29-49.**

"empty" middle ring (usually one size larger than the distal rings) to link the two fixation blocks.
- Preconstruct the frame before surgery to reduce the time spent in the operating room.
- Use the smallest diameter rings that leave sufficient space for swelling after surgery because smaller rings give a more mechanically stable construct. There should be one fingerbreadth of space between the distal ring and the anterior thigh and two fingerbreadths posteriorly at the largest diameter of the posterior calf muscles. The distalmost ring can be a ⅝-inch ring to allow more knee flexion after surgery. This is especially important if there is to be a simultaneous lengthening of the ipsilateral tibia with proximal tibial rings. (Full rings would touch each other after relatively little knee flexion, limiting knee mobility.)
- Connect the bottom two rings initially with two 20-mm or 40-mm threaded hexagonal sockets for better stability, one positioned directly anteriorly and one directly posteriorly. With newer carbon fiber rings, it is possible to "cut out" the back portion of the distal ring as needed to improve knee flexion and to prevent impingement against a tibial construct. Appropriate reinforcement to the nearest ring is required before the carbon fiber ring is cut. In small patients, there may be room distally for only one ring and a drop wire.
- Plan the frame so that the central connection bolts are centered directly over the anterior and posterior midlines.
- Choose two parallel arcs to match the contour of the proximal lateral thigh, usually a 90-degree arc most proximally and a 120-degree arc below it; this causes less impingement of the proximal end of the fixator against the lower abdomen and pelvis during hip flexion.
- Connect the two arcs with two 40-mm hexagonal sockets. The reach of the 120-degree arc can be extended by attaching two oblique supports off the first and last holes on the arc.
- Attach the oblique support to the empty middle ring, which does not hold any wires, but allows a more even 360-degree push-off between the distal and proximal fixation blocks.
- Connect the empty middle ring to the distal fixation block with two threaded rods, one placed anteriorly and one medially, to align the empty ring with the distal ring block anteriorly and medially where the soft-tissue sleeve of the thigh is minimal, and the larger, empty ring placed laterally and posteriorly where extra skin clearance is required. It may be necessary later to build out from the distal block laterally and posteriorly with short connection plates to have additional threaded rods or graduated telescopic rods in these locations.
- For placement of reference wires, position the patient supine with a folded sheet under the ipsilateral buttock. A radiolucent table that splits at the lower extremities, allowing removal of the part of the table under the involved leg, is helpful. Place the foot on a Mayo stand or other small table to permit flexion and extension of the knee and hip to allow assessment of acceptable placement of the wires in the soft tissues around the knee.
- Use fluoroscopy to guide insertion of the distal reference wire. In the distal femur, use 1.8-mm wires, and in the proximal femur, use 5-mm conical self-drilling, self-tapping screws. If preferred, other heavy-gauge half-pins, especially those designed to be predrilled, can be substituted. When using conical pins, be careful not to back them out once they have been inserted, or they will loosen.
- Under fluoroscopic control, insert as the distal reference wire an olive wire from lateral to medial, almost perpendicular to the mechanical axis of the femur, parallel to the knee joint, but slightly higher on the medial side at the level of the adductor tuberosity.
- For the proximal reference pin, insert a half-pin just distal to the level of the greater trochanter, parallel to an imaginary line drawn from the tip of the greater trochanter to the center of the femoral head, normally within 3 degrees of parallel to the axis of the knee joint.
- The distal reference wire should be perpendicular to the mechanical axis of the femur, not perpendicular to the anatomic axis (Fig. 29-118A). This is important because lengthening should occur along the mechanical axis rather than the shaft axis. Failure to adhere to this principle disrupts the normal mechanical axis and causes medialization of the knee.
- Secure the preassembled frame to the top reference pin and bottom reference wire and ensure that clearance between the skin and the frame is adequate, and that all connections are tight.
- Tension the wires to 130 kg of force after fixing the olive end of the wire to the distal ring. Ensure adequate soft-tissue clearance and use the frame as a guide to insert the proximal half-pin secured with either a monopin fixation clamp or a buckle clamp (Fig. 29-118B and C).
- For fixation, insert two oblique smooth wires on the distal ring and one medial olive wire and an oblique smooth wire on the ring above.
- Some important technical points must be remembered while inserting the wires. When inserting a wire from the anterior to the posterior thigh, first flex the knee 45 degrees as the wire penetrates the anterior skin. Then flex the knee 90 degrees as the wire penetrates the quadriceps muscle. Drill the wire through the femur just to the opposite cortex. Tap the wire through the soft tissue, keeping the knee fully extended as the wire traverses the hamstrings; flex the knee to 45 degrees as the wire exits the skin.
- After each wire has been inserted, move the knee from full extension to 90 degrees of flexion. The wire should "float" in the soft tissue and should not be pulled by the muscle or cause tenting of the skin. This technique of wire placement helps minimize skin irritation and joint contractures.
- If a wire does not exit directly in the plane of the ring, build the ring up to the level of the wire with washers or posts. Do not bend the wire in any plane to make it lie closer to the ring.
- In the proximal arc, add one more pin anteriorly, on the opposite side of the arc, to avoid the reference pin. Do not insert this pin any more medially than the anterior superior iliac spine, or the femoral nerve will be at risk.

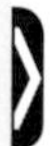

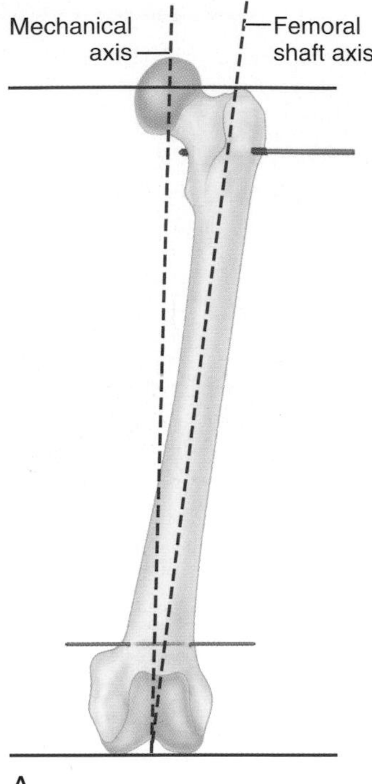

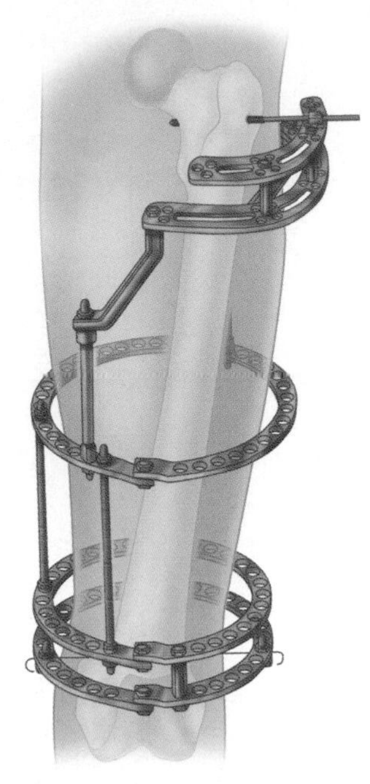

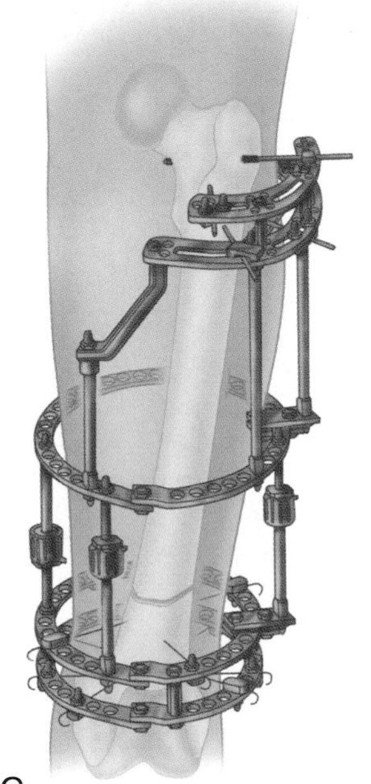

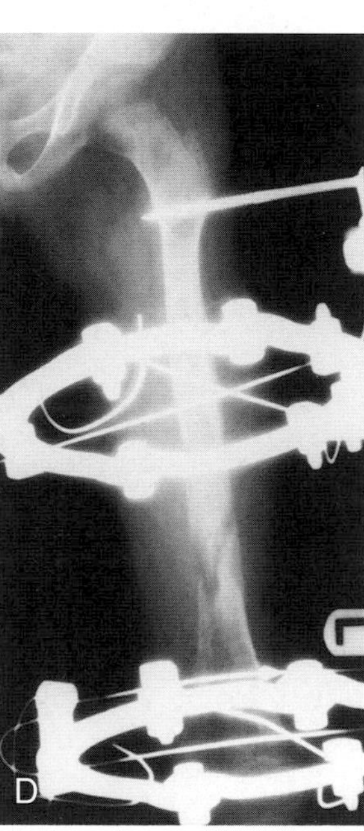

FIGURE 29-118 Application of Ilizarov frame (see text). **A,** Frame is applied perpendicular to mechanical axis, not femoral shaft axis. Distally, reference wire is placed parallel to femoral condyles. Proximally, reference pin is drilled perpendicular to mechanical axis. **B,** Ilizarov femoral lengthening frame is constructed on proximal and distal reference pins. Middle ring is larger in diameter than distal two rings to accommodate conical shape of thigh. **C,** Completed femoral frame. Graduated telescopic distractors are placed in alternating up-down position for greater stability. Olive wires add greater stability to construct. "Empty" middle ring serves as even push-off point. **D,** Modified Ilizarov frame in place after femoral corticotomy for lengthening. **SEE TECHNIQUE 29-49.**

- On the second arc, place two additional pins, one on each side of the arc, in the oblique plane between the two top pins. The ideal mechanical placement of wires and pins should approach 90 degrees when viewed axially, within anatomic limits. A 90-degree fixation spread within a given ring or fixation block resists bending moments in a more uniform manner. Olive wires add mechanical strength to the construct but should not be overused. The olive wires function as fulcrums, acting on the bone to resist or correct axial deviation. Lengthening around the knee tends to angulate into valgus, whereas lengthening near the ankle and hip tends to angulate into varus. All sites are prone to anterior angulation. The olive wires in the femoral construct are placed strategically to resist valgus angulation. An additional olive wire can be placed opposite the lateral olive wire of the distal ring to lock the distal ring into place, if desired. More recently, an alternative method of distal ring fixation has been used, consisting of one transverse reference wire and two half-pins, one posteromedial and one posterolateral.
- For corticotomy, remove the anterior and medial connecting rods from between the empty ring and the distal fixation block.
- Make a ½-inch incision in the lateral skin just proximal to the distal fixation block. Incising the fascia lata transversely makes the lengthening process easier and diminishes the tendency for valgus angulation.
- Dissect bluntly down to the femur with Mayo scissors and insert a small, sharp periosteal elevator down to the lateral cortex of the femur.
- With a knife, make a longitudinal incision through the periosteum and use the elevator to strip a thin, 1-cm wide section of periosteum anterior and posterior, as much as can be reached.
- Transect the lateral cortex with a ½-inch osteotome; cut the anterior and posterior cortices, including the linea aspera, with a ¼-inch osteotome. Do not violate the medullary canal. Alternatively, make the corticotomy as described by DeBastiani (Fig. 29-117).
- To prevent medial cortex comminution and fracture extension into the distal wires, predrill three 3.2-mm holes in the medial cortex, inserting the drill from the lateral wound.
- Fracture the most medial cortex by bending the femur. Ensure that the fragments show enough motion to indicate complete corticotomy, but do not widely displace them.
- Reduce the fracture and align the proximal and distal fixation blocks parallel to each other.
- Use four upright, threaded rods or short, graduated, telescopic tubes to connect the distal fixation block to the empty ring (Fig. 29-118C). Complete the frame by adding components until there are four connectors between every arc or ring in the frame (Fig. 29-118D).
- Close the skin over a drain if needed and apply a pressure dressing to the lateral wound.
- Dress the wire and pin sites with sponges. Apply rubber stoppers to each wire and pin site before attaching them to the frame. The stoppers help maintain slight pressure on the pin dressings and minimize pin-skin interface motion, which is a prelude to pin site infection. Wrap the

proximal four pins tightly with stretch gauze to minimize skin motion over these pins.

POSTOPERATIVE CARE. Physical therapy and protected weight bearing with crutches are begun immediately. Knee flexion of at least 45 to 75 degrees is encouraged, but the knee is splinted in extension at night. Lengthening is begun at 4 to 6 days after surgery, depending on the age of the child, and progresses at a rate of 0.25 mm four times daily. The patient and family are taught how to lengthen before discharge from the hospital, and a record of lengthening should be maintained. Although lengthening at precisely every 6 hours is desirable, it is far more practical to lengthen at breakfast, lunch, dinner, and bedtime. A preoperative lateral view of the knee is essential to help judge early signs of subluxation, especially during large lengthenings in patients with congenital deficiencies of the femur. Radiographs should be made 7 to 10 days after lengthening is begun to ensure distraction of the corticotomy. If insufficient regenerated bone is present after 4 to 6 weeks, the rate of distraction can be adjusted.

When the desired length has been achieved, the fixator is kept in place until there is corticalization of the regenerated bone. Some surgeons "train" the regenerated bone before fixator removal by placing it under slight compression or by retensioning the wires. Weight bearing and fixator stability are crucial factors in producing healthy regenerated bone. At the time of fixator removal, the knee can be manipulated if necessary, but only before removal of the device. Protected weight bearing and vigorous physical therapy are continued, and activity is increased gradually. When lengthening is complete, knee motion typically is limited to about 40 degrees, but after the frame is removed, motion usually is regained at the rate of 10 to 15 degrees a month.

The Ilizarov frame and application can be modified to correct deviation of the mechanical axis or deformity of the proximal femur. Hinges can be placed at the lengthening corticotomy site to effect angular correction. Proximal deformities can be immediately corrected by percutaneous osteotomy between the two proximal arcs. The arcs are initially angulated relative to one another, the osteotomy is performed, and the arcs are immediately brought into parallel alignment to effect the desired correction. Rotational corrections are best done acutely through a proximal (subtrochanteric) osteotomy at the time of initial frame application. The Taylor Spatial Frame also may be used for distraction osteogenesis (see Chapter 54).

FEMORAL LENGTHENING OVER INTRAMEDULLARY NAIL (PRECICE)

TECHNIQUE 29-50

(STANDARD, HERZENBERG, AND GREEN)

- Venting of the femur is done as described for tibial lengthening (see Technique 29-46).

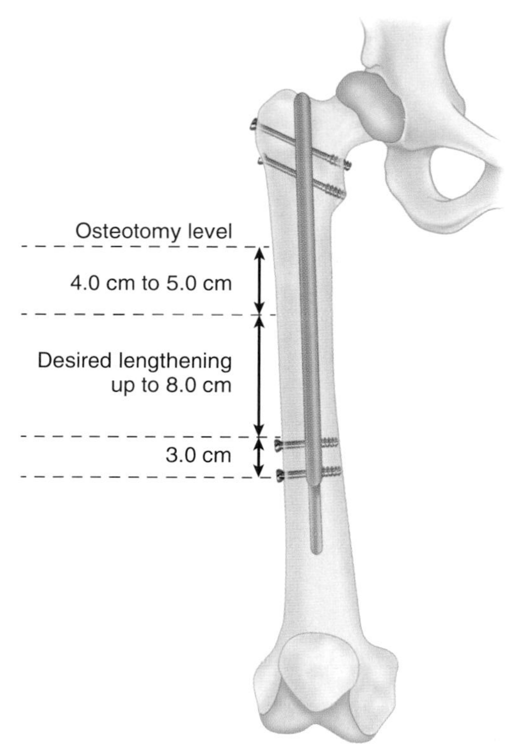

FIGURE 29-119 Osteotomies for femoral lengthening with intramedullary skeletal kinetic distractor (see text). (From Cole JD: Intramedullary skeletal kinetic distractor: femoral surgical technique: technique manual, Orthofix, McKinney, Tex.) **SEE TECHNIQUE 29-50.**

- Place the patient supine or in the lateral decubitus position, depending on surgeon preference and prepare and drape the leg from the anterior superior iliac spine to the proximal tibia.
- Make an osteotomy at the junction of the proximal and middle thirds of the femur unless preexisting bony deformity requires particular positioning of the osteotomy for acute angular correction. As with the tibial technique, do not make the osteotomy in the proximal or distal metaphyseal areas (Fig. 29-119).
- Trochanteric and piriformis entry nails are available. Piriformis entry should be used only on skeletally mature patients because of the risk of osteonecrosis. Alternatively, retrograde nailing combined with distally placed corticotomy can be used (Fig. 29-120).
- Make a 7- to 10-mm incision proximal to the greater trochanter; continue dissection until the tip of the greater trochanter can be palpated. Divide the fibers of the iliotibial band exactly in the middle of the trochanter.
- Check the dimensions of the trochanter by palpation to locate the insertion in the midline; the ideal position is in the piriformis fossa, close to its lateral wall, just medial to the greater trochanter. To avoid injury to the circumflex femoral artery, ensure that the insertion site is not too medial.
- Using a Kirschner wire and cannulated reamer, create the entry to the piriformis fossa just medial to the trochanter, insert the reamer 1 to 2 cm, and check its position with

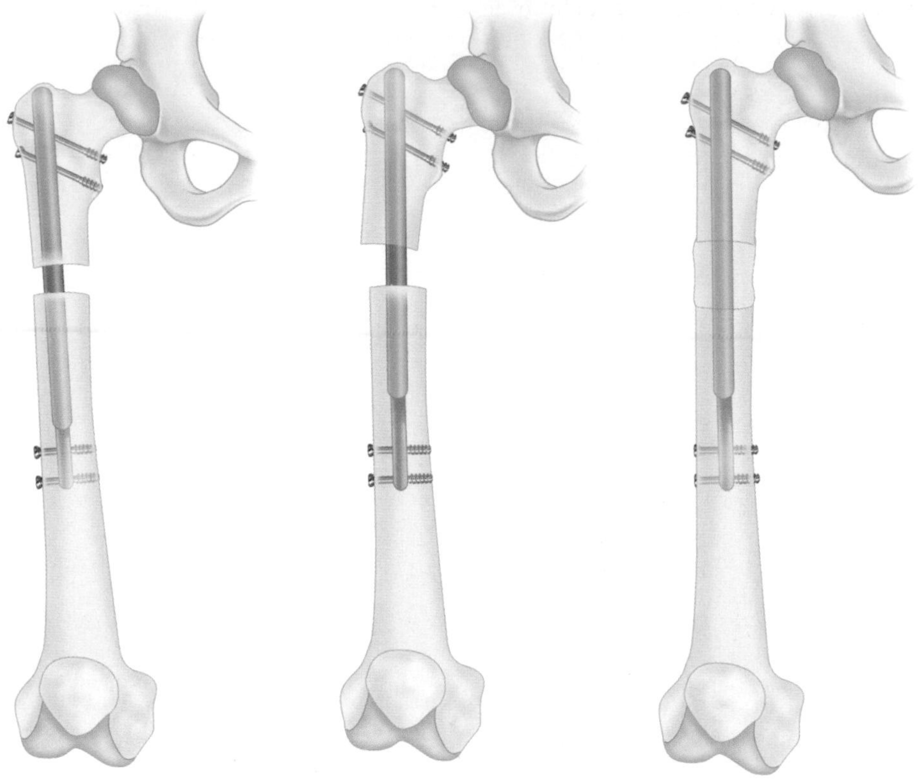

FIGURE 29-120 Retrograde femoral nail. **SEE TECHNIQUE 29-50.**

image intensification to ensure that the tip of the reamer is directly in line with the axis of the diaphysis in the frontal and the sagittal planes.

- When correct position is verified, using gentle pressure and rotational movement, advance the reamer into the femoral canal for 3 to 4 cm, keeping the straight part of the handle in line with the diaphysis.
- Position the guidewire centrally and drive it down until its tip sits in the subchondral bone exactly on the roof of the intercondylar notch, midway between the femoral condyles.
- Starting with an 8-mm reamer, ream the medullary canal with increasingly larger reamers (0.5-mm increments) until a width of 2 mm larger than the proposed lengthener diameter has been obtained.
- Insert the PRECICE nail to the level of the corticotomy.
- Perform the corticotomy as described for the tibial nail (See Technique 29-46).
- Insert the distal and proximal locking screws as described for the tibial nail (see Technique 29-46).

INTRAOPERATIVE EXTERNAL REMOTE CONTROL (ERC) DISTRACTION

- Perform intraoperative external remote control distraction as described for the tibial nail (see Technique 29-46).
- Remove the drill guide and close the incisions in usual fashion. Generally, suction drainage is needed in only the proximal incision (entry portal). Apply a compression dressing and an elastic bandage wrapped around the hip, starting from the foot, to avoid wound seroma.

POSTOPERATIVE CARE. The drain is removed at 24 to 48 hours after surgery. Partial weight bearing with crutches is allowed after 1 week; full weight bearing is not allowed until cortication of the regenerated bone is visible in three of four cortices during the end of the consolidation phase. Isometric exercises are begun early, and gentle knee mobilization can be initiated at about 4 days. Lengthening is initiated 5-7 days after surgery (see Postoperative Care for Technique 29-46).

Complications of Lengthening. All types of limb-lengthening devices and techniques have some complications in common, but certain complications are more or less likely to occur with a given device.

Pin Track Infection. The most common problem is pin track infection, which can be minimized by careful pin insertion. Thin wires should be inserted through the skin directly at the level that the wire enters bone to prevent tenting of the skin. At the end of the procedure, moving the nearby joints through a full range of motion identifies skin tenting over wires, and the sites can be released with a scalpel. The thin transfixion wires may cause fewer problems than the large half-pins, but skin and muscle motion over any wire or pin should be minimized by special dressing techniques. For thin-wire fixators, commercially available 1-inch foam cubes with a slit are placed around the pin site. The slit is stapled to hold the cube in place. Finally, a clip or previously applied rubber stopper is lowered onto the foam to apply mild pressure on the skin. Excessive pressure should be avoided, however, because it can cause ulcerations, especially over bony prominences. For large pins, especially in the thigh, surgical gauze can be wrapped snugly around two or more neighboring pins to apply pressure to the skin around the pins. All wire and pin care should include daily sterilization with an antiseptic, such as povidone-iodine (Betadine) or chlorhexidine gluconate (Hibistat), but only a small amount (1 mL per pin) should be used to avoid skin irritation. If the skin becomes irritated, the solution can be diluted, or a nonirritating antibiotic ointment, such as polymyxin B sulfate-neomycin sulfate (Neosporin), can be used.

At the first sign of pin track infection, broad-spectrum antibiotics should be given, local pin care should be intensified, and the pin site should be incised to promote drainage if necessary. If the infection does not improve with these measures, the pin may have to be removed. If pin removal jeopardizes the stability of the frame, a replacement pin should be inserted. With the Ilizarov apparatus, this is relatively simple: a wire can be placed in a nearby hole or dropped off the ring on a post to avoid the infected pin site. With monolateral fixators, insertion of a replacement pin away from the infected site is more difficult. The Orthofix supplemental screw device can be useful for inserting additional half-pins off-axis. Severe infection usually requires curettage of the pin track and bone.

Muscular Problems. The most difficult complications that occur during lengthening are related to the muscles. Theoretically, the bones can be lengthened by any amount, but the muscles have a limited ability to stretch. Typically, the muscles that cause the most problems are the triceps surae during tibial lengthening and the quadriceps or hamstrings during femoral lengthening. Decreased knee flexion or obligate lateral patellar dislocation with knee flexion after femoral lengthening may require a quadricepsplasty if therapy alone proves insufficient to achieve the desired range of motion. Knee flexion contracture is common during tibial lengthening and can be prevented with prophylactic splinting, especially at night. Custom orthoses or commercially available Dynasplints (Dynasplint Systems, Severna Park, Md) are helpful, and vigorous, frequent physical therapy is crucial. Prophylactic treatment should be started within 1 week of the original surgery. For tibial lengthenings of more than 4 to 5 cm, the foot should be fixed in neutral position by applying a posterior splint for monolateral fixators or by placing two wires in the heel and connecting them to a ring attached to the frame of a thin-wire circular fixator. The heel pins should be removed as soon as possible after lengthening is complete (provided that the knee is not contracted) to allow the subtalar and ankle joints to regain motion. Lengthening of the Achilles tendon should be considered if residual contracture persists. Any preoperative contracture of the Achilles tendon should be corrected before or during tibial lengthening.

Joint Problems. Joint subluxation or dislocation has been reported during femoral lengthening, especially if either the hip or the knee joint is unstable before surgery (as is frequently the case in patients with PFFD). In patients with congenital deformities, prophylactic tenotomies of the rectus femoris proximally, the adductors, and sometimes the hamstrings can be useful. For hips with varus deformities, corrective valgus osteotomy should be delayed until after lengthening. As a general rule, the hip radiograph should show a center-edge angle of at least 15 to 20 degrees before femoral lengthening is considered; otherwise, a preliminary pelvic osteotomy may be necessary. The cruciate ligaments generally are deficient in patients with PFFD, making knee subluxation more likely, and prophylactic fixation of the knee joint with a mobile hinge is possible with the Ilizarov apparatus. A posteriorly dislocated tibia can be slowly pulled anteriorly with a mobile Ilizarov hinge on a rail to reduce the dislocation and allow knee motion. With monolateral fixators, these options are unavailable. For hip subluxation, traction and bed rest usually are sufficient.

Neurovascular Problems. Neurovascular complications usually are related to faulty pin placement, but may result from stretching during lengthening. If the rate of distraction is 1 mm/d, neurovascular tissues almost always are able to stretch to accommodate the lengthening. Decreasing or temporarily stopping the distraction usually is sufficient. If a cutaneous nerve is tented over a wire or pin, removal of the pin is indicated. Peroneal nerve dysfunction that occurs during tibial lengthening should be treated by nerve decompression at the fibular head, extending proximally 5 to 7 cm and distally into the anterior compartment.

Bony Problems. Bony complications of distraction osteogenesis include premature consolidation and delayed consolidation. In Wagner lengthening, common problems are deep infection, pseudarthrosis, plate breakage, and malunion. With distraction osteogenesis by either the Ilizarov or the DeBastiani technique, delayed or premature consolidation usually can be resolved without compromising a satisfactory result. Premature consolidation is caused by an excessive latency period. For femoral lengthening in children, a latency period of 5 days is recommended, and for tibial lengthening, 7 days is recommended. For older patients and patients with compromised vascularity to the limb, longer latency periods may be appropriate. Premature consolidation of the fibula in tibial lengthenings can be prevented by using a standard open osteotomy of the fibula instead of a corticotomy. In some reports of premature consolidation, patients reported successively difficult lengthening until finally a "pop" was felt, followed by brief but intense pain, indicating spontaneous rupture through the consolidated regenerated bone. The bone ends should be brought back to the level of apposition before the rupture, and after a brief latency period, lengthening is resumed. Failure to "back up" can result in cyst formation and nonunion.

Delayed consolidation is more common with diaphyseal lengthening than with metaphyseal corticotomy. Contributing factors include frame instability, overly vigorous corticotomy with excessive periosteal stripping, and a distraction rate that is too rapid, especially after too brief a latency period. Gigli saw osteotomies in thick diaphyseal cortical bone can lead to delayed healing. Underlying medical or nutritional problems and lack of exercise are other contributing factors. In addition to correcting these factors, distraction can be slowed or stopped, the bone can be compressed, or the bone can be alternately compressed and lengthened. Walking and normal use of the limb should always be encouraged. In adults and older children, the best regenerated bone develops in patients who are active and use analgesics sparingly. Autologous cancellous bone grafting of the gap is a final resort, although recent studies have demonstrated some efficacy with an injection of autologous bone marrow aspirate combined with platelet rich plasma.

Extra precautions should be taken during the preparation and draping of the fixator because the pin sites may harbor bacteria. With Wagner lengthening, bone grafting of the gap is expected, but it is easier to drape the monolateral fixators out of the sterile operative site.

Malunion and Axial Deviation. Malunion and axial deviation can be avoided with careful preoperative planning to prevent the introduction of deformity during the lengthening. It is important to remember that intramedullary devices lengthen along the anatomic axis of the bone rather than the mechanical axis of the limb, and this should be taken into consideration when planning the rod insertion, osteotomy level, and direction of initial osteotomy displacement. Malunion also can occur with bending of the regenerate. This often can be avoided by maintaining the rod or external device until adequate consolidation has occurred.

REFERENCES

ANOMALIES OF THE TOES

Choo AD, Mubarak SJ: Longitudinal epiphyseal bracket, *J Child Orthop* 7:449, 2013.

Hop MJ, van der Biezen JJ: Ray reduction of the foot in the treatment of macrodactyly and review of the literature, *J Foot Ankle Surg* 50:434, 2011.

Morrell NT, Fitzpatrick J, Szalay EA: The use of the Tsuge procedure for pedal macrodactyly: relevance in pediatric orthopedics, *J Pediatr Orthop B* 23:260, 2014.

Seok HH, Park JU, Kwo ST: New classification of polydactyly of the foot on the basis of syndactylism, axis deviation, and metatarsal extent of extra digit, *Arch Plast Surg* 40:232, 2013.

ANOMALIES OF THE FOOT

CONGENITAL METATARSUS ADDUCTUS

Paton RW, Choudry Q: Neonatal foot deformities and their relationship to developmental dysplasia of the hip: an 11-year prospective, longitudinal, observational study, *J Bone Joint Surg* 91:655, 2009.

Sankar WN, Weiss J, Skaggs DL: Orthopaedic conditions in the newborn, *J Am Acad Orthop Surg* 17:112, 2009.

CLUBFOOT

Agarwal A, Gupta N: Does initial Pirani score and age influence number of Ponseti casts in children? *Int Orthop* 38:569, 2014.

Ahmed AA: The use of the Ilizarov method in management of relapsed club foot, *Orthopedics* 33:881, 2010.

Al-Aubaidi Z, Lundgaard B, Pedersen NW: Anterior distal tibial epiphysiodesis for the treatment of recurrent equinus deformity after surgical treatment of clubfeet, *J Pediatr Orthop* 31:716, 2011.

Bhargava SK, Tandon A, Prakash M, et al: Radiography and sonography of clubfoot: a comparative study, *Indian J Orthop* 46:229, 2012.

Bor N, Coplan JA, Herzenberg JE: Ponseti treatment for idiopathic clubfoot: minimum 5-year followup, *Clin Orthop Relat Res* 467:1263, 2009.

Bor N, Herzenberg JE, Frick SL: Ponseti management of clubfoot in older infants, *Clin Orthop Relat Res* 444:224, 2006.

Changulani M, Garg N, Bruce CE: Neurovascular complications following percutaneous tendoachilles tenotomy for congenital idiopathic clubfoot, *Arch Orthop Trauma Surg* 127:429, 2007.

Chu A, Labar AS, Sala DA, et al: Clubfoot classification: correlation with Ponseti cast treatment, *J Pediatr Orthop* 30:695, 2010.

Edmondson MC, Oliver MC, Slack R, Tucson KW: Long-term follow-up of the surgically corrected clubfoot, *J Pediatr Orthop B* 16:204, 2007.

El-Adwar KL, Taha Kotb H: The role of ultrasound in clubfoot treatment: correlation with the Pirani score and assessment of the Ponseti method, *Clin Orthop Relat Res* 468:2495, 2010.

El-Deeb KH, Ghoneim AS, El-Adwar KL, Khalil AA: Is it hazardous or mandatory to release the talocalcaneal interosseous ligament in clubfoot surgery? A preliminary report, *J Pediatr Orthop* 27:517, 2007.

El-Mowafi H, El-Alfy B, Refai M: Functional outcome of salvage of residual and recurrent deformities of clubfoot with Ilizarov technique, *Foot Ankle Surg* 15:3, 2009.

Faizan M, Jilani LZ, Abbas M, et al: Management of idiopathic clubfoot by Ponseti technique in children presenting after one year of age, *J Foot Ankle Surg* 54:967, 2015.

Faulks S, Richards BS: Clubfoot treatment: Ponseti and French functional methods are equally effective, *Clin Orthop Relat Res* 467:1278, 2009.

Ferreira RC, Costa MT: Recurrent clubfoot—approach and treatment with external fixation, *Foot Ankle Clin* 14:435, 2009.

Ferreira RC, Costo MT, Frizzo GG, de Fonseca Filho FF: Correction of neglected clubfoot using the Ilizarov external fixator, *Foot Ankle Int* 27:266, 2006.

Freedman JA, Watts H, Otsuka NY: The Ilizarov method for the treatment of resistant clubfoot: is it an effective solution?, *J Pediatr Orthop* 26:432, 2006.

Ganger R, Radler C, Handlbauer A, Grill F: External fixation in clubfoot treatment—a review of the literature, *J Pediatr Orthop B* 21:52, 2012.

Gao R, Tomlinson M, Walker C: Correlation of Pirani and Dimeglio scores with number of Ponseti casts required for clubfoot correction, *J Pediatr Orthop* 34:639, 2014.

Goksan SB, Bursali A, Bilgili F, et al: Ponseti technique for the correction of idiopathic clubfeet presenting up to 1 year of age. A preliminary study in children with untreated or complex deformities, *Arch Orthop Trauma Surg* 126:15, 2006.

Graf A, Hassani S, Krzak J, et al: Long-term outcome evaluation in young adults following clubfoot surgical release, *J Pediatr Orthop* 30:379, 2010.

Gray K, Barnes E, Gibbons P, et al: Unilateral versus bilateral clubfoot: an analysis of severity and correlation, *J Pediatr Orthop B* 23:397, 2014.

Gray K, Gibbons P, Little D, Burns J: Bilateral clubfeet are highly correlated: a cautionary tale for researchers, *Clin Orthop Relat Res* 472:3517, 2014.

Harnett P, Freeman R, Harrison WJ, et al: An accelerated Ponseti versus the standard Ponseti method: a prospective randomised controlled trial, *J Bone Joint Surg* 93:404, 2011.

Hassan FO, Jabaiti S, El tamimi T: Complete subtalar release for older children who had recurrent clubfoot deformity, *Foot Ankle Surg* 16:38, 2010.

Hegazy M, Nasef NM, Abel-Ghani H: Results of treatment of idiopathic clubfoot in older infants using the Ponseti method: a preliminary report, *J Pediatr Orthop B* 18:76, 2009.

Hsu WK, Bhatia NN, Raskin A, Otsuka NY: Wound complications from idiopathic clubfoot surgery: a comparison of the modified Turco and the Cincinnati treatment methods, *J Pediatr Orthop* 27:329, 2007.

Hsu LP, Dias LS, Swaroop VT: Long-term retrospective study of patients with idiopathic clubfoot treated with posterior medial-lateral releases, *J Bone Joint Surg* 95:e27, 2013.

Hui C, Joughin E, Nettel-Aguirre A, et al: Comparison of cast materials for the treatment of congenital idiopathic clubfoot using the Ponseti method: a prospective randomized controlled trial, *Can J Surg* 57:247, 2014.

Janicki JA, Narayanan UG, Harvey BJ, et al: Comparison of surgeon and physiotherapist-directed Ponseti treatment of idiopathic clubfoot, *J Bone Joint Surg* 91:1101, 2009.

Jowett CR, Morcuende JA, Ramachandran M: Management of congenital talipes equinovarus using the Ponseti method: a systematic review, *J Bone Joint Surg* 93:1160, 2011.

Karol LA: Continuous passive motion after surgery in infants with clubfoot led to greater short-term but not long-term improvement relative to standard immobilization, *J Bone Joint Surg* 88:1167, 2006.

Kuo KN, Smith PA: Correcting residual deformity following clubfoot releases, *Clin Orthop Relat Res* 467:1326, 2009.

Mahan ST, Spencer SA, Kasser JR: Satisfactory patient-based outcomes after surgical treatment for idiopathic clubfoot: includes surgeon's individualized technique, *J Pediatr Orthop* 34:631, 2014.

Maripuri SN, Gallacher PD, Bridgens J, et al: Ponseti casting for club foot—above—or below-knee?: A prospective randomised clinical trial, *Bone Joint J* 95B:1570, 2013.

McKay SD, Dolan LA, Morcuende JA: Treatment results of late-relapsing idiopathic clubfoot previously treated with the Ponseti method, *J Pediatr Orthop* 32:406, 2012.

Merrill LJ, Gurnett CA, Siegel M, et al: Vascular abnormalities correlate with decreased soft tissue volumes in idiopathic clubfoot, *Clin Orthop Relat Res* 469:1442, 2011.

Morcuende JA, Abbasi D, Dolan LA, Ponseti IV: Results of an accelerated Ponseti protocol for clubfoot, *J Pediatr Orthop* 25:623, 2005.

Morgenstein A, Davis R, Talwalkar V, et al: A randomized clinical trial comparing reported and measured wear rates in clubfoot bracing using a novel pressure sensor, *J Pediatr Orthop* 2014. [Epub ahead of print].

Mubarak SJ, Van Valin SE: Osteotomies of the foot for cavus deformities in children, *J Pediatr Orthop* 29:294, 2009.

Parada SA, Baird GO, Auffant RA, et al: Safety of percutaneous tendoachilles tenotomy performed under general anesthesia on infants with idiopathic clubfoot, *J Pediatr Orthop* 29:916, 2009.

Pittner DE, Klingele KE, Beebe AC: Treatment of clubfoot with the Ponseti method: a comparison of casting materials, *J Pediatr Orthop* 28:250, 2008.

Prem H, Zenios M, Farrell R, Day JB: Soft tissue Ilizarov correction of congenital talipes equinovarus—5 to 10 years postsurgery, *J Pediatr Orthop* 27:220, 2007.

Saghieh S, Bashoura A, Berjawi G, et al: The correction of the replapsed club foot by closed distraction, *Strategies Trauma Limb Reconstr* 5:127, 2010.

Scher DM, Feldman DS, van Bosse HJ, et al: Predicting the need for tenotomy in the Ponseti method for correction of clubfeet, *J Pediatr Orthop* 24:349, 2004.

Shack N, Eastwood DM: Early results of a physiotherapist-delivered Ponseti service for the management of idiopathic congenital talipes equinovarus foot deformity, *J Bone Joint Surg* 88:1085, 2006.

Silvani S: The Ponseti technique for treatment of talipes equinovarus, *Clin Podiatr Med Surg* 23:119, 2006.

Steinman S, Richards BS, Faulks S, Kaipus K: A comparison of two nonoperative methods of idiopathic clubfoot correction: the Ponseti method and the French functional (physiotherapy) method. Surgical technique, *J Bone Joint Surg* 91(Suppl 2):299, 2009.

Terrazas-Lagargue G, Morcuende JA: Effect of cast removal timing in the correction of idiopathic clubfoot by the Ponseti method, *Iowa Orthop J* 27:24, 2007.

Tripathy SK, Saini R, Sudes P, et al: Application of the Ponseti principle for deformity correction in neglected and relapsed clubfoot using the Ilizarov fixator, *J Pediatr Orthop B* 20:26, 2011.

Van Bosse HJ: Treatment of the neglected and relapsed clubfoot, *Clin Podiatr Med Surg* 30:513, 2013.

Xu RJ: A modified Ponseti method for the treatment of idiopathic clubfoot: a preliminary report, *J Pediatr Orthop* 31:317, 2011.

Yong SM, Smith PA, Kuo KNK: Dorsal bunion after clubfoot surgery: outcome of reverse Jones procedure, *J Pediatr Orthop* 27:814, 2007.

Zhang W, Richards BS, Faulks ST, et al: Initial severity rating of idiopathic clubfeet is an outcome predictor at age two years, *J Pediatr Orthop B* 21:16, 2012.

CONGENITAL VERTICAL TALUS

Aslani H, Sadigi A, Tabrizi A, et al: Primary outcomes of the congenital vertical talus correction using the Dobbs method of serial casting and limited surgery, *J Child Orthop* 6:307, 2012.

Chalayon O, Adams A, Dobbs MB: Minimally invasive approach for the treatment of nonisolated congenital vertical talus, *J Bone Joint Surg* 94:e73, 2012.

David MG: Simultaneous correction of congenital vertical talus and talipes equinovarus using the Ponseti method, *J Foot Ankle Surg* 50:494, 2011.

Dobbs MB, Purcell DB, Nunley R, Morcuende JA: Early results of a new method of treatment for idiopathic congenital vertical talus. Surgical technique, *J Bone Joint Surg* 89(Suppl 2):111, 2007.

Eberhardt O, Fernandez FF, Wirth T: The talar axis-first metatarsal base angle in CVT treatment: a comparison of idiopathic and nonidiopathic cases treated with the Dobbs method, *J Child Orthop* 6:491, 2012.

Kruse L, Gurnett CA, Hootnick D, Dobbs MB: Magnetic resonance angiography in clubfoot and vertical talus: a feasibility study, *Clin Orthop Relat Res* 467:1250, 2009.

Merrill LJ, Gurnett CA, Connolly AM, et al: Skeletal muscle abnormalities and genetic factors related to vertical talus, *Clin Orthop Relat Res* 469:1167, 2011.

Thometz JG, Zhu H, Liu XC, et al: MRI pathoanatomy study of congenital vertical talus, *J Pediatr Orthop* 30:360, 2010.

Wright J, Coggings D, Maizen C, Ramachandran M: Reverse Ponseti-type treatment for children with congenital vertical talus: comparison between idiopathic and teratological patients, *Bone Joint J* 96B:274, 2014.

TARSAL COALITION

Bauer T, Golano P, Hardy P: Endoscopic resection of a calcaneonavicular coalition, *Knee Surg Sports Traumatol Arthrosc* 18:669, 2010.

Crim J: Imaging of tarsal coalition, *Radiol Clin North Am* 46:1017, 2008.

Guignand D, Journeau P, Mainrad-Simard L, et al: Child calcaneonavicular coalitions: MRI diagnostic value in a 19-case series, *Orthop Traumatol Surg Res* 97:67, 2011.

Hetsroni I, Nyska M, Mann G, et al: Subtalar kinematics following resection of tarsal coalition, *Foot Ankle Int* 29:1088, 2008.

Lemley F, Berlet G, Hill K, et al: Current concepts review: Tarsal coalition, *Foot Ankle Int* 27:1163, 2006.

Masquijo JJ, Jarvis J: Associated talocalcaneal and calcaneonavicular coalitions in the same foot, *J Pediatr Orthop B* 19:507, 2010.

Mubarak SJ, Patel PN, Upasani VV, et al: Calcaneonavicular coalition: treatment by excision and fat graft, *J Pediatr Orthop* 29:418, 2009.

Nalaboff KM, Schweitzer MD: MRI of tarsal coalition: frequency, distribution, and innovative signs, *Bull NYU Hosp Jt Dis* 66:14, 2008.

Skwara A, Zounta V, Tibesku CO, et al: Plantar contact stress and gait analysis after resection of tarsal coalition, *Acta Orthop Belg* 75:654, 2009.

Upasani VV, Chambers RC, Mubarak SJ: Analysis of calcaneonavicular coalitions using multi-planar three-dimensional computed tomography, *J Child Orthop* 2:301, 2008.

Zaw H, Calder JD: Tarsal coalitions, *Foot Ankle Clin* 15:349, 2010.

CONGENITAL ANGULAR DEFORMITIES OF THE LEG AND CONGENITAL PSEUDARTHROSIS

Cho TJ, Choi IH, Lee KS, et al: Proximal tibial lengthening by distraction osteogenesis in congenital pseudarthrosis of the tibia, *J Pediatr Orthop* 27:915, 2007.

Fabeck L, Ghafil D, Gerroudj M, et al: Bone morphogenetic protein 7 in the treatment of congenital pseudarthrosis of the tibia, *J Bone Joint Surg* 88:116, 2006.

Inan M, ElRassi G, Riddle EC, Kumar SJ: Residual deformities following successful initial bone union in congenital pseudoarthrosis of the tibia, *J Pediatr Orthop* 26:393, 2006.

Johnston CE 2nd: Congenital pseudarthrosis of the tibia: results of technical variations in the Charnley-Williams procedure, *J Bone Joint Surg* 84A:1799, 2002.

Kaufman SD, Fagg JA, Jones S, et al: Limb lengthening in congenital posteromedial bow of the tibia, *Strategies Trauma Lim Reconstr* 7:147, 2012.

Lee Y, Sinocropi SM, Lee FS, et al: Treatment of congenital pseudarthrosis of the tibia with recombinant human bone morphogenetic protein-7 (rhBMP-7). A report of five cases, *J Bone Joint Surg* 88:627, 2006.

Richards BS, Oetgen ME, Johnston CE: The use of rhBMP-2 for the treatment of congenital pseudarthrosis of the tibia: a case series, *J Bone Joint Surg* 92:177, 2010.

Thabet AM, Paley D, Kocaoglu M, et al: Periosteal grafting for congenital pseudarthrosis of the tibia: a preliminary report, *Clin Orthop Relat Res* 446:2981, 2008.

Vander Have KL, Hensinger RN, Caird M, et al: Congenital pseudarthrosis of the tibia, *J Am Acad Orthop Surg* 16:228, 2008.

CONSTRICTIONS OF THE LEG

Choulakian MY, Williams HB: Surgical correction of congenital constriction band syndrome: replacing Z-plasty with direct closure, *Can J Plast Surg* 16:221, 2008.

Das SP, Sahoo P, Mohanty R, Das S: One-stage release of congenital constriction band in lower limb from new born to 3 years, *Indian J Orthop* 44:198, 2010.

Gabos PG: Modified technique for the surgical treatment of congenital constriction bands of the arms and legs of infants and children, *Orthopedics* 29:401, 2006.

Habenicht R, Hülsemann W, Lohmeyer JA, Mann M: Ten-year experience with one-step correction of constriction rings by complete circular resection and linear circumferential skin closure, *J Plast Reconstr Aesthet Surg* 66:1117, 2013.

Mutaf M, Sunay M: A new technique for correction of congenital constriction rings, *Ann Plast Surg* 57:646, 2006.

CONGENITAL HYPEREXTENSION AND DISLOCATION OF THE KNEE, CONGENITAL DISLOCATION OF THE PATELLA

Johnston CE 2nd: Simultaneous open reduction of ipsilateral congenital dislocation of the hip and knee assisted by femoral diaphyseal shortening, *J Pediatr Orthop* 31:732, 2011.

Oetgen ME, Walick KS, Tulchin K, et al: Functional results after surgical treatment for congenital knee dislocation, *J Pediatr Orthop* 30:216, 2010.

Paton RW, Bonshahi AY, Kim WY: Congenital and irreducible non-traumatic dislocation of the patella—a modified soft tissue procedure, *Knee* 11:117, 2004.

Shah NR, Limpaphayom N, Dobbs MB: A minimally invasive treatment protocol for the congenital dislocation of the knee, *J Pediatr Orthop* 29:720, 2009.

Stewart D, Cheema A, Szalay EA: Dual 8-plate technique is not as effective as ablation for epiphysiodesis about the knee, *J Pediatr Orthop* 33:843, 2013.

Sud A, Kumar N, Mehtani A: Femoral shortening in the congenital dislocation of the knee joint: results of mid-term follow-up, *J Pediatr Orthop B* 22:440, 2013.

Tercier S, Shah H, Joseph B: Quadricepsplasty for congenital dislocation of the knee and congenital quadriceps contracture, *J Child Orthop* 6:397, 2012.

Wada A, Fujii T, Takamura K, et al: Congenital dislocation of the patella, *J Child Orthop* 2:119, 2008.

CONGENITAL LONG BONE DEFICIENCIES

TIBIAL AND FIBULAR HEMIMELIA, PROXIMAL FEMORAL FOCAL DEFICIENCY

Birch JG, Lincoln TL, Mack PW, Birch CM: Congenital fibular deficiency: a review of thirty years' experience at one institution and a proposed classification system based on clinical deformity, *J Bone Joint Surg* 93B:1144, 2011.

Carvalho DR, Santos SC, Oliveira MD, Speck-Martins CE: Tibial hemimelia in Langer-Giedion syndrome in 8q23.1-q24.12 interstitial deletion, *Am J Med Genet A* 155A:2784, 2011.

Catagni MA, Radwan M, Lovisetti L, et al: Limb lengthening and deformity correction by the Ilizarov technique in type III fibular hemimelia: an alternative to amputation, *Clin Orthop Relat Res* 469:1175, 2010.

Cho TJ, Baek GH, Lee HR, et al: Tibial hemimelia-polydactyly-five –fingered hand syndrome associated with a 404 G>A mutation in a distant sonic hedgehog cis-regulator (ZRS): a case report, *J Pediatr Orthop B* 22:219, 2013.

Clinton R, Birch JG: Congenital tibial deficiency: a 37-year experience at 1 institution, *J Pediatr Orthop* 35:385, 2015.

Crawford DA, Tompkins BJ, Baird GO, Caskey PM: The long-term function of the knee in patients with fibular hemimelia and anterior cruciate ligament deficiency, *J Bone Joint Surg* 94:328, 2012.

Mascarenhas R, Simon D, Forsythe B, Harner CD: ACL reconstruction in a teenage athlete with fibular hemimelia, *Knee* 21:613, 2014.

Wada A, Fujii T, Takamura K, et al: Limb salvage treatment for congenital deficiency of the tibia, *J Pediatr Orthop* 26:226, 2006.

Wada A, Nakamura T, Fujii T, et al: Limb salvage treatment for Gollop-Wolfgang complex (femoral bifurcation complete tibial hemimelia, and hand ectrodactyly), *J Pediatr Orthop B* 22:457, 2013.

Weber M: New classification and score for tibial hemimelia, *J Child Orthop* 2:169, 2008.

Zarzycki D, Jasiewicz B, Kacki W, et al: Limb lengthening in fibular hemimelia type II: can it be an alternative to amputation?, *J Pediatr Orthop B* 15:147, 2006.

LIMB-LENGTH DISCREPANCY

Burghardt RD, Herzenberg JE, Specht SC, Paley D: Mechanical failure of the intramedullary skeletal kinetic distractor in limb lengthening, *J Bone Joint Surg* 93:6839, 2011.

Burghardt RED, Specht SC, Herzenberg JE: Mechanical failures of eight-PlateGuided Growth System for temporary hemiepiphysiodesis, *J Pediatr Orthop* 30:594, 2010.

Cha SM, Shin HD, Kim KC, Song JH: Plating after tibial lengthening: unilateral monoaxial external fixator and locking plate, *J Pediatr Orthop B* 22:571, 2013.

Escott BG, Ravi B, Weathermon AC, et al: EO low-dose radiography: reliable and accurate upright assessment of lower-limb lengths, *J Bone Joint Surg* 95A:e1831, 2013.

Gordon JE, Manske MC, Lewis TR, et al: Femoral lengthening over a pediatric femoral nail: results and complications, *J Pediatr Orthop* 33:730, 2013.

Harbacheuski R, Fragomen AT, Rozbruch SR: Does lengthening and then plating (LAP) shorten duration of external fixation?, *Clin Orthop Relat Res* 470:2012, 1771.

Inan M, Chan G, Littleton AG, et al: Efficacy and safety of percutaneous epiphysiodesis, *J Pediatr Orthop* 28:648, 2008.

Iobst CA, Dahl MT: Limb lengthening with submuscular plate stabilization: a case series and description of the technique, *J Pediatr Orthop* 27:504, 2007.

Kenawey M, Krettek C, Liodakis E, et al: Leg lengthening using intramedullary skeletal kinetic distraction: results of 57 consecutive applications, *Injury* 42:150, 2011.

Khoury JG, Tavares JO, McConnell S, et al: Results of screw epiphysiodesis for the treatment of limb length discrepancy and angular deformity, *J Pediatr Orthop* 27:623, 2007.

Kocaoglu M, Eralp L, Bilen FE, Balci HI: Fixator-assisted acute femoral deformity correction and consecutive lengthening over an intramedullary nail, *J Bone Joint Surg* 91:152, 2009.

Kristiansen LP, Steen H, Reikeras O: No difference in tibial lengthening index by use of Taylor spatial frame or Ilizarov external fixator, *Acta Orthop* 77:772, 2006.

Lee DH, Ryu KJ, Kim JW, et al: Bone marrow aspirate concentrate and platelet-rich plasma enhanced bone healing in distraction osteogenesis of the tibia, *Clin Orthop Relat Res* 472:3789, 2014.

Lee DH, Ryu KJ, Song HR, Han SH: Complications of the intramedullary skeletal kinetic distractor (ISKD) in distraction osteogenesis, *Clin Orthop Relat Res* 472:3852, 2014.

Martin BD, Cherkashin AM, Tulchin K, et al: Treatment of femoral lengthening-related knee stiffness with a novel quadricepsplasty, *J Pediatr Orthop* 33:446, 2013.

Oh CW, Shetty GM, Song JR, et al: Submuscular plating after distraction osteogenesis in children, *J Pediatr Orthop B* 17:265, 2008.

Oh CW, Song HR, Kim JW, et al: Limb lengthening with a submuscular locking plate, *J Bone Joint Surg* 91:1394, 2009.

Park HW, Kim HW, Kwak YH, et al: Ankle valgus deformity secondary to proximal migration of the fibula in tibial lengthening with use of the Ilizarov external fixator, *J Bone Joint Surg* 93:294, 2011.

Popkov D, Popkov A, Haumont T, et al: Flexible intramedullary nail use in limb lengthening, *J Pediatr Orthop* 30:910, 2010.

Poutawera V, Stott NS: The reliability of computed tomography scanograms in the measurement of limb length discrepancy, *J Pediatr Orthop B* 19:42, 2010.

Sabharwal S, Shao C, McKeon JJ, et al: Computed radiographic measurement of limb-length discrepancy. Full-length standing anteroposterior radiograph compared with scanogram, *J Bone Joint Surg* 88:2243, 2006.

Sabharwal S, Zhao C: Assessment of lower limb alignment: supine fluoroscopy compared with a standing full-length radiograph, *J Bone Joint Surg* 90:43, 2008.

Sabharwal S, Zhao C, McKeon J, et al: Reliability analysis for radiographic measurement of limb length discrepancy: full-length standing anteroposterior radiograph versus scanogram, *J Pediatr Orthop* 27:46, 2007.

Schiedel F, Elsner U, Gosheger G, et al: Prophylactic titanium elastic nailing (TEN) following femoral lengthening (lengthening then rodding) with one or two nails reduces the risk for secondary interventions after regenerate fractures: a cohort study in monolateral vs. bilateral lengthening procedures, *BMC Musculoskelet Disord* 14:302, 2013.

Vitale MA, Choe JC, Sesko AM, et al: The effect of limb length discrepancy on health-related quality of life: is the "2 cm rule" appropriate?, *J Pediatr Orthop B* 15:1, 2006.

The complete list of references is available online at ***expertconsult.inkling.com****.*

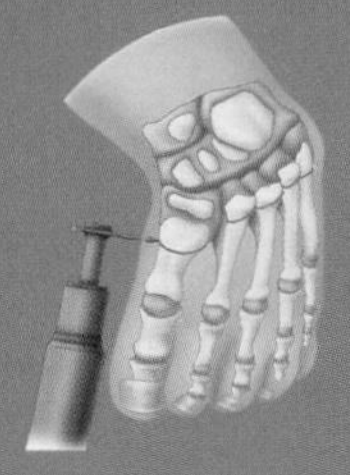

CHAPTER 30

CONGENITAL AND DEVELOPMENTAL ABNORMALITIES OF THE HIP AND PELVIS

Derek M. Kelly

DEVELOPMENTAL DYSPLASIA OF THE HIP

Developmental dysplasia of the hip generally includes subluxation (partial dislocation) of the femoral head, acetabular dysplasia, and complete dislocation of the femoral head from the true acetabulum. In a newborn with true congenital dislocation of the hip, the femoral head can be dislocated and reduced into and out of the true acetabulum. In an older child, the femoral head remains dislocated and secondary changes develop in the femoral head and acetabulum.

Historically, the incidence of developmental dysplasia of the hip has been estimated to be approximately 1 in 1000 live births. A metaanalysis of the literature estimated the incidence of developmental dysplasia of the hip (DDH) revealed by physical examination done by pediatricians to be 8.6 per 1000; for orthopaedic screening, 11.5 per 1000; and for ultrasound examination, 25 per 1000. The estimated odds ratio for DDH for breech delivery was 5.5, for female sex, 4.1 and for positive family history, 1.7. Ultrasound screening of 18,060 hips detected 1001 that deviated from normal (incidence of 55.1 per 1,000); however, only 90 hips remained abnormal at repeat examinations at 2 and 6 weeks, for a true DDH incidence of 5 per 1000. None of the other hips with "sonographic DDH" developed true DDH during 12-month follow-up. The left hip is more commonly involved than the right, and bilateral involvement is more common than involvement of the right hip alone.

Several risk factors should arouse suspicion of developmental dysplasia of the hip. The disorder is more common in girls than in boys—in many series five times more common. Breech deliveries constitute 3% to 4% of all deliveries, and the incidence of developmental dysplasia of the hip is significantly increased in this patient population. MacEwen and Ramsey in a study of 25,000 infants found the combination of female infants and breech presentation to result in developmental dysplasia of the hip in one out of 35 such births. Developmental dysplasia of the hip is more common in firstborn children than in subsequent siblings. A family history of developmental dysplasia of the hip increases the likelihood of this condition to approximately 10%. Ethnic background plays some role in that developmental dysplasia of the hip is more common in white children than in black children. Other reported examples include the high incidence among Navajo Indians and the relatively low incidence among Chinese.

A strong association also exists between developmental dysplasia of the hip and other musculoskeletal abnormalities, such as congenital torticollis, metatarsus adductus, and talipes calcaneovalgus. The coexistence rate of congenital muscular torticollis and DDH is approximately 8%, with boys nearly five times as likely to have both as girls. The relationship between DDH and clubfoot is controversial; however, multiple studies have demonstrated very little association between the presence of clubfoot and DDH. We recommend careful screening by performing hip physical examination in every infant who has a clubfoot deformity. Although we do not perform ultrasound routinely on all these babies, we have a low threshold to obtain a screening hip ultrasound evaluation in this patient population.

Several theories regarding the cause of developmental dysplasia of the hip have been proposed, including mechanical factors, hormone-induced joint laxity, primary acetabular dysplasia, and genetic inheritance. Breech delivery, with the mechanical forces of abnormal flexion of the hips, can easily be seen as a cause of dislocation of the femoral head. The most common intrauterine position places the left hip of the fetus against the maternal sacrum. This could partially explain the increased incidence of DDH in the left hip. Postnatal mechanical factors also could play a role. An increased incidence of developmental dysplasia of the hip has been reported in cultures that swaddle infants with the hip in constant extension.

Several authors have proposed ligamentous laxity as a contributing factor in developmental dysplasia of the hip. The theory is that the influence of the maternal hormone relaxin, which produces relaxation of the pelvis during delivery, may cause enough ligamentous laxity in the child in utero and during the neonatal period to allow dislocation of the femoral head. This theory has credibility because relaxin has been shown to cross the placenta, and DDH is more common in females who are presumably more susceptible to the influences of relaxin.

Wynne-Davies described a familial occurrence of a "shallow" acetabulum, defined as a "dysplasia trait," in proposing primary acetabular dysplasia as one of the risk factors for developmental dysplasia of the hip. The risk of a genetic influence was noted by Ortolani, who reported a 70% incidence of a positive family history in children with developmental dysplasia of the hip.

DIAGNOSIS AND CLINICAL PRESENTATION

The clinical presentation of developmental dysplasia of the hip varies according to the age of the child. In newborns (<6 months old), it is especially important to perform a careful clinical examination because radiographs are not always reliable in making the diagnosis of developmental dysplasia in this age group.

The infant should be calm, relaxed, and pacified during the examination, and only one hip should be examined at a time. The examiner places his or her hand around the infant's knees so that the thumb lies on the inner thigh and the index and long fingers lie at the level of the greater trochanter. The Ortolani test is performed by gently abducting the flexed hip while applying an anteromedially directed force to the greater trochanter to detect any reduction of the femoral head into the true acetabulum. The provocative maneuver of Barlow detects any potential subluxation or posterior dislocation of the femoral head by direct pressure on the longitudinal axis of the femur while the hip is in adduction. A palpable, rather than an audible, clunk is felt as the femoral head reduces into or subluxes out of the acetabulum (Fig. 30-1).

A child may be born with acetabular dysplasia without dislocation of the hip, and the latter may develop weeks or months later. Westin et al. reported the late development of dislocation of the hip in children with normal neonatal clinical and radiographic examinations; they termed this *developmental dysplasia* as opposed to *congenital dysplasia* of the hip as it was previously known.

As the child reaches age 6 to 18 months, several factors in the clinical presentation change. When the femoral head is dislocated and the ability to reduce it by abduction has disappeared, several other clinical signs become obvious. The first and most reliable is a decrease in the ability to abduct the dislocated hip because of a contracture of the adductor musculature (Fig. 30-2A). Asymmetric skin folds are commonly mentioned as a sign to look for, but this sign is not always reliable because normal children may have asymmetric skin folds and children with dislocated hips may have symmetric folds. In general, the rate of DDH is much higher in hips with at least one abnormal clinical finding than in hips without any. Limitation of abduction and asymmetric skin folds are the two most common findings.

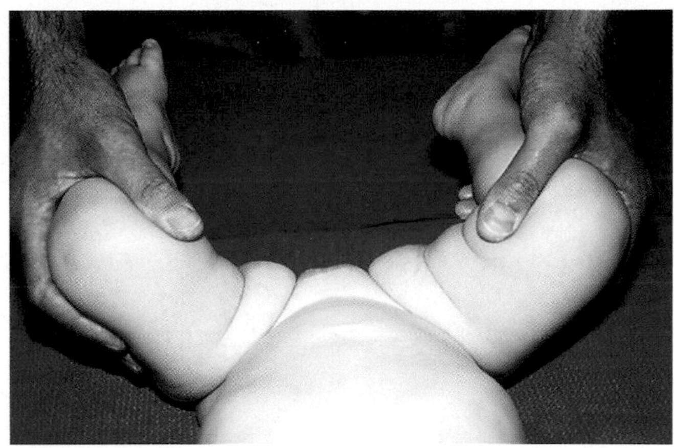

FIGURE 30-1 Ortolani maneuver for routine screening of congenital dislocation of hip. Examiner gently stabilizes infant's left hip and lower extremity and places left hand around right thigh and index and middle fingers over greater trochanter.

The Galeazzi sign is noted when the femoral head becomes displaced not only laterally but also proximally, causing an apparent shortening of the femur on the side of the dislocated hip (Fig. 30-2B). Bilateral dislocations may appear symmetrically abnormal.

In a child of walking age with an undetected dislocated hip, families describe a "waddling" type of gait, indicating dislocation of the femoral head and a Trendelenburg gait pattern. Parents also may describe difficulty in abducting the hip during diaper changes.

SCREENING

The American Academy of Pediatrics recommends routine screening examination of all infants but does not recommend routine ultrasound evaluation of all newborns. Referral to an orthopaedist is recommended with a positive newborn examination or a positive result at 2-week follow-up examination. Ultrasound is recommended for physical examination findings or risk factors that raise suspicion for DDH when the Ortolani and Barlow tests are negative.

The American Academy of Orthopedic Surgeons developed clinical practice guidelines in 2014 for the detection and nonoperative management of pediatric developmental dysplasia of the hip in infants up to 6 months of age. Their recommendations related to screening and imaging include:

1. Moderate evidence supports not performing universal ultrasound screening of newborn infants.
2. Moderate evidence supports performing an imaging study before 6 months of age in infants with one or more of the following risk factors: breech presentation, family history, or history of clinical instability.
3. Limited evidence supports that the practitioner might obtain an ultrasound in infants younger than 6 weeks of age with a positive instability examination to guide the decision to initiate brace treatment.
4. Limited evidence supports the use of an anteroposterior pelvic radiograph instead of an ultrasound to assess DDH in infants beginning at 4 months of age.

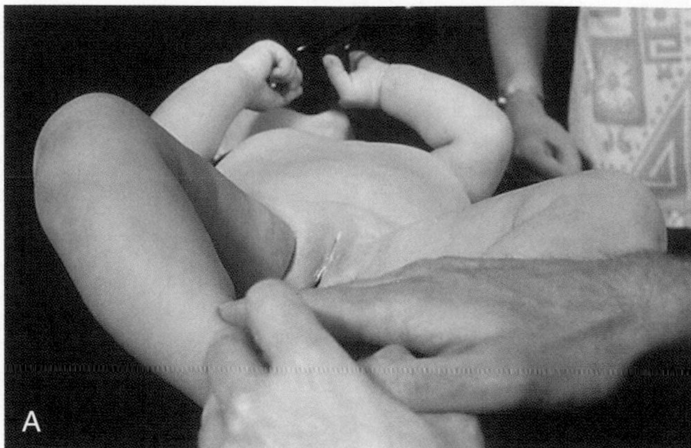
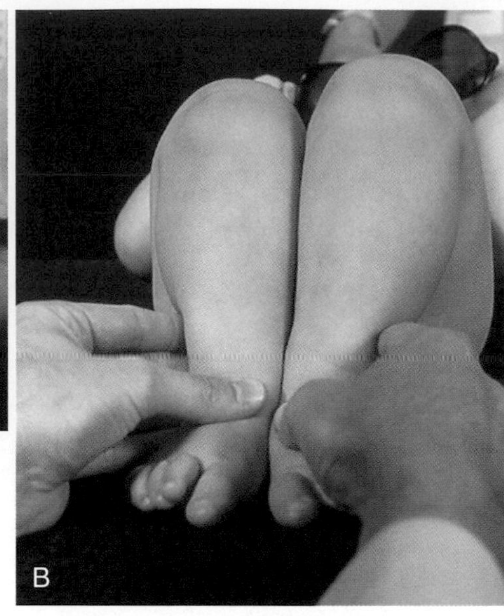

FIGURE 30-2 Clinical signs of congenital dislocation of hip in 13-month-old infant. **A,** Decrease in abduction of right hip with adduction contracture. **B,** Positive Galeazzi sign with apparent shortening of right lower extremity.

5. Limited evidence supports that a practitioner reexamine infants previously screened as having a normal hip examination on subsequent visits prior to 6 months of age.
6. Limited evidence supports that the practitioner perform serial physical examinations and periodic imaging assessments (ultrasound or radiograph based on age) during management for unstable infant hips.

IMAGING

Many reports have evaluated the use of ultrasound screening of newborns for early diagnosis of developmental dysplasia of the hip. The most comprehensive accounts of the anatomy of the infant hip by ultrasound are by Graf of Austria, who described the ultrasonographic anatomy of the newborn hip and devised an ultrasonographic classification for hip dysplasia (Fig. 30-3). Although ultrasound is noninvasive and relatively simple to use, many authors have emphasized that the examination is highly observer dependent and that it is easy to overdiagnose "dysplasia." In addition, ultrasound findings before 6 weeks of age can be questionable because of ligamentous laxity in the early newborn period; treatment before 6 weeks of age should be based on physical examination rather than ultrasound findings alone. Ultrasound diagnosis of "acetabular dysplasia" with a stable hip examination in the early postnatal period may result in unnecessary treatment. Nevertheless, ultrasound can be a useful adjunct to the physical examination and often is helpful in measuring and documenting the response of the hip to Pavlik harness treatment.

Although radiographs are not always reliable in making the diagnosis of developmental dysplasia of the hip in newborns, screening radiographs may reveal any severe acetabular dysplasia or findings of a teratologic dislocation. As a child with a dislocated hip ages and the soft tissues become contracted, radiographs become more reliable and helpful in diagnosis and treatment (Fig. 30-4). The most commonly used lines of reference are the vertical line of Perkins and the horizontal line of Hilgenreiner, both used to assess the position of the femoral head. In addition, the Shenton line is disrupted in an older child with a dislocated hip. Normally, the metaphyseal beak of the proximal femur lies within the inner lower quadrant of the reference lines noted by Perkins and Hilgenreiner. The acetabular index in a newborn generally is 30 degrees or less. Any significant increase in this measurement may be a sign of acetabular dysplasia.

TREATMENT

The treatment of developmental dysplasia of the hip or DDH is age related and tailored to the specific pathologic condition. Five age-related treatment groups have been designated: newborn (birth to 6 months old), infant (6 to 18 months old), toddler (18 to 36 months old), child (3 to 8 years old), and adolescent and young adult (>8 years old). There can be overlap in these age groups that requires modification of treatment plans.

NEWBORN (BIRTH TO 6 MONTHS)

From birth to approximately 6 months old, treatment is directed at stabilizing the hip that has a positive Ortolani or Barlow test or reducing the dislocated hip with a mild-to-moderate adduction contracture. When the diagnosis has been made, either clinically or radiographically, it is essential to carefully evaluate the direction of dislocation, the stability, and the reducibility of the hip before treatment. A success rate of 85% to 95% has been reported in children treated in the Pavlik harness during the first few months of life. As the child ages and soft-tissue contractures develop, along with secondary changes in the acetabulum, the success rate of the Pavlik harness decreases. Attention to detail is required in the use of this harness because the potential complications include osteonecrosis of the femoral head, although this appears to occur in less than 1% of patients.

When properly applied and maintained, the Pavlik harness is a dynamic flexion-abduction orthosis that can produce excellent results in the treatment of dysplastic and

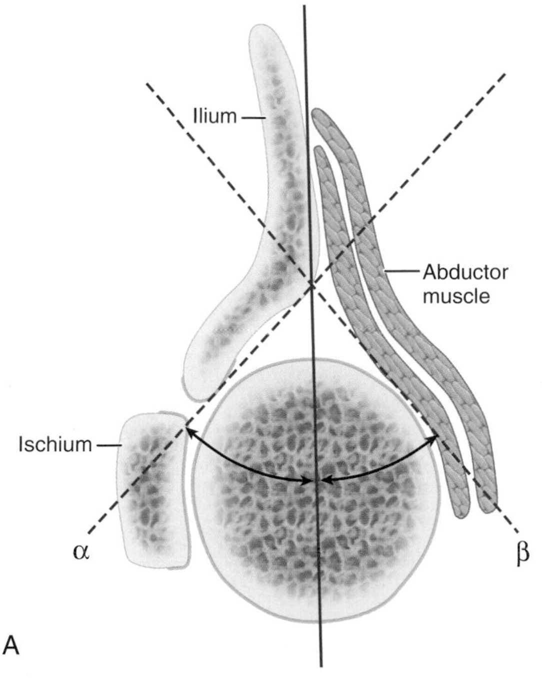

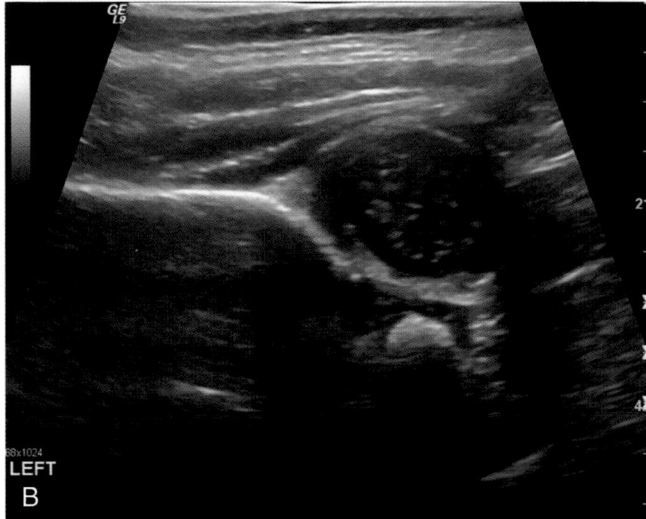

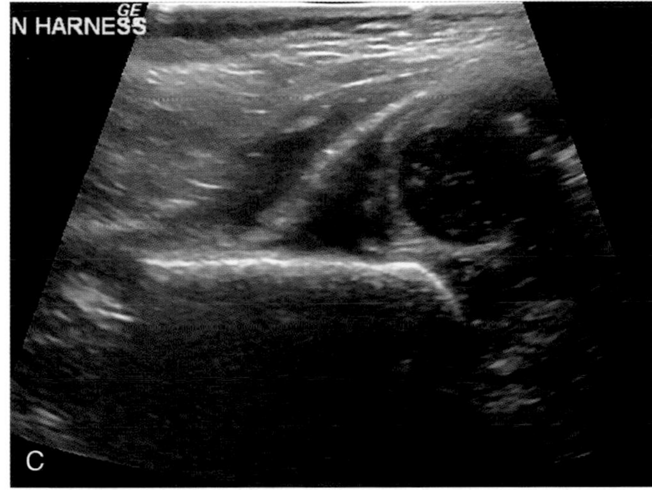

FIGURE 30-3 **A,** Image is rotated 90 degrees clockwise to resemble a hip in the anteroposterior plane in a standing or supine child. Angle α is formed by the intersection of the baseline and the acetabular roofline; it is normally less than 60 degrees. Angle β is formed by the intersection of the baseline and the inclination line; it is normally less than 55 degrees. In a normal hip the baseline should bisect the femoral head. **B,** Ultrasound appearance of a normal hip: α angle of 60 degrees and baseline bisects the femoral head. **C,** Dislocated hip.

dislocated hips in infants during the first few months. The harness is difficult to use in children who are crawling or who have fixed soft-tissue contractures and a fixed hip dislocation. If a teratologic dislocation is present, the Pavlik harness should not be used.

The Pavlik harness consists of a chest strap, two shoulder straps, and two stirrups. Each stirrup has an anteromedial flexion strap and a posterolateral abduction strap. The harness is applied with the child supine and in a comfortable undershirt. The chest strap is fastened first, allowing enough room for three fingers to be placed between the chest and the harness. The shoulder straps are adjusted to maintain the chest strap at the nipple line. The feet are placed in the stirrups one at a time. The hip is placed in flexion (90 to 110 degrees), and the anterior flexion strap is tightened to maintain this position. Finally, the lateral strap is loosely fastened to limit adduction, not to force abduction. Excessive abduction to ensure stability is unacceptable. The knees should be 3 to 5 cm apart at full adduction in the harness (Fig. 30-5).

A radiograph of the patient in the harness can help to confirm that the femoral neck is directed toward the triradiate cartilage, but a radiograph is not routinely necessary. During the first few weeks of harness wear, when the hip feels stable clinically, ultrasound evaluation is appropriate to confirm reduction of the hip.

Four basic patterns of persistent dislocation have been observed after application of the Pavlik harness: *superior, inferior, lateral,* and *posterior.* If the dislocation is superior, additional flexion of the hip is indicated. If the dislocation is inferior, a decrease in flexion is indicated. A lateral dislocation in the Pavlik harness should be observed initially. As long as the femoral neck is directed toward the triradiate cartilage, as confirmed by radiograph or ultrasound, the head may gradually reduce and "dock" into the acetabulum. A persistent posterior dislocation is difficult to treat, and Pavlik

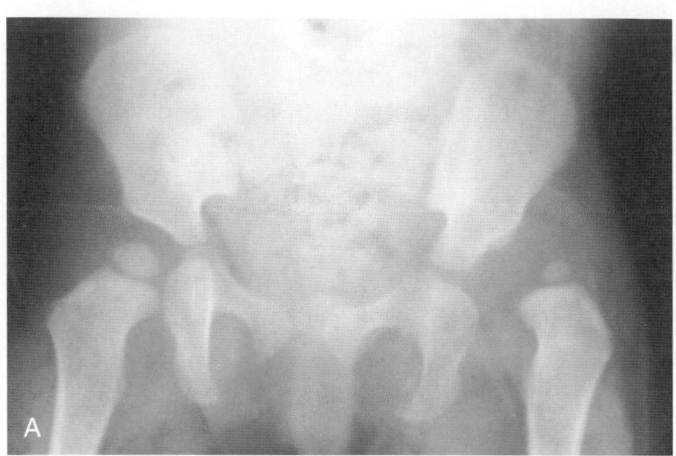

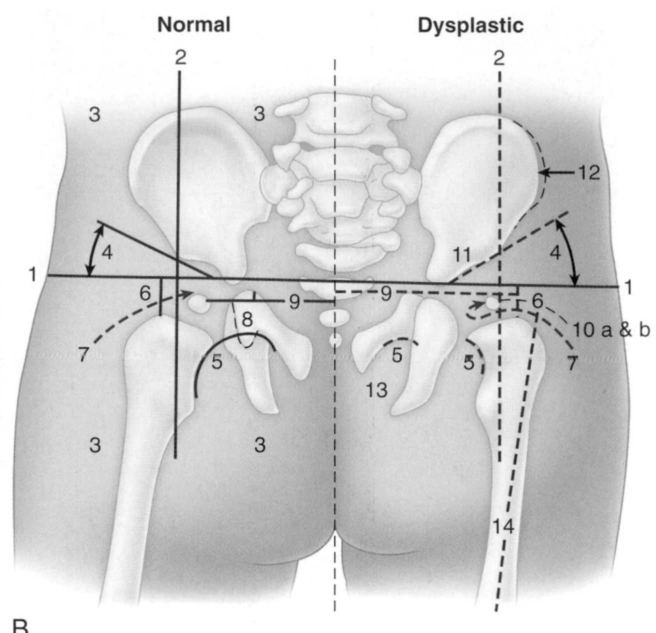

FIGURE 30-4 **A,** Congenital dislocation of left hip in 13-month-old infant. **B,** Radiographic signs of congenital hip dislocation. 1, horizontal line (Hilgenreiner line); 2, vertical line (Perkins line); 3, quadrants (formed by lines 1 and 2); 4, acetabular index (Kleinberg and Lieberman); 5, Shenton line; 6, upward displacement of femoral head; 7, lateral displacement of femoral head; 8, U FIGURE of teardrop shadow (Kohler); 9, Y coordinate (Ponseti); 10, capital epiphyseal dysplasia (a, delayed appearance of center of ossification of femoral head; b, irregular maturation of center of ossification); 11, bifurcation (furrowing of acetabular roof in late infancy (Ponseti); 12, hypoplasia of pelvis (ilium); 13, delayed fusion (ischiopubic juncture); 14, adduction attitude of extremity.

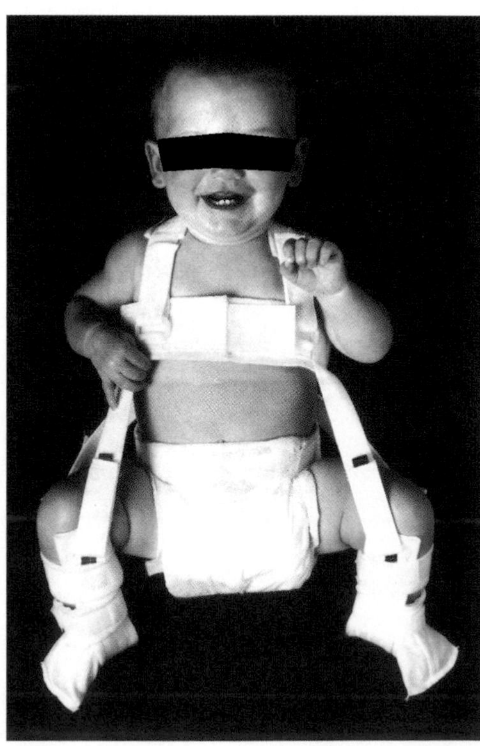

FIGURE 30-5 Properly applied Pavlik harness (see text). (Courtesy of Wheaton Brace, Carol Stream, IL.)

harness treatment frequently is unsuccessful and should be discontinued. Posterior dislocation is usually accompanied by tight hip adductor muscles and may be diagnosed by palpation of the greater trochanter posteriorly.

If any of these patterns of dislocation or subluxation persist for more than 3 to 6 weeks, treatment in the Pavlik harness should be discontinued and a new program initiated; in most patients, this consists of closed or open reduction and casting. The Pavlik harness should be worn full-time until stability is attained, as determined by negative Barlow and Ortolani tests. During this time, the patient is examined at 1- to 2-week intervals and the harness straps are adjusted to accommodate growth. The family is instructed in care of the child in the harness, including bathing, diapering, and dressing.

Quadriceps function should be noted at each examination to detect a femoral nerve palsy, and families should be instructed to remove the legs from the brace daily to ensure that the infant is able to actively extend the knee against gravity. If a femoral nerve palsy develops, the brace should be discontinued until full motor function returns. The duration of treatment depends on the patient's age at diagnosis and the degree of hip instability. There are very few guidelines for brace discontinuation. Recommendations vary from abrupt discontinuation of the Pavlik harness 6 weeks after clinical stability has been obtained, to weaning of up to 2 hours per week until the brace is worn only at night, to transitioning to a nighttime abduction orthosis for additional weeks or months.

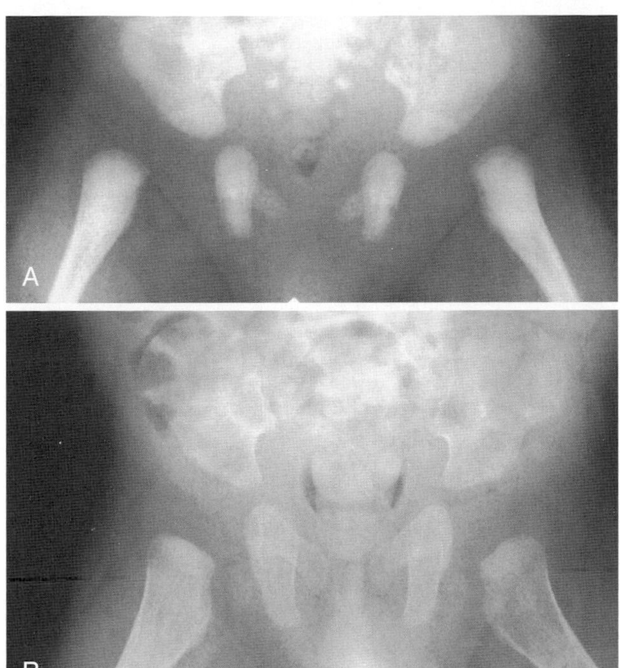

FIGURE 30-6 **A,** Developmental dislocation of hip in 2-month-old boy. **B,** At 5 months of age after reduction in Pavlik harness.

Radiographic or ultrasound documentation can be used throughout the treatment period to verify the position of the hip. Ultrasonographic evaluation is useful at the following times: immediately after the initiation of treatment, after any major adjustment in the harness, when the hip examination is stable after beginning Pavlik harness treatment, and 6 weeks after the hip stabilizes clinically or at the time weaning begins. Radiographs are useful at 6 months old, and also at 1 year old (Fig. 30-6).

Suggested risk factors for Pavlik harness failure include absent Ortolani sign at initial evaluation (irreducible dislocation), bilateral hip dislocations, the development of a femoral nerve palsy during Pavlik treatment, an acetabular angle of 36 degrees or more on a radiograph, irreducible hips, initial coverage of less than 20% (as determined by ultrasound), and delay of Pavlik harness treatment beyond 7 weeks of age. Failure of Pavlik harness management of developmental dislocation of the hip commonly indicates a need for closed or open reduction and a more dysplastic acetabulum.

In multiple series of dislocated hips reduced with the use of the Pavlik harness, the more severe the dislocation, the higher the rates of failed reduction and osteonecrosis, emphasizing the need for gentle reduction and progression to further treatment when the harness fails. Long-term follow-up of patients with Pavlik harness treatment is necessary because many patients have changes in the acetabulum at long-term follow-up despite normal radiographs at 3-year and 5-year follow-up examinations.

INFANT (6 TO 18 MONTHS)

When a child reaches crawling age (4 to 6 months old), success with the Pavlik harness decreases significantly. A 6- to 18-month-old infant with a dislocated hip is likely to require either closed or open reduction.

Children in this age group are often seen initially with a shortened extremity, limited passive abduction, and a positive Galeazzi sign. If the child is walking, a Trendelenburg gait may be present. Radiographic changes include delayed ossification of the femoral head, lateral and proximal displacement of the femoral head, and a shallow, dysplastic acetabulum.

With persistent dysplasia, the femoral head eventually moves superiorly and laterally with weight bearing. The capsule becomes permanently elongated, and anteriorly the psoas tendon may obstruct reduction of the femoral head into the true acetabulum. The limbus acetabuli may hypertrophy along the periphery of the acetabulum, and the ligamentum teres hypertrophies and elongates. The femoral head becomes reduced in size with posteromedial flattening, and coxa valga and excessive anteversion are noted. The true acetabulum is characteristically shallow and at surgery appears small because of the anterior capsular constriction, the hypertrophied limbus, and constriction of the deep acetabular ligament.

Treatment in this age group may include preoperative traction, adductor tenotomy, and closed reduction and arthrogram or open reduction in children with a failed closed reduction. Femoral shortening may be needed in a hip with a high proximal dislocation. Preoperative traction, adductor tenotomy, and gentle reduction with an acceptable "safe zone" are especially helpful in the prevention of osteonecrosis of the femoral head.

PREOPERATIVE TRACTION

The role of preliminary traction in reducing the incidence of osteonecrosis and in improving reduction is controversial. Disagreement exists about whether skin or skeletal traction should be used, whether home or in-hospital traction is preferable, the amount of weight that should be used, the most beneficial direction of pull, and the duration of traction. Although controversial, some suggest that, if traction decreases the risk of osteonecrosis even slightly, the use of a home skin traction program in children with compliant and educated parents spares the expense of hospitalization and allows the child to stay in traction in a home environment. Skeletal traction is not indicated, and primary femoral shortening is now routinely used in older children. The objectives of traction or primary femoral shortening are to bring the laterally and proximally displaced femoral head down to and below the level of the true acetabulum to allow a more gentle reduction with less risk of osteonecrosis.

ADDUCTOR TENOTOMY

A percutaneous adductor tenotomy under sterile conditions can be performed for a mild adduction contracture. For a more severe adduction contracture or one of long duration, an open adductor tenotomy through a small transverse incision is preferable (see Technique 33-1).

ARTHROGRAPHY AND CLOSED REDUCTION

Arthrography and gentle closed reduction are accomplished with the child under general anesthesia.

The interposition of soft tissue in the acetabulum may be suggested by lateralization of the femoral head. Because the radiograph of the hip in an infant or young child cannot yield all the information desired in diagnosing or treating DDH, arthrography is helpful in determining (1) whether mild dysplasia is present, (2) whether the femoral head is subluxated or dislocated, (3) whether manipulative reduction has been or can be successful, (4) to what extent any soft-tissue structures within the acetabulum may interfere with complete reduction of the dislocation, (5) the condition and position of the acetabular labrum (the limbus), and (6) whether the acetabulum and femoral head are developing normally during treatment. Because arthrograms are not always easy to interpret, the surgeon must be thoroughly familiar with the normal and abnormal signs they may reveal and with the technique of making arthrograms.

An arthrogram of the hip is beneficial in all children, regardless of age, who are given a general anesthetic for closed reduction, unless closed reduction is obviously impossible. It is most helpful to determine when manipulative reduction is unstable or when the femoral head is not concentrically seated within the acetabulum. The most important factor that determines outcome of closed treatment of developmental hip dislocation is the quality of the initial reduction. Proposed criteria for accepting a reduction are a medial dye pool of 5 mm or less and maintenance of reduction in an acceptable "safe zone."

The use of image intensification in arthrography makes insertion of the needle much easier. The danger of damaging the articular surfaces by the needle is decreased, and the possibility of injecting the contrast medium directly into the ossific nucleus, the physis, or the medial circumflex artery is prevented.

The findings of the clinical examination and of arthrography at the time of attempted closed reduction determine if the hip will be stable or may require open reduction. A clinical finding that usually indicates an acceptable closed reduction is the sensation of a "clunk" as the femoral head reduces in the true acetabulum. The "safe zone" concept of Ramsey, Lasser, and MacEwen can be used in determining the zone of abduction and adduction in which the femoral head remains reduced in the acetabulum. A wide safe zone (minimum of 20 degrees, preferably 45 degrees) (Fig. 30-7) is desirable, and a narrow safe zone implies an unstable or unacceptable closed reduction. A careful clinical evaluation of the reduction should be made before and after adductor tenotomy and before the arthrogram because when the hip capsule is distended with dye, clinical examination becomes more difficult. An increase in the knee flexion angle (popliteal angle) is another indicator of a successful closed reduction.

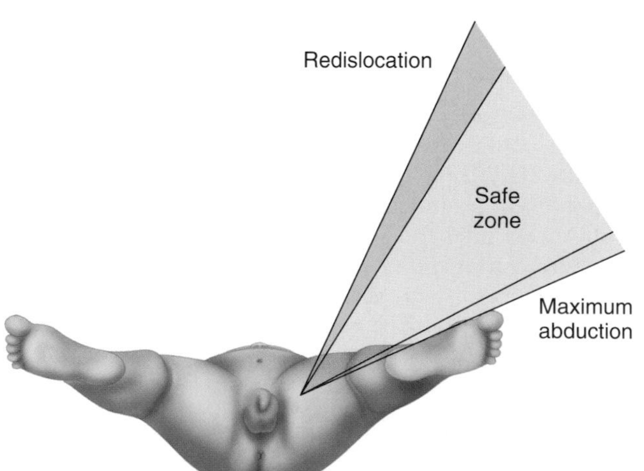

FIGURE 30-7 Safe zone used to determine acceptability of closed reduction of congenital dislocation of hip.

ARTHROGRAPHY OF THE HIP IN DDH

TECHNIQUE 30-1

- Place the child supine after a general anesthetic has been administered. Perform sterile preparation and draping of the hip.
- With a gloved fingertip, locate the hip joint immediately inferior to the middle of the inguinal ligament and one fingerbreadth lateral to the pulsating femoral artery (Fig. 30-8). Alternatively, insert the needle medially, just behind the adductor longus.
- With the assistance of image intensification, insert a 22-gauge spinal needle, to which is attached a 5-mL syringe filled with normal saline solution, until it enters the hip joint; resistance is met as the needle passes through the joint capsule.
- Inject the saline solution into the joint; this is easy at first but becomes more difficult as the joint becomes distended and the hip gradually flexes.
- Release the plunger of the syringe; if the joint has been successfully entered, the saline solution that is under pressure in it reverses the plunger and fluid escapes into the syringe.
- Aspirate the saline solution from the joint and remove the syringe from the needle.
- Fill the syringe with 5 mL of a 25% strength Hypaque solution and inject 1 to 3 mL through the needle into the joint with image intensification.
- Rapidly withdraw the needle and, while the hip is still unreduced, have an arthrogram made at that point if image intensification is unavailable.
- Before developing it, gently reduce the hip into a stable position and have a second arthrogram made.
- Maintain reduction until both arthrograms have been developed and evaluated. Alternatively, use image intensification to evaluate the reduction and safe zone. When arthrograms are to be made of both hips, insert a needle into each, ensuring that both are within the joints before either joint is injected. Inject both hips as described here and make arthrograms of both.

See Video 30-1.

APPLICATION OF A HIP SPICA CAST

After confirmation of a stable reduction, a hip spica cast is applied with the hip joint in 95 degrees of flexion and 40 to 45 degrees of abduction. Salter advocated this "human position" as best for maintaining hip stability and minimizing the risk of osteonecrosis. Kumar described an easily reproducible and simple technique for applying a hip spica

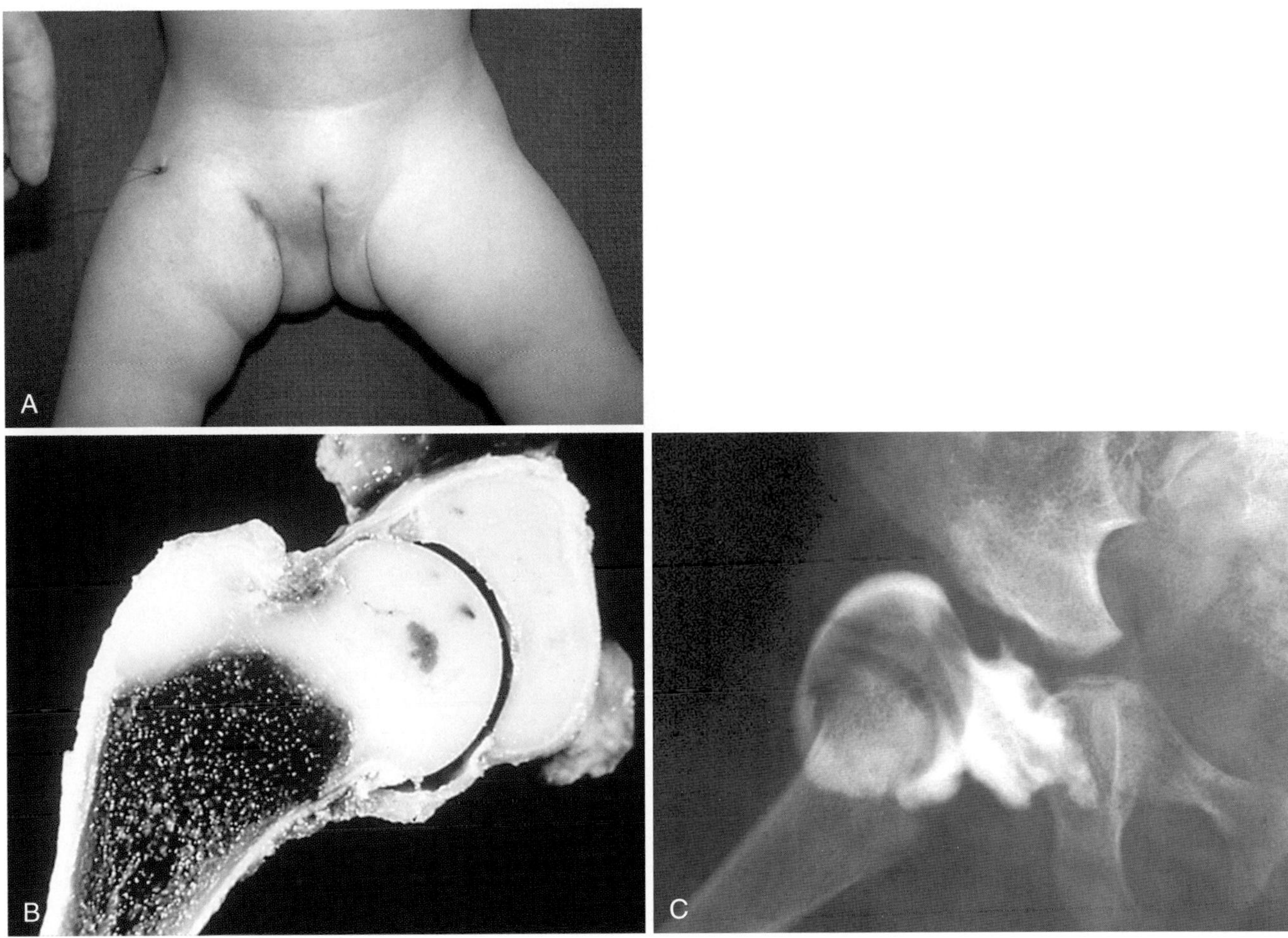

FIGURE 30-8 **A,** Insertion of 22-gauge spinal needle one fingerbreadth lateral to femoral artery and immediately inferior to anterior superior iliac spine for arthrography. **B,** In necropsy specimen, areas of hip in which dye may be easily injected-beneath acetabular labrum, in medial or lateral capsular pouch, and at junction of ossified and cartilaginous portion of femoral head. **C,** Irreducible hip with medial dye pool. (Courtesy of John Ogden, MD.) **SEE TECHNIQUE 30-1.**

cast. Fiberglass can be used in place of plaster, but the technique is described in its original form.

TECHNIQUE 30-2

(KUMAR)

- Place the anesthetized child on the spica frame. Abduct the hip to 40 to 45 degrees and flex it to about 95 degrees (Fig. 30-9A). The amount of hip flexion and abduction required to keep the hip in the most stable position should be determined clinically and checked by radiographs.
- After the correct position of flexion and abduction for stability is determined, place a small towel in front of the abdomen.
- Cover the pelvis and extremities with stockinette. Roll 2-inch (5-cm) Webril from the level of the nipples down to the ankles (Fig. 30-9B). Pad around the bony points with 2-inch (5-cm) standard felt. Apply the first pad over the proximal end of the spica, near the nipple line (Fig. 30-9C).
- Start a second piece of the same size felt at the level of the right groin and carry it posteriorly across the gluteal fold, over the right iliac crest, in front of the abdomen, over the lateral aspect of the left thigh, and to the left inguinal area (Fig. 30-9C).
- Apply a third piece of felt over the knee (Fig. 30-9C) and a fourth piece above the ankle over the distal leg. Place similar pieces of felt over the opposite knee and leg.
- Apply the plaster in two sections—a proximal section from the nipple line to the knees and a distal section from the knees to the ankles.
- Apply a single layer of 4-inch (10-cm) plaster roll from the nipple line to the level of the knees on both sides. Apply four or five plaster splints back to front from the nipple line to the back of the sacrum to reinforce the back of the cast. At the same time, apply a short, thick splint over the anterolateral aspect of the inguinal area (Fig. 30-9D).
- Apply another splint. Starting from the right inguinal area, carry it posteriorly across the gluteal region, the iliac crest, the front of the abdomen, and back the same way

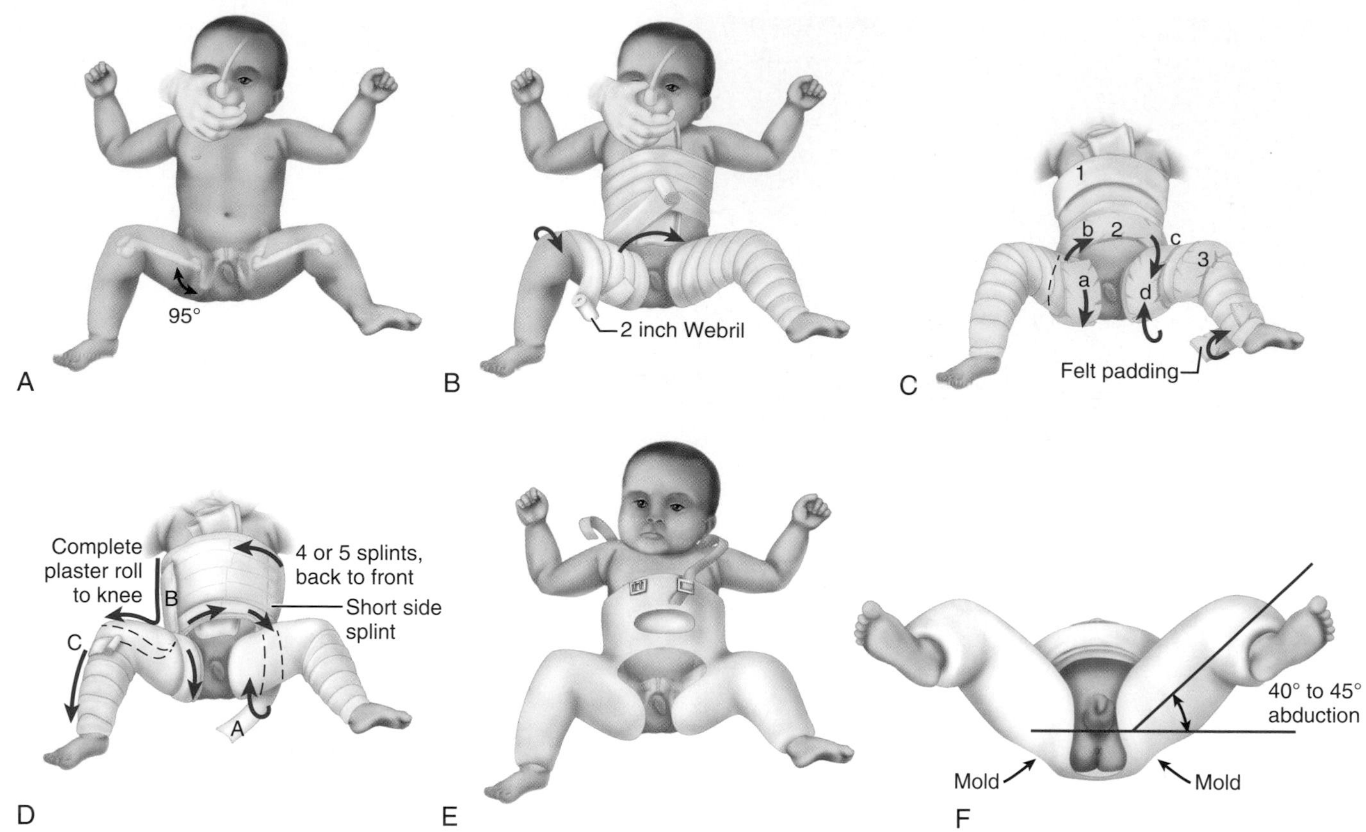

FIGURE 30-9 **A-F, Technique of application of hip spica cast for congenital dislocation of hip. Note positioning of patient in "human" position.** (Redrawn from Kumar SJ: Hip spica application for the treatment of congenital dislocation of the hip, J Pediatr Orthop 1:97, 1981.) **SEE TECHNIQUE 30-2.**

on the opposite thigh (Fig. 30-9D). This is a reinforcing splint that attaches the thigh to the upper segment.

- Apply another long splint from the level of the knee across the anterolateral aspect of the inguinal area and up the chest wall (Fig. 30-9D). This splint is one of the main anchors of the thigh to the body segment.
- Follow this by a roll of 4-inch (10-cm) plaster from the nipple line to the knees. This completes the proximal section of the spica.
- Complete the cast from the knees down to the ankles. Do this by applying on both sides a single roll of 3-inch (7.5-cm) plaster from the knee to the ankle level and reinforcing this by two splints over the medial and lateral aspects of the thigh, knee, and leg.
- Follow this by another roll of 3-inch (7.5-cm) plaster. Shoulder straps can be considered to prevent pistoning of the child in the cast but usually are unnecessary with a snug cast (Fig. 30-9E).
- Because the cast is reinforced laterally around the hips, a wide segment can be removed from the front of the hips without weakening the cast. This permits better radiographs of the hips (Fig. 30-9E).

The final view of the spica cast from inferiorly should appear as shown in Figure 30-9F, with about 40 to 45 degrees of abduction. The amount of abduction is determined by the position of hip stability. Excessive abduction should be avoided. We have found that the hips are always flexed less than they appear to be and are abducted more than they appear. A gentle cast mold over the greater trochanter can aid in maintaining hip reduction.

POSTOPERATIVE CARE. Spica cast immobilization is continued for 3 to 4 months. The cast can be changed at the midpoint with the patient under general anesthesia. Radiographs or arthrograms can be obtained to ensure that the femoral head is reduced anatomically into the acetabulum. Clinical and radiographic follow-up is essential until the hip is considered normal. CT or MRI is useful in the postoperative assessment of reduction. A comparison of MRI and CT in the evaluation of reduction of DDH found sensitivity of 100% for both CT and MRI and specificity of 96% for CT and 100% for MRI. CT required less time (3 minutes) than MRI (10 minutes) and was less expensive, but exposes the child to ionizing radiation. In contrast to routine radiography, a cast does not alter the image of an axial CT or MRI (Figs. 30-10 and 30-11), but because of the radiation exposure the number of cuts should be limited. Fast hip sequences can allow for acquisition of MRI data without additional anesthesia.

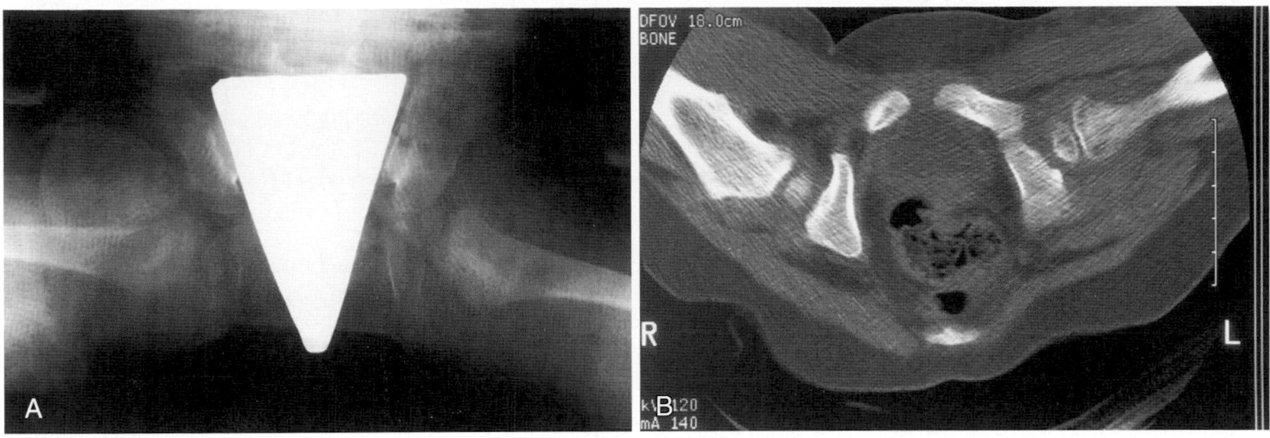

FIGURE 30-10 **A,** Anteroposterior radiograph of pelvis obtained with patient in hip spica cast after closed reduction. Note difficulty in assessing position of femoral head. **B,** CT scan of pelvis to confirm bilateral reduction of femoral head into true acetabulum.

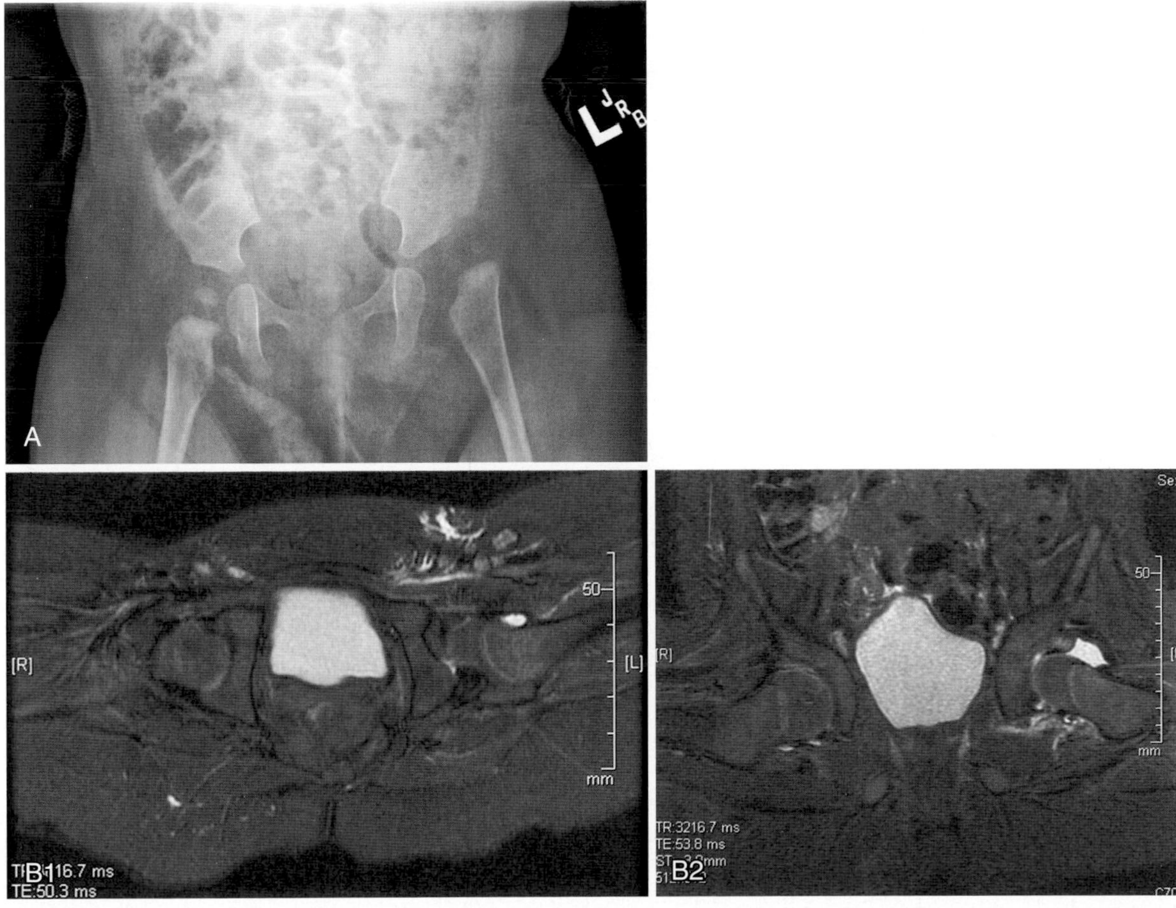

FIGURE 30-11 **A,** Plain anteroposterior view of a 9-month-old girl with persistent hip dislocation. **B,** Axial and coronal MRI of hip after arthrogram, successful closed reduction, and spica cast application.

OPEN REDUCTION

In children in whom efforts to reduce a dislocation without force have failed, open reduction is indicated to correct the interposed soft-tissue structures and to reduce the femoral head concentrically in the acetabulum. This surgical option is indicated by pathology rather than by age because open reduction may be required in children younger than 6 months and closed reduction occasionally can be successful in children 18 months of age. Open reduction can be performed through an anterior, anteromedial, or medial approach; the choice depends on the experience of the surgeon and the particular dislocation.

The anterior approach requires more anatomic dissection but provides greater versatility because the pathologic condition in the anterior and lateral aspects is easily reached and pelvic osteotomy can be performed through this approach if necessary. The anteromedial approach described by Weinstein and Ponseti is actually an anterior approach to the hip through an anteromedial incision. The hip is approached in the interval between the pectineus muscle and the femoral neurovascular bundle. This approach is recommended for children 24 months old or younger. Access to the lateral structures for dissection or osteotomy is impossible with this approach.

The medial (Ludloff) approach utilizes the interval between the iliopsoas and the pectineus. This approach places the medial circumflex vessels at a higher risk and has been reported to be associated with a higher incidence of osteonecrosis (10% to 20%) in some studies and similar rates of osteonecrosis in others. Although the medial approach allows removal of the impediments to reduction, it does not allow capsulorrhaphy and is, therefore, generally recommended in infants 6 to 18 months old.

ANTERIOR APPROACH

TECHNIQUE 30-3

(BEATY; AFTER SOMERVILLE)

- Make an anterior bikini incision from the middle of the iliac crest to a point midway between the anterior superior iliac spine and the midline of the pelvis. The anterior superior iliac crest should be at the midpoint of the incision, which can be placed 1 cm below the iliac crest (Fig. 30-12A).
- Carry sharp dissection through the subcutaneous tissue to the deep fascia.
- Identify and enter the interval between the sartorius and tensor fasciae latae muscles, protecting the lateral femoral cutaneous nerve by retracting it with a Penrose drain during the entire procedure. The presence of inguinal lymph nodes in the most medial dissection indicates the proximity of the neurovascular bundle.
- Detach the iliac apophysis from the ilium, beginning at the anterior superior iliac spine and extending 4 cm posteriorly along the ilium. Alternatively, the iliac apophysis can be split sharply.
- Subperiosteally dissect the tensor fasciae latae laterally to expose the ilium and the full extent of the anterolateral capsule.
- Identify the origin of the sartorius muscle at the anterior superior iliac crest, divide it, and allow it to retract distally.
- Dissect the tensor fasciae latae origin to the anterior inferior iliac spine.
- Place a retractor along the medial aspect of the anterior inferior iliac spine onto the superior pubic ramus.
- Identify the psoas tendon in its groove on the superior pubic ramus, and perform a recession tenotomy to facilitate placement of a right-angle retractor in the groove on the superior pubic ramus normally occupied by the iliopsoas tendon. The retractor protects the psoas muscle and neurovascular bundle anteriorly and assists in medial exposure.
- Identify the origins of the direct and oblique heads of the rectus femoris muscle and perform a tenotomy approximately 1 cm distal to the anterior inferior iliac spine (Fig. 30-12B). Tag the distal segment and allow the tendon to retract distally.
- Identify the capsule of the hip joint anteriorly, medially, and laterally. A large amount of redundant capsule may be present laterally in the region of a false acetabulum.
- Make a T-shaped incision from the most medial aspect of the capsule to the most lateral and continue the incision along the anterior border of the femoral head and neck (Fig. 30-12C). For more exposure, use Kocher clamps to retract the capsule.
- Identify the femoral head and the ligamentum teres; detach the ligamentum teres from the femoral head and place on it a Kocher clamp. Trace the ligamentum teres to the true acetabulum and excise with a rongeur or sharp dissection any pulvinar in the true acetabulum (Fig. 30-12D).
- Gently expose the bony articular surface of the acetabulum with its circumferential cartilage.
- Expose the acetabulum laterally, superiorly, medially, and inferiorly to the level of the deep transverse acetabular ligament, which should be divided to enlarge the most inferior aspect of the acetabulum. Enlarge the entrance to the acetabulum by excision of the fat from the innermost aspect of the acetabulum until the entrance is large enough to allow reduction of the femoral head without difficulty.
- After reducing the femoral head into the acetabulum, move the hip through a complete range of motion (including flexion, extension, adduction, and abduction) to determine the "safe zone" of reduction.
- If the reduction is concentric and stable, reduce the femoral head and close the capsule, suturing the lateral flap of the T-shaped incision as far medially as possible to eliminate any redundant capsule in the region of the false acetabulum (Fig. 30-12F). An adequate capsulorrhaphy significantly improves stability of the hip. Place sutures in the tips of the "T" and along the superior border of the acetabulum.
- When capsulorrhaphy is completed, suture the rectus femoris tendon to its origin and the iliac apophysis to the fascia of the tensor fasciae latae along the iliac crest.
- Close the superficial fascial layers, the subcutaneous tissues, and the skin. Apply a double spica cast with the hips in 90 to 100 degrees of flexion and 40 to 55 degrees of abduction.

POSTOPERATIVE CARE. Radiography, CT, or MRI can be used to confirm reduction of the femoral head into the acetabulum. The spica cast is changed in the operating room at 5 to 6 weeks with final removal at 10 to 12 weeks. Sequential radiographs are used to assess development of the femoral head and acetabulum (Fig. 30-12G and H); these are obtained on a regular basis until the child reaches skeletal maturity.

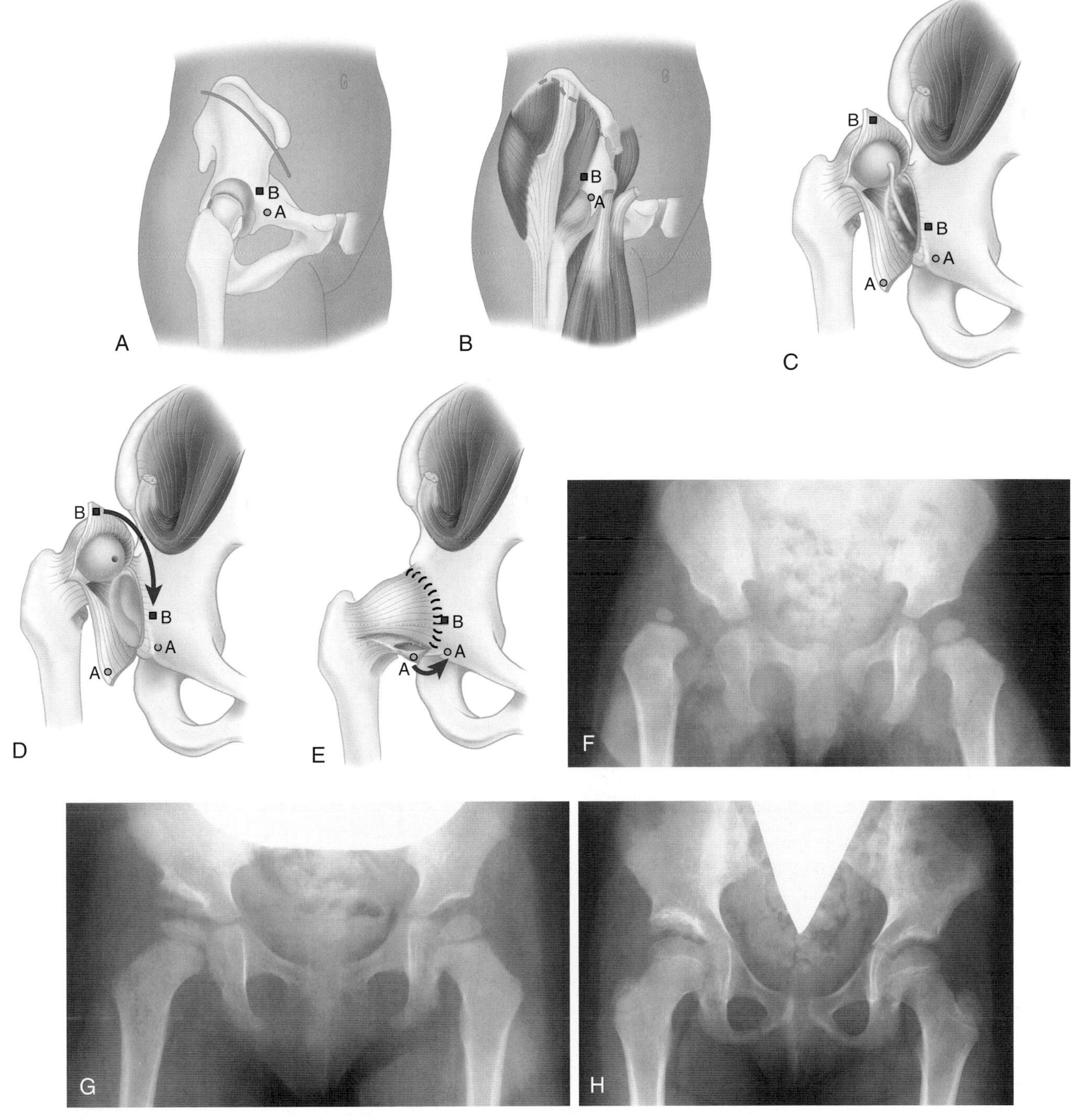

FIGURE 30-12 Technique of anterior open reduction in congenital dislocation of hip. **A,** Bikini incision. **B,** Division of sartorius and rectus femoris tendons and iliac epiphysis. **C,** T-shaped incision of capsule. **D,** Capsulotomy of hip and use of ligamentum teres to find true acetabulum. **E,** Reduction and capsulorrhaphy after excision of redundant capsule. **F,** Developmental dislocation of right hip. **G,** After anterolateral open reduction. **H,** At age 7 years; note remodeling of femoral head and acetabulum. **SEE TECHNIQUE 30-3.**

ANTEROMEDIAL APPROACH

TECHNIQUE 30-4

(WEINSTEIN AND PONSETI)

- With the patient supine, prepare and drape the affected extremity and hemipelvis free to allow full motion of the hip and knee. With the hip flexed to 70 degrees and in unforced abduction, identify the neurovascular bundle and the superior and inferior borders of the adductor longus muscle.
- Make an incision from the inferior border of the adductor longus to just inferior to the femoral neurovascular bundle in the groin crease.
- Incise the skin and subcutaneous tissues down to the deep fascia and incise the fascia over the adductor longus in the direction of the muscle fibers.
- Isolate the adductor longus, section it at its origin, and allow it to retract.
- Follow the anterior branch of the obturator nerve proximally to its entrance into the thigh under the pectineus muscle. Gently retract superiorly the neurovascular bundle. Keep the anterior branch of the obturator nerve in sight, open the sheath overlying the pectineus muscle, and identify its superior and inferior borders.
- Identify and bluntly dissect the interval between the pectineus muscle and the femoral neurovascular bundle.
- Isolate the iliopsoas tendon in the inferior aspect of the wound, section it sharply, and allow it to retract.
- With gentle retraction of the neurovascular bundle superiorly and the pectineus muscle inferiorly, isolate the hip joint capsule by blunt dissection.
- Make a small incision in the anteromedial capsule parallel to the anterior acetabular margin.
- Grasp the ligamentum teres with a Graham hook and bring it into the wound.
- Extend the capsular incision along the ligamentum teres to its insertion on the femoral head. Rotate the leg to bring this attachment into view.
- If the ligamentum teres is hypertrophied or elongated, excise it to make reduction easier. Grasp the stump of the ligamentum teres with a Kocher clamp and identify the interval between the ligament and the anteroinferomedial aspect of the joint capsule; mark this interval with a pair of scissors. Retract the pectineus muscle and sharply incise the anteromedial margin of the capsule.
- Section the ligamentum teres at its base along with the transverse acetabular ligament to open up the "horseshoe" of the acetabulum and increase its diameter. Remove all pulvinar with a pituitary rongeur.
- Reduce the femoral head into the acetabulum and move the hip through a range of motion to test the stability of the reduction.
- Irrigate the wound copiously, leave the joint capsule open, and approximate the deep fascia with running absorbable sutures.
- Close the subcutaneous tissues and skin with absorbable sutures.
- Apply a spica cast with the hip in a position of maximal stability in flexion and mild abduction.

POSTOPERATIVE CARE. The cast is worn for 10 to 12 weeks. If radiographs show satisfactory position of the hip 4 to 6 weeks after surgery, the portion of the cast below the knee is removed to allow knee motion and some hip rotation. After removal of the total cast, an abduction brace is worn full time for 4 to 8 weeks; then it is worn only at night and during naps for 1 to 2 years, until normal acetabular development is evident (Fig. 30-13).

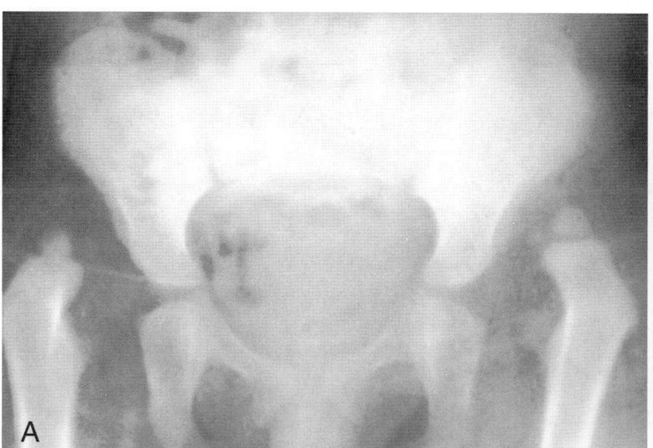

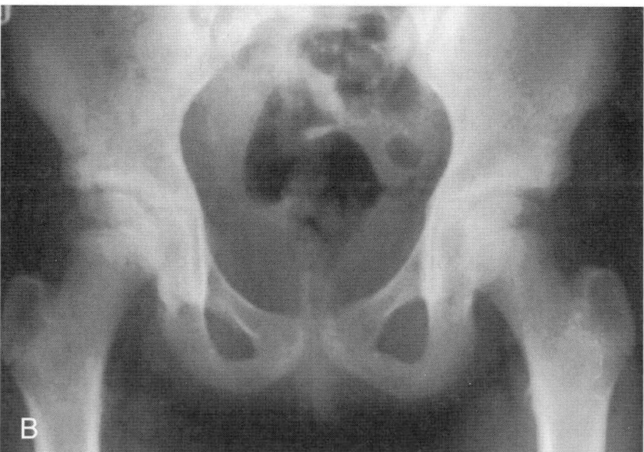

FIGURE 30-13 Anteromedial open reduction. **A,** Bilateral congenital dislocation of hip in 32-month-old girl. **B,** At 12 years of age, there is normal development of femoral head and acetabulum bilaterally. (Courtesy of Stuart Weinstein, MD.) **SEE TECHNIQUE 30-4.**

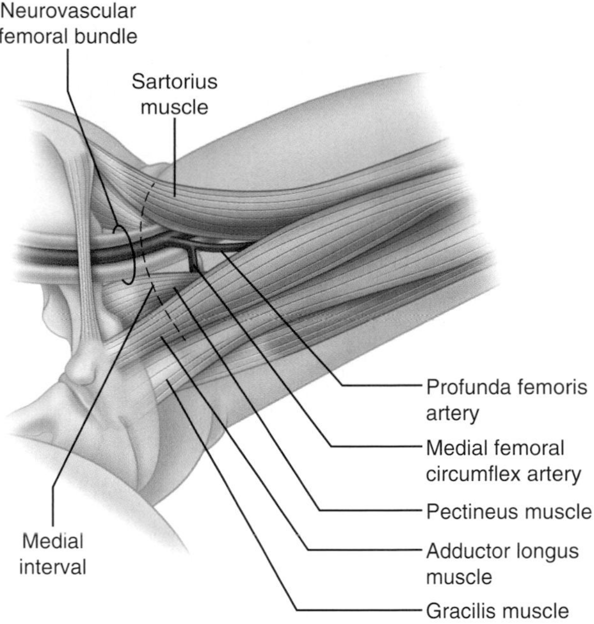

FIGURE 30-14 Incision for medial (Ludloff) approach and open reduction. **SEE TECHNIQUE 30-5.**

MEDIAL APPROACH

TECHNIQUE 30-5

(LUDLOFF)

- Make a transverse incision centered at the anterior margin of the adductor longus, approximately 1 cm distal and parallel to the inguinal ligament (Fig. 30-14).
- Open the fascia along the superior border of the adductor longus. Isolate this muscle, divide it close to its insertion on the pelvis, and retract it distally to expose the adductor brevis muscle in the inferior part of the wound and the pectineus muscle in the superior part of the wound.
- Identify the branches of the anterior obturator nerve on the surface of the adductor brevis muscle and with blunt dissection follow this nerve beneath the pectineus muscle. Free the posterior border of the pectineus muscle proximally to its insertion on the pelvis.
- Place a retractor beneath the pectineus muscle and retract it superiorly. Identify by palpation the lesser trochanter and the iliopsoas tendon. Open the fascial layer surrounding the tendon, pull the tendon into the wound with a right-angle clamp, and sharply divide it.
- With blunt dissection clear the pericapsular fat from the capsule. Dissect free the small branch of the medial circumflex artery that crosses the capsule inferiorly and preserve it.
- Incise the capsule in the direction of the femoral neck. Identify the transverse acetabular ligament and section it.
- If needed for reduction, perform additional release of the capsule. Reduce the hip in 90 to 100 degrees of flexion and 40 to 60 degrees of abduction.
- When the optimal position is determined, close the deep fascia and skin in routine fashion and apply a double spica cast.
- Consider obtaining three-dimensional imaging after cast application to confirm reduction of the femoral head.

POSTOPERATIVE CARE. Postoperative care is similar to that after closed reduction and varies according to the age of the child. Generally, 8 to 12 weeks of cast immobilization is sufficient.

CONCOMITANT OSTEOTOMY

The use of a concomitant osteotomy of the ilium, acetabulum, or femur at the time of open reduction remains controversial. Innominate osteotomy, acetabuloplasty, proximal femoral varus derotation osteotomy, or femoral shortening osteotomy might increase the stability of open reduction. However, in younger children (<12 months), acetabular remodeling potential could render these procedures unnecessary. Conversely, inadequate remodeling after open reduction may necessitate a return to the operating room at a later date for a bony procedure.

Zadeh et al. used concomitant osteotomy at the time of open reduction to maintain stability of the reduction in which the following test of stability after open reduction was used.

1. Hip stable in neutral position—no osteotomy
2. Hip stable in flexion and abduction—innominate osteotomy
3. Hip stable in internal rotation and abduction—proximal femoral derotational varus osteotomy
4. "Double-diameter" acetabulum with anterolateral deficiency—Pemberton-type osteotomy

Aside from the need for osteotomy at the time of open reduction to maintain stability, there also are concerns about residual acetabular dysplasia. Better results have been reported in children younger than 30 months of age who were treated with combined open reduction and Salter osteotomy than in those treated with a staged procedure.

Concomitant osteotomy, particularly a femoral shortening osteotomy with or without derotation, should be done at the time of open reduction when necessary to maintain a safe, stable reduction. If open reduction is stable without an osteotomy, a bony procedure for residual deformity should be considered at the time of the open reduction in an older child (>18 months) and used with caution even in younger infants when needed.

TERATOLOGIC DISLOCATIONS

A teratologic dislocation of the hip is one that occurs at some time before birth, resulting in significant anatomic distortion and resistance to treatment. It often occurs with other conditions, such as arthrogryposis, Larsen syndrome, myelomeningocele, and diastrophic dwarfism.

The anatomic changes in teratologic dislocations are much more advanced than the changes in a typical developmental hip dislocation in a child of the same age. The acetabulum is small, with an oblique or flattened shape; the ligamentum teres is thickened, and the femoral head is of variable size and may be flattened on the medial side

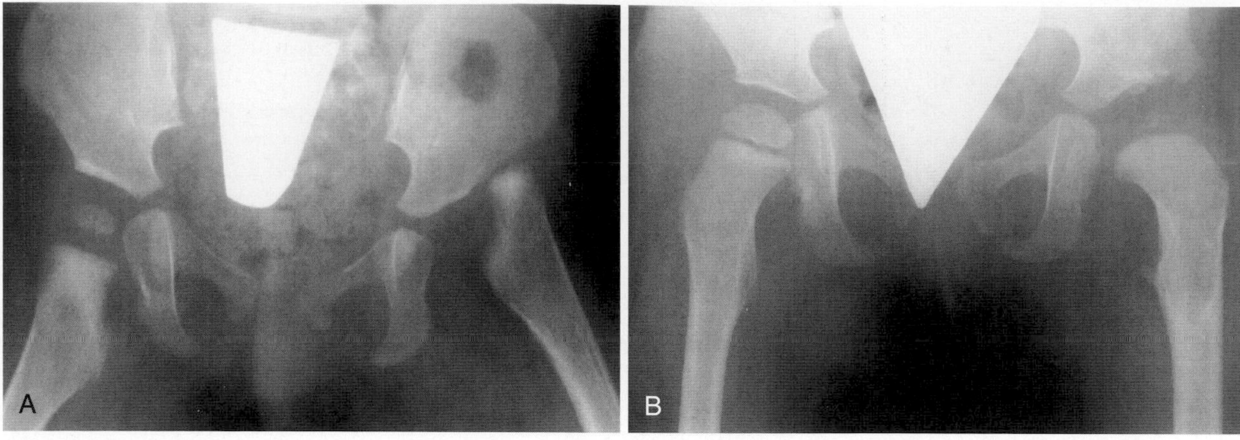

FIGURE 30-15 **A,** Teratologic dislocation of left hip in 18-month-old girl. **B,** Appearance at 3 years of age after primary femoral shortening, anterior open reduction, and innominate osteotomy.

(Fig. 30-15). The hip joint is usually stiff and irreducible, and radiographs show superolateral displacement.

Most authors agree that closed reduction is ineffective and that open reduction is necessary, but indications for treatment are unclear. Most agree that unilateral dislocations should be treated more aggressively than bilateral dislocations, and the ambulatory potential of the patient is probably the most important consideration in deciding whether to treat bilateral dislocations. The difficulty of successfully treating teratologic dislocations is reflected in the results of Gruel et al., who found that of the 27 hips in their series, 44% had poor results and 70% had complications. Osteonecrosis occurred in 48% of hips, redislocation occurred in 19%, and subluxation occurred in 22%. Anterior open reduction and femoral shortening produced the best results with the fewest complications, whereas the worst results and most complications occurred in the hips treated by closed reduction.

Although multiple procedures may be required, good results can be obtained and a stable hip can be achieved in properly selected patients. Open reduction through a medial approach has been recommended for children 3 to 6 months old combined with surgical correction of congenital contractures of the knee and foot. In older children, primary femoral shortening and anterior open reduction, with or without pelvic osteotomy, is preferred.

OSTEONECROSIS

The most serious complication associated with treatment of developmental dysplasia of the hip in early infancy is the development of osteonecrosis. Estimated rates of osteonecrosis vary widely, ranging from less than 5% to almost 50%. Proposed risk factors for osteonecrosis include open reduction with concomitant osteotomies, redislocation after surgical correction, or the need for secondary procedure after initial closed or open reduction. Some authors have suggested that osteonecrosis is more frequent when reduction is done before the appearance of the ossific nucleus of the femoral head, whereas others have stated that waiting until the ossific nucleus appears does not seem to affect the development of osteonecrosis. Luhmann et al. found that delaying reduction of a dislocated hip until the appearance of the ossific nucleus more than doubled the need for future surgery. Despite a slight increase in the rate of osteonecrosis after reduction of hips without an ossific nucleus, they advocated early reduction to optimize development of the hip with the minimal number of operations.

Potential sequelae of osteonecrosis include femoral head deformity, acetabular dysplasia, lateral subluxation of the femoral head, relative overgrowth of the greater trochanter, and limb-length inequalities; osteoarthritis is a common late complication. Bucholz and Ogden and Kalamchi and MacEwen proposed classification systems based on morphologic changes in the capital femoral epiphysis, the physis, and the proximal femoral metaphysis (Fig. 30-16). These classifications are useful in determining proper treatment and prognosis for a particular patient; however, the proper classification may not be identifiable on radiographs until the child is 4 to 6 years old. The Bucholz and Ogden classification system and its prognostic ability has been brought into question by an interrater reliability study; the authors concluded that a new classification scheme is needed. A simplification of the Kalamchi and MacEwen classification scheme has been proposed that combines Groups II, III, and IV into a single Group B. By classifying osteonecrosis cases into Group A or Group B, the authors were able to demonstrate that the type of reduction (closed with traction versus open without femoral shortening) was a factor in the development of osteonecrosis.

Treatment should be directed toward the clinical problems associated with each radiographic classification group. Many patients do not require any treatment during adolescence and young adulthood. In a few, femoral head deformity and acetabular dysplasia, predisposing the hip joint to incongruity and persistent subluxation, can be treated with femoral osteotomy or appropriate pelvic osteotomy or both.

Children with osteonecrosis after treatment of developmental dislocation of the hip should be followed to maturity with serial orthoradiographs. Significantly better results have been reported in patients treated early (1 to 3 years after the ischemic insult) with innominate osteotomy than in patients treated later (5 to 10 years after the ischemic insult) and patients without pelvic osteotomy. Patients treated early also

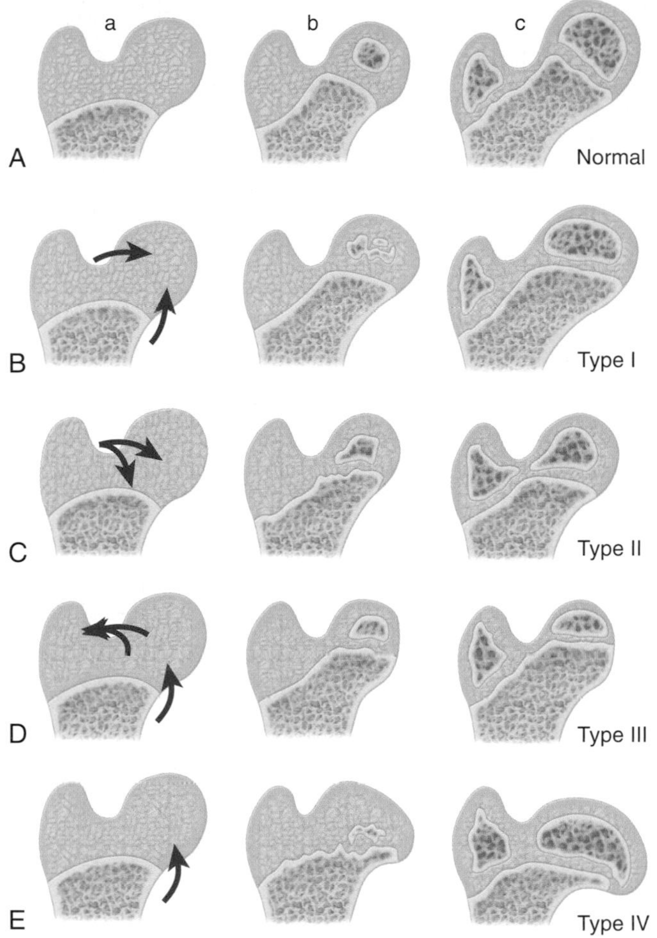

FIGURE 30-16 Bucholz and Ogden classification of osteonecrosis of femoral head in congenital dislocation of hip. **A,** Normal femoral head at 2 months (a), 1 year (b), and 9 years (c) of age. **B,** Type I: a, sites of temporary vascular occlusion; b, irregular ossification in secondary center; c, normal epiphyseal contour, slight decrease in height of capital femoral ossification center. **C,** Type II: a, probable primary site of vascular occlusion; b, metaphyseal and epiphyseal irregularities; c, premature fusion of lateral metaphysis and epiphysis. **D,** Type III: a, sites of temporary vascular occlusion; b, impaired longitudinal growth of capital femoral epiphysis; c, irregularly shaped femoral head. **E,** Type IV: a, sites of temporary vascular occlusion; b, impaired longitudinal and latitudinal growth; c, premature epiphyseal closure. (Redrawn from Bucholz RW, Ogden JA: Patterns of ischemic necrosis of the proximal femur in nonoperatively treated congenital hip disease. In The hip: proceedings of the Sixth Open Scientific Meeting of the Hip Society, St Louis, Mosby, 1978.)

had less pain and fewer gait disturbances and required fewer additional procedures for limb-length inequality or greater trochanteric overgrowth. Early innominate osteotomy has been suggested to induce spherical remodeling of the femoral head, with a resultant congruous hip joint, whereas with later osteotomy the femoral head was already deformed, with little potential for remodeling. Significant limb-length inequality can be corrected by appropriate techniques, usually a well-timed epiphysiodesis. Symptomatic overgrowth of the greater trochanter can be treated in older patients with greater trochanteric advancement, which increases the abductor muscle resting length and increases the abductor lever arm (Fig. 30-17).

TROCHANTERIC ADVANCEMENT

TECHNIQUE 30-6

(LLOYD-ROBERTS AND SWANN)

- Approach the trochanter through a long lateral incision. Place a Gigli saw deep to the gluteus medius and minimus muscles and divide the trochanter at its base. Alternately, remove the lateral two thirds of the greater trochanter with an oscillating saw or large osteotome. Protect the lateral ascending cervical artery medial to the piriformis fossa.
- Mobilize the gluteus muscles anteriorly and posteriorly as they are dissected off the joint capsule and strip them for a short distance from the ilium above.
- Displace the detached trochanter with its attached muscles distally to the lateral cortex of the femur while the hip is abducted.
- Bevel the femoral cortex to help reduce tension and improve placement of the trochanter.
- Secure the trochanter to the femur with screws and suture the femoral periosteum and vastus lateralis muscle. The top of the greater trochanter now should be positioned at the level of the center of the femoral head on an anteroposterior radiograph. The trochanter usually requires advancement anteriorly and distally.

POSTOPERATIVE CARE. The hip is protected by a spica cast in abduction for 3 to 6 weeks. A physical therapy program is begun for rehabilitation of the hip abductor musculature.

TODDLER (18 TO 36 MONTHS)

Because of widespread screening of newborns, it is becoming less common for DDH to go undetected beyond the age of 1 year. An older child with this condition has a wide perineum, shortened lower extremity, and hyperlordosis of the lower spine as a result of femoropelvic instability. For these children with well-established hip dysplasia, open reduction with femoral or pelvic osteotomy, or both, often is required. Persistent dysplasia can be corrected by a redirectional proximal femoral osteotomy in very young children. If the primary dysplasia is acetabular, pelvic redirectional osteotomy alone is more appropriate. Many older children require femoral and pelvic osteotomies, however, if significant deformity is present on both sides of the joint.

FEMORAL OSTEOTOMY IN DYSPLASIA OF THE HIP

Surgeons who recommend femoral osteotomies advise an operation on the pelvic side of the joint only after (1) the femoral head has been concentrically seated in the dysplastic acetabulum by such an osteotomy, (2) the joint has failed to

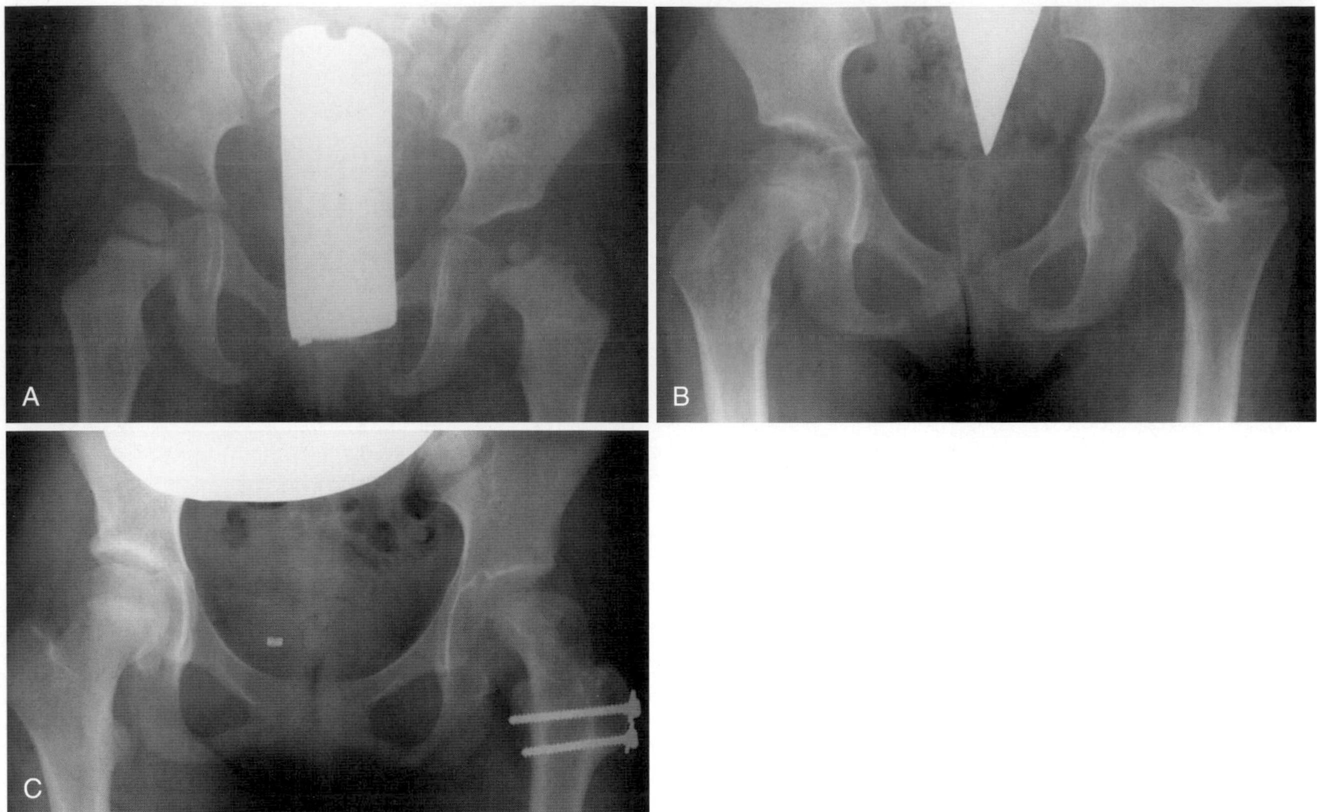

FIGURE 30-17 **A,** Osteonecrosis of left femoral head in 4-year-old girl after closed reduction of left congenital dislocation of hip at 6 months of age. **B,** At 10 years of age, now type II osteonecrosis with premature lateral epiphyseal arrest and relative trochanteric overgrowth is present. **C,** At 13 years of age, after transfer of trochanter distally and anteriorly.

develop satisfactorily, and (3) the growth potential of the acetabulum no longer exists. Opinions differ widely as to the age at which the acetabulum loses its ability to develop satisfactorily over a femoral head concentrically located, although 8 years appears to be most frequently cited upper age limit after which little benefit is derived from femoral osteotomy alone. Femoral osteotomy is most frequently indicated with primary femoral shortening, but the technique is included here for completeness.

VARUS DEROTATIONAL OSTEOTOMY OF THE FEMUR IN HIP DYSPLASIA, WITH PEDIATRIC HIP SCREW FIXATION

TECHNIQUE 30-7

- Place the patient supine on a radiolucent operating table. Image intensification in the anteroposterior projection is desirable.
- Prepare and drape the affected extremity, leaving the unaffected leg draped free to allow intraoperative radiographs or imaging.
- Make a lateral incision from the greater trochanter distally 8 to 12 cm, incise the iliotibial band, and reflect the vastus lateralis muscle to expose the lateral aspect of the femur.
- Make a transverse line in the femoral cortex with an osteotome to mark the level of the osteotomy at the level of the lesser trochanter or slightly distal. Correct positioning of the osteotomy can be verified with image intensification.
- Make a longitudinal orientation line on the anterior femoral cortex to determine correct rotation.
- Drill a hole just distal to the greater trochanter and check its placement with the image intensifier.
- This osteotomy can be stabilized with a pediatric hip screw, an angled blade plate, or a proximal femoral locking plate. The description presented uses a pediatric hip screw.
- Place an appropriate guide pin of the proper length in the femoral neck with the aid of an adjustable angle guide (see Fig. 36-106A).
- Check the placement of the guide pin with image intensification. When the guide pin is placed, use a percutaneous direct measuring gauge to determine the lag screw length.
- Set the adjustable positive stop on the combination reamer for the lag screw length determined by the percutaneous direct measuring gauge.
- Place the reamer over the guide pin and ream until the positive stop reaches the lateral cortex (see Fig. 36-106C).

It is prudent to check periodically the fluoroscopic image during reaming to ensure that the guide pin is not inadvertently advancing proximally into the epiphysis.

- Set the adjustable positive stop on the lag screw tap to the same length that was reamed. Tap until the positive stop reaches the lateral cortex. Screw the appropriate intermediate compression screw over the guide pin (see Fig. 36-106D and E).
- Take the plate chosen during preoperative planning and insert its barrel over the barrel guide and onto the back of the lag screw. The plate angle ultimately determines the final hip angle.
- Remove the barrel guide and insert a compressing screw to prevent the plate from disengaging during the reduction maneuver. Use the slotted screwdriver for the pediatric compressing screw or the hex screwdriver for the intermediate compressing screw. If the plate obscures the osteotomy site, loosen the screw and rotate the side plate.
- Make the osteotomy cut at the transverse line on the cortex in a transverse or oblique direction, depending on the correction desired. If rotational, in addition to angular, correction is desired, complete the osteotomy through the medial cortex. Using the longitudinal mark in the femoral cortex as a guide, rotate the femur as needed to correct femoral anteversion (usually 15 to 30 degrees). Because the deformity is more rotational than angulatory, evaluate the position of the femur with radiographs or image intensification before continuing with varus correction. To achieve varus angulation, remove an appropriate wedge of bone from the medial cortex to effect a neck-shaft angle of 120 to 135 degrees.
- To achieve compression, insert a drill or tap guide into the distal portion of the most distal compression slot. Drill through the medial cortex. If less compression is required, follow the same steps just detailed in the distal portion of either the second or the third distal slots for 2.5 mm of compression.
- Select the appropriate length bone screw and insert it using the screwdriver. Use the self-holding sleeve to keep the screw from disengaging from the screwdriver (see Fig. 36-106F).
- Finally, in the most proximal slot, the intermediate combination drill/tap guide can be angled proximally so that the drill and ultimately the bone screw cross the osteotomy line. Positioning the proximal bone screw in this way can provide additional stability at the osteotomy site.
- Insert screws into any remaining screw holes.
- The lag screw can be inserted farther to provide more compression. To insert the lag screw for approximately 5 mm of compression, stop when the lateral cortex is midway between the two depth calibrations (see Fig. 36-106G). To insert the lag screw for approximately 10 mm of compression, stop when the second depth calibration meets the lateral cortex (see Fig. 36-106H).
- Confirm the position of the fixation device and the proximal and distal fragments with an anteroposterior radiograph or image intensification.
- Irrigate the wound and close it in layers, inserting a suction drain if needed. Apply a one and one half spica cast.

POSTOPERATIVE CARE. The spica cast is worn for 8 to 12 weeks until union of the osteotomy occurs. The internal fixation can be removed at 12 to 24 months if desired.

CHILD (3 TO 8 YEARS)

The management of untreated developmental dislocation of the hip in a child older than 3 years of age is difficult. Even when surgical reduction is achieved and when bony corrections have been made, secondary procedures are common in this age group. By this age, adaptive shortening of the periarticular structures and structural alterations in the femoral head and the acetabulum have occurred. Dislocated hips in this age group require open reduction. Preoperative skeletal traction should not be used as the only means of achieving reduction because of the high frequencies of osteonecrosis (54%) and redislocation (31%) reported with its use alone. Femoral shortening aids in the reduction and decreases the potential for complications but is technically demanding, as is treatment of the dislocated hip, in this older age group.

PRIMARY FEMORAL SHORTENING

Since the early 1990s, the combination of primary open reduction and femoral shortening, usually with pelvic osteotomy, has been an accepted method of treatment of DDH in older children. This approach avoids expensive in-hospital traction, obtains predictable reduction, and results in a lower rate of osteonecrosis (Figs. 30-18 and 30-19).

Primary femoral shortening, anterior open reduction, and capsulorrhaphy, with or without pelvic osteotomy as indicated, have been recommended in children 3 years old or older. Certain circumstances, such as teratologic hip dislocation or a failed traction program, may make the procedure appropriate for younger children. A completely dislocated hip in an older child becomes fixed in a position superior to the true acetabulum. The degree of this superior migration ranges from severe subluxation (inferior head still adjacent to labrum), to dislocation with formation of a false acetabulum just superior to the true acetabulum, to severe dislocation with the femoral head high in the abductor musculature without formation of a false acetabulum. The extent of proximal migration determines the degree of deformation of the capsule and the extent of soft-tissue reconstruction required to correct the deformity.

The capsular abnormality in a developmentally dislocated hip must be recognized and corrected to achieve successful open reduction. The methods for bony correction are well defined, perhaps because the techniques can be clearly illustrated and documented radiographically, but the soft-tissue abnormalities and methods for their correction are not well described. As a result, a hip that appears reduced immediately after surgery may subluxate or redislocate with weight bearing even though the bony procedure appears radiographically faultless.

The dislocation of the hip leads to adaptive enlargement of the hip capsule, with the capsule becoming nearly twice the normal size in the completely dislocated hip. The ligamentum teres hypertrophies and often becomes a partial weight-bearing structure. In older children, this ligament occasionally avulses from the femoral head, retracting and

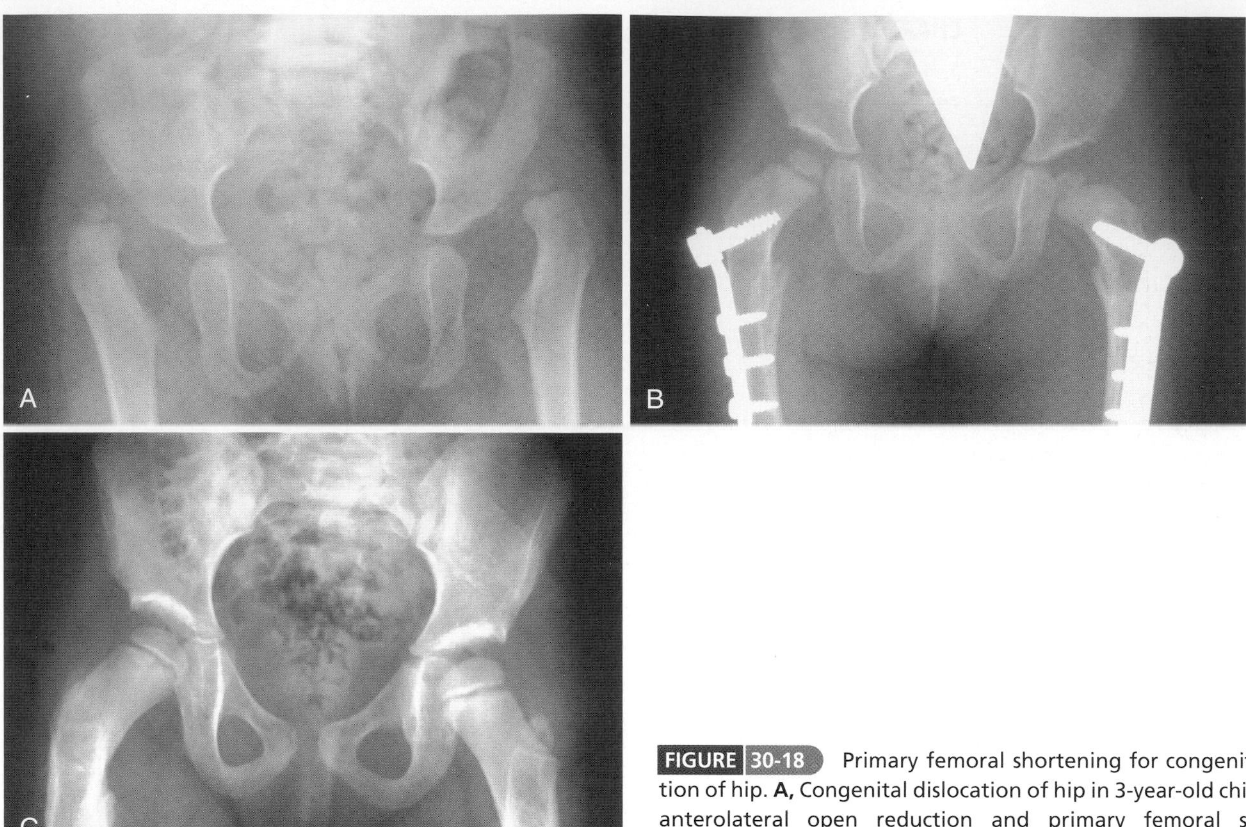

FIGURE 30-18 Primary femoral shortening for congenital dislocation of hip. **A,** Congenital dislocation of hip in 3-year-old child. **B,** After anterolateral open reduction and primary femoral shortening. **C,** Appearance of hip at 6 years of age.

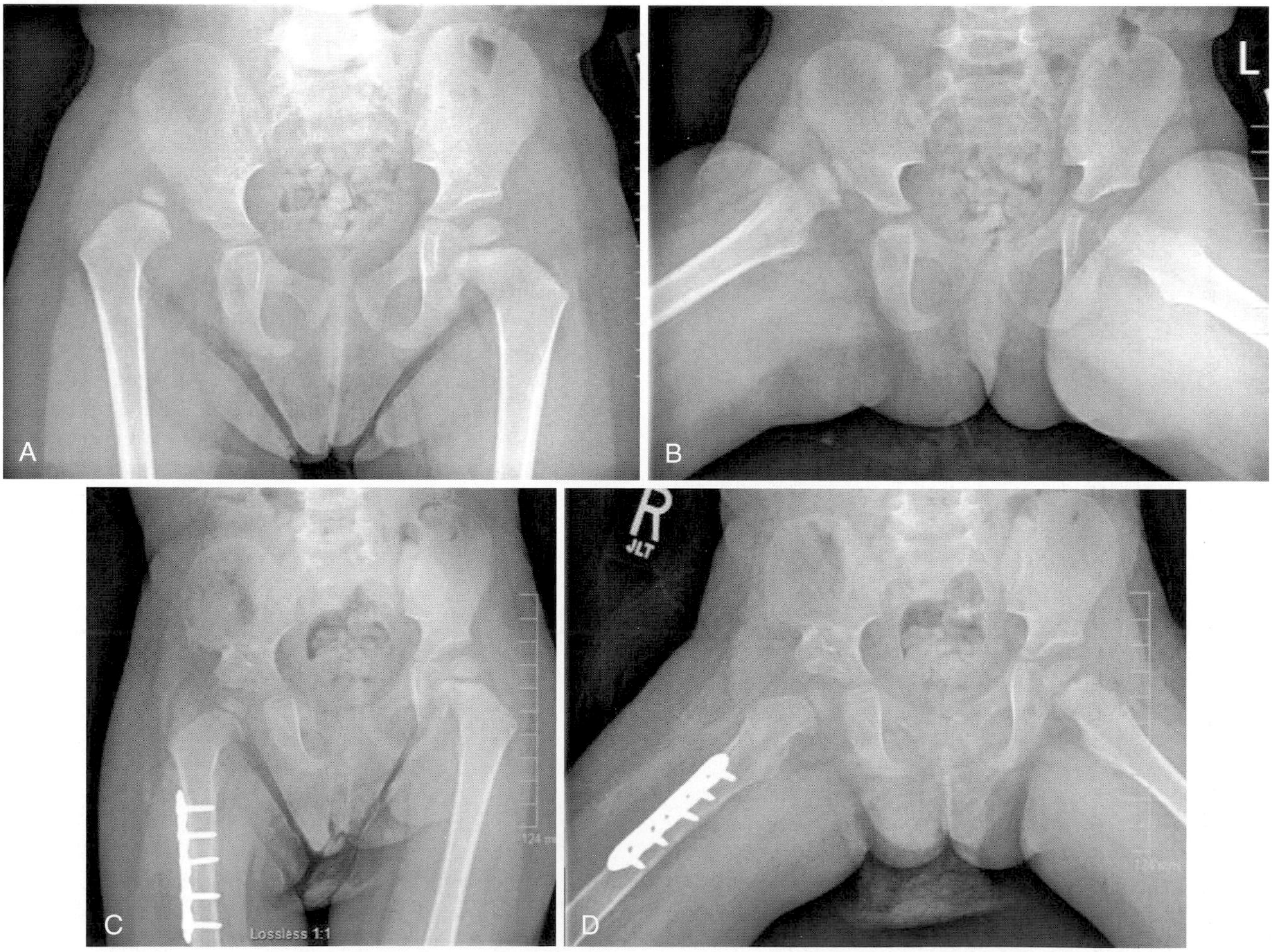

FIGURE 30-19 **A** and **B,** Four-year-old child with dislocated hip and severe dysplasia. **C** and **D,** Postoperative radiographs 3 months after primary femoral shortening, open reduction with capsulorrhaphy, and Pemberton acetabuloplasty.

reattaching to the inferior capsule and forming a mass of tissue that may impede reduction. The fibrocartilaginous labrum is flattened superolaterally, with the attached hypertrophied capsule protruding into the overlying abductor muscle mass, which adheres to the displaced capsule. If the capsule is not separated adequately from the adherent overlying muscles, reduction is difficult and the chance of redislocation is increased.

In a high, severely dislocated hip, the abductor muscles have contracted, and occasionally, despite prior traction or femoral shortening, these contracted muscles and fascia make it difficult to pull the proximal femur distal enough to reduce the femoral head fully. In rare instances, this requires release of the piriformis insertion or release of the anteriormost gluteus minimus fibers, or both, to allow adequate distal movement of the femoral head after femoral shortening. The middle and inferior portions of the capsule predictably are constricted by the overlying psoas tendon. The transverse acetabular ligament, crossing the base of the horseshoe-shaped true acetabulum, is contracted and thickened.

The following description of the technique for primary femoral shortening is a modification of the techniques described by Klisíc et al. and by Wenger and includes anterior open reduction (Technique 30-3) and varus derotational osteotomy (see Technique 30-7) along with soft-tissue management. These techniques should be reviewed carefully before primary femoral shortening is performed (Fig. 30-20).

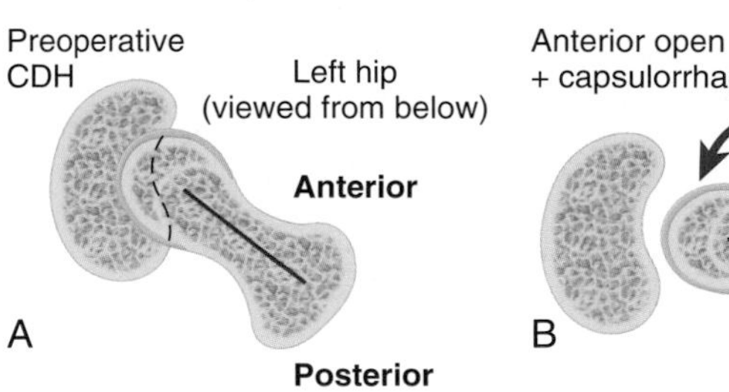

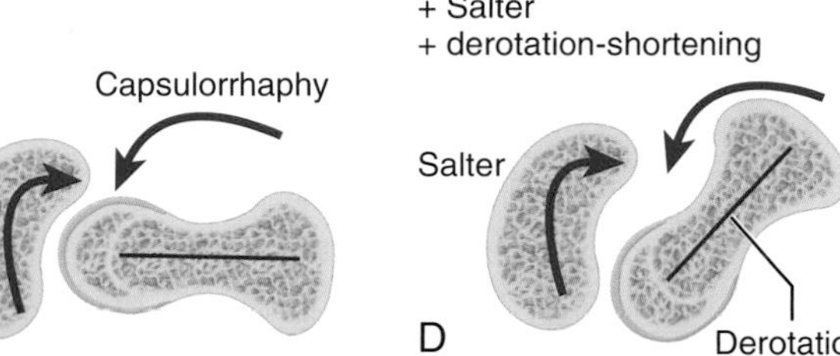

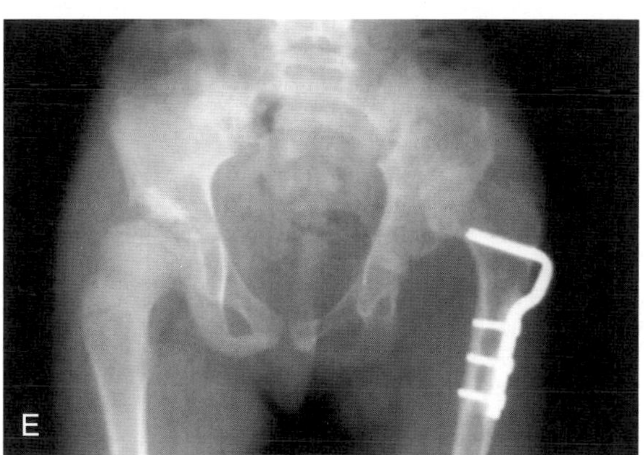

FIGURE 30-20 **A,** Anteverted femur and acetabulum in preoperative developmental dislocation of hip. **B,** Redirection of femoral neck by snug anterior capsulorrhaphy. **C,** Capsulorrhaphy and Salter innominate osteotomy. **D,** Capsulorrhaphy, Salter innominate osteotomy, and full femoral derotation. Combined in excess, this sequence can produce posterior dislocation. **E,** Open reduction, primary femoral shortening, derotation osteotomy, and Salter osteotomy produced fixed posterior hip dislocation in 5-year-old girl. (**A-D** redrawn from Wenger DR: Congenital hip dislocation: techniques for primary open reduction including femoral shortening, Instr Course Lect 38:343, 1989.) **SEE TECHNIQUE 30-8.**

PRIMARY FEMORAL SHORTENING

TECHNIQUE 30-8

- Place the patient supine on the operating table with a small radiolucent pad beneath the affected hip. Prepare and drape the extremity in the usual manner to allow exposure of the pelvis and femur.
- Two incisions are made—an anterior ilioinguinal incision and a straight lateral incision, as described for anterior open reduction (see Technique 30-3) and for femoral osteotomy (see Technique 30-11).
- Through the anterior ilioinguinal incision, perform anterior open reduction as described in Technique 30-3, continuing the dissection to the point where capsulorrhaphy normally would be performed.
- Proceed to the femoral shortening. Make a straight lateral incision from the tip of the greater trochanter to the distal third of the femoral shaft.
- If varus correction is not needed, the femoral shortening and derotation can be performed at the level of the femoral shaft rather than the intertrochanteric level. This shaft osteotomy can be stabilized with a one third tubular plate or a standard compression plate.
- Expose the shaft by dissection through the tensor fasciae latae muscle, iliotibial band, and vastus lateralis muscle.
- Make a transverse mark on the femoral shaft at the level of the lesser trochanter to indicate the osteotomy site, and make a longitudinal mark on the anterior border of the proximal shaft to orient derotation of the femur.
- Insert a lag screw into the femoral neck in the usual manner.
- Estimate the amount of shortening that will be necessary from preoperative radiographs, measuring from the most proximal aspect of the femoral head to the triradiate cartilage. The amount of shortening generally required varies from 1 to 3 cm. Conversely, the correct amount of bony resection can be "dialed in" as bone is removed until the femoral head can be reduced into the acetabulum without undue tension.
- Perform an osteotomy of the femur slightly distal to the lag screw in the femoral neck.

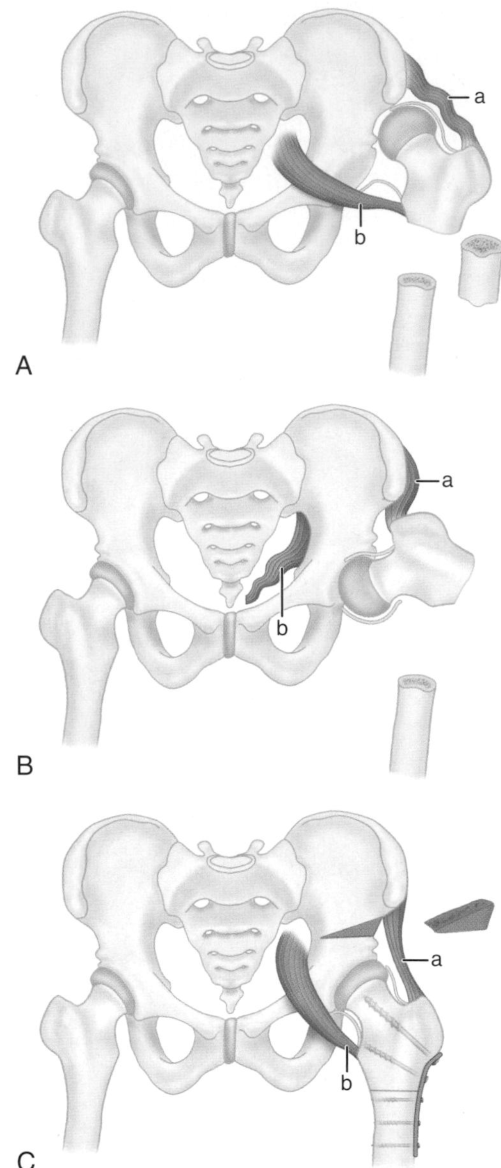

FIGURE 30-21 Technique for open reduction, primary femoral shortening, and Salter osteotomy. **A,** Femoral head is dislocated. Gluteal muscles (a) are retracted and slightly shortened. Iliopsoas muscle (b) is intact. Capsule is interposed between femoral head and ilium. Segment of femur is resected. **B,** Proximal femur is abducted; iliopsoas tendon (b) is divided. Capsule is incised on inferior surface parallel to femoral neck. **C,** Operation is complete. Gluteal muscles (a) are tight. Iliopsoas muscle (b) is reattached. Salter osteotomy is completed with graft in place. Femoral fragments are fixed with pediatric hip screw. **SEE TECHNIQUE 30-8.**

- Make a second osteotomy at the appropriate distance distal to the first. Angle this osteotomy to allow varus and derotation of the femur as necessary.
- Remove the measured segment of the femoral shaft (Fig. 30-21).
- Carefully incise subperiosteally the iliopsoas attachment to the lesser trochanter and the capsule attached to the medial femoral neck, avoiding the medial circumflex artery.
- Gently reduce the femoral head into the acetabulum, using the lag screw in the femoral neck as a lever. Derotation of the proximal fragment of 15 to 45 degrees usually is required.
- Appose the two segments of the femur and attach a side plate to the screw in the femoral neck and fix it to the distal femoral shaft. Use radiographs or image intensification to evaluate the femoral shortening and reduction of the femoral head.
- At this point, a Salter or Pemberton osteotomy, if indicated to correct acetabular dysplasia, can be performed. A thorough and meticulous capsulorrhaphy should be performed as previously described. The most lateral flap of the capsule should be transposed medially to eliminate the redundant capsule of the false acetabulum.
- Irrigate both wounds and close them in the usual manner. Suction drains can be inserted if necessary.
- Apply a spica cast with the extremity in neutral rotation and slight flexion and abduction.

POSTOPERATIVE CARE. The drains are removed 24 to 48 hours after surgery. The spica cast is removed at 8 to 12 weeks. Sequential radiographs are obtained to evaluate development of the femoral head and acetabulum. Although uncommon, limb-length discrepancy should be evaluated annually by clinical evaluation and radiography.

PELVIC OSTEOTOMY

Operations on the pelvis, alone or combined with open reduction, are useful in developmental dysplasia or dislocation of the hip to ensure or to increase stability of the joint. The operations most often used are (1) osteotomy of the innominate bone (Salter), (2) acetabuloplasty (Pemberton), (3) osteotomies that free the acetabulum (Steel triple innominate osteotomy or Ganz acetabular osteotomy), (4) shelf operation (Staheli), and (5) innominate osteotomy with medial displacement of the acetabulum (Chiari). In an older child, one of these operations can be combined with femoral osteotomy to correct femoral and acetabular abnormalities.

Osteotomy of the innominate bone, an operation devised by Salter, is useful only when any subluxation or dislocation has been reduced or can be reduced by open reduction at the time of osteotomy in a child 18 months to 6 years old. The entire acetabulum together with the pubis and ischium is rotated as a unit, with the symphysis pubis acting as a hinge. The osteotomy is held open anterolaterally by a wedge of bone, and the roof of the acetabulum is shifted more anteriorly and laterally. The osteotomy is contraindicated in patients with nonconcentric hips or severe dysplasia.

Acetabuloplasty is also useful only when any subluxation or dislocation has been reduced or can be reduced by open reduction at the time of operation in children at least 18 months old. In acetabuloplasty, the inclination of the acetabular roof is decreased by an osteotomy of the ilium made superior to the acetabulum. Pemberton described a *pericapsular osteotomy of the ilium* in which the osteotomy is made through the full thickness of the bone from just superior to the anterior inferior iliac spine anteriorly to the triradiate cartilage posteriorly; the triradiate cartilage acts as a hinge on which the acetabular roof is rotated anteriorly and laterally. This procedure decreases the volume of the acetabulum and produces joint incongruity that requires remodeling.

Osteotomies that free the acetabulum have been devised by Steel, Eppright, and Ganz. These operations free part of the pelvis, creating a movable segment of bone that includes the acetabulum. They are indicated in older children, adolescents, and skeletally mature adults with residual dysplasia and subluxation in whom remodeling of the acetabulum can no longer be anticipated. These operations are useful because they place articular cartilage over the femoral head. The shelf operation and the operation of Chiari interpose capsular fibrous tissue between the femoral head and the reconstructed acetabulum.

In the triple innominate osteotomy (Steel), the ischium, the superior pubic ramus, and the ilium superior to the acetabulum all are divided and the acetabulum is repositioned and stabilized by a bone graft and metal pins. In the pericapsular dial osteotomy of the acetabulum (Eppright), the entire acetabulum superiorly, posteriorly, inferiorly, and anteriorly is freed by osteotomy and as a single segment of bone is redirected to cover the femoral head appropriately. The Bernese periacetabular osteotomy (Ganz) creates a free acetabular segment through a series of osteotomies in the ischium, superior pubic ramus, and ilium while preserving the posterior column of the pelvis.

The *shelf* procedure (Staheli) is useful for subluxations and dislocations that have been reduced and in which no other osteotomy would establish a congruous joint with apposition of the articular cartilage of the acetabulum to the femoral head. In a classic shelf operation, the acetabular roof is extended laterally, posteriorly, or anteriorly, either by a graft or by turning distally over the femoral head the acetabular roof and part of the lateral cortex of the ilium superior to it.

Innominate osteotomy with medial displacement of the acetabulum, an operation devised by Chiari for patients older than 4 years old, is a modified shelf operation that places the femoral head beneath a surface of bone and joint capsule and corrects the pathologic lateral displacement of the femur. An osteotomy is made at the level of the acetabulum, and the femur and the acetabulum are displaced medially. The inferior surface of the proximal fragment forms a roof over the femoral head. General recommendations for all of these osteotomies are summarized in Table 30-1.

TABLE 30-1

Recommended Osteotomies for Congenital or Developmental Dislocation of the Hip

OSTEOTOMY	AGE	INDICATIONS
Salter innominate osteotomy	18 months-6 years	Congruous hip reduction; <10-15 degrees correction of acetabular index required
Pemberton acetabuloplasty	18 months-10 years	>10-15 correction of acetabular index required; small femoral head, large acetabulum
Steel or Ganz osteotomy	Late adolescence to skeletal maturity	Residual acetabular dysplasia; symptoms; congruous joint
Shelf procedure or Chiari osteotomy	Adolescence to skeletal maturity	Incongruous joint; symptoms; other osteotomy not possible

SALTER INNOMINATE OSTEOTOMY

During open reduction of developmental dislocations of the hip, Salter observed that the entire acetabulum faces more anterolaterally than normal. When the hip is extended, the femoral head is insufficiently "covered" anteriorly, and when it is adducted, there is insufficient coverage superiorly. Salter's osteotomy of the innominate bone redirects the entire acetabulum so that its roof "covers" the femoral head anteriorly and superiorly. If indicated to correct acetabular dysplasia, any dislocation or subluxation must be reduced concentrically before this operation is performed; if not, open reduction is done at the time of osteotomy. During the operation, any contractures of the adductor or iliopsoas muscles are released by tenotomy, and, in dislocations when the capsule is elongated, a capsulorrhaphy is done.

Salter recommended his osteotomy in the primary treatment of developmental dislocation of the hip in children 18 months to 6 years old and in the primary treatment of developmental subluxation in early adulthood. He also recommended it in the secondary treatment of any residual or recurrent dislocation or subluxation after other methods of treatment within the age limits described (Fig. 30-22).

The following are prerequisites for the success of this operation:

1. The femoral head must be positioned opposite the level of the acetabulum. This may require a period of traction before surgery or primary femoral shortening.
2. Contractures of the iliopsoas and adductor muscles must be released. This is indicated in subluxations and dislocations. Open reduction is performed for hip dislocation but usually is unnecessary for hip subluxation.
3. The femoral head must be reduced into the depth of the true acetabulum completely and concentrically. This generally requires careful open reduction and excision of any soft tissue, exclusive of the labrum, from the acetabulum.
4. The joint must be reasonably congruous.
5. The range of motion of the hip must be good, especially in abduction, internal rotation, and flexion.

In a cadaver study, Birnbaum et al. identified several structures that are at risk of injury during a Salter innominate osteotomy:

1. The lateral femoral cutaneous nerve may be injured during an anterior approach. Ensuring that the skin including the lateral femoral cutaneous nerve is pulled anteriorly avoids this.
2. The nutrient vessels to the tensor fasciae latae muscle can be injured if retraction is too prolonged.

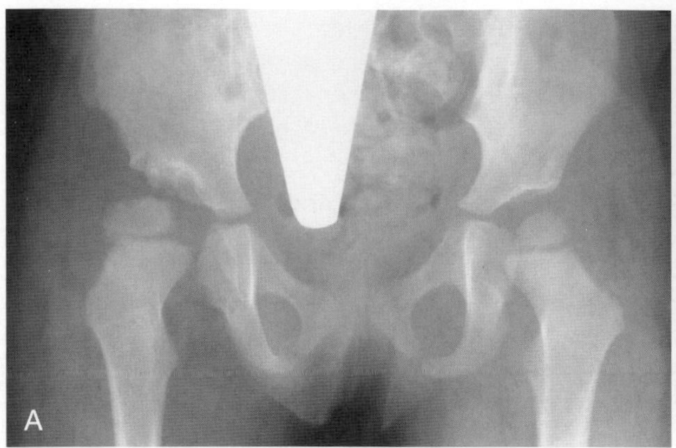

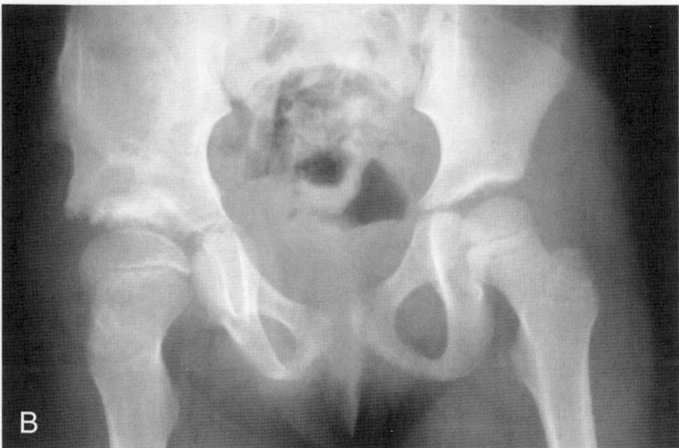

FIGURE 30-22 Salter osteotomy for congenital dislocation of hip. **A,** Residual acetabular dysplasia and subluxation of right hip in 4-year-old girl in whom open reduction had been performed at 9 months of age. **B,** One year after repeat open reduction and Salter innominate osteotomy.

3. The sciatic nerve can be crushed or irritated by an inadequate subperiosteal approach during the pull on the Hohmann retractor.
4. An inadequate subperiosteal application of the medial Hohmann retractor can damage the obturator nerve.
5. Too prolonged retraction of the iliopsoas muscle can cause compression of the femoral nerve.

Because of the narrow spatial connection between the anatomic pathways and the osteotomy area, strict subperiosteal dissection and careful use of retractors are essential to prevent nerve and vessel injuries.

INNOMINATE OSTEOTOMY INCLUDING OPEN REDUCTION

TECHNIQUE 30-9

(SALTER)

- Place the patient supine on the operating table with the thorax on the affected side elevated by a radiolucent sandbag. Drape the trunk on the affected side to the midline anteriorly and posteriorly and to the lower rib cage superiorly. Drape the lower extremity so that it can be moved freely during the operation.
- Release the adductor muscles by subcutaneous or open tenotomy.
- Make a skin incision beginning just inferior to the middle of the iliac crest, extending anteriorly to just inferior to the anterior superior iliac spine and continuing to about the middle of the inguinal ligament. Decrease bleeding by applying pressure with sponges to the wound edges.
- Bluntly dissect between the tensor fasciae latae muscle laterally and the sartorius and rectus femoris medially and expose the anterior superior iliac spine.
- Dissect the rectus femoris from the underlying joint capsule and release its reflected head.
- Make a deep incision separating the iliac apophysis along the crest from the posterior end of the skin incision to the anterior superior iliac spine anteriorly and then turning distally to the anterior inferior iliac spine.
- Reflect the lateral part of the iliac apophysis and the periosteum from the lateral surface of the iliac crest in a continuous sheet inferiorly to the superior edge of the acetabulum and posteriorly to the greater sciatic notch.
- Free any adhesions of the joint capsule from the lateral surface of the ilium and from any false acetabulum.
- Expose the capsule anteriorly and laterally by dissecting bluntly the interval between it and the abductor muscles.
- Pack the dissected spaces with large sponges to control bleeding and to increase the interval between the reflected periosteum and the sciatic notch.
- If concentric reduction of the femoral head into the acetabulum is impossible, open the capsule superiorly and anteriorly, parallel with and about 1 cm distal to the rim of the acetabulum.
- Excise the ligamentum teres if it is hypertrophied.
- Gently reduce the femoral head into the acetabulum. Never excise the limbus. Incise the distal flap of capsule at right angles to the first incision, creating a T-shaped incision, and resect the inferolateral triangular flap so created. Test the stability of the joint; if the head becomes displaced superiorly from the acetabulum when the hip is adducted or anteriorly when it is extended or externally rotated, osteotomy of the innominate bone is performed.
- Allow the hip to redislocate and then strip the medial half of the iliac apophysis from the anterior half of the iliac crest and strip the periosteum from the medial surface of the ilium posteriorly and inferiorly to expose the entire medial aspect of the bone to the sciatic notch.
- Pack the surfaces exposed with sponges to control the loss of blood and to enlarge the interval between the periosteum and the bone.
- Expose the tendinous part of the iliopsoas muscle at the level of the pelvic brim. With scissors, separate the tendinous part from the muscular part and divide the former while protecting the muscle.

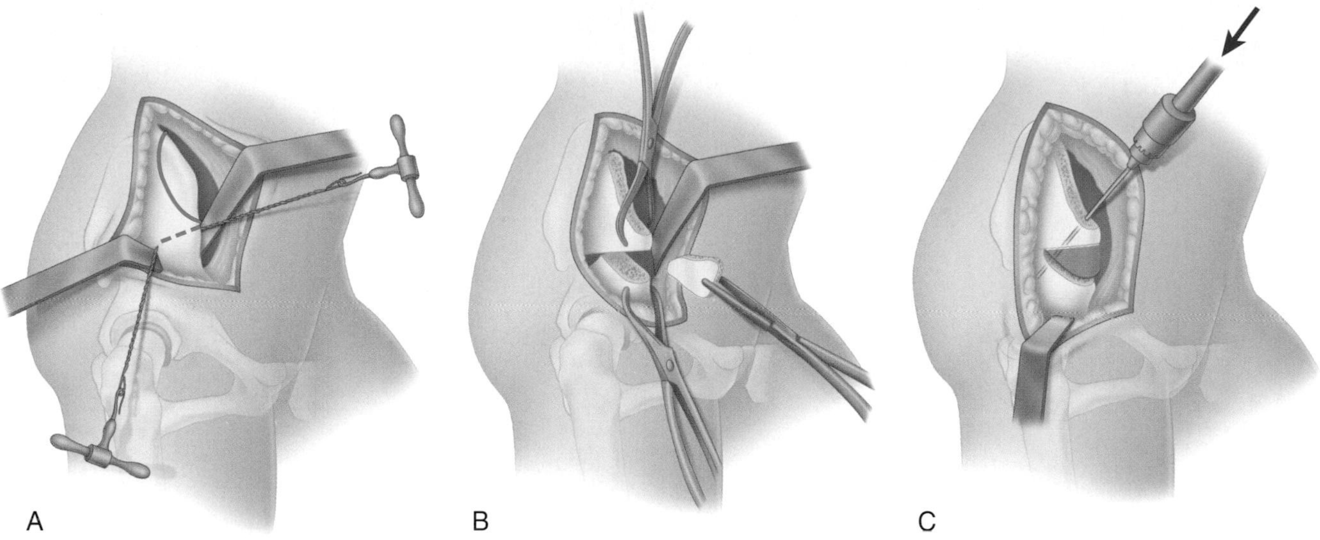

FIGURE 30-23 A-C, Salter technique of osteotomy of innominate bone, including open reduction. **SEE TECHNIQUE 30-9.**

- Pass a curved forceps subperiosteally medial to the ilium into the sciatic notch and with it grasp one end of a Gigli saw. Gently retract the curved forceps to pass the Gigli saw into the sciatic notch.
- Retract the tissues medially and laterally from the ilium and divide the bone with the saw in a straight line from the sciatic notch to the anterior inferior iliac spine.
- Remove a full-thickness graft from the anterior part of the iliac crest (Fig. 30-23A) and trim it to the shape of a wedge. If a primary femoral shortening was performed concurrently, the removed femoral bone segment can be used as structural autograft bone. Make the base of the wedge about as wide as the distance between the anterior superior and anterior inferior iliac spines.
- With towel clips, grasp each fragment of the osteotomized ilium.
- Insert a curved elevator into the sciatic notch and, by levering it anteriorly and by exerting traction on the towel clip that grasps the inferior fragment, shift this fragment anteriorly, inferiorly, and laterally to open the osteotomy anterolaterally. Ensure that the osteotomy remains closed posteriorly (Fig. 30-23B). Placing the limb in a figure-of-four position makes displacement of the distal fragment easier.
- Do not apply traction in a cephalad direction on the proximal fragment because this may dislocate the sacroiliac joint.
- Insert the bone graft into the osteotomy and release the traction on the inferior fragment.
- Drill a strong Kirschner wire through the remaining superior part of the ilium, through the graft, and into the inferior fragment (Fig. 30-23C). Ensure that the Kirschner wire does not enter the acetabulum but that it does traverse all three fragments.
- Drill a second Kirschner wire parallel with the first, using the same precautions.
- Reduce the femoral head again into the acetabulum and reevaluate its stability. Reduction should now be stable with the hip either in adduction or in slight external rotation.
- While closing the wound, have an assistant hold the knee flexed and the hip slightly abducted, flexed, and internally rotated.
- Obliterate any residual pocket of capsule by performing a capsulorrhaphy.
- Move the distal half of the lateral flap of capsule medially beyond the anterior inferior iliac spine. This brings the capsular edges together and increases the stability of reduction by keeping the hip internally rotated. Repair the capsule with interrupted sutures.
- Suture the sartorius and rectus femoris tendons to their origins.
- Suture together over the iliac crest the two halves of the iliac apophysis.
- Cut the Kirschner wires so that their anterior ends lie within the subcutaneous fat.
- Close the skin with a continuous subcuticular suture.
- With the hip held in the same position as during closure, apply a single spica cast.

POSTOPERATIVE CARE. At 8 to 12 weeks, the spica cast is removed and, with the patient under general or local anesthesia, the Kirschner wires are also removed. The positions of the osteotomy and of the hip are checked by radiographs.

PEMBERTON ACETABULOPLASTY

The term *acetabuloplasty* designates operations that redirect the inclination of the acetabular roof by an osteotomy of the ilium superior to the acetabulum followed by levering of the roof inferiorly. Pemberton devised an acetabuloplasty that he called *pericapsular osteotomy of the ilium,* in which an osteotomy is made through the full thickness of the ilium, using the triradiate cartilage as the hinge around which the

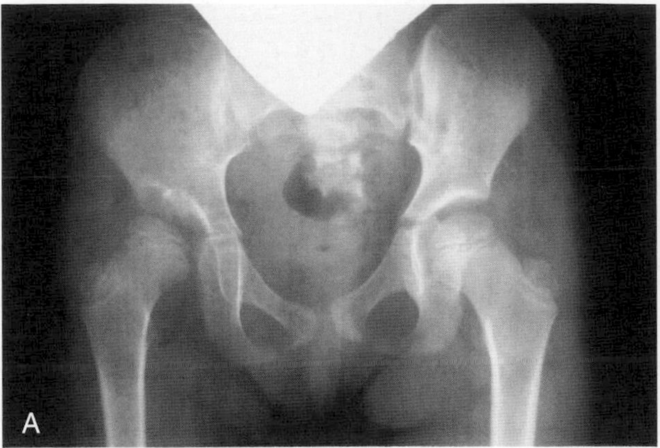

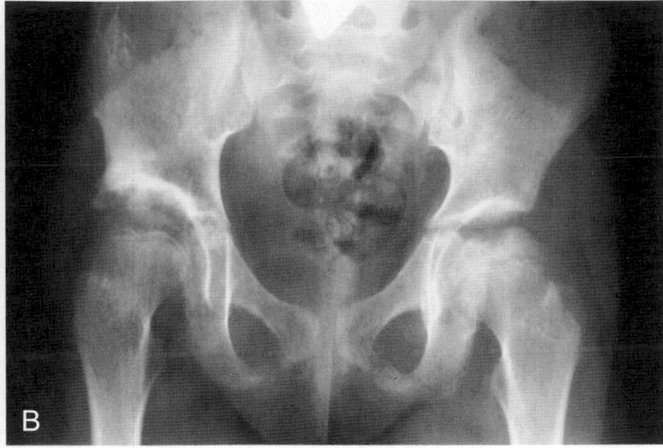

FIGURE 30-24 Pemberton acetabuloplasty. **A,** Symptomatic residual acetabular dysplasia in 8-year-old girl after treatment of congenital dislocation of right hip. **B,** After Pemberton acetabuloplasty.

acetabular roof is rotated anteriorly and laterally. After a review of 115 hips in 91 patients followed for at least 2 years after surgery, Pemberton recommended this procedure for any dysplastic hip in patients between the age of 1 year and the age when the triradiate cartilage becomes too inflexible to serve as a hinge (about 12 years old in girls and 14 years old in boys), provided that any subluxation or dislocation has been reduced or can be reduced at the time of osteotomy (Fig. 30-24).

One advantage of pericapsular over innominate osteotomies is that internal fixation is not always required, and a second, although minor, operation (implant removal) is avoided. A greater degree of correction can be achieved with less rotation of the acetabulum in the pericapsular osteotomy because the fulcrum, the triradiate cartilage, is nearer the site of desired correction; however, Pemberton's operation is technically more difficult to perform. In addition, it alters the configuration and capacity of the acetabulum and can result in an incongruous relationship between it and the femoral head; consequently, some remodeling of the acetabulum is required.

PERICAPSULAR OSTEOTOMY OF THE ILIUM

TECHNIQUE 30-10

(PEMBERTON)

- Place the patient supine with a small radiolucent sandbag beneath the affected hip and expose the hip through an anterior iliofemoral approach.
- Make the superior part of the incision distal to and parallel with the iliac crest and extend it from the anterior superior iliac spine anteriorly to the middle of the crest posteriorly. Extend the distal part of the incision from the anterior superior iliac spine inferiorly for 5 cm parallel with the inguinal crease.
- Beginning at the crest, strip the gluteus and the tensor fasciae latae muscles subperiosteally from the anterior third of the ilium distally to the joint capsule and posteriorly until the greater sciatic notch is exposed.
- With a sharp elevator, separate the iliac apophysis with its attached abdominal muscles from the anterior third of the iliac crest and strip the muscles subperiosteally from the medial aspect of the ilium until the sciatic notch is again exposed.
- Open the capsule of the hip and remove any soft tissue that restricts reduction.
- Reduce the hip under direct vision and ensure that it is well seated; redislocate it until the osteotomy has been made and propped open with a graft.
- Insert two flat retractors subperiosteally into the sciatic notch—one along the medial surface of the ilium and one along the lateral surface to keep the anterior third of the ilium exposed medially and laterally. Image intensification can be helpful in visualizing the location and direction of the osteotomy.
- With a narrow curved osteotome, cut through the lateral cortex of the ilium as follows. Start slightly superior to the anterior inferior iliac spine and curve the osteotomy posteriorly about 1 cm proximal to and parallel with the joint capsule until the osteotome is seen to be well anterior to the retractor resting in the sciatic notch. Image intensification aids in confirming correct placement of the osteotomy.
- From this point when driven farther, the blade of the osteotome disappears from sight, and it is important to direct its tip sufficiently inferiorly so that it does not enter the sciatic notch but instead enters the ilioischial rim of the triradiate cartilage at its midpoint.
- After directing the osteotome properly, drive it 1.5 cm farther to complete the osteotomy of the lateral cortex of the ilium.

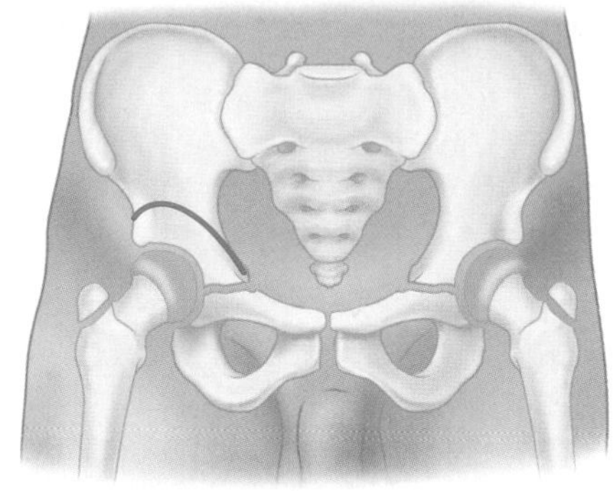

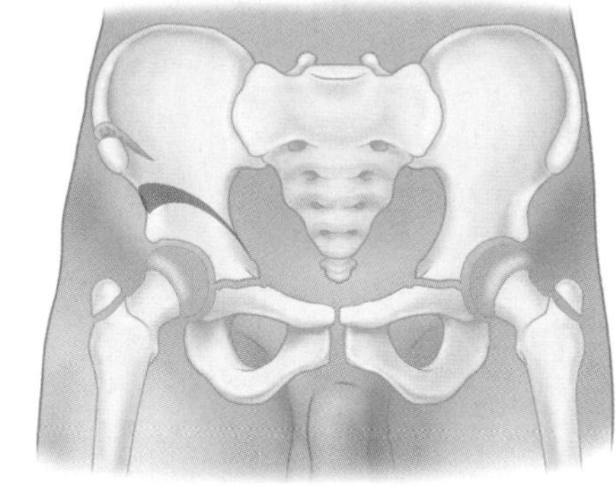

FIGURE 30-25 Pemberton pericapsular osteotomy. **A,** Line of osteotomy beginning slightly superior to anterior inferior iliac spine and curving into triradiate cartilage. **B,** Completed osteotomy with acetabular roof in corrected position and wedge of bone impacted into open osteotomy site. **SEE TECHNIQUE 30-10.**

- With the same osteotome, make a corresponding cut in the medial cortex of the ilium, starting anteriorly at the same point just superior to the anterior inferior iliac spine. Direct this cut posteriorly parallel with that in the lateral cortex until it reaches the triradiate cartilage (Fig. 30-25A).
- The direction in which the acetabular roof becomes displaced after the osteotomy is controlled by varying the position of the posterior part of the osteotomy of the medial cortex. The more anterior this part of the osteotomy, the less the acetabular roof rotates anteriorly; conversely, the more posterior this part of the osteotomy, the more the acetabular roof rotates anteriorly.
- After completing the osteotomy of the two cortices, insert a wide curved osteotome into the anterior part of the osteotomy and lever the distal fragment distally until the anterior edges of the two fragments are at least 2 to 3 cm apart.
- The acetabular roof should be turned inferiorly far enough to correct the dysplasia. The exact degree of correction can be difficult to determine. Some overcorrection is advisable, but overcorrection could result in impingement during flexion and internal rotation.
- Cut a narrow groove in the anteroposterior direction in each raw surface of the ilium.
- Resect a wedge of bone from the anterior part of the ilium including the anterior superior iliac spine; with a lamina spreader, separate the osteotomy fragments and place the wedge of bone in the grooves made in the surfaces of the ilium; drive the wedge into place and firmly impact it. The acetabular roof should remain fixed in the corrected position (Fig. 30-25B). Alternatively, a segment of femur can be used when a concurrent primary femoral shortening procedure has been performed (Fig 30-26).
- Hold the correction with a Kirschner wire, if necessary.
- If the hip has remained dislocated during the osteotomy, reduce it at this time.
- Perform a meticulous capsulorrhaphy for additional soft-tissue stability.
- Suture the iliac apophysis over the remaining ilium and close the wound.

POSTOPERATIVE CARE. With the hip in neutral position (or in slight abduction and internal rotation, if this has been found the most favorable position for closure of the wound), a spica cast is applied from the nipple line to the toes on the affected side and to above the knee on the opposite side. At 8 to 12 weeks, the cast is removed and the osteotomy is checked by radiographs.

STEEL OSTEOTOMY

The Pemberton pericapsular osteotomy is limited by the mobility of the triradiate cartilage, and hinging on this cartilage can cause premature physeal closure. Although the Salter innominate osteotomy can be used in older patients, its results depend on the mobility of the symphysis pubis, and the amount of femoral head coverage is limited. Other, more complex osteotomies, such as those of Steel and Eppright, can provide more correction and improve femoral head coverage.

In the *triple innominate osteotomy* developed by Steel, the ischium, the superior pubic ramus, and the ilium superior to the acetabulum all are divided, and the acetabulum is repositioned and stabilized by a bone graft and pins. The objective of this procedure is to establish a stable hip in anatomic position for dislocation or subluxation of the hip in older children when this is impossible by any one of the other osteotomies (Fig. 30-27). For the operation to be successful, the articular surfaces of the joint must be congruous or become so when the acetabulum has been redirected so that a functional, painless range of motion is achieved and a Trendelenburg gait is absent. Steel reviewed 45 patients in whom 52 of his osteotomies had been performed. The results were satisfactory in 40 hips and unsatisfactory in 12. The unsatisfactory hips were painful and easily fatigued; in two, the Trendelenburg test was positive, and in one, significant motion had been lost.

Lipton and Bowen modified the Steel osteotomy by (1) resecting 1.0 to 1.5 cm of bone after the ischial osteotomy to facilitate medialization and rotation of the acetabulum, (2) resecting a triangular wedge of bone from the outer cortex

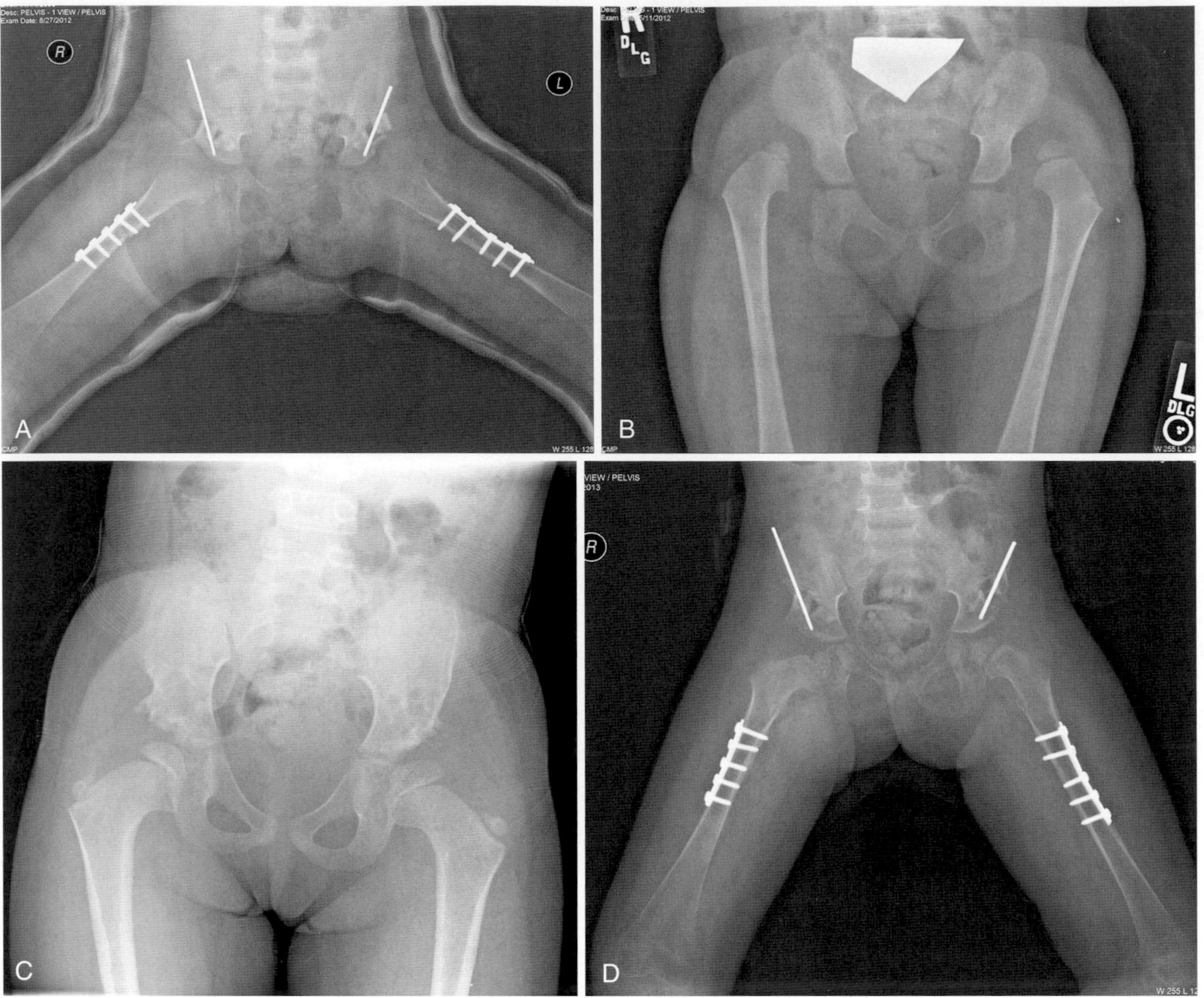

FIGURE 30-26 **A,** Preoperative image demonstrating bilateral hip dislocations in a 2-year-old patient. **B,** Anteroposterior pelvic view after staged open reductions, capsulorrhaphies, primary femoral shortenings, and Pemberton acetabuloplasties using resection femoral segment for pelvic bone grafting. **C,** Postoperative anteroposterior pelvis after spica cast removal. **D,** Two-year follow-up view reveals healing and maintenance of hip reduction. Some residual dysplasia exists, particularly on the left hip. **SEE TECHNIQUE 30-10.**

of the proximal part of the ilium to create a slot that serves as an abutment into which the distal posterior aspect of the ilium fits, and (3) using two 7.3-mm cannulated screws instead of Steinmann pins for fixation of the iliac osteotomy. The procedure is done through two incisions: an ischial incision and a bikini-type iliofemoral incision. Primary advantages of this technique include better coverage of the femoral head by articular cartilage of the acetabulum, better hip joint stability for weight bearing, and no need for spica cast immobilization. Disadvantages include the technical difficulty of the procedure; it does not change the size of the acetabulum, and it distorts the pelvis such that natural childbirth may be impossible in adulthood. Femoral shortening may be performed, and, if necessary, any contracted muscles around the hip are released surgically.

Using three-dimensional CT, Frick et al. identified excessive (>10 degrees) external rotation of the acetabulum after triple innominate osteotomy in five hips, which included two with pubic osteotomy nonunions, two with ischial nonunions, and one with marked external rotation of the leg. They cautioned that the surgical technique for triple innominate osteotomy should be designed to avoid excessive external rotation of the acetabular fragment, which can result in (1) excessive external rotation of the lower limb, (2) decreased posterior coverage, (3) increased gaps at the pubic and ischial osteotomy sites with resultant higher rates of nonunion, and (4) lateralization of the joint center. Technique modifications by Frick et al. include avoidance of the figure-of-four maneuver to mobilize the acetabulum (they believe this promotes external rotation of the acetabulum); strict attention to the intraoperative landmarks of the proximal ilium and anterior inferior iliac spine, keeping the anterior inferior iliac spine in line with the plane of the proximal ilium to prevent external rotation; and use of a temporary Schanz screw in the acetabular segment to serve as a handle to guide the acetabulum into the correct position. Careful

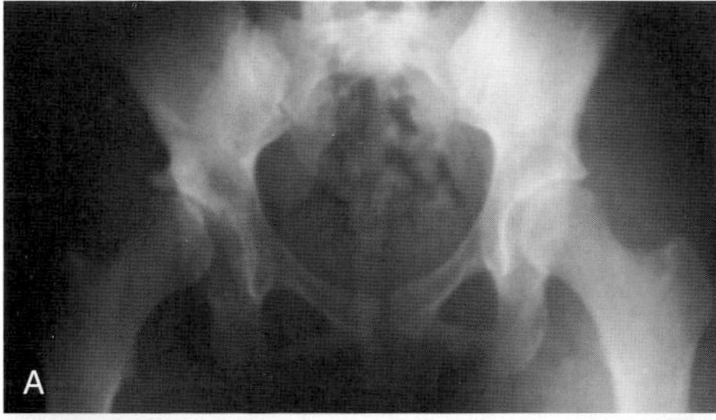

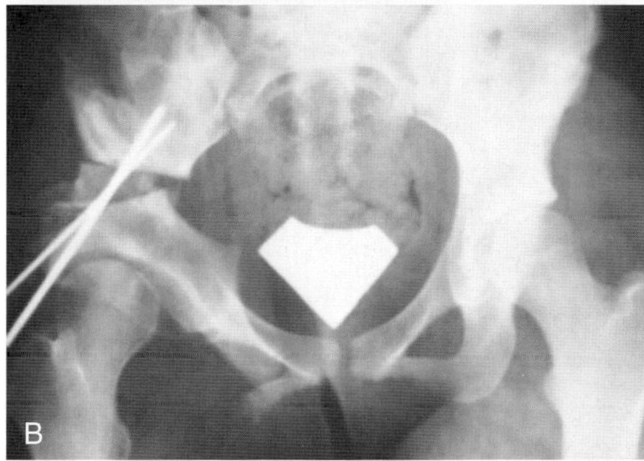

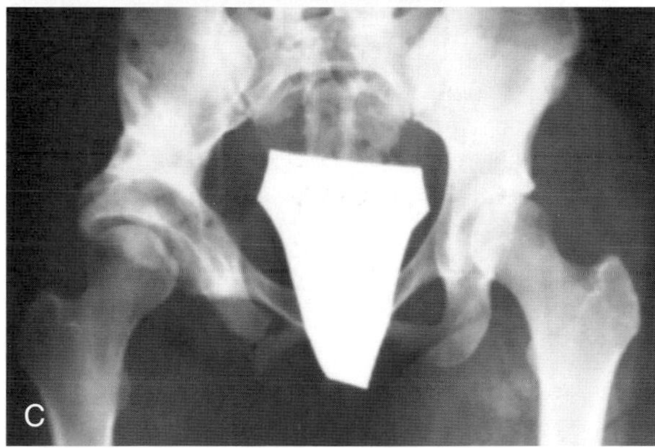

FIGURE 30-27 Steel triple innominate osteotomy. **A,** Sixteen-year-old girl with painful right hip, subluxation, and acetabular dysplasia. **B,** After Steel osteotomy. **C,** One year after surgery. (Courtesy of Randal Betz, MD, and Howard Steel, MD.)

evaluation of the transverse plane acetabular position before and after provisional fixation is recommended to aid in preventing rotational malunions.

TRIPLE INNOMINATE OSTEOTOMY

TECHNIQUE 30-11

(STEEL)

- Place the patient supine on the operating table and flex the hip and knee 90 degrees. Keep the hip in neutral abduction, adduction, and rotation.
- Drape the posterior aspect of the proximal thigh and the buttock, leaving the ischial tuberosity exposed.
- Make a transverse incision perpendicular to the long axis of the femoral shaft 1 cm proximal to the gluteal crease.
- Retract the gluteus maximus muscle laterally and expose the hamstring muscles at their ischial origin.
- By sharp dissection, free the biceps femoris, the most superficial muscle in the area, from the ischium and expose the interval between the semimembranosus and the semitendinosus muscles. The sciatic nerve lies far enough laterally not to be endangered.
- Insert a curved hemostat in the interval between the origins of the semimembranosus and the semitendinosus deep to the ischium and into the obturator foramen.
- Elevate the origins of the obturator internus and externus and bring the tip of the hemostat out at the inferior margin of the ischial ramus. Ensure that the hemostat remains in contact with the bone during its passage deep to the ramus.
- With an osteotome directed posterolaterally and 45 degrees from the perpendicular, divide completely the ischial ramus. Allow the origin of the biceps femoris to fall into place.
- Suture the gluteus maximus to the deep fascia and close the skin.
- Change gowns, gloves, and instruments, and begin in the iliopubic area the second stage of the operation. As an alternative, the superior and inferior pubic rami can be dissected and divided through a medial adductor approach. If a posterior incision was chosen, however, proceed with a full skin preparation medially to the midline and superiorly to the costal margin and drape the extremity free.
- Through an anterior iliofemoral approach, reflect the iliac and gluteal muscles from the wing of the ilium.
- Detach the sartorius and the lateral attachments of the inguinal ligament from the anterior superior iliac spine and reflect them medially.
- Reflect the iliacus and psoas muscles subperiosteally from the inner surface of the pelvis; this protects the femoral neurovascular bundle.
- Divide the tendinous part of the origin of the iliopsoas and expose the pectineal tubercle. Detach the pectineus muscle subperiosteally from the superior pubic ramus and expose the bone 1 cm medial to the pubic tubercle.
- Pass a curved hemostat superior to the superior pubic ramus into the obturator foramen near the bone. With this hemostat, penetrate the obturator fascia so that the tip of the hemostat is brought out inferior to the ramus. If the bone is especially thick, pass a second hemostat inferior to the ramus and direct it superiorly to contact the first one.
- Direct an osteotome posteromedially and 15 degrees from the perpendicular and perform an osteotomy of the pubic ramus.
- The obturator artery, vein, and nerve are protected by the hemostat. Using the technique as described by Salter for innominate osteotomy, divide the ilium with a Gigli saw. When this osteotomy has been completed, free the periosteum and fascia from the medial wall of the pelvis to free the acetabular segment (Fig. 30-28).

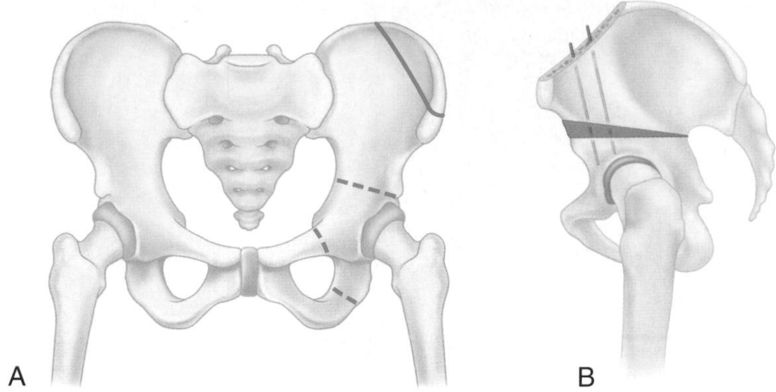

FIGURE 30-28 Steel triple innominate osteotomy. **A,** Osteotomies to be performed in iliac wing and superior and inferior pubic rami. Note wedge of bone to be taken as graft from superiormost portion of ilium. **B,** Lateral view showing graft in place and fixation with two Kirschner wires. **SEE TECHNIQUE 30-11.**

- If the femoral head is subluxated or dislocated, open the capsule at this time and remove any tissue obstructing reduction. Reduce the femoral head as near as possible to the center of the triradiate cartilage and close the capsule.
- With a towel clip, grasp the anterior inferior iliac spine and rotate the acetabular segment in the desired direction, usually anteriorly and laterally, until the femoral head is covered. In an older child, use a lamina spreader to open the osteotomy because the sacroiliac joint usually is more stable in this age group and is not likely to be subluxated.
- With the acetabular fragment in proper position, stabilize it with a triangular bone graft removed from the superior rim of the ilium.
- Transfix the graft with two pins that penetrate the inner wall of the ilium.
- Allow the pectineus and iliopsoas muscles to fall into place.
- Reattach the sartorius and the lateral end of the inguinal ligament to the anterior superior iliac spine and close the wound in layers.

POSTOPERATIVE CARE. A spica cast is applied with the hip in 20 degrees of abduction, 5 degrees of flexion, and neutral rotation. At 8 to 10 weeks, the cast and pins are removed and active and passive motion of the hip are started. All three osteotomies usually unite by 12 weeks after surgery, at which time progressive weight bearing on crutches is started.

DEGA OSTEOTOMY

In 1969, Dega described a transiliac osteotomy for the treatment of residual acetabular dysplasia secondary to developmental hip dysplasia or dislocation. This incomplete transiliac osteotomy involves osteotomy of the anterior and middle portions of the inner cortex of the ilium, leaving an intact hinge posteriorly consisting of the intact posteromedial iliac cortex and sciatic notch.

Because of the variable hinge location, the Dega osteotomy can be done with either an open or a closed triradiate cartilage, although it is usually done before closure of the triradiate cartilage. This osteotomy is only one component of the comprehensive, complicated surgery required to treat severe developmental dysplasia of the hip in children of walking age. It must be accompanied by a satisfactory open reduction and an appropriate correction of proximal femoral deformity when needed (Fig. 30-29).

TRANSILIAC (DEGA) OSTEOTOMY

TECHNIQUE 30-12

(GRUDZIAK AND WARD)

- Position the patient supine with the involved hip tilted up 30 to 40 degrees by a bump placed at the midlumbar level.
- Make an extended anterolateral incision starting 1 cm inferior and posterior to the anterior superior iliac spine and extending distally over the proximal part of the femur, centered over the greater trochanter (Fig. 30-30A). Alternatively, this procedure can be performed through a standard ilioinguinal approach at the time of open reduction of the hip.
- Develop the interval between the tensor fasciae latae muscles posteriorly and the sartorius muscle anteriorly and release the sartorius from its origin on the anterior superior iliac spine.
- Sharply reflect the abductor muscles off of the lateral wall of the ilium just distal to the iliac apophysis, but do not split the apophysis itself. Completely separate the abductor muscles and periosteum from the ilium and the hip capsule back to the sciatic notch, which is fully exposed, and insert an adult-size blunt Hohmann retractor into the notch. Do not dissect either the muscles or the periosteum off of the inner wall of the ilium.
- Separate the reflected head of the rectus femoris muscle from the hip capsule and incise it. Detach the tendon of

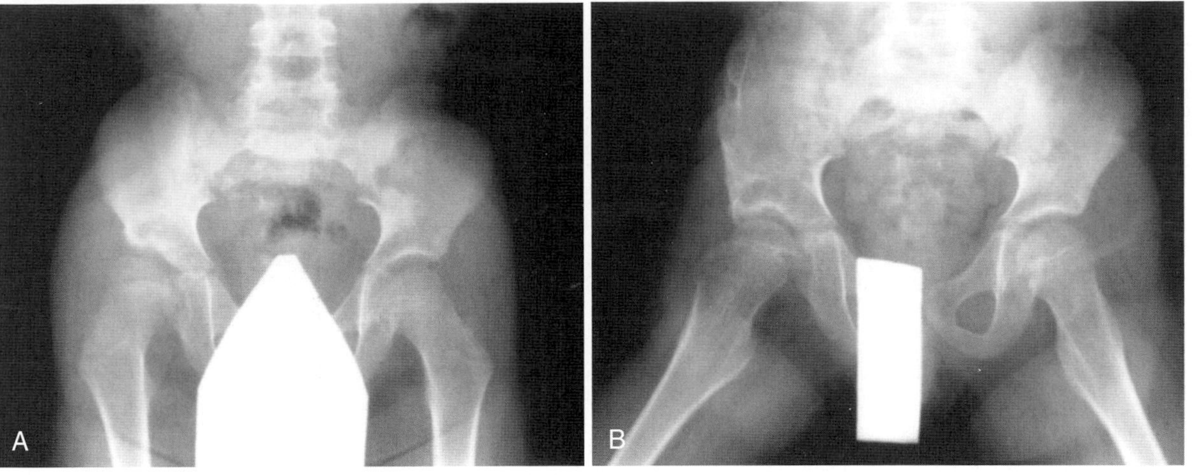

FIGURE 30-29 Before (A) and after (B) Dega transiliac osteotomy.

the straight head of the rectus femoris muscle from the anterior inferior iliac spine only when necessary for proper exposure of the capsule.

- Isolate the tendinous portion of the iliopsoas muscle from the capsule and transect it either over the anteromedial aspect of the capsule just distal to the pelvic brim or more distally near its insertion.
- If required, reduce the hip and perform a femoral osteotomy with shortening and rotation to correct excessive anteversion.
- Make the Dega osteotomy to decrease acetabular dysplasia and to enhance containment of the femoral head.
- Mark the orientation of the osteotomy on the lateral cortex of the ilium (Fig. 30-30B). The direction of the osteotomy is curvilinear when viewed from the lateral cortex, starting just above the anterior inferior iliac spine, curving gently cephalad and posteriorly to reach a point superior to the midpoint of the acetabulum, and then continuing posteriorly to end 1.0 to 1.5 cm in front of the sciatic notch. The most cephalad extent of the osteotomy is in the middle of the acetabulum, at a point on the ilium determined by the steepness of the acetabulum. Very steep acetabular inclinations require a correspondingly higher midpoint.
- Insert a guidewire under fluoroscopic control at the most cephalad point of the curvilinear marking line, directing it caudally and medially to ensure that the osteotomy exits at the appropriate level just above the horizontal limb of the triradiate cartilage.
- Use a straight ¼-inch or ½-inch osteotome to make the bone cut, which extends obliquely medially and inferiorly, paralleling the guidewire to exit through the inner cortex just above the iliopubic and ilioischial limbs of the triradiate cartilage (Fig. 30-30C), leaving the posterior one third of the inner cortex intact (Fig. 30-30D).
- If predominantly anterior coverage is desired, cut the medial (inner) cortex over the anterior and middle portion, leaving only the posterior sciatic notch hinge intact.
- If more lateral coverage is desired, leave more of the medial cortex intact, resulting in a posteromedial hinge based on the posteromedial inner cortex and the entire sciatic notch. Generally, approximately one fourth to one third of the inner pelvic cortex is left intact posteriorly. With experience, the osteotomy cut might be done safely without fluoroscopic guidance, as in Dega's original description; however, we prefer to use fluoroscopy.
- Use a ½-inch osteotome to gently lever open the osteotomy site either anteriorly or laterally in a controlled manner (Fig. 30-30E). A small lamina spreader also is useful for this maneuver. Often, while the osteotomy site is being opened, the osteotomy cut on the outer cortex of the ilium propagates toward the sciatic notch as a greenstick fracture. Because the posterior portion of the inner cortex is still intact, however, the outer cortical greenstick fracture does not weaken the recoil and stability at the osteotomy site.
- Keep the osteotomy site open by inserting two correctly sized bone grafts (Fig. 30-30F). Fashion the grafts from a bicortical segment of iliac crest bone, or, alternatively, if femoral shortening has been done, use the segment of the femur that was removed.
- If there is a substantial gap at the osteotomy site, an autogenous femoral or iliac crest graft may be insufficient. Under these circumstances, the height of the graft can be increased by using freeze-dried fibular allograft cut into trapezoidal sections.
- The correct graft height is determined by simply noting the opening of the osteotomy gap created by the lamina spreader or the levering osteotome. In developmental dysplasia, acetabular deficiency is most pronounced anteriorly, mandating placement of the larger graft more anteriorly. Wedge a smaller graft more posteriorly, just in front of the intact sciatic notch. Ensure that both grafts are of an appropriate height and that the amount of correction of the dysplastic acetabulum provides enough coverage of the femoral head.
- After the grafts have been inserted, they are stable because of the inherent recoil at the osteotomy site produced by the intact sciatic notch. Metallic internal fixation is unnecessary. Variations in the graft size and placement,

extent of the outer and inner cortical cuts, and thickness of the acetabular fragment make it possible to reorient and reshape the acetabulum. The more posterior the extent of the outer cortical cut, and the greater the amount of the inner cortex left intact, the more lateral the tilt of the acetabulum. A more cephalad starting point and a steeper osteotomy angle produce more lateral coverage. A more extensive cut through the inner cortex allows for more anterior coverage of the hip. Finally, the closer the osteotomy is to the acetabulum, the thinner and more pliable is the acetabular fragment, theoretically allowing for more reshaping and less redirection to occur. These three-dimensional changes in the osteotomy are difficult to quantify, as is the true anatomic nature of a dysplastic hip. An experienced orthopaedic surgeon who is familiar with the spectrum of dysplastic hip pathology and who applies the principles described should be able to perform an osteotomy, however, that is precisely suited to the unique pathology of a given dysplastic hip.

- When the osteotomy is done, satisfactory femoral head coverage can be appreciated and the hip should be stable during flexion and rotation.
- After closure, apply a one and one-half spica cast with the hip in neutral extension, approximately 20 degrees of internal rotation and 20 to 30 degrees of abduction.

POSTOPERATIVE CARE. The cast is worn for 8 to 12 weeks, depending on the healing of the osteotomy site. After the cast is removed, progressive walking and range of motion are begun but no formal physical therapy is prescribed.

GANZ (BERNESE) PERIACETABULAR OSTEOTOMY

Ganz et al. developed a triplanar periacetabular osteotomy for adolescents and adults with dysplastic hips that require correction of congruency and containment of the femoral head. If significant degenerative changes involving the weight-bearing surface of the femoral head are present, a proximal femoral osteotomy can be added to provide uninvolved acetabular and proximal femoral weight-bearing surfaces (Fig. 30-31). The reported advantages of periacetabular osteotomy are as follows: (1) only one approach is used; (2) a large amount of correction can be obtained in all directions, including the medial and lateral planes; (3) blood supply to the acetabulum is preserved; (4) the posterior column of the hemipelvis remains mechanically intact, allowing immediate crutch walking with minimal internal fixation; (5) the shape of the true pelvis is unaltered, permitting normal child delivery; and (6) it can be combined with trochanteric osteotomy if needed. Although technically more demanding in previously operated hips, the periacetabular osteotomy has been shown to provide similar radiographic and functional results as periacetabular osteotomy in patients without prior hip surgery (Fig. 30-32). The technique for Ganz periacetabular osteotomy is described in Chapter 6.

SHELF OPERATIONS

Shelf procedures commonly have been performed to enlarge the volume of the acetabulum; however, pelvic redirectional and displacement osteotomies have largely replaced this type of operation. The redirectional osteotomies are inappropriate in hips in which the femoral head and acetabulum are misshapen but still congruent because redirection can cause incongruity.

Staheli described a slotted acetabular augmentation procedure to create a congruous acetabular extension in which the size and position of the augmentation can be easily controlled. A deficient acetabulum that cannot be corrected by redirectional pelvic osteotomy is the primary indication for this operation. Contraindications include dysplastic hips with spherical congruity suitable for redirectional osteotomy, hips requiring concurrent open reduction that must have supplementary stability, and patients unsuited for spica cast immobilization.

SLOTTED ACETABULAR AUGMENTATION

TECHNIQUE 30-13

(STAHELI)

- Before surgery, determine the center-edge angle of Wiberg from anteroposterior standing pelvic radiographs and superimpose a normal center-edge angle (about 35 degrees) on the image. Measure the additional width necessary to extend the existing acetabulum to achieve the normal angle (Fig. 30-33). This determines the width of the augmentation; this measurement added to the depth of the slot gives the total graft length.
- Position the patient supine on a radiolucent operating table with a small bump under the affected hip.
- Make a straight bikini-line skin incision 1 cm below and parallel to the iliac crest.
- Expose the hip joint through a standard iliofemoral approach.
- Divide the tendon of the reflected head of the rectus femoris muscle anteriorly and displace it posteriorly. If the capsule is abnormally thick (>6 mm), thin it by "fileting" with a scalpel.
- The placement of the acetabular slot is the most critical part of the procedure; the slot must be created *exactly at the acetabular margin*. Determine the position of the slot by placing a probe into the joint to palpate the position of the acetabulum. Place a drill in the selected site and verify correct position with image intensification. The floor of the slot should be acetabular articular cartilage and little bone; the end and roof of the slot should be cancellous bone. The slot should be 1 cm deep.
- Make the slot by drilling a series of holes with a $\frac{5}{32}$-inch (4.5-mm) bit and join them with a narrow rongeur. Determine the length of the slot intraoperatively by the need for coverage. If excessive femoral anteversion is present, extend the slot anteriorly. If the acetabulum is deficient posteriorly, extend the slot in that direction.
- Take thin strips of cortical and cancellous bone from the lateral surface of the ilium; cut these as long as possible.
- Extend the shallow decortication inferiorly from the iliac crest to the superior margin of the slot to ensure rapid

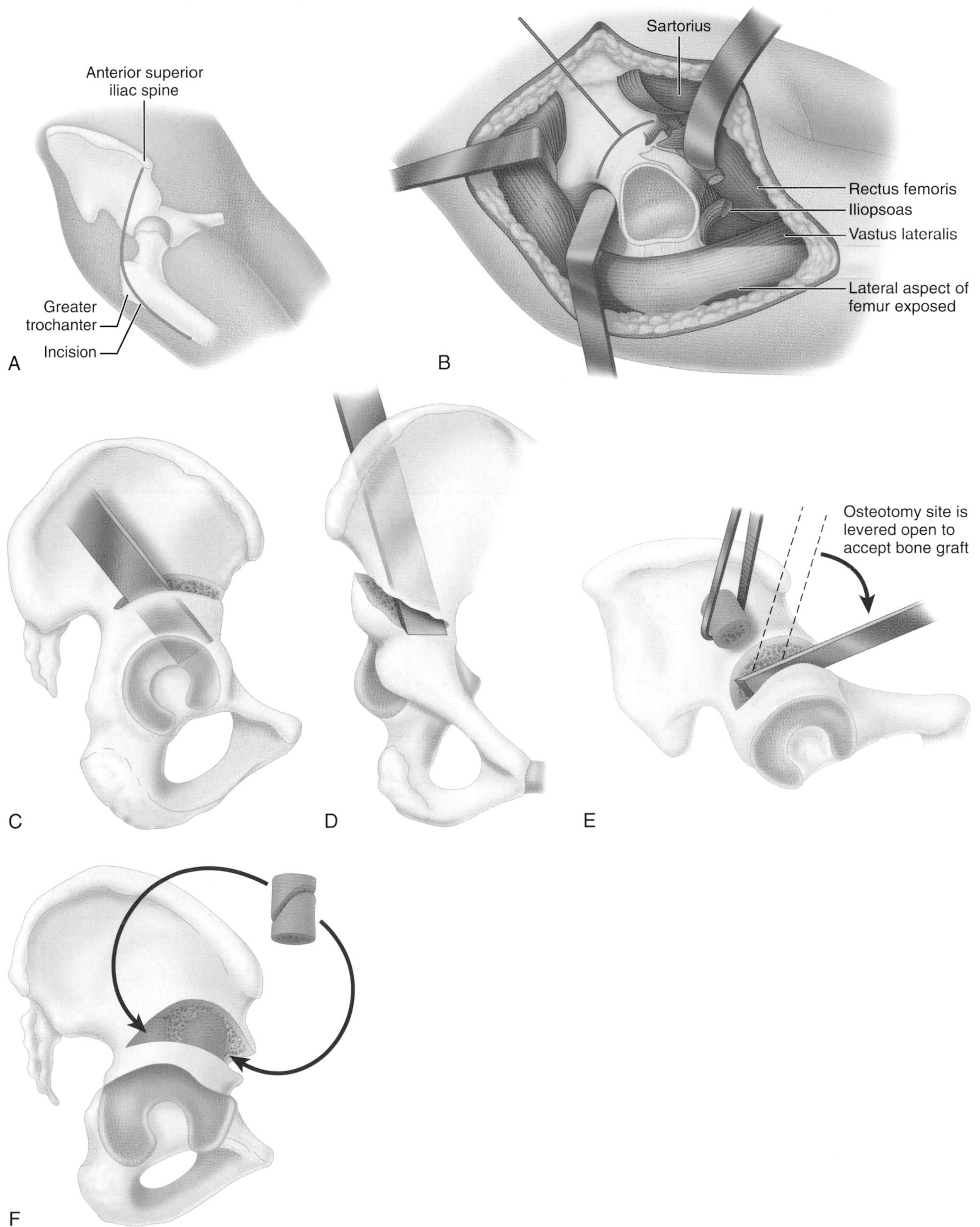

FIGURE 30-30 Dega osteotomy (see text). **A,** Skin incision. **B,** Osteotomy line is marked on lateral cortex of ilium; guidewire is inserted to exit just above horizontal limb of triradiate cartilage. **C,** Osteotome penetrates inner cortex. **D,** View from inner side of pelvis shows intact posteromedial cortical hinge; length of intact inner cortex depends on amount of anterior and lateral coverage desired. **E,** Osteotomy is levered open with osteotome or small lamina spreader. **F,** Larger graft is inserted anteriorly; posterior graft should be smaller to avoid loosening anterior graft. (Redrawn from Grudziak JS, Ward WT: Dega osteotomy for the treatment of congenital dysplasia of the hip, J Bone Joint Surg 83A:845, 2001.) **SEE TECHNIQUE 30-12.**

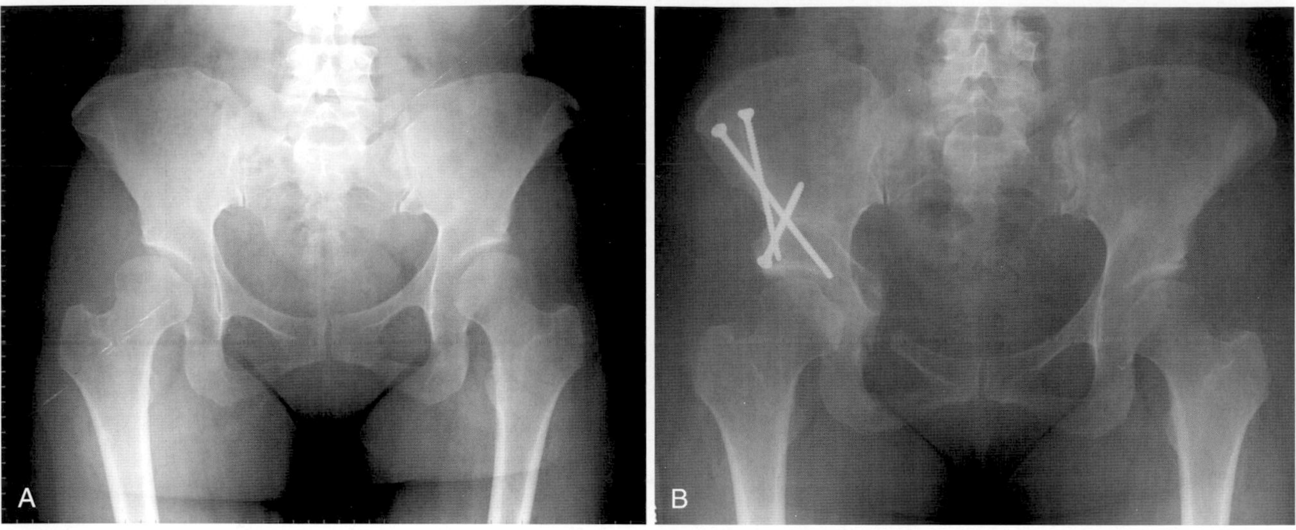

FIGURE 30-31 **A,** Twenty-eight-year-old woman with painful bilateral acetabular dysplasia. **B,** After Ganz osteotomy of right hip. (Courtesy of James Guyton, MD.)

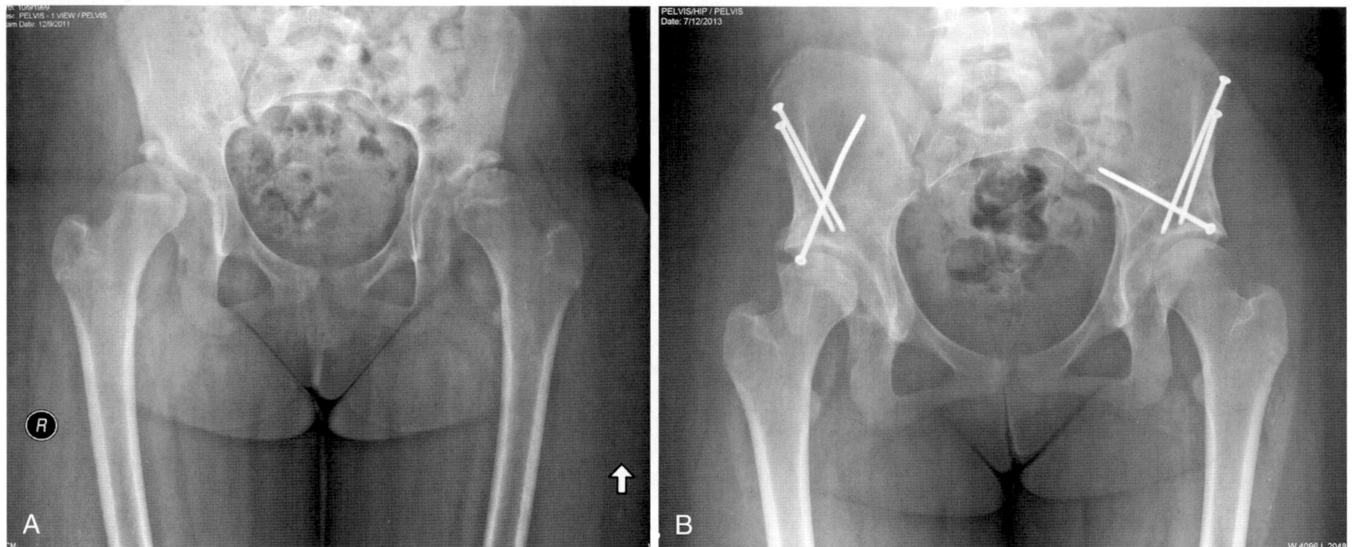

FIGURE 30-32 Preoperative **(A)** and postoperative **(B)** views of adolescent bilateral hip dysplasia in a 14-year-old girl. The patient was treated with bilateral, staged periacetabular osteotomies.

fusion of the graft to the ilium. Do not remove the inner table of the ilium because this may change the contour of the pelvis.

- Measure the depth of the slot and add this to the width of the augmentation as determined preoperatively.
- Select thin strips (1 mm) of cancellous bone and cut them into rectangles about 1 cm wide and of the appropriate length. Assemble these rectangular pieces on a moist sponge, cutting enough to provide a single layer the length of the augmentation.
- Apply the first layer radially from the slot with the concave side down to provide a congruous extension.
- Select longer cancellous strips for the second layer and cut them to the length of the extension. Place these at right angles to the first layer and parallel to the acetabulum. They may be a little thicker (2 mm), especially the most lateral strip, to provide a well-defined lateral margin of the extension. Both layers must be of appropriate width and length. The augmentation should not extend too far anteriorly to avoid blocking hip flexion.
- Secure these two layers of cancellous grafts by bringing the reflected head of the rectus femoris forward over the grafts and suturing it in its original position. A capsular flap can be substituted if this tendon is unavailable.
- Cut the remaining grafts into small pieces and pack them above, but not beyond, the initial layer. They are held in place by the reattached abductor muscles.

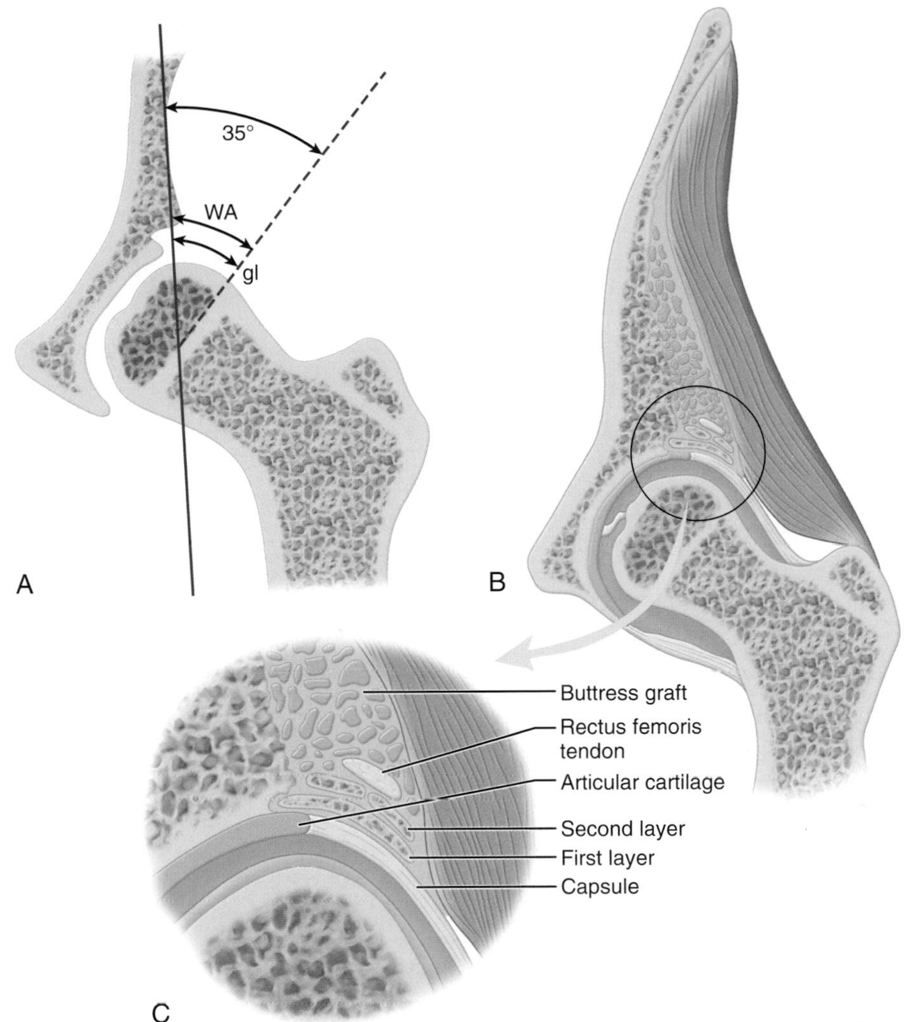

FIGURE 30-33 Slotted acetabular augmentation of Staheli. **A,** Width of augmentation (WA) is determined preoperatively from standing anteroposterior radiograph of pelvis. Center-edge angle and 35-degree angle are drawn. Graft length (gl) is sum of WA and slot depth. **B,** Objective of procedure is to provide congruous extension of acetabulum. **C,** Details of extension. **SEE TECHNIQUE 30-13.**

- Confirm the position and width of the graft by radiographs.
- After closure, apply a single hip spica cast with the hip in 15 degrees of abduction, 20 degrees of flexion, and neutral rotation.

POSTOPERATIVE CARE. The cast is removed after 6 weeks, and crutch walking is permitted with partial weight bearing on the affected side until the graft is incorporated, usually at 3 to 4 months (Fig. 30-34).

CHIARI OSTEOTOMY

The Chiari osteotomy is a capsular interposition arthroplasty and should be considered only in situations in which other reconstructions are impossible, such as when the femoral head cannot be centered adequately in the acetabulum or in painfully subluxated hips with early signs of osteoarthritis. This procedure deepens the deficient acetabulum by medial displacement of the distal pelvic fragment and improves superolateral femoral coverage.

The Chiari procedure is an operation that places the femoral head beneath a surface of cancellous bone with the capacity for regeneration and corrects the lateral pathologic displacement of the femur. An osteotomy of the pelvis is performed at the superior margin of the acetabulum, and the pelvis inferior to the osteotomy along with the femur is displaced medially (Fig. 30-35). The superior fragment of the osteotomy then becomes a shelf, and the capsule is interposed between it and the femoral head.

After using this operation on more than 600 patients, 400 of whom had been observed for more than 2 years, Chiari recommended the operation in the following situations: (1) for congenital subluxations in patients 4 to 6 years old or older, including adults (including subluxations that persist after conservative treatment of dislocations and subluxations previously not treated); (2) for untreated congenital dislocations in patients older than 4 years old, soon after open or closed reduction; (3) for dysplastic hips with osteoarthritis;

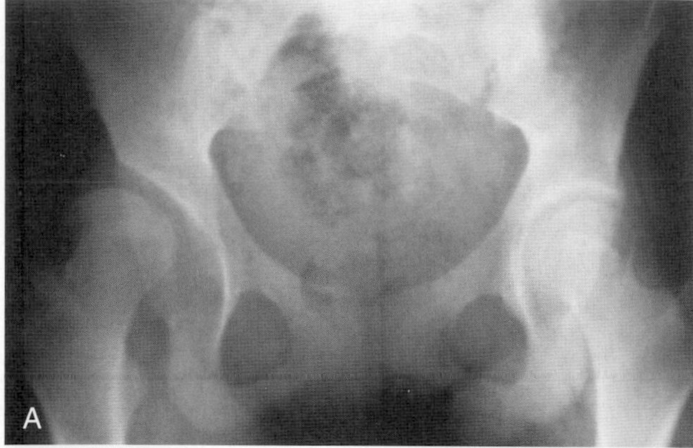

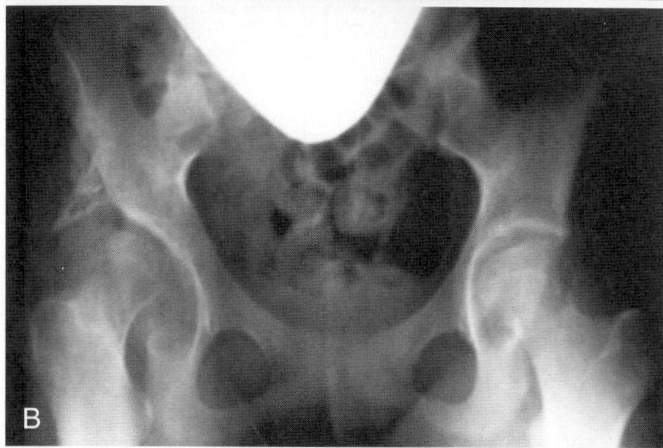

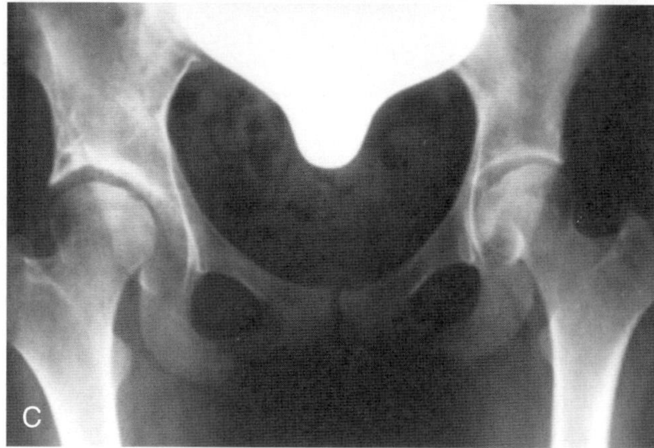

FIGURE 30-34 Staheli slotted acetabular augmentation. **A,** Fourteen-year-old girl with painful right acetabular dysplasia. **B,** Four months after operation. **C,** One year after operation, excellent graft incorporation. (Courtesy of Lynn Staheli, MD.)

(4) for paralytic dislocations caused by muscular weakness or spasticity; and (5) for coxa magna after Perthes disease or osteonecrosis after treatment of congenital dysplasia. These indications are broader than the indications usually accepted by most pediatric orthopaedists. For children younger than about 10 years old, the osteotomy is not recommended in subluxations or in dislocations that can be reduced surgically or conservatively and in which osteotomy of the innominate bone, acetabuloplasty, or osteotomies that free the acetabulum would result in a competent acetabulum. Some surgeons recommend the operation for patients older than 10 years who have symptomatic early subluxation of the hip with acetabular dysplasia too severe to be treated by other pelvic osteotomies; for them, innominate osteotomy with medial displacement is preferred to a shelf operation.

Chiari's operation is a capsular arthroplasty because the capsule is interposed between the newly formed acetabular roof and the femoral head. Because the biomechanics of the hip are improved by displacing the hip nearer the midline, a Trendelenburg limp often is eliminated.

TECHNIQUE 30-14

- Place the patient supine on a fracture table with the feet attached to the traction plate. Slightly abduct and externally rotate the affected hip.
- Make an anterolateral bikini-line incision about 10 cm long. Develop the interval between the tensor fasciae latae and the sartorius muscles and laterally retract the former.
- Incise the iliac apophysis in line with the iliac crest. With a periosteal elevator, detach the lateral half of the apophysis along with the tensor fasciae latae muscle and the anterior part of the gluteus medius muscle.
- Dissect these muscles subperiosteally and retract them posteriorly.
- Insert a periosteal elevator between the capsule of the hip and the gluteus minimus.
- Dissect subperiosteally posteriorly to the point where the pelvis curves inferiorly.
- With a curved periosteal elevator, dissect subperiosteally farther posteriorly until the sciatic notch is reached. Replace this elevator with a flexible metal ribbon retractor 3 cm wide. This completes the dissection posteriorly.
- Return anteriorly to the medial aspect of the ilium. With a periosteal elevator, strip the iliacus muscle and the underlying periosteum posteriorly to the sciatic notch.
- When the sciatic notch is reached, replace the elevator with a flexible metal ribbon retractor that touches and overlaps the ribbon retractor already in the notch.
- With curved scissors, separate the rectus muscle and its reflected head from the capsule of the hip joint. Divide the reflected head.
- The osteotomy should be made with a Hohmann retractor precisely between the insertion of the capsule and the reflected head of the rectus, following the capsular insertion in a curved line and ending distal to the anterior inferior iliac spine anteriorly and in the sciatic notch posteriorly. Do not open or damage the capsule of the joint.
- After the line of the osteotomy has been determined, start the osteotomy with a straight, narrow osteotome, opening the lateral table of the ilium along this line.
- Determine the exact position of the osteotome at the beginning by image intensification or by radiographs. Direct the osteotomy superiorly approximately 20 degrees toward the inner table of the ilium (Fig. 30-36A). Change the position of the osteotome as necessary to make the osteotomy curve superiorly. Do not direct the osteotomy more than 20 degrees superiorly because it might enter the sacroiliac joint.
- When the osteotomy has been completed, displace the hip medially by releasing the traction on the extremity and by forcing the limb into abduction. The distal fragment

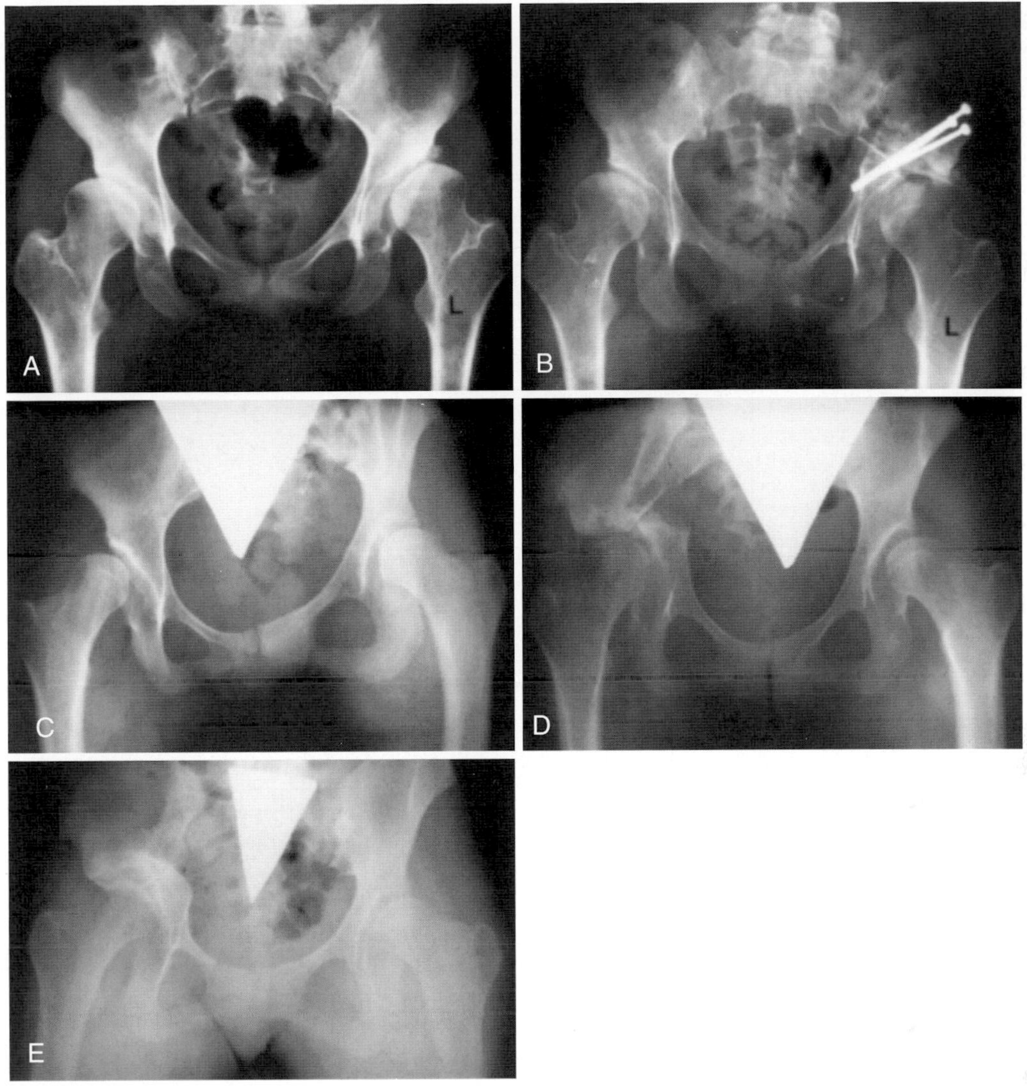

FIGURE 30-35 Chiari osteotomy. **A,** Young adult with painful, bilateral acetabular dysplasia, greater on left than on right. **B,** After Chiari osteotomy of left hip. Note optional internal fixation and medial bone grafting. **C,** Bilateral acetabular dysplasia in 12-year-old girl. **D,** After surgery, right hip is completely displaced. **E,** One year after Chiari osteotomy. (**A** and **B** courtesy of Randal Betz, MD.)

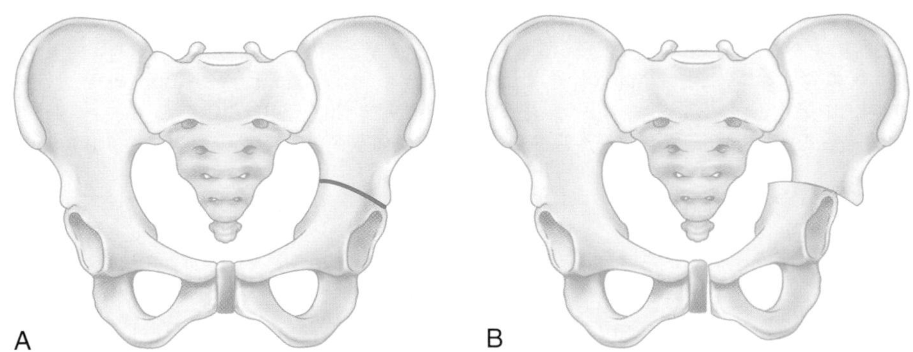

FIGURE 30-36 Chiari medial displacement osteotomy. **A,** Line of osteotomy extending from immediately superior to lip of acetabulum into sciatic notch. Osteotomy can be curved to facilitate femoral head coverage. **B,** Completed osteotomy with medial displacement of distal fragment for interpositional capsular arthroplasty. **SEE TECHNIQUE 30-14.**

displaces medially, hinging at the symphysis pubis (Fig. 30-36B). If the adductor muscles are extremely relaxed, however, it may be necessary to manipulate the head manually or to displace the distal fragment with an instrument. Ensure that the distal fragment is displaced far enough medially (if necessary, 100% of the width of the ilium) so that the proximal fragment completely covers the femoral head.

- Internal fixation can be inserted to secure and maintain adequate displacement.
- After the displacement has been completed, decrease the abduction of the limb to about 30 degrees.
- If the capsule is loose, perform a capsulorrhaphy.
- Check the position of the hip and the osteotomy by image intensification or by radiographs.
- Replace and suture the iliac apophysis and close the wound.
- Apply a spica cast with the hip in 20 to 30 degrees of abduction, neutral rotation, and neutral extension.

POSTOPERATIVE CARE. In children and adults, the cast is removed at 6 to 8 weeks, and active and passive exercises of the hip are started. Partial weight bearing on crutches is allowed and progressed as tolerated.

ADOLESCENT AND YOUNG ADULT (>8 YEARS)

In children older than 8 years old or in young adults in whom the femoral head cannot be repositioned distally to the level of the acetabulum, only palliative salvaging operations are possible. Rarely, a femoral shortening combined with a pelvic osteotomy could be considered, but the chances of creating a hip to last a lifetime are minimal. Reduction of a unilateral dislocation should be strongly considered, even in children 6 years old. After some years, degenerative arthritic changes develop in the hip joint. When these changes cause enough pain or limitation of motion to require additional surgery, a reconstructive operation, such as a total hip arthroplasty, may be indicated at the appropriate age. Arthrodesis is now rarely indicated for old unreduced dislocations and is contraindicated for bilateral dislocations. In bilateral dislocations in this age group, the hips should be left unreduced (Fig. 30-37), and total hip arthroplasties may be done during adulthood. Degenerative joint disease is more likely to develop in early adulthood in a dislocated hip with a false acetabulum in the wing of the ilium than in a dislocated hip without formation of a false acetabulum. Patients with reduced femoral heads but painful acetabular dysplasia can be treated with an appropriate pelvic osteotomy (Table 30-1).

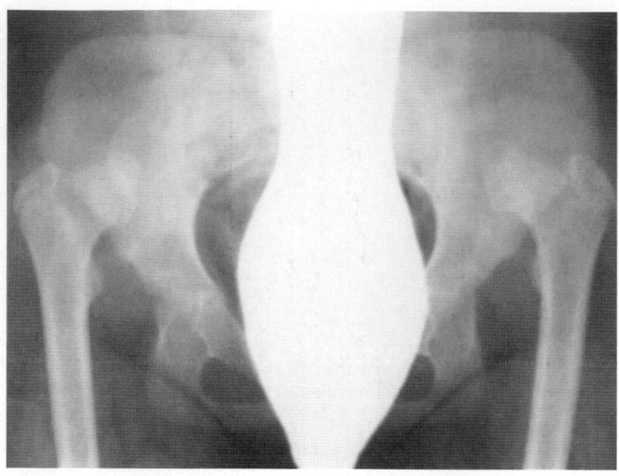

FIGURE 30-37 Bilateral untreated congenital dislocation of hip in 12-year-old girl.

CONGENITAL AND DEVELOPMENTAL COXA VARA

The term *congenital coxa vara* has been applied to two types of coxa vara seen in infancy and childhood. The first type is present at birth, is rare, and is associated with other congenital anomalies, such as proximal femoral focal deficiency or anomalies in other parts of the body such as cleidocranial dysostosis. The second type, usually not discovered until the child is walking, is more common than the first and is associated with no other abnormality.

Coxa vara, often bilateral, is characterized by a progressive decrease in the angle between the femoral neck and shaft, a progressive shortening of the limb, and the presence of a defect in the medial part of the neck (Fig. 30-38). Microscopically, the tissue in this defect consists of cartilage and resembles an abnormal physis; the arrangement of its cells is irregular and ossification within it is atypical. The adjacent metaphyseal bone is osteoporotic, its trabeculae being atrophic, and occasionally it contains large groups of cartilage cells. When walking is begun, the forces that the femoral neck must withstand are increased, and because the neck is weak, varus deformity gradually develops.

As the patient becomes older and heavier, the deformity increases until the greater trochanter eventually lies superior to the femoral head; pseudarthrosis of the femoral neck may develop. In adults, the trochanter may come to lie several inches superior to the femoral head, and if pseudarthrosis is present, the femoral head may be widely separated from the femoral neck. After age 8 years, the likelihood of obtaining a hip that would function normally rapidly diminishes.

The treatment of choice for correction of developmental coxa vara is subtrochanteric osteotomy to place the femoral neck and head in an appropriate valgus position with the shaft of the femur. Surgery can be delayed until the child is 4 or 5 years old to make internal fixation easier. Surgical treatment is indicated when coxa vara deformity is progressive, painful, unilateral, or associated with leg-length discrepancy or when the Hilgenreiner-epiphyseal (H-E) angle is greater than 60 degrees (Fig. 30-39). Surgery also is indicated when the neck-shaft angle is 110 degrees or less. The subtrochanteric osteotomy is fixed internally with either a blade plate or screw and plate combination (Fig. 30-40). Although biomechanically this may provide enough rigid internal fixation to eliminate the need for postoperative immobilization, a spica cast can be worn until union is complete.

Regardless of the method of osteotomy, the deformity can recur, so children should be examined periodically after surgery until their growth is complete. The risk of recurrence can be lessened by improving the H-E angle to less than 38

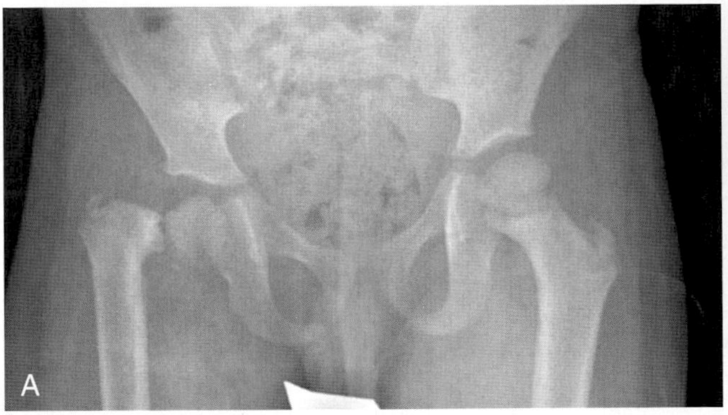

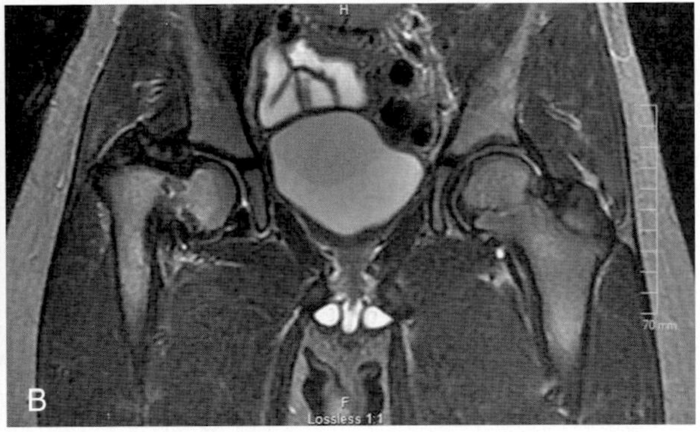

FIGURE 30-38 **A,** Plain anteroposterior radiograph of a 4-year-old boy with congenital coxa vara of the right hip. **B,** Coronal MRI section of the same patient demonstrates irregularity and widening of the physis.

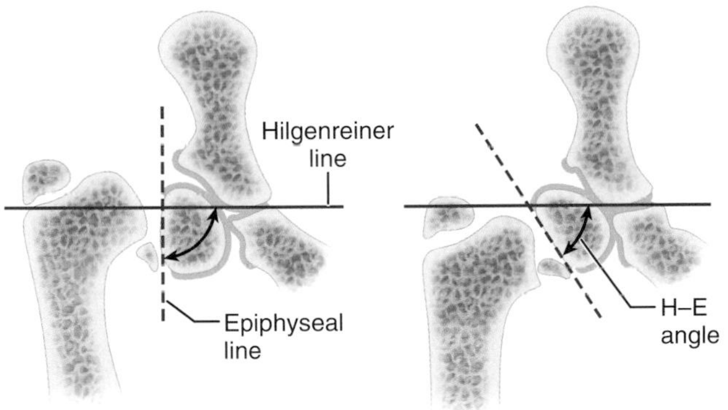

H–E Angle
<45° Good prognosis
45°–59° Monitor closely for progression
>60° Poor prognosis; high risk of progression; surgery is indicated

FIGURE 30-39 Hilgenreiner-epiphyseal (H-E) angle of more than 60 degrees is an indication for surgical treatment of congenital coxa vara.

degrees. In addition to monitoring for recurrence of the varus deformity, a significant number of children with coxa vara have associated femoral hypoplasia and limb-length discrepancy, which also require monitoring and may ultimately require limb length equalization.

VALGUS OSTEOTOMY FOR DEVELOPMENTAL COXA VARA

TECHNIQUE 30-15

- Perform an adductor tenotomy through a small medial incision.
- Expose the greater trochanter and proximal shaft of the femur through an 8- to 10-cm lateral, longitudinal incision.
- If a screw and side plate device is used for internal fixation, insert the screw in the midline of the femoral neck as determined by image intensification or anteroposterior and lateral radiographs. Insert the screw as close as possible to the trochanteric apophysis without entering it. If possible, center the screw in the femoral neck distal to the abnormal physis. If this is technically impossible, center the screw in the femoral head.
- Make a transverse osteotomy slightly distal to the screw at about the level of the lesser trochanter.
- If necessary, take a small lateral wedge of bone to correct the neck-shaft angle to 140 to 150 degrees.
- Fix the side plate to the femoral shaft in the usual manner.
- Irrigate the wound and close it in layers, inserting irrigation-suction drainage if desired.
- Apply a one and one-half spica cast.

POSTOPERATIVE CARE. The cast is removed at 8 to 12 weeks, when radiographic union of the osteotomy has occurred. Regular follow-up includes assessment of possible recurrence of the deformity and the development of progressive limb-length discrepancy that requires additional treatment.

EXSTROPHY OF THE BLADDER

Exstrophy of the bladder occurs as a result of a congenital failure of fusion of the tissues of the midline of the pelvis. The major anomaly is a maldevelopment of the lower part of the abdominal wall and the anterior wall of the bladder so that the anterior surface of the posterior wall of the bladder is exposed to the exterior. Hernias and other defects of the anterior abdominal wall also may be present more proximally. As noted by O'Phelan, however, the orthopaedic surgeon becomes involved in treatment because of the diastasis of the symphysis pubis, the lateral flare of the innominate bones, and the resultant lateral displacement and external rotation of the acetabula. Other orthopaedic anomalies may be present along with exstrophy of the bladder, including congenital dislocation or dysplasia of the hip and myelomeningocele.

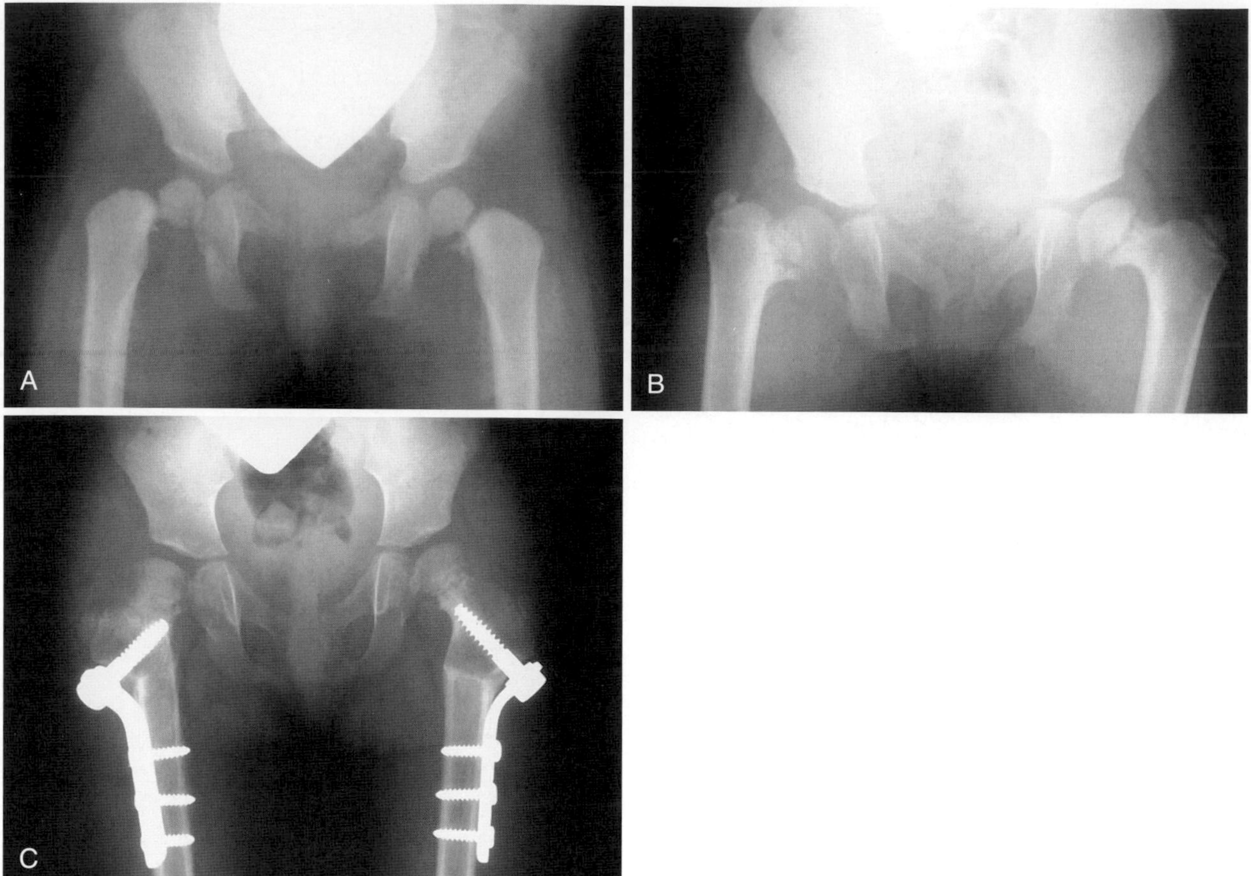

FIGURE 30-40 Congenital coxa vara. **A,** Two-year-old girl with congenital coxa vara. **B,** Preoperative radiograph shows neck-shaft angle of less than 90 degrees bilaterally at age 5 years. **C,** After bilateral subtrochanteric osteotomies and internal fixation with pediatric hip screw.

ANTERIOR ILIAC OSTEOTOMIES AND APPROXIMATION OF THE SYMPHYSIS PUBIS

Because most of the urologic structures are present or bifid, reconstruction is possible. Unless the symphysis pubis is approximated, however, urologic reconstruction is followed by complications such as the formation of fistulas or recurrences. These complications seem to be caused by tension placed on the soft tissues during closure, and this tension can be relieved by repair of the symphysis pubis. There is some controversy, as some authors have reported successfully bladder closure and repair without pelvic osteotomies. However, failure to address the abnormal morphology of the pelvis can have other consequences for the child such as a wide-based, waddling, externally rotated gait. O'Phelan described the results of bilateral posterior iliac osteotomies and approximation of the symphysis (Fig. 30-41). More recently, Sponseller et al. recommended bilateral anterior iliac osteotomies, with internal or external fixation, citing advantages of increased mobility of the pubis, less intraoperative blood loss, and increased correction and avoidance of turning of the patient while under anesthesia for repeat preparation. Postoperative traction was unnecessary in most of their patients. Wound dehiscence or bladder prolapse occurred in 4% of patients, and the only important complication of the osteotomies was transient palsy of the left femoral nerve in seven children. Children who were older at the time of the osteotomy maintained better correction over time. In a later report, Okubadejo, et al. reviewed the records of 624 patients who had bladder exstrophy repair and found that orthopaedic complications occurred in 26 (4%). They divided the complications into five categories: bony complications at the osteotomy site (19%), neurologic complications at the osteotomy site (50%), complications of traction (15%), deep infection (8%), and late infection (8%).

In their report on bladder exstrophy, Kasat and Borwankar identified 11 important factors in obtaining a successful primary closure: (1) proper patient selection, (2) a staged approach, (3) anterior approximation of the pubic bones with placement of the bladder and urethra in the true pelvis, (4) posterior bilateral iliac osteotomies when indicated, (5) double-layered closure of the bladder, (6) 2 weeks of proper ureteric catheter drainage, (7) prevention of infection, (8) prolonged and proper postoperative immobilization, (9) prompt treatment of bladder prolapse, (10) prevention of abdominal distention postoperatively, and (11) ruling out bladder outlet obstruction before removing the bladder catheter.

The three steps are performed as one operative procedure: (1) the anterior iliac osteotomies; (2) repair of the

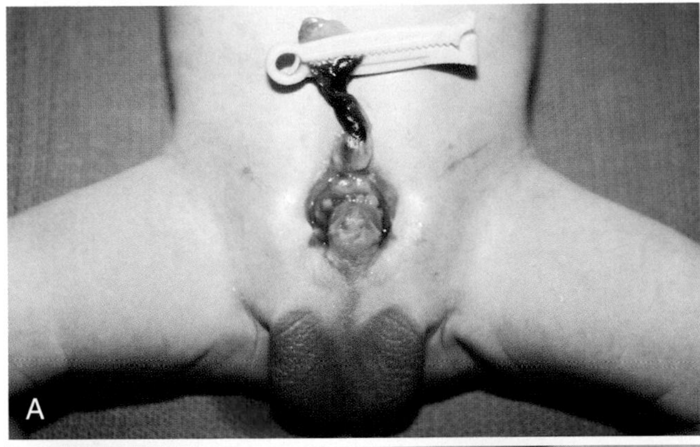

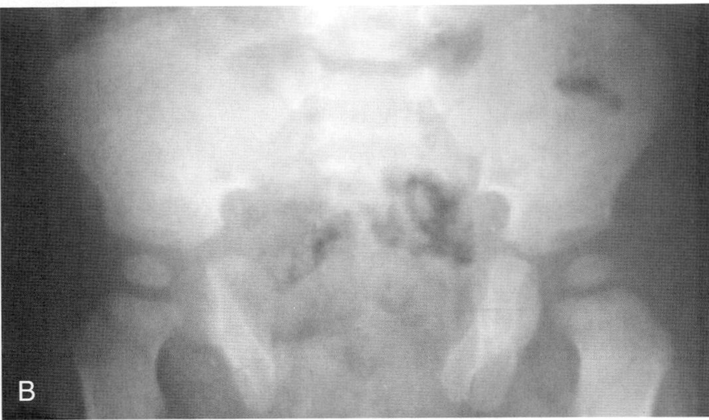

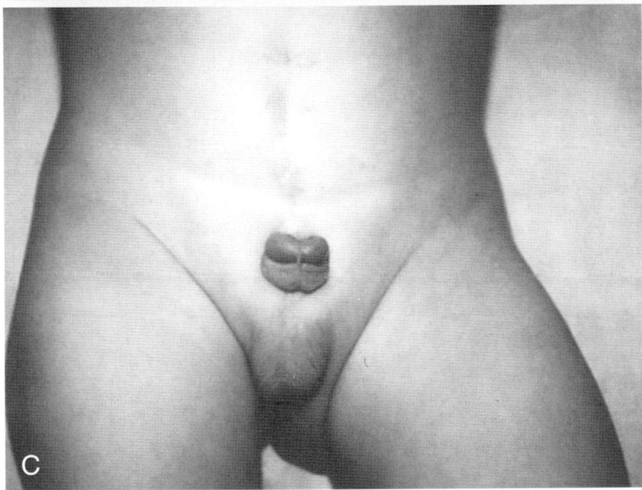

FIGURE 30-41 **A,** Congenital exstrophy of bladder in newborn boy. **B,** Note pubic diastasis on radiograph at 1 year of age. **C,** After bilateral posterior iliac osteotomies and anterior reconstruction.

anterior structures by a urologic surgeon; and (3) repair of the symphysis pubis. A heavy, nonabsorbable suture or biodegradeable implants can be substituted for wire fixation. Although described for treatment of older children or children with recurrent deformities, we prefer this technique for early initial treatment and for older children (Fig. 30-42).

BILATERAL ANTERIOR ILIAC OSTEOTOMIES

TECHNIQUE 30-16

(SPONSELLER, GEARHART, AND JEFFS)

- Place the patient supine on the operating table and circumferentially prepare and drape the entire body below the umbilicus. Elevate the sacrum on folded towels.
- Make an anterior iliofemoral approach to the pelvis, similar to that used for a Salter osteotomy; both sides can be exposed simultaneously.
- Widely expose the medial iliac cortex and carefully elevate the periosteum posteriorly around the sciatic notch, using curved elevators and gauze sponges.
- With a Gigli saw, perform Salter innominate osteotomies. If the saw is difficult to pass, it can be threaded through on a leader of umbilical tape. In children younger than 6 months old, use an oscillating saw because the force applied to the Gigli saw can cause preferential separation of the triradiate cartilage.
- Make the osteotomies from 5 mm above the anterior inferior iliac spine to the most cranial portion of the sciatic notch to leave a sizable inferior segment for internal fixation.
- Rotate the freed ischiopubic segments 30 to 45 degrees to bring the pubic rami together.
- In children older than 6 months, a small external fixator, such as that used in the upper extremity, can be used with 2-mm pins for fixation. Increase the pin size to 4 mm for children 4 to 10 years old and to 5 mm for children older than 10 years old.
- Insert two pins in each iliac wing and two in each distal fragment. Predrilling may be necessary to prevent splitting of the bone in small infants.
- Place one distal fragment pin from the anterior inferior iliac spine to the notch, parallel and 5 to 10 mm inferior to the osteotomy, ensuring that the pin engages the deep posterior cortex of the notch.

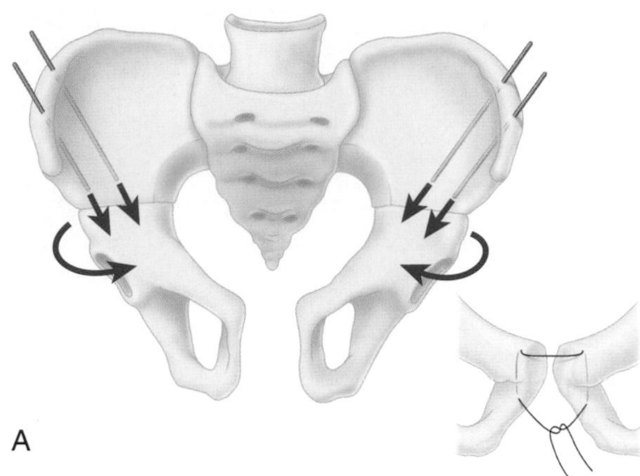

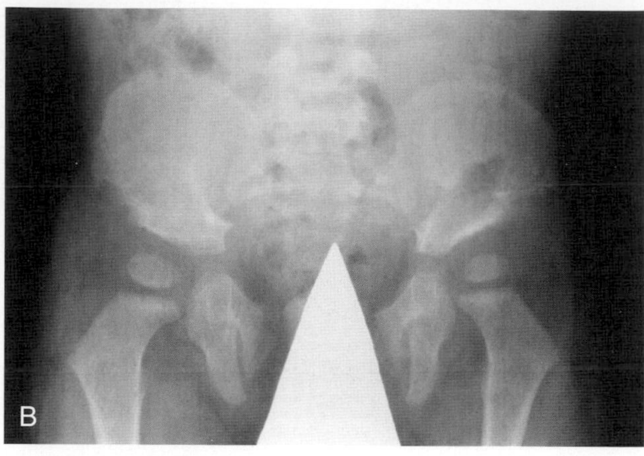

FIGURE 30-42 **A,** Technique for reconstruction in exstrophy of bladder (see text). *Inset* shows suturing of pubic bones. **B,** Postoperative radiograph after bilateral anterior Salter innominate osteotomies.

- Insert another threaded pin just below this pin but externally angled 30 degrees.
- Close the wounds.
- Have the urologic surgeon prepare the operative field and identify the abnormal bladder and urethral structures.
- Use a single suture of 2-0 nylon in a horizontal mattress stitch to suture the pubic bones; tie it anterior to the neourethra and bladder neck while an assistant rotates the greater trochanters medially.
- Place heavy sutures of polyglactin in the rectus fascia just superficial to the pubic closure.
- After the pelvic ring is closed anteriorly, apply the external fixator. Good subperiosteal exposure is mandatory to ensure accurate pin placement away from the hip and triradiate cartilage.
- The procedure can be modified to exclude external fixation by fixing both osteotomies with Kirschner wires and applying a spica cast to be worn for 8 to 12 weeks., or by applying a biodegradeable plate and screws to the symphysis rather than a wire or suture.

POSTOPERATIVE CARE. Light Buck traction or a spica cast can be used for 1 to 2 weeks to maintain comfort and bed rest. This is mandatory in children younger than 1 year old because they have relatively less cortical bone for fixation, but older children can be discharged from the hospital earlier if good external fixation is obtained. External fixation is continued for 4 weeks in children younger than 2 years and for 6 weeks in older children. Gradual resumption of activities is then allowed. No formal physical therapy program is necessary, but a walker is helpful during the first week of ambulation in older children.

REFERENCES

DEVELOPMENTAL DYSPLASIA OF THE HIP

Agus H, Bozoglan M, Kalenderer Ö, et al: How are outcomes affected by performing a one-stage combined procedure simultaneously in bilateral developmental hip dysplasia? *Int Orthop* 38(6):1219, 2014.

Alexiev VA, Harcke HT, Kumar SJ: Residual dysplasia after successful Pavlik harness treatment: early ultrasound predictors, *J Pediatr Orthop* 26:16, 2006.

American Academy of Orthopaedic Surgeons: *Detection and nonoperative management of pediatric developmental dysplasia of the hip in infants up to six months of age. Evidence-based clinical practice guideline.* http://www.aaos.org/Research/guidelines/DDHGuidelineFINAL.pdf.

Arslan H, Sucu E, Ozkul E, et al: Should routine pelvic osteotomy be added to the treatment of DDH after 18 months? *Acta Orthop Belg* 80:205, 2014.

Bolland BJ, Wahed A, Al-Halloa S, et al: Late reduction in congenital dislocation of the hip and the need for secondary surgery: radiologic predictors and confounding variables, *J Pediatr Orthop* 30:676, 2010.

Borowski A, Thawrani D, Grissom L, et al: Bilaterally dislocated hip treated with the Pavlik harness are not at a higher risk for failure, *J Pediatr Orthop* 29:661, 2009.

Carmichael KD, Longo A, Yngve D, et al: The use of ultrasound to determine timing of Pavlik harness discontinuation in treatment of developmental dysplasia of the hip, *Orthopedics* 31:988, 2008.

Carney BT, Vanek EA: Incidence of hip dysplasia in idiopathic clubfoot, *J Surg Orthop Adv* 15:71, 2006.

Chang CH, Yang WE, Kao HK, et al: Predictive value for femoral head sphericity from early radiographic signs in surgery for developmental dysplasia of the hip, *J Pediatr Orthop* 31:240, 2011.

Chin MS, Betz BW, Halanski MA: Comparison of hip reduction using magnetic resonance imaging or computed tomography in hip dysplasia, *J Pediatr Orthop* 31:525, 2011.

Chou DT, Ramachandran M: Prevalence of developmental dysplasia of the hip in children with clubfoot, *J Child Orthop* 7(4):263, 2013.

Cooke SJ, Rees R, Edwards DL, et al: Ossification of the femoral head at closed reduction for developmental dysplasia of the hip and its influence on the long-term outcome, *J Pediatr Orthop B* 19:22, 2010.

De Hundt M, Viemmix F, Bais JM, et al: Risk factors for developmental dysplasia of the hip: a metaanalysis, *Eur J Obstet Gynecol Reprod Biol* 165:8, 2012.

De La Rocha A, Sucato DJ, Tulchin K, Podeszwa DA: Treatment of adolescents with a periacetabular osteotomy after previous pelvic surgery, *Clin Orthop Relat Res* 470:2583, 2012.

El-Sayed MM: Single-stage open reduction, Salter innominate osteotomy, and proximal femoral osteotomy for the management of developmental dysplasia of the hip in children between the ages of 2 and 4 years, *J Pediatr Orthop B* 18:188, 2009.

Ertürk C, Altay MA, Isikan UE: Femoral segment graft is suitable alternative to stabilize pelvic osteotomies in developmental dysplasia of the hip: a comparative study, *J Pediatr Orthop B* 21:200, 2012.

Firth GB, Robertson SJ, Schepers A, Fatti L: Developmental dysplasia of the hip: open reduction as a risk factor for substantial osteonecrosis, *Clin Orthop Relat Res* 468:2485, 2010.

Forlin E, Munhoz da Cunha LA, Figueiredo DC: Treatment of developmental dysplasia of the hip after walking age with open reduction, femoral shortening, and acetabular osteotomy, *Orthop Clin North Am* 37:149, 2006.

Fox AE, Paton RW: The relationship between mode of delivery and developmental dysplasia of the hip in breech infants: a four-year prospective cohort study, *J Bone Joint Surg* 92B:1695, 2010.

Fujii M, Nakashima Y, Yamamoto T, et al: Acetabular retroversion in developmental dysplasia of the hip, *J Bone Joint Surg Am* 92:895, 2010.

Garras DN, Crowder TT, Olson SA: Medium-term results of the Bernese periacetabular osteotomy in the treatment of symptomatic developmental dysplasia of the hip, *J Bone Joint Surg* 89B:721, 2007.

Gholve PA, Flynn JM, Garner MR, et al: Predictors for secondary procedures in walking DDH, *J Pediatr Orthop* 32:282, 2012.

Gould SW, Grissom LE, Niedzielski A, et al: Protocol for MRI of the hips after spica cast placement, *J Pediatr Orthop* 32:504, 2012.

Heesakkers NA, Witbreuk MM, Beeselaar PP, Van Der Sluijs JA: Retrospective radiographic evaluation of treatment results of developmental dysplasia of the hip in walking-age children, *J Pediatr Orthop B* 22:427, 2013.

Joiner ER, Andras LM, Skaggs DL: Screening for hip dysplasia in congenital muscular toricollis: is physical exam of enough? *J Child Orthop* 8:114, 2014.

Kaneko H, Kitoh H, Mishima K, et al: Long-term outcome of gradual redution using overhead traction for developmental dysplasia of the hip over 6 months of age, *J Pediatr Orthop* 33:628, 2013.

Karami M, Fitoussi F, Ilharreborde B, et al: The results of Chiari pelvic osteotomy in adolescents with a brief literature review, *J Child Orthop* 2:63, 2008.

Karlen JW, Skaggs DL, Ramachandran M, Kay RM: The Dega osteotomy: a versatile osteotomy in the treatment of developmental and neuromuscular hip pathology, *J Pediatr Orthop* 29:676, 2009.

Kawaguchi AT, Otsuka NY, Delgado ED, et al: Magnetic resonance arthrography in children with developmental hip dysplasia, *Clin Orthop Relat Res* 374:234, 2000.

Kitoh H, Kawasumi M, Ishiguro N: Predictive factors for unsuccessful treatment of developmental dysplasia of the hip by the Pavlik harness, *J Pediatr Orthop* 29:552, 2009.

Kotnis R, Spiteri V, Little C, et al: Hip arthrography in the assessment of children with developmental dysplasia of the hip and Perthes' disease, *J Pediatr Orthop B* 17:114, 2008.

Laborie LB, Engesaeter IO, Lehmann TG, et al: Screening strategies for hip dysplasia: long-term outcome of a randomized controlled trial, *Pediatrics* 132:492, 2013.

Lipton GE, Guille JT, Altiok H, et al: A reappraisal of the Ortolani examination in children with developmental dysplasia of the hip, *J Pediatr Orthop* 27:27, 2007.

López-Carreno E, Carillo H, Gutiérrez M: Dega versus Salter osteotomy for the treatment of developmental dysplasia of the hip, *J Pediatr Orthop B* 17:213, 2008.

Mahan ST, Katz JN, Kim YJ: To screen or not to screen? A decision analysis of the utility of screening for developmental dysplasia of the hip, *J Bone Joint Surg* 91A:1705, 2009.

Mahan ST, Yazdy MM, Kasser JR, Werler MM: Is it worthwhile to routinely ultrasound screen children with idiopathic clubfoot for hip dysplasia? *J Pediatr Orthop* 33:847, 2013.

Molony DC, Harty JA, Burke TE, D'Souza LG: Popliteal angle as an indicator for successful closed reduction of developmental dysplasia of the hip, *J Orthop Surg (Hong Kong)* 19:46, 2011.

Morsi E: Acetabuloplasty for neglected dislocation of the hip in older children, *J Bone Joint Surg* 89B:372, 2007.

Murhaghan ML, Browne RH, Socato DJ, Birch J: Femoral nerve palsy in Pavlik harness treatment for developmental dysplasia of the hip, *J Bone Joint Surg* 93A:493, 2011.

Nakamura J, Kamegaya M, Saisu T, et al: Treatment for developmental dysplasia of the hip using the Pavlik harness: long-term results, *J Bone Joint Surg* 89B:230, 2007.

Oh CW, Guille JT, Kumar SJ, et al: Operative treatment for type II avascular necrosis in developmental dysplasia of the hip, *Clin Orthop Relat Res* 434:86, 2005.

Oh CW, Joo SY, Kumar SJ, Macewen GD: A radiological classification of lateral growth arrest of the proximal femoral physis after treatment for developmental dysplasia of the hip, *J Pediatr Orthop* 29:331, 2009.

Ok IY, Kim SJ, Ok JH: Operative treatment of developmental hip dysplasia in children aged over 8 years, *J Pediatr Orthop B* 16:256, 2007.

Omeroglu H, Ucar DH, Tümer Y: A new, objective radiographic classification system for the assessment of treatment results in developmental dysplasia of the hip, *J Pediatr Orthop B* 15:77, 2006.

Ortiz-Neira CL, Paolucci EO, Donnon T: A meta-analysis of common risk factors associated with the diagnosis of developmental dysplasia of the hip in newborns, *Eur J Radiol* 81:e344, 2012.

Paton RW, Choudry QA, Jugdey R, Hughes S: Is congenital talipes equinovarus a risk factor for pathological dysplasia of the hip? A 21-year prospective, longitudinal observational study, *Bone Joint J* 96-B:1553, 2014.

Perry DC, Tawfig SM, Roche A, et al: The association between clubfoot and developmental dysplasia of the hip, *J Bone Joint Surg* 92B:1586, 2010.

Portinaro NM, Pelillo F, Cerutti P: The role of ultrasonography in the diagnosis of developmental dysplasia of the hip, *J Pediatr Orthop* 27:247, 2007.

Pospischill R, Weninger J, Ganger R, et al: Does open reduction of the developmental dislocated hip increase the risk of osteonecrosis? *Clin Orthop Relat Res* 470:250, 2012.

Ramani N, Patil MS, Mahna M: Outcome of surgical management of developmental dysplasia of hip in children between 18 and 24 months, *Indian J Orthop* 48:458, 2014.

Rampal V, Sabourin M, Erdeneshoo E, et al: Closed reduction with traction for developmental dysplasia of the hip in children aged between one and five years, *J Bone Joint Surg* 90B:858, 2008.

Rhodes AM, Clarke NM: A review of environmental factors implicated in human developmental dysplasia of the hip, *J Child Orthop* 8:375, 2014.

Roposch A, Liu LQ, Hefti F, et al: Standardized diagnostic criteria for developmental dysplasia of hip in early infancy, *Clin Orthop Relat Res* 469:3451, 2011.

Roposch A, Odeh O, Doria AS, Wedge JH: The presence of an ossific nucleus does not protect against osteonecrosis after treatment of developmental dysplasia of the hip, *Clin Orthop Relat Res* 469:2838, 2011.

Roposch A, Stöhr KK, Dobson M: The effect of the femoral head ossific nucleus in the treatment of developmental dysplasia of the hip: a meta-analysis, *J Bone Joint Surg* 91A:911, 2009.

Roposch A, Wedge JH, Riedl G: Reliability of Bucholz and Ogden classification for osteonecrosis secondary to developmental dysplasia of the hip, *Clin Orthop Relat Res* 40:3499, 2012.

Sabharwal S, Zhao C: The hip-knee-ankle angle in children: reference values based on a full-length standing radiograph, *J Bone Joint Surg* 91A:2461, 2009.

Sankar WN, Neubuerger CO, Moseley CF: Femoral head sphericity in untreated developmental dislocation of the hip, *J Pediatr Orthop* 29:885, 2009.

Sankar WN, Neubuerger CO, Moseley CF: Femoral anteversion in developmental dysplasia of the hip, *J Pediatr Orthop* 30:558, 2010.

Sankar WN, Tany EY, Moseley CF: Predictors of the need for femoral shortening osteotomy during open treatment of developmental dislocation of the hip, *J Pediatr Orthop* 29:868, 2009.

Sankar WN, Young CR, Ling AG, et al: Risk factors for failure after open reduction for DDH: a matched cohort analysis, *J Pediatr Orthop* 31:232, 2011.

Sardelli M, Tashjian RZ, MacWilliams BA: Functional elbow range of motion for contemporary tasks, *J Bone Joint Surg Am* 93:471, 2011.

Schwend RM, Schoenecker P, Richards BS, et al: Screening the newborn for developmental dysplasia of the hip: now what do we do? *J Pediatr Orthop* 27:607, 2007.

Senaran H, Bowen JR, Harcke HT: Avascular necrosis rate in early reduction after failed Pavlik harness treatment of developmental dysplasia of the hip, *J Pediatr Orthop* 27:192, 2007.

Sewell MD, Eastwood DM: Screening and treatment in developmental dysplasia of the hip-where do we go from here? *Int Orthop* 35:1359, 2011.

Shorter D, Hong T, Osborn DA: Cochrane review: screening programmes for developmental dysplasia of the hip in newborn infants, *Evid Base Child Health* 8:11, 2013.

Snyder M, Harcke HT, Domzalski M: Role of ultrasound in the diagnosis and management of developmental dysplasia of the hip: an international perspective, *Orthop Clin North Am* 37:141, 2006.

Spence G, Hocking R, Wedge JH, Roposch A: Effect of innominate and femoral varus derotation osteotomy on acetabular development in developmental dysplasia of the hip, *J Bone Joint Surg* 91A:2622, 2009.

Stevenson DA, Mineau G, Kerber RA, et al: Familial predisposition to developmental dysplasia of the hip, *J Pediatr Orthop* 29:463, 2009.

Subasi M, Arslan H, Cebesoy O, et al: Outcome in unilateral or bilateral DDH treated with one-stage combined procedure, *Clin Orthop Relat Res* 466:830, 2008.

Swaroop VT, Mubarak SJ: Difficult-to-treat Ortolani-positive hip: improved success with new treatment protocol, *J Pediatr Orthop* 29:224, 2009.

Tarassoli P, Gargan MF, Atherton WG, Thomas SR: The medial approach for the treatment of children with developmental dysplasia of the hip, *Bone Joint J* 96B:406, 2014.

Vallamshetla VRP, Mughal E, O'Hara JN: Congenital dislocation of the hip: a re-appraisal of the upper age limit for treatment, *J Bone Joint Surg* 88B:1076, 2006.

van der Sluius JA, De Gier L, Verbeke JI, et al: Prolonged treatment with the Pavlik harness in infants with developmental dysplasia of the hip, *J Bone Joint Surg* 91B:1090, 2009.

von Heideken J, Green DW, Burke SW, et al: The relationship between developmental dysplasia of the hip and congenital muscular torticollis, *J Pediatr Orthop* 26:805, 2006.

Walton MJ, Isaacson Z, McMillan D, et al: The success of management with the Pavlik harness for developmental dysplasia of the hip using a United Kingdom screening programme and ultrasound-guided supervision, *J Bone Joint Surg* 92B:1013, 2012.

Wenger DR: Surgical treatment of developmental dysplasia of the hip, *Instr Course Lect* 63:313, 2014.

Westacott DJ, Mackay ND, Watson A, et al: Staged weaning versus immediate cessation of Pavlik harness treatment for developmental dysplasia of the hip, *J Pediatr Orthop B* 23:103, 2014.

White KK, Sucato DJ, Agrawal S, Browne R: Ultrasonographic findings in hips with a positive Ortolani sign and their relationship to Pavlik harness failure, *J Bone Joint Surg Am* 92:113, 2010.

Wu KW, Wang TM, Huang SC, et al: Analysis of osteonecrosis following Pemberton acetabuloplasty in developmental dysplasia of the hip: long-term results, *J Bone Joint Surg* 92A:2083, 2010.

Xu RJ, Li WC, Ma CX: Slotted acetabular augmentation with concurrent open reduction for developmental dysplasia of the hip in older children, *J Pediatr Orthop* 30:554, 2010.

Zamzam MM, Khosshal KI, Abak AA, et al: One-stage bilateral open reduction through a medial approach in developmental dysplasia of the hip, *J Bone Joint Surg* 91B:113, 2009.

CONGENITAL AND DEVELOPMENTAL COXA VARA

Chotigavanichaya C, Leeprakobboon D, Eamsobhana P, Kaewpornsawan K: Results of surgical treatment of coxa vara in children: valgus osteotomy with angle blade plate fixation, *J Media Assoc Thai* (Suppl 9):S78, 2014.

Fassier F, Sardar Z, Aarabi M, et al: Results and complications of a surgical technique for correction of coxa vara in children with osteopenic bones, *J Pediatr Orthop* 28:799, 2008.

Günther CM, Komm M, Jansson V, Heimkes B: Midterm results after subtrochanteric end-to-side valgization osteotomy in severe infantile coxa vara, *J Pediatr Orthop* 33:353, 2013.

Oh CW, Thacker MM, Mackenzie WG, et al: Coxa vara: a novel measurement technique in skeletal dysplasias, *Clin Orthop Relat Res* 447:125, 2006.

Ranade A, McCarthy JJ, Davidson RS: Acetabular changes in coxa vara, *Clin Orthop Relat Res* 466:1688, 2008.

EXSTROPHY OF THE BLADDER

Jones D, Parkinson S, Hosalkar HS: Oblique pelvic osteotomy in the exstrophy/epispadias complex, *J Bone Joint Surg* 88B:799, 2006.

Kajbafzadeh AM, Talab SS, Elmi A, et al: Use of biodegradable plates and screws for approximation of symphysis pubis in bladder exstrophy: applications and outcomes, *Urology* 77:1248, 2011.

Mushtag I, Garriboli M, Smeulders N, et al: Primary bladder exstrophy closure in neonates: challenging the traditions, *J Urol* 193, 2014.

Nehme A, Oakes D, Perry MJ, et al: Acetabular morphology in bladder exstrophy complex, *Clin Orthop Relat Res* 458:125, 2007.

Satsuma S, Kobayashi D, Yoshiya S, et al: Comparison of posterior and anterior pelvic osteotomy for bladder exstrophy complex, *J Pediatr Orthop B* 15:141, 2006.

Shnorhavorian M, Song K, Samil pa I, et al: Spica casting compared to Bryant's traction after complete primary repair of exstrophy: safe and effective in a longitudinal cohort study, *J Urol* 184:669, 2010.

Wild AT, Sponseller PD, Stec AA, Gearhart JP: The role of osteotomy in surgical repair of bladder exstrophy, *Semin Pediatr Surg* 20:71, 2011.

The complete list of references is available online at ***expertconsult.inkling.com****.*

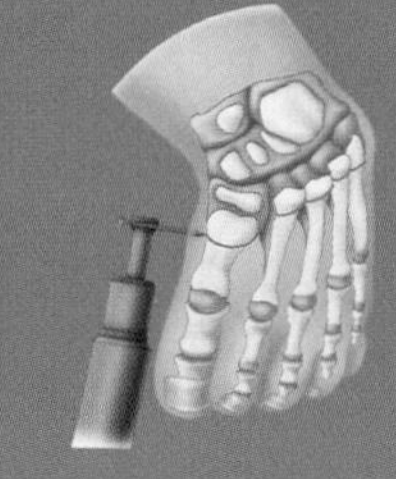

CHAPTER 31

CONGENITAL ANOMALIES OF THE TRUNK AND UPPER EXTREMITY

Benjamin M. Mauck

This chapter discusses congenital elevation of the scapula, congenital torticollis, and congenital pseudarthrosis of the clavicle, radius, and ulna. Congenital anomalies of the hand and certain other anomalies of the forearm are discussed in Chapter 79. Congenital conditions of the spine are discussed in Chapters 43 and 44.

CONGENITAL ELEVATION OF THE SCAPULA (SPRENGEL DEFORMITY)

First described by Eulenberg in 1863, Sprengel deformity is characterized as a congenital upward elevation of the scapula in relation to the thoracic cage. The scapula is commonly hypoplastic and misshapen (Fig. 31-1). Other congenital anomalies may be present, such as cervical ribs, malformations of ribs, and anomalies of the cervical vertebrae (Klippel-Feil syndrome); rarely, one or more scapular muscles are partly or completely absent. The presence of this deformity can often indicate abnormalities in other organ systems. The severity of the functional impairment typically is related to the severity of the deformity (Table 31-1). If the deformity is mild, the scapula is only slightly elevated and is a bit smaller than normal and its motion is only mildly limited; however, if the deformity is severe, the scapula is very small and can be so elevated that it almost touches the occiput. The patient's head is often deviated toward the affected side. The primary limitation of shoulder motion is abduction secondary to diminished scapulothoracic motion. In about half of patients, an extra ossicle, the omovertebral bone, is present; this is a rhomboidal plaque of cartilage and bone lying in a strong fascial sheath that extends from the superior angle of the scapula to the spinous process, lamina, or transverse process of one or more lower cervical vertebrae. Recognition of this abnormality is essential to surgical management. A similar osseous structure has also been reported extending from the medial border of the scapula to the occiput. Sometimes a well-developed joint is found between the omovertebral bone and the scapula; sometimes it is attached to the scapula by fibrous tissue only. A solid osseous ridge between the spinous processes and the scapula is rare.

Radiographic workup is essential to surgical planning. Plain radiographs should be obtained to assess the level of the scapula in relation to vertebrae and in comparison to the contralateral side. Radiographs also can help recognize the presence of associated abnormalities such as the omovertebral bone.

In a morphometric analysis using three-dimensional CT, Cho et al. found that most of the affected scapulae in 15 patients with Sprengel deformity had a characteristic shape, with a decrease in the height-to-width ratio. An inverse relationship was found between scapular rotation and superior displacement; no significant difference was found in glenoid version. Cho et al. suggested that the point of tethering of the omovertebral connection, when present, may determine the shape, rotation, and superior displacement of the scapula and that three-dimensional CT can be helpful in delineating the deformity and planning scapuloplasty.

If deformity and impairment are mild, no treatment is indicated; if they are more severe, surgery may be indicated, depending on the age of the patient and the severity of any associated deformities. Because the deformity is more than just simple scapular elevation, the results of surgical treatment of Sprengel deformity can vary. The long-term function of the shoulder and cosmetic appearance must be carefully measured against the surgical risk and natural history of the deformity. A 26-year review of 22 patients with Sprengel deformity treated by either observation or surgical repair suggested that surgically treated patients had almost 40 degrees more abduction than their nonsurgical counterparts, with a subjective improvement in cosmesis.

An operation to bring the scapula inferiorly to near its normal position is ideally attempted soon after 3 years of age, because the operation becomes more difficult as the child grows. In older children, an attempt to bring the scapula inferiorly to its normal level can injure the brachial plexus.

Numerous operations have been described to correct Sprengel deformity. Green described surgical release of muscles from the scapula along with excision of the supraspinatus portion of the scapula and any omovertebral bone. The scapula is moved inferiorly to a more normal position, and the muscles are reattached. Other modifications include suturing the scapula into a pocket in the latissimus dorsi after

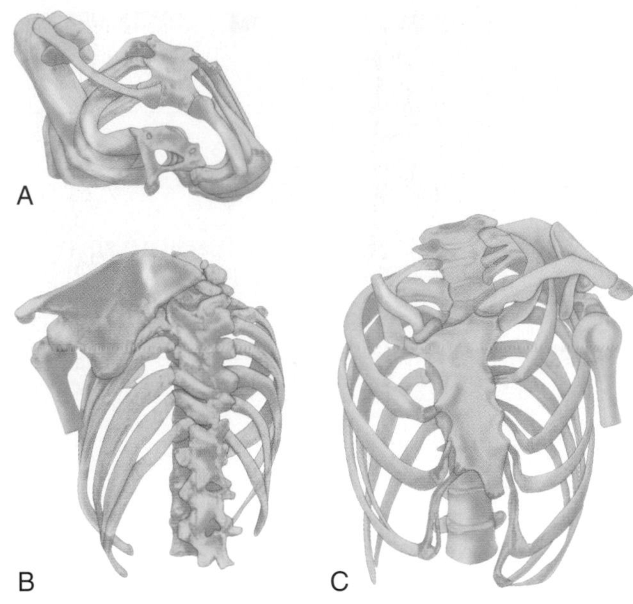

FIGURE 31-1 Elevated, malrotated, and malformed scapula with bony connection to the spine. **A,** Axial. **B,** Posterior. **C,** Anterior. (Redrawn from: Harvey EJ, Bernstein M, Desy NM, et al. Sprengel deformity: pathogenesis and management, J Am Acad Orthop Surg 20:177, 2012.)

TABLE 31-1

Cavendish Classification

Grade 1	Very mild	Shoulders are level; deformity not visible when patient is dressed
Grade 2	Mild	Shoulders are almost level; deformity is visible as a lump in the web of neck when patient is dressed
Grade 3	Moderate	Shoulders elevated 2-5 cm; deformity easily seen
Grade 4	Severe	Shoulder grossly elevated; superior angle of scapula lies near occiput

(Information from Cavendish ME: Congenital elevation of the scapula, J Bone Joint Surg 54:395, 1972.)

rotating the scapula and moving it caudad to a more normal position, and avoiding dissection of the serratus anterior muscle so that mobilization is begun immediately postoperatively. Wada et al. performed a morphometric analysis and reported 23 scapulae in 22 patients treated with the modified Green procedure. At 4-year follow-up the patients demonstrated a 63-degree increase in range of motion.

Woodward, in 1961, described transfer of the origin of the trapezius muscle to a more inferior position on the spinous processes. Greitemann et al. recommended the Woodward procedure for patients with impaired function; for patients with only cosmetic problems, resection of part of the superior angle of the scapula was preferred. They suggested that better results are obtained with the Woodward procedure because (1) the muscles are incised farther from the scapula, which lowers the risk of formation of a scar-keloid that may fix the scapula in poor position; (2) a larger mobilization is possible; and (3) the postoperative scar is not as thick as with Green's procedure. Borges et al. added excision of the prominent superomedial border of the scapula to the Woodward procedure. In a series of patients with long-term follow-up at an average of 14.7 years, Walstra et al. demonstrated improvement of Cavendish grade 3 to 1 or 2 and significant improvement in overall shoulder abduction and improved contrast; Disability of the Arm, Shoulder, and Hand (DASH) and Simple Shoulder Test (SST) scores also improved. No long-term complications were reported. We generally prefer the Woodard procedure (see later) (Fig. 31-2).

To improve function of the shoulder and the cosmetic appearance, Mears developed a procedure that includes partial resection of the scapula, removal of any omovertebral communication, and release of the long head of the triceps from the scapula. In the eight patients in whom this technique was used, average flexion improved from 100 to 175 degrees and abduction improved from 90 to 150 degrees. In two patients, hypertrophic scars formed at the curvilinear incision; this problem was eliminated by the use of a transverse incision in subsequent patients. Mears observed that a contracture of the long head of the triceps seems to represent a significant inhibition to full abduction in patients with Sprengel deformity and that release of this contracture allows increased abduction. Early postoperative active and active-assisted motion exercises of the shoulder are used to improve function.

Brachial plexus palsy is the most severe complication of surgery for Sprengel deformity. The scapula in this deformity is hypoplastic compared with the normal scapula. During surgery, attention should be directed to placing the spine of the scapula at the same level as that on the opposite side, rather than aligning exactly the inferior angles of the scapulae. To avoid brachial plexus palsy, several authors recommended morcellation of the clavicle on the ipsilateral side as a first step in the operative treatment of Sprengel deformity. This is not a routine part of surgical treatment but is recommended in severe deformity or in children who show signs of brachial plexus palsy after surgical correction. In patients older than 8 years of age, a 2-cm midclavicular osteotomy is recommended to decompress the brachial plexus and first rib before scapular resection. In a younger patient, a 1-cm resection osteotomy is considered for severe deformity. Others have suggested the use of intraoperative somatosensory evoked potentials to monitor brachial plexus function during surgical correction.

WOODWARD OPERATION

TECHNIQUE 31-1

- Place the patient prone on the operating table and prepare and drape both shoulders so that the involved shoulder girdle and the arm can be manipulated and the uninvolved scapula can be inspected in its normal position.
- Make a midline incision from the spinous process of the first cervical vertebra distally to that of the ninth thoracic

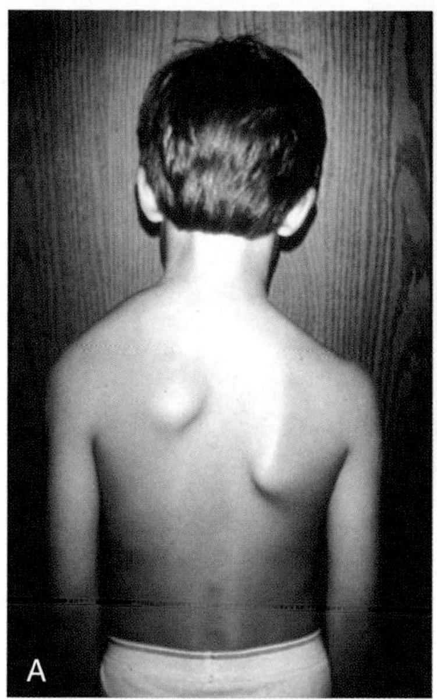

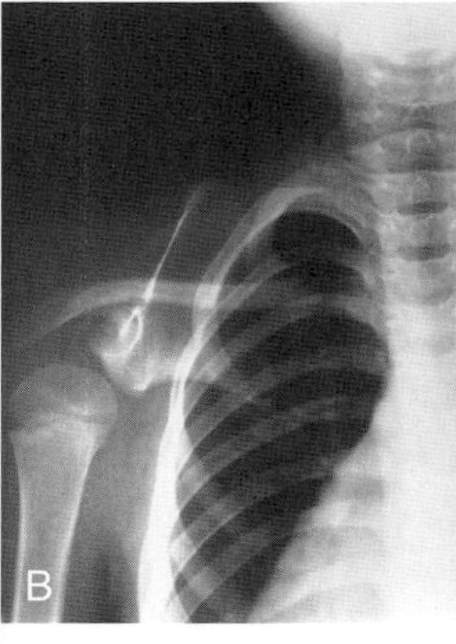

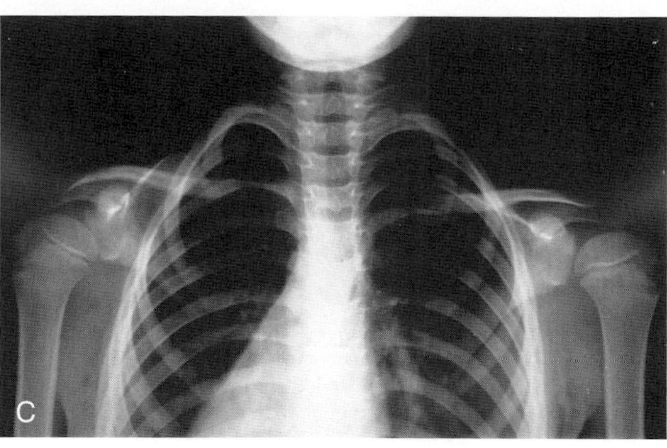

FIGURE 31-2 **A,** Sprengel deformity (left sided) in 5-year-old boy. **B,** Posteroanterior radiograph shows congenital elevation of left scapula. **C,** Posteroanterior radiograph after Woodward procedure.

vertebra (Fig. 31-3A). Undermine the skin and subcutaneous tissues laterally to the medial border of the scapula.

- Identify the lateral border of the trapezius in the distal end of the incision and by blunt dissection separate it from the underlying latissimus dorsi muscle.
- By sharp dissection, free the fascial sheath of origin of the trapezius from the spinous processes.
- Identify the origins of the rhomboideus major and minor muscles and by sharp dissection free them from the spinous processes.
- Free the rhomboids and the superior part of the trapezius from the muscles of the chest wall anterior to them.
- Retract the freed sheet of muscles laterally to expose any omovertebral bone or fibrous bands attached to the superior angle of the scapula.
- By extraperiosteal dissection, excise any omovertebral bone, or if the bone is absent, excise any fibrous band or contracted levator scapulae; avoid injuring the spinal accessory nerve, the nerves to the rhomboids, and the transverse cervical artery.
- If the supraspinous part of the scapula is deformed, resect it along with its periosteum; this releases the levator scapulae (if not already excised), allowing the shoulder girdle to move more freely (Fig. 31-3B).
- Divide transversely the remaining narrow attachment of the trapezius at the level of the fourth cervical vertebra.
- Displace the scapula along with the attached sheet of muscles distally until its spine lies at the same level as that of the opposite scapula (Fig. 31-3C).
- While holding the scapula in this position, reattach the aponeuroses of the trapezius and rhomboids to the spinous processes at a more inferior level.
- In the distal part of the incision, create a fold in the origin of the trapezius and either excise the excess tissue or incise the fold and overlap and suture in place the resultant free edges.

POSTOPERATIVE CARE. A Velpeau bandage is applied and is worn for about 2 weeks. Active and passive range-of-motion exercises are begun.

MORCELLATION OF THE CLAVICLE

TECHNIQUE 31-2

- Make a straight incision over the clavicle extending from 1.5 cm lateral to the sternoclavicular joint to 1.5 cm medial to the acromioclavicular joint.
- Expose the clavicle subperiosteally.
- Divide the bone 2 cm from each end, remove it, and cut it into small pieces (morcellate).
- Replace the pieces in the periosteal tube and close the tube with interrupted sutures.
- Close the subcutaneous tissues and skin in a routine manner.

CONGENITAL MUSCULAR TORTICOLLIS

Congenital muscular torticollis (CMT) is caused by fibromatosis within the sternocleidomastoid muscle. A mass either is palpable at birth or becomes so, usually during the first 2 weeks. Congenital muscular torticollis is more common on

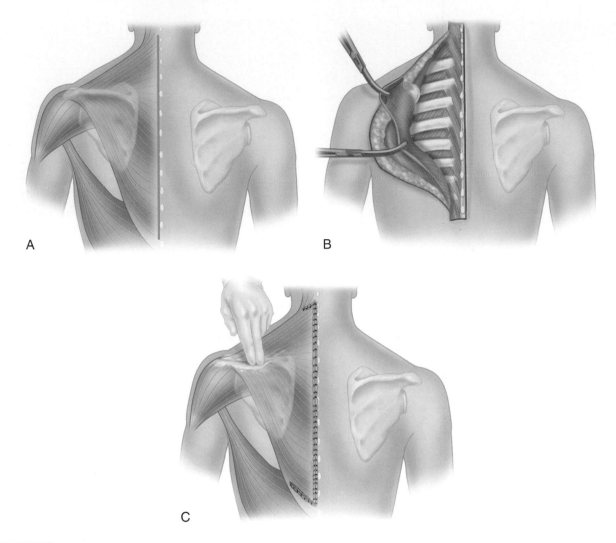

FIGURE 31-3 Woodward operation for congenital elevation of scapula. **A,** Elevation of scapula, extensive origin of trapezius, and skin incision are shown. **B,** Skin has been incised in midline. Origins of trapezius and of rhomboideus major and minor have been freed from spinous processes, and these muscles have been retracted laterally. Levator scapulae, any omovertebral bone, and any deformed superior angle of scapula are to be excised. **C,** Remaining narrow attachment of trapezius superiorly has been divided at level of C4. Scapula and attached sheet of muscles have been displaced inferiorly, and aponeuroses of trapezius and rhomboids have been reattached to spinous processes at more inferior level. A redundant fold of trapezius aponeurosis is formed inferiorly. Fold of trapezius aponeurosis has been incised, and resultant free edges have been overlapped and sutured in place. Free superior edge of trapezius also has been sutured. (Modified from Woodward JW: Congenital elevation of the scapula: correction by release and transplantation of muscle origins: a preliminary report, J Bone Joint Surg 43A:219, 1961.) **SEE TECHNIQUE 31-1.**

the right side than on the left side. It may involve the muscle diffusely, but more often it is localized near the clavicular attachment of the muscle. The mass attains maximal size within 1 or 2 months and may remain the same size or become smaller; usually, it diminishes and disappears within 1 year. If it fails to disappear, the muscle becomes permanently fibrotic and contracted and causes torticollis, which also is permanent unless treated (Fig. 31-4).

Although CMT has been recognized for centuries, its cause remains unclear. Clinical studies have shown that infants with CMT are more often the product of a difficult delivery and have an increased incidence of associated musculoskeletal disorders, such as metatarsus adductus, developmental dysplasia of the hip, and talipes equinovarus. There is a reported incidence of congenital dislocation of the hip or

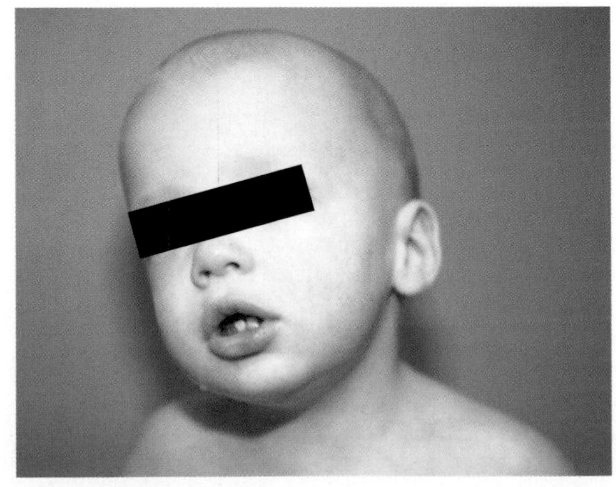

FIGURE 31-4 Congenital torticollis in 14-month-old boy.

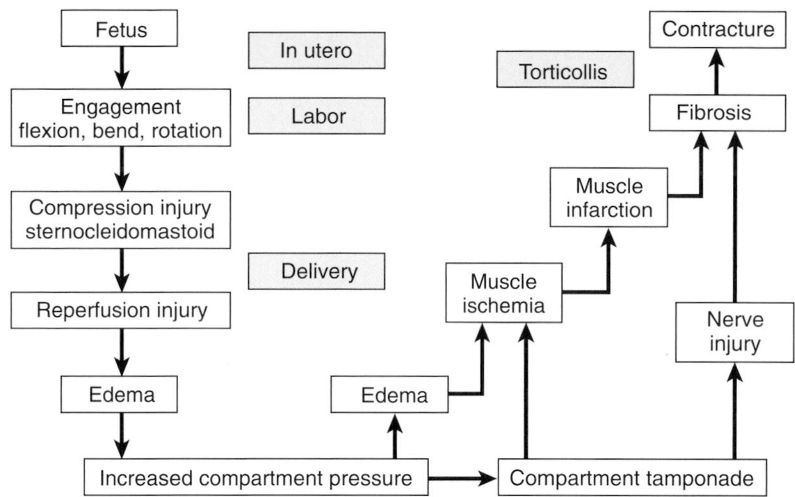

FIGURE 31-5 Pathophysiology of congenital muscular torticollis proposed by Davids, Wenger, and Mubarak, who suggested that congenital muscular torticollis may represent the sequela of intrauterine or perinatal compartment syndrome.

dysplasia of the acetabulum ranging from 7% to 20% in children with CMT. Careful hip screening and, if necessary, ultrasound evaluation are indicated.

Various hypotheses of the cause of CMT include malposition of the fetus in utero, intrauterine constraint, birth trauma, infection, and vascular injury. Davids et al. found that MRI of 10 infants with CMT showed signals in the sternocleidomastoid muscle similar to signals observed in the forearm and leg after compartment syndrome. Further investigation included cadaver dissections and injection studies that defined the sternocleidomastoid muscle compartment; pressure measurements of three patients with CMT that confirmed the presence of this compartment in vivo; and clinical review of 48 children with CMT that showed a relationship between birth position and the side affected by contracture. These findings led the authors to postulate that CMT may represent the sequela of an intrauterine or perinatal compartment syndrome (Fig. 31-5).

A palpable nodule is typically present in the affected sternocleidomastoid muscle at birth or within the first few weeks of life. The patient may also have associated plagiocephaly and facial asymmetry. The presence of the characteristic fibrotic nodule typically confirms the diagnosis, rendering further radiographic evaluation unnecessary in most cases. When the diagnosis remains in doubt, cervical spine radiographs are appropriate. Finally, some authors have advocated ultrasonography for the evaluation and management of congenital muscular torticollis.

When CMT is seen in early infancy, it is impossible to tell whether or not the mass causing it will disappear spontaneously. Lin and Chou reported that ultrasonography was useful in predicting which infants would require surgical treatment. Those patients in whom fibrotic change was limited to only the lower third of the sternocleidomastoid muscle recovered without surgery, whereas 35% of patients with whole muscle involvement required surgical release.

Only conservative treatment is indicated during infancy. The parents should be instructed to stretch the sternocleidomastoid muscle by manipulating the infant's head manually. The child's chin is rotated toward the shoulder on the side of the affected sternocleidomastoid muscle while the head is tilted toward the opposite shoulder. Excising the lesion during early infancy is unjustified; surgery should be delayed until evolution of the fibromatosis is complete, and then, if necessary, the muscle can be released at one or both ends. CMT typically resolves with a home stretching program during the first year of life. Some authors suggest a strong correlation between sternocleidomastoid (5-cm) thickness to duration and response to stretching exercises. Canale et al. found that CMT did not resolve spontaneously if it persisted beyond the age of 1 year. Children who were treated during the first year of life had better results than children treated later, and an exercise program was more likely to be successful if the restriction of motion was less than 30 degrees and there was no facial asymmetry or if the facial asymmetry was noted only by the examiner. Nonoperative therapy after age 1 year was rarely successful. Regardless of the type of treatment, established facial asymmetry and limitation of motion of more than 30 degrees at the beginning of treatment usually precluded a good result.

Any permanent torticollis slowly becomes worse during growth. The head becomes inclined toward the affected side and the face toward the opposite side. If the deformity is severe, the ipsilateral shoulder becomes elevated and the frontooccipital diameter of the skull may become less than normal. Such severe deformity could and should be prevented by surgery during early childhood. Ideally, surgery is performed just before school age so that sufficient growth remains for remodeling of facial asymmetry while giving enough time for the growth of the structures to make surgical dissection and release easier. Many patients are first seen only after the deformities have become fixed, and the remaining growth potential is insufficient to correct them (Fig. 31-6). Nevertheless, many authors have suggested that surgical release in older children can be successful and should be attempted even if the child presents later. The clinical results are significantly less successful in children who have finished growth than in children who still have growth remaining; however, most patients have marked improvement in neck motion and head tilt, with satisfactory functional and

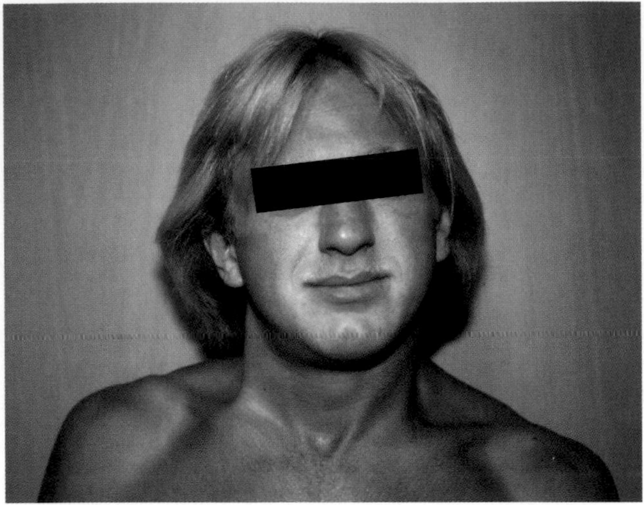

FIGURE 31-6 Untreated torticollis *(right)* in 19-year-old man; note limited rotation and plagiocephaly.

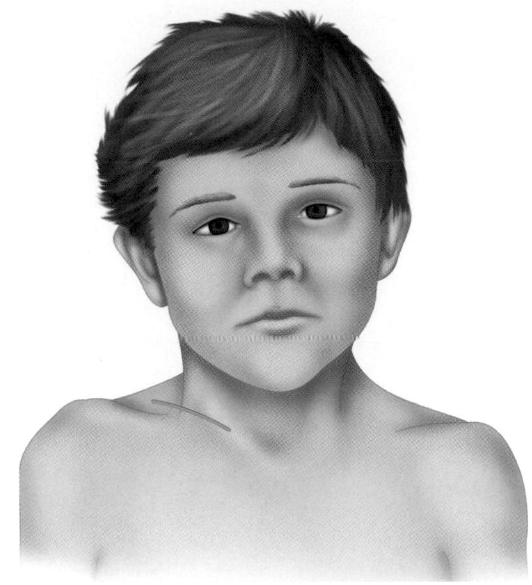

FIGURE 31-7 Unipolar release for torticollis. Note line of skin incision.

cosmetic results. Lee et al. reported marked improvement in craniofacial deformity after surgical release in 80 patients with CMT. Improved results were demonstrated if the release was performed before the patient reached 5 years of age. Most significant changes appeared to occur within the first year postoperatively.

Several operations have been devised to release the sternocleidomastoid muscle at the clavicle. Unipolar release of the muscle distally is appropriate for mild deformity. Bipolar release proximally and distally may be indicated for moderate and severe torticollis. Endoscopic release of the sternocleidomastoid muscle has been described, with suggested advantages of precise division of the muscle fibers, preservation of the neurovascular structures, and an inconspicuous scar; we have no experience with this technique and no large series have been reported.

UNIPOLAR RELEASE

Open unipolar tenotomy of the sternocleidomastoid muscle could be followed by tethering of the scar to the deep structures, reattachment of the clavicular head or the sternal head of the sternocleidomastoid muscle, loss of contour of the muscle, failure to correct the tilt of the head, or failure of facial asymmetry to correct. Tethering of the scar to the deep structures is more common in younger patients; therefore, the operation should be postponed until after 4 years of age.

TECHNIQUE 31-3

- Make an incision 5 cm long just superior to and parallel to the medial end of the clavicle (Fig. 31-7) and deepen it to the tendons of the sternal and clavicular attachments of the sternocleidomastoid muscle.
- Incise the tendon sheath longitudinally and pass a hemostat or other blunt instrument posterior to the tendons.
- By traction on the hemostat, draw the tendons outside the wound and superior and inferior to the hemostat; clamp them and resect 2.5 cm of their inferior ends. If it is contracted, divide the platysma muscle and adjacent fascia.
- With the child's head turned toward the affected side and the chin depressed, explore the wound digitally for any remaining bands of contracted muscle or fascia; and if any are found, divide them under direct vision until the deformity can, if possible, be overcorrected.
- If after this procedure overcorrection is not possible, make a small transverse incision inferior to the mastoid process and carefully divide the muscle near the bone. Avoid damaging the spinal accessory nerve.
- Close the wound and apply a bulky dressing that holds the head in the overcorrected position.

POSTOPERATIVE CARE. At 1 week postoperatively, physical therapy, including manual stretching of the neck to maintain the overcorrected position, is begun. Manual stretching should be continued three times daily for 3 to 6 months; the use of plaster casts or braces usually is unnecessary (Fig. 31-8).

BIPOLAR RELEASE

Surgical correction in children with severe deformity or after failed operation usually requires a bipolar release of the sternocleidomastoid muscle. Ferkel et al. described a modified bipolar release and Z-plasty of the muscle for use in these circumstances. This approach lessens the sunken or hollow appearance of the distal end of the sternocleidomastoid that often occurs with a simple tenotomy, thereby giving the patient a better cosmetic result.

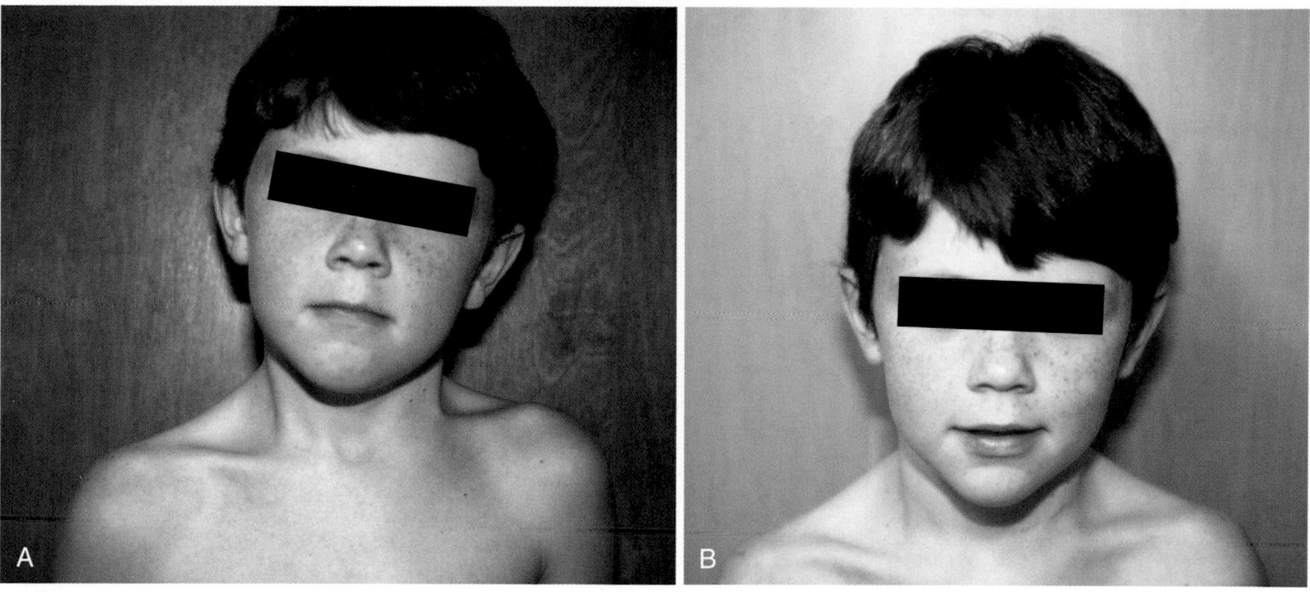

FIGURE 31-8 Seven-year-old boy with left congenital muscular torticollis. **A,** Before unipolar supraclavicular release. **B,** After unipolar release; note scar superior to clavicle in transverse line of skin crease. **SEE TECHNIQUE 31-3.**

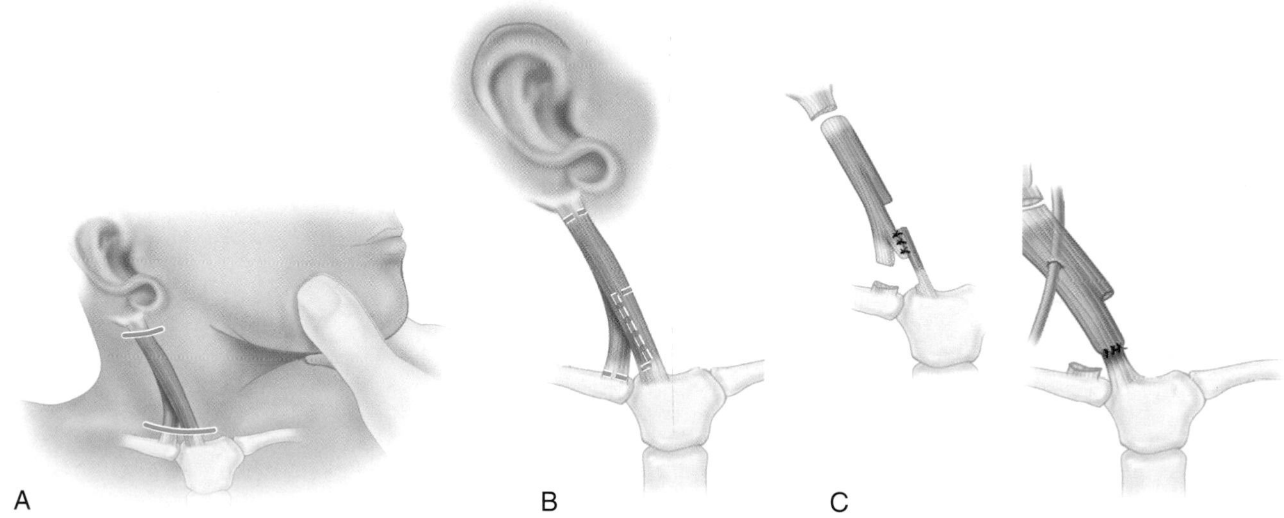

FIGURE 31-9 Bipolar Z-plasty operation for torticollis. **A,** Skin incisions. **B,** Clavicular and mastoid attachments of sternocleidomastoid muscle are cut, and Z-plasty is performed on sternal origin. **C,** Completed operation; note preservation of medial portion of sternal attachment. (Redrawn from Ferkel RD, Westin GW, Dawson EG, et al: Muscular torticollis: a modified surgical approach, J Bone Joint Surg 65A:894, 1983.) **SEE TECHNIQUE 31-4.**

TECHNIQUE 31-4

(FERKEL ET AL.)

- Make a short transverse proximal incision behind the ear (Fig. 31-9A) and divide the sternocleidomastoid muscle insertion transversely just distal to the tip of the mastoid process. With this limited incision, the spinal accessory nerve is avoided, although the possibility that the nerve may take an anomalous route should be considered.
- Make a distal incision 4 to 5 cm long in line with the cervical skin creases, a fingerbreadth proximal to the medial end of the clavicle and the sternal notch.
- Divide the subcutaneous tissue and platysma muscle, exposing the clavicular and sternal attachments of the sternocleidomastoid muscle. Carefully avoid the anterior and external jugular veins and the carotid vessels and sheath during the dissection.
- Cut the clavicular portion of the muscle transversely and perform a Z-plasty on the sternal attachment so as to preserve the normal V-shaped contour of the sternocleidomastoid muscle in the neckline (Fig. 31-9B). Alternatively, release the clavicular head directly from the clavicle while transecting the sternal head proximal to its insertion by 1 to 2 cm. Then suture the two ends together side to side or end to end (Fig. 31-9C).

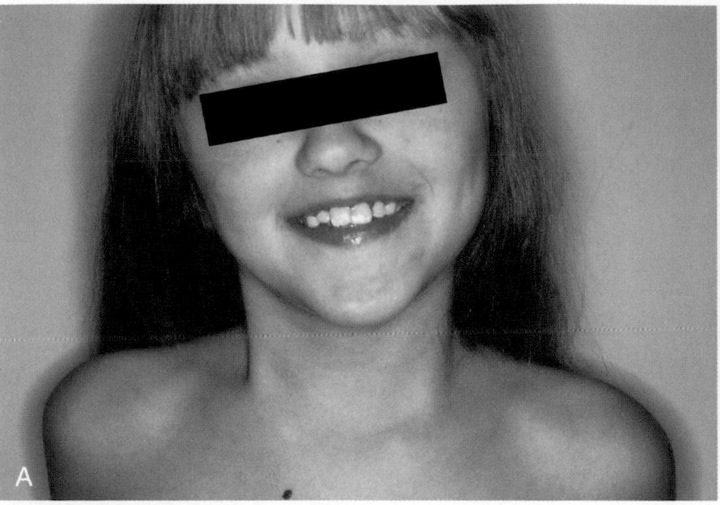

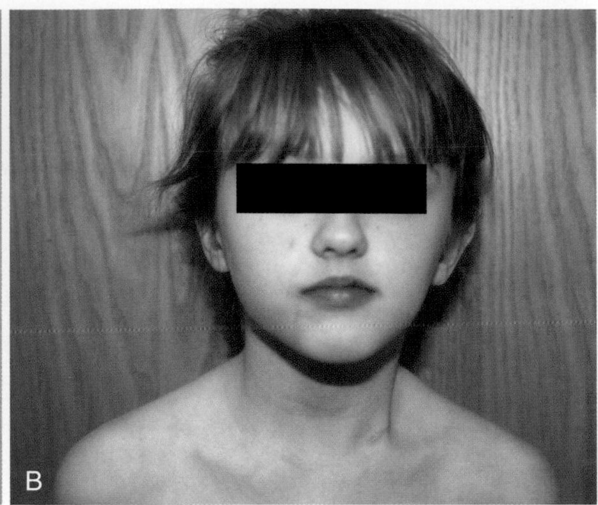

FIGURE 31-10 Bipolar release for congenital torticollis. **A,** Severe congenital torticollis (right side) in 8-year-old girl. **B,** After bipolar release. **SEE TECHNIQUE 31-4.**

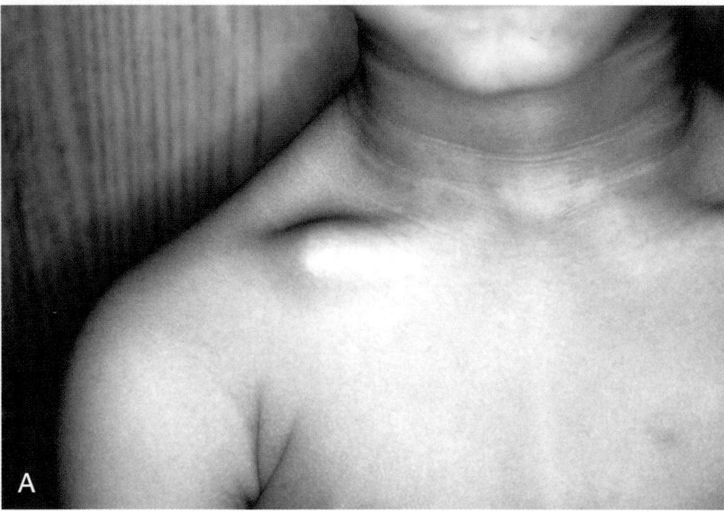

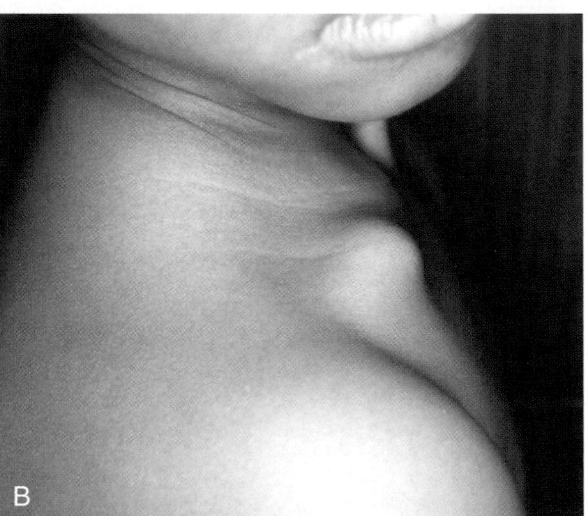

FIGURE 31-11 Congenital pseudarthrosis of clavicle. **A,** Subcutaneous prominence in middle third of right clavicle in 4-year-old child. **B,** Lateral view.

- Obtain the desired degree of correction by manipulating the head and neck during the release.
- Release of additional contracted bands of fascia or muscle occasionally is necessary before closure.
- Close both wounds with subcuticular sutures.

POSTOPERATIVE CARE. Physical therapy, consisting of stretching, muscle strengthening, and active range-of-motion exercises, is instituted in the early postoperative period. Head-halter traction or a cervical collar also can be used during the first 6 to 12 weeks after surgery (Fig. 31-10).

CONGENITAL PSEUDARTHROSIS OF THE CLAVICLE

Congenital pseudarthrosis of the clavicle is rare. Several theories concerning its cause have been proposed. Because the clavicle develops in two separate masses by medial and lateral ossification centers, pseudarthrosis could be explained by failure of ossification of the precartilaginous bridge that would normally connect the two ossification centers. Alternatively, direct pressure from the subclavian artery on the immature clavicle may be the cause. Congenital pseudarthrosis of the clavicle occurs almost invariably on the right; bilateral involvement occurs in approximately 10% of patients. In a series of 60 unilateral lesions, 59 were on the right, and in the one patient with a pseudarthrosis on the left, dextrocardia was found. Pseudarthrosis of the clavicle is present at birth and usually is in the middle third of the clavicle (Fig. 31-11). Differential diagnoses include cleidocranial dysostosis and rarely nonunion after clavicular fracture.

Congenital pseudarthrosis of the clavicle may require treatment, not because of pain or hypermobility of the shoulder girdle but usually because of an unacceptable appearance or occasionally because of pain in adolescent patients. Sales de Gauzy et al. described thoracic outlet syndrome in an adolescent with congenital pseudarthrosis of the clavicle. Hyperabduction of the arm caused compression of the subclavian artery by the medial end of the lateral clavicular fragment. After resection of the pseudarthrosis, iliac bone grafting, and plate fixation, the patient was pain free with total functional recovery. Although congenital pseudarthrosis of the clavicle is asymptomatic in childhood, surgical treatment can restore normal morphology and prevent functional or vascular problems in adolescence and adulthood. Spontaneous union is unknown, and consequently any desired union requires surgical treatment. Most surgeons agree that the ideal time for grafting is between ages 3 and 5 years. Although grafting can be done at any age, with increasing patient age, successful grafting becomes less likely. Simple resection is not recommended because it results in prominent, painful bone ends, prominence of the ends during movements of the shoulder, and asymmetry of the shoulder girdles. Simple resection of the fibrous pseudarthroses and sclerotic bone ends, followed by careful dissection and preservation of the periosteal sleeve to maintain continuity, and approximation of bone ends, without bone grafting or internal fixation has been shown to be successful in children younger than the age of 6 years. Nevertheless, most authors recommend excision of the pseudarthrosis, bone grafting, and fixation with a small reconstruction plate or an intramedullary Kirschner wire.

Union is easier to obtain in congenital pseudarthrosis of the clavicle than in that of the tibia. Almost any type of bone grafting suitable for traumatic nonunion of the clavicle has been satisfactory in pseudarthrosis, but open reduction and internal fixation with plate and screws and autogenous iliac bone grafting have produced the best results with higher rates of union, less time to union, and fewer complications when compared with Kirschner wire fixation. This is especially true if performed in older children (Fig. 31-12).

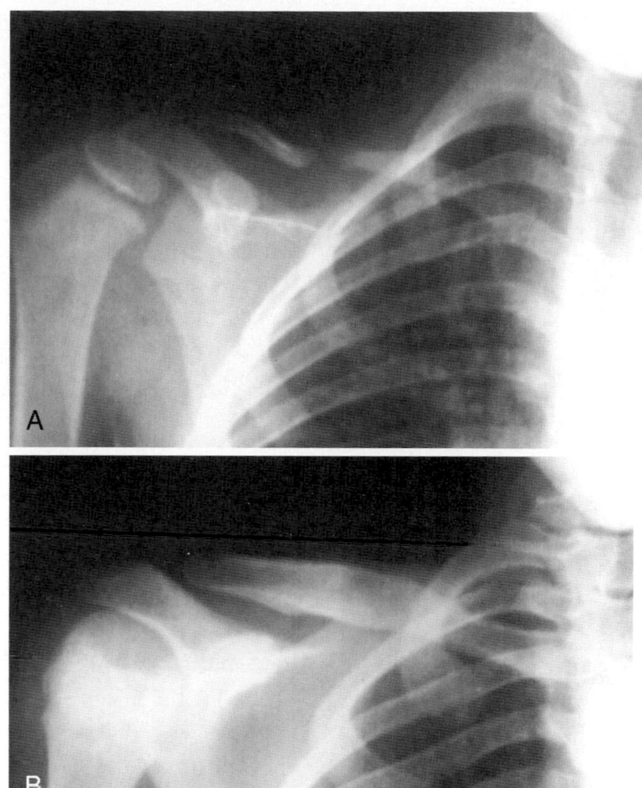

FIGURE 31-12 **A,** Congenital pseudarthrosis of right clavicle before plating and bone grafting. **B,** At 7 years of age after plate removal.

OPEN REDUCTION AND ILIAC BONE GRAFTING FOR CONGENITAL PSEUDARTHROSIS OF THE CLAVICLE

TECHNIQUE 31-5

- Make a transverse 3-inch (7.5-cm) incision centered over the body of the clavicle, approximately a fingerbreadth above the superior border of the bone.
- Carry sharp dissection through the subcutaneous tissue to expose the clavicle medially and laterally in the central third in the area of the pseudarthrosis.
- Expose the bone subperiosteally, protecting the underlying neurovascular structures.
- Debride the site of the pseudarthrosis of all fibrous and cartilaginous tissue down to normal bone medially and laterally.
- Bend a four-hole plate (semitubular, dynamic compression, or acetabular reconstruction) to fit the contours of the bone.
- Fix the plate to the clavicle in the usual manner.
- Obtain autogenous iliac grafts and place them on the superior, inferior, and posterior aspects of the pseudarthrosis.
- Close the wound in layers and the skin with subcuticular sutures.

POSTOPERATIVE CARE. A collar and cuff sling is worn for 2 to 3 weeks. The plate can be removed at 12 to 24 months or when radiographic union occurs.

CONGENITAL DISLOCATION OF THE RADIAL HEAD

Congenital dislocation of the radial head is rare but should be suspected when the radial head has been dislocated for a long time, there is no evidence that the ulna has been fractured, and the radial head appears abnormally small and misshapen. The radiographic findings are fairly characteristic. The radial shaft is abnormally long, and the ulna usually is abnormally bowed. The radial head is dislocated, frequently posteriorly but sometimes anteriorly; is rounded, showing little if any depression for articulation with the capitellum; and usually is smaller than normal. Occasionally, there is an area of ossification in the tissues around the radial head. The capitellum also may be small, and the radial notch of the ulna that should articulate with the radial head may be small or absent (Fig. 31-13). Although bilaterality has been listed in older studies as a criterion for diagnosis of congenital dislocation of the radial head, more recent reports have confirmed the existence of unilateral dislocations. Congenital

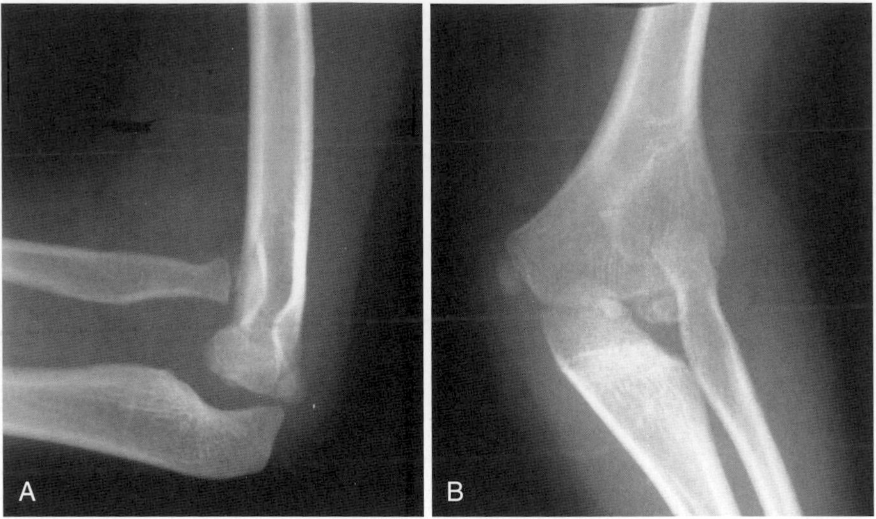

FIGURE 31-13 Congenital dislocation of radial head. **A,** Lateral view. **B,** Anteroposterior view.

dislocation of the radial head may be familial, especially on the paternal side, and may be associated with chondroosteodystrophy, achondroplasia, hypochondroplasia, Larsen syndrome, and nail-patella syndrome.

A congenitally dislocated radial head is irreducible manually or surgically because of adaptive changes in the soft tissues and the absence of normal surfaces for articulation with the ulna and humerus. Consequently, open reduction of the dislocation and reconstruction of the annular ligament in childhood are not advised. Any impairment of function usually is caused by restriction of rotation of the forearm; in children, physical therapy to improve this motion is the only treatment indicated. If pain persists into adulthood, the radial head and neck can be excised. Any resection of the radial head should be postponed until growth is complete, but even then it may not improve motion because of the contractures of the soft tissues. Nevertheless, excision of the radial head should be considered for pain in an older patient and may achieve some improvement in range of motion. Bengard et al. reviewed intermediate and long-term follow-up of both operatively and nonoperatively treated patients with congenital radial head dislocation. The authors showed that operatively treated patients had significant reduction in pain and improved overall satisfaction with minimal gains of motion. However, over 25% of operatively treated patients required additional surgery for wrist pain. Furthermore, nonoperatively treated patients had no loss of motion, development of pain, or the need for further surgical intervention.

CONGENITAL PSEUDARTHROSIS OF THE RADIUS

Congenital pseudarthrosis of the radius is extremely rare. In patients with neurofibromatosis, the pseudarthrosis develops from a cyst in the radius, and patients usually have skin manifestations of neurofibromatosis or a strong family history of the disease.

In each instance reported, pseudarthrosis of the radius occurred in the distal third of the bone and the distal fragment was quite short. Because the lesion is near the distal radial physis, the ends of the bone are attenuated and the ulna is relatively long. The treatment of choice is dual-onlay bone grafting. This operation restores length, provides a viselike grip on the osteoporotic distal fragment, increases the size of the distal end of the proximal fragment, and usually results in satisfactory union (Fig. 31-14).

Others have reported good results after complete resection of the involved radius, with the surrounding periosteum and soft tissue, and free vascularized fibular transfer. This operation can be delayed until skeletal maturity, with the arm supported by a forearm brace until surgery is performed. Alternatively, vascularized fibular grafting has been performed in younger patients, but obtaining stable internal fixation can be challenging in this group. Plate and screw fixation risks damage to the vascular supply of the periosteum around the fibular graft, but unstable fixation with only intramedullary and crossed Kirschner wires might lead to delayed union. In their review of the English-language literature, Witoonchart et al. found that free vascular fibular grafting obtained the best union rate among the reported procedures: it was successful in 18 of 19 ulnar or radial pseudarthroses reported. Vascular fibular grafting is described in Chapter 63.

CONGENITAL PSEUDARTHROSIS OF THE ULNA

Congenital pseudarthrosis of the ulna also is extremely rare. It typically occurs in the patients with neurofibromatosis, and associated congenital pseudarthrosis of the radius is not uncommon. Ulnar pseudarthrosis produces angulation of the radius, shortening of the forearm, and dislocation of the radial head (Fig. 31-15).

Various treatment methods have been described for congenital ulnar pseudarthrosis, including nonvascularized bone grafting with and without internal fixation, creation of a one-bone forearm, free vascularized fibular grafting, and the Ilizarov compression-distraction technique. Bone grafting of

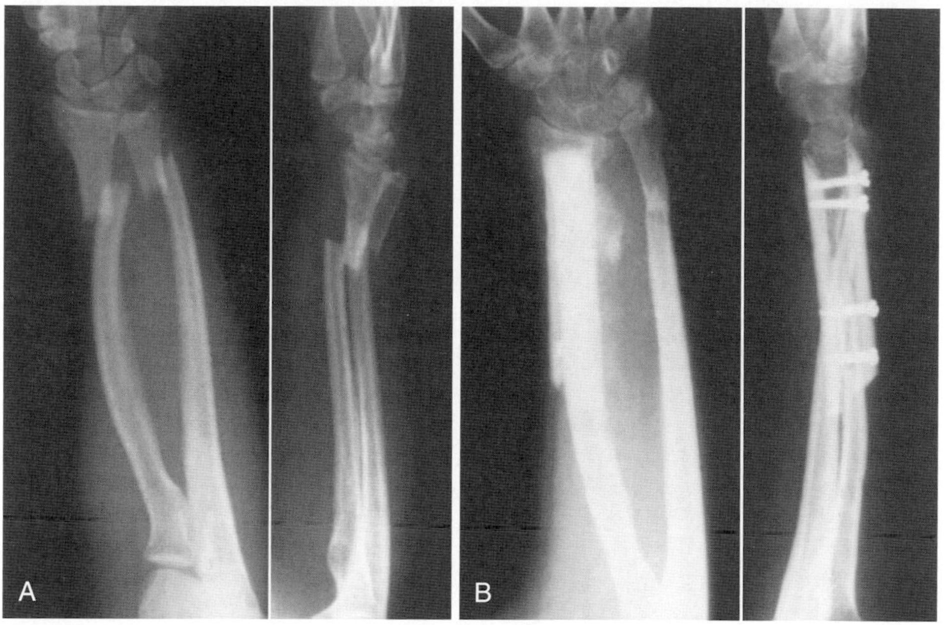

FIGURE 31-14 Congenital pseudarthrosis of radius. **A,** Closed fractures of radius and ulna in child with manifestations of neurofibromatosis. **B,** Union of radius after dual-onlay bone grafting.

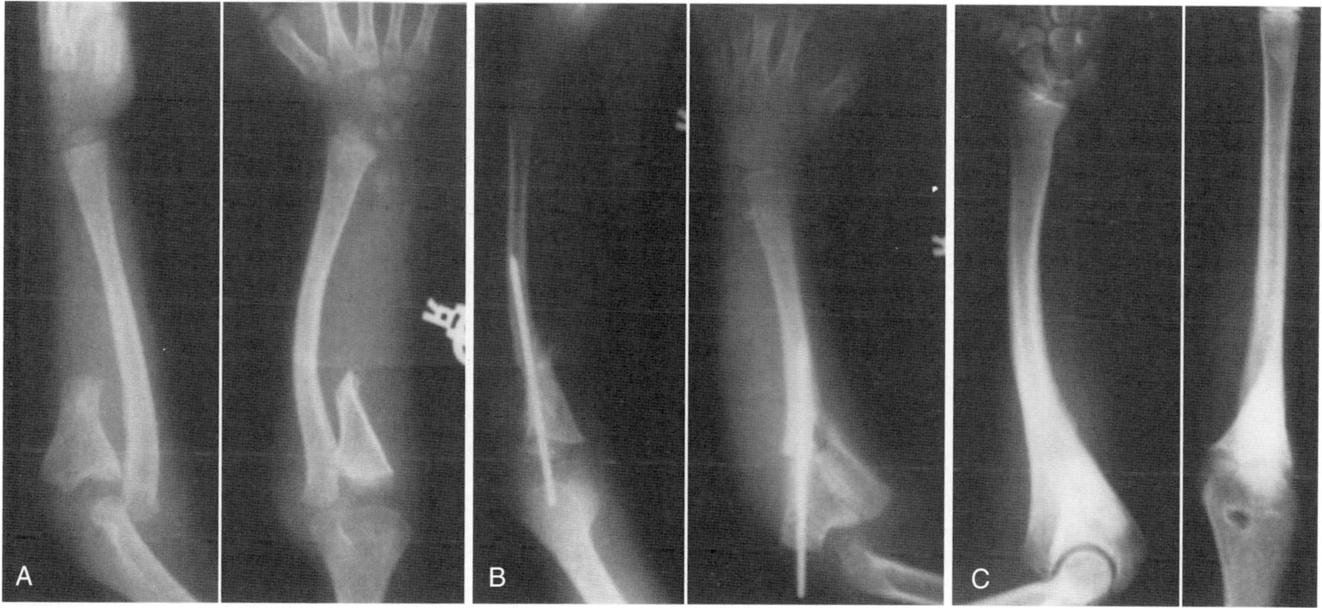

FIGURE 31-15 Congenital pseudarthrosis of ulna with dislocation of radial head. **A,** Before surgery. **B,** After excision of radial head, creation of synostosis between proximal radius and ulna and fixation with medullary nail. **C,** Final appearance of one-bone forearm.

congenital pseudarthrosis of the ulna usually has failed, but because significant bowing of the radius develops in very young children, early surgery is indicated. If the pseudarthrosis has developed through a cystic lesion, early curettage of the cyst, internal fixation of the bone, and bone grafting usually are successful. In established pseudarthrosis with tapering of the ends of the bone, the distal ulna should be excised early to relieve its tethering effect on the radius; then the forearm is fitted with a suitable brace. If the radial head dislocates, it should be excised, and a synostosis (one-bone forearm) should be produced between the radius and ulna (Fig. 31-16). Osteotomy of the distal radius to correct bowing also may be indicated. Use of the Ilizarov device has been reported in patients with small pseudarthrosis "gaps" and bony fragments of acceptable quality. Bae et al. reported successful free vascularized fibular grafting in four children with congenital ulnar pseudarthrosis. In two of the children (3 and 5 years old), the proximal fibular epiphysis was included in the graft and continued growth was present at 6 and 3 years, respectively, after surgery.

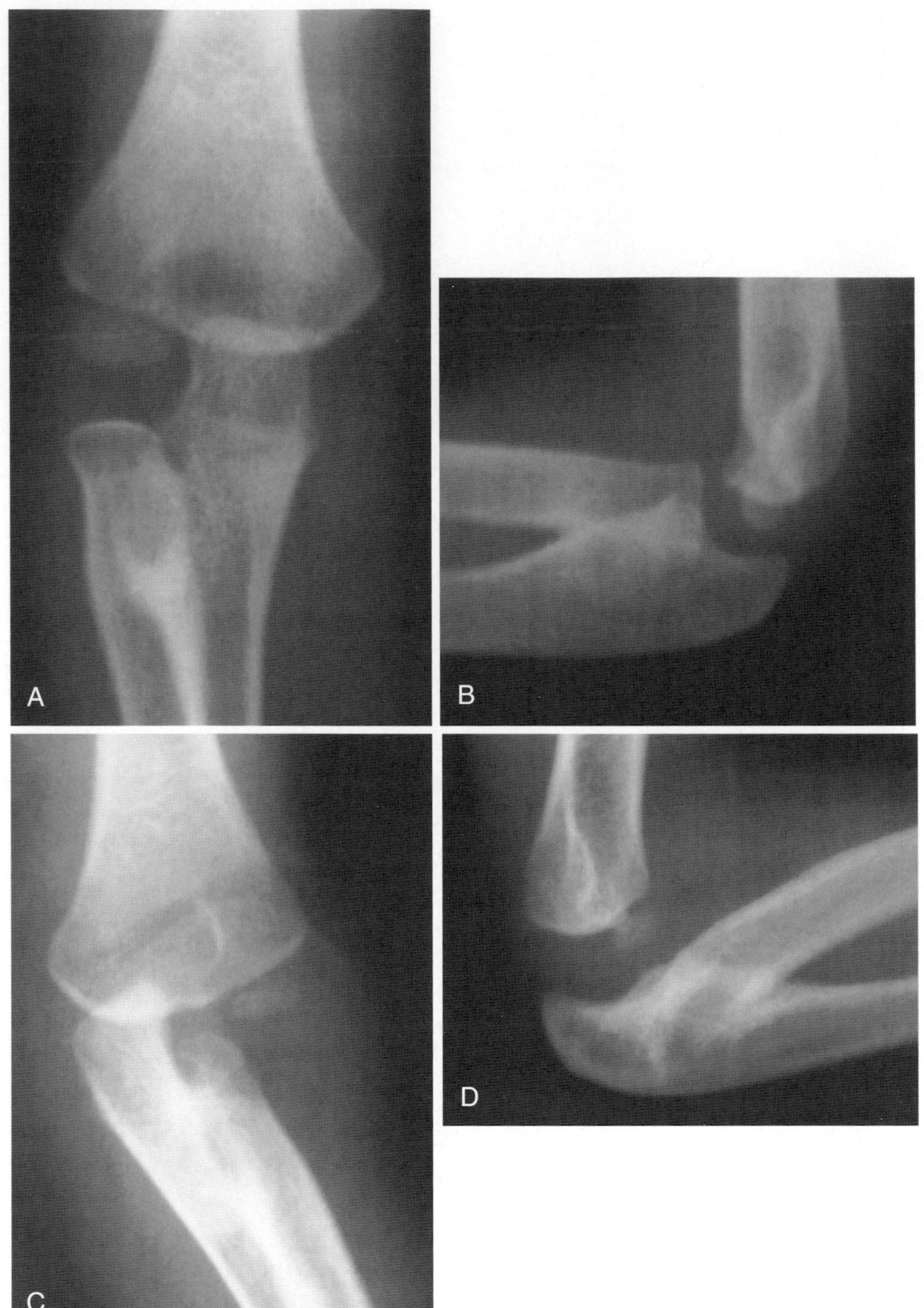

FIGURE 31-16 Congenital radioulnar synostosis. **A** and **B,** First type: proximal radius and ulna are fused for 3 cm, and radius is enlarged. **C** and **D,** Second type: radius is dislocated posteriorly and laterally.

CONGENITAL RADIOULNAR SYNOSTOSIS

Congenital radioulnar synostosis usually involves the proximal ends of the radius and ulna, most often fixing the forearm in pronation. It is more often bilateral than unilateral. Familial predisposition is frequent, and the deformity seems to be transmitted on the paternal side of the family. Wilkie noted two types. In the first type, the medullary canals of the radius and ulna are joined. The proximal end of the radius is malformed and is fused to the ulna for several centimeters (Fig. 31-16). The radius is longer and larger than the ulna, and its shaft arches anteriorly more than normally. In the second type, the radius is fairly normal, but its proximal end is dislocated either anteriorly or posteriorly and is fused to the proximal ulnar shaft; the fusion is neither as extensive nor as intimate as in the first type. Wilkie stated that the second type often is unilateral and that sometimes another deformity, such as a supernumerary thumb, absence of the thumb, or syndactylism, also is present.

Two other classifications classify the deformity based on the presence or absence of an associated radial head

BOX 31-1

Classifications of Congenital Radioulnar Synostosis

Tachdjian

Type I: Absent radial head, osseous fusion proximally
Type II: Radial head dislocation, osseous fusion proximally
Type III: Fibrous synostosis proximally preventing forearm rotation

Cleary and Omer

Type I: Fibrous synostosis
Type II: Osseous synostosis, reduced radial head
Type III: Osseous synostosis, posteriorly dislocated radial head
Type IV: Osseous synostosis, anteriorly dislocated radial head

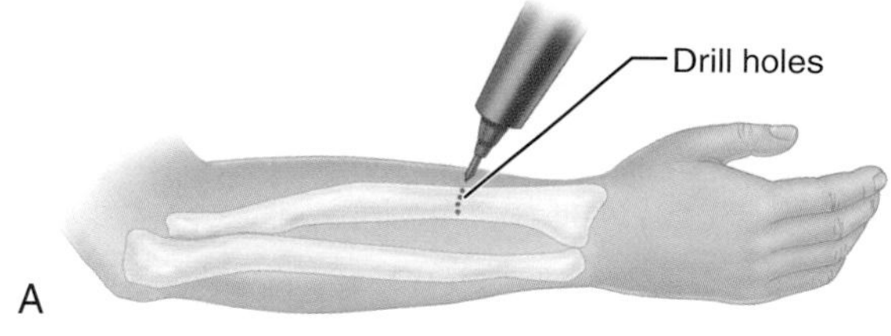

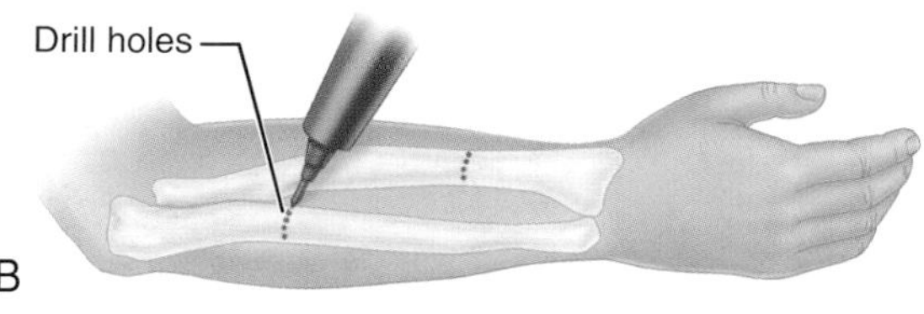

FIGURE 31-17 Correction of congenital radioulnar synostosis with percutaneous drill-assisted osteotomies of radius **(A)** and ulna **(B)**. Ten days later, forearm is manipulated to more functional position. **SEE TECHNIQUE 31-6.**

dislocation and the existence of a fibrous or osseous synostosis (Box 31-1). These two classification systems highlight the association with radial head dislocation that might represent a spectrum of disease beginning in the early embryologic period. Early embryologic development of radioulnar synostosis also explains its association with many other congenital syndromes such as Apert syndrome, Klinefelter syndrome, Carpenter syndrome, arthrogryposis, and others.

Congenital radioulnar synostosis is difficult to treat. The fascial tissues are short and their fibers are abnormally directed, the interosseous membrane is narrow, and the supinator muscles may be abnormal or absent. The anomalies in the forearm may be so widespread that sometimes no rotation would be possible, even if the radius and ulna were separated and the interosseous membrane split throughout its length. Additionally, patient and parent expectations of improved motion after surgical treatment often lead to disappointment if surgery is attempted. Simply excising the fused part of the radius never improves function. It is inadvisable to perform any operation with the hope of obtaining pronation and supination. Surgery is not recommended for most patients because the deformity typically is not disabling enough to justify an extensive operation. Motion of the shoulder, especially when the elbow is extended, compensates well for the deformity in most children.

Osteotomy occasionally is indicated in children with bilateral hyperpronation, but the exact position of the forearm is controversial. Some have suggested positioning one forearm in neutral rotation to assist in hygiene. However, modern widespread use of keyboards and hand-held communication devices makes slight pronation more attractive in developed nations. In Asian cultures, it has been suggested that eating habits of holding a bowl in the nondominant hand may necessitate slight supination.

Seitz et al. reported the use of a small external fixation device after derotational osteotomy in a 2-year-old child with congenital radioulnar synostosis. They cited as advantages to this technique precise rotational correction, adequate stabilization, and avoidance of cast immobilization.

Lin et al. described a two-stage technique for correction of severe forearm rotational deformities, including congenital radioulnar synostosis. Percutaneous drill-assisted osteotomies of the radius and the ulna are performed and are followed 10 days later by manipulation of the forearm into the desired functional position. No internal or external fixation is used; long arm cast immobilization is used for 6 to 8 weeks. These authors reported functional improvement in 25 of 26 forearms, including all 12 forearms with congenital radioulnar synostosis. Although the range of motion was not significantly changed, the arc of motion was in a more functional hand position. Rotational osteotomy performed in a single stage has been described with the addition of segmental bone resection. Early results have shown promise as a safe technique. Here we describe a two-stage osteotomy.

RADIAL AND ULNAR OSTEOTOMIES FOR CORRECTION OF CONGENITAL RADIOULNAR SYNOSTOSIS (TWO-STAGE)

TECHNIQUE 31-6

(LIN ET AL.)

- Under tourniquet control, make a 1- to 2-cm incision over the dorsolateral ridge of the distal third of the radius (Fig. 31-17A).
- Expose the bone subperiosteally and mark the osteotomy site with several fine drill holes that penetrate both cortices.
- Make a second small incision over the subcutaneous aspect of the proximal third of the ulna and similarly expose and drill this bone (Fig. 31-17B).
- Use a sharp osteotome to complete the division of the radius and then the ulna.
- Make no attempt at this point to change the position of the arm.
- Deflate the tourniquet and obtain adequate hemostasis. Irrigate the wounds and close them with subcuticular sutures. Place a long arm cast over sterile dressings.

- Ten days later, remove the cast with the patient under general anesthesia and supinate or pronate the forearm into the desired position.
- Obtain anteroposterior and lateral radiographs to confirm bony apposition and alignment. Generally, affected dominant extremities should be placed in 20 to 30 degrees of pronation and nondominant extremities should be placed in 20 degrees of supination.
- Check pulses carefully after manipulation and monitor the extremity closely to detect signs of compartment syndrome.
- Apply a long arm cast, which is worn for 6 to 8 weeks to allow complete healing of the osteotomies.

Kanaya and Ibaraki described a technique for mobilization of congenital radioulnar synostosis with use of a free vascularized fascia-fat graft to prevent recurrent ankylosis. The graft was obtained from the lateral aspect of the ipsilateral arm, and the authors reported minimal donor site morbidity and no difficulty with closure. The seven patients in whom this procedure was done all had marked improvements in supination and pronation; at an almost 4-year average follow-up, no patients had recurrent ankylosis or loss of the flap. Kanaya and Ibaraki found that adding a radial osteotomy to the procedure prevented dislocation of the radial head and increased the arc of motion (83 degrees in patients with osteotomy compared with 40 degrees in patients without osteotomy). We have no experience with this technique.

REFERENCES

CONGENITAL ELEVATION OF THE SCAPULA

Andrault G, Salmeron F, Laville JM: Green's surgical procedure in Sprengel's deformity: cosmetic and functional results, *Orthop Traumatol Surg Res* 95:330, 2009.

Harvey EJ, Bernstein M, Desy NM, et al: Sprengel deformity: pathogenesis and management, *Am Acad Orthop Surg* 20:177, 2012.

Masquijo JJ, Bassini O, Paganini F, et al: Congenital elevation of the scapula: surgical treatment with Mears technique, *J Pediatr Orthop* 29:269, 2009.

Wada A, Nakamura T, Fujii T, et al: Sprengel deformity: morphometric assessment and surgical treatment by the modified Green procedure, *J Pediatr Orthop* 34:55, 2014.

Walstra FE, Alta TD, van der Eijken JW, et al: Long-term follow-up of Sprengel's deformity treated with the Woodward procedure, *J Shoulder Elbow Surg* 22:752, 2013.

Zhang AM, Zhang J, Lu ML, et al: Partial scapulectomy for congenital elevation of the scapula, *Clin Orthop Relat Res* 457:171, 2007.

CONGENITAL MUSCULAR TORTICOLLIS

Do TT: Congenital muscular torticollis: current concepts and review of treatment, *Curr Opin Pediatr* 18:26, 2006.

Han JD, Kim SH, Lee SJ, et al: The thickness of the sternocleidomastoid muscle as a prognostic factor for congenital muscular torticollis, *Ann Rehabil Med* 35:361, 2011.

Herman MJ: Torticollis in infants and children: common and unusual cause, *Instr Course Lect* 55:647, 2006.

Lee YT, Cho SK, Yoon K, et al: Risk factors for intrauterine constraint are associated with ultrasonographically detected severe fibrosis in early congenital muscular torticollis, *J Pediatr Orthop* 46:514, 2011.

Minihane KP, Grayhack JJ, Simmons TD, et al: Developmental dysplasia of the hip in infants with congenital muscular torticollis, *Am J Orthop (Belle Mead NJ)* 37:E155, 2008.

Petronic I, Brdar R, Cirovic D, et al: Congenital muscular torticollis in children: distribution, treatment duration, and outcome, *Eur J Phys Rehabil Med* 46:153, 2010.

Shim JS, Jang HP: Operative treatment of congenital torticollis, *J Bone Joint Surg* 90:934, 2008.

Tatli B, Aydinli N, Caliskan M, et al: Congenital muscular torticollis: evaluation and classification, *Pediatr Neurol* 34:41, 2006.

von Heideken J, Green DW, Burke SW, et al: The relationship between developmental dysplasia of the hip and congenital muscular torticollis, *J Pediatr Orthop* 26:805, 2006.

CONGENITAL PSEUDARTHROSES OF THE CLAVICLE, RADIUS, AND ULNA

Beals RK, Sauser DD: Nontraumatic disorders of the clavicle, *J Am Acad Orthop Surg* 14:205, 2006.

Chandran P, George H, James LA: Congenital clavicular pseudarthrosis: comparison of two treatment methods, *J Child Orthop* 5:1, 2011.

Currarino G, Herring JA: Congenital pseudarthrosis of the clavicle, *Pediatr Radiol* 39:1343, 2009.

Duyrga Nagaraju K, Vidyadhara S, Raja D, Rajasekaran S: Congenital pseudarthrosis of the ulna, *J Pediatr Orthop B* 16:150, 2007.

CONGENITAL DISLOCATION OF THE RADIAL HEAD

Bengard MJ, Calfee R, Steffen JA, Goldfarb CA: Intermediate-term to long-term outcome of surgically and nonsurgically treated congenital, isolated radial head dislocation, *J Hand Surg [Am]* 37:2495, 2012.

Gogoi P, Dutta A, Sipani AK, Daolagupu AK: Congenital deficiency of distal ulna and dislocation of the radial head treated by single bone forearm procedure, *Case Rep Orthop* 2014:2014, Article ID 526719, 4 pages, doi:10.1155/2014/526719.

Song KS, Ramnani K, Cho CH: Long term follow-up of open realignment procedure for congenital dislocation of the radial head, *J Hand Surg Eur* 36:161, 2011.

CONGENITAL RADIOULNAR SYNOSTOSIS

Dalton JF 4th, Manske PR, Walter JC, et al: Ulnar nonunion after osteoclasis for rotational deformities of the forearm, *J Hand Surg* 31A:973, 2006.

Elliott AM, Kibria L, Reed MH: The developmental spectrum of proximal radioulnar synostosis, *Skeletal Radiol* 39:49, 2010.

Ezaki M, Oishi SN: Technique of forearm osteotomy for pediatric problems, *J Hand Surg [Am]* 37:2400, 2012.

Hung NN: Derotational osteotomy of the proximal radius and the distal ulna for congenital radioulnar synostosis, *J Child Orthop* 2:481, 2008.

Hwang JH, Kim HW, Lee DH, et al: One-stage rotational osteotomy for congenital radioulnar synostosis, *J Hand Surg Eur* 40:855, 2015.

Kasten P, Rettig O, Loew M, et al: Three-dimensional motion analysis of compensatory movements in patients with radioulnar synostosis performing activities of daily living, *J Orthop Sci* 14:307, 2009.

Shingade VU, Shingade RV, Ughade SN: Results of single-staged rotational osteotomy in a child with congenital proximal radioulnar synostosis: subjective and objective evaluation, *J Pediatr Orthop* 34:63, 2014.

The complete list of references is available online at ***expertconsult.inkling.com***.

CHAPTER 32

OSTEOCHONDROSIS OR EPIPHYSITIS AND OTHER MISCELLANEOUS AFFECTIONS

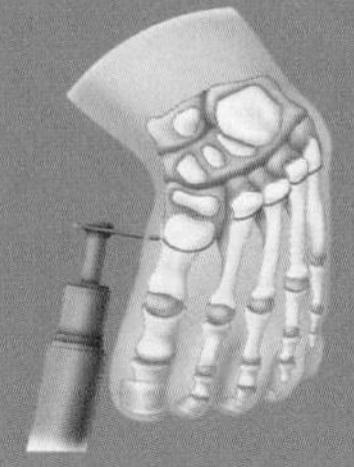

S. Terry Canale

OSTEOCHONDROSIS OR EPIPHYSITIS

The terms *osteochondrosis* and *epiphysitis* designate disorders of actively growing epiphyses. The disorder may be localized to a single epiphysis or occasionally may involve two or more epiphyses simultaneously or successively. The cause generally is unknown, but evidence indicates a lack of vascularity that may be the result of trauma, infection, or congenital malformation.

In some epiphyses, osteochondrosis is distinctive enough to be recognized easily as a distinct clinical entity. Osteochondrosis of some intraarticular epiphyses may closely resemble other diseases, however, and requires careful diagnostic study. Multiple epiphyseal dysplasia may closely resemble Legg-Calvé-Perthes disease of the hip. Radiographs of the ankle should be examined for the lateral narrowing or wedging of the distal tibial epiphysis that is characteristic of multiple epiphyseal dysplasia. In Legg-Calvé-Perthes disease the bone age usually lags 1 to 2 years behind the chronologic age, whereas the bone age usually is normal in multiple epiphyseal dysplasia.

Histologic studies of excised specimens have indicated that Osgood-Schlatter disease is traumatic in origin but not associated with loss of vascularity and should not be grouped with the osteochondroses. Only disorders of the epiphyses that sometimes require surgical treatment, including Osgood-Schlatter disease, are discussed in this chapter.

TRACTION EPIPHYSITIS OF THE FIFTH METATARSAL BASE (ISELIN DISEASE)

In the German literature in 1912, Iselin described a traction epiphysitis of the base of the fifth metatarsal occurring in young adolescents at the time of appearance of the proximal epiphysis of the fifth metatarsal. This secondary center of ossification is a small, shell-shaped fleck of bone oriented slightly obliquely with respect to the metatarsal shaft and located on the lateral plantar aspect of the tuberosity (Fig. 32-1). Anatomic studies have shown that this bone is located within the cartilaginous flare onto which the peroneus brevis inserts. It usually is not visible on anteroposterior or lateral radiographs but can be seen on the oblique view. It appears in girls at about age 10 years and in boys at about age 12 years; fusion occurs about 2 years later.

Iselin disease causes tenderness over a prominent proximal fifth metatarsal. Weight bearing produces pain over the lateral aspect of the foot. Participation in sports requiring running, jumping, and cutting, causing inversion stresses on the forefoot, is a common factor. The affected area over the

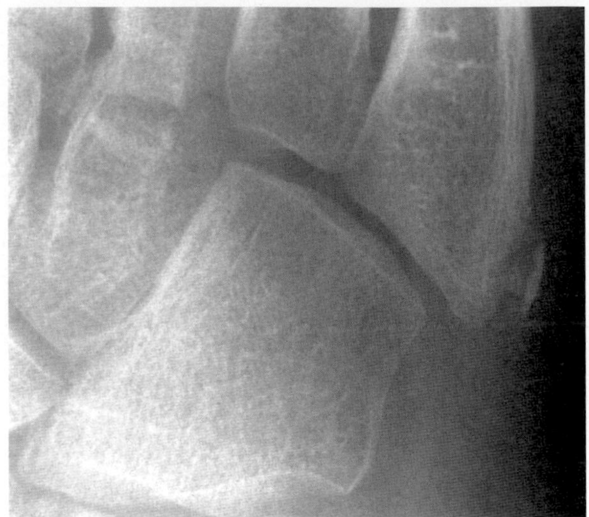

FIGURE 32-1 Ossification of epiphysis on fifth metatarsal shaft.

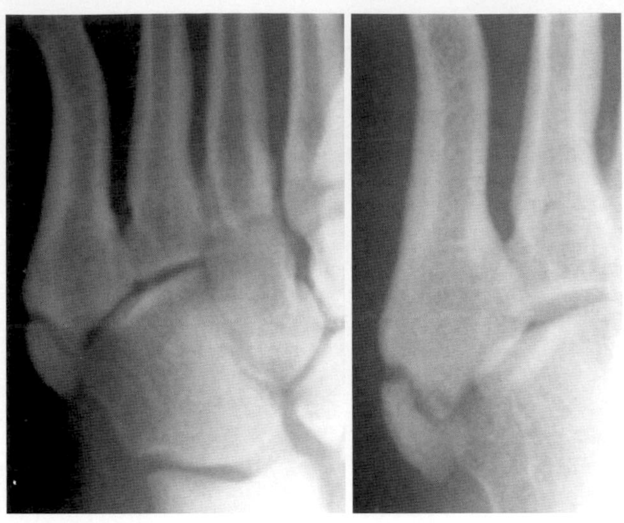

FIGURE 32-3 Nonunion of fifth metatarsal as result of Iselin disease.

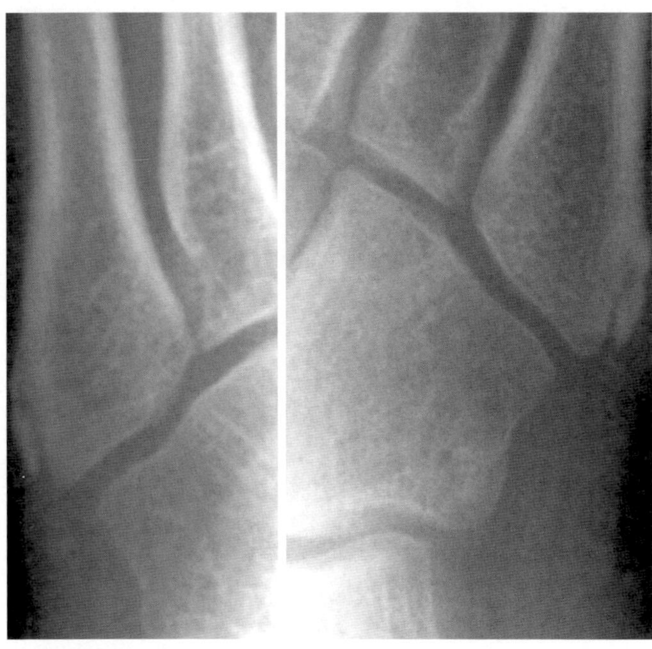

FIGURE 32-2 Enlargement and fragmentation of epiphysis (Iselin disease).

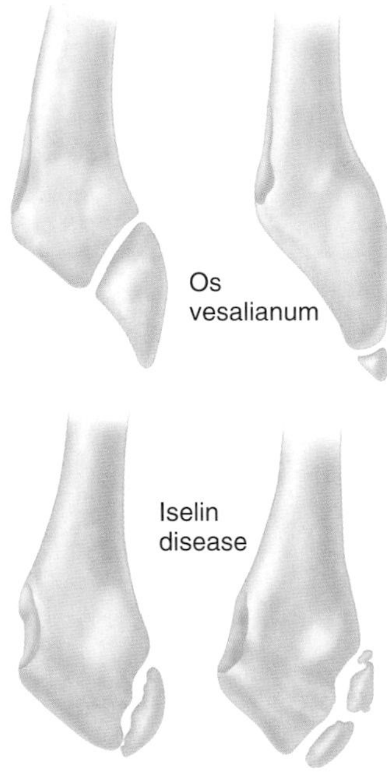

FIGURE 32-4 Os vesalianum must be distinguished from Iselin disease.

tuberosity is larger on the involved side, with soft-tissue edema and local erythema. The area is tender to palpation at the insertion of the peroneus brevis, and resisted eversion and extreme plantar flexion and dorsiflexion of the foot elicit pain. Oblique radiographs show enlargement and often fragmentation of the epiphysis (Fig. 32-2) and widening of the cartilaginous-osseous junction. Technetium-99m bone scanning shows increased uptake over the epiphysis. Nonunion of the fifth metatarsal (Fig. 32-3) has been reported in several adults as a result of Iselin disease and failure of fusion of the epiphysis.

The united epiphysis should not be mistaken for a fracture, and a fracture should not be mistaken for the epiphysis. Os vesalianum, a sesamoid in the peroneus brevis (Fig. 32-4), and traction epiphysitis with widening of the epiphysis also must be distinguished from Iselin disease.

Treatment is aimed at prevention of recurrent symptoms. For acute symptoms, initial treatment should decrease the stress reaction and acute inflammation caused by overpull of the peroneus brevis tendon. For mild symptoms, limitation of sports activity, application of ice, and administration of nonsteroidal antiinflammatory medication usually are sufficient. For severe symptoms, cast

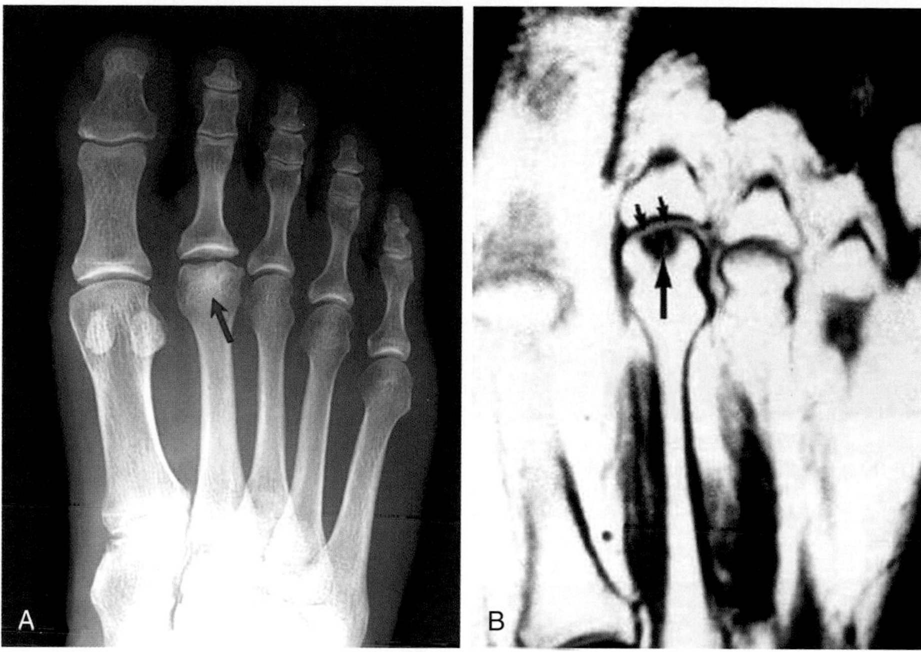

FIGURE 32-5 Freiberg disease. **A**, Elongated second metatarsal enduring stress. **B**, Chronic damage is shown by low-signal intensity on T1 MRI. (From Shane A, Reeves C, Wobst G, Thurston P: Second metatarsophalangeal joint pathology and Freiberg diseases, Clin Podiatr Med Surg 30:313, 2013.)

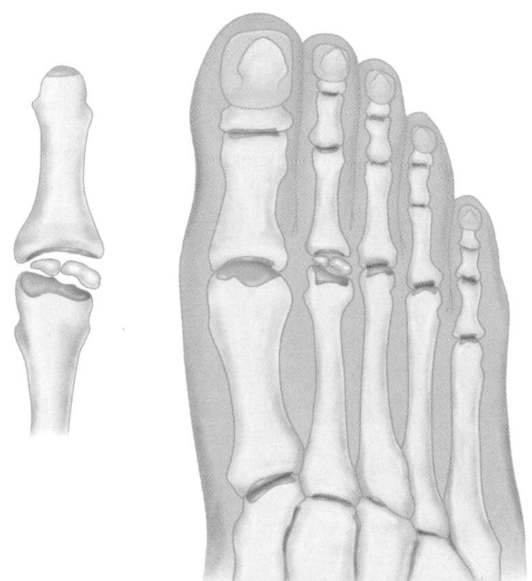

FIGURE 32-6 Freiberg infraction of second metatarsal with two loose bodies.

immobilization may be required. Occasionally, for chronic symptoms, an arch support that wraps around the base of the fifth metatarsal is used. Internal fixation of the epiphysis is not indicated.

OSTEOCHONDROSIS OF THE METATARSAL HEAD (FREIBERG INFRACTION)

Freiberg infraction usually occurs in the head of the second metatarsal but also may occur in the third (Fig. 32-5), fourth, and fifth metatarsals. Surgery is not recommended during the acute stage, which may persist for 6 months to 2 years. It may be indicated later because of pain, deformity, and disability. Occasionally, a loose body is present (Fig. 32-6), and simply removing it may relieve the symptoms. Other procedures used include scraping the sclerotic area and replacing it with cancellous bone (Smillie procedure), osteochondral plug transplantation (Fig. 32-7), dorsal wedge osteotomy, temporary joint spacer, and total joint arthroplasty (Fig. 32-8). The surgical treatment of this disorder is discussed in Chapter 83.

OSTEOCHONDROSIS OF THE NAVICULAR (KÖHLER DISEASE)

Osteochondrosis of the tarsal navicular originally was described by Köhler in 1908. Ossification centers of the navicular appear between the ages of 1.5 and 2 years in girls and 2.5 and 3 years in boys. Abnormalities of ossification vary from minor irregularities in the size and shape of the navicular to gross changes indistinguishable from osteochondrosis. These abnormal ossifying nuclei are more common in late-appearing ossification centers of the navicular. The blood supply to the navicular consists of numerous penetrating vessels in children and adults. The development of the ossific nucleus is associated most frequently with a single artery, but the incorporation of other penetrating vessels as part of the vascular supply varies; occasionally a single vessel is the sole supply until the age of 4 to 6 years. Delayed ossification has been suggested to be the earliest event in the changes leading to irregular ossification because the lateness of ossification of the navicular subjects it to more pressure than the bony structures can withstand. Abnormal ossification may be a response of the unprotected, growing nucleus to normal stresses of weight bearing. If osseous vessels are compressed as they pass through the junction between cartilage and bone, ischemia results and leads to reactive hyperemia and pain.

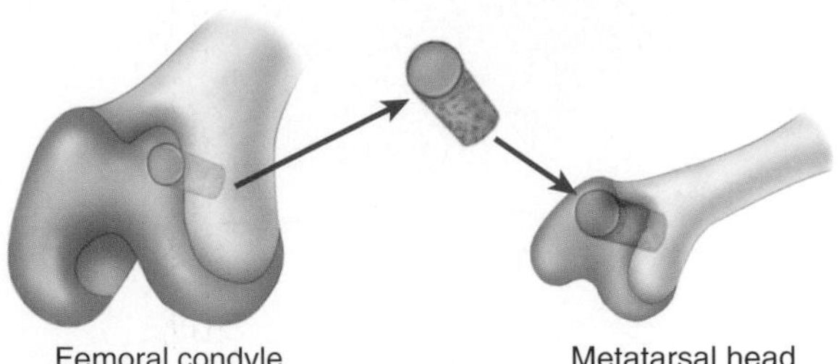

FIGURE 32-7 **Diagram of harvested osteochondral plug from a non-weight-bearing site on the upper lateral femoral condyle of the ipsilateral knee, and transplantation of the plug to the bone in the second metatarsal head.** (Redrawn from Miyamoto W, Takao M, Uchio Y, et al: Late-stage Freiberg disease treated by osteochondral plug transplantation: a case series, Foot Ankle Int 29:950, 2008.)

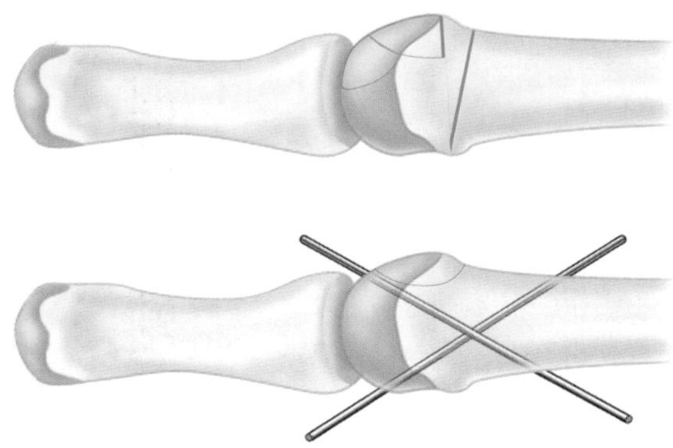

FIGURE 32-8 Osteotomy for Freiberg infraction. **A,** Osteotomy of bony wedge. **B,** Closure and fixation of osteotomy.

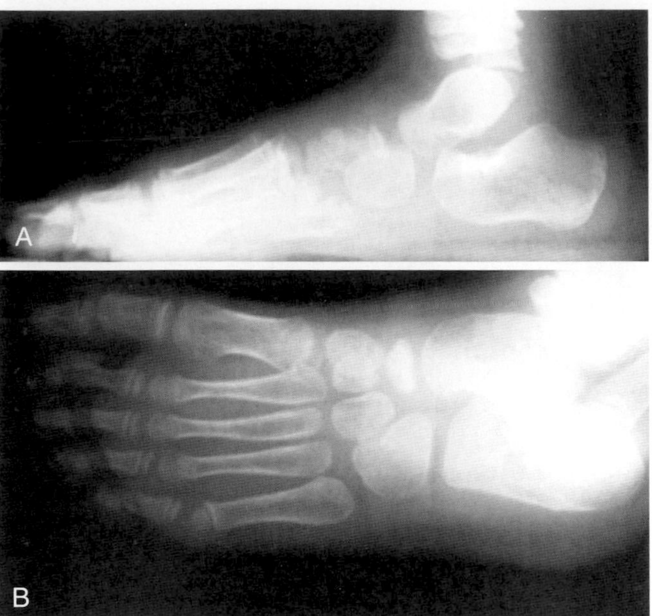

FIGURE 32-9 Lateral **(A)** and oblique **(B)** radiographs show smaller and more sclerotic navicular characteristic of Köhler disease.

The diagnosis of Köhler disease is a clinical one requiring the presence of pain and tenderness in the area of the tarsal navicular associated with radiographic changes of sclerosis and diminished size of the bone (Fig. 32-9). The appearance of multiple ossification centers without an increase in density should not be confused with Köhler disease, and radiographic findings similar to Köhler disease in an asymptomatic foot should be considered an irregularity of ossification.

Cast immobilization has been reported to produce quicker resolution of symptoms. This is a self-limiting condition, and operative treatment rarely is indicated.

Pain and disability occasionally develop after osteochondrosis when the navicular becomes distorted and sclerotic, the head of the talus becomes flattened, the articular surfaces of the two bones become fibrillated, and osteophytes form along the margin of the articular surfaces. Surgery is indicated when disabling symptoms persist. Arthrodesis is the only operation of value, and the calcaneocuboid joint is included because most of its function is lost when the talonavicular joint is fused. The midtarsal joints (talonavicular and calcaneocuboid) can be arthrodesed by a technique similar to that used for deformities in poliomyelitis (see Chapter 34). The results of this operation usually are excellent; most patients become symptom free but may notice loss of lateral movements of the foot. When symptoms arise from the naviculocuneiform joints also, these joints should be included in the fusion. Here arthrodesis is difficult to secure; metallic internal fixation and inlay grafts of autogenous cancellous bone are helpful.

OSTEOCHONDRITIS OF THE ANKLE

Osteochondritis of the ankle in adults is discussed in Chapter 89. The natural history of this lesion in children with open physes seems to be similar to that of osteochondrosis of the knee in that, with immobilization, the lesion heals in most children. Bauer et al., in a long-term (≥20 years) follow-up study of 30 children with osteochondritis of the ankle, found that only one patient developed severe arthritis. Only minor radiographic changes occurred in the rest of the patients, in contrast to osteochondritis of the knee, in which osteoarthritis is frequent. Two of the lesions in their series were located on the joint surfaces of the distal tibia, a site previously unreported. Bauer et al. noted that the lesions in children are indistinguishable from those in adults; however, because the lesions in children heal, there may be some variance in ossification of the talus (Fig. 32-10). Regardless of the cause, the initial treatment should be nonoperative.

EPIPHYSITIS OF THE TIBIAL TUBEROSITY (OSGOOD-SCHLATTER DISEASE)

Surgery rarely is indicated for Osgood-Schlatter disease; the disorder usually becomes asymptomatic without treatment or with simple conservative measures, such as the restriction of activities or cast immobilization for 3 to 6 weeks. Two distinct groups have been identified: (1) patients who before treatment had radiographic fragmentation and who had separated ossicles or abnormally ossified tuberosities at follow-up and (2) patients who before treatment had soft-tissue swelling without radiographic fragmentation and who were

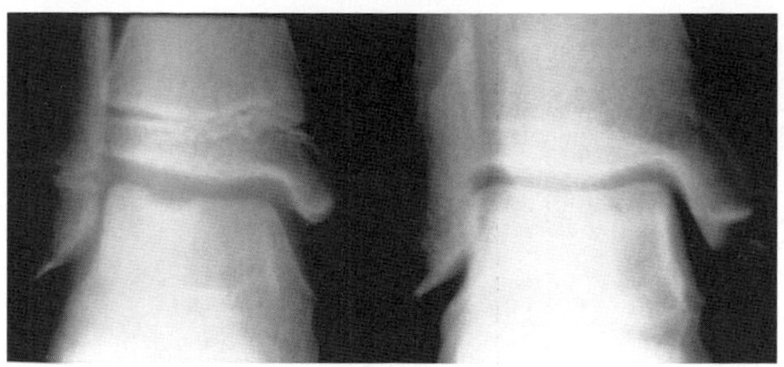

FIGURE 32-10 *Left,* Osteochondritis dissecans in child with open distal tibial physes. *Right,* Three years later, physes closed, patient was asymptomatic, and osteochondritis dissecans lesion was no longer present.

asymptomatic at follow-up. A strong association has been noted between Osgood-Schlatter disease and patella alta, and, in particular, a shortened rectus femoris has been noted. The increase in patellar height may require an increase in the force by the quadriceps to achieve full extension, which could be responsible for the apophyseal lesion. It can be argued, however, that the patella alta is the result of chronic avulsion of the bony tuberosity. Robertsen et al. noted on histologic examination a pseudarthrosis covered with cartilage and no sign of inflammation. They suggested that persistent symptoms of Osgood-Schlatter disease for more than 2 years warrant exploration. Krause et al. concluded that symptoms of Osgood-Schlatter disease resolve spontaneously in most patients and that patients who continue to have symptoms are likely to have distorted tibial tuberosities associated with fragmentation of the apophysis on initial radiographs. Lynch and Walsh described premature fusion of the anterior part of the upper tibial physis in two patients with Osgood-Schlatter disease who were treated nonoperatively, and they recommended screening for this rare complication.

Surgery may be considered if symptoms are persistent and severely disabling; however, tibial sequestrectomy (removal of the fragments) may relieve acute symptoms, but long-term results are no better than conservative treatment. Insertion of bone pegs into the tibial tuberosity (Bosworth procedure) is simple and almost always relieves the symptoms; however, an unsightly prominence remains after this operation and is rarely used. This technique can be found in the 12th edition of Campbell's Operative Orthopaedics. The bony prominence can be excised (ossicle resection and tibial tubercleplasty) through a longitudinal incision in the patellar tendon or arthroscopic removal of the ossicle and tibial tubercle debridement. Reported complications of Osgood-Schlatter disease whether treated surgically or not, include subluxations of the patella, patella alta, nonunion of the bony fragment to the tibia, and premature fusion of the anterior part of the epiphysis with resulting genu recurvatum. Because of the possibility of genu recurvatum, surgery should be delayed until the apophysis has fused. We have removed only the ossicle with satisfactory results; we believe the entire tuberosity should be excised only if it is significantly enlarged and the apophysis is closed. The amount to be excised (debrided) should be determined preoperatively as described by Pihlajamäki et al. (Fig. 32-11).

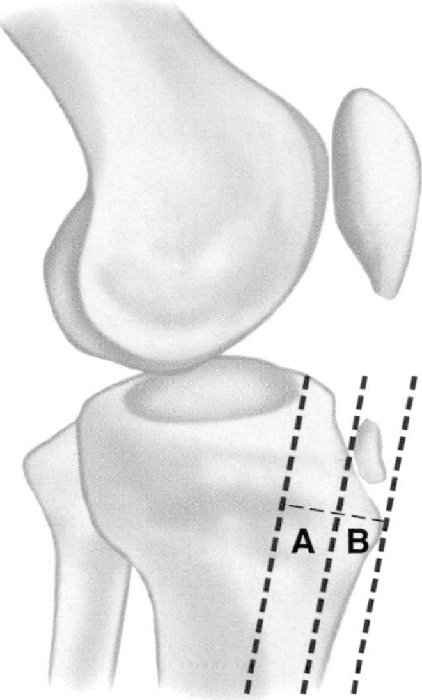

FIGURE 32-11 The tibial tuberosity index assesses the relative thickness of the tuberosity on radiographs. The line through the base of the tibial tuberosity is parallel to the midvertical tibial line. The midvertical tibial line is determined by measuring the middle of the projection of the tibia from four points located at various vertical levels of the cortex of the proximal part of the tibial cortex. The height of the tuberosity is measured from the line running parallel to the midvertical tibial line and passing through the base of the tuberosity. The base of the tubercle is determined by adjusting the line through the estimated base of the tibial tuberosity so that it is parallel to the midvertical tibial line and delineates the tibial tuberosity from the anterior tibial cortex. The tibial tuberosity index is the ratio of the distance from the top of the tuberosity *(dotted line farthest to the right)* to the parallel line of the anterior tibial cortex *(middle dotted line **B**)* to the distance from the top of the tibial tuberosity to the tibial midline *(dotted line farthest to the left **A** + **B**)*. The tibial tuberosity index is calculated by dividing the length of the horizontal line B by the sum of the horizontal lines A and B. (Redrawn from Pihlajamäki HK, Mattila VM, Parviainen M, et al: Long-term outcome after surgical treatment of unresolved Osgood-Schlatter disease in young men, J Bone Joint Surg 91A:2350, 2009.)

TIBIAL TUBEROSITY AND OSSICLE EXCISION

TECHNIQUE 32-1

(PIHLAJAMÄKI ET AL.)

- Place the patient supine on the operating table.
- Make a vertical 5-cm incision over the center of the distal part of the patellar tendon, 1 cm proximal to the tibial tuberosity, and over the center of the tibial tuberosity (Fig. 32-12A).
- Divide the distal patellar tendon longitudinally and elevate the tendon laterally and medially to expose the superior part of the tibial tuberosity (Fig. 32-12B and C).

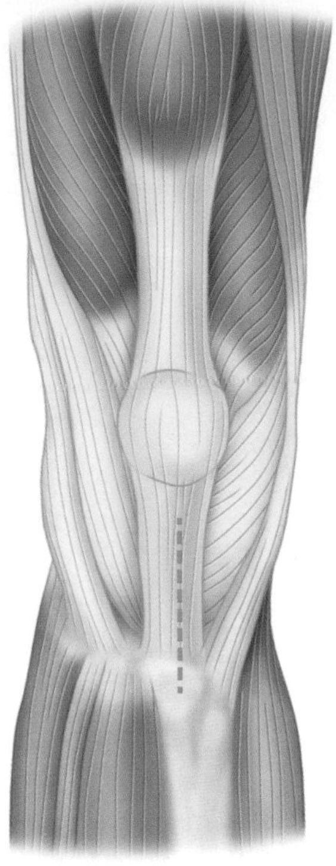

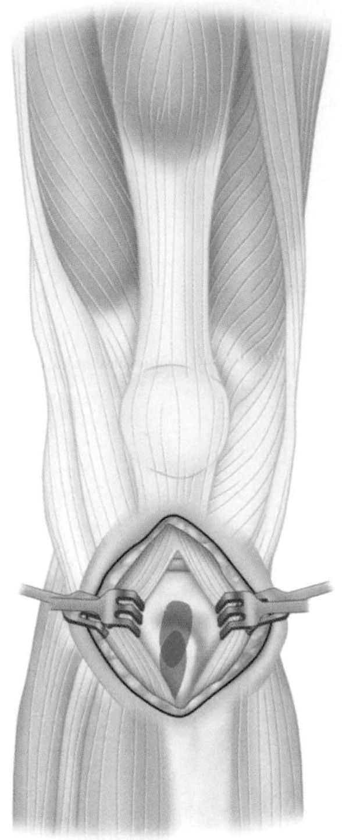

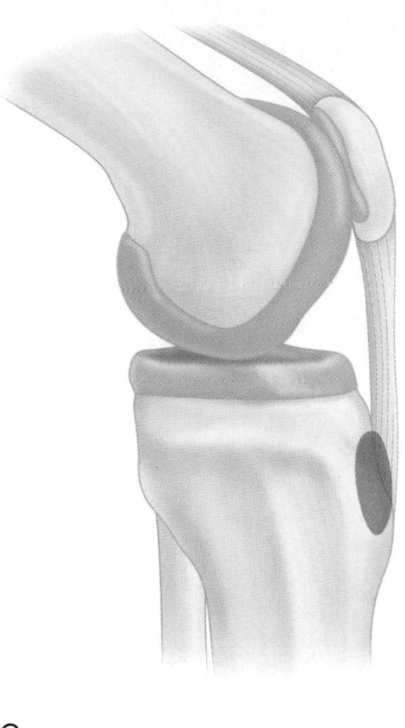

FIGURE 32-12 Pihlajamäki et al. technique for Osgood Schlatter disease. **A,** Skin incision. **B** and **C,** Patellar tendon is split and retracted to expose tibial tuberosity. (Redrawn from Pihlajamäki HK, Visuri TI: Long-term outcome after surgical treatment of unresolved Osgood-Schlatter disease in young men. Surgical Technique, J Bone Joint Surg 92(Suppl 1):258, 2010.) **SEE TECHNIQUE 32-1.**

- With an osteotome and rongeur, remove the prominent tibial tuberosity and, if present, the posterior intratendinous ossicles, which may be firmly attached to the patellar tendon. Remove the osteocartilaginous fragments with or without resecting the tibial tuberosity prominence. Make sure all fragments are removed.
- Resect the tibial tuberosity down to the insertion of the tendon and smooth with a file (Fig. 32-12D and E). Drilling is unnecessary. Try not to disturb the peripheral and distal margins of the patellar tendon insertion.
- Close the wound in layers and apply a light compressive dressing to the whole limb.
- As an alternative, a 5-cm transverse incision can be made, centered over a point 1 cm proximal to the tibial tuberosity (Fig. 32-13A). In this technique, the lateral soft tissue attachments are released longitudinally, leaving the patellar tendon intact. It is then elevated to remove the osteocartilaginous fragments (Fig. 32-13B and C). The rest of the procedure is as described above, with care taken to not disturb the lateral and distal margins of the patellar tendon insertion.

POSTOPERATIVE CARE. On the first day after surgery, quadriceps-setting exercises are started and crutches are used for a short period of time. Adequate quadriceps function should be emphasized, but all strenuous activity should be avoided for 6 to 12 weeks.

EXCISION OF UNUNITED TIBIAL TUBEROSITY FRAGMENT FOR OSGOOD-SCHLATTER DISEASE

TECHNIQUE 32-2

(FERCIOT AND THOMSON)

- Make a longitudinal incision centered over the tibial tuberosity.
- Expose the patellar tendon and incise it longitudinally (Fig. 32-14). Elevate the tendon laterally and medially and excise any loose fragments of bone and enough tibial cortex, cartilage, and cancellous bone to remove any bony prominence completely. Do not disturb the peripheral and distal margins of the insertion of the patellar tendon.
- Close the wound.

POSTOPERATIVE CARE. A cylinder walking cast is applied and worn for 2 to 3 weeks. Exercises are then begun.

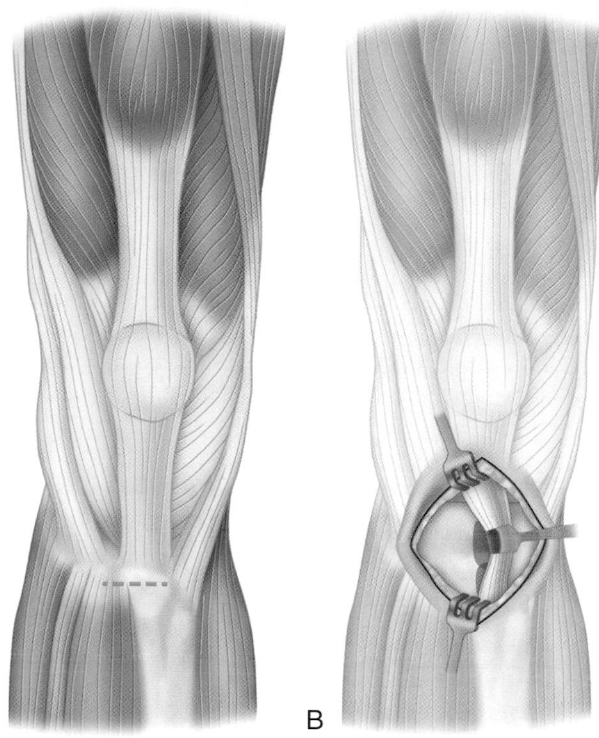

FIGURE 32-13 Pihlajamäki et al. alternative technique for Osgood Schlatter disease. **A,** Skin incision. **B,** Longitudinal incision in lateral soft tissue attachments of patellar tendon, which is elevated to expose tibial tuberosity. (Redrawn from: Pihlajamäki HK, Visuri TI: Long-term outcome after surgical treatment of unresolved Osgood-Schlatter disease in young men. Surgical Technique, J Bone Joint Surg 92(Suppl 1):258, 2010.) **SEE TECHNIQUE 32-1.**

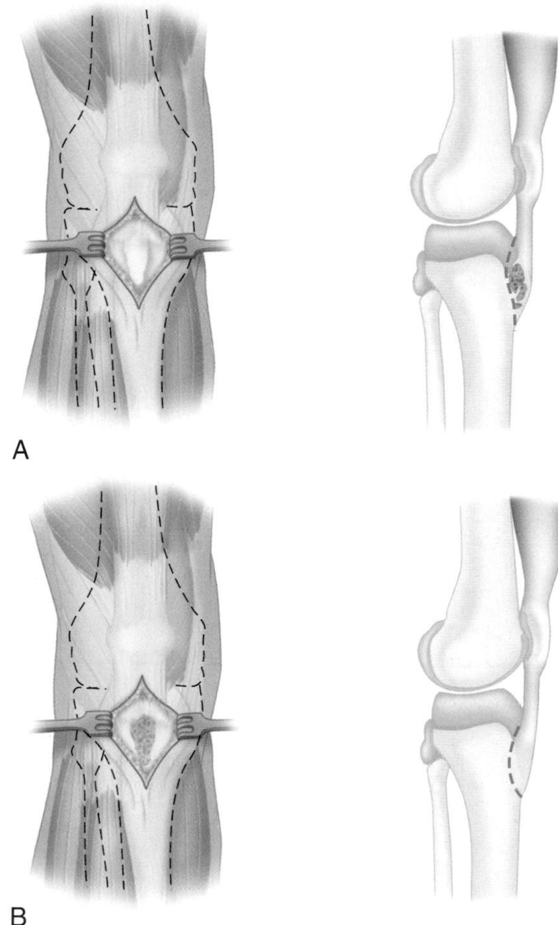

FIGURE 32-14 Ferciot and Thomson excision of ununited tibial tuberosity. **A,** Tibial tuberosity has been exposed. **B,** Bony prominence has been excised. **SEE TECHNIQUE 32-2.**

ARTHROSCOPIC OSSICLE AND TIBIAL TUBEROSITY DEBRIDEMENT FOR OSGOOD-SCHLATTER DISEASE

TECHNIQUE 32-3

- Make standard knee arthroscopy portals.
- To improve the view of the anterior interval, raise the location of the inferomedial and lateral parapatellar tendon portals slightly.
- Using a mechanical shaver and radiofrequency ablation device, perform an anterior interval release. Viewing the meniscal anterior horns and intermeniscal ligament and staying anterior to these structures, aggressively debride into the anterior tibial slope.
- Shell out the bony lesions from their soft-tissue attachments.
- Remove small and loose fragments with a pituitary rongeur; remove larger fragments with an arthroscopic burr. Extending the knee and taking tension off the patellar tendon facilitate the debridement along the anterior tibial slope.

POSTOPERATIVE CARE. Patients are allowed full weight bearing and unrestricted range of motion after surgery.

OSTEOCHONDRITIS DISSECANS OF THE KNEE

Osteochondritis dissecans of the knee usually is unilateral and may be painful. Although there are no specific physical findings diagnostic of osteochondritis dissecans of the knee, MRI is a highly sensitive method for detection of unstable osteochondritis dissecans. Several recent studies of instability, comparing MRI with arthroscopic findings have reported less specificity and sensitivity than previously thought with MRI, noting that MRI alone should not be used to determine lesion stability. The presence of an underlying high-signal intensity line between the lesion and underlying bone, a cystic area, or a focal articular defect indicates instability and may help in preoperative planning. Osteochondritis dissecans of the knee in children should not be confused with anomalous ossification centers. Because these ossification centers may be present in both condyles and in both knees, comparison radiographs of the affected and unaffected knees are advised (Fig. 32-15). MRI findings seem to be different for anomalous ossification centers and osteochondritis dissecans.

Osteochondritis dissecans of the knee in children with open physes usually heals when treated with cast immobilization. This treatment is preferable to excising the fragment early in life and creating a crater (Fig. 32-16). If gross detachment is present, results generally are better after operative than after conservative treatment. Lesions with increased size, associated swelling, and mechanical symptoms are less likely to heal.

Nonoperative treatment always should be considered in patients with open physes (Fig. 32-17); specific indications for operative treatment of osteochondritis dissecans in children are prolonged pain without evidence of healing during a 6-month period, an unhealed lesion in which symptoms persist after physeal closure, a sclerotic lesion in the crater (unstable lesion), and a troublesome loose body (Fig. 32-18). In skeletally mature individuals, surgery is necessary to evaluate the lesion and implement treatment. Kraus et al. noted that up to 12 months of conservative treatment might be successful if the cyst-like lesions are less than 1.3 mm in length as seen on an MRI.

Whether the lesion is drilled (retrograde or transarticular), excised, curetted, replaced and pinned, including loose fragments, or bone grafted depends on the size, stability, and weight-bearing nature of the lesion, which can be determined only at surgery (Fig. 32-19). A discussion of surgical procedures, indications, and complications in children and adolescents can be found in the chapter on knee injuries (Chapter 45).

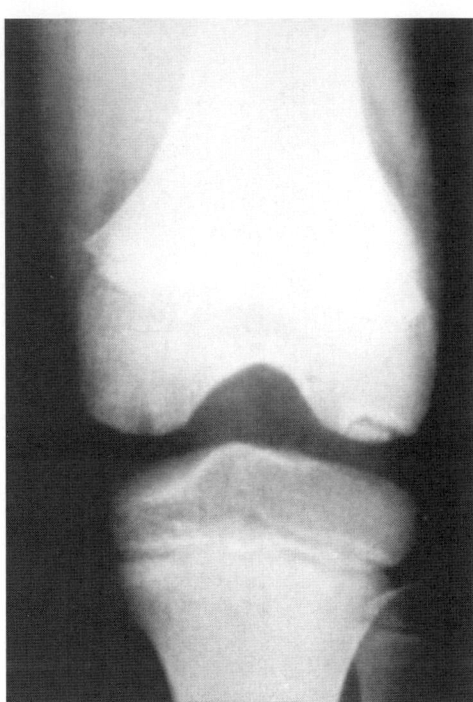

FIGURE 32-15 Bilateral (medial and lateral) anomalous ossification centers in posterior aspect of femoral condyles (not osteochondritis dissecans).

EXTRAARTICULAR DRILLING FOR STABLE OSTEOCHONDRITIS DISSECANS OF THE KNEE

TECHNIQUE 32-4

(DONALDSON AND WOJTYS)

- Place the patient supine and examine the knee arthroscopically to determine the stability of the articular cartilage.
- Make 1- to 2-cm incisions over the affected femoral condyle distal to the femoral physis. For medial lesions, the incision should be just anterior to the medial collateral ligament, and for lateral lesions it should be just anterior to the lateral collateral ligament.
- With the lower extremity in the anatomic position and the knee in full extension, drill appropriate-size Kirschner wires into the lesion from proximal to distal, avoiding the physis. Direct the Kirschner wires toward the lesion in the anteroposterior plane. Anteroposterior lateral C-arm imaging should be used to guide the drilling into the defect so as not to penetrate the knee joint or violate the articular cartilage. The success of the procedure is related

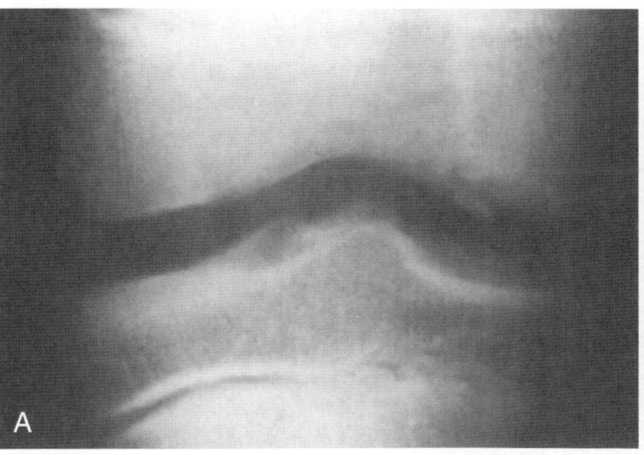

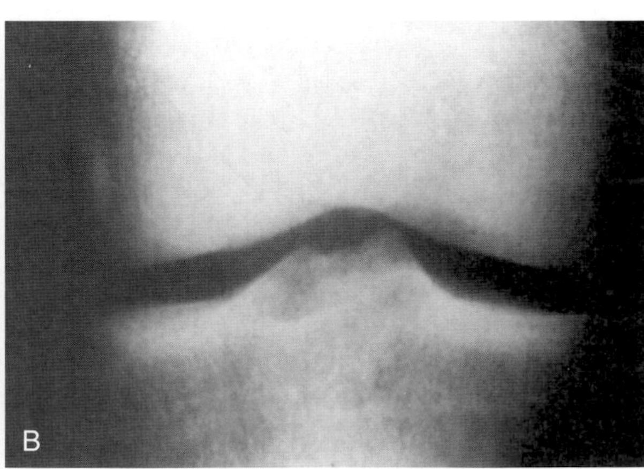

FIGURE 32-16 **A,** Osteochondritis dissecans of medial femoral condyle in child with open physis. **B,** Four years later, physis is closed and lesion has healed.

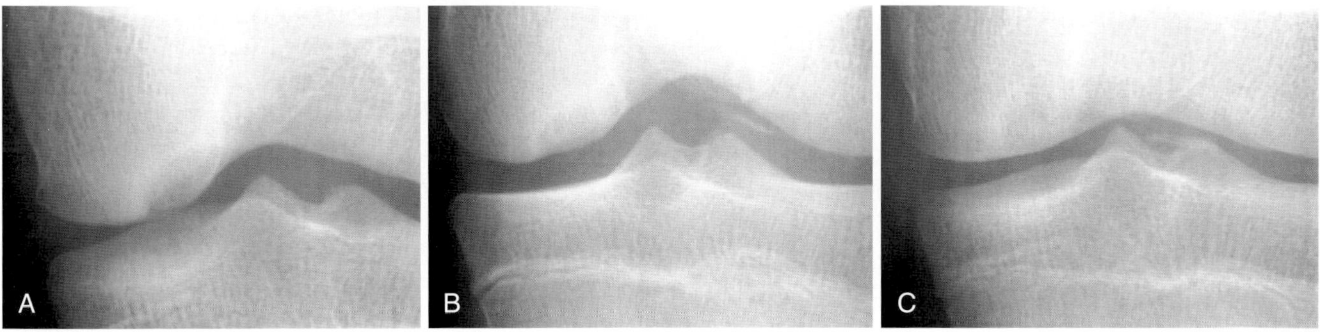

FIGURE 32-17 **A,** Osteochondritis dissecans of medial femoral condyle treated with knee immobilizer in 13-year-old child with physis still open. **B,** At 3-month follow-up, defect appears to be healing; possible osteochondral loose body is noted. **C,** At 5-month follow-up, patient is asymptomatic with healed lesion on radiograph and loose body that is asymptomatic.

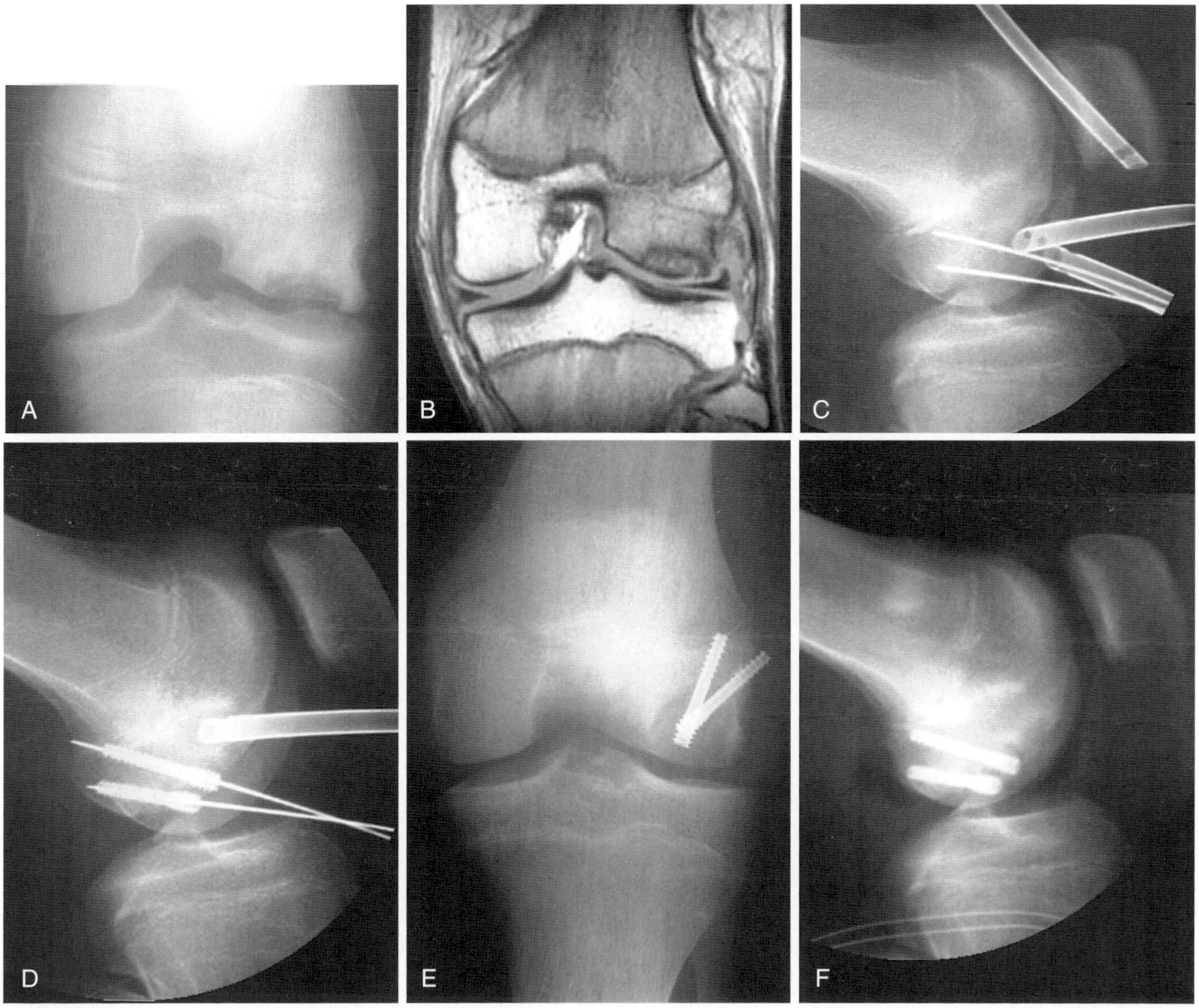

FIGURE 32-18 **A** and **B,** Large osteochondritis dissecans defect on lateral femoral condyle seen on radiograph and MR image. Chondroblastoma was ruled out in this patient with physes still open. **C** and **D,** After 9 months of unsuccessful conservative treatment, arthroscopy and Herbert screw fixation were performed. At time of arthroscopy, lesion was hinged but attached. This procedure requires use of image intensifier for correct guide pin placement and to avoid the physis with the Herbert screws. **E** and **F,** Postoperative anteroposterior and lateral radiographs with Herbert screws in acceptable position.

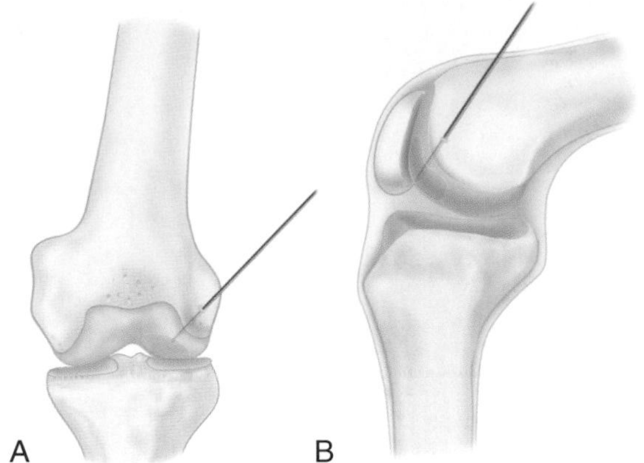

FIGURE 32-19 Anteroposterior **(A)** and lateral **(B)** illustration showing pin placement in osteochondritis dissecans of the knee in skeletally immature patients. (Redrawn from Donaldson LD, Wojtys EM: Extraarticular drilling for stable osteochondritis dissecans in the skeletally immature knee, J Pediatr Orthop 28:831, 2008.) **SEE TECHNIQUE 32-4.**

to perforating the cortical shell of the lesion. If this is not done, revascularization probably will not occur.

POSTOPERATIVE CARE. The knee is wrapped in a soft dressing after surgery. Motion is encouraged and the patients are kept at toe-touch weight bearing on crutches for 6 weeks. Physical therapy should be focused on range-of-motion exercises and low-resistance strength training.

OSTEOCHONDRITIS DISSECANS OF THE PATELLA

Osteochondritis dissecans of the patella is a rare entity that affects the subchondral bone and articular surface and the cartilage overlying the surface of the patella. It may appear as an elliptical fragment within a crater. It rarely occurs bilaterally. It is frequently painful and quite debilitating. Boys age 10 to 15 are most commonly affected.

Osteochondritis dissecans of the patella should be differentiated from a dorsal defect of the patella so that surgical treatment is not carried out on an asymptomatic defect (Table 32-1). The differences between the two are subtle but present. In contrast to osteochondritis dissecans of the patella (Fig. 32-20A), a dorsal defect is a simple, asymptomatic, subchondral defect in the superolateral portion of the patella that does not involve the articular cartilage and usually is an incidental finding on radiograph (Fig. 32-21A and B). A sclerotic border occasionally is present, and 20% to 40% of the time it occurs bilaterally. Safran et al. stated that MRI definitively shows that the dorsal defect does not involve the articular surface compared with osteochondritis dissecans (Figs. 32-20C and D and 32-21C and D). A bone scan also can help differentiate between the two. In osteochondritis dissecans of the patella, the bone scan is exceptionally "hot" (Fig. 32-20B) compared with dorsal defects in which it is "cold."

Treatment of osteochondritis dissecans of the patella, especially in young children whose physes are still open, is nonoperative if possible. Several of our patients have had a painful patella after excision of the fragment. Restriction of activities and immobilization for a time are recommended to avoid surgical excision. If conservative treatment fails, the lesion can be drilled, and if it is loose but still in the crater, the lesion can be internally fixed with a small-diameter Herbert screw. We have had little luck with poly-L-lactic acid pins in this area. If a defect and an old loose body are present, the loose body should be removed and the crater debrided and drilled. If the loose body appears to have viable subchondral bone, the crater should be freshened and the loose body placed within the crater and internally fixed.

TABLE 32-1

Differentiation of Osteochondritis Dissecans of the Patella from Dorsal Defect of the Patella

OSTEOCHONDRITIS DISSECANS OF THE PATELLA	DORSAL DEFECT OF THE PATELLA
Usually symptomatic	Usually asymptomatic
Separation of chondral or osteochondral fragment from subchondral bone	Incidental finding on radiograph
Involves articular cartilage	Does not involve articular cartilage
Rarely bilateral	Round subchondral defect in superolateral portion of patella; occasionally sclerotic border; 20-40% bilateral occurrence
Bone scan hot	Bone scan cold

Peters et al. used arthroscopic chondroplasty, removal of loose bodies, and retinacular release in 37 patients with mechanical symptoms (24 patellar and 13 trochlear groove). The average age of their patients was 15 years, and 54% had open physes. Most patients improved after surgery, but patients with articular cartilage loss had persistent patellofemoral crepitus and discomfort. In our experience, the results after chondroplasty of the patella have been unsatisfactory.

OSTEOCHONDROSIS OF THE CAPITELLUM (OSTEOCHONDRITIS DISSECANS)

Little Leaguer's elbow is a term that has been used loosely to describe changes in the elbow secondary to baseball pitching and usually limited to the capitellum, radial head, or medial epicondyle. We have seen osteochondrosis and osteochondritis dissecans of the capitellum. The cause of both is obscure and is not limited to throwing a baseball. A relationship may or may not exist between osteochondrosis and osteochondritis dissecans of the capitellum (Fig. 32-22).

Most patients with osteochondritis dissecans of the capitellum report symptoms of elbow pain and stiffness that are aggravated by activity and relieved by rest. Reports of locking or catching of the joint suggest the presence of loose bodies within the joint. Anteroposterior and lateral radiographs should be obtained, and comparison views of the contralateral elbow are helpful to identify subtle changes in the capitellum, surrounded by subchondral sclerosis demarcated by a

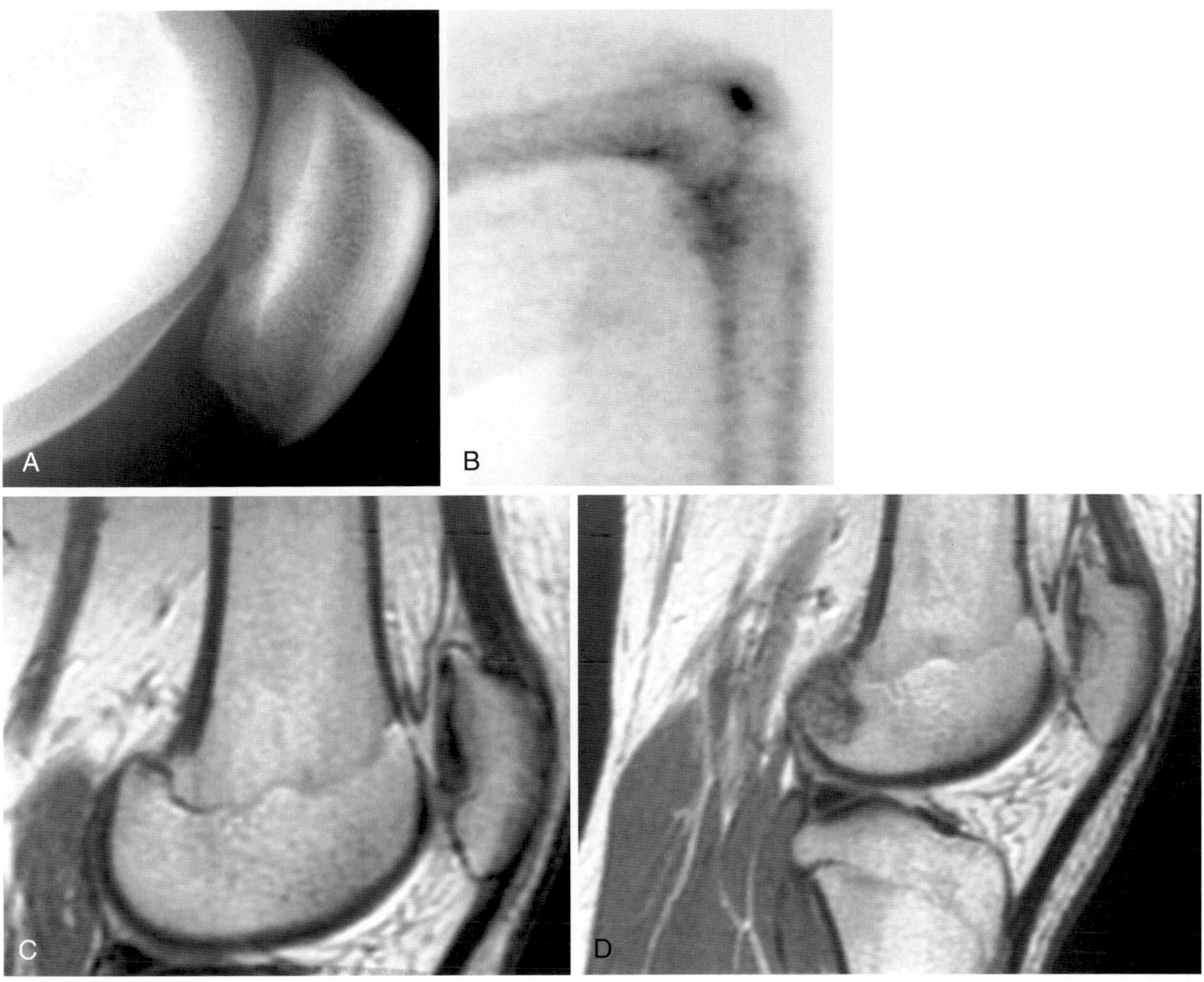

FIGURE 32-20 Osteochondritis dissecans of patella. **A,** Lateral radiograph. **B,** Bone scan. **C** and **D,** MR images showing osteocartilaginous fragment including articular cartilage within crater.

characteristic semilunar rarefied zone (crescent signs); older lesions may have a sclerotic border. Loose bodies may be seen in the joint. Magnetic resonance imaging often identifies early changes of marrow edema before changes are seen on plain radiographs. Recent studies revealed that MRI could reliably predict instability of an elbow lesion.

OCD of the elbow is most frequently classified by the radiographic findings:

Ia	Intact/stable	Intact articular cartilage, no loss of subchondral stability
Ib	Intact/unstable	Intact articular cartilage, unstable subchondral bone with impending collapse
II	Open unstable	Cartilage fracture, collapse or partial displacement of subchondral bone
III	Detached	Loose cartilaginous fragments within the joint

Also, lesions can be classified as contained or uncontained. Compared with elbows that have contained osteochondritis dissecans lesions, elbows with uncontained lesions are more broad and shallow, have greater flexion contractures, and higher rates of joint effusion. If a loose body is not present, nonsurgical treatment usually is satisfactory, especially if the lesion seems stable (type Ia). Resting the joint for 3 to 6 weeks with the use of a hinged elbow brace to eliminate excessive stress usually allows return to activity in 3 to 6 months. Indications for operative treatment include persistent symptoms, symptomatic loose bodies, fracture of the articular cartilage, and displacement of the osteochondral lesion. Operative management may involve excision of loose bodies or partially attached lesions, chondroplasty with osteochondral autogenous graft (mosaicplasty) or subchondral drilling, or internal fixation of a loose fragment. Mixed results have been reported for all of these techniques, with rates of poor results up to 50%.

In more recent literature, the surgical results seem to be better, especially concerning motion, because of arthroscopic techniques. Arthroscopic procedures include partial synovectomy, excision of loose bodies, drilling the crater or the intact lesion, microfracture, internally fixing the unstable viable fragment (mosaicplasty) with bioabsorbable pins, and osteotomy of the capitellum. Although the arthroscopic results seem to be better than nonarthroscopic techniques, no procedure, as noted by Byrd and Jones, ensures return to a

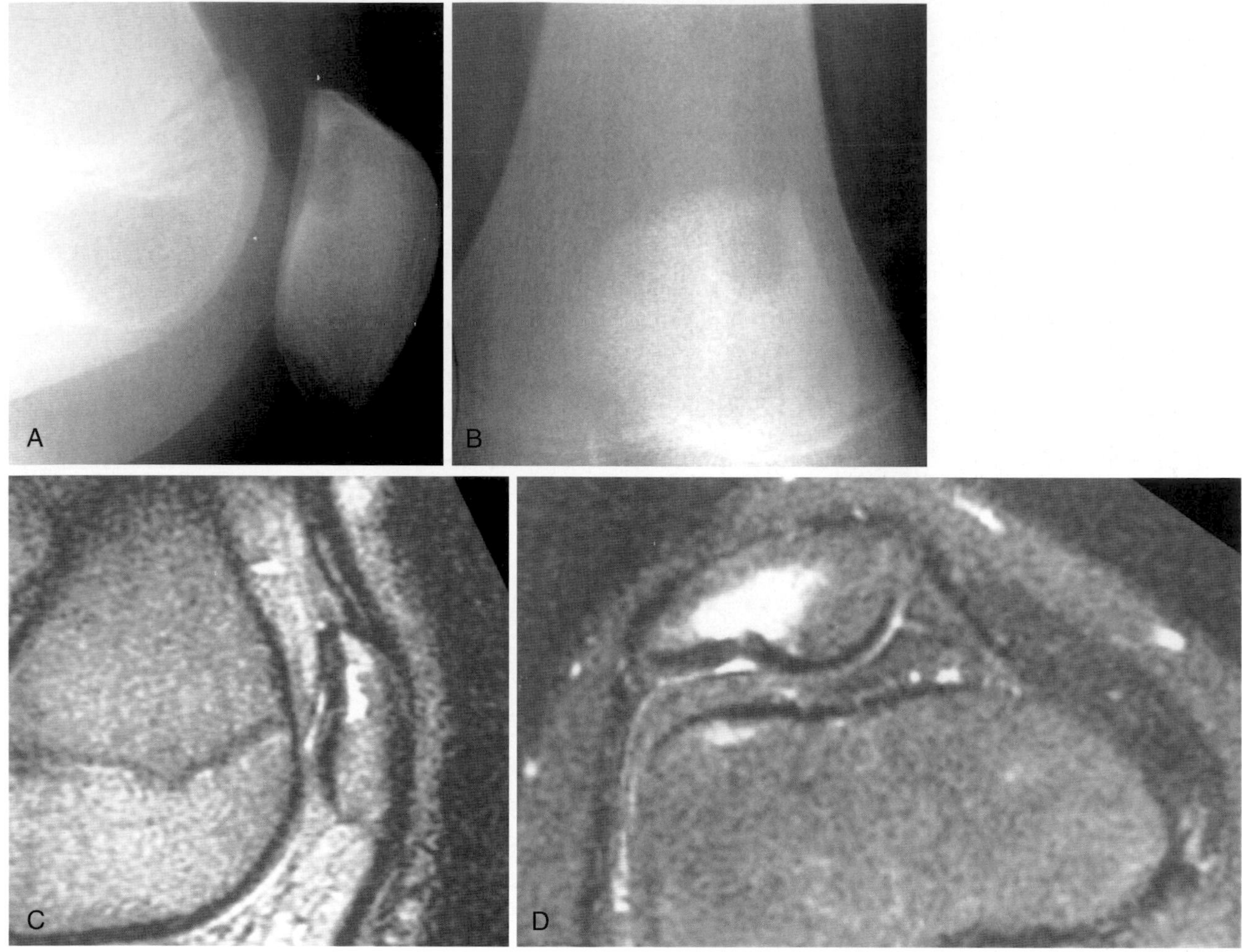

FIGURE 32-21 **A** and **B,** Radiographs of dorsal defect of patella in superolateral quadrant. **C** and **D,** MRI reveals dorsal defect of patella with cystic defect noted but not involving articular cartilage.

throwing sport, such as baseball, and the prognosis should be guarded especially if the lesion is large, widespread, or unstable. Arthroscopy and especially an elbow arthrogram or MRI may be indicated when a loose body is suspected but not seen on plain radiographs. Arthroscopy of the elbow is described in Chapter 52.

RECONSTRUCTION OF THE ARTICULAR SURFACE WITH OSTEOCHONDRAL PLUG GRAFTS FOR OSTEOCHONDROSIS OF THE CAPITELLUM

TECHNIQUE 32-5

(TAKAHARA ET AL.)

ARTHROSCOPIC FRAGMENT REMOVAL

- After administering general anesthesia, place the patient supine.
- Inject 10 to 20 mL of 1% lidocaine with epinephrine into the elbow joint. A tourniquet usually is not necessary.
- Flex the shoulder 90 degrees and elevate the elbow until the upper arm is almost vertical. Maintain this position with skin traction applied from the forearm to the overhead bar.
- Confirm the suitable position and direction of the portals with a 23-gauge needle. Create posterior, posterolateral, anteromedial, and anterolateral portals with a sharp blade.
- Bluntly release the subcutaneous tissues avoiding the cutaneous nerves.
- Widen the portals with the use of step-up cannulas.
- Insert a 4-mm-diameter, 30-degree oblique arthroscope to remove the loose bodies.

OPEN APPROACH FOR FRAGMENT REMOVAL

- For a posterolateral approach, place the upper arm on the operative bed with the shoulder in abduction and the elbow fully flexed.
- Make a 4- to 6-cm posterolateral oblique skin incision on a line from the posterior edge of the lateral epicondyle to the posterior aspect of the radioulnar joint.

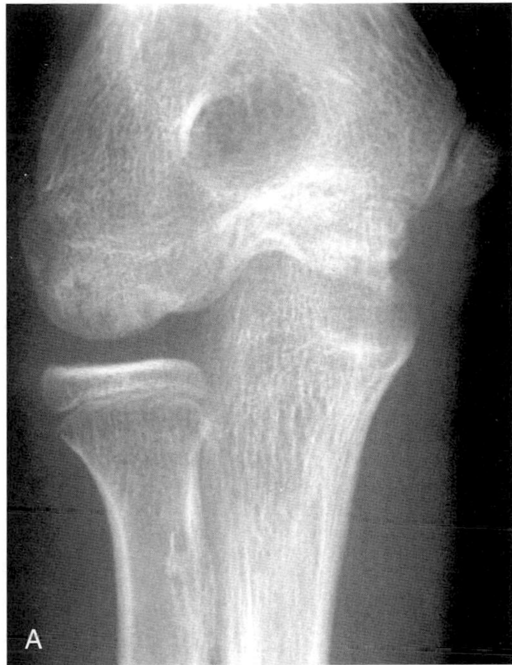

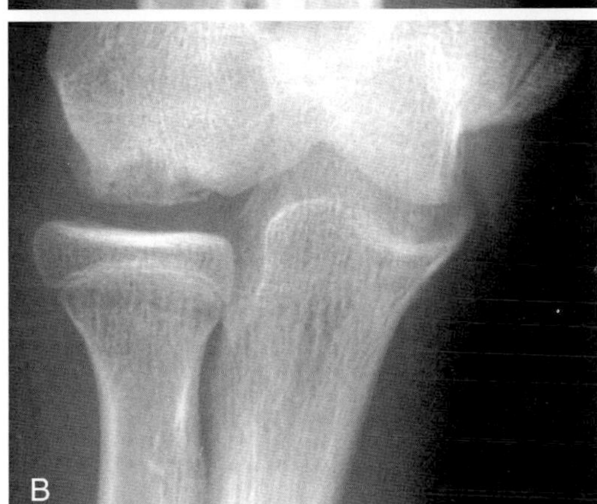

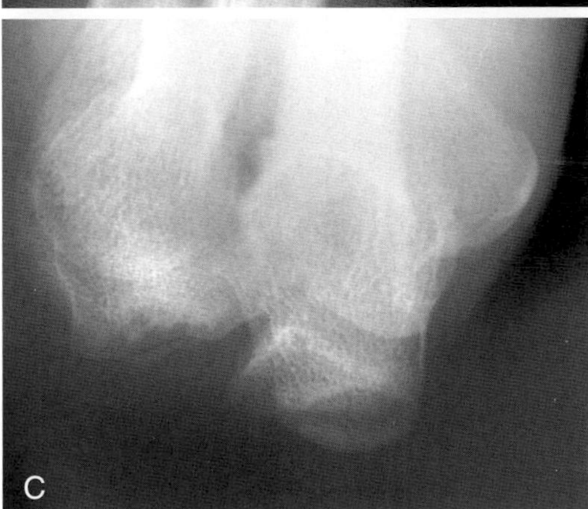

FIGURE 32-22 **A,** Osteochondrosis of capitellum. Anteroposterior **(B)** and Jones **(C)** views 1 year later show evidence of some consolidation, but osteochondritis dissecans appears to be forming.

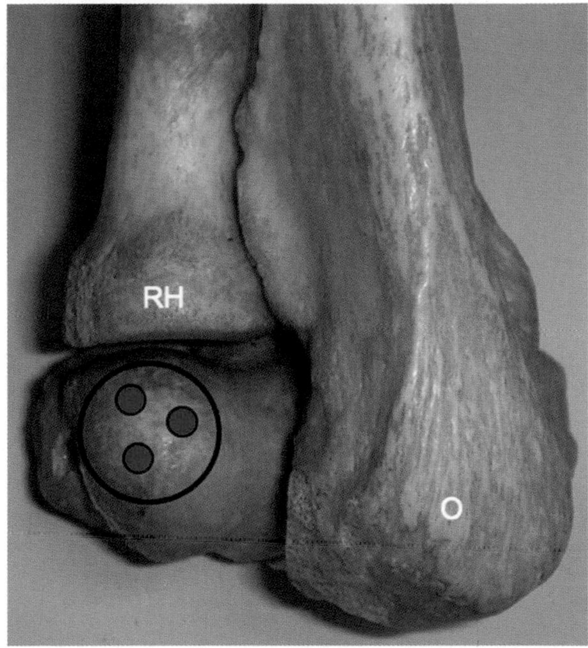

FIGURE 32-23 Reconstruction of the articular surface of the humeral capitellum using osteochondral plug grafts from the lateral femoral condyle. (From Takahara M, Mura N, Sasaki J, et al: Classification, treatment, and outcome of osteochondritis dissecans of the humeral capitellum, *J Bone Joint Surg* 90A:47, 2008.) **SEE TECHNIQUE 32-5.**

- After inflating the tourniquet, incise the skin and fascia. Develop the intermuscular plane between the extensor carpi ulnaris and anconeus muscles or muscle fibers.
- Incise the capsule over the capitellar lesion and elongate the incision from the posterior edge of the lateral epicondyle to the posterior aspect of the radioulnar joint.
- Perform a limited local synovectomy.

RECONSTRUCTION USING BONE PLUG GRAFTS

- After removal of loose fragments arthroscopically or through an open approach, harvest cylindrical osteochondral bone plugs from the lateral part of the lateral femoral condyle at the level of the patellofemoral joint, keeping the tube harvester at a 90-degree angle to the articular surface. One to three plugs may be necessary depending on the size of the defect.
- Prepare the recipient bed.
- Place the osteochondral plugs toward the center of the capitellum to obtain stable fixation. Take care not to damage the capitellar physis or the distal part of the femur in skeletally immature patients (Fig. 32-23). Because the thickness of hyaline cartilage and its surface curvature differ between the elbow and the knee, insert the plugs to match the spherical articular surface of the capitellum. The articular surface of the osteochondral plug graft should be slightly depressed rather than prominent relative to the capitellar surface, and the step-off should be less than 1 mm. Rarely is shaving the articular surface of the osteochondral plug graft necessary. Reconstructing the entire capitellar defect is not necessary.

TABLE 32-2

Stages of Legg-Calve-Perthes (Waldenström)

Initial	■ Infarction produces a smaller, sclerotic epiphysis with medial joint space widening	■ Radiographs may remain occult for 3-6 months
Fragmentation	■ Femoral head appears to fragment or dissolve ■ Result of a revascularization process and bone resorption producing collapse and subsequent increased density	■ Hip related symptoms are most prevalent ■ Lateral pillar classification based on this stage
Reossification	■ Ossific nucleus undergoes reossification as new bone appears as necrotic bone is resorbed	■ May last up to 18 months
Healing or remodeling	■ Femoral head remodels until skeletal maturity	■ Begins once ossific nucleus is completely reossified trabecular pattern returns

POSTOPERATIVE CARE. Immobilize the elbow for 1 to 2 weeks and protect the knee from vigorous flexion for 3 weeks. Physical therapy should focus on reducing pain and swelling and regaining range of motion. Three months after the procedure, gentle elbow exercises against resistance are progressed to full resistance at 4 months. Throwing is allowed at 4 to 5 months if there is no pain and elbow range of motion has returned to preoperative levels. The patient is released for full sports activity at 6 to 8 months.

LEGG-CALVÉ-PERTHES DISEASE

The cause of Legg-Calvé-Perthes disease is unknown but has provoked considerable controversy. Previously, some authors thought that an inherited thrombophilia promoted thrombotic venous occlusion in the femoral vein causing bone death in the femoral head and ultimately leading to Legg-Calvé-Perthes disease. More recent studies have not found an inherited hypercoagulability or a deficiency in protein C activity, however, indicating that inherited thrombophilia is not associated with the osteonecrosis of Legg-Calvé-Perthes disease. Although research continues, it seems that coagulation disorders are not etiologic factors in Legg-Calvé-Perthes disease. As noted by Hosalkar and Mulpuri, even after 100 years the etiology of Legg-Calvé-Perthes disease remains unclear and its treatment is still controversial.

DIAGNOSIS

Differentiating an irritable hip with transient synovitis from the acute symptoms of Legg-Calvé-Perthes disease can be difficult. Distinguishing characteristics involve the sex and age of the patient and the duration of symptoms. Irritable hip syndrome occurs twice as frequently in boys as in girls, whereas Legg-Calvé-Perthes disease occurs three times more frequently in boys than in girls. The average age of patients with irritable hips is 3 years, and the average age of patients with Legg-Calvé-Perthes disease is 7 years. Children with irritable hips have an average duration of symptoms of 6 days, whereas children with Legg-Calvé-Perthes disease have symptoms present for an average of 6 weeks. Radiographic changes of the femoral head (condensation and sclerosis) generally are delayed but occur 6 weeks after initial symptoms. Therefore a follow-up radiograph should be obtained at 6 weeks (Table 32-2).

TABLE 32-3

Catterall Classification

Group I	■ Involvement of the anterior epiphysis only
Group II	■ Involvement of the anterior epiphysis with a clear sequestrum
Group III	■ Only a small part of the epiphysis is not involved
Group IV	■ Total head involvement ■ Based on degree of head involvement ■ At-risk signs (indicate a more severe disease course) Gage sign—V-shaped radiolucency in the lateral portion of the epiphysis and/or adjacent metaphysis Calcification lateral to the epiphysis Lateral subluxation of the femoral head Horizontal proximal femoral physis Metaphyseal cyst—added later to the original four at-risk signs described by Catterall

Meyer dysplasia can be easily mistaken for Legg-Calvé-Perthes disease and lead to unnecessary diagnostic procedures and treatment. Meyer dysplasia has been found to be more common in boys younger than 4 years old and more likely to be bilateral. Characteristic findings included delayed or smaller ossification centers on radiograph, a separated or cracked epiphysis, cystic changes, and mild pain and limping. Condensation, subchondral fractures, fragmentation, and subluxation usually are not present with Meyer dysplasia.

■ CLASSIFICATION

When the diagnosis is established, the primary aim of treatment of Legg-Calvé-Perthes disease is containment of the femoral head within the acetabulum. If this is achieved, the femoral head can re-form in a concentric manner by what Salter has termed *biologic plasticity.*

Historically, Catterall et al. classified patients with this disease into groups according to the amount of involvement of the capital femoral epiphysis: group I, partial head or less than half head involvement; groups II and III, more than half head involvement and sequestrum formation; and group IV, involvement of the entire epiphysis (Table 32-3). They noted

TABLE 32-4

Salter-Thompson Classification

Class A	■ Crescent sign involves < 1/2 of femoral head
Class B	■ Crescent sign involves > 1/2 of femoral head
Based on radiographic crescent sign	

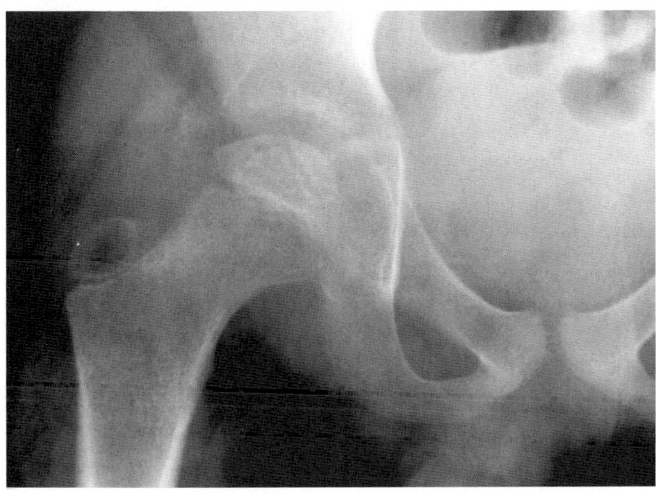

FIGURE 32-24 Type B subchondral fracture involving more than 50% of femoral head.

that certain radiographic signs described as "head at risk" correlated positively with poor results, especially in patients in groups II, III, and IV. These head-at-risk signs include (1) lateral subluxation of the femoral head from the acetabulum, (2) speckled calcification lateral to the capital epiphysis, (3) diffuse metaphyseal reaction (metaphyseal cysts), (4) a horizontal physis, and (5) the Gage sign, a radiolucent V-shaped defect in the lateral epiphysis and adjacent metaphysis. Catterall recommended containment by femoral varus derotational osteotomy for older children in groups II, III, and IV with head-at-risk signs. Contraindications include an already malformed femoral head and delay of treatment of more than 8 months from onset of symptoms. Surgery is not recommended for any group I children or any child without the head-at-risk signs.

Salter and Thompson advocated determining the extent of involvement by describing the extent of a subchondral fracture in the superolateral portion of the femoral head. If the extent of the fracture (line) is less than 50% of the superior dome of the femoral head, the involvement is considered type A, and good results can be expected (Table 32-4). If the extent of the fracture is more than 50% of the dome, the involvement is considered type B, and fair or poor results can be expected (Fig. 32-24). According to Salter and Thompson, this subchondral fracture and its entire extent can be observed radiographically earlier and more readily than trying to determine the Catterall classification (8.1 months average). According to these authors, if the femoral head is graded as type B, probably an operation such as an innominate osteotomy should be carried out. The extent of the subchondral fracture line, when present, has been suggested to be more accurate in

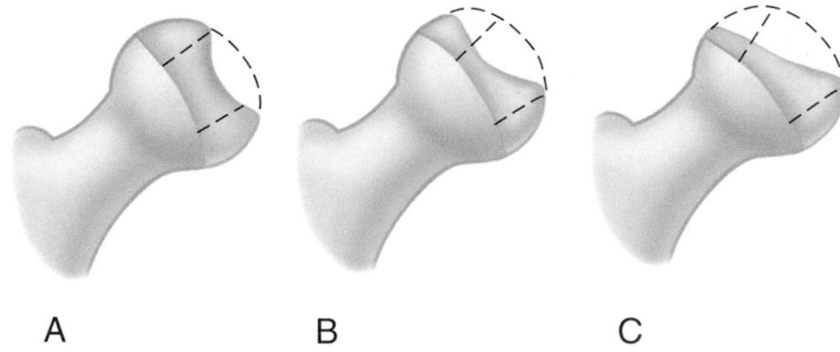

FIGURE 32-25 A-C, Lateral pillar classification based on height of lateral pillar.

predicting the extent of necrosis than is the extent of necrosis seen on MRI. In our experience, however, subchondral fractures are present early in the course of the disease in only a third of patients, and although this classification is a reliable indicator in the group with fractures, it has little to offer in early treatment decisions for the other two thirds of patients.

Presently, the most used classification is by Herring et al. (Table 32-5). They described a classification based on the height of the lateral pillar: group A, no involvement of the lateral pillar; group B, at least 50% of lateral pillar height maintained; and group C, less than 50% of lateral pillar height maintained (Fig. 32-25). A statistically significant correlation was found between the final outcome (Stulberg classification) and the loss of pillar height. Patients in group A had uniformly good outcomes; patients in group B who were younger than 8 to 9 years old at onset had good outcomes, but patients older than age 8 to 9 years had less favorable results; patients in group C had the worst results, with most having aspherical femoral heads, regardless of age at onset or type of treatment. Reproducibility of this classification system was confirmed by 78% of members of the study group who used it. A patient with a pillar group B may progress to a pillar group C or may be in a "gray" area and designated as pillar group B/C. Herring et al. noted that the advantages of this classification are (1) it can be applied easily during the active stages of the disease and (2) the high correlation between the lateral pillar height and the amount of femoral head flattening at skeletal maturity allows accurate prediction of the natural history and treatment methods. Price has challenged the concept that a lateral pillar sign allows accurate prediction of the natural history and treatment. He noted that the sign may change from A to C in the course of the disease and that containment may no longer be beneficial. The lateral pillar sign may help guide treatment for some patients; however, a prognostic indicator to assist decision making in the early stages of the disease may be necessary.

■ BILATERAL INVOLVEMENT

Concerning bilaterality, reports in the literature indicate that patients with bilateral Legg-Calvé-Perthes disease have more severe involvement than patients with unilateral disease because most have a Catterall III or IV or a Herring B or C classification, and 48% rate as a Stulberg 4 or 5 at skeletal maturity. Bilateral involvement can be confused with multiple epiphyseal dysplasia of the hip. Radiographs of the other joints and a wrist radiograph to determine bone age (which is delayed in Legg-Calvé-Perthes disease) help to distinguish

TABLE 32-5

Lateral Pillar (Herring) Classification		
Group A	▪ Lateral pillar maintains full height with no density changes identified	▪ Uniformly good outcome
Group B	▪ Maintains >50% height	▪ Poor outcome in patients with bone age > 6 years
Group B/C Border	▪ Lateral pillar is narrowed (2-3 mm) or poorly ossified with approximately 50% height	▪ Recently added to increase consistency and prognosis of classification
Group C	▪ Less than 50% of lateral pillar height is maintained	▪ Poor outcomes in all patients
▪ Determined at the beginning of fragmentation stage ▪ Usually occurs 6 months after the onset of symptoms ▪ Based on the height of the lateral pillar of the capital femoral epiphysis on anteroposterior imaging of the pelvis ▪ Has best interobserver agreement ▪ Designed to provide prognostic information ▪ Limitation is that final classification is not possible at initial presentation due to the fact that the patient needs to have entered into the fragmentation stage radiographically		

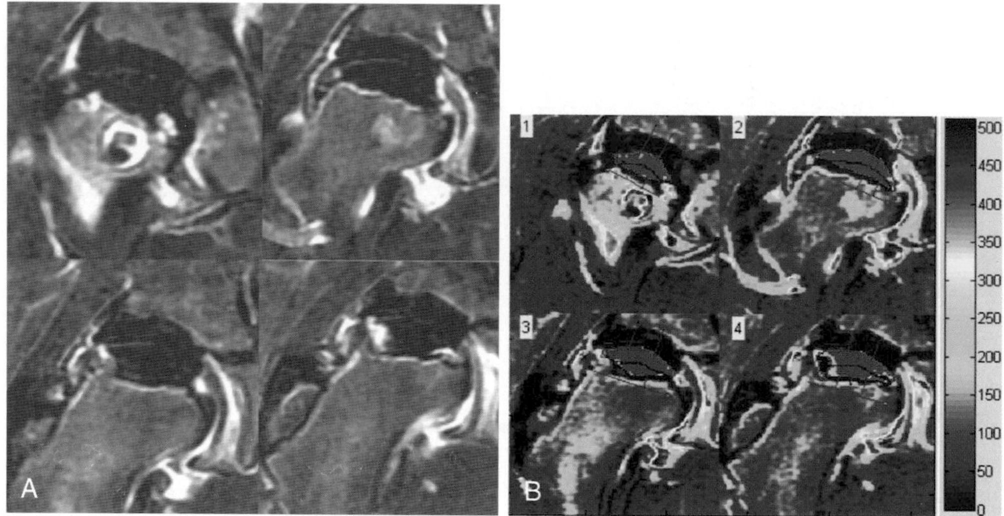

FIGURE 32-26 **A,** Perfusion MRI at initial disease showing lack of perfusion (*black area*) in most of the epiphysis except in gray area in lateral aspect (*right lower panel*). **B,** Corresponding HipViasc images showing level of perfusion in epiphysis. Blue as shown on color scale indicates absence of perfusion. (From Kim HKW, et al. Perfusion MRI in early stage of Legg-Calvé-Perthes disease to predict lateral pillar involvement, J Bone Joint Surg 96A:1152, 2014).

the two. Concerning sex, boys and girls who have the same Catterall classification or lateral pillar classification at the time of initial evaluation can be expected to have similar outcomes according to the classification system of Stulberg, Cooperman, and Wallensten.

IMAGING EVALUATION

In the past, diagnosis often was delayed because plain radiographic changes are not apparent until 6 weeks or more from the clinical onset of Legg-Calvé-Perthes disease. Scintigraphy and MRI can establish the diagnosis much earlier. In the past, we have used a bone scan to try to determine early how much of the femoral head is involved. We compared the uptake with that of the contralateral hip, and if the uptake was decreased less than 50% compared with the opposite femoral head early in the course of the disease, the disease was considered to be a Catterall group I or II. If the uptake was decreased more than 50%, the disease was a Catterall group III or IV, Salter type B, or lateral pillar type C.

MRI also seems to be superior to scintigraphy for depicting the extent of involvement in the early or evolutionary stage of Legg-Calvé-Perthes disease. MRI has become standard at our institution to determine the extent of involvement, the classification, and treatment planning. A limitation of both the Catterall and lateral pillar classifications is that a definitive prediction cannot be made until well into mid-fragmentation stage, thus delaying treatment during this wait and see period (4 to 6 months). Gadolinium-enhanced subtraction MRI (perfusion MRI) has been used at the initial fragmentation (earlier) stage to determine the extent of lateral pillar involvement, thereby allowing initiation of constraint treatment (Fig. 32-26). Although no serious complications have been reported with perfusion MRI for Perthes, approximately 50% of children have to be sedated or given general anesthesia. The Perthes Study Group reported promising results using MRI perfusion for early classification of lateral pillar signs. However, the routine use of perfusion MRI has been challenged by some authors (Schoenecker et al.) who believe that knowing early the extent of head and pillar involvement may not be that essential in treatment or ultimate results.

TREATMENT

Treatment depends on where the child is in the course of the disease. Most treatment is during the active process (early fragmentation). The problem again is to determine early the severity or ultimate involvement of the femoral head (Caterall II, IV, lateral pillar B/C, C, Salter-Thompson B). Treatment in the residual phase is reconstructive to prevent a malformed hip from progressing to osteoarthritis at an early age.

Many procedures have been described for both the active and residual phases of the disease. We have utilized a variety of treatments over the past 40 years and have reported our non-containment results. We also have used abduction orthoses for constraint, varus osteotomy, and a Salter, Pemberton, or pelvic osteotomy when indicated, all with a vigorous hip range of motion program. Whether we altered the natural history in our patients is debatable, but we have learned that approximately 84% satisfactory results can be obtained from nonconstraint and nonoperative treatment.

In the early stage (active phase), our current treatment protocol for children age 4 years and older begins with explaining to the parents the natural history and expected duration of the disease (24 to 36 months). Children 2 to 3 years old can be observed and do not need aggressive treatment. Once synovitis resolves, a daily home physical therapy program, including active and active-assisted range-of-motion and muscle stretching exercises to the hip and knee, is recommended to try to maintain a normal hip range of motion.

Loss of motion at any time indicates a significant change in prognosis. If loss of motion is significant, and subluxation laterally is occurring, bed rest, skin traction, progressive passive and active physical therapy, abduction exercises, and pool therapy, if possible, are indicated. If there is no improvement, we recommend closed reduction with the patient under general anesthesia and percutaneous adductor longus tenotomy, followed by an ambulatory abduction cast (Petrie) for 6 weeks or more.

We rarely recommend surgery for Legg-Calvé-Perthes in the active phase of the disease because of the complications possible after major hip surgery, whether it be a varus derotational osteotomy or an innominate osteotomy. If surgery is indicated during the active phase of the disease, the procedure to use is controversial. Historically, Salter, Thompson, Canale et al., Coleman, and others achieved “containment” by pelvic osteotomy above the hip joint, whereas Axer, Craig, Somerville, and Lloyd-Roberts et al. advocated varus derotational osteotomy. More recently, many studies have emphasized the importance of the timing and the indications for surgery, rather than the type of procedure, recommending that operative intervention be done in the early fragmentation stage before re-formation of a malformed femoral head can occur.

Operative treatment may not produce better results than nonoperative treatment in younger patients but, in general, better results have been reported in older children treated operatively than in children treated nonoperatively when femoral head involvement was severe (lateral pillar B, B/C).

Varus derotational osteotomy and innominate osteotomy have advantages and disadvantages. Varus derotational osteotomy theoretically allows more coverage; however, if too much correction (varus) occurs, and if the capital femoral physis closes prematurely as a result of the disease, excessive varus deformity may persist. Theoretically, a mild increase in length can occur with innominate osteotomy, whereas mild shortening may occur with a varus osteotomy. Compression of an already compromised femoral head also can occur with innominate osteotomy. A second operation to remove hardware is required after both procedures, and both have complications similar to any large operation on the hip. Neither procedure has been shown to accelerate the healing process of the disease. Although numerous authors recommend one procedure over the other, until there is conclusive evidence of superiority, it seems that the choice should be dictated by the surgeon’s familiarity and expertise with a particular procedure.

Shelf arthroplasty (lateral labral support) has been advocated for severe Legg-Calvé-Perthes disease (Catterall III or IV; lateral pillar B, BC,C) in the early stages (fragmentation), with incorporation of the shelf graft into the pelvis as a result of continued growth of the lateral acetabular structures. Although acetabular coverage and size may be increased in children younger than 8 years old, these changes are seen at short-term follow-up, and the amount of coverage at long-term follow-up is similar to that obtained by innominate osteotomy.

Distraction of the hip joint (arthrodiastasis) by an external fixator for an average of 4 months has been described in older children with active and severe Legg-Calvé-Perthes disease. Many complications, such as pin breakage and pin track infections, have been reported with this procedure, and presently its use seems to be limited to the most severe cases.

MRI before surgery is mandatory to determine (1) if any flattening of the femoral head is already present that would contraindicate most osteotomies of any type and (2) how much subluxation is present and how much surgical containment is necessary.

A combined osteotomy (pelvic osteotomy and varus femoral osteotomy) used as a salvage procedure for severe Legg-Calvé-Perthes disease has the theoretical advantage of obtaining maximal femoral head containment while avoiding the complications of either procedure alone, such as limb shortening, extreme neck-shaft varus angulation, and associated abductor weakness. Recently, Stevens et al. described guided growth of the trochanteric apophysis using a “tether” with an eight-plate and soft-tissue release as part of a non-osteotomy management strategy for select children with progressive symptoms and related radiographic changes (Fig. 32-27).

In the residual-stage, indications for reconstructive surgery in Legg-Calvé-Perthes disease are (1) a malformed head causing femoroacetabular impingement or “hinge” abduction in which surgical hip dislocation or hip arthroscopy can be used for osteochondroplasty (cheilectomy) or a

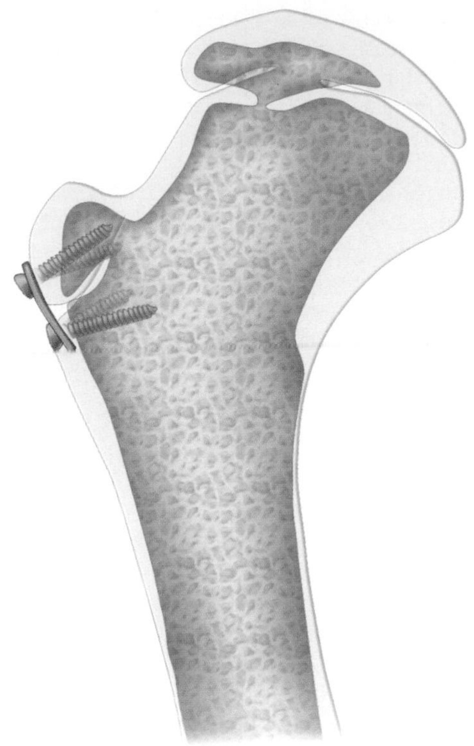

FIGURE 32-27 Tethering of greater trochanter and lack of change to neck-shaft angle after guided growth technique of trochanteric apophysis with soft-tissue release. (Redrawn from Stevens PM, Anderson LA, Gililland JM, Novais E: Guided growth of trochanteric apophysis combined with soft-tissue release for Legg-Calvé-Perthes disease, Strat Traum Lim Recons 9:37, 2014.)

varus, valgus, or femoral head osteotomy can be performed; (2) coxa magna for which a shelf augmentation would provide coverage; (3) a large malformed femoral head with subluxation laterally, for which a pelvic osteotomy may be considered; and (4) capital femoral physeal arrest for which trochanteric advancement or arrest can be performed for relative lengthening of the femoral neck. External fixation across the pelvis and hip has been used to reduce the femoral head to avoid hinge abduction and persistent subluxation. All of these are procedures for an already malformed hip, and when used a high percentage of unsatisfactory results should be expected.

INNOMINATE OSTEOTOMY

The advantages of innominate osteotomy (Figs. 32-28 and 32-29) include anterolateral coverage of the femoral head, lengthening of the extremity (possibly shortened by the avascular process), and avoidance of a second operation for plate removal. The disadvantages of innominate osteotomy include the inability sometimes to obtain adequate containment of the femoral head, especially in older children; an increase in acetabular and hip joint pressure that may cause further avascular changes in the femoral head; and an increase in leg length on the operated side compared with the normal side that may cause a relative adduction of the hip and uncover the femoral head. Innominate osteotomy as described by Salter is included in the discussion of congenital deformities (see Chapter 30). Salter's procedure includes iliopsoas release. Other pelvic osteotomies such as the Pemberton osteotomy (Chapter 30), the Dega osteotomy (Chapter 30), the Bernese osteotomy (Chapter 6), or the Ganz periacetabular osteotomy (Chapter 6) if needed in the residual phase can be used.

INNOMINATE OSTEOTOMY FOR LEGG-CALVÉ-PERTHES DISEASE

TECHNIQUE 32-6

(CANALE ET AL.)

- Through a Smith-Petersen approach to the hip (see Technique 1-60), release the sartorius, tensor fasciae latae, and rectus femoris and expose the anterior inferior iliac spine.
- Release the psoas tendon from its insertion and dissect subperiosteally on the inner and outer walls of the ilium down to the sciatic notch. Using retractors in the sciatic notch, with a right-angle clamp pass a Gigli saw through the notch. With the saw, carefully cut horizontally and anteriorly through the ilium as close as possible to the capsular attachment of the acetabulum.
- Maximally flex the knee and flex and abduct the hip to open the osteotomy. Use a towel clip to pull the distal fragment of the osteotomy anteriorly and laterally.
- Take a full-thickness quadrilateral graft 2 × 3 cm from the wing of the ilium according to the size of the space produced by opening the osteotomy (Fig. 32-29). Predrill or precut the outline of the graft on the surfaces of the ilium to prevent fracture of the inner and outer cortices. Shape the quadrilateral graft carefully to fit the space produced and impact it into the osteotomy site.
- Use one or more threaded pins for fixation and leave the ends subcutaneous so that they can be removed later with local or general anesthesia.
- Use the center-edge angle of Wiberg in the weight-bearing position at this time to assess by radiography the coverage and containment of the femoral head.

POSTOPERATIVE CARE. The patient is immobilized for 10 to 12 weeks in a spica cast before the pins are removed. Range-of-motion exercises and full weight-bearing ambulation are started, and radiographic evaluation is repeated.

LATERAL SHELF PROCEDURE (LABRAL SUPPORT)

Except in the active stage of the disease, lateral shelf acetabuloplasty can be used for older children who are not candidates for femoral osteotomy because of insufficient remodeling capacity and the likelihood that shortening of the femur would cause a persistent limp. Recently, it has been suggested to be indicated in the active early stages. Proponents of doing the labral support procedure early argue that it has three beneficial effects: (1) lateral acetabular growth stimulation, (2) prevention of subluxation, and (3) shelf resolution after

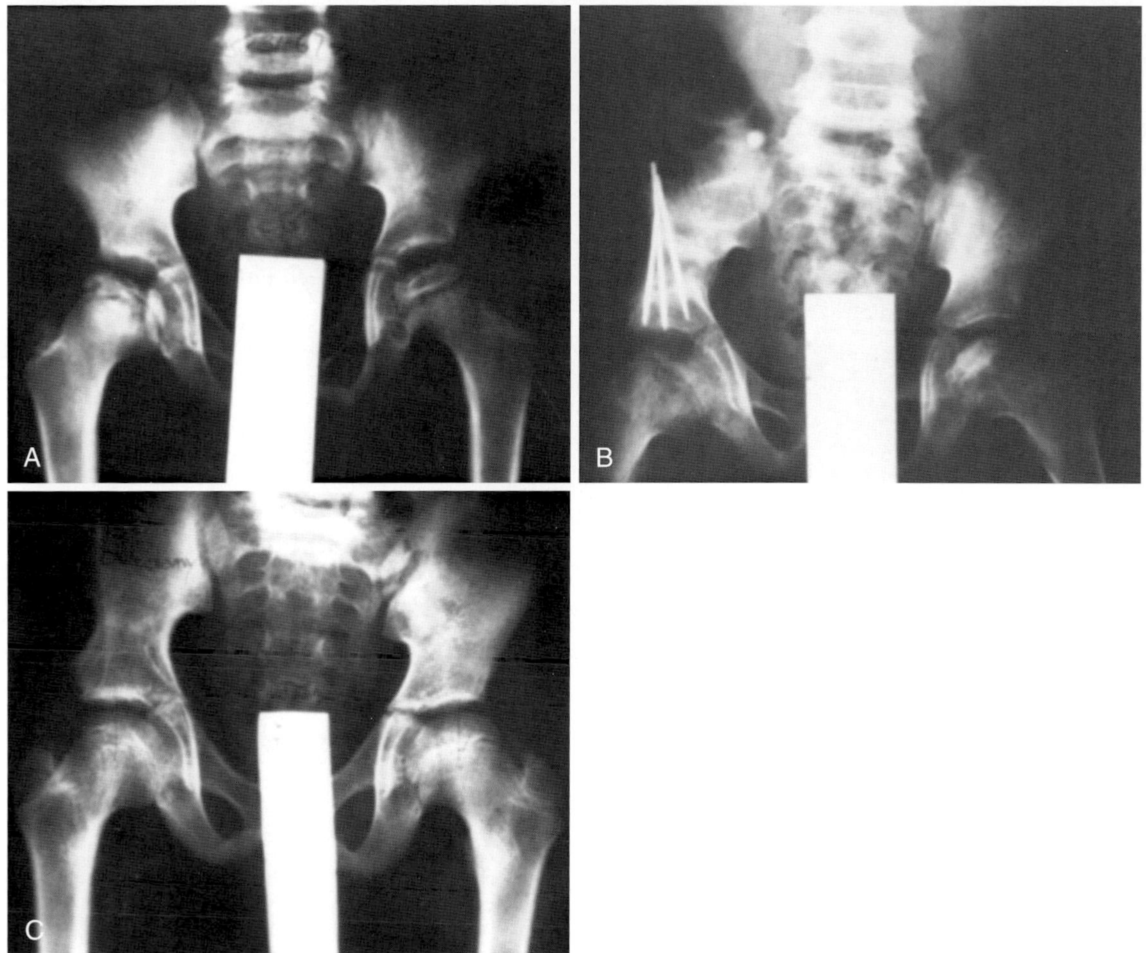

FIGURE 32-28 Innominate osteotomy for Legg-Calvé-Perthes disease. **A,** Seven-year-old child with bilateral Catterall group III involvement with "head-at-risk" signs of lateral calcification (subluxation) and metaphyseal cyst on left. **B,** Eight weeks after innominate osteotomy with fixation using three pins. **C,** Three years after innominate osteotomy. Femoral head is contained without evidence of subluxation. Center-edge angle is 28 degrees, and femoral head is concentric but slightly enlarged.

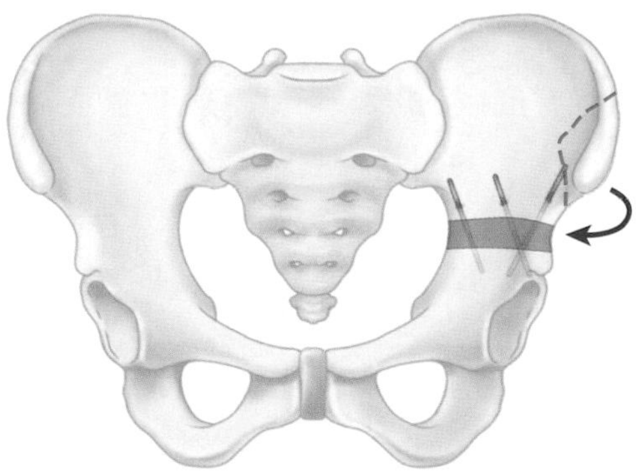

FIGURE 32-29 Innominate osteotomy using quadrangular graft (see text) for Legg-Calvé-Perthes disease. (From Canale ST, d'Anca AF, Cotler JM, et al: Use of innominate osteotomy in Legg-Calvé-Perthes disease, J Bone Joint Surg 54A:25, 1972.) **SEE TECHNIQUE 32-6**.

femoral epiphyseal reossification. Advocates of the shelf procedure in active disease report results as good as those after varus osteotomy or innominate osteotomy of Salter. It is simple to perform (mini-incision with or without a dry arthroscope) and does not induce a permanent deformity in the proximal femur or acetabulum.

LATERAL SHELF PROCEDURE (LABRAL SUPPORT) FOR LEGG-CALVÉ-PERTHES DISEASE

TECHNIQUE 32-7

(WILLETT ET AL.)

- Make a curved incision below the iliac crest, passing 1.5 cm below the anterior superior iliac spine to avoid the lateral cutaneous nerve of the thigh. Strip the glutei subperiosteally from the outer table of the ilium to the level

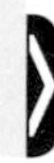

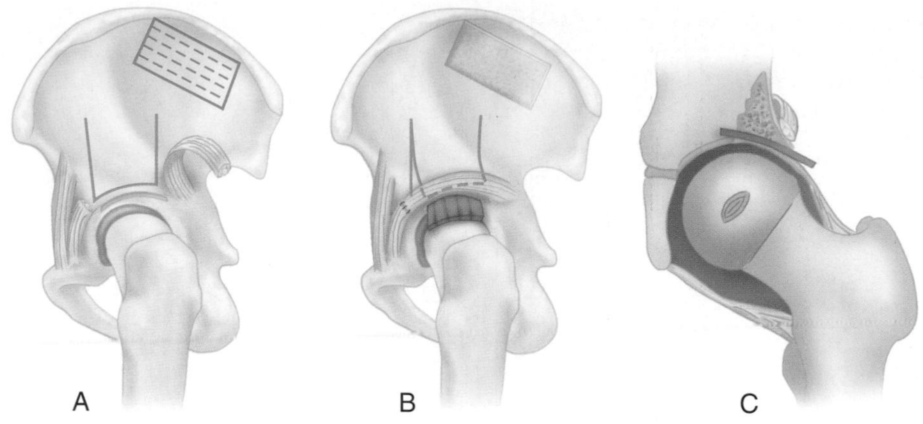

FIGURE 32-30 **A-C,** Operative technique for lateral shelf acetabuloplasty (see text) in Legg-Calvé-Perthes disease. **SEE TECHNIQUE 32-7.**

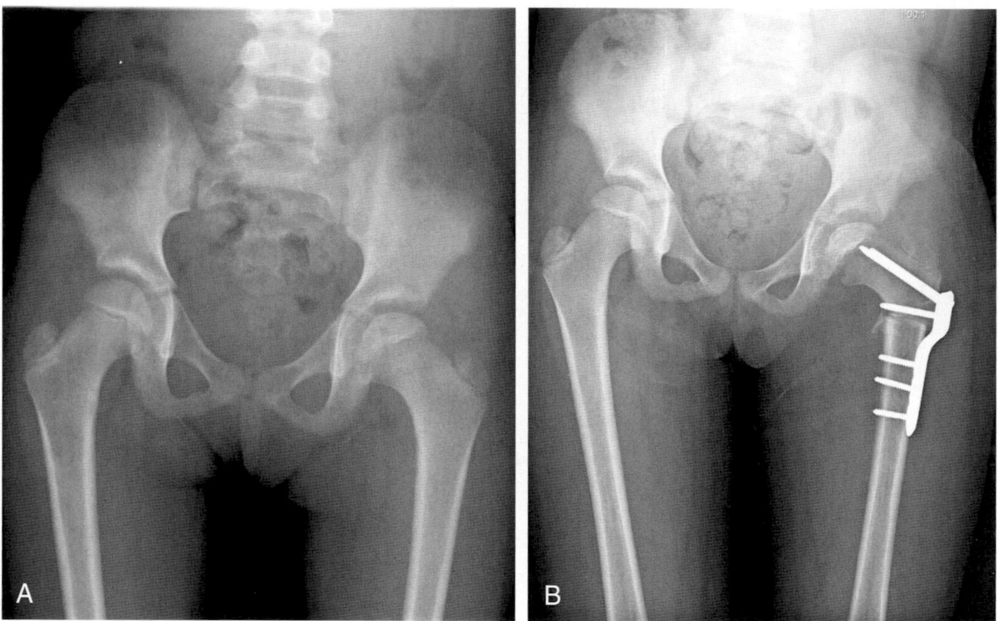

FIGURE 32-31 Legg-Calvé-Perthes disease. **A,** Preoperative radiograph. **B,** After varus osteotomy and fixation.

of insertion of the joint capsule. Mobilize and divide the reflected head of the rectus femoris.

- Create a trough in the bone immediately above the insertion of the capsule (Fig. 32-30A). Raise a bony flap 3 cm wide × 3.5 cm long superiorly from the outer cortex of the ilium.
- Cut strips of cancellous graft from the ilium above the flap and insert them into the trough so that they form a canopy on the superior surface of the hip joint (Fig. 32-30B). Pack the web-shaped space between the flap and the graft canopy with cancellous bone graft (Fig. 32-30C).
- Repair the reflected head of the rectus femoris over the created shelf.
- Close the wound in the usual manner and apply a spica cast.

POSTOPERATIVE CARE. The spica cast is worn for 8 weeks. Protective weight bearing in a single spica cast is continued for 6 additional weeks.

VARUS DEROTATIONAL OSTEOTOMY

The advantages of varus derotational osteotomy of the proximal femur include the ability to obtain maximal coverage of the femoral head, especially in an older child, and the ability to correct excessive femoral anteversion with the same osteotomy (Fig. 32-31). The disadvantages of varus derotational osteotomy include excessive varus angulation that may not correct with growth (especially in an older child), further shortening of an already shortened extremity, the possibility of a gluteus lurch produced by decreasing the length of the lever arm of the gluteal musculature, the possibility of nonunion of the osteotomy, and the requirement of a second operation to remove the internal fixation. Premature closure of the capital femoral physis may cause further varus deformity. Aksoy et al. reported poor results in children with pillar group C hips, especially after the age of 9 years. A varus derotational osteotomy is the procedure of choice when containment of the femoral head is necessary but cannot be achieved with a brace for psychosocial or other reasons, when the child is 8 to 10 years old and without leg-length inequality, when on arthrogram or MRI most of the femoral head is uncovered and the angle of Wiberg is decreased, and when there is a significant amount of femoral anteversion. An anteroposterior radiograph of the pelvis is taken with the lower extremities in internal rotation and parallel to each other (no abduction). If satisfactory containment of the femoral head is noted, derotational osteotomy alone is carried out. The degree of derotation is roughly estimated from the amount of internal rotation of the extremity, but further adjustments are made during the operation.

When internal rotation is seriously limited and remains so preoperatively after 4 weeks of bed rest with traction, varus osteotomy is carried out with the addition of extension that is produced by a slight backward tilt of the proximal fragment. When internal rotation is sufficient, abduction of the extremity brings about the desired containment of the femoral head. The degree of abduction is expressed by the angle formed by the shaft of the femur and a vertical line parallel to the midline of the pelvis. This angle represents the desired angle of the osteotomy (see Technique 32-8). Herring et al. stated that contrary to conventional belief greater varus angulation does not necessarily produce better preservation of the femoral head after osteotomy. Their recommendation was to achieve 0-15 degrees of varus correction for hips that are in the early stages of Perthes.

Reliable information on acetabular containment of the femoral head, the size of the head, the flattening of the epiphysis, and the width of the medial joint space can be obtained from preoperative arthrography or MRI. The osteocartilaginous head of the femur should be covered adequately by the acetabular roof as the femur is abducted and the flattened segment of the femoral head is rotated into the depths of the acetabular fossa. We use a varus (medial closing wedge) osteotomy fixed with an adolescent or pediatric hip screw (Fig. 32-32). According to the recent literature, fracture after plate removal for osteotomies is 5% in patients with Perthes. These data suggest that the time to hardware removal should be extended beyond radiographic union to at least 6 months or more after the osteotomy.

VARUS DEROTATIONAL OSTEOTOMY OF THE PROXIMAL FEMUR FOR LEGG-CALVÉ-PERTHES DISEASE

TECHNIQUE 32-8

(STRICKER)

- Place the patient supine on the operating table with a radiograph cassette holder beneath the patient. Image intensification, positioned in the anteroposterior projection, is desirable. Prepare and drape the affected extremity, leaving it free to allow for intraoperative radiographs or imaging.
- Make a lateral incision from the greater trochanter distally 8 to 12 cm and reflect the vastus lateralis to expose the lateral aspect of the femur.
- Identify the femoral insertion of the gluteus maximus and make a transverse line in the femoral cortex with an osteotome to mark the level of the osteotomy at the level of the lesser trochanter or slightly distal (Fig. 32-32A). Correct positioning of the osteotomy site can be verified with image intensification.
- After the lateral portion of the trochanter and the proximal lateral femur have been exposed, place a guide pin outside the capsule, anterior to the neck. Using the fluoroscopic image, determine the direction of the neck. Set the adjustable angle guide to 120 degrees and position it against the lateral cortex. Attach the guide to the shaft with the plate clamp. Insert the guide pin through the cannulated portion of the adjustable angle guide and into the femoral neck (Fig. 32-32B). Predrilling the lateral cortex with the twist drill can aid in placing the guide pin. Ensure that the guide pin is placed in the center of the femoral neck within 5 mm of the proximal femoral physis without violating it or the trochanteric apophysis (Fig. 32-32C, inset 1). Verify guide pin placement in the anteroposterior and lateral views on the image.
- When the guide pin is placed within 5 mm of the physis, use the percutaneous direct measuring gauge to determine the lag screw length (Fig. 32-32C, inset 2).
- Set the adjustable positive stop on the combination reamer to the lag screw length determined by the percutaneous direct measuring gauge. Place the reamer over the guide pin and ream until the positive stop reaches the lateral cortex (Fig. 32-32D). Do not violate the physis. It is prudent to check the fluoroscopic image periodically during reaming to ensure that the guide pin is not inadvertently advancing into the femoral epiphysis.
- Set the adjustable positive stop on the lag screw tap to the same length that was reamed. Tap until the positive stop reaches the lateral cortex.
- Insert the selected lag screw into the distal end of the insertion/removal wrench. Place it over the guide pin and into the reamed or tapped hole. The lag screw is at the proper depth when (1) the insertion or removal wrench's first depth marking is flush with the lateral cortex (Fig. 32-32E), and (2) the handle of the insertion or removal wrench is perpendicular to the shaft of the femur, with the longitudinal key line facing proximally. This positioning ensures that the plate barrel and lag screw shaft are properly keyed for rotational stability (Fig. 32-32F). Remove the guide pin when the lag screw is at the appropriate length.
- With the lag screw in place, perform the osteotomy (20-degree transverse osteotomy is illustrated). Make the cut as proximal as possible, just below the lag screw entry point, because the proximal metaphyseal bone usually heals better than the cortical subtrochanteric bone. In addition, the correction of the proximal femoral deformity

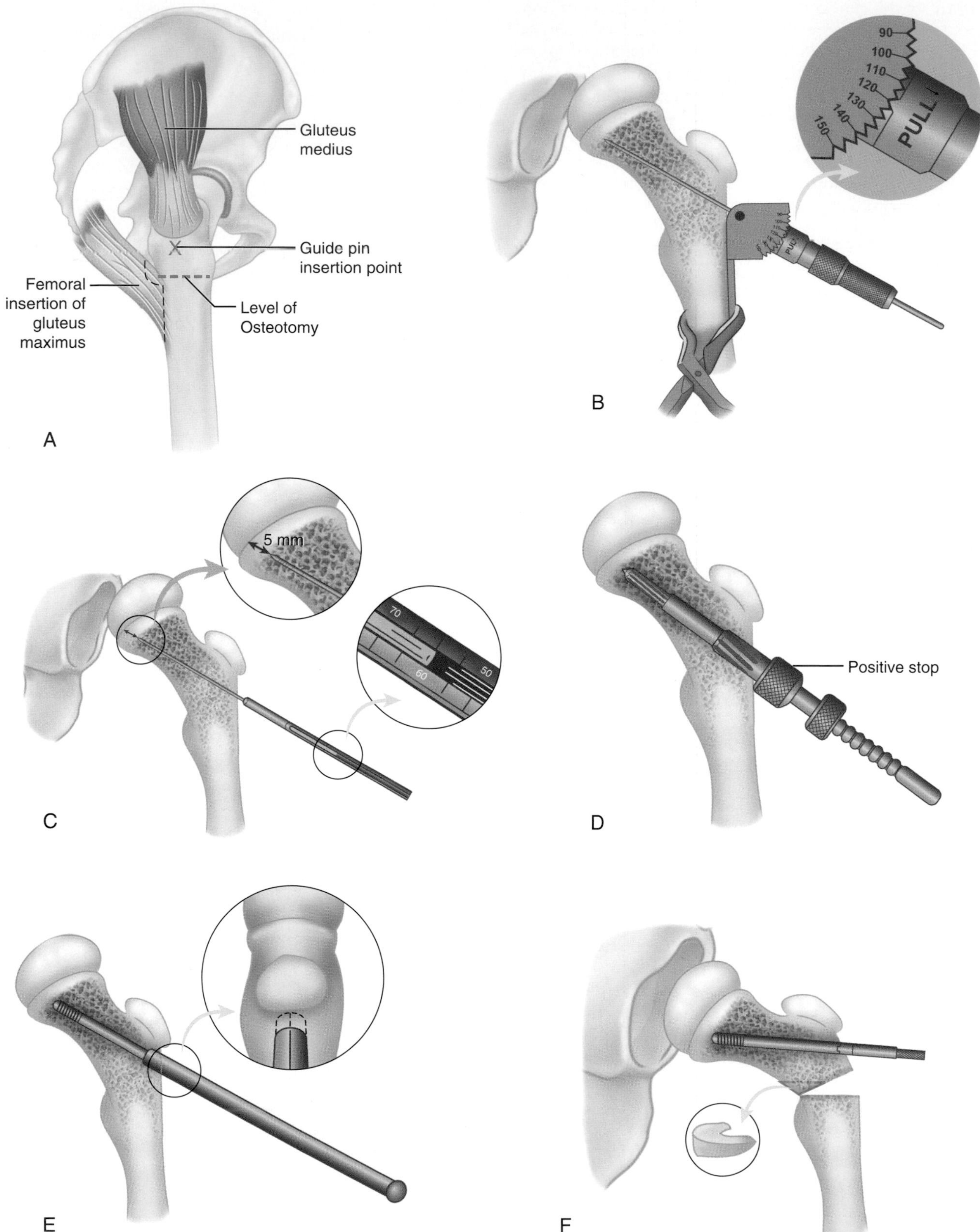

FIGURE 32-32 Varus derotational osteotomy (see text) in Legg-Calvé-Perthes disease. **A,** Level of osteotomy. **B** and **C,** Insertion of guide pin. **D,** Reaming of femur. **E,** First depth marking flush with lateral cortex. **F,** Removal of wedge to customize fit.

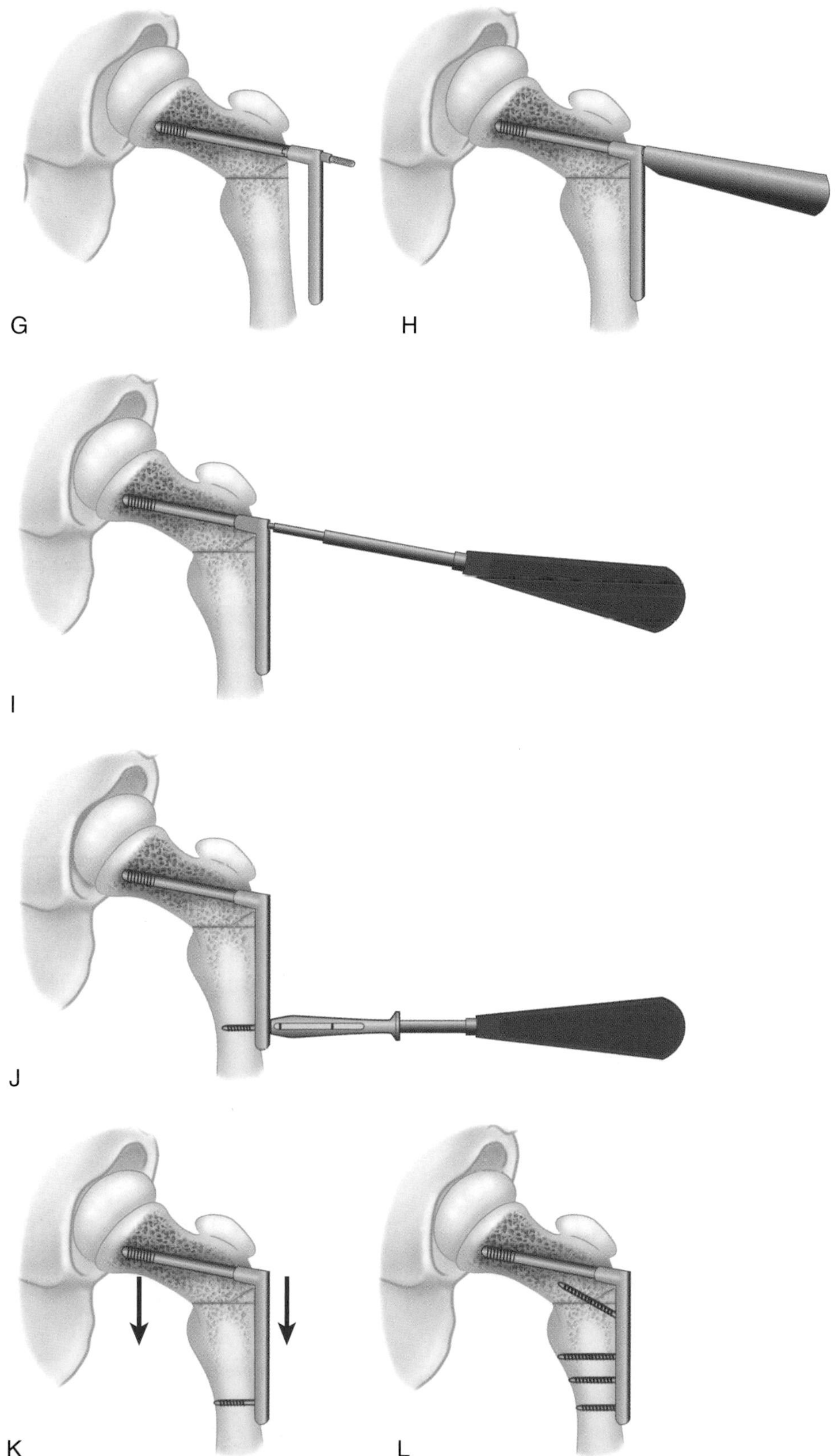

FIGURE 32-32, cont'd **G-I,** Plate and compression screw application. **J-L,** Insertion of bone screws. (Redrawn from Stricker S: Intermediate and pediatric osteotomy systems: technique manual, Memphis, Smith & Nephew Orthopaedics, 2005.) **SEE TECHNIQUE 32-8**.

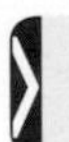

is best accomplished close to the deformity (i.e., as close to the femoral head as possible).

- Insert the barrel guide into the back of the implanted lag screw to help position the proximal femur. The desired correction can be accomplished by tilting the head into valgus or, in this case, varus, removing wedges to customize the fit if needed (Fig. 32-32G). Iliopsoas tenotomy or recession also may facilitate positioning of the osteotomy.
- Take the plate chosen during preoperative planning (100 degrees × 76 mm × four holes in this case) and insert its barrel over the barrel guide and onto the back of the lag screw (Fig. 32-32H). If necessary, insert the cannulated plate tamper over the barrel guide and tap it several times to seat the plate fully (Fig. 32-32I).
- Remove the barrel guide and insert a compressing screw to prevent the plate from disengaging during the reduction maneuver. Use the slotted screwdriver for the pediatric compressing screw or the hex screwdriver for the intermediate compressing screw (Fig. 32-32J).
- Reduce the osteotomy and secure the plate to the femur using the plate clamp. Check the rotational position of the lower extremity in extension.
- A range of 2.5 to 6.5 mm of femoral shaft compression is possible with the use of an intermediate osteotomy hip screw. To achieve 6.5 mm of compression, insert the drill guide end of the intermediate combination drill or tap guide into the distal portion of the most distal compression slot. Drill through to the medial cortex using the twist drill. If less compression is required, follow the same steps detailed previously in the distal portion of either the second or third distal slots for 2.5 mm of compression. If no compression is needed, follow the same steps listed previously except begin by placing the intermediate combination drill/tap guide in the proximal portion of the slot instead of the distal portion used for compression.
- Insert the tap guide end of the intermediate combination drill or tap guide into the slot and insert the bone screw tap.
- Insert the depth gauge through the slot and into the drilled or tapped hole. Ensure that the nose of the guide is inserted fully into the plate's slot. Insert the needle of the depth gauge and hook it on the medial cortex. Read the bone screw length measurement directly off of the depth gauge.
- Select the appropriate length bone screw and insert it using the hex screwdriver. Use the self-holding sleeve to keep the screw from disengaging from the screwdriver. In cases in which compression is being applied, the bone screw abuts the inclined distal aspect of the slot as it is being seated, forcing the plate and the attached proximal fragment slightly distally until resisted by compression of the osteotomy (Fig. 32-32K). Follow the same steps for the remaining two slots.
- In the most proximal slot, the intermediate combination drill or tap guide can be angled proximally so that the drill, and ultimately the bone screw, crosses the osteotomy line. Positioning the proximal bone screw in this way can provide additional stability at the osteotomy site (Fig. 32-32L).
- Irrigate the wound and close in layers, inserting a suction drain if needed. Apply a one and one-half spica cast.

POSTOPERATIVE CARE. The spica cast is worn for 8 to 12 weeks, until union is achieved. The internal fixation can be removed 12 to 24 months after the osteotomy if desired.

LATERAL OPENING WEDGE OSTEOTOMY

Axer described a lateral opening wedge osteotomy for children 5 years of age and younger in which a prebent plate is used to hold the cortices apart laterally the measured amount. The defect laterally fills in rapidly in young children, but the open wedge may result in delayed union or nonunion in children older than 5 years. Because few children younger than 5 years are operated on for Legg-Calvé-Perthes disease in the United States, indications for this procedure are rare.

REVERSED OR CLOSING WEDGE TECHNIQUE FOR LEGG-CALVE-PERTHES DISEASE

TECHNIQUE 32-9

- After calculating from Table 32-6 the height of the base of the wedge to be removed, hold the extremity in internal rotation at the hip and mark a wedge. Close the wedge if a reverse wedge is being used.
- Take a wedge half the height over the anterior surface of the femur with the base medially.
- Remove the wedge with an oscillating saw, rotate the distal fragment externally to the desired degree, turn the bone wedge 180 degrees, and insert it in the osteotomy with its base lateral or reversed. Because its base now is lateral, the varus angle obtained equals the angle that would be obtained with complete removal of a full-height bone wedge medially.
- Fix the bone fragments with the prebent plate as previously described with all cortices in contact. When the reversed bone wedge is not stable enough, fix it to the distal or proximal fragment with small Kirschner wires.

POSTOPERATIVE CARE. A double spica plaster cast is applied and removed after 6 weeks or when union is confirmed by radiography. The child is encouraged to walk, in water initially if increased joint stiffness is noted. No restrictions are imposed on the child except for follow-up every 3 months in the first year.

ARTHRODIASTASIS

The rationale behind arthrodiastasis is that distraction of the joint not only widens but also unloads the joint space, reduces the pressure on the femoral head, allows fibrous repair of articular cartilage defects, and preserves congruency of the femoral head. The articulated fixator allows 50 degrees of hip flexion. Recent reports have described significant

TABLE 32-6

Calculating Height of Base of Wedge to be Removed for Varus Osteotomy*

DESIRED ANGULATORY CHANGE (DEGREES)	FEMORAL SHAFT WIDTH AT OSTEOTOMY SITE (mm)												
	10	*12.5*	*15*	*17.5*	*20*	*22.5*	*25*	*27.5*	*30*	*32.5*	*35*	*37.5*	*40*
10	1.5	2	2.5	3	3.5	4	4.5	5	5.5	6	6.5	7	7.5
15	2	3	4	4.5	5	6	6.5	7.5	8	9	10	10.5	11.5
20	3	4	5	6	7	8	9	10	11	12	13	14	15
25	4.5	5	6.5	7.5	9	10	11.5	12.5	14	15	16	17.5	18.5
30	5.5	6.5	8	10	11.5	12.5	14	15.5	17	18.5	20	22	23
35	6.5	8	10	12	13.5	14	17	18.3	21	22	24	26	27.5
40	8	10	12.5	14.5	16.5	18.5	20	23	25	27	29	31.5	33.5

Credited to Orkan and Roth. Data from Axer A: Personal communication, 1978.

*The height of the base of the wedge in millimeters is read at the junction of the horizontal axis (desired degrees of angulatory change) and the vertical axis (width of the femoral shaft at the osteotomy site).

complications with this procedure; it should not be taken lightly and used only for the most severely involved hips with severe subluxation.

ARTHRODIASTASIS FOR LEGG-CALVÉ-PERTHES DISEASE

TECHNIQUE 32-10

(SEGEV ET AL.)

- Place the patient supine on a transparent operating table. Obtain a hip arthrogram medially to assess cartilage architecture and the extent of hinged abduction.
- Tenotomize the adductor and iliopsoas tendons through a medial approach.
- Using image intensification, insert a 1.6-mm Kirschner wire into the femoral head at the center of rotation of the hip while keeping the leg in 15 degrees of abduction with the patella pointing forward.
- Using the articulated body for the hip Orthofix external fixation device (Bussolengo, Italy; Fig. 32-33), apply it onto the Kirschner wire and attach a standard model "kit body" to the hinge distally.
- Fix the proximal part to the supraacetabular area with a T-clamp using two or three 5- to 6-mm Orthofix screws. The procedure is done using a template that is replaced by the aforementioned parts.
- Immediately distract the joint space 4 to 5 mm under image intensification. Continue distraction at 1 mm per day until the Shenton line is overcorrected.

POSTOPERATIVE CARE. Flexion and extension exercises are encouraged with the fixator in place, and the patient is kept non–weight bearing. The fixator is left in place for 4 to 5 months until lateral pillar reossification appears. The fixator is removed in the operating room, and a hip arthrogram is obtained. After removal of the frame, the patient continues protective non–weight bearing and intensive physical therapy and hydrotherapy for an additional 6 weeks. At this stage, full weight bearing is allowed with continued physiotherapy for another 6 months.

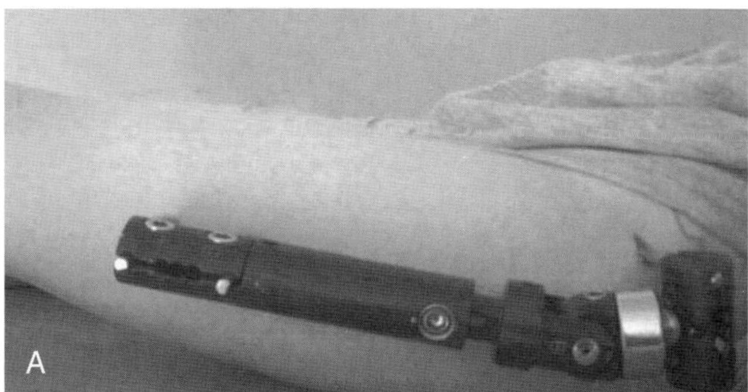

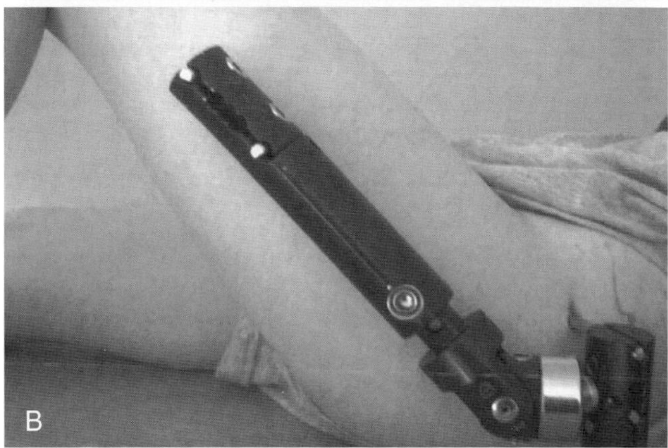

FIGURE 32-33 **A and B, Hinged external fixator (Orthofix, Bussolengo, Italy) for arthrodiastasis in Legg-Calvé-Perthes disease.** (From Maxwell SL, Lappin KJ, Kealey WD, et al: Arthrodiastasis in Perthes' disease, J Bone Joint Surg 86B:244, 2004. Copyright British Editorial Society of Bone and Joint Surgery.) **SEE TECHNIQUE 32-10.**

RECONSTRUCTIVE SURGERY

■ OSTEOCHONDROPLASTY (CHEILECTOMY)

Hip arthroscopy and surgical dislocation of the hip have been used to treat certain types of femoral acetabular impingement (FAI) and other intraarticular lesions caused by Perthes disease. One type of FAI develops in the malformed femoral head; terms such as pincer and cam effect are now replacing terms such as hinge-abduction and "trench." These newer techniques, surgical hip dislocation and arthroscopy, can eliminate intraarticular deformity and other lesions, such as labral tears, osteochondral or chondral lesions, loose bodies, or a torn ligamentum teres, and at the same time they can be combined with previously described extraarticular (extra capsular) procedures that provide coverage of the femoral head, increase acetabular coverage, or change the configuration of the femoral neck by advancing the greater trochanter.

Surgical dislocation of the femoral head has been used to treat FAI, and contrary to previous opinion can be done safely with few or no complications including osteonecrosis, myositis ossificans, or decreased motion secondary to soft-tissue reaction and scarring. Ganz and others popularized this technique and have performed chondroplasties, labral chondral tear or impingement excision, greater trochanteric advancement, and downsizing osteotomy of the mushroomed femoral head. Care must be taken, however, to protect the lateral epiphyseal arteries that are present in a narrow anatomic window on the femoral neck, but as noted by Millis, these are fewer in number in Legg-Calvé-Perthes disease.

Arthroscopy of the hip has become more refined and thus allows osteochondroplasty (cheilectomy) of the hip for FAI (cam and pincer lesions), loose bodies, and chondral and osteochondral defects (OCD). Although arthroscopy is easier to perform than surgical dislocation and is less traumatic, it is not as extensive. Techniques for hip arthroscopy are found in Chapter 51. A combined approach of hip arthroscopy and limited open osteochondroplasty by Clohisy and others is described in Chapter 6.

OSTEOCHONDROPLASTY SURGICAL DISLOCATION OF THE HIP

Ganz, after reviewing the anatomy of the medial circumflex artery, described a technique of surgical dislocation of the hip without compromising the blood supply to the femoral head. Surgical hip dislocation should probably not be carried out when the head is in the early fragmentation phase of the disease. Most of the pathology can be identified at surgery; however, MRI may be helpful as well as hip abduction, adduction, and flexion radiographs to assess for FAI and anterior coverage of the femoral osteotomy. A dynamic, three-dimensional reformation CT scan can be obtained to determine the extent of FAI. The approach for surgical hip dislocation as described by Ganz et al. is in Chapter 6. Ganz's algorithm for surgical treatment (Fig. 32-34) offers a structured way to identify the problem and the surgical treatment to correct structural abnormalities.

TECHNIQUE 32-11

GANZ

- Complete the approach for surgical dislocation of the hip (see Chapter 6), including an osteotomy of the greater trochanter.
- Reevaluate range of motion for intraarticular sources of FAI, such as femoral neck asphericity or acetabular rim prominence. Trim the head and neck as necessary, starting with the femoral head. Trim the acetabular rim if any FAI persists.
- Check for any impingement of the lesser trochanter (with the ischium or posterior acetabulum).
- Determine the exact location of the chondral damage on the femoral head by dividing the head into eight sections, four anterior, and four posterior (Fig. 32-35). Include articular cartilage lesions, labral lesions, OCD lesions, and incongruent protrusions that were resected.
- Check functional radiographs intraoperatively to determine any joint incongruity and to determine if a proximal femoral osteotomy needs to be performed. Indications for a valgus osteotomy is a nonspherical femoral head with good congruency in an adducted view.
- Check the amount of correction that could be obtained by a pelvic acetabular osteotomy. An indication for a pelvic acetabular osteotomy is an associated secondary acetabular dysplasia (defined as a lateral center-edge angle of less than 25 degrees).
- Perform trochanteric advancement for relative lengthening of the femoral neck (see Technique 32-12).
- Perform a valgus osteotomy (Figure 32-36) or a pelvic acetabular osteotomy (Technique 32-6) as indicated.
- Reduce the hip and place in a neutral position in a soft splint.

POSTOPERATIVE CARE. Remove suction drains at 48 hours. Mobilize the patient with crutches and partial weight bearing (15 kg). Restrict active and passive abduction and adduction to protect the trochanteric osteotomy. Use low-molecular-weight heparin for 8 weeks to avoid deep vein thrombosis.

VALGUS EXTENSION OSTEOTOMY

One residual of Legg-Calvé-Perthes disease is a malformed femoral head with resulting hinged abduction. Hinged abduction of the hip is an abnormal movement that occurs when the deformed femoral head fails to slide within the acetabulum. A trench is formed laterally, adjacent to a large uncovered portion of the deformed head anterolaterally. With the aid of image intensification, Snow et al. recognized late anterior impingement of the femoral head in four patients with Legg-Calvé-Perthes disease, all of whom had late-onset pain triggered by internal rotation. Three of the four patients were found to have articular surface damage and osteochondral projections at the area of anterior impingement. Arthroscopic debridement and proximal femoral osteotomies relieved symptoms in all four patients. More recently, Raney et al. described valgus subtrochanteric osteotomy for malformed femoral heads with hinge abduction. All were classified Catterall III and IV with previous failed treatment. At 5-year follow-up, 62% had satisfactory results. We use a valgus extension osteotomy, as described by Catterall, fixed with a pediatric screw and side plate (Fig. 32-36) to relieve this obstruction.

Sequelae of Legg-Calvé-Perthes n=53

- Femoral pathomorphology n=53 (100%)
  - Intraarticular n=53 (100%)
    - Cam n=39 (74%) → SHD ± resection n=38 (72%)
    - Femoral head induced piner n=14 (26%) → SHD ± resection ± head/neck reduction n=13 (25%)
    - Functional retrotorsion n=20 (38%) → SHD ± resection ± valgus/flexion osteotomy n=16 (30%)
  - Extraarticular n=47 (89%)
    - Greater trochanter n=47 (89%) → SHD ± relative neck lengthening n=42 (79%)
    - Lesser trochanter n=4 (8%) → SHD ± distalization n=3 (6%)
- Acetabular pathomorphology n=43 (81%)
  - Dysplasia n=25 (47%) → PAO n=11 (21%)
  - Acetabular retroversion n=29 (55%) → Rim trimming ± anteverting PAO n=21 (40%)
  - Incongruity n=20 (38%) → ± Femoral osteotomy ± acetabular osteotomy n=8 (15%)

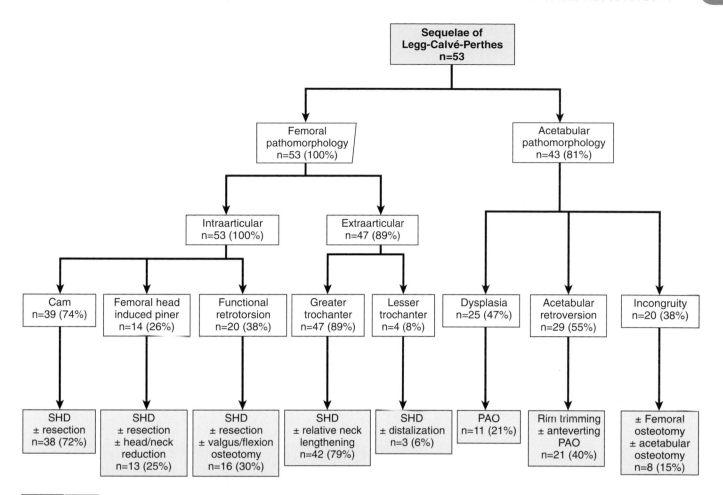

FIGURE 32-34 Morphologic analysis with corresponding surgical treatment algorithm of hips with pathomorphologic sequelae of Legg-Calvé-Perthes disease. SHD, surgical hip dislocation; PAO, periacetabular osteotomy. (From: Albers CE, Steppacher SD, Ganz R, Siebenrock KA: Joint-preserving surgery improves pain, range of motion, and abductor strength after Legg-Calvé-Perthes disease. Clin Orthop Relat Res 470:2450, 2012.)

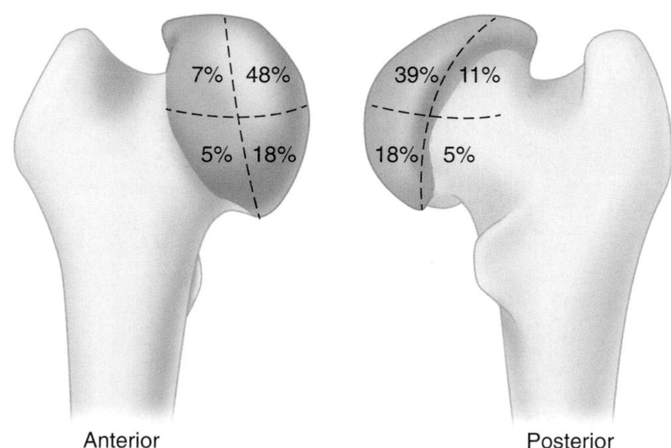

FIGURE 32-35 Numbers represent frequency of chondral damage found in each of the eight sectors in study by Albers et al. (From Albers CE, Steppacher SD, Ganz R, Siebenrock KA: Joint-preserving surgery improves pain, range of motion, and abductor strength after Legg-Calvé-Perthes disease. Clin Orthop Relat Res 470:2450, 2012.) **SEE TECHNIQUE 32-11.**

VALGUS FLEXION INTERNAL ROTATION OSTEOTOMY

Kim and Wenger, using three-dimensional CT in Legg-Calvé-Perthes disease, noted "functional retroversion" rather than femoral anteversion. As a result, they recommended a valgus flexion, internal rotation femoral osteotomy plus a simultaneous acetabuloplasty in patients with severe femoral head deformity. The combined procedure (1) corrects the functional coxa vara and hinge abduction (valgus osteotomy); (2) establishes a more normal articulation between the posteromedial portion of the true femoral head and the acetabulum, while moving the anterolateral protruding portion of the femoral head away from the anterolateral acetabular margin (valgus-flexion osteotomy); (3) corrects external rotation deformity of the distal limb (internal rotation osteotomy); and (4) improves joint congruity and anterolateral femoral head coverage in hips with associated acetabular dysplasia.

SHELF PROCEDURE

If the hip is congruous, a Staheli or Catterall shelf augmentation procedure (see Chapter 30) is performed for coxa magna and lack of acetabular coverage for the femoral head.

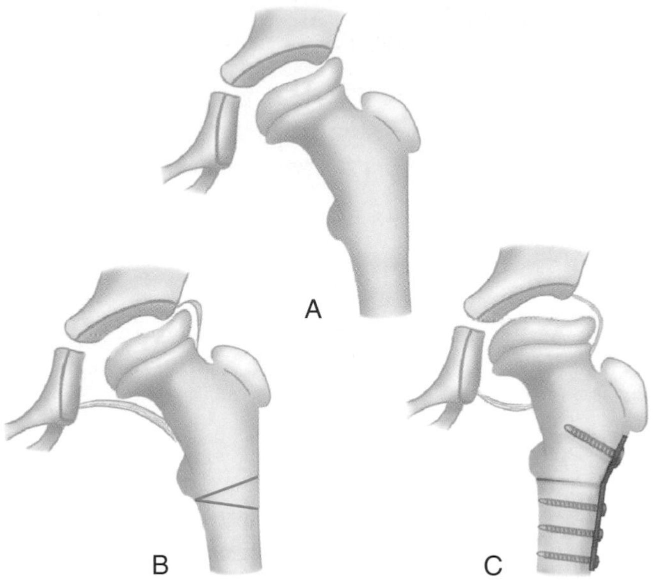

FIGURE 32-36 A-C, Valgus osteotomy to reduce hinge abduction and increase flexion of hip; osteotomy is fixed with pediatric screw and side plate.

CHIARI OSTEOTOMY

We have used the pelvic osteotomy described by Chiari as a salvage procedure to accomplish coverage of a large flattened femoral head in an older child when the femoral head is subluxating and painful (Fig. 32-37). It is described in detail in Chapter 30.

TROCHANTERIC OVERGROWTH

Although trochanteric overgrowth can be caused by numerous conditions, including osteomyelitis, fracture, and congenital dysplasia, it occurs in Legg-Calvé-Perthes disease when the disease causes premature closure of the capital femoral physis. Whatever the mechanism, the result is the same: arrest of longitudinal growth of the femoral neck with continuation of growth of the greater trochanter (Fig. 32-38). According to Wagner, the functional consequences are always the same: elevation (overgrowth) of the trochanter decreases tension and mechanical efficiency of the pelvic and trochanteric muscles; shortening of the femoral neck moves the greater trochanter closer to the center of rotation of the hip, decreasing the lever arm and mechanical advantage of the muscles, and impairing muscular stabilization of the hip; the line of pull of the muscles becomes more vertical, increasing the pressure forces concentrated over a diminished area of hip joint surface; and impingement of the trochanter on the

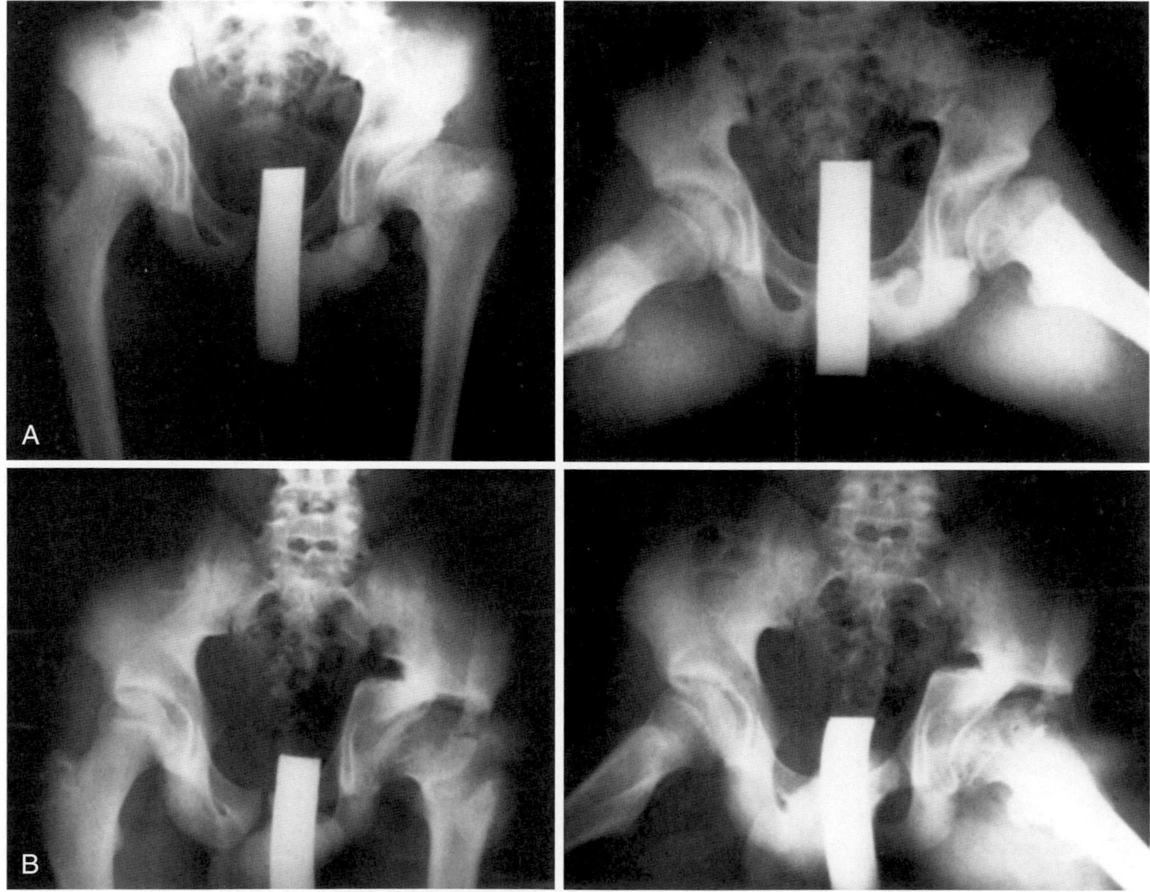

FIGURE 32-37 Chiari osteotomy for residual Legg-Calvé-Perthes disease. **A,** Residual Legg-Calvé-Perthes disease (coxa plana) and subluxation in hip on right. **B,** Eight months after Chiari osteotomy with good coverage of femoral head.

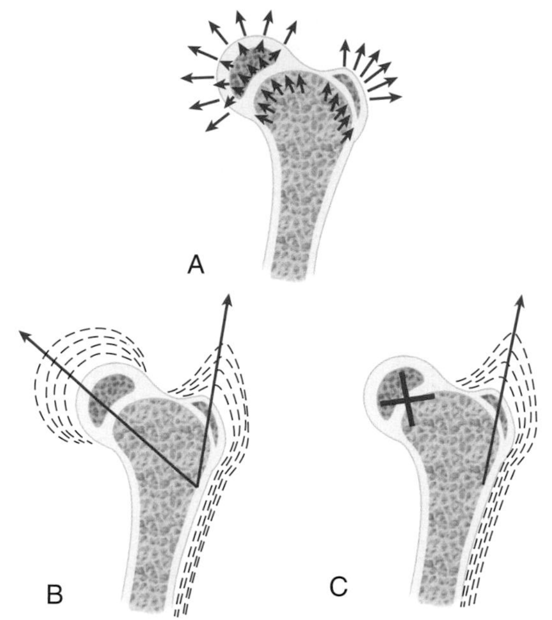

FIGURE 32-38 **A** and **B**, Growth of proximal femur; *arrows* indicate site and direction of growth. **C**, If growth potential is impaired, longitudinal growth is arrested but greater trochanter continues to grow.

rim of the acetabular roof during abduction limits range of motion. Macnicol and Makris described a "gearstick" sign of trochanteric impingement that is useful in the preoperative evaluation. This sign is based on the observation that hip abduction is limited by impingement of the greater trochanter on the ilium when the hip is extended but full abduction is possible when the hip is fully flexed. The "gear stick" sign is especially useful for differentiating between trochanteric impingement and other causes of limited abduction. Transfer of the greater trochanter distally restores normal tension to the trochanteric muscles and improves mechanical efficiency, puts a more horizontal pull on the pelvic and trochanteric muscle action to distribute forces over the hip joint more uniformly, and increases the length of the femoral neck to increase abduction and decrease acetabular impingement.

Premature closure of the proximal femoral physis often occurs after Legg-Calvé-Perthes disease and may limit abduction and produce gluteal insufficiency. Trochanteric advancement has been advocated for the late treatment of Legg-Calvé-Perthes disease and is thought to improve gluteal efficiency and increase the range of abduction, which was limited by impingement of the trochanter on the ilium. With surgical dislocation of the hip, the greater trochanter is routinely osteotomized. If trochanteric advancement is necessary, Ganz, Mills and Novales have described an extended retinacular soft-tissue flap that protects the blood supply to the femoral head and allows for a relative lengthening of the femoral neck. The greater trochanter is advanced distally such that its tip is in line with the center of the femoral head. Fixation is secured with two or three 3.5- or 4.5-mm screws (see Technique 32-12). Alternative methods of treatment include abduction valgus osteotomy of the femur and trochanteric epiphysiodesis. Trochanteric epiphyseodesis does not appear to change the radiographic appearance but according to some authors reduces the Trendelenburg gait.

TROCHANTERIC ADVANCEMENT FOR TROCHANTERIC OVERGROWTH

TECHNIQUE 32-12

(WAGNER)

- With the patient supine, approach the hip through a lateral incision. Incise the fascia lata longitudinally and release the vastus lateralis from the greater trochanter.
- Retract the gluteus medius muscle posteriorly, and insert a Kirschner wire superiorly, parallel to the femoral neck and greater trochanteric physis and pointing toward the trochanteric fossa (Fig. 32-39A). Confirm the placement of the guidewire by image intensification. Internally rotating the hip slightly aids placement of the wire and allows better imaging.
- Make the osteotomy parallel to the Kirschner wire with a low-speed oscillating saw, completing it proximally with a flat osteotome (Fig. 32-39B). Pry open the osteotomy until the medial cortex fractures (Fig. 32-39C and D).
- Mobilize the greater trochanter first cephalad, and with dissecting scissors remove any adhesions, joint capsule, and soft tissue flush with the medial surface of the trochanter, sparing the blood vessels in the trochanteric fossa (Fig. 32-39E).
- When the greater trochanter is freed, transfer it distally and laterally. If excessive anteversion is present, it also can be transferred anteriorly.
- Using an osteotome, freshen the lateral femoral cortex to which the trochanter is to be attached. Place the trochanter against the lateral femoral cortex and check the position with image intensification. According to Wagner, the tip of the greater trochanter should be level with the center of the femoral head, and the distance between them should be 2 to 2.5 times the radius of the femoral head.
- When proper position is confirmed, fix the greater trochanter with two screws inserted in a cephalolateral to caudad direction (Fig. 32-39F). These screws, with washers, should compress an area of bony contact between the trochanter and femur. Bury the screw heads by retracting all soft tissues to prevent soft-tissue necrosis and local mechanical irritation from occurring postoperatively. Wagner uses a supplemental strong tension band suture that he believes helps absorb tensile forces from the pelvic and trochanteric muscles and prevents trochanteric avulsion; we have not found this suture to be necessary.
- No postoperative immobilization is required if the patient is compliant and the fixation is secure.

POSTOPERATIVE CARE. Ambulation on crutches is begun at 7 days, but active exercises of the pelvic and trochanteric muscles are not permitted until 3 weeks. Sitting upright and flexing the hip also should be avoided because overpull of the gluteus medius muscle may cause loss of fixation.

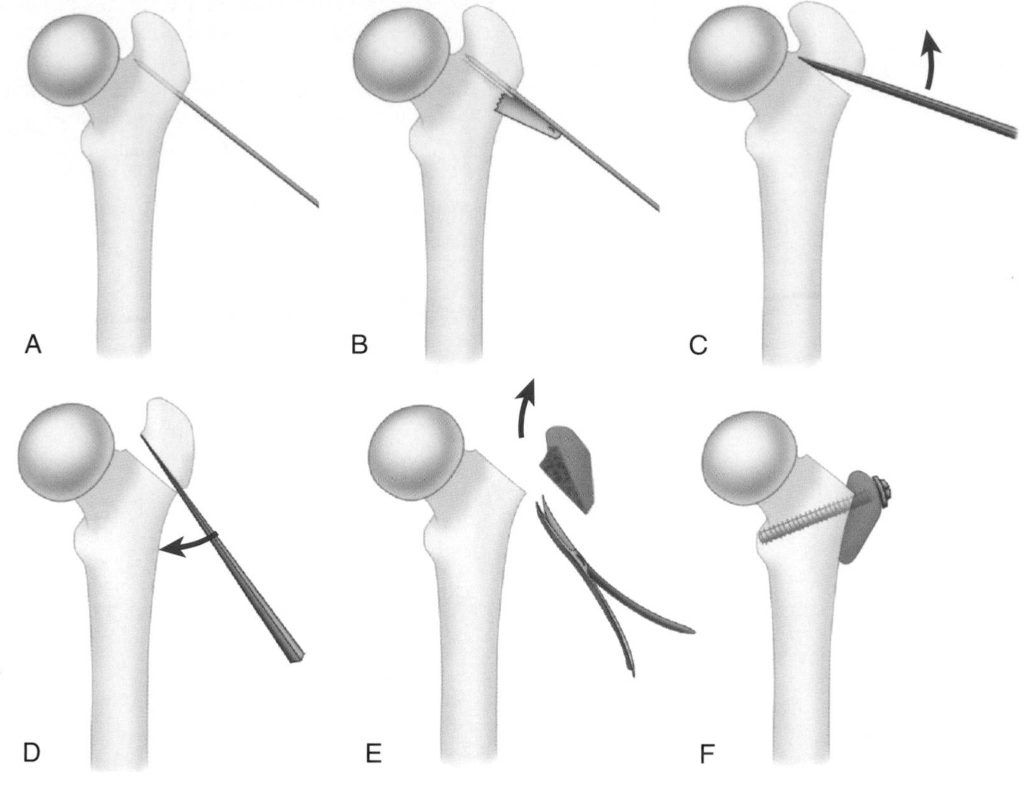

FIGURE 32-39 **A-F,** Trochanteric advancement for trochanteric overgrowth (see text). **SEE TECHNIQUE 32-12.**

TROCHANTERIC ADVANCEMENT FOR TROCHANTERIC OVERGROWTH

TECHNIQUE 32-13

(MACNICOL AND MAKRIS)

- Approach the greater trochanter through a straight lateral incision under lateral image intensification.
- With a power saw, divide the base of the trochanter in line with the upper border of the femoral neck. Mobilize the trochanteric fragment and the gluteal muscles from their distal soft-tissue attachment.
- Remove a thin wedge of bone from the posterolateral femoral cortex (Fig. 32-40) to provide a cancellous bone bed for the transferred trochanter and to ensure that the trochanter does not project too far laterally. Any undue prominence would cause friction of the fascia lata and produce discomfort and bursitis.
- Fix the trochanter with two compression screws to prevent rotation of the fragment and to allow early partial weight bearing.

POSTOPERATIVE CARE. A spica cast is not used, but patients walk with crutches by the end of the first post-operative week. Exercises to promote movement are introduced gradually, but upright sitting, abduction, flexion, and internal rotation are not forced.

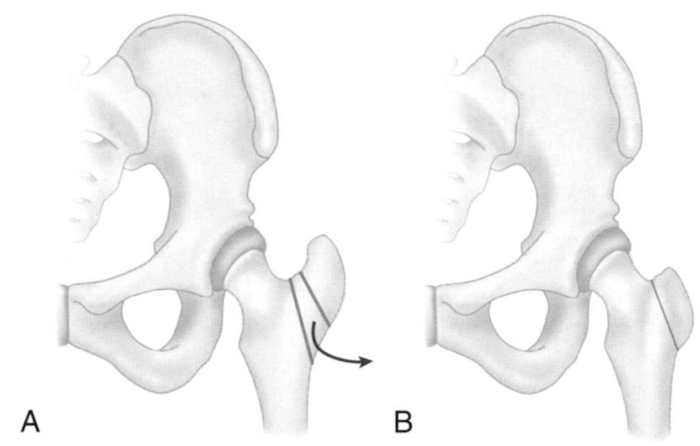

FIGURE 32-40 **A and B, After initial osteotomy of greater trochanter, trapezoidal wedge of bone is removed.** (Redrawn from Macnicol MF, Makris D: Distal transfer of the greater trochanter, J Bone Joint Surg 73B:838, 1991.) **SEE TECHNIQUE 32-13.**

GREATER TROCHANTERIC EPIPHYSIODESIS FOR TROCHANTERIC OVERGROWTH

TECHNIQUE 32-14

- Approach the physis of the greater trochanter through a lateral incision and determine its location and orientation by inserting a Keith needle. If necessary, use radiographs to confirm its position.

- Use a small drill bit to outline the four corners of a rectangle that spans the lateral portion of the greater trochanteric epiphysis. Remove this lateral rectangle of cortical bone with osteotomies.
- Curet the physis, reverse the rectangle of bone, and replace it in its bed.
- Internal fixation is unnecessary.

POSTOPERATIVE CARE. Postoperative cast immobilization is not required unless curettage has been so vigorous that the physis of the greater trochanter has been excessively disrupted. Weight bearing is progressed as tolerated.

OSTEOCHONDRITIS DISSECANS OF THE HIP

Osteochondritis dissecans of the hip occurs most frequently after Legg-Calvé-Perthes disease; it rarely occurs as an isolated entity, although a recent report speculated that it might be caused by FAI. In children, loose bodies secondary to Legg-Calvé-Perthes disease, osteonecrosis of sickle cell disease, and multiple epiphyseal dysplasia have to be ruled out before this can be established as an isolated diagnosis. In adults, idiopathic osteonecrosis, Gaucher disease, and occult trauma, such as a torn acetabular labrum, have to be considered in the differential diagnosis.

Unless the fragment interferes with hip mechanics, treatment of osteochondritis dissecans of the hip after Legg-Calvé-Perthes disease should be conservative (Fig. 32-41).

In an asymptomatic child with osteochondritis dissecans of the hip, restriction of activity and prolonged observation are indicated to allow healing and revascularization.

Operative treatment is indicated for severe lesions with disabling symptoms. The choice of operative procedure depends on the extent and location of the lesion, the age and activity expectations of the patient, and the presence of degenerative joint changes. Surgical dislocation of the hip as described by Ganz and others may be necessary (see Chapter 6). Good results have been reported in small series of patients who had open or arthroscopic excision of the fragment, internal fixation of the fragment, curettage or drilling, and arthroscopic removal of loose osteocartilaginous fragments. Recently, fresh stored osteochondral grafts have been used as well. None of these procedures is recommended if severe osteoarthritic changes are present, and a procedure to redirect the femoral head (e.g., valgus extension osteotomy) is preferred.

In addition to removal of an osteochondritis lesion, arthroscopy of the hip may be indicated for synovial biopsy, removal of loose bodies, removal of debris and inspection of the labrum after fracture-dislocation, and partial or total synovectomy. If the lesion is not anterior or anterolateral, it is difficult to see, and longitudinal traction should be used to increase the visibility of posterior or posterolateral lesions. A fracture table and image intensification are helpful in judging the correct amount of distraction and joint penetration. Anterior portals are used most often, but the lateral portals may be necessary for more posteriorly located lesions. Arthroscopy of the hip is described in Chapter 51.

HEMOPHILIA

Elective surgery for patients with classic hemophilia (factor VIII deficiency), hemophilia A and Christmas disease (factor IX deficiency), or hemophilia B has become possible and reasonable with the availability of factor VIII and factor IX concentrates. Previously, only lifesaving surgery was performed and mortality was high. Wound hematomas with massive sloughs and infection were common. Catastrophic complications can be minimized only by expert management and strict control of the clotting mechanism, and surgery in patients with hemophilia must not be undertaken casually. Bracing and casting techniques, such as the spring-loaded Dynasplint, can be used along with physical therapy to protect joints or to stretch soft-tissue contractures. These measures may be as important as hematologic management in avoiding surgery.

The current popularity of home therapy for hemophilic patients with self-administration of factor VIII or IX as soon as periarticular stiffness and pain occur may result in a lower incidence of degenerative arthritis and in fewer indications for major reconstructive procedures. Factor given prophylactically from age 1 or 2 years through adolescence (preventing the factor VIII concentration from decreasing to <1 of normal) seems to prevent hemophilic arthropathy, and only minor joint defects have been noted. The National Hemophiliac Foundation recommends prophylactic factor; however, prophylactic factor given daily has to be given intravenously, which increases the possibility of contamination and infection. Also, the use of ultrasound to determine early soft-tissue bleeds has been recommended to aid in the use of prophylactic factor.

Three changes have been noted regarding surgery in hemophiliacs: (1) decrease in the need for surgery, (2) increase in the age of the patient, and (3) changes in types of operations. The indications for surgery include the following:

1. Chronic, progressive hypertrophic synovial enlargement from repeated hemarthrosis that cannot be controlled by adequate factor replacement; preferably, synovectomy is done before the cartilage becomes thin and at least some of the articular cartilage is preserved. Timely synovectomy also may decrease the incidence of hemorrhage into the joint. This can be done by intraarticular radioisotope injection, arthroscopically, or with an open procedure.
2. Severe soft-tissue contractures that have not responded to nonoperative measures (e.g., a knee flexion contracture that is so severe that serial casting or a turn-buckle casting technique causes subluxation of the knee joint); supracondylar osteotomy of the femur has been beneficial in this instance, provided that 70 to 80 degrees of knee motion remains and the contracture is not so severe that correction would result in excessive traction on the neurovascular bundle in the popliteal space. For correction of a knee flexion contracture of less than 45 degrees after conservative measures have failed, good results have been reported with hamstring release and posterior transverse capsulotomy. Correction by osteotomy of a contracture of more than 50 to 60 degrees probably should be done in stages and preferably after physeal closure.

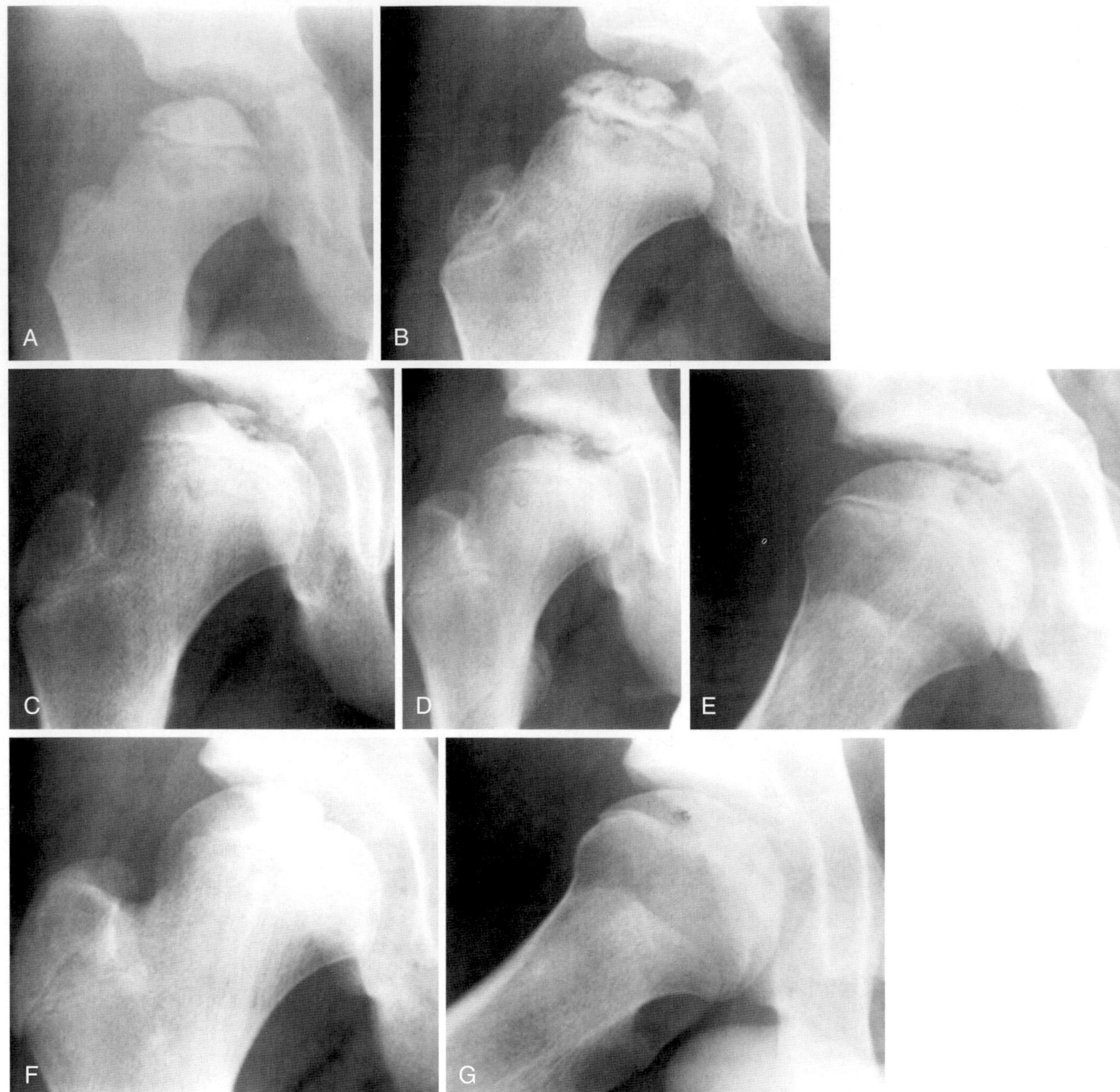

FIGURE 32-41 Osteochondritis dissecans of hip. **A,** Onset of Legg-Calvé-Perthes disease in 6-year-old patient. **B,** Fourteen months later, fragmentation and reossification stage. **C,** Persistent defect 5 years after onset. **D,** Osteochondritic lesion at 7 years with some evidence of healing. **E,** Lateral radiograph during same period shows osteochondritic lesion. Note air arthrogram with smooth cartilage surface. **F,** At 8 years defect is healing. **G,** Lateral radiograph at same time shows no evidence of defect.

3. A bony deformity severe enough to require osteotomy.
4. An expanding hematoma (pseudotumor) that continues to enlarge despite adequate factor replacement and possibly radiation therapy.
5. Useless or chronically infected extremities (amputation).
6. Severe arthritic changes with incapacitating pain and hemorrhage (total joint arthroplasty) (Fig. 32-42).

Successful surgery in hemophilia depends on a close working relationship between the orthopaedist and an experienced hematologist. All hematologic aspects of the patient's care must be the responsibility of the hematologist, including a hematologic team consisting of a hematologic nurse, surgeon, and physical therapist.

The hemorrhagic disorder must be diagnosed accurately before surgery is contemplated. Correct replacement of coagulation factors cannot be undertaken without precise identification and quantitation of the missing factor. Adequate reserve supplies of concentrate must be available in advance, and the supporting laboratory must be able to perform unlimited assays for the factor. It also is essential to determine within a few days of the operation whether the patient has developed an inhibitor against his or her deficient factor because the inhibitor hinders hematologic therapy and may

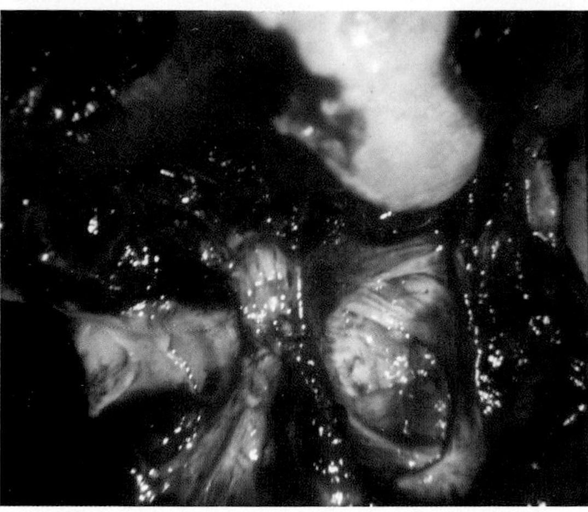

FIGURE 32-42 Damaged knee joint with hemophilia (factor VIII deficiency). *Upper right,* Marked destruction and erosion of articular surface of femoral condyle. *Center,* Anterior cruciate ligament and intercondylar notch. Tibial plateaus are grossly eroded, and articular surfaces and menisci are destroyed by invasion of synovium.

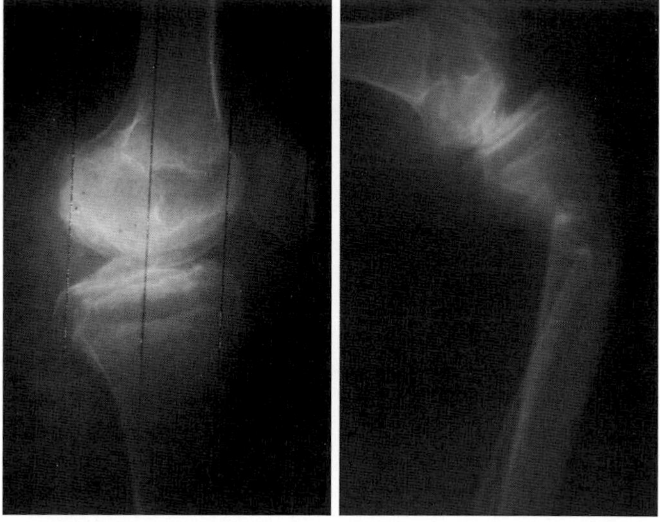

FIGURE 32-43 Late complications of hemophilic arthropathy. Note osteopenia and resulting fractures owing to manipulation.

eliminate the possibility of elective or semielective surgery. A bypass agent (described below) should be available at the time to counteract an inhibitor. In addition, a factor assay should be obtained at the time of surgery. The hematocrit should be measured for several days after surgery, especially in blood groups A, B, and AB, because a Coombs-positive hemolytic anemia may develop. The patient's HIV and hepatitis status should be known before surgery. In patients with HIV or hepatitis, the extent of involvement should be investigated. T lymphocyte counts and other parameters should be known to determine the ability to heal and the potential for infection. Fortunately, HIV and hepatitis that were prevalent in the 1990s have almost disappeared in the hemophiliac population because of the use of "clean" factor.

Post and Telfer emphasized meticulous surgical technique and detailed preoperative evaluation in this surgery. They recommended (1) as many procedures at one surgical session as the patient can tolerate—this reduces the times that the patient is at risk of bleeding complications and hepatitis and reduces the high cost of the concentrate and the possibility of inducing an inhibitor; (2) meticulous aseptic technique and pneumatic tourniquets whenever possible; (3) tight, careful wound closure to avoid dead space; (4) avoidance of electrocautery because of the tendency of the coagulated areas to slough after surgery; (5) wound suction in deep wounds for a minimum of 24 hours; (6) no aspirin or other medications postoperatively that inhibit platelet function; and (7) as far as possible, no intramuscular injections postoperatively for pain relief.

When coagulation is controlled with hematologic therapy, wound slough or infection usually does not occur. Pain relief and a substantial decrease in recurrent bleeding into joints usually result.

With the availability of factor, elective orthopaedic surgery can be safely performed utilizing a multidisciplinary team approach; however, an inhibitor is a life-threatening risk factor and a major risk factor for infection. Factor VII and IX "bypassing" agents have been used to counteract inhibitors and obtain hemostatic control after surgery. With the use of recombinant activated factor VII (RFVIIa) and plasma activated prothrombin complex concentrates (pd-APCC), elective orthopaedic surgery is a viable option for hemophiliac patients with inhibitors. For minor surgery (100%) and for major surgery (85-100%) coagulation, a bolus of the RFVIIa usually is given with continuous infusion. This "inhibitor" surgery should not be taken lightly and should only be performed with an experienced hematologist team at a specialized hemophiliac center.

TOTAL JOINT ARTHROPLASTY

Synovectomy or total knee arthroplasty (see Chapter 7) may be cost effective in that the cost of hematologic maintenance (concentrate) is markedly lower after surgery. Total knee arthroplasty should be considered only if hemophilic arthritis is advanced and range of motion is adequate because the arthroplasty is unlikely to increase motion. Careful examination of the quadriceps mechanism and correction of any flexion contracture of more than 30 degrees are recommended before surgery. We also suspect that late complications similar to those seen in rheumatoid arthritis would develop because of disuse osteopenia (Fig. 32-43). Because most candidates for total knee arthroplasty in hemophilic arthropathy are relatively young, all other means of relieving the symptoms should be attempted first, such as hyaluronic acid injection (viscosupplementation) in milder disease, radiosynovectomy, or arthroscopic synovectomy. Most often, both knees are involved, and bilateral arthroplasties are indicated, although arthrodesis of one knee and total knee arthroplasty of the other is a reasonable alternative to bilateral arthroplasty, provided that motion in the knee selected for arthroplasty is 80 to 90 degrees preoperatively.

Reports in the literature, although not conclusive, state that hemophiliac patients are less prone to venous thrombosis because of their disease than the normal population, and the same is true for those undergoing major orthopaedic surgery, including synovectomy and total joint replacement. Even so, a postoperative compression device, early ambulation, and joint mobilization with physical therapy are recommended. Routine use of antithrombotic agents prophylactically is controversial and not recommended in the face of an inhibitor. The exception is the hemophiliac patient undergoing major orthopaedic surgery with risk factors for venous thrombosis, such as a history of venous thromboembolism, obesity, malignancy, and varicose veins, or women with von Willebrand disease taking oral contraception. If prophylaxis is for venous thrombosis, enoxaparin has been used successfully.

Surgical infection in this patient population is related to lack of meticulous technique and the amount and length of time factor is given. Most series report an 8% infection rate if factor is given less than 2 weeks and much lower than 8% if given for 2 weeks with the patient 100% "covered." Continuous factor should be given for 2 weeks after total knee or total hip arthroplasty at 100%.

Total hip arthroplasty (see Chapter 7) is an appropriate operation for disabling hemophilic hip arthropathy. In the shoulder or elbow, we have little or no experience with arthroplasty in these joints in hemophiliacs. In the ankle, there are several small series in the literature of total ankle arthroplasty being done in hemophiliacs with encouraging results.

SYNOVECTOMY

Although synovectomy of joints can decrease pain and the number of bleeding episodes in patients with hemophilia, it does not seem to alter the course of joint destruction. We performed 16 synovectomies of the knee in 14 children, adolescents, and young adults with hemophilia. Pain was eliminated or decreased in all patients, and the number of bleeding episodes dramatically decreased in all patients at 3-year follow-up. Some knee motion was lost in five patients. At long-term follow-up (average 9 years) of nine of these patients (11 knees), decreases in pain and frequency of bleeding episodes were sustained, but arthropathy had progressed in all 11 knees, and 8 knees had lost motion compared with short-term follow-up. A disturbing finding in this group of patients was that at long-term follow-up all nine were either HIV positive or had developed acquired immunodeficiency syndrome (AIDS). Fortunately, HIV contaminated factor has virtually been eliminated.

Both open and arthroscopic synovectomies of the knee in patients with "classic" hemophilia can reduce hemarthrosis; however, the arthroscopic procedure seems to be less complete but have less morbidity. Although arthroscopy may require a longer operative time, it requires shorter hospitalization and less factor replacement.

The elbow is a frequent site (second only to the knee) of repeated hemorrhage followed by enlargement of the radial head and degenerative arthritis of the radiocapitellar and ulnar-trochlear articulations. We have been pleased with the pain relief resulting from synovectomy of the elbow joint and excision of the radial head. Improvement in flexion and extension of the elbow cannot be expected, but increased forearm rotation frequently results.

Synovectomy also has proved beneficial for hemophilic arthropathy of the ankle. Open synovectomy or arthroscopic synovectomy can be performed (see Chapter 50) because removal of the posterior synovial tissue from the crypts of the malleoli is difficult and may injure the articular cartilage even with the use of the posterolateral portal and distraction of the joint arthroscopically may be difficult.

Ankle, knee, and elbow arthroscopic synovectomy are described in Chapters 50 to 52.

Radionuclide synovectomy, or synoviorthesis (destruction of synovial tissue by intraarticular injection of a radioactive agent), has produced encouraging results. The procedure has little morbidity and can be done on an outpatient basis in the radiology department. The isotope appears to shrink the outer layer of synovium, decreasing pain, bleeding, and the recurrence rate.

Improved range of motion and decreased frequency of hemorrhage have been reported in nearly 80% of adult patients treated with synoviorthesis of the elbow or knee using chromic phosphate P32 and 0.5 to 1 mCi of yttrium-90 silicate, depending on the joint involved. New isotopes using Holmium-166-chitosan 186Re complex have been advocated. In situations where radioisotopes are not available, chemical synovectomy can be used with rifampicin. Two to three injections may be necessary (at 6-month intervals), and if not successful then a surgical synovectomy should be performed. Synoviorthesis appears to be most effective when done early, before the synovium enlarges. Because most recurrent joint hemorrhages begin in early childhood, this procedure would be useful in the prevention of bony joint damage in children with hemophilia who have developed chronic hemarthrosis or synovitis. The long-term effects on joints in children, such as premature physeal closure or irritation, are not known. Most of the literature recommends radioisotope synovectomy at age 12 or older using yttrium-90 at a dose of 90 mBq in children, viscosupplementation with stearic acid and joint lavage, or Holmium-16-chitosan complex. If not effective, chemical synovectomy with rifampicin can be used. If needed earlier than 12 years, a surgical synovectomy should be performed. The long-term effects on joints in children, such as premature physeal closure or tumor formation, are unknown, however. Two patients with hemophilia who developed acute lymphoblastic leukemia after radionuclide synovectomy have been reported.

In our experience, short-term results of radionuclide synovectomy of the ankle and knee in children and adults have been encouraging because the nuclide seems to be able to penetrate posteriorly; however, the recurrence rate (need for a second synoviorthesis) seems to be higher than for open or arthroscopic synovectomy.

SYNOVECTOMY OF THE KNEE IN HEMOPHILIA

TECHNIQUE 32-15

- Inflate a pneumatic tourniquet around the thigh.
- Through a medial parapatellar incision (see Technique 1-38), remove as much synovium from the knee capsule as possible. Removal of all synovium from the lateral gutter is extremely difficult, and considerable hemorrhage usually occurs in this area.
- Remove synovium from the medial joint space, including over and around the medial meniscus and collateral

ligament. Remove synovium from the intercondylar notch and anterior cruciate ligament and finally from the lateral joint space.
- Release the tourniquet and obtain meticulous hemostasis with electrocautery; this may require more time than the removal of the synovium.
- Tightly close the capsule and soft tissues in layers to obliterate any dead space; insert a closed suction drainage tube.
- If the medial capsule is redundant, oversew it to prevent recurrent dislocation of the patella.

POSTOPERATIVE CARE. The knee is immobilized for 24 hours, then motion is initiated with the aid of the physical therapist and a continuous passive motion machine, if available. The drain is removed at 48 hours under adequate clotting factor replacement. Physical therapy is continued for 6 weeks; the continuous passive motion machine can be used at home.

ARTHROSCOPIC SYNOVECTOMY

Arthroscopic synovectomy is described in Chapter 51.

SYNOVIORTHESIS FOR TREATMENT OF HEMOPHILIC ARTHROPATHY

TECHNIQUE 32-16

- Replacement therapy for hemostasis at the time of the synoviorthesis is the same as that used for minor operations. For patients in whom an inhibitor is present, synoviorthesis is sometimes done without preparation for hemostasis.
- Using aseptic technique, anesthetize the skin with 2% procaine (without epinephrine) with a 23-gauge needle. Note free flow of procaine indicating the introduction of the needle into the intraarticular space.
- Withdraw synovial fluid when possible.
- Inject 2 to 5 mL of contrast medium and with radiography ensure there is no obvious leak from the synovial space. Inject colloidal chromic phosphate P32 (Phosphocol P32) intraarticularly.
- Use 1 mCi for knees and 0.5 mCi for other joints.
- Flush the needle with 2% lidocaine and remove.
- Apply a sterile plastic bandage and an appropriate immobilizer.

POSTOPERATIVE CARE. The patient can bear weight immediately, but activity should be decreased for 48 hours.

OPEN ANKLE SYNOVECTOMY

Transfusion of the missing clotting factor (factor VIII or IX) is based on the previously described protocol. Approximately 2 hours before the operation, the patient is given a transfusion to increase the level of the deficient clotting factor to close to 100%. Open synovectomy of the ankle is done through anteromedial, anterolateral, and posterior incisions.

OPEN ANKLE SYNOVECTOMY IN HEMOPHILIA

TECHNIQUE 32-17

(GREENE)
- Place a sandbag underneath the ipsilateral buttock to facilitate positioning of the ankle for the anterior portion of the synovectomy.
- Make an anteromedial incision 3 cm long just medial to the anterior tibial tendon.
- Retract the anterior tibial tendon laterally and retract the branches of the saphenous vein medially.
- Make a longitudinal incision in the joint capsule. Preserve the capsule even though it is stretched and attenuated by the underlying hypertrophic synovial tissue because its presence may facilitate postoperative rehabilitation. Free the joint capsule from the adherent synovial tissue by sharp dissection.
- Remove all visible synovial tissue. Use small pituitary rongeurs to remove folds of synovial tissue that extend into the crypts between the talus and the medial malleolus.
- Make a 3-cm long anterolateral incision centered just lateral to the peroneus tertius tendon and retract this tendon medially.
- Open the joint capsule longitudinally and excise the synovial tissue in the same manner described for the anteromedial incision.
- Resect the folds of synovial tissue interposed between the talus and the lateral malleolus.
- Remove the sandbag beneath the ipsilateral buttock and place it beneath the contralateral buttock before making the posterior incision. Make a posterior incision approximately twice as long as the anterior incision and center it between the medial malleolus and the Achilles tendon. Open the sheath of the posterior tibial tendon so that it can be retracted adequately. Dissect the other posterior tendons and the neurovascular structures away from the posterior portion of the capsule of the ankle joint.
- Place a retractor lateral to the flexor hallucis muscle and medial to the posterior tibial tendon, permitting retraction of the soft-tissue structures located posterior to the ankle joint. This provides full exposure of the posterior portion of the capsule. Incise the capsule horizontally from the medial malleolus to the distal end of the fibula.
- Dissect the insertion of synovial tissue on the talus and the distal end of the tibia. Use pituitary rongeurs to remove any residual folds of synovial tissue lying in the crypts of the malleoli. If the synovium cannot be removed from the capsule, or the capsule appears intimately involved, removal of large sections of the capsule may be necessary. According to Greene, postoperative rehabilitation may be impeded by extensive scar reaction in the posterior capsule.

- When the synovectomy has been completed, deflate the pneumatic tourniquet and secure hemostasis meticulously.
- Repair the anterior portion of the capsule but leave the posterior portion open and place a drain. Close the wounds in a standard fashion and immobilize the ankle joint in a neutral position with a bulky dressing augmented by a plaster of Paris splint.

POSTOPERATIVE CARE. Patients who have factor VIII deficiency should receive continuous transfusion therapy, and patients with factor IX deficiency should be given a bolus of factor IX every 12 hours. Transfusion should be continued throughout the hospital stay (7 to 10 days). After discharge, transfusion is given three times a week for 4 weeks. This regimen keeps the deficient clotting factor level sufficiently elevated to minimize the risk of a spontaneous hemarthrosis during the immediate postoperative period while the soft-tissue reaction is resolving. The drain is removed on the first postoperative day, and active range-of-motion exercises with the aid of hydrotherapy are begun on postoperative day 2. Initially, weight bearing is not permitted. Also, the ankle is intermittently splinted in a neutral position until range of motion of the ankle from neutral dorsiflexion to 25 degrees of plantar flexion is obtained. The hematologist and the surgeon determine discharge from the hospital. Walking with crutches with touch-down weight bearing is continued for approximately 5 weeks after discharge from the hospital.

ARTHRODESIS

Arthrodesis of the ankle (see Chapter 11), shoulder (see Chapter 13), and knee (see Chapter 8) has been satisfactory in small series of patients with hemophilia. The use of internal fixation rather than external fixators that require transcutaneous pins is recommended to reduce bleeding and infection around the pins (Fig. 32-44). Fixed flexion contractures can be corrected by removing appropriate bone wedges at the time of arthrodesis.

OSTEOTOMY

For hemophilic patients with symptomatic bony deformities, osteotomies may be necessary. In patients with symptomatic genu varum deformities, proximal valgus closing wedge osteotomies may be done (see Chapter 9).

COMPLICATIONS OF HEMOPHILIA

A rare, yet disabling and frequently life-threatening complication, iliac hemophilic pseudotumor occurs in 1% to 2% of patients with factor VIII deficiency. Two types of pseudotumors have been identified: one occurs primarily in the femur or pelvis in adults and has an exceptionally poor prognosis, and one occurs more distally in the extremities in children and has a better prognosis. Recommended treatment includes factor replacement, immobilization, close observation, and avoidance of cyst aspiration. Operative resection for the adult-type pseudotumor may be life threatening, and amputation should be considered. Preoperative consideration of the tumor size and degree of infiltration is crucial in operative management. Early excision eliminates the possibility of endogenous infection. Partial resection of huge tumors that leave the lateral wall intact for compression and recovery of function may be preferable to excision of the entire wall, leaving a huge dead space that allows massive hematoma and sepsis. Several studies have shown early promising results using radiation for pseudotumors that are inaccessible or inappropriate for resection.

In addition to involvement of various joints, nerve lesions are common in patients with hemophilia. Katz et al. described 81 such peripheral nerve lesions. The femoral nerve was the most commonly involved, followed by the median nerve and the ulnar nerve. In 49% of the lesions, the nerves had full motor and sensory recovery after significant bleeds. In 34%, a residual sensory deficit (normal motor) was present, and in 16% persistent motor and sensory deficits were present. Patients who had inhibitors to factor VIII were significantly less likely to recover full motor or sensory function than patients who did not have antibodies, and time to full motor recovery in these patients was significantly longer.

Hemophilia-related AIDS was first reported in the United States in 1981. Current estimates of the percentage of hemophilic patients with HIV antibodies range from 30% to 90%. Before 1985, it was estimated that 90% of patients seen in hemophiliac clinics were HIV positive, and a large percentage of patients also had laboratory evidence of hepatitis. The Centers for Disease Control and Prevention estimated that 9000 hemophiliacs, or 45% of the hemophiliac population, contracted AIDS and that 1900 patients died as the result of AIDS. The screening for the presence of HIV in blood and blood products for transfusion since 1985 and the development of monoclonal antibodies to factor VIII and of synthetically derived blood products have decreased the rate of transmission markedly. Because of this increased risk of HIV infection in hemophilic patients, albeit now small, orthopaedic surgeons treating these patients should observe not only the universal precautions recommended by the Centers for Disease Control and Prevention but also the recommendations of the American Academy of Orthopaedic Surgeons Task Force on AIDS and Orthopaedic Surgery.

RICKETS, OSTEOMALACIA, AND RENAL OSTEODYSTROPHY

Rickets is the bony manifestation of altered vitamin D, calcium, and phosphorus metabolism in a child; osteomalacia is the adult form. There are multiple causes of rickets and osteomalacia, but, regardless of the cause of the abnormal metabolism, children with rickets have similar long bone and trunk deformities.

Because vitamin D deficiency has become less common in the United States, rickets and osteomalacia are not often considered as differential diagnoses in patients who have extremity pain or deformity. According to Clark et al., the children now at greatest risk for vitamin D deficiency are "white, breastfed, protected from the sun, and obese." Rickets can manifest as atypical muscle pain, a pathologic fracture, or slipped capital femoral epiphysis. The orthopaedist should remain familiar with the radiographic and laboratory findings that accompany these diseases. When treating patients

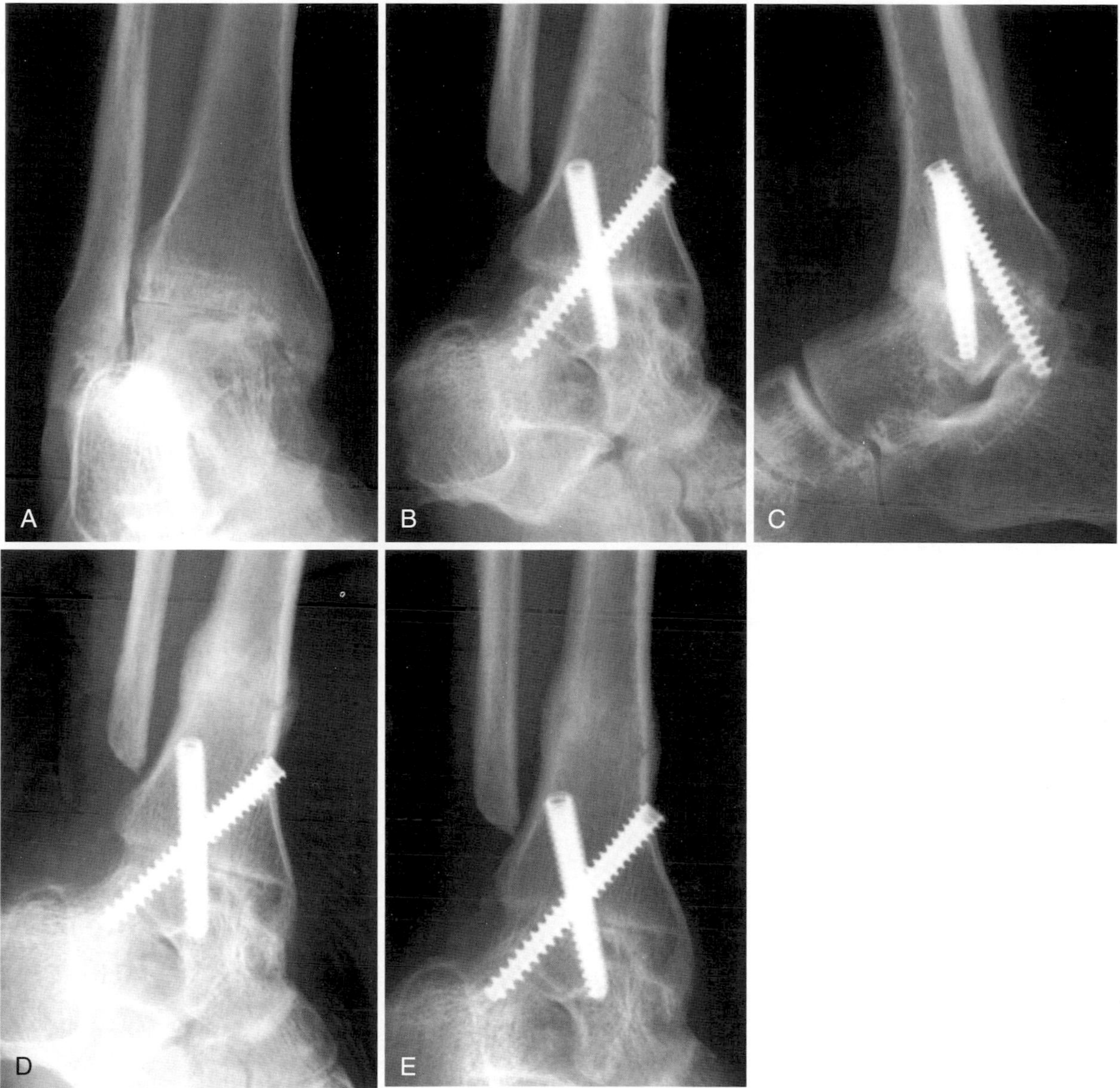

FIGURE 32-44 A, Preoperative radiograph of severe hemophilic arthropathy and painful swollen ankle. B and C, Postoperative radiographs of cross-threaded screw fixation. At 6 months, distal tibial pain and stress fracture are noted. D, At 12 months, stress fracture callus is noted but no pain. E, At 24 months, there is solid fusion. Stress fracture has resolved.

with rickets, osteomalacia, or renal dystrophy, the orthopaedist always must be concerned about the effect treatment may have on impaired calcium homeostasis.

In very young children with deformity, treatment of the metabolic defect supplemented by corrective splinting or bracing may correct the deformity (Fig. 32-45). In prepubertal children or adolescents, medical management and bracing usually do not correct an established deformity, and early osteotomy is indicated to ensure that the joints are in a position of function if they became stiff.

Before surgery, management of the metabolic defect with vitamin D, phosphorus, and calcium or other appropriate measures should be done for several months. If the disease is not controlled metabolically, the deformity is likely to recur after corrective osteotomy. Treatment with large doses of vitamin D should be discontinued for at least 3 weeks before surgery, however, because otherwise hypercalcemia is likely to occur with immobilization.

If a water-soluble preparation of vitamin D, such as dihydrotachysterol, is used instead of cholecalciferol that is stored in the liver, the period without medication before surgery can be shortened. In addition, in hypophosphatemic vitamin D–resistant rickets, if the disease is controlled by using inorganic phosphate plus 50,000 U or less of vitamin D per day, symptoms of hypercalcemia during the immediate postoperative period are less likely to occur, even if the preoperative vitamin D medication is not discontinued. We recommend stopping the administration of vitamin D 3 weeks before surgery, however, because hypercalcemia can cause severe symptoms of anorexia, nausea, vomiting, weight loss, confusion, and seizures. Mobilization of the patient as quickly as possible after surgery to allow early resumption of medical treatment

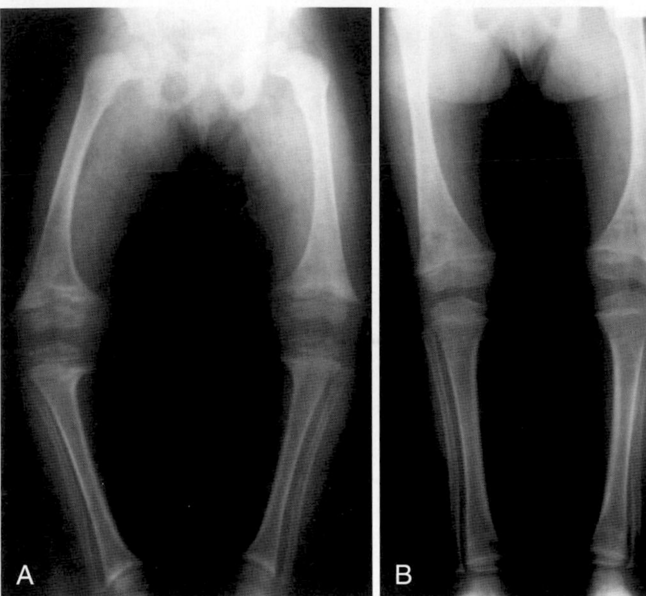

FIGURE 32-45 Vitamin D–deficient rickets. **A,** Standing radiograph of young child with nutritional rickets from vitamin D deficiency. **B,** Same child 18 months later after treatment with vitamin D and braces.

would prevent delayed mineralization of the healing osteotomy and avoid recurrence of deformity with continued growth. When deformity is severe in older children, and there has been no previous medical treatment, after complete diagnostic studies are made, and if the patient does not have azotemic osteodystrophy, it may be better to proceed with the surgery with the patient in a less than homeostatic but compensated metabolic condition rather than to load the patient preoperatively with high doses of vitamin D, calcium, and phosphorus and run the risk of hypercalcemia and extraosseous calcification, especially in the kidney.

With azotemic osteodystrophy, expert preoperative and postoperative medical management is essential and ideally is done by a special team trained in the treatment of chronic renal failure. Correction of anemia, adequate hydration, uremia control, and electrolyte balance are required for safe administration of anesthesia. Peritoneal dialysis or hemodialysis may be required before surgery. If attention is given to detail, children with azotemic osteodystrophy can undergo orthopaedic surgery successfully. Requisites for surgery are a reasonable life expectancy, an intelligent and motivated patient and parents, demonstrated improvement of bone lesions on medical management, deformities that can be corrected with one or two orthopaedic procedures, and the likelihood that the surgery would significantly reduce the patient's disability. Surgery for children with renal osteodystrophy and knee deformities is feasible, but careful surgical planning and preoperative metabolic stabilization are essential. Use of an external fixator can allow precise correction of the deformities without interruption of medical management. Patients with resistant hypertension usually have short life expectancies and should not be considered as surgical candidates. In addition, when parathyroid autonomy is present and not controlled by parathyroidectomy and medical treatment, surgery is not indicated.

The deformities that require surgical correction most often are genu varum and genu valgum. In genu varum, usually the femur, tibia, and fibula all are deformed, often the latter two more severely; there is not only lateral bowing but also internal torsion. Osteotomy of the tibia and the fibula near the apex of the most severe bowing usually is required. Sometimes osteotomy of the femur also is necessary (Fig. 32-46). Osteotomies can be done bilaterally at one operation.

In genu valgum, most of the bowing usually is in the femur, and a severe deformity in older children and in adults can be corrected by supracondylar osteotomy of the femur. The goal of tibial and femoral osteotomies should be correction of deformity and alignment so that the plane of each knee joint is perfectly horizontal with the patient standing.

The techniques of osteotomy are described in Chapter 9.

TIBIA VARA (BLOUNT DISEASE)

Erlacher is credited with the first description of tibia vara and internal tibial torsion (1922), but it was Blount's article in 1937 that prompted recognition of this disorder. Blount described tibia vara as "an osteochondrosis similar to coxa plana and Madelung deformity but located at the medial side of the proximal tibial epiphysis." Currently, tibia vara is considered an acquired disease of the proximal tibial metaphysis, however, rather than an epiphyseal dysplasia or osteochondrosis. The exact cause is unknown, but enchondral ossification seems to be altered. Suggested causative factors include infection, trauma, osteonecrosis, and a latent form of rickets, although none of these has been proved. A combination of hereditary and developmental factors is the most likely cause. Weight bearing must be necessary for its development because it does not occur in nonambulatory patients, and the relationship of early walking and obesity to Blount disease has been clearly documented. Because of the "obesity epidemic" and vitamin D deficiency in children in the United States, it has been speculated that the number of cases of Blount disease will rise.

Although the exact cause of tibia vara is controversial, the clinical and radiographic findings are consistent. The abnormality is characterized by varus and internal torsion of the tibia and genu recurvatum. Blount distinguished, according to age at onset, two types of tibia vara: infantile, which begins before 8 years of age, and adolescent, which begins after 8 years of age but before skeletal maturity. The infantile form is difficult to differentiate from physiologic bowing common in this age group, especially before the age of 2 years. Infantile tibia vara is bilateral and symmetric in approximately 60% of affected children; physiologic bowing is almost always bilateral. In Blount disease, the varus deformity increases progressively, whereas physiologic bowing tends to resolve with growth.

Although not nearly as common as the infantile form, adolescent Blount disease has been divided into two types: (1) an adolescent form occurring between ages 8 and 13 years caused by partial closure of the physis after trauma or infection and (2) "late-onset" tibia vara that occurs in obese children, especially black children, between ages 8 and 13, without a distinct cause. The marked similarity of histologic changes that occur in patients with late-onset tibia vara and

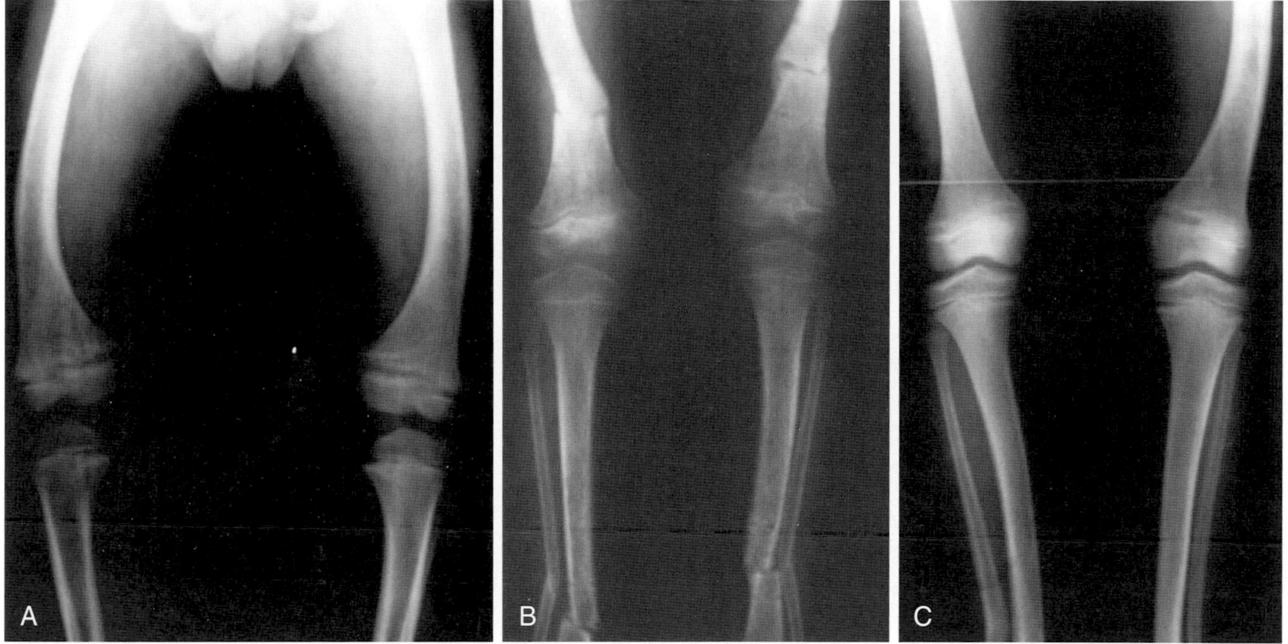

FIGURE 32-46 Vitamin D–resistant rickets. **A,** Child before treatment has deformities in distal femurs. Tibias are not shown in this film. **B,** Three months after valgus osteotomies of distal femurs and tibias using pins incorporated in plaster above and below osteotomy sites. **C,** Two years after osteotomies vitamin D–resistant rickets is well controlled with large doses of vitamin D, calcium, and phosphorus. No deformities have recurred.

in patients with infantile tibia vara and slipped capital femoral epiphysis suggests a common cause for these conditions.

In tibia vara, characteristically the medial half of the epiphysis as seen on radiographs is short, thin, and wedged; the physis is irregular in contour and slopes medially. The proximal metaphysis forms a projection medially that is often palpable, but this projection is not diagnostic of tibia vara. Medial metaphyseal fragmentation *is* pathognomonic for the development of a progressive tibia vara. The angular deformity occurs just distal to the projection. MRI studies reveal other soft-tissue abnormalities: (1) increased thickness of the chondroepiphysis of the proximal medial aspect of the tibia, (2) increased height and width of the medial meniscus (increased sign in the posterior horn), and (3) abnormal medial femoral epiphysis.

Langenskiöld noted progression of epiphyseal changes and the deformity through six stages with growth and development (Fig. 32-47). At stage VI, the medial portion of the epiphysis fuses at a 90-degree downward angle.

Normally, the tibiofemoral angle progresses from pronounced varus before the age of 1 year to valgus between ages 1.5 and 3 years. Several authors have suggested that deviation from normal tibiofemoral angle development indicates Blount disease, and the metaphyseal-diaphyseal angle is an early indicator of Blount disease. In one study, most children with metaphyseal-diaphyseal angles of 11 degrees or more developed Blount disease, whereas children with angles of less than 11 degrees had physiologic bowing that resolved with growth. This measurement is not an absolute prognosticator of Blount disease, but a metaphyseal-diaphyseal angle of more than 11 degrees warrants close observation (Fig. 32-48). Because of rotation, the Drennan angle is believed by some to be unreliable, although excellent interobserver reliability has been noted, and other angle measurements have been suggested: MRI to predict late resolution of tibial bowing, length of the fibula compared with the tibia, and the severity of proximal tibial angulation compared with distal femoral angulation. Although other angles of the femur and

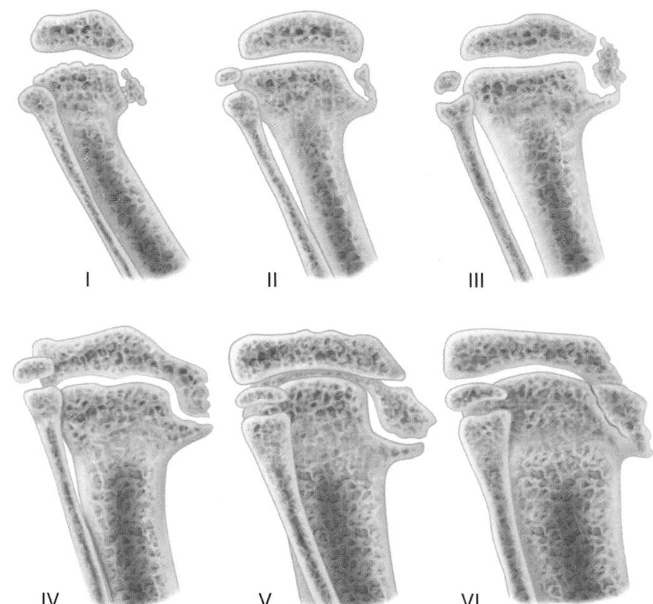

FIGURE 32-47 Diagram of radiographic changes seen in infantile type of tibia vara and their development with increasing age. (From Langenskiöld A, Riska EB: Tibia vara (osteochondrosis deformans tibiae): a survey of seventy-one cases, J Bone Joint Surg 46A:1405, 1964.)

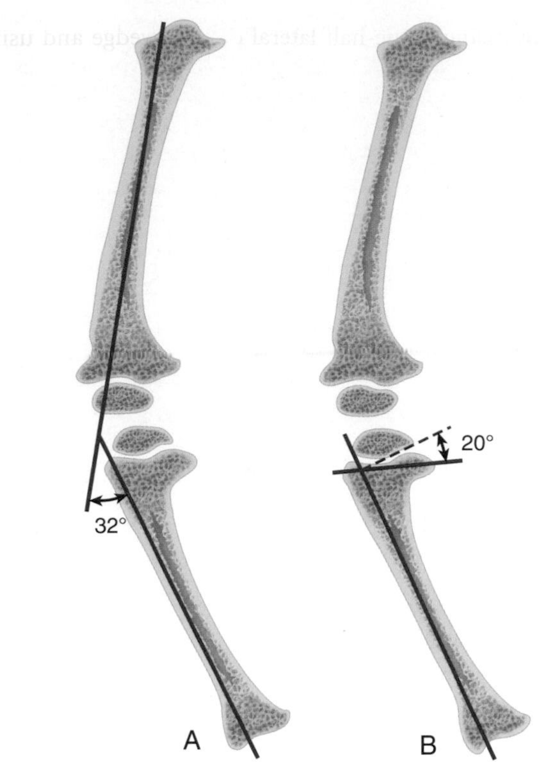

FIGURE 32-48 **A,** Tibiofemoral angle is formed by lines drawn along longitudinal axes of tibia and femur. **B,** Metaphyseal-diaphyseal angle is formed by line drawn perpendicular to longitudinal axis of the tibia and line drawn through two beaks of metaphysis to determine transverse axis of tibial metaphysis. (Redrawn from Levine A, Drennan J: Physiological bowing and tibia vara: the metaphyseal-diaphyseal angle in measurement of bowleg deformities, J Bone Joint Surg 64A:1158, 1982.)

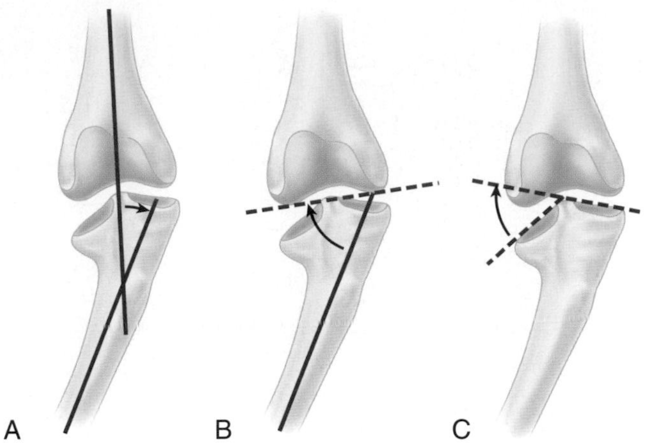

FIGURE 32-49 **A,** Angle formed by femoral shaft and tibial shaft. **B,** Angle formed by femoral condyle and tibial shaft. **C,** Depression of medial plateau of tibia. (From Schoenecker PL, Johnston R, Rich MM, et al: Elevation of the medial plateau of the tibia in the treatment of Blount disease, J Bone Joint Surg 74A:351, 1992.)

tibia at the knee can be determined (Fig. 32-49), when the deformity is present, most authors agree that the mechanical axis of the limb, as it relates to the tibiofemoral angle on radiographs, should be the most functional measurement of the amount of deformity present (Fig. 32-50).

Kline et al. described femoral varus as a significant deformity of late-onset Blount disease. They showed an average deformity of 10 degrees of femoral varus more than the calculated ideal femoral-tibial joint angle. This represented 34% to 76% of the genu varum deformity of the affected limbs. Gordon and Schoenecker recommended that calculations be made on standing long-film radiographs to determine the amount of excessive femoral varus and that this should be corrected by femoral osteotomy or epiphyseodesis at the time of tibial osteotomy to avoid a subsequent compensatory deformity.

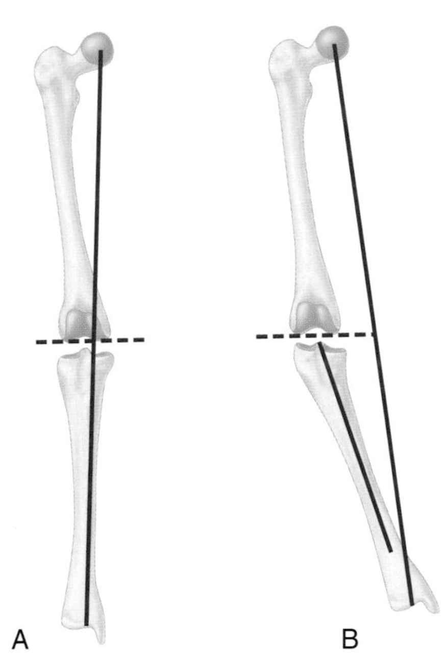

FIGURE 32-50 Mechanical axis of limb as it relates to angle formed by femoral condyle and tibial shaft. **A,** Normal alignment. Angle formed by femoral condyle and tibial shaft is approximately 90 degrees. **B,** Tibia vara. Angle formed by femoral condyle and tibial shaft is less than 90 degrees. (From Schoenecker PL, Johnston R, Rich MM, et al: Elevation of the medial plateau of the tibia in the treatment of Blount disease, J Bone Joint Surg 74A:351, 1992.)

Focal fibrocartilaginous dysplasia has been reported as a cause of tibia vara in a few patients. Bell described the characteristic radiographic appearance and unilateral nature of this lesion of the proximal medial metaphysis. Later reports suggest that this generally is a self-limiting condition that corrects spontaneously (Fig. 32-51) and that severe progression should be documented before valgus osteotomy is done. The proximal tibial physis has the potential to correct the deformity in the adjacent metaphysis, depending on the age of the patient and the severity of the deformity. Osteotomy is indicated only for significant deformity in an older child when spontaneous correction no longer can be expected. Infantile tibia vara resulting from slipping of the proximal tibial epiphysis has been described. It appears to be an atraumatic "slip" of the proximal tibial epiphysis on the metaphysis in severely obese children. Radiographically, the condition is

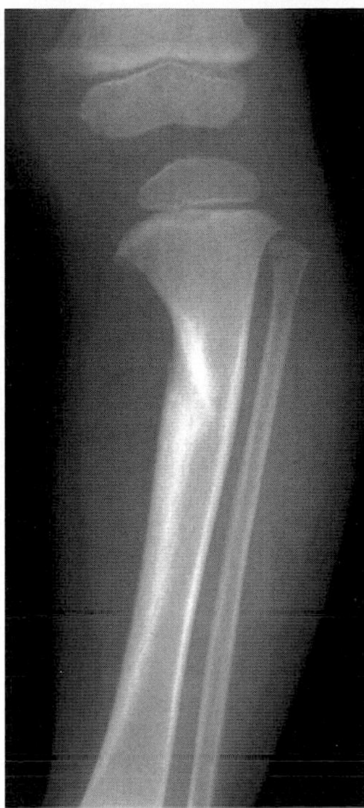

FIGURE 32-51 Fibrocartilaginous dysplasia in proximal tibia with resultant varus deformity simulating "bowlegs" of Blount disease.

characterized by a dome-shaped metaphysis, an open growth plate, and disruption of the continuity between the lateral borders of the epiphysis and metaphysis, with inferomedial translation of the proximal tibial epiphysis. It is important to recognize this entity because of the differences in treatment between it and conventional Blount disease.

The treatment of Blount disease depends on the age of the child and the severity of the varus deformity. Generally, observation is indicated for children between ages 2 and 5 years, but progressive deformity usually requires osteotomy. Recurrence of the deformity is not as frequent after osteotomy at an early age as after osteotomy when the child is older, with recurrence rates of about 80% reported in older children compared with less than 20% in younger children. Beaty et al. reported that early osteotomy (2 to 4 years old) produced the best results, with only one of their 10 patients having recurrence of the deformity. Conversely, of 12 patients in whom osteotomy was done after age 5 years, 10 (83%) had recurrence of the deformity necessitating repeated osteotomy. They recommended valgus osteotomies of the proximal tibia and fibula with mild overcorrection in young children.

Rab described a proximal tibial osteotomy for Blount disease in which a single-plane oblique cut allows simultaneous correction of varus and internal rotation and permits postoperative cast wedging if necessary to obtain appropriate position. More recently, Laurencin et al., in an effort to avoid neurovascular and physeal complications, described an oblique incomplete closing wedge osteotomy fixed with a lateral tension plate. Greene also described a chevron osteotomy in which opening and closing wedges can be made so that the limb-length deformity present in moderate to severe tibia vara is not increased. He prefers a crescent-shaped osteotomy, using a one-half lateral closing wedge and using the graft medially in an opening wedge to maintain length. Internal fixation of the graft often is necessary.

One cause of recurrence of the deformity after osteotomy is a physeal bar. Greene listed the following criteria for deciding if CT studies should be done preoperatively to determine if a bony bar is present: (1) age older than 5 years, (2) medial physeal slope of 50 to 70 degrees, (3) Langenskiöld grade IV radiographic changes, (4) body weight greater than the 95th percentile, and (5) black girls who meet the previous criteria. Bony bridge resection should be considered in children with remaining growth potential and can be done in conjunction with tibial osteotomy if angulation is significant.

In children older than age 9 years with more severe involvement, osteotomy alone, with bony bar resection, or with epiphysiodesis of the lateral tibial and the fibular physes may be indicated. Medial physeal bar resection alone has been reported to be effective when premature closure of the physis is evident, but significant angular deformity would not be corrected by bar resection alone. Lateral tibial epiphysiodesis can be done, with or without osteotomy, after the age of 9 years but before skeletal maturity. In unilateral involvement, epiphysiodesis of the uninvolved leg may be indicated to correct leg-length discrepancy. Several reports in the literature have described lateral guided growth correction (manipulation) with temporary epiphysiodesis for infantile Blount disease with tension band plates (eight-plate technique). The results have been satisfactory in selected patients but with the following observations: (1) recurrence of the deformity after plate removal is secondary to a slower growth rate of the medial physis; (2) mechanical failure of the tension band plate screws can occur in those who are obese, and, if in doubt, four screws or two eight-plates can be used; and (3) tension band plates are as effective as staple hemiepiphysiodesis for guided correction of growth with respect to rate of correction and complications.

For older patients in whom bracing and tibial osteotomy have failed to prevent progressive deformity, and when the risk of abnormal spontaneous medial epiphysiodesis is great, as evidenced by severe disorderly enchondral ossification, an intraepiphyseal osteotomy to correct severe joint instability and a valgus metaphyseal osteotomy to correct the varus angulation may be indicated.

An essential element of this procedure is reconstruction of the horizontal level of the medial tibial plateau. This method is for considerable depression of the medial femoral condyle within the defect of the tibial epiphyseal bone and when there is the possibility of a bony bridge between the metaphysis and epiphysis of the medial tibia. In addition to elevation of the depressed medial tibial plateau, metaphyseal valgus osteotomy may be needed to correct alignment of the tibia (Fig. 32-52).

Zayer described a hemicondylar tibial osteotomy through the epiphysis, but not through the physis, into the intercondylar notch (Fig. 32-53). This method corrects the medial slope of the tibial epiphysis while avoiding the physis. Because obesity, unequal limb lengths, and femoral deformity often are present in patients with Blount disease, external fixation, including the Taylor spatial frame, may be indicated to achieve stability after osteotomy and immediate correction and seems to be an excellent method of treating an extremely obese patient for whom unilateral or especially bilateral

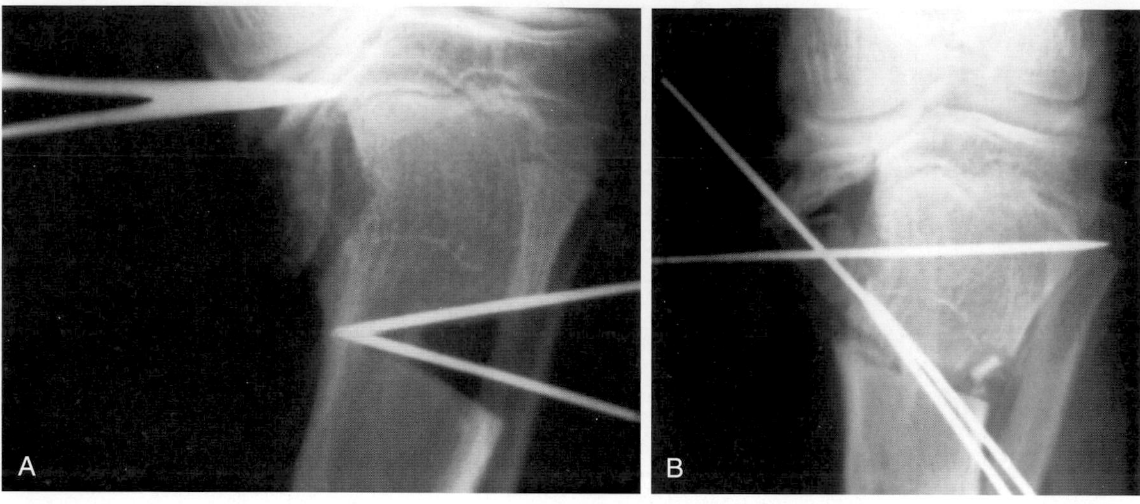

FIGURE 32-52 Severe Blount disease. **A,** Closing wedge metaphyseal osteotomy. **B,** Epiphyseal elevation. **SEE TECHNIQUE 32-20.**

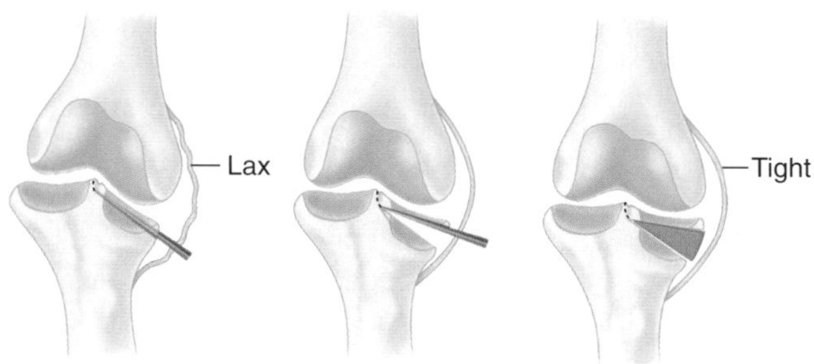

FIGURE 32-53 Hemicondylar osteotomy. (From Zayer M: Hemicondylar tibial osteotomy in Blount's disease: a report of two cases, Acta Orthop Scand 63:350, 1992.)

casting is impractical. A uniplanar external fixator also can be used especially for isolated frontal one-plane deformities with satisfactory results. The advantages seem to be ease of application, adjustability, early weight bearing, the ability to lengthen the extremity, and avoiding a second operation to remove the hardware (Fig. 32-54). The Ilizarov technique is effective for correction of deformity and lengthening if needed in adolescent patients. This technique allows adjustment of limb alignment postoperatively, if necessary, to obtain a perfect mechanical axis. Fixation of the tibia is achieved through four proximal and four distal wires that are affixed to rings and tensioned. Half-pin modifications also can be used.

OSTEOTOMIES

The oblique osteotomy described by Rab begins at a point distal to the tibial tubercle, proximal to the posterior tibial metaphysis, and just distal to the physis and is done through a cosmetic transverse incision. Fasciotomy and fibular osteotomy are done through a separate incision. Because rigid internal fixation is not used, postoperative adjustments through cast wedging are possible.

Correction is obtained by rotating around the face of the oblique osteotomy and can be described best by considering the individual cuts in their anatomic planes (Fig. 32-55). Correction of a purely rotational deformity requires an osteotomy in the transverse plane, whereas purely varus or valgus correction requires osteotomy in the frontal (coronal) plane. An oblique osteotomy, directed from anterodistal to posteroproximal, splits the difference between the transverse and frontal planes. Rotation with its two faces in contact corrects varus and internal rotation. Osteotomy cuts that are more vertical (frontal) correct more varus than internal rotation. More horizontal (transverse) cuts do the opposite. According to Rab, patients with Blount disease have almost equal amounts of varus and internal rotation and in practice a 45-degree upward osteotomy provides adequate correction in most patients. He reported simultaneous correction of varus deformity of 44 degrees and internal rotation of 30 degrees. A quick estimate of the osteotomy angle when different degrees of external rotation and valgus correction are required is provided in Figure 32-56. A mathematic model of the osteotomy rotations is shown in Figure 32-57.

METAPHYSEAL OSTEOTOMY FOR TIBIA VARA

TECHNIQUE 32-18

(RAB)

- Prepare and drape the patient in the usual manner and apply and inflate a tourniquet.
- Make a transverse incision at the lower pole of the tibial tubercle (Fig. 32-58A). Make a Y-shaped incision in the periosteum and dissect periosteally (including the pes anserinus insertion medially) until malleable or Blount retractors can be placed behind the tibia (Fig. 32-58B). Elongate the periosteal incision distally, if necessary, to obtain subperiosteal protection posteriorly.
- Place a small Steinmann pin at a 45-degree angle 1 cm distal to the tibial tubercle and advance it under image intensifier control until it passes just into the posterior

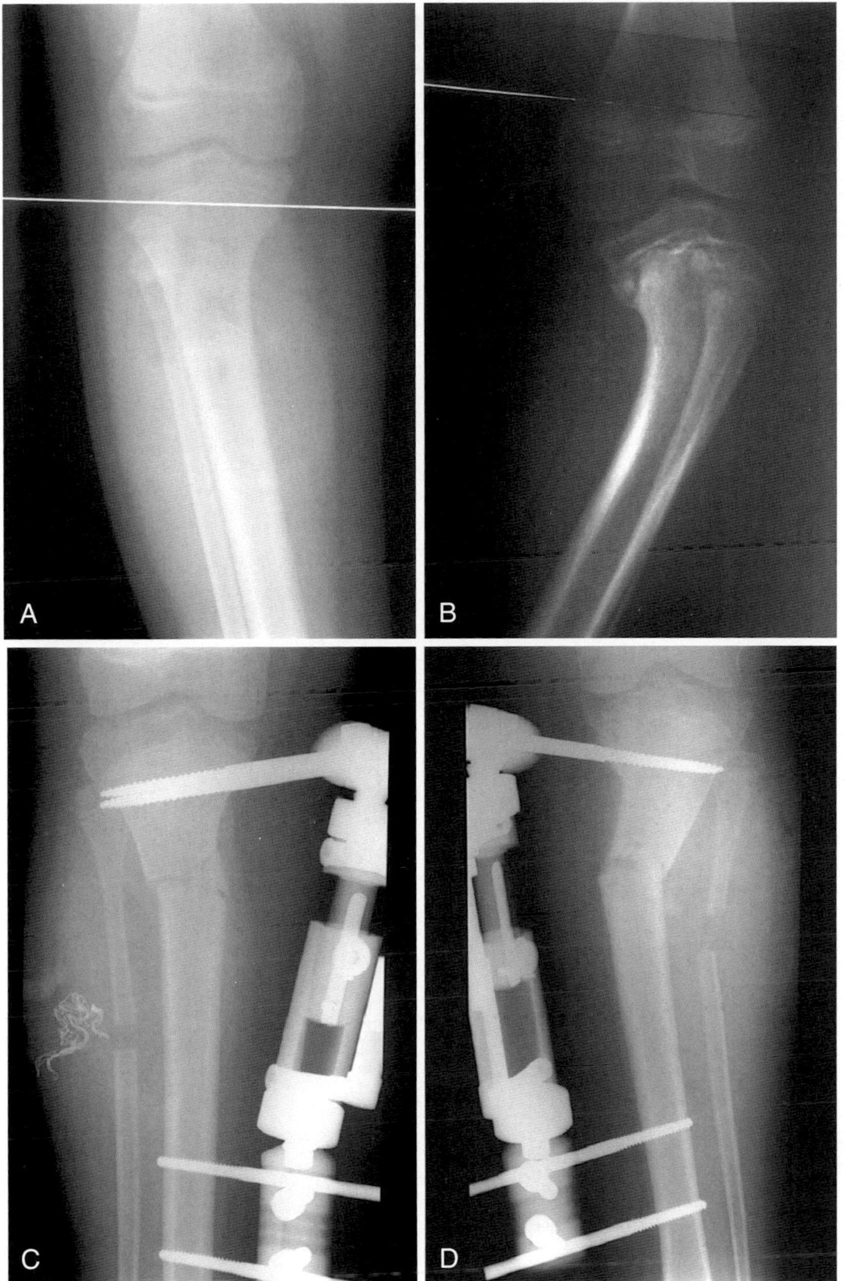

FIGURE 32-54 **A** and **B,** Anteroposterior radiographs of severe bilateral tibia vara in obese adolescent. **C** and **D,** Radiographs of unilateral frame external fixators after metaphyseal osteotomies.

cortex (Fig. 32-58C). Ensure the pin is distal to the physis at the posterior cortex on the image intensifier view. Measure the pin length and use a marking pen or Steri-strip to mark the same length on the osteotomes and sagittal saw blades (Fig. 32-58D). This serves as a reminder of the saw depth and can indicate if a lateral image intensifier exposure is appropriate.

- With the saw and osteotome, carefully make the osteotomy cut immediately distal to the Steinmann pin, checking frequently with image intensification (Fig. 32-58E). As the cut nears completion, it may be helpful to make some of the cut from the anteromedial side of the tibia where subperiosteal exposure is better.
- Make a second small incision over the midfibula and excise a 1- to 2-cm subperiosteal segment of the fibula. Move the tibial osteotomy back and forth to free some of the posterior periosteum from the fragments.
- Drill a hole in the anteroposterior direction across the osteotomy cut lateral to the tibial tubercle. Rotate the osteotomy on its face by external rotation and valgus rotation (in Blount disease), overcorrecting if necessary. Through the drill hole, secure the osteotomy with a single 3.5-mm cortical or cancellous lag screw overdrilled anteriorly (Fig. 32-58F). Do not overtighten this screw.
- Perform a subcutaneous fasciotomy between the two incisions and release the tourniquet. Check for return of

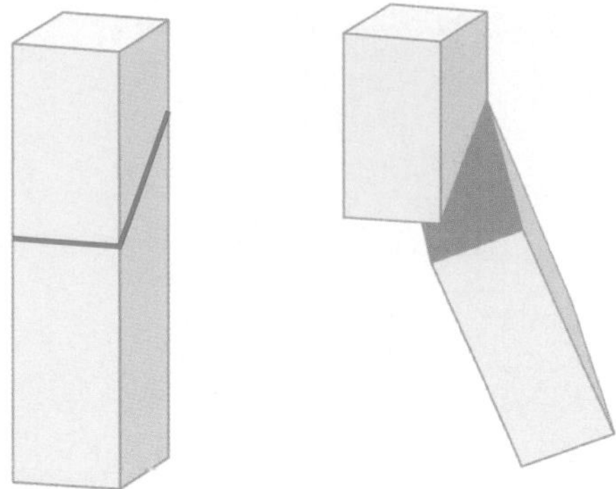

FIGURE 32-55 Principle of oblique osteotomy for tibia vara. Rotation around face of cut produces valgus and external rotation.

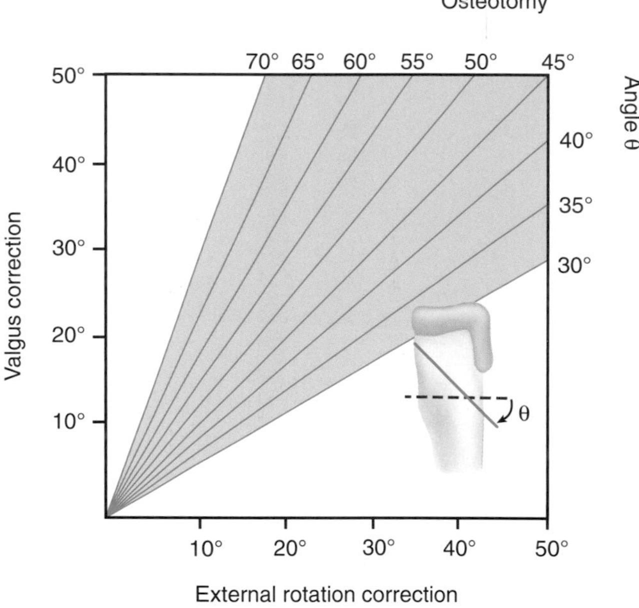

FIGURE 32-56 Nomogram for calculation of angle of oblique osteotomy for tibia vara. Desired valgus correction is found on vertical axis, and desired rotational correction is found on horizontal axis; intersection indicates osteotomy angle from horizontal as shown *(inset).* (Redrawn from Rab GT: Oblique tibial osteotomy for Blount's disease (tibia vara), J Pediatr Orthop 8:715, 1988.) **SEE TECHNIQUE 32-20**.

pulses, especially in the dorsalis pedis artery. Obtain hemostasis and close the wound over suction drains with fine absorbable subcutaneous and subcuticular sutures. Check both extremities for correct clinical alignment, which is crucial at this stage. The single screw is loose enough to allow adjustment of the osteotomy position by cast wedging if necessary. Apply a long leg, bent-knee cast.

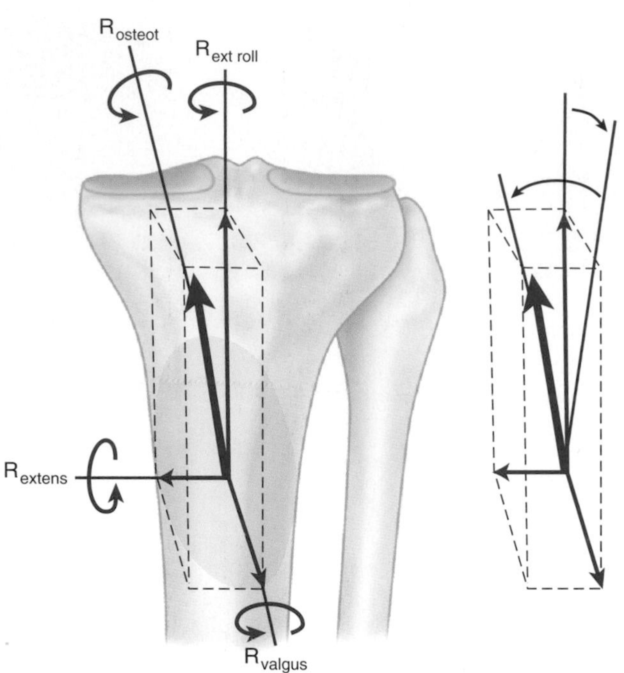

FIGURE 32-57 Mathematic description of osteotomy rotations. Vectors represent rotation in frontal, transverse, and sagittal planes, and R_{osteot} is actual rotation around face of osteotomy cut. Vectors describing rotation are normal to (at right angles to) plane of osteotomy cut.

POSTOPERATIVE CARE. The cast is changed at 4 weeks, and weight bearing is allowed as tolerated if callus is visible on radiograph. The cast is worn for 8 weeks or until union is evident radiographically.

Greene described an opening-closing chevron osteotomy that is a modification of the dome osteotomy and has the advantage of providing greater stability and minimal changes in leg length. Theoretical disadvantages are a slightly longer period of cast immobilization, which may be necessary to incorporate the wedge segment, and loss of correction caused by loss of fixation.

CHEVRON OSTEOTOMY FOR TIBIA VARA

TECHNIQUE 32-19

(GREENE)

- Before surgery, make a paper template that outlines the desired lateral wedge.
- Place the patient supine on the operating table with a sandbag under the ipsilateral hip to improve exposure of the fibula. Prepare the leg from the toes to the proximal thigh. Preparing the foot allows more accurate evaluation of the tibial torsion and allows evaluation of the dorsalis pedis and posterior tibial pulses when the tourniquet is deflated.

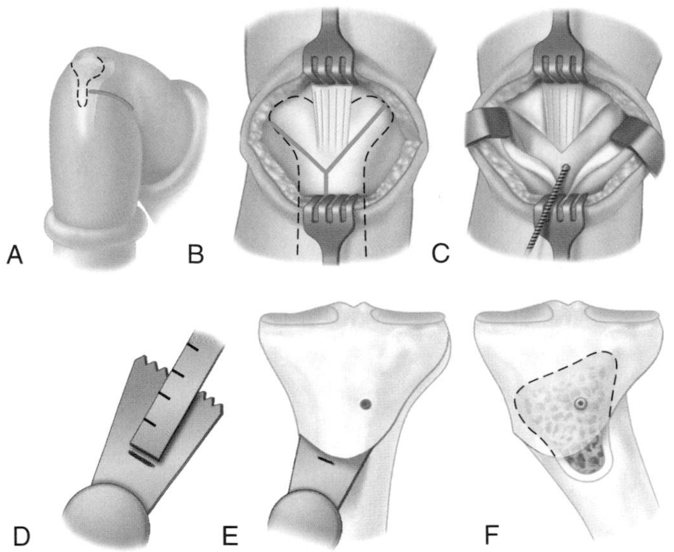

FIGURE 32-58 Oblique tibial osteotomy (see text) for tibia vara. **A,** Transverse incision at tibial tubercle. **B,** Y-shaped periosteal incision. **C,** Insertion of Steinmann pin after subperiosteal exposure. **D,** Marking of saw and osteotomies to avoid overpenetration. **E,** Oblique cut beneath pin. **F,** Rotation of osteotomy and fixation with single lag screw. **SEE TECHNIQUE 32-18.**

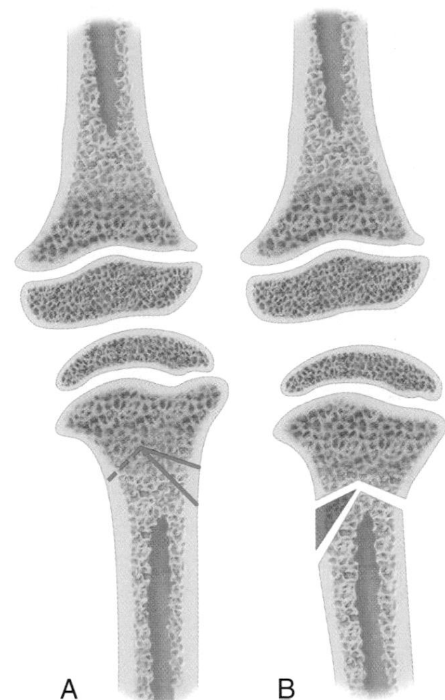

FIGURE 32-59 Opening-closing chevron osteotomy for tibia vara. **A,** Osteotomy cuts. **B,** Lateral wedge is inserted medially. (From Greene WB: Infantile tibia vara, J Bone Joint Surg 75A:130, 1993.) **SEE TECHNIQUE 32-19.**

FIBULAR OSTEOTOMY

- Expose the middle third of the fibula through the interval between the lateral and posterior compartments. Sharply incise the periosteum of the fibula and carefully elevate the periosteum circumferentially to prevent injury to the adjacent peroneal vessels.
- Remove a 1-cm segment of the fibula with a reciprocating saw. Cut the fibula obliquely, from superolateral to inferomedial. This allows the distal portion of the fibula to slide past the proximal fragment as the leg is brought from a varus to a valgus position.

TIBIAL OSTEOTOMY

- Make a hockey-stick incision 4 to 5 cm distal to the tibial tubercle staying medial and lateral to the anterior spine of the tibia. Extend the incision to the tibial tubercle and curve it laterally toward the Gerdy tubercle. Sharply incise the periosteum immediately adjacent to the anterior compartment muscles. Incise the periosteum transversely just distal to the tibial tubercle, and elevate it circumferentially so that curved retractors can be placed to protect the posterior soft tissues. Because of its triangular shape, more care is required at the posterolateral and posteromedial edges of the tibia to ensure that dissection remains subperiosteal.
- Outline the osseous cuts on the anterior surface of the tibia with an osteotome or cautery (Fig. 32-59). The apex of the osteotomy should be just distal to the tibial tubercle. Drill a hole from anterior to posterior at this point to minimize the risk of extending the osteotomy beyond the desired location. Complete the osteotomy with an oscillating saw and remove the lateral wedge.
- Swing the distal tibia into the desired position of valgus and external rotation. Insert the lateral wedge medially in a position that maintains the correction.
- Depending on the age of the child, the degree of obesity, and the stability of the osteotomy, a single pin or two crossed pins may be used for fixation if necessary. Use smooth or threaded pins and predrill the diaphysis to make pin insertion easier and more accurate. Any pin used for fixation should cross the osteotomy and exit through the proximal cortex without crossing the physis.
- Release the tourniquet and check the circulation in the foot. If circulation is satisfactory and correction is adequate on radiographs, bury the ends of the pins beneath the skin to prevent pin track infection and skin ulceration. Perform subcutaneous fasciotomy in the anterolateral compartment.
- Close the fibular and tibial incisions, leaving the fascia open, and close the skin with subcuticular sutures. Apply a long leg, bent-knee cast with the knee flexed 45 degrees and the ankle in the neutral position.

POSTOPERATIVE CARE. No weight bearing is allowed for the first 4 weeks after surgery. The cast is changed at 4 weeks, and, if healing is satisfactory on radiographs, the pins are removed and weight bearing is begun. Usually 8 to 10 weeks of immobilization is necessary, depending on the age of the child. The osteotomy must be protected long enough to minimize the risk of fracture that accompanies a quick resumption of vigorous play activity.

EPIPHYSEAL AND METAPHYSEAL OSTEOTOMY FOR TIBIA VARA

TECHNIQUE 32-20

(INGRAM, CANALE, BEATY)

- Determine preoperatively the amount of wedge to be removed from the epiphyseal and metaphyseal areas (see Fig. 32-52) and whether a graft is to be taken from the fibula or tibia.
- Prepare and drape the patient in the usual manner and apply and inflate a tourniquet.
- Expose the proximal tibia through a longitudinal incision approximately 10 cm long at the lateral border of the bone in the area of the physis. Carry the dissection through the soft tissue to expose the physis (Fig. 32-60B). Continue subperiosteal exposure distally and place reverse retractors in the metaphyseal area of the bone into the area of the tibial collateral ligament attachment on the tibia. Make a short incision in the proximal third of the lateral compartment and carry soft-tissue dissection down to the fibula, avoiding the peroneal nerve.
- Remove a segment of the fibula approximately 1.5 cm long. If a graft is to be used beneath the tibial plateau, a longer segment of fibula may be required.
- Fasciotomy can be done through this incision or through the tibial incision. With an osteotome and mallet, make an osteotomy through the physis, resecting any bony bar (Fig. 32-60C). Complete the osteotomy from the periphery to the center of the knee anteriorly to posteriorly, avoiding vessels and nerves posteriorly. Place an elevator in the osteotomy site and gently pry open and elevate the medial tibial plateau until it is as nearly parallel as possible to the lateral tibial plateau (Fig. 32-60D). If there is any offset of the osteotomy in the middle of the joint, arthrotomy can be done to inspect the joint; the abundant soft tissue and cartilage in the area of the tibial eminence act as a hinge, preventing any offset.
- Cut the appropriate closing lateral wedge in the metaphysis and insert two parallel Steinmann pins. Place the wedge of bone (or bone graft from the fibula) beneath the elevated tibial plateau (Fig. 32-60E); apply compression if desired (Fig. 32-60E).
- Insert crossed Steinmann pins through the epiphysis and proximal tibial graft.
- Close the wound and apply a long leg, bent-knee cast incorporating the pins in the plaster (Fig. 32-60F) or in an external fixator apparatus.

POSTOPERATIVE CARE. The pins in the osteotomy site are removed at 6 weeks, and the pins in the medial plateau are removed at 12 weeks. Cast immobilization is discontinued at 12 weeks, and range-of-motion exercises are begun.

INTRAEPIPHYSEAL OSTEOTOMY FOR TIBIA VARA

TECHNIQUE 32-21

(SIFFERT, STØREN, JOHNSON ET AL.)

- With the knee in extension, begin a medial longitudinal incision at the medial femoral epicondyle, extend it distally and anteriorly, and end it 2 cm medial and distal to the tibial tuberosity. (Siffert prefers a transverse incision along the medial joint line, curved distally to the tibial tuberosity.) Take care to preserve the infrapatellar branch of the saphenous nerve at the inferior aspect of the wound.
- Open the knee joint through a capsular incision anterior to the medial collateral ligament. The medial meniscus may be found hypertrophied; we try to preserve it. The capsular incision allows inspection of the articular surface of the tibia as the osteotomy is made.
- With a scalpel, make a circumferential incision through the epiphyseal cartilage down to the primary ossification center of the proximal tibial epiphysis, extending from the posteromedial corner of the tibia to the anteromedial corner; make the incision midway between the articular surface and the prominent vascular ring of vessels penetrating the epiphysis just proximal to the physis.
- Using a 3/4-inch (18-mm), gently curved osteotome, make an osteotomy through the medial aspect of the primary ossification center of the epiphysis. Because of the abnormal slope of the medial tibial plateau, the osteotomy parallels the articular surface medially and should reach the subchondral bone in the intercondylar area adjacent to the anterior cruciate ligament (Fig. 32-61). Gently elevate this segment, bringing the medial tibial plateau congruent with the medial femoral condyle and level with the lateral tibial plateau. Siffert stated this should correct the genu recurvatum that is frequently present.
- Insert small cortical grafts from the medial proximal tibia (or bank bone) into the opened osteotomy. Because the articular depression usually is more posterior than anterior, grafts of different sizes and shapes are needed to maintain articular congruity and contact throughout a normal range of motion. It is important that the grafts be placed only in the opened wedge of the epiphyseal bone and not in the cartilage medially.

Andrade and Johnston described a more extensive operation using dental burrs and methyl methacrylate pin construct for fixation. They emphasized the importance of elevating the depression (Fig. 32-62). A medially based opening wedge osteotomy of the proximal tibia also may be required to correct varus of the tibia. A proximal fibular osteotomy is needed, and through the lateral incision required for the fibular osteotomy we recommend a subcutaneous fasciotomy,

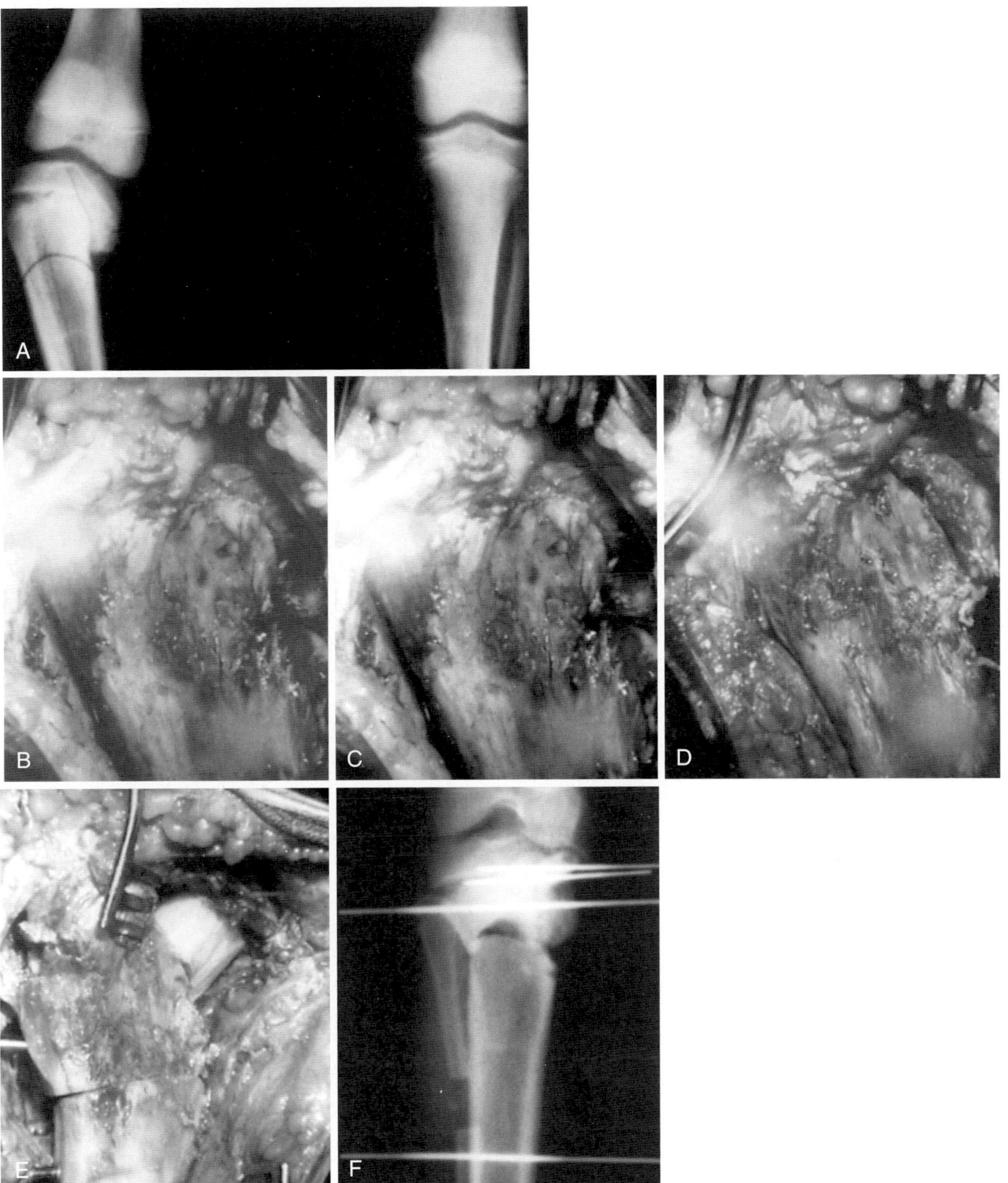

FIGURE 32-60 Epiphyseal and metaphyseal osteotomy for tibia vara. **A,** Severe Blount disease with physis slipped 90 degrees. **B,** Exposure of physis. **C,** Osteotomy. **D,** Elevation of medial tibial plateau. **E,** Placement of bone graft under compression. **F,** Cast incorporating pins in plaster. **SEE TECHNIQUE 32-20.**

taking care to protect the superficial peroneal nerve as it penetrates the deep investing fascia of the lower leg to become subcutaneous. We also insert a smooth Steinmann pin proximal and distal to the osteotomy of the proximal tibia, and with these incorporated in a long leg cast the position of the osteotomy is maintained without a graft. A cortical graft also can be used in an opening wedge and is held with crossed Steinmann pins. The technique of osteotomy of the proximal tibia is described in Chapter 9.

A lateral epiphysiodesis can be done with any of the osteotomies by extending the subperiosteal dissection proximally to expose the physis. A curet or dental burr can be used to excise the cartilaginous physis. The technique for epiphysiodesis is described in Chapter 29.

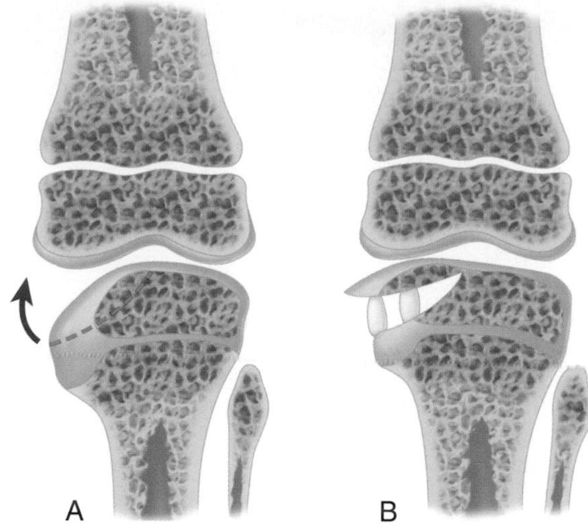

FIGURE 32-61 Correction of intraarticular component of Blount disease by osteotomy of epiphysis. **A,** Incision made into epiphyseal cartilage at its midportion medially. Curved osteotomy directed laterally and proximally to subchondral intercondylar region paralleling articular surface. **B,** Osteotomized tibial condyle elevated on its intercondylar cartilage hinge to position of congruity with femur; bone struts are placed into gap to maintain contact in all planes of motion and to tighten medial ligament. (From Siffert RS: Intraepiphyseal osteotomy for progressive tibia vara: case report and rationale of management, J Pediatr Orthop 2:81, 1982.) **SEE TECHNIQUE 32-21**.

HEMIELEVATION OF THE EPIPHYSIS OSTEOTOMY WITH LEG LENGTHENING USING AN ILIZAROV FRAME FOR TIBIA VARA

TECHNIQUE 32-22

(JONES ET AL., HEFNEY ET AL.)

STAGE 1

- Place the patient supine and apply a tourniquet.
- Make a J-shaped skin incision on the medial side of the knee for subperiosteal exposure of the proximal tibia.
- Place a ring-handled retractor subperiosteally behind the knee to protect the neurovascular structures.
- Determine the level of the proposed osteotomy using image intensification and insert a Kirschner wire into the midline of the tibia anteriorly just below the tibial spine. Place a second Kirschner wire into the medial aspect of the proximal tibia (distal to the first wire) to mark the distal extent of the osteotomy (usually at the metaphyseal-diaphyseal junction). Predrill the osteotomy in line with the Kirschner wires, verifying the position of the drill holes using image intensification.
- Close the skin temporarily.
- Insert three 4-mm or 5-mm half-pins, depending on the size of the patient, into the fragment of the medial tibial plateau, parallel to the medial joint line as determined by an intraoperative arthrogram and three-dimensional CT (Fig. 32-63). If there is a posterior slope, pins should be placed parallel to it from anterior to posterior. The skin wound can be reopened and the osteotomy completed with Lambotte osteotomes, leaving the articular cartilage intact proximally. Examine the osteotomy clinically and radiographically.
- Attach a half-ring of appropriate size to the three half-pins orientated parallel to the joint line in the anteroposterior and mediolateral planes. Apply a two-ring frame distally perpendicular to the long axis of the tibia and attach to the half ring using anterior and posterior hinges. Place the hinges opposite the intact articular cartilage at the proximal end of the osteotomy. In the presence of a posterior slope, based on CT, the posterior hinge acts as a distraction hinge to elevate the posterior slope while the anterior hinge is fixed. Position the anterior hinge carefully in the midline over the tibial spine. The hinge must lie over the cartilage-bone junction because the osteotomy hinges here. Two threaded rods, mounted medially, act as motors. Use a 4-mm half-pin and an olive wire at each level for distal ring fixation.

STAGE 2

- The second stage is done after the medial plateau and the regenerate bone consolidates.
- Remove or adjust the Ilizarov frame for lengthening; if necessary, correct rotational deformities. Correct any residual varus.
- In patients with open physes, epiphysiodesis of the proximal fibular and lateral tibial physes should be done with the use of image intensification to prevent recurrence of deformity. The tibia should be lengthened by the amount equal to the anticipated shortening (using a Moseley graph) and the measured leg-length difference.
- Perform a fibular osteotomy at the level of the tibial osteotomy through a longitudinal skin incision using an oscillating saw.
- Using image intensification, mark the site of the proposed tibial osteotomy, and place a Gigli saw subperiosteally with two mini skin incisions.
- Add a half-ring to the existing half-ring over the medial plateau to convert it to a full ring. Attach the proximal tibial using olive wires. Attach the proximal ring block to the existing distal ring block by threaded rods for simple lengthening or derotation devices for correction of rotation if necessary.
- Complete the tibial osteotomy with the Gigli saw and suture the skin incisions.

POSTOPERATIVE CARE. The leg is kept elevated, and a radiograph of the tibia is obtained. Distraction is started 3 to 5 days later under the supervision of a physiotherapist. Weight bearing is allowed as tolerated.

Janoyer et al. used an Orthofix (Gentilly, France) external fixator prototype, which is composed of an upper epiphyseal articulating ring. This allows medial plateau elevation in the orthogonal slope with a posteromedial axis of 10 to 20 degrees. Early results were good with similar complications as other

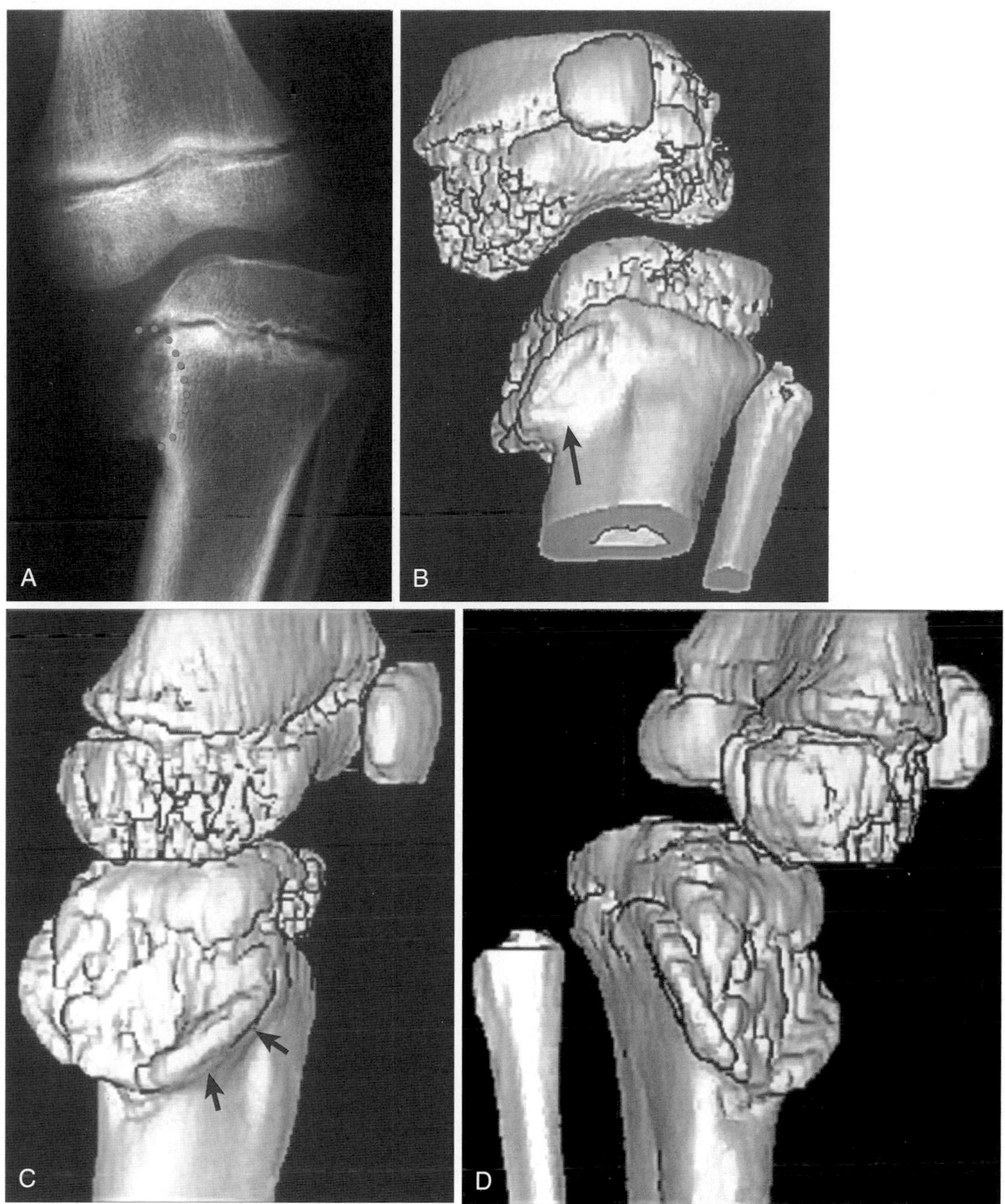

FIGURE 32-62 Medial epiphysiolysis for stage IV infantile tibia vara. **A,** Metaphyseal bone and Blount lesion to be excised is outlined. **B,** Three-dimensional reconstruction from CT showing extent of abnormally depressed epiphyseal bone anteriorly. *Arrow* indicates cleft on the anterior surface of the metaphysis where initial resection for epiphysiolysis begins. **C** and **D,** Lateral and posterolateral views of the metaphyseal beak. (From Andrade N, Johnston CE: Medial epiphysiolysis in severe infantile tibia vara, J Pediatr Orthop 26:652, 2006.)

external fixation devices. Van Huyssteen reported a medial plateau elevating tibial osteotomy with lateral epiphyseodesis (performed delayed or concomitantly) for late presenting Blount disease (Fig. 32-64). The advantage of this procedure is that all deformities can be corrected in one operation.

NEUROVASCULAR COMPLICATIONS OF HIGH TIBIAL OSTEOTOMY

Neurovascular complications after an osteotomy for genu varum result most commonly from vascular occlusion or peroneal nerve palsy. Stretching of the anterior tibial artery occurs at the interosseous membrane with varus correction (as for genu valgum), and compression of the artery occurs with valgus correction (as for genu varum). Regardless of the cause, early recognition is mandatory. Immediate diagnosis with return of the extremity to the preoperative position of deformity is beneficial regardless of the cause, especially because the causative factors may not be clearly evident in each patient. Sensory loss on the dorsum of the foot and loss of active dorsiflexion of the foot without pain usually are caused

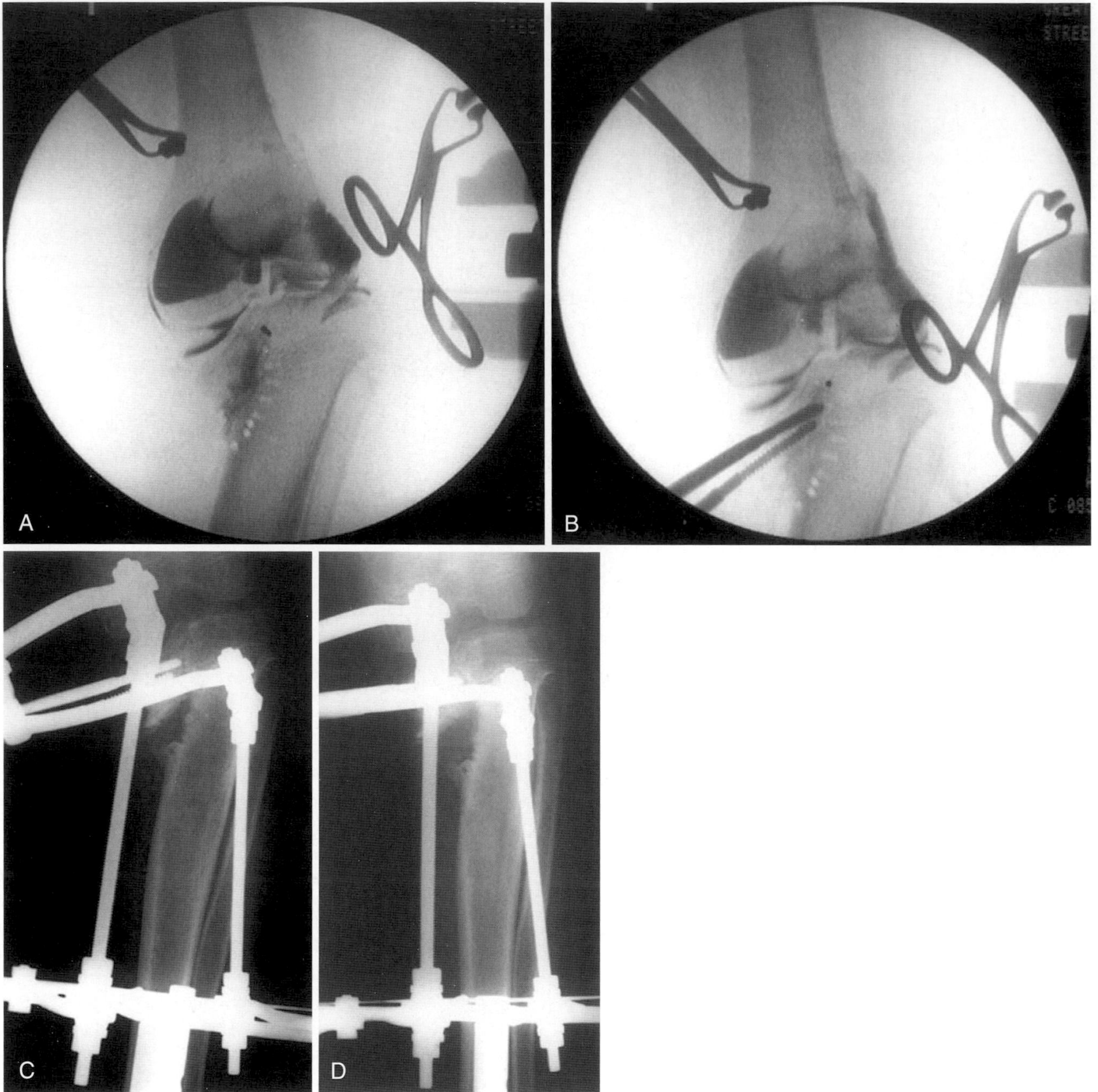

FIGURE 32-63 Hemiplateau elevation for infantile tibia vara. **A,** Intraoperative arthrogram using image intensifier showing drill holes marking proposed osteotomy site. **B,** Two half-pins inserted into fragment of medial tibial plateau parallel to true medial knee joint line. **C** and **D,** Completed osteotomy with elevation of hemiplateau under way using Ilizarov frame. (From Jones S, Hosalkar HS, Hill RA, et al: Relapsed infantile Blount's disease treated by hemiplateau elevation using the Ilizarov frame, J Bone Joint Surg 85B:565, 2003. Copyright British Editorial Society of Bone and Joint Surgery.) **SEE TECHNIQUE 32-22**.

by paralysis of the common peroneal nerve. Decrease in dorsiflexion and severe pain on plantar flexion of the toes are the most common clinical signs of occlusion of the artery or of an anterior compartment syndrome (see Chapter 48). Matsen and Staheli outlined appropriate treatment for each as follows:

1. For traction on the peroneal nerve (more common with varus correction), remove the cast and return the leg to the preoperative position. Remove all pressure on the peroneal nerve, loosen all dressings from the thigh to the toes, and observe closely.
2. For anterior compartment syndrome, remove the cast and return the leg to the preoperative position. Loosen all dressings from the thigh to the toes. If improvement does not occur immediately, fasciotomy without delay is mandatory.
3. For anterior tibial artery occlusion, remove the cast and return the leg to the preoperative position. Loosen all dressings from the thigh to the toes, and observe closely. If immediate improvement is not evident, consider arteriography followed by appropriate surgery.

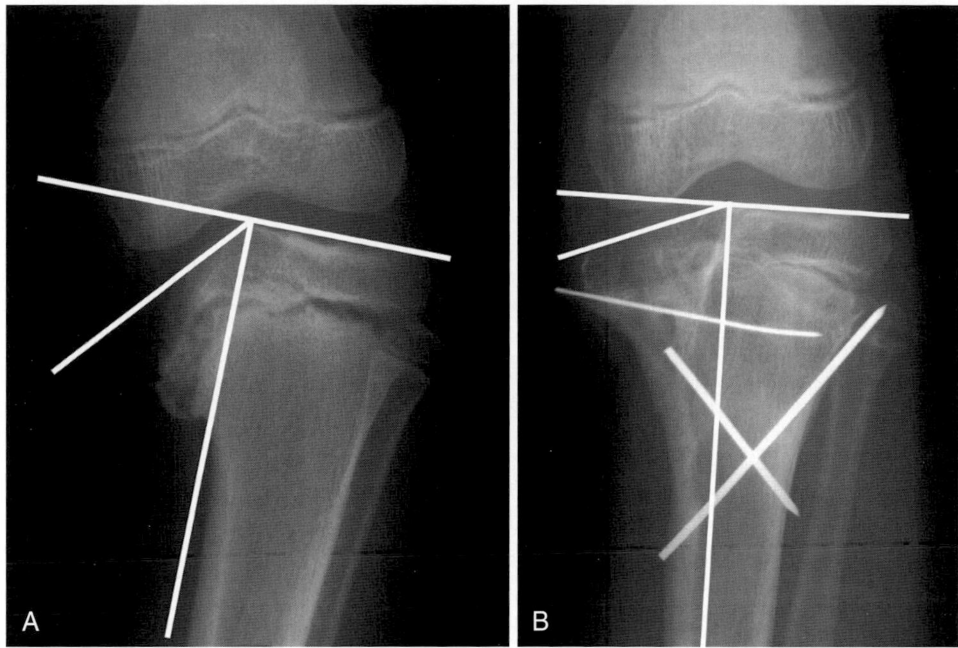

FIGURE 32-64 Anteroposterior radiographs of left knee in 12-year-old boy with stage V Blount disease. **A,** Preoperative radiograph showing angle of depression of medial tibial plateau of 50 degrees and tibial varus angle of 95 degrees. **B,** At 10 months after surgery note recurrent mechanical varus of 5 degrees; the angle of depression of the medial tibial plateau was maintained at 25 degrees but the tibial varus angle increased to 90 degrees because of fusion of the medial tibial physis with an open lateral physis. (From van Huyssteen AL, Olesak M, Hoffman EB: Double-elevating osteotomy for late-presenting infantile Blount's disease. J Bone Joint Surg 87B:710, 2005. Copyright British Editorial Society of Bone and Joint Surgery.)

CONGENITAL AFFECTIONS

Most affections of bone seemingly of congenital origin may respond favorably to surgery. The surgical treatment of enchondromatosis (Ollier disease) and of hereditary multiple exostoses is described in Chapter 25.

OSTEOGENESIS IMPERFECTA

Osteogenesis imperfecta is a disease apparently of the mesodermal tissues with abnormal or deficient collagen that has been shown in bone, skin, sclerae, and dentin. The so-called diagnostic triad of blue sclerae, dentinogenesis imperfecta, and generalized osteoporosis in a patient with multiple fractures or bowing of the long bones usually is used clinically. There is no specific laboratory test for this disease other than skin biopsy and DNA testing. Multiple wormian bones around the base of the skull are a major finding only in the congenital type of osteogenesis imperfecta. Osteogenesis imperfecta congenita is characterized at birth by multiple fractures, bowing of the long bones, short extremities, and generalized osteoporosis. The most used classification noted in the literature is by Sillence who originally classified the disease into four types, although it is likely that osteogenesis imperfecta is a continuum (Table 32-7). Since Sillence's classification, additional types have been added. Ninety percent of patients are type I or IV. Although many children with osteogenesis imperfecta have blue sclerae, the only two characteristics that are present in all patients with osteogenesis imperfecta are fractures and generalized osteoporosis.

Orthopaedic surgery is most involved with the bowing of the long bones in osteogenesis imperfecta tarda type 1, in which progressively increasing deformities may cause deterioration in activity of these children from walkers to sitters and from braceable to unbraceable. Healing of fractures and osteotomies usually is satisfactory, although the healed bone may be no stronger than the original. Hyperplastic callus occasionally is seen after fractures and osteotomies, although difficult and persistent nonunions have been noted. Because of frequently frail and disabling bone and joint deformities and fractures that preclude ambulation, a comprehensive rehabilitation program with long leg bracing has been suggested to result in a high level of functional activity with an acceptable level of risk of fracture in children with osteogenesis imperfecta. Results of surgery in these patients have been inconsistent, with frequent complications reported. Patients should be examined for scoliosis before surgical procedures are undertaken because thoracic scoliosis of greater than 60 degrees has severe adverse effects on pulmonary function in patients with osteogenesis imperfecta, which may partly explain the increased pulmonary morbidity in adult patients with osteogenesis imperfecta and scoliosis compared with that in the general population. Besides pulmonary problems other anesthetic complications can occur such as difficulty in positioning the patient, malignant hyperthermia, basilar invagination, cardiac abnormalities, or bleeding from platelet dysfunction. Although a transfusion rate of 14% was noted in one series of patients with osteogenesis imperfecta treated with intramedullary rods, the blood loss was described as low and manageable.

TABLE 32-7

Sillence Classification of Osteogenesis Imperfecta (Simplified)

TYPE	INHERITANCE	SCLERAE	FEATURES
Type I	Autosomal dominant	Blue	Mildest form. Presents at preschool age (tarda). Hearing deficit in 50%. Divided into type A and B based on tooth involvement
Type II	Autosomal recessive	Blue	Lethal in perinatal period
Type III	Autosomal recessive	Normal	Fractures at birth. Progressively short stature. Most severe survivable form
Type IV	Autosomal dominant	Normal	Moderate severity. Bowing bones and vertebral fractures are common. Hearing normal. Divided into type A and B based on tooth involvement
Type V			Hypertrophic callus after fracture. Ossification of IOM between radius and ulna and tibia and fibula
Type VI			Moderate severity. Similar to type IV
Type VII			Associated with rhizomelia and coxa vara

Type V, VI, VII have been added to the original classification system (these have no type I collagen mutation but have abnormal bone on microscopy and a similar phenotype).

The use of bisphosphonates has been shown to reduce osteoclast-mediated bone resorption. Intravenous administration of bisphosphonates, such as pamidronate, zoledronate, and risedronate, has been shown to decrease bone pain and incidence of fracture and to increase bone density and level of ambulation with minimal side effects. Increase in size of vertebral bodies and thickening of cortical bone also have been reported. There are no standardized guidelines for initiating bisphosphonate treatment in children. Recent data suggest that both intravenous or oral bisphosphonates are effective, but which medication and dosing regimens are optimal and how long patients should be treated have not been established. Recently, pamidronate has been recommended for use in combination with surgery both preoperatively and postoperatively. Because of the recently described long-term complications of bisphosphonates (atypical femoral fracture, breast cancer), its efficacy in patients with osteogenesis imperfecta and its prolonged use have been called into question. In the recent literature, almost an equal number of reports find it beneficial as unbeneficial. While the answer is unknown, bisphosphonates have raised the enthusiasm for surgery in patients with osteogenesis imperfecta. Besides fracture procedures (e.g. intramedullary rods) elective procedures, such as total joint arthroplasty and, spine surgery, including scoliosis surgery, are being reported.

MULTIPLE OSTEOTOMIES, REALIGNMENT, AND MEDULLARY NAIL FIXATION

The most successful surgical method of treating the deformities of osteogenesis imperfecta is based on the work of Sofield and Millar who used a method of multiple osteotomies, realignment of fragments, and medullary nail fixation for long bones (Fig. 32-65). This operation and its modifications are now widely used when surgical treatment of fresh fractures is indicated and for correction of bowing and as prophylaxis to allow a child more activity without repeated fractures. Historically, Sofield and Millar reported no disturbances in growth when the smooth medullary nail penetrated the physis. Almost routinely, the bone grows beyond the end of the nail, usually distally because the bones of the lower extremities are the ones most commonly treated surgically. The bone extending beyond the end of the medullary nail tends to angulate, and the nail itself tends to cut out and allow deformity and a tendency to fracture at the end of the nail. Routine central placement of the rod across the physis has been recommended to add length to the rod and postpone the problem of the rod becoming too short. Determining the correct rod diameter from preoperative radiographs is imprecise because it is not possible to obtain perfectly anteroposterior and lateral radiographs in these patients because of distortions of bony anatomy, and often the radiographs overestimate the diameter of the medullary canal. A more accurate method is repeat fluoroscopic examinations in multiple planes during surgery to obtain views of the medullary canal at different levels. The important points of treatment include adequate reduction of the ends of the long bones, proper placement of the rod in the metaphysis and epiphysis (Fig. 32-66), use of a hook on the femoral rods to prevent migration, use of a rod of adequate length, and incorporation of corrective forces in postoperative casts and braces.

In infants with a severe form of osteogenesis imperfecta, the operative technique has been modified significantly from those presented earlier in the literature. Early intramedullary stabilization even soon after birth may be justified in selected patients with severe osteogenesis imperfecta to improve possibilities for motor development and make later insertion of telescoping rods easier. Closed and semi-closed techniques appear to be superior to open fragmentation because they are relatively easy and save time, operative trauma is less, morbidity is lower, and several bones can be stabilized in one session. A possible solution to the rapid growing away from the nails seems to be early stabilization with simple nonexpandable implants and, around the age of 4 years, insertion of telescoping nails.

Bailey and Dubow used a telescoping medullary rod with small flanges at its distal and proximal ends that are fixed within the bony epiphysis or cortex of the bone. With growth, the rod elongates and allows the entire length of the long bone to remain reinforced for several years by the same internal

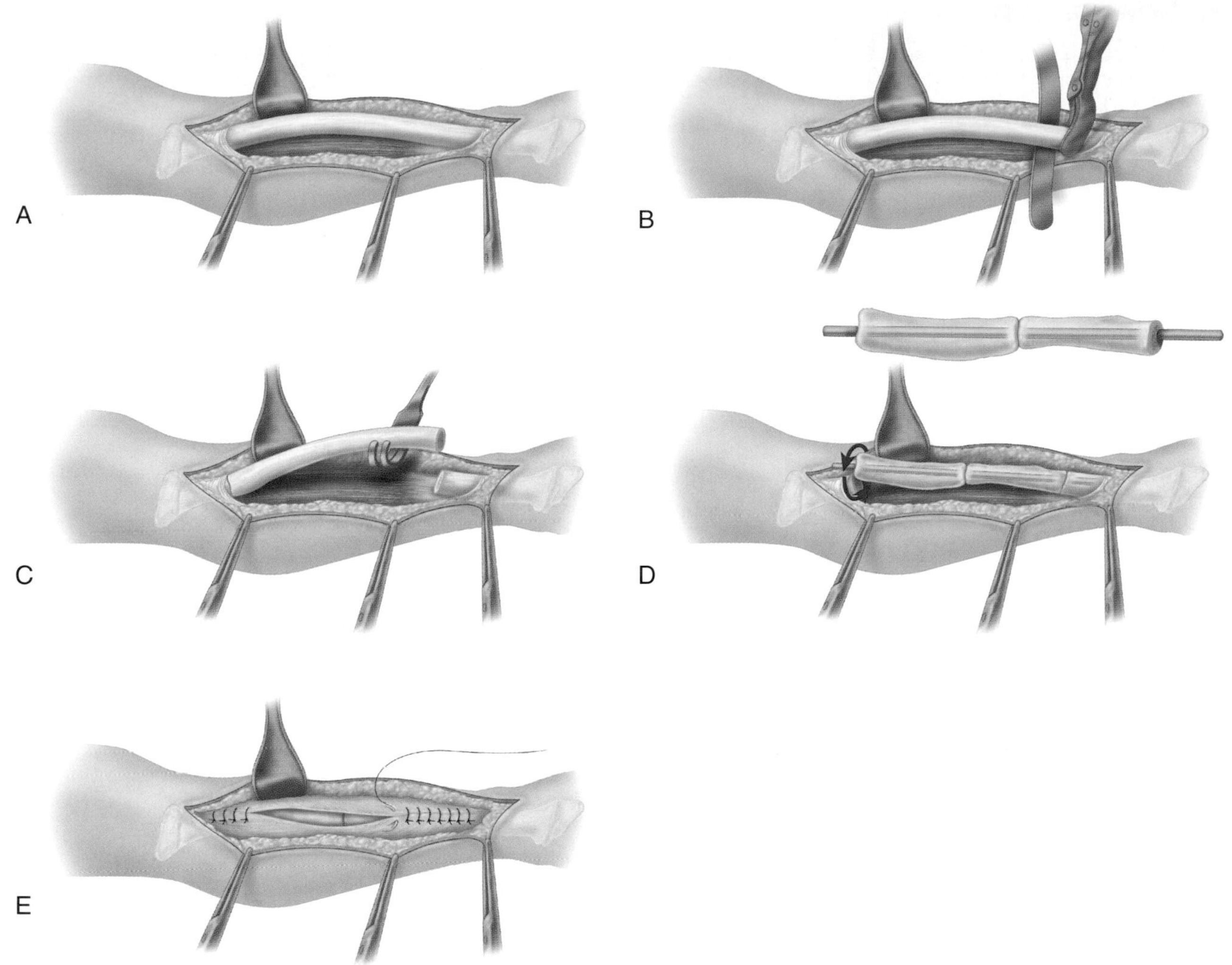

FIGURE 32-65 **A-E,** Technique for fragmentation and realignment of bone and insertion of medullary nail. **A-C,** Exposure and removal of shaft. **D,** Osteotomies. **E,** Closure. (From Sofield HA, Millar EA: Fragmentation, realignment, and intramedullary rod fixation of deformities of the long bones in children: a 10-year appraisal, J Bone Joint Surg 41A:1371, 1959.)

support. Of the several types of medullary rods that we have used in patients with this disease, these telescoping rods have produced the best results. Despite frequent complications, expandable nails can correct angular deformities, decrease the number of fractures, and allow most previously nonambulatory children to walk.

In comparisons of Bailey-Dubow expandable rods with nonelongating rods, the complication rates for the Bailey-Dubow rod have been slightly higher, but the reoperation rates for the nonelongating rods have been greater. The most common complication for both types of nails is migration. Generally, complications, reoperations, replacements, and number of nail migrations have not been found to be significantly different between the two types of nails (Fig. 32-67). The replacement rate also was higher for nonelongating rods. Of the Bailey-Dubow complications, 34% involved the T-piece and were potentially avoidable. Recently, a distal interlocked telescoping rod has been advocated to avoid the problems of the T-piece.

Complications reported with the telescoping rod include fracture at the tip of the rod, proximal migration secondary to angular deformity, and eccentric rod positioning at the distal physis. Even so, the telescoping rod appears to be superior to the nontelescoping rod. In one study, the 3-year survival rate of the telescoping rod was 92.9% compared with 7.2% of the nontelescoping rod, and the reoperation rate was 7.2% compared with 31.6%, respectively. For these reasons we have been using the Fassier-Duval elongating intramedullary rod system.

For the tibia, to allow use of the longest possible medullary rod, Williams reported a technique in which an extension is screwed onto the distal end of the rod and is pushed through the distal tibia and out the sole of the foot. After the fragments of the tibia are realigned, the nail is reinserted in a retrograde fashion until the distal end lies just proximal to the surface of the ankle joint. The extension is unscrewed, leaving the rod extending only into the distal tibial epiphysis.

MODIFIED SOFIELD-MILLAR OPERATION IN THE FEMUR AND TIBIA IN OSTEOGENESIS IMPERFECTA

TECHNIQUE 32-23

(LI ET AL.)

- Place the patient supine, and elevate the side to be operated.
- Use image intensification to guide the entry of the nail and to monitor the progress of the osteotomies.
- Expose the tip of the greater trochanter and ream as for closed insertion of an intramedullary nail. Insert a reamer of the same size as the femoral canal through the greater trochanter.
- Stop the reamer at the first site of the angulation of the femur (Fig. 32-68) and confirm with image intensification.
- Make a small lateral incision about 2 cm in length to expose a small portion of the femur.
- Incise the periosteum longitudinally, elevate, and protect it.
- Remove a small lateral wedge of bone to correct the angulation using a bone cutter or oscillating saw. Leave the medial cortex intact to provide stability.
- Reduce the deformity and advance the nail more distally.
- Usually, a second block occurs, and the procedure should be repeated. Normally, two osteotomies are sufficient to correct the deformity and to allow the nail to be passed through to the condylar region. Occasionally, a third osteotomy may be necessary.
- The end of the rod ideally should be in the middle of the femoral condyles.
- Suture the periosteum if possible, close the wound, and apply a hip spica cast.
- For the tibia, the entry site is just behind the patellar tendon; otherwise, the procedure is the same as for the femur.

POSTOPERATIVE CARE. A long leg plaster cast is applied. The patient should be immobilized for 6 weeks and allowed to bear weight as soon as possible.

The internal fixation device used in this procedure consists of a hollow tube or sleeve with a solid rod that telescopes inside. For the femur, it is used with one end anchored within the distal portion of the distal femoral epiphysis immediately adjacent to the knee joint and the proximal end in the superior portion of the neck at its junction with the greater trochanter. In the tibia, each end is in a bony epiphysis adjacent to a joint.

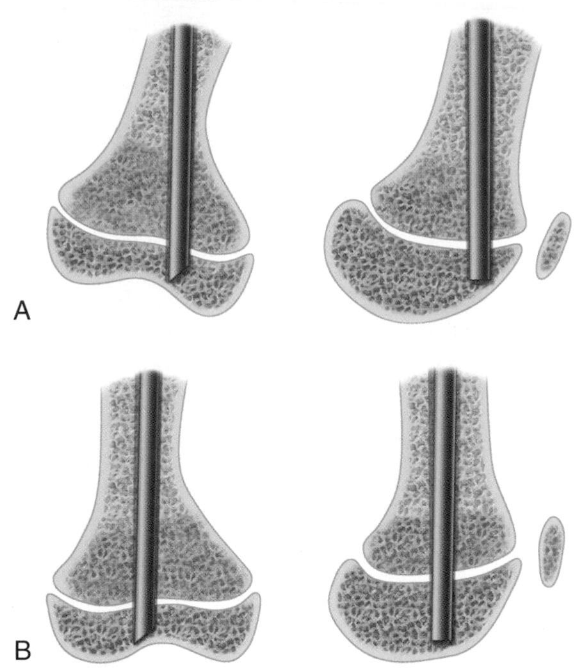

FIGURE 32-66 Medullary rod positioning in osteotomies for osteogenesis imperfecta. **A,** Incomplete reduction with poor position of rod. Rod is not centrally placed and is anterior in epiphysis. Physis is still tilted on both projections. **B,** Complete reduction of end fragments and good central positioning of medullary rod. (From Tiley F, Albright JA: Osteogenesis imperfecta: treatment by multiple osteotomy and intramedullary rod insertion, J Bone Joint Surg 55A:701, 1973.)

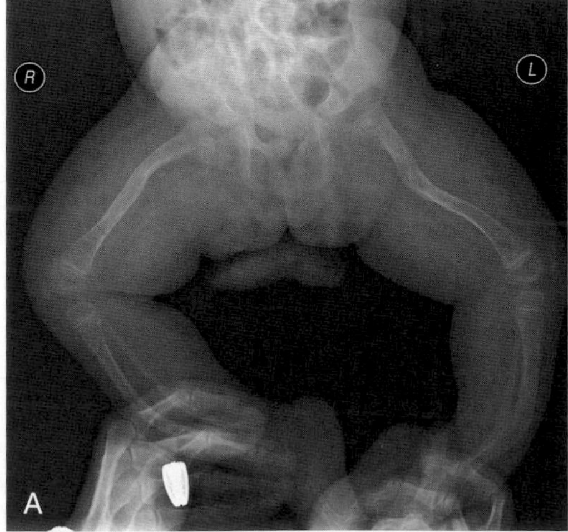

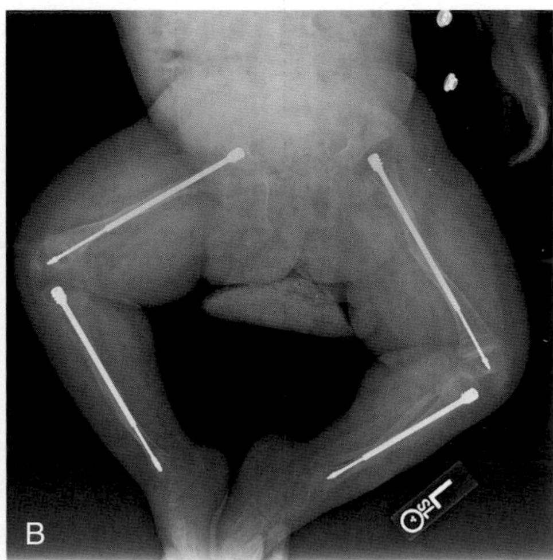

FIGURE 32-67 **A,** Preoperative radiograph of patient with osteogenesis imperfecta. **B,** After osteotomies of femur and tibia and insertion of elongating intramedullary rods.

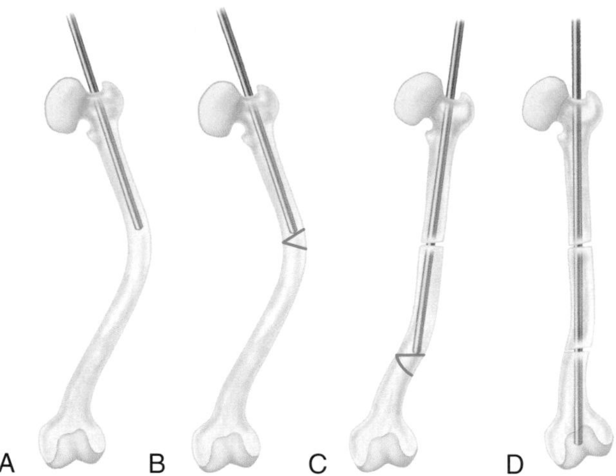

FIGURE 32-68 Modified Sofield-Millar procedure. **A,** Intramedullary rod passed to point of angulation under image intensification. **B,** Osteotomy carried out with minimal exposure and rod passed farther distally. **C,** Second osteotomy carried out at next site of angulation. **D,** Final correction. (From Li YH, Chow W, Leong JCY: The Sofield-Millar operation in osteogenesis imperfecta, J Bone Joint Surg 82B:11, 2000. Copyright British Editorial Society of Bone and Joint Surgery.) **SEE TECHNIQUE 32-23.**

OSTEOTOMY AND MEDULLARY NAILING WITH A TELESCOPING ROD IN THE FEMUR FOR OSTEOGENESIS IMPERFECTA

TECHNIQUE 32-24

(BAILEY AND DUBOW)

- Approach the femur subperiosteally as with the Sofield technique. Expose the intercondylar notch of the femur through a parapatellar incision, and for the tibia use a similar incision proximally and a transverse medial incision through the deltoid ligament distally to displace the talus and enter the ankle joint. The approach to the proximal part of the femur may require only a small incision placed directly over the end of the tubular sleeve as it is drilled proximally through the medullary canal and out the superior aspect of the neck just medial to the base of the greater trochanter.
- After osteotomies have been made in the metaphyses of the involved bone, make the multiple osteotomies as with the Sofield technique so that the segments can be lined up with insertion of the rod. The rod when collapsed should reach from the proximal to the distal end of the entire bone less 2 cm to allow a margin for error and for impaction of the shaft segments after the surgery.
- Fit the tubular sleeve with the special detachable drill point and drill through the medullary canal of one metaphysis, through the bony epiphysis, and into the joint; repeat this at the opposite end of the bone.
- After drilling the medullary canal of all the fragments with the same drill point attached to the tubular sleeve, replace the drill point with the T-shaped flange that screws on the end of the tubular sleeve. At the other end of the bone, insert the obturator rod across the joint through the articular cartilage and into the canal that was drilled in the metaphysis. Thread the fragments of the shaft on the sleeve portion of the rod and place the other metaphysis in position with the obturator up inside the tubular sleeve. Manually kink with compression the T-shaped flange so that it does not loosen. Gamble et al. and Janus et al. recommended the following: avoid loosening of the T junction of the obturator portion by scoring the T-piece before its insertion into the sleeve or stoutly crimping the sleeve after insertion of the T-piece; place the T below the subchondral bone or below the periosteal-perichondral surface but not so deep that it migrates into the medullary canal. After insertion, turn the T-piece 90 degrees in the direction of insertion to help prevent backout.
- Countersink the T-shaped end of the obturator through the articular cartilage and into the bony portion of the distal epiphysis. The sleeve end of the rod is similarly impacted into the joint cartilage of the proximal tibia or at the proximal end of the femur against the base of the trochanter.
- After radiographs are taken, close the periosteum around the fragments and then close the remainder of the operative wounds.

POSTOPERATIVE CARE. The patient is immobilized in a hip spica (femur) or long leg cast (tibia) until the osteotomies have healed (Fig. 32-69).

MODIFIED ROD WITH INTERLOCKING OBTURATOR FOR OSTEOGENESIS IMPERFECTA

TECHNIQUE 32-25

(CHO ET AL.)

- Perform multilevel osteotomies to realign the limb segment along the rod. Percutaneous osteotomies are preferred, but if intramedullary reaming is needed for a narrow or obliterated medullary cavity or resection of a substantial wedge of bone is needed to correct an acute angulation, open osteotomies are necessary.
- Insert a Kirschner wire through the medullary canal of the osteotomy fragments.
- Cut the sleeve to an appropriate length and insert over the Kirschner wire in an antegrade direction. It is important to ensure that the distal tip of the sleeve points to the center of the distal epiphysis on both anteroposterior and lateral projections of radiographs.

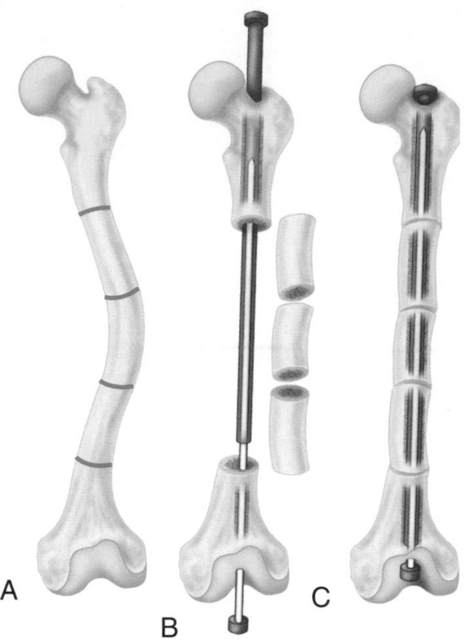

FIGURE 32-69 Elongating medullary rods in treatment of osteogenesis imperfecta. **A,** Multiple osteotomies are performed. **B,** Proximal and distal joints are entered, and each half of rod is inserted. **C,** Fragments are threaded onto rod halves, which are telescoped together, and T-pieces on each end are gently rotated and sunk beneath articular surface. Sleeve and rod (obturator) should be longer than illustrated, and each should be almost as long as the bone. (From Marafioti RL, Westin GW: Elongating intramedullary rods in the treatment of osteogenesis imperfecta, J Bone Joint Surg 59A:467, 1977.) **SEE TECHNIQUE 32-24**.

- Replace the Kirschner wire with the obturator, which is advanced antegrade inside the sleeve into the distal epiphysis. The rotational orientation of the hole at its distal end can be controlled and adjusted with the use of an obturator-impactor.
- Using a free-hand technique, anchor the obturator in the distal epiphysis with a Kirschner wire and advance using gentle tapping.
- Cut the wire to an appropriate length and push deep, preferably within the osseous epiphysis.
- In the femur, adjust the sleeve position so that the T-piece abuts the greater trochanter cartilage within the gluteal muscles. In the tibia, bury the T-piece of the sleeve within the osseous epiphysis. If a 3-mm sleeve is used, through which the obturator cannot pass, assemble the sleeve and obturator and then insert as one piece through the osteotomy fragments. When the sleeve reaches its destination, advance the obturator into the distal epiphysis and transfix as described above.

POSTOPERATIVE CARE. The limb is immobilized with a long leg splint for 4 to 6 weeks postoperatively (Fig. 32-70).

FASSIER-DUVAL TELESCOPING ROD (PEGA MEDICAL, INC., LAVAL, QUEBEC, CANADA)

This expandable rod is designed for children with osteogenesis imperfecta to prevent or stabilize fractures or correct deformity of the long bones during growth. It is indicated for children 18 months of age or older. It has been designed for use in the femur, tibia, and humerus. The main advantage is its easy placement and better fixation in the physis of long bones. As compared with other expandable rods, an open or percutaneous osteotomy technique can be employed for the femur. For patients with large bones and thin cortices, a percutaneous technique is recommended. For the tibia an open osteotomy technique is recommended.

FASSIER-DUVAL TELESCOPING ROD, FEMUR

TECHNIQUE 32-26

OPEN OSTEOTOMY

- Through a posterolateral approach, expose the femur subperiosteally.
- Perform an osteotomy under C-arm guidance (Fig. 32-71A and B).
- With a cannulated reamer, ream the proximal fragment or drill up to the greater trochanter over a small-diameter guidewire. The diameter of the reamer should be 0.25 to 0.35 mm larger than the diameter of the nail implant size chosen. Prepare the distal fragment in same fashion. If the guidewire does not reach the distal epiphysis, perform a second osteotomy after reaming the intermediate fragment (Fig. 32-71C)
- Insert a male-size Kirschner wire retrograde from the direction of the osteotomy through the proximal fragment (Fig. 32-71D).
- Make a second incision at the buttock to allow the extremity of the Kirschner wire to exit proximally (Fig. 32-71E).

PERCUTANEOUS OSTEOTOMY

- If a percutaneous technique for osteotomy is chosen, insert a small diameter guidewire through the greater trochanter into the apex of the deformity. Ream the femur to the appropriate size with a cannulated reamer (Fig. 32-71F).
- Through a 0.5-cm incision perform the first osteotomy in the convexity of the deformity just distal to the reamer (Fig. 32-71G).
- Apply counterpressure at the osteotomy site and with gentle manipulation progressively correct the deformity. When the bone is straightened, push the guidewire distally and advance the reamer accordingly (Fig. 32-71H).
- Push the guidewire distally to the apex of the second deformity, then perform a second osteotomy as described for the first osteotomy until the length of the medullary canal has been reamed to just before the physis (Fig. 32-71I).

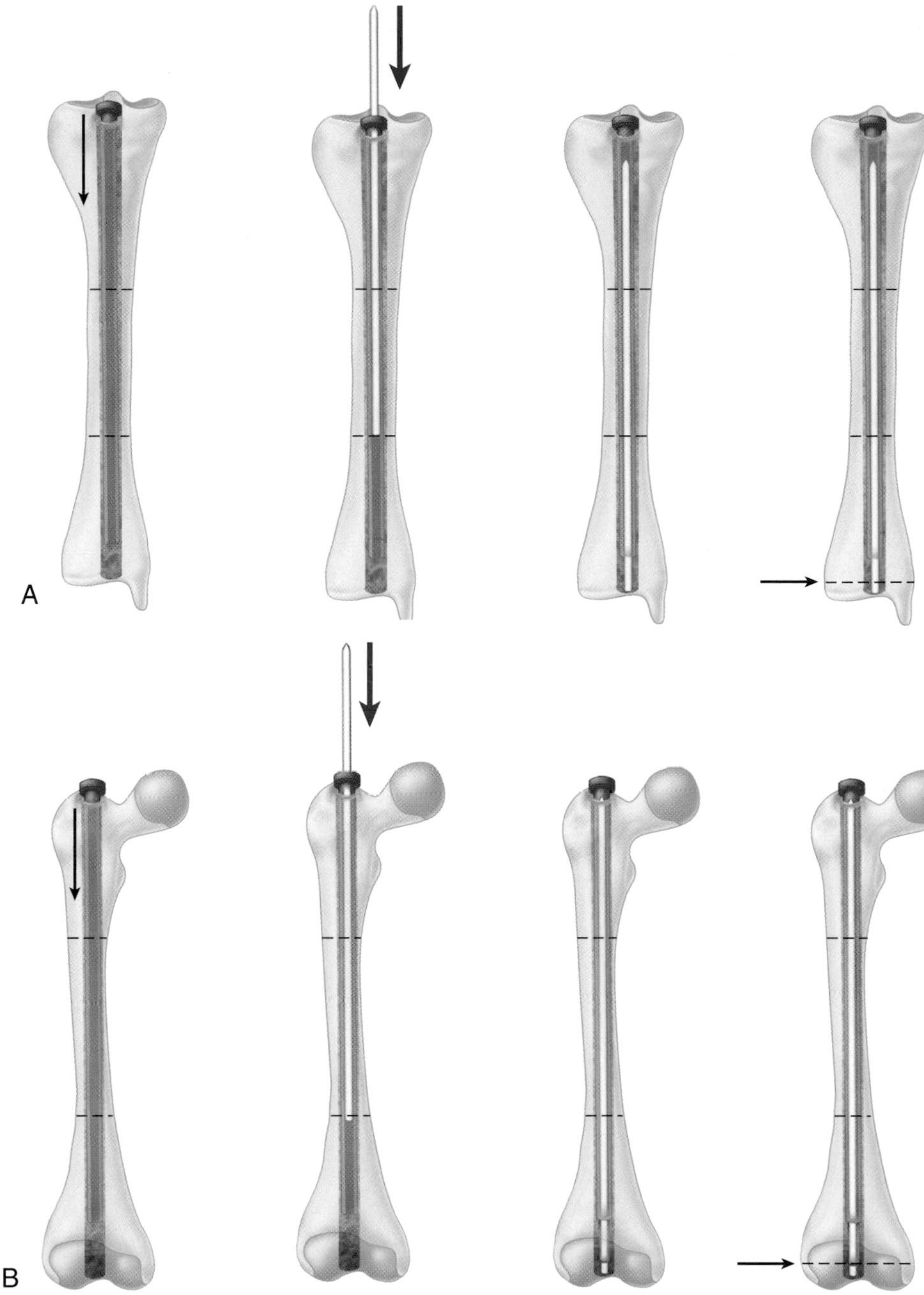

FIGURE 32-70 **Schematic of surgical procedure for insertion of interlocking telescopic rod in the tibia (A) and the femur (B). The obturator is inserted within the sleeve in an antegrade manner and is transfixed at the distal epiphysis.** (Redrawn from Cho T-J, et al: Interlocking telescopic rod for patients with osteogenesis imperfecta, *J Bone Joint Surg* 89A:1028, 2007.) **SEE TECHNIQUE 32-25**.

TELESCOPING ROD INSERTION

- After a corrective osteotomy is completed, estimate the length of the bone from the greater trochanter to the distal growth plate. Based on the height of the distal epiphysis as measured on an anteroposterior radiograph, choose a long (L) or short (S) nail.
- Cut the length of the female hollow component to size. Do not cut the male solid nail until after the components have been implanted.
- Remove the wire and place the male solid nail in the driver, making sure that the wings of the male solid nail are fitted into the male driver slot. These drivers lock the male component to facilitate maneuvering the nail upon insertion. Lock the male implant component after it is inserted inside the male driver by simply rotating the eccentric ring to the locked position.
- Push the male solid nail distally after reduction of the osteotomy(ies) and screw it into the distal epiphysis. Verify with fluoroscopy that the distal thread is positioned beyond the physis (Fig. 32-71J through L). Center the distal tip of the nail on anteroposterior and lateral views on the distal femoral epiphysis. Once the male implant

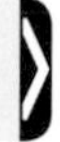

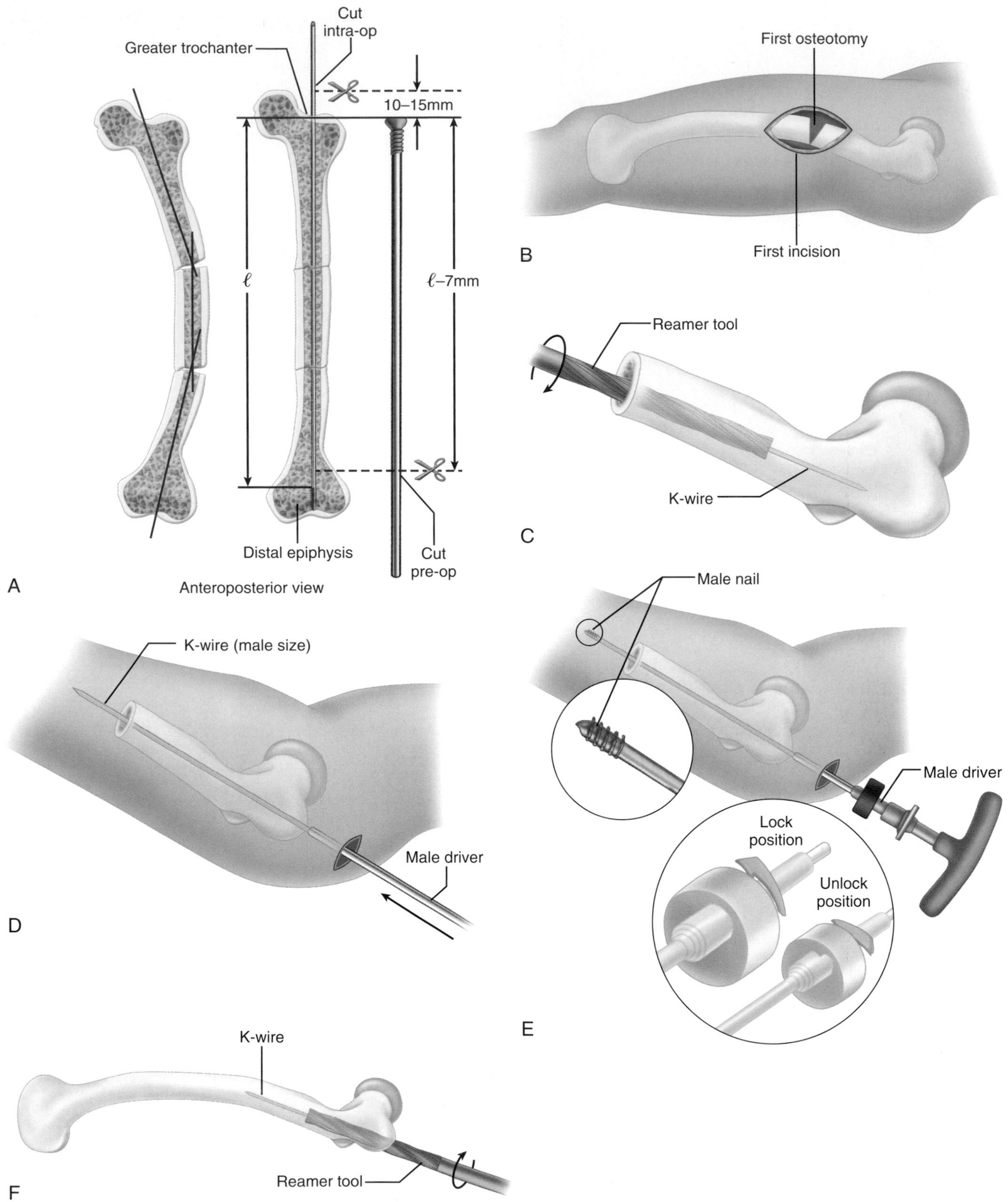

FIGURE 32-71 Fassier-Duvall telescopic intramedullary rod system (Pega Medical, Laval, Quebec, Canada). **SEE TECHNIQUE 32-26.**

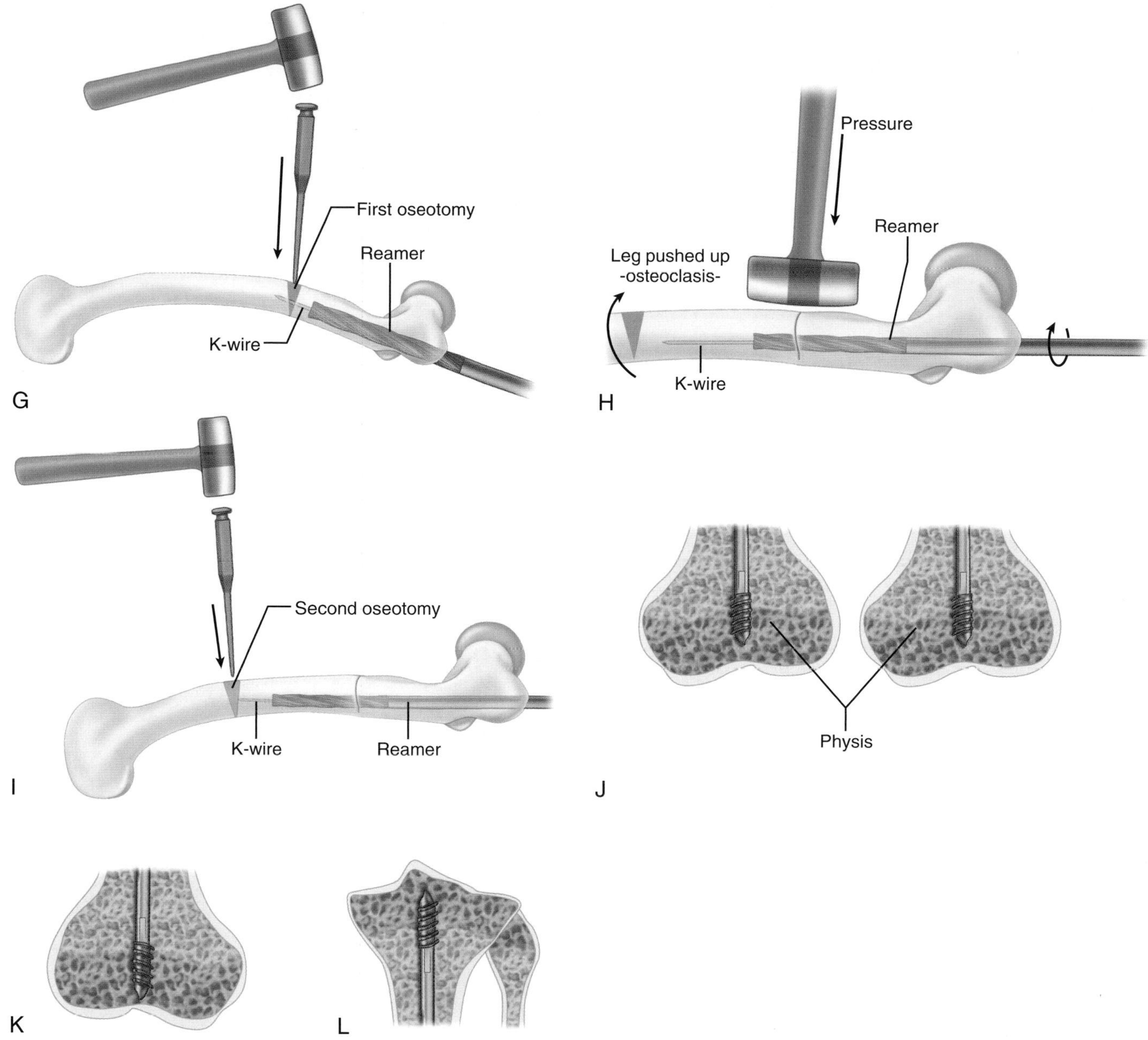

FIGURE 32-71, cont'd

Continued

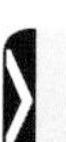

component has been screwed into the distal epiphysis, unlock the implant by rotating the eccentric ring and remove the male driver (Fig. 32-71M). Use the pushrod to reduce stress to the nail fixation while withdrawing the driver.

- Screw the female hollow nail into the greater trochanter with the appropriate driver. The threaded portion of the nail is inserted into bone (at least one or two threads), and the nonthreaded part of the female head is inserted in the nonossified part of the greater trochanter (Fig. 32-71N).
- Remove the female driver.
- Cut the solid nail (male) at this time, leaving a stub 10 to 15 mm above the female head for future growth (Fig. 32-71O). Check the smoothness of the cut end of the male nail with an appropriately sized probe.
- Close the incisions.

POSTOPERATIVE CARE. The limb is immobilized until the osteotomies heal.

OSTEOTOMY AND MEDULLARY NAILING WITH TRIGEN NAIL

In an older child in whom disturbance of the physis would not cause a significant growth problem, a small-diameter medullary nail can be used, with or without proximal or distal

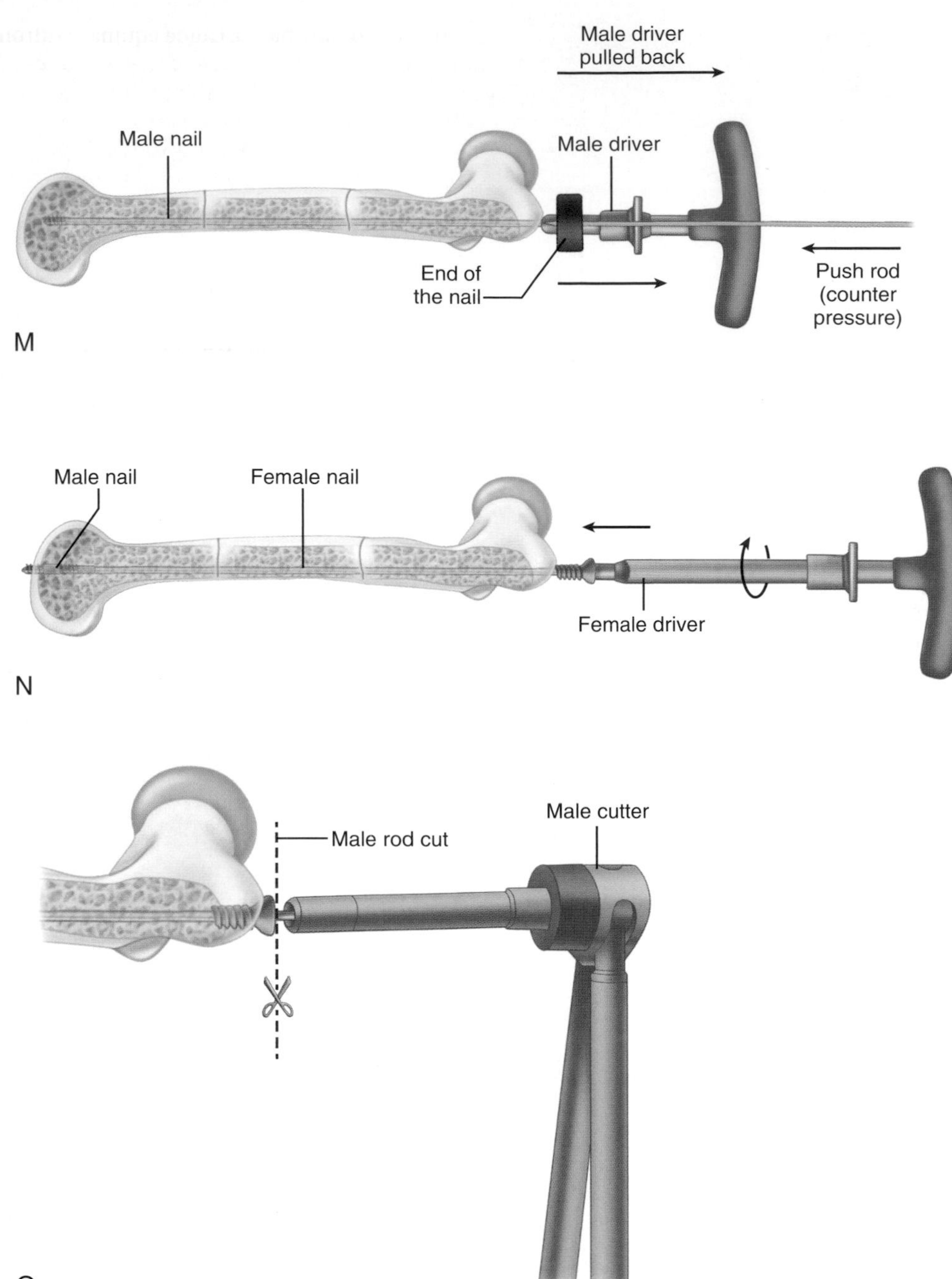

FIGURE 32-71, cont'd

locking. The TriGen nail is available in an 8-mm diameter, and we have used this successfully in several older children with osteogenesis imperfecta. The guidewire is passed, in a closed manner, proximally to the point of angulation (Fig. 32-72A). Through a small incision, an osteotomy is made at this site where the guidewire is impeded (Fig. 32-72B). The medullary nail is inserted in a closed manner and locked proximally and distally. The nail should extend as far distally as possible to prevent fracture distal to it. The technique for insertion of an interlocking medullary rod is described in Chapter 54.

DWARFISM (SHORT STATURE)

Dwarfism with disproportionate shortness of the trunk or extremities has many different causes and is commonly difficult to classify, but certain orthopaedic problems are common to many of these patients. The main areas of concern to orthopaedic surgeons are atlantoaxial instability, hip dysplasia, and malalignment of the lower extremities.

Cervical myelopathy and anomalies of the cervical spine are especially common in dwarfs with a disproportionately short trunk and are rare in achondroplasia. Dwarfs with a short trunk may exhibit a rudimentary or absent odontoid

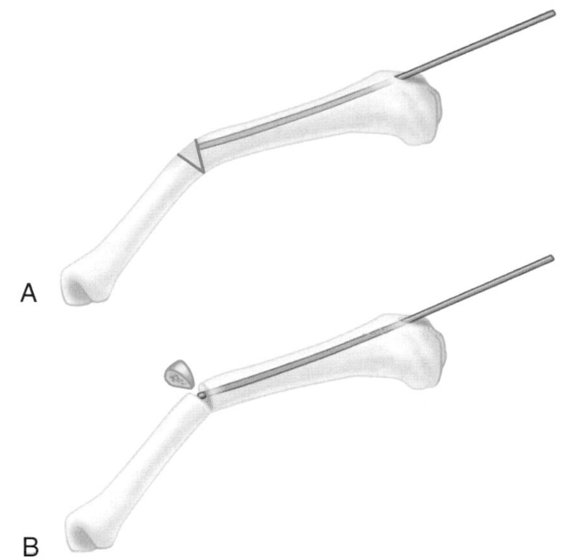

FIGURE 32-72 Osteotomy and medullary nailing (see text). **A,** Guidewire passed to point of angulation. **B,** Osteotomy.

process with ligamentous laxity and resultant atlantoaxial instability.

The first symptoms of myelopathy are a decrease in physical endurance and an early fatigue without neurologic deficit. Neurologic signs may develop later. Cord compression occurs because of bony displacement, ligamentous instability, and hypertrophy of the posterior longitudinal ligament. Often the spinal cord shifts laterally within the canal and accounts for the unilateral neurologic signs and symptoms. Cord compression also can occur at the foramen magnum (achondroplastic dwarfs) or secondary to severe cervical kyphosis from ligamentous laxity. The diagnosis of atlantoaxial instability can be made from lateral flexion and extension radiographic views or with cineradiography. Cervical fusion generally is indicated only when (1) there are obvious clinical signs of compression myelopathy or (2) there is obliteration of the subarachnoid space around the cord in flexion or extension as seen on gas myelography. Atlantoaxial instability shown on radiographs or cineradiography is not in itself an indication for surgery, and prophylactic bracing is not indicated (see Chapter 40).

Kyphosis or scoliosis occurs commonly in short-trunk dwarfs, but with the exception of diastrophic dwarfs, the scoliosis usually is mild and does not require surgery. Severe scoliosis is common in diastrophic dwarfs, and surgical correction and fusion seem to be the only reasonably effective treatment. With profound hypotonia, ligamentous laxity, and a collapsing spine, fusion may be necessary for stability while sitting.

Ligamentous laxity can cause kyphosis in achondroplasia. Severe progressive kyphoscoliosis with a posteriorly displaced vertebral body occasionally occurs in achondroplasia and in a variety of dwarfs. For neurologic deficit, anterior decompression and fusion are best and are followed by posterior fusion when the deformity is greater than 60 degrees.

In the *lumbar spine,* profound lordosis, bulging intervertebral discs, and a narrowed spinal canal are characteristic of achondroplasia. By the third decade of life, many of these patients complain of low back pain, have nerve root signs, and occasionally have a cauda equina syndrome and claudication. Laminectomy, cord and nerve root decompression, disc excision, and spinal fusion ultimately may be needed to relieve symptoms in some patients.

The *hip joint* in many dwarfing syndromes is spared compared with the remainder of the lower extremity. Multiple epiphyseal dysplasia and spondyloepiphyseal dysplasia involve the epiphysis and may cause severe, early crippling arthritis. Hip fusion usually is not indicated in dwarfs for three reasons: (1) with extremely short stature, mobility is crucial for activities of daily living such as dressing and stepping up stairs; (2) hip fusion may increase low back pain that already may be present from lumbar lordosis; and (3) hip fusion would shorten further a patient of already short stature. We have performed total hip arthroplasty in dwarfs with severe arthritis. Careful planning is necessary because nonstandard size femoral and acetabular components almost always are necessary. Bilateral dislocation of the hips is commonly seen in Morquio syndrome and usually is not vigorously treated (Fig. 32-73).

Two other conditions, *coxa vara* and *coxa valga,* occur in a substantial percentage of dwarfs. Coxa valga is commonly seen with Morquio syndrome, and coxa vara is commonly seen with spondyloepiphyseal dysplasia (Fig. 32-74). Varus and valgus osteotomies of the hips of patients with bone dysplasias should be done only rarely and after much study because of probable instability. Intertrochanteric osteotomies for severe coxa valga should be reserved for proven hip instability resulting from the valgus deformity, and for severe coxa vara they should be reserved for a waddling gait and cartilaginous defects. Varus and valgus osteotomies of the hip are described in Chapters 30 and 33.

A substantial percentage of dwarfs have *genu varum* or *genu valgum.* In general, dwarfs with disproportionately short trunks have genu valgum, whereas dwarfs with disproportionately short extremities have genu varum. Angulation may be the result of ligamentous laxity, bowing of the proximal tibia and distal femur, or, as is characteristic of achondroplastic dwarfs, bowing of the distal tibia.

The deformity usually is progressive with an ultimate length discrepancy between the fibula and the tibia. Foot placement is in a forced varus or valgus position depending on the direction of angulation at the knees. Osteotomy at or near the site of the deformity is our preferred treatment. When operating on recurrent genu valgum, such as in Ellis-Van Creveld, the surgeon should be prepared to release the lateral structures such as the iliotibial band and tighten the medial structures by reefing the vastus medialis. We have tried to control the deformity in young children with ambulatory "knock-knee" or "bowleg" braces. These braces are heavy and cumbersome and may promote ligamentous laxity, but in several patients we have been able to stop the progression or improve the deformity (Fig. 32-75). At a later age, we have performed an osteotomy without recurrence of the angulation.

Because of the disproportionate length of the extremities, especially the lower, limb lengthening has been attempted by several methods. Formerly, the most often used method in the United States was that popularized by Wagner, which combines osteotomy with slow distraction (see Chapter 29). The Ilizarov and DeBastiani techniques have been reported to achieve greater lengthening with fewer complications. More recently, tibial lengthening over an intramedullary nail

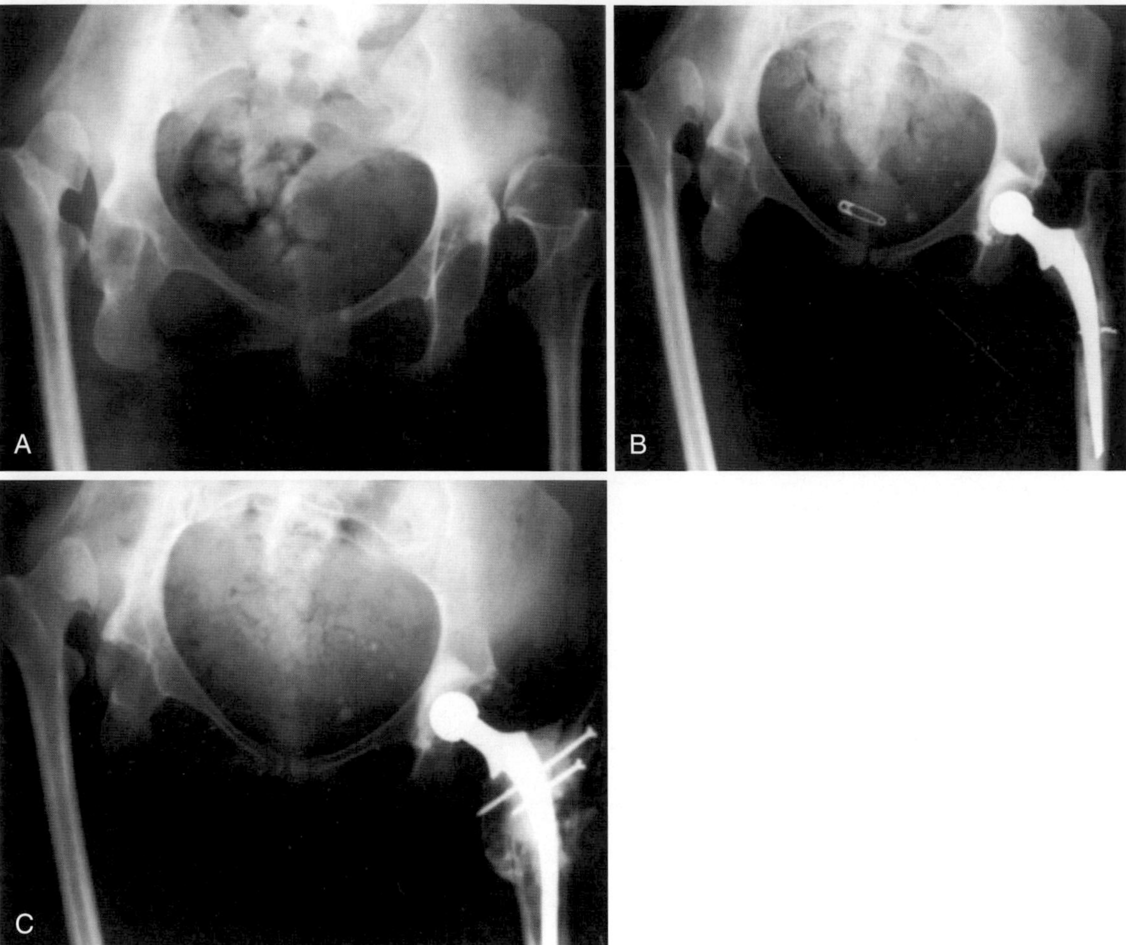

FIGURE 32-73 **A,** Adult patient with Morquio disease with bilateral dislocated hips. Left hip was painful and disabling. **B,** Appearance after total hip arthroplasty using custom-designed femoral component with small stem. Despite this, femoral shaft proximally was fractured during insertion. **C,** Appearance after revision of total hip arthroplasty with second custom-designed long-stem femoral component and anchoring screws in methylmethacrylate. Result was satisfactory.

with the use of an external fixator has shown to result in new bone formation equal to the conventional Ilizarov technique, however, with fewer complications and less time required for internal fixation. The frequency of complications and the lengthy immobilization period associated with limb lengthening by any method caused some authors in the past to discourage its use, however, especially in dwarfs. Limb lengthening should be attempted only in informed, cooperative patients committed to the lengthy procedure and with realistic expectations of the result. As the lengthening procedures have been better perfected and the complications fewer, disproportionate extremity dwarfs are commonly having lower extremity lengthenings done. In the recent literature, large series have been described with good results with the following observations: (1) lengthening should be started in children early but not before the age of 9 years, (2) premature physeal arrest (closure) of the distal femur and proximal tibia in extensive lengthening should be included in the preoperative calculations and counseling, and (3) humeral lengthenings compared with femoral lengthenings seem to have fewer complications, and callus forms at a higher rate. Humeral hybrid monolateral fixators can be used that are less bulky and allow patients to perform activities of daily living.

TIBIAL LENGTHENING OVER AN INTRAMEDULLARY NAIL WITH EXTERNAL FIXATION IN DWARFISM

TECHNIQUE 32-27

(PARK ET AL.)

- To be treated with lengthening over an intramedullary nail, the tibial medullary diameter must be at least 8 mm.
- Insert an AO tibial nail with a diameter 1 mm smaller than that of the tibial isthmus. To make passage less traumatic, remove irregularities on the endosteal surface with a single pass of a reamer.
- Insert two proximal interlocking screws in a mediolateral direction.
- Parallel to the nail, apply a preconstructed Ilizarov frame with two rings connected with telescoping rods.
- Insert two proximal tensioned wires posterior to the nail. At least one wire at each ring should pass the fibular head

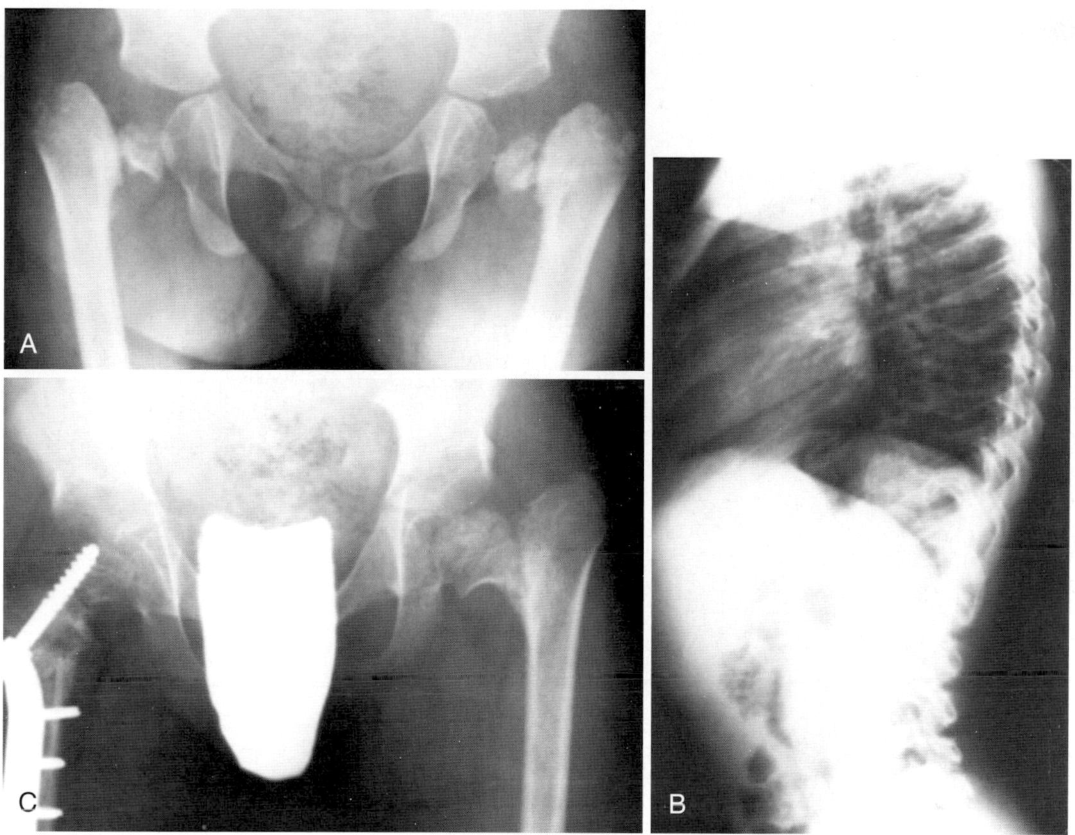

FIGURE 32-74 Spondyloepiphyseal dysplasia. **A,** Severe bilateral coxa vara deformity. **B,** Platyspondyly in same patient. **C,** After valgus osteotomy of right hip using Coventry lag screw. Cartilaginous defect is now more horizontal and under compression rather than shear.

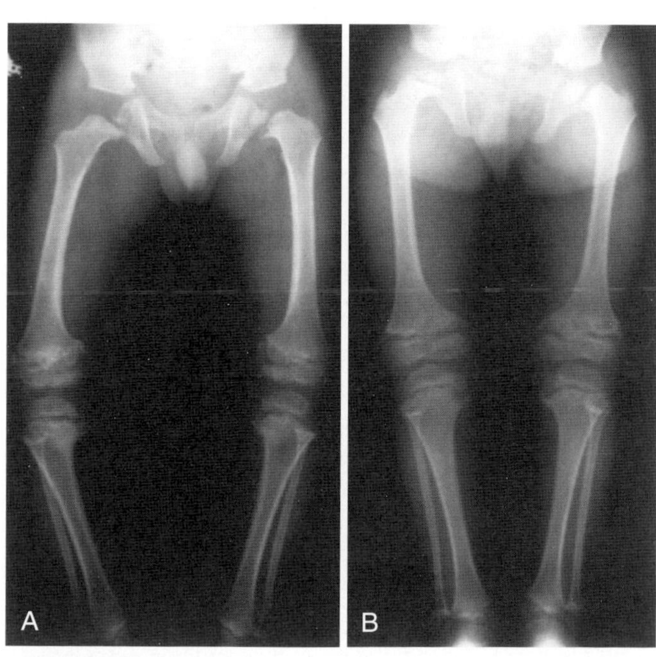

FIGURE 32-75 Multiple epiphyseal dysplasia. **A,** Radiograph obtained while weight bearing in 4-year-old boy showing delayed ossification of capital femoral epiphyses, coxa vara, and femoral and tibial bowing. **B,** Appearance 1 year after treatment in ambulatory bowleg braces. Femoral and tibial bowing is markedly improved.

or the distal part of the fibula to prevent migration of a fibular segment during lengthening.

- Perform a tibial corticotomy at the metaphyseal-diaphyseal junction with a technique utilizing multiple drill holes.
- Initiate lengthening 7 to 10 days postoperatively at a rate of 0.25 mm four times daily at each distraction site. Obtain radiographs every week during the distraction phase and every 4 weeks during the consolidation phase. Callus formation is determined to have occurred when new bone formation is seen in the distraction gap on lateral radiographs.
- When the desired length has been achieved, insert two distal interlocking screws and one distal tibiofibular transfixing screw after consolidation of the fibula.

POSTOPERATIVE CARE. Patients are allowed to bear weight with the use of two crutches (Fig. 32-76).

TRAUMATIC PHYSEAL ARREST FROM BRIDGE OF BONE

Physeal arrest after fracture in young children can produce significant limb shortening and angulatory deformity. Angulation osteotomies, epiphysiodesis of the involved epiphysis, and epiphysiodesis of the contralateral epiphysis are worthwhile and time-honored procedures to reduce angular deformity and limb-length discrepancy.

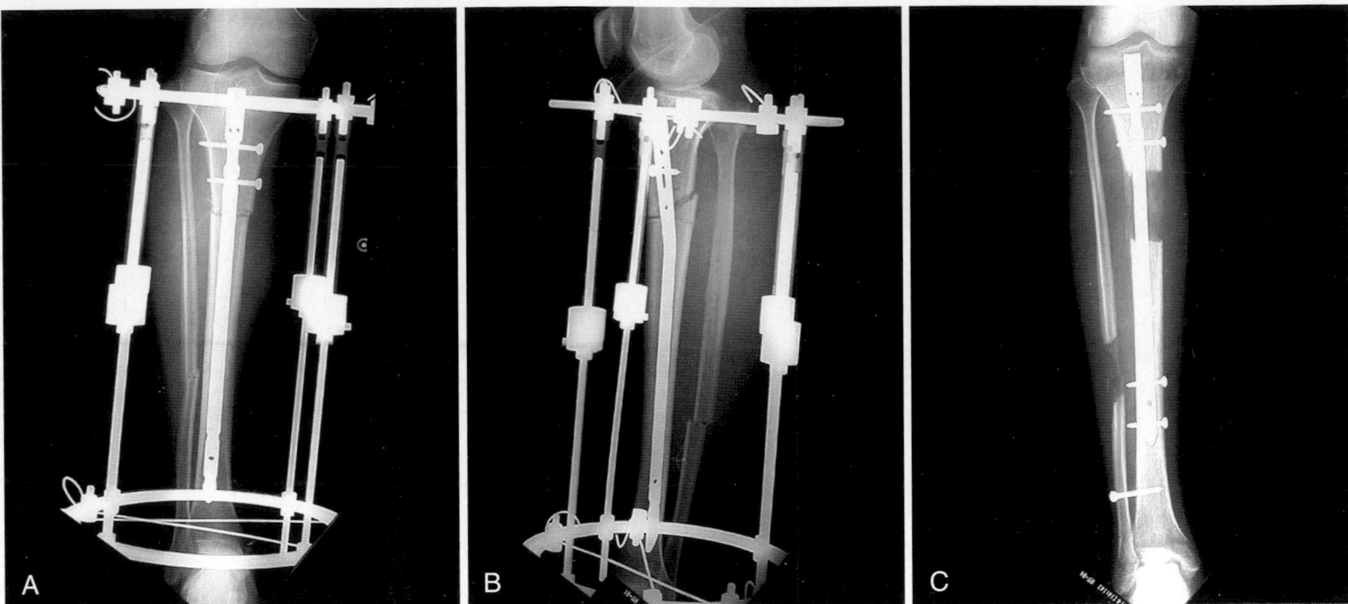

FIGURE 32-76 **A and B, Immediate postoperative anteroposterior and lateral radiographs demonstrating tibial lengthening over an intramedullary nail. C, After gradual lengthening, two distal interlocking screws and one distal tibiofibular transfixing screw are inserted. The external fixator is removed.** (From Park HW, et al: Tibial lengthening over an intramedullary nail with use of the Ilizarov external fixator for idiopathic short stature. J Bone Joint Surg 90:1970, 2008.) **SEE TECHNIQUE 32-27.**

Bright and Langenskiöld described resection of small, localized bony bridges (after fracture across a physis) that produced angular deformity or limb-length discrepancy. They recommended this procedure for a young child with a significant deformity caused by a bony bridge across less than one half of the physis of a bone that is peripheral and accessible. Tomograms, CT, and MRI are helpful in determining the extent of the bony bridge. Three-dimensional reconstruction to produce a three-dimensional model has been described to show the extent and to help in preoperative "mapping" of the bar.

After resection, Langenskiöld filled the space with fat and Bright used Silastic 382. Although the physis apparently does not regenerate in the area where the bony bridge was resected, the remaining normal physeal cartilage cells surrounding this area can produce bone in a more linear and orderly fashion than before. In a rabbit model, Lee et al. compared the results of interposition with physeal grafts, free fat, and Silastic after epiphysiodesis for correction of partial growth arrest. Clinical, radiographic, and histologic studies showed physeal grafts (from the iliac crest) to be superior to Silastic in correcting angular deformity and contributing to the longitudinal growth of the tibia after resection of a large, peripherally situated bony bridge. Interposition of fat produced the worst results. We have resected a bony bridge in conjunction with an angulation osteotomy and used fat or silicone to fill the resected area.

Depending on the location of the physis and the amount of the deformity, we agree with MacEwen (personal communication) that bony bridge resection usually does not correct a significant angular deformity, but that the resection may decrease the number of osteotomies necessary during the growth of a young child by decreasing the rate of recurrence of the angular deformity.

Ingram at this clinic described a technique for osteotomy at the level of the bony bridge adjacent and parallel to the physis. With this technique, the bridge does not have to be peripheral. When the osteotomy is opened, the white, sclerotic bridge of bone can be differentiated easily from the normal cancellous metaphyseal bone with or without a magnifying optical loupe or microscope. The bridge is resected with a dental burr, leaving only the normal physis and cancellous bone of the epiphysis and the metaphysis. A free graft of fat or a piece of silicone is placed in the defect, and the osteotomy is secured after insertion of a wedge of bone to correct deformity.

BONY BRIDGE RESECTION FOR PHYSEAL ARREST

TECHNIQUE 32-28

(LANGENSKIÖLD)

- Before the operation, exact localization and estimation of the size of the bony bridge by MRI, CT, and tomography in at least two planes are essential (Fig. 32-77A and B). More than half of the physis should be normal, and the bony bridge should be peripheral, causing a progressive angular deformity or progressive discrepancy of leg length or both.
- Expose the periphery of the physis by a suitable approach near the bony bridge. Use a tourniquet for a bloodless field for localization of the cartilaginous plate, which may be thin when close to the bridge. Use of a microscope or binocular loupe makes the procedure easier.

- Define the most peripheral part of the bony bridge and remove the overlying periosteum. Remove the bony bridge until the normal periphery of the physis is reached on both sides of the bridge and until the cartilaginous plate can be seen around the whole cavity. It is essential that no part of the bridge be left and that normal physeal cartilage not be removed unnecessarily.
- Release the tourniquet, and while hemostasis is occurring, secure a piece of fat from the subcutaneous tissue, preferably from the gluteal fold, to fill the cavity. After cessation of bleeding, fill the cavity with the autogenous fat. When the resected cavity is irregular, divide the fat transplant into several pieces to ensure complete filling.
- To keep the autogenous fat in place, suture ligament, muscle, or subcutaneous tissue over the defect. Close the wound in layers without drainage.

BONY BRIDGE RESECTION AND ANGULATION OSTEOTOMY FOR PHYSEAL ARREST

TECHNIQUE 32-29

(INGRAM)

- Accompanying a bony bridge there is usually not only angular deformity but also shortening, and an opening wedge osteotomy usually is indicated to gain length.
- Perform the osteotomy on the same side of the bone as the bony bridge causing the angular deformity (Fig. 32-77A and B). Expose the metaphyseal area of the bone without damaging the periphery of the physis on the side of the bone where the bridge is located.
- After subperiosteal exposure, place a guide pin in the metaphysis parallel to the physis and just adjacent to it, using either radiographic control or image intensifier fluoroscopy. The guide pin should penetrate or lie just adjacent to the bony bridge (Fig. 32-77C).
- Perform an osteotomy at the level of the guide pin and open the osteotomy site wide with a laminar spreader. Using a small dental burr, resect completely the white sclerotic bony bridge, using an operating microscope or a magnifying loupe for improved vision (Fig. 32-77D). Carry the resection through the physis, ensuring that all of the bony bridge is resected and that normal physeal cartilage appears on all sides of the cavity. This can be facilitated with the use of a dental mirror.
- After adequate resection, obtain hemostasis and fill the area with autogenous fat obtained from the subcutaneous tissue at the incision or with a silicone implant. Correct the angular deformity appropriately by inserting a wedge of autogenous bone into the osteotomy and secure the osteotomy with smooth pins (Fig. 32-77E).
- Close the wound in layers and apply a sterile dressing and a plaster splint.

POSTOPERATIVE CARE. Weight bearing and activities should be limited until the osteotomy has completely healed and the pins are removed.

Peripheral and linear bars are more easily approached and identified than are central bars. The normal perichondral ring at the perimeter of the healthy physis is replaced by periosteum over the bar and is easily stripped. Peripheral bar resection involves scooping out the bar but leaving the residual healthy physis intact. This requires knowing where the bar meets the physis at the perimeter of the bone and the depth that the bar reaches into the physis.

PERIPHERAL AND LINEAR PHYSEAL BAR RESECTION FOR PHYSEAL ARREST

TECHNIQUE 32-30

(BIRCH ET AL.)

- Carefully expose the peripheral junction of the bar and the healthy perichondral ring at one, or preferably both, edges of the bar. This junction serves as an excellent starting point for removing the bar. Use fluoroscopy to ensure that the resection remains at the level of the physis and does not drift into the metaphysis or epiphysis (Fig. 32-78A).
- Continue resection until the physis is visible from each edge of healthy perichondrium and throughout the depth of the cavity (Fig. 32-78B). As an alternative, identify the bar with periosteal stripping and fluoroscopic guidance and develop a cavity directed toward the physis until it is identified (Fig. 32-78C). Extend this cavity peripherally until healthy perichondrium is identified at either end of the bar.
- Fill the defect with autogenous fat from the area or from a small incision in the buttocks or groin.

Central bars can be approached from the metaphyseal marrow cavity through a metaphyseal cortical window or an osteotomy. Arthroscopically assisted central bar resection has been described using the scope to identify the normal cartilage after dental burr resection in the defect.

CENTRAL PHYSEAL BAR RESECTION FOR PHYSEAL ARREST

TECHNIQUE 32-31

(PETERSON)

- For bars extending completely across the physis, evaluate tomographic maps to determine surgical approach and ensure complete removal (Fig. 32-79). Approach centrally located bars (Fig. 32-80A) through the metaphysis or epiphysis. Because the bar is not readily accessible through

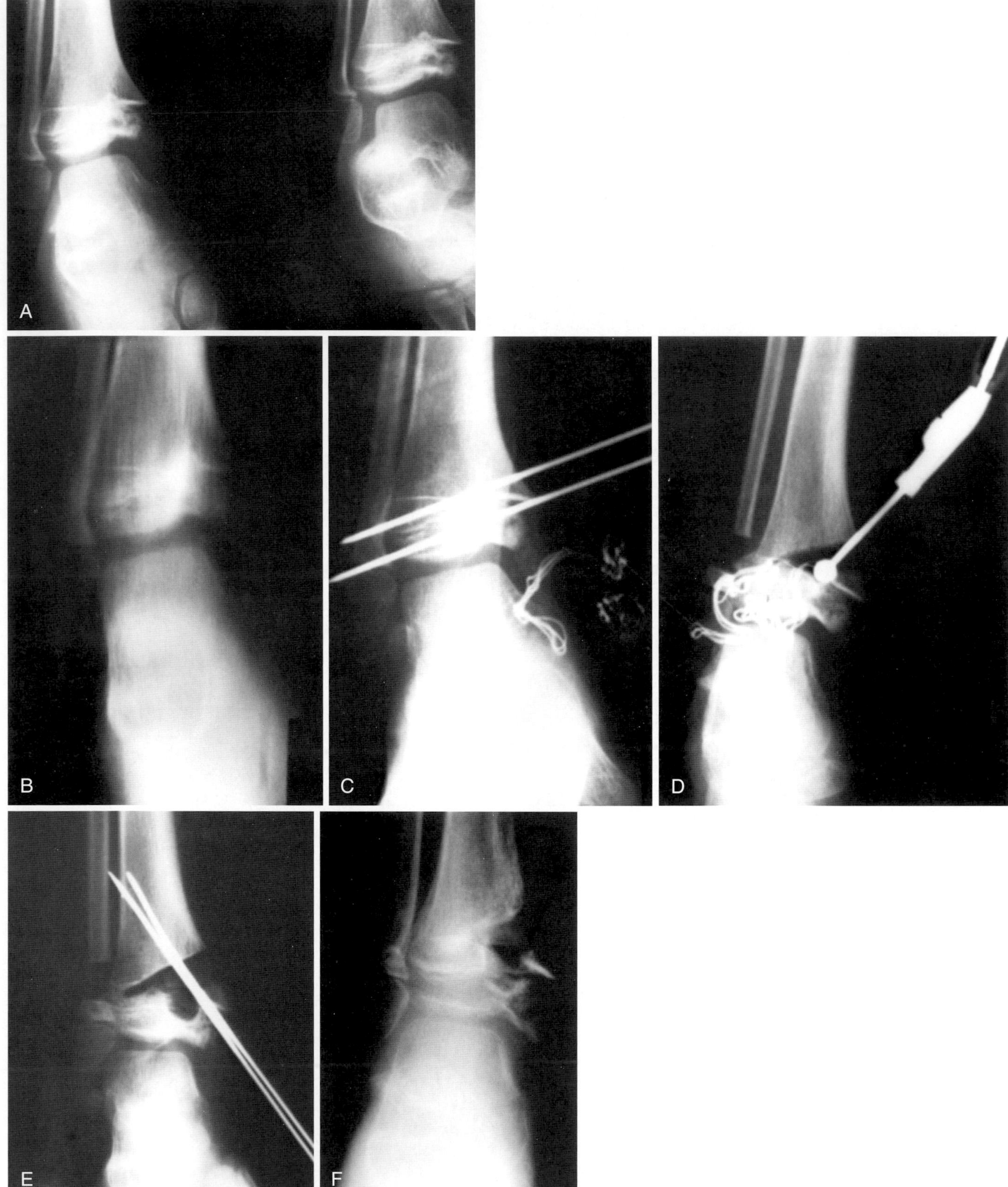

FIGURE 32-77 Traumatic epiphyseal arrest from bridge of bone. **A** and **B,** Anteroposterior radiographs and tomogram of lesion resulting from trauma to medial aspect of the distal tibial epiphysis. **C-E,** Steps in operative technique of Ingram for excision of bony bar and wedge osteotomy of distal tibia (see text). **F,** Radiograph showing correction of deformity and defect at bony bridge site. (**C-F** from Canale ST, Harper MC: Biotrigonometric analysis and practical applications of osteotomies of tibia in children, Instr Course Lect 30:85, 1981.) **SEE TECHNIQUES 32-28 AND 32-29**.

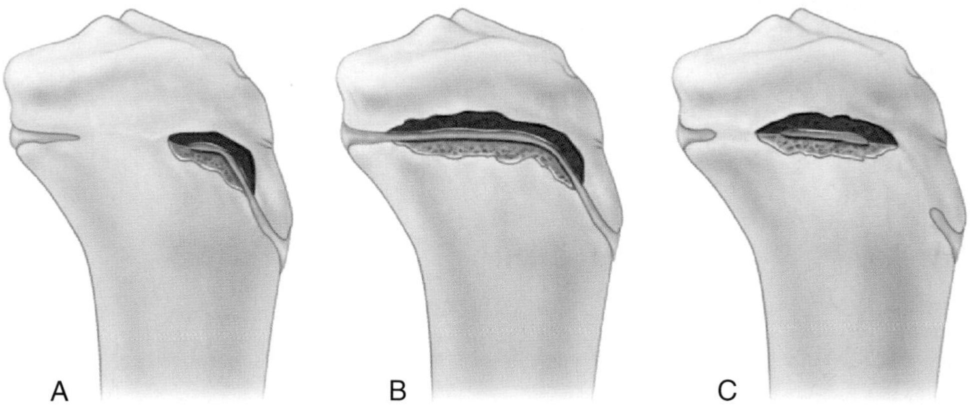

FIGURE 32-78 Peripheral bar resection (see text). **A,** Fluoroscopy ensures that resection remains at level of physis. **B,** Resection continues until physis is visible throughout depth of cavity. **C,** An alternative method for exposure is periosteal stripping with fluoroscopic guidance. (Redrawn from Birch JG: Technique of partial physeal bar resection, Op Tech Orthop 3:166, 1993.) **SEE TECHNIQUES 32-30 AND 31**.

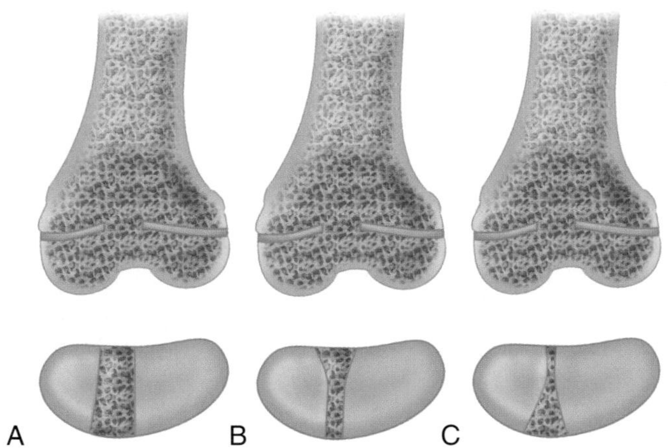

FIGURE 32-79 **A-C,** Elongated bar extending from anterior to posterior surfaces. Although all three have same appearance on anteroposterior view *(top row),* they have different contours on transverse sections *(bottom row)* (see text).

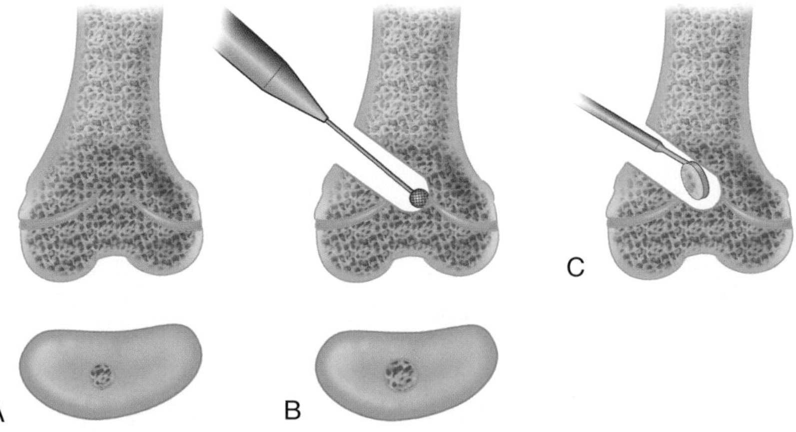

FIGURE 32-80 **A,** Central bar with peripheral growth results in "tenting" or "cupping" of physis (see text). **B,** Excision of central bar through window in metaphysis (see text). **C,** Examination of entire physis with dental mirror (see text). **SEE TECHNIQUE 32-31**.

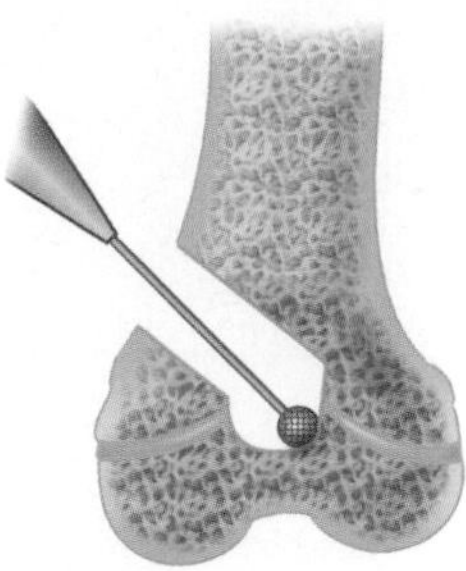

FIGURE 32-81 Smoothing metaphyseal bone surface (see text). **SEE TECHNIQUE 32-31.**

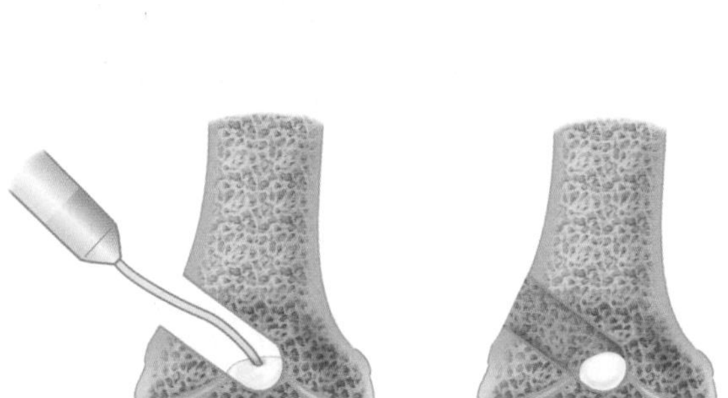

FIGURE 32-82 **A,** Insertion of Cranioplast with syringe (see text). **B,** Bone graft filling remainder of defect (see text). **SEE TECHNIQUE 32-31.**

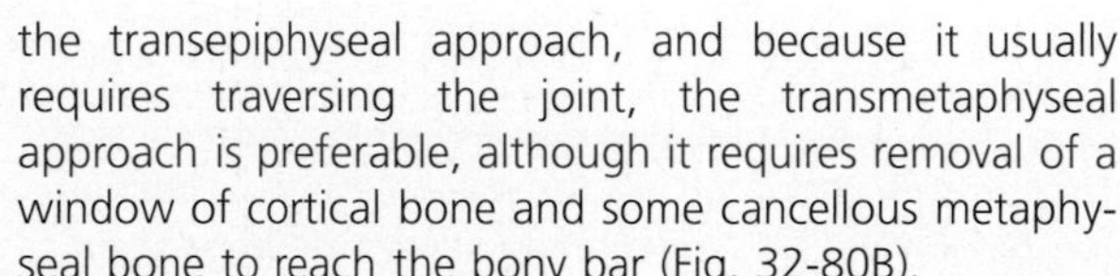

the transepiphyseal approach, and because it usually requires traversing the joint, the transmetaphyseal approach is preferable, although it requires removal of a window of cortical bone and some cancellous metaphyseal bone to reach the bony bar (Fig. 32-80B).

- After removal of the entire bar with a high-speed burr, inspect the normal physis with a small dental mirror (Fig. 32-80C). The sides of the cavity should be flat and smooth (Fig. 32-81).
- Place metal markers, such as surgical clips, in the metaphysis and epiphysis to aid in accurate measurement of subsequent growth of the involved physis. Place these markers in cancellous bone, not in contact with the cavity, and in the same longitudinal plane proximally and distally to the defect.
- In a large cavity that is gravity dependent, pour liquid Cranioplast into the defect. If the cavity is not gravity dependent, place the Cranioplast in a syringe and push it into the defect through a short polyethylene tube (Fig. 32-82A) or allow the Cranioplast to set partially and push it like putty into the defect. Allow as little Cranioplast as possible to remain in the metaphysis. After the Cranioplast has set, fill the remainder of the metaphyseal cavity with cancellous bone (Fig. 32-82B). The contour of the cavity also is important. Bar formation is less likely when the interposition material remains in the epiphysis (Fig. 32-83A) than when the epiphysis grows away from it (Fig. 32-83B).

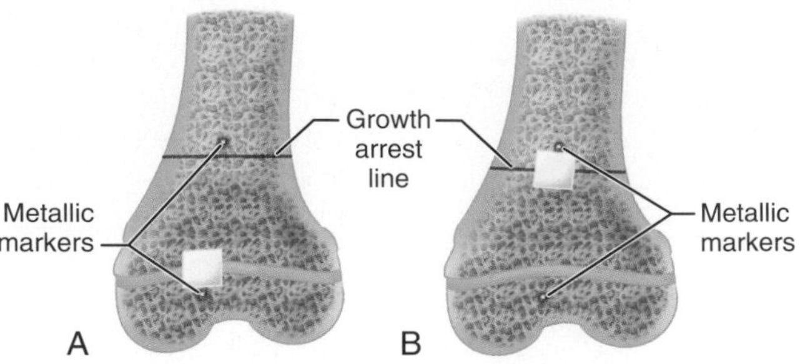

FIGURE 32-83 **A,** Plug growing away from proximal marker and growth arrest line (see text). **B,** Plug remaining with metaphysis as epiphysis grows (see text). **SEE TECHNIQUE 32-31.**

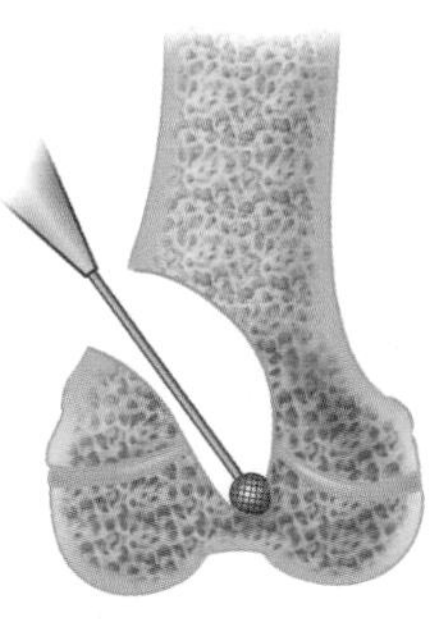

FIGURE 32-84 Undermining of epiphysis (see text). **SEE TECHNIQUE 32-31.**

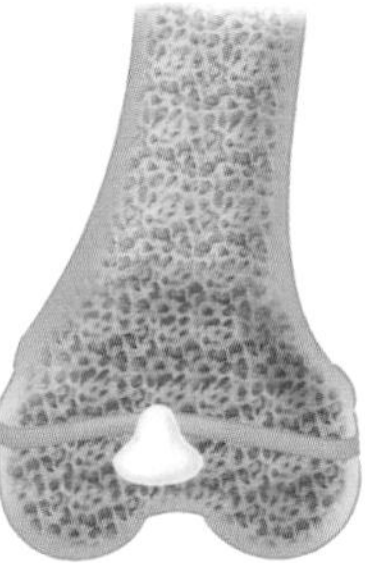

FIGURE 32-85 "Collar button" contour of plug to act as anchor (see text). **SEE TECHNIQUE 32-31.**

- Methods of keeping the plug in the epiphysis include drilling holes in the cavity (undermining) (Fig. 32-84) and enlarging the cavity (Fig. 32-85).

POSTOPERATIVE CARE. Joint motion is begun immediately. If osteotomy has not been done, no cast or other immobilization is necessary. Weight bearing is encouraged on the day of surgery or as soon as comfort permits. Follow-up with scanograms continues until maturity.

REFERENCES

FREIBERG DISEASE; OSTEOCHONDROSIS OF THE ANKLE, KNEE, AND ELBOW; AND OSGOOD-SCHLATTER DISEASE

Abouassaly M, Peterson D, Salci L, et al: Surgical management of osteochondritis dissecans of the knee in the paediatric population: a systematic review addressing surgical techniques, *Knee Surg Sports Traumatol Arthrosc* 22:1216, 2014.

Adachi N, Deie M, Nakamae A, et al: Functional and radiographic outcome of stable juvenile osteochondritis dissecans of the knee treated with retroarticular drilling without bone grafting, *Arthroscopy* 25:145, 2009.

Adachi N, Deie M, Nakamae A, et al: Functional and radiographic outcomes of unstable juvenile osteochondritis dissecans of the knee treated with lesion fixation using bioabsorbable pins, *J Pediatr Orthop* 35:82–88, 2015.

Al-Ashhab MEA, Kandel WA, Rizk AS: A simple surgical technique for treatment of Freiberg's disease, *The Foot* 23:29, 2013.

Brownlow HC, O'Connor-Read LM, Perko M: Arthroscopic treatment of osteochondritis dissecans of the capitellum, *Knee Surg Sports Traumatol Arthrosc* 14:198, 2006.

Boughanem J, Riaz R, Patel RM, Sarwark JF: Functional and radiographic outcomes of juvenile osteochondritis dissecans of the knee treated with extra-articular retrograde drilling, *Am J Sports Med* 39:2212, 2011.

Camp CL, Krych AJ, Stuart MJ: Arthroscopic preparation and internal fixation of an unstable osteochondritis dissecans lesion of the knee, *Arthrosc Tech* 2:3461, 2013.

Chambers HG, Shea KG, Anderson AF, et al: American Academy of Orthopaedic Surgeons clinical practice guideline on: the diagnosis and treatment of osteochondritis dissecans, *J Bone Joint Surg* 94A:1322, 2012.

Czyrny Z: Osgood-Schlatter disease in ultrasound diagnostics—a pictorial essay, *Med Ultrason* 12:323, 2010.

DeBerardino TM, Branstetter JG, Owens BD: Arthroscopic treatment of unresolved Osgood-Schlatter lesions, *Arthroscopy* 23:1127, 2007.

De Lucena GL, dos Santos Gomes C, Guerra RO: Prevalence and associated factors of Osgood-Schlatter syndrome in a population-based sample of Brazilian adolescents, *Am J Sports Med* 39:415, 2011.

Donaldson LD, Wojtys EM: Extraarticular drilling for stable osteochondritis dissecans in the skeletally immature knee, *J Pediatr Orthop* 28:831, 2008.

Gomoll AH, Flik KR, Hayden JK, et al: Internal fixation of unstable Cahill type-2C osteochondritis dissecans lesions of the knee in adolescent patients, *Orthopedics* 30487, 2007.

Heywood CS, Benke MT, Brindle K, Fine KM: Correlation of magnetic resonance imaging to arthroscopic findings of stability in juvenile osteochondritis dissecans, *Arthroscopy* 27:194, 2011.

Itsubo T, Murakami N, Uemura K, et al: Magnetic resonance imaging staging to evaluate the stability of capitellar osteochondritis dissecans lesions, *Am J Sports Med* 42:1972–1977, 2014.

Iwasaki N, Kamishima T, Kato H, et al: A retrospective evaluation of magnetic resonance imaging effectiveness on capitellar osteochondritis dissecans among overhead athletes, *Am J Sports Med* 40:624, 2012.

Iwasaki N, Kato H, Ishikawa J, et al: Autologous osteochondral mosaicplasty for capitellar osteochondritis dissecans in teenaged patients, *Am J Sports Med* 34:1233, 2006.

Iwasaki N, Kato H, Ishikawa J, et al: Autologous osteochondral mosaicplasty for osteochondritis dissecans of the elbow in teenage athletes, *J Bone Joint Surg* 91:2359, 2009.

Jans LB, Ditchfield M, Anna G, et al: MR imaging findings and MR criteria for instability in osteochondritis dissecans of the elbow in children, *Eur J Radiol* 81:1306, 2012.

Jones KJ, Wiesel BB, Sankar WN, Ganley TJ: Arthroscopic management of osteochondritis dissecans of the capitellum: mid-term results in adolescent athletes, *J Pediatr Orthop* 30:8, 2010.

Kessler JI, Weiss JM, Nikizad H, et al: Osteochondritis dissecans of the ankle in children and adolescents: demographics and epidemiology, *Am J Sports Med* 42:2165–2167, 2014.

Khoury J, Jerushalmi J, Loberant N, et al: Kohler disease: diagnoses and assessment by bone graphy, *Clin Nucl Med* 32:179, 2007.

Kida Y, Morihara T, Kotoura Y, et al: Prevalence and clinical characteristics of osteochondritis dissecans of the humeral capitellum among adolescent baseball players, *Am J Sports Med* 42:1963–1971, 2014.

Kijowski R, Blankenbaker DG, Shinki K, et al: Juvenile versus adult osteochondritis dissecans of the knee: appropriate MR imaging criteria for instability, *Radiology* 248:571, 2008.

Kocher MS, Czarnecki JJ, Andersen JS, Micheli LJ: Internal fixation of juvenile osteochondritis dissecans lesions about the knee, *Am J Sports Med* 35:712, 2007.

Kosaka M, Nakase J, Takahashi R, et al: Outcomes and failure factors in surgical treatment for osteochondritis dissecans of the capitellum, *J Pediatr Orthop* 33:719, 2013.

Krause M, Hapfelmeier A, Möller M, et al: Healing predictors of stable juvenile osteochondritis disecans knee lesions after 6 and 12 months of nonoperative treatment, *Am J Sports Med* 41:2384, 2013.

Lam KY, Siow HM: Conservative treatment for juvenile osteochondritis dissecans of the talus, *J Orthop Surg (Hong Kong)* 20:176, 2012.

Lebolt JR, Wall EJ: Retroarticular drilling and bone grafting of juvenile osteochondritis dissecans of the knee, *Arthroscopy* 23:794, 2007.

Lykissas MG, Wall EJ, Nathan S: Retro-articular drilling and bone grafting of juvenile knee osteochondritis dissecans: a technical description, *Knee Surg Sports Traumatol Arthrosc* 22:274, 2014.

Magnussen RA, Carey JL, Spindler KP: Does operative fixation of an osteochondritis dissecans loose body result in healing and long-term maintenance of knee function? *Am J Sports Med* 37:754, 2009.

Matsuura T, Kashiwaguchi S, Iwase T, et al: Conservative treatment for osteochondrosis of the humeral capitellum, *Am J Sports Med* 36:868, 2008.

Michael JW, Wurth A, Eysel P, König DP: Long-term results after operative treatment of osteochondritis dissecans of the knee joint—30 year results, *Int Orthop* I32:217, 2008.

Miyamoto W, Takao M, Uchio Y, et al: Late-stage Freiberg disease treated by osteochondral plug transplantation: a case series, *Foot Ankle Int* 29:950, 2008.

Murphy RT, Pennock AT, Bugbee WD: Osteochondral allograft transplantation of the knee in the pediatric and adolescent population, *Am J Sports Med* 42:635, 2014.

Nierenberg G, Falah M, Keren Y, Eidelman M: Surgical treatment of residual Osgood-Schlatter disease in young adults: role of the mobile osseous fragment, *Orthopedics* 34:176, 2011.

Pengas IP, Assiotis A, Kokkinakis M, et al: Knee osteochondritis dissecans treated by the AO hook fixation system: a four year follow-up of an alternative technique, *Open Orthop J* 8:209, 2014.

Pennock AT, Bomar JD, Chambers HG: Extra-articular, intraepiphyseal drilling for osteochondritis dissecans of the knee, *Arthrosc Tech* 2:e231, 2013.

Pihlajamäki HK, Mattila VM, Parviainen M, et al: Long-term outcome after surgical treatment of unresolved Osgood-Schlatter disease in young men, *J Bone Joint Surg* 91A:2350, 2009.

Pihlajamäki HK, Visuri TI: Long-term outcome after surgical treatment of unresolved Osgood-Schlatter disease in young men. Surgical Technique, *J Bone Joint Surg* 92(Suppl 1):258, 2010.

Rosenberger RE, Fink C, Bale RJ, et al: Computer-assisted minimally invasive treatment of osteochondritis dissecans of the talus, *Oper Orthop Traumatol* 18:300, 2006.

Sabo MT, McDonald CP, Ferreira LM, et al: Osteochondral lesions of the capitellum do not affect elbow kinematics and stability with intact collateral ligaments: an in vitro biomechanical study, *J Hand Surg [Am]* 36:74, 2011.

Salci L, Ayeni O, Abouassaly M, et al: Indications for surgical management of osteochondritis dissecans of the knee in the pediatric population: a systematic review, *J Knee Surg* 27:147, 2014.

Samora WP, Chevillet J, Adler B, et al: Juvenile osteochondritis dissecans of the knee: predictors of lesion stability, *J Pediatr Orthop* 32:1, 2012.

Satake H, Takahara M, Harada M, Maruyama M: Preoperative imaging criteria for unstable osteochondritis dissecans of the capitellum, *Clin Orthop Relat Res* 471:1137, 2013.

Sato K, Nakamura T, Toyama Y, Ikegami H: Costal osteochondral grafts for osteochondritis dissecans of the capitulum humeri, *Techn Hand Upper Extr Surg* 12:85, 2008.

Shane A, Reeves C, Wobst G, Thurston P: Second metatarsophalangeal joint pathology and Freiberg disease, *Clin Podiatr Med Surg* 30:313, 2013.

Shi LL, Bae DS, Kocher MS, et al: Contained versus uncontained lesions in juvenile elbow osteochondritis dissecans, *J Pediatr Orthop* 32:221, 2012.

Shimada K, Tanaka H, Matsumoto T, et al: Cylindrical costal osteochondral autograft for reconstruction of large defects of the capitellum due to osteochondritis dissecans, *J Bone Joint Surg* 94A:992, 2012.

Tabaddor RR, Banffy MB, Andersen JS, et al: Fixation of juvenile osteochondritis dissecans lesions of knee using poly 96L/4D-lactide copolymer bioabsorbable implants, *J Pediatr Orthop* 30:14, 2010.

Takahara M, Mura N, Sasaki J, et al: Classification, treatment, and outcome of osteochondritis dissecans of the humeral capitellum. Surgical technique, *J Bone Joint Surg* 90A:47, 2008.

Takeba J, Takahashi T, Hino K, et al: Arthroscopic technique for fragment fixation using absorbable pins for osteochondritis dissecans of the humeral capitellum: a report of 4 cases, *Knee Surg Sports Traumatol Arthrosc* 18:831, 2010.

Tatebe M, Hirata H, Shinohara T, et al: Pathomechanical significance of radial head subluxation in the onset of osteochondritis dissecans of the radial head, *J Orthop Trauma* 26:e4, 2012.

Thacker MM, Dabney KW, Mackenzie WG: Osteochondritis dissecans of the talar head: natural history and review of the literature, *J Pediatric Orthop* 21:373, 2012.

Tis JE, Edmonds EW, Bastrom T, Chambers HG: Short-term results of arthroscopic treatment of osteochondritis dissecans in skeletally immature patients, *J Pediatr Orthop* 32:226, 2012.

Van den Ende KI, McIntosh AL, Adams JE, Steinmann SP: Osteochondritis dissecans of the capitellum: a review of the literature and a distal ulnar portal, *Arthroscopy* 27:122, 2011.

Wall EJ, Vourazeris J, Myer GD, et al: The healing potential of stable juvenile osteochondritis dissecans knee lesions, *J Bone Joint Surg* 90A:2655, 2008.

Webb JE, Lewallen LW, Christophersen C, et al: Clinical outcome of internal fixation of unstable juvenile osteochondritis dissecans lesions of the knee, *Orthopedics* 36:31444, 2013.

Weiss JM, Jordan SS, Andersen JS, et al: Surgical treatment of unresolved Osgood-Schlatter disease. Ossicle resection with tibial tubercleplasty, *J Pediatr Orthop* 27:844, 2007.

Wulf CA, Stone RM, Giveans MR, Lervick GN: Magnetic resonance imaging after arthroscopic microfracture of capitellar osteochondritis dissecans, *Am J Sports Med* 40:2549, 2012.

Yamamoto Y, Ishibashi Y, Tsuda E, et al: Oteochondral autograft transplantation for osteochondritis dissecans of the elbow in juvenile baseball players. Minimum 2-year follow-up, *Am J Sports Med* 34:714, 2006.

Yonetani Y, Tanaka Y, Shiozaki Y, et al: Transarticular drilling for stable juvenile osteochondritis dissecans of the medial femoral condyle, *Knee Surg Sports Traumatol Arthrosc* 20:1528, 2012.

LEGG-CALVÉ-PERTHES DISEASE

Albers CE, Steppacher SD, Ganz R, et al: Joint-preserving surgery improves pain, range of motion, and abductor strength after Legg-Calvé-Perthes disease, *Clin Orthop Relat Res* 470:2450, 2012.

Anderson LA, Erickson JA, Severson EP, Peters CL: Sequelae of Perthes disease: treatment with surgical hip dislocation and relative femoral neck lengthening, *J Pediatr Orthop* 30:758, 2010.

Arkader A, Sankar WN, Amorim RM: Conservative versus surgical treatment of late-onset Legg-Calvé-Perthes disease: a radiographic comparison at skeletal maturity, *J Child Orthop* 3:21, 2009.

Baunin C, Sanmartin-Viron D, Accadbled F, et al: Prognosis value of early diffusion MRI in Legg-Calvé-Perthes disease, *Orthop Traumatol Surg Res* 100:317, 2014.

Beer Y, Smorgick Y, Oron A, et al: Long-term results of proximal femoral osteotomy in Legg-Calvé-Perthes disease, *J Pediatr Orthop* 28:819, 2008.

Boutault JR, Baunin C, Bérard E, et al: Diffusion MRI of the neck of the femur in Legg-Calvé-Perthes disease: a preliminary study, *Diagn Interv Imaging* 94:78, 2013.

Bowen JR, Guille JT, Jeong C, et al: Labral support shelf arthroplasty for containment in early stages of Legg-Calvé-Perthes disease, *J Pediatr Orthop* 31(Suppl 2):S206, 2011.

Bulut M, Demirts A, Ucar BY, et al: Salter pelvic osteotomy in the treatment of Legg-Calvé-Perthes disease: the medium-term results, *Acta Orthop Belg* 80:56, 2014.

Carsi B, Judd J, Clarke NM: Shelf acetabuloplasty for containment in the early stages of Legg-Calvé-Perthes disease, *J Pediatr Orthop* 35:151–156, 2015.

Castaneda P, Haynes R, Mijares J, et al: Varus-producing osteotomy for patients with lateral pillar type B and C Legg-Calvé-Perthes disease followed to skeletal maturity, *J Child Orthop* 2:373, 2008.

Chang JH, Kuo KN, Huang SC: Outcomes in advanced Legg-Calvé-Perthes disease treated with the Staheli procedure, *J Surg Res* 168:237, 2011.

Chiarapattanakom P, Thanacharoenpanich S, Pakpianpairoj C, Liupolvanish P: The remodeling of the neck-shaft angle after proximal femoral varus osteotomy for the treatment of Legg-Calvé-Perthes syndrome, *J Med Assoc Thai* 95(Suppl 10):S135, 2012.

Citlak A, Kerimoglu S, Baki C, Aydin H: Comparison between conservative and surgical treatment in Perthes disease, *Arch Orthop Trauma Surg* 132:87, 2012.

Clohisy JC, North JD, Schoenecker PL: What are the factors associated with acetabular correction in Perthes-like hip deformities? *Clin Orthop Relat Res* 470:3439, 2012.

Clohisy JC, Ross JR, North JD, et al: What are the factors associated with acetabular correction in Perthes-like hip deformities, *Clin Orthop Relat Res* 470:3439, 2012.

Conroy E, Sheehan E, O'Connor P, et al: Triple pelvic osteotomy in Legg-Calvé-Perthes disease using a single anterolateral incision: a 4-year review, *J Pediatr Orthop B* 19:323, 2010.

Domzalski ME, Glutting J, Bowen R, Littleton AG: Lateral acetabular growth stimulation following a labral support procedure in Legg-Calvé-Perthes disease, *J Bone Joint Surg* 88A:1458, 2006.

Du J, Lu A, Dempsey M, et al: MR perfusion index as a quantitative method of evaluation epiphyseal perfusion in Legg-Calvé-Perthes disease and correlation with short-term radiographic outcome: a preliminary study, *J Pediatr Orthop* 33:707, 2013.

Eamsobhana P, Kaewporsawan K: Combined osteotomy in patients with severe Legg-Calvé-Perthes disease, *J Med Assoc Thai* 95(Suppl 10):S128, 2012.

Edmonds EW, Heyworth BE: Osteochondritis dissecans of the shoulder and hip, *Clin Sports Med* 33:285, 2014.

Forster MC, Kumar S, Rajan RA, et al: Head-at-risk signs in Legg-Calvé-Perthes disease: poor inter- and intra-observer reliability, *Acta Orthop* 77:413, 2006.

Freeman CR, Jones K, Byrd JWT: Hip arthroscopy for Legg-Calvé-Perthes disease: minimum 2-year follow-up, *Arthroscopy* 29:666, 2013.

Ghanem I, Haddad E, Haidar R, et al: Lateral shelf acetabuloplasty in the treatment of Legg-Calvé-Perthes disease: improving mid-term outcome in severely deformed hips, *J Child Orthop* 4:13, 2010.

Glard Y, Katchburian MV, Jadquemier M, et al: Genu valgum in Legg-Calvé-Perthes disease treated with femoral varus osteotomy, *Clin Orthop Relat Res* 467:1587, 2009.

Grzegorzewski A, Synder M, Kmiec K, et al: Shelf acetabuloplasty in the treatment of severe Legg-Calvé-Perthes disease: good outcomes at midterm follow-up, *Biomed Res Int* 2013:859483, 2013. [Epub 2013 Nov 27].

Hailer YD, Haag AC, Nilsson O: Legg-Calvé Perthes disease: quality of life, physical activity, and behavior pattern, *J Pediatr Orthop* 34:514, 2014.

Hailer YD, Montgomery SM, Ekbom A, et al: Legg-Calvé-Perthes disease and risks for cardiovascular diseases and blood diseases, *Pediatrics* 125:e1308, 2010.

Hardesty CK, Liu RW, Thompson GH: The role of bracing in Legg-Calvé-Perthes disease, *J Pediatr Orthop* 31(Suppl 2):S178, 2011.

Hosalkar H, Munhoz da Cunha AL, Baldwin K, et al: Triple innominate osteotomy for Legg-Calvé-Perthes disease in children: does the lateral coverage change with time? *Clin Orthop Relat Res* 470:2402, 2012.

Javid M, Wedge JH: Radiographic results of combined Salter innominate and femoral osteotomy in Legg-Calvé-Perthes disease in older children, *J Child Orthop* 3:229, 2009.

Joo SY, Lee KS, Koh IH, et al: Trochanteric advancement in patients with Legg-Calvé-Perthes disease does not improve pain or limp, *Clin Orthop Relat Res* 466:927, 2008.

Kim HK, da Cunha AM, Browne R, et al: How much varus is optimal with proximal femoral osteotomy to preserve the femoral head in Legg-Calvé-Perthes disease? *J Bone Joint Surg* 93A:341, 2011.

Kim HK, Kaste S, Dempsey M, Wilkes D: A comparison of non-contrast and contrast-enhanced MRI in the initial stage of Legg-Calvé-Perthes disease, *Pediatr Radiol* 43:1166, 2013.

Kim HT, Gu JK, Bae SH, et al: Does valgus femoral osteotomy improve femoral head roundness in severe Legg-Calvé-Perthes disease? *Clin Orthop Relat Res* 471:1021, 2013.

Kim HT, Oh MH, Lee JS: MR imaging as a supplement to traditional decision-making in the treatment of LCP disease, *J Pediatr Orthop* 31:246, 2011.

Kim WC, Hiroshima K, Imaeda T: Multicenter study for Legg-Calvé-Perthes disease in Japan, *J Orthop Sci* 11:333, 2006.

Kitoh H, Kaneko H, Mishima K, et al: Prognostic factors for trochanteric overgrowth after containment treatment in Legg-Calvé-Perthes disease, *J Pediatr Orthop B* 22:432, 2013.

Kosashvili Y, Raz G, Backstein D, et al: Fresh-stored osteochondral allografts for the treatment of femoral head defects: surgical technique and preliminary results, *Int Orthop* 37:1001, 2013.

Laklouk MA, Hosny GA: Hinged distraction of the hip joint in the treatment of Perthes disease: evaluation at skeletal maturity, *J Pediatr Orthop B* 21:386, 2012.

Larson AN, Sucato DJ, Herring JA, et al: A prospective multicenter study of Legg-Calvé-Perthes disease: functional and radiographic outcomes of nonoperative treatment at a mean follow-up of twenty years, *J Bone Joint Surg* 94:584, 2012.

Lee ST, Vaidya SV, Song HR, et al: Bone age delay patterns in Legg-Calvé-Perthes disease: an analysis using the Tanner and Whitehouse 3 method, *J Pediatr Orthop* 27:198, 2007.

Leunig M, Ganz R: Relative neck lengthening and intracapital osteotomy for severe Perthes and Perthes-like deformities, *Bull NYU Hosp Joint Dis* 69:S62, 2011.

Moya-Angeler J, Abril JC, Rodriguez IV: Legg-Calvé-Perthes disease: role of isolated adductor tenotomy? *Eur J Orthop Surg Traumatol* 8:921, 2013.

Myers GJC, Mathur K, O'Hara J: Valgus osteotomy: a solution for late presentation of hinge abduction in Legg-Calvé-Perthes disease, *J Pediatr Orthop* 28:169, 2008.

Nakamura J, Kamegaya M, Saisu T, et al: Outcome of patients with Legg-Calvé-Perthes onset before 6 years of age, *J Pediatr Orthop* 35:144–150, 2015.

Nguyen NA, Klein G, Dogbey G, et al: Operative versus nonoperative treatments for Legg-Calvé-Perthes disease: a meta-analysis, *J Pediatr Orthop* 32:697, 2012.

Novais EN: Application of the surgical dislocation approach to residual hip deformity secondary to Legg-Calvé-Perthes disease, *J Pediatr Orthop* 33:S62, 2013.

Oh CW, Rodriguez A, Guille JT, Bowen JR: Labral support shelf arthroplasty for the early stages of severe Legg-Calvé-Perthes disease, *Am J Orthop* 39:26, 2010.

Onishi E, Ikeda N, Ueo T: Degenerative osteoarthritis after Perthes' disease: a 36-year follow-up, *Arch Orthop Trauma Surg* 131:701, 2011.

Park MS, Chung CY, Lee KM, et al: Reliability and stability of three common classifications for Legg-Calvé-Perthes disease, *Clin Orthop Relat Res* 470:2376, 2012.

Price CT: The lateral pillar classification for Legg-Calvé-Perthes disease, *J Pediatr Orthop* 27:5, 2007.

Rich MM, Schoenecker PL: Management of Legg-Calvé-Perthes disease using an A-frame orthosis and hip range of motion: a 25-year experience, *J Pediatr Orthop* 33:112, 2013.

Rosenfeld SB, Herring JA, Chao JC: Legg-Calvé-Perthes disease: a review of cases with onset before six years of age, *J Bone Joint Surg* 89A:2712, 2007.

Ross JR, Nepple JJ, Baca G, et al: Intraarticular abnormalities in residual Perthes and Perthes-like hip deformities, *Clin Orthop Relat Res* 470:2968, 2012.

Rowe SM, Jung ST, Cheon SY, et al: Outcome of cheilectomy in Legg-Calvé-Perthes disease: minimum 25-year follow-up of five patients, *J Pediatr Orthop* 26:204, 2006.

Sankar WN, Castaneda TS, Hont T, et al: Feasibility and safety of perfusion MRI for Legg-Calvé-Perthes disease, *J Pediatr Orthop* 2014. [Epub ahead of print].

Sankar WN, Flynn JM: The development of acetabular retroversion in children in Legg-Calvé-Perthes disease, *J Pediatr Orthop* 28:440, 2008.

Sankar WN, Thomas S, Castaneda P, et al: Feasibility and safety of perfusion MRI for Legg-Calvé-Perthes disease, *J Pediatr Orthop* 34:679–682, 2014.

Schaaf AC, Weiner DS, Steiner RP, et al: Fracture incidence following plate removal in Legg-Calvé-Perthes disease: a 32-year study, *J Child Orthop* 2:381, 2008.

Schoenecker PL: Do we need another gold standard to assess acute Legg-Calvé-Perthes disease? *J Bone Joint Surg* 96A(1):e125, 2014.

Shah H, Siddesh ND, Joseph B, Nair SN: Effect of prophylactic trochanteric epiphyseodesis in older children with Perthes' disease, *J Pediatr Orthop* 29:889, 2009.

Sharma S, Shewale S, Sibinski M, Sherlock DA: Legg-Calvé-Perthes disease affecting children less than eight years of age: a paired outcome study, *Int Orthop* 33:231, 2009.

Shore BJ, Millis MB, Kim YJ: Vascular safe zones for surgical dislocation in children with healed Legg-Calvé-Perthes disease, *J Bone Joint Surg* 94A:721, 2012.

Shore BJ, Novais EN, Millis MB, Kim Y-J: Low early failure rates using a surgical dislocation approach in healed Legg-Calvé-Perthes disease, *Clin Orthop Relat Res* 470:2441, 2012.

Siebenrock KA, Pwell JN, Ganz R: Osteochondritis dissecans of the femoral head, *Hip Int* 20:489, 2010.

Sink E, Zaltz I, Session Participants: Report of break-out session: management of sequelae of Legg-Calvé-Perthes disease, *Clin Orthop Relat Res* 470:3462, 2012.

Tannast M, Hanke M, Ecker TM, et al: LCPD: reduced range of motion resulting from extra- and intraarticular impingement, *Clin Orthop Relat Res* 470:2431, 2012.

Terjesen T, Wiig O, Svenningsen S: Varus femoral improves sphericity of the femoral head in older children with severe form of Legg-Calvé-Perthes disease, *Clin Orthop Relat Res* 470:2394, 2012.

Thompson GH: Salter osteotomy in Legg-Calvé-Perthes disease, *J Pediatr Orthop* 31(Suppl 2):S192, 2011.

Van Campenhout A, Moens P, Fabry G: Serial bone graphy in Legg-Calvé-Perthes disease: correlation with the Catterall and Herring classification, *J Pediatr Orthop B* 15:6, 2006.

Volpon JB: Comparison between innominate osteotomy and arthrodistraction as a primary treatment for Legg-Calvé-Perthes disease: a prospective controlled trial, *Int Orthop* 36:1899, 2012.

Yoo W, Choi IH, Moon HJ, et al: Valgus femoral osteotomy for noncontainable Perthes hips: prognostic factors of remodeling, *J Pediatr Orthop* 33:650, 2013.

Wright DM, Perry DC, Bruce CE: Shelf acetabuloplasty for Perthes disease in patients older than eight years of age: an observational cohort study, *J Pediatr Orthop B* 22:96, 2013.

HEMOPHILIA

Bai Z, Zhang E, He Y, et al: Arthroscopic ankle arthrodesis in hemophilic arthropathy, *Foot Ankle Int* 34:1147, 2013.

Barg A, Elsner A, Hefti D, Hintermann B: Haemophilic arthropathy of the ankle treated by total ankle replacement: a case series, *Haemophilia* 16:647, 2010.

Bluth BE, Fong YJ, Houman JJ, et al: Ankle fusion in patients with haemophilia, *Haemophilia* 19:432, 2013.

Carulli C, Matassi F, Civinini R, et al: Intra-articular injections of hyaluronic acid induce positive clinical effects in knees of patients affected by haemophilic arthropathy, *Knee* 20:36, 2013.

Caviglia H, Candela M, Galatro G, et al: Elective orthopaedic surgery for haemophilia patients with inhibitors: single centre experience of 40 procedures and review of the literature, *Haemophilia* 17:910, 2011.

Chevalier Y, Dargaud Y, Lienhart A, et al: Seventy-two total knee arthroplasties performed in patients with haemophilia using continuous infusion, *Vox Sang* 104:135, 2013.

Cho YJ, Kim KI, Chun YS, et al: Radioisotope synoviorthesis with Holmium-166-chitosan complex in haemophilic arthropathy, *Haemophilia* 16:640, 2010.

De Almeida AM, de Rezende MU, Cordeiro FG, et al: Arthroscopic partial anterior synovectomy of the knee on patients with haemophilia, *Knee Surg Sports Traumatol Arthrosc* 23:785–791, 2015.

Dell'Era L, Facchini R, Corona F: Knee synovectomy in children with juvenile idiopathic arthritis, *J Pediatr Orthop B* 17:128, 2008.

Giangrande PL, Wilde JT, Madan B, et al: Consensus protocol for the use of recombinant activated factor VI (eptacog alfa (activated); NovoSeven] in elective orthopaedic surgery in haemophilic patients with inhibitors, *Haemophilia* 15:501, 2009.

Goddard NJ, Mann HA, Lee CA: Total knee replacement in patients with end-stage haemophilic arthropathy: 25-year results, *J Bone Joint Surg* 92B:1085, 2010.

Hirose J, Takedani H, Koibuchi T: The risk of elective orthopaedic surgery for haemophilia patients: Japanese single-centre experience, *Haemophilia* 19:951, 2013.

Johnson JN, Shaughnessy WJ, Stans AA, et al: Management of knee arthropathy in patients with vascular malformations, *J Pediatr Orthop* 29:380, 2009.

Lambert T, Auerswald G, Benson G, et al: Joint disease, the hallmark of haemophilia: what issues and challenges remain despite the development of effective therapies? *Thromb Res* 133:967, 2014.

Melchiorre D, Linari S, Innocenti M, et al: Ultrasound detects joint damage and bleeding in haemophilic arthropathy: a proposal of a score, *Haemophilia* 17:112, 2011.

Ozelo MC: Surgery in patients with hemophilia: is thromboprophylaxis mandatory? *Thromb Res* 130(Suppl 1):S23, 2012.

Poenaru DV, Patrascu JM, Andor BC, Popa I: Orthopaedic and surgical features in the management of patients with haemophilia, *Eur J Orthop Surg Traumatol* 24:685, 2014.

Rangarajan S, Austin S, Goddard NJ, et al: Consensus recommendations for the use of FEIBA(®) in haemophilia A patients with inhibitors undergoing elective orthopaedic and non-orthopaedic surgery, *Haemophilia* 19:294, 2013.

Raza S, Kale G, Kim D, et al: Thromboprophylaxis and incidence of venous thromboembolism in patients with hemophilia A or B who underwent high-risk orthopedic surgeries, *Clin Appl Thromb Hemost* 2014. [Epub ahead of print].

Rezazadeh S, Haghighat A, Mahmoodi M, et al: Synviorthesis induced by rifampicin in hemophilic arthropathy: a report of 24 treated joints, *Ann Hematol* 90:963, 2011.

Rodriguez-Merchan EC: Hemophilic synovitis of the knee: radiosynovectomy or arthroscopic synovectomy? *Expert Rev Hematol* 7:507, 2014.

Rodriguez-Merchan EC: Haemophilic synovitis of the elbow: radiosynovectomy, open synovectomy or arthroscopic synovectomy? *Thromb Res* 132:15, 2013.

Rodriguez-Merchan EC: Intra-articular injections of hyaluronic acid (viscosupplementation) in the haemophilic knee, *Blood Coagul Fibrinolysis* 23:580, 2012.

Rodriguez-Merchan EC, De La Corte-Rodriguez H, Jiminez-Yuste V: Is radiosynovectomy (RS) effective for joints damaged by haemophilia with articular degeneration in simple radiography (ADSR)? *Expert Rev Hematol* 7:507, 2014.

Rodriguez-Merchan EC: Orthopaedic problems about the ankle in hemophilia, *J Foot Ankle Surg* 51:772, 2012.

Rodriguez-Merchan EC: Special features of total knee replacement in hemophilia, *Epert Rev Hematol* 6:337, 2013.

Siboni SM, Biguzzi E, Solimeno LP, et al: Orthopaedic surgery in patients with von Willebrand disease, *Haemophilia* 20:133, 2014.

Silva M, Luck JV Jr: Radial head excision and synovectomy in patients with hemophilia, *J Bone Joint Surg* 89:2156, 2007.

Takedani H, Kawahara H, Kajiwara M: Major orthopaedic surgeries for haemophilia with inhibitors using rFVIIa, *Haemophilia* 16:290, 2010.

Tsukamoto S, Tanaka Y, Matsuda T, et al: Arthroscopic ankle arthrodesis for hemophilic arthropathy: two case reports, *Foot (Edinb)* 21:103, 2011.

Westberg M, Paus AC, Holme PA, Tjonnfjord GE: Haemophilic arthropathy: long-term outcomes in 107 primary total knee arthroplasties, *Knee* 21:147, 2014.

Wong JM, Mann HA, Goddard NJ: Perioperative clotting factor replacement and infection in total knee arthroplasty, *Haemophilia* 18:607, 2012.

RICKETS, OSTEOMALACIA, AND RENAL OSTEODYSTROPHY

Clarke NM, Page JE: Vitamin D deficiency: a paediatric orthopaedic perspective, *Curr Opin Pediatr* 24:46, 2012.

Dipaolo CP, Bible JE, Biswas D, et al: Survey of spine surgeons on attitudes regarding osteoporosis and osteomalacia screening and treatment for fractures, fusion surgery, and pseudoarthrosis, *Spine J* 9:537, 2009.

Eralp L, Kocaoglu M, Toker B, et al: Comparison of fixator-assisted nailing versus circular external fixator for bone realignment of lower extremity angular deformity in rickets disease, *Arch Orthop Trauma Surg* 131:581, 2011.

Fucentese SF, Neuhaus TJ, Ramseier LE, Ulrich Exner G: Metabolic and orthopedic management of X-linked vitamin D-resistant hypophosphatemic rickets, *J Child Orthop* 2:285, 2008.

Larson AN, Trousdale RT, Pagnano MW, et al: Hip and knee arthroplasty in hypophosphatemic rickets, *J Arthroplast* 25:1099, 2010.

Mataliotaks G, Lykissas MG, Mavrodontidis AN, et al: Femoral neck fractures secondary to renal osteodystrophy. Literature review and treatment algorithm, *J Musculoskelet Neuronal Interact* 9:130, 2009.

Petje G, Meizer R, Radler C, et al: Deformity correction in children with hereditary hypophosphatemic rickets, *Clin Orthop Relat Res* 466:3078, 2008.

Veilleux LN, Cheung M, Ben Amor M, Rauch F: Abnormalities in muscle density and muscle function in hypophosphatemic rickets, *J Clin Endocrinol Metab* 97:E1492, 2012.

Veilleux LN, Cheung MS, Glorieux FH, Rauch F: The muscle-bone relationship in X-linked hypophosphatemic rickets, *J Clin Endocrinol* 98:E990, 2013.

TIBIA VARA

Andrade N, Johnston CE: Medial epiphysiolysis in severe infantile tibia vara, *J Pediatr Orthop* 26:652, 2006.

Burghardt RD, Specht SC, Herzenberg JE: Mechanical failures of eight-plate guided growth system for temporary hemiepiphysiodesis, *J Pediatr Orthop* 30:594, 2010.

Bushnell BD, May R, Campion ER, et al: Hemiepiphyseodesis for late-onset tibia vara, *J Pediatr Orthop* 29:285, 2009.

Clarke SE, McCarthy JJ, Davidson RS: Treatment of Blount disease: a comparison between the multiaxial correction system and other external fixators, *J Pediatr Orthop* 29:103, 2009.

Feldman DS, Madan SS, Ruchelsman DE, et al: Accuracy of correction of tibia vara: acute versus gradual correction, *J Pediatr Orthop* 26:794, 2006.

Gary J, Richards BS: Infantile tibia vara: correction of recurrent varus deformity following epiphyseolysis, *Orthopedics* 31:503, 2008.

Gkiokas A, Brilakis E: Management of neglected Blount disease using double corrective tibia osteotomy and medial plateau elevation, *J Child Orthop* 6:411, 2012.

Gordon JE, King DJ, Luhmann SJ, et al: Femoral deformity in tibia vara, *J Bone Joint Surg* 88A:380, 2006.

Hefny H, Salaby H, El-kawy S, et al: A new double elevating osteotomy in management of severe neglected infantile tibia vara using the Ilizarov technique, *J Pediatr Orthop* 26:233, 2006.

Ho-Fung V, James C, Delgado J, et al: MRI evaluation of the knee in children with infantile Blount disease: tibial and extra-tibial findings, *Pediatr Radiol* 43:1316, 2013.

Janoyer M, Jabbari H, Rouvillain JL, et al: Infantile Blount's disease treated by hemiplateau elevation and epiphyseal distraction using a specific external fixator preliminary report, *J Pediatr Orthop* 16B:273, 2007.

Khanfour AA: Does Langenskiold staging have a good prognostic value in late onset tibia vara? *J Orthop Surg Res* 7:23, 2012.

Lavelle WF, Shovlin J, Drvaric DM: Reliability of the metaphyseal-diaphyseal angle in tibia vara as measured on digital images by pediatric orthopaedic surgeons, *J Pediatr Orthop* 28:695, 2008.

Laville JM, Wiart Y, Salmeron F: Can Blount's disease heal spontaneously? *Orthop Traumatol Surg Res* 96:531, 2010.

Li Y, Spencer SA, Hedequist D: Proximal tibial osteotomy and Taylor Spatial Frame application for correction of tibia vara in morbidly obese adolescents, *J Pediatr Orthop* 33:276, 2013.

Masrouha KZ, Sraj S, Lakkis S, Saghieh S: High tibial osteotomy in young adults with constitutional tibial vara, *Knee Surg Sports Traumatol Arthrosc* 19:89, 2011.

McCarthy JJ, MacIntyre NR, Hooks B, Davidson RS: Double osteotomy for the treatment of severe Blount disease, *J Pediatr Orthop* 29:115, 2009.

McIntosh AL, Hanson CM, Rathjen KE: Treatment of adolescent tibia vara with hemiepiphysiodesis: risk factors for failure, *J Bone Joint Surg* 91A:2873, 2009.

Montgomery CO, Young KL, Austen M, et al: Increased risk of Blount disease in obese children and adolescents with vitamin D deficiency, *J Pediatr Orthop* 30:879, 2010.

Oh CW, Kim SJ, Park SK, et al: Hemicallotasis for correction of varus deformity of the proximal tibia using a unilateral external fixator, *J Orthop Sci* 16:44, 2011.

Sabharwal S, Wenokor C, Mehta A, Zhao C: Intra-articular morphology of the knee joint in children with Blount disease: a case-control study using MRI, *J Bone Joint Surg* 94A:883, 2012.

Sabharwal S, Zhao C, Sakamoto SM, McClemens E: Do children with Blount disease have lower body mass index after lower limb realignment? *J Pediatr Orthop* 34:213, 2014.

Sanghrajka AP, Hill RA, Murnaghan CF, et al: Slipped upper tibial epiphysis in infantile tibial vara. Three cases, *J Bone Joint Surg* 94B:1288, 2012.

Scott AC: Treatment of infantile Blount disease with lateral tension band plating, *J Pediatr Orthop* 32:29, 2012.

Segal LS, Crandall RC: Tiba vara deformity after below knee amputation and synostosis formation in children, *J Pediatr Orthop* 29:120, 2009.

Tavares JO, Molinero K: Elevation of medial tibial condyle for severe tibia vara, *J Pediatr Orthop* 15B:362, 2006.

Wiemann JM 4th, Tryon C, Szalay EA: Physeal stapling versus 8-plate hemiepiphysiodesis for guided correction of angular deformity about the knee, *J Pediatr Ortho* 29:481, 2009.

OSTEOGENESIS IMPERFECTA

Aarabi M, Rauch F, Hamdy RC, Fassier F: High prevalence of coxa vara in patients with severe osteogenesis imperfecta, *J Pediatr Orthop* 26:24, 2006.

Aglan MS, Hosny L, El-Houssini R, et al: A scoring system for the assessment of clinical severity in osteogenesis imperfecta, *J Child Orthop* 6:29, 2012.

Anissipour AK, Hammerberg KW, Caudill A, et al: Behavior of scoliosis during growth in children with osteogenesis imperfecta, *J Bone Joint Surg* 96A:237, 2014.

Bajpai A, Kabra M, Gupta N, et al: Intravenous pamidronate therapy in osteogenesis imperfecta: response to treatment and factors influencing outcome, *J Pediatr Orthop* 27:225, 2007.

Biggin A, Briody JN, Ormshaw E, et al: Fracture during intravenous bisphosphonate treatment in a child with osteogenesis imperfecta: an argument for a more frequent, low-dose treatment regimen, *Horm Res Paediatr* 81:204, 2014.

Cho T-J, Choi IH, Chung CY, et al: Interlocking telescopic rod for patients with osteogenesis imperfecta, *J Bone Joint Surg* 89A:2018, 2007.

Cho TJ, Kim JB, Lee JW, et al: Fracture in long bones stabilised by telescopic intramedullary rods in patients with osteogenesis imperfecta, *J Bone Joint Surg* 93B:634, 2011.

Chow W, Negandhi R, Kuong E, To M: Management pitfalls of fractured neck of femur in osteogenesis imperfecta, *J Child Orthop* 7:195, 2013.

Dwan K, Phillipi CA, Steiner RD, Basel D: Bisphosphonate therapy for osteogenesis imperfecta, *Cochrane Database Syst Rev* (7):CD005088, 2014.

El-Adl G, Khalil MA, Enan A, et al: Telescoping versus nontelescoping rods in the treatment of osteogenesis imperfecta, *Acta Orthop Belg* 75:200, 2009.

El Sobky MA, Hanna AAZ, Basha NE, et al: Surgery versus surgery plus pamidronate in the management of osteogenesis imperfecta patients: a comparative study, *J Pediatr Orthop B* 15:222, 2006.

Hatz D, Esposito PW, Schroeder B, et al: The incidence of spondylolysis and spondylolisthesis in children with osteogenesis imperfecta, *J Pediatr Orthop* 31:655, 2011.

Kim RH, Scuderi GR, Dennis DA, Nakano SW: Technical challenges of total knee arthroplasty in skeletal dysplasia, *Clin Orthop Relat Res* 469:69, 2011.

Kocher S, Dichtel L: Osteogenesis imperfecta misdiagnosed as child abuse, *J Pediatr Orthop B* 20:440, 2011.

Krishnan H, Patel NK, Skinner JA, et al: Primary and revision total hip arthroplasty in osteogenesis imperfecta, *Hip Int* 23:303, 2013.

Lee K, Park MS, Yoo WJ, et al: Proximal migration of femoral telescopic rod in children with osteogenesis imperfecta, *J Pediatr Orthop* 35:178–184, 2015.

Mesfin A, Nesterenko SO, Al-Hourani KG, et al: Management of hangman's fractures and a subaxial compression fracture in two children with osteogenesis imperfecta, *J Surg Orthop Adv* 22:326, 2013.

Nicolaou N, Agrawal Y, Padman M, et al: Changing pattern of femoral fractures in osteogenesis imperfecta with prolonged use of bisphosphonates, *J Child Orthop* 6:21, 2012.

Oakley I, Reece LP: Anesthetic implications for the patient with osteogenesis imperfecta, *AANA J* 78:47, 2010.

Pichard CP, Robinson RE, Skolasky RL, et al: Surgical blood loss during femoral rodding in children with osteogenesis imperfecta, *J Child Orthop* 3:301, 2009.

Poyrazoglu S, Guonoz H, Darendeliler F, et al: Successful results of pamidronate treatment in children with osteogenesis imperfecta with emphasis on the interpretation of bone mineral density for local standards, *J Pediatr Orthop* 28:483, 2008.

Ruck J, Dahan-Oliel N, Montpetit K, et al: Fassier-Duval femoral rodding in children with osteogenesis imperfecta receiving bisphosphonates: functional outcomes at one year, *J Child Orthop* 5:217, 2011.

Vitale MG, Matsumoto H, Kessler MH, et al: Osteogenesis imperfecta: determining the demographics and the predictors of death from an inpatient population, *J Pediatr Orthop* 27:228, 2007.

Wagner R, Luedke C: Total knee arthroplasty with concurrent femoral and tibial osteotomies in osteogenesis imperfecta, *Am J Orthop* 43:37, 2014.

Yilmaz G, Hwang S, Oto M, et al: Surgical treatment of scoliosis in osteogenesis imperfecta with cement-augmented pedicle screw instrumentation, *J Spinal Disord Tech* 27:174, 2014.

DWARFISM

Inan M, Chan G, Bowen JR: Correction of angular deformities of the knee by percutaneous hemiepiphysiodesis, *Clin Orthop Relat Res* 456:164, 2006.

Kim SJ, Agashe V, Song SH, et al: Comparison between upper and lower limb lengthening in patients with achondroplasia: a retrospective study, *J Bone Joint Surg* 94B:128, 2012.

Kim SJ, Balce GC, Agashe MV, et al: Is bilateral lower limb lengthening appropriate for achondroplasia? Midterm analysis of the complications and quality of life, *Clin Orthop Relat Res* 470:616, 2012.

Launay F, Younsi R, Pithioux M, et al: Fracture following lower limb lengthening in children: a series of 58 patients, *Orthop Traumatol Surg Res* 99:72, 2013.

Malot R, Park KW, Song SH, et al: Role of hybrid monolateral fixators in managing humeral length and deformity correction, *BMJ Case Rep* 2013. pii:bcr2013008793.

Marsh JS, Polzhofer GK: Arthroscopically assisted central physeal bar resection, *J Pediatr Orthop* 26:255, 2006.

Park HW, Yang KH, Lee KS, et al: Tibial lengthening over an intramedullary nail with use of the Ilizarov external fixator for idiopathic short stature, *J Bone Joint Surg* 90:1970, 2008.

Song SH, Agashe MV, Huh YJ, et al: Physeal growth arrest after tibial lengthening in achrondroplasia: 23 children followed to skeletal maturity, *Acta Orthop* 83:282, 2012.

Song SH, Kim SE, Agashe MV, et al: Growth disturbance after lengthening of the lower limb and quantitative assessment of physeal closure in skeletally immature patients with achondroplasia, *J Bone Joint Surg* 94B:556, 2012.

Weiner DS, Jonah D, Leighley B, et al: Orthopaedic manifestations of chondroectodermal dysplasia: the Ellis-van Creveld syndrome, *J Child Orthop* 7:465, 2013.

TRAUMATIC EPIPHYSEAL ARREST FROM BRIDGE OF BONE

Kang HG, Yoon SJ, Kim JR: Resection of a physeal bar under computer-assisted guidance, *J Bone Joint Surg* 92B:1452–1455, 2010.

Marsh JS, Polzhofer GK: Arthroscopically assisted central physeal bar resection, *J Pediatr Orthop* 26:255–259, 2006.

The complete list of references is available online at ***expertconsult.inkling.com****.*

PART X

NERVOUS SYSTEM DISORDERS IN CHILDREN

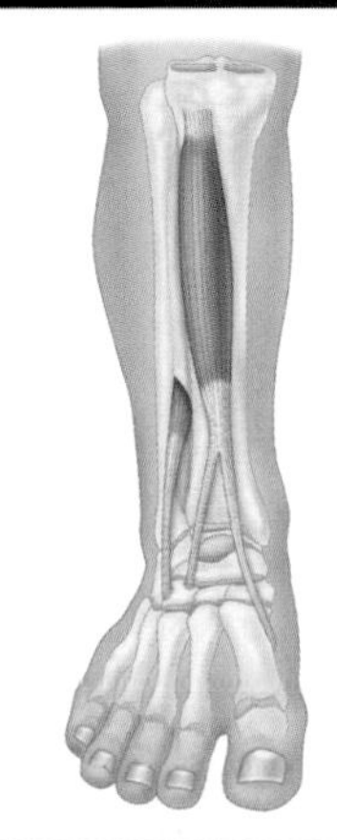

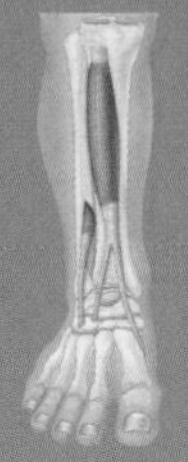

CHAPTER 33

CEREBRAL PALSY

Jeffrey R. Sawyer, David D. Spence

ETIOLOGY

Cerebral palsy is a heterogeneous disorder of movement and posture that has a wide variety of presentations, ranging from mild motor disturbance to severe total body involvement. Because of this variability in clinical presentation and the absence of a definitive diagnostic test, defining exactly what cerebral palsy is has been difficult and controversial. It is generally agreed that there are three distinctive features common to all patients with cerebral palsy: (1) some degree of motor impairment, which distinguishes it from other conditions, such as global developmental delay or autism; (2) an insult to the developing brain, making it different from conditions that affect the mature brain in older children and adults; and (3) a neurologic deficit that is nonprogressive, which distinguishes it from other motor diseases of childhood, such as the muscular dystrophies. In 2004 the International Executive Committee for the Definition of Cerebral Palsy revised the definition of cerebral palsy to state: Cerebral palsy (CP) describes a group of permanent disorders of the development of movement and posture, causing activity limitation, that are attributed to nonprogressive disturbances that occurred in the developing fetal or infant brain. The motor disorders of cerebral palsy often are accompanied by disturbances of sensation, perception, cognition, communication, and behavior, by epilepsy, and by secondary musculoskeletal problems.

The insult to the brain is believed to occur between the time of conception and age 2 years, at which time a significant amount of motor development has already occurred. A similar injury to the brain after age 2 years can have a similar effect, however, and often is called cerebral palsy. By 8 years of age, most of the development of the immature brain is complete, as is gait development, and an insult to the brain results in a more adult-type clinical picture and outcome.

Although the neurologic deficit is permanent and nonprogressive, the effect it can have on the patient is dynamic, and the orthopaedic aspects of cerebral palsy can change dramatically with growth and development. Growth, along with altered muscle forces across joints, can lead to progressive loss of motion, contracture, and eventually joint subluxation or dislocation, resulting in degeneration that may require orthopaedic intervention.

Children with cerebral palsy constitute the largest group of pediatric patients with neuromuscular disorders in the United States. The prevalence of cerebral palsy varies around the world according to the amount and quality of prenatal care, the socioeconomic condition of the parents, the environment, and the type of obstetric and pediatric care the mother and child receive. The determination of the true prevalence also is difficult because many children are not diagnosed until age 2 or 3 years; this most often occurs in socioeconomic groups that have decreased access to medical care. In the United States, the occurrence is approximately two per 1000 live births; there are approximately 25,000 new patients with cerebral palsy each year, and approximately 400,000 children with cerebral palsy at any given time. The United States experienced an initial decrease in the number of affected children in the 1950s and 1960s as a result of better understanding and treatment of maternal-fetal Rh incompatibility and improvements in obstetric techniques. More recently, the prevalence of cerebral palsy was thought to be increasing because of the increased survival of premature and low-birth-weight infants; however, two large population-based studies showed that the improved survival of these infants has not contributed to the increase in prevalence of cerebral palsy in the United States. Worldwide, the prevalence ranges from 0.6 to 7.0 cases per 1000 live births. The cost of operative treatment in children with cerebral palsy is substantial. In 1997, there were an estimated 37,000 operative procedures performed, with the most common being gastrostomy tube placements, soft-tissue releases, fundoplications, spinal fusions, and hip osteotomies. These procedures accounted for 50,000 hospital days and $150 million in charges.

Injury to the developing brain can occur at any time from gestation to early childhood and typically is categorized as prenatal, perinatal, or postnatal. Contrary to popular belief, fewer than 10% of injuries that result in cerebral palsy occur during the birth process, with most occurring in the prenatal period. A wide variety of risk factors for cerebral palsy have been identified in the prenatal period, including risk factors inherent to the fetus (most commonly genetic disorders), factors inherent to the mother (seizure disorders, mental retardation, and previous pregnancy loss), and factors inherent to the pregnancy itself (Rh incompatibility, polyhydramnios, placental rupture, and drug or alcohol exposure). External factors, such as TORCH syndrome (toxoplasmosis, other agents, rubella, cytomegalovirus, herpes simplex), also can lead to cerebral palsy in the prenatal period. Occurrences in the absence of any known risk factors may be caused by some yet unknown factor during this critical time in brain development. Several more recent studies have suggested a possible role of chorioamnionitis as one of these factors.

Cerebral palsy in the perinatal period, from birth until a few days after birth, typically is associated with asphyxia or trauma that occurs during labor. Oxytocin augmentation, umbilical cord prolapse, and breech presentation all have been associated with an increased occurrence of cerebral palsy. Only 10% of cases of cerebral palsy occur during this time period, and most patients with cerebral palsy have no history of asphyxia. Although cerebral palsy is often associated with low Apgar scores during this period, many neonates have low scores because of other conditions, such as genetic disorders, that are completely unrelated to asphyxia. Low-birth-weight infants (<1500 g) are at dramatically increased risk of cerebral palsy, with an incidence of 60 per 1000 births compared with two per 1000 births in infants of normal weight. This increased incidence is believed to be caused by the fragility of the periventricular blood vessels, which are highly susceptible to physiologic fluctuations during pregnancy (Fig. 33-1). These fluctuations, which include hypoxic episodes, placental pathology, maternal diabetes, and infection, can injure these vessels and lead to subsequent intraventricular hemorrhages. These injuries are graded on a scale from I to IV (Table 33-1), with an increased incidence of neurologic consequences such as hydrocephalus and cerebral palsy in grade III (bleeding into ventricles with dilation) and grade IV (bleeding into brain substance). In addition, the periventricular area, which is important for motor control, is especially susceptible from the 26th to the 32nd week of pregnancy. If this area is injured, diplegia usually results. Often, a synergistic combination of events leads to brain injury and

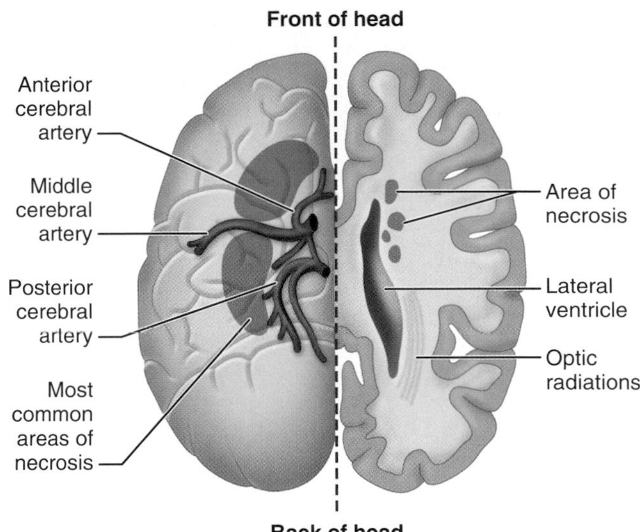

FIGURE 33-1 Periventricular leukomalacia. Cross-sectional view shows blood vessels that supply brain with blood *(left)* and brain structures *(right)*. Area surrounding ventricles contains "white matter" that includes descending neuronal pathways of motor control system. This area, especially farther forward in brain, is susceptible to damage in premature infants because of relative paucity of blood vessels. Fluctuations in blood flow, blood oxygen, or blood glucose levels can cause damage in this area, resulting in disturbance of motor control system and subsequent (usually spastic) cerebral palsy.

TABLE 33-1

Grading of Periventricular Lesions

Grade	Description
I	Bleeding confined to germinal matrix
II	Bleeding extends into ventricles
III	Bleeding into ventricles with dilation
IV	Bleeding into brain substance

Adapted from Pellegrino L, Dormans JP: Definitions, etiology, and epidemiology of cerebral palsy. In Pellegrino L, Dormans JP, editors: Caring for children with cerebral palsy: a team-based approach, Baltimore, 1998, Paul Brookes.

the subsequent development of cerebral palsy. Pregnancies involving multiple births also are at increased risk for cerebral palsy, primarily because of their association with premature delivery.

Although most children born with cerebral palsy are delivered at full term, full-term infants are at a much lower risk of developing cerebral palsy than are premature infants. Hypoxic-ischemic encephalopathy, which is characterized by hypotonia, decreased movement, and seizures, is a common cause of cerebral palsy during the postnatal period. Meconium aspiration and persistent fetal circulation with true ischemia are the most common causes of hypoxic-ischemic encephalopathy. Infections such as encephalitis and meningitis, most commonly caused by group B *Streptococcus* and herpes, can lead to cerebral palsy during this period. Traumatic brain injury from accidents or child abuse also accounts for a significant number of cases of cerebral palsy that develop in the postnatal period. Improvements in obstetric care have dramatically decreased the frequency of iatrogenic brain injury.

CLASSIFICATION

Because of the wide variability in presentation and types of cerebral palsy, various classification schemes have been described. Traditionally, cerebral palsy has been classified by the clinical physiologic picture, the region of the body affected, or the neuroanatomic region of the brain that was injured. More recently, the Gross Motor Functional Classification System (GMFCS) has been adopted as the most widely used classification scheme; this system stratifies children based on function at various ages.

TABLE 33-2

Geographic Classification of Cerebral Palsy

TYPE	DESCRIPTION	INVOLVEMENT
Monoplegia	One extremity involved, usually lower	
Hemiplegia	Both extremities on same side involved Usually upper extremity involved more than lower extremity	
Paraplegia	Both lower extremities equally involved	
Diplegia	Lower extremities more involved than upper extremities Fine-motor/sensory abnormalities in upper extremity	
Quadriplegia	All extremities involved equally Normal head/neck control	
Double hemiplegia	All extremities involved, upper more than lower	
Total body	All extremities severely involved No head/neck control	

GEOGRAPHIC CLASSIFICATION

The anatomic region of the body affected with the movement disorder should be identified as shown in Table 33-2. Often, it is difficult to classify completely the pattern of involvement geographically because some extremities may be only subtly involved and a patient's pattern of involvement can change over time. This classification is useful, however, in describing general patterns of involvement.

■ MONOPLEGIA

Monoplegia is very rare and usually occurs after meningitis. Most patients diagnosed with monoplegia actually have hemiplegia with one extremity only very mildly affected.

■ HEMIPLEGIA

In hemiplegia, one side of the body is involved, with the upper extremity usually more affected than the lower extremity. Patients with hemiplegia, approximately 30% of patients with cerebral palsy, typically have sensory changes in the affected extremities as well. Severe sensory changes, especially in the upper extremity, are a predictor of poor functional outcome after reconstructive surgery. Hemiplegic patients also may have a leg-length discrepancy, with shortening on the affected side, which can be treated with contralateral epiphysiodesis or leg lengthening.

■ DIPLEGIA

Diplegia is the most common anatomic type of cerebral palsy, constituting approximately 50% of all cases. Patients with diplegia have motor abnormalities in all four extremities, with the lower extremities more affected than the upper. The close proximity of the lower extremity tracts to the ventricles most likely explains the more frequent involvement of the lower extremities with periventricular lesions (Fig. 33-1). This type of cerebral palsy is most common in premature infants; intelligence usually is normal. Most children with diplegia walk eventually, although walking is delayed usually until around age 4 years.

■ QUADRIPLEGIA

In quadriplegia, all four extremities are equally involved and many patients have significant cognitive deficiencies that make care more difficult. Head and neck control usually is present, which helps with communication, education, and seating. Treatment goals for patients with quadriplegia include a straight spine and level pelvis, located mobile hips with 90 degrees of flexion for sitting and 30 degrees of extension for pivoting, plantigrade feet that can fit in shoes, and an appropriate wheelchair.

■ TOTAL BODY

Patients with total body involvement typically have profound cognitive deficits in addition to loss of head and neck control. These patients usually require full-time assistance for activities of daily living and specialized seating systems to assist with head positioning. Drooling, dysarthria, and dysphagia also are common and complicate care.

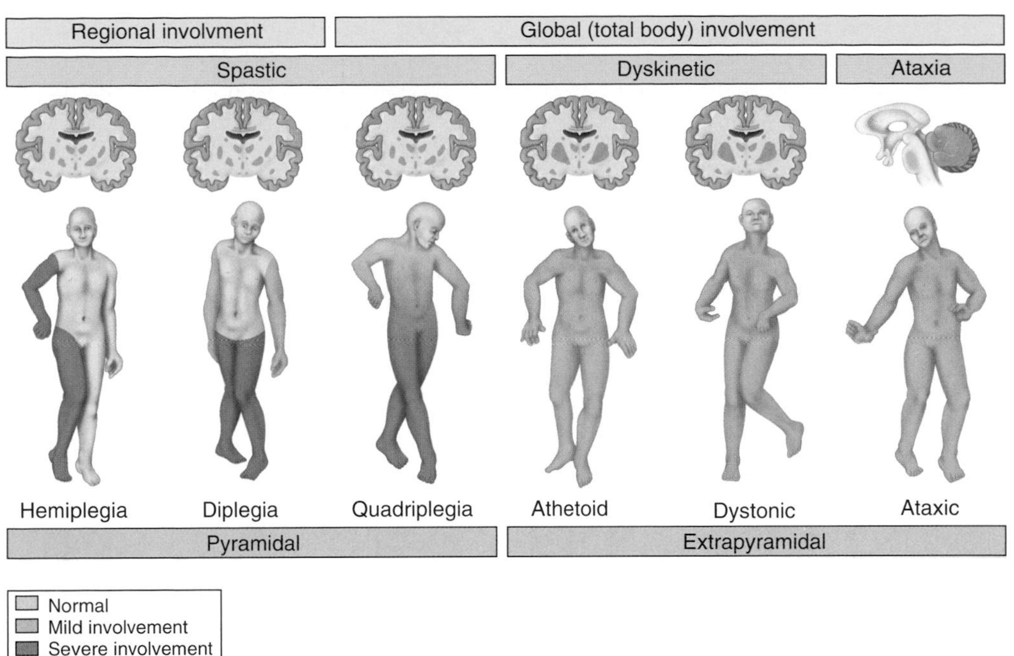

FIGURE 33-2 Classification of cerebral palsy. Although overlaps in terminology exist, cerebral palsy can be classified according to distribution (regional versus global involvement, hemiplegic, diplegic, quadriplegic), physiologic type (spastic, dyskinetic/dystonic, dyskinetic/athetoid, ataxic), or presumed neurologic substrate (pyramidal, extrapyramidal). (Redrawn from Pellegrino L: Cerebral palsy. In Batshaw ML, editor: Children with disabilities, ed 4, Baltimore, 1997, Paul H. Brookes.)

OTHER TYPES

Some patients have a double hemiplegia pattern as a result of bleeding in both hemispheres of the brain. It often is difficult to differentiate this from diplegia or quadriplegia; however, in double hemiplegia, the upper extremities typically are more involved than the lower.

Paraplegia is very rare and is characterized by bilateral lower extremity involvement with (in contrast to diplegia) completely normal gross and fine motor skills in the upper extremity. Many patients diagnosed with paraplegia actually are diplegic with very mildly involved upper extremities. Although occasionally mentioned, triplegia, the involvement of three extremities, probably does not exist. With careful examination, most patients believed to have triplegia actually have subtle motor deficits of the least involved limb.

PHYSIOLOGIC CLASSIFICATION

Most patients with cerebral palsy have recognizable patterns of movement that also can be classified. A basic understanding of normal brain development is important to understanding the various types. During the first trimester, the immature brain separates into the gross structures, including the cerebrum, cerebellum, and medulla. Neurons begin to form in the second trimester, and the total number of neurons an individual eventually has are present at the end of this time frame. Any neurons lost from this point forward are irreplaceable. Synaptic connections and myelination begin during the third trimester and continue through adolescence in a highly organized fashion. As these synapses develop and myelinization continues, primitive reflexes disappear and more mature motor patterns arise. Because of this continued development after birth, many injuries to the newborn nervous system go unrecognized until the absence of expected patterns can be detected. Different pathways of the brain are myelinated at different times; therefore spastic diplegia usually is not detected until 8 to 10 months of age; hemiplegia, 20 months of age; and athetoid cerebral palsy, after 24 months of age. Keep this in mind because a child's pattern may change over time.

Physiologically, cerebral palsy can be divided into a spastic type, which affects the corticospinal (pyramidal) tracts, and an extrapyramidal type, which affects the other regions of the developing brain. The extrapyramidal types of cerebral palsy include athetoid, choreiform, ataxic, rigid, and hypotonic (Fig. 33-2).

SPASTIC

Spastic is the most common form of cerebral palsy, constituting approximately 80% of cases, and usually is associated with injury to the pyramidal tracts in the immature brain. Spasticity, or the velocity-dependent increase in muscle tone with passive stretch, is caused by an exaggeration of the normal muscle passive stretch reflex. Booth showed histologically that this altered muscle function leads to the deposition of type I collagen in the endomysium of the affected muscle, leading to thickening and fibrosis, the degree of which correlated to the severity of the spasticity. Often, patients have simultaneous cocontraction of normally antagonistic muscle groups leading to fatigue, loss of dexterity and coordination, and balance difficulties. Joint contractures, subluxation, and degeneration are common in patients with spastic cerebral palsy.

ATHETOID

Athetoid cerebral palsy is caused by an injury to the extrapyramidal tracts and is characterized by dyskinetic, purposeless movements that may be exacerbated by environmental stimulation. The clinical picture varies based on the level of excitement of the patient. In pure athetoid cerebral palsy, joint contractures are uncommon; the results of soft-tissue releases, in contrast to those seen in spastic cerebral palsy, are unpredictable, and the procedures have a high complication rate. With the improvements in prevention of Rh incompatibility leading to kernicterus, the incidence of athetoid cerebral palsy is decreasing. Dystonia, characterized by increased overall tone and distorted positioning in response to voluntary movements, or hypotonia also can occur with athetoid cerebral palsy.

CHOREIFORM

Choreiform cerebral palsy is characterized by continual purposeless movements of the patient's wrists, fingers, toes, and ankles. This continuous movement can make bracing and sitting difficult.

RIGID

Patients with rigid cerebral palsy are the most hypertonic of all cerebral palsy patients. This hypertonicity occurs in the absence of hyperreflexia, spasticity, and clonus, which are common in spastic cerebral palsy. These patients have a "cogwheel" or "lead pipe" muscle stiffness that often requires surgical release. When a surgical release is done, it is essential not to overweaken the muscle, which would cause the opposite deformity to occur.

ATAXIC

Ataxic cerebral palsy is very rare and probably is the most often misdiagnosed type. It is characterized by the disturbance of coordinated movement, most commonly walking, as a result of an injury to the developing cerebellum. It is important to distinguish true ataxia from spasticity because with treatment many children with ataxia are able to improve their gait function without surgery. Overaggressive tendon lengthening in patients with ataxia can lead to iatrogenic weakness, which further interferes with gait function.

HYPOTONIC

Hypotonic cerebral palsy is characterized by weakness in conjunction with low muscle tone and normal deep tendon reflexes. Many children who ultimately develop spastic or ataxic cerebral palsy pass through a hypotonic stage lasting 1 or 2 years before the true nature of their brain injury becomes apparent. Persistent hypotonia can lead to difficulties with sitting balance, head positioning, and communication.

MIXED

Many patients with cerebral palsy have features of more than one type and are referred to as having mixed cerebral palsy. Patients with mixed cerebral palsy usually show signs of pyramidal and extrapyramidal deficits. The final clinical appearance is determined by the relative components of spasticity, athetosis, and ataxia. Surgical releases in this group can be less predictable, especially when a large athetoid or ataxic component is present.

FUNCTIONAL CLASSIFICATION

In recent years, newer classification systems have been developed based on function. Functional classifications systems are able to grade individuals based on their abilities instead of their deficiencies and promote the concepts of the World Health Organization's International Classification of Functioning, Disability, and Health, which focuses on activity and participation. The first widely accepted functional classification was the Gross Motor Function Classification System (GMFCS) (Box 33-1). Initially described by Palisano et al., this five-level ordinal grading system has been found to be a reliable and stable method of classification and prediction of motor function for children under the age of 12 years. It has since been expanded and revised to include children 12 to 18 years of age. It takes into account functional limitations for assistive devices, such as walkers and wheelchairs, and the quality of movement based on age. The emphasis of this scale is on self-initiated movement and walking and sitting function. The GMFCS has been shown to be predictive of hip dislocation.

The impact and acceptance of the GMFCS led to the introduction of the Manual Abilities Classification System (MACS) (Table 33-3). This five-level ordinal system was developed to be similar to the GMFCS but is intended to assess how a child with cerebral palsy uses his or her hands to perform activities of daily living. It also has been validated by multiple studies, and interrater reliability has been found to be good to excellent among healthcare professionals and care providers for children 4 to 18 years of age. Also similar to the GMFCS, the MACS remains stable over time with little change after the age of 4 years.

DIAGNOSIS

History and physical examination are the primary tools in making the diagnosis of cerebral palsy. The history should include a thorough investigation of the pregnancy and delivery. With the exception of several rare conditions, such as familial spastic paraparesis and congenital ataxia, there is no known genetic component to cerebral palsy. Ancillary studies, such as radiographs, hematologic studies, chromosomal analysis, computed tomography (CT), magnetic resonance imaging, and positron emission tomography, rarely are needed to make the diagnosis but may be helpful in determining the type and extent of cerebral palsy present. Diagnosis of cerebral palsy before 2 years of age can be difficult. One study found that 55% of children diagnosed with cerebral palsy by 1 year of age did not meet the criteria by 7 years of age. Transient dystonia of prematurity is a condition characterized by increased tone in the lower extremities between 4 and 14 months old and often is confused with cerebral palsy. This is a self-limiting condition and resolves without treatment. In addition, African-American children tend to have higher muscle tone than other ethnic groups, which also can lead to a misdiagnosis of cerebral palsy.

Knowledge of normal motor developmental milestones and primitive reflexes allows identification of children who are delayed in their motor development. Motor development usually occurs in a cephalad-to-caudal pattern, starting with swallowing and sucking, which are present at birth, and proceeding to sphincter control, which occurs at 24 to 36 months

BOX 33-1

Gross Motor Functional Classification System (GMFCS)

Level I

- **Up to 2 Years of Age:** Infants start to learn to sit on the floor and use both hands to play with and manipulate objects. Infants are also capable of crawling and pulling themselves up, and by 18 months, can walk.
- **Ages 2 to 4:** Children can successfully sit on the floor with no assistance. They may also begin to stand without adult assistance and walk. Walking is typically preferred over crawling.
- **Ages 4 to 6:** Children can sit in a chair and get up from a chair without assistance. They can also move to the floor from a chair without assistance, walk freely without assistance, and begin to run and jump.
- **Ages 6 to 12:** Children can run, walk, jump, and climb stairs without assistance; balance and coordination may be lacking still.

Level II

- **Up to 2 Years of Age:** Infants may begin to sit on the floor but only with adult assistance or by relying on their hands for support. They may begin to crawl on hands and knees or "creep" on their belly.
- **Ages 2 to 4:** Children can sit on the floor but require assistance, especially if they're using their hands to manipulate and grab objects. Reciprocal patterns are used when crawling on hands and knees, and children can walk either with assistive devices or by holding onto furniture or other sturdy objects.
- **Ages 4 to 6:** Children can now sit in a chair without assistance but need assistance from standing to moving to the floor, such as a sturdy table or surface. Additionally, they can walk for short distances without support and can climb stairs as long as they are holding the rails for support. However, they cannot skip, run, or jump.
- **Ages 6 to 12:** Children can walk both indoors and outdoors with little to no assistance but will need help with walking in crowds, in unfamiliar settings, and on inclined surfaces. They still need rails when climbing steps and only possess minimal abilities for gross motor skills, such as running, jumping, and skipping.

Level III

- **Up to 2 Years of Age:** Infant can roll and creep in a forward position while on their stomachs but will need assistance with sitting via lower back support.
- **Ages 2 to 4:** Children can sit on the floor unsupported but typically in the "W" position: rotated hips and knees. They also can crawl on their hands and knees, usually without moving the legs. Crawling tends to be the preferred method of moving around.
- **Ages 4 to 6:** Children can sit upright on a chair but require trunk support if using their hands. Additionally, they can lift themselves from the chair with the assistance of sturdy furniture, such as a table, and can climb stairs with adult help. They can also walk while using a mobility device for assistance.
- **Ages 6 to 12:** With a mobility device for assistance, children walk both outdoors and indoors. They may be able to climb stairs without adult assistance but with the use of handrails. If they are traveling long distances or walking on uneven or inclined distances, they will either need to be carried or use a wheelchair.

Level IV

- **Up to 2 Years of Age:** Infants can roll from back to stomach and vice versa but can only sit upright with trunk assistance.
- **Ages 2 to 4:** When placed on the floor, children can sit up, but will need to use their hands and arms for support. In most instances, they will need adaptive equipment for both sitting and standing, but crawling on their hand and knees, stomach creeping, and/or rolling are the preferred methods of moving.
- **Ages 4 to 6:** Children can sit on a chair with trunk support and can move from the chair by holding onto a sturdy surface. They can walk short distances, but adult supervision is highly recommended as they may have problems turning and keeping their balance.
- **Ages 6 to 12:** Children will maintain the same mobility from age 6, but they may rely more on wheelchairs and walk-assisting devices, especially at school or in the community.

Level V

- **Up to 2 Years of Age:** Voluntary control of movements are physically impaired and, in turn, the infant cannot hold his or her head and trunk without support. They also need assistance in rolling over.
- **Ages 2 to 4:** All areas of motor function are still limited, rendering it difficult for the child to sit without assistance, to crawl, or achieve any type of independent mobility at all.
- **Ages 4 to 6:** Children can now sit on a chair but will need adaptive equipment to hold them in place. In addition, they will need to be transported, even for daily activities, as they still have no independent mobility.
- **Ages 6 to 12:** Some children may be able to achieve mobility on their own via an electronic wheelchair, but mobility will still be limited to the point where they cannot move on their own, including the inability to support their trunks and bodies. Additional expansive adaptation equipment is used in some instances.

of age (Table 33-4). Primitive reflex patterns of motor activity that are outgrown as part of the normal maturation process persist longer than normal and in some cases permanently in children with cerebral palsy. Other, more mature motor patterns, which are essential for normal ambulation, may be significantly delayed or never appear. By determining which reflexes are present or absent, the child's neurologic age can be determined. By comparing the neurologic age with the chronologic age, a neurologic quotient can be determined, which is useful in determining prognosis and treatment. The presence of these primitive reflexes also can contribute to further deformity.

TABLE 33-3

Manual Ability Classification System (MACS) Levels

LEVEL	DESCRIPTION	COMMENTS
1	Handles objects easily and successfully	At most, limitations in the ease of performing manual tasks requiring speed and accuracy; however, any limitations in manual abilities do not restrict independence in daily activities
2	Handles most objects but with somewhat reduced quality and/or speed	Certain activities may be avoided or be achieved with some difficulty; alternative ways of performance might be used, but manual abilities do not usually restrict independence in daily activities
3	Handles objects with difficulty; needs help to prepare and/or modify activities	Performance is slow and is achieved with limited success regarding quality and quantity; activities are performed independently if they have been set up or adapted
4	Handles a limited selection of easily managed objects in adapted situations	Performs parts of activities with effort and with limited success; requires continuous support and assistance and/or adapted equipment for even partial achievement of the activity
5	Does not handle objects and has severely limited ability to perform even simple actions	Requires total assistance

TABLE 33-4

Early Motor Developmental Milestones

MILESTONE	AVERAGE AGE (MO)	95TH PERCENTILE
Head control	3	6
Independent sitting	6	9
Crawling	8	Variable, some never do
Pull to stand	8	12
Independent walking	12	17

PROGNOSTIC FACTORS

Considerable work has been done investigating prognostic factors for function, including ambulation, in patients with cerebral palsy. The presence of tonic neck reflexes usually is incompatible with independent standing balance and the ability to perform alternating movements of the lower extremities necessary for walking. Sitting independently by 2 years of age is a good predictor of independent ambulation. If a child cannot sit independently by 4 years, it is unlikely he or she will ever walk without assistance. If a child has not learned to walk by 8 years of age, and he or she is not limited by severe contractures, it is unlikely he or she will ever walk at all.

Poor prognostic signs for walking reported by Bleck included (1) an imposable asymmetric tonic neck reflex, (2) persistent Moro reflex, (3) strong extensor thrust on vertical suspension, (4) persistent neck-righting reflex, and (5) absence of normal parachute reaction after 11 months. The persistence of these primitive reflexes is associated with extensive and severe brain damage and a poor prognosis for independent ambulation, self-care, and activities of daily living.

GAIT ANALYSIS

Before the development of computer-based gait analysis systems, careful clinical observation was the primary method of diagnosing gait disturbances in children with cerebral palsy. It is still an essential component in making the diagnosis. This clinical observation is done by repeatedly watching the child walk from the front, sides, and back, studying one component of gait at a time. Attention should be paid to the pelvis, hip, knee, ankle, and foot and to stride length, cadence, rotational alignment, trunk position, and side-to-side differences.

Modern quantitative gait analysis uses high-speed motion picture cameras from different angles, retroreflective markers on the surface of the skin aligned with palpable skeletal landmarks, and force platforms to measure the various components of gait. Kinematic data are provided that are presented in a waveform that represents the three-dimensional motion of the joints during the gait cycle. Electromyographic (EMG) testing, which documents the activation of various muscles during the gait cycle, also is used to determine which muscles are firing in a normal pattern and which are firing out of phase. Other components of quantitative gait analysis include pedobarography (foot pressure) and oxygen consumption measurement. Combined, these give the trained observer an accurate representation of the complex interaction of all of the components of gait. Gait analysis frequently is used in preoperative planning before lower extremity surgery to delineate a patient's specific gait deviations and plan the appropriate intervention. One study found that when experienced observers were given quantitative gait analysis for patients after surgical recommendations had already been made based on clinical observation, the surgical recommendation changed 52% of the time.

Although quantitative gait analysis provides objective data, interpretation of that data seems to be subjective. Only slight-to-moderate agreement has been noted among physicians in identification of soft-tissue and bony problems and in recommendations for treatment. Significant institutional differences in diagnosis and treatment recommendations also have been found. Clinical examination combined with gait analysis has been reported to improve surgical outcome. As noted, postoperative gait analysis may be useful not only in assessing outcomes but also in making further treatment recommendations, including recommendations for bracing, specific physical therapy protocols, and further surgical intervention.

Although quantitative gait analysis techniques continue to improve, their role in the evaluation and treatment of children with cerebral palsy remains controversial. Although gait analysis has been shown to alter decision-making, studies are necessary to determine if these changes lead to improved clinical outcomes. Davids et al. proposed a five-step paradigm for clinical decision making to optimize the walking ability of children with cerebral palsy. The five points are clinical history, physical examination, diagnostic imaging, quantitative gait analysis, and examination under anesthesia. We believe that this type of approach is better than relying on quantitative gait analysis alone in the diagnosis and treatment of children with cerebral palsy.

ASSOCIATED CONDITIONS

Most patients with cerebral palsy have associated impairments that interfere with their daily function, independence, mobility, and overall health. These issues may be more important to the patient, the patient's family, and their caregivers than the child's ambulatory status. These conditions must be taken into account when considering any type of therapeutic intervention. In one study, adults with cerebral palsy ranked what was most important to them, and education and communication were most important, followed by activities of daily living and mobility. Ambulation was ranked fourth. Because of the complex nature of these conditions, a multidisciplinary team approach to patients with cerebral palsy is essential.

The most common associated conditions in patients with cerebral palsy are mental impairment or learning disability (40%); seizures (30%); complex movement disorders (20%); visual impairment (16%); malnutrition and related conditions, such as gastroesophageal reflux, obesity, and undernutrition (15%); and hydrocephalus (14%). Mental impairment and learning disability can range from very mild deficits to severe impairment and inability to live independently. Mental retardation, as defined as an IQ less than 50, occurs in 30% to 65% of children with cerebral palsy, most commonly in quadriplegics. Learning disabilities are worsened by seizure disorders, various medications with central nervous system side effects, and communication difficulties. Bulbar involvement can lead to drooling, dysphagia, and speech difficulties, which can limit cognitive and social development further.

Many children with cerebral palsy (50% in some series) have significant visual difficulties, with 7% having a severe visual defect. Common visual disturbances include myopia, amblyopia, strabismus, visual field defects, and cortical blindness. Visual screening is indicated in all children with cerebral palsy. Hearing loss has been reported to occur in 10% to 25% of children with cerebral palsy, which can exacerbate communication and learning difficulties further. Hearing screenings, similar to visual screenings, should be part of the routine evaluation of patients with cerebral palsy.

Approximately 30% of patients with cerebral palsy also have seizures, most commonly patients with hemiplegia, quadriplegia, or postnatally acquired syndromes. Seizures and the medications used in their management can have profound effects on learning, communication, and ambulation. This has led to renewed interest in alternative medication delivery systems, such as intrathecal baclofen and intramuscular botulinum toxin injections.

Osteopenia with increased risk of fracture also is common in children with cerebral palsy, especially children who are more severely affected. Fractures often can be difficult to diagnose, especially in nonverbal patients. The use of whole-body technetium bone scanning can be helpful to identify occult fractures in these patients. The nonoperative and operative treatment of these fractures has a high complication rate and usually interferes with the child's social and school activities and can make it difficult for caretakers. Significant femoral osteopenia (bone mineral density Z-score of < -2) has been identified in nearly 80% of children with cerebral palsy and 97% of nonstanders. Femoral fractures can occur especially in nonambulatory patients with severe involvement. Although these can be treated nonoperatively, there is a high rate of malunion requiring surgery and increased cast-related complications. Bisphosphonates and growth hormone have been shown in small studies to be safe and effective in increasing bone mineral density in children with cerebral palsy, but large multicenter trials are lacking. Severe medical problems, such as aspiration pneumonia and profound feeding problems, can lead to malnutrition, immune suppression, and metabolic abnormalities. Gastroesophageal reflux often can be managed medically and with positioning, but fundoplication may be necessary. Enteral feeding augmentation often is necessary because of swallowing dysfunction and the risk of aspiration pneumonia. This can be done with a gastrostomy or jejunostomy tube. Patients with protein malnutrition have been shown to be at increased risk of postoperative infection.

Emotional problems add to these associated conditions. The child's self-image plays an important role, especially in adolescence, when the differences between the affected child and peers become more apparent. Communication difficulties also may affect self-image at this stage. The attitudes of the parents, siblings, treatment team, and community are important to help the child or young adult maximize his or her independence and function. As young adulthood is reached, concerns about employment, self-care, sexual function, marriage, childbearing, and caring for aging parents may become emotional stressors.

TREATMENT

Because of the heterogeneous nature of cerebral palsy, it is difficult to make generalized statements regarding treatment, and it is best to have an individualized approach to each patient and his or her needs. In some centers, a multidisciplinary team approach (including physical, occupational, and speech therapy; orthotics; nutrition; social work; orthopaedics; and general pediatrics) has been successful. Four basic treatment principles exist. The first is that although the central nervous system injury, by definition, is nonprogressive, the deformities caused by abnormal muscle forces and contractures are progressive. The second, which can be a source of frustration, is that the treatments currently available correct the secondary deformities only and not the primary problem, which is the brain injury. The third is that the deformities typically become worse during times of rapid growth. For some patients, it may be beneficial to delay surgery until after a significant growth spurt to decrease the risk of recurrence. When determining the timing of surgery, consider the fact that most children with cerebral palsy have an advanced skeletal age compared with chronologic age by approximately 2 years and a significantly advanced age compared with normal controls of both sexes. The highest correlation between advanced bone age was found in quadriplegics and in boys with GMFCS level III and girls with a body mass index of less than 15. The fourth is that operative or nonoperative treatment should be done to minimize the negative effect it has on the patient's socialization and education. It is important to be aware of these timing issues when considering any form of treatment in this patient population. For most patients a combined approach using nonoperative and operative methods is more beneficial than one form of treatment alone.

NONOPERATIVE TREATMENT

Nonoperative modalities, such as medication, splinting and bracing, and physical therapy, commonly are used as primary treatment or in conjunction with other forms of treatment such as surgery. A wide variety of medications have been used to treat cerebral palsy. The three most common agents are diazepam and baclofen, which act centrally, and dantrolene, which acts at the level of skeletal muscle. Baclofen mimics the action of γ-aminobutyric acid, a powerful inhibitory neurotransmitter centrally and peripherally, whereas diazepam potentiates the activity of γ-aminobutyric acid. These medications can be difficult to use because of wide variability in effectiveness among children and a narrow therapeutic window. Because these drugs increase inhibitory neurotransmitter activity, common systemic side effects include sedation, balance difficulties, and cognitive dysfunction, which can have a dramatic detrimental effect on ambulation, education, and communication.

Dantrolene acts at the level of skeletal muscle and decreases muscle calcium ion release. It has an affinity for fast twitch muscle fibers and selectively decreases abnormal muscle stretch reflexes and tone. Dantrolene is used less frequently than other medications because some patients taking it develop profound weakness, and there is a risk of hepatotoxicity with long-term use. Because of the systemic side effects of these medications, there is a renewed interest in alternative drug delivery systems, such as intrathecal baclofen and intramuscular botulinum toxin injections.

Baclofen, in addition to inhibiting abnormal monosynaptic extensor activity and polysynaptic flexor activity, has been shown to decrease substance P levels, which limits nociception. Baclofen has been shown to penetrate the blood-brain barrier poorly, and it has a short half-life (3 to 4 hours). This requires gradual titration of medication and the use of extremely high systemic levels to obtain a central effect of spasticity reduction. Intrathecal injection of baclofen requires 1/30 the dose of oral baclofen to achieve a similar or better response. Injecting baclofen intrathecally with an implantable programmable pump dramatically decreases the dose required to affect spasticity and decreases some of the side effects such as sedation. This pump typically is implanted subcutaneously in the abdominal wall and requires refilling approximately every 2 to 3 months (Fig. 33-3). A meta-analysis of 14 studies of intrathecal baclofen management found that it reduced lower extremity spasticity, seemed to improve function and ease of care, and had manageable complications. Baclofen also works at the level of the spinal cord to slow abnormal spinal reflexes and decrease motor neuron drive, which can reduce spasticity further. Careful monitoring is required to prevent overdosage, which can cause a decrease in trunk tone, weakness, and sedation. Complications from intrathecal baclofen include catheter and pump infection or malfunction, spinal fluid leak, respiratory depression, drug reactions, and oversedation. Ten to 20 percent of patients require further surgery or pump removal. There also have been concerns about the progression of scoliosis in patients who receive intrathecal baclofen therapy. One study, however, comparing curve magnitude progression in patients with and without the use of intrathecal baclofen showed no differences in curve progression between the groups. Until longer-term studies can be done, this treatment method is indicated for patients whose spasticity significantly interferes with self-care and quality of life and in whom other modalities have failed.

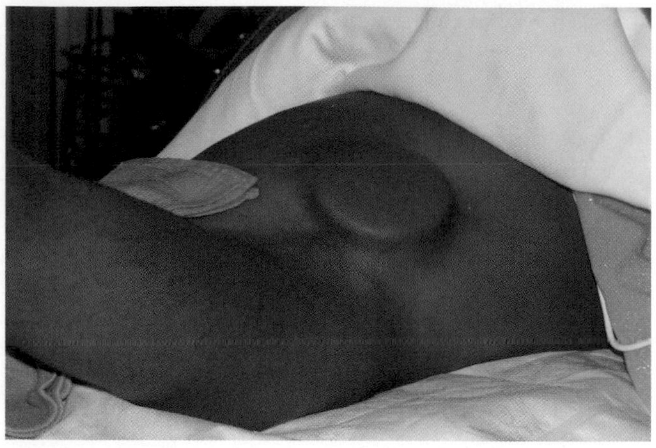

FIGURE 33-3 Continuous intrathecal baclofen infusion. Baclofen is injected through skin to reservoir, which is located within surgically placed pump beneath skin of abdomen. The pump, which is about size of hockey puck, is programmable using device placed against skin and over pump. Medication is continuously infused through catheter that tunnels under skin and is inserted directly into spinal canal; baclofen mixes with spinal fluid, directly affecting spinal cord and decreasing spasticity.

Botulinum toxin is a potent neurotoxin, of which there are seven serotypes, produced by *Clostridium botulinum*. Botulinum toxin type A (BTX-A) (Botox, Dysport) has been used to weaken muscles selectively in patients with cerebral palsy. BTX-A injected directly into the muscle acts at the level of the motor end plate, blocking the release of the neurotransmitter acetylcholine and inhibiting muscle contraction. Because it can diffuse 2 to 3 cm in the tissues, it is easier to achieve the desired effect with BTX-A than with other agents, such as phenol or alcohol, which require more accurate injection. It also is safer than these other agents because it binds selectively to the neuromuscular junction and not to other surrounding tissues. This effect begins approximately 24 hours after injection and lasts 2 to 6 months. Care must be taken to prevent systemic injection of this toxin, which in large enough doses can cause respiratory depression and death. The maximal safe dose of BTX-A based on primate data is 36 to 50 units per kilogram of body weight; however, most studies report doses of less than 20 units/kg. BTX-A has been shown to be effective when used in conjunction with other modalities, such as physical therapy or serial casting. The most common side effects are local pain and irritation from the injection. The most common use of BTX-A is as an adjuvant to a bracing, casting, or physical therapy treatment program over a finite period. It is beneficial in young patients in whom there is a need to delay surgery. It also has been used to predict the results of tendon-lengthening surgery; however, this is controversial. BTX-A also has been shown to improve energy expenditure with walking and has been reported to improve upper extremity function and self-care, but the results are highly variable. With long-term use, efficacy may decrease because of the production of antibodies to the toxin; it is recommended that injections be done 3 to 4 months apart and only when other methods have failed. Contraindications to BTX-A therapy include known resistance or antibodies, fixed deformity or contracture, concurrent use of aminoglycoside antibiotics, failure of previous response, and certain neurologic conditions such as myasthenia gravis.

Physical therapy is an essential component in the treatment of patients with cerebral palsy. Physical therapy typically is used as a primary treatment modality and in conjunction with other modalities, such as casting, bracing, BTX-A, and surgery. The therapist plays a crucial role in all aspects of care, including identifying children who may have cerebral palsy, treating their spasticity and contractures, fabricating splints and simple braces, providing family education and follow-up, acting as a liaison with the school and other health care providers, and implementing home stretching and exercise programs with the patients and their families. Because of the variability in patients with cerebral palsy, an individualized approach to therapy is necessary. Goals for ambulatory patients include strengthening of weakened muscles, contracture prevention, and gait and balance training; for severely affected individuals, goals are improvements in sitting balance, hygiene, and ease of care for caregivers. The parents should be encouraged from the beginning to take an active role in the child's therapy program.

Objective data in the literature supporting or disputing the use of physical therapy in patients with cerebral palsy are few because most studies involve small groups of heterogeneous patients who are not randomized. Unanswered questions include what types of therapeutic modalities should be used, by whom, and for how long. There are no clear data to support lifelong physical therapy, although many parents request this. Lifelong physical therapy may be detrimental to the child and the family financially, developmentally, socially, and emotionally.

Bracing, as with physical therapy and medication, typically is used in conjunction with other modalities. Bracing in patients with cerebral palsy most commonly is used to prevent or slow progression of deformity. The most commonly used braces for the treatment of cerebral palsy include ankle-foot orthoses, hip abduction braces, hand and wrist splints, and spinal braces or jackets. A patient-centered approach should be used. The goals of bracing for an ambulatory child differ from the goals for a child with severe involvement. Bracing of the lower extremities, most commonly with ankle-foot orthoses, is common in patients with cerebral palsy. These have been shown to improve gait function and decrease crouch during walking, even in the absence of surgery in ambulatory children. The goals of bracing in a severely affected child include facilitating shoe wear, preventing further progression of contractures, improving wheelchair positioning, and assisting standing programs. The use of floor-reaction ankle-foot orthoses, which use a plantar flexion–knee extension couple to help eliminate crouched-knee gait and improve stance phase knee extension, has dramatically decreased the need for bracing above the knee with knee-ankle-foot orthoses.

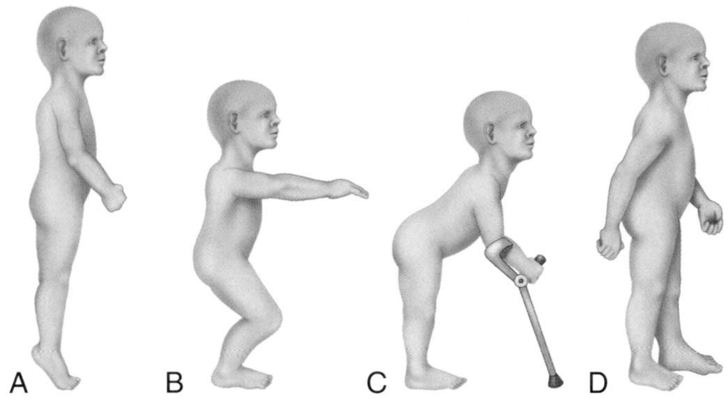

FIGURE 33-4 "Birthday surgery" should be avoided in favor of simultaneous multilevel surgery. **A** and **B,** Young child with diplegia and toe-walking **(A)** undergoes isolated heel cord lengthening, which increases crouch gait **(B)**. **C,** One year later, he has isolated hamstring lengthening and develops hip flexion contracture. **D,** One year later, he has hip flexor release to allow him to ambulate in upright position. (Redrawn from Rang M: Neuromuscular disease. In Wenger DR, Rang M, editors: The art of pediatric orthopaedics, New York, 1993, Raven Press.)

OPERATIVE TREATMENT

Operative treatment typically is indicated when contractures or deformities decrease function, cause pain, or interfere with activities of daily living. Because many patients with cerebral palsy have significant comorbidities, operative treatment carries with it an increased risk of complications compared with the general population. Preoperative consultation with the patient's pediatrician, pulmonologist, and other members of the care team can help optimize the patient's condition before surgery. Surgical procedures should be scheduled to minimize the number of hospitalizations and interference with school and social activities. "Birthday surgery," or multiple procedures performed at different times, as described by Rang, should be avoided whenever possible (Fig. 33-4). Although comparison studies of staged and single-event multilevel surgery are lacking, the use of single-event multilevel surgery has become the most common method to minimize a patient's exposure to repeated hospitalizations and rehabilitation. Newer techniques, such as percutaneous muscle lengthening and osteotomies, show promise in terms of decreased blood loss, operative time, and return to mobilization, but further research is necessary.

Up to 30% of patients with cerebral palsy have been shown to be malnourished, which increases the risk of postoperative wound healing problems and infection. In a study of 1746 patients with cerebral palsy, Minas et al. found underweight to be an independent predictor of increased complications after osteotomies and spine surgery, with no independent increased risk in overweight or obese patients. A serum albumin level less than 35 g/L and a blood lymphocyte count of less than 1.5 g/L have been associated with a significant increase in the risk of postoperative infection. Determination of a patient's nutritional status and improving it before surgery may decrease the overall complication rate.

It is essential to ensure that parental and patient concerns and expectations are discussed before operative intervention. Parents of younger children and children with more severe manifestations show higher levels of concern about surgery. The top preoperative concerns are the duration of rehabilitation, immediate postoperative pain, general anesthesia, and cost. Postoperative parental satisfaction has been shown to be correlated with a higher GMFCS level (level I), unilateral involvement, and younger age at the time of surgery.

Operative treatment of deformities related to cerebral palsy can be divided into several groups, including procedures to (1) correct static or dynamic deformity, (2) balance muscle power across a joint, (3) reduce spasticity (neurectomy), and (4) stabilize uncontrollable joints. Often, procedures can be combined; for example, an adductor tendon release can be done at the time of pelvic osteotomy for hip subluxation.

Flexible static and dynamic deformities typically are corrected with a muscle-tendon lengthening procedure; capsulotomies and osteotomies are reserved for more severe or rigid deformities. Over time, spasticity causes a relative shortening of the musculotendinous unit, leading to abnormal joint motion and loading and, if left untreated, degenerative changes. Operative lengthening of the musculotendinous unit causes a relative weakening of the muscle with restoration of more normal forces and motion across the joint. Lengthening can be done using a recession or release of the muscular aponeurosis at the musculotendinous junction, a Z-plasty within the substance of the tendon itself, or a complete tenotomy depending on the circumstances. Recessions tend to avoid complications that can occur with overlengthening and subsequent weakness that can occur with tenotomy or Z-plasty. More severe deformities usually cannot be corrected with soft-tissue release alone and typically require osteotomy.

Balancing muscle forces across any joint can be difficult and is even more difficult in patients with cerebral palsy because of the decreased control of voluntary muscle function, lowered threshold of stretch reflexes, increased frequency of cocontraction of antagonistic muscle groups, and inability to learn to use the transferred muscle in an altered location or function. In addition, muscles that are spastic throughout the gait cycle typically remain spastic after transfer. Often, the goal of tendon transfer in this patient population is either to remove a deforming or out-of-phase muscle force away from a joint or to act as a passive tendon sling.

Neurectomy, by a variety of mechanical and chemical methods, has been proposed as a way to decrease the muscle forces acting across a joint. A primary concern about neurectomy is the overweakening of the affected muscle, leading to uncontrolled antagonistic function and development of a secondary opposite deformity. Because of these concerns, neurectomy is not commonly performed. If neurectomy is considered, a trial can be conducted by temporarily disrupting nerve function using a local anesthetic such as lidocaine to determine if neurectomy will have the desired effect.

With continued abnormal muscle forces applied across a joint, pathologic changes to the joint can occur, including subluxation, dislocation, and cartilaginous degeneration. Joint stabilization procedures, such as osteotomies, usually combined with soft-tissue releases, have produced good long-term results. For severe joint destruction, procedures such as arthrodesis, especially in the foot, and resection arthroplasty, especially in the hip, have been shown to be beneficial. Joint replacement, which was initially contraindicated in patients with neuromuscular diseases such as cerebral palsy, also has been used in this population with end-stage arthritis with good functional improvement and pain relief. Joint replacement should be done only in carefully selected patients and in a center with experience with this type of procedure.

NEUROSURGICAL INTERVENTION

Selective dorsal root rhizotomy is a technique to reduce spasticity and balance muscle tone in carefully selected patients. In patients with cerebral palsy, the normal central nervous system inhibitory control of the gamma efferent system is deficient, leading to the exaggerated stretch reflex response. In addition, the ability to coordinate movement, mediated by the alpha motor neurons, is abnormal. Stimulatory afferent input from the muscle spindle travels to the spinal cord through the dorsal rootlets. The goal of selective dorsal rhizotomy is to identify the rootlets carrying excessive stimulatory information and section them to reduce the stimulatory input from the dorsal sensory fibers.

The indications for rhizotomy are variable, and further work is necessary to develop more uniform consensus guidelines. Three randomized trials of rhizotomy, with and without physical therapy, compared with physical therapy alone showed improvement in both groups, but slightly more in the rhizotomy group. There also is some limited evidence to show that rhizotomy decreases the need for orthopaedic procedures as well. The ideal patient for this procedure is a child 3 to 8 years old, GMFCS II or III, with spastic diplegia, voluntary motor and trunk control, pure spasticity, and no fixed contractures. Children who were born preterm or with low birth weight tend to have better results than children who were born full term because they tend to have pure spasticity, whereas children born full term are more likely to have rigidity plus spasticity. In addition, the patient and family should exhibit intelligence and a high level of motivation because this procedure requires extensive physical therapy postoperatively. In the early postoperative period, patients have significant weakness, but when rehabilitation is complete, most patients show significant improvement in lower extremity function, including decreased spasticity in the ankle dorsiflexors, increased strength in the knee flexors/extensors and foot dorsiflexors and plantarflexors, and more efficient ambulation. If surgery is performed in the appropriate patient, gross function can be expected to improve one GMFCS level. Improvements also can occur in upper extremity function, swallowing and speech, bladder function, pain control, and overall happiness, but these are less predictable. In addition, patients have been shown to have a decreased need for adjunct orthopaedic surgical procedures or botulinum toxin injections after rhizotomy. The role of selective posterior rhizotomy is less clear in patients with spastic quadriplegia and hemiplegia, and usually it is not recommended. A 10-year follow-up study showed that peak joint range of motion and ambulatory status occurred 3 years after rhizotomy and then declined gradually. In this cohort, 16 of 19 patients (84%) had a mean of three orthopaedic procedures, indicating that contracture development in cerebral palsy is not mediated entirely by spasticity. Although there is some decline in results with time after rhizotomy, it appears that patients still show statistical improvement in terms of gait mechanics from their preoperative measurements, and the majority of adults who had rhizotomy would recommend the procedure to others.

Complications of selective dorsal root rhizotomy include hip subluxation and dislocation in patients with increased GMFCS level, lumbar hyperlordosis (especially in patients with >60 degrees of lordosis preoperatively), scoliosis, spondylolysis, and spondylolisthesis. It is difficult to determine to what extent these complications are related to the rhizotomy or to the disease progression itself. Progression of coronal and sagittal plane abnormalities has been documented in 25% of patients with scoliosis, 32% of patients with kyphosis, and 36% of patients with hyperlordosis. Approximately half of patients also develop planovalgus foot deformities. One of the most difficult postoperative complications to manage is weakness, either iatrogenic or unrecognized preoperative weakness that becomes apparent after surgery.

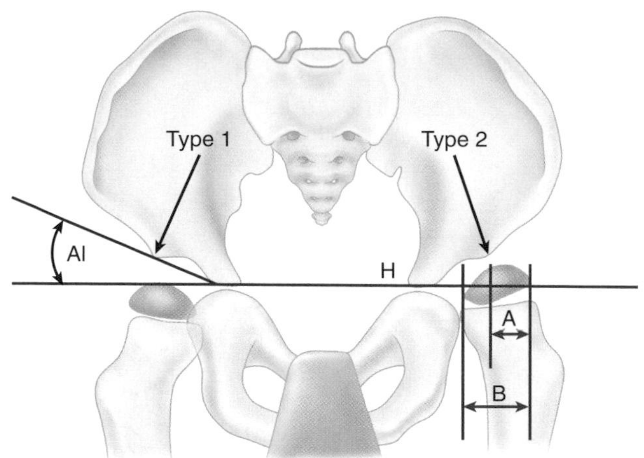

FIGURE 33-5 Subluxated left hip joint. Migration index (MI) is calculated by dividing width of uncovered femoral head *A* by total width of femoral head *B*. Acetabulum is dysplastic (type 2) sourcil, with lateral corner of acetabulum above weight-bearing dome. Normal hip (left side) with acetabular index (AI) indicated. There is normal (type 1) sourcil; lateral corner is sharp and below weight-bearing dome. H, horizontal axis.

HIP

Deformities of the hip in patients with cerebral palsy range from mild painless subluxation to complete dislocation with joint destruction, pain, and impaired mobility. When a hip begins to dislocate, it rarely improves without treatment. Hip pain is one of the main complaints of young adults with cerebral palsy, affecting up to 47% of patients. Most studies show that the risk of hip dislocation is correlated with the GMFCS score. Ninety-two percent of patients with spastic cerebral palsy were found in one study to have some degree of hip deformity, and another study found hip subluxation and dislocation in 60% of dependent sitters.

In most patients, the hip is normal at birth and radiographic changes typically become apparent between 2 and 4 years of age. The cause of this progressive deformity is multifactorial and includes muscle imbalance, retained primitive reflexes, abnormal positioning, and pelvic obliquity. These altered forces across the hip along with decreased weight bearing lead to bony deformities, including acetabular dysplasia, excessive femoral anteversion, increased neck-shaft angle, and osteopenia. Prolonged spasticity of the adductor muscles leads to a relative overpowering of the abductor muscles, causing a growth inhibition of the greater trochanter and producing a relative valgus overgrowth of the proximal femur. In many patients, the apparent increase in neck-shaft angle observed may be caused, however, more by the appearance of increased anteversion on the radiograph than to an actual increase in the neck-shaft angle.

The neck-shaft angle in children with cerebral palsy has been shown to increase with age, and anteversion, which normally decreases with age, does not change in children with cerebral palsy. Increased anteversion is more common in ambulators than nonambulators and does not change significantly after age 6 years.

In a study of the incidence and pathogenesis of structural changes around the hip in patients with cerebral palsy, only 21% were considered normal. Hip subluxation in patients with cerebral palsy can be difficult to detect clinically because of the presence of abnormal muscle forces and contractures, and because early hip subluxation typically is painless. This has led to the development of hip surveillance programs for children with cerebral palsy in which routine clinical and radiographic examinations are performed at intervals based on severity of their cerebral palsy and GMFCS grade, usually every 6 months until 7 to 8 years of age. These programs have been effective in reducing the rate of hip dislocation in these screened populations. A practical radiographic method for quantifying the amount of hip subluxation present was described by Reimers as the "migration percentage." Careful patient positioning, with the patient supine, the hips together, and the patellae facing forward, increases the accuracy of the measurement. The measurement error for an experienced observer using this method is approximately 5 degrees. The migration percentage (Fig. 33-5) is determined by drawing the Hilgenreiner line connecting the two triradiate cartilages and then perpendicular lines at the lateral margins of the bony acetabula. The width of the femoral head uncovered (lateral to the perpendicular line) is divided by the total width of the femoral head and multiplied by 100 to give the migration percentage (Fig. 33-5). The measurement error for an experienced observer using this method is approximately 5 degrees. This index typically is 0 until age 4 years and less than 5% from 4 years until skeletal maturity. A migration of greater than 33% is considered subluxation and greater than 100% as dislocation. Hip subluxation, as measured by the migration percentage, is related to the GMFCS score and has been shown to increase approximately 12% per year in nonambulators as compared with 2% per year in ambulators, with the highest risk being in quadriplegic nonambulators who are younger than 5 years old. More important than the absolute value is the change observed within a given patient.

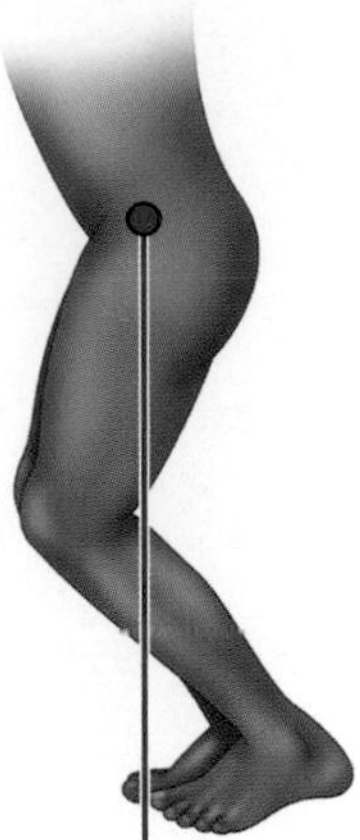

FIGURE 33-6 Typical crouch posture caused by flexion deformities of hips or fixed flexion deformities of knees.

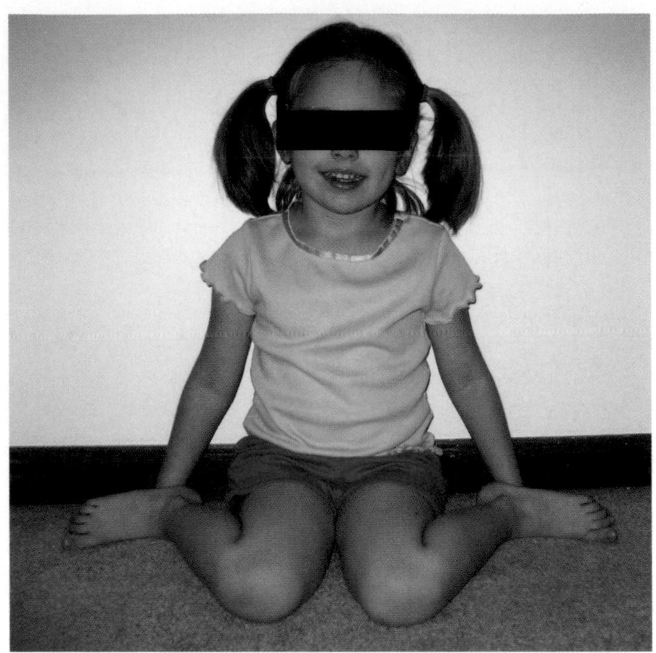

FIGURE 33-7 W position.

FLEXION DEFORMITIES

Crouched gait, or flexion of the hip, with or without flexion contractures around the hip, knee, and ankle, has been well described. Excessive hip flexion brings the center of gravity anteriorly and is compensated for by increased lumbar lordosis, knee flexion, and ankle dorsiflexion (Fig. 33-6). It is important to determine whether the increased hip flexion is the primary deformity or is secondary to other deformities around the lower extremities, such as knee or ankle contractures. If an unrecognized knee flexion contracture is present, hip flexor release can weaken the hip further and increase hip flexion. Careful physical examination is helpful in making this determination. One source of confusion is differentiating flexion-internal rotation deformity of the hip, or "pseudoadduction," from isolated adduction deformity, although often both coexist in the same patient. Children with flexion-internal rotation deformity sit with a wide base of support in the W position: hips flexed 90 degrees and maximally internally rotated, knees maximally flexed, and feet externally rotated (Fig. 33-7). With flexion-internal rotation deformity, femoral anteversion and external tibial torsion are increased, and planovalgus feet are present. With a true adduction contracture, these secondary deformities in the femoral neck, tibia, and feet are absent.

At the time of hip surgery, contractures around the knees and ankles also should be corrected. Single-stage multilevel procedures are preferable to staged single-level procedures. Hip flexion contractures from 15 to 30 degrees usually are treated with psoas lengthening through an intramuscular recession over the pelvic brim, especially in ambulatory children in whom complete iliopsoas release at its insertion may lead to excessive hip flexion weakness and difficulties with clearance of the foot during the swing phase of gait. Contractures of more than 30 degrees may require more extensive releases of the rectus femoris, sartorius, and tensor fasciae latae and the anterior fibers of the gluteus minimus and medius, in addition to the iliopsoas. Because they span two joints, the tensor fasciae latae, rectus femoris, and the anterior fibers of the gluteus medius and minimus may contribute to the flexion deformity. Release of these muscles, because of its extensive nature, is used only for large deformities, and isolated iliopsoas lengthening is better suited for smaller ones.

ADDUCTION DEFORMITIES

Adduction is the most common deformity of the hip in children with cerebral palsy. Adduction contractures can cause various difficulties, including scissoring of the legs during gait, hip subluxation, and, in severely affected children, difficulty with perineal hygiene. For mild contractures, an adductor tenotomy usually is sufficient; more severe contractures often require release of the gracilis and the anterior half of the adductor brevis. Adductor tenotomies usually are done bilaterally to prevent a "windswept" pelvis. Immediately after surgery, a program of physical therapy and abduction bracing is begun.

ADDUCTOR TENOTOMY AND RELEASE

Adductor tenotomy is indicated for a patient with a mild adduction contracture, as indicated by a scissoring gait or early hip subluxation. This procedure should be done early because damage to the developing acetabulum from abnormal hip muscle forces is greatest before 4 years of age. The ideal candidate for soft-tissue lengthening is an ambulatory child younger than 8 years, and preferably younger than 4 years, who has hip abduction of less than 30 degrees and a migration index of less than 50%. Neurectomy of the anterior branch of the obturator nerve should be avoided to prevent iatrogenic hip abduction contracture. Miller et al. reported the results of adductor release in 147 hips (74 children) with hip abduction of less than 30 degrees or migration index of more than 25%. At an average follow-up of 39 months, 54% of hips were classified as good, 34% as fair, and 12% as poor based on the migration index. A longer-term study with an 8-year average follow-up showed that 58% of patients required a second surgical procedure, indicating that, although still beneficial, early soft-tissue release alone may be insufficient to prevent long-term hip subluxation and dislocation. It may delay major bony surgery, however, until the risk of recurrence is decreased.

TECHNIQUE 33-1

- Place the patient supine on the operating table and prepare the area from the toes to the inferior costal margin, isolating the perineum (Fig. 33-8A).
- Identify the adductor longus by palpation and make a 2- to 3-cm transverse incision over the adductor longus tendon approximately 1 cm distal from its origin.
- Dissect through the subcutaneous tissue and identify the adductor longus fascia (Fig. 33-8B).
- Make a longitudinal incision in the adductor fascia, identify the tendinous portion of the adductor longus, and resect it with electrocautery.
- Release with electrocautery any remaining muscle fibers of the adductor longus as necessary. Avoid injury to the anterior branch of the obturator nerve, which is in the interval between the adductor longus and brevis (Fig. 33-8C).
- Gradually abduct the hip and determine the amount of correction obtained. If further correction is required, slowly release the anterior half of the adductor brevis using electrocautery and avoiding injury to the branches of the obturator nerve. Do not release an excessive amount of the adductor brevis and protect the posterior branch of the obturator nerve to prevent an abduction contracture.
- If the gracilis muscle is found to be tight, release it with electrocautery (Fig. 33-8D).
- When the final correction is obtained, close the wound in layers. Take care to close the adductor fascia to help prevent skin dimpling postoperatively (Fig. 33-8E).

POSTOPERATIVE CARE. Postoperatively, the patient is placed in the abducted position. Depending on the patient's functional status, quality of caregivers, and other procedures done, the patient can be immobilized in bilateral long leg casts with an abduction bar or abduction pillow for 1 month. A removable abduction pillow can be used, which allows physical therapy to be started immediately after surgery to help maintain and increase optimally hip range of motion.

ILIOPSOAS RECESSION

Bleck recommended iliopsoas recession when the hip internally rotates during walking or when passive external rotation is absent with the hip in full extension and present when the joint is passively flexed to 90 degrees. This procedure usually is done in conjunction with other soft-tissue releases of the lower extremities. Iliopsoas recession is used more commonly than complete tenotomy at the level of the lesser trochanter to avoid causing excessive hip flexion weakness.

TECHNIQUE 33-2

FIGURE 33-9

- Place the patient supine with a roll under the buttock of the operative side.
- Palpate the course of the femoral artery and mark it on the skin, keeping in mind that the femoral nerve is lateral to it.
- For an isolated iliopsoas recession, make a 5-cm "bikini" incision. This incision can be modified as needed if other procedures are going to be done at the same time. Center the incision medial to and 2 cm below the anterior superior iliac spine.
- Identify and develop the interval between the tensor fasciae latae and sartorius to expose the direct head of the rectus femoris with its origin at the anterior inferior iliac spine. It is not necessary to identify the femoral neurovascular structures.
- Palpate the pelvic brim just medial and inferior to the rectus femoris origin to locate the iliopsoas tendon in a shallow groove.
- Slightly flex the hip to relax the soft-tissue structures around the hip.
- Place a right-angle retractor on the lateral aspect of the iliopsoas muscle and pull the retractor medially and anteriorly, exposing the posteromedial aspect of the muscle and the psoas tendon (Fig. 33-9). The retractor is protecting the femoral nerve, which is medial to it.
- Dissect the surrounding muscle fascia and isolate the tendon from the muscle with a right-angle clamp. Verify that there is enough muscle remaining at that level so that continuity is maintained after tendon release.
- Under direct vision, carefully internally and externally rotate the hip to see the tendon loosen and tighten. If there is any doubt as to the identification of the tendon, use an elevator to dissect around the tendon proximally until its muscle fibers are identified. An electrical nerve stimulator or careful brief stimulation with electrocautery also can be used to help confirm that the tendon has been found and that the femoral nerve has not been mistakenly identified.
- Release the tendinous portion, leaving the muscle fibers in continuity. Extend and internally rotate the hip to separate the tendon ends.
- Close the wound in layers and apply sterile dressings.

POSTOPERATIVE CARE. Patients with an isolated iliopsoas release are started immediately in a physical therapy program emphasizing hip extension and external rotation. Patients, especially those who are unable to cooperate with physical therapy, are placed prone at bed rest to help improve hip extension. This can be modified as needed if other procedures are done at the same time.

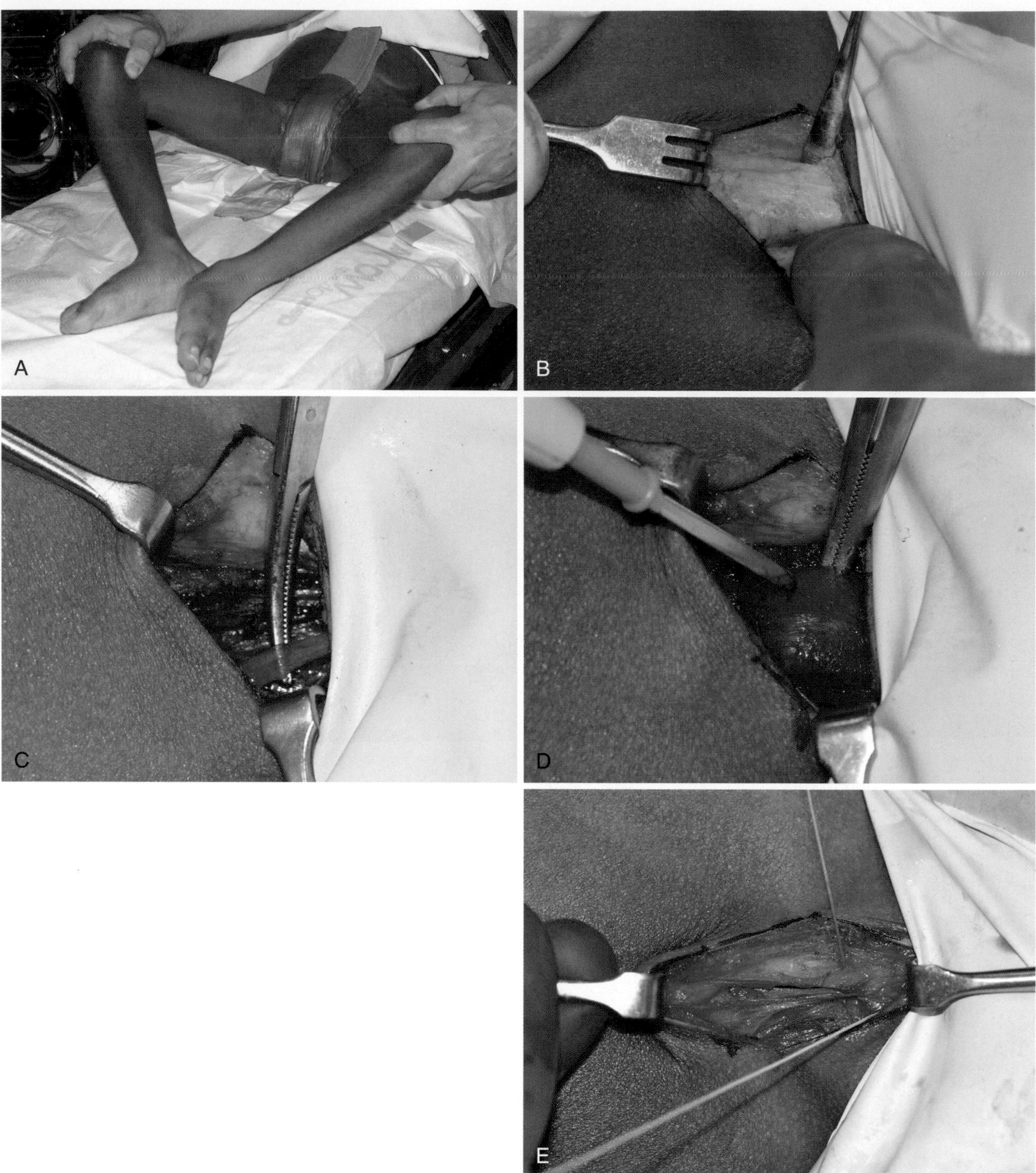

FIGURE 33-8 Adductor tenotomy. **A,** Patient positioning. **B,** Skin incision and subcutaneous dissection to identify adductor longus fascia. **C,** Hemostat placed under anterior branch of obturator nerve. **D,** Release of tight gracilis muscle with electrocautery. **E,** Closure of adductor fascia. **SEE TECHNIQUE 33-1.**

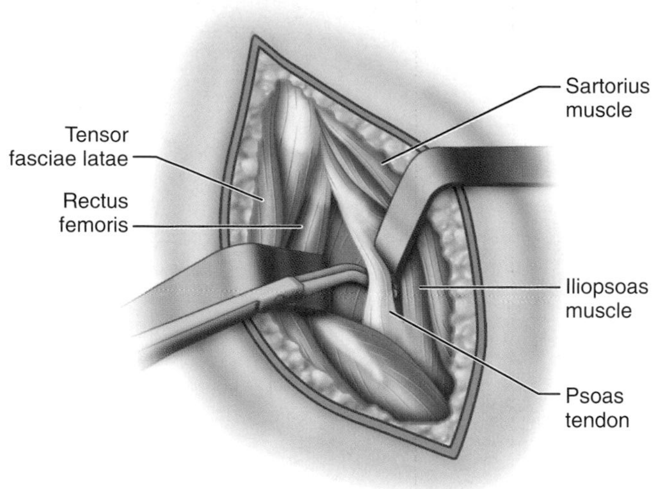

FIGURE 33-9 Skaggs et al. surgical approach for iliopsoas recession. When procedure is done alone, much smaller incision is adequate. **SEE TECHNIQUE 33-2.**

ILIOPSOAS RELEASE AT THE LESSER TROCHANTER

Iliopsoas release at its insertion on the lesser trochanter is better for nonambulatory patients than for ambulatory patients because of the risk of causing excessive hip flexion weakness, which can severely affect an ambulatory patient. It often is done at the same time as another procedure, such as an adductor release or varus derotational osteotomy.

Additional release of the secondary hip flexors including the sartorius and rectus femoris also may be used for severe deformities.

TECHNIQUE 33-3

- Make a transverse incision 1 to 3 cm distal to the inguinal crease. If an adductor release is to be done at the same time, make a longitudinal incision in the adductor longus fascia and transect the adductor longus with electrocautery; perform a myotomy of the gracilis if necessary.
- Resect as much of the adductor brevis as necessary to obtain 45 degrees of abduction.
- Develop the interval between the residual adductor brevis and the pectineus or between the pectineus and the neurovascular bundle until the femur is identified.
- Open the bursa over the iliopsoas and its sheath.
- Place a retractor into the tendon sheath and retract the tendon medially.
- Pass a right-angle clamp under the tendon of the iliopsoas, which can be completely released with electrocautery in a nonambulatory child.
- Release the iliopsoas as far proximally as possible in an ambulatory child to preserve the iliacus muscle attachment to the iliopsoas tendon.

POSTOPERATIVE CARE. Physical therapy is started 2 days after surgery, emphasizing range-of-motion exercises of the hips and knees. Leg-knee immobilizers are used 8 to 12 hours a day for 1 month. Parents are encouraged to have the child sleep prone as much as possible.

SUBLUXATION AND DISLOCATION

Hip dislocation occurs on a continuum from mild subluxation to true dislocation with significant degenerative changes. Because early intervention can be very effective in preventing or delaying the development of dislocation, considerable work has been done to identify hips at risk. Children with risk factors for subluxation or dislocation should be examined and radiographs obtained at 6-month intervals until it can be established that the hips are stable, and then follow-up can be less frequent. Of hip dislocations, 70% to 90% occur in patients with quadriplegia, which necessitates screening for all patients in this high-risk group. Clinically, a hip at risk has contractures of the adductors and flexors. Hips with flexion contractures of more than 20 degrees and abduction of less than 30 degrees are at increased risk of progressive subluxation. Radiographically, a hip at risk has an increased neck-shaft angle and increased femoral anteversion. Acetabular dysplasia and an abnormal migration index also may be present. When a hip at risk is identified, a program of aggressive physical therapy and abduction splinting typically is started, although there are no well-controlled long-term studies to support this. If further progression continues, early operative treatment consisting of soft-tissue release of contracted tendons is indicated. The goal of adductor release is restoration of more than 60 degrees of abduction with the hips flexed and 45 degrees with the hips extended. The release begins sequentially with the complete release of the adductor longus, the anterior half of the adductor brevis, and occasionally the gracilis until the desired range of motion is achieved. Care must be taken not to perform too extensive a release, which can cause an abduction contracture that is extremely difficult to manage. For this reason, neurectomy of the anterior branch of the obturator nerve should not be done. Immediately after adductor release or transfer, a program of physical therapy is begun, emphasizing hip abduction and night splinting for 6 months.

Hip subluxation occurs when more than one third of the femoral head is uncovered and there is a break in the Shenton line. Nonoperative treatment alone at this point is ineffective. In younger children, soft-tissue releases alone may be sufficient, but most patients with hip subluxation require osteotomy in addition to soft-tissue release. Operative correction of femoral valgus and anteversion and acetabular dysplasia is necessary at this stage to prevent further subluxation and dislocation. Plain radiographs and CT scans with three-dimensional reconstruction are necessary to evaluate the proximal femoral and acetabular deformities. Rotational studies using CT can be helpful in quantifying the amount of femoral anteversion and any tibial rotation.

A femoral varus and derotation (external rotation) osteotomy, often combined with femoral shortening, generally is used to reduce the neck-shaft angle to 115 degrees in ambulatory patients and often less in nonambulatory patients. A wide variety of acetabular osteotomies have been used in the treatment of acetabular dysplasia in patients with cerebral palsy, including osteotomies described by Salter, Pemberton, Dega, Ganz, and Steel and salvage-type osteotomies such as the Chiari and shelf. Careful matching of the procedure to the deformity is essential to prevent inadvertent iatrogenic worsening of the deformity. For example, a Salter osteotomy, which redirects the acetabulum anteriorly and laterally, if done in a patient with posterior acetabular deficiency would uncover the femoral head further. Often patients with cerebral palsy have a posterosuperior deficiency for which a Dega osteotomy or shelf procedure is effective. The Dega osteotomy has been shown by CT morphometry to increase anterosuperior, superolateral, and posterosuperior coverage and increase acetabular volume by 68%. Although typically done before the time of triradiate cartilage closure, it has been done in patients with cerebral palsy after triradiate closure with good improvement in subluxation and dislocation radiographically. Postoperatively, patients can be immobilized for a brief time in a spica cast, followed by a period of aggressive rehabilitation that includes physical therapy, bracing, and progressive weight bearing. Because of concerns about the risk of abduction contracture and fracture after cast immobilization, we now avoid casting when possible and use early physical therapy to increase range of motion.

Hip dislocation is common in patients with cerebral palsy, especially in severely affected children. Radiographic abnormalities, such as increased femoral neck-shaft angle and increased internal femoral rotation, have been shown to be correlated with increased GMFCS level. Similar acetabular changes also are seen in patients with dislocated hips having global acetabular defects and smaller acetabular volume than in those with subluxed hips having more posterior acetabular defects and greater acetabular volume. The patient's risk of hip dislocation is related to GMFCS level, with a 0% incidence for patients with grade I and 90% for patients with grade V. The head-shaft angle, which measures the amount of proximal femoral valgus, has been shown to be predictive of hip dislocation: for every 10-degree increase in head-shaft angle, the risk of dislocation increases 1.6-fold. The natural history of the untreated hip in these patients is progressive subluxation associated with bony deformity of the proximal femur and acetabulum. The spastic adductors and hip flexors compress the femoral head against the posterolateral acetabulum and labrum. The capsule and superior rim of the acetabulum cause focal deformation of the femoral head. The indented femoral head locks on the acetabular rim, causing significant cartilage loss and pain. Mathematic models have predicted that a child with spastic hip disease has a six-fold increase in forces across the hip. The acetabulum in affected children usually is normal until about 30 months of age, when a change in the acetabular index is seen. With continued abnormal muscle forces, the hip typically dislocates superolaterally, which has been confirmed by CT studies. Late findings include dislocation of the hip and degenerative changes. Most authors agree that hip subluxation and dislocation should be prevented in all patients who are medically able to tolerate treatment. The treatment of an established dislocation is more controversial. A patient with a long-standing dislocation is not a good candidate for a relocation procedure because of the deformities of the proximal femur and acetabulum, which also may be associated with degenerative changes. Treatment options for hip dislocations in patients with cerebral palsy include observation; relocation procedures on the femur, acetabulum, or both; proximal femoral resection; hip arthrodesis; and, in carefully selected patients, total hip arthroplasty.

A dislocated hip usually is not disabling in a severely affected patient who is neurologically immature, extremely intellectually impaired, bedridden, and institutionalized. Four criteria for open reduction of a dislocated hip are (1) the patient must be moderately mature intellectually; (2) the patient should have at least sitting potential if not walking ability; (3) pelvic obliquity should be minimal or corrected; and (4) dislocation should ideally be unilateral. The heterogeneous literature concerning surgical treatment of dislocated hips in patients with cerebral palsy makes it difficult to compare studies. Because of the variable nature of cerebral palsy, most studies include a wide spectrum of severity of neurologic involvement and a wide variety of procedures used. Varus femoral osteotomy was found in one study to be effective in preventing redislocation and surgery in 84%. The amount of bony deformity present preoperatively, as measured by center-edge angle and migration index, was a predictor of final outcome. Worse results were reported in quadriplegics than in diplegics and hemiplegics.

Good results were reported in 95% of patients at mean 7-year follow-up after a one-stage combined approach that included soft-tissue lengthenings, open reduction with capsulorrhaphy (open if migration index was more than 70 degrees), varus derotational osteotomy, and pericapsular acetabuloplasty. A recent report of 168 hip reconstructions in children with cerebral palsy showed statistically significant improvement in pain relief and function (GMFCS level) with a 10% complication rate. Preoperative migration percentage was correlated with increasing pain and worse outcome while femoral head shape was not. Although most centers favor a one-stage approach, good results have been obtained with femoral osteotomy and later acetabular osteotomy if needed; however, this approach requires a second hospitalization and rehabilitation. Despite these good outcomes, remember that complications following hip osteotomy are common. In one large series, 65% of children with cerebral palsy who had hip osteotomy had at least one postoperative complication, most (83%) of which were medical rather than orthopaedic. Redislocations also can occur, especially in GMFCS IV and V patients in whom the migration percentage was found to increase 2% per year and 3.5% per year in GMFCS IV and V patients, respectively. Long-term follow-up monitoring is necessary.

In a series of patients treated with Chiari osteotomies, 79% of 23 hips were reportedly painless at an average follow-up of 7 years; however, 29% of the hips had a migration index of 30% or greater; resubluxation typically occurred in the first year after surgery.

VARUS DEROTATIONAL OSTEOTOMY

Varus derotational osteotomy, usually combined with soft-tissue releases, is indicated for patients with hip subluxation or dislocation and excessive anteversion and valgus deformity of the proximal femur. Computer models have shown that to normalize the muscle forces across a spastic hip, the psoas, iliacus, gracilis, and adductor longus and brevis must be released. The benefit of a varus derotational osteotomy comes primarily through the bony shortening that acts biomechanically similar to a soft-tissue lengthening. Decreasing the neck-shaft angle and anteversion has little effect on the hip forces. An isolated varus derotational osteotomy, often with femoral shortening, is indicated only when there is mild or no acetabular dysplasia present because, although there is some remodeling potential of the acetabulum, it is variable in patients with cerebral palsy. Acetabular remodeling is better in GMFCS I-III patients and is correlated with the amount of varus produced. Varus derotational osteotomy can be combined with an acetabular osteotomy if significant subluxation and acetabular dysplasia are present. In a prospective gait study of 37 patients, varus derotational osteotomy improved hip external rotation and extension, knee extension strength, and cosmetic appearance and decreased anterior pelvic tilt. Patients who are nonambulatory and patients with a gastrostomy or tracheostomy are at increased risk of postoperative complications, including decubitus ulcers and fractures. The risk of recurrent dislocation is higher in patients with higher GMFCDS levels or insufficient correction of valgus and acetabular dysplasia, and the risk of osteonecrosis is proportional to the patient's age and degree of preoperative subluxation.

The technique of varus derotational osteotomy is described in Chapter 30 (see Technique 30-7).

COMBINED ONE-STAGE CORRECTION OF SPASTIC DISLOCATED HIP (SAN DIEGO PROCEDURE)

TECHNIQUE 33-4

MEDIAL APPROACH (SOFT-TISSUE RELEASE)

- With the patient on a radiolucent table, prepare and drape the hip from the toes to the costal margin.
- Use electrocautery to release the adductor longus and gracilis.
- Release the psoas in the interval between the neurovascular bundle and the pectineus. After the sciatic nerve is carefully identified, release the proximal hamstrings posterior to the adductor magnus. Avoid the sciatic nerve.

ANTERIOR APPROACH (OPEN REDUCTION)

- Make the second incision parallel to the iliac crest using a Salter incision (see Technique 30-3)
- Divide the iliac crest apophysis and strip the iliac wing subperiosteally down to the sciatic notch medially and laterally. Alternatively, the iliac crest apophysis can be elevated instead of split.
- Resect the direct and indirect heads of the rectus femoris and retract them distally to expose the underlying capsule.
- Make a T-capsulotomy, and identify the ligamentum teres.
- Remove the ligamentum teres, cut the contracted transverse acetabular ligament, and clear the acetabulum of any remaining soft tissue.
- Inspect the femoral head to assess deformity and cartilage loss. If more than 50% of the cartilage is lost, reduction may be unsuccessful and other options (e.g., valgus osteotomy or resection of the femoral head) should be considered.

LATERAL APPROACH (FEMORAL OSTEOTOMY)

- Make an incision on the lateral aspect of the proximal femur and perform a lateral exposure.
- Split the tensor fasciae latae and dissect to the lateral aspect of the femur.
- Perform a varus derotational shortening femoral osteotomy at the lesser trochanter. Remove 1 to 2 cm of bone (Fig. 33-10).
- The neck-shaft angle should be decreased to 110 degrees, and anteversion should be corrected to 10 to 20 degrees.
- Fix the femoral osteotomy with an AO blade plate of the appropriate size for the child. Several implant systems have been developed to accommodate infantile, pediatric, and adolescent anatomic variations. Alternatively, a size-appropriate proximal femoral locking plate can be used.

ANTERIOR APPROACH (PERICAPSULAR PELVIC OSTEOTOMY)

- Return to the anterior incision and place five nonabsorbable No. 1 sutures into the capsulotomy for later closure.
- With a straight osteotome, make an osteotomy 0.5 to 1.0 cm above the edge of the acetabulum, on a line drawn between the anterior inferior iliac spine and the sciatic notch. Extend this through the lateral wall of the pelvis, but not through the medial wall (Fig. 33-11). To allow proper bending, both corners should be cut at the anterior and posterior ends of the osteotomy (anterior superior iliac spine and sciatic notch). This is most easily done by using a regular rongeur anteriorly and a large Kerrison rongeur posteriorly in the sciatic notch.
- Use a curved osteotome 1.9 to 2.5 cm wide and an image intensifier to perform the second part of the osteotomy. Direct the osteotome halfway between the articular surface and the medial cortex. Extend the cut medially and distally to the level of the triradiate cartilage. Use gentle downward pressure on the osteotome to open the osteotomy site 1.0 to 1.5 cm (Fig. 33-12).
- Remove a bicortical graft from the iliac crest and shape it into three or four triangular grafts measuring approximately 1 cm at the base. Insert the grafts into the osteotomy, using the largest one for the area of most desired coverage.
- Alternatively, tricortical allograft bone can be used, which gives good structural support to the osteotomy.
- When a stable reduction is obtained, repair the capsule using the sutures placed earlier.
- Close all three wounds in standard fashion and check a radiograph to ensure proper reduction before application of a hip spica cast with the hip in 45 degrees of flexion and 30 degrees of abduction.

POSTOPERATIVE CARE. The patient is placed in a well-padded spica cast, which typically is removed at 6 weeks postoperatively with the patient anesthetized. Physical therapy for range of motion and progressive weight bearing are started after cast removal, but vigorous physical therapy and attempted weight bearing are not advised until 10 weeks after surgery.

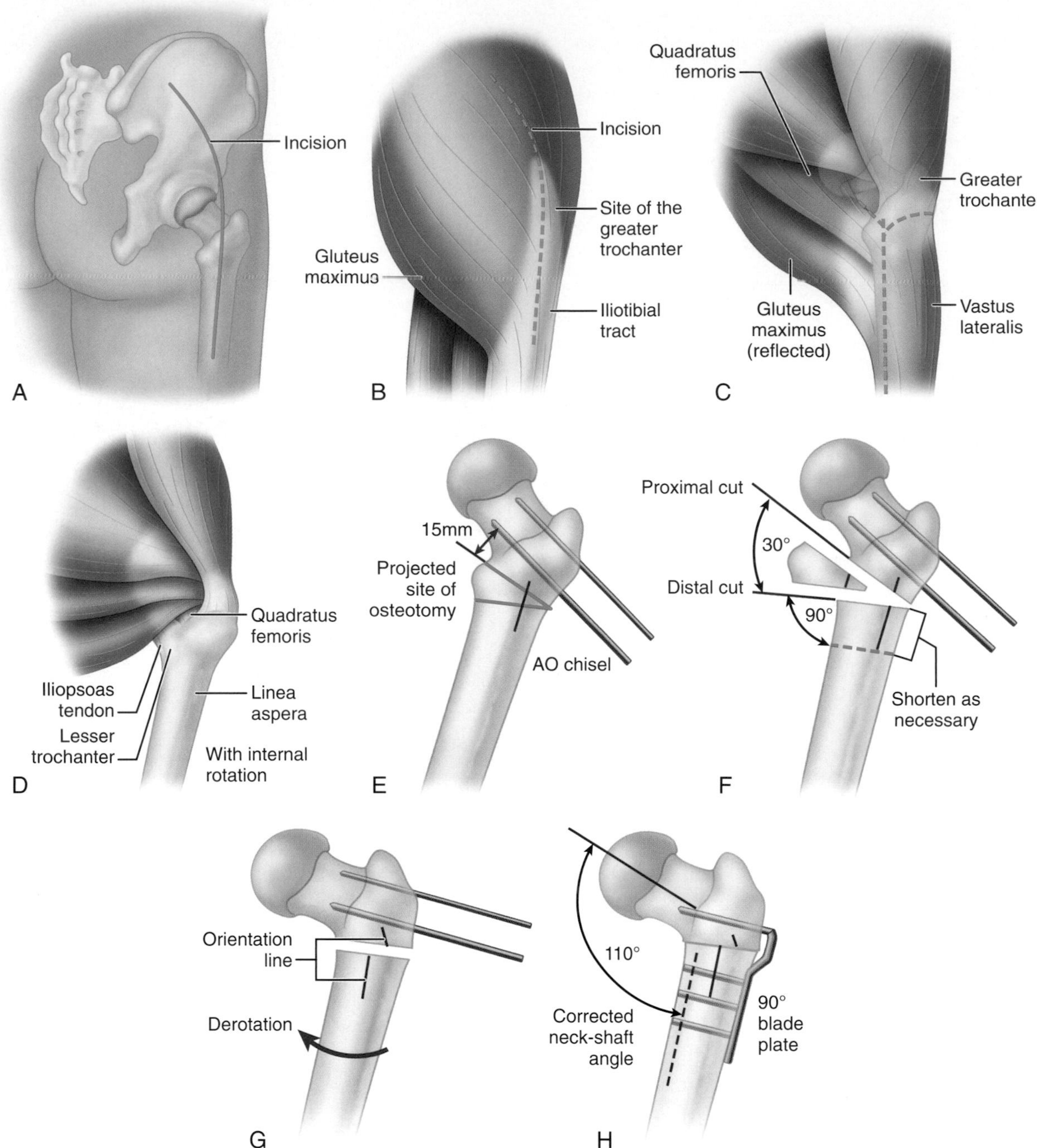

FIGURE 33-10 Root and Siegal varus derotational osteotomy of hip. **A,** Skin incision. **B,** Incision through gluteus maximus and fascia lata (iliotibial tract). **C,** Greater trochanter, quadratus femoris, origin of vastus lateralis, tendinous attachment of gluteus maximus, and linea aspera are identified. **D,** Osteotomy site is exposed in area of lesser trochanter; psoas tendon can be released if necessary. **E,** Guidewire and chisel are inserted in parallel position. *Shaded area* represents wedge to be excised; *scored line* is for reference for later rotation. **F,** Location of osteotomy planes; proximal osteotomy is 15 mm distal to chisel. **G,** Rotation is accomplished by external rotation of femur. **H,** Osteotomy is fixed with AO plate and screws. **SEE TECHNIQUE 33-4.**

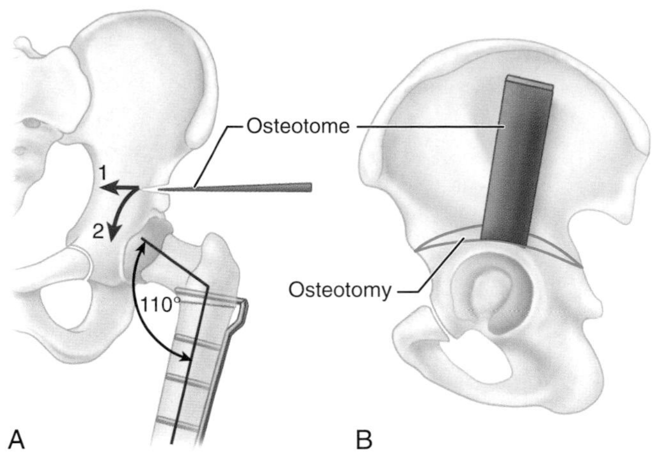

FIGURE 33-11 Mubarak et al. one-stage correction of spastic dislocated hip. **A,** Pericapsular acetabuloplasty is begun approximately 1 cm above lateral margin of acetabulum. **B,** Osteotomy proceeds in line between anterior inferior iliac spine and sciatic notch, penetrating outer wall of ilium only. Bicortical cuts are made at anterior inferior iliac spine and sciatic notch. Straight or slightly curved osteotome extends osteotomy toward triradiate cartilage, avoiding penetration of joint or inner pelvic wall. **SEE TECHNIQUE 33-4.**

Other pelvic osteotomy techniques are discussed in Chapter 30.

Resection arthroplasty, arthrodesis, and total hip arthroplasty have been proposed for the treatment of a painful dislocated hip when a relocation procedure is impossible. Because of the heterogeneous nature of the patients and procedures performed, as well as the lack of large long-term comparison studies, the optimal treatment for the painful dislocated nonreconstructable hip is unclear. The goals of these procedures are pain relief, improved function, and increased ease of care for caregivers. Hip resection arthroplasty, most commonly a Girdlestone intertrochanteric resection, has been used for the treatment of end-stage hip degeneration caused by other conditions, such as osteoarthritis, osteonecrosis, septic arthritis, and slipped capital femoral epiphysis. In patients with cerebral palsy, the use of this type of resection arthroplasty has been modified because of the high rate of postoperative pain from femoral-iliac impingement. Proximal femoral resection, combined with capsular interposition, has been effective. The advantage of this type of resection is that it is technically straightforward, requires less postoperative immobilization and operating room time, and requires no permanent implants, in contrast to other techniques such as relocation procedures and arthrodesis. The use of capsular interposition (Castle and Schneider) has been shown to have a lower complication rate than the

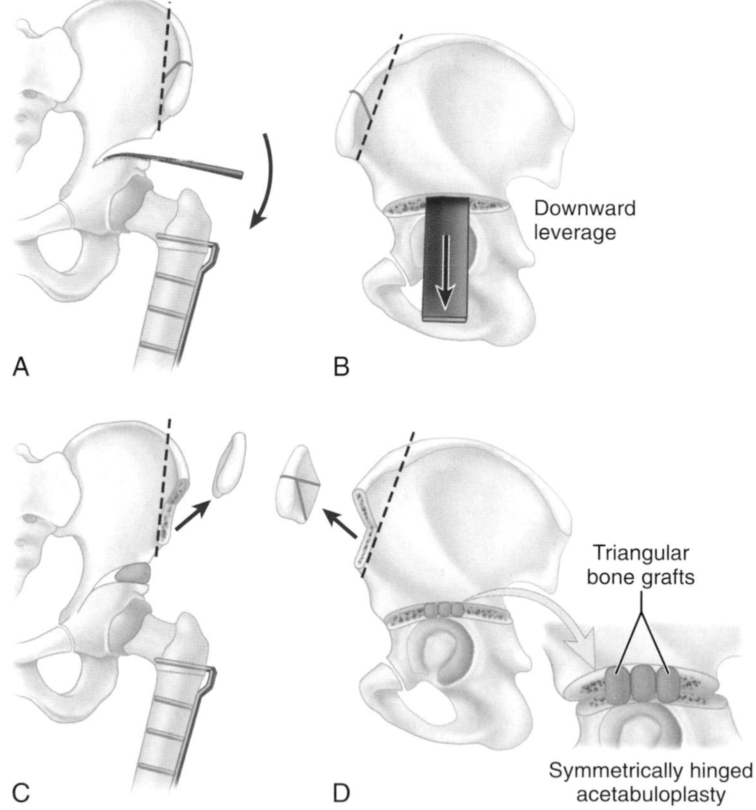

FIGURE 33-12 Mubarak et al. one-stage correction of spastic dislocated hip. Osteotomy stops several millimeters from triradiate cartilage and is hinged open laterally to correct dysplasia. **A,** Tricortical segment of iliac wing is harvested for bone graft. **B,** Trapezoidal segments are fashioned to fit into osteotomy site. **C** and **D,** Three trapezoidal segments of tricortical bone graft are impacted into place to hold osteotomy site open. Elasticity of intact medial cortex holds bone grafts in place; fixation is not required. **SEE TECHNIQUE 33-4.**

interposition of capsule and iliopsoas and gluteal muscles (McCarthy). A study of 34 severely affected institutionalized patients who had proximal femoral resections (56 hips), 33 were able to sit comfortably and have painless perineal care at 2-year follow-up; 79% of patients developed heterotopic ossification postoperatively, but this had little to no effect on overall function. Although initially recommended, the use of postoperative traction following Girdlestone resection has become less common and may not improve outcome.

PROXIMAL FEMORAL RESECTION

TECHNIQUE 33-5

- After administration of general anesthesia, place the patient supine with a sandbag elevating the affected hip.
- Make a straight lateral incision along the proximal femur beginning 10 cm superior to the greater trochanter and ending inferior to the level of the lesser trochanter.
- Split the fascia of the tensor fasciae latae and femoris and extraperiosteally detach the insertions of the vastus lateralis and gluteus medius and minimus from the proximal femur.
- Detach the psoas tendon from the lesser trochanter and complete the exposure of the proximal femur extraperiosteally.
- Incise the periosteum circumferentially around the femur just distal to the insertion of the gluteus maximus or at the proposed level of femoral resection.
- Determine the level of the osteotomy by drawing a line on the preoperative anteroposterior radiograph from the ischium to the femur, parallel to the inferior border of the ischium.
- Divide the short external rotators.
- Incise the capsule circumferentially and free it from the base of the femoral neck.
- Divide the ligamentum teres and remove the proximal femur, using an oscillating saw to make the osteotomy (Fig. 33-13A).
- Test the range of motion of the hip at this point and, if necessary for motion, tenotomize the proximal hamstrings through the same incision after identifying the sciatic nerve. If necessary, also release the adductors.
- Seal the acetabular cavity by oversewing the capsular edges. Alternatively, the iliopsoas can be sutured to the lateral part of the capsule and the abductors to the medial part of the capsule.
- Bring the vastus lateralis lateral to medial over the femoral stump, sewing it into the rectus femoris muscle.
- To decrease the risk of heterotopic ossification, handle tissue carefully, completely excise the periosteum, and irrigate thoroughly.
- Secure meticulous hemostasis and close the wound over a suction drain.

POSTOPERATIVE CARE. Skeletal traction can be applied immediately after surgery and removed daily for gentle exercises. Gentle range-of-motion exercises emphasizing maximal flexion and extension, abduction, and internal and external rotation of the hip are started on the second day after surgery. Over the first 6 weeks of traction, the head of the bed is gradually elevated to prevent posttraction hypotension. Patients are allowed back into a wheelchair as tolerated.

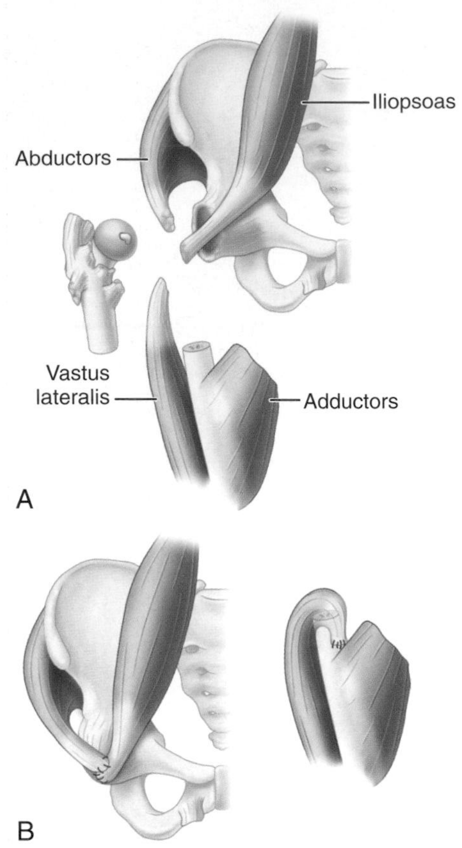

FIGURE 33-13 McCarthy et al. proximal femoral resection. **A,** Extraperiosteal approach, periosteal excision, and release of musculotendinous attachments. **B,** Interpositional arthroplasty-iliopsoas and abductors are sutured to hip capsule, and femoral stump is covered by vastus lateralis. **SEE TECHNIQUE 33-5.**

Redirectional osteotomy also has been proposed as an alternative to resection arthroplasty. This proximal femoral valgus osteotomy places the legs in a more abducted position, which improves perineal hygiene and sitting. The ideal candidate for this procedure is a child with severe hip adduction with minimal or no pain. The osteotomy directs the lesser trochanter into the acetabulum and the femoral head away from the pelvis.

HIP ARTHRODESIS

Hip arthrodesis also can be effective in relieving pain and improving function in carefully selected patients. The ideal candidate is a patient with unilateral disease and no spinal involvement. Hip arthrodesis may be preferable in ambulatory patients because it allows weight bearing, in contrast to proximal femoral resections. In two studies of arthrodesis in patients with cerebral palsy and painful hip dislocation, fusions were obtained in 6 of 8 patients and 11 of 14 hips after the first attempt, resulting in pain relief and improvement in posture. The remainder required repeat arthrodesis. One negative aspect of hip arthrodesis is the need for postoperative casting for 2 months and the complications associated with it.

TECHNIQUE 33-6

- Place the patient supine with a soft pad under the gluteal region.
- Perform an adductor tenotomy as described in Technique 33-1.
- Through a longitudinal lateral incision to the hip, split the gluteal muscles.
- Extend the exposure of the hip joint to allow an iliopsoas tenotomy.
- Resect the pulvinar and ligamentum teres, remove any remaining cartilage from the femoral head and acetabulum, and deepen the dysplastic acetabulum.
- Position the hip in 40 degrees of flexion, 15 degrees of abduction, and neutral rotation. The fixation device used depends on the local bone width and quality, the size of the femoral head and neck, and the desirable degree of hip flexion. Appropriate implants include a 4.5-mm AO-D cerebral palsy plate, AO-Cobra plate, and 6.5-mm cannulated screws.

POSTOPERATIVE CARE. A hip spica cast is worn for 2 months postoperatively. Patients are then started in a progressive range-of-motion and weight-bearing program.

Total hip arthroplasty is an option for patients with cerebral palsy with end-stage hip degeneration. The ideal candidate is an intelligent, independent ambulator with mild soft-tissue contractures. Good midterm results (10 years) have been reported after hip arthroplasty. Another study reported return to preoperative function in all patients, return to prepain function in 88%, and implant survivorship in 95% at 2 years and 85% at 10 years. Increasing the anteversion and inclination of the acetabular component may help increase stability. Although the results of total hip replacement are best in GMFCS I and II patients, surface replacement has been shown to be effective for pain relief in a small series of GMFCS III-V patients.

KNEE

HIP AND KNEE RELATIONSHIPS

Deformities of the knee in patients with cerebral palsy are difficult to evaluate and treat and rarely occur in isolation. Pelvic, hip, knee, ankle, and foot deformities are interrelated. The hip and the knee are tightly coupled because of the muscles that cross both joints, the "two-joint muscles." These muscles include the rectus femoris anteriorly, gracilis medially, and semimembranosus, semitendinosus, and biceps femoris posteriorly. Pathologic conditions that affect these muscles, such as spasticity or contracture, and surgical changes affect the function of both joints. A similar relationship exists between the knee and ankle with the gastrocnemius muscle, which crosses both joints. A patient with cerebral palsy who ambulates with his or her knees flexed may not have hamstrings that are tight or spastic. A patient with a hip flexion contracture ambulates with increased knee flexion to help maintain sagittal balance. Likewise, surgical correction of a knee flexion contracture may lead to spontaneous improvement in hip flexion. Because of these relationships, a careful physical examination of the entire lower extremity is essential when evaluating the knee in patients with cerebral palsy.

FLEXION DEFORMITY

Flexion is the most common knee deformity in patients with cerebral palsy and frequently occurs in ambulatory children. Knee flexion deformities keep the knee from fully extending at the end of the swing phase of gait. This causes the knee to be flexed during stance phase, leading to decreased stride length and increased energy expenditure. Spastic hamstrings, weak quadriceps, or a combination of both can cause isolated knee flexion. It also can result from hip or ankle pathology. Patients with spastic hip flexors or weak hip extensors or both develop compensatory knee flexion that results in crouch gait in which the hips, knees, and ankles are flexed (Fig. 33-14). Patients with weakened gastrocnemius-soleus muscles, from cerebral palsy or more commonly from Achilles tendon overlengthenings, ambulate with knee flexion to accommodate for the relative overpull of the ankle dorsiflexors. Prolonged spasticity and crouched knee gait can lead to true contracture of the knee itself. This is a difficult problem to deal with and has led to the increased use of single-event multilevel surgery

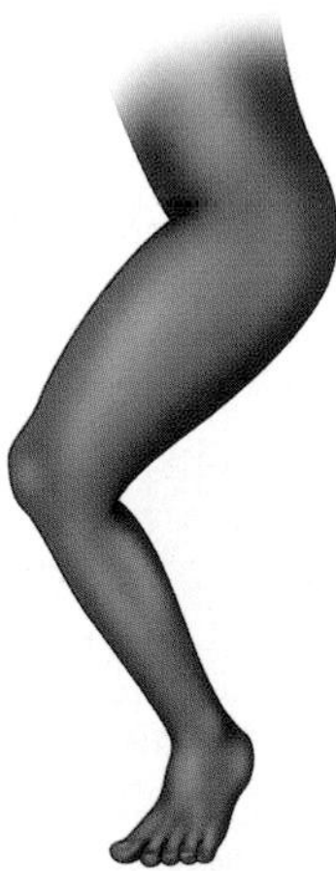

FIGURE 33-14 Typical jump posture caused by plantar flexion deformities of ankles, which require flexion of knees, hip, and lumbar spine to place center of gravity over weight bearing surface.

rather than staged procedures. A wide variety of procedures has been proposed for this, including femoral shortening or distal femoral extension osteotomy with patellar tendon advancement or both. Patellar advancement has been shown to improve gait mechanics better than extension osteotomy alone.

To find the source of the knee flexion, the muscles must be assessed to determine if the deformity is caused by spasticity or contracture or both. Strength testing should be done, although this can be difficult in patients with cerebral palsy. Cerebral palsy is an upper motor neuron disorder in which the brain is geographically affected, causing the body to be regionally affected. This is different from a lower motor neuron injury, such as a peripheral nerve laceration, in which only the innervated muscle or group of muscles is affected. In patients with cerebral palsy, if the hamstrings are affected, most likely the quadriceps are affected to some degree as well. Quadriceps strength, spasticity, and firing pattern should be evaluated throughout the gait cycle. Lengthening, and essentially weakening, the hamstrings in the presence of a spastic rectus femoris can lead to hyperextension deformity of the knee and significant gait disturbance.

Hamstring strength, spasticity, and knee contracture are assessed with the patient prone and supine. With the patient prone, the examiner extends the hips as much as possible and exerts gentle pressure on the calves. The angle that the femur and the tibia make after spasticity has been overcome is the degree of contracture of the soft tissues behind the knee. Next, the patient is placed supine to test hamstring spasticity. The examiner stabilizes the opposite knee in as much extension as possible and raises the leg being examined with the knee straight. If knee extension is limited as the hip is flexed, either medial or lateral hamstring tightness is present (Fig. 33-15). The patient can be examined for medial hamstring spasticity in the supine position with the knees flexed and feet off the table. This relaxes the hamstrings proximally and allows the hip to be abducted if there is no contracture of the adductor muscles. If extension is not possible unless the hip is adducted, there is tightness in the medial hamstrings and gracilis (Fig. 33-16). The amount of equinus in the ankle should be measured with the knee flexed and fully extended (Fig. 33-17). If ankle dorsiflexion improves with knee flexion, there is gastrocnemius spasticity or contracture.

As previously mentioned, quadriceps strength, contracture, and function should be evaluated when examining a patient with knee flexion deformity. Quadriceps strength is best assessed with the patient supine and the feet off the end of the table. The examiner extends the hips and allows the knees to flex passively (Fig. 33-18A) and then asks the patient to extend the knees voluntarily against resistance (Fig. 33-18B). To determine if the rectus femoris is spastic, the examiner turns the patient prone and performs the prone rectus (Ely) test (Fig. 33-19). With the patient prone and the knees extended, the examiner flexes the knees. If the rectus is spastic, the hips flex and the buttocks rise off the table when the rectus is stretched. It is best to do this one side at a time to determine the relative spasticity of each rectus femoris muscle.

Physical therapy and bracing can be used for milder deformities. Serial stretch casting has been shown to be effective as well, but care is necessary to prevent soft-tissue complications or breakdown and neurapraxia. The indications for hamstring lengthening are a straight-leg raise of less than 70 degrees or a popliteal angle of less than 135 degrees in the absence of significant bony deformity. In an ambulatory patient, knee contracture of more than 10 degrees can lead to excessive compensatory hip flexion and ankle dorsiflexion. Care must be taken not to overlengthen the hamstrings because it can lead to excessive weakness and knee hyperextension gait. In hyperextension gait, the femur moves forward over a fixed tibia, which is prevented from moving forward either by a spastic gastrocnemius-soleus or a limited ankle dorsiflexion. Rectus femoris spasticity, which is common in patients with cerebral palsy, also can exacerbate this condition. For this reason, most surgeons begin with lengthening the medial hamstrings by a Z-plasty of the gracilis and semitendinosus tendons and a fractional lengthening of the semimembranosus. If further correction is desired, the biceps femoris laterally can be lengthened using fractional lengthening. Identify the proximal aponeurosis of the semimembranosus anteriorly as it arises from the tendon of the proximal attachment. It is separate and proximal from the distal aponeurosis and should be released at the time of surgery as well.

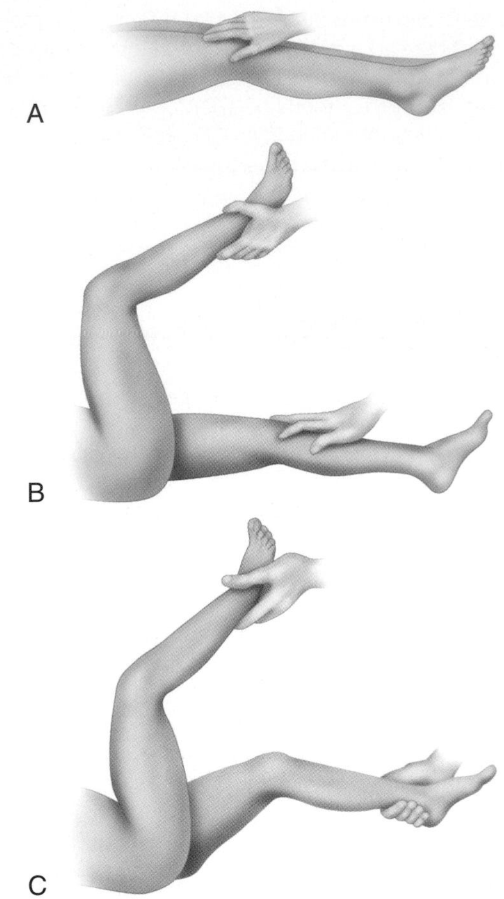

FIGURE 33-15 Testing for hamstring spasticity and contracture. **A,** Patient is supine with hips extended. Pressure is exerted over knees, forcing them into extension. Flexion remaining in knees is absolute knee flexion contracture. **B,** Knee on side to be tested is flexed while opposite knee is stabilized in extension. **C,** Attempted flexion of hip results in more flexion of knee.

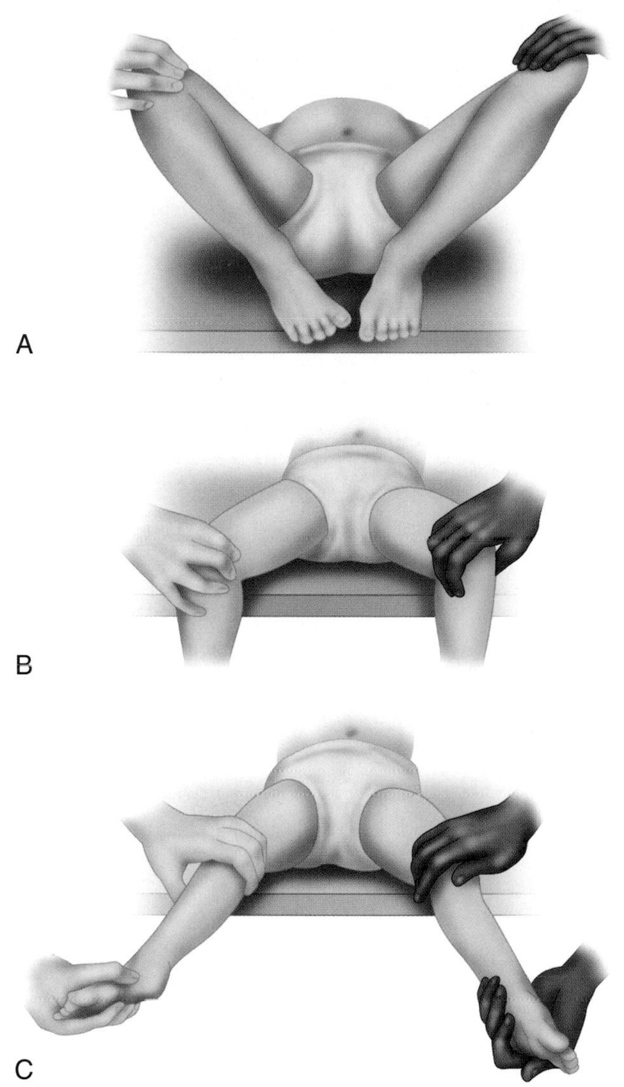

FIGURE 33-16 Testing for adductor and medial hamstring tightness. **A,** Thighs abduct well with hips and knees flexed, indicating no adductor contracture. **B,** With hips extended and knees flexed, hips abduct well. **C,** With hips extended, bringing knees into extension causes thighs to adduct, indicating medial hamstring spasticity.

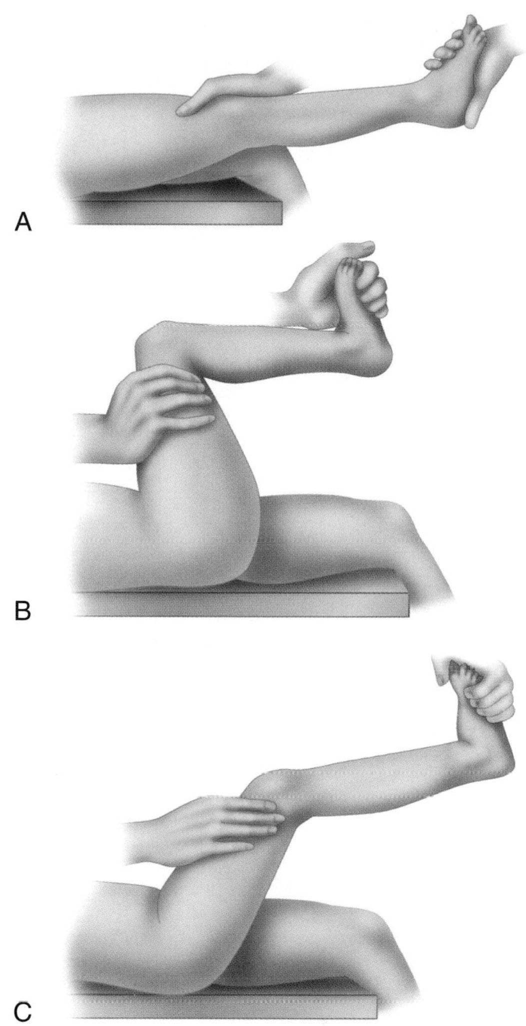

FIGURE 33-17 Testing for gastrocnemius contracture and spasticity. **A,** With knee extended, equinus in ankle is noted. **B,** With knee flexed, ankle is easily dorsiflexed, indicating no soleus contracture. **C,** As knee is extended, ankle dorsiflexion is resisted by tight or spastic gastrocnemius muscles.

FRACTIONAL LENGTHENING OF HAMSTRING TENDONS

Although knee extension in stance phase has been shown to improve dramatically after hamstring lengthening, velocity, stride length, and cadence have not been shown to improve. With spastic hamstrings and quadriceps, knee flexion during swing phase markedly diminishes. In addition, the results of surgery have been reported to deteriorate with time, with reoperation being necessary in up to 17%. Because very little change can be expected from repeat hamstring lengthening in patients with recurrent knee flexion after hamstring lengthening, alternative surgical interventions may be more beneficial. Some improvement in the popliteal angle and knee extension has been noted in patients with combined medial and lateral hamstring lengthenings, however, with greater risk of knee hyperextension and hamstring weakness.

TECHNIQUE 33-7

- Place the patient prone and inflate the thigh tourniquet.
- Make medial and lateral posterior incisions just above the popliteal crease extending 4 to 6 cm proximally. Alternatively, a single midline incision can be used (Fig. 33-20A).
- Divide the subcutaneous tissue and deep fascia in line with the skin incision, protecting the posterior femoral cutaneous nerve in the proximal portion of the wound.
- Expose the semitendinosus tendon, which is the most superficial posteromedial structure and is tendinous at

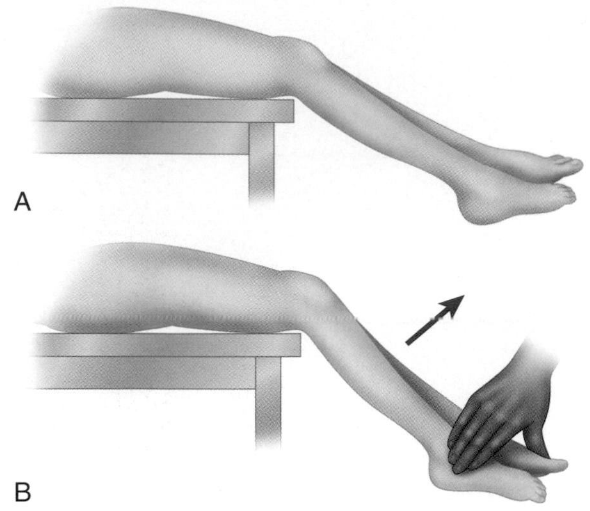

FIGURE 33-18 Testing for quadriceps strength. **A,** With hips extended, knees are allowed to flex off end of table. **B,** Patient voluntarily extends knees from flexed position against resistance.

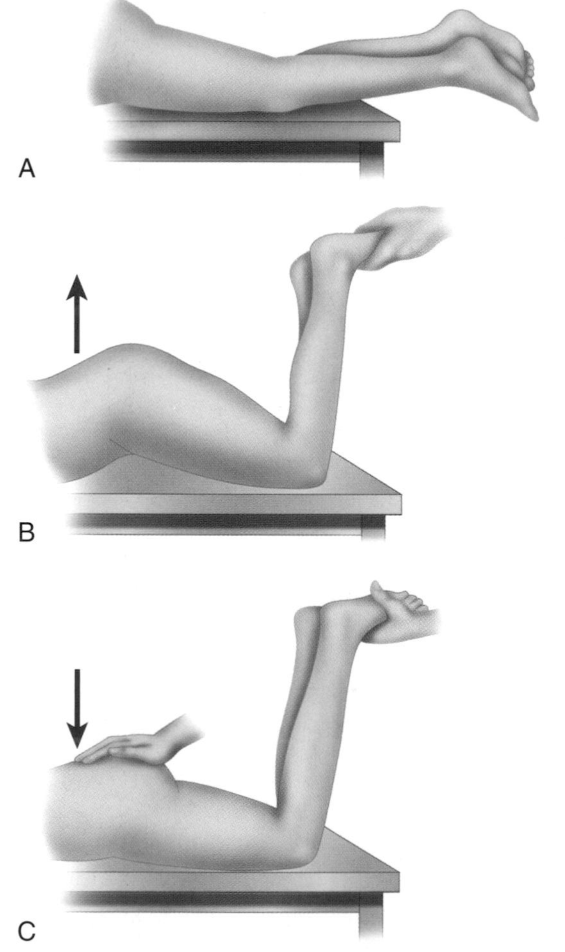

FIGURE 33-19 Prone rectus test. **A,** Patient is prone, and knees are extended. **B,** Flexing knees causes buttocks to rise from table. **C,** Spasticity in rectus is overcome by downward pressure on buttocks.

this level. Incise the tendon transversely or, alternatively, perform a Z-plasty.

- Identify and isolate the semimembranosus and incise its tendon sheath longitudinally. Divide its aponeurosis sharply at two levels, leaving the underlying muscle intact (Fig. 33-20B and C).
- Extend the knee with the hip in extension and the tendinous portion of the semimembranosus slides on the muscle. If further correction is required, identify the biceps femoris tendon laterally and isolate it from the peroneal nerve lying along its medial side. Pass a blunt instrument deep to the biceps femoris tendon, incise its tendinous portion transversely at two levels 3 cm apart, and leave the muscle fibers intact (Fig. 33-21D).
- Perform a similar lengthening maneuver by extending the knee with the hip in extension. Do not forcefully extend the knee with the hip flexed because this may cause a traction injury to the sciatic nerve and risk injury to the peroneal injury.
- Close all tendon sheaths, but do not close the deep fascia (Fig. 33-20E).
- After deflating the tourniquet, obtain hemostasis and close the subcutaneous tissues and skin.
- Apply a long leg cast with the knee in maximal extension.

POSTOPERATIVE CARE. Straight-leg raises are begun immediately postoperatively with the cast on to help stretch the hamstring tendons. The patient may walk with crutches and bear weight as tolerated. After 3 to 4 weeks, the casts are removed and the patient is started on a physical therapy program to maintain, and in some cases improve, range of motion. Nighttime extension splints or knee immobilizers are used for 8 to 12 weeks postoperatively.

COMBINED HAMSTRING LENGTHENING, POSTERIOR CAPSULAR RELEASE

If hamstring lengthening alone is ineffective in achieving the desired range of motion, a posterior capsular release can be used. This most commonly occurs in older children with significant fixed knee flexion contractures. This technique also can be combined with quadriceps shortening to help correct elongation of the infrapatellar tendon caused by chronic quadriceps weakening to obtain improved range of motion.

DISTAL FEMORAL EXTENSION OSTEOTOMY AND PATELLAR TENDON ADVANCEMENT

Because the results of revision hamstring lengthening are poor, the use of a distal femoral extension osteotomy has increased, especially for severe or recurrent knee flexion contractures after hamstring release. Stout et al. described a distal femoral extension osteotomy and patellar tendon advancement for treatment of crouch gait in cerebral palsy and obtained improved function and level of community

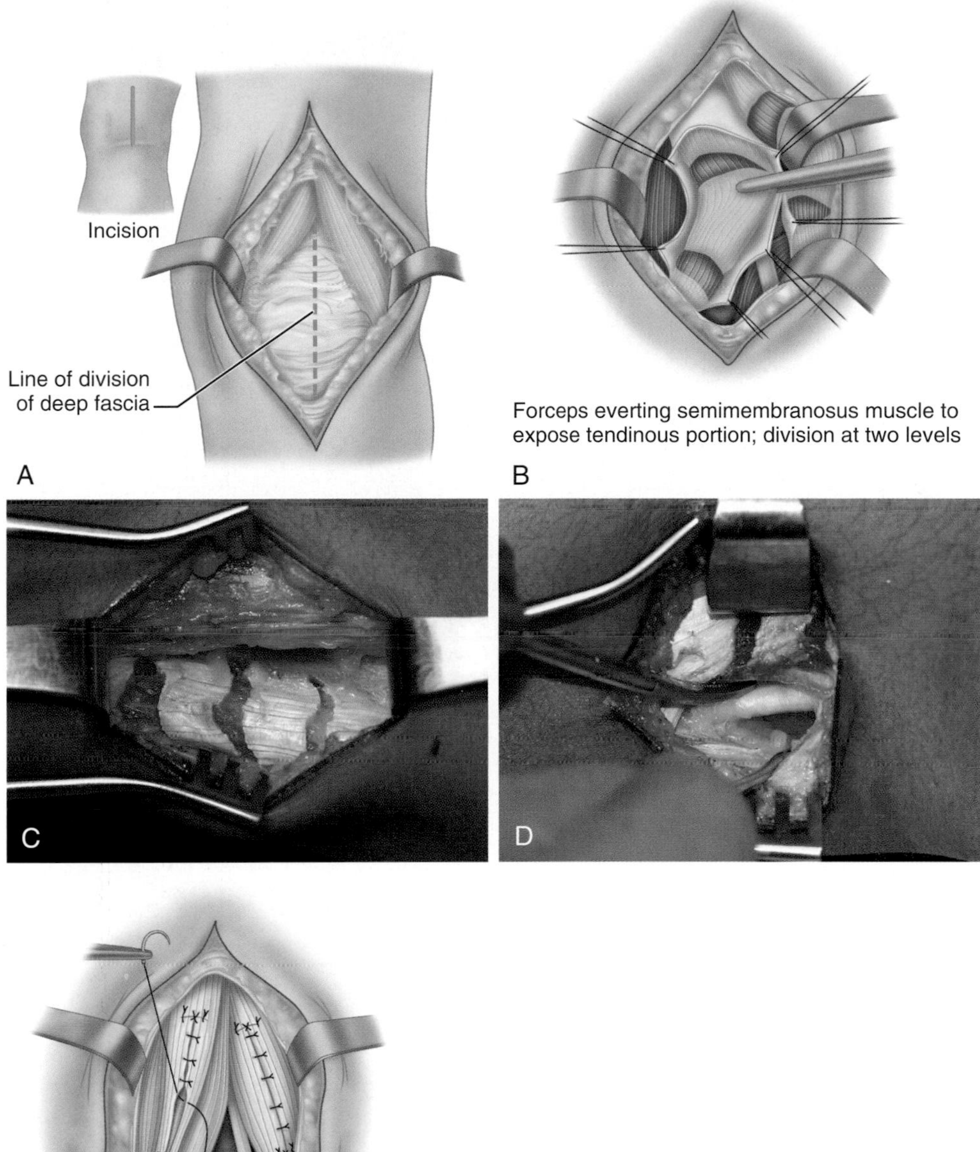

FIGURE 33-20 Fractional lengthening of hamstrings. **A,** Skin incision and incision in deep fascia over back of knee. **B** and **C,** Incisions in semimembranosus. **D,** Incisions in biceps femoris; note hemostat anterior to peroneal nerve. **E,** Tendon sheaths of biceps femoris and semimembranosus are sutured before wound closure. **SEE TECHNIQUE 33-7.**

ambulation. The osteotomy is most commonly fixed with distal femoral plates, but external fixation has also been used. Recurrence of deformity is less likely in patients in whom growth is complete. Patients should be followed closely after surgery because up to 10% of children have a postoperative nerve palsy that is unrelated to the degree of correction. To avoid these complications of acute correction, anterior distal femoral hemiepiphysiodesis has been used in small series to correct fixed knee flexion contractures (Fig. 33-21). This technique requires that patients have significant growth remaining to allow for correction. Immature patients (age <11 years) should be followed for premature closure of the proximal tibial physis leading to decreased posterior slope.

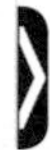

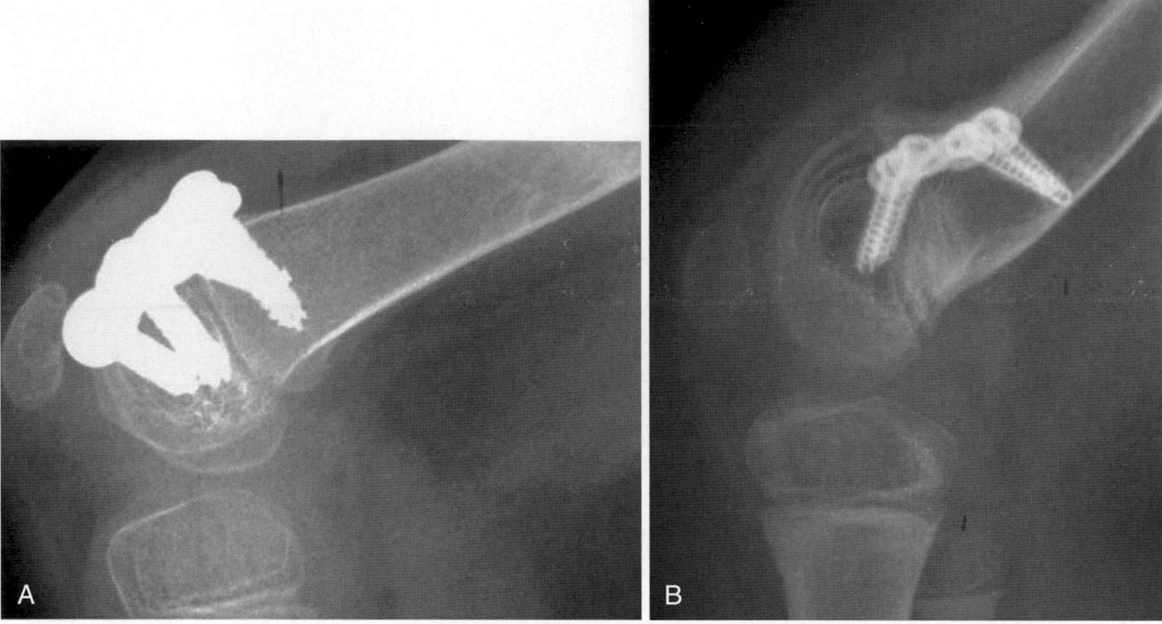

FIGURE 33-21 **A, Patient with cerebral palsy and fixed knee flexion contracture treated with anterior distal femoral epiphysiodesis using 8-plates. B, 20 months after surgery.** (From Al-aubaidi Z, Lundgaard B, Pedersen NW: Anterior distal femoral hemi- epiphysiodesis in the treatment of fixed knee flexion contracture in neuromuscular patients, J Chil Orthop 6:313, 2012.) **SEE TECHNIQUE 33-7**

TECHNIQUE 33-8

(STOUT ET AL.)

- Approach the distal part of the femur posterior to the vastus lateralis.
- Insert a chisel for a 90-degree blade plate just proximal to a guidewire placed at a 90-degree angle to the femoral shaft and just proximal to the physis (or physeal scar) with the angle guide of the chisel parallel to the tibia. This placement avoids varus or valgus displacement of the osteotomy.
- Remove an anterior triangular wedge of bone that matches the degree of contracture. Also, remove any bone protruding posteriorly from the distal fragment (Fig. 33-22). Coronal and transverse plane abnormalities can be corrected simultaneously.
- The type of patellar tendon advancement depends on the skeletal maturity of the patient. If the physis is open, sharply divide the patellar tendon from the tibial tubercle to avoid physeal injury and advance it under a periosteal flap. If the physis is closed, transpose the tibial tubercle with the attached patellar tendon distally and secure it with a compression screw.
- Insert a 16-gauge wire or tension-band wire transversely through the patella and the proximal part of the tibia to protect the repair (Fig. 33-23).

DISTAL TRANSFER OF RECTUS FEMORIS

Stiff knee gait is common in patients with cerebral palsy and is caused by co-contracture of the quadriceps and hamstring muscles or weakness caused by previous hamstring lengthening, or both. Co-spasticity of the hamstrings and quadriceps causes a loss of knee flexion that leads to decreased power and difficulties with foot clearance during the swing phase of gait. Patients with rectus femoris spasticity also have difficulty transitioning from standing to sitting. Dynamic EMG analysis often reveals a rectus femoris muscle that also is abnormally active during swing phase. To help achieve balanced knee function during swing phase, transfer of the distal rectus femoral tendon to the semitendinosus medially or iliotibial band laterally can be done, depending on the presence of malrotation. No functional differences in knee flexion are seen between the transfer sites, and this should then be determined by surgeon preference and concomitant procedures. Ten degrees of malrotation can be corrected depending on the direction of transfer, but larger degrees of malrotation require rotational osteotomy of the affected bone. Gage et al. found significant improvement in swing-phase knee motion and foot clearance when the following criteria were met: (1) hamstring contractures corrected so that the knee can extend fully in midstance, (2) foot plantigrade and stable in stance, and (3) foot in line of progression to generate a moment of sufficient magnitude to maintain knee extension in midstance and terminal stance. In comparison studies of hamstring lengthening with and without rectus femoris transfer, patients

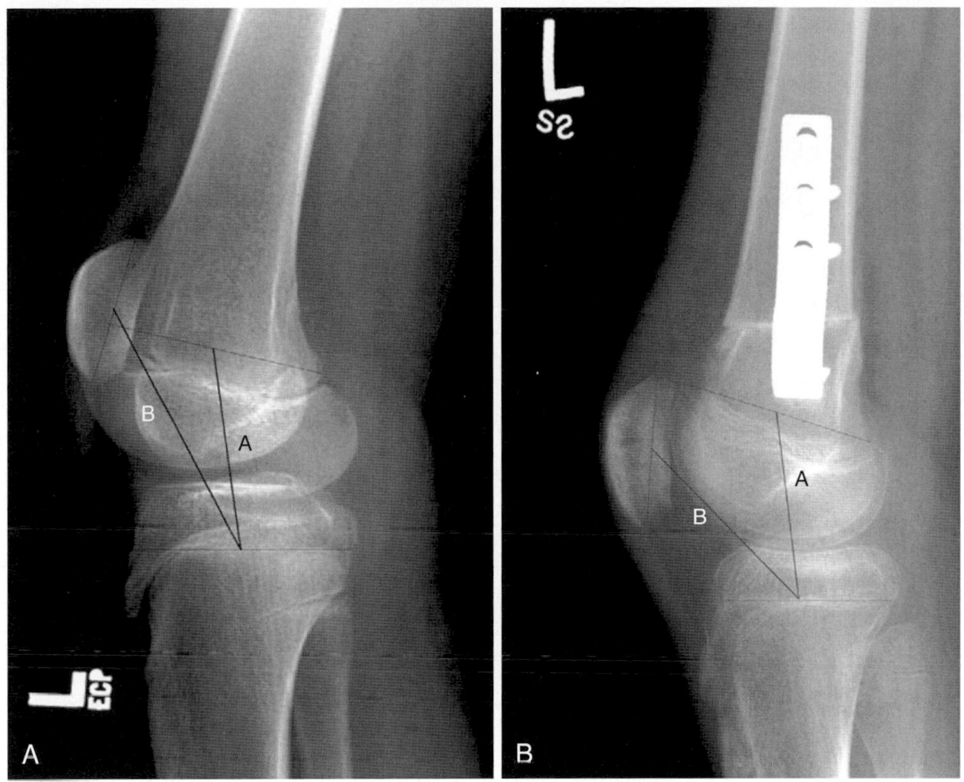

FIGURE 33-22 **A** and **B**, Preoperative and postoperative lateral radiographs of left knee in maximal extension in patient treated with distal femoral extension osteotomy. (From Stout et al: Distal femoral extension osteotomy and patellar tendon advancement to treat persistent crouch gait in cerebral palsy, J Bone Joint Surg 90A:2470, 2008.) **SEE TECHNIQUE 33-8.**

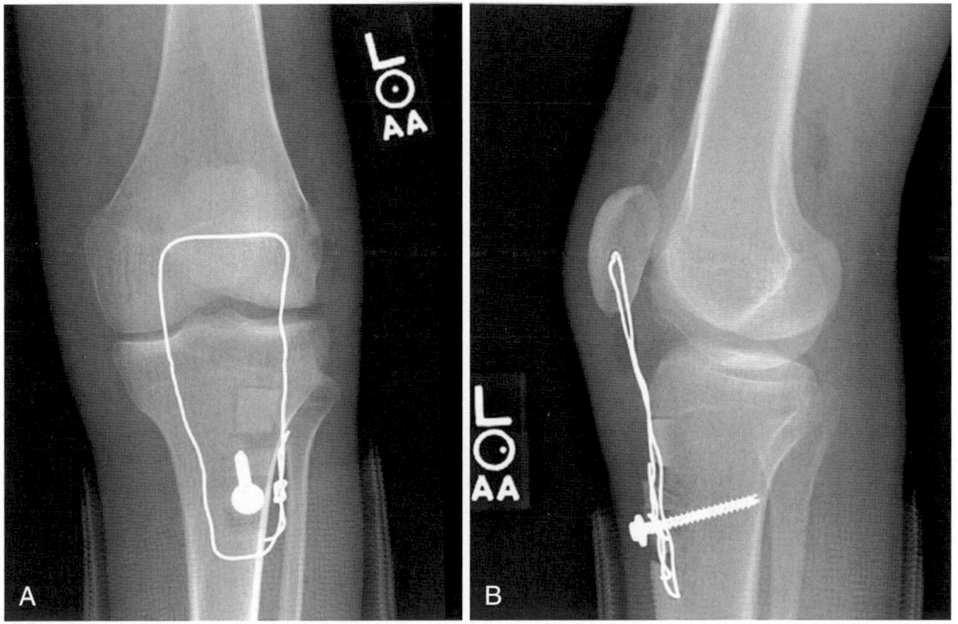

FIGURE 33-23 **A** and **B**, Anteroposterior and lateral radiographs of knee in maximal extension after patellar tendon advancement. (From Stout et al: Distal femoral extension osteotomy and patellar tendon advancement to treat persistent crouch gait in cerebral palsy, J Bone Joint Surg 90A:2470, 2008.) **SEE TECHNIQUE 33-8.**

with rectus femoris transfer had significantly improved foot clearance and gait efficiency, most markedly in GMFCS I and II patients. More improvements than deterioration of results have been reported in ambulatory children at long-term follow-up.

RECTUS FEMORIS TRANSFER

TECHNIQUE 33-9 *FIGURE 33-24*

(GAGE ET AL.)

- With the patient anesthetized and supine, make a longitudinal incision in the anterior thigh, 5 to 6 cm proximal to the superior pole of the patella.
- Identify the rectus femoris tendon proximally as it lies between the vastus medialis and vastus lateralis. Separate the rectus tendon from the remainder of the quadriceps tendon; avoid entering the knee joint. Dissect it free to approximately 3 cm proximal to the patella. Divide the tendon and separate it from the vastus intermedius tendon posteriorly.
- Transfer the freed tendon stump to either the distal stump of the semitendinosus or the iliotibial band depending on whether the desired rotatory effect is lateral rotation (to the iliotibial band) or medial (to the semitendinosus stump).
- For medial transfer to the semitendinosus, divide the semitendinosus 2 to 3 cm proximal to its musculotendinous junction and dissect the distal stump to its insertion at the pes anserinus. Transfer the tendon through the medial intermuscular septum and suture it to the distal end of the rectus femoris tendon.
- For a lateral transfer to the iliotibial band, resect the fibers of the iliotibial band until the remaining fibers are posterior to the knee joint axis. Pass the distal end of the rectus femoris around the iliotibial band and suture it onto itself.

POSTOPERATIVE CARE. If hamstring lengthening also has been done, patients are placed in long leg casts for 3 to 4 weeks. If hamstring lengthening has not been done, cast immobilization is unnecessary; instead, a knee immobilizer is used. The patient is allowed to sit in a reclining wheelchair and is gradually moved to the upright sitting position with the knee fully flexed. Standing with support is allowed on the third day, and the knee immobilizer is removed for passive and active range of motion of the knee. At 4 weeks, the patient is instructed by the physical therapist to begin vigorous exercises to encourage muscle strengthening and gait training. Improvements in gait function typically are seen for 12 months postoperatively.

RECURVATUM OF THE KNEE

Recurvatum of the knee is caused by a relative imbalance between the quadriceps and the hamstrings owing to several factors, including (1) co-spasticity of the quadriceps and hamstrings in which the quadriceps is stronger; (2) weakened hamstrings secondary to previous surgery, overlengthening, or transfer; (3) gastrocnemius-soleus weakness secondary to proximal head recession; and (4) ankle equinus. For a patient with an ankle equinus contracture, the only way to put the feet flat is to compensate with knee recurvatum.

The prone rectus test can be used to test for quadriceps spasticity. If the rectus femoris is tight, it can be lengthened or released in nonambulatory patients and transferred posteriorly in ambulatory children. Recurvatum of the knee caused by excessive hamstring weakness is difficult to treat. Replantation of transferred tendons or shortening of overlengthened

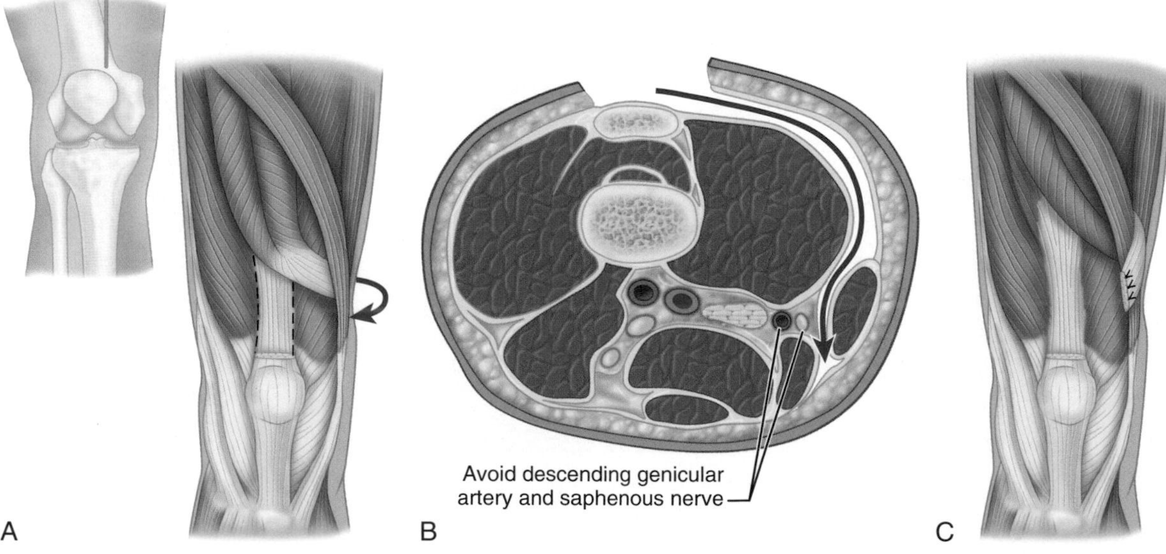
Avoid descending genicular artery and saphenous nerve
A
B
C

FIGURE 33-24 Distal release or transfer of rectus femoris. **A,** Rectus femoris is separated from vastus medialis, vastus lateralis, and vastus intermedius. *Inset,* Longitudinal incision along medial side of distal third of rectus femoris. **B,** Rectus femoris may be transferred through medial intermuscular septum to sartorius if desired. **C,** Rectus femoris is sutured to sartorius. **SEE TECHNIQUE 33-9.**

tendons would not improve functional strength because the muscles have been permanently weakened by the previous surgery.

To determine if recurvatum of the knee is caused by ankle equinus, a short leg cast or ankle orthosis is applied with the ankle in the neutral position. If the knee goes into recurvatum with the foot plantigrade, the recurvatum is not caused by ankle equinus. If ankle equinus does exist, correction of this operatively or nonoperatively is indicated. Significant recurvatum should be treated with bilateral long leg braces with a pelvic band with the knees locked in 20 degrees of flexion and ankle stops at 5 degrees of dorsiflexion. When hip control is achieved, the pelvic band can be removed, but long leg braces often are used for years until a stable knee is obtained. Flexion osteotomy for this condition is not advised.

KNEE VALGUS

Knee valgus in patients with cerebral palsy usually is caused by a hip adduction deformity and rarely occurs independently. It is usually associated with hip internal rotation and flexion of the knees, which can accentuate the appearance of valgus. In most patients, correction of the hip adduction and internal rotation improves the position and appearance of the knee. In these patients, surgery on the knee itself is rarely indicated.

A tight iliotibial band also can cause a knee valgus deformity. The presence of iliotibial band tightness can be determined by having the patient lie on the contralateral side and flex the knee nearest the table to the chest. With the knee flexed, the hip being tested is flexed and abducted, moved from the position of flexion to extension, and then adducted. If the hip does not adduct without flexing, the iliotibial band is tight and usually can be palpated subcutaneously along the distal third of the thigh. The tight band should be resected (see Chapter 34).

PATELLA ALTA

Patella alta is common in patients with cerebral palsy (93% in one study) and usually is associated with crouched gait (Fig. 33-25). Despite this frequent occurrence, the prevalence of anterior knee pain in these patients is approximately 10% to 20%, being more common in older children, females, and possibly those with larger flexion contractures. Patellar subluxation and dislocation are rare; they can be caused by quadriceps spasticity or long-standing knee flexion deformity. Patella alta leads to a decrease in the moment arm of terminal knee extension, which further weakens an already weakened extensor mechanism. This increased tension can lead to repetitive microtrauma to the patellar and quadriceps tendons, causing elongation of these structures and fragmentation and stress fractures of the patella and tibial tubercle; it is thought to be one of the causes of knee pain in patients with cerebral palsy. Because these changes are almost universal in ambulatory patients with cerebral palsy and most patients are pain free, operative treatment rarely is indicated. Often, correction of the flexion deformity of the knee with hamstring lengthening and other associated procedures causes improvement in not only the patella alta but also knee function in general. Operative treatment to correct the underlying pathologic process, which usually is patellar subluxation and dislocation, is helpful in patients in whom conservative treatment has failed.

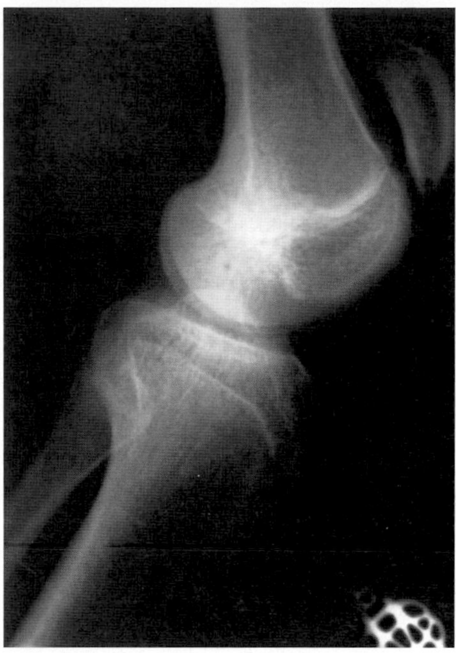

FIGURE 33-25 Patella alta in patient with cerebral palsy.

ROTATIONAL ABNORMALITIES

Rotational abnormalities, either internal or external, can cause significant gait dysfunction in patients with cerebral palsy. These deformities usually occur at multiple levels including the hip or femur, tibia or ankle, and foot. There is no role for bracing in correction of these deformities in patients with cerebral palsy. A thorough rotational evaluation is essential before any operative intervention. A large gait analysis study of 412 children found that the most common cause of internal rotation gait was internal hip rotation followed by internal tibial torsion, and multiple abnormalities were found in almost 50% of affected limbs. Differences were noted between hemiplegic and diplegic patients, with the most common site of internal rotation deformity in diplegics being the hip (57%), tibia (52%), and pelvis (19%) compared with hemiplegics, in whom foot deformities included pes varus (42%) and metatarsus adductus (24%).

These deformities should be corrected at the time of soft-tissue procedures. Minimally invasive percutaneous osteotomies of the femur and supramalleolar tibia have been described.

FOOT

Foot deformities caused by altered or abnormal muscle forces are common in patients with cerebral palsy, with 70% to 90% of children affected. The most common deformity is ankle equinus, with equinovarus and equinovalgus deformities being equally common. In a series of 306 children with cerebral palsy, approximately 50% had normal "side-to-side" balance, 25% had valgus deformities, and 23% had varus deformities. The presence of a bilateral as opposed to a unilateral foot deformity, regardless of the type, has been shown to have a significant effect on overall level of ambulation. A patient's deformity may change over time, especially in young children. For example, in a very young child with a valgus foot deformity, persistent tonic reflexes and abnormal muscle forces may over time cause a varus foot position to develop. Digital deformity is caused by an imbalance between the intrinsic muscles of the foot and extrinsic muscles of the leg (intrinsic plus foot) and can cause hallux valgus, claw toes, and forefoot adduction. Spasticity of the smaller muscles of the foot can lead to other deformities, such as hallux valgus, claw toes, and forefoot adduction. These can occur in isolation but more often occur in association with other deformities related to abnormal extrinsic foot musculature.

EQUINUS DEFORMITY

Equinus deformity is the most common foot deformity in patients with cerebral palsy, affecting 70% of children, of whom approximately 25% develop a deformity severe enough to require operative treatment. Conservative treatment consisting of stretching, bracing, botulinum toxin A (BTX-A), and, occasionally, casting remains the primary form of treatment or means of delaying operative intervention. Ankle-foot orthoses, in addition to preventing or delaying surgical treatment, improve gait function in children with cerebral palsy, although the exact mechanism by which this occurs is unknown and most likely multifactorial. Equinus is caused by spasticity of the gastrocnemius-soleus muscle, which often worsens during periods of rapid growth because of overgrowth of the tibia relative to the gastrocnemius-soleus. Animal models have shown that muscles in mice with hereditary spasticity grow at a slower rate than normal muscle. Ultrasound evaluation of the musculotendinous junction showed that patients with cerebral palsy have longer Achilles tendons and shorter muscle bellies than normal controls. Whereas ankle dorsiflexion increases in operatively treated patients, the muscle-tendon architecture remains abnormal. Bracing, especially at night, to prevent the foot from going into the equinus position is essential. The exact indications for surgery are unclear given the variable nature of cerebral palsy; however, surgery typically is indicated when the ankle cannot be brought into the neutral position in an ambulatory child because ankle kinematics change dramatically with the ankle fixed in more than 10 degrees of dorsiflexion. Other indications include difficulties with hygiene, foot wear, and standing programs in a nonambulatory child.

SURGICAL CORRECTION OF EQUINUS DEFORMITY

Because of the variable nature of cerebral palsy and the fact that numerous procedures and postoperative regimens have been used in the treatment of equinus contracture, it is difficult to compare studies and success rates. In addition, many recurrences are more than 5 years after the initial operation and may not be included in short-term studies. The recurrence rate in the literature ranges from 0% to 50%, depending on the type of patient and the length of follow-up. Younger patients, especially those younger than 3 years, and hemiplegics are most likely to have recurrence. Recurrence in patients older than 6 years is very rare. A study of 243 children with cerebral palsy (mean age, 7.8 years) who had Achilles tendon lengthening showed a recurrence rate of 11% at 10 years. A large meta-analysis showed that age is the most important determinant of recurrence and that overcorrection leading to a calcaneal deformity was more common in diplegics (15%) compared with hemiplegics (1%). Despite numerous techniques used, there did not seem to be a significant difference in outcomes between techniques, although the majority of the studies were level IV evidence.

The gastrocnemius-soleus can be lengthened at either the musculotendinous junction with an aponeurotic recession or at the level of the Achilles tendon through an open or percutaneous approach. For mild to moderate contractures, it is recommended that lengthening be done at the level of the musculotendinous junction; the higher rate of overlengthening seen with the use of open Z-plasty techniques leads to residual weakness. The use of the percutaneous approach has been shown in a small (28 feet) randomized, blinded study to provide rapid healing as demonstrated on ultrasound evaluation of the tendon, shorter operative and hospitalization times, postoperative dorsiflexion, and higher parental satisfaction. Larger studies are necessary to further evaluate this. Overlengthening of the gastrocnemius-soleus should be avoided, especially in an ambulatory child, because it can cause weakness in push-off and crouch gait. Because overlengthening is less common with an aponeurosis recession, this is the most commonly used procedure in ambulatory children, with open Achilles lengthening reserved for patients with severe deformities and for nonambulatory patients. It is important to evaluate patients after release for toe flexion contractures that have been unmasked after Achilles tendon lengthening, because this can lead to abnormal weight bearing on the tips of the toes. This can be treated with simultaneous Z-lengthenings of the flexor digitorum longus and flexor hallucis longus.

OPEN LENGTHENING OF THE ACHILLES TENDON

TECHNIQUE 33-10

(WHITE MODIFICATION)

- Use a posteromedial incision to expose the Achilles tendon from its insertion to approximately 10 cm proximally, preserving the sheath (Fig. 33-26A).
- Divide the posteromedial two thirds of the tendon near its insertion.
- Apply a moderate dorsiflexion force to the foot and divide the medial two thirds of the tendon 5 to 8 cm proximal to the site of the distal division.
- Dorsiflex the foot so that the tendon lengthens to the desired length (Fig. 33-26B).
- The tendon can be sutured in a side-to-side fashion with absorbable suture.
- Carefully close the tendon sheath and subcutaneous tissues to prevent adherence of the tendon to the overlying skin.
- Apply a short leg cast with the ankle in maximal dorsiflexion.

POSTOPERATIVE CARE. The patient is allowed to bear full weight on the leg postoperatively. The cast is left on for approximately 4 weeks. During this time, knee extension is encouraged to maintain the lengthening of the

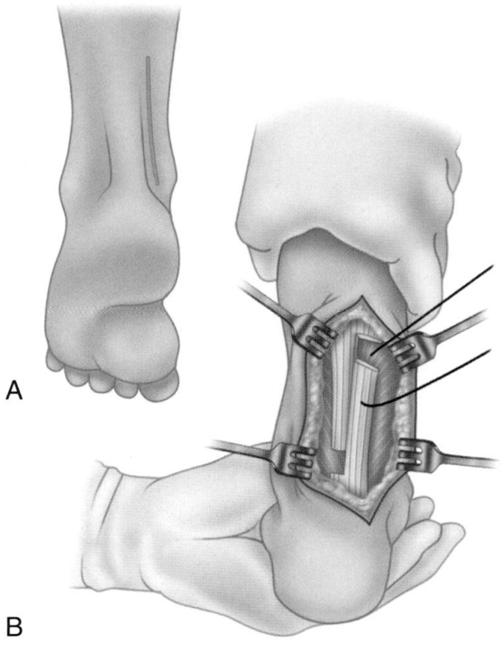

FIGURE 33-26 Sliding lengthening of Achilles tendon. **A,** Posteromedial incision. **B,** Two cuts are made through one half of tendon in opposite directions. Rotation of fibers must be followed accurately. As foot is placed in dorsiflexion, tendon fibers separate. **SEE TECHNIQUE 33-10.**

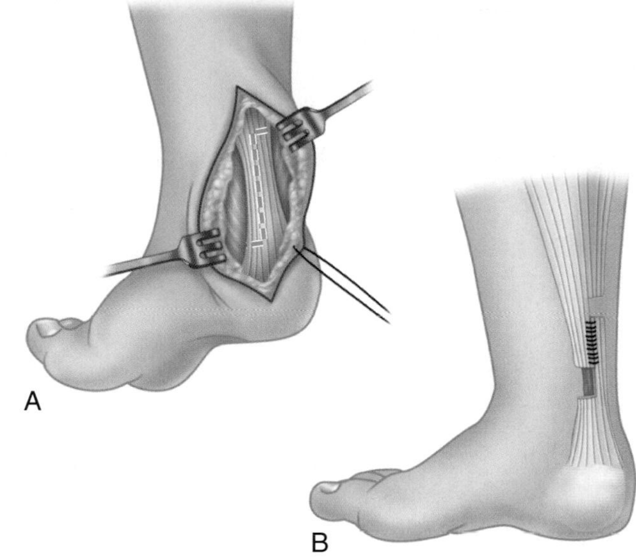

FIGURE 33-27 Z-plasty lengthening of Achilles tendon. **A,** Longitudinal incision, halfway between posterior aspect of medial malleolus and tendon. Longitudinal cut in tendon is brought out proximally in one direction and distally in opposite direction. **B,** Ends are sutured to repair tendon. **SEE TECHNIQUE 33-11.**

gastrocnemius-soleus complex. The cast is removed, and an ankle-foot orthosis is fitted with the ankle in maximal dorsiflexion. Alternatively, a mold for a custom ankle-foot orthosis can be made at the time of the initial procedure so that it is ready at the time of cast removal. This is especially helpful if patient compliance and follow-up are questionable. The patient begins with full-time brace wear, and this is modified depending on the patient's growth remaining and progress in physical therapy.

Z-PLASTY LENGTHENING OF THE ACHILLES TENDON

Rattey et al. reported recurrence of contractures in 18% and 41% of diplegic and hemiplegic patients 10 years after 77 open Z-plasty lengthenings of the Achilles tendon. Children 6 years old or older at the time of lengthening did not have recurrence. Diplegic patients who were operated on before age 4 years and patients who had longitudinal incisions had statistically significantly higher recurrence rates.

TECHNIQUE 33-11

- Make a posteromedial incision midway between the Achilles tendon and the posterior aspect of the medial malleolus. The lower extent of the incision is at the superior border of the calcaneus, and it continues cephalad for 4 to 5 cm (Fig. 33-27A).
- Expose the Achilles tendon with sharp dissection directed posteriorly toward it.
- Incise the sheath of the Achilles tendon longitudinally from the superior to the inferior extent of the incision. Free the tendon from the surrounding tissues.
- Make a longitudinal incision in the center of the Achilles tendon from proximal to distal (Fig. 33-27A).
- Turn the scalpel either medially or laterally distally and divide that half of the tendon transversely. Make the distal cut toward the medial side for a varus deformity and toward the lateral for a valgus deformity.
- Hold this cut portion of the tendon with forceps and bring the scalpel to the proximal portion of the longitudinal incision in the tendon.
- Turn the scalpel opposite the distal cut and divide that half of the tendon transversely to free the Achilles tendon completely.
- Divide the plantaris tendon on the medial aspect of the Achilles tendon transversely.
- Evaluate the passive excursion of the triceps surae muscle using a Kocher clamp to pull the proximal stump of the tendon to its maximally stretched length.
- Allow the tendon to retract halfway back to its resting length and suture it to the distal tendon end at that point (Fig. 33-27B).
- Control tension further by adjusting the foot position: neutral for mild spasticity, 10 degrees of dorsiflexion for moderate involvement, and 20 degrees of dorsiflexion for severe deformity.
- Perform the repair in a side-to-side manner with heavy absorbable sutures.

- Close the wound with absorbable sutures or subcuticular sutures and skin strips and apply a long leg cast.

POSTOPERATIVE CARE. Postoperative care is as described after Technique 33-10.

PERCUTANEOUS LENGTHENING OF THE ACHILLES TENDON

Moreau and Lake found that when done as an outpatient procedure, percutaneous lengthening of the Achilles tendon was quick, inexpensive, and free of complications. Of the 90 legs treated in this fashion, 97% showed improvement in gait function.

TECHNIQUE 33-12

- With the patient prone and the leg prepared to the midthigh to include the toes, extend the knee and dorsiflex the ankle to tense the Achilles tendon so that it is subcutaneous, easily outlined, and away from the neurovascular structures anteriorly.
- Make three partial tenotomies in the Achilles tendon (Fig. 33-28). Make the first medial cut, just at the insertion of the tendon onto the calcaneus, through one half of the width of the tendon. Make the second tenotomy proximally and medially, just below the musculotendinous junction. Make the third laterally through half the width of the tendon midway between the two medial cuts.
- Place the two incisions on the medial side if the heel is in varus as it usually is and on the lateral side if the heel is in valgus.
- Dorsiflex the ankle to the desired angle.
- The incisions do not require closure, only a sterile dressing and a long leg cast with the knee in full extension.

POSTOPERATIVE CARE. The postoperative care is the same as that described for Technique 33-10.

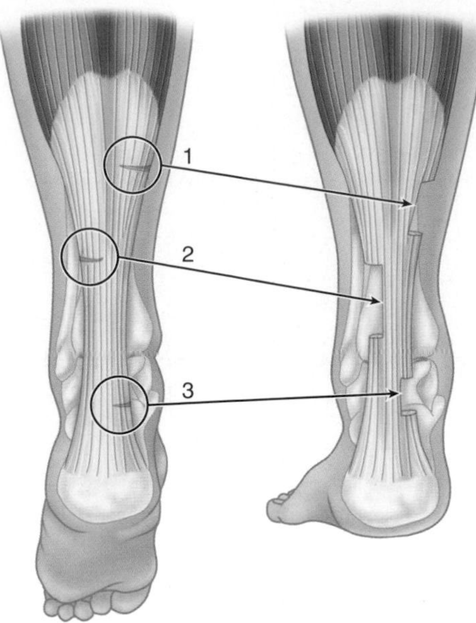

FIGURE 33-28 Incisions for percutaneous Achilles tendon lengthening. Cut ends slide on themselves with forceful dorsiflexion of foot. **SEE TECHNIQUE 33-12.**

LENGTHENING OF THE GASTROCNEMIUS-SOLEUS MUSCLE COMPLEX

Surgical lengthening of the gastrocnemius-soleus complex is commonly performed to treat equinus deformity, either as an isolated procedure or as part of other reconstructive surgery. A variety of surgical procedures have been described to accomplish this lengthening, varying in terms of selectivity, stability, and amount of correction. In a systematic review by Shore et al., 10 different procedures were summarized and grouped by anatomic zone (Fig. 33-29). They concluded that cerebral palsy subtype (hemiplegia or diplegia) and age at index surgery were more important in determining outcomes of surgery than the choice of surgical procedure. In a biomechanical cadaver study, Firth et al. tested six procedures in the three zones and determined that zone 1 procedures were very stable but obtained limited lengthening, zone 2 procedures were stable and obtained more lengthening, and zone

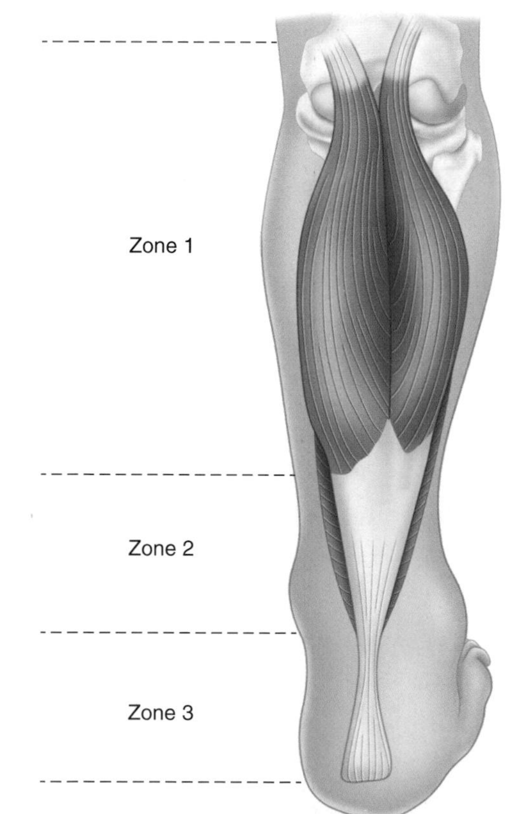

FIGURE 33-29 Three discrete anatomical zones of the gastrocsoleus complex. (Redrawn from Shore BJ, White N, Graham HK: Surgical correction of equinus deformity in children with cerebral palsy: a systematic review, J Child Orthop 4:277, 2010.)

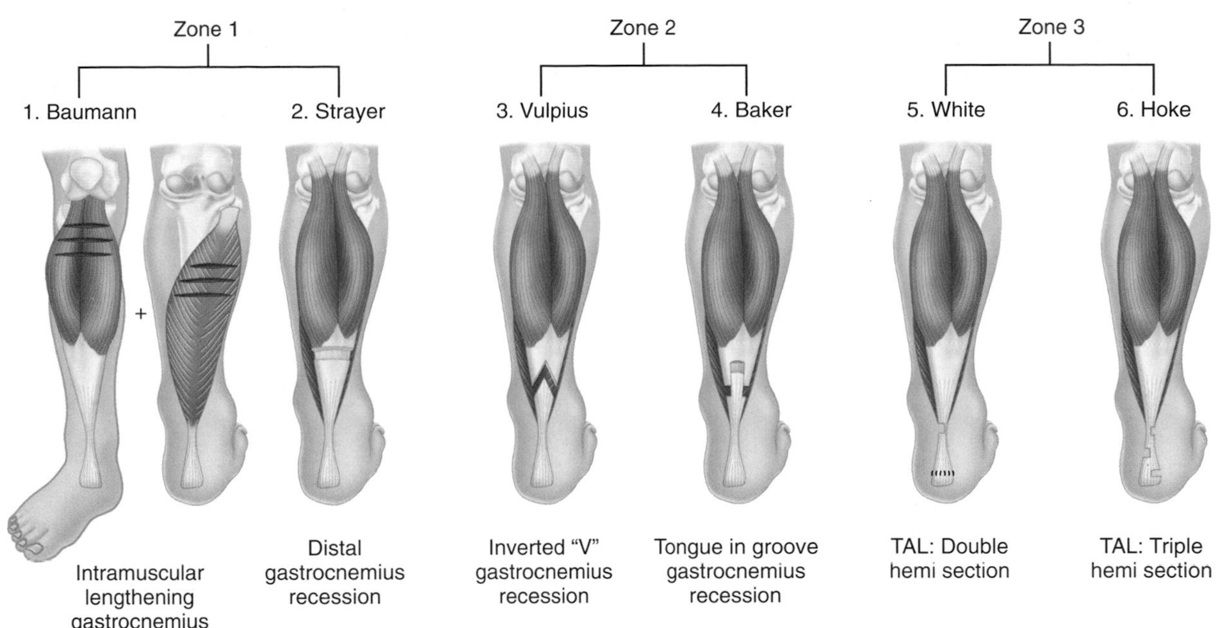

FIGURE 33-30 Six procedures for gastrocnemius-soleus lengthening according to zone (Fig. 32-9). TAL, tendo Achilles lengthening. (Redrawn from Firth BM, McMullean M, Chin T, et al: Lengthening of the gastrocnemius-soleus complex: an anatomical and biomechanical study in human cadavers, J Bone Joint Surg 95:1489, 2013.)

3 procedures were not stable but obtained the most lengthening (Fig. 33-30). The clinical implications of these findings are unclear. In a later clinical study of 40 children with spastic diplegia, Firth et al. found that equinus gait usually could be corrected by conservative procedures in zone 1; severe crouch gait was abolished, calcaneal deformity was infrequent, and the rate of overcorrection was low (2.5%). The procedure chosen should be based on the surgeon's experience and the unique clinical presentation of the patient.

GASTROCNEMIUS-SOLEUS LENGTHENING

TECHNIQUE 33-13

- Make a posterior longitudinal incision over the middle of the calf at the level of the musculotendinous junction, expose the aponeurosis of the gastrocnemius, and make an inverted or transverse incision through it (Fig. 33-31A). Release this in a lateral-to-medial fashion to ensure complete release.
- Release the raphes of the gastrocnemius-soleus and the plantaris tendon (Fig. 33-31B) completely.
- Bring the ankle into slight dorsiflexion, which separates the ends of the tendon (Fig. 33-31C).
- If the aponeurosis of the soleus tendon is contracted and further correction is desired, divide it, but do not disturb the soleus muscle itself.
- Baker modified the Vulpius technique by lengthening the aponeurotic tendon of the gastrocnemius in a tongue-in-groove fashion. We prefer a simple transverse incision, through a slightly posteromedial approach, releasing the plantaris tendon as well.

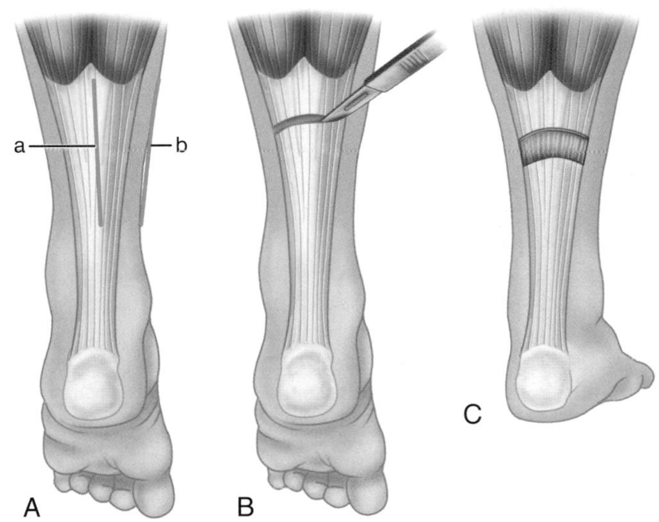

FIGURE 33-31 Gastrocnemius lengthening. **A,** Incision over posterior aspect of calf. **B,** Transverse cut through tendon. **C,** Foot is placed in dorsiflexion to neutral to separate tendon ends. **SEE TECHNIQUE 33-13.**

POSTOPERATIVE CARE. Postoperative care is the same as after Technique 33-10.

VARUS OR VALGUS DEFORMITY

Varus and valgus deformities can occur in patients with cerebral palsy, most commonly in association with an equinus deformity. The direction of deformity depends on the type and severity of cerebral palsy and the overall biomechanics of the affected limb. Computer motion analysis and dynamic EMG have shown that anterior tibial muscle dysfunction alone or in combination with dysfunction of the posterior tibial muscle is more commonly the cause of varus deformity than isolated posterior tibial dysfunction. In hemiplegia the foot deformity has been found to be either equinus or equinovarus, and in diplegia and quadriplegia it was valgus in 64% or varus in 36% of affected children. Although less common, varus deformities are more functionally disabling, more difficult to manage nonoperatively, and easier to correct operatively. Consequently, surgery is done more often and more successfully for varus than for valgus deformities.

The biomechanics of the hip and knee also influence whether a varus or valgus deformity is present. Diplegic patients typically have internally rotated and adducted hips, flexed knees, and external rotation deformity of the tibia. This combination of deformities causes the foot to assume a valgus position. In hemiplegic patients, the internally rotated thigh with the knee coming to full extension in stance phase causes the foot to internally rotate and produce a varus deformity.

EQUINOVARUS DEFORMITY

Varus deformity, which usually is accompanied by equinus, is caused most commonly by an abnormal posterior tibial muscle that is overactive or firing out of phase. The normal posterior tibial muscle is active during stance phase to stabilize the foot and inactive during swing phase. In many children with cerebral palsy, the posterior tibial muscle contracts during swing phase, leading to the varus position of the foot at heel strike. This also may be associated with anterior tibial muscle dysfunction; however, isolated anterior tibial muscle function is less likely to cause a varus deformity of the foot. Gait studies using EMG are helpful in determining which muscles are overactive or out of phase. It is essential to determine which muscles are responsible for the deformity before any attempt at surgical correction. The gastrocnemius-soleus contracture that usually accompanies the varus contracture also contributes to the overall varus deformity of the foot. It also is important to determine whether the deformity is flexible and correctable or rigid because patients with flexible deformities are more likely to be successfully treated nonoperatively with orthotics and shoe modifications and operatively with soft-tissue procedures such as tendon lengthenings, releases, or transfers (usually of the abnormally active muscle). Patients with rigid varus deformities generally require bone procedures, such as calcaneal osteotomy.

LENGTHENING OF THE POSTERIOR TIBIAL TENDON

The posterior tibial tendon can be lengthened in a variety of ways, including open Z-plasty of the tendon itself and various recession procedures, such as step-cut lengthening and intramuscular lengthening. The type of procedure used depends on the severity of the deformity and other procedures being done. A Z-plasty lengthening of the tendon, although it gives a large amount of correction, can cause scarring and tethering of the tendon in its sheath, leading to recurrence of deformity. Recession procedures such as lengthening at the musculotendinous junction have a lower risk of overlengthening and scarring of the tendon sheath. Recession procedures, because the tendon itself is spared, are good for patients at high risk of recurrence or in whom a posterior tibial transfer may be needed in the future.

Z-PLASTY LENGTHENING OF THE POSTERIOR TIBIAL TENDON

TECHNIQUE 33-14

- Make an 8-cm longitudinal incision beginning just above and posterior to the medial malleolus.
- Identify the posterior tibial tendon sheath and incise it, protecting the underlying neurovascular bundle.
- Make an approximately 6-cm long incision in the middle of the posterior tibial tendon sheath. Proximally release the medial half of the tendon and distally release the lateral half of the tendon.
- Bring the foot to the corrected position, including neutral dorsiflexion, and repair the overlapping tendon ends with nonabsorbable suture in a side-to-side fashion.
- Close the tendon sheath with absorbable sutures.
- Close the incision and apply a short leg cast with the foot in a slightly overcorrected position.

POSTOPERATIVE CARE. Weight bearing as tolerated is allowed in the cast for 4 to 6 weeks. The patient is placed in a full-time ankle-foot orthosis for 3 months and a nighttime orthosis for an additional 3 months. Physical therapy and a home stretching program are started immediately after cast removal.

STEP-CUT LENGTHENING OF THE POSTERIOR TIBIAL TENDON

TECHNIQUE 33-15

- Expose the tendon sheath as described previously.
- Just above the medial malleolus, incise the lateral half of the tendon sheath and tendon.
- Move 6 to 8 cm proximally and incise the medial half of the tendon sheath and tendon.
- Manipulate the foot into the corrected position; the tendon slides on itself within the sheath.
- Do not repair the tendon or close the tendon sheath.
- Close the subcutaneous tissue and skin before placing a short leg cast with the foot in a slightly overcorrected (valgus) position.

POSTOPERATIVE CARE. The postoperative care is the same as for Technique 33-14.

MUSCULOTENDINOUS RECESSION OF THE POSTERIOR TIBIAL TENDON

TECHNIQUE 33-16

- Place the patient supine and make a 3-cm longitudinal incision over the posteromedial aspect of the tibia, at the junction between the middle and distal thirds.
- Incise the deep fascia and identify the flexor digitorum longus and retract it posteriorly.
- Identify the posterior tibial musculotendinous junction by placing a hemostat beneath it and observing its action when inverting the foot without flexing the toes.
- Pass a hemostat around the tendinous portion of the musculotendinous junction to isolate it from the surrounding muscle, protecting the neurovascular bundle.
- Divide the tendinous portion of the posterior tibial musculotendinous unit, leaving its muscular fibers intact (Fig. 33-32A).
- Manipulate the foot into an overcorrected position (Fig. 33-32B).
- Close the wound and apply a short leg walking cast.

POSTOPERATIVE CARE. The postoperative care is the same as for Technique 33-14.

SPLIT TENDON TRANSFERS

Depending on the muscles that are out of phase, split tendon transfers of the posterior or anterior tendon can be done. Full tendon transfers should be avoided because of the higher risk of complications and overcorrection of the deformity. Full posterior tibial tendon transfer to the dorsum of the foot has fallen out of favor for these reasons. Seventy-eight percent poor results were reported in one study with full tendon transfer because of unrecognized rigid varus deformity, simultaneous Achilles tendon lengthening leading to calcaneus deformity, lateral transplant of the tendon leading to valgus deformity, and detachment of the transferred tendon at the bone-tendon interface. Preoperatively, it is essential to ensure that the deformity is flexible and to identify the correct tendon to be transferred. A tendon transfer alone is insufficient to correct a rigid deformity. The split transfer not only improves active muscle function during gait but also acts as a dynamic sling, balancing the abnormal forces evenly across the foot.

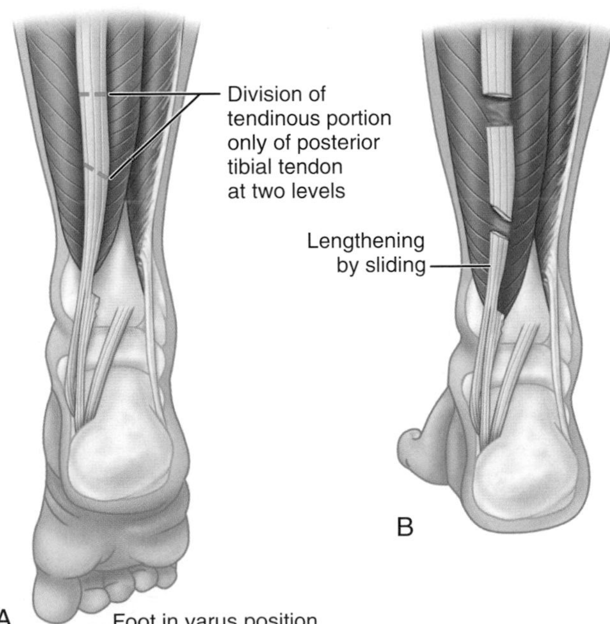

FIGURE 33-32 Sliding lengthening of posterior tibial tendon. **A,** Position of cuts in tendon. **B,** Lengthening by sliding. **SEE TECHNIQUE 33-16.**

SPLIT POSTERIOR TIBIAL TENDON TRANSFER

A study of 37 split posterior tibial tendon transfers in 30 children with cerebral palsy showed that in an average follow-up of 8 years there were 30 excellent, 4 good, and 3 poor results. Results did not deteriorate with time, and most patients were able to ambulate without braces.

TECHNIQUE 33-17

FIGURE 33-33

- Begin the first of two incisions 5 cm proximal and medial to the medial malleolus and extend the incision distally, ending over the navicular.
- Identify the posterior tibial muscle and tendon and the Achilles tendon, which can be lengthened as necessary.
- Identify and protect the neurovascular bundle with a vessel loop throughout the entire procedure.
- Open the anterior aspect of the posterior tibial tendon sheath from the navicular to the musculotendinous junction, preserving the posterior tunnel to prevent dislocation of the tendon.
- Dissect the plantar portion of the posterior tibial tendon from its insertion on the navicular, preserving as much length for transfer as possible.
- Deliver this portion of the tendon into the proximal aspect of the wound and place a nonabsorbable suture in the free end of the tendon.
- Make a second incision over the lateral side of the ankle 2 cm proximal to the lateral malleolus and extend it to the insertion of the peroneus brevis tendon at the base of the fifth metatarsal.
- Open the sheath of the peroneus brevis tendon.
- Through the medial incision, create a tunnel posterior to the tibia and anterior to the neurovascular bundle, directed laterally toward the fibula.
- Pass the free end of the tendon through the tunnel, ensuring that the transferred tendon is posterior to the tibia and fibula and anterior to the neurovascular bundle and toe-flexor tendons to prevent neurovascular and flexor tendon compression during muscle contraction.
- Weave the end of the tendon through the peroneus brevis tendon and suture it to the tendon.

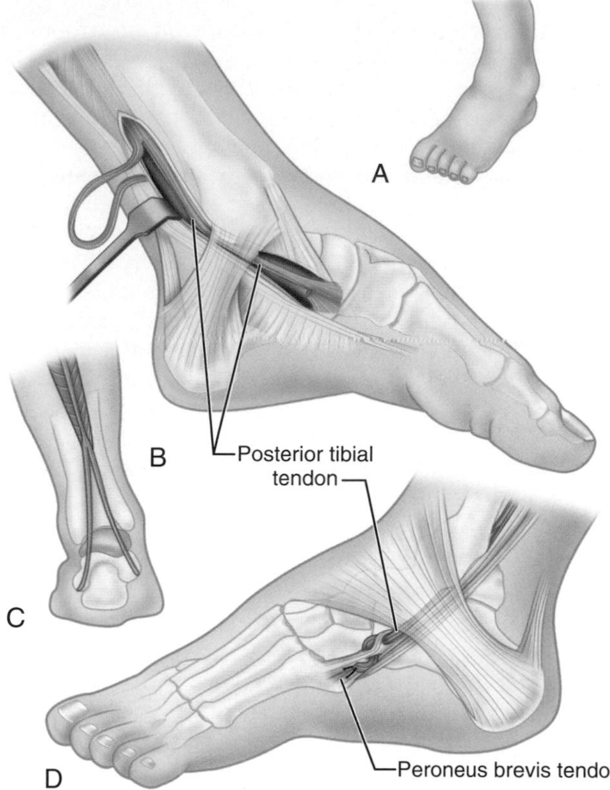

FIGURE 33-33 Kaufer split transfer of posterior tibial tendon for varus deformity. **A,** Foot is in varus position. **B,** Posterior tibial tendon has been split, one half is freed distally, and flexor tendons of toes and neurovascular bundle are retracted posteriorly. **C** and **D,** Freed half of tendon is passed from medial to lateral behind tibia and sutured to peroneus brevis tendon near its insertion. **SEE TECHNIQUE 33-17.**

- Adjust tension on the transferred tendon so that the hindfoot is in neutral with the ankle in neutral dorsiflexion.
- If the Achilles tendon was lengthened with a Z-plasty, repair it at this time.
- Close the wounds in routine fashion and apply a long leg cast with the knee slightly flexed and the foot in neutral.

POSTOPERATIVE CARE. Weight bearing is allowed immediately. The long leg cast is worn for 6 weeks, and then a short leg cast is worn for 2 weeks. An ankle-foot orthosis is prescribed only if patients have weak or absent anterior tibial muscle function preoperatively.

SPLIT ANTERIOR TIBIAL TENDON TRANSFER

A 10-year follow-up of 21 patients who had split anterior tibial tendon transfers found that 19 were community ambulators with improved gait without the use of orthotics. Posterior tibial intramuscular lengthening and Achilles tendon lengthening combined with split anterior tibial tendon transfer was reported to produce excellent or good results in 18 of 20 children. The poor results were in patients with fixed hindfoot deformities and weak anterior tibial tendons preoperatively. A biomechanical study found that for a split tendon transfer the ideal insertion site, biomechanically, is the fourth metatarsal, and for whole tendon transfers it is the third metatarsal.

TECHNIQUE 33-18

(HOFFER ET AL.)

- Three incisions are used for the split anterior tibial tendon transfer.
- With the patient supine, make the first incision medially over the anterior tibial insertion on the medial cuneiform and first metatarsal.
- Identify the anterior tibial tendon, protecting the dorsalis pedis artery, and split the tendon with an umbilical tape (Fig. 33-34B).
- Make a second incision over the anterior aspect of the leg at the musculotendinous junction and identify the anterior tibial tendon; pass the umbilical tape into the second incision (Fig. 33-34C).
- Identify the lateral half of the tendon, release it from its insertion, and secure it with a locking stitch (Fig. 33-34D), preserving as much length as possible, and then pass it into the second incision as well.
- Make the third incision on the foot over the dorsal aspect of the cuboid. Pass the lateral half of the tendon subcutaneously into the third incision and close the first two incisions (Fig. 33-34E).
- Drill a hole into the cuboid, preserving a roof of bone. Pass the lateral slip of tendon through the drill hole and suture it to itself with nonabsorbable suture with the ankle in slight dorsiflexion and hindfoot eversion.
- If this is combined with lengthening of the Achilles tendon or posterior tibial tendon recession, these procedures should be done before the anterior tibial tendon transfer.
- Carefully hold the foot in the corrected position during wound closure and application of a short leg cast (Fig. 33-34F).

POSTOPERATIVE CARE. A short leg cast is worn for 6 weeks, and weight bearing is allowed immediately. An ankle-foot orthosis is worn for 6 months to prevent recurrence.

OSTEOTOMY OF THE CALCANEUS

When the heel becomes fixed in varus, a corrective procedure on the bone is required, combined with a muscle balancing soft-tissue procedure. Osteotomy of the calcaneus as advocated by Dwyer corrects the varus of the heel and, in contrast to a triple arthrodesis, does not impair mobility in the subtalar or midtarsal joints. Opening wedge osteotomies of the calcaneus are not recommended. The skin laterally and medially along the bone is only slightly mobile, and opening wedges put tension on the suture line and tend to cause incisional skin sloughs. The medial calcaneal nerves also may be stretched by an opening wedge osteotomy made from the medial side, causing painful neuromas. For these reasons, a

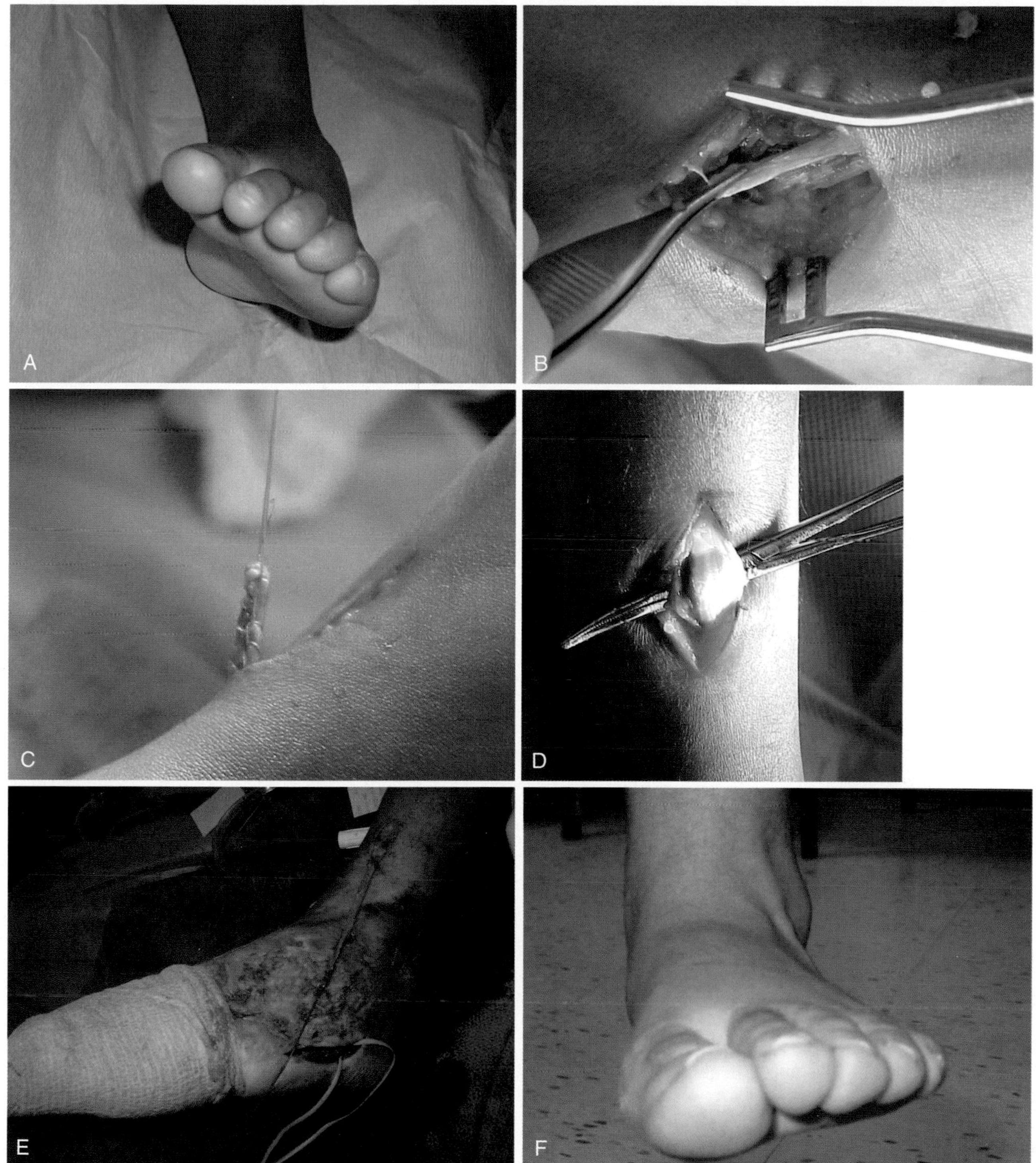

FIGURE 33-34 Transfer of anterior tibial tendon. **A,** Preoperative appearance of foot; note flexible forefoot supination. **B,** Lateral half of anterior tibial tendon is released from insertion, with care to resect as distally as possible to maximize graft length. **C,** Anterior tibial tendon is identified in anterior compartment, and graft is brought into anterior incision. **D,** Tendon is secured with locked nonabsorbable suture. **E,** Lateral slip of tendon is passed subcutaneously into third incision on lateral border of foot. **F,** Corrected position of foot postoperatively; note improved forefoot position and position of transferred tendon. **SEE TECHNIQUE 33-18.**

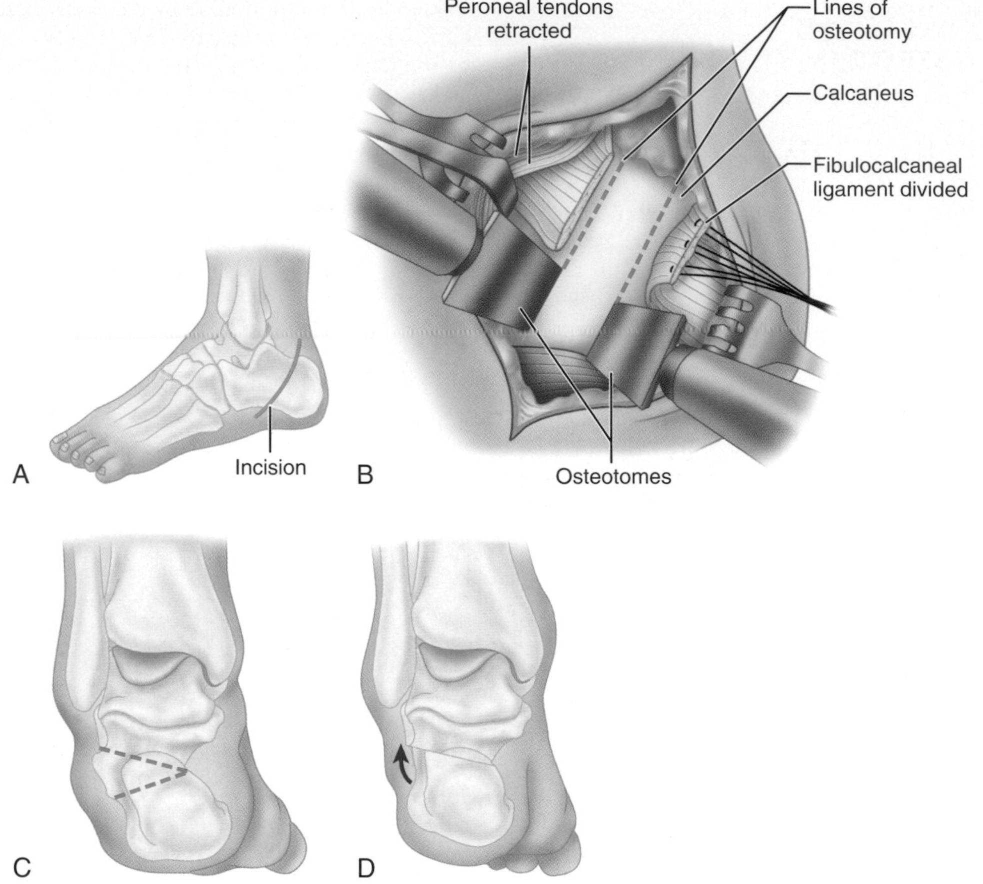

FIGURE 33-35 Dwyer closing wedge osteotomy of calcaneus for varus heel. **A,** Lateral skin incision is made inferior and parallel to peroneal tendons. **B,** Wedge of bone is resected with its base laterally. **C,** Wedge of bone is tapered medially. **D,** Calcaneus is closed after bone has been removed, and varus deformity is corrected to slight valgus. **SEE TECHNIQUE 33-19.**

closing wedge resection osteotomy of the calcaneus is recommended. For varus deformities, the incision is lateral and the base of the wedge of bone removed is lateral. Alternatively, a lateral displacement osteotomy can be used to correct hindfoot varus. Although widely discussed as a treatment option, there are no good long-term outcome studies of this technique or comparisons with Dwyer osteotomy.

Good long-term results have been reported after a modified Dwyer calcaneal osteotomy (Fig. 33-35). A minimum age of 3 years is recommended for this osteotomy. Triple arthrodesis is recommended in children 9 years old or older.

LATERAL CLOSING-WEDGE CALCANEAL OSTEOTOMY

TECHNIQUE 33-19

(DWYER)

- Expose the lateral aspect of the foot through a curved incision parallel and about 1 cm posterior and inferior to the peroneus longus tendon (Fig. 33-35A).
- Retract the superior wound edge until the tendon sheath of the peroneus longus is exposed.
- Strip the periosteum from the superior, lateral, and inferior surfaces of the calcaneus posterior to this tendon.
- Remove a wedge of bone from the calcaneus just inferior and posterior to the tendon and parallel with it (Fig. 33-35B). Make the base of the wedge 8 to 12 mm wide as needed for correction of the deformity and taper the wedge medially to, but not through, the medial cortex of the calcaneus (Fig. 33-35C).
- Manually break the medial cortex and close the gap in the bone. Bring the bony surfaces snugly together by pressing the foot into dorsiflexion against the pull of the Achilles tendon (Fig. 33-35D). Failure to close the gap in the calcaneus indicates that a small piece of bone has been left behind at the apex of the wedge and should be removed. Ensure that the varus deformity has been corrected and that the heel is in the neutral or a slightly varus position. Close the wound and apply a cast from the toes to the tibial tuberosity.

POSTOPERATIVE CARE. The patient is placed in a short leg cast and weight bearing is protected for 4 weeks when possible. Weight bearing is progressed at that time, and cast immobilization is continued until the osteotomy is solid, usually no longer than 8 weeks.

LATERAL DISPLACEMENT CALCANEAL OSTEOTOMY

This technique is described in Chapter 82.

PLANOVALGUS DEFORMITY

Planovalgus is a common foot deformity in children with diplegia and quadriplegia, which, in contrast to equinovarus, rarely causes pain or gait dysfunction. Spasticity of the gastrocnemius-soleus usually is accompanied by overpull of the peroneal muscles or weakness of the foot inverters or both. The gastrocnemius-soleus acts as the primary deforming force. The contracted Achilles tendon acts as a bowstring, preventing dorsiflexion of the ankle. The dorsiflexion observed during gait occurs at the midtarsal joints, causing the calcaneus to evert and removing the sustentaculum tali from its normal supporting position underneath the talus. This, along with abduction of the midtarsal joint, causes the talus to move into a more medial and vertical position. External rotation deformity of the tibia, which is common in patients with diplegia and quadriplegia, also plays a role in this deformity. This altered talar position may cause pain with weight bearing and callus formation over the uncovered talar head. For this reason, gastrocnemius-soleus lengthening should accompany any procedure intended to correct planovalgus.

Most patients can be treated conservatively with shoe modifications or an orthosis to help control the hindfoot eversion. Operative treatment is indicated for patients in whom conservative treatment fails and who have significant deformity that is either painful or limits function. Soft-tissue procedures alone, such as lengthening or transfer of the peroneal tendons, usually are insufficient to correct this deformity. Perry and Hoffer transferred the peroneus longus or brevis into the posterior tibial tendon if either or both were active during stance phase only. Subtalar joint arthroereisis has fallen out of favor because of the unpredictable results and approximately 50% failure rate. Surgical treatment usually consists of calcaneal osteotomy, especially for milder deformities and GMFCS I and II patients, and subtalar arthrodesis for more severe deformities most commonly in GMFCS III-V patients. A 10-year follow-up study of cerebral palsy patients who had either calcaneal lengthening or subtalar fusion showed improvement in both groups; however, patients with poor functional abilities and those who had fusion had less foot pain. Regardless of the procedure, a recent gait study showed that correction of a planovalgus foot deformity led to improvements in knee flexion, especially in patients with milder deformities.

Calcaneal osteotomy, consisting of lateral column lengthening, is effective in the treatment of mild-to-moderate deformities and is more effective in normalizing foot contact pressures than subtalar arthrodesis. It has been shown that preoperative weight bearing lateral radiographs with a less than 35-degree talocalcaneal angle, less than 25-degree talo–first metatarsal angle, and greater than 5 degrees of calcaneal pitch are associated with good outcomes. Although graft failure is rare (5%), it is less common with tricortical allografts than with patellar allografts. Postoperative subluxation of the calcaneocuboid joint is common after lateral column lengthening; however, stabilization of the calcaneocuboid joint at the time of correction has been shown not to reduce the incidence or magnitude of this. It also has been shown to be more effective in ambulatory children; nonambulatory children have a higher recurrence rate. A medial column stabilization consisting of either talonavicular stapling or fusion can be used, especially in GMFCS III-V patients. Medial column arthrodesis has also been shown to be effective in treating recurrent planovalgus deformity following lateral column lengthening.

A review of lateral column lengthening in 31 feet in 20 children with severe hindfoot valgus deformities in whom conservative treatment had failed found satisfactory results in 29 of the 31 feet with good preservation of subtalar motion. This technique is described in Chapter 82.

MEDIAL DISPLACEMENT CALCANEAL OSTEOTOMY

For more severe deformities, a translational osteotomy of the calcaneus can be used. Excellent results were reported in 17 of 18 patients at an average of 42 months after medial displacement calcaneal osteotomy to correct hindfoot valgus. A combined procedure of medial displacement osteotomy, opening wedge cuboid osteotomy, and pronation plantar flexion osteotomy of the medial cuneiform also has shown good restoration of foot position.

TECHNIQUE 33-20

- Place the patient supine and apply a midthigh tourniquet.
- Expose the lateral surface of the calcaneus through an incision beginning near the lateral tuberosity of the Achilles tendon attachment and extending distally and parallel but inferior to the sural nerve.
- By blunt dissection, expose the lateral surface of the calcaneus, reflecting the peroneal tendons and sural nerve superiorly.
- Using the plantar surface of the foot as a guide, place a Kirschner wire along the lateral side of the calcaneus and with a fluoroscopic image determine the appropriate placement of the osteotomy. It should not extend forward into the subtalar or calcaneocuboid joint.
- Make the osteotomy transverse and parallel to the sole of the foot, beginning just posterior to the subtalar joint, and direct it plantarward toward the attachment of the plantar fascia to the calcaneus (Fig. 33-36A). In making the osteotomy, protect the Achilles tendon superiorly and the plantar muscles, nerves, and vessels inferiorly. Do not penetrate the medial periosteum.
- When the osteotomy is complete, slide the inferior fragment medially to align the calcaneus with the tibia.
- Insert a threaded Kirschner wire, directed downward and medially, through the two fragments of calcaneus (Fig. 33-36B).
- Close the wound over suction drainage and apply a short leg cast.

POSTOPERATIVE CARE. The cast is changed at 4 weeks, and the wire is removed. A new short leg cast is placed, and weight bearing is progressed over the next 4 weeks.

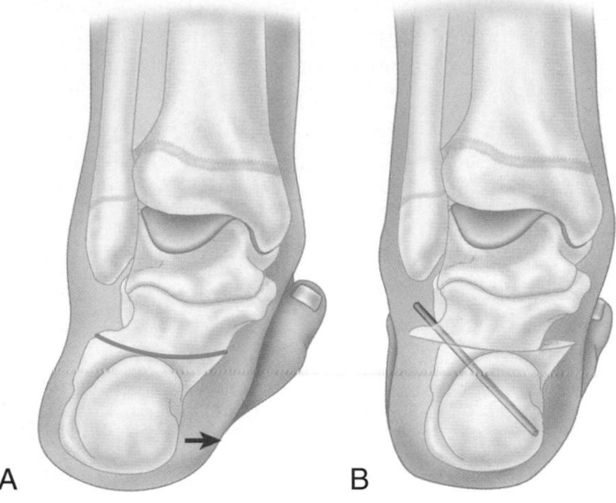

FIGURE 33-36 Medial displacement of calcaneus for hindfoot valgus. **A,** Transverse osteotomy of calcaneus. **B,** Fixation with Kirschner wire after distal fragment has been shifted medially to place calcaneus in weight bearing line of tibia. **SEE TECHNIQUE 33-20.**

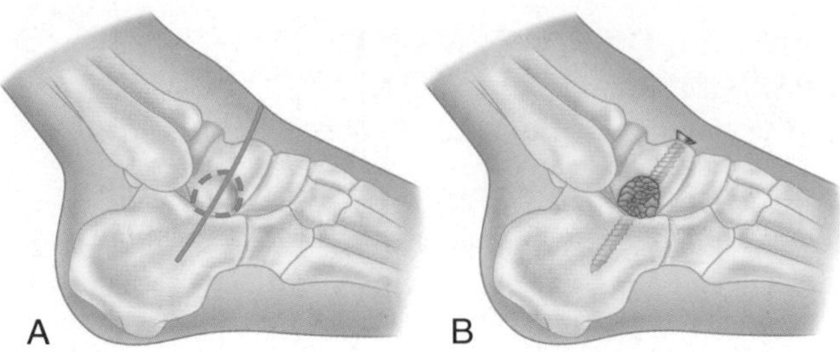

FIGURE 33-37 Dennyson and Fulford technique of extraarticular subtalar arthrodesis using screw and cancellous bone chips. **A,** Skin incision and bone area curetted from lateral side of talus and calcaneus. **B,** Placement of iliac bone chips in side of talus and calcaneus after screw has been inserted across subtalar joint with heel in corrected position. **SEE TECHNIQUE 33-21.**

SUBTALAR ARTHRODESIS

Arthrodesis also has been used in the treatment of calcaneovalgus feet, with the classic procedure being the Grice extraarticular subtalar arthrodesis. It should be noted that although hindfoot alignment is improved this does not treat residual forefoot supination and ankle equinus. Because of high graft failure and pseudarthrosis rates of the initial procedure, a variety of modifications have been proposed. The modifications have been aimed at better retention of the calcaneus beneath the talus with internal fixation and decreased rates of pseudarthrosis. Good results have been reported in 70% of patients at an average follow-up of 5.6 years after Dennyson-Fulford modification of the extraarticular arthrodesis according to Hadley et al. The pseudarthrosis rate has been reported to be 6.4%. A report of 46 children who had bilateral subtalar fusion using an Ollier incision and precut corticocancellous graft found that at mean follow-up of 55 months functional mobility scores improved in all patients, especially GMFS III patients, with no wound complications and fusion in 45. Alternatively, tibiotalocalcaneal arthrodesis has been reported in a small series of patients with severe calcaneovalgus deformity as a salvage procedure.

TECHNIQUE 33-21

- Obliquely incise the skin over the sinus tarsi beginning anteriorly at the middle of the ankle and proceeding laterally to the peroneal tendons (Fig. 33-37A).
- Incise and reflect as one flap the subcutaneous fat and origins of the extensor digitorum brevis muscles.
- By sharp dissection, excise the fat from the sinus tarsi down to bone proximally and distally.
- With a small gouge or burr, remove cortical bone from the apex of the sinus tarsi to expose cancellous bone on the talar neck and the superior surface of the calcaneus. Do not remove the cortical bone from the outer part of the sinus tarsi where a transfixion screw is to pass.
- Dorsally expose the small depression just behind the neck of the talus through a small separate skin incision and by blunt dissection between the neurovascular bundle and the tendons of the extensor digitorum longus.
- Hold the calcaneus in the corrected position and pass an awl posteriorly, inferiorly, and slightly laterally so that it passes through the cortical bone of the talus above and below and through the cortical bone of the calcaneus above and inferolaterally. Use the awl to determine the desired length of a screw needed for fixation into the hole and insert the screw in the hole.
- Alternatively, a cannulated screw can be placed using fluoroscopy (Fig. 33-37B).
- Remove chips of cancellous bone from the iliac crest and pack them into the sinus tarsi and above the bone that has been denuded on the talus and calcaneus.
- Replace the extensor digitorum brevis and close the skin.

POSTOPERATIVE CARE. A short leg cast is applied with careful padding and molding around the heel. This cast is worn for 6 to 8 weeks with the patient kept non–weight bearing. The cast is changed to a short leg walking cast, and gradual weight bearing is begun.

Triple arthrodesis also has been used in the treatment of equinovalgus foot deformities. The addition of a lateral column lengthening as proposed by Horton allows better correction of the flatfoot deformity while offering good pain relief. A long-term study of 21 patients (26 feet) with cerebral palsy and a mean follow-up of 19 years after triple arthrodesis showed that although residual deformity was present in 39% of feet, 62% of patients were pain free and 95% were happy with the operation. The rate of adjacent joint arthritis was 12% tibiotalar and 4% midfoot. After skeletal maturity, all residual deformities in the ankle, hindfoot, and midfoot can be corrected by a triple arthrodesis with appropriate wedge resections (see Chapter 34). Before undertaking a triple arthrodesis in a child with cerebral palsy, the surgeon always

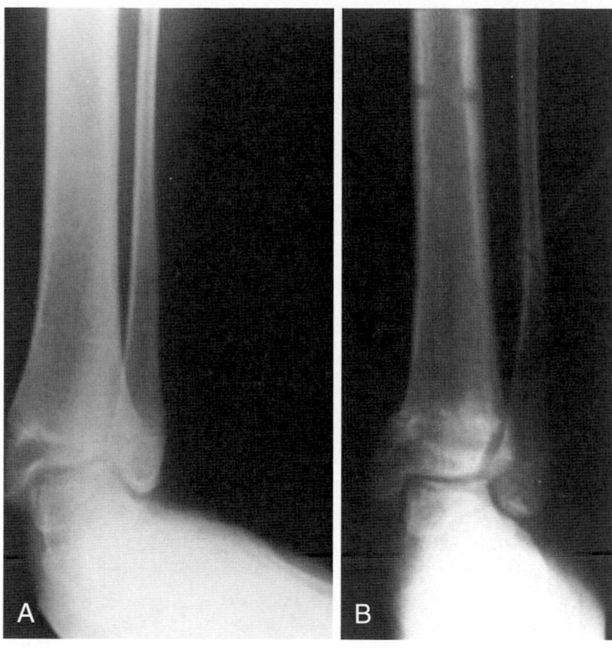

FIGURE 33-38 A, Standing anteroposterior view of ankle shows valgus deformity of ankle joint. B, Alignment of ankle achieved by supramalleolar osteotomy.

should obtain standing anteroposterior radiographs of the ankle. What often appears to be a valgus of the heel may be valgus of the ankle mortise, which should be corrected by a supramalleolar osteotomy and realignment of the ankle, rather than by creation of a secondary compensatory deformity in the subtalar joint (Fig. 33-38). Any external tibial torsion should be recognized before a triple arthrodesis is done because if the ankle joint is externally rotated, the foot will still appear to be in valgus and abduction after the triple arthrodesis.

CALCANEUS DEFORMITY

Pure calcaneus deformity is rare in patients with cerebral palsy and usually is associated with calcaneovalgus. It is most commonly caused by overlengthening or repeated lengthenings of the Achilles tendon. It can develop as a primary deformity when the dorsiflexors of the foot are spastic and the gastrocnemius-soleus is weak. This condition tends to be progressive and unresponsive to bracing. A variety of soft-tissue transfers have been proposed to help correct the deformity, including transfer of the anterior tibial or the peroneal tendons to the calcaneus, with limited success. The best treatment of this condition is prevention of excessive lengthening or denervation of the gastrocnemius-soleus complex.

CRESCENTIC OSTEOTOMY OF THE CALCANEUS

Occasionally, talipes calcaneus is purely in the hindfoot and is accompanied by a cavus deformity in the midfoot. In such instances, a crescentic osteotomy of the calcaneus can be used to lengthen the foot and elevate the base of the heel.

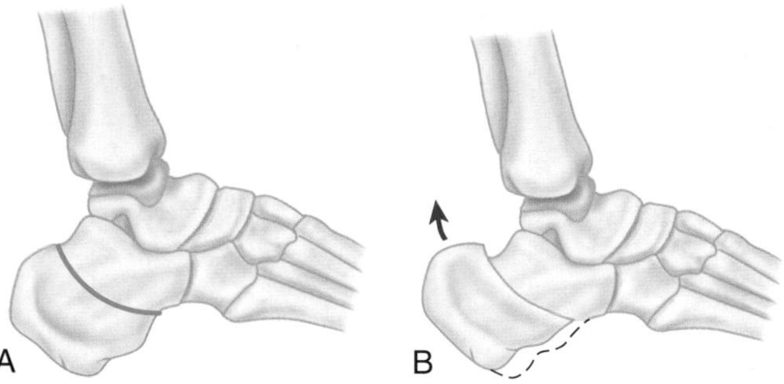

FIGURE 33-39 Samilson technique of crescentic osteotomy of calcaneus. A, Line of osteotomy. B, Displacement of posterior fragment of calcaneus posterosuperiorly. **SEE TECHNIQUE 33-22.**

TECHNIQUE 33-22

- Inflate a midthigh tourniquet and incise the skin laterally over the calcaneus posterior to the subtalar joint and overlying the posterior tuberosity of the calcaneus. The peroneal tendons should lie anterior to the incision, which should parallel them.
- Expose the lateral side of the calcaneus, protect the peroneal tendons, and perform a plantar fasciotomy from the lateral surface of the foot.
- Make a crescentic osteotomy in the calcaneus with a curved saw blade or osteotome (Fig. 33-39A).
- Free the posterior tuberosity of the calcaneus and shift it proximally and posteriorly in the line of the osteotomy to correct the calcaneocavus deformity (Fig. 33-39B).
- Secure the fragments with a Kirschner wire or staple and apply a short leg cast.

POSTOPERATIVE CARE. The cast and staple or Kirschner wire are removed 6 weeks after surgery, and full weight bearing is allowed.

CAVUS DEFORMITY

Cavus deformity is rare in children with cerebral palsy and is typically caused by an imbalance between the extrinsic and intrinsic musculature of the foot. In a review of 33 children in whom 38 osteotomies were done for cavus deformity, only one child (two feet) had cerebral palsy. Cavus deformity can be caused by hindfoot deformity in which the calcaneus is in a dorsiflexed position, or by midfoot deformity, in which the angulation of the foot occurs at the level of the midfoot. Conservative treatment alone rarely is successful in the treatment of this condition. Mild forefoot cavus may respond to plantar fascia release and casting; however, most such deformities require osteotomies as described in Chapter 35. Severe cavus deformities can be treated with triple arthrodesis. One must ensure that the patient does not have significant ankle valgus or external tibial deformity before performing triple arthrodesis.

FOREFOOT ADDUCTION DEFORMITY

Adduction deformity of the forefoot can occur in patients with cerebral palsy as an isolated deformity or in association with other deformities, such as in an incompletely corrected or recurrent clubfoot. In patients with an isolated abductor hallucis contracture, the tight tendon usually can be palpated when the great toe is adducted. Patients with isolated abductor hallucis spasticity have a passively correctable forefoot with the heel and ankle stabilized.

CORRECTION OF FLEXIBLE FOREFOOT ADDUCTUS

If the forefoot is passively correctable, resecting a segment of the muscle and its tendon can be done. In a report of 18 feet treated with this procedure, 16 had no increase in the adduction deformity and 2 developed hallux valgus deformities.

In older children, forefoot adduction that interferes with shoe wear or is painful should be corrected by osteotomy of the metatarsals, realignment, and Kirschner wire fixation as described in Chapter 29. Medial column opening wedge (medial cuneiform) and lateral column closing wedge (cuboid) osteotomies also have been used to treat this condition.

HALLUX VALGUS DEFORMITY

Hallux valgus deformity in patients with cerebral palsy usually is associated with other deformities, such as equinovalgus foot, heel valgus, and external rotation of the tibia. These conditions cause the foot to pronate, forcing the first metatarsophalangeal joint into abduction and creating a hallux valgus deformity. The extensor hallucis tendon may sublux into the first web space and becomes an abductor of the hallux, leading to further deformity.

Any other underlying deformities, such as heel valgus or external rotation of the tibia, should be corrected before surgical correction of the hallux valgus. If the causative deformities are not corrected, recurrence is almost certain, especially if fusion of the first metatarsophalangeal joint is not done. Isolated soft-tissue procedures for hallux valgus in patients with cerebral palsy, because of altered muscle forces, rarely are successful and have a high recurrence rate, and great toe metatarsophalangeal joint fusion is recommended.

First metatarsophalangeal joint fusion has been shown to provide the best overall outcome with functional gains and anatomic correction of the deformity being maintained. Surgical procedures for the correction of hallux valgus are discussed in Chapter 81.

CLAW TOES

Claw toe deformities are common in adolescents and adults with cerebral palsy, although most require only observation and foot wear modifications, such as high toe box shoes. Operative treatment is recommended if the claw toe deformity becomes painful, interferes with foot wear, or interferes with walking. Although neurectomy of the lateral plantar nerve has been proposed, the method most commonly used to treat claw toes is metatarsophalangeal joint capsulotomies and tenotomy of the long toe extensors to the lesser toes, with proximal interphalangeal joint resections or fusions using Kirschner wire fixation until bony fusion occurs. Surgical procedures for claw toes are discussed in Chapter 86.

SPINE-PELVIC OBLIQUITY AND SCOLIOSIS

The combination of hip dislocation, pelvic obliquity, and scoliosis is common in wheelchair-bound patients with cerebral palsy and can cause significant difficulties with pain, sitting balance, and overall independence (Fig. 33-40). In an ambulatory child, spinal deformity and imbalance can make standing erect difficult if not impossible. In a nonambulatory child, scoliosis can lead to abnormal skin pressure areas and decubitus ulcers, seating/positioning difficulties, and, in severe cases, cardiopulmonary compromise. The scoliosis in patients with cerebral palsy is different from that of idiopathic adolescent scoliosis in that the curves tend to be long thoracolumbar C-shaped curves, with or without accompanying pelvic obliquity. The optimal treatment of scoliosis associated with hip dislocation and pelvic obliquity is controversial.

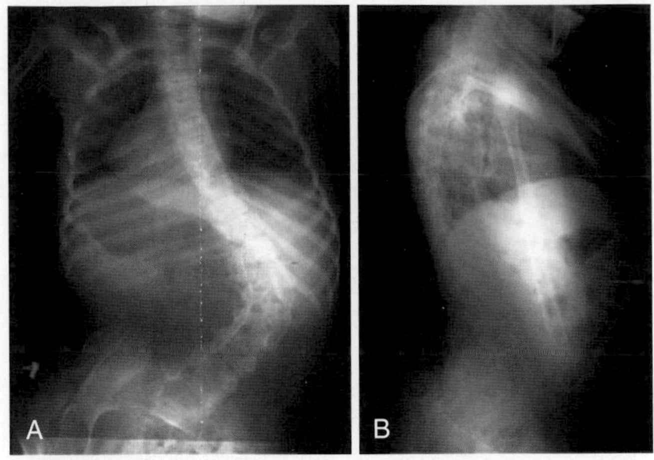

FIGURE 33-40 **A,** Posteroanterior view of spine of patient with spastic quadriplegic cerebral palsy with 73-degree thoracolumbar scoliosis and pelvic obliquity. **B,** Lateral view of spine of same patient shows progressive lumbar lordosis. This deformity was believed to contribute to increased skin pressures and seating difficulties. (From McCarthy JJ, D'Andrea LP, Betz RR, et al: Scoliosis in the child with cerebral palsy, J Am Acad Orthop Surg 14:367, 2006.)

Although pelvic obliquity and scoliosis are common and related to disease severity in patients with cerebral palsy, the relationship between the two is not well established. A review of 500 children with cerebral palsy found no correlation between the frequency of dislocated hips, either bilateral or unilateral, and pelvic obliquity. All degrees of pelvic obliquity were found in children in whom both hips were dislocated. The frequency of hip dislocation on the same side as the elevated hemipelvis had no direct correlation with the degree of pelvic obliquity. In "windswept" hips there was no correlation between the direction of the windswept hips and the direction of the pelvic obliquity. This and other studies have shown that hip pathology is a result of muscle imbalance around the hip and that pelvic obliquity and scoliosis are related to muscle imbalance of the trunk and independent of the position of the hips.

Scoliosis associated with cerebral palsy is related to the severity of motor involvement, with 50% to 75% of quadriplegics affected compared with fewer than 5% of hemiplegics. Compared with curves in idiopathic scoliosis, curves in patients with cerebral palsy tend to occur at a younger age and be more progressive and usually require operative treatment. Orthotic management has been shown to be ineffective in preventing progression of scoliosis but is occasionally used to help improve sitting balance or in efforts to delay surgery in immature patients to allow for further thoracic development. Risk factors for curve progression include GMFCS level, younger age, poor sitting balance, and multiple curves. A study of 182 cerebral palsy patients with scoliosis showed that for GMFCS IV and V patients mean progression of the coronal Cobb angle was 3.4 degrees, thoracic kyphosis was 2.2 degrees, and apical translation was 5.4 mm per year. Curves of more than 30 degrees tend to progress, even after skeletal maturity.

Patients with cerebral palsy also have sagittal plane abnormalities. Hyperkyphosis is the most common deformity, especially in young children with weak spinal extensor muscles. This can significantly interfere with sitting balance and communication and usually is treated with wheelchair modifications, such as adding chest supports or reclining the seat. A soft body orthosis can be used as well. Hyperlordosis occurs less commonly and usually is associated with hip flexion contractures or a rigid thoracic kyphosis. Treatment of the primary deformity usually improves or corrects hyperlordosis.

Operative treatment should be considered for patients in whom scoliosis or pelvic obliquity interferes with overall function, rather than based on the absolute magnitude of the curve. The goals of treatment should be functionally oriented and related to loss of sitting balance, pelvic obliquity, and presence of pain rather than to the degree of curvature. Improvement in pain is one of the most important factors in the improvement in quality of life after spinal surgery. The goals of surgery are to prevent further deformity, provide a well-balanced spine in the coronal and sagittal planes, and correct any underlying pelvic obliquity. Complication rates after scoliosis surgery in patients with cerebral palsy are markedly higher, up to 25% to 50% in some series, than for adolescent idiopathic scoliosis and are often related to comorbidities such as aspiration, poor nutritional status, cardiopulmonary compromise, and increased risk of infection. The incidence of deep wound infection after scoliosis surgery in patients with cerebral palsy may be as high as 10%. Patients with wound breakdown and greater residual curves, greater preoperative white blood cell count, and fusion using unit rods may be at higher risk. *Escherichia coli* and *Pseudomonas aeruginosa* are commonly cultured organisms and, therefore, gram-negative prophylaxis should be considered. Surgical stabilization usually consists of posterior spinal instrumentation with segmental fixation, using screws, hooks, or wires. The use of pedicle screw fixation has become more common and has been shown to be effective in correcting coronal and sagittal deformity and pelvic obliquity. Osteotomies can be used in selected patients with severe focal deformities. Growth-sparing techniques, both rib-based and spine-based, have been shown in small series to be effective in controlling scoliosis while maintaining growth in patients with cerebral palsy; however, complications, especially infection, are frequent. The use of antibiotic-impregnated bone graft may decrease the rate of postoperative infection, and it is becoming more widely used.

Although parental and caretaker satisfaction after spinal fusion in patients with cerebral palsy remains high, it is difficult to find objective criteria that correlate with this. A review of 50 patients with scoliosis and cerebral palsy treated with posterior spinal fusion showed statistically significant improvement in the health-related quality of life (HRQL) scores postoperatively. However, only a weak correlation was found between the magnitude of curve correction and HRQL scores, and no correlation was found between complications and extension of the fusion to the pelvis. Another large study of 84 patients found that although functional improvement postoperatively was limited, satisfaction was high and was thought to be related to sitting balance and cosmesis. Factors in this study associated with less satisfaction included a higher complication rate, greater residual major curve magnitude, and hyperlordosis, which may relate to poorer overall sitting balance. Further study of factors leading to parental and caregiver satisfaction after spinal fusion in patients with cerebral palsy is necessary. A comparison of patients with cerebral palsy who had spinal fusion with patients who did not have fusion found no significant differences in pain, need for pulmonary medication or therapy, the presence of decubitus ulcers, patient function, or time required for daily care. Subjectively, however, most health care workers believed that patients who had undergone fusion were more comfortable.

UPPER EXTREMITY

Many patients with cerebral palsy have involvement of the upper extremities, especially patients with hemiplegia and quadriplegia. A review of 100 cerebral palsy patients found that 83% had upper limb involvement and 69% had reduced hand control. The most common contracture patterns were thumb in palm/clasped hand and shoulder adduction/internal rotation and wrist flexion/pronation. Functionally, 70% of children have limitation of forearm supination, and 63% have limitation of wrist and finger extension in the affected limb(s). The degree of upper extremity deformity is significantly related to GMFCS function in diplegic but not hemiplegic patients. Most patients can be treated nonoperatively with physical therapy, splinting, and BTX-A. Selective dorsal rhizotomy, usually done to reduce lower extremity tone, has been shown to decrease upper extremity tone as well. Despite this high prevalence of deformity and functional limitations, only approximately 5% are surgical candidates. This may be related to the fact that in patients with cerebral palsy the upper extremity movement disorder often is associated with sensory deficits, particularly in proprioception, stereognosis, barognosis, and light touch, and there is seldom normal sensation in the affected hand. This alteration in sensation can cause a complete neglect of the affected extremity. Children who are likely to benefit from upper extremity surgery are highly functioning and have difficulties with activities of daily living, such as dressing and hygiene, or have severe contractures and deformities leading to pain and skin breakdown. Other positive predictors for a good outcome after upper extremity surgery include high motivation, reasonable intelligence, emotional stability, no neglect, good voluntary control, strength, and normal sensation. A randomized study of 39 children with cerebral palsy undergoing upper extremity surgery found that a combination of flexor carpi ulnaris to extensor carpi radialis brevis transfer, pronator teres release, and extensor pollicis brevus rerouting produced more improvement, although modest, than treatment with BTX-A injections or physical therapy. Children with severe spasticity, athetosis, and neglect still may benefit from surgery, which consists of static joint stabilizing procedures such as arthrodesis. The family should be considered so that they have realistic expectations regarding the goals of upper extremity surgery to prevent disappointment with the surgical outcome. Ancillary studies, such as kinetic EMG studies, are useful in evaluating the upper extremity before surgery.

The function of the upper extremity is to position the hand in space to perform a specific activity. If the hand is functional, procedures to correct these deformities may be useful in improving overall function. A review of the results of surgery in 84 upper limbs of 64 patients with cerebral palsy found a statistically significant improvement in functional status, hygiene, and appearance in carefully selected patients at an average follow-up of 4 years.

SHOULDER

Contracture of the shoulder or spasticity of the muscles that control it usually is not sufficiently disabling to justify surgery. The deformity usually is adduction and internal rotation. When surgery is indicated, useful procedures include procedures similar to those performed for brachial plexus palsy (see Chapter 34) and rotational osteotomy of the humerus done at the level of the deltoid tubercle. The use of pectoralis major release alone and combined with latissimus dorsi release for severe deformities may be beneficial in patients with severe cerebral palsy to improve axillary hygiene, bathing, and dressing.

ELBOW

The two groups of patients who have been shown to benefit from surgical procedures around the elbow are highly functioning patients with useful hand function and severely involved patients with significant contractures leading to antecubital fossa skin breakdown. When releasing a flexion contracture around the elbow, avoid acutely extending the elbow fully to prevent stretch injury to the brachial artery and median nerve, which have shortened as well. The addition of partial biceps tendon lengthening has been shown to increase elbow extension better than brachialis fractional lengthening, lacertus fibrosis division, and pretendinous adventitia debridement alone. The improvements gained are maintained in long-term outcome studies. Note that biceps lengthening will weaken it, which is important in patients with underlying supination weakness.

RELEASE OF ELBOW FLEXION CONTRACTURE

A report of 32 anterior elbow releases in patients with cerebral palsy showed no neurovascular injuries and no recurrence of deformity. The indications for this operation are fixed elbow contracture of 45 degrees or more that interferes with the ability to reach forward with a functional forearm and hand. Other procedures that improve forearm supination and hand function by releasing the flexor-pronator muscle origins from the medial capsule result in a mild gain in elbow flexion as well.

TECHNIQUE 33-23

- With the patient supine and the arm fully draped and with or without a tourniquet, approach the antecubital space with a gently curving S-shaped incision over the flexor crease. If necessary, ligate the veins that cross the region.
- Dissect the soft tissue and deep fascia to the muscle belly of the biceps proximally and follow the muscle distally to its tendon and the lacertus fibrosus. Isolate the lacertus fibrosus and resect it (Fig. 33-41A).
- Identify and protect the lateral antebrachial cutaneous nerve as it enters the area between the biceps and the brachialis laterally.
- Retract the nerve laterally and then flex the elbow partially and free the biceps tendon down to its insertion on the tuberosity of the proximal radius.
- Divide the biceps tendon for a Z-plasty lengthening (Fig. 33-41B). The musculofascial surface of the brachialis muscle can be seen under it. The radial nerve lies lateral to the brachialis muscle, and the brachial artery and median nerve lie medial to it. Identify and protect these structures.
- Extend the elbow maximally and circumferentially incise the aponeurotic tendinous fibers of the brachialis muscle at its distal end at one or two levels (Fig. 33-41C).
- Maximally extend the elbow and, if necessary, perform an anterior elbow capsulotomy. Allow the tourniquet to deflate and secure hemostasis.
- Extend the elbow and repair the previously divided biceps tendon (Fig. 33-41D).
- Ensure the integrity of the median nerve and brachial artery.
- Close only the subcutaneous tissue and skin and immobilize the arm in a well-padded cast with the elbow maximally, but not forcefully, extended and the forearm fully supinated. Bivalve the cast.

POSTOPERATIVE CARE. The arm is elevated for 48 hours, and finger motion is encouraged. At 5 days, flexion and extension exercises out of the cast are begun. For 6 weeks after surgery, the arm is replaced in the cast when the exercise period has been completed. Nighttime splinting is continued for 6 months. Maximal elbow extension usually is obtained 3 to 5 months postoperatively.

FOREARM, WRIST, AND HAND

Deformities of the forearm, wrist, and hand are described in Chapter 72 in the discussion of the hand in patients with cerebral palsy.

ADULTS WITH CEREBRAL PALSY

Because of the tremendous advances in the care given to patients with cerebral palsy, a generation of children who in the past would have been institutionalized now have been integrated into the family and society. These advances have been relatively recent, and more is becoming known about adults with cerebral palsy and the long-term outcomes of treatment. Population-based studies have shown that adults with cerebral palsy can live independently and maintain a high level of function. Long-term outcome studies of adults with cerebral palsy have found that for individuals who are

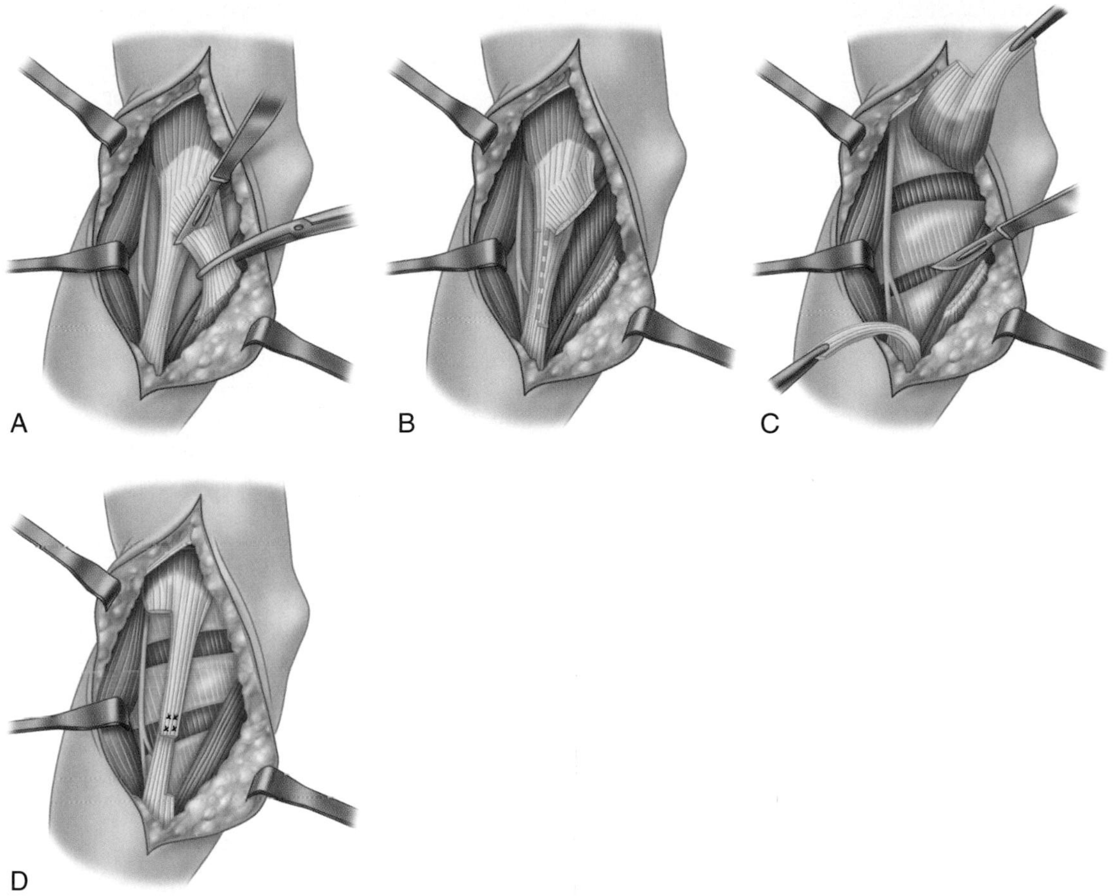

FIGURE 33-41 Mital elbow flexion release. **A,** Lacertus fibrosus is severed through incision in antecubital space. **B,** Tendon of insertion of biceps muscle is lengthened by Z-plasty. **C,** Fascia covering brachialis muscle anteriorly is cut at two levels. **D,** Z-plasty in biceps tendon is sutured after elbow is extended. **SEE TECHNIQUE 33-23.**

mobile as young adults there is a marked decline in ambulation with age, with fatigue and falls having a negative impact on quality of life. Approximately 25% of ambulatory adults with cerebral palsy will experience a gait decline sooner than their nondisabled peers, especially older patients with bilateral motor impairment, with more frequent use of assistive devices and higher levels of pain and/or fatigue. The exact cause of this decline is unknown but likely is multifactorial. Skills such as feeding, speech, and ability to order meals in public are well preserved. In one long-term study, 18% of 60-year olds lived independently and 41% resided in facilities providing higher-level medical care. Long-term survival rates were moderately worse than the general population, especially in nonambulatory patients. In a review of 819 adults with cerebral palsy, 33% of patients (77% controls) had education beyond secondary school, 29% (82% controls) were competitively employed, and 5% had specially created jobs. Social outcome studies have found a higher rate of unemployment in patients with other comorbidities, such as seizures, self-care limitations, and cognitive and communication impairments, with no substantial impact of severity of motor involvement on employment rate. Although more likely to be single and living with parents, 14% to 28% of patients with cerebral palsy without intellectual impairment were in a long-term partnership or had established their own families.

Many patients with cerebral palsy return for orthopaedic care in their thirties and forties when compensatory mechanisms they have relied on in the past begin to fail. This transition from care in the pediatric setting to the adult setting can be challenging for patients and physicians because of a lack of communication between the two systems, fear of the new system, and different treatment styles for adults and children. Common orthopaedic problems for adults with cerebral palsy include fatigue, knee instability that arises from long-standing ankle equinus, degenerative hip disease, flatfoot deformity, and scoliosis. Osteopenia also is frequently present in adults with cerebral palsy, which can predispose them to fractures. A patient-centered approach, just as with children, should be used in treating an adult with cerebral palsy. Not all deformities require treatment, and attention should be focused on the deformities that cause pain or interfere with independent function.

ADULT STROKE PATIENTS

Considerable literature exists regarding the orthopaedic evaluation and treatment of patients who have had cerebrovascular accidents, especially with the incidence of cerebrovascular accidents and the survival rate increasing. The development a multidisciplinary team approach incorporating early physical and occupational therapy, bracing, standing, use of BTX-A and the gait analysis has led to marked improvement in the treatment of adult stroke patients.

LOWER EXTREMITY

Of patients who have had a stroke, 65% to 75% recover enough function in their lower extremities to permit ambulation. This is because the lower extremity does not depend as much on sensation for its function as does the upper extremity and the activities necessary for walking are gross motor functions that are enhanced by primitive postural reflexes. Most patients with residual hemiparesis require the use of an external support and a brace to ambulate independently.

Orthotic positioning and range-of-motion exercises of the lower extremity begin in the early phases of recovery when the primary goal is prevention of fixed contractures. This treatment extends through the period of motor recovery and gait training to the time when the neurologic deficit becomes stationary and a definitive brace to aid in ambulation is required. In the early phase, the paralysis usually is flaccid and deformities occur as a result of poor positioning. Passive range-of-motion exercises help prevent undesirable patterning of movements, which often occurs in the recovery phase. Equinus deformity should be prevented by appropriate splinting and frequent range-of-motion exercises. Preventing deformity of the lower extremity is greatly assisted by having the patient stand and walk as soon as his or her medical condition permits. The use of BTX-A has become more common and has been shown to improve range of motion, lower extremity function, and ability to perform activities of daily living. Electrical stimulation can be used to help maintain strength and keep joints mobilized, and as a sensorimotor educational tool to increase the awareness of the sensation of muscle contractions, especially in the anterior tibial and peroneal muscles. In the early phase, this can be done with cutaneous stimulation; later in recovery, electrodes can be placed directly on a motor nerve with stimulation controlled through an externally placed transmitter. Various pharmacologic agents have been used in the treatment of spasticity, including baclofen, oral muscle relaxants, anticonvulsants, and cannabis, with limited success because of the variable nature of stroke patients, side effects, and the fact that these are systemic treatments for targeted dysfunctional muscle groups.

Motor recovery occurs during the first 3 to 4 months, and the quality of gait can change dramatically during that time. To become a functional ambulator, the patient must obtain adequate spontaneous improvement to allow voluntary control of the hip and knee. Bracing may be necessary to help achieve this goal; however, many of the braces used to stabilize the knee can be difficult to apply and manage and can negatively affect the ability to ambulate. When maximal motor recovery has been obtained and the gait function has stabilized, definitive bracing can be done.

Neurophysiologic studies have shown that there are seven neurologic sources of motion, two of which are sophisticated components of normal function (selective control and habitual control) and five are primitive forms of control. These primitive forms, which are present and suppressed in the normal state, become expressed as overt sources of motion (locomotor pattern, verticality, limb synergy, fast stretch, slow stretch) following a stroke.

Selected control is the normal ability to move one joint independently of another, to contract an isolated muscle, or to select a desired combination of motions. *Habitual control* is the normal automatic performance of a learned skill, such as walking.

Primitive *locomotor patterns* are mass movements of flexion and extension. The patient can initiate or terminate the movements but cannot otherwise modify them. If the knee is extended, the ankle also is automatically plantar flexed and the hip is extended. The opposite movements occur in knee flexion. This voluntary motion is preserved after a loss of cortical control and presumably is controlled by the midbrain. *Control of verticality* is a vestibular function and is an antigravity mechanism. When the body is erect, the extensor muscles have more tone than when the body is supine; additionally, standing creates a more intense stimulus than does sitting. In the upper extremity, the flexor muscles respond in this manner. Primitive *limb synergy* is the result of a multisegmental spinal cord reflex, tying the action of the extensor muscles to the posture of the limb. When the knee is extended, the tone of the soleus and the gastrocnemius is greatly increased, making both muscles much more sensitive to stretch than when the knee is flexed. Similarly, the tone in the antagonistic muscles may be inhibited. This activity confuses the results in the Silfverskiöld test used to differentiate contracture of the gastrocnemius from that of the soleus. The *fast stretch reflex,* characterized by the familiar clonic response, is caused by an intermittent burst of muscle activity. It is initiated by the velocity sensors in the muscle spindles. The *slow stretch reflex* is characterized by rigidity, a clinical term for continuous muscle reaction to stretch and often misinterpreted as contracture. This reflex disappears under anesthesia when length-change sensors in the muscle spindles are inactive. Primitive locomotor patterns and control of verticality, and stretch reflex activity, are especially troublesome to stroke patients.

In addition to motor problems, stroke patients frequently have impaired sensation. Impaired proprioception is especially important because it causes a delay or hesitancy in making a voluntary motor response. The duration of this delay indicates the time it takes to process the central nervous signals, and if the delay is too great, walking may not be a reasonable goal.

Gait analysis and various standing tests, including double limb support, hemiparetic single limb stance, and hemiparetic limb flexion, are useful if determining whether or not the patient can walk and if orthopaedic surgery is necessary.

Surgery should be deferred until at least 6 months after the stroke. Most patients make a rapid spontaneous recovery during the first 6 to 8 weeks. They subsequently strengthen these gains and learn to live with their disability. Progress in control of the limb occurs, and this typically is the result of extensive therapy. Patients with better early functional scores maintain better function at 6 months than those with lower scores. By 6 to 9 months after a stroke, patients have obtained maximal spontaneous improvement and must come to realize the permanence of their residual deficits. Surgical intervention, which usually is soft-tissue release, is indicated if it is likely to improve function or hygiene or decrease pain, and occasionally, improve cosmesis. The goals of surgery must be clearly explained to prevent unrealistic expectations. Although improvement in a single deficit may be expected, restoration of normal function in the extremity is almost impossible.

HIP

Scissoring gait secondary to adductor spasticity can be corrected by soft-tissue release. To determine whether or not the hip adductors are necessary for hip flexion in a patient, a diagnostic block of the obturator nerve before surgery is performed. If the effect of the nerve block is prolonged, it can be repeated once or twice, and occasionally the results are permanent.

Surgical release of a hip flexion contracture rarely is indicated in stroke patients because the decrease in hip flexion power may make the patient unable to walk. When gait EMG shows continuous activity of the hip flexors and medial hamstrings, releasing the iliopsoas and adductor longus and medial hamstring transfer to the femur sometimes allow the limb to assume an upright position.

KNEE

Flexion contractures of the knee can be treated operatively if the patient has adequate power in the gluteus maximus and quadriceps muscles to extend the hip when the hamstrings are lengthened. One study reported that 43% of 30 patients obtained ambulation ability after hamstring release, and 17% gained the ability to transfer. Caution was recommended in patients with severe peripheral vascular disease because of an increased risk of complications as a result of poor wound healing and risk of neurovascular injury.

Stiff knee gait, caused by increased activity of the rectus femoris during the swing phase of gait, can cause difficulties with foot clearance for stroke patients. A meta-analysis of the effect of chemodenervation of the rectus femoris on stiff knee gait showed that it does lead to improved peak knee flexion during swing phase. Release of the rectus femoris from the patella by excision of its distal segment can improve knee flexion by 15 to 20 degrees.

FOOT

Talipes equinovarus is the most common foot deformity in a stroke patient. Other deformities can occur, such as equinus without varus, varus of the forefoot, footdrop, planovalgus foot, and in-curling of the toes. Early physical therapy, use of ankle foot orthoses, and BTX-A have been shown to be effective in preventing equinus deformity and improving gait function in some patients.

TALIPES EQUINUS

The goal **of** surgery is to correct talipes equinus in the midswing and midstance phases while preserving heel lift support in the terminal stance phase and accepting a flat-footed contact with the floor. This goal can be accomplished with a closed subcutaneous triple hemisection of the Achilles tendon. The distal cut is made medially, proximal to the insertion of the tendon; the next is made 2.5 cm proximal to the first through the lateral half of the tendon; and the final one is made 2.5 cm proximal to the second through the medial half of the tendon. After surgery, the foot is immobilized in a cast in a slight equinus position so that walking does not overstretch the tendon. Patients can bear weight on the cast for 4 weeks before cast removal.

TALIPES EQUINOVARUS

Talipes equinovarus is common in stroke patients because of weakness in the foot dorsiflexors and evertors or spasticity of their antagonists. The goal of surgery is either to provide a plantigrade foot that can be braced in a nonambulatory patient or to rid an ambulator of braces. In the presence of moderate action of the anterior tibial muscle without the assistance of the toe extensors, the equinus deformity is corrected by rebalancing the foot to eliminate the varus deformity. The anterior and posterior tibial, soleus, flexor hallucis longus, and flexor digitorum longus, despite their swing phase and stance phase action, can be active well into the other phase and often are active continuously. They also can be inactive. A varus deformity in either swing or stance phase can be caused by any one or a combination of these muscles being abnormal, in contrast to varus deformity in patients with cerebral palsy. The posterior tibial muscle-tendon unit rarely is the deforming force in a stroke patient.

CORRECTION OF TALIPES EQUINOVARUS

Soft-tissue releases and tendon transfers can be used in adults to help balance the muscle forces across the foot. Historically, this has been done by transferring three fourths of the anterior tibial tendon to the third cuneiform, the flexor hallucis longus tendon to the same area, with the flexor digitorum longus tendon released and the posterior tibial tendon undisturbed (Fig. 33-42). Significant improvement in patient autonomy, ability to ambulate independently, and increased ability to wear normal shoes have been reported after this procedure. Similar results have been reported with the use of a split anterior tendon transfer alone in 132 feet in which improvements were made in walking distance and shoewear.

TECHNIQUE 33-24

- Make a 2-cm incision on the medial border of the foot over the navicular.
- Identify and expose the insertion of the anterior tibial tendon.
- Separate and detach the lateral three fourths of the tendon from the medial one fourth.
- Bring the detached part out through an incision made 2 cm proximal to the ankle and route it subcutaneously to the dorsal surface of the third cuneiform.
- Expose the cuneiform, drill converging holes in the bone and use a curet to construct a tunnel. Loop the free part of the tendon through this tunnel to be anchored later.
- Through a separate 4-cm incision in the arch of the foot, use electrocautery to release the plantar flexors of the toes.
- Through a posterior incision at the level of the ankle, identify the flexor hallucis longus tendon at its tunnel, detach it, and pass it anteriorly through a large window made in the interosseous membrane.
- Insert this tendon through the tunnel in the third cuneiform opposite to the direction of the anterior tibial tendon.

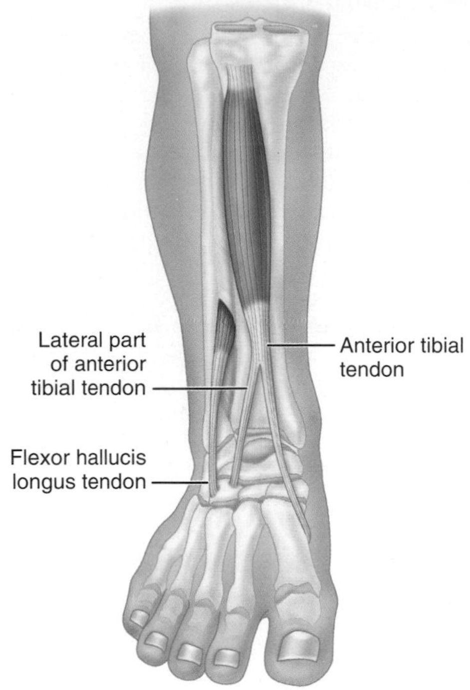

FIGURE 33-42 Technique of Perry et al. to correct equinovarus deformity in stroke patients. Lateral three fourths of anterior tibial tendon and flexor hallucis longus tendon are transferred to third cuneiform. Flexor digitorum longus is released (see text). **SEE TECHNIQUE 33-24.**

- Lengthen the Achilles tendon as described in Technique 33-10.
- With the ankle in the neutral position and the foot slightly everted, sew the two tendons to themselves as loops and to each other.
- The flexor digitorum longus can be transferred instead of the flexor hallucis longus if the toe flexors are active in the swing phase of gait.

POSTOPERATIVE CARE. Because the Achilles tendon has been lengthened, a cast is applied with the foot in slight plantar flexion. At 6 weeks, the cast is removed and the foot is protected with a locked ankle brace for an additional 6 months. Because the muscles in a hemiplegic patient pull strongly or not at all, several months are necessary for the scar to mature enough not to yield under tension.

Satisfactory results have been reported in adult hemiplegics with talipes equinovarus using a procedure that consists of triple sectioning of the Achilles tendon, open Z-plasty lengthening and suturing of the posterior tibial tendon just proximal to the medial malleolus, transfer of one half of the anterior tibial tendon to the third cuneiform, and transverse division of the flexor digitorum brevis and the flexor digitorum longus tendons at the base of each toe.

VARUS FOOT

The anterior tibial muscle usually is the deforming force in a patient with forefoot varus. A split anterior tibial tendon transfer (see Technique 33-18) is the procedure of choice for this condition as long as a fixed hindfoot varus is not present. A short leg walking cast is worn for 6 weeks. An ankle-foot orthosis is used when walking to protect the muscle transfer for an additional 6 months.

PLANOVALGUS

If pes planus preceded the stroke, in rare cases a planovalgus deformity can occur after the stroke. Spasticity of the triceps surae pulls the calcaneus laterally, and the peroneals may be hyperactive with no opposing posterior tibial muscle function during stance phase. If walking is impeded by pain, surgical correction is indicated. As in equinus deformity, the treatment involves lengthening of the Achilles tendon with a triple-level hemitenotomy. The distal hemisection in the Achilles tendon is performed in the lateral half of the tendon to reduce the valgus placement or thrust of the tendon on the calcaneus.

If the peroneals are hyperactive during stance phase, the peroneus brevis can be transferred medially into the posterior tibial tendon to support the medial border of the foot or the peroneus longus and brevis can be lengthened. A triple arthrodesis ultimately is required if an ankle-foot orthosis does not control the deformity.

TOE FLEXION

Toe flexion occurs at the metatarsophalangeal joint and is different from the claw toe deformity in most neurologic disorders in which the extensors are hyperactive. Toe curling or toe flexion in a stroke patient occurs from overactivity of the long toe flexors. These can be released by tenotomies of the toe flexor tendons at the level of the metatarsophalangeal joint.

UPPER EXTREMITY

The prognosis for recovering normal function in the upper extremity in stroke patients is poor, and approximately one third are left with a permanently functionless limb. The most important reason for this is that the patterns of neuromuscular activity in the normally functioning upper extremity are highly sophisticated and complex and are modified by multiple sophisticated somatosensory impulses. Permanent impairment in motor and sensory function in the upper extremity is incurable, and permanent impairment of function is to be expected. Upper limb recovery after stroke is adaptive and consists of training the individual to accomplish activities of daily living as a one-handed person. For patients who show sufficient neurologic recovery, additional training for development of assistive function is indicated.

The orthopaedic surgeon may release contractures, weaken spastic muscles that cause imbalance and deformity, and transfer functioning muscle units to attempt to restore some balance to the affected extremity. These operations also can relieve persistent pain, which causes further immobility and lack of participation in other areas of rehabilitation.

SHOULDER

Some stroke patients report pain localized precisely to the shoulder and specifically to the adductor and internal rotator groups. In others, a hemicorporeal type of diffuse discomfort is present and is untreatable by present methods. Patients with the first type of pain develop progressively decreasing ranges of motion despite intensive conservative treatment. They also have an exaggerated stretch reflex on rapid external rotation of the shoulder, abduction of less than 45 degrees, and internal rotation of less than 15 degrees. Modalities such as suprascapular nerve blocks, joint injection, use of BTX-A, and therapy/taping programs are of minimal benefit. Surgery is recommended only for patients who have a reasonable potential for rehabilitation. A review of 34 adults with spastic hemiparesis who had fractional lengthening of the pectoralis major, latissimus dorsi, and teres major had improvements in their spasticity scores, shoulder range of motion, especially external rotation, as well as pain relief and a high degree of satisfaction with the outcome.

RELEASE OF INTERNAL ROTATION CONTRACTURE OF THE SHOULDER

In a comparison study, patients who had internal rotation contracture release showed significant improvement in motion in 10 of 13 patients. Of 12 control patients with similar symptoms not treated by surgery, none had a spontaneous resolution of the painful joint contracture.

TECHNIQUE 33-25

- Make an anterior deltopectoral approach to the shoulder.
- Identify the subscapularis tendon and cauterize the vascular bundle at its distal edge. Excise this tendon, but preserve the anterior capsule of the shoulder joint.
- Palpate the tendon of the pectoralis major and, with scissors passed distally along the humerus, cut its tendinous insertion.

POSTOPERATIVE CARE. A sling is worn on the arm, and a program of assisted range-of-motion exercises is begun within the first few days of surgery. Reciprocal pulley exercises are begun within the first 5 days. It is important to supervise the patient's participation in the exercises.

FRACTIONAL LENGTHENING OF PECTORALIS MAJOR, LATISSIMUS DORSI, TERES MAJOR

TECHNIQUE 33-26

- With the patient in the beachchair position with a bolster between the scapula, make a deltopectoral approach (see Technique 1-87) to expose the pectoralis major tendon.
- Divide the tendon as it overlaps the muscle belly on the undersurface.
- Identify the brachial plexus and retract it medially.
- Identify the insertions of the latissimus dorsi and teres major in the interval between the short head of the biceps and the deltoid.
- Lengthen the tendons at the musculotendinous junction.
- The long head of the triceps can be lengthened if further correction of elbow extension is desired.
- Place a drain and close in layers.

POSTOPERATIVE CARE. A sling is worn on the arm for comfort, and a program of assisted range-of-motion exercises is begun within the first few days of surgery.

ELBOW

Fixed flexion of the elbow seriously impairs function of the upper extremity. Some patients with mild spasticity may benefit from the early use of BTX-A in conjunction with physical therapy. For those who do not respond to nonoperative measures and who have reasonable functional goals, surgical release of the elbow can be considered. A review of 42 patients with elbow flexion deformities showed improvements in active and passive range of motion with a low rate of superficial wound problems at a mean of 6 years after anterior release and fractional myotendinous elbow flexor lengthening.

PHENOL NERVE BLOCK

Phenol injection into motor nerves in adults and children with spastic hemiplegia produced early improvement in 17 of 18 patients. Unfortunately, the results deteriorated over 6 months, with 2 patients having recurrence of the deformity within 1 year. The 6-month window allows time to begin treatment programs aimed at decreasing contractures and to train weakened muscles before the spasticity returns. In addition, patients who receive nerve ablation can have sensory loss that can lead to painful dysesthesia. For these reasons, as well as the reversible nature of BTX-A, the use of phenol nerve block is decreasing.

FUNCTIONAL ELECTRICAL NERVE STIMULATION

Functional electrical stimulation allows restoration of function in paralyzed muscles by electrical stimulation. The aim is to have functional muscle control occur during stimulation, but occasionally a carryover occurs, and the muscle comes under voluntary control. Functional electrical stimulation theoretically depends on a single stimulation, such as heel lift, being transferred through an antenna to an electrical implant, which fires another signal to the nerve supply to the muscles, such as the peroneal nerve, to perform a function, such as dorsiflexion to the foot. The device needs to be small and cosmetically acceptable, and the activity should be under some degree of voluntary control; otherwise too much stimulation may occur. Functional electrical stimulation is used in the upper and lower extremities, around the foot and ankle to suppress spasticity, to correct scoliosis, for electrophrenic respiration, and for bladder control. There remains a need for external control of motor unit gradation, for synergistic activity in other muscles, and for some proprioceptive kinesthetic feedback.

REFERENCES

GENERAL

Akerstedt A, Risto O, Odman P, Oberg B: Evaluation of single event multilevel surgery and rehabilitation in children and youth with cerebral palsy—a 2-year follow-up study, *Disabil Rehabil* 32:530, 2010.

Akpinar P, Tezel CG, Eliasson AC, et al: Reliability and cross-cultural validation of the Turkish version of Manual Ability Classification System (MACS) for children with cerebral palsy, *Disabil Rehabil* 32:1910, 2010.

Ali O, Shim M, Fowler E, et al: Growth hormone therapy improves bone mineral density in children with cerebral palsy: a preliminary pilot study, *J Clin Endocrinol Metab* 92:932, 2007.

Bajelidze G, Beilthur MV, Littleton AG, et al: Diagnostic evaluation using whole-body technetium bone scan in children with cerebral palsy and pain, *J Pediatr Orthop* 28:112, 2008.

Gannotti ME, Gorton GE 3rd, Nahorniak MT, Masso PD: Walking abilities of young adults with cerebral palsy: changes after multilevel surgery and adolescence, *Gait Posture* 32:46, 2010.

Gollapudi K, Feeley BT, Otsuka NY: Advanced skeletal maturity in ambulatory cerebral palsy patients, *J Pediatr Orthop* 27:295, 2007.

Imms C, Carlin J, Eliasson AC: Stability of caregiver-reported manual ability and gross motor function classifications of cerebral palsy, *Dev Med Child Neurol* 52:153, 2010.

Kanellopoulos AD, Mavrogenis AF, Mitsiokapa EA, et al: Long lasting benefits following the combination of static night upper extremity splinting with botulinum toxin A injections in cerebral palsy children, *Eur J Phys Rehabil Med* 45:501, 2009.

Lee SH, Chung CY, Park MS, et al: Parental satisfaction after single-event multilevel surgery in ambulatory children with cerebral palsy, *J Pediatr Orthop* 29:398, 2009.

Minhas SV, Chow I, Otsuka NY: The effect of body mass index on postoperative morbidity after orthopaedic surgery in children with cerebral palsy, *J Pediatr Orthop* 2015 Apr 17. [Epub ahead of print].

Park MS, Chung CY, Lee KM, et al: Issues of concern before single event multilevel surgery in patients with cerebral palsy, *J Pediatr Orthop* 30:489, 2010.

Saraph V, Zwick EB, Steinwender G, et al: Leg lengthening as part of gait improvement surgery in cerebral palsy: an evaluation using gait analysis, *Gait Posture* 23:83, 2006.

Svehlik M, Steinwender G, Kraus T, et al: The influence of age at single-event multilevel surgery on outcome in children with cerebral palsy who walk with flexed knee gait, *Dev Med Child Neurol* 53:730, 2011.

Thompson N, Stebbins J, Seniorou M, et al: The use of minimally invasive techniques in multi-level surgery for children with cerebral palsy: preliminary results, *J Bone Joint Surg* 92B:1442, 2010.

Westbomb L, Bergsrand L, Wagner P, Nordmark E: Survival at 19 years of age in a total population of children and young people with cerebral palsy, *Dev Med Child Neurol* 53:808, 2011.

NEUROSURGICAL TREATMENT

Armstron RW: The first meta-analysis of randomized controlled surgical trials in cerebral palsy (2002), *Dev Med Child Neurol* 50:244, 2008.

Carraro E, Zeme S, Ticcinelli V, et al: Multidimensional outcome measure of selective dorsal rhizotomy in spastic cerebral palsy, *Eur J Paediatr Neurol* 18:704, 2014.

Cole GF, Farmer SE, Roberts A, et al: Selective dorsal rhizotomy for children with cerebral palsy: the Oswestry experience, *Arch Dis Child* 92:781, 2007.

Criswell SR, Crowner BE, Racette BA: The use of botulinum toxin therapy for lower-extremity spasticity in children with cerebral palsy, *Neurosurg Focus* 21:e1, 2006.

Dudley RW, Parolin M, Gagnon B, et al: Long-term functional benefits of selective dorsal rhizotomy for spastic cerebral palsy, *J Neurosurg Pediatr* 12:142, 2013.

Grunt S, Fieggen AG, Vermeulen RJ, et al: Selection criteria for selective dorsal rhizotomy in children with spastic cerebral palsy: a systematic review of the literature, *Dev Med Child Neurol* 56:302, 2014.

Hurvitz EA, Marciniak CM, Daunter AK, et al: Functional outcomes of childhood dorsal rhizotomy in adults and adolescents with cerebral palsy, *J Neurosurg Pediatr* 11:380, 2013.

Langerak NG, Lamberts RP, Fleggen AG, et al: A prospective gait analysis study in patients with diplegic cerebral palsy 20 years after selective dorsal rhizotomy, *J Neurosurg Pediatr* 1:180, 2008.

Lundkvist A, Hagglund G: Orthopaedic surgery after selective dorsal rhizotomy, *J Pediatr Orthop B* 15:244, 2006.

Park TS, Johnston JM: Surgical techniques of selective dorsal rhizotomy for spastic cerebral palsy, *Neurosurg Focus* 21:E7, 2006.

Ramachandran M, Eastwood DM: Botulinum toxin and its orthopaedic applications, *J Bone Joint Surg* 88B:981, 2006.

Tedroff K, Löwing K, Jacobson DN, Aström E: Does loss of spasticity matter? A 10-year follow-up after selective dorsal rhizotomy in cerebral palsy, *Dev Med Child Neurol* 53:724, 2011.

HIP

Bayusentono S, Choi Y, Chung CY, et al: Recurrence of hip instability after reconstructive surgery in patients with cerebral palsy, *J Bone Joint Surg* 96:1527, 2014.

Boldingh EJ, Bouwhuis CB, van der Heijden-Maessen HC, et al: Palliative hip surgery in severe cerebral palsy: a systematic review, *J Pediatr Orthop B* 23:86, 2014.

Braatz F, Staude D, Klotz MC, et al: Hip-joint congruity after Dega osteotomy in patients with cerebral palsy: long-term results, *Int Orthop* 2015 Oct 10. [Epub ahead of print].

Chang CH, Chen YY, Wang CJ, et al: Dynamic displacement of the femoral head by hamstring stretching in children with cerebral palsy, *J Pediatr Orthop* 30:475, 2010.

Chang FM, Ma J, Pan Z, et al: Acetabular remodeling after a varus derotational osteotomy in children with cerebral palsy, *J Pediatr Orthop* 36(2):198–204, 2016.

Chung CY, Park MS, Choi IH, et al: Morphometric analysis of acetabular dysplasia in cerebral palsy, *J Bone Joint Surg* 88B:243, 2006.

Cobelijic G, Bajin Z, Lesic A, et al: A radiographic and clinical comparison of two soft-tissue procedures for paralytic subluxation of the hip in cerebral palsy, *Int Orthop* 33:503, 2009.

Dartnell J, Gough M, Paterson JM, Norman-Taylor F: Proximal femoral resection without post-operative traction for the painful dislocated hip in patients with cerebral palsy: a review of 79 cases, *Bone Joint J* 96B:701, 2014.

DiFazio R, Vessey JA, Miller P, et al: Postoperative complications after hip surgery in patients with cerebral palsy: a retrospective matched cohort study, *J Pediatr Orthop* 36:56, 2016.

El Hage S, Rachkidi R, Noun Z, et al: Is percutaneous adductor tenotomy as effective and safe as the open procedure, *J Pediatr Orthop* 30:485, 2010.

Fucs PM, Yamada HH: Hip fusion as hip salvage procedure in cerebral palsy, *J Pediatr Orthop* 34(Suppl 1):S32, 2014.

Hachache B, Eid T, Ghosn E, et al: Is percutaneous proximal gracilis tenotomy as effective and safe as the open procedure? *J Child Orthop* 9(6):477–481, 2015.

Hägglund G, Alriksson-Schmidt A, Lauge-Pedersen H, et al: Prevention of dislocation of the hip in children with cerebral palsy: 20-year results of a population-based prevention programme, *Bone Joint J* 96B:2014, 1546.

Hermanson M, Hägglund G, Riad J, Wagner P: Head-shaft angle is a risk factor for hip displacement in children with cerebral palsy, *Acta Orthop* 86:229, 2015.

Huh K, Rethlefsen SA, Wren TA, Kay RM: Surgical management of hip subluxation and dislocation in children with cerebral palsy: isolated VDRO or combined surgery? *J Pediatr Orthop* 31:858, 2011.

Khalife R, Ghanem I, El Hage S, et al: Risk of recurrent dislocation and avascular necrosis after proximal femoral varus osteotomy in children with cerebral palsy, *J Pediatr Orthop B* 19:32, 2010.

Koi PS, Jameson PG 2nd, Chang TL, Sponseller PD: Transverse-plane pelvic asymmetry in patients with cerebral palsy and scoliosis, *J Pediatr Orthop* 31:277, 2011.

Krebs A, Strobl WM, Grill F: Neurogenic hip dislocation in cerebral palsy: quality of life and results after hip reconstruction, *J Child Orthop* 2:125, 2008.

Lanert P, Risto O, Hägglund G, Wagner P: Hip displacement in relation to age and gross motor function in children with cerebral palsy, *J Child Orthop* 8:129, 2014.

Lovejoy SA, Tylkowski C, Oeffinger D, et al: The effects of hamstring lengthening on hip rotation, *J Pediatr Orthop* 27:142, 2007.

Morton RE, Scott B, McClelland V, Henry A: Dislocation of the hips in children with bilateral spastic cerebral palsy, 1985-2000, *Dev Med Child Neurol* 48:555, 2006.

Raphael BS, Dines JS, Akerman M, Root L: Long-term followup of total hip arthroplasty in patients with cerebral palsy, *Clin Orthop Relat Res* 468:1845, 2010.

Riccio AI, Carney CD, Hammell LC, et al: Three-dimensional computed tomography for determination of femoral anteversion in a cerebral palsy model, *J Pediatr Orthop* 35:167, 2015.

Robb JE, Brunner R: A Dega-type osteotomy after closure of the triradiate cartilage in non-walking patients with severe cerebral palsy, *J Bone Joint Surg* 88B:933, 2006.

Robin J, Graham HK, Selber P, et al: Proximal femoral geometry in cerebral palsy: a population-based cross-sectional study, *J Bone Joint Surg* 90B:1372, 2008.

Rodda JM, Graham HK, Nattrass GR, et al: Correction of severe crouch gait in patients with spastic diplegia with use of multilevel orthopaedic surgery, *J Bone Joint Surg* 88A:2653, 2006.

Rutz E, Gaston MS, Tirosh O, Brunner R: Hip flexion deformity improves without psoas-lengthening after surgical correction of fixed knee flexion deformity in spastic diplegia, *Hip Int* 22:379, 2012.

Rutz E, Vavken P, Camathias C, et al: Long-term results and outcome predictors in one-stage hip reconstruction in children with cerebral palsy, *J Bone Joint Surg* 97:500, 2015.

Ruzbarsky JJ, Beck NA, Baldwin KD, et al: Risk factors and complications in hip reconstruction for nonambulatory patients with cerebral palsy, *J Child Orthop* 7:487, 2013.

Sankar WN, Spiegel DA, Gregg JR, Sennett BJ: Long-term follow-up after one-stage reconstruction of dislocated hips in patients with cerebral palsy, *J Pediatr Orthop* 26:1, 2006.

Shore B, Spence D, Graham H: The role for hip surveillance in children with cerebral palsy, *Curr Rev Musculoskelet Med* 5:126, 2012.

Soo B, Howard JJ, Boyd RN, et al: Hip displacement in cerebral palsy, *J Bone Joint Surg* 88A:121, 2006.

Terjesen T: Development of the hip joints in unoperated children with cerebral palsy: a radiographic study of 76 patients, *Acta Orthop* 77:125, 2006.

Zhang S, Wilson NC, Mackey AH, Stott NS: Radiological outcome of reconstructive hip surgery in children with gross motor function classification system IV and V cerebral palsy, *J Pediatr Orthop B* 23:430, 2014.

KNEE

Al-Aubaidi Z, Lundgaard B, Pedersen NW: Anterior distal femoral hemiepiphysiodesis in the treatment of fixed knee flexion contracture in neuromuscular patients, *J Child Orthop* 6:313, 2012.

Blumetti FC, Morais Filho MC, Kawamura CM, et al: Does the GMFCS level influence the improvement in knee range of motion after rectus femoris transfer in cerebral palsy? *J Pediatr Orthop B* 24:433, 2015.

Brunner R, Camathias C, Gaston M, Rutz E: Supracondylar osteotomy of the paediatric femur using the locking compression plate: a refined surgical technique, *J Child Orthop* 7:571, 2013.

Choi Y, Lee SH, Chung CY, et al: Anterior knee pain in patients with cerebral palsy, *Clin Orthop Surg* 6:426, 2014.

Inan M, Sarikaya IA, Yildirim E, Güven MF: Neurological complications after supracondylar femoral osteotomy in cerebral palsy, *J Pediatr Orthop* 35:290, 2015.

Klatt J, Stevens PM: Guided growth for fixed knee flexion deformity, *J Pediatr Orthop* 28:626, 2008.

Lee SY, Kwon SS, Chung CY, et al: Rectus femoris transfer in cerebral palsy patients with stiff knee gait, *Gait Posture* 40:76, 2014.

Leet AI, Shirley ED, Barker C, et al: Treatment of femur fractures in children with cerebral palsy, *J Child Orthop* 3:253, 2009.

McMulkin ML, Gordon AB, Caskey PM, et al: Outcomes of orthopaedic surgery with and without an external femoral derotational osteotomy in children with cerebral palsy, *J Pediatr Orthop* 2015 Apr 1. [Epub ahead of print].

Novacheck TF, Stout JL, Gage JR, Schwartz MH: Distal femoral extension osteotomy and patellar tendon advancement to treat persistent crouch gait in cerebral palsy. Surgical technique, *J Bone Joint Surg* 91A(Suppl 2):271, 2009.

Patthanacharoenphon C, Maples DL, Saad C, et al: The effects of patellar tendon advancement on the immature proximal tibia, *J Child Orthop* 7:139, 2013.

Rethlefsen SA, Nguyen DT, Wren TA, et al: Knee pain and patellofemoral symptoms in patients with cerebral palsy, *J Pediatr Orthop* 35:519, 2015.

Rethlefsen SA, Yasmeh S, Wren TA, Kay RM: Repeat hamstring lengthening for crouch gait in children with cerebral palsy, *J Pediat Orthop* 33:501, 2013.

Scully WF, McMulkin ML, Baird GO, et al: Outcomes of rectus femoris transfer in children with cerebral palsy: effect of transfer site, *J Pediatr Orthop* 33:303, 2013.

Senaran H, Holden C, Dabney KW, et al: Anterior knee pain in children with cerebral palsy, *J Pediatr Orthop* 27:12, 2007.

Skiak E, Karakasli A, Basci O, et al: Distal femoral derotational osteotomy with external fixation for correction of excessive femoral anteversion in patients with cerebral palsy, *J Pediatr Orthop B* 24:425, 2015.

Stout JL, Gage JR, Schwartz MH, Novacheck TF: Distal femoral extension osteotomy and patellar tendon advancement to treat persistent crouch gait in cerebral palsy, *J Bone Joint Surg* 90A:2470, 2008.

Westberry DE, Davids JR, Jacobs JM, et al: Effectiveness of serial stretch casting for resistant or recurrent knee flexion contractures following hamstring lengthening in children with cerebral palsy, *J Pediatr Orthop* 26:109, 2006.

FOOT AND ANKLE

Adams SB Jr, Simpson AW, Pugh LI, Stasikelis PJ: Calcaneocuboid joint subluxation after calcaneal lengthening for planovalgus foot deformity in children with cerebral palsy, *J Pediatr Orthop* 29:170, 2009.

Boffeli TJ, Collier RC: Surgical treatment guidelines for digital deformity associated with intrinsic muscle spasticity (intrinsic plus foot) in adults with cerebral palsy, *J Foot Ankle Surg* 54:985, 2015.

Danino B, Erel S, Kfir M, et al: Are gait indices sensitive enough to reflect the effect of ankle foot orthosis on gait impairment in cerebral palsy diplegic patients? *J Pediatr Orthop* 2015 Mar 6. [Epub ahead of print].

Ettl V, Wollmerstedt N, Kirschner S, et al: Calcaneal lengthening for planovalgus deformity in children with cerebral palsy, *Foot Ankle Int* 30:398, 2009.

Firth GB, McMullan M, Chin T, et al: Lengthening of the gastrocnemius-soleus complex: an anatomical and biomechanical study in human cadavers, *J Bone Joint Surg* 95:1489, 2013.

Firth BG, Passmore E, Sangeux M, et al: Multilevel surgery for equinus gait in children with spastic diplegic cerebral palsy. Medium-term follow-up with gait analysis, *J Bone Joint Surg* 95:931, 2013.

Handelsman JE, Weinberg J, Corso S: Management of long toe flexor spasticity in the equinus foot in cerebral palsy, *J Pediatr Orthop B* 16:185, 2007.

Houx L, Lempereur M, Rémy-Néris O, Brochard S: Threshold of equinus which alters biomechanical gait parameters in children, *Gait Posture* 38:582, 2013.

Huang CN, Wu KW, Hunag SC, et al: Medial column stabilization improves the early result of calcaneal lengthening in children with cerebral palsy, *J Pediatr Orthop B* 22:233, 2013.

Jaddue DA, Abbas MA, Sayed-Noor AS: Open versus percutaneous tendo-Achilles lengthening in spastic cerebral palsy with equinus deformity of the foot in children, *J Surg Orthop Adv* 19:196, 2010.

Kadhim M, Holmes L Jr, Church C, et al: Pes planovalgus deformity surgical correction in ambulatory children with cerebral palsy, *J Child Orthop* 6:217, 2012.

Kadhim M, Holmes L Jr, Miller F: Long-term ourcome of planovalgus foot surgical correction in children with cerebral palsy, *J Foot Ankle Surg* 52:697, 2013.

Kadhim M, Miller F: Crouch gait changes after planovalgus foot deformity correction in ambulatory children with cerebral palsy, *Gait Posture* 39:793, 2014.

Kadhim M, Miller F: Pes planovalgus deformity in children with cerebral palsy: review article, *J Pediatr Orthop B* 23:400, 2014.

Lee IH, Chung CY, Lee KM, et al: Incidence and risk factors of allograft bone failure after calcaneal lengthening, *Clin Orthop Relat Res* 473:1765, 2015.

Michlitsch MG, Rethlefsen SA, Kay RM: The contributions of anterior and posterior tibialis dysfunction to varus foot deformity in patients with cerebral palsy, *J Bone Joint Surg* 88A:1764, 2006.

Narayanan UG: The role of gait analysis in the orthopaedic management of ambulatory cerebral palsy, *Curr Opin Pediatr* 19:38, 2007.

Park KB, Park HW, Lee KS, et al: Changes in dynamic foot pressure after surgical treatment of valgus deformity of the hindfoot in cerebral palsy, *J Bone Joint Surg* 90A:1712, 2008.

Rethlefsen SA, Healty BS, Wren TA, et al: Causes of intoeing gait in children with cerebral palsy, *J Bone Joint Surg* 88A:2175, 2006.

Ries AJ, Novacheck TF, Schwartz MH: The efficacy of ankle-foot orthoses on improving the gait of children with diplegic cerebral palsy: a multiple outcome analysis, *PM R* 7:922, 2015.

Shore BJ, Smith KR, Riazi A, et al: Subtalar fusion for pes valgus in cerebral palsy: results of a modified technique in the setting of single event multilevel surgery, *J Pediatr Orthop* 33:431, 2013.

Shore BJ, White N, Kerr Graham H: Surgical correction of equinus deformity in children with cerebral palsy: a systematic review, *J Child Orthop* 4:277, 2010.

Trehan SK, Ihekweazu UN, Root L: Long-term outcomes of triple arthrodesis in cerebral palsy patients, *J Pediatr Orthop* 35:751, 2015.

Wren TA, Chatwood AP, Rethlefsen SA, et al: Achilles tendon length and medial gastrocnemius architecture in children with cerebral palsy and equinus gait, *J Pediatr Orthop* 30:479, 2010.

Zeifang F, Breusch SJ, Döderlein L: Evans calcaneal lengthening procedure for spastic flexible flatfoot in 32 patients (46 feet) with a followup of 3 to 9 years, *Foot Ankle Int* 27:500, 2006.

SPINE

Abol Oyoun N, Stuecker R: Bilateral rib-to-pelvis Eiffel Tower VEPTR construct for children with neuromuscular scoliosis: a preliminary report, *Spine J* 14:1183, 2014.

Bohtz C, Meyer-Heim A, Min K: Changes in health-related quality of life after spinal fusion and scoliosis correction in patients with cerebral palsy, *J Pediatr Orthop* 31:668, 2011.

Borkhuu B, Borowski A, Shah SA, et al: Antibiotic-loaded allograft decreases the rate of acute deep wound infection after spinal fusion in cerebral palsy, *Spine* 33:2300, 2008.

Hasler CC: Operative treatment for spinal deformities in cerebral palsy, *J Child Orthop* 7:419, 2013.

Lee SY, Chung CY, Lee KM, et al: Annual changes in radiographic indices of the spine in cerebral palsy patients, *Eur Spine J* 2015 Jan 9. [Epub ahead of print].

Lonstein JE, Koop SE, Novachek TF, Perra JH: Results and complications after spinal fusion for neuromuscular scoliosis in cerebral palsy and static encephalopathy using Luque Galveston instrumentation: experience in 93 patients, *Spine* 37:583, 2012.

McElroy MJ, Sponseller PD, Dattilo JR, et al: Growing rods for the treatment of scoliosis in children with cerebral palsy: a critical assessment, *Spine* 37:E1504, 2012.

Mensch S, Penning C: Comment on Watanabe K, Lenke LG, Daubs MD, et al: Is spine deformity surgery in patients with spastic cerebral palsy truly beneficial? *Spine* 34:2222–2232, 2009; Spine 35:E621, 2010; author reply E621.

Modi HN, Hong JY, Mehta SS, et al: Surgical correction and fusion using posterior-only pedicle screw construct for neuropathic scoliosis in patients with cerebral palsy: a three-year follow-up study, *Spine* 34:1167, 2009.

Mohamed A, Koutharawu DN, Miller F, et al: Operative and clinical markers of deep wound infection after spine fusion in children with cerebral palsy, *J Pediatr Orthop* 30:851, 2010.

Sewell MD, Malagelada F, Wallace C, et al: A preliminary study to assess whether spinal fusion for scoliosis improves carer-assessed quality of life for children with GMFCS level IV or V cerebral palsy, *J Pediatr Orthop* 2015 Mar 3. [Epub ahead of print].

Shilt JS, Lai LP, Cabrerar MN, et al: The impact of intrathecal baclofen on the natural history of scoliosis in cerebral palsy, *J Pediatr Orthop* 28:684, 2008.

Sponseller PD, Jain A, Shah SA, et al: Deep wound infections after fusion in children with cerebral palsy: a prospective cohort study, *Spine* 38:2023, 2013.

Sponseller PD, Shah SA, Abel MF, et al: Infection rate of spine surgery in cerebral palsy is high and impairs results: multicenter analysis of risk factors and treatment, *Clin Orthop Relat Res* 468:711, 2010.

Tsirikos AI, Mains E: Surgical correction of spinal deformity in patients with cerebral palsy using pedicle screw instrumentation, *J Spinal Disord Tech* 25:401, 2012.

UPPER EXTREMITY

Barus D, Kozin SH: The evaluation and treatment of elbow dysfunction secondary to spasticity and paralysis, *J Hand Ther* 19:192, 2006.

Domzalski M, Inan M, Littleton AG, Miller F: Pectoralis major release to improve shoulder abduction in children with cerebral palsy, *J Pediatr Orthop* 27:457, 2007.

Gigante P, McDowell MM, Bruce SS, et al: Reduction in upper-extremity tone after lumbar selective dorsal rhizotomy in children with spastic cerebral palsy, *J Neurosurg Pediatr* 12:588, 2013.

Gong HS, Cho HE, Chung CY, et al: Early results of anterior elbow release with and without biceps lengthening in patients with cerebral palsy, *J Hand Surg [Am]* 39:902, 2014.

Koman LA, Smith BP, Williams R, et al: Upper extremity spasticity in children with cerebral palsy: a randomized, double-blind, placebo-controlled study of the short-term outcomes of treatment with botulinum A toxin, *J Hand Surg [Am]* 38:435, 2013.

Leafblad ND, Van Heest AE: Management of the spastic wrist and hand in cerebral palsy, *J Hand Surg [Am]* 40:1035, 2015.

Makki D, Duodu J, Nixon M: Prevalence and pattern of upper limb involvement in cerebral palsy, *J Child Orthop* 8:215, 2014.

Park ES, Sim EG, Rha DW: Effect of upper limb deformities on gross motor and upper limb functions in children with spastic cerebral palsy, *Res Dev Disabil* 32:2389, 2011.

Smitherman JA, Davids JR, Tanner S, et al: Functional outcomes following single-event multilevel surgery of the upper extremity for children with hemiplegic cerebral palsy, *J Bone Joint Surg* 93A:655, 2011.

Van Heest AE, Bagley A, Molitor F, James MA: Tendon transfer surgery in upper-extremity cerebral palsy is more effective than botulinum toxin injections or regular ongoing therapy, *J Bone Joint Surg* 97:529, 2015.

ADULTS WITH CEREBRAL PALSY

Frisch D, Msall ME: Health, functioning, and participation of adolescents and adults with cerebral palsy: a review of outcomes research, *Dev Disabil Res Rev* 18:84, 2013.

Hemming K, Hutton JL, Pharoah PO: Long-term survival for a cohort of adults with cerebral palsy, *Dev Med Child Neurol* 48:90, 2006.

Lariviere-Bastien D, Bell E, Majnemer A, et al: Perspectives of young adults with cerebral palsy on transitioning from pediatric to adult healthcare systems, *Semin Pediatr Neurol* 20:154, 2013.

Michelsen SI, Uldall P, Hansen T, Madsen M: Social integration of adults with cerebral palsy, *Dev Med Child Neurol* 48:643, 2006.

Morgan P, McGinley J: Gait function and decline in adults with cerebral palsy: a systematic review, *Disabil Rehabil* 36:1, 2014.

Morgan PE, Soh SE, McGinley JL: Health-related quality of life of ambulant adults with cerebral palsy and its association with falls and mobility decline: a preliminary cross sectional study, *Health Qual Life Outcomes* 12:132, 2014.

Oetgen ME, Ayyala H, Martin BD: Treatment of hip subluxation in skeletally mature patients with cerebral palsy, *Orthopedics* 38:e248, 2015.

Opheim A, McGinley JL, Olsson E, et al: Walking deterioration and gait analysis in adults with spastic bilateral cerebral palsy, *Gait Posture* 37:165, 2013.

Reddihough DS, Jiang B, Lanigan A, et al: Social outcomes of young adults with cerebral palsy, *J Intellect Dev Disabil* 38:215, 2013.

Vogtle LK, Malone LA, Azuero A: Outcomes of an exercise program for pain and fatigue management in adults with cerebral palsy, *Disabil Rehabil* 36:818, 2014.

ADULT STROKE PATIENTS

Anakwenze OA, Namdari S, Hsu JE, et al: Myotendinous lengthening of the elbow flexor muscles to improve active motion in patients with elbow spasticity following brain injury, *J Shoulder Elbow Surg* 22:318, 2013.

Appel C, Perry L, Jones F: Shoulder strapping for stroke-related upper limb dysfunction and shoulder impairments: systematic review, *Neurorehabilitation* 35:191, 2014.

Bakheit AM: The pharmacological management of post-stroke muscle spasticity, *Drugs Aging* 29:941, 2012.

Carda S, Invernizzi M, Baricich A, Cisari C: Casting, taping or stretching after botulinum toxin type A for spastic equinus foot: a single-blind randomized trial on adult stroke patients, *Clin Rehabil* 25:1119, 2011.

Jeon WH, Park GW, Jeong HJ, Sim YJ: The comparison of effects of suprascapular nerve block, intra-articular steroid injection, and a combination therapy on hemiplegic shoulder pain: pilot study, *Ann Rehabil Med* 38:167, 2014.

Marciniak CM, Harvey RL, Gagnon CM, et al: Does botulinum toxin type A decrease pain and lessen disability in hemiplegic survivors of stroke with shoulder pain and spasticity? A randomized, double-blind, placebo-controlled trial, *Am J Phys Med Rehabil* 91:1007, 2012.

Mercer VS, Freburger JK, Yin Z, Preisser JS: Recovery of paretic lower extremity loading ability and physical function in the first six months after stroke, *Arch Phys Med Rehabil* 95:2014, 1547.

Namdari S, Alosh H, Baldwin K, et al: Outcomes of tendon fractional lengthenings to improve shoulder function in patients with spastic hemiparesis, *J Shoulder Elbow Surg* 21:691, 2012.

Otom AH, Al-Khawaja IM, Al-Quliti KW: Botulinum toxin type-A in the management of spastic equinovarus deformity after stroke. Comparison of 2 injection techniques, *Neurosciences (Riyadh)* 19:199, 2014.

Rosales RL, Kong KH, Goh KJ, et al: Botulinum toxin injection for hypertonicity of the upper extremity within 12 weeks after stroke: a randomized controlled trial, *Neurorehabil Neural Repair* 26:812, 2012.

Rousseaux M, Daveluy W, Kozlowski O, Allart E: Onabotulinumtoxin-A injection for disabling lower limb flexion in hemiplegic patients, *Neurorehabilitation* 35:25, 2014.

Tenniglo MJ, Nederhand MJ, Prinsen EC, et al: Effect of chemodenervation of the rectus femoris muscle in adults with a stiff knee gait due to spastic paresis: a systematic review with a meta-analysis in patients with stroke, *Arch Phys Med Rehabil* 95:576, 2014.

Vogt JC, Bach G, Cantini B, Perrin S: Split anterior tibial tendon transfer for varus equinus spastic foot deformity. Initial clinical findings correlate with functional results: a series of 132 operated feet, *Foot Ankle Surg* 17:178, 2011.

The complete list of references is available online at ***expertconsult.inkling.com.***

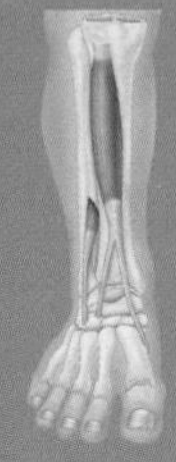

CHAPTER 34

PARALYTIC DISORDERS

William C. Warner Jr., James H. Beaty

POLIOMYELITIS

Acute anterior poliomyelitis is a viral infection localized in the anterior horn cells of the spinal cord and certain brainstem motor nuclei. One of three types of poliomyelitis viruses is usually the cause of infection, but other members of the enteroviral group can cause a condition clinically and pathologically indistinguishable from poliomyelitis. Viral transmission is primarily fecal-oral, and initial invasion by the virus occurs through the gastrointestinal and respiratory tracts and spreads to the central nervous system through a hematogenous route. Although most individuals in an endemic area are infected with poliovirus, only 0.5% of infected individuals develop paralytic poliomyelitis.

Since the introduction and extensive use of the poliomyelitis vaccine, the incidence of acute anterior poliomyelitis has decreased dramatically. In 1988, there were an estimated 350,000 cases; in 2013, fewer than 400 cases were reported. Currently, it most often affects children younger than 5 years old in developing tropical and subtropical countries and unimmunized individuals. In 2014, only three countries (Afghanistan, Nigeria, and Pakistan) were classified as polio-endemic by the WHO. Isolated outbreaks of poliomyelitis occurred in North America and Europe in the 1990s.

Administration of three doses of the Sabin oral polio vaccine, containing all three types of attenuated virus, can prevent the disease. The use of the live attenuated virus vaccine remains controversial. Live oral poliovirus vaccine (OPV) may immunize contacts who have not been vaccinated; however, this carries a risk of developing vaccine-associated paralytic polio, which has been estimated at 1 case per 2.5 million doses. Outbreaks of paralytic poliomyelitis in the United States have been associated with the use of live poliovirus vaccine. The implementation of an all-inactive polio vaccine (IPV) schedule in the United States in 2000 has eliminated indigenous acquired vaccine-associated poliomyelitis. Despite the safety and efficacy of the IPV, OPV remains the vaccine of choice for global eradication in many parts of the world where logistical issues and the higher cost of IPV prohibit its use and in places where inadequate sanitation necessitates an optimal mucosal barrier to wild-type poliovirus circulation. Challenges to the complete eradication of polio include the transmission of wild-type viruses in endemic areas, outbreaks related to vaccine-related polioviruses, and excretion of vaccine-related viruses in vaccines with B-cell immunodeficiencies.

PATHOLOGIC FINDINGS

When the poliomyelitis virus invades the body through the oropharyngeal route, it multiplies in the alimentary tract lymph nodes and spreads through the blood, acutely attacking the anterior horn ganglion cells of the spinal cord, especially in the lumbar and cervical enlargements. How the virus penetrates the blood-brain barrier and why the virus has a predilection for the anterior horn cell is under investigation. The incubation period is 6 to 20 days. The anterior horn motor cells may be damaged directly by viral multiplication or toxic by-products of the virus or indirectly by ischemia, edema, and hemorrhage in the glial tissues surrounding them. Destruction of the spinal cord occurs focally and randomly, and within 3 days, Wallerian degeneration is evident throughout the length of the individual nerve fiber. Macrophages and neutrophils surround and partially remove necrotic ganglion cells, and the inflammatory response gradually subsides. Within the muscle, axonal "sprouting" occurs when nerve cells from surviving motor units develop new axons, which innervate muscle cells that have lost their lower motor neuron, thus expanding the size of the motor unit. After 4 months, residual areas of gliosis and lymphocytic cells fill the area of destroyed motor cells in the spine. Reparative neuroglial cells proliferate. Continuous disease activity has been reported in spinal cord segments 20 years after disease onset.

The number of individual muscles affected by the resultant flaccid paralysis and the severity of paralysis vary; the clinical weakness is proportional to the number of lost motor units. Weakness is clinically detectable only when more than 60% of the nerve cells supplying the muscle have been destroyed. Muscles innervated by the cervical and lumbar spinal segments are most often affected, and paralysis occurs twice as often in the lower extremity muscles as in upper extremity muscles. In the lower extremity, the most commonly affected muscles are the quadriceps, glutei, anterior tibial, medial hamstrings, and hip flexors; in the upper extremity, the deltoid, triceps, and pectoralis major are most often affected.

The potential for recovery of muscle function depends on the recovery of damaged, but not destroyed, anterior horn cells. Most clinical recovery occurs during the first month after the acute illness and is almost complete within 6 months, although limited recovery may occur for about 2 years. A muscle paralyzed at 6 months remains paralyzed.

CLINICAL COURSE AND TREATMENT

Approximately 95% of patients infected with poliovirus remain asymptomatic. Nonspecific findings such as fever and sore throat occur in 4% to 8% of people infected. Between 0.5% and 2% of patients will progress to poliomyelitis. The course of poliomyelitis can be divided into three stages: acute, convalescent, and chronic. General guidelines for treatment are described here. Specific indications and techniques for operative procedures are discussed in specific sections.

ACUTE STAGE

The acute stage generally lasts 7 to 10 days, and up to 95% of all anterior horn cells may be infected. Symptoms range from mild malaise to generalized encephalomyelitis with widespread paralysis. With upper spinal cord involvement, diaphragmatic dysfunction and respiratory compromise can be life threatening. A high index of suspicion of this is necessary, especially in patients with shoulder involvement, given the close proximity of their respective anterior horn cells. In younger children, systemic symptoms include listlessness, sore throat, and a slight temperature elevation; these may resolve, but recurrent symptoms, including hyperesthesia or paresthesia in the extremities, severe headache, sore throat, vomiting, nuchal rigidity, back pain, and limitation of straight-leg raising, culminate in characteristically asymmetrical paralysis. In older children and adults, symptoms include slight temperature elevation, marked flushing of the skin, and apprehension; muscular pain is common. Muscles are tender even to gentle palpation. Superficial reflexes usually are absent first, and deep tendon reflexes disappear when the muscle group is paralyzed. Differential diagnoses include Guillain-Barré syndrome and other forms of encephalomyelitis. In rare cases, transverse myelitis can follow receipt of OPV.

Treatment of poliomyelitis in the acute stage generally consists of bed rest, analgesics, and anatomic positioning of the limbs to prevent contractures. Gentle, passive range-of-motion exercises of all joints should be performed several times daily.

CONVALESCENT STAGE

The convalescent stage begins 2 days after the temperature returns to normal and continues for 2 years. It has been estimated that approximately half of the infected anterior horn cells survive the initial infection, and muscle power improves spontaneously during this stage, especially during the first 4 months and more gradually thereafter. Treatment during this stage is similar to that during the acute stage. Muscle strength should be assessed monthly for 6 months and then every 3 months. Physical therapy should emphasize muscle activity in normal patterns and development of maximal capability of individual muscles. Muscles with more than 80% return of strength recover spontaneously without specific therapy. According to Johnson, an individual muscle with less than

30% of normal strength at 3 months should be considered permanently paralyzed.

Vigorous passive stretching exercises and wedging casts can be used for mild or moderate contractures. Surgical release of tight fascia and muscle aponeuroses and lengthening of tendons may be necessary for contractures persisting longer than 6 months. Orthoses should be used until no further recovery is anticipated.

■ CHRONIC STAGE

The chronic stage of poliomyelitis usually begins 24 months after the acute illness. During this time, the orthopaedist attempts to help the patient achieve maximal functional activity by management of the long-term consequences of muscle imbalance. Goals of treatment include correcting any significant muscle imbalances and preventing or correcting soft-tissue or bony deformities. Static joint instability usually can be controlled indefinitely by orthoses. Dynamic joint instability eventually results in a fixed deformity that cannot be controlled with orthoses. Young children are more prone than adults to develop bony deformity because of their growth potential. Soft-tissue surgery, such as tendon transfers, should be done in young children before the development of any fixed bony changes; bony procedures for correcting a deformity usually can be delayed until skeletal growth is near completion.

TENDON TRANSFERS

Tendon transfers are indicated when dynamic muscle imbalance results in a deformity that interferes with ambulation or function of the upper extremities. Surgery should be delayed until the maximal return of expected muscle strength in the involved muscle has been achieved. The objectives of a tendon transfer are (1) to provide active motor power to replace function of a paralyzed muscle or muscles, (2) to eliminate the deforming effect of a muscle when its antagonist is paralyzed, and (3) to improve stability by improving muscle balance.

Tendon transfer shifts a tendinous insertion from its normal attachment to another location so that its muscle can be substituted for a paralyzed muscle in the same region. In selecting a tendon for transfer, the following factors must be carefully considered:

1. *Strength.* The muscle to be transferred must be strong enough to accomplish what the paralyzed muscle did or to supplement the power of a partially paralyzed muscle. A muscle to be transferred should have a rating of *good* or *better* because a transferred muscle loses at least one grade in power after transfer.
2. *Efficiency.* The transferred tendon should be attached as close to the insertion of the paralyzed tendon as possible and should be routed in as direct a line as possible between the muscle's origin and its new insertion.
3. *Excursion.* The tendon to be transferred should have a range of excursion similar to the one it is reinforcing or replacing. It should be retained in its own sheath or into the sheath of another tendon or it should be passed through tissues, such as subcutaneous fat, that would allow it to glide. Routing a tendon through fascial or osseous tunnels can lead to scarring and decreased excursion.
4. *Neurovascular.* The nerve and blood supply to the transferred muscle must not be impaired or traumatized in making the transfer.
5. *Articular.* The joint on which the muscle is to act must be in a satisfactory position; any contractures must be released before the tendon transfer. A transferred muscle cannot be expected to correct a fixed deformity.
6. *Tension.* The transferred tendon must be securely attached under tension slightly greater than normal. If tension is insufficient, excursion is used in removing slack in the musculotendinous unit, rather than in producing the desired function.

Muscle transfers, whenever possible, should occur between agonistic muscles that are phasic, or active at the same time in the gait cycle. The anterior muscles of the leg are predominantly swing-phase muscles, and the posterior muscles, or flexors, are stance-phase muscles; in the thigh, the quadriceps is characteristically a stance-phase muscle, and the hamstrings are swing-phase muscles. In general, phasic transfers retain their preoperative phasic activities and regain their preoperative duration of contraction and electrical intensity. In contrast, nonphasic muscle transfers often retain their preoperative phasic activity and fail to assume the action of the muscles for which they are substituted and are not recommended. Some nonphasic transfers are capable of phasic conversion; however, phasic conversion is somewhat unpredictable and requires extensive postoperative physical therapy. Phasic conversion is not related to the use of splints and/or braces or time between disease onset and muscle transfer.

The ideal muscle for tendon transfer would have the same phasic activity as the paralyzed muscle, would be of about the same size in cross section and of equal strength, and could be placed in proper relationship to the axis of the joint to allow maximal mechanical effectiveness. Not all of these criteria can be met in every instance.

Paralytic deformities from muscle paralysis can be dynamic or static, and often both types are present. The extent to which the paralytic deformity is dynamic or static should be determined because a static deformity can be controlled with a brace in a growing child or with arthrodesis in an adult. A dynamic deformity is more likely to be appropriate for tendon transfer in children and adults. In a growing child with dynamic deformity, recurrence is possible with arthrodesis alone; in a child with static deformity, however, recurrence after arthrodesis is rare. In a growing child with dynamic deformity, an appropriate tendon transfer with minimal external support redistributes muscle power, preventing permanent deformity until the patient is old enough for an arthrodesis.

ARTHRODESIS

A relaxed or flail joint is stabilized by restricting its range of motion. Although a properly constructed brace may control a flail joint, a reconstructive operation that would not only eliminate the need for a brace but also improve function may be more effective. Arthrodesis is the most efficient method of permanent stabilization of a joint. Tenodeses that use flexor or extensor tendons to stabilize joints of the fingers (see Chapters 66 and 71) are notable exceptions, as are tenodeses of the peroneus longus or Achilles tendon in paralytic calcaneal deformity; results are satisfactory here because the pull of gravity and body weight usually are not enough to overstretch the tendons.

Because the lower extremities are designed primarily to support the weight of the body, it is important that their joints are stable and their muscles have sufficient power. When the control of one or more joints of the foot and ankle is lost because of paralysis, stabilization may be required. In the upper extremity, reach, grasp, pinch, and release require more mobility than stability and more dexterity than power. An operation to limit or obliterate motion in a joint of an upper extremity should be performed only after careful study of its advantages and disadvantages and of its general effect on the patient, especially in normal daily activity. Because of the high prevalence of lower extremity weakness in patients with poliomyelitis and because many patients use ambulatory assistive devices, any surgical treatment that affects the upper extremity can have a dramatic impact on ambulation as well. Arthrodesis of the shoulder is useful for some patients but has certain cosmetic and functional disadvantages that must be weighed. Arthrodesis of the elbow is rarely indicated in poliomyelitis. Arthrodesis of the wrist, although useful for some patients, may increase the disability of other patients. A patient who must use a wheelchair or crutches and has a wrist that is fused in the "optimal" position (for grasp and pinch) may be unable to rise from a chair or to manipulate crutches because he or she cannot shift the body weight to the palm of the hand with the wrist extended.

FOOT AND ANKLE

Because the foot and ankle are the most dependent parts of the body and are subjected to significant amounts of stress, they are especially susceptible to deformity from paralysis. The most common deformities of the foot and ankle include claw toes, cavovarus foot, dorsal bunion, talipes equinus, talipes equinovarus, talipes cavovarus, talipes equinovalgus, and talipes calcaneus. When the paralysis is of short duration, these dynamic deformities are not fixed and may be evident only on contraction of unopposed muscles or on weight bearing; later, as a result of muscle imbalance, habitual posturing, growth, and abnormal weight-bearing alignment, a permanent deformity can occur from contracture of the soft tissues and eventual osseous changes.

Ambulation requires a stable plantigrade foot with even weight distribution between the heel and forefoot and no significant fixed deformity. In the foot, muscle transfer is performed to prevent contracture formation, balance the muscles responsible for dorsiflexion and plantarflexion and for inversion and eversion, and reestablish as normal a gait as possible. Arthrodesis to correct deformity or stabilize the joints usually should be delayed until about age 10 to 12 years to allow for adequate growth of the foot.

TENDON TRANSFERS

Tendon transfers around the foot and ankle after 10 years of age can be supplemented by arthrodesis to correct fixed deformities, to establish enough lateral stability for weight bearing, and to compensate in part for the loss of function in the evertor and invertor muscles of the foot. When tendon transfers and arthrodesis are combined in the same operation, the arthrodesis should be performed first.

Transfer of a tendon usually is preferable to excision, not only to preserve function but also to prevent further atrophy of the leg. When the paralysis is severe enough to require arthrodesis, there usually is some weakness of the dorsiflexor or plantar flexor muscles. In this case, the invertor or evertor muscles can be transferred to the midline of the foot anteriorly or posteriorly into the calcaneus and Achilles tendon. In the rare instance when a muscle function is discarded, 7 to 10 cm of its tendon should be excised to prevent scarring of the tendon ends by fibrous tissue. In addition to arthrodesis and tendon transfers, any deformities of the leg, such as excessive tibial torsion, genu varum, or genu valgum (bowlegs), should be corrected because otherwise they might cause recurrence of the foot deformity.

PARALYSIS OF SPECIFIC MUSCLES

Isolated muscles may be paralyzed in patients with poliomyelitis, but more often combinations of muscles are affected. The specific muscle or muscles involved and the resulting muscle imbalance should be determined before treatment is started. Common deformities caused by muscle imbalance in the foot and ankle are described, according to the muscles involved. The exact pattern of muscle paralysis and the specific deformity that occurs must be carefully determined before any surgical intervention is undertaken.

ANTERIOR TIBIAL MUSCLE

Severe weakness or paralysis of the anterior tibial muscle results in loss of dorsiflexion and inversion power and produces a slowly progressive deformity (equinus and cavus or varying degrees of planovalgus) that is first evident in the swing phase of gait. The extensors of the long toe, which usually assist dorsiflexion, become overactive in an attempt to replace the paralyzed anterior tibial muscle, causing hyperextension of the proximal phalanges and depression of the metatarsal heads. A cavovarus deformity occasionally results from unopposed activity of the peroneus longus combined with an active posterior tibial muscle.

Passive stretching and serial casting can be tried before surgery to correct the equinus contracture. Posterior ankle capsulotomy and Achilles tendon lengthening occasionally are required and are combined with anterior transfer of the peroneus longus to the base of the second metatarsal. The peroneus brevis is sutured to the stump of the peroneus longus to prevent a dorsal bunion. As an alternative, the extensor digitorum longus can be recessed to the dorsum of the midfoot to supply active dorsiflexion. Claw toe deformity is managed by transfer of the long toe extensors into the metatarsal necks (see Chapter 86).

Plantar fasciotomy and release of intrinsic muscles may be necessary before tendon surgery for a fixed cavovarus deformity. In this situation, the peroneus longus is transferred to the base of the second metatarsal and the extensor hallucis longus is transferred to the neck of the first metatarsal. The claw toe deformity frequently recurs because of reattachment of the extensor hallucis longus; this can be prevented by suturing its distal stump to the extensor hallucis brevis.

ANTERIOR AND POSTERIOR TIBIAL MUSCLES

If the anterior tibial and the posterior tibial muscles are paralyzed, development of hindfoot and forefoot equinovalgus is more rapid and the deformity becomes fixed as the Achilles tendon and peroneal muscles shorten. This deformity may be similar to congenital vertical talus on a standing lateral radiograph, but the apparent vertical talus is not confirmed when a plantarflexion lateral view is obtained. Serial casting is used before surgery to stretch the tight Achilles tendon and to avoid weakening the gastrocnemius-soleus. If the peroneal muscles are normal, and both tibial muscles are paralyzed, one of the peroneal muscles must be transferred. Because of its greater excursion, the peroneus longus is transferred to the base of the second metatarsal to replace the anterior tibial and one of the long toe flexors replaces the posterior tibial. The peroneus brevis is sutured to the distal stump of the peroneus longus tendon.

POSTERIOR TIBIAL MUSCLE

Isolated paralysis of the posterior tibial muscle is rare but can result in hindfoot and forefoot eversion. The flexor hallucis longus and the flexor digitorum longus have been used for tendon transfers in this situation. Through a posteromedial incision, the intrinsic plantar muscles are dissected sharply from their calcaneal origin and one of the long toe flexors is exposed and divided. If the flexor digitorum longus is used, it is dissected from its tendon sheath posterior and proximal to the medial malleolus, rerouted through the posterior tibial sheath, and attached to the navicular. In rare cases, as an alternative, the extensor hallucis longus can be transferred posteriorly through the interosseous membrane and then through the posterior tibial tunnel.

For children 3 to 6 years old, Axer recommended bringing the conjoined extensor digitorum longus and peroneus tertius tendons through a transverse tunnel in the talar neck and suturing the tendon back onto itself. For fixed equinus deformity, lengthening of the Achilles tendon may be required before tendon transfer. For severe valgus, Axer recommended transfer of the peroneus longus into the medial side of the talar neck and transfer of the peroneus brevis into the lateral side. Isolated transfer of the peroneus brevis should not be done because it can cause a forefoot inversion deformity. After surgery, cast immobilization is continued for 6 weeks, followed by 6 months of orthosis wear.

ANTERIOR TIBIAL, TOE EXTENSOR, AND PERONEAL MUSCLES

Progressively severe equinovarus deformity develops when the posterior tibial and gastrocnemius-soleus are unopposed. The posterior tibial muscle increases forefoot equinus and cavus deformity by depressing the metatarsal head and shortening the medial arch of the foot. Further equinus and varus deformity results from contracture of the gastrocnemius-soleus, which acts as a fixed point toward which the plantar intrinsic muscles pull and increase forefoot adduction.

Stretching by serial casting may be attempted, but lengthening of the Achilles tendon usually is required. Radical soft-tissue release of the forefoot cavus deformity also may be necessary. Anterior transfer of the posterior tibial to the base of the third metatarsal or middle cuneiform can be supplemented by anterior transfer of the long toe flexors. Arthrodesis usually is not required; the deformity can be controlled by physical therapy and orthoses. A bony tunnel can be made through the base of the third metatarsal or the middle cuneiform, with suture of the transfer to a button over a felt pad placed on the non–weight-bearing area of the plantar surface of the foot.

PERONEAL MUSCLES

Isolated paralysis of the peroneal muscles is rare in patients with poliomyelitis but can cause severe hindfoot varus deformity because of the unopposed activity of the posterior tibial muscle. The calcaneus becomes inverted, the forefoot is adducted, and the varus deformity is increased by the action of the invertor muscles during gait. The unopposed anterior tibial activity can cause a dorsal bunion. In this situation, the anterior tibial muscle can be transferred laterally to the base of the second metatarsal; however, isolated transfer of the anterior tibial muscle can result in overactivity of the extensor hallucis longus, causing hyperextension of the hallux and development of a painful callus under the first metatarsal head. In children younger than 5 years of age, lengthening of the extensor hallucis longus tendon may be required. In children older than 5 years, the extensor hallucis longus should be transferred to the first metatarsal neck before the bony deformity becomes fixed.

PERONEAL AND LONG TOE EXTENSOR MUSCLES

Paralysis of the peroneal muscles and long toe extensors causes a less severe equinovarus deformity that can be treated by transfer of the anterior tibial tendon to the base of the third metatarsal or the middle cuneiform.

GASTROCNEMIUS-SOLEUS MUSCLES

The gastrocnemius-soleus is a strong muscle group in the body, lifting the entire body weight with each step. Paralysis of the gastrocnemius-soleus, leaving the dorsiflexors unopposed, causes a rapidly progressive calcaneal deformity. Adequate tension of the Achilles tendon is important to the normal function of the long toe flexors and extensors and to the intrinsic foot muscles. If the gastrocnemius-soleus is weak, the posterior tibial, the peroneal muscles, and the long toe flexors cannot effectively plantarflex the hindfoot; however, they can depress the metatarsal heads and cause an equinus deformity. Shortening of the intrinsics and plantar fascia draws the metatarsal heads and the calcaneus together, similar to a bowstring. The long axes of the tibia and the calcaneus coincide, negating any residual power in the gastrocnemius-soleus.

Keeping the foot in slight equinus during the acute stage of poliomyelitis helps prevent overstretching of the gastrocnemius-soleus, and the position is maintained in the convalescent stage. If the gastrocnemius-soleus is weak, early walking is discouraged. Serial standing radiographs should be obtained frequently, especially in children younger than 5 years old, because of the rapid development of the deformity.

Surgical correction is indicated to prevent development of calcaneal deformity and to restore hindfoot plantarflexion. In the acute stage, the only absolute indication for tendon transfer in children younger than 5 years old is a progressive calcaneal deformity.

The combination of muscles transferred posteriorly depends on the residual strength of the gastrocnemius-soleus and the pattern of remaining muscle function. If the motor strength of the gastrocnemius-soleus is fair, posterior transfer of two or three muscles may be sufficient for normal gait. If the gastrocnemius-soleus is completely paralyzed, as many muscles as are available should be transferred. Plantar fasciotomy and intrinsic muscle release are required before tendon transfer in fixed forefoot cavus deformity.

The anterior tibial muscle can be transferred posteriorly 18 months after the acute stage of poliomyelitis. This can be done as an isolated procedure if the lateral stabilizers are balanced and the strong toe extensors can be used for dorsiflexion. In more severe deformity, transfer of the toe extensors to the metatarsal heads and fusion of the interphalangeal joints may be required to prevent claw toe deformity.

POSTERIOR TRANSFER OF ANTERIOR TIBIAL TENDON

TECHNIQUE 34-1

(DRENNAN)

- Take care to obtain maximal length of the anterior tibial tendon, which may have shortened because of the calcaneal deformity of the interosseous membrane.
- Split the insertion of the Achilles tendon longitudinally and develop osteoperiosteal flaps on the calcaneal tuberosity.
- Place the foot in maximal plantarflexion to ensure that the transfer is attached under appropriate tension. If necessary to obtain adequate plantarflexion, release other dorsal soft structures, including the ankle joint capsule, or lengthen the long toe extensors. If the attenuated Achilles tendon requires shortening, use a Z-plasty technique, resecting the redundant tendon from the proximal part.
- Attach the transferred anterior tibial tendon to the tuberosity of the calcaneus and to the distal stump of the Achilles tendon, which has retained its normal attachment to the calcaneal tuberosity.
- Close the wound in normal fashion and apply a long leg cast with the foot in the plantarflexed position. The cast is worn for 5 weeks, and a brace is worn for an additional 4 months.

If the invertors and evertors are balanced, a pure calcaneocavus deformity develops. Posterior transfer of only one set of these muscles causes instability and deformity. If the gastrocnemius-soleus strength is fair, transfer of the peroneus brevis and posterior tibial to the heel is sufficient to control the calcaneal deformity and allow normal gait. Lateral imbalance requires transposition of the acting invertor or evertor to the heel. Both peroneals are transferred to the heel for calcaneovalgus deformity, and the posterior tibial and flexor hallucis longus can be transferred for cavovarus deformity.

Westin and Defiore recommended tenodesis of the Achilles tendon to the fibula for paralytic calcaneovalgus deformity (Fig. 34-1). They used a T-shaped incision in the periosteum instead of a drill hole, with imbrication of the distal segment of the sectioned tendon below the periosteum. For mobile calcaneal deformities, Makin recommended transfer of the peroneus longus into a groove cut in the posterior calcaneus, without disturbance of the origin or insertion of the tendon. The tendon is freed proximal to the lateral malleolus and at the cuboid groove, and the foot is maximally plantarflexed, allowing the peroneus longus to displace posteriorly into the calcaneal groove, where it eventually unites with the bone.

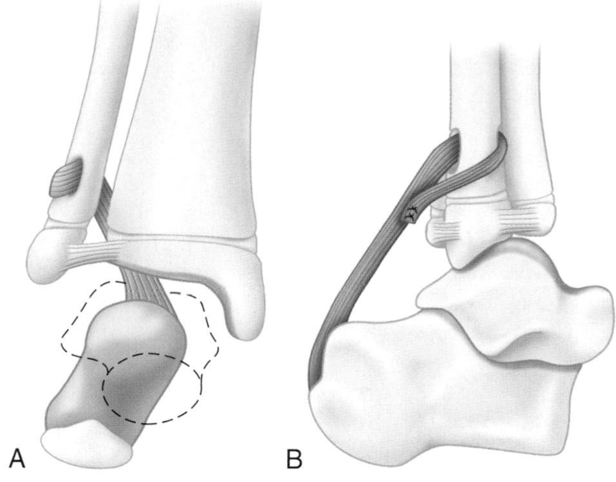

FIGURE 34-1 Anterior **(A)** and lateral **(B)** views of tenodesis of Achilles tendon to fibula.

Extraarticular subtalar arthrodesis may be required as a second procedure.

In rare cases, if no invertors or evertors are present for transfer, the hamstrings can be used to replace the gastrocnemius-soleus. Prerequisites for this procedure include complete paralysis of the gastrocnemius-soleus, strong medial hamstrings or biceps femoris muscles, and strong ankle dorsiflexors and quadriceps muscles. The insertions of the semitendinosus and gracilis and occasionally the semimembranosus are mobilized, passed subcutaneously, and attached to the sagittally incised Achilles tendon. A mattress suture at the proximal end of the Achilles tendon prevents this incision from extending proximally. The tendons are sutured with the knee flexed to 25 degrees and the foot in plantarflexion.

FLAIL FOOT

When all muscles distal to the knee are paralyzed, equinus deformity results because of passive plantarflexion. The intrinsic muscles may retain some function, leading to forefoot equinus or cavoequinus deformity. Radical plantar release, sometimes combined with plantar neurectomy, usually controls this deformity. Midfoot wedge resection may be required for the forefoot equinus deformity in older patients.

DORSAL BUNION

In a dorsal bunion deformity, the shaft of the first metatarsal is dorsiflexed and the great toe is plantarflexed; it usually results from muscle imbalance, although occasionally there may be other causes. In its early stages, the deformity is not fixed but is present only on weight bearing, especially walking. If the muscle imbalance is not corrected, the deformity becomes fixed, although it remains more pronounced on weight bearing.

Usually, only the metatarsophalangeal joint of the great toe is flexed, and on weight bearing the first metatarsal head is displaced upward; the longitudinal axis of the metatarsal shaft can be horizontal, or its distal end can even be directed slightly upward. The first cuneiform also can be tilted upward. A small exostosis can form on the dorsum of the metatarsal head. When flexion of the great toe is severe enough, the metatarsophalangeal joint can subluxate and the dorsal part of the cartilage of the metatarsal head eventually can degenerate. The plantar part of the joint capsule and the flexor hallucis brevis muscle can become contracted.

Two types of muscle imbalance can cause a dorsal bunion. The more common dorsiflexes the first metatarsal, and the plantarflexion of the great toe is secondary. The less common plantarflexes the great toe, and dorsiflexion of the first metatarsal is secondary.

The most common imbalance is between the anterior tibial and peroneus longus muscles; normally, the anterior tibial muscle raises the first cuneiform and the base of the first metatarsal, and the peroneus longus opposes this action. When the peroneus longus is weak or paralyzed or has been transferred elsewhere, the first metatarsal can be dorsiflexed by a strong anterior tibial muscle or by a muscle substituting for it. When the first metatarsal is dorsiflexed, the great toe becomes actively plantarflexed to establish a weight-bearing point for the medial side of the forefoot and to assist push-off in walking. Weakness of the dorsiflexor muscles of the great toe also may favor the development of this position of the toe. Many dorsal bunions develop after ill-advised tendon transfers for residual poliomyelitis. In such patients, the opposing actions of the peroneus longus and anterior tibial muscles on the first metatarsal were considered in the transfers. Before any transfer of the peroneus longus tendon, the effect of its loss on the first metatarsal must be carefully considered. When the anterior tibial is paralyzed and tendon transfer is feasible, the peroneus longus tendon or the tendons of the peroneus longus and peroneus brevis should be transferred to the third cuneiform, rather than to the insertion of the anterior tibial; as an alternative, the peroneus brevis tendon can be transferred to the insertion of the anterior tibial, leaving the peroneus longus tendon undisturbed. We believe that when the peroneus longus tendon is transferred, the proximal end of its distal segment should be securely fixed to bone at the level of division. When the gastrocnemius-soleus group is weak or paralyzed, and the anterior tibial and peroneus longus muscles are strong, the peroneus longus should not be transferred to the calcaneus unless the anterior tibial is transferred to the midline of the foot. A dorsal bunion does not always follow ill-advised tendon transfers, however, because the muscle imbalance may not be severe enough to cause it. When the deformity is progressive, surgery may simply consist of transferring the anterior tibial (or the previously transferred peroneus longus) to the third cuneiform; correcting the deformity itself may be unnecessary. When the deformity is fixed, however, surgery must correct not only the muscle imbalance but also the deformity.

The second and less common muscle imbalance that can cause a dorsal bunion results from paralysis of all muscles controlling the foot except the gastrocnemius-soleus group, which may be of variable strength, and the long toe flexors, which are strong. These strong toe flexors help steady the foot in weight bearing and sustain the push-off in walking. The flexor hallucis longus assumes a large share of this added function and with active use, the great toe may be almost constantly plantarflexed; the first metatarsal head is displaced upward to accommodate it. A strong flexor hallucis brevis muscle also may help produce the deformity.

There are other, less common causes for the deformity. It can develop in conjunction with a hallux rigidus in which dorsiflexion of the first metatarsophalangeal joint is painful. The articular surfaces become irregular, and the plantar part of the joint capsule gradually contracts; proliferation of bone on the dorsum of the first metatarsal head often becomes pronounced and blocks dorsiflexion of the joint. When walking, the patient may unconsciously supinate the foot and plantarflex the great toe to protect the weight-bearing pad of the great toe. A dorsal bunion also is sometimes seen in a severe congenital flatfoot with a rocker bottom deformity (see Chapter 29). Transfer of the flexor hallucis longus to the neck of the first metatarsal, combined with bony correction by plantar closing wedge osteotomy of the first metatarsal when necessary, currently is our preferred technique for correction of dorsal bunions (Chapter 29, Technique 29-19). A strong unopposed anterior tibial tendon that contributes to forefoot supination is an indication for addition of a split anterior tibial tendon transfer.

BONY PROCEDURES (OSTEOTOMY AND ARTHRODESIS)

The object of arthrodesis in patients with poliomyelitis is to reduce the number of joints the weakened or paralyzed muscles must control. The structural bony deformity must be corrected before a tendon transfer is performed. Stabilizing procedures for the foot and ankle are traditionally of five types: (1) calcaneal osteotomy, (2) extraarticular subtalar arthrodesis, (3) triple arthrodesis, (4) ankle arthrodesis, and (5) bone blocks to limit motion at the ankle joint. These procedures can be performed singly or in combination with other procedures. The choice of operations depends on the age of the patient and the particular deformity that must be corrected.

CALCANEAL OSTEOTOMY

Calcaneal osteotomy (see Chapter 34) can be performed for correction of hindfoot varus or valgus deformity in growing children. For cavovarus deformity, it can be combined with release of the intrinsic muscles and the plantar fascia, and for calcaneovarus deformity, with posterior displacement calcaneal osteotomy. Fixed valgus deformity may require medial displacement osteotomy in a plane parallel to the peroneal tendons.

DILLWYN-EVANS OSTEOTOMY

The Dillwyn-Evans osteotomy can be used for talipes calcaneovalgus deformity as an alternative to triple arthrodesis in children 8 to 12 years old. This osteotomy, the reverse of the original technique used in clubfeet, lengthens the calcaneus by a transverse osteotomy of the calcaneus and the insertion of a bone graft to open a wedge and lengthen the lateral border of the foot (Fig. 34-2).

SUBTALAR ARTHRODESIS

Paralytic equinovalgus deformity results from paralysis of the anterior tibial and posterior tibial and the unopposed action of the peroneals and gastrocnemius-soleus. The calcaneus is everted and displaced laterally and posteriorly. The sustentaculum tali no longer functions as the calcaneal buttress for

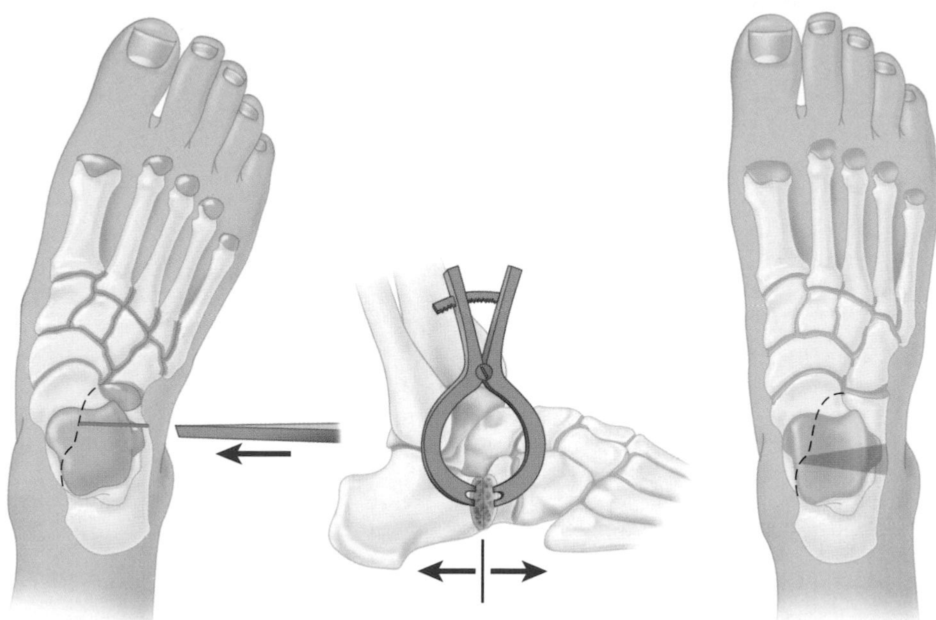

FIGURE 34-2 Dillwyn-Evans procedure.

the talar head, which shifts medially and into equinus. Hindfoot and forefoot equinovalgus deformities develop rapidly and, with growth, become fixed and require bony correction.

Grice and Green developed an extraarticular subtalar fusion to restore the height of the medial longitudinal arch in patients 3 to 8 years old. Ideally, this procedure is performed when the valgus deformity is localized to the subtalar joint and when the calcaneus can be manipulated into its normal position beneath the talus. Careful clinical and radiographic examinations should determine whether the valgus deformity is located primarily in the subtalar joint or the ankle joint. If the forefoot is not mobile enough to be made plantigrade when the hindfoot is corrected, the procedure is contraindicated. The most common complications of the Grice and Green arthrodesis are varus deformity and increased ankle joint valgus because of overcorrection. Bone infection, pseudarthrosis, graft resorption, and degenerative arthritis of the metatarsal joints also have been reported.

Dennyson and Fulford described a technique for subtalar arthrodesis in which a screw is inserted across the subtalar joint for internal fixation and an iliac crest graft is placed in the sinus tarsi. Because the screw provides internal fixation, maintenance of the correct position does not depend on the bone graft.

SUBTALAR ARTHRODESIS

TECHNIQUE 34-2

(GRICE AND GREEN)

- Make a short curvilinear incision on the lateral aspect of the foot directly over the subtalar joint.
- Carry the incision down through the soft tissues to expose the cruciate ligament overlying the joint. Split this ligament in the direction of its fibers and dissect the fatty and ligamentous tissues from the sinus tarsi.
- Dissect the short toe extensors from the calcaneus and reflect them distally. The relationship of the calcaneus to the talus now can be determined, and the mechanism of the deformity can be demonstrated.
- Place the foot in equinus and then invert it to position the calcaneus beneath the talus. A severe, long-standing deformity may require division of the posterior subtalar joint capsule or removal of a small piece of bone laterally from beneath the anterosuperior calcaneal articular surface.
- Insert an osteotome or broad periosteal elevator into the sinus tarsi and block the subtalar joint to evaluate the stability of the graft and its proper size and position.
- Prepare the graft beds by removing a thin layer of cortical bone from the inferior surface of the talus and the superior surface of the calcaneus (Fig. 34-3).
- Now make a linear incision over the anteromedial surface of the proximal tibial metaphysis, incise the periosteum, and take a block of bone large enough for two grafts (usually 3.5 to 4.5 cm long and 1.5 cm wide). As alternatives to tibial bone, take a short segment of the distal fibula or a circular segment of the iliac crest.
- Cut the grafts to fit the prepared beds. Use a rongeur to shape the grafts so that they can be countersunk into the cancellous bone to prevent lateral displacement.
- With the foot held in a slightly overcorrected position, place the grafts in the sinus tarsi. Evert the foot to lock the grafts in place.
- If a segment of the fibula or iliac crest is used, a smooth Kirschner wire can be used to hold the graft in place for

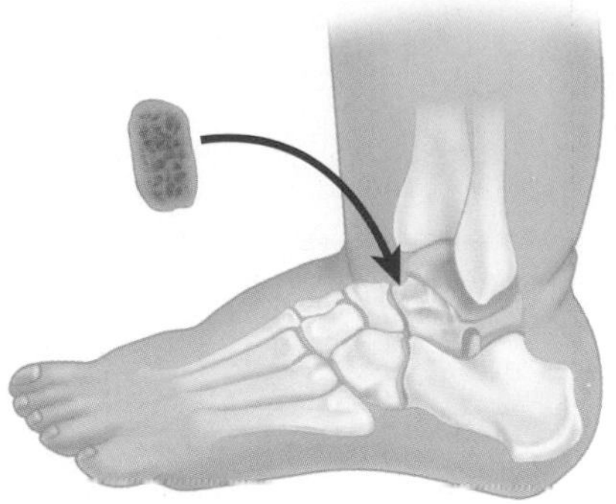
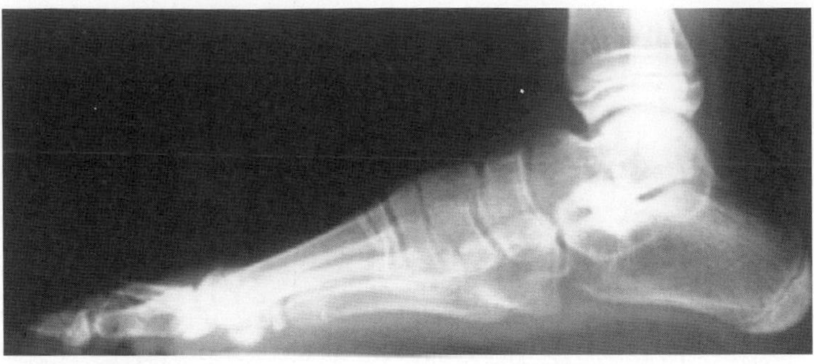

FIGURE 34-3 Grice-Green subtalar fusion. Preparation of graft bed and placement of graft in lateral aspect of subtalar joint. **SEE TECHNIQUE 34-2.**

12 weeks. A screw can be inserted anteriorly from the talar neck into the calcaneus for rigid fixation.

- Apply a long leg cast with the knee flexed, the ankle in maximal dorsiflexion, and the foot in the corrected position.

POSTOPERATIVE CARE. After 12 weeks of non–weight-bearing, the long leg cast is removed and a short-leg walking cast is applied and worn for an additional 4 weeks.

SUBTALAR ARTHRODESIS

TECHNIQUE 34-3

(DENNYSON AND FULFORD)

- Make an oblique incision in the line of the skin creases, centered over the sinus tarsi and extending from the middle of the front of the ankle proximally and laterally to the peroneal tendons (Fig. 34-4A).
- Raise the origin of the extensor digitorum brevis, along with a pad of subcutaneous fat, proximally and reflect it distally to expose the sinus tarsi.
- Remove the fat from the sinus tarsi by sharp dissection close to the bone and, with a narrow gouge, remove cortical bone from the apex of the sinus tarsi to expose cancellous bone on the undersurface of the talar neck and on the nonarticular area in the upper calcaneal surface (Fig. 34-4B). Do not remove cortical bone from the outer part of the sinus tarsi in the area through which the screw will pass.
- Expose the depression on the superior surface of the talar neck by blunt dissection between the tendon of the extensor digitorum longus and the neurovascular bundle.
- Hold the calcaneus in its correct position and pass a bone awl from this depression through the neck of the talus and across the sinus tarsi to enter the upper surface of the calcaneus toward the lateral side until it pierces the cortex of the calcaneus at its inferolateral border (Fig. 34-4C). The awl must pass through cortical bone on both the superior and inferior surfaces of the talar neck and on the superior and inferolateral surfaces of the calcaneus.
- Determine the length of the awl that is within the bones and insert a minifragment cancellous screw of the same length. Tighten the screw until its head is seated into the superior surface of the talus.
- Pack chips of cancellous bone from the iliac crest into the apex of the sinus tarsi (Fig. 34-4D).
- Replace the extensor digitorum brevis and close the wound.
- Apply a long leg, non–weight-bearing cast.

POSTOPERATIVE CARE. The long leg cast is removed at 6 to 8 weeks, and a short leg walking cast is applied and worn for an additional 4 to 6 weeks.

TRIPLE ARTHRODESIS

The most effective stabilizing procedure in the foot is triple arthrodesis (Fig. 34-5): fusion of the subtalar, calcaneocuboid, and talonavicular joints. Triple arthrodesis limits motion of the foot and ankle to plantarflexion and dorsiflexion. It is indicated when most of the weakness and deformity are at the subtalar and midtrial joints. Triple arthrodesis is performed (1) to obtain stable and static realignment of the foot, (2) to remove deforming forces, (3) to arrest progression of deformity, (4) to eliminate pain, (5) to eliminate the use of a short leg brace or to provide sufficient correction to allow fitting of a long leg brace to control the knee joint, and (6) to obtain a more normal-appearing foot. Generally, triple arthrodesis is reserved for severe deformity in children 12 years old and older; occasionally, it may be required in children 8 to 12 years old with progressive, uncontrollable deformity.

The exact technique of triple arthrodesis depends on the type of deformity, and this should be determined before surgery. A paper tracing can be made from a lateral radiograph of the ankle, and the components of the subtalar joint are divided into three sections: the tibiotalar and calcaneal components and another component comprising all the bones of the foot distal to the midtarsal joint. These are

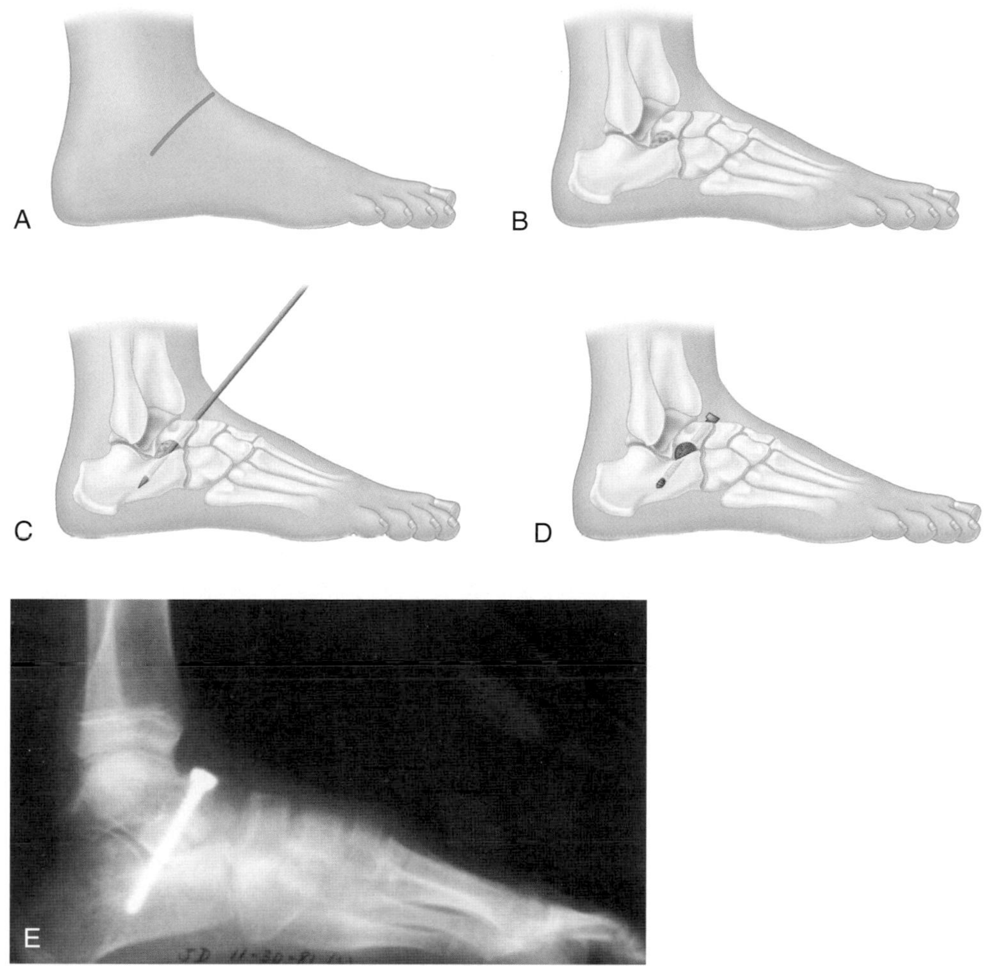

FIGURE 34-4 Subtalar arthrodesis with internal fixation. **A,** Oblique incision over sinus tarsi. **B,** Exposure of sinus tarsi, cancellous bone of calcaneus, and talus. **C,** Steinmann pin is placed across subtalar joint entering talus as far distal as possible with foot held in corrected position. **D,** Screw is placed across subtalar joint from talar neck into calcaneus; sinus tarsi is filled with iliac crest bone graft. **E,** Radiograph of corrected foot with screw in place. **SEE TECHNIQUE 34-3.**

reassembled with the foot in the corrected position so that the size and shape of the wedges to be removed can be measured accurately.

In talipes equinovalgus, the medial longitudinal arch of the foot is depressed, the talar head is enlarged and plantarflexed, and the forefoot is abducted. Raising the talar head and shifting the sustentaculum tali medially beneath the talar head and neck restores the arch. A medially based wedge consisting of a portion of the talar head and neck is excised (Fig. 34-5C). When the hindfoot valgus deformity is corrected, the forefoot tends to supinate; this is controlled by midtarsal joint resection with a medially based wedge. An additional medial incision may be required for resection of the talonavicular joint.

In talipes equinovarus, the enlarged talar head lies lateral to the midline axis of the foot and blocks dorsiflexion. A laterally based subtalar wedge, combined with midtarsal joint resection, places the talar head slightly medial to the midline axis of the foot (Fig. 34-5D).

In talipes calcaneocavus, the arthrodesis should allow posterior displacement of the foot at the subtalar joint. After stripping of the plantar fascia, a wedge-shaped or cuneiform section of bone is removed to allow correction of the cavus deformity, and a wedge of bone is removed from the subtalar joint to correct the rotation of the calcaneus (Fig. 34-5D).

The muscle balance of the foot and ankle determines how much the foot should be displaced posteriorly. Posterior displacement of the foot transfers its fulcrum (the ankle) anteriorly to a position near its center and lengthens its posterior lever arm; this is especially important when the gastrocnemius-soleus group is weak.

TRIPLE ARTHRODESIS

TECHNIQUE 34-4

- Make an oblique incision centered over the sinus tarsi in line with the skin creases on the lateral side of the foot, beginning dorsolaterally at the lateral border of the tendons of the long toe extensors at the level of the talonavicular joint (Fig. 34-5A). Continue the incision

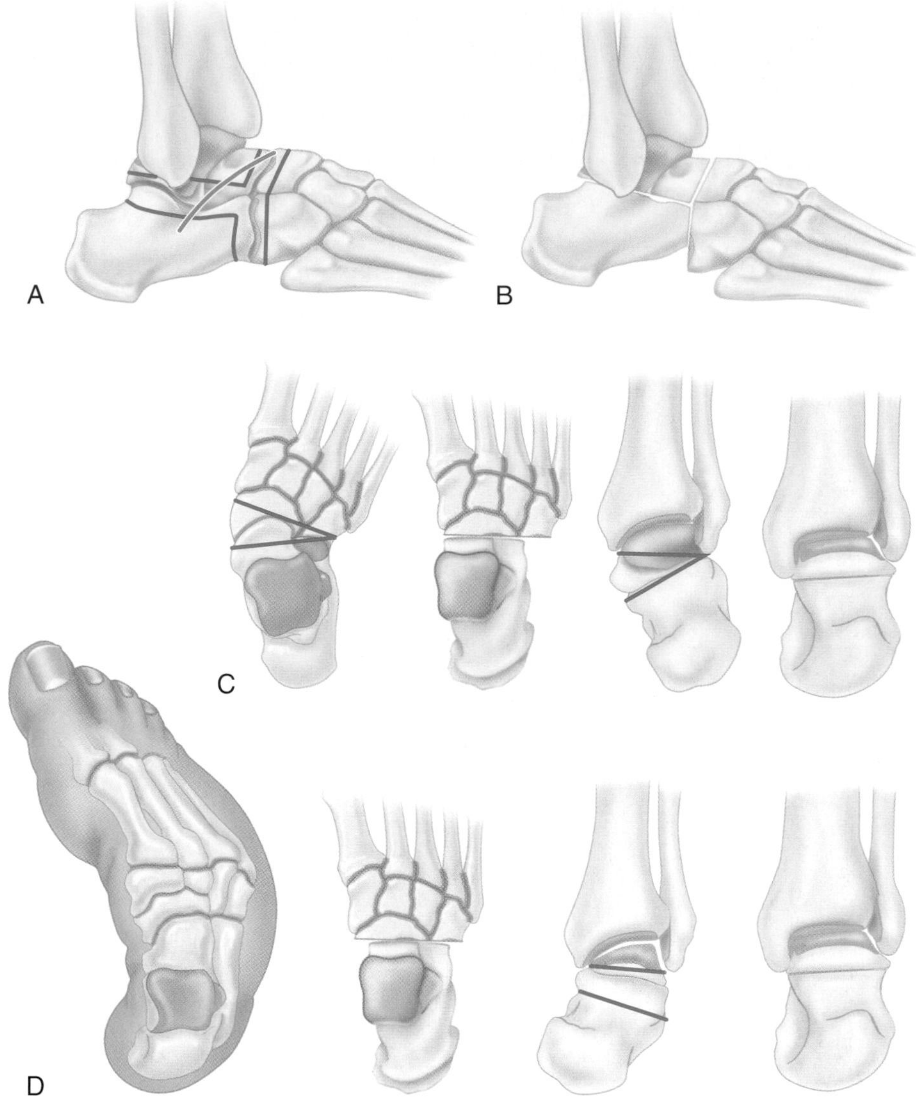

FIGURE 34-5 Triple arthrodesis. **A,** Oblique incision in sinus tarsi to expose subtalar, talonavicular, and calcaneocuboid joints. **B,** Cartilage and cortical bone removed from all joint surfaces; appropriate wedges are removed if necessary. **C,** Wedges necessary for correction of valgus deformity. **D,** Wedges necessary for correction of varus deformity. **SEE TECHNIQUES 34-4 AND 34-5.**

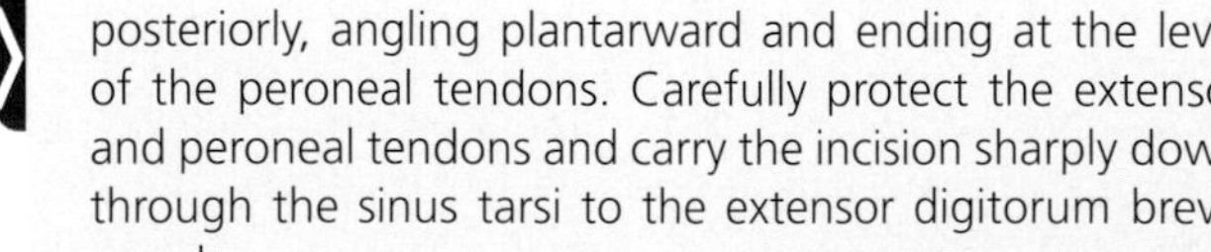

posteriorly, angling plantarward and ending at the level of the peroneal tendons. Carefully protect the extensor and peroneal tendons and carry the incision sharply down through the sinus tarsi to the extensor digitorum brevis muscle.

- Reflect the origin of this muscle distally along with the fat in the sinus tarsi.
- Clean the remainder of the sinus tarsi of all tissue to expose the subtalar and calcaneocuboid joints and the lateral portion of the talonavicular joint.
- Incise the capsules of the talonavicular, calcaneocuboid, and subtalar joints circumferentially to obtain as much mobility as possible. If this release allows the foot to be placed in a normal position, removal of large bony wedges is not required. If correction is impossible after soft-tissue release, appropriate bone wedges are removed (Fig. 34-5C and D).
- Identify the anterior articular process of the calcaneus and excise it at the level of the floor of the sinus tarsi for better exposure of all joints.
- To make this osteotomy, use an osteotome placed parallel to the plantar surface of the foot; preserve the bone for grafting.
- With an osteotome remove the articular surfaces of the calcaneocuboid joint to expose cancellous bone.
- Remove an equal amount from both bones unless wedge correction of a bone deformity is required (Fig. 34-5B).
- Remove the distal portion of the head of the talus with $\frac{1}{4}$-inch and $\frac{1}{2}$-inch straight and curved osteotomes. Remove only enough bone to expose the cancellous bone of the talar head unless a medial wedge is required to correct a fixed deformity. A small lamina spreader can be inserted for better exposure. A second medial incision

may be necessary to expose the most medial portion of the talonavicular joint.

- Remove the proximal articular surface and subchondral bone of the navicular and shape and roughen the surfaces for a snug fit with the talus.
- Excise the articular surfaces of the sustentaculum tali and the anterior facet of the subtalar joint.
- Approach the subtalar joint and completely remove its articular surfaces. For better exposure of the posterior portion, use the small lamina spreader to expose the subtalar joint. Remove appropriate wedges from this joint if necessary; otherwise, make the joint resections parallel to the articular surfaces.
- Cut the removed bone into small pieces to be used for bone grafting. Place most of the bone graft around the talonavicular joint and in the depth of the sinus tarsi.
- Correction is maintained with internal fixation, usually smooth Steinmann pins or Kirschner wires.
- Close the muscle pedicle of the extensor digitorum brevis over the sinus tarsi to reduce the dead space.
- Close the wound over a suction drain and apply a well-padded, short leg cast.

POSTOPERATIVE CARE. Considerable bleeding from the drain and through the wound itself can be expected. The foot should be elevated to minimize swelling. The drain is removed at 24 to 48 hours. Walking with crutches or a walker, with touch-down weight bearing on the operated foot, is allowed as tolerated. The cast and pins or wires are removed at 6 to 8 weeks, and a short leg walking cast is applied and worn until union is complete, usually 4 weeks more.

CORRECTION OF CAVUS DEFORMITY

TECHNIQUE 34-5

- Perform a medial radical plantar release to correct the contracted soft tissues bridging the longitudinal arch. Then forcibly correct the cavus deformity as much as possible.
- Expose the calcaneocuboid, talonavicular, and subtalar joints through the incision described earlier.
- With an osteotome, remove from the talonavicular and calcaneocuboid joints a wedge-shaped or cuneiform section of bone with its base anterior and large enough to correct the cavus deformity that remains after the plantar fascial stripping.
- Dorsiflex the forefoot and appose the raw surfaces to see if the cavus is corrected; if so, expose the subtalar joint and remove from it a wedge of bone with its base posterior to correct the deformity or rotation of the calcaneus (see Fig. 34-5D). Be sure that all bone surfaces fit together well and that the foot is in satisfactory position before closing the wound.

POSTOPERATIVE CARE. Correction usually is maintained with Steinmann pins or Kirschner wires. A cast is applied, and firm pressure is exerted on the sole of the foot while the plaster is setting to stretch the plantar structures as much as possible. When internal fixation is not used, the cast and sutures are removed at 10 to 14 days, the foot is inspected, and radiographs are made. If the position is not satisfactory, the foot is manipulated with the patient under general anesthesia. A new cast, snug but properly padded, is then applied and is molded to the contour of the foot; this cast is removed at 12 weeks.

COMPLICATIONS OF TRIPLE ARTHRODESIS

The most common complication of triple arthrodesis is pseudarthrosis, especially of the talonavicular joint. The additional stress on the ankle joint caused by loss of mobility of the hindfoot can lead to the development of degenerative arthritis. Excessive resection of the talus can cause osteonecrosis, especially in adolescents; this usually is evident on radiographs 8 to 12 weeks after triple arthrodesis. Ligamentous laxity around the ankle joint may require ankle fusion. Muscle imbalance after hindfoot stabilization can lead to forefoot deformity; unopposed function of the anterior tibial or peroneal muscles is the most common cause of this complication and should be corrected by tendon transfer. Residual deformity usually is caused by insufficient correction at surgery, inadequate immobilization, pseudarthrosis, or muscle imbalance.

TALECTOMY

Talectomy provides stability and posterior displacement of the foot and generally is recommended for children 5 to 12 years old when the deformity is not correctable by arthrodesis. Talectomy limits motion of the ankle joint, especially dorsiflexion, and creates a tibiotarsal ankylosis. Posterior displacement of the foot places the distal tibia over the center of the weight-bearing area, producing even weight distribution and good lateral stability. Appearance usually is satisfactory, pain is relieved, and special shoes or orthoses are not required.

The most common cause of failure of talectomy is muscle imbalance, usually the presence of a strong anterior or posterior tibial muscle. Intrinsic muscle activity can cause contracture of the plantar fascia, resulting in a forefoot equinus deformity. In children younger than 5 years old, recurrence of the deformity is frequent, and pain is common in individuals older than 15 years, especially with inadequate excision of the entire talus. Tibiocalcaneal arthrodesis can be performed for failed talectomy and most commonly is indicated because of persistent pain. The technique of talectomy is described in Chapter 29.

LAMBRINUDI ARTHRODESIS

The Lambrinudi arthrodesis is recommended for correction of isolated fixed equinus deformity in patients older than 10 years. Retained activity in the gastrocnemius-soleus, combined with inactive dorsiflexors and peroneals, causes the footdrop deformity. The posterior talus abuts the

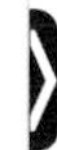

undersurface of the tibia, and the posterior ankle joint capsule contracts to create a fixed equinus deformity. In the Lambrinudi procedure, a wedge of bone is removed from the plantar distal part of the talus so that the talus remains in complete equinus at the ankle joint while the remainder of the foot is repositioned to the desired degree of plantarflexion. Tendon resection or transfer may be necessary to prevent varus or valgus deformity if active muscle power remains. The Lambrinudi arthrodesis is not recommended for a flail foot or when hip or knee instability requires a brace. A good result depends on the strength of the dorsal ankle ligaments. If anterior subluxation of the talus is noted on a weight-bearing lateral radiograph, a two-stage pantalar arthrodesis is recommended. Complications of the Lambrinudi arthrodesis include ankle instability, residual varus or valgus deformities caused by muscle imbalance, and pseudarthrosis of the talonavicular joint.

TECHNIQUE 34-6

(LAMBRINUDI)

- With the foot and ankle in extreme plantarflexion, make a lateral radiograph and trace the film. Cut the tracing into three pieces along the outlines of the subtalar and midtarsal joints; from these pieces the exact amount of bone to be removed from the talus can be determined with accuracy before surgery. In the tracing, the line representing the articulation of the talus with the tibia is left undisturbed but that corresponding to its plantar and distal parts is to be cut so that when the navicular and the calcaneocuboid joint are later fitted to it the foot will be in 5 to 10 degrees of equinus relative to the tibia (Fig. 34-6) unless the extremity has shortened; more equinus may then be desirable.
- Expose the sinus tarsi through a long, lateral curved incision.
- Section the peroneal tendons by a Z-shaped cut, open the talonavicular and calcaneocuboid joints, and divide the interosseous and lateral collateral ligaments of the ankle to permit complete medial dislocation of the tarsus at the subtalar joint.
- With a small power saw (more accurate than a chisel or osteotome), remove the predetermined wedge of bone from the plantar and distal parts of the neck and body of the talus. Remove the cartilage and bone from the superior surface of the calcaneus to form a plane parallel with the longitudinal axis of the foot.
- Next make a V-shaped trough transversely in the inferior part of the proximal navicular and denude the calcaneocuboid joint of enough bone to correct any lateral deformity.
- Firmly wedge the sharp distal margin of the remaining part of the talus into the prepared trough in the navicular and appose the calcaneus and talus. Take care to place the distal margin of the talus well medially in the trough; otherwise, the position of the foot will not be satisfactory. The talus is now locked in the ankle joint in complete equinus, and the foot cannot be further plantarflexed.
- Insert smooth Kirschner wires for fixation of the talonavicular and calcaneocuboid joints.

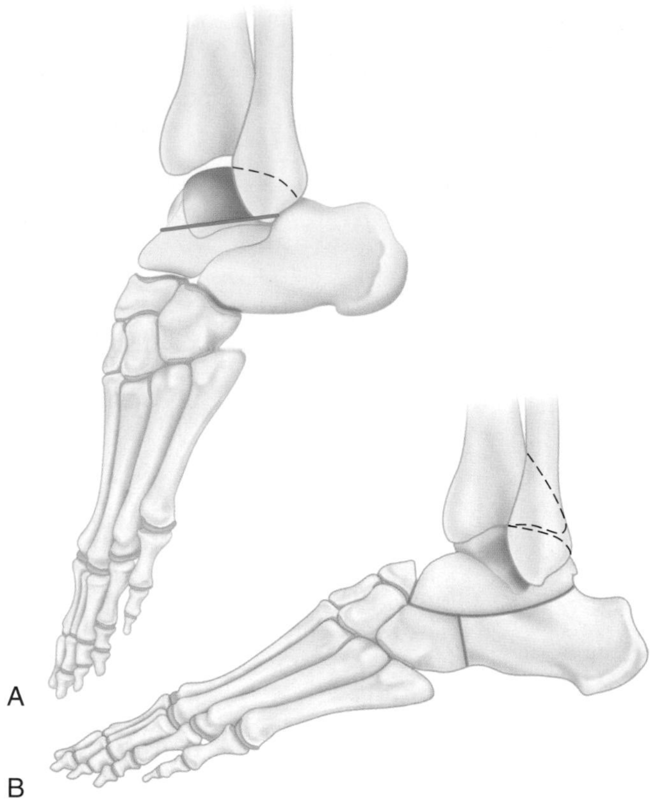

FIGURE 34-6 Lambrinudi operation for talipes equinus. **A,** *Colored area* indicates part of talus to be resected. **B,** Sharp distal margin of remaining part of talus has been wedged into prepared trough in navicular, and raw osseous surfaces of talus, calcaneus, and cuboid have been apposed. **SEE TECHNIQUE 34-6.**

- Suture the peroneal tendons, close the wound in the routine manner, and apply a cast with the ankle in neutral or slight dorsiflexion.

POSTOPERATIVE CARE. The cast and sutures are removed at 10 to 14 days, and the position of the foot is evaluated by radiographs. If the position is satisfactory, a short leg cast is applied, but weight bearing is not allowed for another 6 weeks, after which a short leg walking cast is applied and is worn until fusion is complete, usually at 3 months.

ANKLE ARTHRODESIS

Ankle fusion may be indicated for a flail foot or for recurrence of deformity after triple arthrodesis. Compression arthrodesis (see Chapter 11) generally is recommended for older children and adolescents. Subcutaneous plantar fasciotomy and lengthening of the Achilles tendon can be performed initially, followed by ankle arthrodesis.

PANTALAR ARTHRODESIS

Pantalar arthrodesis is fusion of the tibiotalar, talonavicular, subtalar, and calcaneocuboid joints. For flail feet with paralyzed quadriceps, pantalar arthrodesis may be indicated to eliminate the need for long leg braces. The ideal patient for this operation is one with a flail foot and ankle and normal muscles around the hip and knee. Absolute prerequisites for this procedure include a strong gluteus maximus to initiate toe-off during gait and a normally aligned knee with full extension or a few degrees of hyperextension.

The ankle should be fused in 5 to 10 degrees of plantarflexion to produce the backward thrust on the knee joint necessary for stable weight bearing. Excessive plantarflexion of the ankle results in pain and increased pressure under the metatarsal heads; acceptable plantarflexion should be confirmed with a lateral radiograph during surgery. Pantalar arthrodesis can be done in two stages: the first in the foot and the second in the ankle because it is difficult to achieve and maintain proper position of the foot and the ankle at the same time. Provelengios et al. described one-stage pantalar arthrodesis in 24 patients (average age, 20 years) with a Steinmann pin used to stabilize the ankle and subtalar joints. At an average follow-up of 37 years, 22 of the 24 patients were satisfied with their outcomes. The position of the fused ankle did not correlate with the development of ipsilateral knee pain. More recently, the authors modified their technique by using a circular external fixator to stabilize all four joints. Complications of pantalar arthrodesis include pseudarthrosis, painful plantar callosities caused by unequal weight distribution, and excessive heel equinus, which causes increased pressure on the forefoot. Provelengios et al. reported a complication rate of 46%, but all were minor wound or skin problems.

TENDON TRANSFER TECHNIQUES

TALIPES EQUINOVARUS

Talipes equinovarus caused by poliomyelitis is characterized by equinus deformity of the ankle, inversion of the heel, and, at the midtarsal joints, adduction and supination of the forefoot. When the deformity is of long duration there also is a cavus deformity of the foot; clawing of the toes may develop secondary to substitution of motor patterns. In paralytic talipes equinovarus, the peroneal muscles are paralyzed or severely weakened but the posterior tibial muscle usually is normal; the anterior tibial may be weakened or normal. The gastrocnemius-soleus is comparatively strong but becomes contracted by a combination of motor imbalance, growth, gravity, and posture. Treatment depends on the age of the patient, the forces causing the deformity, the severity of the deformity, and its rate of increase.

Anterior transfer of the posterior tibial tendon removes a dynamic deforming force and aids active dorsiflexion of the foot; however, transfer alone rarely restores active dorsiflexion. Rerouting of the tendon anterior to the medial malleolus diminishes its plantarflexion power and lengthens the posterior tibial muscle; the deformity may not be corrected, however, because the muscle retains its varus pull. The entire tendon can be transferred through the interosseous membrane to the middle cuneiform, or the tendon can be split, with the lateral half transferred to the cuboid.

ANTERIOR TRANSFER OF POSTERIOR TIBIAL TENDON

TECHNIQUE 34-7

(BARR)

- Make a skin incision on the medial side of the ankle beginning distally at the insertion of the posterior tibial tendon and extending proximally over the tendon just posterior to the malleolus and from there proximally along the medial border of the tibia for 5.0 to 7.5 cm.
- Free the tendon from its insertion, preserving as much of its length as possible.
- Split its sheath and free it in a proximal direction until the distal 5.0 cm of the muscle has been mobilized. Carefully preserve the nerves and vessels supplying the muscle.
- Make a second skin incision anteriorly; begin it distally at the level of the ankle joint and extend it proximally for 7.5 cm just lateral to the anterior tibial tendon. Carry the dissection deep between the tendons of the anterior tibial muscle and the extensor hallucis longus, carefully preserving the dorsalis pedis artery; expose the interosseous membrane just proximal to the malleoli.
- Cut a generous window in the interosseous membrane but avoid stripping the periosteum from the tibia or fibula.
- Pass the posterior tibial tendon through the window between the bones, taking care that it is not kinked, twisted, or constricted and that the vessels and nerves to the muscle are not damaged. Pass the tendon beneath the cruciate ligament, which can be divided if necessary to relieve pressure on the tendon.
- Expose the third cuneiform or the base of the third metatarsal through a transverse incision 2.5 cm long.
- Retract the extensor tendons, sharply incise the periosteum over the bone in a cruciate fashion, and fold back osteoperiosteal flaps.
- Drill a hole through the bone in line with the tendon and large enough to receive it; anchor it in the bone with a pull-out wire. Be sure that the button on the plantar surface of the foot is well padded.
- Suture the osteoperiosteal flaps to the tendon with two figure-of-eight nonabsorbable sutures.
- Close the incision and apply a plaster cast to hold the foot in calcaneovalgus position.

Instead of the long medial incision used by Barr, we make a short longitudinal one to free the posterior tibial tendon at its insertion and withdraw it through another incision 5 cm long at the musculotendinous junction just posterior to the subcutaneous border of the tibia (Fig. 34-7). The tendon also can be anchored to bone by passing it through a hole drilled in the bone, looping it back, and suturing it to itself with nonabsorbable sutures.

POSTOPERATIVE CARE. The cast is removed at 3 weeks, the wounds are inspected, the sutures are removed, and a short leg walking cast is applied with the foot in the neutral position and the ankle in slight dorsiflexion. Six weeks after surgery the cast is removed, and

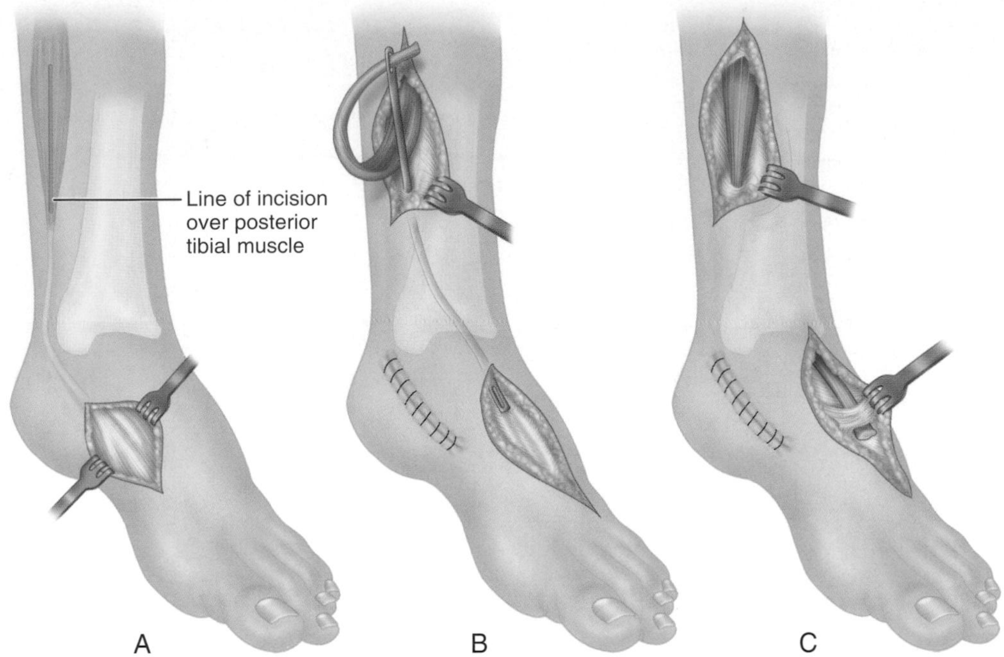

FIGURE 34-7 Ober anterior transfer of posterior tibial tendon. **A,** Insertion of posterior tibial tendon has been exposed. Note line of skin incision over muscle. **B,** Tendon has been freed from its insertion, and muscle has been dissected from tibia. **C,** Tendon and muscle have been passed through anterior tibial compartment to dorsum of foot, and tendon has been anchored in third metatarsal. **SEE TECHNIQUES 34-7 AND 34-8.**

a program of rehabilitative exercises is started that is continued under supervision until a full range of active resisted function is obtained. The transfer is protected for 6 months by a double-bar foot-drop brace with an outside T-strap.

ANTERIOR TRANSFER OF POSTERIOR TIBIAL TENDON

TECHNIQUE 34-8

(OBER)

- Through a medial longitudinal incision 7.5 cm long, free the posterior tibial tendon from its attachment to the navicular (Fig. 34-7).
- Make a second longitudinal medial incision 10 cm long centered over the musculotendinous junction of the posterior tibial tendon and muscle.
- Withdraw the tendon from the proximal wound and free the muscle belly well up on the tibia.
- Strip the periosteum obliquely on the medial surface of the tibia so that when the tendon is moved into the anterior tibial compartment only the belly of the muscle will come in contact with denuded bone. The tendon must not be in contact with the tibia.
- Make a third incision over the base of the third metatarsal, draw the posterior tibial tendon from the second into the third incision, and anchor its distal end in the base of the third metatarsal.

POSTOPERATIVE CARE. Postoperative care is the same as after Technique 34-7.

SPLIT TRANSFER OF ANTERIOR TIBIAL TENDON

TECHNIQUE 34-9

- Make a 2- to 3-cm longitudinal incision dorsomedially over the medial cuneiform (Fig. 34-8A).
- Identify the anterior tibial tendon and split it longitudinally in the midportion. Detach the lateral half of the tendon from its insertion, preserving as much length as possible, and continue the split proximally to the extent of the incision.
- Make a second 2- to 3-cm incision anteriorly over the distal tibia, identify the tibialis anterior tendon sheath, and split it longitudinally.
- Continue the split in the anterior tibial tendon proximally into this incision and up to the musculotendinous

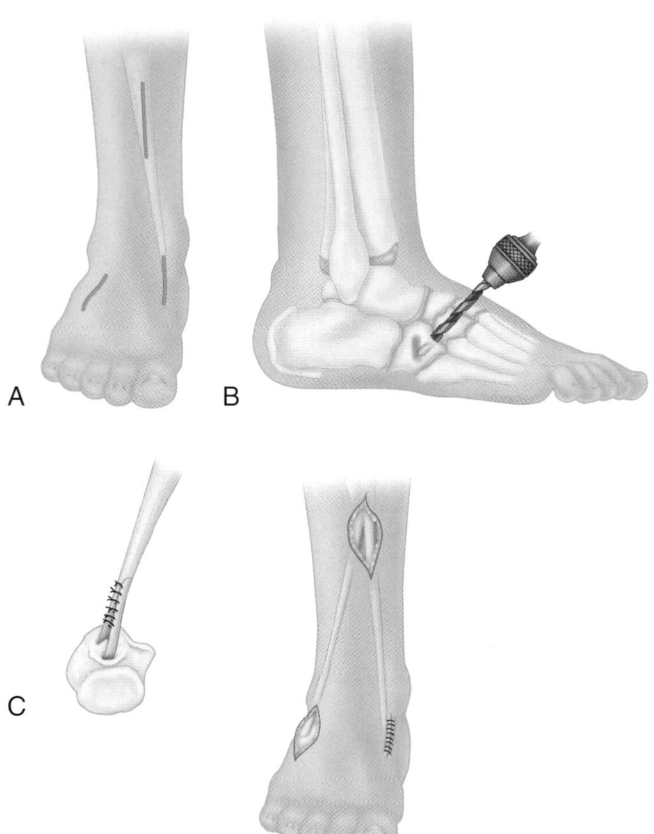

FIGURE 34-8 Split transfer of anterior tibial tendon. **A,** Three incisions: longitudinal over insertion of anterior tibial tendon and longitudinally over distal leg and over cuboid. **B,** Two holes are drilled in cuboid. **C,** Split portion of anterior tibial tendon is pulled into one hole and out the other and sutured to itself. **D,** New split portion of tendon in its redirected position. **SEE TECHNIQUE 34-9.**

junction. Umbilical tape can be used to continue the split in the tendon. Place the tape into the split and bring its two ends into the proximal incision. Before the lateral half of the tendon is detached, continue the split to the musculotendinous junction by pulling on the tape.

- Once the split in the tendon is complete, detach the lateral half and bring it into the proximal wound.
- Make a third 2- to 3-cm longitudinal incision over the cuboid on the dorsolateral aspect of the foot.
- Drill two holes in the cuboid, placing them as far away from each other as possible so that they meet well within the body of the cuboid (Fig. 34-8B). Enlarge the holes with a curet if necessary, but be certain to leave a bridge of bone between the two holes.
- Pass the split lateral portion of the anterior tibial tendon distally through the subcutaneous tunnel from the proximal incision to the dorsolateral incision over the cuboid.
- Attach a nonabsorbable suture to the end of the tendon and pass it into one hole in the cuboid and out the other (Fig. 34-8C).
- Hold the foot in dorsiflexion, pull the tendon tight, and suture the free end to the proximal portion of the tendon under moderate tension (Fig. 34-8D).
- As an alternative, drill a hole in the cuneiform through the plantar cortex, pass the tendon through this hole, and anchor it on the plantar aspect of the foot with a suture over felt and a button.

POSTOPERATIVE CARE. A short leg cast is worn for 6 weeks. An ankle-foot orthosis may be needed for 6 months.

SPLIT TRANSFER OF THE POSTERIOR TIBIAL TENDON

The split transfer of the posterior tibial tendon technique is used more often for patients with cerebral palsy and is described in Chapter 33.

TALIPES CAVOVARUS

Paralytic talipes cavovarus can be caused by an imbalance of the extrinsic muscles or by persistent function of the short toe flexors and other intrinsic muscles when the foot is otherwise flail. Treatment of the cavus foot is discussed in Chapter 86.

TALIPES EQUINOVALGUS

Talipes equinovalgus usually develops when the anterior and posterior tibial muscles are weak, the peroneus longus and peroneus brevis are strong, and the gastrocnemius-soleus is strong and contracted. The gastrocnemius-soleus pulls the foot into equinus and the peroneals into valgus position; when the extensor digitorum longus and the peroneus tertius muscles are also strong, they help to pull the foot into valgus position on walking. Structural changes in the bones and ligaments follow the muscle imbalance; eventually, the plantar calcaneonavicular ligament becomes stretched and attenuated, the weight-bearing thrust shifts to the medial border of the foot, the forefoot abducts and pronates, and the head and neck of the talus become depressed and prominent on the medial side of the foot.

Treatment of this deformity in a skeletally immature foot is difficult. Subtalar arthrodesis and anterior transfer of the peroneus longus and brevis tendons usually suffice until skeletal maturity is reached; if necessary, a triple arthrodesis can then be done. Failure to transfer the tendons is the usual cause of recurrence.

Paralysis of the anterior tibial muscle alone usually causes only a moderate valgus deformity that is more pronounced during dorsiflexion of the ankle and may disappear during plantarflexion. Treatment of this deformity may require transfer of the peroneus longus to the first cuneiform, transfer of the extensor digitorum longus, or the Jones procedure (see Chapter 86). Paralysis of the posterior tibial alone can cause a planovalgus deformity. Normally, this muscle inverts the foot during plantarflexion; when it is paralyzed, a valgus deformity develops. Because most of the functions of the foot are performed during plantarflexion, loss of the posterior tibial is a severe impairment. Treatment of this deformity may involve transfer of the peroneus longus tendon, the flexor digitorum longus, the flexor hallucis longus, or the extensor hallucis longus. Paralysis of the anterior tibial and the posterior tibial muscles results in an extreme deformity similar to rocker-bottom flatfoot. For this deformity, a transfer to replace the posterior tibial is necessary, followed by another to replace the anterior tibial if necessary. Extraarticular subtalar arthrodesis may be indicated for equinovalgus deformity in children 4 to 10 years old. The equinus must be corrected by Achilles tendon lengthening at surgery to allow the calcaneus to be brought far enough distally beneath the talus to correct the deformity. The technique of Grice and Green (see Technique 34-2) or preferably of Dennyson and Fulford (see Technique 34-3) can be used. Talipes equinovalgus in skeletally mature patients usually requires triple arthrodesis (see Technique 34-4) and lengthening of the Achilles tendon, followed in 4 to 6 weeks by appropriate tendon transfers.

PERONEAL TENDON TRANSFER

TECHNIQUE 34-10

- Expose the tendons of the peroneus longus and peroneus brevis through an oblique incision paralleling the skin creases at a point midway between the distal tip of the lateral malleolus and the base of the fifth metatarsal.
- Divide the tendons as far distally as possible, securely suture the distal end of the peroneus longus to its sheath to prevent the development of a dorsal bunion, and free the tendons proximally to the posterior border of the lateral malleolus. (When they are to be transferred at the time of arthrodesis, they can be divided through a short extension of the routine incision, as shown in Figure 34-5.)
- Make a second incision 5 cm long at the junction of the middle and distal thirds of the leg overlying the tendons. Gently withdraw the tendons from their sheaths, taking care not to disrupt the origin of the peroneus brevis muscle.
- The new site of insertion of the peroneal tendons is determined by the severity of the deformity and the existing muscle power. When the extensor hallucis longus is functioning and is to be transferred to the neck of the first metatarsal, the peroneal tendons should be transferred to the lateral cuneiform; when no other functioning dorsiflexor is available, they should be transferred to the middle cuneiform anteriorly.
- Expose the new site of insertion of the tendons through a short longitudinal incision.
- Retract the tendons of the extensor digitorum longus and make a cruciate or H-shaped cut in the periosteum of the recipient bone.
- Raise and fold back osteoperiosteal flaps and drill a hole in the bone large enough to receive the tendons. Then bring the tendons out beneath the cruciate crural ligament into this incision and anchor them side by side and under equal tension through a hole drilled in the bone, either by suturing them back on themselves or by securely fixing them to bone using a platform staple.
- As an alternative, drill a hole through the middle cuneiform and pull the tendons through the hole and then through a button on the plantar aspect of the foot.
- When there is significant clawing of the great toe, the extensor hallucis longus tendon should be transferred to the neck of the first metatarsal and then the interphalangeal joint is fused (Jones procedure, see Chapter 86).
- Residual clawing of the lateral four toes usually is of little or no significance after transfer of the peroneal and extensor hallucis longus tendons.

PERONEUS LONGUS, FLEXOR DIGITORUM LONGUS, OR FLEXOR OR EXTENSOR HALLUCIS LONGUS TENDON TRANSFER

TECHNIQUE 34-11

(FRIED AND HENDEL)

- In this operation the tendon of the peroneus longus, flexor digitorum longus, flexor hallucis longus, or extensor hallucis longus can be transferred to replace a paralyzed posterior tibial muscle.
- When the peroneus longus tendon is to be transferred, make a longitudinal incision 5 to 8 cm long laterally over the shaft of the fibula.
- After incising the fascia of the peroneal muscles, inspect them; if their color does not confirm their preoperative grading, the transfer will fail.
- Now make a second incision along the lateral border of the foot over the cuboid and the peroneus longus tendon.
- Free the tendon, divide it as far distally in the sole of the foot as possible, suture its distal end in its sheath, and withdraw the tendon through the first incision.
- By blunt dissection create a space between the gastrocnemius-soleus and the deep layer of leg muscles; from here make a wide tunnel posterior to the fibula and to the deep muscles and directed to a point proximal and posterior to the medial malleolus.
- Now make a small incision at this point and draw the peroneus longus tendon through the tunnel; it now emerges where the posterior tibial tendon enters its sheath.
- Make a fourth incision 5 cm long over the middle of the medial side of the foot centered below the tuberosity of the navicular.
- Free and retract plantarward the anterior border of the abductor hallucis muscle and expose the tuberosity of the navicular and the insertion of the posterior tibial tendon; proximal to the medial malleolus open the sheath of this tendon and into it introduce and advance a curved probe until it emerges with the tendon at the sole of the foot.
- Using the probe, pull the peroneus longus tendon through the same sheath, which is large enough to contain this second tendon.
- Drill a narrow tunnel through the navicular, beginning on its plantar surface lateral to the tuberosity and emerging through its anterior surface.

- Pull the peroneus longus tendon through the tunnel in an anterior direction and anchor it with a Bunnell pull-out suture. Also suture it to the posterior tibial tendon close to its insertion.
- Close the wounds and apply a short leg cast with the foot in slight equinus and varus position.
- When the flexor digitorum longus tendon is to be transferred, make the incision near the medial malleolus as just described but extend it for about 7 cm.
- Free the three deep muscles and observe their color; if it is satisfactory, make the incision on the medial side of the foot as just described.
- Free and retract the short plantar muscles and expose the flexor digitorum longus tendon as it emerges from behind the medial malleolus.
- Free the tendon as far distally as possible, divide it, and withdraw it through the first incision; now pass it through the sheath of the posterior tibial tendon and anchor it in the navicular as just described.
- When the flexor hallucis longus tendon is to be transferred, use the same procedure as described for the flexor digitorum longus.
- When the extensor hallucis longus tendon is to be transferred, cut it near the metatarsophalangeal joint of the great toe.
- Suture its distal end to the long extensor tendon of the second toe.
- Withdraw the proximal end through an anterolateral longitudinal incision over the distal part of the leg.
- Open the interosseous membrane widely, make the incision near the medial malleolus as previously described, and with a broad probe draw the tendon through the interosseous space and through the sheath of the posterior tibial tendon to the insertion of that tendon.
- Then continue with the operation as described for transfer of the peroneus longus tendon.

POSTOPERATIVE CARE. A short leg walking cast is applied. At 6 weeks the walking cast is removed, a splint is used at night, and muscle reeducation is started.

TALIPES CALCANEUS

Talipes calcaneus is a rapidly progressive paralytic deformity that results when the gastrocnemius-soleus is paralyzed and the other extrinsic foot muscles, especially the muscles that dorsiflex the ankle, remain functional. Mild deformity in skeletally immature patients should be treated conservatively with braces or orthoses until the rate of progression of the deformity can be determined. For rapidly progressing deformities, especially in young children, early tendon transfers are recommended. The goal of surgery in the skeletally immature foot is to stop progression of the deformity or to correct severe deformity without damaging skeletal growth; arthrodesis may be necessary after skeletal maturity. If muscles of adequate power are available, tendons should be transferred early to improve function and avoid progressive deformity. If adequate muscles are unavailable, tenodesis of the Achilles tendon to the fibula may be appropriate.

The calcaneotibial angle (Fig. 34-9) is formed by the intersection of the axis of the tibia with a line drawn along

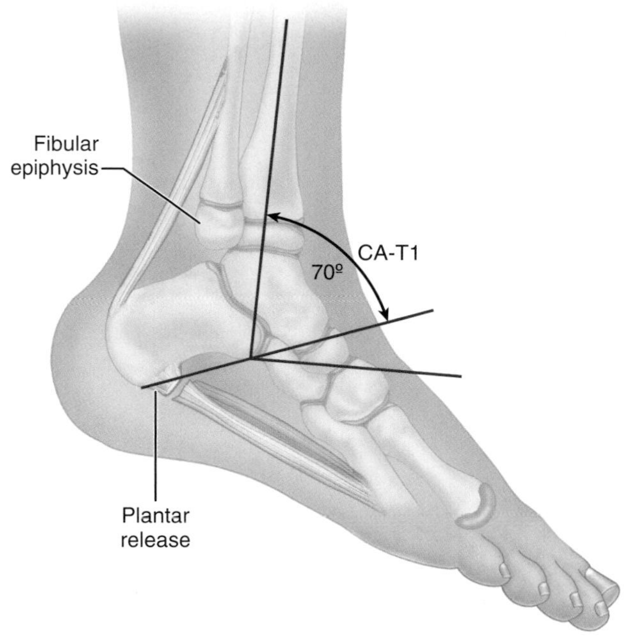

FIGURE 34-9 Measurement of calcaneotibial angle (see text).

the plantar aspect of the calcaneus. Normally, this angle measures between 70 and 80 degrees; in equinus deformity it is greater than 80 degrees, and in calcaneal deformity it is less than 70 degrees. When the tenodesis is fixed at 70 degrees or more at the time of surgery, a tendency to develop a progressive equinus deformity with growth has been noted. Progressive equinus also is directly related to the patient's age at surgery: the younger the patient, the greater the calcaneotibial angle and the more likely the development of progressive equinus deformity with subsequent growth.

In skeletally mature feet, initial surgery for talipes calcaneus consists of plantar fasciotomy and triple arthrodesis that corrects the calcaneus and the cavus deformities; the arthrodesis should displace the foot as far posteriorly as possible to lengthen its posterior lever arm (the calcaneus) and reduce the muscle power required to lift the heel. Six weeks after arthrodesis, the tendons of the peroneus longus and peroneus brevis and the posterior tibial tendon are transferred to the calcaneus; and when the extensor digitorum longus is functional, it can be transferred to a cuneiform and then the anterior tibial tendon can be transferred to the calcaneus.

TENODESIS OF THE ACHILLES TENDON

TECHNIQUE 34-12

(WESTIN)

- With the patient supine and tilted toward the nonoperative side, apply and inflate a pneumatic tourniquet.
- Make a posterolateral longitudinal incision just behind the posterior border of the fibula beginning 7 to 10 cm above

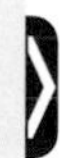

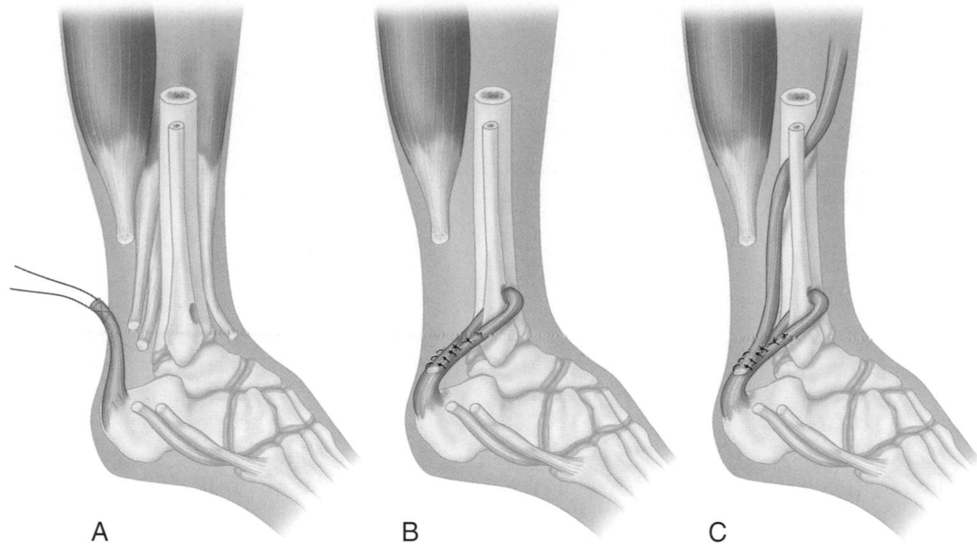

FIGURE 34-10 Calcaneal tenodesis. **A,** After division of Achilles tendon, tenotomy of peroneus brevis and longus, and detachment of anterior tibial tendon from its insertion, transverse hole is made in fibula 2 cm proximal to epiphysis. **B,** Achilles tendon is passed through hole in fibula and sutured to itself. **C,** If necessary, anterior tibial tendon can be passed through interosseous membrane and attached to calcaneus. **SEE TECHNIQUE 34-12.**

the tip of the lateral malleolus and extending distally to the insertion of the Achilles tendon on the calcaneus.

- Expose the tendon and section it transversely at the musculotendinous junction, usually 6 cm from its insertion. Stevens advised that the tendon be split eccentrically, leaving the lateral one fifth to prevent retraction. Transect the medial four fifths proximally.
- Expose the peroneus brevis and longus tendons, and if they are completely paralyzed or spastic, excise them. Expose the distal fibula, taking care not to damage the distal fibular physis.
- About 4 cm proximal to the distal physis, use a fine drill bit to make a transverse hole in an anteroposterior direction. Make the hole large enough for the Achilles tendon to pass through it easily (Fig. 34-10A).
- If the tendon is too large, trim it longitudinally for about 2.5 cm. Bring the tendon through the hole and suture it to itself under enough tension to limit ankle dorsiflexion to 0 degrees (Fig. 34-10B). Do not suture the tendon with the foot in too much equinus because of the possibility of causing a fixed equinus deformity.
- In patients with active anterior tibial tendons, simultaneous transfer of this tendon through the interosseous membrane to the calcaneus is indicated to avoid stretching of the Achilles tendon after surgery (Fig. 34-10C).

POSTOPERATIVE CARE. Weight bearing is allowed in a short leg cast with the ankle in 5 to 10 degrees of equinus. The cast is removed at 6 weeks, and an ankle-foot orthosis is fitted with the ankle in neutral position. Any residual cavus deformity is corrected by plantar release 3 to 6 months after tenodesis.

In skeletally mature feet, initial surgery for talipes calcaneus consists of plantar fasciotomy and triple arthrodesis that corrects both the calcaneus and cavus deformities; the arthrodesis should displace the foot as far posteriorly as possible to lengthen its posterior lever arm (the calcaneus) and reduce the muscle power required to lift the heel. Six weeks after arthrodesis, the tendons of the peroneus longus and peroneus brevis and the posterior tibial muscles are transferred to the calcaneus, and when the extensor digitorum longus is functional, it can be transferred to a cuneiform and then the anterior tibial muscle can be transferred to the calcaneus.

POSTERIOR TRANSFER OF PERONEUS LONGUS, PERONEUS BREVIS, AND POSTERIOR TIBIAL TENDONS

TECHNIQUE 34-13

- Expose the peroneus longus and peroneus brevis tendons through an oblique incision 2.5 cm long midway between the tip of the lateral malleolus and the base of the fifth metatarsal.
- Divide the tendons as far distally as possible and securely suture the distal end of the peroneus longus tendon to its sheath.
- Bring the tendons out through a second incision overlying the peroneal sheath at the junction of the middle and distal thirds of the leg.

- If desired, suture the peroneus brevis at its musculotendinous junction to the peroneus longus tendon and discard the distal end of the peroneus brevis tendon.
- Expose the posterior tibial tendon through a short incision over its insertion; free its distal end and gently bring it out through a second incision 2.5 cm long at its musculotendinous junction 5 cm proximal to the medial malleolus.
- Reroute all three tendons subcutaneously to and out of a separate incision lateral and anterior to the insertion of the Achilles tendon.
- Drill a hole in the superior surface of the posterior part of the calcaneus just lateral to the midline of the bone and enlarge it enough to receive the tendons; anchor the tendons in the hole with a large pull-out suture while holding the foot in equinus and the heel in the corrected position. An axial pin also can be inserted into the calcaneus and left in place for 6 weeks.
- With interrupted figure-of-eight sutures, fix the tendons to the Achilles tendon near its insertion; then close the wounds.

POSTOPERATIVE CARE. The foot is immobilized in a long leg cast with the ankle in plantarflexion and the knee at 20 degrees. The pull-out sutures and cast (and axial pin, if used) are removed at 6 weeks, and physical therapy is started. Weight bearing is not allowed until active plantarflexion is possible and dorsiflexion to the neutral position has been regained. The foot is protected for at least 6 more months by a reverse 90-degree ankle stop brace and an appropriate heel elevation.

POSTERIOR TRANSFER OF POSTERIOR TIBIAL, PERONEUS LONGUS, AND FLEXOR HALLUCIS LONGUS TENDONS

TECHNIQUE 34-14

(GREEN AND GRICE)

- Place the patient prone for easier access to the heel.
- First, expose the posterior tibial tendon through an oblique incision 3 or 4 cm long from just inferior to the medial malleolus to the plantar aspect of the talonavicular joint; open its sheath and divide it as close to bone as possible for maximal length.
- Remove the epitenon from its distal 3 or 4 cm, scarify it, and insert a 1-0 or 2-0 braided nonabsorbable suture into its distal end.
- When the flexor hallucis longus tendon also is to be transferred, expose it through this same incision where it lies posterior and lateral to the flexor digitorum longus tendon.
- At the proper level for the desired tendon length, place two braided nonabsorbable sutures in the flexor hallucis longus tendon and divide it between them; suture the distal end of this tendon to the flexor digitorum longus tendon.
- Second, make a longitudinal medial incision, usually about 10 cm long, over the posterior tibial muscle, extending distally from the junction of the middle and distal thirds of the leg.
- Open the medial compartment of the leg and identify the posterior tibial and flexor hallucis longus muscle bellies.
- Using moist sponges, deliver the tendons of these two muscles into this wound.
- Third, make an incision parallel to the bottom of the foot from about a fingerbreadth distal to the lateral malleolus to the base of the fifth metatarsal.
- Expose the peroneus longus and peroneus brevis tendons throughout the length of the incision and divide that of the peroneus longus between sutures as far distally as possible in the sole of the foot and free its proximal end to behind the lateral malleolus.
- Place a suture in the peroneus brevis tendon, detach it from its insertion on the fifth metatarsal, and suture it to the distal end of the peroneus longus tendon.
- Make a lateral longitudinal incision over the posterior aspect of the fibula at the same level as the medial incision and deliver the peroneus longus tendon into it.
- Make a posterolateral transverse incision 6 cm long over the calcaneus in the part of the heel that neither strikes the ground nor presses against the shoe. Deepen the incision, reflect the skin flaps subcutaneously, and expose the Achilles tendon and calcaneus.
- Beginning laterally, partially divide the Achilles tendon at its insertion and reflect it medially, exposing the calcaneal apophysis.
- With a 9/64-inch (3.57-mm) drill bit, make a hole through the calcaneus beginning in the center of its apophysis and emerging through its plantar aspect near its lateral border. Enlarge the hole enough to receive the three tendons and ream its posterior end to make a shallow facet for their easier insertion.
- Next, through the medial wound on the leg (the second incision), incise widely the intermuscular septum between the medial and posterior compartments; insert a tendon passer through the wound and along the anterior side of the Achilles tendon to the transverse incision over the calcaneus. Thread the sutures in the ends of the posterior tibial and flexor hallucis longus tendons through the tendon passer and deliver the tendons at the heel.
- Through the lateral wound on the leg (the fourth incision), open widely the intermuscular septum between the medial and posterior compartments in this area and pass the peroneus longus tendon to the heel.
- Pass all tendons through smooth tissues in a straight line from as far proximally as possible to avoid angulation.
- With a twisted wire probe, bring the tendons through the hole in the calcaneus; suture them to the periosteum and ligamentous attachments where they emerge.
- When the dorsiflexors are weak, suture them under enough tension to hold the foot in 10 to 15 degrees of equinus, and when they are strong, suture them in about 30 degrees of equinus. Also suture the tendons to the apophysis at the proximal end of the tunnel and to each other with 2-0 or 3-0 sutures.

- Replace the Achilles tendon posterior to the transferred tendons and suture it in its original position.
- Close the wounds and apply a long leg cast with the foot in equinus.

POSTOPERATIVE CARE. At 3 weeks, the cast is bivalved and exercises are started with the leg in the anterior half of the cast; the bivalved cast is reapplied between exercise periods. At first, dorsiflexion exercises are not permitted, but, later, guided reciprocal motion is allowed. The exercises are gradually increased, and at 6 weeks the patient is allowed to stand but not to bear full weight on the foot. The periods of partial weight-bearing on crutches are increased, depending on the effectiveness of the transfer, the cooperation of the patient, and the ability to control his or her motions. Usually at 6 to 8 weeks a single step is allowed, using crutches and an elevated heel; later more steps are allowed, using crutches and a plantarflexion spring brace with an elastic strap posteriorly. Crutches are used for 6 to 12 months.

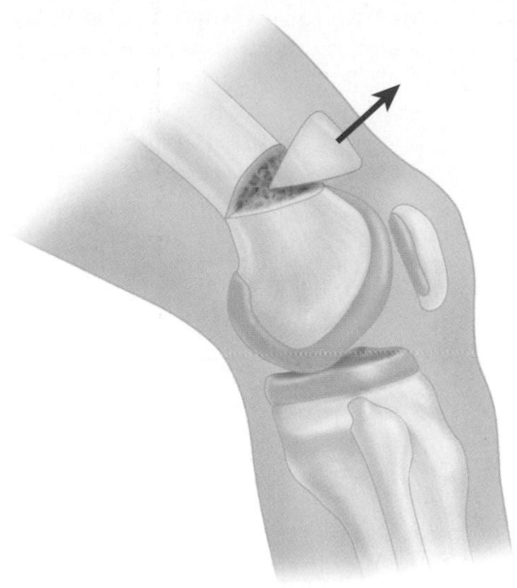

FIGURE 34-11 Supracondylar extension osteotomy of femur for fixed knee flexion deformity in older child.

KNEE

The disabilities caused by paralysis of the muscles acting across the knee joint include (1) flexion contracture of the knee, (2) quadriceps paralysis, (3) genu recurvatum, and (4) flail knee.

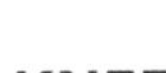

■ FLEXION CONTRACTURE OF THE KNEE

Flexion contracture of the knee can be caused by a contracture of the iliotibial band; contracture of this band can cause not only flexion contracture but also genu valgum and an external rotation deformity of the tibia on the femur. Flexion contracture also can be caused by paralysis of the quadriceps muscle when the hamstrings are normal or only partially paralyzed. When the biceps femoris is stronger than the medial hamstrings, there may be genu valgum and an external rotation deformity of the tibia on the femur; often the tibia subluxates posteriorly on the femur.

Contractures of 15 to 20 degrees or less in young children can be treated with posterior hamstring lengthening and capsulotomy. More severe contractures usually require a supracondylar extension osteotomy of the femur (Fig. 34-11).

Flexion contractures of more than 70 degrees result in deformity of the articular surfaces of the knee. In a growing child with poliomyelitis, a decrease in pressure and a tendency toward posterior subluxation cause increased growth on the anterior surface of the proximal tibia and distal femur. The quadriceps expansion adheres to the femoral condyles, and the collateral ligaments are unable to glide easily. Severe knee flexion contractures in growing children can be treated by division of the iliotibial band and hamstring tendons, combined with posterior capsulotomy. Skeletal traction after surgery is maintained through a pin in the distal tibia; a second pin in the proximal tibia pulls anteriorly to avoid posterior subluxation of the tibia. Long-term use of a long leg brace may be required to allow the joint to remodel. Supracondylar osteotomy may be required as a second-stage procedure in older patients near skeletal maturity.

■ QUADRICEPS PARALYSIS

Disability from paralysis of the quadriceps muscle is severe because the knee may be extremely unstable, especially if there is even a mild fixed flexion contracture. When there is slight recurvatum, the knee may be stable if the gastrocnemius-soleus is active.

Tendons usually are transferred around the knee joint to reinforce a weak or paralyzed quadriceps muscle; transfers are unnecessary for paralysis of the hamstring muscles because, in walking, gravity flexes the knee as the hip is flexed. Several muscles are available for transfer to the quadriceps tendon and patella: the biceps femoris, semitendinosus, sartorius, and tensor fasciae latae. When the power of certain other muscles is satisfactory, transfer of the biceps femoris has been the most successful. Transfer of one or more of the hamstring tendons is contraindicated unless one other flexor in the thigh and the gastrocnemius-soleus, which also acts as a knee flexor, are functioning. If a satisfactory result is to be expected after hamstring transfer, the power not only of the hamstrings but also of the hip flexors, the gluteus maximus, and the gastrocnemius-soleus must be fair or better; when the power of the hip flexor muscles are less than fair, clearing the extremity from the floor may be difficult after surgery. Transfer of the tensor fasciae latae and sartorius muscles, although theoretically more satisfactory, is insufficient because these muscles are not strong enough to replace the quadriceps.

Ease in ascending or descending steps depends on the strength of the hip flexors and extensors. Strong hamstrings are necessary for active extension of the knee against gravity after the transfer; however, a weak medial hamstring can be transferred to serve as a checkrein on the patella to prevent it from dislocating laterally. A normal gastrocnemius-soleus is desirable because it aids in preventing genu recurvatum and remains as an active knee flexor after surgery; it may not always prevent genu recurvatum, however, which can result from other factors. Recurvatum after hamstring transfers can be kept to a minimum if (1) strength in the gastrocnemius-soleus is fair or better; (2) the knee is not immobilized in hyperextension after surgery; (3) talipes equinus, when present, is corrected before weight bearing is resumed; (4) postoperative bracing is used to prevent knee hyperextension; and (5) physical therapy is begun to promote active knee extension.

TRANSFER OF BICEPS FEMORIS AND SEMITENDINOSUS TENDONS

TECHNIQUE 34-15

- Make an incision along the anteromedial aspect of the knee to conform to the medial border of the quadriceps tendon, the patella, and the patellar tendon.
- Retract the lateral edge of the incision and expose the patella and the quadriceps tendon.
- Incise longitudinally the lateral side of the thigh and leg from a point 7.5 cm distal to the head of the fibula to the junction of the proximal and middle thirds of the thigh.
- Isolate and retract the common peroneal nerve, which is near the medial side of the biceps tendon.
- With an osteotome, free the biceps tendon, along with a thin piece of bone, from the head of the fibula. Do not divide the lateral collateral ligament, which lies firmly adherent to the biceps tendon at its point of insertion.
- Free the tendon and its muscle belly proximally as far as the incision will permit; free the origin of the short head of the biceps proximally to where its nerve and blood supplies enter so that the new line of pull of the muscle may be as oblique as possible.
- Create a subcutaneous tunnel from the first incision to the lateral thigh incision and make it wide enough for the transferred muscle belly to glide freely.
- To further increase the obliquity of pull of the transferred muscle, divide the iliotibial band, the fascia of the vastus lateralis, and the lateral intermuscular septum at a point distal to where the muscle will pass.
- Beginning distally over the insertion of the medial hamstring tendons into the tibia, make a third incision longitudinally along the posteromedial aspect of the knee and extend it to the middle of the thigh.
- Locate the semitendinosus tendon; it inserts on the medial side of the tibia as far anteriorly as its crest and lies posterior to the tendon of the sartorius and distal to that of the gracilis. Divide the insertion of the semitendinosus tendon and free the muscle to the middle third of the thigh.
- Reroute this muscle and tendon subcutaneously to emerge in the first incision over the knee.
- Make an I-shaped incision through the fascia, quadriceps tendon, and periosteum over the anterior surface of the patella and strip these tissues medially and laterally. With an 11/64-inch (4.36-mm) drill bit, make a hole transversely through the patella at the junction of its middle and proximal thirds; if necessary, enlarge the tunnel with a small curet.

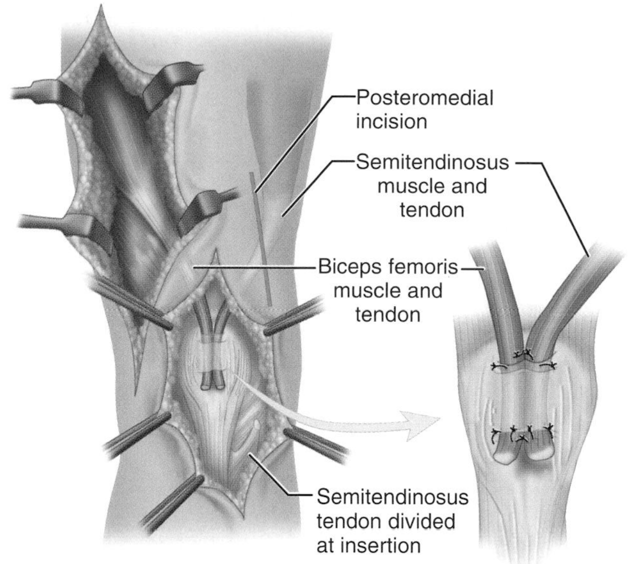

FIGURE 34-12 Transfer of semitendinosus and biceps femoris tendons to patella for quadriceps paralysis. **SEE TECHNIQUE 34-15.**

- Place the biceps tendon in line with and anterior to the quadriceps tendon, the patella, and the patellar tendon.
- Suture the biceps tendon to the patella with the knee in extension or hyperextension.
- When only the biceps tendon is transferred, close the soft tissues over the anterior aspect of the patella and the transferred tendon. With interrupted sutures, fix the biceps tendon to the medial side of the quadriceps tendon.
- When the semitendinosus also is transferred, place it over the biceps and suture the two together with interrupted sutures; place additional sutures proximally and distally through the semitendinosus, quadriceps, and patellar tendons.
- Alternatively, detach the insertion of the semitendinosus from the tibia through an incision 2.5 cm long and bring it out through a posteromedial incision 7.5 cm long over its musculotendinous junction (Fig. 34-12). Incise the enveloping fascia to prevent acute angulation of the muscle and pass the tendon subcutaneously in a straight line to the patellar incision.

POSTOPERATIVE CARE. With the knee in the neutral position, a long leg cast is applied. To prevent swelling, the extremity is elevated by raising the foot of the bed rather than by using pillows; otherwise, flexion of the hip may put too much tension on the transferred tendons. At 3 weeks, physical therapy and active and passive exercises are started. Knee flexion is gradually developed, and the hamstring muscles are reeducated. At 8 weeks, weight bearing is started, with the extremity supported by a controlled dial knee brace locked in extension. Knee motion is gradually allowed in the brace when the muscles of the transferred tendons are strong enough to extend the knee actively against considerable force. To prevent overstretching or strain of the muscles, a night splint is worn for at least 6 weeks and the brace for at least 12 weeks.

GENU RECURVATUM

In genu recurvatum the deformity is the opposite of that in a flexion contracture and the knee is hyperextended. Mild genu recurvatum can cause some disability, but when the quadriceps is severely weakened or paralyzed, such a deformity is desirable because it stabilizes the knee in walking. Severe genu recurvatum is significantly disabling, however.

Genu recurvatum from poliomyelitis is of two types: that caused by structural articular and bone changes stemming from lack of power in the quadriceps and that caused by relaxation of the soft tissues around the posterior aspect of the knee. In the first type, the quadriceps lacks the power to lock the knee in extension; the hamstrings and gastrocnemius-soleus usually are normal. The pressures of weight bearing and gravity cause changes in the tibial condyles and in the proximal third of the tibial shaft. The condyles become elongated posteriorly; their anterior margins are depressed compared with their posterior margins; and the angle of their articular surfaces to the long axis of the tibia, which is normally 90 degrees, becomes more acute. The proximal third of the tibial shaft usually bows posteriorly, and partial subluxation of the tibia may gradually occur. In the second type, the hamstrings and the gastrocnemius-soleus muscles are weak. Hyperextension of the knee results from stretching of these muscles, often followed by stretching of the posterior capsular ligament.

The prognosis after correction of the first type of recurvatum is excellent. The skeletal deformity is corrected first, and then one or more hamstrings can be transferred to the patella. Irwin described an osteotomy of the proximal tibia to correct the first type of genu recurvatum caused by structural bone changes. Storen modified the Campbell osteotomy by immobilizing the fragments of the tibia with a Charnley clamp.

OSTEOTOMY OF THE TIBIA FOR GENU RECURVATUM

TECHNIQUE 34-16

(IRWIN)

- Through a short longitudinal incision, remove a section of the shaft of the fibula about 2.5 cm long from just distal to the neck.
- Pack the defect with chips from the sectioned piece of bone.
- Close the periosteum and overlying soft tissues.
- Through an anteromedial incision, expose and, without entering the joint, osteotomize the proximal fourth of the tibia as follows: With a thin osteotome or a power saw, outline a tongue of bone but leave it attached to the anterior cortex of the distal fragment. At a right angle to the longitudinal axis of the knee joint and parallel to its lateral plane, pass a Kirschner wire through the distal end of the proposed proximal fragment before the tibial shaft is divided. Complete the osteotomy with a Gigli saw, an osteotome, or a power saw.
- Lift the proximal end of the distal fragment from its periosteal bed and remove from it a wedge of bone of predetermined size, its base being the posterior cortex.
- Replace the tongue of bone in its recess in the proximal fragment and push the fragments firmly together.
- Suture the periosteum, which is quite thick in this area, firmly over the tongue of bone; this is enough fixation to keep the fragments in position until a cast can be applied.

The osteotomy can be fixed with percutaneous Kirschner wires, an external fixator, or, in adults, rigid plate fixation. Figure 34-13 shows correction of genu recurvatum by the Campbell technique.

SOFT-TISSUE OPERATIONS FOR GENU RECURVATUM

Another type of genu recurvatum results from stretching of the posterior soft tissues. The prognosis is less certain after correction of this type of deformity; no muscles are available for transfer, the underlying cause cannot be corrected, and the deformity can recur. An operation on the soft tissues, triple tenodesis of the knee, has been described for correcting paralytic genu recurvatum. If the deformity is 30 degrees or less, prolonged bracing of the knee in flexion usually prevents an increase in deformity. When the deformity is severe, however, bracing is ineffective, the knee becomes unstable and weak, the gait is inefficient, and, in adults, pain is marked. The three following principles must be considered if operations on the soft tissues for genu recurvatum are to be successful:

1. The fibrous tissue mass used for tenodesis must be sufficient to withstand the stretching forces generated by walking; all available tendons must be used.
2. Healing tissues must be protected until they are fully mature. The operation should not be undertaken unless the surgeon is sure that the patient will conscientiously use a brace that limits extension to 15 degrees of flexion for 1 year.
3. The alignment and stability of the ankle must meet the basic requirements of gait. Any equinus deformity must be corrected to at least neutral. If the strength of the soleus is less than good on the standing test, this defect must be corrected by tendon transfer, tenodesis, or arthrodesis of the ankle in the neutral position.

TRIPLE TENODESIS FOR GENU RECURVATUM

The operation for triple tenodesis for genu recurvatum consists of three parts: proximal advancement of the posterior capsule of the knee with the joint flexed 20 degrees, construction of a checkrein in the midline posteriorly using the tendons of the semitendinosus and gracilis, and creation of two diagonal straps posteriorly using the biceps tendon and the anterior half of the iliotibial band.

TECHNIQUE 34-17

(PERRY, O'BRIEN, AND HODGSON)

- Place the patient prone, apply a tourniquet high on the thigh, and place a large sandbag beneath the ankle to flex the knee about 20 degrees.

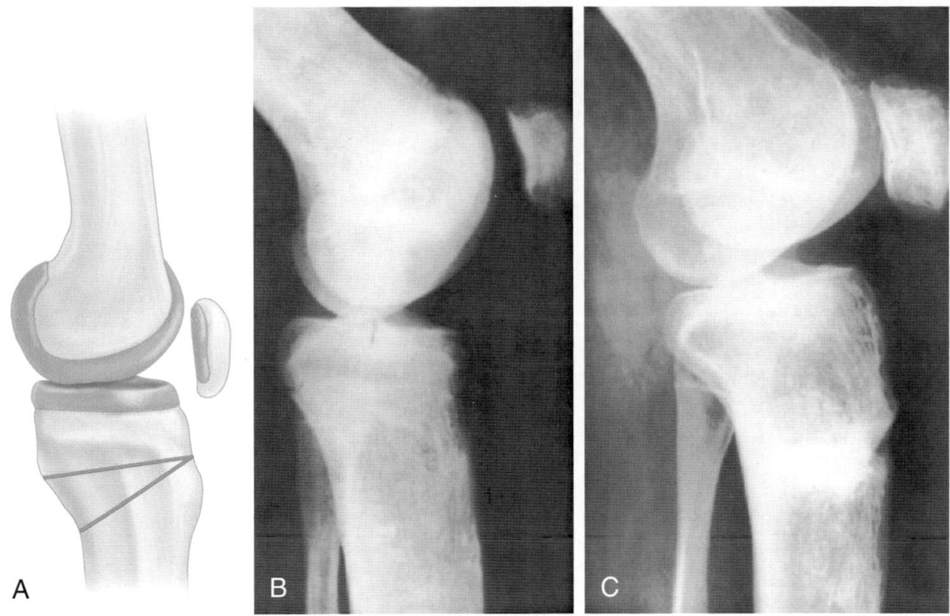

FIGURE 34-13 Closing wedge osteotomy for genu recurvatum. **A,** Wedge of bone removed from tibia. **B,** Recurvatum secondary to anterior tilt of tibial plateau. **C,** Five months after operation. **SEE TECHNIQUE 34-16.**

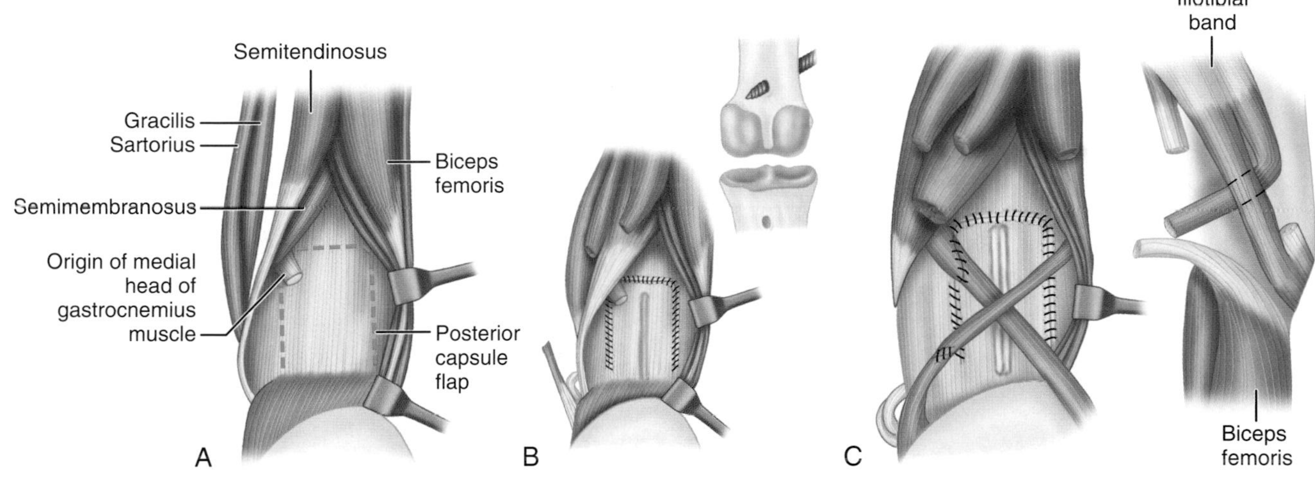

FIGURE 34-14 Perry, O'Brien, and Hodgson operation for genu recurvatum. **A,** Origin of medial head of gastrocnemius has been released, leaving proximal strap. Broad flap of posterior capsule is released for future advancement. **B,** Semitendinosus and gracilis tendons are divided at musculotendinous junctions. Each is passed through tunnel in tibia, then across exterior of joint, and then through tunnel in femur. Flap of posterior capsule is advanced and sutured snugly with knee flexed 20 degrees. **C,** Cross straps are made with biceps femoris and iliotibial band. **SEE TECHNIQUE 34-17.**

- Make an S-shaped incision beginning laterally parallel to and 1 cm anterior to the biceps tendon; extend it distally 4 cm to the transverse flexion crease of the knee, carry it medially across the popliteal fossa, and extend it distally for 4 or 5 cm overlying or just medial to the semitendinosus tendon.
- Identify the sural nerve and retract it laterally. Then identify the tibial nerve and the popliteal artery and vein and protect them with a soft rubber tape. Next, identify and free the peroneal nerve and protect it in a similar manner. Retract the neurovascular bundle laterally and identify the posterior part of the joint capsule.
- Detach the medial head of the gastrocnemius muscle in a step-cut fashion, preserving a long, strong proximal strap of the Z to be used in the tenodesis (Fig. 34-14A).
- Next, use a knife to detach the joint capsule from its attachment to the femur just proximal to the condyles and the intercondylar notch.

- Detach the tendons of the gracilis and semitendinosus at their musculotendinous junctions and suture their proximal ends to the sartorius. Be sure to divide these tendons as far proximally as possible because all available length will be needed.
- Next, drill a hole in the tibia beginning at a point in the midline posteriorly inferior to the physis and emerging near the insertion of the pes anserinus; take care to avoid the physis.
- Drill a hole in the femur beginning in the midline posteriorly proximal to the femoral physis and emerging on the lateral aspect of the distal femur (Fig. 34-14B).
- Draw the tendons of the gracilis and semitendinosus through the hole in the tibia, pass them posterior to the detached part of the capsule, and pull them through the hole in the femur to emerge on the lateral aspect of the distal femur; suture the tendons to the periosteum here under moderate tension with heavy nonabsorbable sutures with the knee flexed 20 degrees.
- Advance the free edge of the joint capsule proximally on the femur until all slack has disappeared and suture it to the periosteum in its new position using nonabsorbable sutures.
- Detach the biceps tendon from its muscle, rotate it on its fibular insertion, pass it across the posterior aspect of the joint deep to the neurovascular structures, and anchor it to the femoral origin of the medial head of the gastrocnemius under moderate tension (Fig. 34-14C).
- Detach the anterior half of the iliotibial band from its insertion on the tibia, pass it deep to the intact part of the band, the biceps tendon, and the neurovascular structures, and suture it to the semimembranosus insertion on the tibia under moderate tension.
- If one of the tendons being used is of an active muscle, split that tendon and use only half of it in the tenodesis, leaving the other half attached at its insertion.
- Close the wound in layers and use suction drainage for 48 hours. Apply a well-padded cast from groin to toes with the knee flexed 30 degrees to prevent tension on the sutures.

POSTOPERATIVE CARE. The cast is removed at 6 weeks, and a long leg brace that was fitted before surgery is applied. The brace is designed to limit extension of the knee to 15 degrees of flexion. Full weight bearing is allowed in the brace, and at night a plaster shell is used to hold the knee flexed 15 degrees. Twelve months after surgery the patient is readmitted to the hospital and the flexion contracture of the knee is corrected gradually to neutral by serial plaster casts; unprotected weight bearing is then permitted. It is important that the soft tissues are completely healed before being subjected to excessive stretching caused by unprotected weight bearing or by wedging plaster casts.

FLAIL KNEE

When the knee is unstable in all directions, and muscle power sufficient to overcome this instability is unavailable for tendon transfer, either a long leg brace with a locking knee joint must be worn or the knee must be fused. Fusion of the knee in a good position not only permits a satisfactory gait but also improves it by eliminating the weight of the brace; fusion of the knee causes inconvenience while sitting. One option is to defer fusion until the patient is old enough to weigh its advantages and disadvantages before a final decision is made. For patients who are heavy laborers and would have trouble maintaining a brace, the advantages of being free of a brace outweigh the advantages of being able to sit with the knee flexed in a brace; in these patients, an arthrodesis is indicated. Others who sit much of the time may prefer to use a brace permanently. When both legs are badly paralyzed, one knee can be fused and the other stabilized with a brace.

Before an arthrodesis is performed, a cylinder cast can be applied on a trial basis, immobilizing the knee in the position in which it would be fused; this allows the patient to make an informed decision concerning the advantages and disadvantages of arthrodesis of the knee. The techniques of knee fusion are described in Chapter 8.

TIBIA AND FEMUR

Angular and torsional deformities of the tibia and femur are more often caused by conditions other than poliomyelitis, such as congenital abnormalities, metabolic disorders, or trauma, and the various osteotomies used for their treatment are discussed in Chapters 29 and 36.

HIP

Paralysis of the muscles around the hip can cause severe impairment. This impairment may include flexion and abduction contractures of the hip, hip instability and limping caused by paralysis of the gluteus maximus and medius muscles, and paralytic hip dislocation.

FLEXION AND ABDUCTION CONTRACTURES OF THE HIP

An abduction contracture is the most common deformity associated with paralysis of the muscles around the hip; it usually occurs in conjunction with flexion and external rotation contractures of varying degrees. Less often, a contracture of the hip may occur that consists of adduction with flexion and internal rotation. When contractures of the hip are severe and bilateral, locomotion is possible only as a quadruped; the upright position is possible after the contractures have been released.

Spasm of the hamstrings, hip flexors, tensor fasciae latae, and hip abductors is common during the acute and convalescent stages of poliomyelitis. Straight-leg raising usually is limited. The patient assumes the frog position, with the knees and hips flexed and the extremities completely externally rotated. When this position is maintained for even a few weeks, secondary soft-tissue contractures occur; a permanent deformity develops, especially when the gluteal muscles have been weakened. The deformity puts the gluteus maximus at a disadvantage and prevents its return to normal strength. If the faulty position is not corrected, growth of the contracted soft tissues would fail to keep pace with bone growth and the deformity would progressively increase. If positioning in bed is correct while muscle spasm is present, and if the joints are carried through a full range of motion at regular intervals after the muscle spasm disappears, contractures can be prevented and soft tissues can be kept sufficiently long and elastic to meet normal functional demands.

The large expanse of the tensor fasciae latae must be recognized before the deforming possibilities of the iliotibial band can be appreciated. Proximally, the fascia lata arises from the coccyx, the sacrum, the crest of the ilium, the inguinal ligament, and the pubic arch and invests the muscles of the thigh and buttock. Either the superficial or the deep layer is attached to most of the gluteus maximus muscle and to all of the tensor fasciae latae muscle. All of the attachments of the fascia converge to form the iliotibial band on the lateral side of the thigh.

Contracture of the iliotibial band can contribute to the following deformities:

1. *Flexion, abduction, and external rotation contracture of the hip.* The iliotibial band lies lateral and anterior to the hip joint, and its contracture can cause flexion and abduction deformity. The hip is externally rotated for comfort and, if not corrected, the external rotators of the hip contract and contribute to a fixed deformity.
2. *Genu valgum and flexion contracture of the knee.* With growth, the contracted iliotibial band acts as a taut bowstring across the knee joint and gradually abducts and flexes the tibia.
3. *Limb-length discrepancy.* Although the exact mechanism has not been clearly defined and may be related more to the loss of neurologic and muscle function, a contracted iliotibial band on one side may be associated with considerable shortening of that extremity after years of growth.
4. *External tibial torsion, with or without knee joint subluxation.* Because of its lateral attachment distally, the iliotibial band gradually rotates the tibia and fibula externally on the femur; this rotation may be increased if the short head of the biceps is strong. When the deformity becomes extreme, the lateral tibial condyle subluxates on the lateral femoral condyle and the head of the fibula lies in the popliteal space.
5. *Secondary ankle and foot deformities.* With external torsion of the tibia, the axes of the ankle and knee joints are malaligned, causing structural changes that may require surgical correction.
6. *Pelvic obliquity.* When the iliotibial band is contracted, and the patient is supine with the hip in abduction and flexion, the pelvis may remain at a right angle to the long axis of the spine (Fig. 34-18). When the patient stands, however, and the affected extremity is brought into the weight-bearing position (parallel to the vertical axis of the trunk), the pelvis assumes an oblique position: The iliac crest is low on the contracted side and high on the opposite side. The lateral thrust forces the pelvis toward the unaffected side. The trunk muscles on the affected side lengthen, and the muscles on the opposite side contract. An associated lumbar scoliosis can develop. If not corrected, the two contralateral contractures (i.e., the band on the affected side and the trunk muscles on the unaffected side) hold the pelvis in this oblique position until skeletal changes fix the deformity (Fig. 34-19).
7. *Increased lumbar lordosis.* Bilateral flexion contractures of the hip pull the proximal part of the pelvis anteriorly; for the trunk to assume an upright position, a compensatory increase in lumbar lordosis must develop.

A flexion and abduction contracture of the hip can be minimized or prevented in the early convalescent stage of poliomyelitis. The patient should be placed in bed with the hips in neutral rotation, slight abduction, and no flexion. All joints must be carried through a full range of passive motion several times daily; the hips must be stretched in extension, adduction, and internal rotation. To prevent rotation, a bar similar to a Denis Browne splint is useful, especially when a knee roll is used to prevent a genu recurvatum deformity; the bar is clamped to the shoe soles to hold the feet in slight internal rotation. The contracture is carefully watched for in the acute and early convalescent stages; if found, it must be corrected before ambulation is allowed.

Secondary adaptive changes occur soon after the iliotibial band contracts, and the resulting deformity, regardless of its duration or of the patient's age, cannot be corrected by conservative measures; on the contrary, attempts at correction with traction only increase the obliquity and hyperextension of the pelvis and cannot exert any helpful corrective force on the deformity.

Simple fasciotomies around the hip and knee may correct a minor contracture, but recurrence is common; they do not correct a severe contracture. For abduction and external rotation contractures, a complete release of the hip muscles (Ober-Yount procedure) is indicated. For severe deformities, complete release of all muscles from the iliac wing with transfer of the crest of the ilium (Campbell technique) is indicated.

COMPLETE RELEASE OF HIP FLEXION, ABDUCTION, AND EXTERNAL ROTATION CONTRACTURE

TECHNIQUE 34-18

(OBER; YOUNT)

- With the patient in a lateral position, make a transverse incision medial and distal to the anterior superior iliac spine, extending it laterally above the greater trochanter.
- Divide the iliopsoas tendon distally and excise 1 cm of it.
- Detach the sartorius from its origin in the anterior superior iliac spine, detach the rectus from the anterior inferior iliac spine, and divide the tensor fasciae latae from its anterior border completely posteriorly (Fig. 34-15).
- Detach the gluteus medius and minimus and the short external rotators from their insertions on the trochanter.
- Retract the sciatic nerve posteriorly and then open the hip capsule from anterior to posterior, parallel with the acetabular labrum.
- Close the wound over a suction drain and apply a hip spica cast with the hip in full extension, 10 degrees of abduction, and, if possible, internal rotation.
- For the Yount procedure, expose the fascia lata through a lateral longitudinal incision just proximal to the femoral condyle.
- Divide the iliotibial band and fascia lata posteriorly to the biceps tendon and anteriorly to the midline of the thigh at a level 2.5 cm proximal to the patella.
- At this level, excise a segment of the iliotibial band and lateral intermuscular septum 5 to 8 cm long.

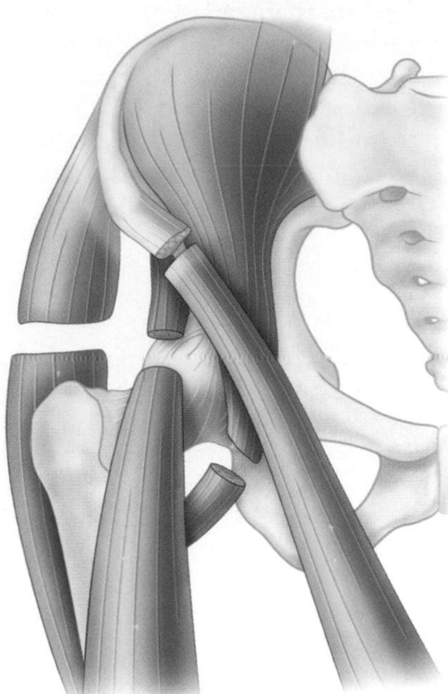

FIGURE 34-15 Complete release of flexion-abduction-external rotation contracture of hip. **SEE TECHNIQUE 34-18.**

- Before closing the wound, determine by palpation that all tight bands have been divided.

POSTOPERATIVE CARE. The cast is removed at 2 weeks, and a long leg brace with a pelvic band is fitted with the hip in the same position.

COMPLETE RELEASE OF MUSCLES FROM ILIAC WING AND TRANSFER OF CREST OF ILIUM

TECHNIQUE 34-19

(CAMPBELL)

- Incise the skin along the anterior one half or two thirds of the iliac crest to the anterior superior spine and then distally for 5 to 10 cm on the anterior surface of the thigh.
- Divide the superficial and deep fasciae to the crest of the ilium.
- Strip the origins of the tensor fasciae latae and gluteus medius and minimus muscles subperiosteally from the wing of the ilium down to the acetabulum (Fig. 34-16A).
- Free the proximal part of the sartorius from the tensor fasciae latae.
- With an osteotome, resect the anterior superior iliac spine along with the origin of the sartorius muscle and allow both to retract distally and posteriorly.

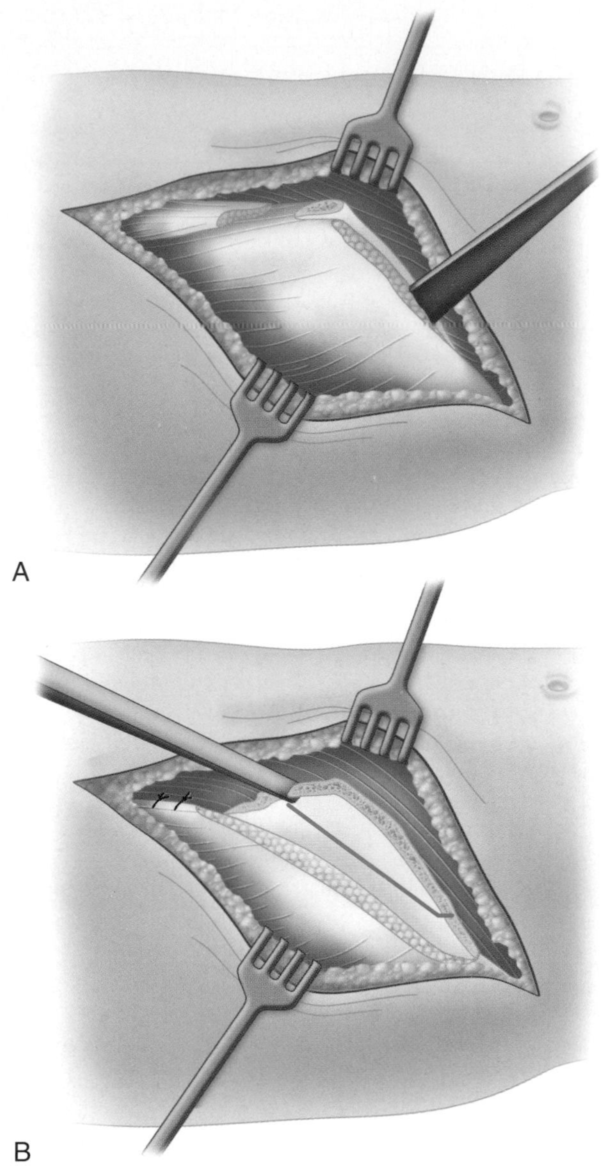

FIGURE 34-16 Campbell transfer of crest of ilium for flexion contracture of hip. **A,** Origins of sartorius, tensor fasciae latae, and gluteus medius muscles are detached from ilium. **B,** Redundant part of ilium is resected. **SEE TECHNIQUE 34-19.**

- Denude the anterior border of the ilium down to the anterior inferior iliac spine. Free subperiosteally the attachments of the abdominal muscles from the iliac crest (or resect a narrow strip of bone with the attachments). Strip the iliacus muscle subperiosteally from the inner table.
- Free the straight tendon of the rectus femoris muscle from the anterior inferior iliac spine and the reflected tendon from the anterior margin of the acetabulum, or simply divide the conjoined tendon of the muscle. Releasing these contracted structures often will allow the hip to be hyperextended without increasing the lumbar lordosis; this is a most important point because, in this situation, correction may be more apparent than real.

- If the hip cannot be hyperextended, other contracted structures must be divided. If necessary, divide the capsule of the hip obliquely from proximally to distally and, as a last resort, free the iliopsoas muscle from the lesser trochanter by tenotomy.
- After the deformity has been completely corrected, resect the redundant part of the denuded ilium with an osteotome (Fig. 34-16B).
- Suture the abdominal muscles to the edge of the gluteal muscles and tensor fasciae latae over the remaining rim of the ilium with interrupted sutures. Suture the superficial fascia on the medial side of the incision to the deep fascia on the lateral side to bring the skin incision 2.5 cm posterior to the rim of the ilium.
- To preserve the iliac physis in a young child, modify the procedure as follows. Free the muscles subperiosteally from the lateral surface of the ilium.
- Detach the sartorius and rectus femoris as just described and, if necessary, release the capsule and iliopsoas muscle. Stripping the muscles from the medial surface of the ilium is unnecessary.
- Now with an osteotome remove a wedge of bone from the crest of the ilium distal to the physis from anterior to posterior; its apex should be as far posterior as the end of the incision and its base anterior and 2.5 cm or more in width, as necessary to correct the deformity.
- Then displace the crest of the ilium distally to contact the main part of the ilium and fix it in place with sutures through the soft tissues.

POSTOPERATIVE CARE. When the deformity is mild, the hip is placed in hyperextension and about 10 degrees of abduction, and a spica cast is applied on the affected side and to above the knee on the opposite side. After 3 or 4 weeks the cast is removed, and the hip is mobilized. Support may be unnecessary during the day when the patient is on crutches; however, Buck extension or an appropriate splint should be used at night.

PARALYSIS OF THE GLUTEUS MAXIMUS AND MEDIUS MUSCLES

One of the most severe disabilities from poliomyelitis is caused by paralysis of the gluteus maximus or the gluteus medius or both; the result is an unstable hip and an unsightly and fatiguing limp. During weight bearing on the affected side when the gluteus medius alone is paralyzed, the trunk sways toward the affected side and the pelvis elevates on the opposite side (the "compensated" Trendelenburg gait). When the gluteus maximus alone is paralyzed, the body lurches backward. The strength of the gluteal muscles can be shown by the Trendelenburg test. When a normal person bears weight on one extremity and flexes the other at the hip, the pelvis is held on a horizontal plane and the gluteal folds are on the same level; when the gluteal muscles are impaired, and weight is borne on the affected side, the level of the pelvis on the normal side drops lower than that on the affected side; when the gluteal paralysis is severe, the test cannot be made because balance on the disabled extremity is impossible.

Because no apparatus would stabilize the pelvis when one or both of these muscles is paralyzed, function can be improved only by transferring muscular attachments to replace the gluteal muscles when feasible. These operations are only relatively successful. When the gluteal muscles are completely paralyzed, normal balance is never restored. Although the gluteal limp can be lessened, it remains; however, when the paralysis is only partial, the gait can be markedly improved.

POSTERIOR TRANSFER OF THE ILIOPSOAS FOR PARALYSIS OF THE GLUTEUS MEDIUS AND MAXIMUS MUSCLES

For weakness of the hip abductors the tendon of the iliopsoas muscle can be transferred to the greater trochanter. Although it is a more extensive operation, the iliopsoas tendon and the entire iliacus muscle can be transferred posteriorly when the gluteus maximus and gluteus medius are paralyzed. Open adductor tenotomy should always precede iliopsoas transfer.

TECHNIQUE 34-20

(SHARRARD)

- Place the patient on the operating table slightly tilted toward the nonoperative side. Through a transverse incision overlying the adductor longus, expose and divide the adductor muscles.
- Expose the lesser trochanter and detach it from the femur (Fig. 34-17A). Then clear the psoas muscle as far proximally as possible.
- Make a second incision just below and parallel to the iliac crest.
- Detach the crest with the muscles of the abdominal wall and open the psoas muscle sheath. Locate the insertion of the muscle with a fingertip.
- Through the first incision, grasp the lesser trochanter with a Kocher forceps and pull it upward, within the psoas sheath and into the upper operative area (Fig. 34-17B).
- Next expose the sartorius muscle and divide it in its proximal half. Allow the muscle to remain in the cartilaginous portion of the anterior superior iliac spine, which is retracted medially.
- Identify the direct head of the rectus femoris muscle and divide it at its origin in the anterior inferior iliac spine. Identify the reflected head of the rectus femoris muscle, dissect it free from the hip capsule, and elevate it posteriorly.
- If the hip is dislocated, open the capsule anteriorly and laterally, parallel to the labrum, excise the ligamentum teres, and remove any hypertrophic pulvinar.
- Reduce the hip joint.
- Make a hole through the iliac wing just lateral to the sacroiliac joint. Make an oval with its long axis longitudinal, its width slightly more than one third of that of the iliac wing, and its length 1 1/2 times as long as its width.
- Pass the iliopsoas tendon and the entire iliacus muscle through the hole (Fig. 34-17C). Pass a finger from the gluteal region distally and posteriorly into the bursa deep

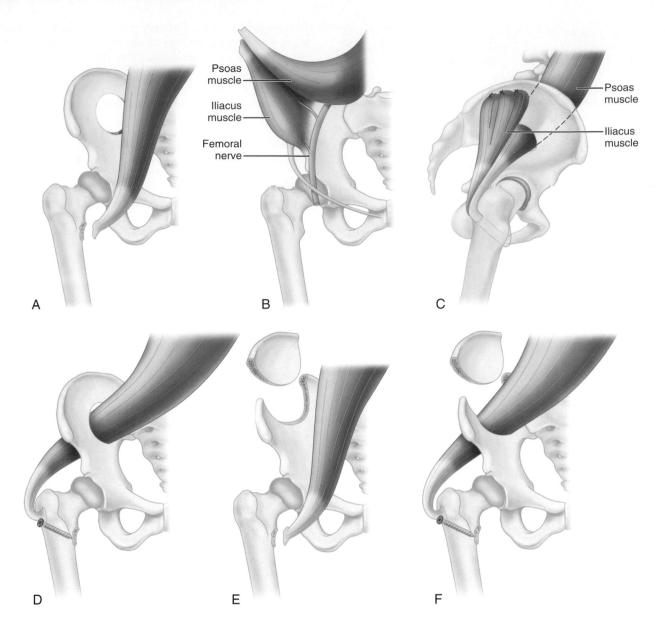

FIGURE 34-17 Sharrard transfer of iliopsoas muscle. **A,** Iliopsoas tendon is released from lesser trochanter. **B,** Tendon and lesser trochanter are detached, iliacus and psoas muscles are elevated, origin of iliacus is freed, and hole is made in ilium. **C,** Iliopsoas tendon is passed from posterior to anterior through hole in greater trochanter. **D,** Iliopsoas muscle and lesser trochanter are secured to greater trochanter with screw. **E** and **F,** Modification of technique in which muscle and tendon are redirected laterally through notch in ilium and inserted into greater trochanter, as described by Weisinger et al. **SEE TECHNIQUE 34-20.**

to the gluteus maximus tendon and identify by touch the posterolateral aspect of the greater trochanter. By referring to this point, expose the corresponding anterior aspect of the greater trochanter by dissecting through the fascia.

- With awls and burs and from anteriorly to posteriorly, make a hole through the greater trochanter until it is big enough to receive the tendon.
- While the hip is held in abduction, extension, and neutral rotation, pass the end of the tendon through the buttock and from posteriorly to anteriorly through the tunnel in the greater trochanter (Fig. 34-17C).
- Secure the psoas and lesser trochanter to the greater trochanter with sutures or a screw (Fig. 34-17D).
- Suture the origin of the iliacus muscle to the ilium inferior to the crest.
- For severe coxa valga or anteversion that requires more than 20 to 30 degrees of abduction for stability, a varus derotation osteotomy with internal fixation can be performed before insertion and suturing of the iliopsoas tendon in the greater trochanter.
- As an alternative, cut a "gutter," or notch, into the posterior lateral iliac crest rather than a window in the ilium. The muscle and its tendon can be redirected laterally

through the notch and inserted into the greater trochanter (Fig. 34-17 E and F). This is technically simpler because the iliacus muscle is not transferred to the outside of the pelvis.

POSTOPERATIVE CARE. The hip is immobilized for 6 weeks in an abduction spica cast.

PARALYTIC DISLOCATION OF THE HIP

If a child contracts poliomyelitis before age 2 years, and the gluteal muscles become paralyzed but the flexors and adductors of the hip do not, the child may develop a paralytic dislocation of the hip before he or she is grown. That the combination of imbalance in muscle power, habitually faulty postures, and growth is important in producing deformity is illustrated nowhere better than in this situation. Generally, children with paralytic dislocation of the hip have normal strength of the flexors and adductors but paralysis of the gluteal muscles. Unless this muscle imbalance is corrected, dislocation is likely to recur regardless of other treatment. Dislocation also can develop because of fixed pelvic obliquity, in which the contralateral hip is held in marked abduction, usually by a tight iliotibial band or a structural scoliosis. If the pelvic obliquity is not corrected, the hip gradually subluxates and eventually dislocates. Weakness of the abductor musculature retards the growth of the greater trochanteric apophysis. The proximal femoral capital epiphysis continues to grow away from the greater trochanter and increases the valgus deformity of the femoral neck; femoral anteversion also may be increased; and the hip becomes mechanically unstable and gradually subluxates. The uneven pressure in the acetabulum causes an increased obliquity in the acetabular roof.

The goals of treatment of paralytic hip dislocations are reduction of the femoral head into the acetabulum and restoration of muscle balance. The bony deformity should be corrected before or at the time of any muscle-balancing procedures. Reduction of the hip in young children can often be achieved by simple abduction, sometimes aided by open adductor tenotomy and traction. Traction can be used to bring the femoral head opposite the acetabulum before closed reduction is attempted. If the hip cannot be reduced by traction, open reduction and adductor tenotomy may be required, in combination with primary femoral shortening, varus derotation osteotomy of the femur, and appropriate acetabular reconstructions (see Chapter 30). Hip arthrodesis rarely is indicated and should be used as the last alternative for treatment of a flail hip that requires stabilization or of an arthritic hip in a young adult that cannot be corrected with total hip arthroplasty. The Girdlestone procedure is the final option for failed correction of the dislocation.

LEG-LENGTH DISCREPANCY

Leg-length discrepancies are common in patients with poliomyelitis owing to a variety of factors, including abnormal limb growth, abnormal muscle forces, and joint contractures. At skeletal maturity, most patients have discrepancies in the range of 4 to 7 cm and many have associated lower extremity deformities, most commonly of the foot.

Leg lengthening in general and especially in neuromuscular patients is associated with a high complication rate. In patients with poliomyelitis, lengthening is a longer process (approximately 1 cm per 2 months) than in other patients because of associated muscular atrophy and hypoplasia of bone. This delayed consolidation places patients at increased risks of pin track infection, pin loosening, and joint contracture. Because of abnormal muscle forces, these patients also are at greater risk for joint contractures. Use of an intramedullary nail for tibial lengthening in patients with poliomyelitis has been reported to decrease mean healing time compared with lengthening without a nail. A high rate of recurrent foot deformity was found with the use of Ilizarov lengthening, and triple arthrodesis was recommended rather than contracture release. Poliomyelitis patients with leg-length discrepancy alone have been found not have a higher level of ambulatory function than those with leg-length discrepancy and associated angular deformity. Leg lengthening improved ambulatory function at various distances only when combined with angular correction. Leaving a small residual length discrepancy was recommended to allow for clearance of the weak limb from the ground.

TOTAL JOINT ARTHROPLASTY

Total joint arthroplasty in neuromuscular patients also is associated with increased complication rates. Several small series and case studies have reported relatively short follow-up of total joint arthroplasty in patients with poliomyelitis. Improvements in knee range of motion, pain, and function have been reported after total knee arthroplasty, but further study and longer follow-up are necessary to fully establish the efficacy and safety of total joint arthroplasty in patients with poliomyelitis.

TRUNK

To understand the deformities and disabilities that may occur when the muscles of the trunk and hips are affected by poliomyelitis requires knowledge of the normal actions and interactions of these muscles. Irwin described the actions of the hip abductors and of the lateral trunk muscles during weight bearing as follows.

The different muscle groups, bone levers, and weight-bearing thrusts have a symmetric and triangular relationship, as shown in Figures 34-18 and 34-19. The line *BC* represents the abductor muscles of the hip; *AB,* the femoral head, neck, and trochanter, which provide a lever for the abductor muscles; *AC,* the weight-bearing thrust on the femoral head; *DF* and *CF,* the lateral trunk muscles; *CE,* the bone lever of the pelvis through which the trunk muscles act; and *FE,* the weight-bearing thrust through the midline of the pelvis from above. When the body is balanced, the triangles above and below the pelvis are symmetric.

During normal walking, the abductors of the hip on the weight-bearing side pull downward on the pelvis and the lateral trunk muscles on the opposite side pull upward; these two sets of muscles hold the pelvis at a right angle to the longitudinal axis of the trunk. The femoral head on the weight-bearing side serves as the fulcrum. The point of fixation of the trunk muscles (the ribs and spine) is less stable than that of the abductor muscles. When *DF* elevates the pelvis, *CF* must provide counterfixation; *CF* depends on the abductors of the hip, *BC,* for counterfixation. With each step,

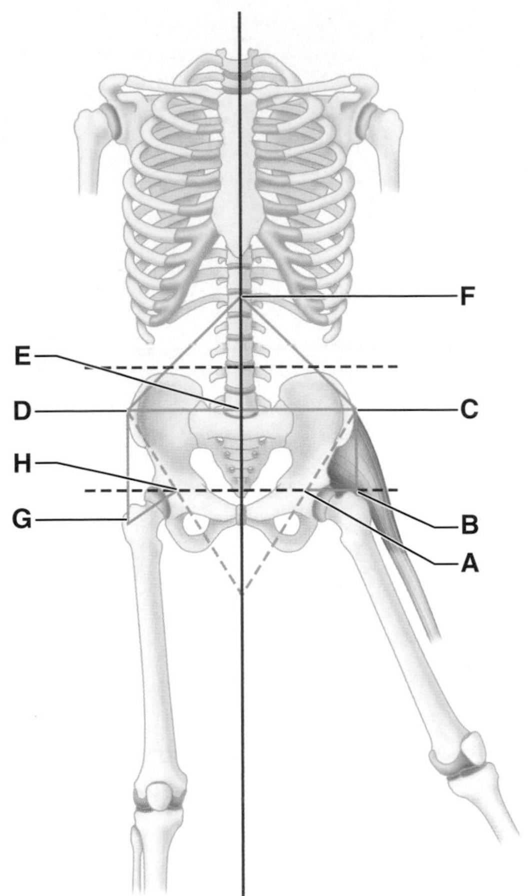

FIGURE 34-18 Most true fixed pelvic obliquities are initiated by contractures below iliac crest (see text).

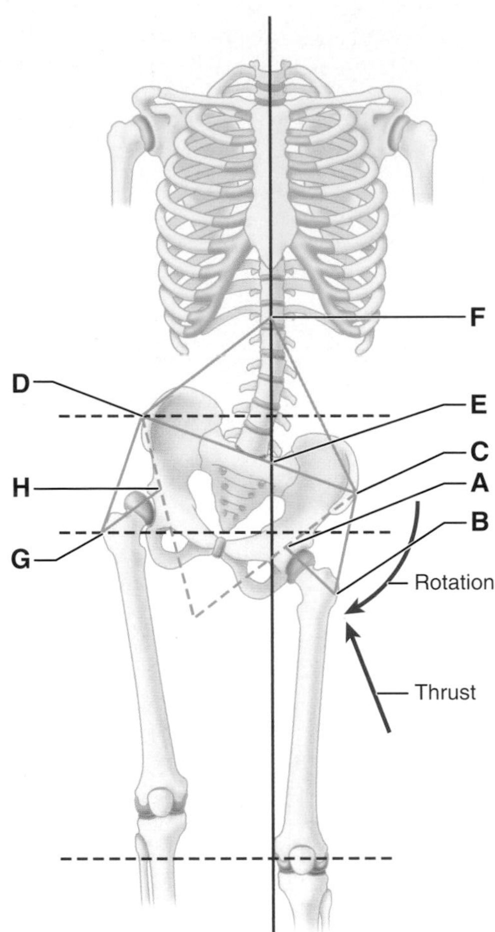

FIGURE 34-19 Abnormal mechanical relationships are created when contracted hip is brought down into weight-bearing position (see text).

the femur on the weight-bearing side is the central point of action for this coordinated system of fixation and counterfixation. Each part of the system depends on the others for proper pelvic balance during walking.

PELVIC OBLIQUITY

When there is an abduction contracture of the hip, line *BC* is shortened; as the affected extremity is placed in the weight-bearing position, the femur, acting through the contracted abductor group, *BC,* depresses the pelvis on that side. During this motion, the affected extremity and the pelvis act as a unit; the pelvis is displaced by the lateral thrust toward the opposite side, and the normal symmetry of the pelvis in relation to the weight-bearing thrust from above is altered. This thrust from above, *FE,* now closely approaches the affected hip, and the pelvis is tilted obliquely. The adducted position of the unaffected hip elongates the abductor muscles, *DG,* to about the same extent that the abductors on the affected side, *BC,* have been shortened, so even when the abductors, *DG,* are normal, their contractility and efficiency are diminished. The demand on these weakened muscles is increased by the increase in the length of line *DE.*

The trunk muscles also are affected by this asymmetry. The lateral trunk muscles, *CF,* become elongated, and their efficiency is impaired. The elongation of the abductors, *DG,* alters their interrelation with the lateral trunk muscles, *DF,* in providing a fixed point for contraction of the lateral trunk muscles, *CF.* The lateral trunk muscles, *CF,* normally elevate the pelvis on that side, but their position now prevents efficient function. Shortening of the lever, *EC,* places the trunk muscles, *CF,* at a further disadvantage. All these alterations in function and structure disrupt the mechanics of walking. When the contracted lateral trunk muscles, *DF,* and contracted hip abductors, *BC,* hold the pelvis in this position long enough, its obliquity becomes fixed through adaptive changes in the spine.

When pelvic obliquity is associated with paralysis of the legs severe enough to require two long leg braces, walking is even more difficult. When the quadriceps is strong on the side of the abduction contracture (the apparently long extremity), the brace can be unlocked to allow knee flexion, and walking becomes possible, although with a marked limp. When the brace on the affected side cannot be unlocked, and the heel on the opposite side (the apparently short extremity) is not elevated, the affected extremity must be widely abducted in walking; otherwise, weight is borne only on the affected extremity and the opposite one becomes almost useless.

TREATMENT

Most pelvic obliquities arise from contractures distal to the iliac crest, and a few arise from unilateral weakness of the abdominal and lateral trunk muscles. When contractures are absent distal to the iliac crest, a pelvic obliquity should not be considered a true one but one secondary to scoliosis.

The early origin of a true pelvic obliquity from contracture of the iliotibial band has already been discussed. Before starting treatment, the degree of fixation of the lumbar scoliosis should be determined by radiographs. When the deformity is mild and the lumbar scoliosis is not fixed, the pelvic obliquity is corrected by treating the flexion and abduction contracture of the hip (see Technique 34-18). When the pelvic obliquity is moderately severe and the lumbar scoliosis is fixed, the scoliosis is corrected first by instrumentation, as described in Chapter 44. After this treatment has been completed, the contractures around the hip are released.

For adults with arthritic changes in the lumbar spine that make correction impossible, the weight borne on the adducted extremity (the apparently short one) can be shifted nearer the midline by valgus osteotomy; a severe unilateral weakness of the gluteus medius also can be treated in this way. This procedure may enable a patient to walk who could not do so before. When the pelvic obliquity is extreme and the femoral head of the abducted extremity (the apparently long one) is almost within the center of gravity, varus osteotomy of the femur is indicated. The osteotomy usually is made at the level of the lesser trochanter, and the fragments are immobilized by appropriate internal fixation.

SERRATUS ANTERIOR PARALYSIS

The following procedures were devised to treat serratus anterior paralysis:

1. Fascial transplant to anchor the inferior angle of the scapula to the inferior border of the pectoralis major
2. Multiple fascial transplants extending from the vertebral border of the scapula to the fourth, fifth, sixth, and seventh thoracic spinous processes
3. Transfer of the teres major tendon from the humerus to the fifth and sixth ribs
4. Transfer of the coracoid insertion of the pectoralis minor muscle to the vertebral border of the scapula
5. Transfer of the coracoid insertion of the pectoralis minor to the inferior angle of the scapula
6. Transfer of the pectoralis minor to distal third of the scapula

TRAPEZIUS AND LEVATOR SCAPULAE PARALYSIS

The following procedures are used to treat trapezius and levator scapulae paralysis:

1. Fascial transplants extending from the spine of the scapula to the cervical muscles and to the first thoracic spinous process; also, anchoring of the inferior angle of the scapula to the adjacent paraspinal muscles for stability
2. Transplant of two fascial strips, one extending from the vertebral border of the scapula just proximal to its spine to the sixth cervical spinous process and the other from a point 6 cm distal to the first transplant to the third thoracic spinous process
3. Fascial transplant extending from the middle of the vertebral border of the scapula to the spinous process of the second and third thoracic vertebrae and transfer of the insertion of the levator scapulae muscle lateralward on the spine of the scapula to a point adjacent to the acromion

PARALYTIC SCOLIOSIS

The treatment of paralytic scoliosis is discussed in Chapter 44.

SHOULDER

The disability caused by paralysis of the muscles around the shoulder can be diminished to some extent by tendon and muscle transfers or by arthrodesis of the joint; the pattern and severity of the paralysis determine which method is most appropriate. Neither procedure is indicated, however, unless the hand, forearm, and elbow have remained functional or have already been made so by reconstructive surgery.

Tendons and muscles are transferred to substitute for a paralyzed deltoid muscle or to reinforce a weak one. For these operations to be successful, power must be fair or better in the serratus anterior, the trapezius, and the short external rotators of the shoulder (for the trapezius transfer, power must be fair or better in the pectoralis major, the rhomboids, and the levator scapulae). When the short external rotators are below functional level, the latissimus dorsi or teres major can be transferred to the lateral aspect of the humerus to reinforce them (Harmon). When the supraspinatus is below functional level, the levator scapulae (preferred), sternocleidomastoid, scalenus anterior, scalenus medius, or scalenus capitis can be transferred to the greater tuberosity. When the subscapularis is below functional level, the pectoralis minor or the superior two digitations of the serratus anterior or the latissimus dorsi or teres major posteriorly can be transferred to the lesser tuberosity to a point exactly opposite the insertion of the subscapularis (here the action is backward, although identical to that of the subscapularis after elevation > 90 degrees). Arthrodesis of the shoulder may be indicated when the paralysis around the joint is extensive, provided that power in at least the serratus anterior and the trapezius is fair or better.

TENDON AND MUSCLE TRANSFERS FOR PARALYSIS OF THE DELTOID

Transfer of the insertion of the trapezius is the most satisfactory operation for complete paralysis of the deltoid. Resecting a part of the spine of the scapula and including it in the transfer permits fixation of the transfer with screws after the muscle is pulled like a hood over the head of the humerus (Fig. 34-20). In a technique modification, the superior and middle trapezius is completely mobilized laterally from its origin and the transfer is made 5 cm longer without endangering its nerve or blood supply; this added length greatly increases leverage of the transfer on the humerus. The entire insertion of the trapezius is freed by resecting the lateral clavicle, the acromion, and the adjoining part of the scapular spine; these are anchored to the humerus by screws (Fig. 34-21).

Saha developed a functional classification of the muscles around the joint and recommended careful assessment of their strength before surgery.

1. *Prime movers:* the deltoid and clavicular head of the pectoralis major, which in lifting exert forces in three directions at the junction of the proximal and middle thirds of the humeral shaft axis.
2. *Steering group:* the subscapularis, the supraspinatus, and the infraspinatus. These muscles exert forces at the junction of the axes of the humeral head and neck and

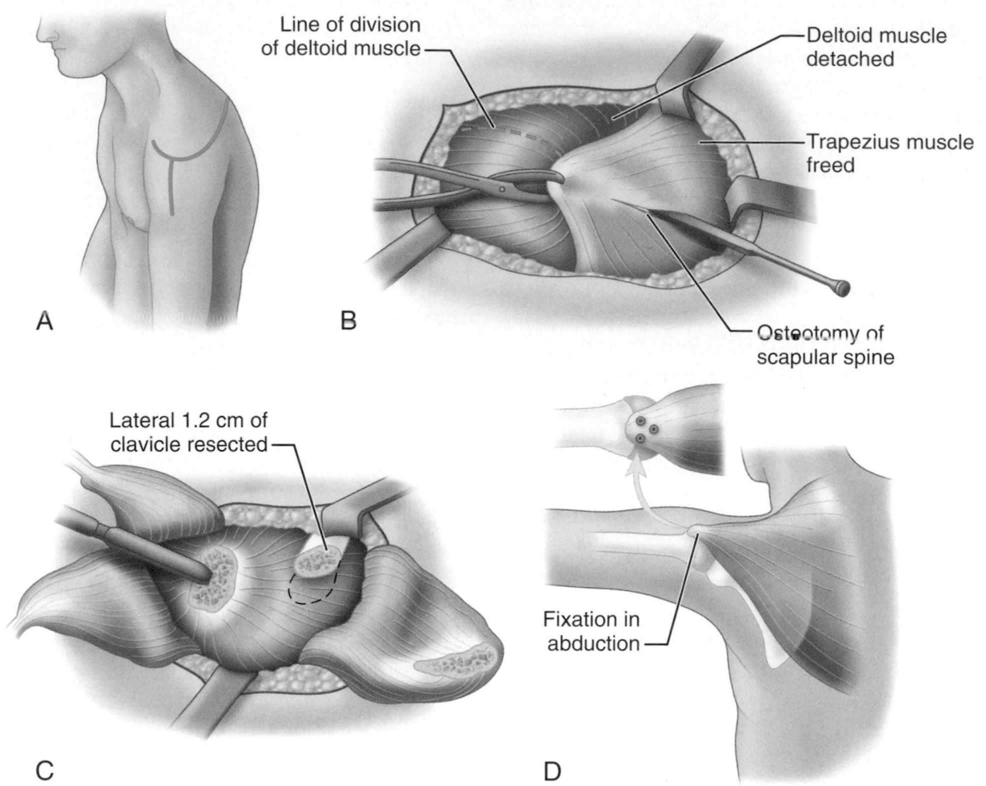

FIGURE 34-20 Bateman trapezius transfer for paralysis of deltoid. **A,** Skin incision. **B,** Spine of scapula is osteotomized near its base in obliquely distal and lateral plane. *Broken line* indicates division of deltoid. **C,** Atrophic deltoid has been split, deep surface of acromion and spine and corresponding area on lateral aspect of humerus have been roughened, and lateral end of clavicle has been resected. **D,** Acromion has been anchored to humerus as far distally as possible with two or three screws. **SEE TECHNIQUE 34-21.**

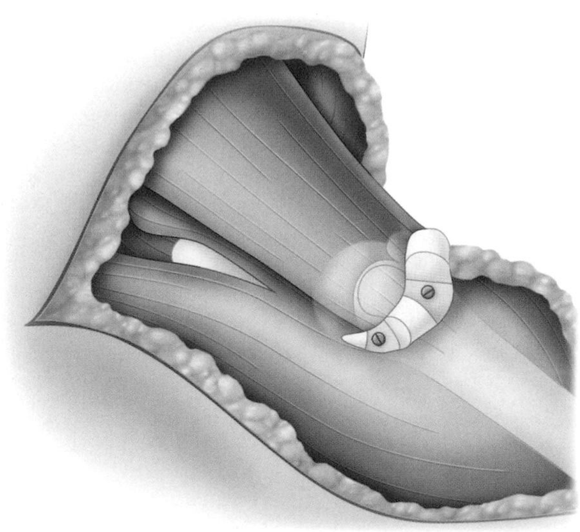

FIGURE 34-21 Saha trapezius transfer for paralysis of deltoid. Entire insertion of trapezius along with attached lateral end of clavicle, acromioclavicular joint, and acromion and adjoining part of scapular spine have been anchored to lateral aspect of humerus distal to tuberosities by two screws. **SEE TECHNIQUE 34-22.**

humeral shaft. As the arm is elevated, the humeral head, by rolling and gliding movements, constantly changes its point of contact with the glenoid cavity. Although these muscles exert a little force in lifting the arm, their chief function is stabilizing the humeral head as it moves in the glenoid.

3. *Depressor group:* the pectoralis major (sternal head), latissimus dorsi, teres major, and teres minor. These muscles are intermediately located and exert their forces on the proximal fourth of the humeral shaft axis. During elevation, they rotate the shaft, and in the last few degrees of this movement, they depress the humeral head. They exert only minimal steering action on the head. Absence of their power would cause no apparent disability except that performance of the limb in lifting weights above the head would be diminished.

The classic methods of transferring a single muscle (or even several muscles to a common attachment) to restore abduction of the shoulder do not consider the functions of the steering muscles. When the steering muscles are paralyzed and a single muscle has been transferred to restore functions only of the deltoid, the arm cannot be elevated more than 90 degrees and scapulohumeral motion is significantly disturbed. For paralysis of the deltoid, the entire insertion of the trapezius can be transferred to the humerus to replace the anterior and middle parts of the muscle; however, the subscapularis, the supraspinatus, and the infraspinatus must be carefully evaluated. When any two are paralyzed, their functions also must be restored because otherwise the effectiveness of the transferred trapezius as an elevator of the shoulder would be greatly reduced. As already mentioned, for paralysis of the subscapularis, either the pectoralis minor or the superior two digitations of the serratus anterior can be transferred because either can be rerouted and anchored to the lesser tuberosity; as an alternative procedure, the latissimus dorsi or the teres major can be transferred posteriorly to a point exactly opposite the lesser tuberosity. For paralysis of the supraspinatus, the levator scapulae, sternocleidomastoid, scalenus anterior, scalenus medius, or scalenus capitis can be transferred to the greater tuberosity; of these, the levator scapulae is the best because of the direction and length of its fibers. When suitable transfers are unavailable, the insertion of the trapezius can be anchored more anteriorly or posteriorly on the humerus to restore internal or external rotation. Contractures of unopposed muscles around the shoulder rarely are severe enough to cause extreme disability; most can be corrected at the time of transfer or arthrodesis.

TRAPEZIUS TRANSFER FOR PARALYSIS OF DELTOID

TECHNIQUE 34-21

(BATEMAN)

- With the patient prone, approach the shoulder through a T-shaped incision (Fig. 34-20A); extend the transverse part around the shoulder over the spine of the scapula and the acromion and end it just above the coracoid process; extend the longitudinal limb distally over the lateral aspect of the shoulder and upper arm for 6 cm.
- Mobilize the flaps, split the atrophic deltoid muscle, and expose the joint.
- Free the undersurface of the acromion and spine of the scapula of soft tissue and osteotomize the spine of the scapula near its base in an obliquely distal and lateral plane; thus, a broad cuff of the trapezius is freed but still attached to the spine and the acromion.
- Resect the lateral 2 cm of the clavicle, taking care to avoid damaging the coracoclavicular ligament.
- Roughen the deep surface of the acromion and spine, abduct the arm to 90 degrees, and at the appropriate level on the lateral aspect of the humerus roughen a corresponding area.
- With firm traction, bring the muscular cuff laterally over the humeral head and anchor the acromion to the humerus as far distally as possible with two or three screws (Fig. 34-20D). Immobilize the arm in a shoulder spica cast with the shoulder abducted to 90 degrees.

POSTOPERATIVE CARE. Immobilization is continued for 8 weeks, but at 4 to 6 weeks the arm and shoulder part of the spica is bivalved to allow some movement. When the transplanted acromion has united with the humerus, the arm is placed on an abduction humeral splint and is gradually lowered to the side and the muscle is reeducated by exercises.

TRAPEZIUS TRANSFER FOR PARALYSIS OF DELTOID

TECHNIQUE 34-22

(SAHA)

- Make a saber-cut incision (Fig. 34-21) convex medially; begin it anteriorly a little superior to the inferior margin of the anterior axillary fold at about its middle, extend it superiorly, then posteriorly, and finally inferiorly, and end it slightly inferior to the base of the scapular spine and 2.5 cm lateral to the vertebral border of the scapula.
- Mobilize the skin flaps and expose the trapezius medially to 2.5 cm medial to the vertebral border of the scapula; expose the acromion, the capsule of the acromioclavicular joint, the lateral third of the clavicle, and the entire origin of the paralyzed deltoid muscle.
- Detach and reflect laterally the origin of the deltoid and locate the anterior border of the trapezius.
- Identify the coronoid ligament and divide the clavicle just lateral to it.
- Palpate the scapular notch, identify the acromion and the adjoining part of the scapular spine, and with a Gigli saw and beveling posteriorly, resect the spine.
- Elevate the insertion of the trapezius along with the attached lateral end of the clavicle, the acromioclavicular joint, and the acromion and adjoining part of the scapular spine. Then free the trapezius from the superior border of the remaining part of the scapular spine medially to the base of the spine where the inferior fibers of the muscle glide over the triangular area of the scapula. Next free from the investing layer of deep cervical fascia the anterior border of the trapezius and raise the muscle from its bed for rerouting.
- Denude the inferior surfaces of the bones attached to the freed trapezius insertion; with forceps, break these bones in several places but leave intact the periosteum on their superior surfaces. Denude also the area on the lateral aspect of the proximal humerus selected for attachment of the transfer.
- With the shoulder in neutral rotation and 45 degrees of abduction, anchor the transfer by two screws passed through fragments of bone and into the proximal humerus (Fig. 34-21).
- When suitable transfers are unavailable to replace any paralyzed external or internal rotators, anchor the muscle a little more anteriorly or posteriorly. Transfers for paralysis of the subscapularis, supraspinatus, or infraspinatus are discussed later; when indicated, they should be performed at the time of trapezius transfer.

POSTOPERATIVE CARE. A spica cast is applied with the shoulder abducted 45 degrees, neutrally rotated, and flexed in the plane of the scapula. At 10 days the sutures

are removed and radiographs are made to be sure that the humeral head has not become dislocated inferiorly. At 6 to 8 weeks, the cast is removed and active exercises are started.

TRANSFER OF DELTOID ORIGIN FOR PARTIAL PARALYSIS

TECHNIQUE 34-23

(HARMON)

- Make a U-shaped incision 20 cm long extending from the middle third of the clavicle laterally and posteriorly around the shoulder just distal to the acromion to the middle of the spine of the scapula.
- Raise flaps of skin and subcutaneous tissue proximally and distally.
- Detach subperiosteally from its origin the active posterior part of the deltoid and free it distally from the deep structures for about one half its length, being careful not to injure the axillary nerve and its branches.
- Expose subperiosteally the lateral third of the clavicle, transfer the muscle flap anteriorly, and anchor it against the clavicle with interrupted nonabsorbable sutures through the adjacent soft tissues (Fig. 34-22).

POSTOPERATIVE CARE. A shoulder spica cast is applied, holding the arm abducted 75 degrees. At 3 weeks, part of the cast is removed for massage and active exercise. At 6 weeks, the entire cast is removed and an abduction humeral splint is fitted to be worn for at least 4 months; supervised active exercises are continued during this time.

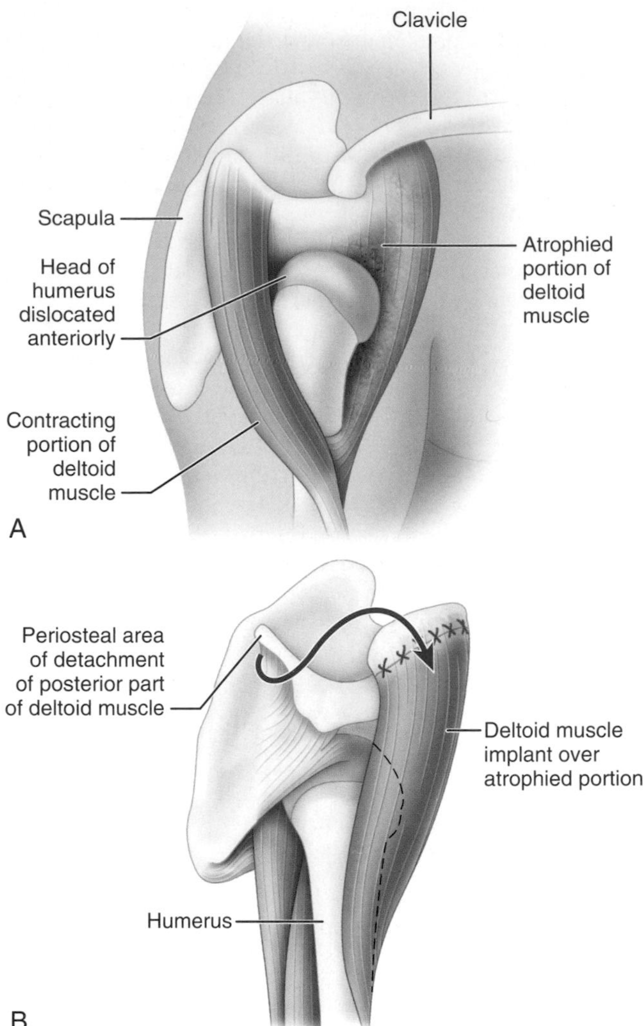

FIGURE 34-22 Harmon transfer of origin of deltoid for partial paralysis. **A,** Posterior part of deltoid is functioning; middle and anterior parts are paralyzed. **B,** Transferred posterior part of deltoid is overlying atrophic anterior part. When transfer contracts, it prevents anterior dislocation of shoulder and exerts more direct abduction force than in its previous posterior location. **SEE TECHNIQUE 34-23.**

TENDON AND MUSCLE TRANSFERS FOR PARALYSIS OF THE SUBSCAPULARIS, SUPRASCAPULARIS, SUPRASPINATUS, OR INFRASPINATUS

When two of these three muscles are paralyzed, their functions must be restored by suitable transfers; this is just as necessary as the trapezius transfer for paralysis of the deltoid. Without the function of these muscles or their substitutes the effectiveness of the transferred trapezius in elevating the shoulder would be markedly reduced. Muscles suitable for transfer are muscles whose distal ends can be carried to the tuberosities of the humerus and whose general directions of pull correspond to those of the muscles they are to replace. The transfers should be rerouted close to the end of the axis of the humeral head and neck, or the desired functions will not be restored. The nerve and blood supply to any transferred muscle must be protected. Currently, the most commonly performed transfers are transfer of the latissimus dorsi or teres major or both and posterior transfer of the pectoralis minor to the scapula. These transfers, when indicated, are done at the same time as the Saha trapezius transfer for paralysis of the deltoid. Consequently, in each instance, the sabercut incision would have been made, the lateral end of the clavicle and the acromion and adjoining part of the scapular spine would have been elevated, and the superior and middle trapezius would have been mobilized as already described.

TRANSFER OF LATISSIMUS DORSI OR TERES MAJOR OR BOTH FOR PARALYSIS OF SUBSCAPULARIS OR INFRASPINATUS

TECHNIQUE 34-24

(SAHA)

- Elevate the arm about 130 degrees. Then make an incision in the posterior axillary fold beginning in the upper arm about 6.5 cm inferior to the crease of the axilla and extending to the inferior angle of the scapula, crossing the crease in a zigzag manner.

- Expose and free the insertion of the latissimus dorsi and raise the muscle from its bed, taking care to preserve its nerve and blood supply.
- If the transfer is to be reinforced by the teres major, free and raise both muscles.
- Fold the freed insertion on itself and close its margins by interrupted sutures; place in its end a strong mattress suture.
- With a blunt instrument, open the interval between the deltoid and long head of the triceps.
- Identify the tubercle at the inferior end of the greater tuberosity, carry the end of the transfer to this tubercle, and while holding the limb in neutral rotation, anchor the transfer there by interrupted sutures.

ARTHRODESIS

When paralysis around the shoulder is extensive, arthrodesis may be the procedure of choice, especially when there is a paralytic dislocation, the muscles of the forearm and hand are functional, and the serratus anterior and trapezius are strong. Motion of the scapula compensates for lack of motion in the joint. Normal function of the forearm and hand is a prerequisite.

The position of the shoulder for arthrodesis is similar to that recommended for any shoulder fusion (see Chapter 13). The angle of abduction should be determined on the basis of the clinical presentation of the arm's position in relation to the body. This angle traditionally is obtained by measuring the angle between the vertebral border of the scapula and the humerus; however, this frequently is difficult to determine on radiographs. The position of the arm in shoulder arthrodesis should be established with the arm at the side of the body, with enough abduction of the arm clinically determined from the side of the body to clear the axilla (15 to 20 degrees) and enough forward flexion (25 to 30 degrees) and internal rotation (40 to 50 degrees) to bring the hand to the midline of the body. An additional 10 degrees of abduction should be obtained in children with poliomyelitis when no internal fixation is used. When both shoulders must be fused, their positions should allow the patient to bring the hands together. A weak or flail shoulder should be fused in only slight abduction. A study of 11 patients (average age, 15 years) with 13 shoulder arthrodesis reported great variability in the position of fusion, but improved function in all patients. The authors concluded that the position of arthrodesis and the resulting arc of motion were less important than stability of the glenohumeral joint. Care must be taken to preserve the proximal humeral physis in skeletally immature patients. The techniques for shoulder arthrodesis are described in Chapter 13.

ELBOW

Most operations for paralysis of the muscles acting across the elbow are designed to restore active flexion or extension of the joint. Operations to correct deformity or operations to stabilize the joint, such as posterior bone block or arthrodesis, rarely are necessary.

MUSCLE AND TENDON TRANSFERS TO RESTORE ELBOW FLEXION

Several methods of restoring active elbow flexion are available. Here, as elsewhere, the actual and the relative power of the remaining muscles must be accurately determined before a transfer procedure is chosen. Also, because the function of the hand is more important than flexion of the elbow, these operations should not be done when the muscles controlling the fingers are paralyzed, unless their function has been or can be restored by tendon transfers. Several methods of restoring elbow flexion have been described: (1) flexorplasty (Steindler), (2) anterior transfer of the triceps tendon (Bunnell and Carroll), (3) transfer of part of the pectoralis major muscle (Clark), (4) transfer of the sternocleidomastoid muscle (Bunnell), (5) transfer of the pectoralis minor muscle (Spira), (6) transfer of the pectoralis major tendon (Brooks and Seddon), and (7) transfer of the latissimus dorsi muscle (Hovnanian).

FLEXORPLASTY

Flexorplasty consists of transferring the common origin of the pronator teres, the flexor carpi radialis, the palmaris longus, the flexor digitorum sublimis, and the flexor carpi ulnaris muscles from the medial epicondylar region of the humerus proximally about 5 cm. Its chief disadvantage is the frequent development of a pronation deformity of the forearm.

Flexorplasty is indicated when the biceps brachii and brachialis are paralyzed, and the group of muscles arising from the medial epicondyle are fair or better in strength. The best results are obtained when the elbow flexors are only partially paralyzed and the finger and wrist flexors are normal. The strength in active flexion and the range of motion of the elbow after surgery do not compare favorably with that of the normal elbow, but the usefulness of the arm is nonetheless increased. When only the flexor digitorum sublimis is active, the elbow can be flexed only if the fingers are strongly flexed; this interferes with the function of the hand, and another method should be used to restore elbow flexion. Unsuccessful results from this procedure usually are caused by overestimating the strength of the muscles to be transferred. A practical way to test them is to hold the patient's arm at a right angle to the body, rotate it to eliminate the influence of gravity, and determine whether the muscles to be transferred can flex the elbow in this position; if not, this type of transfer would fail and another should be used.

TECHNIQUE 34-25

(BUNNELL)

- Make a curved longitudinal incision over the medial side of the elbow beginning 7.5 cm proximal to the medial epicondyle and extending distally posterior to the medial condyle and thence anteriorly on the volar surface of the forearm along the course of the pronator teres muscle.
- Locate the ulnar nerve posterior to the medial epicondyle and retract it posteriorly.

- Detach en bloc the common origin of the pronator teres, flexor carpi radialis, palmaris longus, flexor digitorum sublimis, and flexor carpi ulnaris from the medial epicondyle close to the periosteum. Free these muscles distally for 4 cm and prolong the common muscle origin with a free graft of fascia lata.
- Advance this origin 5 cm up the lateral side rather than the medial side of the humerus (Fig. 34-23); this results in a moderate, although not complete, correction of the tendency of the transfer to pronate the forearm.
- Should a pronation deformity persist after this procedure, it can be corrected by transferring the tendon of the flexor carpi ulnaris around the ulnar margin of the forearm into the distal radius.
- Apply a cast with the elbow in acute flexion and the forearm midway between pronation and supination.

POSTOPERATIVE CARE. At 2 weeks the cast is replaced by a splint that holds the arm in this same position for at least 6 weeks; physical therapy and active exercises are then started and are gradually increased to strengthen the transferred muscles.

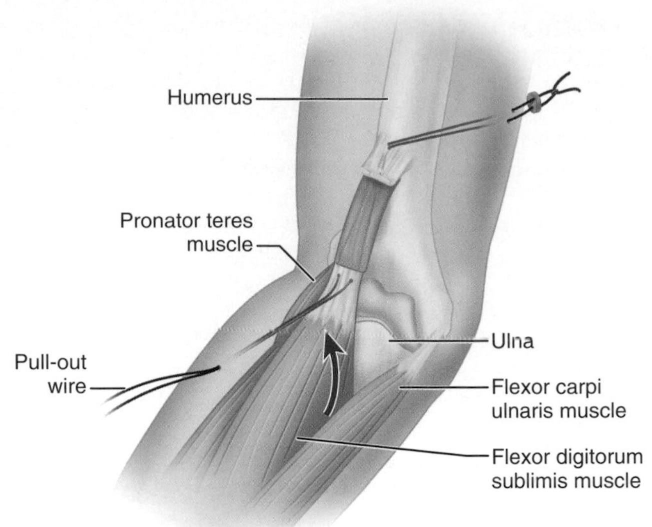

FIGURE 34-23 Bunnell modification of Steindler flexorplasty. Common muscle origin is transferred laterally on humerus by means of fascial transplant. **SEE TECHNIQUE 34-25.**

ANTERIOR TRANSFER OF THE TRICEPS

Anterior transfer of the triceps tendon can be done to regain active elbow flexion. One disadvantage of this transfer is that the triceps tendon would not reach the tuberosity of the radius; a short graft of fascia or a tendon graft must be used to complete the transfer.

TECHNIQUE 34-26

(BUNNELL)

- Through a posterolateral incision expose the triceps tendon and divide it at its insertion.
- Dissect it from the posterior aspect of the distal fourth of the humerus and transfer it around the lateral aspect.
- Make an anterolateral curvilinear incision and retract the brachioradialis and pronator teres muscles to expose the tuberosity of the radius.
- Prolong the triceps tendon by a graft of fascia lata that is 4 cm long and wide enough to make a tube.
- Attach it to the roughened tuberosity of the radius with a steel pull-out suture passed to the dorsum of the forearm via a hole drilled through the tuberosity and the neck of the radius (Fig. 34-24).
- Flex the elbow, gently pull the suture taut to snug the tendon against the bone, and tie the suture over a padded button.
- Apply a cast with the elbow in acute flexion and the forearm midway between pronation and supination.
- Carroll described a similar method of triceps transfer in which the tendon is passed superficial to the radial nerve and through a longitudinal slit in the biceps tendon and is sutured under tension with the elbow in flexion.

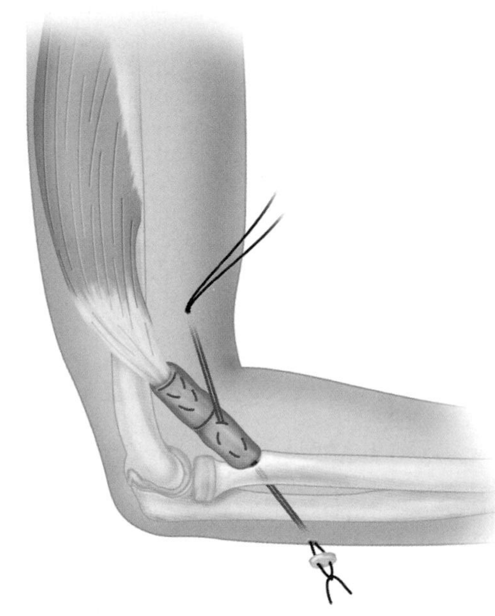

FIGURE 34-24 Bunnell anterior transfer of triceps for paralysis of biceps. Triceps tendon elongated by short graft of fascia or tendon, routed laterally, and inserted into tuberosity of radius by pull-out suture. **SEE TECHNIQUE 34-26.**

POSTOPERATIVE CARE. At 2 weeks the cast is replaced by a splint that holds the arm in the same position for at least 6 weeks. The pull-out wire is removed at 4 weeks. Physical therapy and active exercises are begun at 6 weeks and are gradually increased.

TRANSFER OF THE PECTORALIS MAJOR TENDON

Brooks and Seddon described an operation to restore elbow flexion in which the entire pectoralis major muscle is used as the motor and its tendon is prolonged distally by means of the long head of the biceps brachii. This transfer is contraindicated unless the biceps is completely paralyzed; they recommended it when flexorplasty is not applicable, when the distal part of the pectoralis major is weak but the proximal part is strong, or when both parts of the muscle are so weak that the entire muscle is needed for transfer. To avoid undesirable movements of the shoulder during elbow flexion after this procedure, muscular control of the shoulder and scapula must be good, or an arthrodesis of the shoulder should be performed.

TECHNIQUE 34-27

(BROOKS AND SEDDON)

- Make an incision from the distal end of the deltopectoral groove distally to the junction of the proximal and middle thirds of the arm.
- Detach the tendon of insertion of the pectoralis major as close to bone as possible and by blunt dissection mobilize the muscle from the chest wall proximally toward the clavicle (Fig. 34-25A).
- Retract the deltoid laterally and superiorly and expose the tendon of the long head of the biceps as it runs proximally into the shoulder joint; sever this tendon at the proximal end of the bicipital groove and withdraw it into the wound.
- By blunt and sharp dissection free the belly of the long head of the biceps from that of the short head and ligate and divide all vessels entering it.
- Make an L-shaped incision at the elbow with its transverse limb in the flexor crease and its longitudinal limb extending proximally along the medial border of the biceps muscle.
- Mobilize the long head of the biceps by dividing its remaining neurovascular bundles so that the tendon and muscle are completely freed distally to the tuberosity of the radius; withdraw the tendon and muscle through the distal incision (Fig. 34-25B and C). (When the muscle belly is adherent to the overlying fascia, free it by sharp dissection.)
- Replace the long head of the biceps in its original position, and through the proximal incision pass its tendon and muscle belly through two slits in the tendon of the pectoralis major; loop the long head of the biceps on itself so that its proximal tendon is brought into the distal incision.
- Then, using nonabsorbable sutures, suture the end of the proximal tendon through a slit in the distal tendon (Fig. 34-25D) and suture the tendon of the pectoralis major to the long head of the biceps at their junction.
- Close the incisions and apply a posterior plaster splint with the elbow in flexion.

POSTOPERATIVE CARE. At 3 weeks, the splint is removed and muscle reeducation is started. Care must be taken to extend the elbow gradually so that active flexion of more than 90 degrees is preserved. It may be 2 or 3 months before full extension is possible.

TRANSFER OF THE LATISSIMUS DORSI MUSCLE

Hovnanian described a method of restoring active elbow flexion by transferring the origin and belly of the latissimus dorsi to the arm and anchoring the origin near the radial tuberosity. This transfer is possible because the neurovascular bundle of the muscle is long and easily mobilized (Fig. 34-26A); a similar transfer in which the origin is anchored to the olecranon to restore active extension also is possible.

TECHNIQUE 34-28

(HOVNANIAN)

- Place the patient on his or her side with the affected extremity upward. Start the skin incision over the loin and extend it superiorly along the lateral border of the latissimus dorsi to the posterior axillary fold, distally along the medial aspect of the arm, and finally laterally to end in the antecubital fossa (Fig. 34-26B). Carefully expose the dorsal and lateral aspects of the latissimus dorsi, leaving its investing fascia intact.
- Free the origin of the muscle by cutting across its musculofascial junction inferiorly and its muscle fibers superiorly. Then gradually free the muscle from the underlying abdominal and flank muscles.
- Divide the four slips of the muscle that arise from the inferior four ribs and the few arising from the angle of the scapula.
- Carefully protect the neurovascular bundle that enters the superior third of the muscle. To prevent injury of the vessels to the latissimus dorsi, ligate their branches that anastomose with the lateral thoracic vessels. Identify and gently free the thoracodorsal nerve that supplies the muscle; its trunk is about 15 cm long and runs from the apex of the axilla along the deep surface of the muscle belly.
- Next prepare a bed in the anteromedial aspect of the arm to receive the transfer.
- Carefully swing the transfer into this bed without twisting its vessels or nerve. To prevent kinking of the vessels, divide the intercostobrachial nerve and the lateral cutaneous branches of the third and fourth intercostal nerves; also free as necessary any fascial bands.
- Now suture the aponeurotic origin of the muscle to the biceps tendon and the periosteal tissues about the radial tuberosity and then suture the remaining origin to the sheaths of the forearm muscles and to the lacertus fibrosus (Fig. 34-26C).
- Close the wound in layers and bandage the arm against the thorax with the elbow flexed and the forearm pronated.

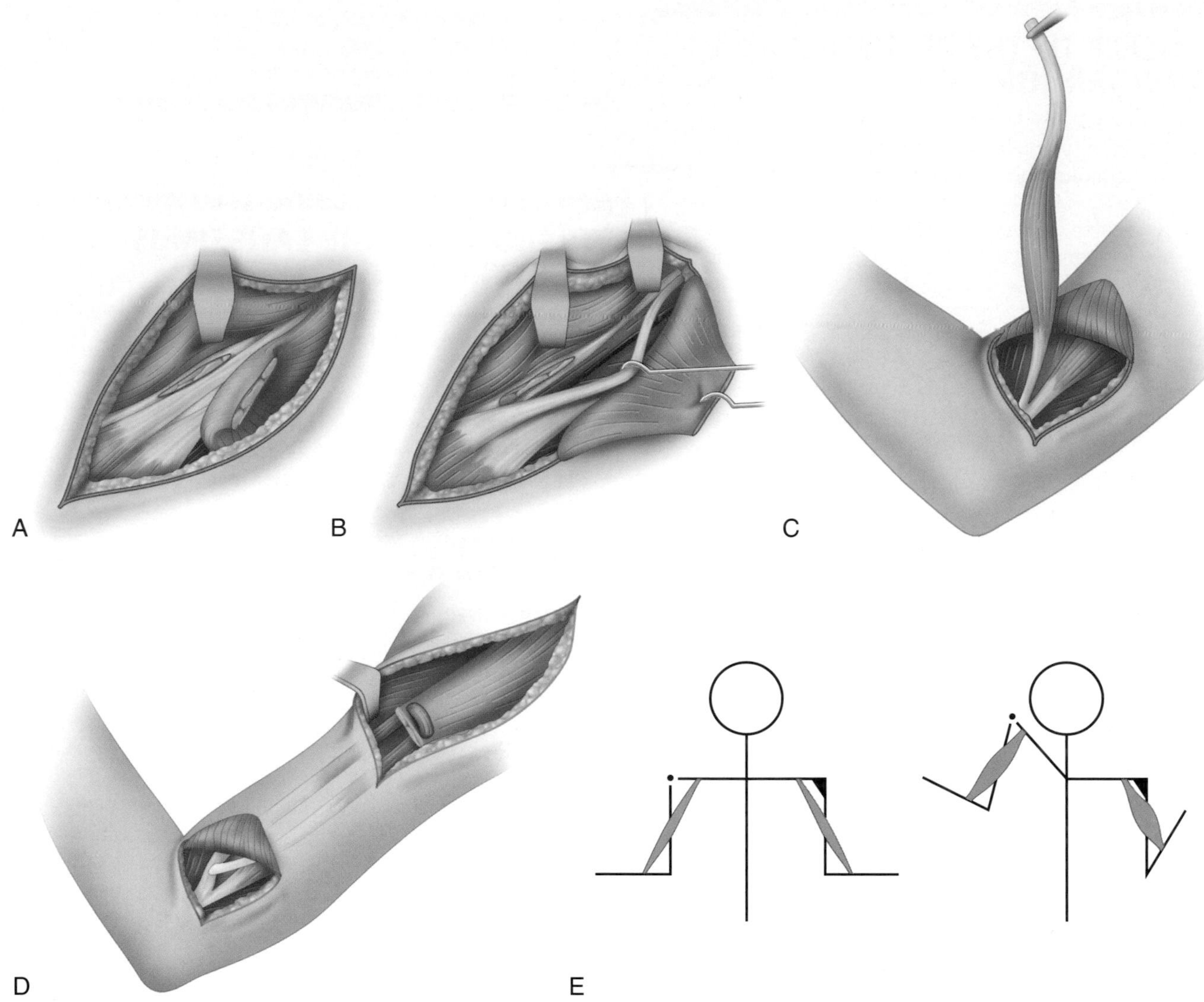

FIGURE 34-25 Brooks-Seddon transfer of pectoralis major tendon for paralysis of elbow flexors. **A,** Insertion of pectoralis major is detached as close to bone as possible. **B,** Tendon of long head of biceps is exposed and divided at proximal end of bicipital groove. **C,** Tendon and muscle of long head of biceps are completely mobilized distally to tuberosity of radius by dividing all vessels and nerves that enter muscle proximal to elbow. **D,** Long head of biceps is passed through two slits in pectoralis major, is looped on itself so that its proximal tendon is brought into distal incision, and is sutured through slit in its distal tendon. **E,** To avoid undesirable movements of shoulder during elbow flexion after this transfer, muscular control of shoulder and scapula must be good, or shoulder must be fused. Left shoulder shown is flail; right has been fused. When transfer on left contracts, some of its force is wasted because of lack of control of shoulder, but, on right, transfer moves only elbow. **SEE TECHNIQUE 34-27.**

POSTOPERATIVE CARE. Exercises of the fingers are encouraged early. At 3 or 4 weeks, the bandage is removed and passive and active exercises of the elbow are started.

MUSCLE TRANSFERS FOR PARALYSIS OF THE TRICEPS

Weakness or paralysis of the triceps muscle usually is considered of little importance because gravity would extend the elbow passively in most positions that the arm assumes. A good triceps is essential, however, to crutch walking or to shifting the body weight to the hands during such activities as moving from a bed to a wheelchair. A functioning triceps allows the patient to perform these activities by locking the elbow in extension. To place the hand on top of the head when the patient is erect, the triceps must be strong enough to extend the elbow against gravity; thrusting and pushing motions with the forearm also require a functional triceps. In other activities, strong active extension of the elbow is relatively unimportant compared with strong active flexion.

POSTERIOR DELTOID TRANSFER (MOBERG PROCEDURE)

Moberg described an operation to transfer the posterior third of the deltoid muscle to the triceps to restore active elbow extension in the quadriplegic patient. Patients with complete

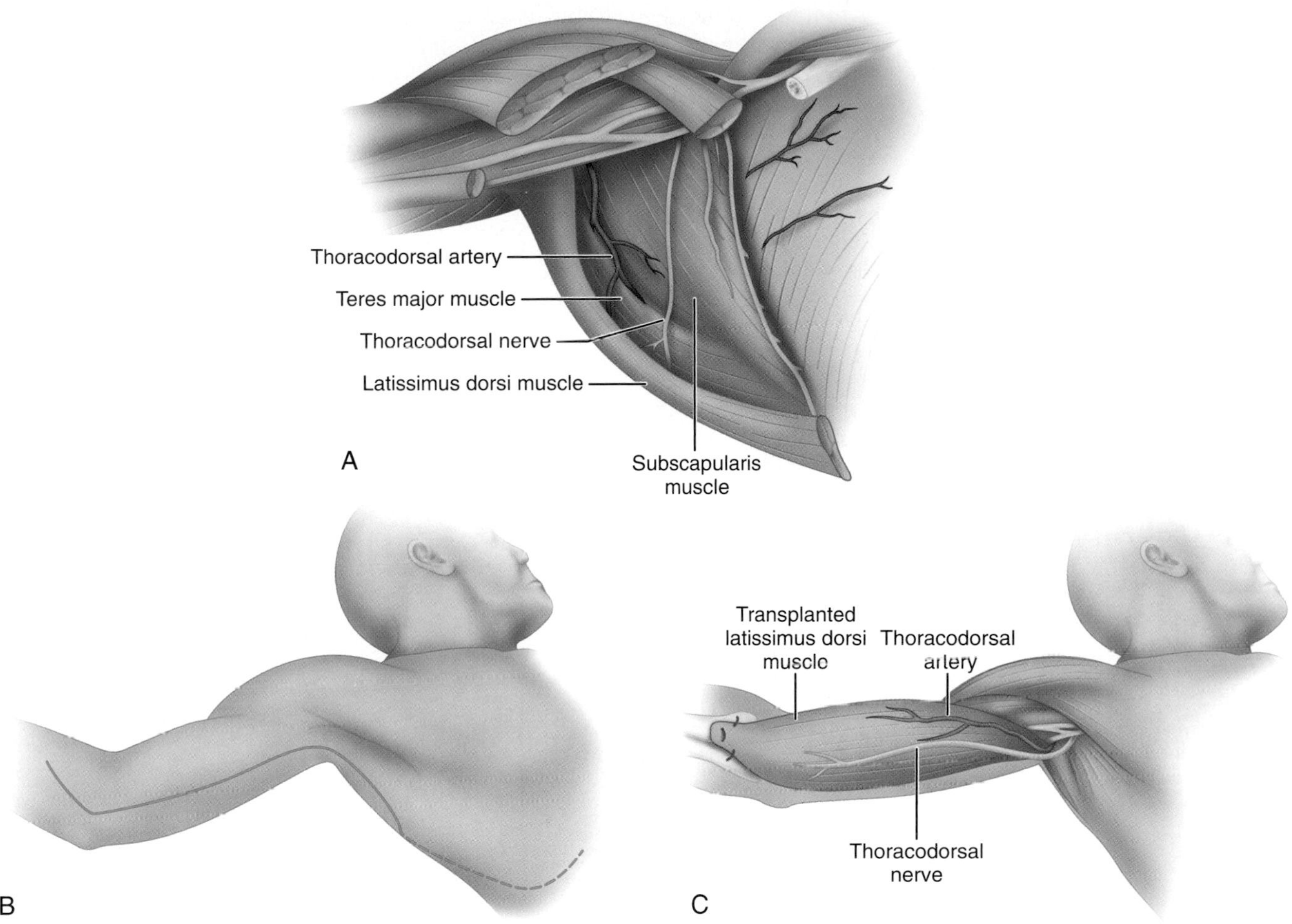

FIGURE 34-26 Hovnanian transfer of latissimus dorsi muscle for paralysis of biceps and brachialis muscles. **A,** Normal anatomy of axilla; note that thoracodorsal nerve and artery are long and can be easily mobilized. **B,** Skin incision. **C,** Origin and belly of latissimus dorsi have been transferred to arm, and origin has been sutured to biceps tendon and to other structures distal to elbow joint. **SEE TECHNIQUE 34-28.**

quadriplegia at the functioning level of C5 or C6 have active elbow flexion, shoulder flexion and abduction, and possibly wrist extension. Elbow extension is by gravity only, without triceps function (C7). Active extension is impossible. Ambulation is not a realistic goal in such patients. Rather, improved strength, mobility, and function and improved ability to reach overhead, to perform personal hygiene and grooming, to relieve ischial pressure from the wheelchair, to achieve driving ability and wheelchair use, and to eat and control eating utensils are sought.

The Moberg procedure has been modified by the construction of tendinoperiosteal tongues proximally and distally instead of using the free tendon grafts from the foot. The posterior belly of the deltoid muscle is freed, along with the most distal insertion of the muscle and including a strip of periosteum 1.0 × 3.0 cm, continuous with the muscle and its insertion. A tongue of the triceps tendon 1.5 to 2.0 cm wide is developed by parallel incisions and including a continuous strip of periosteum similar to that for the deltoid, if possible.

The length of the tendinoperiosteal tongues should be such that with the elbow extended and the arm adducted their deep surfaces should appose when the triceps tendon is folded over 180 degrees. The angle of tendinous reflection is reinforced by a narrow sheet of Dacron wrapped around the grafts and sutured to the tongues and to itself.

FOREARM

Operations on the forearm after poliomyelitis consist of tenotomy, fasciotomy, and osteotomy to correct deformities and tendon transfers to restore function.

■ PRONATION CONTRACTURE

Deformities of the forearm seldom are disabling enough in themselves to warrant surgery; the most common exception is a fixed pronation contracture from imbalance between the supinators and pronators. When the pronator teres is not strong enough to transfer to replace the paralyzed supinators, correcting the contracture alone is indicated, provided that there is active flexion of the elbow. When the pronators of the forearm and the flexors of the wrist are active, however, function can be improved not only by correcting the pronation contracture but also by transferring the flexor carpi ulnaris (see Chapter 72).

Fixed supination deformity develops from muscle imbalance in which usually the pronators and finger flexors are weak and the biceps and wrist extensors are strong. The soft tissues, such as the interosseous membrane, contract; the bones become deformed, and eventually the radioulnar joints may dislocate. A fixed supination deformity combined with weak shoulder abduction markedly limits an otherwise functional hand. Recommended procedures for this deformity include rerouting of the biceps tendon (Zancolli) and manual osteoclasis of the middle thirds of the radius and ulna (Blount). The latter is recommended for children younger than 12 years old with insufficient muscle power for tendon transfer.

REROUTING OF BICEPS TENDON FOR SUPINATION DEFORMITIES OF FOREARM

TECHNIQUE 34-29

(ZANCOLLI)

- If full passive pronation is already possible before surgery, omit the first part of the operation. Otherwise, make a longitudinal incision on the dorsum of the forearm over the radial shaft (Fig. 34-27A, *1*).
- By blunt dissection, expose the interosseous membrane and retract the dorsal muscles radialward to protect the posterior interosseous nerve (Fig. 34-27B).
- Divide the interosseous membrane throughout its length close to the ulna. If the dorsal ligaments of the distal radioulnar joint are contracted, extend the incision distally and perform a capsulotomy of this joint.
- If necessary, release the supinator muscle after identifying and protecting the posterior interosseous nerve in the proximal part of the incision. At this point in the operation full passive pronation of the forearm should be possible.
- Now make a second incision; begin it on the medial aspect of the arm proximal to the elbow and extend it distally to the flexion crease of the joint, then laterally across the joint in the crease, and then distally over the anterior aspect of the radial head (Fig. 34-27A, *2*).
- Identify and retract the median nerve and brachial artery.
- Divide the lacertus fibrosus and expose the insertion of the biceps tendon on the radial tuberosity.
- Now divide the biceps tendon by a long Z-plasty (Fig. 34-27C).
- Reroute the distal segment of the tendon around the radial neck medially, then posteriorly, and then laterally so that traction on it will pronate the forearm (Fig. 34-27D).

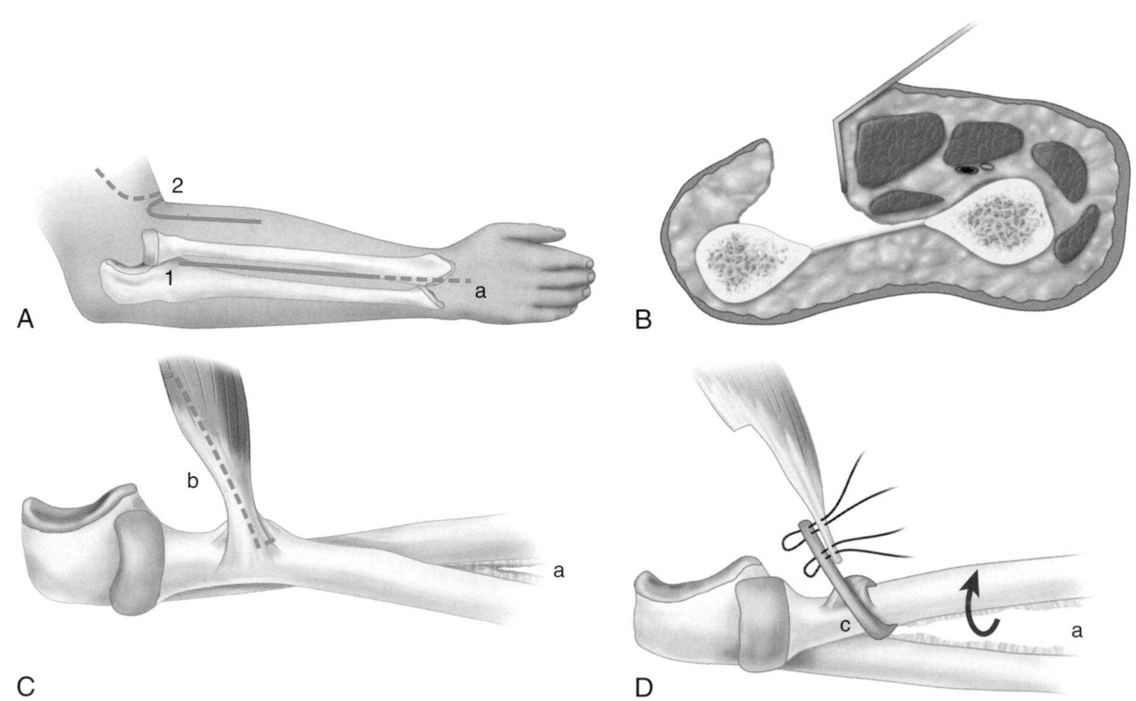

FIGURE 34-27 Zancolli rerouting of biceps tendon for supination deformity of forearm. **A,** 1, Dorsal skin incision *(dotted line)* is extended distally to *a* when distal radioulnar joint requires capsulotomy. 2, Anterior incision to expose biceps tendon and radial head. **B,** Exposure of interosseous membrane by retracting dorsal muscles radially (see text).**C,** Line at *b* shows Z-plasty incision to be made in biceps tendon. Interosseous membrane has been divided at *a*. **D,** At *c*, biceps tendon has been divided by Z-plasty, distal segment has been rerouted around radial neck medially, and ends of tendon are being sutured together. Traction on tendon will now pronate forearm as indicated by *arrow*. **SEE TECHNIQUE 34-29.**

- Place the ends of the biceps tendon side-by-side and suture them together under tension that will maintain full pronation and yet allow extension of the elbow.
- If the radial head is subluxated or is dislocated, reduce it if possible and hold it in place by capsulorrhaphy of the radiohumeral joint; if the radial head cannot be reduced, excise it and transfer the proximal segment of the biceps tendon to the brachialis tendon.
- Close the incisions and apply a cast with the elbow flexed 90 degrees and the forearm moderately pronated.

POSTOPERATIVE CARE. At about 3 weeks the cast and sutures are removed and passive and active exercises are begun.

WRIST AND HAND

The treatment of disabilities of the wrist and hand caused by paralysis is discussed in Chapter 71.

MYELOMENINGOCELE

EPIDEMIOLOGY

Myelomeningocele is a complex congenital malformation of the central nervous system. Advances in medicine, surgery, and allied health services have reduced the mortality rates in patients born with severe defects of the central nervous system. The challenge for orthopaedic surgeons is to assist these patients in attaining the best possible function within their anatomic and physiologic limitations. With advances in technology such as gait analysis, as well as the use of evidence-based medicine and multispecialty care models, significant changes in the management of patients with myelomeningocele are occurring.

Myelomeningocele is the most common of the spectrum of conditions described as spina bifida. Myelomeningocele is a severe form of spinal dysraphism that also includes meningocele, lipomeningocele, and caudal regression syndrome. *Neural tube defect* is a broader term that includes myelomeningocele, anencephaly, and encephalocele. A myelomeningocele is a saclike structure containing cerebrospinal fluid and neural tissue (Fig. 34-28A). The herniation of the spinal cord and its meninges through a defect in the vertebral canal results in variable neurologic defects depending on the location and severity of the lesion. A meningocele is a cystic distention of the meninges through unfused vertebral arches, but the spinal cord remains in the vertebral canal. Most lesions are posterior, but rarely an anterior or lateral meningocele may occur. Neurologic deficits are not as common as in myelomeningocele. *Spina bifida occulta* is a term that refers to a defect in the posterior vertebral elements that includes the spinous process and often part of the lamina, most commonly of the fifth lumbar and first sacral vertebrae. Spina bifida occulta occurs in approximately 10% of asymptomatic adult spines and is often an incidental finding on plain radiographs that is rarely associated with neurologic involvement.

The nervous system develops by the formation of a tubular structure (neurulation). Closure of this tube is

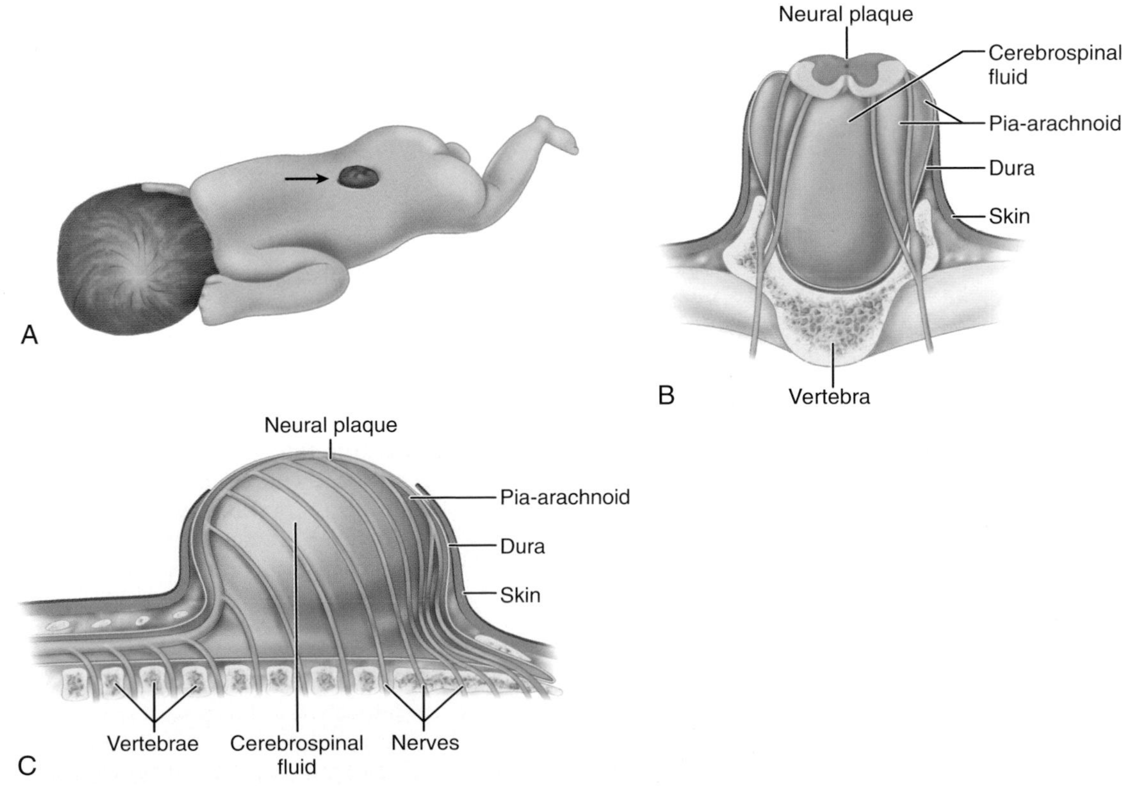

FIGURE 34-28 **A,** Infant with myelomeningocele. Lesion may be small extension **(B)** or large sessile protrusion **(C)**.

completed by closure of the cranial and caudal neuropores between day 26 to 28 of gestation. Myelomeningocele and anencephaly occur because of abnormalities during this phase of closure of the neural tube. Conditions such as meningocele, lipomeningocele, and diastematomyelia occur from abnormalities during the canalization phase from day 28 to 48 of gestation and are referred to as *postneurulation defects*.

The myelomeningocele is formed by the protrusion of dura and arachnoid through the defect in the vertebral arches. The spinal cord and nerve roots are carried out through this defect (Fig. 34-28B and C). These lesions can occur at any level along the spinal column but occur most commonly in the lower thoracic and lumbosacral regions. The skin over a myelomeningocele is almost always absent. The neural placode is covered by a thin membrane (arachnoid) that breaks down in a couple of days, leaving an ulcerated granulating surface. The superficial surface of the neural placode represents the everted interior of the neural tube. The ventral surface represents what should have been the outside of a closed neural tube. Because of this pathologic anatomy, the nerve roots arise from the ventral part of the neural placode. The pedicles are everted and lie almost horizontal in the coronal plane. The affected lamina are hypoplastic and everted, and the paraspinal muscles are everted with the pedicles and lie in an anterior position. These muscles act as flexors of the spine instead of functioning normally as extensors because of their anterior position.

The incidence of myelomeningocele in the United States is 0.6 to 0.9 per 1000 births and would likely be higher, but an estimated 23% of pregnancies with myelomeningocele are terminated. The overall incidence of infants born with neural tube defects is decreasing, which is most likely related to better prenatal screening and the use of folic acid supplementation before conception and during the first month of pregnancy. Testing for elevated levels of maternal serum α-fetoprotein between 16 and 18 weeks of gestation can detect 75% to 80% of affected pregnancies. If the maternal serum α-fetoprotein is found to be elevated, ultrasound examination, ultrafast MRI, and amniocentesis for α-fetoprotein and acetylcholinesterase may be needed to confirm a possible neural tube defect. Ultrasound is a sensitive and efficient test to determine the presence and location of a neural tube defect. If no abnormalities are found on ultrasound examination, an amniocentesis is recommended to evaluate for α-fetoprotein and acetylcholinesterase. With this prenatal screening program, there has been a reported decrease in birth prevalence of anencephaly from 100% to 80% and birth prevalence of myelomeningocele from 80% to 60%. Other studies have shown a 60% to 100% reduction in the risk of neural tube defects when adequate levels of folate are taken by pregnant women. The U.S. Food and Drug Administration recommends that all women of childbearing age receive 0.4 mg folate before conception and during early pregnancy. The Centers for Disease Control and Prevention also recommends that women who are at high risk (i.e., women who have given birth to a prior affected child or who have a first-degree relative with a neural tube defect) receive 4 mg of folate daily.

Genetic factors also play a role in myelomeningocele. There is a greater incidence of neural tube defects, including myelomeningocele, in siblings of affected children, in the range of 2% to 7%. There also is a higher frequency in twins than in single births. For a couple who has a child with myelomeningocele the chance that a subsequent child will be affected by a major malformation of the central nervous system is approximately 1 in 14. With over 100 known genes that affect neurulation and the low frequency of occurrence in the population, the determination of the exact molecular defect(s) remains difficult.

ASSOCIATED CONDITIONS

The natural history of myelomeningocele has changed over the past several decades because of advances in medical treatment. Patients born with myelomeningocele often died of urinary tract infection, renal failure, meningitis, and sepsis. With early neurosurgical and urologic intervention, patients born with myelomeningocele are surviving into adult life, with about 65% having normal intelligence. Myelomeningocele was believed to be nonprogressive, but studies have shown progressive neurologic deterioration can occur, manifested by increasing levels of paralysis and decreasing upper extremity function. Hydrocephalus and associated hydrosyringomyelia, Arnold-Chiari malformation, and tethered cord syndrome have been associated with progressive neurologic deterioration.

■ HYDROCEPHALUS

Hydrocephalus is a dilation of the ventricles of the brain from excessive cerebrospinal fluid. Before closure of the myelomeningocele defect, the ventricles are decompressed by their direct communication to the persistently open central canal of the cord. Of children with myelomeningocele, 80% to 90% have hydrocephalus that requires cerebrospinal shunting. Chakarborty et al. described new protocols aimed at reducing shunt placement rates in myelomeningocele patients. Using these protocols, the shunt rate in infants with myelomeningocele was decreased to 60%.

The incidence of hydrocephalus is related to the neurologic level of the lesion, with patients with thoracic and upper lumbar lesions having a higher incidence than those with lower lumbar and sacral level lesions. Early treatment of hydrocephalus has improved the early mortality rate and, more importantly, improved the long-term intellectual development of these children. If the hydrocephalus is not treated, the increased fluid pressure results in atrophy of the brain, hydromyelia, and syringomyelia. Children who do not require shunting have a better prognosis for upper extremity function and trunk balance than children who require shunting. Shunt malfunctions, manifested by signs of acute hydrocephaly such as nausea, vomiting, and severe headaches, do occur. In older children, the diagnosis may be more difficult because the shunt malfunction may be associated with increased irritability, decreased perceptual motor function, short attention span, intermittent headaches, increasing scoliosis, and increased level of paralysis.

■ HYDROSYRINGOMYELIA

Hydrosyringomyelia is an accumulation of fluid in the enlarged central canal of the spinal cord. This usually is the result of hydrocephalus or an alteration in the normal cerebrospinal fluid dynamics. Hydrosyringomyelia can cause three problems in patients with myelomeningocele: (1) an increasing level of paralysis of the lower extremities, often associated with an increase in spasticity of the lower extremity, (2) progressive scoliosis, and (3) weakness in the hands and upper extremities. This condition can be diagnosed with MRI; early treatment may reverse some of the neurologic loss and scoliosis.

■ ARNOLD-CHIARI MALFORMATION

Arnold-Chiari malformation (caudal displacement of the posterior lobe of the cerebellum) is a consistent finding in patients with myelomeningocele. Type II Arnold-Chiari malformation is seen most often in children with myelomeningocele and is characterized by displacement of the medulla oblongata into the cervical neural canal through the foramen magnum. This malformation causes dysfunction of the lower cranial nerves, resulting in weakness or paralysis of vocal cords and difficulty in feeding, crying, and breathing. Sometimes, these symptoms are episodic, which makes diagnosis difficult. In childhood, symptoms may consist of nystagmus, stridor, swallowing difficulties, and a depressed cough reflex. Spastic weakness of the upper extremities also may be present. Placement of a ventriculoperitoneal shunt to control hydrocephalus often resolves brainstem symptoms, and surgical decompression of the Arnold-Chiari malformation is unnecessary unless the neurologic symptoms are not relieved by shunting. In these rare cases, the posterior fossa and upper cervical spine require surgical decompression.

■ TETHERED SPINAL CORD

MRI shows signs of tethering of the spinal cord in most children with myelomeningocele, but only 20% to 30% have clinical manifestations. Clinical signs vary, but the most consistent are (1) loss of motor function, (2) development of spasticity in the lower extremities, primarily the medial hamstrings and ankle dorsiflexors and evertors, (3) development of scoliosis before age 6 years in the absence of congenital anomalies of the vertebral bodies, (4) back pain and increased lumbar lordosis in an older child, and (5) changes in urologic function. Deterioration in somatosensory evoked potentials of the posterior tibial nerve has been used to document deterioration of lower extremity function and a clinically significant tethered cord. MRI evaluation should be performed in any child suspected of having a tethered cord syndrome. Because dermal elements are left attached during initial closure, a dermal cyst often is seen in association with a tethered cord. If clinical signs are documented, surgical treatment is indicated to prevent further deterioration of the motor function and to diminish the progress of spasticity and scoliosis. It is important to make an early diagnosis and start treatment because surgical release of the tethered cord rarely provides complete return of lost function.

■ OTHER SPINAL ABNORMALITIES

Vertebral bone anomalies, such as a defect in segmentation and failure of formation of vertebral bodies, may cause congenital scoliosis, kyphosis, and kyphoscoliosis. Other spinal anomalies the treating physician should be aware of are duplication of the spinal cord and diastematomyelia. Diastematomyelia may cause progressive loss of neurologic function.

■ UROLOGIC DYSFUNCTION

Almost all children with myelomeningocele have some form of bladder dysfunction, with most having bladder paralysis. Chronic renal failure and sepsis from urinary tract infections were the most common causes of delayed mortality in patients with myelomeningocele before modern urologic treatment methods. The goal of urologic management is to achieve continence at an appropriate age, decompress the upper urinary tract to prevent renal failure, and prevent urinary tract infections. The mainstay of treatment is clean intermittent catheterization to prevent hydronephrosis and maintain bladder compliance and capacity. Antibiotic prophylaxis and anticholinergic medication to reduce infection and vesicoureteral reflux may be beneficial. Screening examinations, consisting of voiding cystometrograms and renal sonograms, are routinely done every 6 to 12 months. Surgical options for patients in whom medical treatment is unsuccessful include vesicostomy, a diversion of the bladder to the lower abdominal wall to facilitate catheterization, and bladder augmentation in which a segment of the ileum is added to the bladder to increase capacity and reduce bladder pressure. The orthopaedist must be aware of the effects any orthopaedic surgery may have on the need for self-catheterization and any possible urinary diversion procedures.

■ BOWEL DYSFUNCTION

Most patients with myelomeningocele have innervation of the bowel and anus that results in dysmotility, poor sphincter control, and often fecal incontinence. Constipation and fecal impaction resulting from decreased bowel motility can cause increased intraabdominal pressure that leads to ventriculoperitoneal shunt malfunction. Oral laxatives, suppositories, or enemas can be used to achieve continence and avoid fecal impaction by promoting regular fecal elimination. If these are unsuccessful, the Malone antegrade continence enema (MACE) procedure is an option: the appendix and cecum are used to create a stoma through which the colon can be irrigated. In one study evaluating the results of the MACE procedure in 108 patients with myelomeningocele, approximately 85% achieved continence.

■ LATEX HYPERSENSITIVITY

Latex hypersensitivity has been noted in children with myelomeningocele, with a reported incidence of 3.8% to 38%. The hypersensitivity is a type 1 immunoglobulin E (IgE)-mediated response to residual free protein found in latex products. Tosi et al. reported a serologic prevalence of hypersensitivity in 38% of at-risk patients but a clinical prevalence of 10%. A detailed history is the most sensitive way to detect individuals at risk for latex reaction. It is recommended that all patients with myelomeningocele be treated "latex free" during surgery with avoidance of latex gloves and latex-containing accessories (catheters, adhesives, tourniquets, and anesthesia equipment) (Box 34-1). High-risk patients or those with known hypersensitivity reactions can be treated prophylactically with corticosteroids and/or antihistamines before medical procedures (Table 34-1).

■ MISCELLANEOUS MEDICAL ISSUES

Depending on the severity of involvement, children with myelomeningocele are at risk for depression, as well as cognitive dysfunction and learning difficulties. Obesity also is a problem for children with myelomeningocele both medically and functionally. This is especially true in nonambulatory

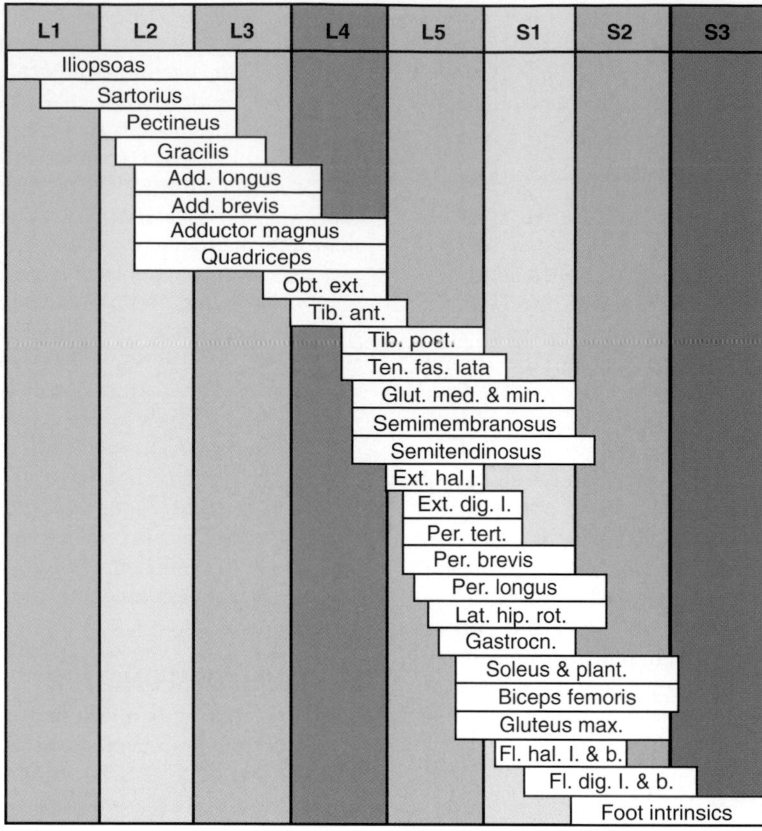

FIGURE 34-29 Neurosegmental innervation of lower limb muscles.

BOX 34-1

Latex-Avoidance Protocol

- Use of nonlatex gloves by surgical, anesthesia, and nursing personnel
- Avoidance of any known latex product in the sterile field by the surgeon
- Use of plastic anesthesia facemask for preoxygenation and positive-pressure ventilation
- Use of nonlatex anesthetic reservoir bag for positive-pressure ventilation
- Use of nonlatex tourniquet for intravenous catheter placement
- Use of nonlatex blood pressure cuff/tubing, electrocardiogram leads, and stethoscope
- Use of nonlatex tape
- Intravenous injection via stopcock rather than rubber injection port

From Birmingham PK, Dsida RM, Grayhack JJ, et al: Do latex precautions in children with myelodysplasia reduce intraoperative allergic reactions? J Pediatr Orthop 16:799, 1996.

children in whom it may be difficult to increase caloric expenditure. Small changes in body weight can have a dramatic impact on ambulation because of the increased demands placed on already weak muscles by the additional body weight. It is exceptionally rare for an obese nonambulatory child to lose weight and regain ambulation.

CLASSIFICATION

The most commonly used classification of myelomeningocele is based on the neurologic level of the lesion (Fig. 34-29); however, there are several difficulties with this classification system, including performing isolated muscle testing in young children, differences in classification systems, and differences in the affected neurologic level compared with the anatomic defect. In addition, not all patients have these distinct levels of paralysis. Some patients may not have symmetric levels for each extremity, and some may be flaccid, whereas others may have some associated spasticity in the involved lower extremities.

Despite these limitations, patients with myelomeningocele can be grouped into four distinct levels: thoracic level, upper lumbar level, lower lumbar level, and sacral level. This classification assists in predicting the patient's natural history and expected deformities that may need intervention. Patients can be placed into one of four groups according to the level of the lesion and resultant muscle function. Patients with thoracic level lesions have no active hip flexion and no voluntary muscle control in the lower extremities. Patients with upper lumbar level lesions have variable power with hip flexion and adduction (L1-2) and quadriceps function (L3). Patients with lower lumbar level lesions have active knee flexion against gravity (hamstring power), anterior tibial function (L4), and extensor hallucis longus function (L5). Patients with sacral level lesions have weakness of the peroneals and intrinsic muscles of the foot but have some active toe flexor function and hip extensor and abductor power.

TABLE 34-1

Prophylaxis for Latex Allergy

	DOSE (mg/kg)	MAXIMUM (mg)
HIGH-RISK GROUP		
A. Patient is admitted 24 hr before scheduled procedure		
B. The following medications are administered intravenously before surgery and for 72 hr postoperatively, administered every 6 hr (minimum, two doses)		
	DOSE (mg/kg)	**MAXIMUM (mg)**
Methylprednisolone	1	50
Diphenhydramine	1	50
Cimetidine	5	300
C. Attempt to eliminate all latex-containing materials from the operating room environment		
MODERATE-RISK GROUP		
A. Patient may be treated as outpatient		
B. Oral medications are begun 24 hr before surgery		
	DOSE (mg/kg)	**MAXIMUM (mg)**
Prednisone	1	50
Diphenhydramine	1	50
C. The following medications are given every 6 hr for 24 hr before surgery with minimum of two doses		
	DOSE (mg/kg)	**MAXIMUM (mg)**
Prednisone	1	50
Diphenhydramine	1	50
Cimetidine	5	50
D. Attempt to eliminate all latex-containing materials from the operating room environment		
LOW-RISK GROUP		
A. Patient may be treated as outpatient		
B. Oral therapy is begun 12 hr before surgery		
	DOSE (mg/kg)	**MAXIMUM (mg)**
Prednisone	1	50
Diphenhydramine	1	50
C. The following medications are given 1 hr before surgery		
	DOSE (mg/kg)	**MAXIMUM (mg)**
Prednisone	1	50
Diphenhydramine	1	50
D. Attempt to eliminate all latex-containing materials from the operating room environment		

From Dormans JP, Templeton J, Schreinder MS, et al: Intraoperative latex anaphylaxis in children: classification and prophylaxis of patients at risk, J Pediatr Orthop 17:622, 1997.

The sensory level has been suggested to be a better way to define the level of paralysis because muscles that can communicate with the brain through sensory feedback are functional but muscles that cannot become flaccid or spastic, functioning only by reflex. A sensory level classification also may be more reproducible between different observers.

The functional classification described by Swaroop and Dias is useful in determining a child's prognosis for ambulation and bracing. Patients are divided into four groups based on lesion level and accompanying functional and ambulatory capacity (Table 34-2).

The Functional Mobility Scale (FMS) also has been used to evaluate the functional ability of children with neuromuscular disorders. This scale is simple and fast, rating the child's mobility on a scale of 1 to 6 (1 = wheelchair, 2 = walker, 3 = two crutches, 4 = one crutch, 5 = independent on level surfaces, 6 = independent on all surfaces) over three different distances: home (5 meters), school (50 meters), and community (500 meters). Additional advantages of the FMS include the ability to systematically compare children affected with different neuromuscular diseases and the fact that this is more a true measure of the child's functional abilities than isolated motor or sensory testing.

ORTHOPAEDIC EVALUATION

Orthopaedic evaluation of children with myelomeningocele should include the following:

1. *Serial sensory and motor examinations:* Evaluate the neurologic level of function; this may be difficult before 4 years of age.
2. *Sitting balance:* Indicates central nervous system function; if significant support is required for sitting, the probability of ambulation is significantly decreased.
3. *Upper extremity function:* Assesses ability to use assistive devices; decreased grip strength and atrophy of the thenar musculature are indications of hydromyelia.
4. *Spine evaluation:* Clinical evaluation and yearly radiographs are needed to detect development of scoliosis and/or kyphosis and lumbar hyperlordosis.
5. *Hip evaluation:* Range of motion, stability, contractures, pelvic obliquity
6. *Knee evaluation:* Range of motion, alignment, contractures, and spasticity
7. *Rotational evaluation:* Including internal/external tibial torsion
8. *Ankle evaluation:* Range of motion, valgus deformity
9. *Foot evaluation:* Foot deformities including congenital vertical talus, skin breakdown
10. *Mobility and bracing evaluation:* Changes in mobility that have remained stable; braces fitting properly and in good condition
11. *Miscellaneous:* Depression, obesity, school performance

GAIT EVALUATION

Advances in the quality and use of gait analysis have produced useful information about gait function and energy expenditure in patients with myelomeningocele. Most patients with myelomeningocele, especially those with higher level involvement, have multilevel three-dimensional deformities. These deformities can be difficult to assess on isolated clinical examination. Gait analysis allows assessment of the patient in real time during ambulation, which can be helpful diagnostically and in planning treatment strategies. Gait analysis has shown that hip abductor strength is one of the most important determinants of ambulatory kinematics and ability; that pelvic obliquity, determined by hip abductor strength, has the strongest correlation to oxygen cost during gait; and that children tend to self-select both velocity and dynamics to maintain a comfortable level of exertion. Gait studies also have shown increased dynamic knee flexion in patients with myelomeningocele compared with static examination. Patients with low

TABLE 34-2

Functional Classification of Myelomeningocele

GROUP	NEUROLOGIC LEVEL OF LESION	PREVALENCE (%)	FUNCTIONAL CAPACITY	AMBULATORY CAPABILITY	FUNCTIONAL MOBILITY SCALE
Thoracic/high lumbar	L3 or above	30	No functional quadriceps (≤ grade 2)	During childhood, require bracing to level of pelvis for ambulation (RGO, HKAFO) 70%-99% require wheelchair for mobility in adulthood	1,1,1
Low lumbar	L3 – L5	30	Quadriceps, medial hamstring ≥ grade 3 No functional activity (≤ grade 2) of gluteus medius and maximus, gastrocsoleus	Require AFOs and crutches for ambulation 80%-95% maintain community ambulation in adulthood	3,3,1
High sacral	S1 – S3	30	Quadriceps, gluteus medius ≥ grade 3 No functional activity (≤ grade 2) of gastrocsoleus	Require AFOs for ambulation 94%-100% maintain community ambulation in adulthood	6,6,6
Low sacral	S3 – S5	5-10	Quadriceps, gluteus medius, gastrocsoleus ≥ grade 3	Ambulate without braces or support 94%-100% maintain community ambulation in adulthood	6,6,6

From Swaroop VT, Dias L: Myelomeningocele. In Weinstein SL, Flynn JM, editors: Lovell and Winter's Pediatric Orthopaedics, ed 7, Philadelphia, Wolters Kluwer, 2014.
AFO, Ankle-foot orthosis; HKAFO, hip-knee-ankle-foot orthosis; RGO, reciprocal gait orthosis.

lumbar level lesions have a walking velocity that is 60% of normal, and patients with high sacral level lesions have a walking velocity approximately 70% of normal.

PRINCIPLES OF ORTHOPAEDIC MANAGEMENT

Orthopaedic management should be tailored to meet specific goals during childhood, taking into account the expected function in adulthood. The goal for a child with myelomeningocele is to establish a pattern of development for the child that is as near normal as possible. Ambulation is not the goal for every child. Despite the best medical and surgical care, about 40% of children with myelomeningocele are unable to walk as adults. An evidence-based review found that neurosegmental level is the primary determinant of walking ability and physical function. Other factors believed to play a lesser role in the ability to ambulate in children with myelomeningocele include cognitive ability, physical therapy, compliant parents, clubfoot deformity, scoliosis, increased age, back pain, and lack of motivation. Often, the goal of orthopaedic treatment is a stable posture in braces or in a wheelchair. Surgery may be more detrimental than helpful, causing long-term disability. Before aggressive orthopaedic treatment is instituted, the lifetime prognosis for the patient should be considered. Only 30% of all patients with myelomeningocele are functionally independent, and only 30% of adults with myelomeningocele are employed full time or part time. Almost all patients with L2 or higher level lesions use a wheelchair, and more than two thirds of patients with lower-level lesions (L3-5) use a wheelchair at least part of the time.

Most children achieve their maximal level of ambulation around age 4 to 6 years. If a child with myelomeningocele is not standing independently by about age 6 years, walking is unlikely. Prerequisites for walking include a spine balanced over the pelvis; absence of hip and knee contractures (or only mild contractures); and plantigrade, supple, braceable feet with the center of gravity centered over them. An extension posture at the hip and knee can be maintained with minimal support from leg and arm muscles, whereas a flexion posture tends to be a collapsing posture (Fig. 34-30). At least 80% of children with myelomeningocele have some impairment of their upper extremities; effective ambulation with low energy consumption and minimal bracing is possible in only about 50% of adult patients. Although ambulation into adolescence and adulthood is unlikely, children who walk tend to be more mobile than children who never walk and they have fewer fractures and skin pressure sores. If a child has functioning quadriceps and medial hamstring muscles, good sitting balance, and upper extremity function, all efforts should be made to achieve ambulation.

NONOPERATIVE MANAGEMENT

Almost all children with myelomeningocele except those with low sacral level lesions will require some type of orthotic device. Orthotic treatment goals include maintenance of motion, prevention of deformity, assistance with ambulation/mobility, and the protection of insensate skin. Bracing and splinting vary with the degree of motor deficit and trunk balance, and each child should be carefully evaluated using a team approach. Children 12 to 18 months old may benefit from the use of a standing frame for upright positioning, and for children older than 2 years, a parapodium that supports the spine and allows a swing-to or swing-through gait with crutches or a walker may be beneficial. An ankle-foot orthosis is used in children with low lumbar or sacral level lesions and fair quadriceps muscle function. The ankle-foot orthosis

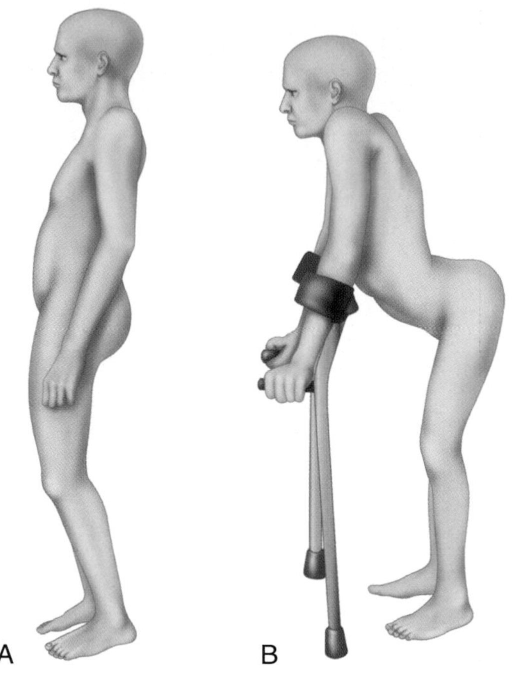

FIGURE 34-30 A, Extension posture with hips and knees extended, feet plantigrade; posture aimed for regardless of bracing necessary. B, Flexion posture at the hips imposes lumbar lordosis and patient uses both arms for weight bearing and loses other, more valuable function.

should be rigid enough to provide ankle and foot stabilization and to maintain the ankle at 90 degrees. A knee-ankle-foot orthosis may be indicated for a child with a lumbar level lesion and weak quadriceps function to prevent abnormal valgus of the knee during the stance phase of gait. Children with high-level lesions often have excessive anterior pelvic tilt and lumbar lordosis and require a pelvic band, either a conventional hip-knee-ankle-foot orthosis or a reciprocating gait orthosis. The reciprocating gait orthosis also can be used in patients with upper lumbar lesions, allowing them to be upright and assisting them in attempts at ambulation. This brace is started around the age of 2 and provides the ability to walk in a reciprocal fashion by dynamically coupling the flexion of one hip to the simultaneous extension of the contralateral hip. For the reciprocating orthosis to be effective, the patient should have good upper extremity strength, sitting (trunk) balance, and active hip flexion. Energy expenditure for children in reciprocal gait orthoses and traditional hip-knee-foot orthoses are similar; however, children with hip-knee-foot orthoses have a faster gait velocity. A child can be tapered from a reciprocal gait orthosis to a hip-knee-foot orthoses if he or she develops enough upper body strength to use crutches safely.

The use of newer materials such as carbon fiber may provide an alternative to patients who do not benefit from current braces. Carbon fiber ankle-foot orthoses have been shown to increase energy return and ankle plantarflexion motion, positive work, and stride length compared with standard materials.

■ OPERATIVE MANAGEMENT

Orthopaedic deformities in children with myelomeningocele are caused by (1) muscle imbalance resulting from the neurologic abnormality, (2) habitually assumed posture, and (3) associated congenital malformations. Surgical correction of deformities may be indicated. Most surgical procedures in patients with myelomeningocele are performed during the first 15 years of life. When surgical correction is indicated, the deformity should be completely and permanently corrected.

Principles of orthopaedic management include:

1. Multiple procedures should be done simultaneously to minimize repeated anesthetic exposures.
2. Cast immobilization, especially in recumbency, should be minimized owing to the risk of osteopenia and pathologic fracture.
3. The orthopaedic treatment program must be integrated with the total treatment program.
4. The absence of sensation, osteopenia, and the increased risk of infection secondary to urinary tract problems must be constantly considered.
5. Hospitalization must be kept at a minimum.
6. The demands on the family in terms of time, effort, expense, and separation must be minimized.

FOOT

Approximately 75% of children with myelomeningocele have foot deformities that can seriously limit function. These deformities can take many forms including clubfoot, acquired equinovarus, varus, metatarsus adductus, equinus, equinovalgus, vertical talus, talipes calcaneus, calcaneovalgus, calcaneovarus, calcaneocavus, cavus, cavovarus, supination, pes planovalgus, and toe deformities.

The goal of orthopaedic treatment of foot deformities is a plantigrade, painless, mobile, braceable foot. Muscle-balancing procedures that remove deforming muscular forces are more reliable than tendon transfer procedures. Often tendon excision is more reliable than tendon lengthening or transfer. Bone deformities should be corrected by appropriate osteotomies that preserve joint motion. Arthrodesis should be avoided if possible because most feet in patients with myelomeningocele are insensate, which can lead to neuropathic problems including joint destruction and pressure sores.

Manipulation and casting should be used with caution in these patients to avoid pressure sores and iatrogenic fractures. Most foot deformities eventually require surgical correction if correction of the deformity is needed to improve function. Despite surgical correction, there is a relatively high recurrence rate of the deformity because of the deforming neurologic forces present.

■ EQUINUS DEFORMITY

Equinus usually is an acquired deformity that may be prevented or delayed by bracing and splinting. Depending on the ambulatory function of the patient, an Achilles tendon lengthening, tenotomy, or resection can be performed. Equinus is seen more frequently in children with high lumbar or thoracic level lesions. For mild deformities, excision of 2 cm of the Achilles tendon through a vertical incision usually is sufficient. Alternatively, a percutaneous Achilles tendon lengthening may be performed. Often the long toe flexors must be released to prevent persistent toe flexion deformities that can result in pressure sores. For more severe deformity, radical posterior release is required, including excision of all the tendons contributing to the equinus and extensive capsulotomies of the ankle and subtalar joints. In rare cases, salvage procedures such as osteotomy or talectomy may be required for a symptomatic deformity.

CLUBFOOT

Clubfoot is present at birth in approximately 30% to 50% of children with myelomeningocele. The deformity usually is rigid and resembles that of arthrogryposis multiplex congenita and differs markedly from idiopathic clubfoot. It is characterized by severe rigidity, supination-varus deformity, rotational malalignment of the calcaneus and talus, subluxation of the calcaneocuboid and talonavicular joints, and often a cavus component. Internal tibial torsion often is present. With the increased use of the Ponseti clubfoot casting technique, infants with myelomeningocele are being treated with this method. Some patients can be successfully treated with this technique, but the complication and recurrence rates are much higher than in idiopathic clubfoot. A 68% early relapse rate and a 25% surgical release rate have been reported in children with myelomeningocele treated with this method. Even with adequate surgical correction, recurrence of the clubfoot deformity is frequent.

Surgery can be done between 10 and 12 months of age. Radical posteromedial-lateral release through the Cincinnati incision (see Chapter 29) is recommended. If there is significant equinus, a variety of techniques have been described to help prevent posterior soft-tissue and incision breakdown including the use of medial and posterior incisions (Carroll), a modification of the Cincinnati incision that includes a complete circumferential skin release (Noonan et al.), and a modified V-Y plasty (Lubicky and Altiok) (Fig. 34-31). Another method to avoid undue tension on the incision posteriorly is to immobilize the foot postoperatively in an undercorrected position until the wound is healed. Two weeks later, when the incision has healed, the cast can be changed and the foot can be placed in a corrected position safely.

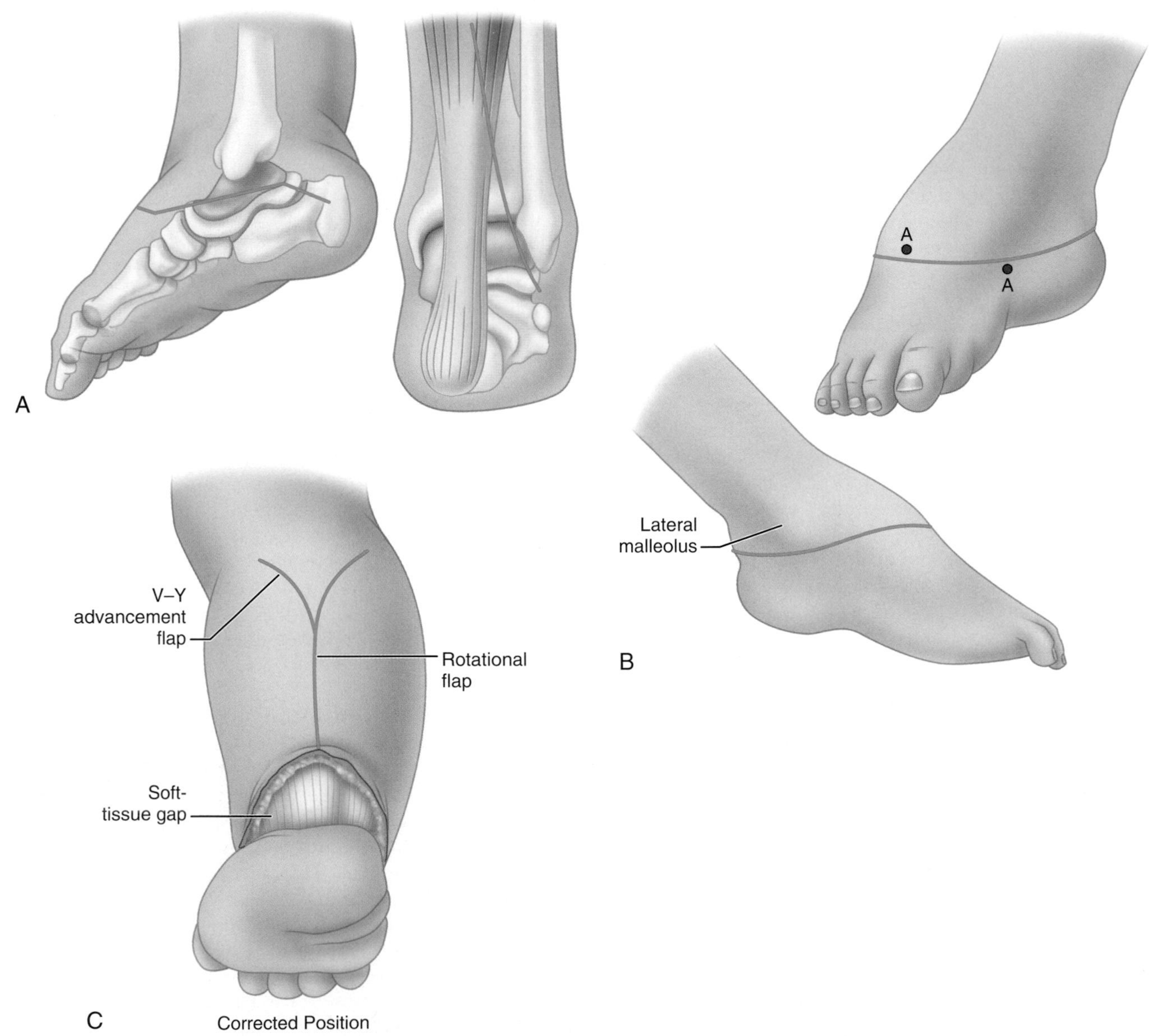

FIGURE 34-31 Incisions used for clubfoot correction. **A,** Carroll two-incision technique. **B,** Modification of the Cincinnati incision by Noonan et al. **C,** V-Y advancement flap technique of Lubicky and Altiok.

Tenotomies instead of tendon lengthening should be done to minimize any recurrence with growth. If the anterior tibial tendon is active, simple tenotomy should be performed to prevent recurrent supination deformity. In older children, the imbalance between the medial and lateral columns of the foot may be so severe that it cannot be corrected by soft-tissue release alone. Closing wedge osteotomy of the cuboid (see Chapter 29), lateral wedge resection of the distal calcaneus (Lichtblau procedure; see Chapter 29), or calcaneocuboid arthrodesis (Dillwyn-Evans procedure; Fig. 34-2) may be required to shorten the lateral column. Talectomy (see Chapter 29) is indicated as a salvage procedure for a severely deformed rigid clubfoot in an older child. The talus should be completely removed because any fragment left behind would resume its growth and cause recurrence of the deformity. The Achilles tendon may need to be resected after talectomy to prevent further equinus. Talectomy would correct the hindfoot deformity, but any adduction deformity should be corrected by shortening of the lateral column through the same incision. Severe forefoot deformities require midtarsal or metatarsal osteotomies (see Chapter 29).

V-O PROCEDURE

Verebelyi and Ogston described a decancellation procedure to correct residual clubfoot deformity in patients with myelomeningocele. This procedure consists of removing as much cancellous bone as possible from the talus and the cuboid. This leaves a hollow shell of bone and more space for correction. The foot is manipulated into calcaneus and valgus, which, because of collapse of the talus and cuboid bone, would lead to correction of the residual deformity. In selected patients, this procedure may be preferable to talectomy for correction of severe rigid clubfoot deformity.

TECHNIQUE 34-30

- Make an oblique incision on the dorsolateral aspect of the foot to expose the cuboid and the talus.
- Retract the peroneal tendons and sural nerve plantarly and protect them while retracting the extensor digitorum brevis dorsally.
- Cut a square window in the cuboid with a 1/4-inch osteotome and remove all cancellous bone with a curet.
- Along the lateral talus, cut a rectangular window with the longer dimension parallel to the long axis of the talus and curet the cancellous contents of the body, neck, and head.
- Confirm the removal of all cancellous bone, with fluoroscopy or radiography, especially at the posterior aspect of the talus.
- Obtain correction by collapsing the empty cartilaginous shells of the cuboid and talus. If satisfactory correction is not obtained, remove lateral wedges from the cuboid or the talar neck.
- If necessary, perform a percutaneous heel cord lengthening.
- Close the wounds routinely, and apply a short leg cast, monovalved for swelling.

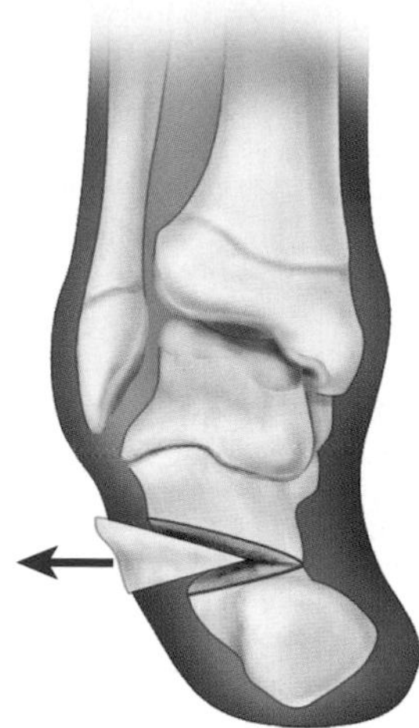

FIGURE 34-32 Lateral closing wedge osteotomy of calcaneus for isolated varus deformity of hindfoot.

POSTOPERATIVE CARE. After the swelling has subsided, the cast is reinforced and initially changed at 1 to 10 days, maintaining the foot in a neutral or slightly overcorrected position. At 4 weeks after surgery, at the time of the second cast change, a mold is made of the foot in a slightly overcorrected position for an ankle-foot orthosis. When the cast is removed at 6 weeks, the orthosis is worn usually until skeletal maturity.

VARUS DEFORMITY

Isolated varus deformity of the hindfoot is rare; it is usually associated with adduction deformity of the forefoot, cavus deformity, or supination deformity. Imbalance between the invertors and evertors should be evaluated carefully. For isolated, rigid hindfoot varus deformity, a closing wedge osteotomy is indicated. After removal of the lateral wedge (Fig. 34-32), the calcaneus should be translated laterally, if needed to increase correction.

CAVOVARUS DEFORMITY

Cavovarus deformities occur mainly in children with sacral level lesions. The cavus is the primary deformity that causes the hindfoot varus. The Coleman test (see Chapter 35) helps to determine the rigidity of the varus deformity. For a supple deformity, radical plantar release (see Chapter 35) is indicated to correct the cavus deformity, without hindfoot bone surgery. If the varus deformity is rigid despite plantar release with or without midtarsal osteotomy, a closing wedge osteotomy (see Chapter 86) is indicated. Any muscle balance must be corrected before the bony procedures or at the same time. Triple arthrodesis (see Technique 34-4) rarely is indicated as a salvage procedure and should be used with caution in myelomeningocele patients.

SUPINATION DEFORMITY

Supination deformity of the forefoot occurs most frequently in children with L5 to S1 level lesions and is caused by the unopposed action of the anterior tibial muscle when the peroneus brevis and peroneus longus are inactive. Adduction deformity also can be present. If the muscle imbalance is not corrected, the deformity becomes fixed. If the deformity is supple, simple tenotomy of the anterior tibial tendon is adequate. Simple tenotomy usually is the preferred treatment method for patients with myelomeningocele, but a tendon transfer may be indicated in selective situations. If there is some gastrocnemius-soleus activity and no spasticity, the anterior tibial tendon can be transferred to the midfoot in line with the third metatarsal. Split anterior tibial tendon transfer (see Technique 34-9) occasionally can be used, with the lateral half of the tendon inserted in the cuboid. Osteotomy of the first cuneiform or the base of the first metatarsal may be required for residual bone deformity.

CALCANEAL DEFORMITY

Approximately one third of children with myelomeningocele have calcaneal deformities, most frequently children with L4 and L5 lesions. The most common form is a calcaneovalgus deformity caused by the active anterior leg muscles and inactive posterior muscles. Spasticity of the evertors and dorsiflexors may cause calcaneal deformity in children with high-level lesions. Untreated calcaneal deformity produces a bulky, prominent heel that is prone to pressure sores and makes shoe wear difficult. Patients also lose toe-off power and develop an increased crouched gait. If the deformity is supple, as usually is the case, manipulation and splinting can bring the foot to a neutral position, but this rarely gives permanent correction. Muscle imbalance can be corrected early by simple tenotomy of all ankle dorsiflexors, as well as the peroneus brevis and peroneus longus. After anterolateral release in some patients, spasticity develops in the gastrocnemius-soleus muscle, causing an equinus deformity that requires tenotomy of the Achilles tendon or posterior release. Posterior transfer of the anterior tibial tendon has been reported to give good results. This often is combined with other soft-tissue and bony procedures to balance the foot. In older children with severe structural deformities, tendon transfers or tenotomies seldom achieve correction and bone procedures are indicated.

ANTEROLATERAL RELEASE

TECHNIQUE 34-31

- With the patient supine, apply and inflate a pneumatic tourniquet.
- Make a transverse incision about 2.5 cm long 2.0 to 3.0 cm above the ankle joint (Fig. 34-33A). Alternatively, an anterior lazy-S incision may be made. With sharp dissection, divide the superficial fascia to expose the tendons of the extensor hallucis longus, extensor digitorum communis, and tibialis anterior.
- Divide each tendon and excise at least 2.0 cm of each (Fig. 34-33B).
- Locate the peroneus tertius tendon in the lateralmost part of the wound and divide it.
- Make a second longitudinal incision above the ankle joint lateral and posterior to the fibula (Fig. 34-33A).

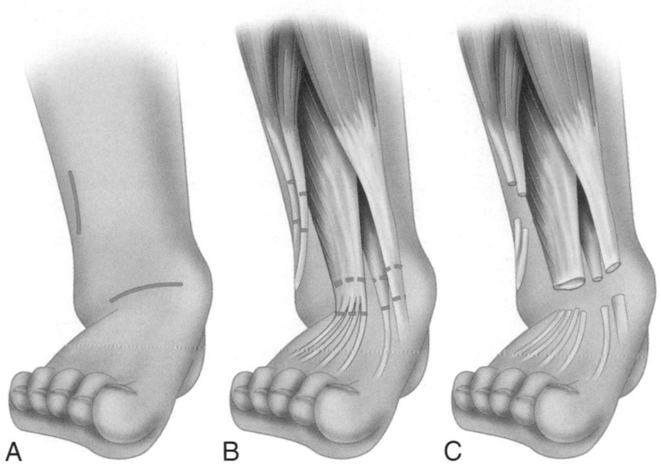

FIGURE 34-33 Anterolateral release for calcaneal deformity (see text). **A,** Transverse and longitudinal incisions. **B** and **C,** Excision of portion of tendons and tendon sheaths. **SEE TECHNIQUE 34-31.**

- Identify and divide the peroneus brevis and longus tendons and excise a section of each (Fig. 34-33C). Close the wounds, and apply a short leg walking cast.

POSTOPERATIVE CARE. The cast is worn for 10 days, and then an ankle-foot orthosis is fabricated for night wear.

TRANSFER OF THE ANTERIOR TIBIAL TENDON TO THE CALCANEUS

TECHNIQUE 34-32

- With the patient supine, make an incision in the dorsal aspect of the foot at the level of the insertion of the anterior tibial tendon at the base of the first metatarsal.
- Carefully detach the tendon from its insertion and free it as far proximally as possible.
- Make a second incision on the anterolateral aspect of the leg, just lateral to the tibial crest and 3 to 5 cm above the ankle joint.
- Free the tendon as far distally as possible and bring it up into the proximal wound (Fig. 34-34A).
- Expose the interosseous membrane and make a wide opening in it (Fig. 34-34B).
- Make a third transverse incision posteriorly at the level of the insertion of the Achilles tendon into the calcaneus.
- Using a tendon passer, bring the anterior tibial tendon through the interosseous membrane, from anterior to posterior, down to the level of this incision (Fig. 34-34C).
- Drill a large hole in the calcaneus, starting posteriorly and medially and exiting laterally and plantarward.
- Pass a Bunnell suture through the tendon and use a Keith needle to draw the tendon through the hole. A button

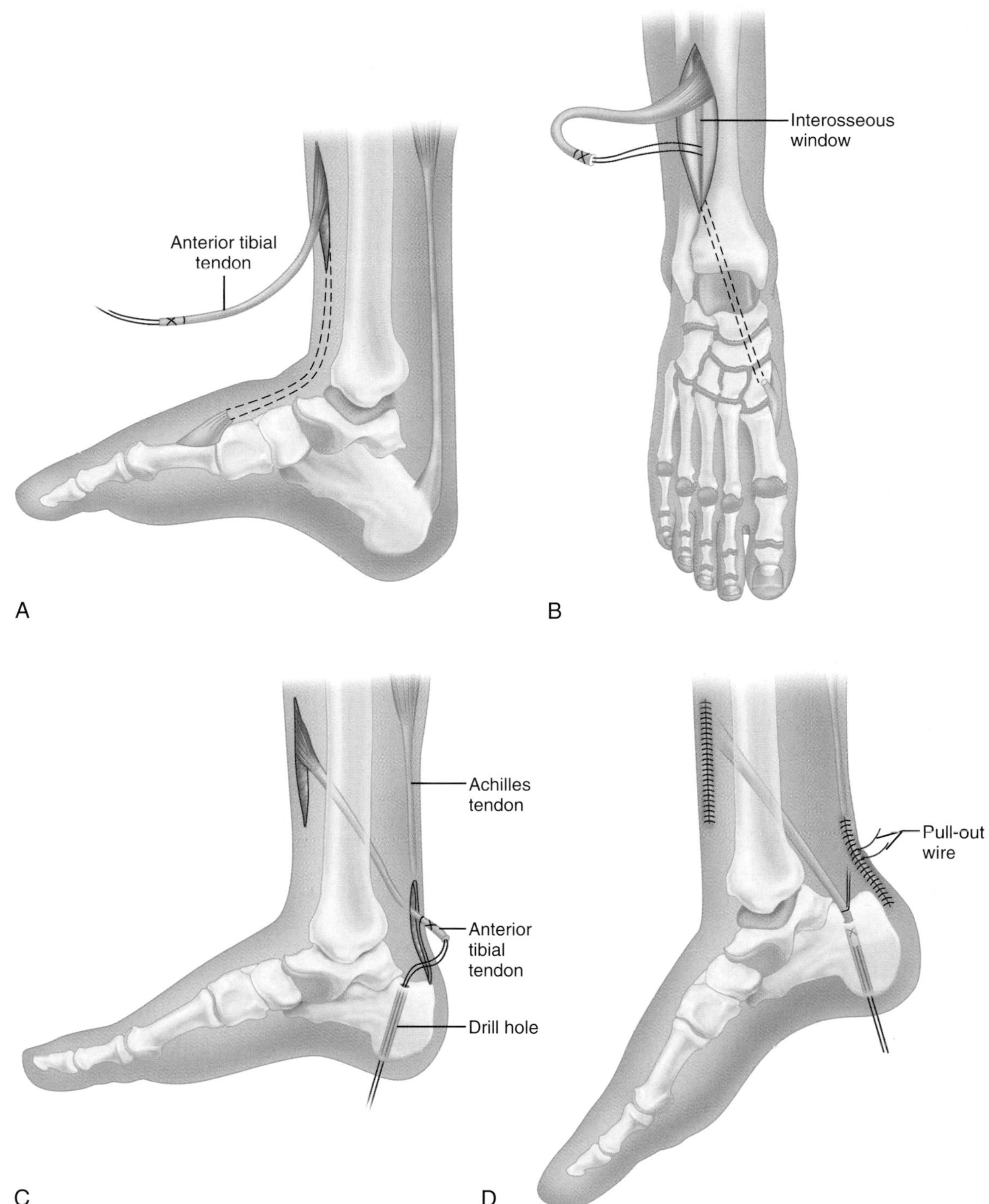

FIGURE 34-34 **A,** Anterior tibial tendon is divided distally and passed subcutaneously to the proximal incision. **B,** A 4 × 1.5 cm window is created in the interosseous membrane. **C,** The anterior tibial tendon is transferred posteriorly through the interosseous membrane. **D,** The transferred tendon is fixed to the calcaneus with a Bunnell suture or suture anchor. (Redrawn from Georgiadis GM, Aronson DD: Posterior transfer of the anterior tibial tendon in children who have a myelomeningocele, J Bone Joint Surg 72A:392, 1990.) **SEE TECHNIQUE 34-32.**

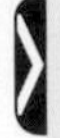

suture is not recommended because of pressure sores. Suture the tendon to the surrounding soft tissues to the level of its entrance into the calcaneus and to the Achilles tendon (Fig. 34-34D). Alternatively, a suture anchor can be used to secure the transferred tendon. The length of tendon is often not enough to secure the transfer to the calcaneus. When this occurs the transferred anterior tibial tendon can be sutured directly into the Achilles tendon.

- Close the wounds and apply a short leg cast.

HINDFOOT VALGUS

Valgus deformity at the ankle joint and external rotation deformity of the tibia and fibula frequently can exacerbate a hindfoot valgus deformity. Initially, this can be controlled with a well-fitted orthosis, but as the child becomes taller and heavier, control of the deformity is more difficult, pressure sores develop over the medial malleolus and the head of the talus, and surgical treatment is indicated. Clinical and radiographic measurements of the hindfoot valgus should be obtained; more than 10 mm of "lateral shift" of the calcaneus is significant. The Grice extraarticular arthrodesis (see Technique 34-2) is the classic treatment for this problem, but frequently reported complications include resorption of the graft, nonunion, varus overcorrection, and residual valgus. A 19-year follow-up of 35 feet treated with the Grice arthrodesis found significant improvement in visual analog scale (VAS) satisfaction scores and, although there was some mild increase in ankle valgus, 83% of patients were satisfied with their outcome. Medial displacement osteotomy has been recommended for correction of hindfoot valgus so that arthrodesis of the subtalar joint can be avoided (see Chapter 11). The combination of hindfoot and ankle valgus should be considered; if the ankle deformity is more than 10 to 15 degrees, closing wedge osteotomy or hemiepiphysiodesis of the distal tibial epiphysis is recommended in addition to the calcaneal osteotomy.

VERTICAL TALUS

Vertical talus deformities occur in approximately 10% of children with myelomeningocele. The deformity is characterized by malalignment of the hindfoot and midfoot. The talus is almost vertical, the calcaneus is in equinus and valgus, the navicular is dislocated dorsally on the talus, and the cuboid may be subluxated dorsally in relation to the calcaneus. Two types of vertical talus, developmental and congenital, occur in children with myelomeningocele. Neither the developmental nor the congenital type can be corrected by conservative methods. In developmental vertical talus, the foot is more supple and the talonavicular dislocation can be reduced by plantarflexion of the foot. In congenital vertical talus, manipulation and serial casting may partially correct the soft-tissue contractures in preparation for a complete posteromedial-lateral release (see Chapter 29), which should be performed when the child is ready to stand in braces, usually between 12 and 18 months old. The anterior tibial tendon can be resected or transferred into the neck of the talus. Occasionally, an extraarticular subtalar arthrodesis is needed to stabilize the subtalar joint. Dobbs et al. described a technique for correction of vertical talus in which serial manipulation and casting are followed by closed or open reduction of the talus and pin fixation. Percutaneous Achilles tenotomy is required to correct the equinus deformity. This method has been used successfully in children from birth to 4 years of age; the upper age limit at which this technique can be successful has not been defined.

PES CAVUS DEFORMITY

Cavus deformity, alone or with clawing of the toes or varus of the hindfoot, occurs most often in children with sacral level lesions. It may cause painful callosities under the metatarsal heads and difficulty with shoe wear. Plantarflexion of the first ray must be corrected for successful correction of the deformity. Although several procedures have been recommended for this deformity, few have been reported in patients with myelomeningocele. For an isolated cavus deformity with no hindfoot varus, radical plantar release is indicated. When varus deformity is present, medial subtalar release (see Chapter 29) is indicated. After surgery, a short leg cast is applied, and 1 to 2 weeks later the deformity is gradually corrected by cast changes every week or every other week for 6 weeks. In older children with rigid cavus deformities, anterior first metatarsal closing wedge osteotomy (see Chapter 86) is indicated in addition to radical plantar release. Opening wedge midfoot osteotomies also can be performed to correct the cavus. For residual varus deformity, a Dwyer closing wedge osteotomy of the calcaneus (see Chapter 33) is recommended.

TOE DEFORMITIES

Claw toe or hammer toe deformities occur more often in children with sacral level lesions and can cause problems with shoe and orthotic fitting. For flexible claw toe deformities, simple tenotomy of the flexors at the level of the proximal phalanx usually is sufficient. Rigid claw toe deformities can be treated with partial resection of the interphalangeal joint or arthrodesis. The Jones procedure (tendon suspension; see Chapter 86) is indicated when clawing of the great toe is associated with a cavus deformity. Arthrodesis of the proximal interphalangeal joint (see Chapter 86) or tenodesis of the distal stump of the extensor pollicis longus to the extensor pollicis brevis is recommended with the Jones procedure, although arthrodesis would hold up better than a tenodesis. The Hibbs transfer (see Chapter 35) can be performed to treat clawing of the lesser toes.

ANKLE

Progressive valgus deformity at the ankle or in combination with hindfoot valgus occurs most frequently in children with low lumbar level lesions. The strength of the gastrocnemius-soleus muscle is diminished or absent, and excessive laxity of the Achilles tendon allows marked passive ankle dorsiflexion. The medial malleolus is bulky, the head of the talus is shifted medially, and pressure ulcerations in these areas are common. The calcaneovalgus deformity usually appears early, but problems with orthotic fitting do not arise until the child is about 6 years old. Fibular shortening is common in children with L4, L5, or higher-level lesions. In the paralytic limb, abnormal shortening of the fibula and lateral malleolus causes a valgus tilt of the talus, with subsequent valgus deformity at the ankle (Fig. 34-35). Shortening of the fibula alters the normal distribution of forces on the distal tibial articular surface and increases compression forces on the lateral portion of the tibial epiphysis, further inhibiting growth, whereas decreased compression on the medial portion of the tibial epiphysis accelerates growth. This imbalance causes the lateral wedging that produces a valgus inclination of the talus. The degree of lateral wedging of the tibial epiphysis correlates with the degree of fibular shortening.

To evaluate valgus ankle deformity in children with myelomeningocele accurately, three factors must be determined: (1) the degree of fibular shortening, (2) the degree of valgus tilt of the talus in the ankle mortise, and (3) the amount of "lateral shift" of the calcaneus in relation to the weight-bearing axis of the tibia. Fibular shortening can be evaluated by measuring the distance between the distal fibular physis and the dome of the talus. In the normal ankle joint, the distal fibular physis is 2 to 3 mm proximal to the dome of the talus in children 4 years old (Fig. 34-36A). Between ages 4 and 8 years, the physis is at the same level as the talar dome (Fig. 34-36B), and in children older than 8 years, it is 2 to 3 mm distal to the talar dome (Fig. 34-36C). Differences of more than 10 mm from these values are considered significant. The valgus tilt of the talus can be measured accurately on anteroposterior, weight-bearing radiographs. The lateral shift of the calcaneus is more difficult to determine, and radiographic techniques have been developed for evaluating ankle valgus and hindfoot alignment. If the talar tilt exceeds 10 degrees, the x-ray tube should be tilted appropriately to obtain a true lateral weight-bearing view of the foot. On this view, the weight-bearing axis of the tibia is drawn and the distance from this line to the center of the calcaneus is measured. On an anteroposterior weight-bearing view, the beam should be directed horizontally to preserve the coronal relationship in both dimensions. The foot is positioned in slight dorsiflexion by placing a hard foam wedge under the plantar surface, but not under the calcaneus, and by positioning the cassette behind the foot and ankle. The normal lateral shift of the calcaneus is 5 to 10 mm (Fig. 34-37A); if the center of the calcaneus is more than 10 mm lateral to the weight-bearing line, excessive valgus is present (Fig. 34-37B). This technique is useful to determine before surgery if the valgus deformity is at the ankle or subtalar level.

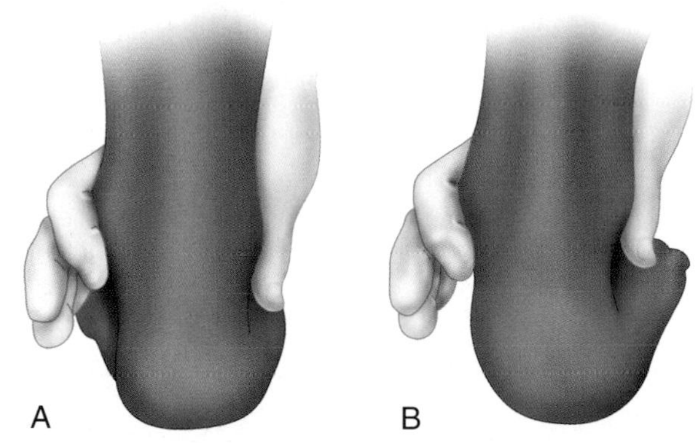

FIGURE 34-35 **A,** Posterior view of right foot of normal child with correct alignment of malleoli and hindfoot. **B,** In child with myelomeningocele, medial malleolus is prominent and lateral malleolus is shortened, causing valgus deformity of ankle.

Operative treatment is indicated when the ankle valgus deformity causes problems with orthotic fitting and cannot be relieved with orthoses. Achilles tenodesis is indicated for valgus talar tilt between 10 and 25 degrees in patients 6 to 10 years old (Fig. 34-1). Other procedures to correct ankle valgus caused by bone deformities include hemiepiphysiodesis for mild deformity in children with remaining growth and supramalleolar derotation osteotomy for severe angular deformity. Medial sliding osteotomy of the calcaneus may be indicated if the valgus deformity is in the subtalar joint and calcaneus.

HEMIEPIPHYSIODESIS OF THE DISTAL TIBIAL EPIPHYSIS

Hemiepiphysiodesis of the distal tibial epiphysis is indicated in young children with valgus deformities of less than 20 degrees and mild fibular shortening. Through a medial incision at the ankle, the medial aspect of the epiphysis is exposed and epiphysiodesis is performed by a percutaneous or an open method (Fig. 34-38). The growth arrest of the medial physis combined with continued growth of the lateral side gradually corrects the lateral wedging of the tibial epiphysis.

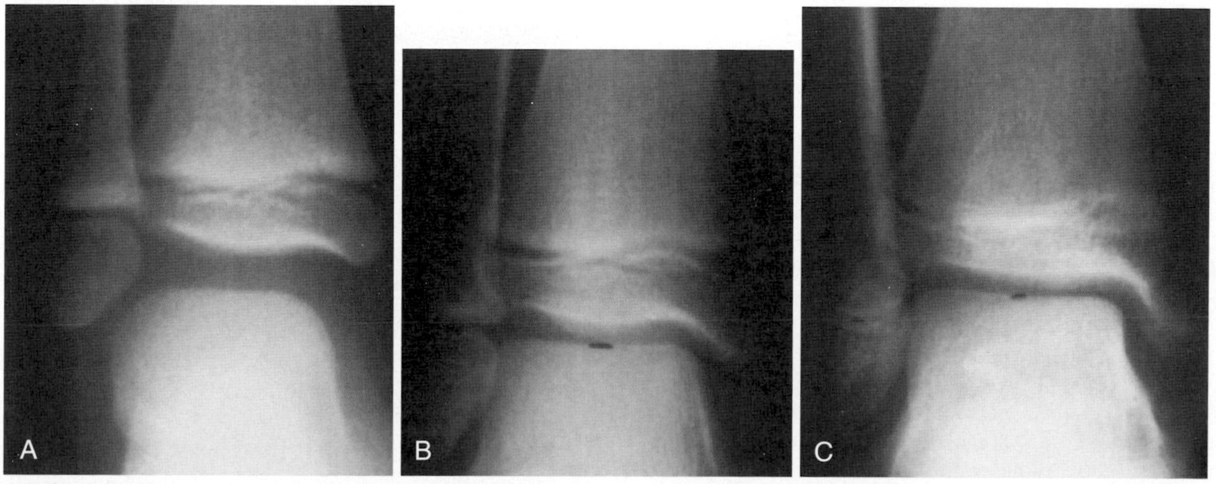

FIGURE 34-36 Normal position of distal fibular physis. **A,** Proximal to dome of talus in children up to 4 years of age. **B,** Level with dome of talus in children between 4 and 8 years of age. **C,** Distal to dome of talus in children older than 8 years of age.

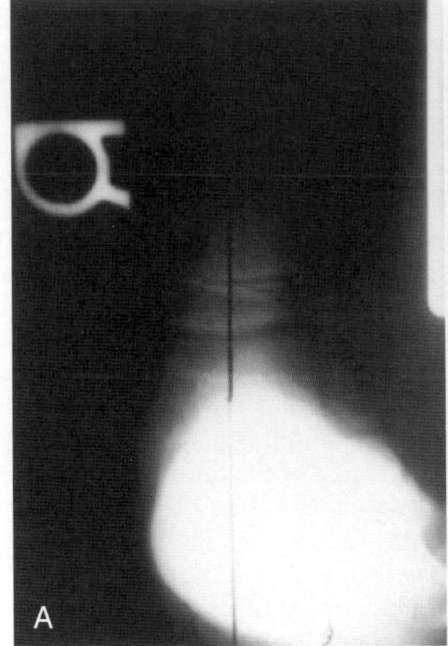
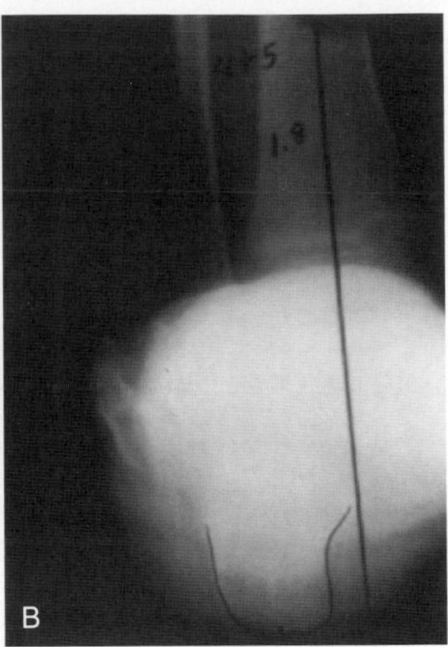

FIGURE 34-37 Radiographic technique for evaluation of ankle valgus. **A,** Normal shift of calcaneus is 5 to 10 mm. **B,** Lateral shift of 15 to 18 mm indicates excessive valgus.

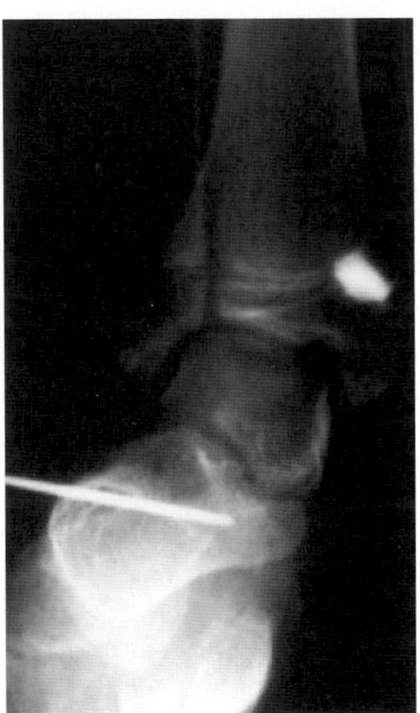

FIGURE 34-38 Radiopaque dye shows extent of medial hemiepiphysiodesis of distal tibial epiphysis.

If overcorrection occurs, the epiphysiodesis should be completed laterally. This procedure does not correct any rotational component of the deformity, and derotation osteotomy of the distal tibia and fibula may be required.

SCREW EPIPHYSIODESIS

Good results have been obtained with screw epiphysiodesis for correction of ankle valgus, which involves placing a vertical 4.5-mm screw across the medial malleolar physis to slow medial growth, allowing gradual correction of ankle valgus (median rate of correction of 0.59 degree per month). If the single screw is removed, growth resumes and the deformity will recur. This procedure is recommended in children older than 6 years (Fig. 34-39).

TECHNIQUE 34-33

- Place the patient supine.
- Make a 3-mm stab wound over the medial malleolus. Use image intensification to properly position the incision.
- Insert a guide pin from the 4.5-mm cannulated screw set into the medial malleolus and advance it proximally and medially across the distal tibial physis. Confirm the position of the guide pin by image intensification. The guide pin should be as vertical as possible in the medial one fourth of the medial distal tibial physis in the anteroposterior plane. In the sagittal plane the guide pin should cross the physis through its middle third.
- Place a tap over the guide pin and tap the bone across the physis. Insert a fully threaded, cannulated screw over the guide pin until it is completely seated.

SUPRAMALLEOLAR VARUS DEROTATION OSTEOTOMY

Supramalleolar osteotomy is recommended for children older than 10 years of age with low lumbar level lesions, severe fibular shortening (>10 to 20 mm), valgus tilt of more than 20 degrees, and external tibial torsion.

TECHNIQUE 34-34

- With the patient supine, make an anterior longitudinal incision at the distal third of the leg. Expose the distal tibia and identify the epiphysis.
- Make a second incision over the distal third of the fibula and perform an oblique osteotomy beginning laterally and extending distally and medially, depending on the degree of valgus to be corrected.

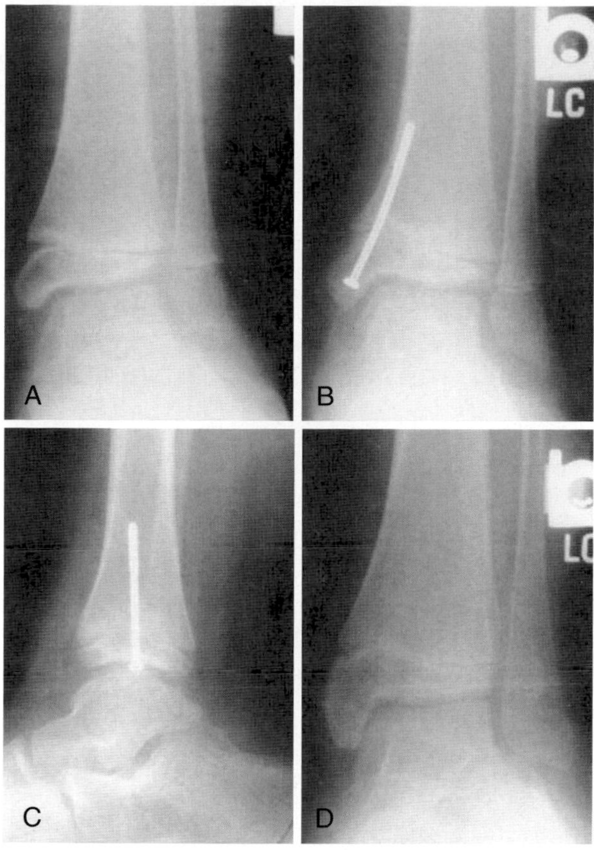

FIGURE 34-39 **A,** Preoperative standing anteroposterior radiographs of ankle in an 8-year, 6-month-old boy with symptomatic flexible pes planus. Note valgus alignment of tibiotalar axis (11 degrees valgus), increased fibular station (station 1), and distal tibial epiphyseal wedging (index 0.55). Standing anteroposterior **(B)** and lateral **(C)** radiographs 1 year, 3 months after placement of transphyseal medial malleolar screw. Tibiotalar axis is improved (3 degrees varus), whereas fibular station and epiphyseal wedging are unchanged. Note position of screw in both planes, subtle distal tibial metaphyseal deformity, and obliquity of physis created by screw. **D,** Standing anteroposterior radiograph of ankle 1 year, 4 months after screw removal. With release of medial tether and resumption of complete physeal growth, ankle valgus recurred (6 degrees valgus). (From Davids JR, Valadie AL, Ferguson RL, et al: Surgical management of ankle valgus in children: use of a transphyseal medial malleolar screw, J Pediatr Orthop 17:3, 1997.) **SEE TECHNIQUE 34-33.**

- Make the medial-based wedge osteotomy as distal on the tibia as possible (Fig. 34-40A).
- At the time of correction of the valgus, rotate the distal fragment internally to correct external tibial torsion.
- Use two Kirschner wires to temporarily hold the fragments in place and obtain radiographs to evaluate correction of the valgus deformity. The talus should be horizontal and the lateral malleolus lower than the medial malleolus.
- Staples or Kirschner wires (Fig. 34-40C) or, in patients nearing skeletal maturity, a plate and screws (Fig. 34-40B) can be used for internal fixation.
- Close the wounds and apply a long leg cast with the ankle and foot in neutral.

POSTOPERATIVE CARE. Partial weight bearing with crutches is allowed immediately. At 3 weeks, the cast is changed to a below-knee cast and full weight-bearing is allowed. The Kirschner wires can be removed at 8 to 12 weeks.

Rotational deformities of the lower extremity can cause functional problems in patients with myelomeningocele. Out-toeing can result either from an external rotation deformity of the hip or from external tibial torsion and can lead to abnormal knee stress, primarily valgus, as well as difficulties with brace fitting. Internal rotation osteotomies should be considered in children with 20 degrees or more of tibial torsion that interferes with gait. In-toeing can cause difficulties with foot clearance during swing phase of gait. In-toeing frequently occurs in patients with L4 or L5 lesions because of an imbalance between the medial and lateral hamstrings. The hamstrings tend to remain active during the stance phase of gait and, when the biceps femoris is paralyzed, the muscle imbalance produces an in-toeing gait. Another cause for in-toeing is residual internal tibial torsion.

Rotation deformity of the hip and external and internal tibial torsion can be corrected by derotation osteotomies. Dynamic in-toeing gait can be corrected by transferring the semitendinosus laterally to the biceps tendon.

KNEE

Knee deformities are common in patients with myelomeningocele and can cause significant difficulties in maintaining ambulatory function. Deformities of the knee in patients with myelomeningocele are of four types: (1) flexion contracture, (2) extension contracture, (3) valgus deformity, and (4) varus deformity.

FLEXION CONTRACTURE

Flexion contractures are more common than extension contractures. About half of children with thoracic or lumbar level lesions have knee flexion contractures. Contractures of 20 degrees are common at birth, but most correct spontaneously. Knee flexion contractures may become fixed because of (1) the typical position assumed when supine—hips in abduction, flexion, and external rotation; knees in flexion; and feet in equinus; (2) gradual contracture of the hamstring and biceps muscles, with contracture of the posterior knee capsule from quadriceps weakness and prolonged sitting; (3) spasticity of the hamstrings that may occur with the tethered cord syndrome; and (4) hip flexion contracture or calcaneal deformity in the ambulatory patient. Knee flexion contractures of more than 20 degrees can interfere with an effective bracing and standing program and ambulation in an ambulatory patient. Patients who are nonambulatory may tolerate larger degrees of flexion contractures as long as it does not interfere with transfers and sitting balance. Radical flexor release usually is required for contractures of 20 to 30 degrees, especially in children who walk with below-knee orthoses. Supracondylar extension osteotomy of the femur (Fig. 34-11) generally is required for contractures of more than 30 to 45 degrees in older children who are community ambulators and

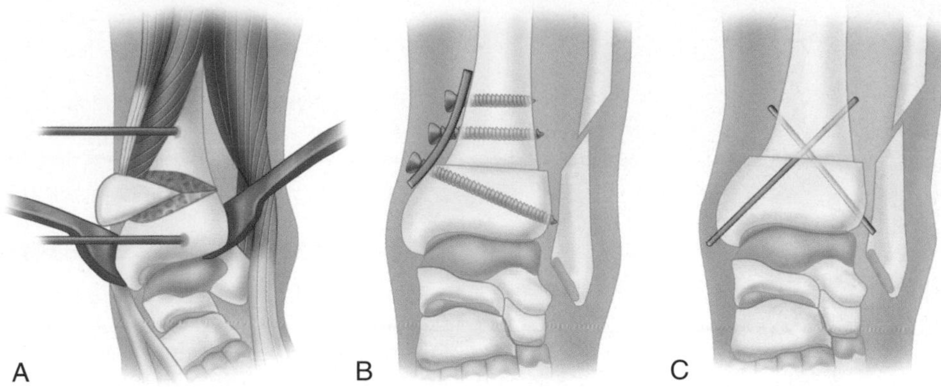

FIGURE 34-40 Supramalleolar varus derotation osteotomy for severe ankle valgus deformity in adolescents. **A,** Removal of medial bone wedge from distal tibial metaphysis. **B,** Fixation of osteotomy with plate and screws. **C,** Fixation with crossed wires. **SEE TECHNIQUE 34-34.**

in whom radical flexor release was unsuccessful. If a hip flexion contracture is present, hip and knee contractures should be corrected at the same time. Spiro et al. reported that anterior femoral epiphysiodesis by stapling is an effective and safe method for the treatment of fixed knee flexion deformity in growing children and adolescents with spina bifida. No surgical treatment is indicated in older children who are not community ambulators if the contracture does not interfere with mobility and sitting balance.

RADICAL FLEXOR RELEASE

TECHNIQUE 34-35

- Make a medial and a lateral vertical incision just above the flexor crease. Alternatively, a vertical midline incision just above the flexor crease can be used. Z- or S-shaped incisions that cross the flexor crease should be avoided because of difficulty with skin closure after a radical flexor release.
- In a child with a high-level lesion, identify and divide the medial hamstring tendons (semitendinosus, semimembranosus, gracilis, and sartorius).
- Resect part of each tendon (Fig. 34-41A).
- Laterally, identify, divide, and resect the biceps tendon and the iliotibial band.
- In a child with a low lumbar-level lesion, intramuscularly lengthen the biceps and semimembranosus to preserve some flexor power.
- Free the origin of the gastrocnemius from the medial and lateral condyles, exposing the posterior knee capsule, and perform an extensive capsulectomy (Fig. 34-41B).
- If full extension is not obtained, divide the medial and lateral collateral ligaments and the posterior cruciate ligament (Fig. 34-41C).
- Close the wound over a suction drain and apply a long leg cast with the knee in full extension. If the flexion contracture is greater than 45 degrees, because of the possibility of vascular problems the first cast should be

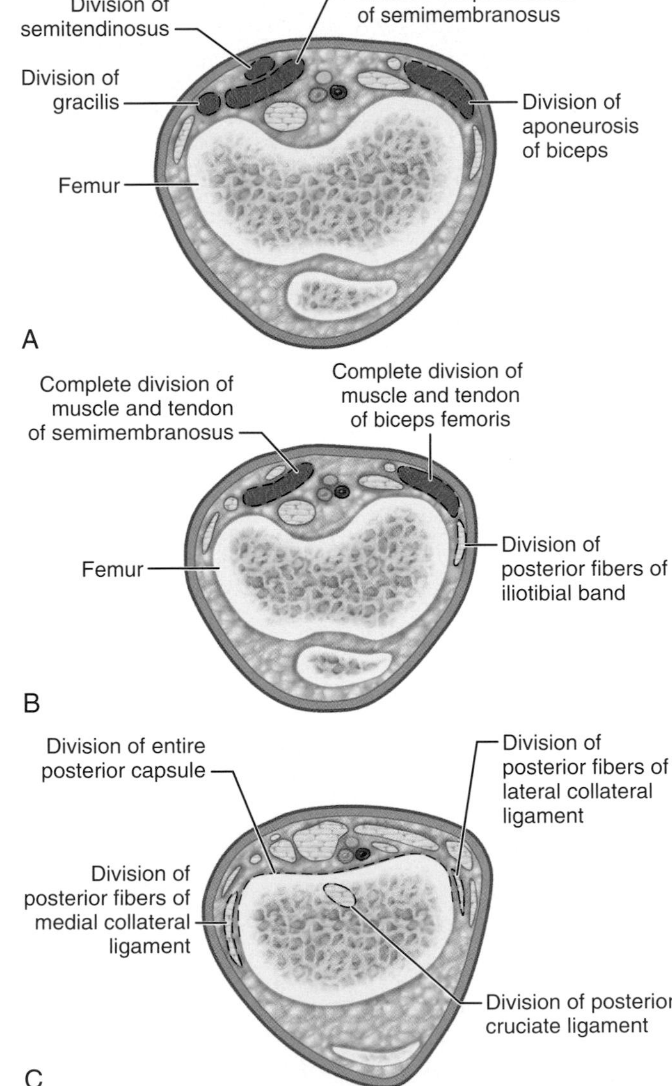

FIGURE 34-41 Release of flexor tendons for flexion contracture of knee. **A,** Minimal procedure. **B,** Additional optional procedures above joint level. **C,** Additional optional procedures at joint level. **SEE TECHNIQUE 34-35.**

applied with the knee in 20 to 30 degrees of flexion and gradually brought to full extension through serial cast changes.

POSTOPERATIVE CARE. The cast is removed at 14 days, and a long leg splint is used at night. For children with low lumbar level lesions, intensive physical therapy for strengthening of the quadriceps mechanism is imperative after cast removal.

EXTENSION CONTRACTURE

Knee extension contractures can occur in patients with myelomeningocele. Approximately two thirds have no useful muscle function in the lower extremities, one third of which are caused by unopposed quadriceps function from paralytic hamstring muscles. Extension contractures usually are bilateral and frequently are associated with other congenital anomalies, such as dislocation of the ipsilateral hip, external rotation contracture of the hip, equinovarus deformity of the foot, and occasionally valgus deformity of the knee. Knee extension contracture can impair ambulation and make wheelchair sitting and transfers difficult. Serial casting, attempting to flex the knee to at least 90 degrees, is successful in some patients. If this does not correct the contracture, lengthening of the quadriceps mechanism is indicated. The most common procedure to correct this deformity is a V-Y quadriceps lengthening, capsular release, and posterior displacement of the hamstring muscles (Fig. 34-42). This usually is done by 1 year of age. Other methods of lengthening have been described, including "anterior circumcision," in which all of the structures in front and at the side of the knee are divided by subcutaneous tenotomy, subcutaneous release of quadriceps tendon, Z-plasty of the extensor mechanism combined with anterior capsulotomy, and subcutaneous release of the patellar ligament.

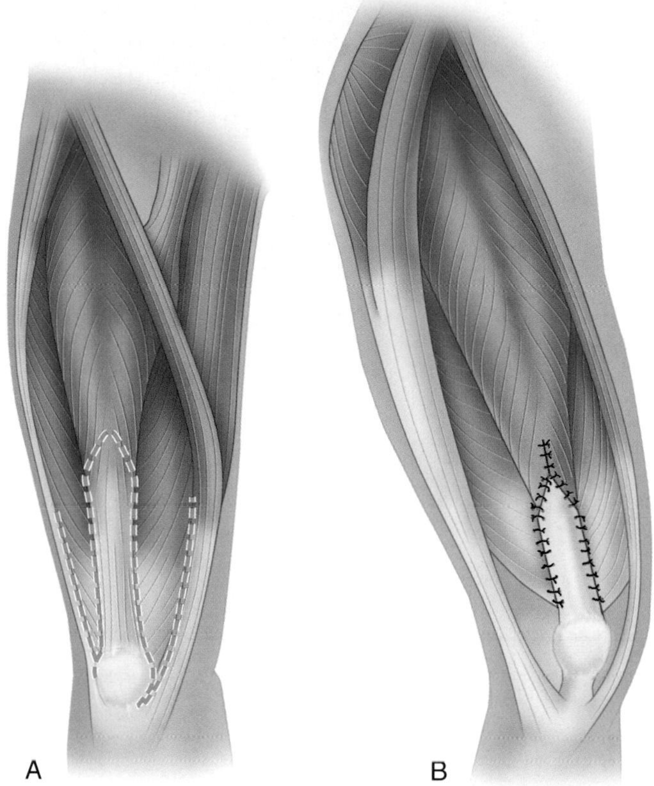

FIGURE 34-42 V-Y quadricepsplasty for hyperextension contracture of the knee. **A,** Detachment of rectus femoris tendon from muscle of rectus femoris, vastus medialis, and vastus lateralis muscles; vastus medialis and lateralis muscles are separated from iliotibial band, lateral hamstrings, medial hamstrings, and sartorius muscles. **B,** When knee is flexed, hamstring muscles and tensor fascia lata slip posterior to knee axis, restoring normal function. Quadriceps muscles are repaired in lengthened position.

VARUS OR VALGUS DEFORMITY

Varus or valgus deformity of the knee can occur in patients with myelomeningocele and can result from abnormal trunk mechanics that lead to abnormal knee mechanics or from malunion of a supracondylar fracture of the femur or proximal metaphyseal fracture of the tibia. In ambulatory patients, valgus knee instability is more common. This is caused by several reasons in ambulatory patients. Weak quadriceps, gastrocnemius-soleus muscles, and hip abductors cause the knee to go into valgus as the patient displaces the hemipelvis laterally during stance phase. The amount of knee valgus is proportional to the degree of neurologic impairment. This deformity also can be associated with excessive femoral anteversion or excessive external tibial torsion. Both increase the valgus or adductor stresses at the knee during the stance phase of gait (Fig. 34-43). This eventually leads to increased joint laxity and degenerative changes around the knee. Nonoperative treatment consists of the use of forearm crutches to decrease the Trendelenburg gait. Bracing with a knee-ankle-foot orthosis can be used to stabilize the knee, but often they are too bulky and not well accepted by an ambulatory patient. Deformities that interfere with bracing and mobility require supracondylar or tibial osteotomy with internal fixation to correct the deformity. Hemiepiphysiodesis, stapling, or an eight-hole plate across the physis also may be used for correction if the angular deformity is recognized early.

HIP

Treatment recommendations for deformities and instability around the hip in children with myelomeningocele have changed owing, in part, to the use of gait analysis. Deformities or instability of the hip in children with myelomeningocele can be caused by muscle imbalance, congenital dysplasia, habitual posture, or a combination of these three. Nearly half of children with myelomeningocele have hip subluxation or dislocation, which correlates poorly with overall hip function and ambulatory potential. Many authors found that the presence of a concentric reduction did not lead to improvements in hip range of motion, ability to ambulate, and decreased pain. The goal of current treatment protocols is to maintain hip range of motion through contracture prevention and release rather than obtaining anatomic concentric reduction.

Abduction or adduction contractures of the hip can cause infrapelvic obliquity that can interfere with ambulation and bracing. Hip flexion contractures with associated lumbar lordosis and knee flexion contracture may cause more disability than mobile dislocated hips. Because of the different levels of

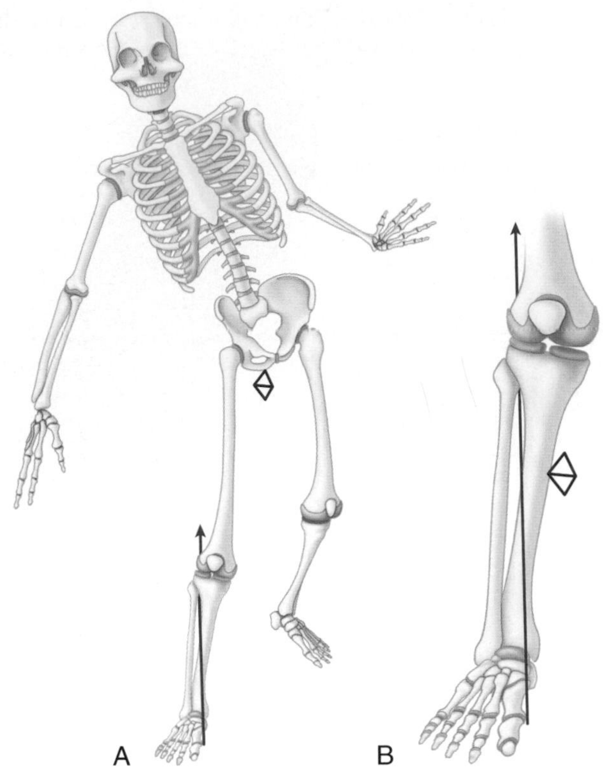

FIGURE 34-43 **A,** Maximal coronal plane movement and posteromedial position of ground reaction force in relation to knee joint center. **B,** Close-up of ground reaction force during maximal coronal plane displacement of trunk. (From Gupta RT, Vankoski S, Novak RA, Dias LS: Trunk kinematics and the influence on valgus knee stress in persons with high sacral level myelomeningocele, J Pediatr Orthop 25:89, 2005.)

paralysis and the combination of mixed and flaccid paralysis, treatment must be individualized for each patient. An evidence-based review of hip surgery in patients with myelomeningocele found that there was no benefit to surgical treatment of dislocated hips and that walking ability was related to the degree of contracture present. The only subgroup that might benefit from surgery is children with myelomeningocele below L4 with a unilateral hip dislocation. Children in this group may have a worsened Trendelenburg gait secondary to leg-length discrepancy; however, this remains controversial. Gait analysis has shown that walking speed is unaffected by the presence of a hip dislocation in patients with low-level myelomeningocele, and gait symmetry more closely correlates to the absence of joint contractures or the presence of symmetric contractures rather than the status of the hip itself.

In addition, the complication rate for surgical reduction of the hip in patients with myelomeningocele can be very high, ranging from 30% to 45%. Complications include loss of motion, pathologic fractures, worsening ambulatory function, and worsening neurologic deficits.

FLEXION CONTRACTURE

Flexion deformity of the hip occurs most frequently in children with high lumbar or thoracic level lesions. The proposed causes for a hip flexion contracture are unopposed action of the hip flexors (iliopsoas, sartorius, and rectus femoris), habitual posture from long periods of lying supine or sitting, and spasticity of the hip flexors. Hip flexion contractures must be distinguished from the physiologic flexion position, and the amount of hip flexion should be determined by the Thomas test. Because of a tendency to improve, hip flexion deformities rarely should be surgically treated before 24 months of age. A hip flexion contracture of 20 to 30 degrees usually can be accommodated. Increased lumbar lordosis and knee flexion often are associated with hip flexion contractures and may make a stable upright posture difficult. Surgical release is indicated for contractures that interfere with bracing, walking, or obtaining an upright posture when hip flexion contractures are greater than 30 degrees. Knee flexion contractures, which commonly occur with the hip contractures, should be corrected at the same time as the hip contracture.

Anterior hip release involves release of the sartorius, rectus femoris, iliopsoas, and tensor fasciae latae muscles; the anterior hip capsule; and the iliopsoas tendon. This procedure should adequately correct flexion contractures of 60 degrees. If deformity remains after release, subtrochanteric extension osteotomy is indicated.

ANTERIOR HIP RELEASE

TECHNIQUE 34-36

- Make a "bikini-line" skin incision slightly distal and parallel to the iliac crest, extending it obliquely along the inguinal crease.
- Identify and protect the neurovascular bundle medially.
- Identify the iliopsoas tendon as far distally as possible and divide it transversely.
- Detach the sartorius muscle from its origin on the superior iliac crest.
- Identify the rectus insertion in the anterior inferior iliac crest and detach it.
- Laterally, identify the tensor fasciae latae muscle and, after carefully separating it from the fascia, divide the fascia transversely completely posterior to the anterior border of the gluteal muscles to expose the anterior hip capsule.
- If any residual flexion contracture remains, open the joint capsule transversely about 2 cm from the acetabular labrum.
- Place a suction drain in the wound, suture the subcutaneous tissue with interrupted sutures and approximate the skin edges with subcuticular nylon sutures.
- Apply a hip spica cast or a total body splint with the hip in full extension, 10 degrees of abduction, and neutral rotation.
- In children with low lumbar level lesions this release greatly reduces hip flexor power and may impair mobility. A free tendon graft, using part of the tensor fasciae latae, can be used to reattach the sartorius to the anterior superior iliac crest, and the rectus tendon can be sutured distal to the sartorius muscle in the hip capsule.

POSTOPERATIVE CARE. Early weight bearing for 2 to 3 hours a day is encouraged. The spica cast is removed at 4 to 6 weeks. If a splint is used, it can be removed for range-of-motion exercises after the wounds are healed.

FLEXION-ABDUCTION–EXTERNAL ROTATION CONTRACTURE

Flexion-abduction-external rotation contractures are common in children with thoracic level lesions and complete paralysis of the muscles of the lower extremity. Continuous external rotation of the hip in the supine position causes contractures of the posterior hip capsule and short external rotator muscles; this occurrence may be decreased by the use of night splints (total body splints) and range-of-motion exercises. Complete hip release (see Technique 34-18) is indicated only when the deformity interferes with bracing. If both hips are contracted, as is often the case, both should be corrected at the same time.

EXTERNAL ROTATION CONTRACTURE

Isolated external rotation contracture of the hip occasionally occurs in children with low lumbar level lesions. Initially, bracing and physical therapy help improve the external rotation contracture. If the external hip rotation persists after the child is 5 or 6 years old, a subtrochanteric medial rotation osteotomy (see Chapter 33) is indicated.

ABDUCTION CONTRACTURE

Isolated unilateral abduction contracture is a common cause of pelvic obliquity, scoliosis, and difficulty in sitting and ambulation. It generally is caused by contracture of the tensor fasciae latae, but it may occur after iliopsoas transfer. It is common in children with high-level lesions, and early splinting and physical therapy may decrease the risk of its occurrence. Fascial release is indicated when the abduction contracture causes pelvic obliquity and scoliosis and interferes with function or bracing.

FASCIAL RELEASE

TECHNIQUE 34-37

- Incise the skin along the anterior one half or two thirds of the iliac crest to the anterior superior iliac spine.
- Divide all thigh fascial and tendinous structures around the anterolateral aspect of the hip; fascia lata, fascia over the gluteus medius and gluteus minimus, and tensor fasciae latae.
- Do not divide the muscle tissue, only the enveloping fascial structures.
- Fasciotomy of the fascia lata distally, as described by Yount (see Technique 34-18), also may be required.
- Close the wound over a suction drain and apply a hip spica cast with the operated hip in neutral abduction and the opposite hip in 20 degrees of abduction, enough to permit perineal care.

POSTOPERATIVE CARE. The cast is removed at 2 weeks, and a total body splint is fitted.

ADDUCTION CONTRACTURE

Adduction contractures are common with dislocation or subluxation of the hip in children with high-level lesions because of spasticity and contracture of the adductor muscles. Surgery is indicated when the contracture causes pelvic obliquity and interferes with sitting or walking. Adductor release may be combined with operative treatment of hip subluxation or dislocation.

ADDUCTOR RELEASE

TECHNIQUE 34-38

- Make a transverse inguinal incision 2 to 3 cm long just distal to the inguinal crease over the adductor longus tendon.
- Open the superficial fascia to expose the adductor longus tendon.
- Using electrocautery, divide the tendon close to its insertion on the pubic ramus.
- If necessary, divide the muscle fibers of the gracilis proximally and completely divide the adductor brevis muscle fibers, taking care to protect the anterior branch of the obturator nerve. At least 45 degrees of abduction should be possible.
- Close the wound over a suction drain

POSTOPERATIVE CARE. A brace or cast that holds the hip in 25 to 30 degrees of abduction can be used post- operatively. If a cast is used, it is removed at 2 weeks, and a splint is fitted with the hip in 25 degrees of abduction.

HIP SUBLUXATION AND DISLOCATION

True developmental hip dislocation is rare in patients with myelomeningocele and occurs in children with sacral level lesions without muscle imbalance. Treatment should follow standard conservative methods (Pavlik harness, closed reduction, and spica cast immobilization). Teratologic dislocations usually occur in children with high-level lesions. Initial radiographs show a dysplastic acetabulum, with the head of the femur displaced proximally; these dislocations should not be treated initially.

Paralytic subluxation or dislocation is the most common type, occurring in 50% to 70% of children with low-level (L3 or L4) lesions. Dislocation occurs most frequently during the first 3 years of life because of an imbalance between abduction and adduction forces. Dislocations in older children usually are caused by contractures or spasticity of the unopposed adductors and flexors associated with a tethered cord syndrome or hydromyelia.

Reduction of hip dislocations in children with myelomeningocele is generally not recommended. Maintaining a level pelvis and flexible hips seems more important than reduction of the hip dislocation. The goal of treatment should be maximal function, rather than radiographic reduction. Soft-tissue release alone is indicated in patients without functional quadriceps muscles because only occasionally do they remain community ambulators as adults. Open reduction is appropriate only for rare children with sacral level involvement who have strong quadriceps muscles bilaterally, normal trunk balance, and normal upper extremity function. Bilateral or unilateral hip dislocation or subluxation in children with high-level lesions does not require extensive surgical treatment, but soft-tissue contractures should be corrected.

If treatment is undertaken for hip subluxation or dislocation in the rare patient who may benefit from it, the principles of paralytic hip surgery should be adhered to as follows: (1) obtain reduction of the hip into the acetabulum, (2) correct any residual bony deformity, and (3) balance the deforming muscle forces to prevent recurrence. The two most common procedures to balance the deforming muscle forces in an unstable hip in patients with myelomeningocele have been transfer of the iliopsoas muscle (Sharrad or Mustard procedure) and transfer of the external oblique muscle. Iliopsoas transfer with adductor release, capsulorrhaphy, and acetabuloplasty can be done in addition to open reduction. The Sharrad iliopsoas transfer through the posterolateral ilium (see Technique 34-21) is most often used. Iliopsoas transfer is controversial, with reported success rates ranging from 20% to 95%. Alternative procedures include transfer of the external oblique muscle to the greater trochanter (see Technique 34-19) in conjunction with femoral osteotomy and posterolateral transfer of the tensor fasciae latae with transfer of the adductor and external oblique muscles.

TRANSFER OF ADDUCTORS, EXTERNAL OBLIQUE, AND TENSOR FASCIAE LATAE

TECHNIQUE 34-39

(PHILLIPS AND LINDSETH)

- Place the patient supine and expose the adductor muscles through a transverse incision beginning just anterior to the tendon of the adductor longus and extending posteriorly to the ischium.
- Incise the fascia longitudinally and detach the tendons of the gracilis, adductor longus and brevis, and the anterior third of the magnus from the pubis.
- Carry the dissection posteriorly to the ischial tuberosity and suture the detached origins of the adductor muscles to the ischium with nonabsorbable sutures. Take care not to disrupt the anterior branch of the obturator nerve that supplies the adductor muscles.
- Transfer the external abdominal oblique muscle to the gluteus medius tendon or preferably to the greater trochanter, as described by Thomas, Thompson, and Straub.
- Make an oblique skin incision extending from the posterior third of the iliac crest to the anterior superior iliac spine (Fig. 34-44A).
- Curve the incision distally and posteriorly to the junction of the proximal and middle third of the femur.
- With sharp and blunt dissection, raise skin flaps to expose the fascia of the leg from the lateral border of the sartorius to the level of the greater trochanter.
- Expose the external oblique similarly from the iliac crest to the posterior superior iliac spine and from its costal origin to the pubis (Fig. 34-44B).
- Make two incisions approximately 1 cm apart in the aponeurosis of the external oblique parallel to the Poupart ligament and join them close to the pubis at the external ring.
- Extend the superior incision proximally along the medial border of the muscle belly until the costal margin is reached.
- Free the muscle from the underlying internal oblique by blunt dissection until the posterior aspect is reached in the Petit triangle.
- Elevate the muscle fibers from the iliac crest by cutting from posterior to anterior along the crest.
- Close the defect that remains in the aponeurosis of the external oblique beginning at the pubis and extending as far laterally as possible.
- Fold the cut edges of the muscle and aponeurosis over and suture with a single suture at the muscle-tendinous junction.
- Weave a heavy, nonabsorbable suture through the aponeurosis in preparation for transfer (Fig. 34-44C).
- Attention is then directed to the tensor fasciae latae.
- Detach the origin of the tensor fasciae latae from the ilium.
- Separate the muscle along its anterior border from the sartorius down to its insertion into the iliotibial band.
- Divide the iliotibial band transversely to the posterior part of the thigh.
- Carry the incision in the iliotibial band proximally to the insertion of the oblique fibers of the tensor fasciae latae and the tendon of the gluteus maximus. Take care to preserve the superior gluteal nerve and arteries beneath the gluteus medius muscle approximately 1 cm distal and posterior to the anterior superior iliac spine (Fig. 34-44D).
- Abduct the hip and fold the origin of the tensor fasciae latae back on itself to the limit allowed by the neurovascular bundle and then suture it to the ilium with nonabsorbable sutures so that its origin overlies the gluteus medius muscle. Do not attach the distal end to the gluteus maximus tendon until the end of the procedure.
- The hip, proximal femur, and ilium are now easily accessible for indicated corrective procedures such as open reduction of the hip, capsular plication, proximal femoral osteotomy, and acetabular augmentation. The origins of the rectus femoris and the psoas tendon are not routinely divided, although they can be released at this time if there is a hip flexion contracture.
- With the patient maximally relaxed or paralyzed, transfer the tendon of the external oblique to the greater trochanter.
- Drill a hole in the greater trochanter and pass the tendon of the external oblique from posterior to anterior and suture it back on itself. The muscle should reach the greater trochanter and should follow a straight line from the rib cage to the trochanter; if it does not, the borders of the muscle should be inspected to ensure that they are free from all attachments (Fig. 34-44D).
- Weave the distal end of the tensor fasciae latae through the tendon of the gluteus maximus while the hip is abducted approximately 20 degrees.

POSTOPERATIVE CARE. A hip spica cast is applied postoperatively with the hips in extension and abducted 20 degrees. The child is encouraged to stand in the cast to prevent osteopenia. The cast is removed 1 month after surgery, and physical therapy is started. The patient is returned to the braces used before the operation. Any modification in bracing is made as indicated on follow-up.

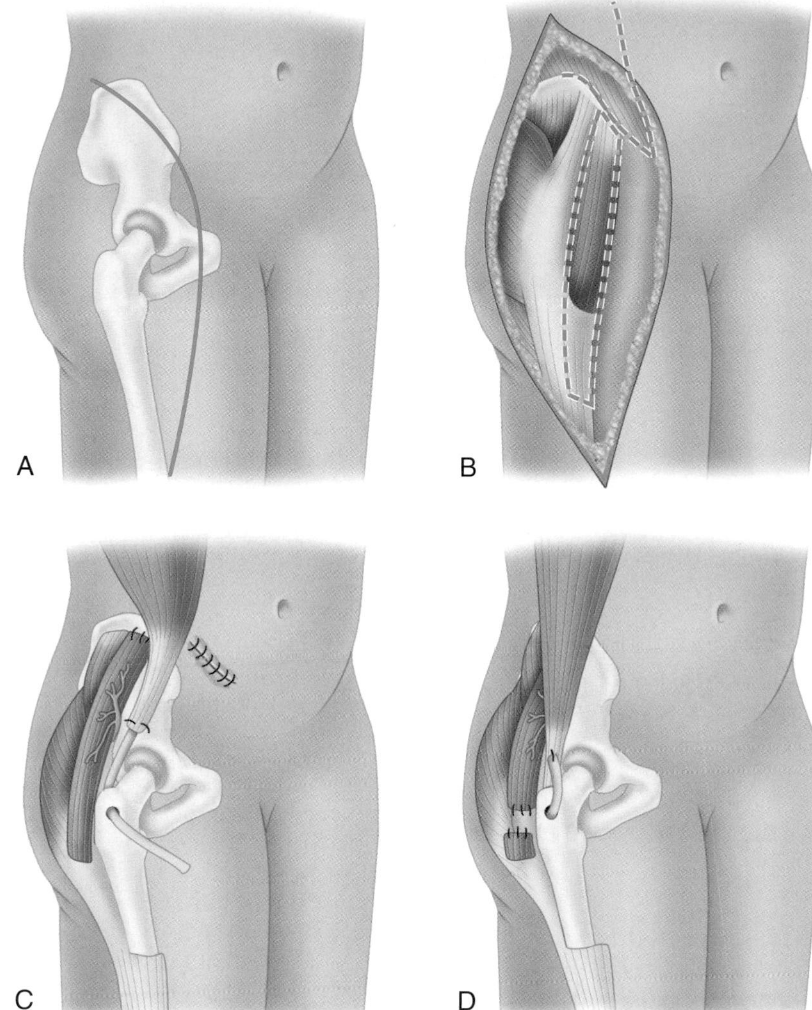

FIGURE 34-44 Transfer of adductors, external oblique, and tensor fasciae latae. **A,** Skin incision. **B,** Skin flaps are elevated to expose fascia of leg and external oblique muscle. **C,** Cut edges of external oblique muscle and aponeurosis are folded over and sutured. Defect in aponeurosis is sutured. Origin of tensor fasciae latae on ilium is detached, with care being taken to preserve neurovascular bundle. Remainder of muscle is prepared for transfer. **D,** Tendon of external oblique is transferred to greater trochanter from posterior to anterior. Distal end of tensor fasciae latae is woven through tendon of gluteus maximus. **SEE TECHNIQUE 34-39.**

For severe acetabular dysplasia, a shelf procedure or Chiari pelvic osteotomy (see Chapter 30) can be done at the same time as the transfer. If more than 20 to 30 degrees of abduction is necessary to maintain concentric reduction of the hip, a varus femoral osteotomy is indicated. Even with these procedures to correct acetabular dysplasia there is a high failure rate if muscle-balancing procedures are not included as part of the procedure.

PROXIMAL FEMORAL RESECTION AND INTERPOSITION ARTHROPLASTY

Severe joint stiffness is one of the most disabling results of hip surgery in patients with myelomeningocele. If the hip is stiff in extension, the child cannot sit; if it is stiff in flexion, the child cannot stand; if it is stiff "in between," the child can neither sit nor stand. Resection of the femoral head and neck often is not effective. Proximal femoral resection and interposition arthroplasty is recommended in severely involved multiply handicapped children with dislocated hips and severe adduction contractures of the lower extremity.

TECHNIQUE 34-40

(BAXTER AND D'ASTOUS)

- Position the patient with a sandbag beneath the affected hip.
- Make a straight lateral approach beginning 10 cm proximal to the greater trochanter and extending down to the proximal femur.
- Split the fascia lata.
- Detach the vastus lateralis and gluteus maximus from their insertions and detach them from the greater trochanter.

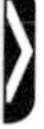

- Identify the psoas tendon and detach its distal insertion on the lesser trochanter to expose extraperiosteally the proximal femur.
- Incise the periosteum circumferentially just distal to the gluteus maximus insertion and transect the bone at this level.
- Divide the short external rotators. Incise the capsule circumferentially at the level of the basal neck.
- Cut the ligamentous teres, remove the proximal femur, and test the range of motion of the hip. If necessary, perform a proximal hamstring tenotomy through the same incision after identifying the sciatic nerve.
- Adductor release also can be performed through a separate groin incision.
- Seal the acetabular cavity by oversewing the capsular edges.
- Cover the proximal end of the femur with the vastus lateralis and rectus femoris muscles.
- Interpose the gluteal muscles between the closed acetabulum and the covered end of the proximal femur to act as a further soft-tissue cushion.
- Close the wound in layers over a suction drain.

POSTOPERATIVE CARE. The operated lower extremity is placed in Russell traction in abduction until the soft tissues have healed, and then gentle range-of-motion exercises are begun. If traction is not tolerated, the patient can be placed in a cast or brace until the soft tissues have healed.

PELVIC OBLIQUITY

Pelvic obliquity is common in patients with myelomeningocele. In addition to predisposing the hip to dislocation, it interferes with sitting, standing, and walking, and it can lead to ulceration under the prominent ischial tuberosity. Pelvic obliquity is an important determinant of ambulatory function, second only to neurologic level of involvement. Gait analysis has shown that pelvic obliquity has the strongest correlation with oxygen cost in ambulatory patients with myelomeningocele and that patients may self-select their walking speed to minimize the pelvic shift in the sagittal and coronal planes during gait. Mayer described three types of pelvic obliquity: (1) infrapelvic, caused by contracture of the abductor and tensor fasciae latae muscles of one hip and contracture of the adductors of the opposite hip; (2) suprapelvic, caused by uncompensated scoliosis resulting from bony deformity of the lumbosacral spine or severe paralytic scoliosis; and (3) pelvic, caused by bony deformity of the sacrum and sacroiliac joint, such as partial sacral agenesis, causing asymmetry of the pelvis. Incidence of infrapelvic obliquity can be decreased by splinting, range-of-motion exercises, and positioning, but when hip contractures are well established, soft-tissue release is required. Occasionally, more severe deformities require proximal femoral osteotomy. Suprapelvic obliquity can be corrected by control of the scoliosis by orthoses or spinal fusion. If severe scoliosis cannot be completely corrected, bony pelvic obliquity becomes fixed.

Obliquity of 20 degrees is sufficient to interfere with walking and to produce ischial decubitus ulcerations; Mayer recommended pelvic osteotomy in this instance. Before osteotomy, hip contractures should be released and the scoliosis should be corrected by spinal fusion. The degree of correction of pelvic obliquity is determined preoperatively from appropriate radiographs of the pelvis and spine (Fig. 34-45A). The maximal correction obtainable with bilateral iliac osteotomies is 40 degrees.

PELVIC OSTEOTOMY

TECHNIQUE 34-41

(LINDSETH)

- The approach is similar to that described by O'Phelan for iliac osteotomy to correct exstrophy of the bladder (see Chapter 30).
- With the child prone, make bilateral, inverted, L-shaped incisions beginning above the iliac crest, proceeding medially to the posterior superior iliac spine, and then curving downward along each side of the sacrum to the sciatic notch.
- Detach the iliac apophysis by splitting it longitudinally starting at the anterior superior iliac spine and proceeding posteriorly (Fig. 34-45B).
- Retract the paraspinal muscles, the quadratus lumborum muscle, and the iliac muscles medially along the inner half of the epiphysis and the inner periosteum of the ilium.
- After the sacral origin of the gluteus maximus has been detached from the sacrum, divide the outer periosteum of the ilium longitudinally just lateral to the posteromedial iliac border, extending from the posterior superior iliac spine down to the sciatic notch.
- Strip the outer periosteum along the gluteus muscles and the outer half of the epiphysis from the outer table of the ilium, taking care to avoid damaging the superior and inferior gluteal vessels and nerves. Retract the soft tissues down to the sciatic notch and protect them by inserting malleable retractors. Next, make bilateral osteotomies approximately 2 cm lateral to each sacroiliac joint. The size of the wedge is determined by the amount of the correction desired and is limited to no more than one third of the iliac crest; the base of the wedge usually is about 2.5 cm long (Fig. 34-45C).
- After the wedge of bone has been removed, correct the deformity by pulling on the limb on the short side and pushing up on the limb on the long side (Fig. 34-45C). Usually this closes the osteotomy on the long side. If upper migration of the ilium onto the sacrum is severe, trim the excess iliac crest.
- Close the wedge osteotomy with two threaded pins or sutures through drill holes.
- Then use a spreader to open the osteotomy on the opposite (short) side sufficiently to receive the graft.
- Use two Kirschner wires to hold the graft in place (Fig. 34-45D).
- Close the wound over suction-irrigation drains and apply a double full-hip spica cast.

POSTOPERATIVE CARE. The cast is worn for 2 weeks. The Kirschner wires are removed when radiographs show sufficient healing of the osteotomy.

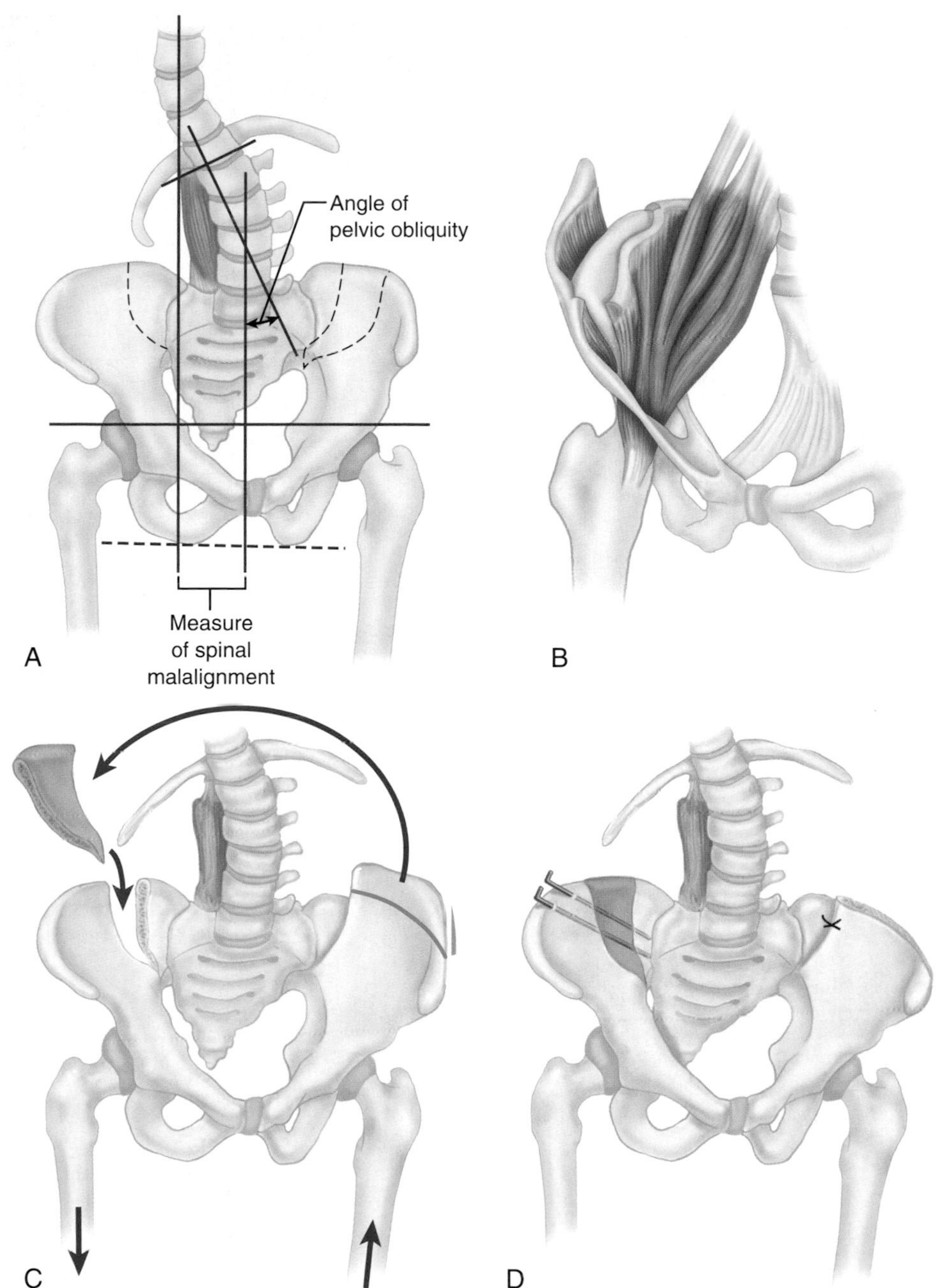

FIGURE 34-45 Pelvic osteotomy for pelvic obliquity, as described by Lindseth. **A,** Preoperative determination of size of iliac wedge to be removed and transferred. **B,** Exposure of ilium. **C,** After bilateral osteotomies and removal of wedge from low side, deformity is corrected. **D,** Transferred iliac wedge is fixed with two Kirschner wires. **SEE TECHNIQUE 34-41.**

SPINE

■ SCOLIOSIS

Paralytic spinal deformities have been reported in 90% of patients with myelomeningocele. Scoliosis is the most common deformity and usually is progressive. The incidence of scoliosis is related to the level of the bone defect and the level of paralysis: 100% with T12 lesions, 80% with L2 lesions, 70% with L3 lesions, 60% with L4 lesions, 25% with L5 lesions, and 5% with S1 lesions. Glard expanded on this concept by dividing patients into four neurosegmental groups based on the spinal deformities that occur within each group. Group 1 (L5 or below) had no spinal deformity, group 2 (L3-L4) had variable deformities, group 3 (L1-L2) was predictive of spinal deformity, and group 4 (T12 and above) was predictive of kyphosis. The curves develop gradually until the child reaches age 10 years and may increase rapidly with the adolescent growth spurt. Raycroft and Curtis differentiated between developmental (no vertebral anomalies) and congenital (structural abnormalities of the vertebral bodies) scoliosis in patients with myelomeningocele. The two types were almost evenly divided in their patients. They suggested muscle imbalance and habitual posturing as causes of developmental scoliosis. Developmental curves occur later than congenital curves, are more flexible, and usually are in the lumbar area with compensatory curves above and below. Several authors have suggested that developmental scoliosis can be caused in some patients by hydromyelia or a tethered cord syndrome, and an early onset of scoliosis (<6 years) frequently occurs in patients with these lesions.

Spinal radiographs should be obtained at least once each year, beginning when the child is 5 years old. If any scoliosis is detected, further evaluation is indicated. MRI should be performed to determine if hydromyelia or a tethered spinal cord is present. The use of a thoracolumbosacral orthosis for daytime wear when the curve is more than 30 degrees may help with sitting balance and may slow curve progression. Bracing slows curve progression and delays surgical intervention but does not halt the progress of most curves. The use of a brace may be challenging because of poor skin and the risk of pressure sores, as well as interference with bowel and bladder care.

Indications for spinal fusion include a progressive increase in angular deformity that cannot be controlled by bracing, unacceptable deformities, and progressive thoracic lordosis. The goals of surgery are to achieve a solid fusion with maximal safe correction, minimize pelvic obliquity, and increase sitting tolerance and independence. These goals must be weighed against the extremely high complication rate of spinal surgery in this patient population; complications include nonunion in up to 40%, deep infection, hardware irritation and resultant skin breakdown, and loss of ambulatory function. In 49 patients who had spinal surgery, sitting balance was improved in 70%, but the ability to ambulate was negatively affected in 67% of patients who had anterior and posterior surgery. Another study found that sitting was the only outcome measure to be improved by spinal surgery, and an evidence-based review concluded that the benefits of spine surgery in this patient population were uncertain. Anterior and posterior surgery was found to provide greater correction with lower pseudarthrosis rates (Fig. 34-46).

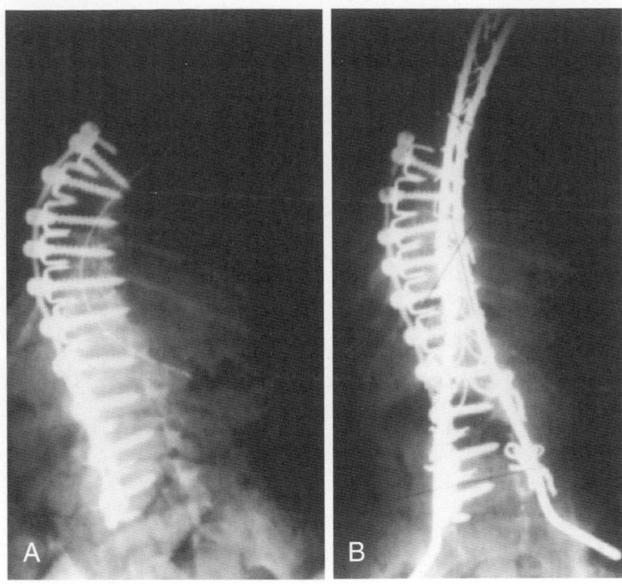

FIGURE 34-46 Correction of severe scoliosis with anterior fusion with Dwyer instrumentation **(A)** followed by posterior fusion with Luque rods **(B)**.

KYPHOSIS

The most severe spinal deformity in patients with myelomeningocele is congenital kyphosis; it occurs in approximately 10% of patients. The kyphosis usually is present at birth and may make sac closure difficult. The curve generally extends from the lower thoracic level to the sacral spine, with its apex in the midlumbar region. The deformity usually is progressive.

KYPHECTOMY

Congenital kyphosis is unresponsive to bracing and usually requires surgery for correction. The goal of treatment of kyphosis is not to obtain a normal spine but to provide sitting balance without the use of the arms and hands for support. Other goals are to increase the lumbar height to allow room for abdominal contents and provide better mechanics for breathing and to prevent pressure sores by reducing the kyphotic prominence.

Kyphectomy is very effective in correcting kyphosis; however, the complication rate is high. Wound and skin breakdown are the most common complications, occurring in up to 50% of patients.

Surgical techniques for spinal fusion in scoliosis and correction of kyphosis are described in Chapter 44. Complications of spinal surgery in patients with myelomeningocele are significantly greater than in patients with idiopathic scoliosis. The most common complication is failure of fusion, which is reported to occur in 40% of patients. Infection rates of 43% also have been reported.

ARTHROGRYPOSIS MULTIPLEX CONGENITA

Arthrogryposis multiplex congenita (multiple congenital contractures) is a physical finding, not a diagnosis, and the term represents a group of unrelated disorders with the common phenotypic characteristic of multiple joint contractures. Arthrogryposis multiplex congenita should be considered a symptom complex that results in this characteristic phenotype that can occur in 300 different disorders. Arthrogryposis usually is a nonprogressive syndrome characterized by deformed, rigid joints that affect two or more areas of the body. The involved muscles or muscle groups are atrophied or absent. The involved extremities appear cylindrical, fusiform, or cone-shaped and have diminished skin creases and subcutaneous tissue. Contracture of the joint capsule and periarticular tissues is present. Dislocation of the joints is common, especially of the hip and knee (Fig. 34-47). Sensation and intellect are normal. The incidence of arthrogryposis has been reported to be 1 in 3000 live births.

More than 300 specific entities can be associated with what has been known as arthrogryposis multiplex congenita; because it is no longer considered a discrete clinical entity, the term *multiple congenital contractures* is preferred. Determining whether a child has normal neurologic function is essential to establish a differential diagnosis. In a child with a normal neurologic examination, arthrogryposis is most

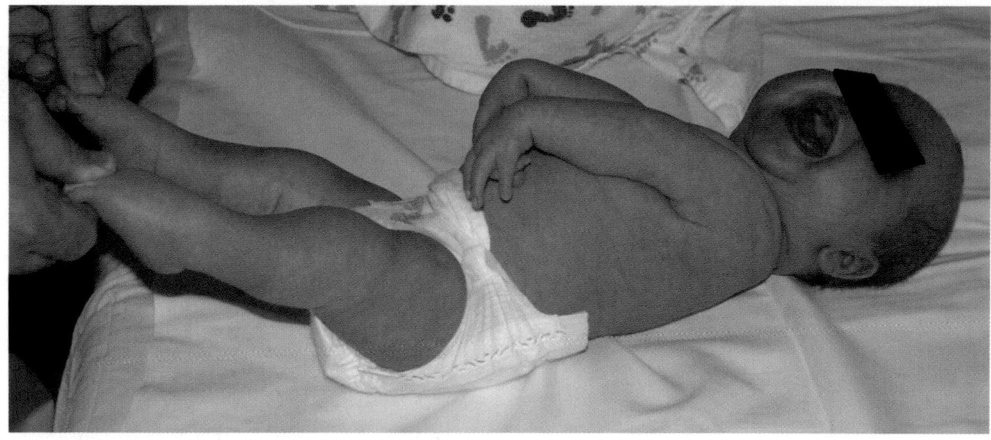

FIGURE 34-47 Newborn with arthrogryposis multiplex congenita. Note orthopaedic conditions: congenital dislocation of knees, teratologic clubfeet, internal rotation contractures of shoulder, extension contractures of elbow, and flexion contractures of wrist.

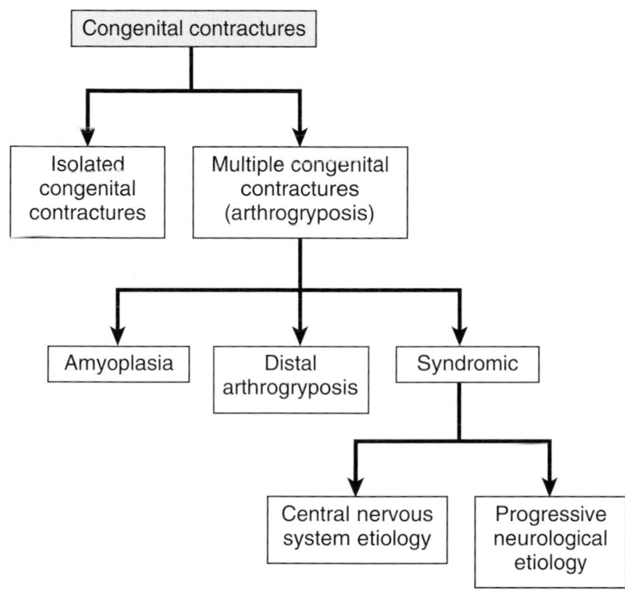

FIGURE 34-48 Types of congenital contractures. (From Bamshad M, Van Heest AE, Pleasure D: Arthrogryposis: a review and update. J Bone Joint Surg 91A(Suppl 4):40, 2009.)

likely caused by amyoplasia, distal arthrogryposis, generalized connective tissue disorder, or fetal crowding. An abnormal neurologic examination indicates that movement in utero was diminished as a result of an abnormality of the central or peripheral nervous system, the motor endplate, or muscle (Fig. 34-48). The deformities may result from neurogenic, myogenic, skeletal, or environmental factors. Genetic evaluation is recommended for patients with arthrogryposis. Limited intrauterine movement is common to all types of arthrogryposis. Histologic analysis shows a small muscle mass with fibrosis and fat between the muscle fibers. Myopathic and neuropathic features often are found in the muscle. The periarticular soft-tissue structures are fibrotic and create a fibrous ankylosis.

Clinical examination is the best modality for establishing the diagnosis of arthrogryposis multiplex congenita. Neurologic assessment, electromyography and nerve conduction studies, serum enzyme tests, DNA testing, and muscle biopsy can help to determine the underlying diagnosis. Radiographic examination assesses the integrity of the skeletal system, especially the presence or absence of dislocated hips or knees, scoliosis, and other skeletal anomalies. The most common lower extremity deformities are rigid clubfoot and fixed extension or flexion contractures of the knees. Major problems in the upper extremity usually are immobile, adducted, and internally rotated shoulders; elbow contractures; severe, fixed palmar flexion and ulnar-deviated deformities of the wrist; and contractures of the metacarpophalangeal and interphalangeal joints. Involvement usually is bilateral but not always symmetric. Scoliosis has been reported to occur in 10% to 30% of patients.

Classic arthrogryposis or amyoplasia usually involves all four extremities. The shoulders are internally rotated and adducted. The elbow usually has an extension contracture, and the wrists are palmar flexed and ulnarly deviated. The fingers often are rigidly flexed with the thumbs adducted. There often is a midline cutaneous hemangioma on the forehead. Patients with distal arthrogryposis have fixed hand and foot contractures, but the major large joints of the arms and legs are spared. Distal arthrogryposis is divided into type I and type II based on the absence or presence of facial abnormalities. In contrast to amyoplasia, which occurs sporadically, distal arthrogryposis is inherited in an autosomal dominant fashion. Genetic analysis has identified 10 distinct types of distal arthrogryposis (Table 34-3).

Current labels and Online Mendelian Inheritance in Man (OMIM) numbers for the distal arthrogryposis syndromes are listed in Table 34-4. Pterygia syndromes have skin webs across the flexion aspects of knees, elbows, and other joints. Multiple pterygias and popliteal pterygia fit into this group.

TREATMENT

Most children with arthrogryposis have a relatively good prognosis; treatment should be focused on obtaining maximal function. Some contractures may seem to worsen with age, but no new joints become involved. At least 25% of affected patients are nonambulatory. An early program of passive stretching exercises for each contracted joint, to be followed by serial splinting with custom thermoplastic splints, is

TABLE 34-3

Common Causes of Arthrogryposis

DISEASE	GENETIC INFLUENCE	ADDITIONAL FACTORS/FINDINGS
Amyoplasia	Sporadic	Usually quadrimelic involvement
Myelomeningocele	Multifactorial	Folic acid deficiency
Larsen syndrome	AD	Joint dislocations, spatulate thumbs, flattened nasal bridge
Distal arthrogryposis type I	AD	Hand, foot involvement
Multiple pterygium syndrome (Escobar syndrome)	AR	Pterygium of upper and lower extremities, neck
Freeman-Sheldon syndrome (whistling face syndrome)	AD	Whistling appearance of face, ulnar deviation of hands, clubfoot, congenital vertical talus
Beal contractural arachnodactyly	AD	Slender limbs with knee, elbow, and hand contractures
Sacral agenesis	Sporadic	Maternal diabetes, exposure to organic solvents, retinoic acid
Diastrophic dysplasia	AR	Clubfoot, hitchhiker's thumb, short stature, scoliosis, hypertrophic pinnae
Metatropic dysplasia	AD, AR	Platyspondylia, kyphosis, scoliosis
Thrombocytopenia–absent radii (TAR) syndrome	AR	Absent radii with thumbs present, knee involvement, thrombocytopenia
Steinert myotonic dystrophy	AD	Myotonia, typical facies
Spinal muscular atrophy	AR	Anterior horn cell degeneration
Congenital muscular dystrophy	AR	Heterogeneous group of diseases, some with central nervous system involvement
Möbius syndrome	Sporadic, AD	Cranial nerve VI, VII palsy; micrognathia, clubfoot

From Bernstein RM: Arthrogryposis and amyoplasia, J Am Acad Orthop Surg 10:417, 2002.
AD, Autosomal dominant; *AR*, autosomal recessive.

TABLE 34-4

Foot Deformities in Patients With Myelomeningocele

LEVEL	CLUBFOOT	CALCANEOVALGUS DEFORMITY	VERTICAL TALUS	NO DEFORMITY
Thoracic	40	8	0	38
L1, L2	22	4	1	13
L3	24	21	9	0
L4	50	4	0	14
L5	11	38	5	20
Sacral	19	4	0	41
Total	166	60	7	135

In patients with asymmetric paralysis, each foot was counted separately.
From Schafer ME, Dias LS: Myelomeningocele: orthopaedic treatment, Baltimore, 1983, Williams & Wilkins.

recommended. Although gains are achieved in extremity function and the need for corrective surgery is reduced, most authors report that any improvement after physical therapy is transient at best and that recurrence of the deformity is likely.

The primary long-term goals of treatment are increased joint mobility and muscle strength and the development of adaptive use patterns that allow walking and independence with activities of daily living. To achieve these goals, correcting lower extremity alignment to make plantigrade standing and walking possible is necessary. Existing joint motion should be preserved and placed in the most functional location. Treatment should also focus on active motion, and tendon-muscle transfers should be done when necessary. In addition, stiff joints should be positioned for functional advantage. Surgical intervention can be divided into early and late treatment. Early treatment should accomplish as much functional improvement as possible in the involved extremities by 6 to 7 years of age. Knee and hip surgery should be done by 6 to 9 months of age. Foot surgery should be done close to the time when the patient normally begins to stand to decrease the incidence of recurrence.

LOWER EXTREMITY

The rigid foot deformity in multiple congenital contractures usually is a clubfoot or congenital vertical talus. The goal of

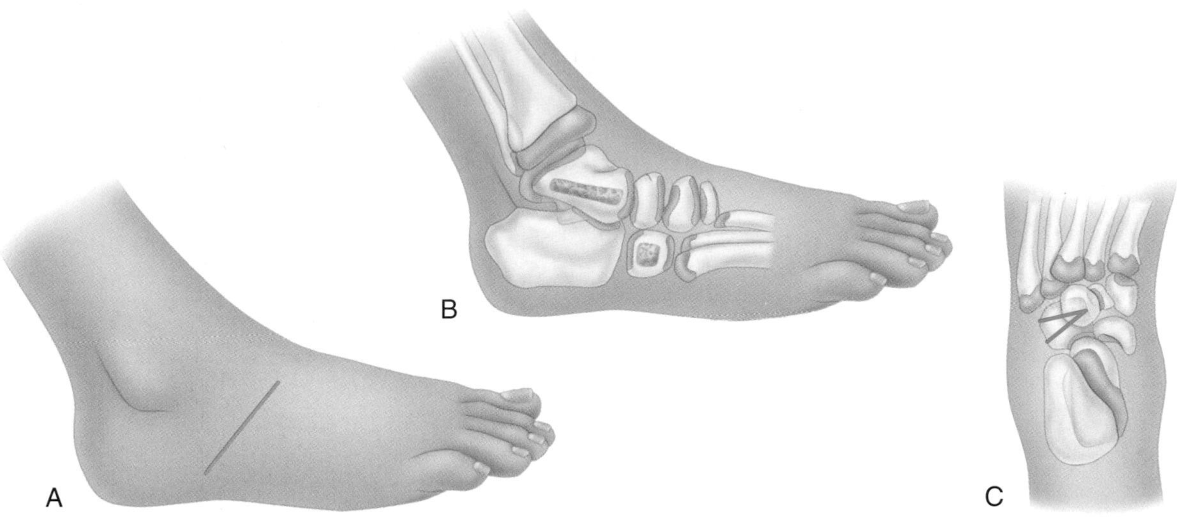

FIGURE 34-49 Cancellectomy of talus and cuboid. **A,** Incision. **B,** Windows in talus and cuboid to expose cancellous bone. **C,** Closing wedge osteotomy in cuboid.

treatment is conversion of the rigid deformed foot into a plantigrade foot. If the valgus foot is plantigrade, treatment usually is not required. The most common foot deformity is clubfoot. The Ponseti method of clubfoot casting has been used successfully in patients with arthrogryposis and clubfeet, but a greater number of casts were required than for idiopathic clubfeet, and the relapse rate was 27% at 2-year follow-up. If casting fails, an extensive posteromedial and posterolateral release (see Chapter 29) is recommended. If the deformity recurs in a young child or is so severe that it cannot be corrected by posteromedial soft-tissue release, talectomy is indicated. Fusion of the calcaneocuboid joint at the time of talectomy may decrease the risk of progressive midfoot adduction. Gross described a technique, similar to that described by Ogston and Kopits for use in myelomeningocele, of cancellectomy of the talus and cuboid in which a window is created in the dorsal cortex of the cuboid and lateral cortex of the neck and body of the talus (Fig. 34-49). All cancellous bone is carefully curetted, and the deformity is corrected by manual manipulation (see Technique 34-30). Triple arthrodesis may be performed for rigid deformity in adolescents. Gradual correction of the deformity with circular-frame external fixators is an alternative method for obtaining a plantigrade foot but is technically demanding.

The two most common deformities around the knee are a flexion contracture and an extension contracture. Initial treatment of flexion contractures is by serial splinting or casting in progressive degrees of extension. Ambulation is possible with a residual knee flexion contracture of 15 to 20 degrees. If complete correction has not been obtained by 6 to 12 months of age, posterior medial and lateral hamstring lengthening and knee capsulotomies are indicated. This should be approached through vertical medial and lateral posterior incisions or an extensile posterolateral Henry incision. S-shaped incisions should be avoided because they place excessive tension on the skin after correction causing subsequent wound breakdown. After a posterior release has been performed, an anterior release of scar tissue may need to be done to obtain correction. Supracondylar extension osteotomy of the distal femur may be required to correct a contracture and allow use of orthoses. Extension osteotomies should be done when the patient is near skeletal maturity if possible to decrease the risk of recurrent deformity with remodeling. If osteotomies are done before skeletal maturity, about 50% of correction is maintained even if the deformity recurs. Often a femoral shortening may need to be combined with an extension osteotomy to protect neurovascular structures. Gradual correction of a knee flexion contracture can be achieved with a circular-frame external fixator, with or without an associated posterior release. This technique is used most often when soft-tissue webbing is associated with a knee flexion contracture.

CORRECTION OF KNEE FLEXION CONTRACTURE WITH CIRCULAR-FRAME EXTERNAL FIXATION

TECHNIQUE 34-42

(VAN BOSSE ET AL.)

APPROXIMATION OF KNEE CENTER OF ROTATION

- On a true lateral projection of the knee, with the distal and posterior femoral condyles superimposed, the intersection of the posterior femoral cortex and the widest anterior-posterior dimension of the femoral condyles gives the best estimate of the knee axis of motion (Fig. 34-50).

POSTERIOR KNEE RELEASE

- Approach the knee through medial and lateral incisions, 5 to 8 cm long, centered over the palpable posterior femoral condyle and parallel to the ground when both the hip and knee are on the operating table (Fig. 34-51A).

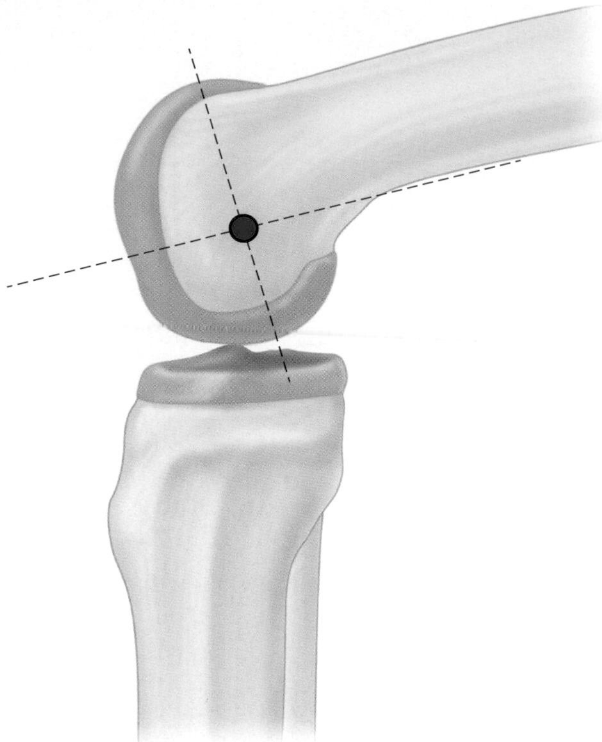

FIGURE 34-50 Estimation of the knee axis of rotation. On a true lateral projection of the knee, with the distal and posterior femoral condyles superimposed, the intersection of the posterior femoral cortex and the widest anteroposterior dimension of the femoral condyles gives the best estimate of knee axis of rotation. (Redrawn from van Bosse HJP, Feldman DS, Anavian J, Sala DA: Treatment of knee flexion contractures in patients with arthrogryposis, J Pediatr Orthop 27:930, 2007.) **SEE TECHNIQUE 34-42.**

- Laterally, incise the iliotibial band in line with the incision and release its posterior half.
- After verifying the safety of the common peroneal nerve, isolate the biceps femoris tendon and transect it proximally.
- With blunt dissection, elevate soft tissues off the knee joint capsule posteriorly until a finger can be run along the posterior aspect of the joint capsule to at least the midpoint.
- Identify the lateral head of the gastrocnemius, running as a tight band just proximal and posterior to the joint capsule; isolate and transect its tendon.
- Make a small capsulotomy posterolaterally and continue it anteriorly to incise the posterior half of the lateral collateral ligament (Fig. 34-51B).
- Use a Freer elevator to retract the posterior soft tissues and cut the posterior capsule along the joint line with Mayo scissors. If the geniculate artery is cut or avulsed, obtain hemostasis by packing the wound for approximately 5 minutes.
- Medially, retract the vastus medialis obliquus anteriorly and transect the semitendinosus and gracilis tendons.
- Deep to the tendons, transect the fascia of the semimembranosus, leaving the muscle belly intact.
- Bluntly elevate the soft tissues off the medial aspect of the posterior capsule and transect the medial head of the gastrocnemius.
- At this point, it should be possible to pass a finger across the entire posterior joint line of the knee, even in small patients.
- Use scissors to advance a posteromedial corner capsulotomy anteriorly, incising the posterior half of the medial collateral ligament, staying cephalad to its attachments to the medial meniscus. Complete the capsulotomy with the scissors (Fig. 34-51C).
- Verify complete release by direct palpation. If the posterior cruciate ligament can be felt as a taut band in the intercondylar notch, release it.
- Close only the skin with absorbable sutures.

APPLICATION OF ILIZAROV FIXATOR

- Attach a femoral frame with two full rings to the femur and position Ilizarov universal joints on either side in line with the knee axis wire.
- Hang a tibial frame from the two universal joints with threaded rods.
- Position a transverse transfixation wire in the proximal tibial ring so that as it is tensioned it pulls the tibia slightly anterior on the femur. This helps counter forces that cause posterior tibial subluxation during contracture correction (Fig. 34-51D).
- Secure the tibial frame to the tibia.
- Distract the joint 5 to 10 mm by lengthening between the universal joints and the tibial frame, avoiding impingement and crushing of the articular cartilage during correction.
- A telescopic rod for correction can be placed posteriorly or anteriorly; the latter is more convenient for seating purposes. Occasionally, the frame is extended to include the foot to simultaneously correct a deformity or prevent ankle equinus during treatment.

POSTOPERATIVE CARE. Approximately 1 week after surgery, correction is begun at 1 to 2 degrees a day, adjusted to the patient's tolerance. Once fully corrected to 0 degrees, the frame is maintained in full extension for an additional 2 to 4 weeks, depending on the ease of initial correction. The frame is removed in the operating room, and a cast is applied with the knee in full extension; the cast is molded to prevent posterior tibial subluxation. The cast is worn for 2 weeks and then replaced with a knee-ankle-foot orthosis (KAFO) with locking knee hinges. Physical therapy is begun for gait training and knee range of motion. The KAFO is worn in full extension for 3 months and is removed only for bathing and physical therapy. After 3 months, it is worn routinely at night and during the day as needed for ambulation.

Anterior distal femoral stapling with 8-plates has been reported by Palocaren et al. to improve flexion deformity and ambulatory capacity in arthrogrypotic patients with knee flexion contractures. This technique is less invasive than soft-tissue releases, distal femoral osteotomies, or frame

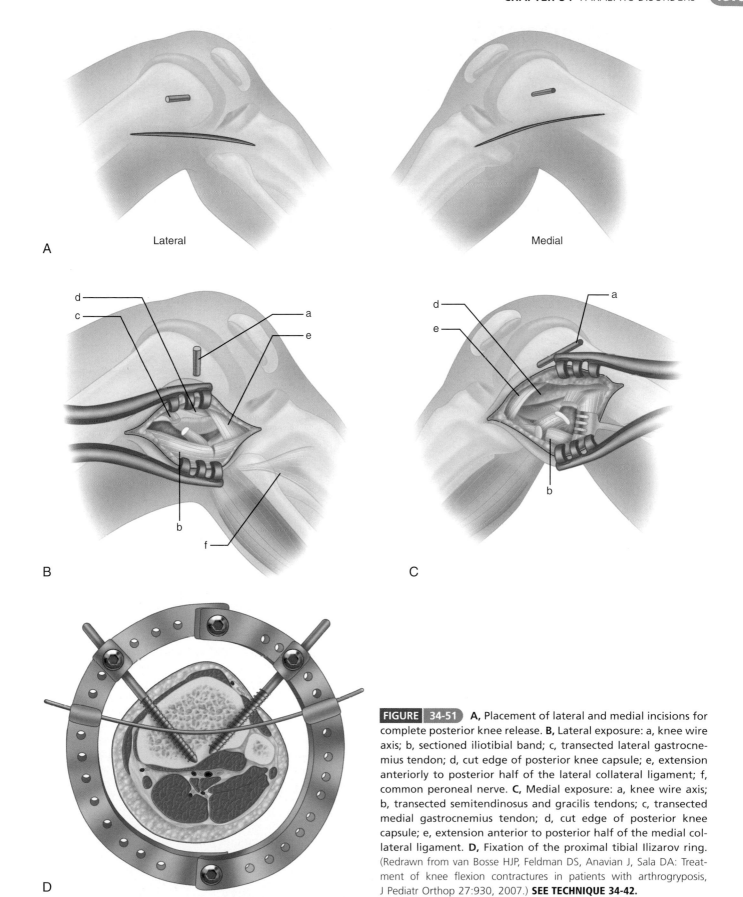

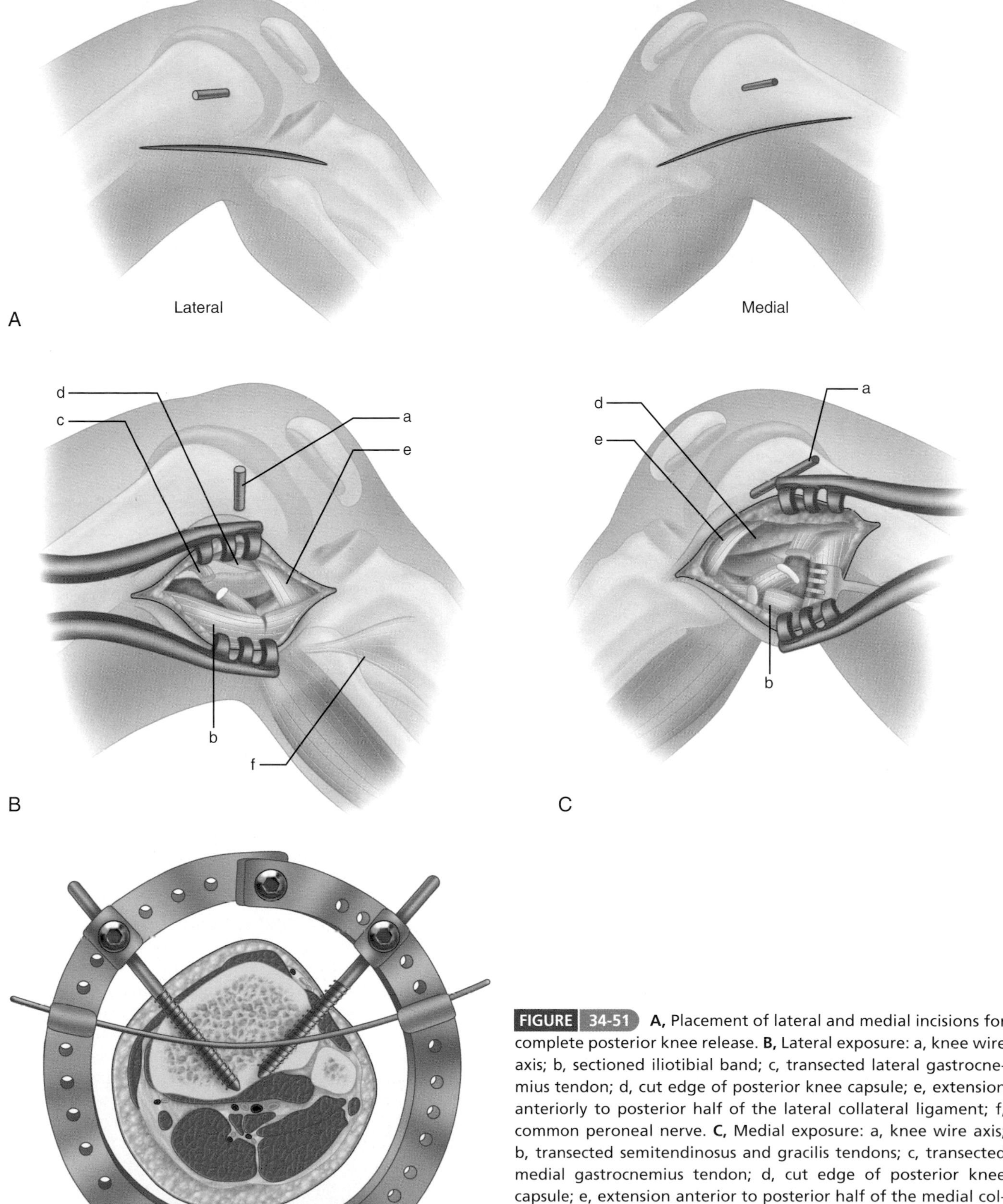

FIGURE 34-51 **A,** Placement of lateral and medial incisions for complete posterior knee release. **B,** Lateral exposure: a, knee wire axis; b, sectioned iliotibial band; c, transected lateral gastrocnemius tendon; d, cut edge of posterior knee capsule; e, extension anteriorly to posterior half of the lateral collateral ligament; f, common peroneal nerve. **C,** Medial exposure: a, knee wire axis; b, transected semitendinosus and gracilis tendons; c, transected medial gastrocnemius tendon; d, cut edge of posterior knee capsule; e, extension anterior to posterior half of the medial collateral ligament. **D,** Fixation of the proximal tibial Ilizarov ring. (Redrawn from van Bosse HJP, Feldman DS, Anavian J, Sala DA: Treatment of knee flexion contractures in patients with arthrogryposis, J Pediatr Orthop 27:930, 2007.) **SEE TECHNIQUE 34-42.**

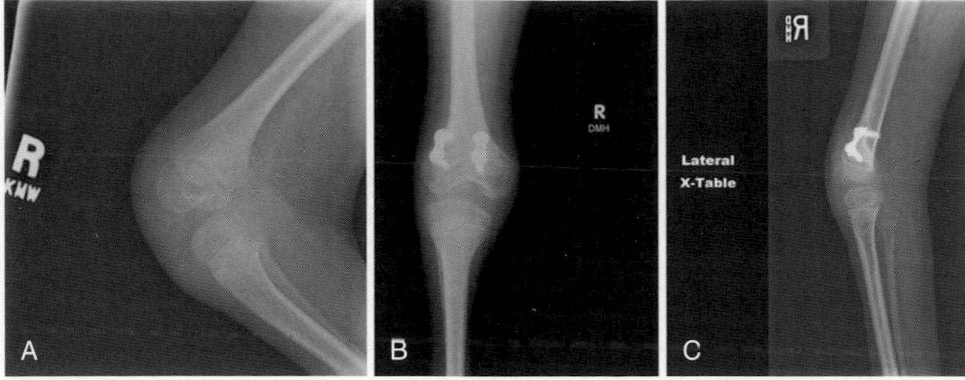

FIGURE 34-52 **A,** Preoperative lateral knee radiograph of a 4-year-old boy with arthrogryposis. **B** and **C,** Two years after anterior stapling of the distal femur with 8-plates. Lateral view shows correction of the flexion deformity and divergence of the screws with growth. (From Palocaren T, Thabet AM, Rogers K, et al: Anterior distal femoral stapling for correcting knee flexion contracture in children with arthrogryposis—preliminary results, J Pediatr Orthop 30:169, 2010.) **SEE TECHNIQUE 34-43.**

distraction and is most beneficial in children with flexion contractures of less than 45 degrees. The stapling can be done as an outpatient procedure, depending on the patient's general health, anesthetic tolerance, and need for concomitant procedures. The timing of stapling is determined by the size of the femoral condyle rather than the chronologic age of the child: the condyle must be large enough to accommodate the smallest screw in the 8-plate set (16 mm).

CORRECTION OF KNEE FLEXION CONTRACTURE WITH ANTERIOR STAPLING

TECHNIQUE 34-43

(PALOCAREN ET AL.)

- Use image intensification to determine the location of the distal femoral physis and make two 3-cm incisions on either side of the patella centered at the level of the physis.
- With image intensifier guidance, place a needle into the physis and thread the central hole in the 8-plate over the needle so that the plate spans the physis.
- Ensure that the plate rests about 2 to 3 mm away from the lateral and medial edges of the patella. If the plate is fixed too close to the patella, knee movement will be restricted and painful.
- Insert two 1.6-mm guidewires through the screw holes in the plate and verify their position with fluoroscopy.
- Place two self-tapping cannulated screws over the guidewires. The screws should be sufficiently long to meet, but not penetrate, the opposite cortex. Take care not to violate the physis or the joint.
- Close the wound in layers and apply a soft dressing. A knee immobilizer can be used for comfort.

POSTOPERATIVE CARE. Ambulation is allowed as tolerated. Follow-up radiographs are obtained at 4 weeks. Patients are followed at 6-month intervals for clinical evaluation of the flexion deformity, stance, and gait. The plates are left in place until the deformity is corrected (Fig. 34-52).

Contracture of the quadriceps mechanism can cause hyperextension of the knee, which is treated initially by serial casting. If the deformity does not respond to conservative treatment by 6 to 12 months of age, surgical correction by quadricepsplasty (see Chapter 45) is recommended. It is important to counsel families that although knee range of motion and function improve in the short term, both function and outcomes decline as the deformities recur with time.

The hip is involved in approximately 80% of patients with multiple congenital contractures. In general, hip deformities should be treated by passive stretching exercises, beginning in infancy. If conservative measures fail, surgical correction of the hip deformity should be delayed until deformities of the knees have been corrected. Mild hip flexion contractures may be accommodated by an increase in lumbar lordosis. Flexion contractures of more than 45 degrees should have surgical release. Developmental hip dysplasia and hip dislocation occur in about two thirds of patients with arthrogryposis. Traditional recommendations are that bilateral teratologic hip dislocations should not be reduced because reduction may not improve function. Good results have been reported, however, with early (3 to 6 months of age) open reduction through a medial approach. If surgical intervention is done between 12 and 36 months of age, a one-stage open reduction, primary femoral shortening, and possible pelvic osteotomy are recommended. Unilateral dislocation of the hip, whether flexible or rigid, should be reduced surgically and placed in a functional position to avoid potential pelvic obliquity and scoliosis. The treatment of bilateral dislocations should be individualized. Good results have been reported in bilateral hip dislocations treated with a medial or anterior approach. If the dislocated hips are treated surgically, postoperative immobilization should be limited to 6 to 8 weeks.

UPPER EXTREMITY

Traditional recommendations for treatment of the upper extremities in children with arthrogryposis were to leave the shoulders internally rotated and adducted, the elbows extended, and the wrist flexed. Most of these children adapted to their disabilities and developed some form of bimanual function. Correction of upper extremity deformities should be delayed until ambulation has been achieved, usually by 3 to 4 years of age. If surgery is delayed until age 8 years, the use patterns are so well established that the child would not adapt as well to surgical correction. The goal of treatment of upper extremity deformities is to provide optimal function of the hand in activities of daily living. Function may be adequate despite severe deformity in children with arthrogryposis; the benefits of surgical intervention must be carefully weighed against the risk of surgery.

The shoulder usually is adducted and internally rotated. Weakness and stiffness around the shoulder do not significantly impair function and usually require no treatment, but the fixed internal rotation of the shoulder becomes a major obstacle for normal elbow and hand function. Proximal humeral rotation osteotomy (see Technique 34-45) may be indicated to correct this internal rotation deformity.

Deformity of the elbow usually means severe limitation of either flexion or extension. The stiff flexed elbow is not a severe impairment, and surgery is not indicated. Fixed extension elbow deformity, especially if bilateral, is a severe functional impairment. The goals for surgery for a fixed extension elbow deformity are to gain functional range of motion and achieve active elbow flexion. Surgical options available for the fixed extended elbow are release of extension contractures, tricepsplasty, triceps transfer (Fig. 34-53), flexorplasty, and pectoralis major transfer. Lengthening of the triceps mechanism and posterior capsulotomy are the most reliable and durable of available surgical procedures. This procedure is indicated when elbow flexion is limited to 45 degrees or less, with a goal to gain functional range of motion around the elbow. Zlotolow and Kozin combined posterior elbow capsular release with external rotation osteotomy of the humerus to place the forearm and hand in a better position for function and optimize hand-to-mouth activities.

POSTERIOR ELBOW CAPSULOTOMY WITH TRICEPS LENGTHENING FOR ELBOW EXTENSION CONTRACTURE

TECHNIQUE 34-44

(VAN HEEST ET AL.)

- For unilateral release, place the patient in a lateral decubitus position; for bilateral release, position the patient supine.
- Apply a tourniquet and approach the elbow through a curvilinear posterior incision (Fig. 34-53A).
- In patients with minimal elbow movement, take care to correctly identify the posterior aspect of the olecranon; severe internal rotation of the limb may cause the medial epicondyle to be mistaken for the olecranon.
- Identify the ulnar nerve in the medial intermuscular septum. Release the cubital tunnel, trace the ulnar nerve to the flexor carpi ulnaris innervation, and place a vessel loop around it for protection during subsequent dissection.
- Once the ulnar nerve has been identified, released, and protected, remove the tourniquet.
- Isolate, mobilize medially and laterally, and lengthen the triceps with either a Z-lengthening or V-Y advancement. Most commonly, the triceps is incised in a "V" fashion so that the central tongue is based on the olecranon and the two lateral limbs include tendon over as great a length as possible, from the proximal muscular portion distally to the olecranon insertion.
- Incise the posterior aspect of the capsule at the tip of the olecranon to allow identification of the joint surface.
- Extend the arthrotomy medially and laterally to allow maximal elbow flexion with a gentle passive stretch. If necessary, extend the capsular release around the medial and lateral sides to include the posterior edges of the medial and lateral collateral ligament.
- Flex the elbow as much as possible (more than 90 degrees) while allowing contact between the distal ends of the lateral triceps limbs and the proximal end of the central tongue of triceps.
- Repair the triceps in an elongated position with nonresorbable or reinforced suture.
- Close the skin, apply a light dressing, and place the arm in a long arm cast or a prefabricated custom hinged elbow brace.

POSTOPERATIVE CARE. The elbow is immobilized in 90 degrees of flexion, with passive range of motion allowed as soon as tolerated. During the first month after surgery, physical therapy is advanced to include hand-to-mouth activities; passive flexion is limited to 90 degrees to protect the triceps lengthening during this time but is then advanced to full passive flexion. The splint or cast is worn for 4 to 6 weeks.

Passive elbow flexion to a right angle is a prerequisite for considering a tendon transfer for active elbow flexion. Triceps transfer can be done to regain elbow flexion, but over time a flexion contracture often occurs. Elbow stability in extension should not be sacrificed with this procedure because it can make the use of crutches, rising from a sitting position, and wheelchair transfers difficult. Procedures to achieve active elbow flexion in an arthrogrypotic patient are triceps transfer, flexorplasty, pectoralis major transfer, latissimus transfer, and free gracilis transfer. These procedures all have been relatively ineffective in maintaining long-term elbow flexion and have significant donor site morbidity.

POSTERIOR RELEASE OF ELBOW EXTENSION CONTRACTURE AND TRICEPS TENDON TRANSFER

TECHNIQUE 34-45

(TACHDJIAN)

- Place the patient laterally.
- Make a midline incision on the posterior aspect of the arm, beginning in its middle half and extending distally

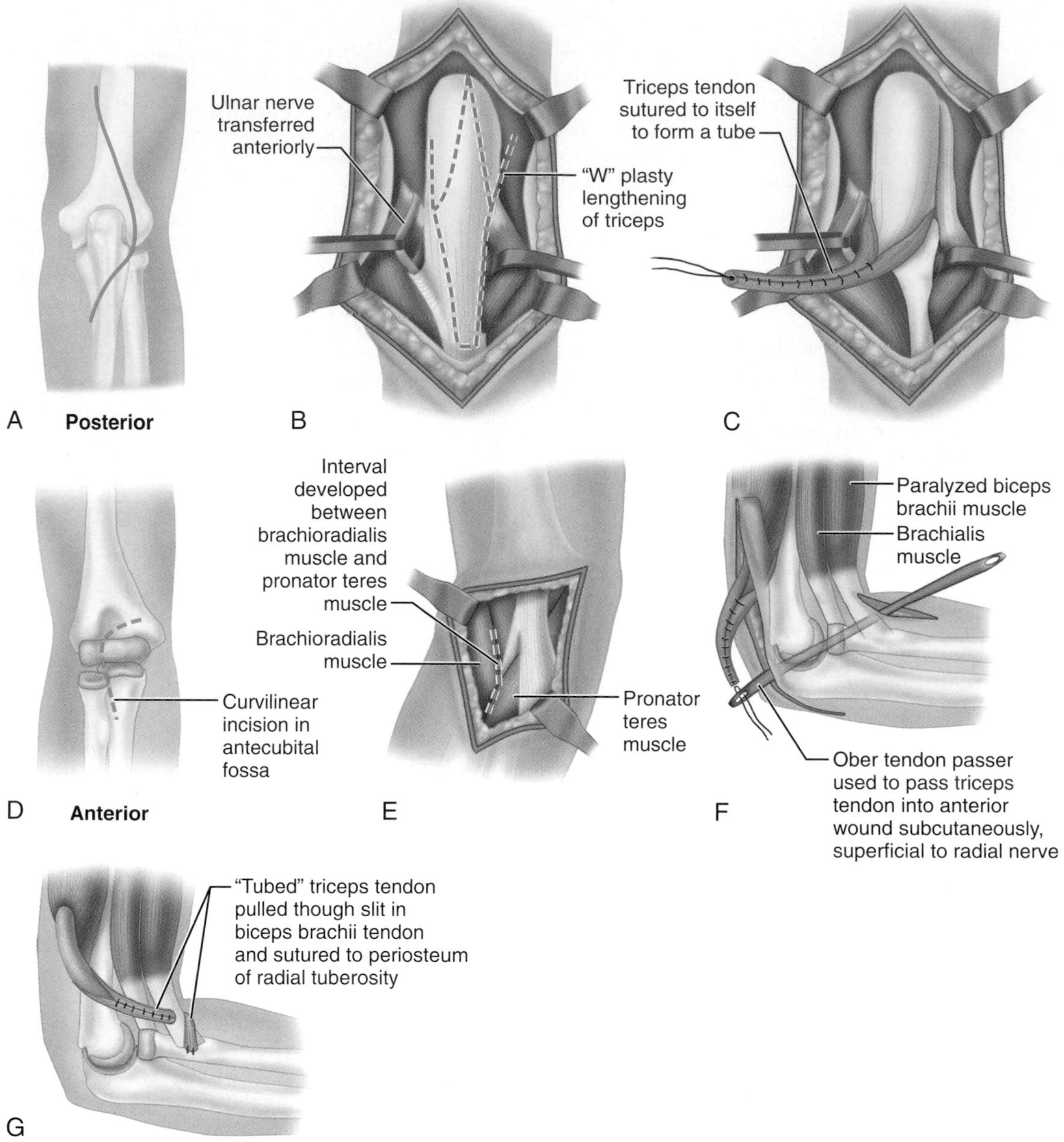

FIGURE 34-53 **Posterior release of elbow extension contracture and triceps tendon transfer to restore flexion.** (Redrawn from Herring JA, editor: Tachdjian's pediatric orthopaedics, ed 3. Philadelphia, 2002, Saunders.) **SEE TECHNIQUES 34-44 AND 34-45.**

to a point lateral to the olecranon process; carry the incision over the subcutaneous surface of the shaft of the ulna for a distance of 5 cm.

- Divide the subcutaneous tissue and mobilize the wound flaps (Fig. 34-53A).
- Identify the ulnar nerve and mobilize it medially to protect it from injury.
- Expose the intermuscular septum laterally.
- Mobilize the ulnar nerve and transfer it anteriorly.
- Lengthen the triceps muscle in a W fashion, leaving a long proximal tongue (Fig. 34-53B).
- Free the triceps muscle and mobilize it proximally as far as its nerve supply permits. The motor branches of the radial nerve to the triceps enter the muscle in the interval between the lateral and medial heads as the radial nerve enters the musculospiral groove.
- Suture the distal portion of the detached triceps to itself to form a tube (Fig. 34-53C).
- Make a curvilinear incision in the antecubital fossa and develop the interval between the brachioradialis and the pronator teres (Fig. 34-53D and E).
- With a tendon passer, pass the triceps tendon into the anterior wound subcutaneously, superficial to the radial nerve (Fig. 34-53F).
- With the elbow in 90 degrees of flexion and the forearm in full supination, either suture the triceps tendon to the

biceps tendon or anchor it to the radial tuberosity by a suture passed through a drill hole (Fig. 34-53G).

- Close the wound in the routine fashion.
- Apply an above-elbow cast with the elbow in 90 degrees of flexion and full supination.

POSTOPERATIVE CARE. Four weeks after surgery the cast is removed and active exercises are begun to develop elbow flexion. Gravity provides extension to the elbow.

Steindler flexorplasty produces elbow flexion by transferring the flexor pronator origin from the medial epicondyle to the anterior humerus (Fig. 34-23). For this procedure to be beneficial, both active wrist flexors and extensors need to be present. This procedure rarely is indicated in children with multiple congenital contractures because the wrist flexors usually are inactive and contracted. An active radial wrist extensor also needs to be present to prevent unacceptable wrist flexion after a flexorplasty. Triceps transfer would allow for early improvement in elbow flexion, but over time flexion contractures may occur and function deteriorates, so one must be cautious in the use of this transfer. Transfer of the long head of the triceps can be used as an alternative (Fig. 34-24). The long head of the triceps has a separate neurovascular pedicle that can be separated from the rest of the triceps. A fascia lata graft often is needed to allow for transfer into the proximal ulna. This transfer often allows for adequate elbow flexion without loss of active elbow extension. Microsurgical transfer of the gracilis muscle to the arm has been reported.

The wrist is usually flexed and in an ulnar-deviated position. Wrist stabilization in the optimal functional position probably is the most beneficial procedure in patients with multiple congenital contractures, but determination of the best position for function must be made carefully. Neutral or mild ulnar deviation and dorsiflexion between 5 and 20 degrees proves to be the most satisfactory position. Procedures described for the arthrogrypotic wrist are tendon transfers, proximal row carpectomy, dorsal radial closing wedge osteotomy of the midcarpus, and wrist fusion. Wrist palmar flexion contracture can be corrected with flexor carpi ulnaris lengthening or transfer to the wrist extensors. This transfer acts more like a tenodesis procedure than a dynamic transfer. Proximal row carpectomy is not often recommended because of the loss of correction and stiffness that occurs with this procedure. In younger patients, a closing wedge osteotomy through the midcarpus can correct the wrist deformity. When the patient is near skeletal maturity, a wrist fusion can be performed by traditional methods.

DORSAL CLOSING WEDGE OSTEOTOMY OF THE WRIST

TECHNIQUE 34-46

(VAN HEEST AND RODRIGUEZ, EZAKI, AND CARTER)

- Through a dorsal approach to the wrist, isolate and protect the digital and wrist extensor tendons, then make a dorsal capsulotomy.
- At the level of the midcarpus, make a dorsal wedge osteotomy sufficient to correct the wrist flexion deformity to at least a neutral position, taking care not to violate the radiocarpal joint and ensuring that finger flexor tightness is not produced by tenodesis.
- Make the proximal cut distal to the radiocarpal joint at the level of the capsular attachment of the proximal carpal row, perpendicular in two planes to the long axis of the forearm.
- Make the distal cut through the distal carpal row, perpendicular in both planes to the long axis of the metacarpus.
- If ulnar deviation correction also is required, resect more bone on the radial side of the dorsal carpal wedge to provide biplanar correction.
- Insert two crossed Kirschner wires to hold the osteotomy closed.

POSTOPERATIVE CARE. The wrist is kept elevated for the first several days after surgery. The cast or splint is changed at 2 to 3 weeks. The wrist is immobilized in a cast or splint for an additional 6 weeks or until union is apparent on radiographs.

Flexion contractures of the fingers are best treated with passive stretching and splinting. Surgical procedures have not had any functional benefit over nonoperative treatment. Thumb-in-palm deformity may respond to appropriate releases. This usually is accomplished with a comprehensive thenar release.

SCOLIOSIS

Scoliosis has been reported to occur in 10% to 30% of patients with multiple congenital contractures, generally associated with neuromuscular weakness or pelvic obliquity. If the deformity is severe and progressive, early surgical intervention is warranted. The indications and techniques for treatment of scoliosis in patients with multiple congenital contractures are the same as those for patients with other neuromuscular disorders (see Chapter 44).

BRACHIAL PLEXUS PALSY

Brachial plexus palsy may be seen after injury to the brachial plexus during birth. Reported incidences range from 0.1% to 0.4% of live births. Despite advances in obstetric care, the incidence of brachial plexus palsy is believed to be increasing because of the increase in high birth weight infants. Numerous risk factors have been identified, including large birth weight, prolonged labor, difficult delivery, forceps delivery, and previous births with brachial plexopathy. Brachial plexus palsy is thought to be caused by a mechanical traction injury during the birth process. Delivery by cesarean section does not exclude the possibility of brachial plexus birth palsy but does decrease the likelihood from 0.2% to 0.02%. Shoulder dystocia is the mechanical factor that results in an upper trunk lesion. A breech delivery often results in a stretch of the lower plexus from traction applied to the trunk with the arm abducted.

Brachial plexus birth palsy was classified by Narakas according to the location of the injury of the brachial plexus

TABLE 34-5

Classification and Prognosis in Obstetric Palsy

TYPE	CLINICAL PICTURE	RECOVERY
I	C5-6	Complete or almost in 1-8 wk
II	C5-6 C7	Elbow flexion: 1-4 wk Elbow extension: 1-8 wk Limited shoulder: 6-30 wk
III	C5-6 C7 C8-T1 (no Horner sign)	Poor shoulder: 10-40 wk Elbow flexion: 16-40 wk Elbow extension: 16-20 wk Wrist: 40-60 wk Hand complete: 1-3 wk
IV	C5-7 C8 T1 (temporary Horner sign)	Poor shoulder: 10-40 wk Elbow flexion: 16-40 wk Elbow extension incomplete, poor: 20-60 wk or nil Wrist: 40-60 wk Hand complete: 20-60 wk
V	C5-7 C7 C8 T1 C8-T1 (Horner sign usually present)	Shoulder and elbow Wrist poor or only extension; poor flexion or none Very poor hand with no or weak flexors and extensors; no intrinsic as above

Modified from Narakas AO: Injuries to the brachial plexus. In Bora FW Jr, editor: The pediatric upper extremity: diagnosis and management, Philadelphia, 1986, Saunders.

(Table 34-5). Group I includes upper plexus lesions involving C5 and C6, the classic Erb palsy. This is the most common type (46% of cases) and has the most favorable prognosis. Group II consists of lesions of C5, C6, and C7. This group is the second most common (30% of cases) but has a worse prognosis than type I. Group III is a total plexus lesion with a flail extremity. This occurs in 20% of patients. Group IV is the most severe form, characterized by global plexopathy with flail extremity and Horner syndrome, which indicates involvement of the sympathetic chain and a probable avulsion injury. Injuries isolated to the C8 and T1 nerve roots (Klumpke palsy) are rare and account for less than 1% of cases of brachial plexus birth palsy.

The likelihood of recovery also is affected by whether the level of nerve injury is preganglionic or postganglionic. The degree and type of postganglionic neural injury were defined by Sunderland as neurapraxia, axonotmesis, and neurotmesis. Neurapraxia is paralysis in the absence of peripheral degeneration. Recovery usually is complete in this type. Axonotmesis is damage to the nerve fiber with complete peripheral degeneration but intact external tissues to provide support for regeneration. Recovery depends on the degree of nerve injury and is more prolonged. Neurotmesis is disruption of the neural and supporting tissues, which carries a poor prognosis. This includes neuroma in continuity, division of the nerve, and anatomic disruption. Preganglionic avulsion injuries cannot spontaneously recover motor function because the nerve roots are avulsed from the spinal cord. These injuries also are associated with loss of motor function of other nerves that arise close to the spinal cord, which can aid in early diagnosis of these injuries. Loss of the phrenic (elevated hemidiaphragm), long thoracic, dorsal scapular, suprascapular, and thoracodorsal nerves (scapular stabilization) and the sympathetic chain with resultant Horner syndrome are suggestive of a preganglionic avulsion injury.

CLINICAL FEATURES

The diagnosis usually is evident at birth. The newborn has decreased spontaneous movement and asymmetry of infantile reflexes such as Moro reflex or asymmetric tonic neck reflex. In upper root involvement, the arm is held in internal rotation and active abduction is limited. The elbow may be slightly flexed or in complete extension. The thumb may be flexed, and occasionally the fingers do not extend. In complete paralysis, the entire arm and hand is flail. Pinching produces no reaction. Vasomotor impairment may be indicated by the relative paleness of the involved extremity. An ipsilateral Horner syndrome consisting of ptosis and a small pupil indicates injury to the T1 cervical sympathetic nerves. This is a major indication for a poor outcome. Radiographs of the shoulder may reveal fracture of the proximal humeral epiphysis or fracture of the clavicle. A clavicular fracture occurs in association with plexus palsy in 10% to 15% of patients. Pseudoparalysis from a clavicular or proximal humeral fracture should resolve within 10 to 21 days. If limited motion persists after 1 month of age, most likely a concomitant brachial plexus palsy is present. A septic shoulder in an infant also can cause a pseudoparalysis, which can be differentiated from a brachial plexus palsy by evidence of systemic illness and resolution of the pseudoparalysis after the infection is treated.

Serial physical examinations of children with brachial plexus birth palsy are needed to access motor function and the development of joint contractures. Treatment will be determined by the return or absence of return of motor function and the development of joint contractures. Passive internal and external rotation of the shoulder should be measured with the arm adducted and also abducted to 90 degrees while stabilizing the scapula against the thorax. Assessing motor function in infants often is an approximation of function by observing spontaneous activity.

Three assessment tools have been described to aid in the clinical evaluation of patients with brachial plexus birth palsy: the Toronto Test Score, the Hospital for Sick Children Active Movement Scale, and the Mallet score (Table 34-6). All have been shown to have positive intraobserver and interobserver reliability with aggregate scores. The Toronto Test Score was designed to determine surgical indications and provide an assessment tool after nerve reconstruction procedures. The Hospital for Sick Children Active Movement Scale is a more comprehensive score that evaluates the entire brachial plexus using 15 different upper extremity movements. The Modified Mallet Classification of Shoulder Function is the most commonly used outcome measure in patients with neonatal brachial plexus palsy (Fig. 34-54). Because this scale is heavily weighted toward external rotation of the shoulder, Abzug et al. added a sixth category—hand to belly button or navel—that adds another assessment of internal rotation. Assessing a child's ability to touch his or her belly button is important

TABLE 34-6

Clinical Evaluation of Patients With Brachial Plexus Birth Palsy

TORONTO TEST SCORE

Elbow flexion	0-2
Elbow extension	0-2
Wrist extension	0-2
Digital extension	0-2
Thumb extension	0-2
Total score	0-10

Each motor function is tested and allocated a numeric value. A score of 0 indicates no function, and a score of 2 indicates normal function. A total score of 3.5 or lower at the age of 3 months or more is considered an indication for microsurgical repair.

Adapted from Michelow BJ, Clarke HM, Curtis CG, et al: The natural history of obstetrical brachial plexus palsy, Plast Reconstr Surg 93:675, 1994.

HOSPITAL FOR SICK CHILDREN ACTIVE MOVEMENT SCALE

Gravity Eliminated	
No contraction	0
Contraction, no motion	1
Motion, < 50% range	2
Motion, > 50% range	3
Full motion	4
Against Gravity	
Motion, < 50% range	5
Motion, > 50% range	6
Full motion	7

Motor function tested: shoulder flexion, shoulder abduction and adduction, shoulder internal and external rotation, elbow flexion and extension, forearm pronation and supination, wrist flexion and extension, finger flexion and extension, thumb flexion and extension.

Adapted from Clarke HM, Curtis CG: An approach to obstetrical brachial plexus injuries. Hand Clin 11:563, 1995.

MODIFIED MALLET CLASSIFICATION OF SHOULDER FUNCTION

	Grade I	Grade II	Grade III	Grade IV	Grade V
Global abduction	None	< 30°	30°-90°	> 90°	Normal
Global external rotation	None	<0°	0°-20°	> 20°	Normal
Hand to neck	None	Not possible	Difficult	Easy	Normal
Hand on spine	None	Not possible	S1	T12	Normal
Hand to mouth	None	Marked trumpet sign	Partial trumpet sign	< 40° of abduction	Normal

Patients are asked to actively perform five different shoulder movements, and each movement is graded on a scale of 1 (no movement) to 5 (normal motion symmetric to the contralateral unaffected side.)

Adapted from Mallet J: Primaute du traitement de l'épaule—méthod d'expression des résultats, Rev Chir Ortho 58S:166, 1972.

to understanding whether a child can perform activities of daily living, such as perineal care and using zippers and buttons.

Characteristic deformities usually develop promptly. The shoulder becomes flexed, internally rotated, and slightly abducted; active abduction of the joint decreases; and external rotation disappears. Abnormal muscle forces across the shoulder lead to early changes in the glenoid. These changes include flattening of the posterior glenoid creating a pseudoglenoid (Fig. 34-55). As the deformity progresses, the glenohumeral joint center becomes more posterior and the glenoid becomes more retroverted and flattened or even convex. This leads to progressive posterior glenohumeral subluxation and eventual dislocation with the humeral head becoming flattened against the glenoid. These advanced glenohumeral changes can occur early and have been described by the age of 2 years.

Evaluation of the brachial plexus neurologic injury may include electrical diagnostic studies, ultrasound, myelography, and MRI. Combined use of MRI and electromyography is helpful because MRI may correlate better than electromyography with physical examination findings. In addition, MRI can help with anatomic localization of the nerve injury and help with surgical planning. Large diverticula and meningoceles indicate root avulsions. Plain radiography, arthrography, CT, and MRI, as well as diagnostic arthroscopy, have been used to determine the nature and severity of glenohumeral deformity. Often plain radiographs show delayed ossification of the proximal humerus. MRI has become more commonly used than CT for evaluation of the glenohumeral joint because of its ability to demonstrate the cartilaginous anatomy as well as the bony anatomy and lack of exposure of the patient to ionizing radiation. Waters et al. measured the glenoscapular angle (the degree of version of the glenoid) and

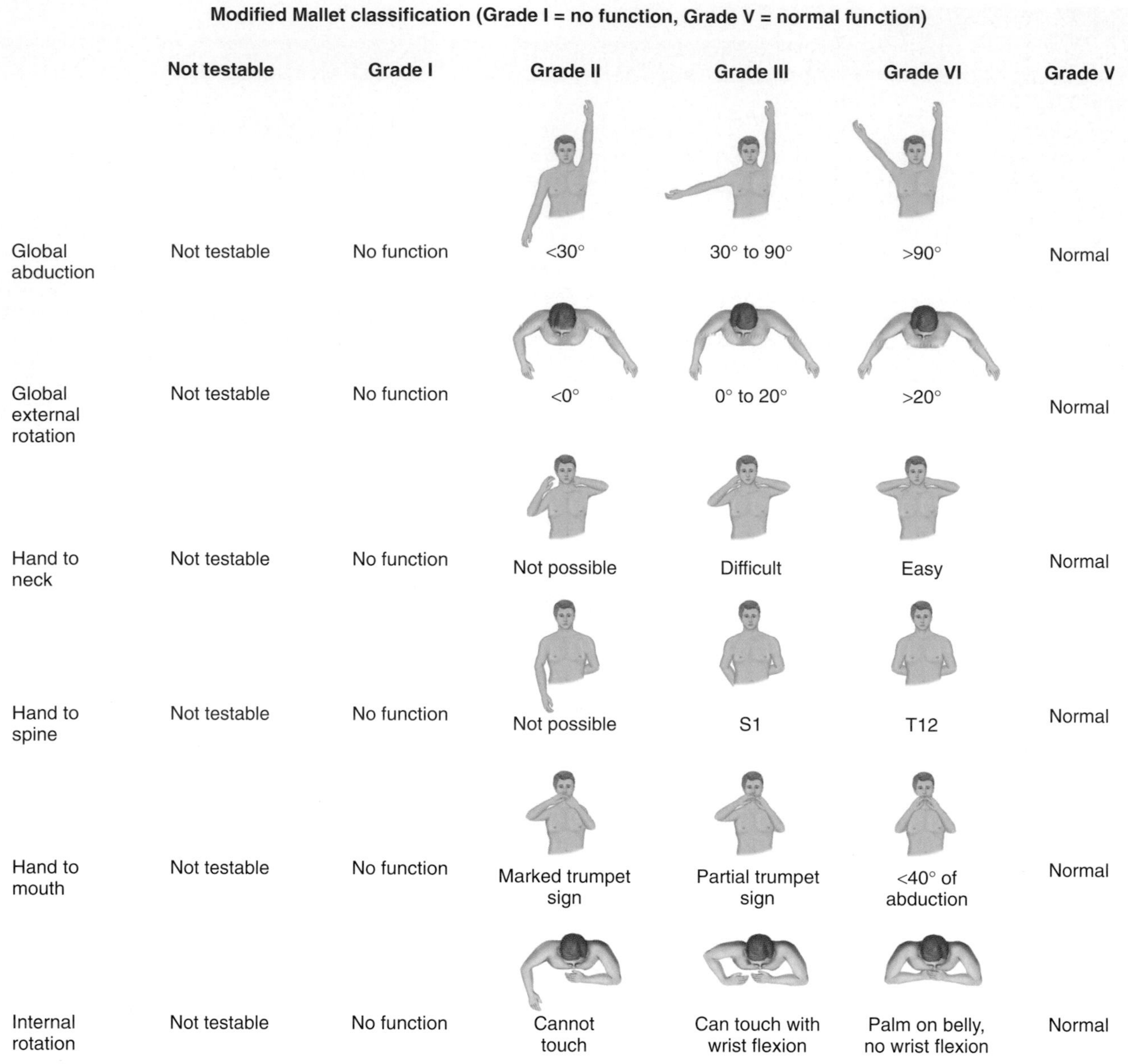

Modified Mallet classification (Grade I = no function, Grade V = normal function)

	Not testable	Grade I	Grade II	Grade III	Grade VI	Grade V
Global abduction	Not testable	No function	<30°	30° to 90°	>90°	Normal
Global external rotation	Not testable	No function	<0°	0° to 20°	>20°	Normal
Hand to neck	Not testable	No function	Not possible	Difficult	Easy	Normal
Hand to spine	Not testable	No function	Not possible	S1	T12	Normal
Hand to mouth	Not testable	No function	Marked trumpet sign	Partial trumpet sign	<40° of abduction	Normal
Internal rotation	Not testable	No function	Cannot touch	Can touch with wrist flexion	Palm on belly, no wrist flexion	Normal

FIGURE 34-54 Modified Mallet classification.

the percentage of the humeral head anterior to it on CT and MR images (Fig. 34-56) and classified the degree of glenohumeral deformity. The degree of deformity noted on the imaging studies can help guide the surgical management of a child with brachial plexus birth palsy. Diagnostic arthrography, although invasive, is the only modality in which dynamic assessment of the joint can be obtained. Often it is performed as part of the surgical reconstruction.

TREATMENT

Varying degrees of clinical presentation and recovery correlate with the extent of injury to the brachial plexus. Most brachial plexus birth palsies are mild injuries with a good prognosis. Most authors report significant recovery within the first 3 months, with slower recovery occurring within the next 6 to 12 months. If no evidence of deltoid or biceps recovery is seen by age 3 months, surgical exploration should be considered.

The aim of treatment in the initial stages is prevention of contractures of muscles and joints. Gentle passive exercises are begun to maintain full range of passive motion of all joints of the upper extremity. Scapular stabilization and passive glenohumeral mobilization in all planes is needed to prevent contractures about the shoulder. Range of motion of the elbow, wrist, and fingers also should be included. Cortical recognition and integration of the affected limb are promoted. Ezaki et al. described the injection of botulinum toxin-A into the internal rotator muscles as an adjunct to surgery to prevent internal rotation contractures and early posterior subluxation or dislocation of the shoulder in infants with neonatal brachial plexus palsy. The use of physical therapy with casting and botulism toxin injections have been shown to be effective in the treatment of elbow flexion contractures; however, recurrence is common and may be a result of noncompliance. Functional bracing may help encourage early hand use.

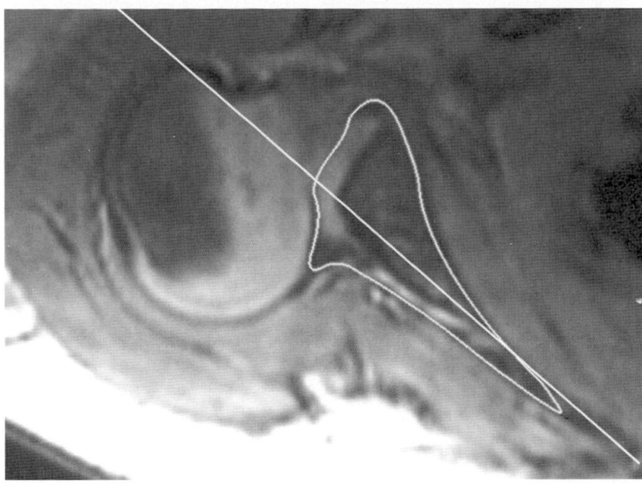

FIGURE 34-55 T2-weighted three-dimensional gradient-echo magnetic resonance image shows a pseudoglenoid. The glenoid contour and the scapular center line are enhanced with line tracings. (From Pearl ML, Edgerton BW, Kazimiroff PA, et al: Arthroscopic release and latissimus dorsi transfer for shoulder internal rotation contractures and glenohumeral deformity secondary to brachial plexus birth palsy, J Bone Joint Surg 88A:564, 2006.)

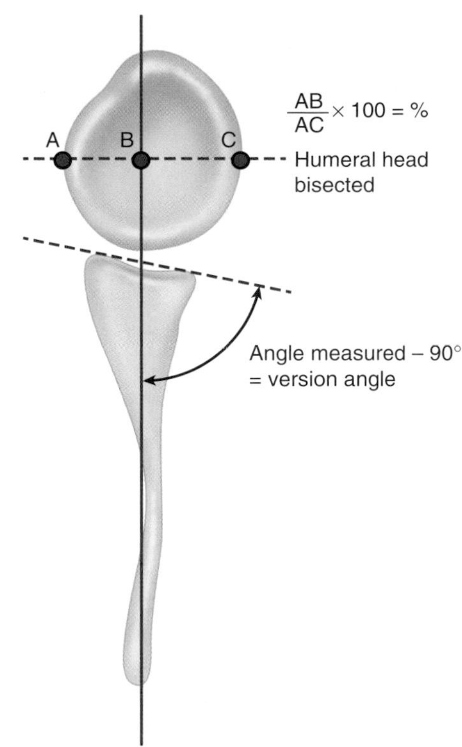

FIGURE 34-56 Measurement of the glenoscapular angle (glenoid version) and the percentage of posterior subluxation of the humeral head. To measure the glenoscapular angle, a line is drawn parallel to the scapula and a second line is drawn tangential to the joint. The second line connects the anterior and posterior margins of the glenoid. On MR images, the cartilaginous margins are used. On CT scans, the osseous margins are used. The intersecting line connects the center point of the first line (approximately the middle of the glenoid fossa) and the medial aspect of the scapula. The angle in the posterior medial quadrant (*arrow*) is measured with a goniometer; 90 degrees is subtracted from this measurement to determine glenoid version. The percentage of posterior subluxation is measured by defining the percentage of the humeral head that is anterior to the same scapular line. The greatest circumference of the head is measured as the distance from the scapular line to the anterior portion of the head. This ratio (the distance to the anterior aspect of the humeral head [*AB*] divided by the circumference of the humeral had [*AC*], multiplied by 100) is the percentage of subluxation. (Redrawn from Waters PM, Smith GR, Jaramillo D: Glenohumeral deformity secondary to brachial plexus birth palsy, J Bone Joint Surg 80A:668, 1998.)

The role and timing of microsurgical intervention in the treatment of brachial plexus birth palsy remain controversial. Microsurgical intervention at approximately 3 months of age is recommended in infants with global plexus palsies and Horner syndrome. These avulsion injuries have a poor prognosis of recovery. Reconstruction is limited to nerve transfers because grafting is not a viable option when the nerve root is avulsed from the spinal cord.

More controversy exists over the management of intraplexus ruptures in which there are varying degrees of injury severity and recovery. Return of antigravity elbow flexion strength is the key factor in determining the need for brachial plexus exploration and nerve reconstruction. Most authors recommend microsurgical intervention if antigravity flexion has not returned by 3 to 9 months of age. Resection and nerve grafting is the most widely used technique for restoring function; however, nerve transfers are gaining popularity as an addition to or in lieu of nerve grafting.

Indications for surgical intervention involving the shoulder are infantile dislocation, persistent internal rotation contracture refractory to physiotherapy, limitation of active abduction and external rotation function with plateauing of neural recovery, and progressive glenohumeral deformity. The general problems that must be corrected are muscle imbalance, soft-tissue contractures, and joint deformity. Surgery generally involves one of four soft-tissue procedures, all of which include some form of contracture release with or without a muscle transfer to augment external rotation: (1) anterior capsular release and Z-plasty lengthening of the subscapularis tendon with or without transfer of muscles for external rotation, (2) pectoralis major release with transfer of the latissimus and teres major as advocated by Hoffer et al., (3) subscapularis slide with or without a latissimus transfer, as described by Carlioz and Brahimi, or (4) arthroscopic release of the internal rotation contracture with or without latissimus transfer. For children with extensive glenohumeral deformity, external rotation osteotomy of the humerus is recommended to place the arm in a more functional position.

Waters recommended that patients with grade I (normal), grade II (mild increase in glenoid retroversion), or mild grade III (slight posterior subluxation) glenohumeral deformities have an anterior musculotendinous lengthening of the pectoralis major and posterior latissimus dorsi and teres major transfer to the rotator cuff. Patients with grade V glenohumeral deformities should have a humeral derotation osteotomy. Follow-up studies have shown that both tendon transfers alone and open reduction most commonly with tendon transfers improve shoulder range of motion; however, patients

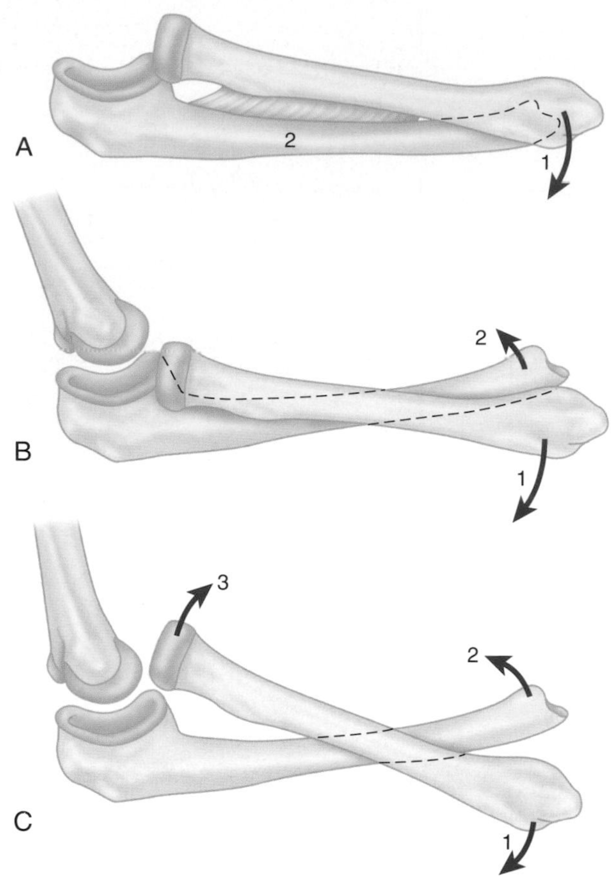

FIGURE 34-57 Physiopathology of supination deformity and progressive deformity with growth. **A,** Simple contracture with supination of the radius (1) and contracture of the interosseous membrane (2). **B,** Volar dislocation of the distal epiphysis of the ulna. **C,** Volar dislocation of the distal ulnar epiphysis and head of the radius *(final picture).*

who have open reduction demonstrate remodeling of the glenoid retroversion and improvement of glenohumeral joint, which is not seen in patients who have tendon transfer alone.

Elbow flexion and forearm supination deformities can occur with a Klumpke palsy (C8-T1) or a mixed brachial plexus lesion. Progressive deformities occur because of weak or absent triceps, pronator teres, and pronator quadratus muscles with an intact biceps muscle. This creates progressive elbow flexion and supination deformity from the unopposed biceps muscle. Radial head dislocation may occur with associated deformity of radius and ulna (Fig. 34-57). The wrist and hand usually are held in extreme dorsiflexion because of the unopposed wrist dorsiflexors. The biceps tendon can be Z-lengthened and rerouted around the radius to convert it from a supinator to a pronator (see Technique 34-29); this improves elbow extension and forearm pronation. In the presence of a supination contracture, a simultaneous interosseous membrane release may be effective. Bony correction of the forearm deformity can be performed more predictably. This can be achieved by forearm osteoclasis or osteotomy and internal fixation. The forearm should be positioned in 20 to 30 degrees of pronation.

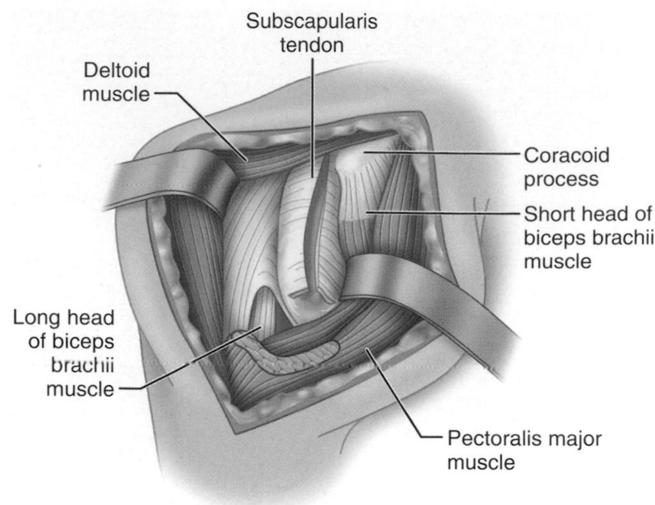

FIGURE 34-58 Anterior shoulder release for internal rotation contracture in brachial plexus palsy. **SEE TECHNIQUE 34-47.**

ANTERIOR SHOULDER RELEASE

TECHNIQUE 34-47

(FAIRBANK, SEVER)

- Make an incision on the anterior aspect of the shoulder in the deltopectoral groove distally from the tip of the coracoid process to a point distal to the tendinous insertion of the pectoralis major muscle; divide this tendon parallel to the humerus.
- Retract the anterior margin of the deltoid laterally and the pectoralis major medially and expose the coracobrachialis muscle.
- With the shoulder externally rotated and abducted, trace the coracobrachialis superiorly to the coracoid process.
- If the coracoid is elongated, resect 0.5 to 1.0 cm of its tip together with the insertions of the coracobrachialis, the short head of the biceps, and the pectoralis minor muscles; this resection increases the range of motion of the shoulder in external rotation and abduction.
- Now locate the inferior edge of the subscapularis tendon at its insertion on the lesser tuberosity of the humerus, elevate it with an elevator (Fig. 34-58A), and divide it completely without incising the capsule. External rotation and abduction of the shoulder then should be almost normal.
- A curved elongation of the acromion may interfere with abduction and with reduction of any mild posterior subluxation of the joint; in this event, either resect this obstructing part or divide the acromion and elevate this part.

POSTOPERATIVE CARE. An abduction splint that holds the shoulder in abduction and mild external rotation is applied and is worn constantly for 2 weeks and intermittently for another 4 weeks. Active exercises are started early and are continued until maximal improvement has occurred.

ROTATIONAL OSTEOTOMY OF THE HUMERUS

TECHNIQUE 34-48

(ROGERS)

- Approach the humerus anteriorly between the deltoid and pectoralis major muscles.
- With the arm abducted, perform an osteotomy 5 cm distal to the joint.
- Under direct vision externally rotate the distal fragment of the humerus the desired amount to correct the internal rotation deformity and ensure that the fragments are then apposed.
- Fix the osteotomy with a compression plate and screws.
- Close the wound.

POSTOPERATIVE CARE. A shoulder immobilizer or a sling is used for approximately 6 weeks with restriction of activities until radiographic healing.

DEROTATIONAL OSTEOTOMY WITH PLATE AND SCREW FIXATION

TECHNIQUE 34-49

(ABZUG ET AL.)

As an alternative, Abzug et al. described performing the derotational osteotomy and plate and screw fixation through a medial approach, which has the advantage of a more cosmetic scar.

- Make a medial incision overlying the intermuscular septum and midshaft of the humerus.
- Protect the superficial nerves, identify the intermuscular septum, and excise it.
- Retract the ulnar posteriorly and the median nerve and brachial artery anteriorly. Do not use loops around the nerves or reverse retractors than can place undue pressure on the nerve.
- Expose the humeral diaphysis.
- Choose a 6- to 8-hole plate, depending on the girth of the humerus, usually 2.7 mm or 3.5 mm. Place the plate over the humerus and insert the proximal three to four bicortical screws through the plate and humerus.
- Incise the periosteum only over the osteotomy site and place a Kirschner wire in the distal humerus below the intended osteotomy site to mark the amount of desired correction. Verify the position of the wire with a goniometer and visual assessment.
- With the wire placed in line with a hole in the plate, remove the plate and make the humeral osteotomy with an oscillating saw.
- Rotate the humerus so that the screw holes and Kirschner wire are aligned and the wire passes through a hole in the plate.
- Using the predrilled screw holes, fix the plate to the proximal fragment, close the osteotomy, and secure the distal fragment with screws using standard compression technique.
- Close the wound in standard fashion and apply a large bulky dressing from the hand to the axilla.

POSTOPERATIVE CARE. No splint is used postoperatively; however, a sling must be worn to prevent stress across the osteotomy site. The dressings are removed and a humeral brace is fabricated 2 to 3 weeks after surgery. The brace is worn for about 1 month until union is confirmed radiographically and clinically.

GLENOID ANTEVERSION OSTEOTOMY AND TENDON TRANSFER

Dodwell et al. described glenoid anteversion osteotomy as an alternative to external rotation humeral osteotomy to stabilize the shoulder and improve function in older children (>4 years of age) with severe glenohumeral dysplasia (Waters type IV or V). All 32 patients in their series had improvement in active external rotation.

TECHNIQUE 34-50

(DODWELL ET AL.)

- Through an L-shaped posterior incision (Fig. 34-59A), elevate the deltoid muscle origin laterally.
- Perform a subscapularis slide by elevating the muscle belly from the anterior aspect of the scapula in an inferior-to-superolateral direction.
- Translate the humeral head anteriorly in external rotation and progressively externally rotate the shoulder to between 70 and 90 degrees in adduction to complete the muscular slide.
- Release the teres major and latissimus dorsi tendons from their insertions on the proximal part of the humerus (Fig. 34-59B). Release any adhesions to ensure adequate excursion of these muscles.
- Approach the posterior aspect of the glenohumeral joint through the infraspinatus and teres minor interval. Detach the infraspinatus tendon from its insertion and clear the scapular neck subperiosteally, taking care to protect the suprascapular neurovascular bundle.
- Make a vertical posterior capsulotomy to visually inspect the joint.
- If the scapulohumeral angle was diminished on preoperative evaluation, indicating insufficient shoulder elevation, recess the tendon of the long head of the triceps origin at the glenoid.
- If a marked Putti sign (scapular rotation with a prominent superomedial corner at the base of the neck) is present, indicating a substantial abduction contracture, perform a lateral slide of the supraspinatus.

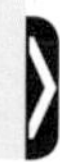

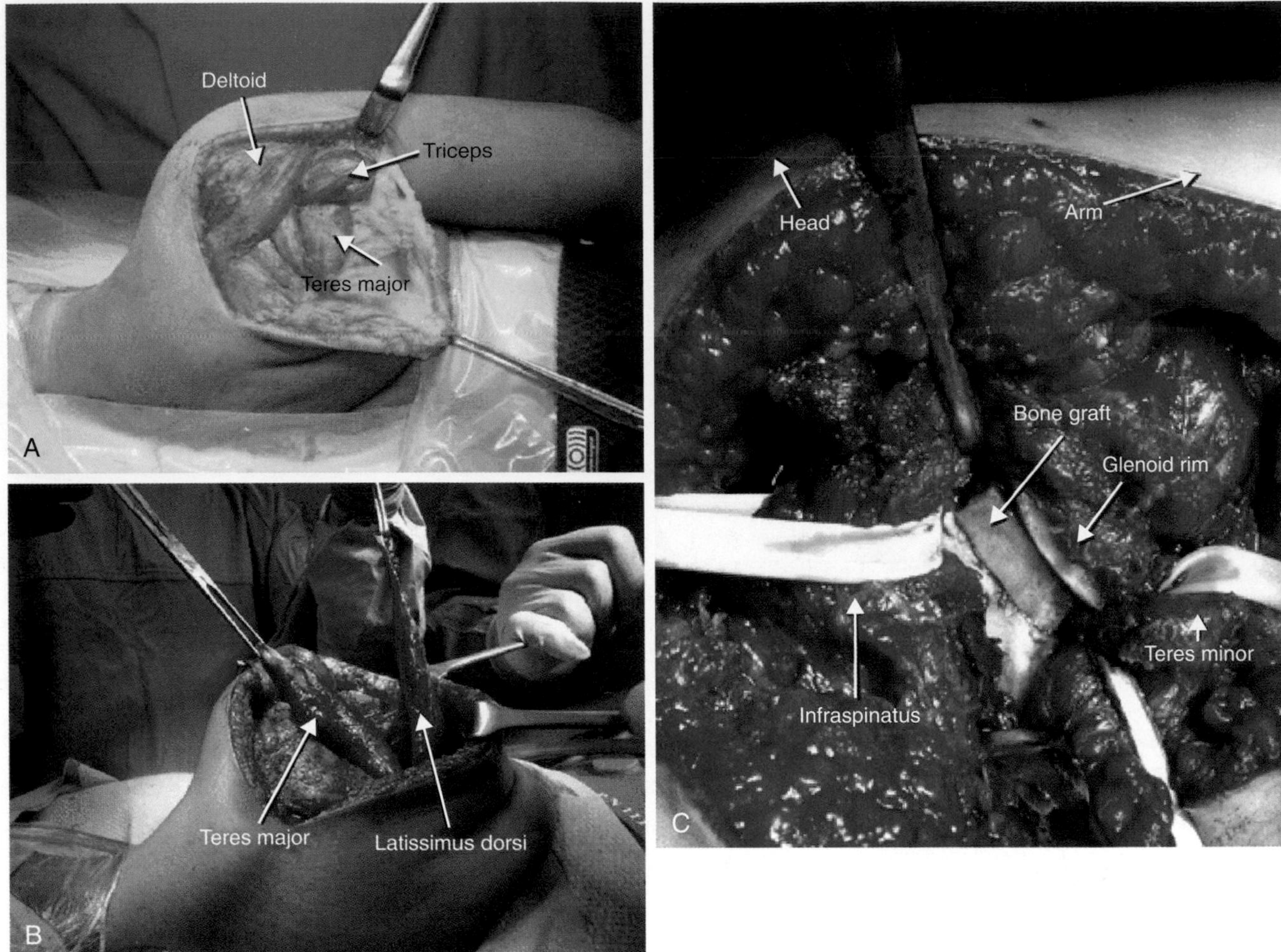

FIGURE 34-59 **A,** L-shaped posterior incision. **B,** Release of the teres major and latissimus dorsi tendons lateral to the long head of the triceps. **C,** Cortical wedge inserted in the osteotomy site. (From Dodwell E, Calaghan J, Anthony A, et al: Combined glenoid anteversion osteotomy and tendon transfers for brachial plexus birth palsy, J Bone Joint Surg 94A:2145, 2012.) **SEE TECHNIQUE 34-50.**

- Harvest a tricortical autograft from the medial aspect of the scapular spine or from the posterior aspect of the acromion. Based on preoperative templating from MR or CT images, determine the length of posterior cortical opening required to correct the glenoid retroversion to neutral, with the hinge point being the anterior cortex, and size the bone graft appropriately.
- Use an osteotome to make a scapular neck osteotomy extending from the lateral aspect of the spinoglenoid notch to the inferior aspect of the scapular neck, staying at least 5 mm medial to the glenoid rim to ensure protection of the glenoid blood supply and avoid osteonecrosis. Deepen the osteotomy to just short of the anterior cortex to retain an intact anterior hinge. Align the osteotomy parallel to the retroverted glenoid surface under direct observation.
- Use a narrow osteotome to lever open the osteotomy site and insert the bone graft (Fig. 34-59C). Gently tamp the graft into place so that it acts as a wedge, opening the cortex of the posterior aspect of the neck, and is stable.
- With the joint in the reduced position, close the capsule without capsulorrhaphy to minimize stiffness in internal rotation. Repair the infraspinatus anatomically. Suture the latissimus dorsi and teres major tendons into a longitudinal bone trough in the region of the greater humeral tuberosity, with the teres major in the inferior aspect of the trough and the latissimus, given its greater excursion, superior. Repair the deltoid to the scapular spine with sutures through bone.
- Apply a shoulder spica cast with the shoulder in maximal external rotation (70 to 90 degrees) and limited (20 to 30 degrees) abduction.

POSTOPERATIVE CARE. The cast is worn for 5 or 6 weeks, at which time a supervised physical therapy program is begun.

RELEASE OF THE INTERNAL ROTATION CONTRACTURE AND TRANSFER OF THE LATISSIMUS DORSI AND TERES MAJOR

When performed before age 6 years, the Sever-L'Episcopo procedure, as modified by Hoffer, improves external rotation of the shoulder by releasing the internal rotation contracture and transferring the latissimus dorsi and teres major posteriorly to provide active external rotation.

TECHNIQUE 34-51

(SEVER-L'EPISCOPO, GREEN)

- Place a sandbag under the upper part of the chest for proper exposure. Prepare and drape in the usual manner. An adequate amount of whole blood should be available for transfusion.
- Make an anterior incision beginning over the coracoid process and extending distally along the deltopectoral groove for 12 cm (Fig. 34-60A).
- Identify the cephalic vein and ligate or retract it with a few fibers of the deltoid muscle.
- With blunt dissection, develop the interval between the pectoral and deltoid muscles. Expose the coracobrachialis, the short head of the biceps, the coracoid process, the insertion of the tendinous portion of the subscapularis, and the insertion of the pectoralis major.
- Detach the short head of the biceps and coracobrachialis from their origin on the coracoid process and reflect downward.
- In the distal part of the wound, expose the insertion of the pectoralis major at its humeral attachment (Fig. 34-60B).
- With a periosteal elevator, reflect the muscle fibers of the pectoralis major medially to expose the tendinous portion of its insertion.
- To perform Z-lengthening, divide the distal half of the tendinous insertion of the pectoralis major immediately on the humeral shaft (Fig. 34-60C).
- Divide the upper half of the tendinous portion of the pectoralis major as far medially as good aponeurotic tendinous material exists, usually 4 to 5 cm from its insertion (Fig. 34-60D). Later, the distal tendon stump will be attached to the proximal tendon left inserted on the humerus, thus providing further length to the pectoralis major. The reattachment of the tendon more proximally permits a greater degree of shoulder abduction but still allows rotary function.
- Apply whip sutures to the tendon still attached to the shaft and to the portion of the tendon attached to the muscle.
- Expose the subscapularis muscle over the head of the humerus. Starting medially with a blunt instrument, separate the subscapularis and elevate it from the capsule. Do not open the shoulder capsule. With a knife, lengthen the subscapularis tendon by an oblique cut (Fig. 34-60E).
- Starting medially, split the tendon into anterior and posterior halves, becoming more superficial laterally and completing the division at the insertion of the subscapularis into the humerus. Again, take care not to open the capsule.
- Once the subscapularis has been divided, the shoulder joint will abduct and externally rotate freely.
- If the coracoid process is elongated, hooked downward and laterally, and limits external rotation, it should be resected to its base. Likewise, if the acromion process is beaked downward and obstructs shoulder abduction, partially resect it.
- Next, identify the insertions of the latissimus dorsi and teres major and expose by separating them from adjacent tissues both anteriorly and posteriorly.
- The attachment of the latissimus dorsi is superior and anterior to that of the teres major. Divide both tendons immediately on bone and suture each tendon with a whip stitch.
- With the patient turned over on the side and with the patient's arm adducted across the chest, make a 7- to 8-cm incision over the deltoid-triceps interval (Fig. 34-60F).
- Retract the deltoid muscle anteriorly and the long head of the triceps posteriorly. Be careful not to damage the radial and axillary nerves.
- Subperiosteally expose the lateral surface of the proximal diaphysis of the humerus.
- Make a 5-cm longitudinal cleft using drills, an osteotome, and a curet.
- Drill four holes from the depth of the cleft coming out on the medial surface of the humeral shaft at the site of the former insertion of the teres major and latissimus dorsi muscles.
- Identify the tendons of the latissimus dorsi and teres major in the anterior wound and deliver them into the posterior incision so that their line of pull is straight from their origins to the proposed site of attachment on the lateral humerus.
- Draw the latissimus dorsi and teres major tendons into the slot in the humerus and tie securely into position with 1-0 silk sutures in the front (Fig. 34-60G and H).
- Suture the subscapularis tendon, which is lengthened "on the flat," at its divided ends to provide maximal lengthening. Suture the pectoralis major in a similar way.
- Reattach the coracobrachialis and short head of the biceps to the base of the coracoid process. If the coracobrachialis and short head of the biceps are short, lengthen them at their musculotendinous junction (Fig. 34-60I and J).
- The lengthened muscles should be of sufficient length to permit complete external rotation in abduction without undue tension.
- Close the wound in the usual manner and immobilize the upper limb in a previously prepared, bivalved shoulder spica cast that holds the shoulder in 90 degrees of abduction, 90 degrees of external rotation, and 20 degrees of forward flexion. Position the elbow in 80 to 90 degrees of flexion.
- Place the forearm and hand in a functional neutral position.

POSTOPERATIVE CARE. Exercises are begun 3 weeks after surgery to develop abduction and external rotation

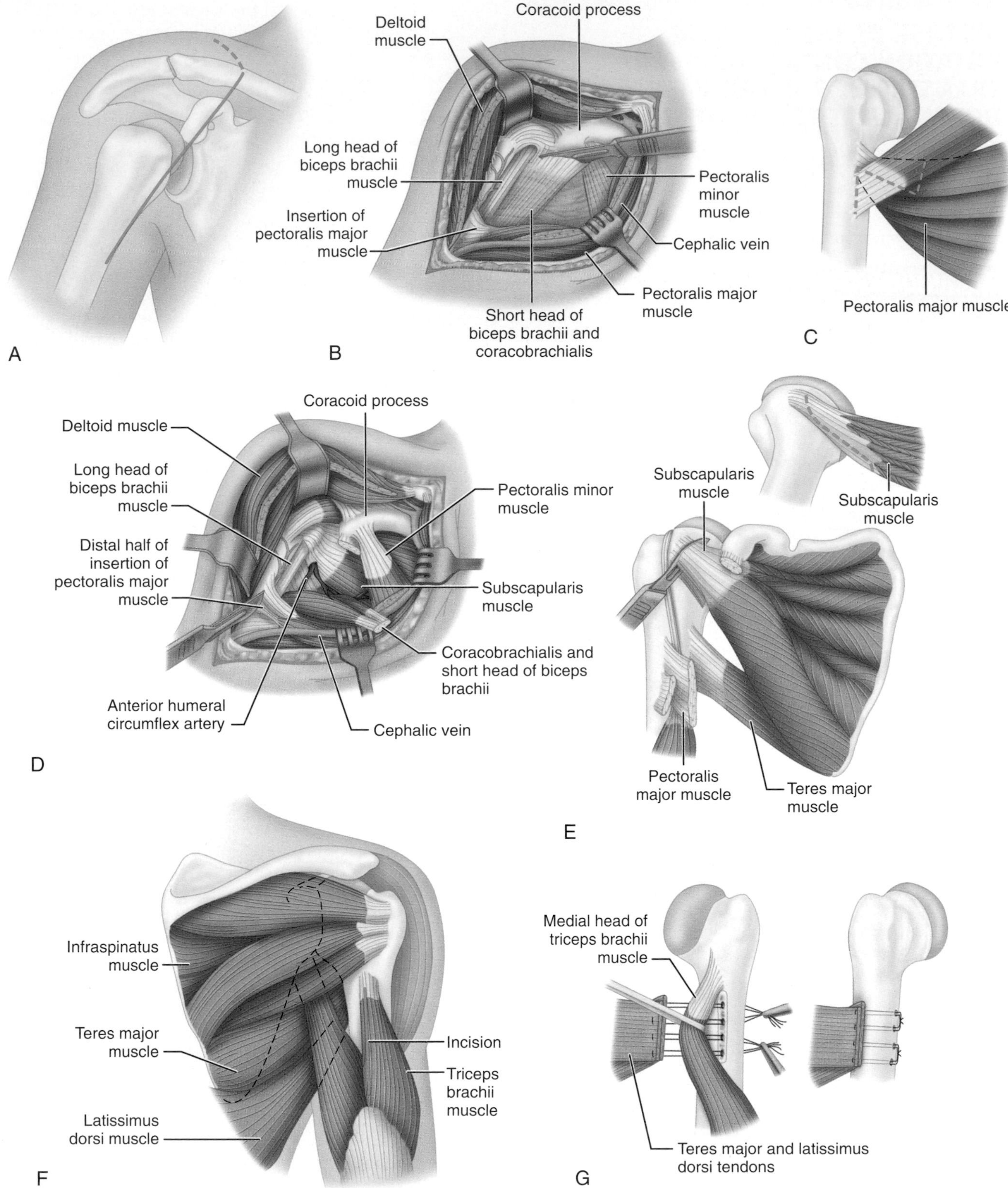

FIGURE 34-60 Sever-L'Episcopo and Green procedure. **A,** Anterior incision. **B,** Exposure of insertion of pectoralis major at humeral attachment. **C,** Incisions of tendinous insertion of pectoralis major for Z-lengthening. **D,** Distal half of tendinous insertion of pectoralis major on shaft of humerus is divided. **E,** Subscapularis is divided by oblique cut. **F,** Incision over deltoid-triceps interval *(back view).* **G,** Teres major and latissimus dorsi tendons are attached to cleft in lateral humerus.

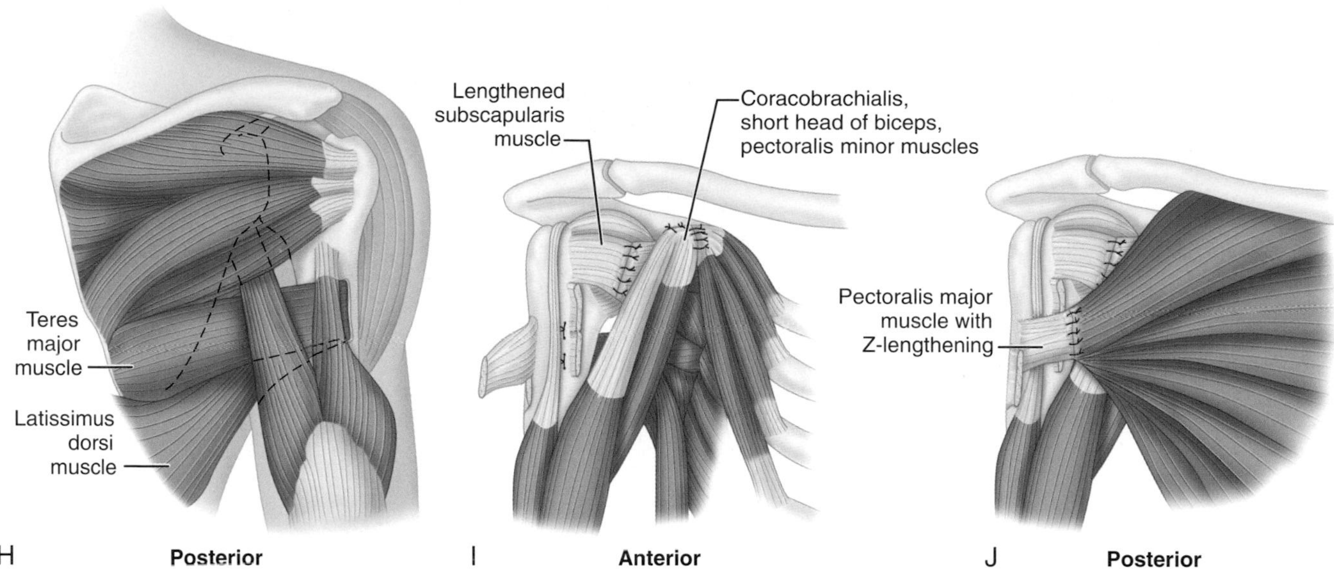

FIGURE 34-60, cont'd **H,** Back view showing reattachment of muscles. **I** and **J,** Front views showing reattachment of muscles. **SEE TECHNIQUE 34-51.**

of the shoulder, as well as shoulder adduction and internal rotation. Particular emphasis is given to developing the function and strength of the transferred muscles. When the arm adducts satisfactorily, a sling is used during the day and the bivalved shoulder spica cast is worn at night. The night support is continued for 3 to 6 more months. Exercises are performed for many months or years to preserve functional range of motion of the shoulder and to maintain muscle control.

Transfer of the latissimus dorsi and the teres major to the rotator cuff has been reported to have a stabilizing effect on the rotator cuff and to increase glenohumeral abduction and external rotation (Fig. 34-61).

Arthroscopic techniques have been developed for release and for release combined with latissimus dorsi transfer (recommended for older children). These procedures have been reported to restore nearly normal passive external rotation and a centered glenohumeral joint at the time of surgery; however, gains in active elevation are minimal and loss of internal rotation, from moderate to severe, occurs in all children after this surgery. Pearl et al. listed the following guidelines for arthroscopic treatment of contractures and deformity secondary to brachial plexus birth palsy:

Arthroscopic release: Children younger than 3 years of age with passive external rotation of less than neutral (0 degrees) with the arm at the side

Arthroscopic release plus latissimus dorsi transfer: Children older than 3 years of age with a similar degree of contracture

Arthroscopic latissimus dorsi transfer without release: Children older than 3 years of age who have no substantial internal rotation contracture but have weakness of external rotation.

ARTHROSCOPIC RELEASE AND TRANSFER OF THE LATISSIMUS DORSI

TECHNIQUE 34-52

(PEARL ET AL.)

- With the patient in a lateral decubitus position, establish a posterior portal (see Chapter 52). Because of contracture and advanced deformity, it may be necessary to abduct the arm to approximately 90 degrees to allow passage of the scope across the glenohumeral joint. A surgical assistant maintains arm position while applying longitudinal traction. Make the posterior portal at the posterior glenohumeral joint line about 1 cm below the level of the posterior part of the acromion. Take care to avoid making the portal too low. A superior position makes it easier to insert the arthroscope over the top of the humeral head to avoid damage to the articular surface.
- Make an anterior portal from outside in, under direct observation through the posterior portal.
- Use an electrocautery device to release the anterior capsular ligaments, including the middle glenohumeral ligament and the anterior portion of the inferior glenohumeral ligament, at their attachment to the glenoid labrum. Basket forceps also are helpful.
- After release of the anterior soft tissues, identify the axillary nerve. Do not release the muscular portion of the subscapularis.
- Release the contracture by tenotomy of the subscapular tendon at its insertion and the overlying joint capsule. In younger children, this should allow full external rotation

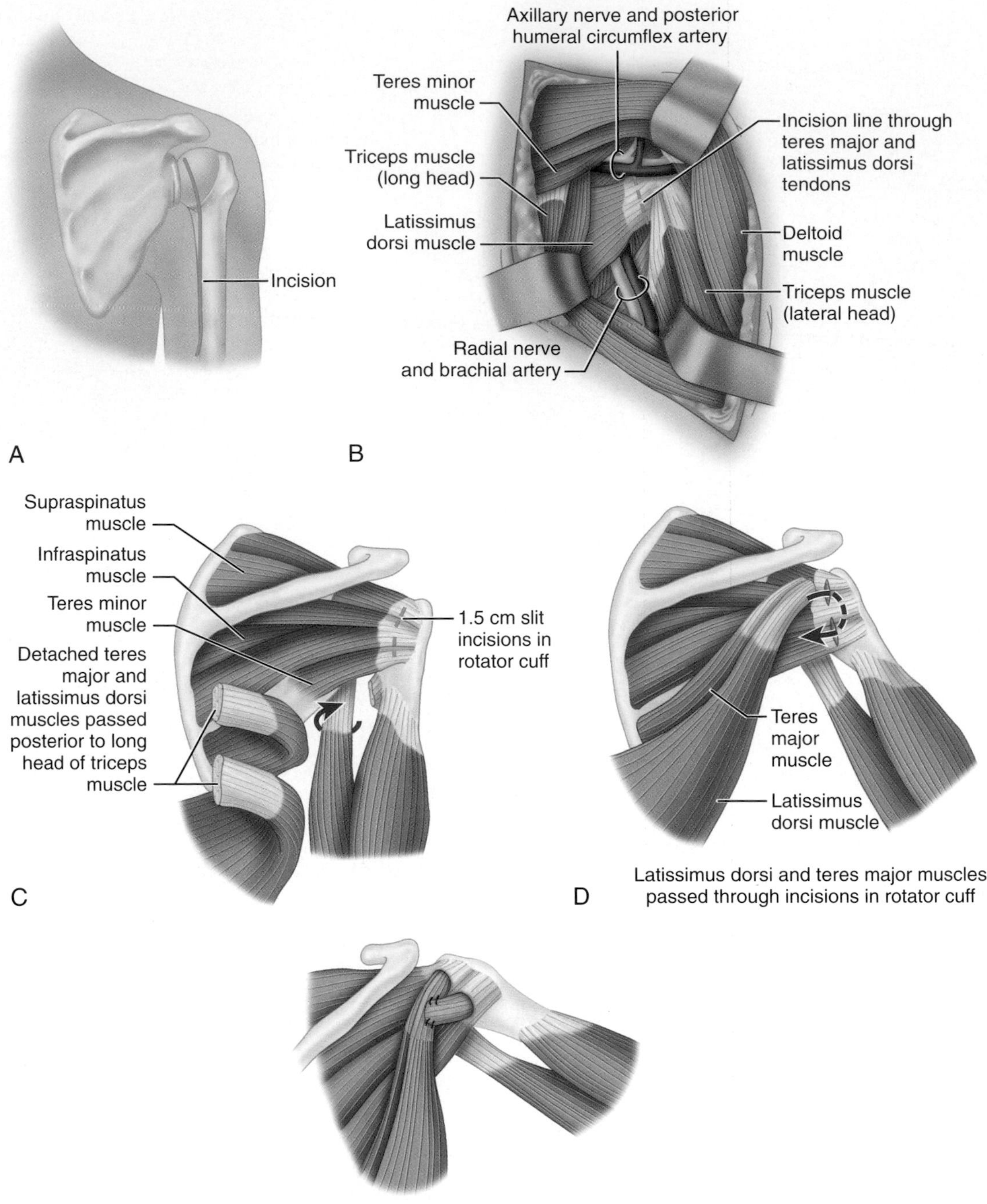

FIGURE 34-61 **Latissimus dorsi and teres major transfer to the rotator cuff.** (Redrawn from Herring JA, editor: Tachdjian's pediatric orthopaedics, ed 3. Philadelphia, 2002, Saunders.)

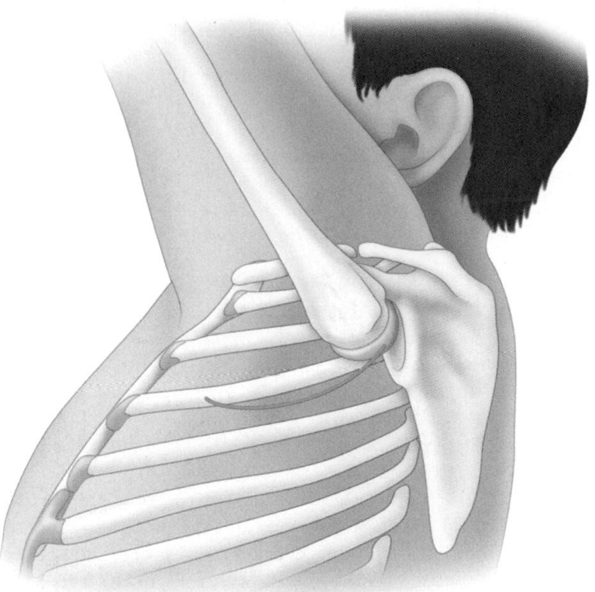

FIGURE 34-62 **Curved incision in the skin lines, just medial to the posterior axillary crease toward the midline of the axilla, for latissimus dorsi transfer in conjunction with arthroscopic contracture release.** (From Pearl ML, Edgerton BW, Kazimiroff PA, et al: Arthroscopic release and latissimus dorsi transfer for shoulder internal rotation contractures and glenohumeral deformity secondary to brachial plexus birth palsy, J Bone Joint Surg 88A:564, 2006.) **SEE TECHNIQUE 34-52.**

(70 to 90 degrees) with the arm at the side. If necessary in older children and those with more severe contractures, release the rotator interval tissue, exposing the base of the coracoid process. Release is not considered complete unless external rotation of 45 degrees or more is obtained.

- If latissimus dorsi transfer is to be done, make a 6- to 8-cm curved incision in the skin lines, just medial to the posterior axillary crease toward the midline of the axilla (Fig. 34-62). In larger children, extend the incision to include the posterior arthroscopic portal.
- Carefully isolate the latissimus dorsi tendon from the teres major (which is left in situ), release it directly from the humerus, and transfer it under the posterior aspect of the deltoid to the greater tuberosity just adjacent to the infraspinatus tendon insertion. Secure the tendon with four No. 2 Ethibond sutures.
- Apply a shoulder spica cast to hold the arm in adduction and full external rotation.

POSTOPERATIVE CARE. The shoulder spica cast is worn for 6 weeks and then modified to be used as a night splint for an additional 6 weeks.

REFERENCES

POLIOMYELITIS

Anderson GA, Thomas BP, Pallapati SC: Flexor carpi ulnaris tendon transfer to the split brachioradialis tendon to restore supination in paralytic forearms, *J Bone Joint Surg* 92B:230, 2010.

Chen D, Chen J, Liu F, Jiang Y: Tibial lengthening using a humeral intramedullary nail combined with a single-plane external fixator for leg discrepancy in sequelae of poliomyelitis, *J Pediatr Orthop B* 20:84, 2011.

Chumakov K, Ehrenfeld E: New generation of inactivated poliovirus vaccines for universal immunization after eradication of poliomyelitis, *Clin Infect Dis* 47:1587, 2008.

de Moraes Barros Fucs PM, Svartman C, de Assumpcao RM: Knee flexion deformity from poliomyelitis treated by supracondylar femoral extension osteotomy, *Int Orthop* 29:380, 2005.

Dutta A: Epidemiology of poliomyelitis—options and update, *Vaccine* 26:5767, 2008.

Emara KM, Khames A: Functional outcome after lengthening with and without deformity correction in polio patients, *Int Orthop* 32:403, 2008.

Fucs PM, Svartman C, Santili C, et al: Results in the treatment of paralytic calcaneus-valgus feet with the Westin technique, *Int Orthop* 31:555, 2007.

Jordan L, Kligman M, Sculco TP: Total knee arthroplasty in patients with poliomyelitis, *J Arthroplasty* 22:543, 2007.

Kraay MJ, Bigach SD: The neuromuscularly challenged patient. Total hip replacement is now an option, *Bone Joint J* 96-B(11 Suppl A):27, 2014.

Lee WC, Ahn JY, Cho JH, Park CH: Realignment surgery for severe talar tilt secondary to paralytic cavovarus, *Foot Ankle Int* 34:1552, 2013.

Miller JD, Pinero JR, Goldstein R, et al: Shoulder arthrodesis for treatment of flail shoulder in children with polio, *J Pediatr Orthop* 31:679, 2011.

Nathanson N, Kew OM: From emergence to eradication: the epidemiology of poliomyelitis deconstructed, *Am J Epidemiol* 172:1213, 2010.

Provelengios S, Papavasiliou KA, Krykos MJ, et al: The role of pantalar arthrodesis in the treatment of paralytic foot deformities. A long-term follow-up study, *J Bone Joint Surg* 91A:575, 2009.

Provelengios S, Papavasiliou KA, Krykos MJ, et al: The role of pantalar arthrodesis in the treatment of paralytic foot deformities. Surgical technique, *J Bone Joint Surg* 92A(Suppl 1):44, 2010.

Rahman J, Hanna SA, Kayani B, et al: Custom rotating hinge total knee arthroplasty in patients with poliomyelitis affected limbs, *Int Orthop* 39:833, 2015.

Rolfe KW, Green TA, Lawrence JF: Corrective osteotomies and osteosynthesis for supination contracture of the forearm in children, *J Pediatr Orthop* 29:406, 2009.

Savolainen-Kopra C, Blomqvist S: Mechanisms of genetic variation in polioviruses, *Rev Med Virol* 20:358, 2010.

Sierra RJ, Schoeniger SR, Millis M, Ganz R: Periacetabular osteotomy for containment of the nonarthritis dysplastic hip secondary to poliomyelitis, *J Bone Joint Surg* 92A:2917, 2010.

Song HR, Myrboh V, Oh CW, et al: Tibial lengthening and concomitant foot deformity correction in 14 patients with permanent deformity after poliomyelitis, *Acta Orthop* 76:261, 2005.

Tigani D, Fosco M, Amendola L, Boriani L: Total knee arthroplasty in patients with poliomyelitis, *Knee* 16:501, 2009.

Wenz W, Bruckner T, Akbar M: Complete tendon transfer and inverse Lambrinudi arthrodesis: preliminary results of a new technique for the treatment of paralytic pes calcaneus, *Foot Ankle Int* 29:683, 2008.

Yoon BH, Lee YK, Yoo JJ, et al: Total hip arthroplasty performed in patients with residual poliomyelitis: does in work?, *Clin Orthop Relat Res* 472:933, 2014.

MYELOMENINGOCELE

Bartonek A, Eriksson M, Guitierrez-Farewik EM: Effects of carbon fibre spring orthoses on gait in ambulatory children with motor disorders and plantarflexor weakness, *Dev Med Child Neurol* 49:615, 2007.

Battibugli S, Gryfakis N, Dias L, et al: Functional gait comparison between children with myelomeningocele: shunt versus no shunt, *Dev Med Child Neurol* 49:764, 2007.

Chakraborty A, Crimmins D, Hayward R, Thompson D: Toward reducing shunt placement rates in patients with myelomeningocele, *J Neurosurg Pediatr* 1:361, 2008.

Chambers HG: Update on neuromuscular disorders in pediatric orthopaedics: Duchenne muscular dystrophy, myelomeningocele, and cerebral palsy, *J Pediatr Orthop* 34(Suppl 1):S44, 2014.

Dobbs MB, Purcell DB, Nunley R, Morcuende JA: Early results of a new method of treatment for idiopathic congenital vertical talus. Surgical technique, *J Bone Joint Surg* 89A(Suppl 2):111, 2007.

Flanagan A, Gorzkowski M, Altiok H, et al: Activity level, functional health, and quality of life in children with myelomeningocele as perceived by parents, *Clin Orthop Relat Res* 469:1230, 2011.

Garg S, Oetgen M, Rathjen K, Richards BS: Kyphectomy improves sitting and skin problems in patients with myelomeningocele, *Clin Orthop Relat Res* 469:1279, 2011.

Gerlach DJ, Gurnett CA, Limpaphayom N, et al: Early results of the Ponseti method for the treatment of clubfoot associated with myelomeningocele, *J Bone Joint Surg* 91A:1350, 2009.

Glard Y, Launay F, Viehweger E, et al: Hip flexion contracture and lumbar spine lordosis in myelomeningocele, *J Pediatr Orthop* 25:476, 2005.

Glard Y, Launay F, Viehweger E, et al: Neurological classification in myelomeningocele as a spine deformity predictor, *J Pediatr Orthop B* 16:287, 2007.

Guille JT, Sarwark JF, Sherk HH, Kumar SJ: Congenital and developmental deformities of the spine in children with myelomeningocele, *J Am Acad Orthop Surg* 14:294, 2006.

Gupta RT, Vankoski S, Novak RA, Dias LS: Trunk kinematics and the influence on valgus knee stress in persons with high sacral level myelomeningocele, *J Pediatr Orthop* 25:89, 2005.

Gutierrez EM, Bartonek A, Haglund-Akerlind Y, Saraste H: Kinetics of compensatory gait in persons with myelomeningocele, *Gait Posture* 21:12, 2005.

Hoiness PR, Kirkhus E: Grice arthrodesis in the treatment of valgus feet in children with myelomeningocele: a 12.8-year follow-up study, *J Child Orthop* 3:283, 2009.

Kelly SP, Bache CE, Graham HK, Donnan LT: Limb reconstruction using circular frames in children and adolescents with spina bifida, *J Bone Joint Surg* 92B:1017, 2010.

Khoshbin A, Vivas L, Law PW, et al: The long-term outcome of patients treated operatively and non-operatively for scoliosis deformity secondary to spina bifida, *Bone Joint J* 96:1244, 2014.

Klatt J, Stevens PM: Guided growth for fixed knee flexion deformity, *J Pediatr Orthop* 28:626, 2008.

Moen TC, Dias L, Swaroop VT, et al: Radical posterior capsulectomy improves sagittal knee motion in crouch gait, *Clin Orthop Relat Res* 469:1286, 2011.

Moen T, Gryfakis N, Dias L, Lemke L: Crouched gait in myelomeningocele: a comparison between the degree of knee flexion contracture in the clinical examination and during gait, *J Pediatr Orthop* 25:657, 2005.

Molto FJL, Garrido IM: Retrospective review of L3 myelomeningocele in three age groups: should posterolateral iliopsoas transfer still be indicated to stabilize the hip, *J Pediatr Orthop* 14B:177, 2005.

Padmanabhan R: Etiolgy, pathogenesis and prevention of neural tube defects, *Congenit Anom (Kyoto)* 46:55, 2006.

Park KB, Park HW, Joo SY, Kim HW: Surgical treatment of calcaneal deformity in a select group of patients with myelomeningocele, *J Bone Joint Surg* 90A:2149, 2008.

Patel J, Walker JL, Talwalkar VR, et al: Correlation of spine deformity, lung function, and seat pressure in spina bifida, *Clin Orthop Relat Res* 469:1302, 2011.

Rowe DE, Jadhav AL: Care of the adolescent with spina bifida, *Pediatr Clin North Am* 55:1359, 2008.

Sibinski M, Synder M, Higgs ZC, et al: Quality of life and functional disability in skeletally mature patients with myelomeningocele-related spinal deformity, *J Pediatr Orthop B* 22:106, 2013.

Spiro AS, Babin K, Lipovas S, et al: Anterior femoral epiphysiodesis for the treatment of fixed knee flexion deformity in spina bifida patients, *J Pediatr Orthop* 30:858, 2010.

Swaroop VT, Dias L: Orthopedic management of spina bifida: I. Hip, knee, and rotational deformities, *J Child Orthop* 3:441, 2009.

Swaroop VT, Dias L: Orthopaedic management of spina bifida: II. Foot and ankle deformities, *J Child Orthop* 5:403, 2009.

Swaroop VT, Dias LS: Strategies of hip management in myelomeningocele: to do or not to do, *Hip Int* 19(Suppl 6):S53, 2009.

Swaroop VT, Dias LS: Myelomeningocele. In Weinstein SL, Flynn JM, editors: *Lovell and Winter's Pediatric Orthopaedics*, ed 7, Philadelphia, 2014, Wolters Kluwer.

Thompson JD, Segal LS: Orthopaedic management of spina bifida, *Dev Disabil Res Rev* 16:96, 2010.

Wolf SI, Alimusaj M, Rettig O, Döderlein L: Dynamic assist by carbon fiber spring AFOs for patients with myelomeningocele, *Gait Posture* 28:175, 2008.

Wright JG: Hip and spine surgery is of questionable value in spina bifida: an evidence-based review, *Clin Orthop Relat Res* 469:1258, 2011.

ARTHROGRYPOSIS MULTIPLEX CONGENITA

Astur N, Flynn JM, Flynn JM, et al: The efficacy of rib-based distraction with VEPTR in the treatment of early-onset scoliosis in patients with arthrogryposis, *J Pediatr Orthop* 34:8, 2014.

Bamshad M, Van Heest AE, Pleasure D: Arthrogryposis: a review and update, *J Bone Joint Surg Am* 91A(Suppl 4):40, 2009.

Beals RK: The distal arthrogryposes: a new classification of peripheral contractures, *Clin Orthop Relat Res* 435:203, 2005.

Bevan WP, Hall JG, Bamshad M, et al: Arthrogryposis multiplex congenita (amyoplasia): an orthopaedic perspective, *J Pediatr Orthop* 27:594, 2007.

Boehm S, Limpaphayom N, Alaee F, et al: Early results of the Ponseti method for the treatment of clubfoot in distal arthrogryposis, *J Bone Joint Surg* 90A:1501, 2008.

Dillon ER, Bjornson KF, Jaffe KM, et al: Ambulatory activity in youth with arthrogryposis: a cohort study, *J Pediatr Orthop* 29:214, 2009.

Eldelman M, Katzman A: Treatment of arthrogrypotic foot deformities with the Taylor Spatial Frame, *J Pediatr Orthop* 31:429, 2011.

Eriksson M, Gutierrez-Farewik EM, Broström E, Bartonek A: Gait in children with arthrogryposis multiplex congenital, *J Child Orthop* 4:21, 2010.

Ezaki M, Carter PR: Carpal wedge osteotomy for the arthrogrypotic wrist, *Tech Hand Up Extrem Surg* 8:224, 2004.

Fassier A, Wicart P, Dubousset J, Seringe R: Arthrogryposis multiplex congenita: long-term follow-up from birth until skeletal maturity, *J Child Orthop* 3:383, 2009.

Fucs PMMB, Svartman C, Cesar de Assumpção RM, Verde SRL: Quadricepsplasty in arthrogryposis (amyoplasia): long-term followup, *J Pediatr Orthop* 14:219, 2005.

Greggi T, Martikos K, Pipitone E, et al: Surgical treatment of scoliosis in a rare disease: arthrogryposis, *Scoliosis* 5:24, 2010.

Ho CA, Karol LA: The utility of knee releases in arthrogryposis, *J Pediatr Orthop* 28:307, 2008.

Kowalczyk B, Lejman T: Short-term experience with Ponseti casting and the Achilles tenotomy method for clubfeet treatment in arthrogryposis multiplex congenita, *J Child Orthop* 2:365, 2008.

Lahoti O, Bell MJ: Transfer of pectoralis major in arthrogryposis to restore elbow flexion: deteriorating results in the long term, *J Bone Joint Surg* 87B:858, 2005.

Morcuende JA, Dobbs MB, Frick SL: Results of the Ponseti method in patients with clubfoot associated with arthrogryposis, *Iowa Orthop J* 28:22, 2008.

Mubarak SJ, Dimeglio A: Navicular excision and cubcid closing wedge for severe cavovarus foot deformities: a salvage procedure, *J Pediatr Orthop* 31:551, 2011.

Palocaren T, Thabet AM, Rogers K, et al: Anterior distal femoral stapling for correction knee flexion contracture in children with arthrogryposis-preliminary results, *J Pediatr Orthop* 30:169, 2010.

van Bosse HJ, Feldman DS, Anavian J, Sala DA: Treatment of knee flexion contractures in patients with arthrogryposis, *J Pediatr Orthop* 27:903, 2007.

Van Heest A, James MA, Lewica A, Anderson KA: Posterior elbow capsulotomy with tricpes lengthening for treatment of elbow extension contracture in children with arthrogryposis, *J Bone Joint Surg* 90A:1517, 2008.

Van Heest A, Rodriguez R: Dorsal carpal wedge osteotomy in the arthrogrypotic wrist, *J Hand Surg Am* 38:265, 2013.

Wada A, Yamaguchi T, Nakamura T, et al: Surgical treatment of hip dislocation in amyoplasia-type arthrogryposis, *J Pediatr Orthop B* 21:381, 2012.

Widman RF, Do TT, Burke SW: Radical soft-tissue release of the arthrogrypotic clubfoot, *J Pediatr Orthop* 14B:111, 2005.

Yang SS, Dahan-Oliel N, Montpetit K, Hamdy RC: Ambulation gains after knee surgery in children with arthrogryposis, *J Pediatr Orthop* 30:863, 2010.

Zlotolow DA, Kozin SH: Posterior elbow release and humeral osteotomy for patients with arthrogryposis, *J Hand Surg Am* 37:1078, 2012.

BRACHIAL PLEXUS

Abid A, Accadbled F, Louis D, et al: Arthroscopic release for shoulder internal rotation contracture secondary to brachial plexus birth palsy: clinical and magnetic resonance imaging results on glenohumeral dysplasia, *J Pediatr Orthop B* 21:305–309, 2012.

Abzug JM, Kozin SH: Evaluation and management of brachial plexus birth palsy, *Orthop Clin North Am* 45:225, 2014.

Abzug JM, Chafetz RS, Gaughan JP, et al: Shoulder function after medial approach and derotational humeral osteotomy in patients with brachial plexus birth palsy, *J Pediatr Orthop* 30:469, 2010.

Al-Qattan MM, Al-Husainan H, Al-Otaibi A, El-Sharkawy MS: Long-term results of low rotation humeral osteotomy in children with Erb's obstetric brachial plexus palsy, *J Hand Surg Eur Vol* 34:486, 2009.

Birch R, Ahad N, Kono H, Smith S: Repair of obstetric brachial plexus palsy: results in 100 children, *J Bone Joint Surg* 87B:1089, 2005.

Breton A, Mainard L, De Gaspéri M, et al: Arthroscopic release of shoulder contracture secondary to obstetric brachial palsy: retrospective study of 18 children with an average follow-up of 4.5 years, *Orthop Traumatol Surg Res* 98:638, 2012.

Chauhan SP, Rose CH, Gherman RB, et al: Brachial plexus injury: a 23-year experience from a tertiary center, *Am J Obstet Gynecol* 192:1795, 2005.

Chen L, Gu YD, Wang H: Microsurgical reconstruction of obstetric brachial plexus palsy, *Microsurgery* 28:108, 2008.

Di Mascio L, Chin KF, Fox M, Sinisi M: Glenoplasty for complex shoulder subluxation and dislocation in children with obstetric brachial plexus palsy, *J Bone Joint Surg* 93B:102, 2011.

Dodwell E, O'Callaghan J, Anthony A, et al: Combined glenoid anteversion osteotomy and tendon transfers for brachial plexus birth palsy: early outcomes, *J Bone Joint Surg* 94A:2145, 2012.

El-Gammal TA, Saleh WR, El-Sayed A, et al: Tendon transfer around the shoulder in obstetric brachial plexus paralysis: clinical and computed tomographic study, *J Pediatr Orthop* 26:641, 2006.

Hale HB, Bae DS, Waters PM: Current concepts in the management of brachial plexus birth palsy, *J Hand Surg Am* 35:332, 2009.

Ho ES, Roy T, Stephens D, Clarke HM: Serial casting and splinting of elbow contractures in children with obstetric brachial plexus palsy, *J Hand Surg* 35A:84, 2010.

Hogendoorn S, van Overvest KL, Watt I, et al: Structural changes in muscle and glenohumeral joint deformity in neonatal brachial plexus palsy, *J Bone Joint Surg* 92A:935, 2010.

Immerman I, Valencia H, DiTaranto P, et al: Subscapularis slide correction of the shoulder internal rotation contracture after brachial plexus birth injury:technique and outcomes, *Tech Hand Surg* 17:52, 2013.

Kozin SH: The evaluation and treatment of children with brachial plexus birth palsy, *J Hand Surg Am* 36:1360, 2011.

Kozin SH, Boardman MJ, Chafetz RS, et al: Arthroscopic treatment of internal rotation contracture and glenohumeral dysplasia in children with brachial plexus birth palsy, *J Shoulder Elbow Surg* 19:102, 2010.

Kozin SH, Chafetz RS, Shaffer A, et al: Magnetic resonance imaging and clinical findings before and after tendon transfers about the shoulder in children with residual brachial plexus birth palsy: a 3-year follow-up study, *J Pediatr Orthop* 30:154, 2010.

Lippert WC, Mehlman CT, Cornwall R, et al: The intrarater and interrater reliability of glenoid version and glenohumeral subluxation measurements in neonatal brachial plexus palsy, *J Pediatr Orthop* 32:378–384, 2012.

Little KJ, Zlotolow DA, Soldado F, et al: Early functional recovery of elbow flexion and supination following median and/or ulnar nerve fascicle transfer in upper neonatal brachial plexus palsy, *J Bone Joint Surg* 96A:215, 2014.

Louden RJ, Broering CA, Mehlman CT, et al: Meta-analysis of function after secondary shoulder surgery in neonatal brachial plexus palsy, *J Pediatr Orthop* 33:656, 2013.

Luo PB, Chen L, Zhou CH, et al: Results of intercostal nerve transfer to the musculocutaneous nerve in brachial plexus birth palsy, *J Pediatr Orthop* 31:884, 2011.

Mehlman CT, DeVoe WB, Lippert WC, et al: Arthroscopically assisted Sever-L'Episcopo procedure improves clinical and radiographic outcomes in neonatal brachial plexus palsy patients, *J Pediatr Orthop* 31:341–351, 2011.

Pearl ML: Shoulder problems in children with brachial plexus birth palsy: evaluation and management, *J Am Acad Orthop Surg* 17:242, 2009.

Pearl ML, Edgerton BW, Kaszimiroff POA, et al: Arthroscopic release and latissimus dorsi transfer for shoulder internal rotation contractures and glenohumeral deformity secondary to brachial plexus birth palsy, *J Bone Joint Surg* 88A:565, 2006.

Reading BD, Laor T, Salisbury SR, et al: Quantification of humeral head deformity following neonatal brachial plexus palsy, *J Bone Joint Surg* 94A:131, 2012.

Sheffler LC, Lattanza L, Hagar Y, et al: The prevalence, rate of progression, and treatment of elbow flexion contracture in children with brachial plexus birth palsy, *J Bone Joint Surg* 94A:403, 2012.

Sibbel SE, Bauer AS, James MA: Late reconstruction of brachial plexus birth palsy, *J Pediatr Orthop* 34(Suppl 1):S57, 2014.

Smith AB, Gupta N, Strober J, Chin C: Magnetic resonance neurography in children with birth-related brachial plexus injury, *Pediatr Radiol* 38:159, 2008.

Terzis JK, Kokkalis ZT: Restoration of elbow extension after primary reconstruction in obstetric brachial plexus palsy, *J Pediatr Orthop* 30:161, 2010.

van Alphen NA, van Doorn-Loogman MH, Maas H, et al: Restoring wrist extension in obstetric palsy of the brachial plexus by transferring wrist flexors to wrist extensors, *J Pediatr Rehabil Med* 6:53, 2013.

van Heest A, Glisson C, Ma H: Glenohumeral dysplasia changes after tendon transfer surgery in children with birth brachial plexus injuries, *J Pediatr Orthop* 30:371, 2010.

Waters PM: Update on management of pediatric brachial plexus palsy, *J Pediatr Orthop* 25:116, 2005.

Waters PM, Bae DS: The early effects of tendon transfers and open capsulorrhaphy on glenohumeral deformity in brachial plexus birth palsy, *J Bone Joint Surg* 90A:2171, 2008.

Waters PM, Bae DS: The early effects of tendon transfers and open capsulorrhaphy on glenohumeral deformity in brachial plexus birth palsy. Surgical technique, *J Bone Joint Surg* 91A(Suppl 2):213, 2009.

Waters PM, Monica JT, Earp BE, et al: Correlation of radiographic muscle cross-sectional area with glenohumeral deformity in children with brachial plexus birth palsy, *J Bone Joint Surg* 91A:2367, 2009.

The complete list of references is available online at ***expertconsult.inkling.com.***

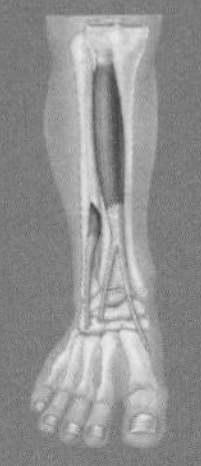

CHAPTER 35

NEUROMUSCULAR DISORDERS

William C. Warner Jr., Jeffrey R. Sawyer

Neuromuscular disease in children includes conditions that affect the spinal cord, peripheral nerves, neuromuscular junctions, and muscles. Accurate diagnosis is essential because the procedures commonly used to treat deformities in patients with neuromuscular disease such as poliomyelitis or cerebral palsy may not be appropriate for hereditary neuromuscular conditions. The diagnosis is made on the basis of clinical history, detailed family history, physical examination, laboratory testing (including serum enzyme studies, especially serum levels of creatine kinase and aldolase), genetic testing, electromyography, nerve conduction velocity studies, and nerve and muscle biopsies. Serum enzyme levels of creatine kinase generally are elevated, but the increase varies dramatically from levels of 50 to 100 times normal in patients with some dystrophic muscle conditions (e.g., Duchenne muscular dystrophy) to only slight increases (one to two times normal) in some patients with congenital myopathy or spinal muscular atrophy.

Nerve or muscle biopsy, or both, is useful for precise diagnosis. The biopsy specimen must be obtained from a muscle that is involved but still functioning, usually the deltoid, vastus lateralis, or gastrocnemius. The biopsy specimen should not be taken from the region of musculotendinous junctions because the normal fibrous tissue septa can be confused with the pathologic fibrosis. Specimens should be about 10 mm long and 3 mm deep and should be fixed in glutaraldehyde in preparation for electron microscopy. The muscle specimen that is to be processed for light microscopy should be frozen in liquid nitrogen within a few minutes after removal. The specimen should not be placed into saline solution or formalin. For nerve biopsy, the sural nerve usually is chosen. This nerve can be accessed laterally between the Achilles tendon and the lateral malleolus just proximal to the level of the tibiotalar joint. The entire width of the nerve should be taken for a length of 3 to 4 cm. Atraumatic technique is essential in either type of biopsy for meaningful results.

Tremendous advances have been made in the understanding of the genetic basis of neuromuscular disorders. Through advances in molecular biology, chromosome locations for various abnormal genes have been identified, characterized, and sequenced (Table 35-1). In certain diseases, such as Duchenne and Becker muscular dystrophy, not only have the genes been localized, cloned, and sequenced but also the biochemical basis for these diseases is now understood. The gene responsible for Duchenne and Becker muscular dystrophy is located in the Xp21 region of the X chromosome. This region is responsible for the coding of the dystrophin protein. Dystrophin testing (dystrophin immunoblotting) can be used as a biochemical test for muscular dystrophy; it also is useful for the differentiation of Duchenne muscular dystrophy from Becker muscular dystrophy. In addition, different types of mutations or variations can be used to predict clinical outcome. For example, Friedrich ataxia is caused by expansion of GAA nucleotide repeats in the frataxin gene intron. The amount of expansion of the GAA repeats correlates with disease severity and progression.

Orthopaedic treatment has been aimed at preventing the worsening of deformities and providing stability to the skeletal system to improve the quality of life for these children. Although a cure may be possible in the future with gene therapy, orthopaedic treatment is still necessary to improve the quality of life for most children no matter how severely impaired. Louis et al. reported 34 surgical procedures performed in individuals with severe multiple impairments to improve sitting posture, care, and comfort. Significant improvement was found in most patients, and no patient was made worse. The priorities of patients with severe neuromuscular diseases are the ability to communicate with other people, the ability to perform many activities of daily living,

TABLE 35-1

Classification of Major Muscular Dystrophies

DISEASE	LOCUS	PROTEIN
X-LINKED RECESSIVE		
Duchenne-Becker dystrophy	Xp21	Dystrophin
Emery-Dreifuss dystrophy	Xp28	Emerin
AUTOSOMAL DOMINANT (AD)		
Myotonic dystrophy	19q	Myotonin
Facioscapulohumeral dystrophy	4q	?
LGMD—1A	5q	?
LGMD—1B	Other	?
AUTOSOMAL RECESSIVE (AR)		
LGMD—2A	15q	Calpain
LGMD—2B	2q	?
LGMD—2C	13q	γ-Sarcoglycan
LGMD—2D	17q	α-Sarcoglycan
LGMD—2E	4q	β-Sarcoglycan
LGMD—2F	5q	δ-Sarcoglycan
CONGENITAL DYSTROPHIES		
Congenital muscular (AR)	6q	Merosin
Fukuyama disease (AR)	9q13	?
CONGENITAL MYOPATHIES		
Central core disease (AD)	19q	Ryanodine receptor
	14q	Myosin
Nemaline rod disease (AD)	1q22	Tropomyosin
Myotubular myopathies	Xq26	?
Distal muscular dystrophy (AD)	14q	?
Oculopharyngeal dystrophy (AD)	14q	?

From Brown RH Jr, Phil D: Dystrophy-associated proteins and the muscular dystrophies, Annu Rev Med 48:457, 1997.

AD, Autosomal dominant; *AR,* autosomal recessive; *LGMD,* limb-girdle muscular dystrophy.

mobility, and ambulation. The role of the orthopaedic surgeon in achieving these goals includes prescribing orthoses for lower extremity control to facilitate transfer to and from wheelchairs, preventing or correcting joint contractures, and maintaining appropriate standing and sitting postures. Treatment must be individualized for each patient. The choice and timing of the procedures depend on the particular disorder, the severity of involvement, the ambulatory status of the patient, and the experience of the physician. This chapter discusses the common neuromuscular disorders in children that frequently require surgical intervention.

TREATMENT CONSIDERATIONS

FRACTURES

Fractures are common in children with neuromuscular disease because of disuse osteoporosis and frequent falls. Larson and Henderson found a significant decrease in bone mineral density on dual-energy x-ray absorptiometry scans in boys with Duchenne muscular dystrophy, with 44% sustaining fractures. James et al. found that 33% of patients with Duchenne or Becker muscular dystrophy had sustained at least one fracture; full-time wheelchair use was a significant risk factor for fracture. Most fractures are nondisplaced metaphyseal fractures that heal rapidly. Minimally displaced metaphyseal fractures of the lower limbs should be splinted so that walking can be resumed quickly. If braces are being used, they can be enlarged to accommodate the fractured limb and allow progressive weight bearing. Displaced diaphyseal fractures can be treated with cast-braces or open reduction and internal fixation, if indicated, to allow walking during fracture healing. Medical treatment of disuse osteopenia may be beneficial in decreasing the frequency of fractures in this patient population.

ORTHOSES

Spinal bracing occasionally may be used to assist with sitting balance. Bracing may slow, but does not prevent, the progression of spinal deformity. Spinal bracing may be accomplished with a polypropylene plastic shell with a soft foam polyethylene lining, in the form of either an anterior and posterior (bivalved) total-contact orthosis or an anterior-opening thoracolumbosacral orthosis with lumbar lordotic contouring. Knee-ankle-foot orthoses provide stability for patients with proximal muscle weakness. A pelvic band with hip and knee locks can be added if necessary. Ankle-foot orthoses help to position the ankle and foot in a plantigrade position in an effort to prevent progressive equinus and equinovarus deformities.

SEATING SYSTEMS

For most children with severe neuromuscular disease, walking is difficult and frustrating, and a wheelchair eventually may be needed. The chair, whether manual or electric, must be carefully contoured. A narrow chair with a firm seat increases pelvic support, and a firm back in slight extension supports the spine. Lateral spine supports built into the chair may help sitting balance but usually do not alter the progression of scoliosis. Specialized seating clinics can provide custom-fitted chairs with numerous options for daily use. These custom-fitted chairs can accommodate most spinal deformities and pelvic obliquity that are present.

DIFFERENTIATION OF MUSCLE DISEASE FROM NERVE DISEASE

In addition to the history, physical examination, and routine laboratory studies, special tests, such as electromyography, muscle tissue biopsy, serum enzyme, and molecular and genetic studies help differentiate the two diseases.

HEMATOLOGIC STUDIES

Serum enzyme assays are extremely helpful, especially the level of serum creatine kinase in the blood. Serum creatine kinase is a sensitive test for showing abnormalities of striated muscle function. Elevation of this enzyme is extremely important in the diagnosis in the early stages of Duchenne muscular dystrophy. Elevation of the creatine kinase parallels the amount of muscle necrosis. There is a significant elevation early in the disease process, but the elevation decreases with time as the muscle is replaced by fat and fibrous tissue. The creatine kinase levels can be elevated 20 to 200 times above normal limits. The level may decline in the later stages of the disease, when the greater muscle mass has already deteriorated and there is less breakdown of muscle mass than in the earlier stages. The levels are higher in Duchenne than in Becker muscular dystrophy; however, there is some overlap between the two diseases. This test is beneficial in detecting the carrier state of Duchenne and Becker muscular dystrophies because creatine kinase is usually elevated in the carrier female. A muscle provocation test also is beneficial in detecting the female carrier state because elevation of creatine kinase levels is greater after strenuous exercise in carrier females than in noncarrier females. Urine creatine is excessive in dystrophic patients in the active stage of muscle breakdown. Any process that causes muscle breakdown, such as excessive exercise, diabetes mellitus, and starvation in which carbohydrate intake is reduced, can cause an excess of creatine in the urine. In myotonic dystrophy, because of the reduced ability of the liver to produce creatine phosphate, the level of creatine in the blood is decreased.

Aldolase is another enzyme that is elevated in patients with muscular dystrophy. Its course is similar to that of creatine kinase enzyme. Aspartate aminotransferase and lactate dehydrogenase values also may be elevated, but these enzymes are nonspecific for muscle disease.

DNA mutation analysis (polymerase chain reaction or DNA blot analysis) can provide a definitive diagnosis of Duchenne or Becker muscular dystrophy. These tests also can help identify the carrier and may allow prenatal diagnosis in some cases. These DNA tests can be done from a small sample of blood or amniotic fluid.

ELECTROMYOGRAPHIC STUDIES

In an electromyogram of normal muscle, resting muscles usually are relatively electrosilent; on voluntary contraction of a normal muscle, the electromyogram shows a characteristic frequency, duration, and amplitude action potential (Fig. 35-1). In a myopathy, the electromyogram shows increased frequency, decreased amplitude, and decreased duration of the motor action potentials. In a neuropathy, it shows decreased frequency and increased amplitude and duration of the action potentials. In a neuropathy, nerve conduction velocities usually are slowed; in a myopathy, the nerve conduction velocities usually are normal. Myotonic dystrophy is characterized by an increase in frequency, duration, and amplitude of the action potentials on needle electrode insertion, which gradually decreases over time. These action potentials when amplified create the "dive bomber" sound that is almost universal in this disease.

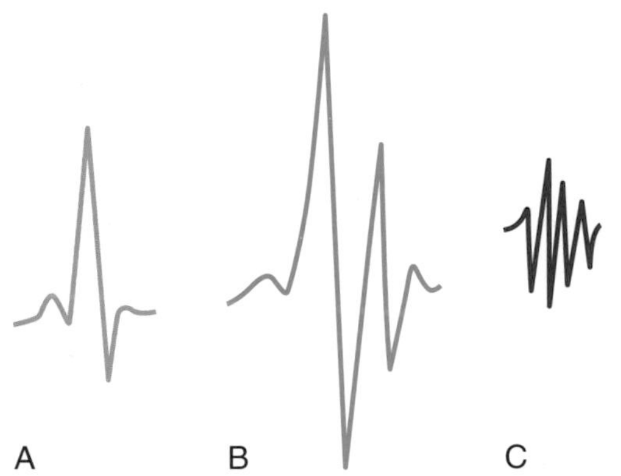

FIGURE 35-1 Motor units seen in electromyography. **A,** Normal triphasic motor unit potential. **B,** Large polyphasic motor units as seen in neurogenic disorders, such as spinal muscular atrophy, in which they also are reduced in number. **C,** Small polyphasic motor units as seen in muscular dystrophy. These usually are of normal number. (Courtesy of Tulio E. Bertorini, MD.)

MUSCLE TISSUE BIOPSY

Interpretation of the muscle tissue biopsy differentiates not only myopathy from neuropathy but also the various types of congenital dystrophy from one another. In addition to the usual hematoxylin and eosin stain, special stains and techniques, such as the Gomori modified trichrome stain, nicotinamide adenine dinucleotide-tetrazolium reductase (NADH-TR) stain, and the alizarin red S stain, are helpful. Electron microscopy also is beneficial.

Histopathologic study of muscle affected by myopathy shows an increased fibrosis in and between muscle spindles, with necrosis of the fibers (Fig. 35-2B). Later, deposition of fat within the fibers occurs, accompanied by hyaline and granular degeneration of the fibers. The number of nuclei is increased with migration of some nuclei to the center of the fibers. Some small groups of inflammatory cells also may be seen, and inflammatory cells are markedly increased in polymyositis. Special histochemical stains that can show muscle fiber type show a preponderance of type I fibers. In normal skeletal muscle, the ratio of type I to type II fibers is 1 : 2 (Fig. 35-2A). In some dystrophies other than the Duchenne type, fiber splitting is apparent. Calcium accumulation in muscle fibers also has been shown.

The microscopic picture in neuropathy is quite different (Fig. 35-2C). There is little or no increase in fibrous tissue, and small, angular, atrophic fibers are present between groups of normal-sized muscle fibers. Special stains that show fiber type show that 80% of the fibers are type II.

An adequate biopsy specimen must be obtained to make a correct diagnosis. An open muscle biopsy usually is performed, but in some cases a needle biopsy in small children has proved satisfactory. Muscles that are totally involved should not be used; biopsy specimens of muscles suspected of early involvement are indicated. The muscle bellies of the gastrocnemius in a patient with Duchenne muscular dystrophy usually are involved early and are a poor site to obtain material for a biopsy, whereas the quadriceps (especially the vastus lateralis at midthigh) and rectus abdominis usually show early involvement without total replacement of the muscle spindles by fibrous tissue or fat. Biopsy specimens of these muscles usually are the most reliable.

When securing a biopsy specimen ensure that the muscle is maintained at its normal length between clamps (Fig. 35-3) or sutures (Fig. 35-4) and that the biopsy specimen has not been violated by a needle electrode during an electromyogram or infiltrated with a local anesthetic before the biopsy. Biopsy needles should have a minimal core diameter of 3 mm.

A second sample of muscle tissue should be taken at the time of biopsy and sent for dystrophin analysis (dystrophin

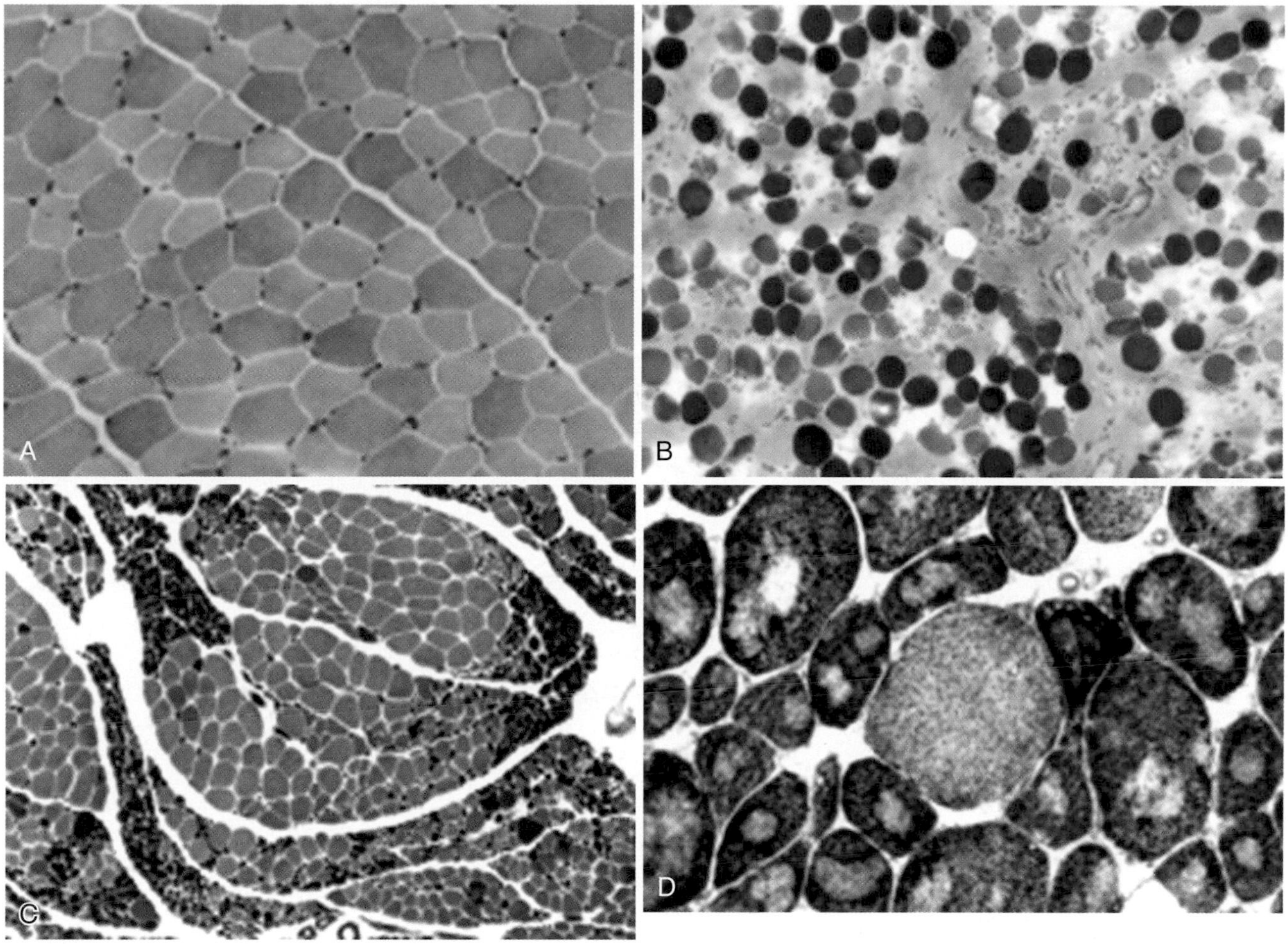

FIGURE 35-2 **A,** Normal muscle biopsy specimen (except for one small angular fiber). Note polygonal shape of myofibrils, normal distribution of type I and type II fibers, and normal connective tissue of endomysium (NADH-TR stain, ×125). **B,** Muscular dystrophy. Fibers are more rounded, some fibers have internalized nuclei, and others are atrophic. One muscle fiber is necrotic and is undergoing phagocytosis. Connective tissue between fibers is increased (hematoxylin & eosin, ×295). **C,** Chronic neurogenic atrophy (juvenile spinal muscular atrophy). Notice grouping of fibers of same type and some atrophic angular fibers. Fat is increased between muscle fascicles (NADH-TR stain, ×125). **D,** Central core disease. Note pale areas of central cores in muscle fibers characteristic of this disease (NADH-TR stain ×200). (Courtesy of Tulio E. Bertorini, MD.)

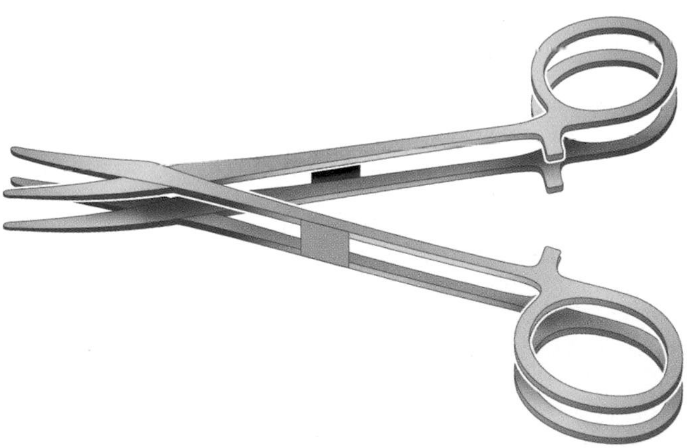

FIGURE 35-3 Two hemostats bound together to preserve length when securing muscle biopsy. (From Cruess RL, Rennie WRJ: Adult orthopaedics, New York, 1984, Churchill Livingstone.) **SEE TECHNIQUE 35-1.**

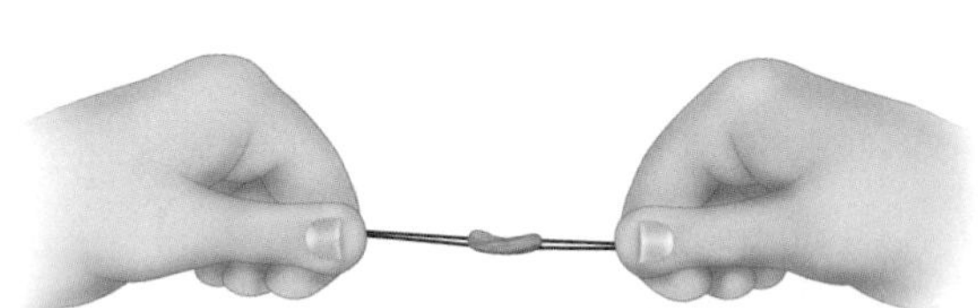

FIGURE 35-4 Muscle length maintained by muscle biopsy done on outer side of previously placed sutures. **SEE TECHNIQUE 35-1.**

immunoblotting). Dystrophin is a muscle protein that has been found to be absent, decreased, or modified in certain types of dystrophy. The measurement and quantification of this protein combined with the clinical picture of certain types of muscular dystrophy have added significantly to the ability to diagnose various dystrophies.

Regional block anesthesia can be used for the biopsy, but a general anesthetic may be necessary. General anesthesia carries the known risk of anesthetic complications, such as malignant hyperthermia.

OPEN MUSCLE BIOPSY

TECHNIQUE 35-1

- Block the area regionally with 1% lidocaine, and make a 1.5-cm incision through the skin and subcutaneous tissues.
- Carefully split the enveloping fascia to expose clearly the muscle bundles from which the biopsy specimen is to be taken.
- Using a special double clamp (Fig. 35-3) or silk sutures approximately 2 cm apart (Fig. 35-4), grasp the muscle and section around the outside of the arms of the clamp or sutures.
- Prevent bleeding within the muscle and take only small biopsy specimens.
- Take more than one specimen because different stains need different preservative techniques; for example, some histochemical changes are best shown on fresh frozen sections that have had special staining. The pathologist should know in advance that a muscle biopsy is to be done so that special fixative techniques, such as freezing with liquid nitrogen, are readily available when the specimen is received.

PERCUTANEOUS MUSCLE BIOPSY

Mubarak, Chambers, and Wenger described percutaneous muscle biopsy in 379 patients. This procedure can be performed in an outpatient clinic with only local anesthesia.

TECHNIQUE 35-2

(MUBARAK, CHAMBERS, AND WENGER)

- Prepare the biopsy site with iodophor paint. Place a fenestrated adhesive drape over the site. Infiltrate the skin and subcutaneous tissue with 5 to 8 mL of 1% lidocaine without epinephrine. When a biopsy specimen of the quadriceps is being obtained, also anesthetize the fascia.
- Check the Bergström biopsy needle to ensure a smooth sliding of the cutter within the trocar. Cut the K-50 tube at an angle and place it into the end of the cutting needle with the other end attached to a 10-mL syringe.
- Use a No. 11 scalpel blade to make a small stab wound in the skin and fascia lata at about the midthigh level.
- Insert the Bergström needle into the muscle, preferably the rectus femoris, at an oblique angle.
- Pull the needle back about one half of its length and have an assistant apply suction with the 10-mL syringe. This allows muscle to be pulled into the cutting chamber.
- Cut by compressing the cutter into the trocar.
- Remove the Bergström apparatus from the thigh. Remove the muscle sample from the chamber with a fine needle and place it on saline-soaked gauze in a Petri dish.
- Through the same incision and track, reinsert the Bergström needle and repeat the procedure until five or six samples have been obtained.
- Close the small wound with 1/4-inch adhesive strips.

POSTOPERATIVE CARE. Dressing sponges are applied and held in place with foam tape to serve as a compressive, but not constricting, bandage for 2 days. The adhesive strips are left in place for 10 days; no perioperative antibiotics or narcotic analgesics are necessary.

MUSCULAR DYSTROPHY

The muscular dystrophies are a group of hereditary disorders of skeletal muscle that produce progressive degeneration of skeletal muscle and associated weakness (Table 35-1). The X-linked dystrophies are more common and include Duchenne muscular dystrophy, Becker muscular dystrophy, and Emery-Dreifuss muscular dystrophy. Limb-girdle muscular dystrophy and congenital muscular dystrophy are the two most common autosomal recessive muscular dystrophies. Facioscapulohumeral muscular dystrophy is inherited as an autosomal dominant trait (Table 35-2).

DUCHENNE MUSCULAR DYSTROPHY

Duchenne muscular dystrophy, a sex-linked recessive inherited trait, occurs in males and in females with Turner syndrome; carriers are female. It is reported to occur in one in 3500 live births. There is a family history in 70% of patients, and the condition occurs as a spontaneous mutation in about 30% of patients.

Duchenne muscular dystrophy is the result of a mutation in the Xp21 region of the X chromosome, which encodes the 400-kd protein dystrophin. Dystrophin is important to the stability of the cell membrane cytoskeleton. In patients with Duchenne muscular dystrophy, the total absence of this transcellular protein results in progressive muscle degeneration and loss of function.

Children with Duchenne muscular dystrophy usually reach early motor milestones at appropriate times, but independent ambulation may be delayed, and many are initially toe-walkers. The disease usually becomes evident between 3 and 6 years of age. Clinical features include large, firm calf muscles; the tendency to toe-walk; a widely based, lordotic stance; a waddling Trendelenburg gait; and a positive Gower test indicative of proximal muscle weakness (Fig. 35-5). The diagnosis usually is obvious by the time the child is 5 or 6 years old (Fig. 35-6). A dramatically elevated level of creatine kinase (50 to 100 times normal) and genetic testing of blood samples confirm the diagnosis. Muscle biopsy shows

TABLE 35-2

Characteristics of the Muscular Dystrophies

TYPE	ONSET	SYMPTOMS	PROGRESSION	INHERITANCE
Duchenne	Early childhood (2-6 years)	Generalized weakness and muscle wasting first affecting muscles of hips, pelvic area, thighs, and shoulders. Calves often enlarged.	Eventually affects all voluntary muscles, as well as heart and breathing. Survival uncommon beyond early thirties.	X-linked recessive
Becker	Adolescence or early adulthood	Similar to Duchenne, but less severe.	Progression is slow and variable, but can affect all voluntary muscles. Survival usually well into mid-to-late adulthood.	X-linked recessive
Emery-Dreifuss	Childhood, usually by 10 years of age	Weakness and wasting of shoulder, upper arm, and calf muscles; joint stiffening; fainting caused by cardiac abnormalities.	Progression is slow; cardiac complications common and may require a pacemaker.	X-linked recessive Autosomal dominant Autosomal recessive
Limb-girdle	Childhood to adulthood	Weakness and wasting first affecting muscles around shoulders and hips.	Progression is slow; cardiac complications common in later stages of disease.	Autosomal dominant Autosomal recessive
Facioscapulohumeral (Landouzy-Dejerine)	Adolescence or early adulthood, usually by 20 years of age	Weakness and wasting of muscles around eyes and mouth, as well as shoulders, upper arms, and lower legs initially; later affects abdominal muscles and hip muscles.	Progression is slow, with periods of rapid deterioration; may span many decades.	Autosomal dominant
Myotonic (Steinert disease)	Congenital form at birth; more common, less severe form in adolescence or adulthood	Weakness and wasting of muscles of face, lower legs, forearms, hands, and neck with delayed relaxation of muscles after contraction. Can affect gastrointestinal system, vision, heart, or respiration. Learning disabilities in some.	Progression is slow, sometimes spanning 50 to 60 years.	Autosomal dominant
Oculopharyngeal	Adulthood, usually forties or fifties	Weakness of muscles of eyelids and throat, later facial and limb muscles. Swallowing problems and difficulty keeping eyes open are common.	Progression is slow.	Autosomal dominant Autosomal recessive
Distal	Childhood to adulthood	Weakness and wasting of muscles of hands, forearm, lower limbs.	Progression is slow, not life-threatening.	Autosomal dominant Autosomal recessive
Congenital	At or near birth	Generalized muscle weakness, possible joint stiffness or laxity; may involve scoliosis, respiratory insufficiency, mental retardation.	Progression is variable; some forms are slowly progressive, and some shorten life span.	Autosomal recessive Autosomal dominant Spontaneous

Data from www.mda.org.

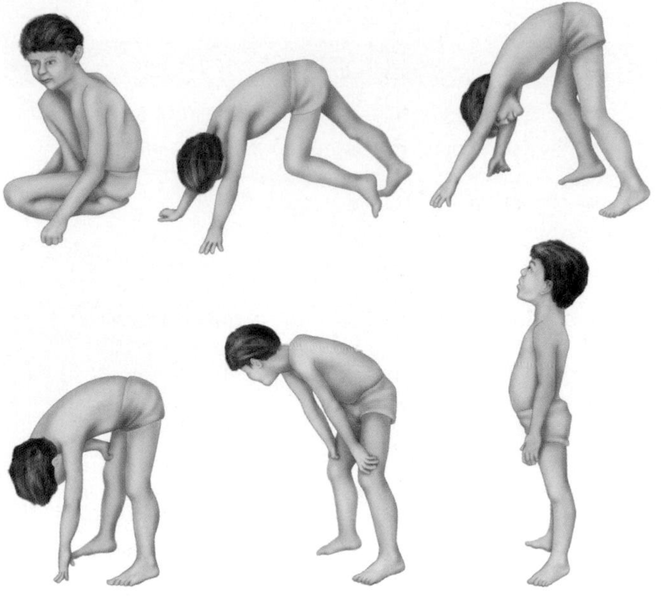

FIGURE 35-5 Gower sign. Child must use hands to rise from sitting position. (Redrawn from Siegel IM: Clinical management of muscle disease, London, 1977, William Heinemann.)

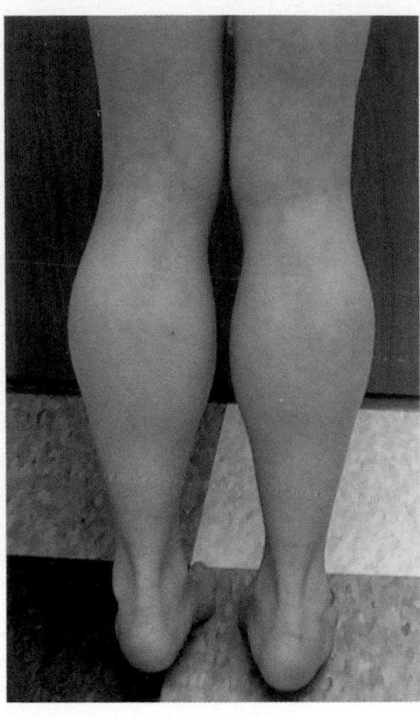

FIGURE 35-7 Calf pseudohypertrophy in muscular dystrophy.

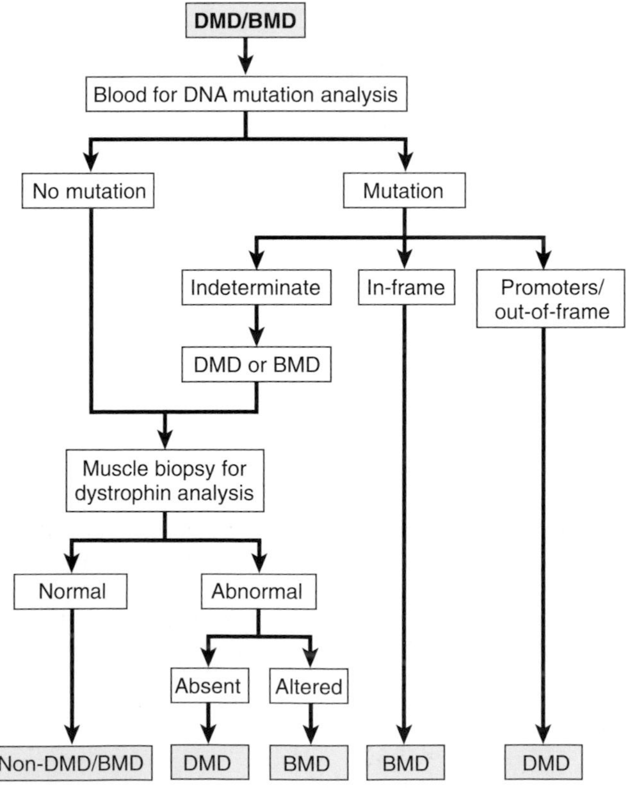

FIGURE 35-6 Flow chart of process for molecular diagnostic evaluation of patients in whom diagnosis of Duchenne muscular dystrophy (DMD) or Becker muscular dystrophy (BMD) is suspected. (From Shapiro F, Specht L: Current concepts review: the diagnosis and orthopaedic treatment of inherited muscular diseases of childhood, J Bone Joint Surg 75A:439, 1993.)

variations in fiber size, internal nuclei, split fibers, degenerating or regenerating fibers, and fibrofatty tissue deposition. Dystrophin testing of the muscle biopsy specimen will help confirm the type of muscular dystrophy but is not 100% confirmatory.

PHYSICAL EXAMINATION

The degree of muscular weakness depends on the age of the patient. Because the proximal musculature weakens before the distal muscles, examination of the lower extremities shows an early weakness of gluteal muscle strength. The weakness in the proximal muscles of the lower extremity can be shown by a decrease in the ability to rise from the floor without assistance of the upper extremities (Gower sign). The calf pseudohypertrophy is caused by infiltration of the muscle by fat and fibrosis, giving the calves the feel of hard rubber (Fig. 35-7). The extrinsic muscles of the foot and ankle retain their strength longer than the proximal muscles of the hip and knee. The posterior tibial muscle retains its strength for the longest time. This pattern of weakness causes an equinovarus deformity of the foot. Weakness of the shoulder girdle musculature can be shown by the Meryon sign, which is elicited by lifting the child with one arm encircling the child's chest. Most children contract the muscles around the shoulder to increase shoulder stability and facilitate lifting. In children with muscular dystrophy, however, the arms abduct because of the lack of adductor muscle tone and severe shoulder girdle muscle weakness until the child eventually slides through the examiner's arms unless the chest is tightly encircled. Later in the disease process, the Thomas test shows hip flexion contracture and the Ober test shows an abduction contracture of the hip.

MEDICAL TREATMENT

The use of prednisone and deflazacort has been shown to preserve or improve strength, prolong ambulation, and slow the progression of scoliosis. Steroids help stabilize cell membranes and decrease inflammation and, therefore, have the potential to inhibit myocyte cell death and decrease the secondary effects associated with cell death. A group of boys treated with daily high-dose deflazacort had a substantially reduced rate of scoliosis compared with boys who elected not to take this medication. Eighty percent of untreated boys developed scoliosis of at least 20 degrees by age 18, whereas fewer than 25% of the boys in the treatment group developed scoliosis. Daily high-dose deflazacort also has been reported to result in long-term maintenance of pulmonary function. The age at which boys became full-time wheelchair users increased by several years over boys who did not use deflazacort. This therapy has significant side effects, including weight gain, osteopenia, behavioral changes, cataracts, and myopathy. The osteopenia may lead to pathologic fractures of the spine and extremities and makes instrumentation of the spine for scoliosis more difficult. Gordon et al. reported that the addition of bisphosphonates to steroid treatment improved survival compared with treatment with steroid alone. More recently, Lebel et al. reported that long-term glucocorticoid treatment substantially reduced the need for spinal surgery in boys who took deflazacort (20%) compared with those who did not (92%). Other medical therapies that have been used but have not shown definite benefit are myoblast transfers, azathioprine, and aminoglycosides. Gene therapy and stem cell therapy may show promise as a treatment for muscular dystrophy but are still investigational.

ORTHOPAEDIC TREATMENT

The goal of orthopaedic treatment is to maintain functional ambulation as long as possible. The specific procedures required differ according to the age of the child and the stage of disease severity (Table 35-3). Between ages 8 and 14 years (median 10 years), children with Duchenne muscular dystrophy typically have a sensation of locking of the joints. Contractures of the lower extremity may require early treatment to prolong the child's ability to ambulate, if even for 1 to 2 years. This requires prevention or retardation of the development of contractures of the lower extremity, which would eventually prohibit ambulation. It is easier to keep patients walking than to induce them to resume walking after they have stopped. When children with Duchenne muscular dystrophy stop walking, they also become more susceptible to the development of scoliosis and severe contractures of the lower extremities. Scoliosis develops in nearly all children with Duchenne muscular dystrophy, usually when they require aided mobility or shortly after becoming wheelchair bound. The use of steroids has been reported to decrease the occurrence of scoliosis in these patients.

For surgical correction of lower extremity contractures, three approaches have been used, as follows:

1. *Ambulatory approach.* The goal of surgery during the late ambulatory phase is to correct any contractures in the lower extremity while the patient is still ambulatory. Rideau recommended early aggressive surgery. His indications for surgery were first appearance of contractures in lower extremities; a plateau in muscle strength, usually around 5 to 6 years of age; and difficulty maintaining upright posture with the feet together. Rideau recommended that surgery be performed before deterioration of the Gower maneuver time or time to rise from the floor. Other surgeons have recommended surgery later in the ambulatory phase, just before the cessation of ambulation.
2. *Rehabilitative approach.* Surgery is performed after the patient has lost the ability to walk but with the intention that walking will resume. Surgery during this stage usually allows for only minimal ambulation with braces.
3. *Palliative approach.* The palliative approach treats only contractures that interfere with shoe wear and comfortable positioning in a wheelchair.

A comparison of ambulation and foot position in three groups of patients with Duchenne muscular dystrophy (those who had surgery to maintain ambulation, those who had surgery to correct and maintain foot position, and those who had no surgery) found that the mean age at cessation of ambulation for those who had surgery was 11.2 years, compared with 10.3 years in those who did not have surgery. Foot position was neutral in 94% of those who had surgery, and none had toe flexion deformities; 96% of those who had surgery reported being able to wear any type of shoes, compared with only 60% of those who had no surgery. In contrast, another study of full-time wheelchair users with Duchenne muscular dystrophy found no significant differences between patients who did and did not have foot surgery with respect to shoe wear, hypersensitivity, or cosmesis. Hindfoot motion was significantly better, but equinus contracture was significantly worse in those who had not had surgery.

Currently, the most common approach is to correct contractures just before the patient has a significant decline in

TABLE 35-3

Orthopaedic Treatment of Duchenne Muscular Dystrophy

STAGE OF MUSCULAR DYSTROPHY	AGES	ORTHOPAEDIC TREATMENT
Stage 1 (Diagnostic stage)	Birth to 5 years of age	No orthopaedic interventions indicated
Stage 2 (Quiescent stage)	5-8 years of age	Achilles tendon lengthening Possible hip and knee releases Fracture treatment
Stage 3 (Loss of ambulation)	9-12 years of age	Contracture releases Achilles tendon lengthening or tenotomy Transfer of posterior tibial muscle to dorsum of foot
Stage 4 (Full-time sitting/development of spinal deformity)	12-16 years of age	Spinal fusion
Stage 5 (Complete dependence and development of respiratory insufficiency)	≥15 years of age	Fracture treatment

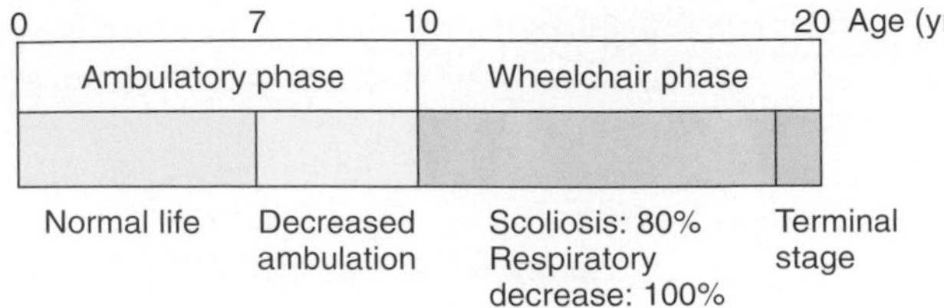

FIGURE 35-8 Graph of natural course of Duchenne muscular dystrophy: age-related stages. (From Rideau Y, Duport G, Delaubier A, et al: Early treatment to preserve quality of locomotion for children with Duchenne muscular dystrophy, Semin Neurol 15:9, 1995.)

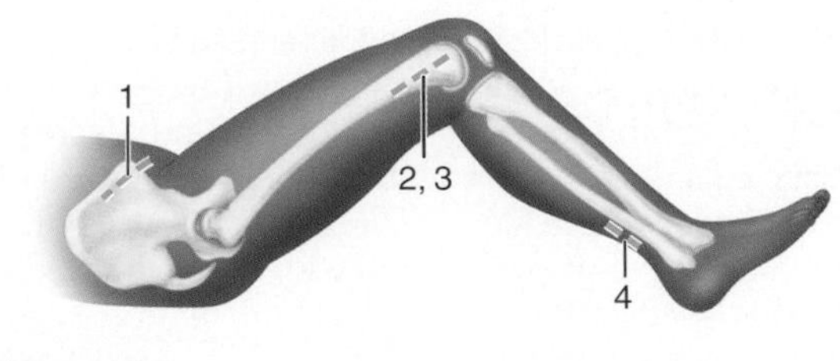

FIGURE 35-9 Tenotomy sites for release of hip flexors (1), tensor fasciae latae and fascia lata (2, 3), and Achilles tendon (4). **SEE TECHNIQUE 35-3.**

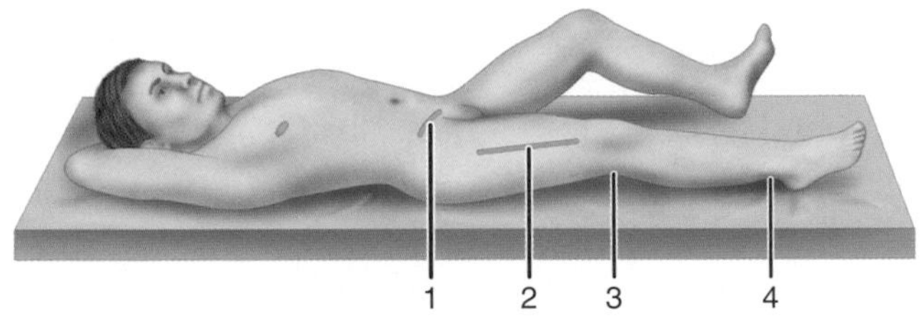

FIGURE 35-10 Surgical sites for musculotendinous releases to reduce bilaterally contractures of the hip (1), thigh (2), knee (3), and ankle (4).

ambulation and before the patient has to use a wheelchair (ambulatory approach) (Fig. 35-8).

Mild equinus contractures of the feet can help force the knee into extension, which helps prevent the knee buckling caused by severe weakness of the quadriceps. Stretching exercises and nightly bracing can be used to prevent the contractures from becoming severe. Flexion and abduction contractures of the hip impede ambulation, however, and should be minimized. Exercises to stretch the hip muscles and lower extremity braces worn at night to prevent the child's sleeping in a frog-leg position are helpful initially. Interestingly, a high level of muscle activity has been suggested to hasten myocyte cell death, indicating that certain exercises could decrease strength.

If surgery is indicated, the foot and hip contractures should be released simultaneously, usually through percutaneous incisions. Ambulation should be resumed immediately after surgery if possible. Polypropylene braces are preferred to long-term casting. Prolonged immobilization must be avoided to prevent or limit the progressive muscle weakness caused by disuse.

PERCUTANEOUS RELEASE OF HIP FLEXION AND ABDUCTION CONTRACTURES AND ACHILLES TENDON CONTRACTURE

TECHNIQUE 35-3

(GREEN)

- With the child supine on the operating table, prepare and drape both lower extremities from the iliac crests to the toes.
- First flex and then extend the hip to be released, holding the hip in adduction to place tension on the muscles to be released; keep the opposite hip in maximal flexion to flatten the lumbar spine.
- Insert a No. 15 knife blade percutaneously just medial and just distal to the anterior superior iliac spine (Fig. 35-9).
- Release the sartorius muscle first and then the tensor fasciae femoris muscle. Push the knife laterally and subcutaneously, without cutting the skin, to release the tensor fasciae latae completely. Bring the knife to the original insertion point and push it deeper to release the rectus femoris completely. Avoid the neurovascular structures of the anterior thigh.
- At 3 to 4 cm proximal to the upper pole of the patella, percutaneously release the fascia lata laterally through a stab wound in its midportion. Push the knife almost to the femur to release the lateral intermuscular septum completely.
- Perform a percutaneous release of the Achilles tendon.
- Apply long leg casts with the feet in neutral position and with the heels well padded to prevent pressure ulcers.

POSTOPERATIVE CARE. The patient is mobilized immediately after surgery. If tolerated, a few steps are allowed. Walker-assisted ambulation is begun as soon as possible; and when transfer is achieved, the patient is placed on a regular bed and physical therapy is continued. The casts are bivalved, and bilateral polypropylene long leg orthoses are fitted as soon as possible. Patients are discharged from the hospital as soon as they can ambulate independently with a walker.

RIDEAU TECHNIQUE

Rideau et al. described a similar technique, but with an open procedure to release the hip flexor contractures and lateral thigh contractures. They also excised the iliotibial band and the lateral intermuscular septum (Fig. 35-10).

TRANSFER OF THE POSTERIOR TIBIAL TENDON TO THE DORSUM OF THE FOOT

In patients with marked overpull of the posterior tibial muscle, Greene found that transfer of the posterior tibial tendon to the dorsum of the foot combined with other tenotomies or tendon lengthening gave better results than posterior tibial tendon lengthening alone. Although transfer of the posterior tibial tendon is technically more demanding and has a higher perioperative complication rate, Greene noted that the patients retained the plantigrade posture of their feet, even after walking ceased. Despite the more extensive surgical procedure, early ambulation of the patients was not impeded.

TECHNIQUE 35-4

(GREENE)

- Place the patient supine; after placing a tourniquet, make a 3-cm incision starting medially at the neck of the talus and extending to the navicular (Fig. 35-11A).
- Open the sheath of the posterior tibial tendon from the distal extent of the flexor retinaculum to the navicular.
- Release the tendon from its bony insertions, preserving as much length as possible.
- Make a second incision 6 to 8 cm long vertically between the Achilles tendon and the medial distal tibia. The Achilles tendon can be lengthened through the same incision if necessary.
- Incise the posterior tibial tendon sheath and pull the distal portion of the tendon through the second operative wound.
- Make a third incision 6 cm long lateral to the anterior crest of the tibia and extend it to the superior extensor retinaculum (Fig. 35-11B).
- Incise the anterior compartment fascia and retract the anterior tibial tendon laterally.
- Carefully incise the interosseous membrane on the lateral aspect of the tibia adjacent to its tibial insertion for a distance of 3 cm. Enlarge the opening by proximal and distal horizontal cuts, extending halfway across the interosseous membrane.
- Pass a curved clamp close to the tibia from the anterior compartment proximally into the second incision. Keep the curved clamp on the tibia to prevent injury to the peroneal vessels.
- After grasping the posterior tibial tendon and pulling it into the third incision, inspect the tendon through the second incision to ensure that it has neither twisted on itself nor ensnared the flexor digitorum longus tendon.
- Make a fourth incision 3 cm long on the dorsum of the foot in the region of the middle cuneiform.
- Incise the periosteum of the middle cuneiform and expose the central portion of the bone.
- Drill a hole 5 to 8 mm to insert the tendon through the middle of the cuneiform.
- Pass a Kelly clamp subcutaneously from the third incision to the fourth incision distally to create a subcutaneous track for the posterior tibial tendon. Pull the tendon through the subcutaneous track with a tendon passer.
- Holding on to the sutures tied to the end of the posterior tibial tendon, pass the tendon into the hole in the middle cuneiform and pass the sutures through the dorsum of the foot with the aid of straight needles. Alternatively,

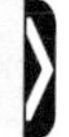

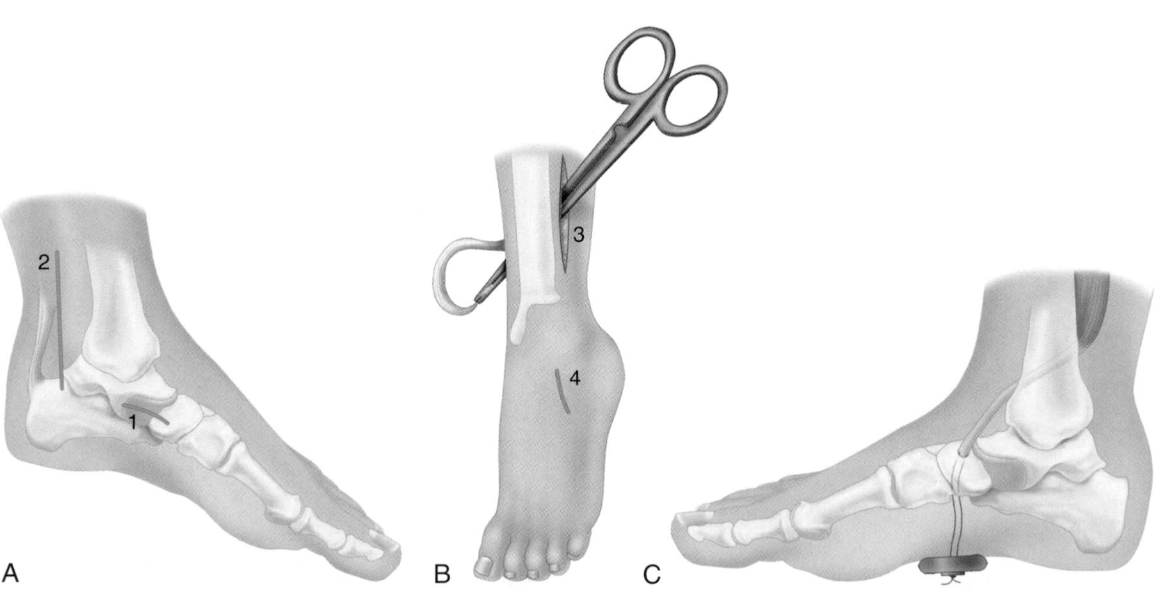

FIGURE 35-11 Posterior tibial tendon transfer. **A,** First and second incisions. **B,** Third and fourth incisions and clamp placement for pulling posterior tibial tendon from posterior to anterior compartment of leg. **C,** Position of transplanted tendon and suture tied over felt pad and button on plantar aspect of foot. **SEE TECHNIQUE 35-4.**

the tendon can be secured to the middle cuneiform with a suture anchor.
- Release the tourniquet and inspect, irrigate, and close the wounds.
- After the wounds have been closed, tie the suture over a felt pad and button on the plantar aspect on the foot with the foot in a neutral position (Fig. 35-11C).
- Apply a long leg cast with the knee extended and the ankle in neutral position.

POSTOPERATIVE CARE. Standing and walking are allowed 24 to 48 hours after surgery. A long leg cast is worn for 4 to 6 weeks, and a knee-ankle-foot orthosis is worn permanently.

TRANSFER OF THE POSTERIOR TIBIAL TENDON TO THE DORSUM OF THE BASE OF THE SECOND METATARSAL

Mubarak described transfer of the posterior tibial tendon to the dorsum of the base of the second metatarsal. Compared with the Greene technique, the more distal placement of the posterior tibial tendon increases the lever arm in dorsiflexion of the ankle and the technique allows easier plantarflexion and dorsiflexion balancing of the ankle at the time of surgery.

TECHNIQUE 35-5

(MUBARAK)
- With the patient supine and a tourniquet in place, make a 3-cm incision over the insertion of the posterior tibial tendon on the navicular.
- Open the sheath of the posterior tibial tendon from the anterior aspect of the medial malleolus to the navicular.
- Release the tendon from the bony insertions, preserving as much length as possible.
- Make a second incision in the posteromedial calf in the region of the myotendinous junction of the posterior tibial tendon. A gastrocnemius recession can be done through this incision if necessary, but excessive lengthening of the triceps surae complex should be avoided to prevent the development of a crouched gait postoperatively.
- Open the posterior tibial tendon sheath and pull the tendon through the sheath into the calf wound.
- At the myotendinous junction of the posterior tibial tendon, incise the tendon transversely halfway through its width. Extend this incision distally to within 0.5 cm of the cut insertion of the tibial tendon.
- Secure the distal aspect of the tendon with a single suture to prevent the longitudinal cut from extending out to the end of the tendon. This procedure effectively doubles the length of the posterior tibial tendon (Fig. 35-12A).
- Make a third incision 6 cm long lateral to the anterior crest of the tibia, extending it to the superior extensor retinaculum.
- Perform an anterior compartment fasciotomy and retract the anterior tibial tendon laterally.
- Incise the interosseous membrane of the lateral aspect of the tibia for a distance of 3 cm.
- Place a Kelly clamp through the anterior compartment wound across the interosseous membrane and into the deep posterior compartment. Grasp the end of the lengthened posterior tibial tendon and bring it through the interosseous membrane into the anterior compartment of the calf (Fig. 35-12B).
- Make another incision, 2 to 3 cm long, over the base of the second metatarsal. Dissect down to the base of the second metatarsal and subperiosteally dissect around the base of the second metatarsal circumferentially.
- Take the elongated posterior tibial tendon and tunnel it subcutaneously into the incision over the dorsum of the second metatarsal. Loop the tendon around the base of

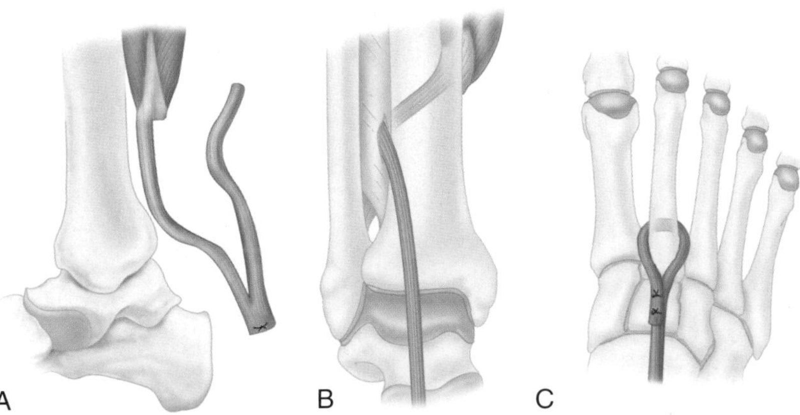

FIGURE 35-12 **A,** Posterior tibial tendon removed from insertion. Length can be effectively doubled by splitting at myotendinous junction to cut end. Secure midpoint at lengthened tendon with suture. **B,** Lengthened tendon is passed through hole in interosseous membrane (posterior to anterior) and subcutaneously across anterior aspect of ankle. **C,** Lengthened tendon is pulled subcutaneously across dorsum of midfoot, looped around base of second metatarsal, and sutured to itself with enough tension to hold ankle in neutral. **SEE TECHNIQUE 35-5.**

the second metatarsal as a sling and suture it to itself with the appropriate tension on the ankle to hold it into a neutral plantarflexion and dorsiflexion (Fig. 35-12C).

- Release the tourniquet and inspect the tibial vessels to ensure that they are not being kinked by the transferred tendon. Irrigate the wounds and close them in a standard fashion.

POSTOPERATIVE CARE. Postoperative care is the same as for transfer of the posterior tibial tendon to the dorsum of the foot (see Technique 35-4).

Equinus contractures can be corrected by a percutaneous Achilles tendon lengthening or an open Achilles tendon lengthening (Chapter 33). If an open procedure is needed because of severe contractures, lengthening or release of the posterior tibial, flexor digitorum, and flexor hallucis longus tendons also may be needed. When these lengthening procedures or releases are done, the child will need an ankle-foot orthosis to continue to stand or ambulate.

Although release of contractures usually allows another 2 to 3 years of ambulation, by age 12 to 13 years most children with Duchenne muscular dystrophy can no longer walk, and spinal deformity becomes the primary problem. Scoliosis affects almost all children with Duchenne muscular dystrophy, and the curve usually is progressive (Fig. 35-13), although with the use of steroids in the medical treatment of Duchenne muscular dystrophy the frequency of scoliosis has decreased. Scoliosis produces pelvic obliquity, which makes sitting increasingly difficult. Bracing and wheelchair spinal-support systems may slow progression of the curve, but spinal fusion ultimately is required for most patients.

When a patient becomes nonambulatory, the scoliosis almost invariably worsens and significant kyphosis develops. Many authors recommend spinal arthrodesis at the onset of scoliosis when the curve is only 20 degrees. Given the natural history of the condition, delaying surgery until the curve reaches 40 or 50 degrees has no advantage and can make surgery more complicated because of the worsening of cardiac and pulmonary function during the delay. Most authors recommend that the forced vital capacity of the lungs be 50% or more of normal to reduce pulmonary complications to an acceptable level, and a forced vital capacity of less than 35% has been cited as a relative contraindication to surgery and as evidence of significant cardiomyopathy. Surgery still can be done when vital capacity is less than 50%, but the risk of pulmonary and cardiac complications increases.

Posterior spinal fusion with segmental instrumentation is the operation of choice. The fusion and instrumentation should extend to the proximal thoracic spine to prevent postoperative kyphosis above the fusion (see Chapter 44). Facet joint arthrodesis should be performed at every level, using autogenous or allograft bone graft as needed. Most authors have recommended that fusion extend to the pelvis.

OTHER VARIANTS OF MUSCULAR DYSTROPHY

BECKER MUSCULAR DYSTROPHY

Becker muscular dystrophy is a sex-linked recessive disorder that has a later onset and a slower rate of muscle deterioration than Duchenne muscular dystrophy. The prevalence of Becker muscular dystrophy based on dystrophin analysis is 2.3 per 100,000. The affected gene in Becker muscular dystrophy is identical to that in Duchenne muscular dystrophy (located at

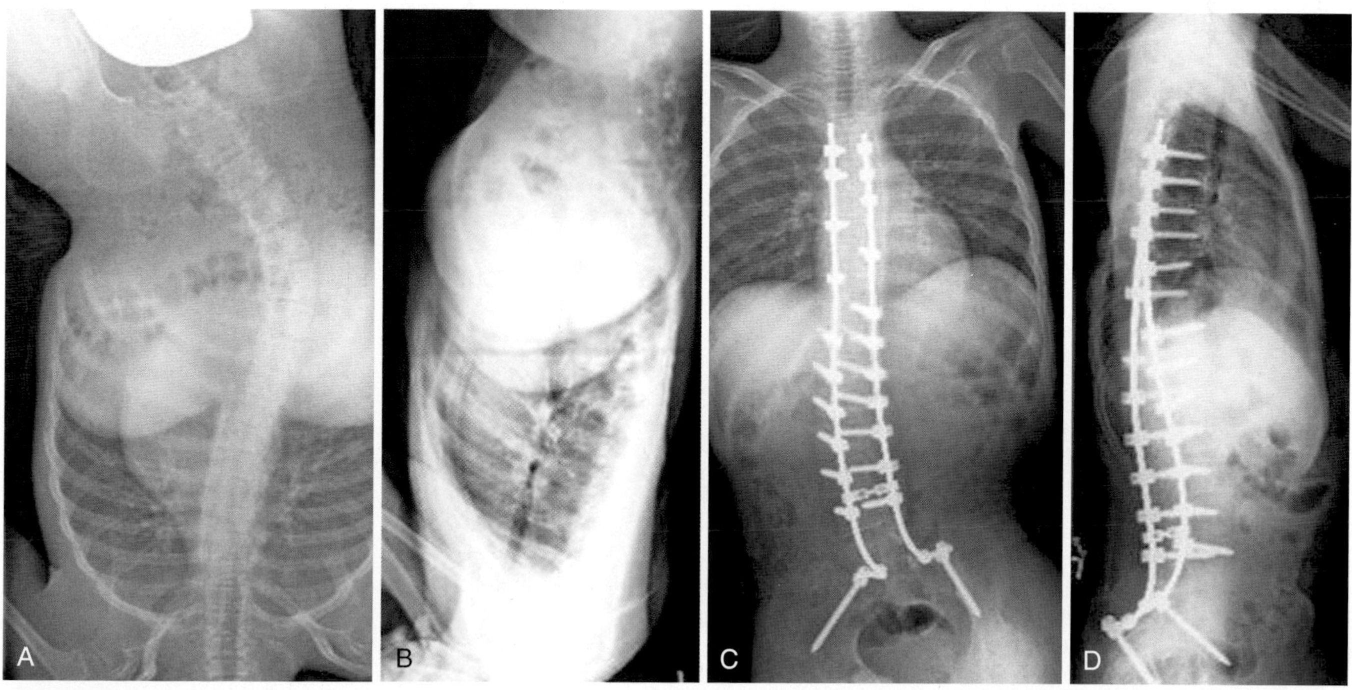

FIGURE 35-13 **A** and **B**, Radiographs of patient with Duchenne muscular dystrophy and scoliosis. **C** and **D**, Postoperative radiographs after posterior fusion and instrumentation to the pelvis.

the Xp21 locus on the X chromosome), but patients with Becker muscular dystrophy show some evidence of a functional intracellular dystrophin. The dystrophin in Becker muscular dystrophy, although present, is altered in size or decreased in amount or both. The severity of the disease depends on the amount of functional dystrophin in the muscles. Genetic studies and dystrophin testing now allow the clinician to better define severe forms of Becker muscular dystrophy. Serum creatine kinase levels are highest before muscle weakness is clinically apparent and can be 10 to 20 times normal levels. Onset of symptoms usually occurs after age 7 years, and patients may live to their mid forties or later. Cardiac involvement is frequent in patients with Becker muscular dystrophy; a high percentage of patients with Becker muscular dystrophy have electrocardiographic abnormalities and cardiomyopathy.

The orthopaedic treatment of Becker muscular dystrophy depends on the severity of the disease. In patients with large amounts of functional dystrophin, orthopaedic procedures frequently are not needed until after childhood, and in patients with more severe forms of the disease, treatment consideration is the same as for Duchenne muscular dystrophy. Contractures of the foot and overpull of the posterior tibial muscle can be treated effectively with Achilles tendon lengthening and posterior tibial tendon transfers with good long-term results. Patients rarely need soft-tissue releases around the hip. Scoliosis is not as common in patients with Becker muscular dystrophy, and no definitive recommendations exist in the literature, so treatment must be individualized.

EMERY-DREIFUSS MUSCULAR DYSTROPHY

Emery-Dreifuss muscular dystrophy is an X-linked recessive disorder, with the fully developed disease seen only in boys, although milder disease has been reported in girls. The gene locus for the most common form of Emery-Dreifuss muscular dystrophy is in the Xq28 region of the X chromosome. This region encodes for a nuclear membrane protein named emerin. Muscle biopsy of patients with Emery-Dreifuss muscular dystrophy shows normal levels of dystrophin but an absence of emerin.

During the first few years of life, patients have muscle weakness, an awkward gait, and a tendency for toe-walking. The full syndrome, usually occurring in the teens, is characterized by fixed equinus deformities of the ankles, flexion contractures of the elbows, extension contracture of the neck, and tightness of the lumbar paravertebral muscles. A significant factor in the diagnosis and treatment of Emery-Dreifuss muscular dystrophy is the presence of cardiac abnormalities, consisting of bradycardia and atrial ventricular conduction defects that can lead to complete heart block. It is important to recognize Emery-Dreifuss muscular dystrophy because of the cardiac abnormalities, which initially are almost always asymptomatic but lead to a high incidence of sudden cardiac death, which may be averted by a cardiac pacemaker. Most patients are able to ambulate until the fifth or sixth decade of life.

Orthopaedic treatment of Emery-Dreifuss muscular dystrophy involves release of the heel cord contractures and other muscles around the foot. This usually requires an Achilles tendon lengthening and a posterior ankle capsulotomy. Anterior transfer of the posterior tibial tendon also may be needed. Elbow flexion contractures usually do not exceed 35 degrees, but contractures of 90 degrees have been reported. Full flexion and normal pronation and supination are maintained. Successful results of release of elbow contractures have not been reported. Contractures around the neck and back should be treated conservatively with range of motion, although full range of motion should not be expected. Scoliosis can occur with this form of muscular dystrophy but has a lower incidence of progression.

LIMB-GIRDLE DYSTROPHY

Limb-girdle dystrophy is an autosomal recessive disorder, although an autosomal dominant pattern of inheritance has been reported in some families. The clinical characteristics are sometimes indistinguishable from those of Becker muscular dystrophy, but normal dystrophin is noted on laboratory examination. The disease usually occurs in the first to fourth decades of life. The initial muscle weakness involves the pelvic or shoulder girdle (Fig. 35-14). Lower extremity weakness usually involves the gluteus maximus, the iliopsoas, and the quadriceps. Upper extremity weakness may involve the trapezius, the serratus anterior, the rhomboids, the latissimus dorsi, and the pectoralis major. Some weakness also may develop in the prime movers of the fingers and wrists. There are two major forms of limb-girdle dystrophy: the more common pelvic girdle type and a scapulohumeral type. Surgery seldom is required in patients with limb-girdle dystrophy. Stabilization of the scapula to the ribs may be required for winging of the scapula, and in rare cases muscle transfers around the wrist may be needed.

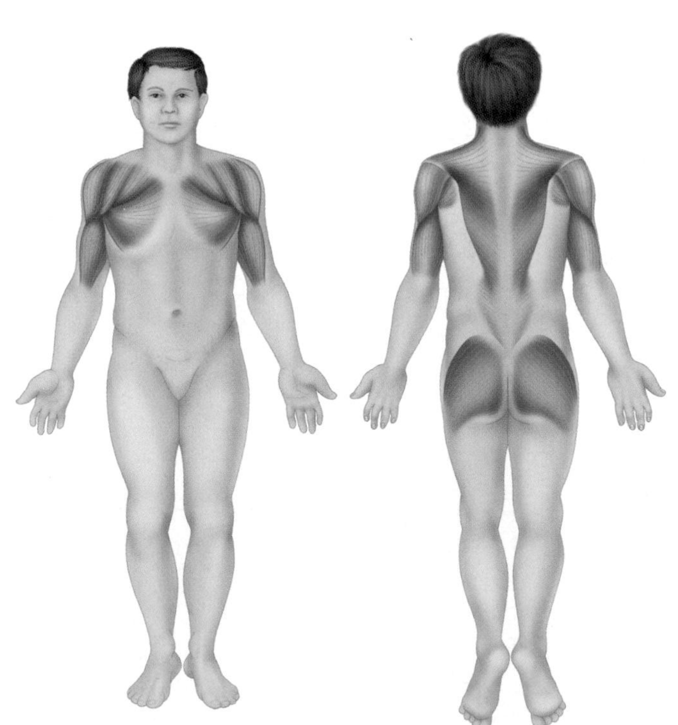

FIGURE 35-14 Pattern of weakness in limb-girdle dystrophy. (Redrawn from Siegel IM: Clinical management of muscle disease, London, 1977, William Heinemann.)

FACIOSCAPULOHUMERAL MUSCULAR DYSTROPHY

Facioscapulohumeral muscular dystrophy is an autosomal dominant condition with characteristic weakness of the facial and shoulder girdle muscles (Fig. 35-15). The affected gene is located on chromosome 4q35. Onset of the disease may be in early childhood, in which case the disease runs a rapid, progressive course, confining most children to a wheelchair by age 8 to 9 years; alternatively, onset may occur in patients 15 to 35 years old, in which case the disease progresses more slowly. The most striking clinical manifestation is facial weakness with an inability to whistle, purse the lips, wrinkle the brow, or blow out the cheeks. The greatest functional impairments are the inability to abduct and flex the arms at the glenohumeral joints and winging of the scapula, both caused by progressive weakness of the muscles that fix the scapula to the thoracic wall, whereas the muscles that abduct the glenohumeral joint remain strong. As the disease progresses, weakness of the lower extremities, especially in the peroneal and the anterior tibial muscles, results in a footdrop that requires the use of an ankle-foot orthosis. Sometimes the quadriceps muscle is involved, requiring expansion of the orthosis to a knee-ankle-foot orthosis. Scoliosis is rare, although increased lumbar lordosis is common.

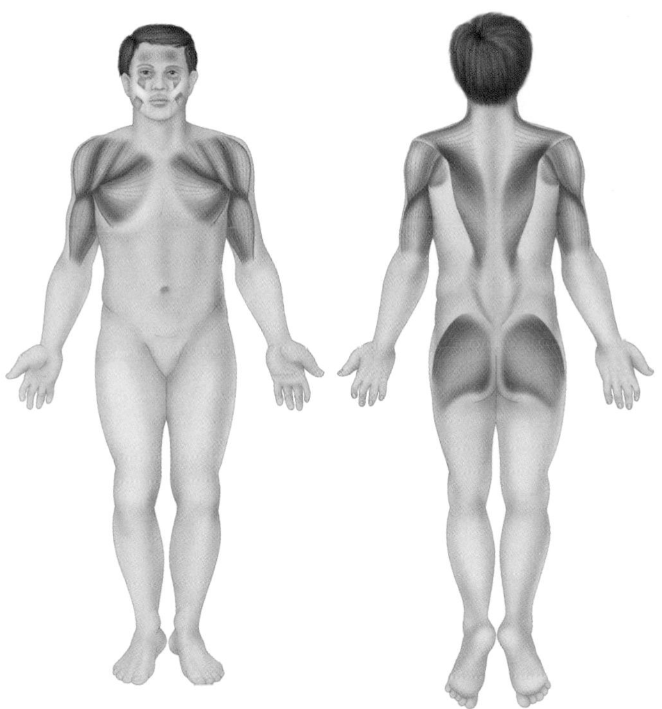

FIGURE 35-15 Pattern of weakness in facioscapulohumeral dystrophy.

The inability to flex and abduct the shoulder functionally usually is treated by stabilization of the scapula, with scapulothoracic arthrodesis. Scapulothoracic fusion with strut grafts or with plates and screws provides a satisfactory fusion of the medial border of the scapula to the posterior thoracic ribs (Fig. 35-16); however, it is associated with significant complications, including pneumothorax, pleural effusion, atelectasis, and pseudarthrosis. Techniques using wires for fixation have been described by Jakab and Gledhill, Twyman et al., and Diab et al. Copeland et al. described a similar fusion technique, but instead of wires they used screws to stabilize the scapula to the fourth, fifth, and sixth ribs (Fig. 35-17).

Cited indications for scapulothoracic fusion include limited shoulder abduction and flexion of more than 90 degrees, scapular winging, and shoulder discomfort; deltoid strength should be at least grade 4 of 5 at the time of surgery. In their 11 procedures in eight patients, the only complication reported by Diab et al. was prominent subcutaneous wires that required trimming in two patients. They noted that scapulothoracic fusion can relieve shoulder fatigue and pain, allow smooth abduction and flexion of the upper extremity, and improve the appearance of the neck and shoulder. Although disease progression affecting the deltoid muscle can cause a loss of abduction, other benefits of the procedure are maintained long term.

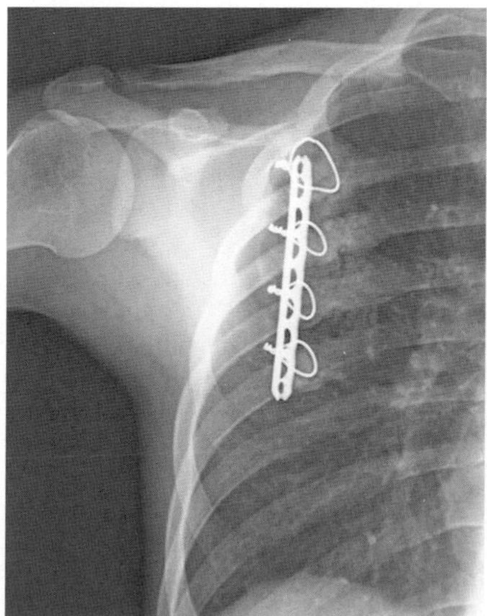

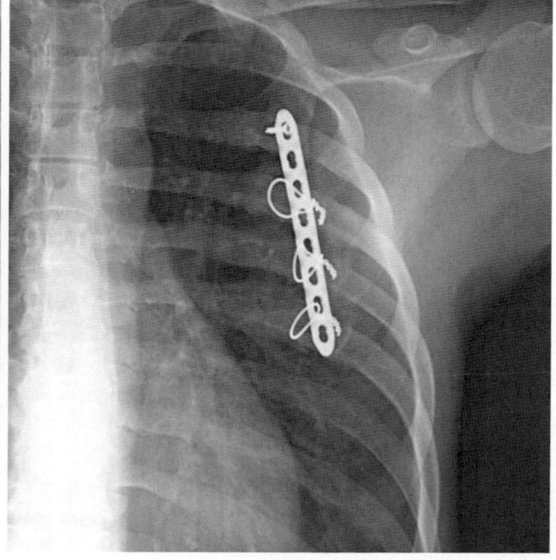

FIGURE 35-16 Bilateral scapulothoracic arthrodesis in a patient with fascioscapulohumeral dystrophy.

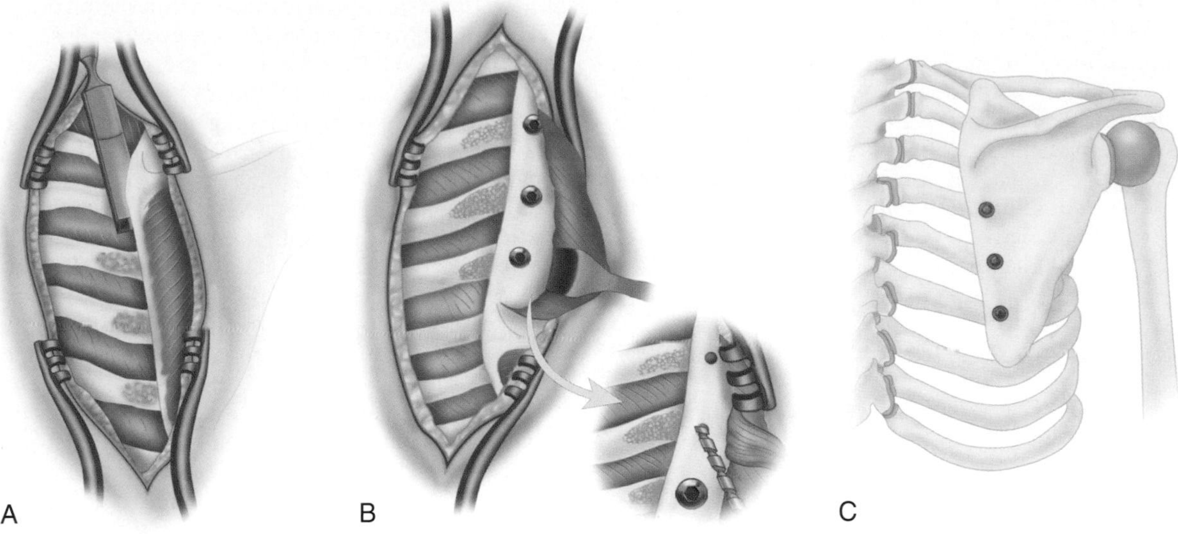

FIGURE 35-17 Copeland technique of scapulothoracic fusion. **A,** Decortication of ribs. **B** and **C,** Drilling and insertion of rib screws after application of cancellous bone graft.

SCAPULOTHORACIC FUSION

TECHNIQUE 35-6

(DIAB ET AL.)

- Place the patient prone, with the forequarter draped free. Abduct the upper limb so that the scapula lies flat against the posterior part of the thorax with its vertebral border externally rotated at an angle of 25 degrees to the midline.
- Make a linear incision over the entire vertebral border of the scapula in the reduced position.
- Cut the trapezius muscle in line with the cutaneous incision.
- Release the levator scapulae and rhomboid major and minor muscles from their sites of insertion on the vertebral border of the scapula and dissect them medially. These muscles usually are atrophic and markedly fibrotic and fatty.
- Reflect the supraspinatus, infraspinatus, and teres major muscles 2 to 3 cm laterally from their sites of origin on the vertebral border of the scapula.
- Expose the posterior surface of the vertebral border of the scapula subperiosteally (Fig. 35-18A).
- Reflect a 4- to 5-cm segment of the origin of the subscapularis laterally from the anteromedial part of the scapula, also in the subperiosteal plane. Excise part of the subscapularis if necessary to expose the deep surface of the vertebral border of the scapula and to permit its apposition against the adjacent ribs.
- In the process of clearing the vertebral border of the scapula subperiosteally, free the insertion of the serratus anterior anteriorly from the whole length of the medial border of the scapula. This should allow the scapula to be placed without tension in a more medial and inferior position against the posterior part of the chest wall. It is important not to attempt to gain even further medial-inferior correction by forceful efforts because doing so might stretch adjacent neurovascular structures and cause a brachial plexus palsy.
- Expose subperiosteally, from the neck to the posterior angle, five ribs at the fusion site, typically the second to the sixth or the third to seventh ribs, taking care to protect the parietal pleura and subcostal neurovascular bundles.
- Harvest an autogenous cancellous bone graft from the posterior iliac crest.
- Use a motorized burr to partially decorticate to bleeding bone the anterior surface of the scapula and the posterior surface of the ribs.
- Place the scapula against the posterior part of the chest wall and mark the points of wire passage from the vertebral border of the scapula to the immediately adjacent ribs. Position the wires with one above the scapular spine, one at the level of the spine, and one below it, with the lowest at the most distal part of the vertebral border (Fig. 35-18B).
- Bend a doubled 16-gauge wire into a C shape and pass it under the rib subperiosteally from superior to inferior; twist the two ends once against the posterior surface of the rib to prevent impingement against the pleura.
- Drill holes along the vertebral border of the scapula, 1.5 to 2.0 cm from its margin, opposite the selected ribs in the supraspinatus and infraspinatus fossae, and through the base of the scapular spine (Fig. 35-18B).
- Apply screws with washers or preferably a dynamic compression plate or a flattened semitubular plate to the posteromedial surface of the scapula to reinforce the thin scapular bone (Fig. 35-18C). Occasionally, if a single contoured plate is too bulky, two plates can be used, with one above and one below the scapular spine.

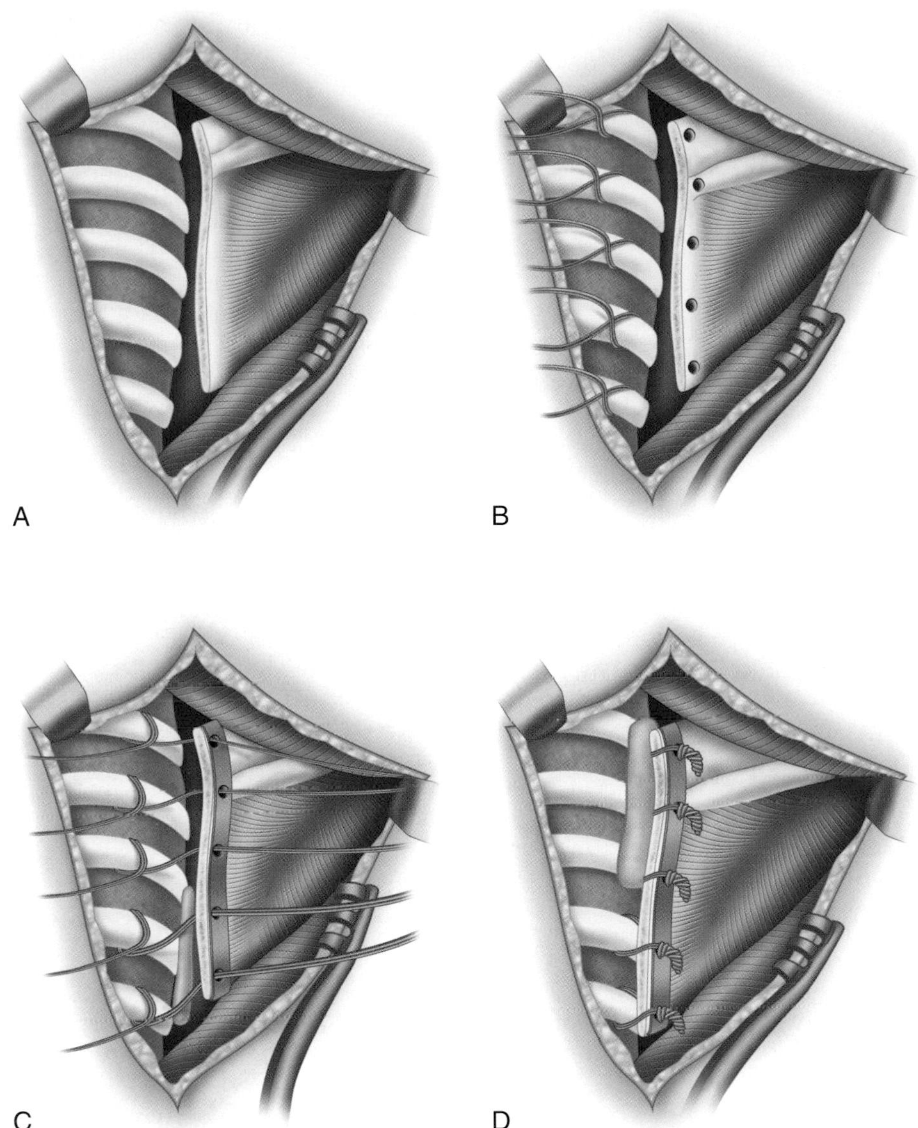

FIGURE 35-18 Technique of Diab et al. for scapulothoracic fusion (see text). **A,** Vertebral border of scapula and ribs are seen after surrounding muscles, fat, fibrous tissues, and periosteum have been cleared. **B,** Five doubled, 16-gauge wires are passed subperiosteally under the ribs and twisted on themselves to prevent impingement on the pleura. Five holes are drilled in medial aspect of scapula, adjacent to planned point of attachment to ribs. **C,** Single plate is bent to conform to shape of scapula, and one end of each wire is passed through drill hole and corresponding plate hole. Bone graft is placed between anterior border of scapula and posterior surface of ribs. **D,** Other end of each wire is pulled to posterior side of scapula and plate and tightened to firmly press scapula against ribs. (Redrawn from Diab M, Darras BT, Shapiro F: Scapulothoracic fusion for facioscapulohumeral muscular dystrophy, J Bone Joint Surg 87A:2267, 2005.) **SEE TECHNIQUE 35-6.**

- Pass one end of each wire from anterior to posterior through the adjacent hole in the vertebral border of the scapula and through the hole in the overlying plate or washers.
- Sandwich the cancellous bone graft between the scapular and costal surfaces, with adjacent ribs bridged by cancellous strips (Fig. 35-18C).
- With the scapula held in its final position, pull the other end of each wire over the posterior part of the plate and tighten the wires sequentially by twisting in a clockwise direction.
- Place any remaining bone graft between the posterior surfaces of the ribs medially and the vertebral border of the scapula (Fig. 35-18D).
- Fill the operative field with crystalloid solution and perform a Valsalva maneuver to detect any relatively large pleural tears.
- Cut and twist the wires to lie flat.
- Close the posterior muscles over the posterior surface of the scapula to provide a tenodesis effect and to cover the implants. Close the thoracic and posterior iliac wounds in a routine fashion.

- In the recovery room, obtain a chest radiograph to check for a developing pneumothorax; clinical symptoms may be masked by postoperative drowsiness or pain medications.

POSTOPERATIVE CARE. The shoulder and upper limb are immobilized in a sling and swathe for 4 weeks. Then the sling alone is used, with daily active range-of-motion exercises of the elbow, forearm, wrist, and hand, but no humeral abduction or flexion is allowed for 4 weeks. Shoulder abduction and flexion are progressed to full active range of motion with weaning from the sling over the next 4 to 8 weeks. At 3 to 4 months after surgery, when the rehabilitation program has led to pain-free clinical abduction and flexion, unrestricted activity is allowed.

INFANTILE FACIOSCAPULOHUMERAL MUSCULAR DYSTROPHY

An early-onset form of facioscapulohumeral muscular dystrophy has been described in which weakness is rapidly progressive and the lower extremities also are affected. Patients become wheelchair bound by the second decade of life. Facial weakness is seen in infancy, and this is followed by sensorineural hearing loss at an average of 5 years of age. A progressive lumbar hyperlordosis develops and is almost pathognomonic for infantile facioscapulohumeral muscular dystrophy. The hyperlordosis leads to fixed hip flexion contractures. Treatment consists of accommodation of the lordosis in the wheelchair. Spinal bracing has been unsuccessful. Spinal fusion may be indicated to assist with sitting balance. Scapulothoracic fusion is usually not indicated in these patients because of the advanced weakness associated with this form of facioscapulohumeral muscular dystrophy.

CONGENITAL DYSTROPHIES

Congenital dystrophies include relatively rare conditions, such as nemaline dystrophy, central core myopathy, myotubular myopathy, congenital fiber disproportion, and multicore and minicore disease. Congenital myopathies and congenital muscular dystrophies usually are defined by the histologic appearance of the muscle biopsy specimen, rather than by specific clinical or molecular criteria. Electron microscopy may be needed to differentiate some of the types. Weakness and contractures at birth can cause hip dislocation, clubfeet, or other deformities. Respiratory weakness and difficulty with feeding and swallowing are common. The clinical appearance is one of dysmorphism, with kyphoscoliosis, chest deformities, a long face, and a high palate. Muscle tissue gradually is replaced with fibrous tissue, and contractures can become severe. Treatment is aimed at keeping the patient ambulatory and preventing contractures by exercises and orthotic splinting. Equinus and varus deformities of the feet may require releases if they interfere with ambulation. Congenital dislocation of the hip and clubfoot deformity are treated conventionally, but recurrence is frequent.

MYOTONIC DYSTROPHY

Myotonic dystrophy is characterized by an inability of the muscles to relax after contraction. It is progressive and usually is present at birth, although it may develop in childhood. Inheritance is most often autosomal dominant but may be autosomal recessive. The genetic defect is located on chromosome 19. In addition to the inability of the muscles to relax, muscle weakness causes the most functional impairment. Other defects include hyperostosis of the skull, frontal and temporal baldness, gonadal atrophy, dysphasia, dysarthria, electrocardiographic abnormalities, and mental retardation. The characteristic clinical appearance is a tent-shaped mouth, facial diplegia, and dull expression. About half of children with myotonic dystrophy have clubfoot deformities, and hip dysplasia and scoliosis may exist. Hip dysplasia is treated conventionally, but because of capsular laxity it may not respond as readily as in other children. Serial casting can correct equinovarus deformity early on, but recurrence is likely, and extensile release usually is required; triple arthrodesis may be required at skeletal maturity because of recurrence despite extensile releases. In patients with marked clubfoot deformity, extensive posteromedial release may be insufficient to correct the deformity and a talectomy may be needed. An ankle-foot orthosis, which frequently is needed for weakness in dorsiflexion, usually can maintain postoperative correction. In some adolescent patients, scoliosis develops and should be treated with the same principles as for the treatment of idiopathic scoliosis. The high incidence of cardiac abnormalities and decreased pulmonary function increases the risk of surgery and may prohibit surgery in these patients.

HEREDITARY MOTOR AND SENSORY NEUROPATHIES

Hereditary motor and sensory neuropathies are a large group of inherited neuropathic disorders. The most common disorder among these neuropathies is Charcot-Marie-Tooth (CMT) disease. The hereditary motor and sensory neuropathies have been classified into seven types; types I, II, and III occur most often in children, and types IV, V, VI, and VII occur in adults (Table 35-4).

CHARCOT-MARIE-TOOTH DISEASE (PERONEAL MUSCULAR ATROPHY)

CMT disease is an inherited degenerative disorder of the central and peripheral nervous systems that causes muscle atrophy and loss of proprioception. It usually is an autosomal dominant trait but can be X-linked recessive or autosomal recessive. The incidence of the various forms of CMT disease ranges from 20 per 100,000 to one per 2500.

Muscle atrophy is steadily progressive in most patients with the autosomal dominant form; less often, the disease arrests completely or manifests intermittently. The recessive forms have an early onset (first or second decade) and are more rapidly progressive. Initial complaints usually are general weakness of the foot and an unsteady gait. Foot problems include pain under the metatarsal heads, claw toes, foot fatigue, and difficulty in wearing regular shoes. Distal loss of proprioception and spinal ataxia are common. CMT disease should be suspected in patients with claw toes, high arches, thin legs, poor balance, and an unsteady gait. Patients also may have hand dysfunction manifested by difficulties with handwriting because of weakness, pain, and

TABLE 35-4

Classification of Hereditary Motor Sensory Neuropathies

TYPE	NAME(S)	INHERITANCE
I	Peroneal atrophy, Charcot-Marie-Tooth disease (hypertrophic form), Roussy-Lévy syndrome (areflexic dystasia)	Autosomal dominant
II	Charcot-Marie-Tooth disease (neuronal form)	Variable
III	Dejerine-Sottas disease	Autosomal recessive
IV	Refsum disease	
V	Neuropathy with spastic paraplegia	
VI	Optic atrophy with peroneal muscle atrophy	
VII	Retinitis pigmentosa with distal muscle weakness and atrophy	

altered sensation, all of which may make the use of assistive ambulatory devices more difficult. In addition to physical examination and family history, electromyograms, which show an increased amplitude in duration of response and slow nerve conduction velocity, typically confirm the diagnosis. Karakis et al. cited several clinical features that are helpful in differentiating CMT disease from idiopathic pes cavus deformities: weakness, unsteady gait, positive family history, sensory deficits, distal atrophy and weakness, absent ankle jerks, and gait abnormalities. In a study of 148 children with bilateral cavus feet, 78% had CMT disease; the frequency increased to 91% if there was a positive family history.

Advances in molecular biology have improved the ability to confirm the diagnosis of CMT disease and to differentiate between variants of the condition. A mutation of the connexin-32 gene has been found to be associated with the most common form of X-linked CMT disease. Type IA CMT disease, or hereditary neuropathy with liability of pressure palsies, has been associated with a duplication or deletion of the peripheral myelin protein 22 gene *(PMP22)*. This association has been found in 70% of patients with type IA CMT disease. Southern blot analysis can be performed in commercial laboratories to confirm the presence or absence of these genetic abnormalities. The use of molecular biology may allow orthopaedic surgeons to make more specific treatment recommendations for patients with the variants of CMT disease.

CAVOVARUS FOOT DEFORMITY

Cavovarus foot deformities are the most common orthopaedic deformities in all types of CMT disease except type II, in which planovalgus foot deformities are most common. CMT disease is the most common neuromuscular cause of cavovarus foot deformity in children, but other causes should be considered when evaluating a child with a cavovarus foot deformity (Box 35-1). This is a complex deformity of the forefoot and hindfoot. Surgery often is required to stabilize the foot. Although there is little question that the cavovarus deformity is caused by muscle imbalance, theories explaining which muscles are involved and how the imbalances produce the rigid cavovarus deformity do not completely account for the clinical deformity. The neuropathic cavovarus deformity of CMT disease has been suggested to be caused by a combination of intrinsic and extrinsic weakness, beginning with weakness of the intrinsic foot muscles and the anterior tibial muscle, with normal strength of the posterior tibial and peroneus longus muscles. The triceps surae also is weak and may be contracted. The forefoot is pulled into equinus relative to the hindfoot, and the first ray becomes plantarflexed (Fig. 35-19). The long toe extensors attempt to assist the weak anterior tibial tendon in dorsiflexion but contribute to metatarsal plantarflexion, and the forefoot is pronated into a valgus position with mild adduction of the metatarsals. Initially, the foot is supple and plantigrade with weight bearing, but as the forefoot becomes more rigidly pronated, the hindfoot assumes a varus position. Weight bearing becomes a "tripod" mechanism, with weight borne on the heel and the first and fifth metatarsal heads.

BOX 35-1

Possible Causes of Cavovarus Foot Deformity

Brain
- Cerebral palsy
- Friedreich ataxia
- Stroke
- Tumor
- Spinocerebellar degeneration

Spinal Cord
- Tumor
- Spinal dysraphism
- Poliomyelitis
- Spinal muscular atrophy

Peripheral Nervous System
- Hereditary sensorimotor neuropathy (e.g., Charcot-Marie-Tooth disease)
- Traumatic peripheral nerve lesion (sciatic nerve)

Muscle and Tendon
- Leg compartment syndrome
- Residual clubfoot deformity
- Peroneus longus tendon laceration
- Duchenne muscular dystrophy

Bone
- Tarsal coalition
- Malunion of talar or calcaneal fracture

Idiopathic

Adapted from Lee MC, Sucato DJ: Pediatric issues with cavovarus foot deformity, Foot Ankle Clin North Am 13:199, 2008.

CLINICAL AND RADIOGRAPHIC EVALUATION

Clinical evaluation of the cavovarus deformity includes determination of the rigidity of the hindfoot varus, usually with the block test of Coleman (Fig. 35-20), and assessment of individual muscle strength and overall balance. Careful examination of the peripheral and central nervous systems is required, including electromyography and nerve conduction velocity studies.

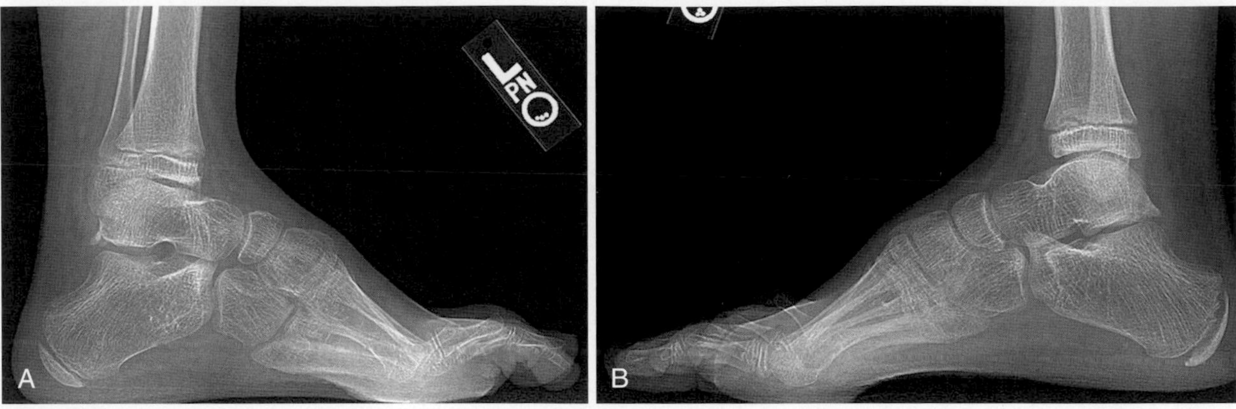

FIGURE 35-19 **A** and **B,** Left and right weight-bearing lateral radiographs of child with Charcot-Marie-Tooth disease demonstrating high arches, clawing of toes, and plantarflexed first metatarsal. Note asymmetry in the two sides. (From Beals TC, Nickish F: Charcot-Marie-Tooth disease and the cavovarus foot, Foot Ankle Clin North Am 13:259, 2008.)

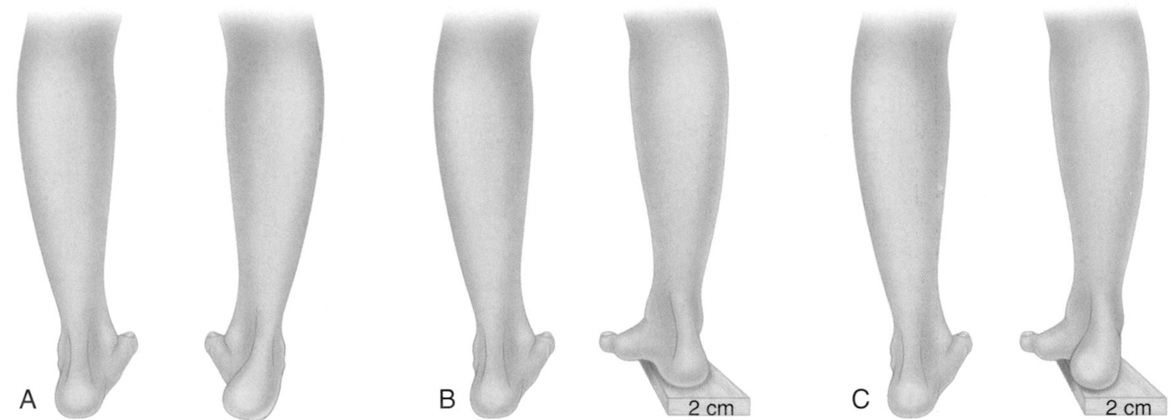

FIGURE 35-20 Coleman block test. **A,** Heel of foot and lateral border are placed on wooden block, allowing head of first metatarsal to drop into plantarflexion. **B,** If hindfoot varus is second to tripod effect of plantarflexed first ray, hindfoot will correct to neutral or valgus alignment. **C,** If hindfoot varus is rigid, it will not correct.

Standard anteroposterior, lateral, and oblique radiographs are the most useful methods for evaluating the child's foot; however, to determine any significant relationships between the bones, it is essential that the anteroposterior and lateral views be made with the foot in a weight-bearing or simulated weight-bearing position. Anteroposterior views document the degree of forefoot adduction. The degree of cavus can be estimated on the lateral view by determining the Meary angle, the angle between the long axis of the first metatarsal and long axis of the talus; the normal angle is 0 degrees. Radiographs using the Coleman block test show the correction of the varus deformity if the hindfoot is flexible.

ORTHOPAEDIC TREATMENT

Treatment is determined by the age of the patient and the cause and severity of the deformity. Medical treatment with high-dose ascorbic acid has been found to be ineffective in altering the natural history of this condition. Nonoperative treatment of the cavovarus foot, including the use of serial casting and botulinum toxin, generally has been unsuccessful. A randomized trial of 4 weeks of night casting found increased ankle dorsiflexion compared with no intervention, but at 8 weeks there was no significant difference. In a randomized trial of botulinum toxin to prevent pes cavus progression, although safe and well-tolerated, the injections did not affect the progression of the deformity.

Surgical procedures are of three types: soft tissue (plantar fascia release, tendon release or transfer), osteotomy (metatarsal, midfoot, calcaneal), and joint stabilizing (triple arthrodesis). Experience in the treatment of foot deformities in CMT disease has shown that early, aggressive treatment when the hindfoot is flexible and early soft-tissue releases can delay the need for more extensive reconstructive procedures. Even in young patients with a fixed hindfoot deformity, limited soft-tissue release, combined with a first metatarsal, midfoot osteotomy or calcaneal osteotomy, or both, can provide a satisfactory functional outcome without sacrificing the hindfoot and midfoot joint motion that is lost after triple arthrodesis. Because of early degenerative changes in the ankle, forefoot, and midfoot, triple arthrodesis should serve as a salvage procedure for patients in whom other procedures were unsuccessful or in patients with untreated fixed deformities (Fig. 35-21).

Younger patients and patients with flexible hindfeet usually respond to plantar releases and appropriate tendon transfers. Faldini et al. reported treatment of 24 flexible cavus feet in 12 patients (age 14 to 28 years) with CMT with a combination of plantar fascia release (Steindler stripping), closed superolateral wedge osteotomy of the cuboid and naviculocuneiform arthrodesis with closed superolateral wedge resection of articular surfaces (midtarsal osteotomy), dorsiflexion osteotomy of the first metatarsal, and extensor hallucis transfer (Jones procedure). Results were graded as excellent in 12 feet, good in 10, and fair in 2. These authors cited as advantages of midtarsal osteotomy correction of the main component of the deformity (excess elevation of the plantar arch) and preservation of the overall range of motion of the foot, which results in a more normal range of motion during walking.

PLANTAR FASCIOTOMY, OSTEOTOMIES, AND ARTHRODESIS FOR CHARCOT-MARIE-TOOTH DISEASE

TECHNIQUE 35-7

(FALDINI ET AL.)

PLANTAR FASCIOTOMY

- Make a 2-cm skin incision on the medial aspect of the heel and identify the plantar fascia.
- Apply tension by dorsiflexing the metatarsophalangeal joint and use a scalpel to completely strip the fascia from its origin. Take care to avoid damage to the lateral plantar artery and nerve and the inferior calcaneal nerve (Fig. 35-22A).

HINDFOOT CORRECTION AND STABILIZATION

- Before correction of the cavus deformity, manually reduce heel varus and stabilize the hindfoot with a 2.5-mm

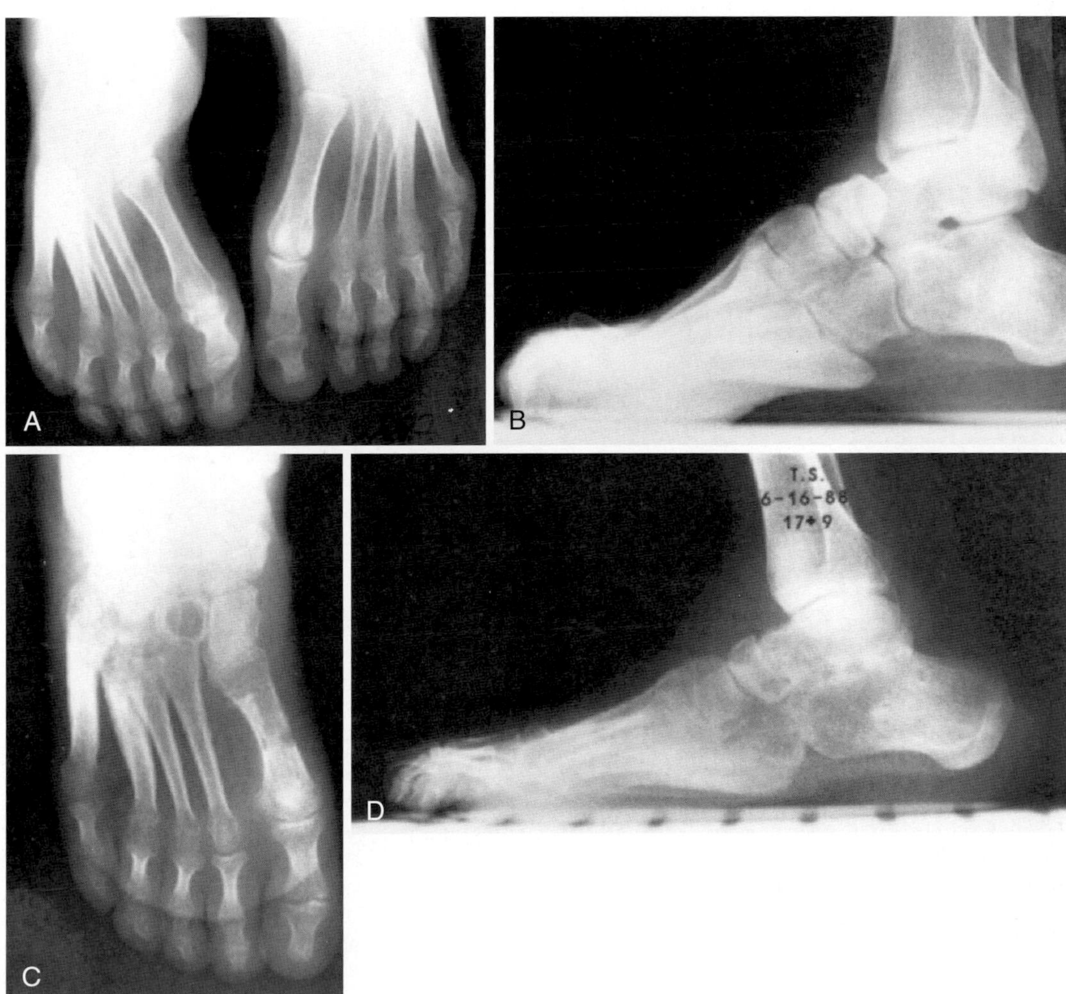

FIGURE 35-21 Cavovarus deformity in Charcot-Marie-Tooth disease. **A** and **B,** Preoperative radiographs. **C** and **D,** After triple arthrodesis, Achilles tendon lengthening, and posterior tibial tendon transfer. (Courtesy of Jay Cummings, MD.)

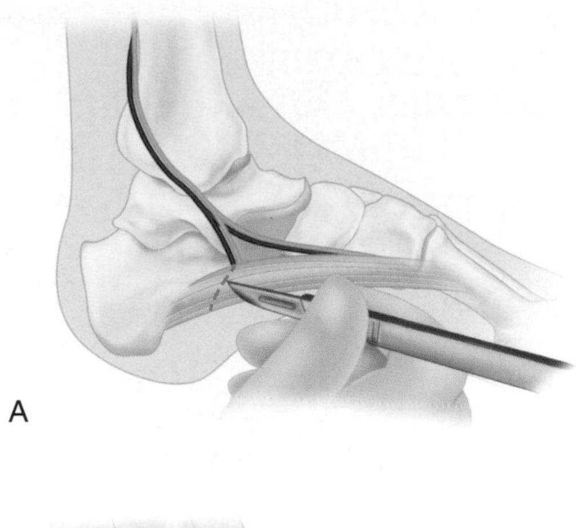

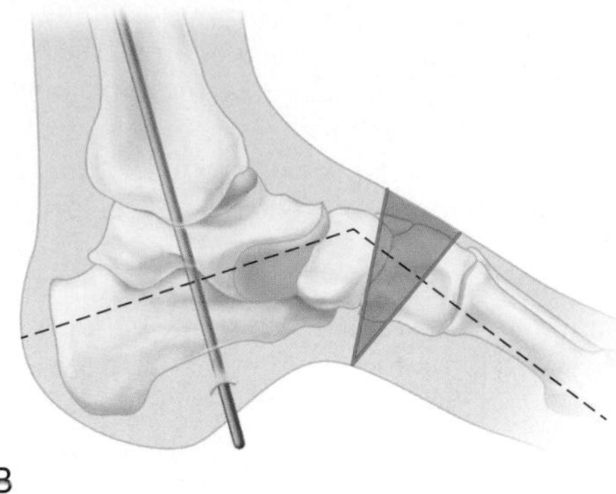

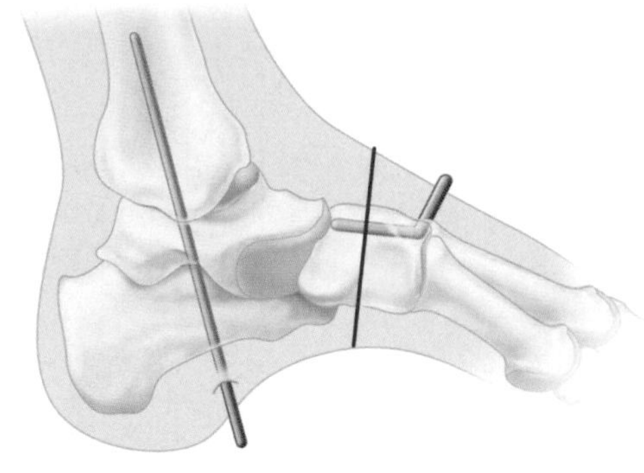

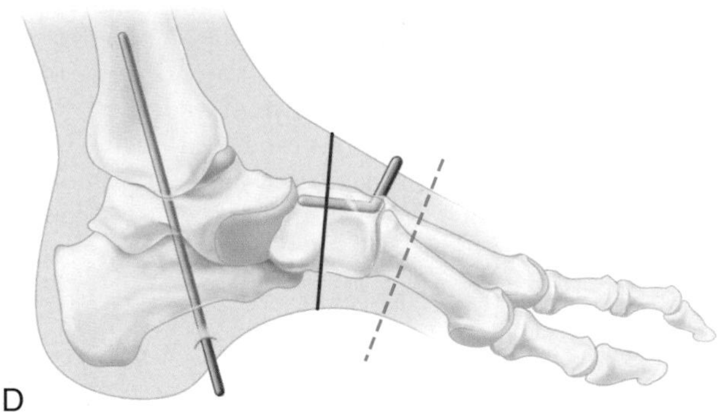

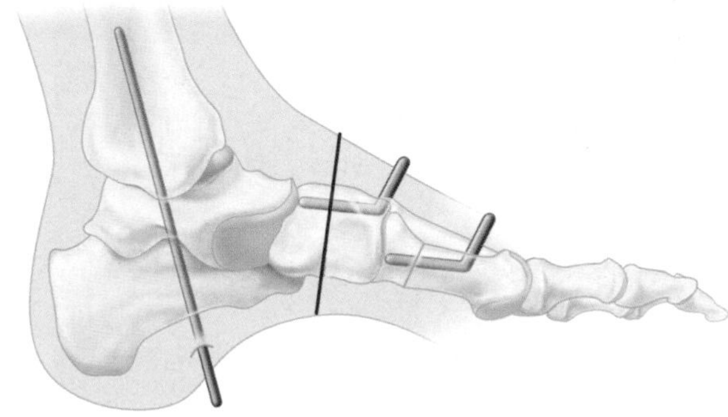

FIGURE 35-22 Treatment of cavus foot deformity in Charcot-Marie-Tooth disease. **A,** Plantar fasciotomy. **B,** Naviculocuneiform wedge resection. **C,** Fixation of arthrodesis with Kirschner wire. **D,** First metatarsal dorsiflexion osteotomy. **E,** Fixation with Kirschner wire. (Redrawn from Faldini C, Traina F, Nanni M, et al: Surgical treatment of cavus foot in Charcot-Marie-Tooth disease: a review of twenty-four cases, J Bone Joint Surg 97A:e30(1-10), 2015.) **SEE TECHNIQUE 35-7.**

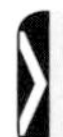

Kirschner wire inserted from the plantar aspect of the calcaneus into the tibia to maintain approximately 5 degrees of heel valgus and 20 degrees of ankle plantarflexion. This allows planning of the midtarsal osteotomy using the stabilized hindfoot as a fixed reference.

- Confirm the correct position of the ankle and correct insertion of the wire with fluoroscopy.

MIDTARSAL OSTEOTOMY

- Make a medial approach, approximately 3.5 cm long and centered slightly distal to the navicular prominence.
- Identify and expose the naviculocuneiform joint, with retraction of the marginal medial vein and the anterior tibial tendon.
- Use an oscillating saw to make a superolateral wedge resection of the articular surfaces.
- Through a lateral approach, also approximately 3.5 cm long, identify the cuboid and retract the extensor digitorum brevis dorsally.
- Expose the cuboid, sparing the calcaneocuboid and cuboid-metatarsal joints.
- Make a superolateral wedge resection of the cuboid to complete the midtarsal osteotomy (Fig. 35-22B).
- Close the naviculocuneiform arthrodesis and the cuboid osteotomy and fix them with a 2.5-mm Kirschner wire (Fig. 35-22C).

DORSIFLEXION OSTEOTOMY OF THE FIRST METATARSAL

- Through the medial approach, identify the base of the first metatarsal and use an oscillating saw to make a complete osteotomy of the meta-diaphysis (Fig. 35-22D).

- Displace the distal stump of the osteotomy in a plantar direction, approximating the dorsal corner of the diaphysis into the base of the metatarsal to obtain dorsiflexion of the ray.
- Fix the osteotomy with a 2-mm Kirschner wire (Fig. 35-22E).

EXTENSOR HALLUCIS TRANSFER

- Through the medial approach, expose the hallux up to the interphalangeal joint and identify the extensor hallucis longus tendon.
- Free the tendon from its retinacular attachment and detach it at the level of the first metatarsophalangeal joint.
- Drill a 3.2-mm hole at the metaphysis of the first metatarsal and pass the tendon through the hole and suture it to itself to form a loop, dorsiflexing the forefoot and applying moderate tension on the tendon transfer (Fig. 35-23A-C).
- Finally, tenodese the distal stump of the extensor longus to the extensor brevis and arthrodese the interphalangeal joint of the hallux, fixing it with a percutaneous Kirschner wire (Fig. 35-23D and E).

POSTOPERATIVE CARE. A non-weight-bearing boot cast is worn for 1 month, then the cast and percutaneous Kirschner wires are removed. An ambulatory boot cast is worn for another month. After its removal, active and passive mobilization of the foot and ankle, proprioceptive exercises, and muscle strengthening are begun.

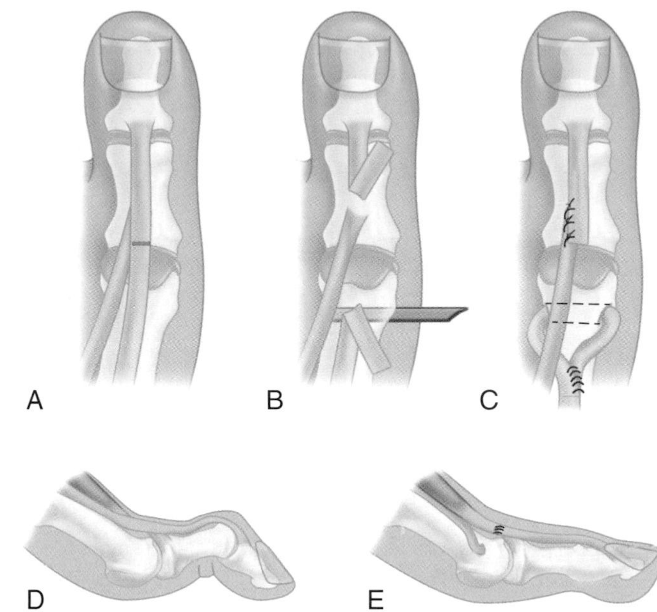

FIGURE 35-23 Treatment of cavus foot deformity in Charcot-Marie-Tooth disease. Extensor hallucis longus transfer (Jones procedure) **A** and **B**, Tendon detached at level of first metatarsophalangeal joint, passed through hole (**C**) and sutured to itself. **D** and **E**, Distal stump of extensor hallucis longus is tenodesed to extensor hallucis brevis. (Redrawn from Faldini C, Traina F, Nanni M, et al: Surgical treatment of cavus foot in Charcot-Marie-Tooth disease: a review of twenty-four cases, J Bone Joint Surg 97A:e30(1-10), 2015.) **SEE TECHNIQUE 35-7.**

In older children with rigid hindfoot deformities, radical plantar-medial release, first metatarsal osteotomy or midfoot osteotomy, and a calcaneal osteotomy usually correct the deformity. In a fixed hindfoot with a prominent calcaneus, a Dwyer lateral closing wedge osteotomy may be preferred to shorten the heel (Chapter 33). If the heel is not prominent, a sliding calcaneal osteotomy (Chapter 33) gives satisfactory results. Mubarak recommended a stepwise approach using joint-sparing osteotomies for rigid feet. These include (1) dorsal closing wedge osteotomy of the first metatarsal, (2) opening plantar wedge osteotomy of the medial cuneiform, (3) cuboid closing wedge osteotomy, and (4) accessory procedures as needed, including second/third metatarsal osteotomy, calcaneal sliding osteotomy, and peroneus longus to brevis transfer. The Ilizarov method also has been used in small series to correct rigid deformities. Although patient satisfaction is improved, there was no significant improvement in pain, function, or range of motion after surgery. Further study is necessary on the use of external fixation in correction of these deformities. Complete navicular excision and cuboid closing wedge osteotomy also can be used as a salvage procedure in severe rigid deformities where fusion is not appropriate.

Approximately 15% of patients with CMT disease require triple arthrodesis (Chapter 34). The Hoke arthrodesis or a modification of it is most often recommended. Appropriate wedge resections correct the hindfoot varus and midfoot component of the cavus deformity; soft-tissue release and muscle balancing are required for the forefoot deformity. In the most severe deformities, a Lambrinudi triple arthrodesis can produce a painless plantigrade foot. Restoration of hindfoot stability with triple arthrodesis and transfer of the posterior tibial tendon anteriorly have been recommended to eliminate the need for a postoperative footdrop brace, with a reported 88% good or excellent results. Achilles tendon lengthening with triple arthrodesis is recommended after correction of the forefoot (Fig. 35-21). Even with surgical correction and improvement in radiographic parameters, careful examination of the feet postoperatively is essential because pedobarometric pressures can remain abnormal in feet that appear corrected radiographically.

Flexible claw toe deformity usually is corrected without additional surgery when the midfoot deformity is corrected. For clawing in a young child without severe weakness of the anterior tibial muscle, the toe extensors can be transferred to the metatarsal necks with tenodesis of the interphalangeal joint of the great toe (Jones procedure). For adolescents or children with severe weakness of the anterior tibial muscle, all the long toe extensors can be transferred to the middle cuneiform with fusion of the interphalangeal joint (Hibbs procedure). For severe deformity, the posterior tibial tendon can be transferred anteriorly to the middle cuneiform instead of the long toe extensors (Technique 35-10).

Surgical procedures usually are staged. The initial procedure is a radical plantar or plantar-medial release, with a dorsal closing wedge osteotomy of the first metatarsal base if necessary. Achilles tendon lengthening should not be performed as part of the initial procedure because the force used to dorsiflex the forefoot would dorsiflex the calcaneus into an unacceptable position. If the hindfoot is flexible and a posterior release is unnecessary, posterior tibial tendon transfer can be done as part of the initial procedure for severe anterior tibial weakness.

RADICAL PLANTAR-MEDIAL RELEASE AND DORSAL CLOSING WEDGE OSTEOTOMY

TECHNIQUE 35-8

(COLEMAN)

- Make a curved incision over the medial aspect of the foot, extending anteriorly from the calcaneus to the base of the first metatarsal (Fig. 35-24A).
- Identify the origin of the abductor hallucis and separate it from its bony and soft-tissue attachments proximally and distally, but leave it attached at its origin and insertion.
- Identify the posterior neurovascular bundle as it divides into medial and lateral branches and enters the intrinsic musculature of the foot.
- Identify the tendinous origin of the abductor at its attachment on the calcaneus between the medial and lateral plantar branches of the nerve and artery and sever it to free the origin of the abductor hallucis.
- Identify the long toe flexors as they course along the plantar aspect of the foot and section the retinaculum of the tendons.
- Sever the origins of the plantar aponeurosis, the abductor hallucis, and the short flexors from their attachments to the calcaneus (Fig. 35-24B), and gently dissect this entire musculotendinous mass distally and extraperiosteally as far as the calcaneocuboid joint.
- If the first metatarsal remains in plantarflexion after this release, make a dorsally based closing wedge osteotomy immediately distal to the physis, removing enough bone to correct the lateral talo/first metatarsal angle to 0 degrees.
- Fix the osteotomy with a smooth Steinmann pin or Kirschner wire.
- Close the wound in routine fashion and apply a short leg cast with the foot in the corrected position.

POSTOPERATIVE CARE. If there is excessive tension on the wound, the foot can be cast in slight plantar flexion. A new cast should be applied at 2 weeks with the foot in a fully corrected position. The pins and cast are removed at 6 to 8 weeks.

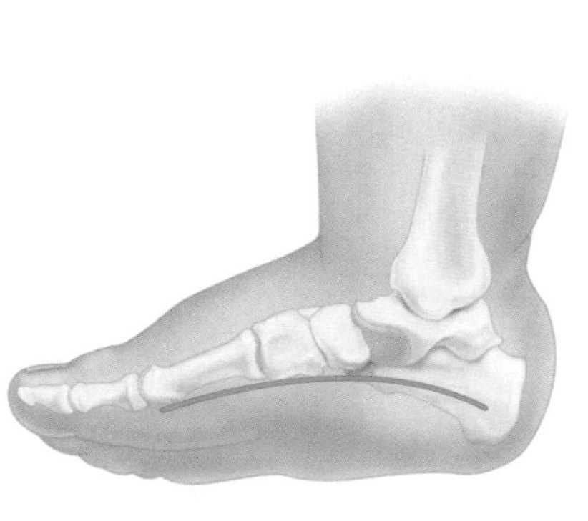
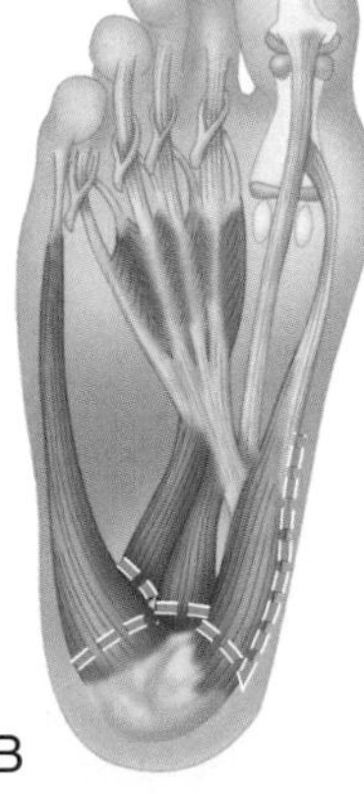

FIGURE 35-24 Radical plantar-medial release and dorsal closing wedge osteotomy for cavovarus deformity. **A,** Incision. **B,** Release of musculotendinous mass. **SEE TECHNIQUE 35-8.**

TRANSFER OF THE EXTENSOR HALLUCIS LONGUS TENDON FOR CLAW TOE DEFORMITY

TECHNIQUE 35-9

(JONES)

- Expose the interphalangeal joint of the great toe through an L-shaped incision (Fig. 35-25).
- Retract the flap of skin and subcutaneous tissue medially and proximally and expose the tendon of the extensor hallucis longus.
- Cut the tendon transversely 1 cm proximal to the joint and expose the joint.
- Excise the cartilage, approximate the joint surfaces, and insert a 5/64-inch intramedullary Kirschner wire or screw for fixation. Clip the wire off just outside the skin.
- Expose the neck of the first metatarsal through a 2.5-cm dorsomedial incision extending distally to the proximal extensor skin crease.
- Dissect free the extensor hallucis longus tendon, but protect the short extensor tendon. Cleanly and carefully excise the sheath of the long extensor tendon throughout the length of the proximal incision.
- Beginning on the inferomedial aspect of the first metatarsal neck, drill a hole transverse to the long axis of the bone to emerge on the dorsolateral aspect of the neck.
- Pass the tendon through the hole and suture it to itself with interrupted sutures.
- The same procedure can be performed on adjacent toes with clawing.
- Close the wounds and apply a short leg walking cast with the ankle in neutral position.

POSTOPERATIVE CARE. Walking with crutches is allowed in 2 to 3 days. At 3 weeks, the cast and skin sutures are removed and a short leg walking cast is applied. At 6 weeks, the walking cast and Kirschner wire are removed and active exercises are begun.

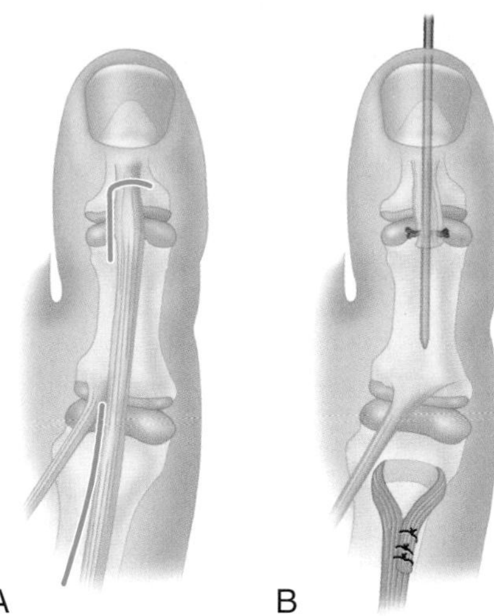

FIGURE 35-25 Transfer of extensor hallucis longus tendon for claw toe deformity (Jones procedure). **A,** Incisions. **B,** Completed procedure. **SEE TECHNIQUE 35-9.**

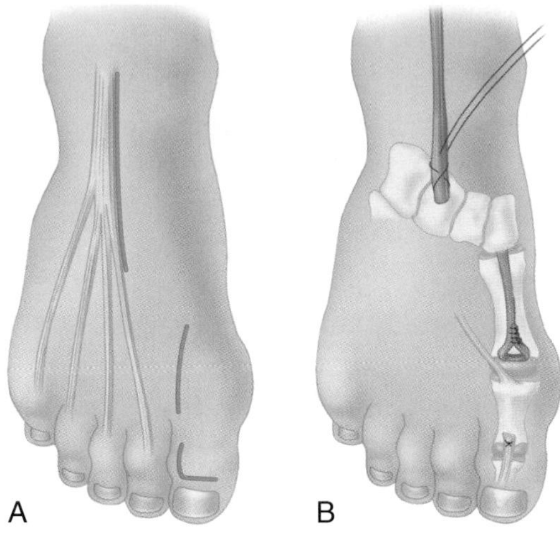

FIGURE 35-26 Transfer of extensor tendons to middle cuneiform for claw toe deformity (Hibbs procedure). **A,** Incisions. **B,** Completed procedure combined with Jones procedure. **SEE TECHNIQUE 35-10.**

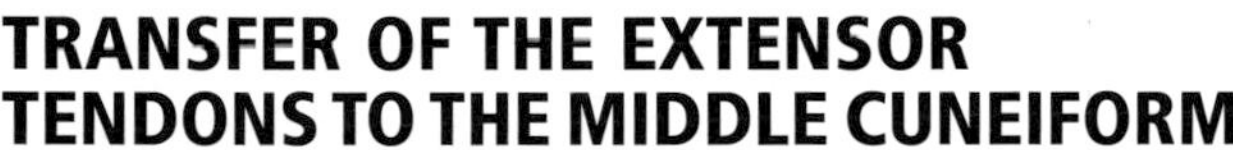

TRANSFER OF THE EXTENSOR TENDONS TO THE MIDDLE CUNEIFORM

TECHNIQUE 35-10

(HIBBS)

- Make a curved incision 7.5 to 10 cm long on the dorsum of the foot lateral to the midline and expose the common extensor tendons (Fig. 35-26).
- Divide the tendons as far distally as feasible, draw their proximal ends through a tunnel in the third cuneiform, and fix them with a nonabsorbable suture.
- As an alternative, use a plantar button and felt with a Bunnell pull-out stitch.
- Close the wounds and apply a plaster boot cast with the foot in the corrected position.

POSTOPERATIVE CARE. The cast and plantar button are removed at 6 weeks.

STEPWISE JOINT-SPARING FOOT OSTEOTOMIES

TECHNIQUE 35-11

(MUBARAK AND VAN VALIN)

FIRST RAY OSTEOTOMIES (OPENING-WEDGE OSTEOTOMY OF THE MEDIAL CUNEIFORM, DORSAL CLOSING-WEDGE OSTEOTOMY OF THE FIRST METATARSAL)

- Initial attention is focused on the first ray. Place a medial incision over the foot at the level of the first metatarsal and first cuneiform.
- Partially release the anterior tibial tendon insertion on the cuneiform.
- Place two needles to identify the midportion of the cuneiform and a position at least 1 cm distal to the first metatarsal physis. Take care not to disrupt the first metatarsal physis, which is proximal.
- Remove a 20- to 30-degree dorsal wedge from the first metatarsal and save it (Fig. 35-27A).
- Perform an opening-wedge osteotomy of the medial cuneiform (if necessary) (Fig. 35-27B) and place the bone wedge from the first metatarsal osteotomy into it and secure it with one or two Kirschner wires.

CUBOID CLOSING-WEDGE OSTEOTOMY

- Make a lateral incision over the cuboid and identify the calcaneocuboid and cuboid–fifth metatarsal joints fluoroscopically. Remove a 5- to 10-mm dorsal wedge of the cuboid and save the wedge (Fig. 35-27C). Secure the osteotomy with a single Kirschner wire.

METATARSAL OSTEOTOMIES

- If the second and third metatarsal heads are now prominent, dorsal closing-wedge osteotomies can be done. Place a single incision between the second and third metatarsals and remove and save dorsal wedges. These osteotomies can each be secured with a single intramedullary Kirschner wire.

ACCESSORY PROCEDURES

- Calcaneal osteotomy, usually a lateral displacement and closing wedge, is done if there is a fixed hindfoot deformity (Fig. 35-28).
- Plantar fasciotomies usually are done through a small incision if the plantar fascia is tight after osteotomies are complete.
- Peroneus longus-to-brevis transfer can be done after the cuboid closing–wedge osteotomy. Identify the peroneus longus on the plantar surface of the cuboid and release

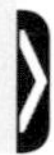

it. Attach the proximal end to the peroneus brevus using nonabsorbable suture.

POSTOPERATIVE CARE. The patient is kept non–weight bearing in a short leg cast that is bivalved to allow for swelling. The pins are removed at approximately 4 weeks after surgery under light sedation, and a walking cast is applied. Patients can fully bear weight 8 weeks after surgery.

In patients with advanced CMT disease, a triple arthrodesis may be necessary to establish a plantigrade foot; however, triple arthrodesis should not be routinely done in younger patients with less severe disease because degenerative changes of the ankle may result. In patients who have not had limited procedures during early adolescence but have major hindfoot, midfoot, and forefoot deformities, a triple arthrodesis may be the only treatment option. In severe deformity, a more extensive procedure, such as a Lambrinudi triple arthrodesis, can be performed. Techniques for triple arthrodesis are outlined in Chapter 34.

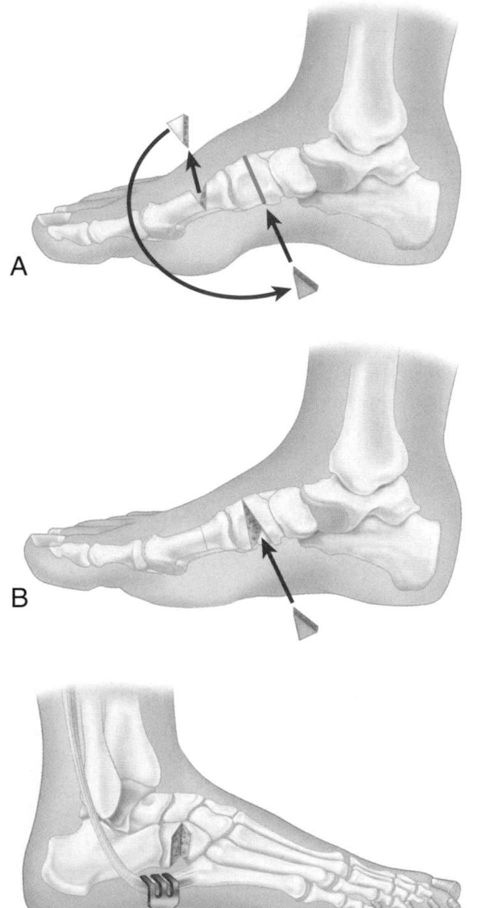

FIGURE 35-27 Stepwise joint-sparing osteotomies for cavus foot deformities (see text). **A,** First metatarsal closing-wedge osteotomy; removed piece will be used in cuneiform. **B,** Medial cuneiform opening-wedge osteotomy. **C,** Cuboid closing-wedge osteotomy, with or without second and third metatarsal osteotomies. (Redrawn from Mubarak SJ, Van Valin SE: Osteotomies of the foot for cavus deformities in children, J Pediatr Orthop 29:294, 2009.) **SEE TECHNIQUE 35-11.**

HIP DYSPLASIA

Hip dysplasia, which usually becomes apparent in the second and third decades of life, has been reported in 6% to 8% of patients with CMT disease. Dysplasia is more likely to occur in hereditary motor and sensory neuropathy type I than in type II. The treating physician should be aware of this association. If hip dysplasia is present, it should be corrected. Novais et al. found that acetabular dysplasia, hip subluxation, acetabular anteversion, coxa valga, and hip osteoarthritis were more severe in patients with CMT than in those with developmental dysplasia and suggested that this should be considered in determining the appropriate surgical strategy. In a series of 19 hips with symptomatic dysplasia in 14 CMT patients, Bernese periacetabular osteotomy successfully corrected radiographic abnormalities, but complications were common, including osteonecrosis of the femoral head, transient complete bilateral peroneal nerve palsy, inferior rami fractures, and heterotopic ossification. Most patients reported improved outcomes, although seven showed signs of radiographic progression of osteoarthritis. A later comparative study by Novais et al. of the Bernese periacetabular osteotomy in patients with hip dysplasia secondary to CMT disease (27 patients) or developmental dysplasia (54 patients) found that the osteotomy obtained improvements in patient-reported outcomes scores and in redirecting the acetabulum in symptomatic

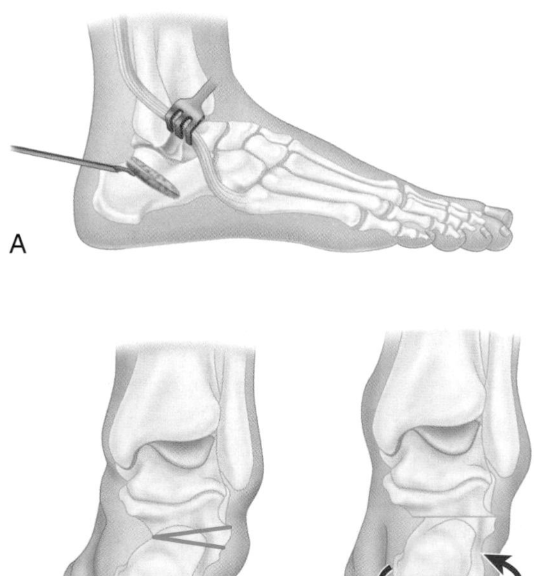

FIGURE 35-28 Stepwise joint-sparing osteotomies for cavus foot deformities (see text). **A,** Calcaneal osteotomy through lateral approach. **B,** Closing and lateral sliding wedge osteotomy. **C,** Closing and sliding wedge osteotomy. (Redrawn from Mubarak SJ, Van Valin SE: Osteotomies of the foot for cavus deformities in children, J Pediatr Orthop 29:294, 2009.) **SEE TECHNIQUE 35-11.**

CMT dysplasia; complications were much more frequent in patients with CMT (33%) than in those with developmental dysplasia of the hip (DDH; 13%).

SPINAL DEFORMITIES

Spinal deformities are present in approximately 25% of all patients with CMT disease. Approximately 75% of these patients have hereditary motor and sensory neuropathy type I with duplication of *PMP22* (peripheral myelin protein gene on chromosome 17). Scoliosis is uncommon in association with CMT disease, occurring in 10% to 30% of young patients, and the curve usually is mild to moderate and often does not require any treatment. In patients with CMT disease, nonoperative treatment with a brace usually is well tolerated and successfully controls the curve in many patients. Generally, spinal deformities in children with CMT disease can be managed by the same techniques used for idiopathic scoliosis (see Chapter 44). Because of the demyelination of the peripheral nerves and degeneration of the dorsal root ganglion and dorsal column of the spinal cord, somatosensory-evoked potentials may be absent.

CHARCOT-MARIE-TOOTH DISEASE VARIANTS

Genetic analysis of patients with the autosomal dominant form of CMT disease shows duplication of chromosome 17. A human peripheral myelin protein gene is contained within the duplication, and an abnormality in this gene encodes a myelin protein, which is the etiologic basis for CMT disease.

Roussy-Lévy syndrome (hereditary areflexic dystasia) is an autosomal dominant disease with the clinical characteristics of classic CMT disease plus a static tremor in the hands. The disease usually begins in infancy and is benign until adolescence. It is characterized by severe alterations in nerve conduction and sensory dysfunction.

Dejerine-Sottas syndrome (familial interstitial hypertrophic neuritis) usually is an autosomal recessive disease but may show an autosomal dominant inheritance with variable penetrance. The disease usually begins in infancy but may not appear until adolescence. Along with the classic pes cavus deformity, marked sensory loss occurs in all four extremities and patients may have clubfoot or kyphoscoliosis.

Refsum disease is an autosomal recessive disorder beginning in childhood or puberty in which the cerebrospinal fluid protein level is increased. The gene responsible for Refsum disease is on chromosome 10. The condition is caused by a defect in phytanoyl-CoA hydroxylase, the enzyme responsible for the degradation of phytanic acid. It is accompanied by retinitis pigmentosa and is characterized by a hypertrophic neuropathy with ataxia and areflexia. Distal sensory and motor loss occurs in the hands and feet. The course is unpredictable, with repeated reactivations and remissions, but the prognosis is poor.

Neuronal-type CMT disease is an autosomal dominant disease with a usually late onset (middle age or later). The small muscles of the hands are not as weak as in other forms of the disease, but the ankle muscles and plantar muscles of the feet are much weaker and more atrophic.

FRIEDREICH ATAXIA

Friedreich ataxia is an autosomal recessive condition characterized by spinocerebellar degeneration. The prevalence of Friedreich ataxia is approximately one in 50,000. The abnormal gene is located on chromosome 9, but the definitive form of Friedreich ataxia is caused by a trinucleotide repeat of GAA, which causes loss of expression of the frataxin protein. This leads to a neuronopathy of the dorsal root ganglion, leading to degeneration of peripheral nerve fibers and the dorsal spinal columns. An ataxic gait usually is the presenting symptom, with onset routinely between 7 and 15 years old. The clinical triad of ataxia, areflexia, and positive Babinski reflex suggests the diagnosis. A definitive diagnosis can be made with DNA testing. The disease is progressive, and almost all patients are wheelchair bound by the first or second decade of life. Patients typically exhibit progressive dysarthria or weakness, decreased vibratory sense in the lower extremities, cardiomyopathy, pes cavus, and scoliosis. Knee jerk and ankle jerk reflexes are lost quite early. Patients usually die in the fourth or fifth decades of life as a result of progressive cardiomyopathy, pneumonia, and aspiration.

The primary concern of the orthopaedist is the correction of foot and spinal deformities. In patients with Friedreich ataxia, the plantar reflex sometimes is so great that when standing is attempted, the feet and toes immediately plantar flex and the posterior tibial tendon pulls the forefoot into equinovarus. If general anesthesia is contraindicated because of myocardial involvement or other medical conditions, tenotomies of the Achilles tendon, the posterior tibial tendon at the ankle, and the toe flexors at the plantar side of the metatarsophalangeal joints can be done with the patient under local anesthesia. Surgery should be delayed in patients who are able to walk and who have deformities that are supple or can be controlled in braces; however, the cavovarus deformities tend to worsen and become rigid. In patients with rigid cavovarus deformity, primary triple arthrodesis provides a solid base of support with a fixed plantigrade foot. Because most patients become wheelchair bound, later development of ankle and midfoot degenerative changes seldom is clinically significant. Posterior tibial tenotomy, lengthening, or transfer should be combined with the triple arthrodesis. Bracing is routinely required after surgery.

In a study of 56 patients with Friedreich ataxia and scoliosis, the curve patterns were similar to those of idiopathic scoliosis, many curves were not progressive, no relationship existed between muscle weakness and the curvature, and the onset of the scoliosis before puberty was the major factor in progression. As opposed to idiopathic scoliosis, however, kyphosis frequently was noted in patients with Friedreich ataxia. The authors recommended that curves of less than 40 degrees should be observed and curves of more than 60 degrees should be treated surgically; treatment of curves between 40 and 60 degrees is based primarily on the patient's age at onset of the disease, age at which the scoliosis was first recognized, and evidence of the curve's progression. Stabilization of the spine should be performed when the curve is greater than 40 to 50 degrees and the patient is no longer ambulatory. A single-stage posterior arthrodesis with segmental instrumentation is the treatment of choice (Chapter 44). The fusion should extend from the upper thoracic spine to the lower region of the lumbar spine.

SPINAL MUSCULAR ATROPHY

Spinal muscular atrophy (SMA) is an inherited degenerative disease of the anterior horn cells of the spinal cord that occurs in one in 20,000 births. It is generally transmitted by an autosomal recessive gene, but other hereditary patterns have been described. Hoffmann (1893) and Werdnig (1894) first described an infantile condition of generalized weakness that resulted in early death from respiratory failure, and in 1956 Kugelberg and Welander described a similar condition of juvenile onset that was less progressive. Spinal muscular atrophy has been classified into three types (Table 35-5).

Although awareness of SMA has increased, diagnostic delay is common because symptoms can vary widely in onset and severity and can resemble other diseases. Early diagnosis of SMA is important because it allows early supportive care and reduction in patient and caregiver stress. A systematic literature review determined that diagnostic delay averaged 6 months for type I, 21 months for type II, and 50 months for type III. A review of families' experiences found that for most people the time between their noticing symptoms and receiving a diagnosis was lengthy, frustrating, and emotional. SMA should be considered in the differential diagnosis in children with any of the clinical characteristics associated with the disease (Table 35-1), and these signs should prompt referral to a pediatric neurologist as well as for a *SMN1* gene deletion test.

In patients with spinal muscular atrophy, the blood creatine kinase or aldolase value is normal or mildly elevated. Electromyography reveals muscle denervation. Nerve conduction velocities are normal. Genetic studies have shown the defective gene to be located on chromosome 5. In 98% of patients with spinal muscular atrophy, deletions of either exon 7 or exon 8 have been identified in the survival motor neuron *(SMN)* gene. A second disease-modifying gene, *SMN2,* also plays a role in the severity of the disease. Advances in molecular biology have now made a test for these genes and their potential deletions commercially available. The three types of spinal muscular atrophy seem to result from different mutations of the same gene.

Clinical characteristics of spinal muscular atrophy include severe weakness and hypotonia, areflexia, fine tremor of the fingers, fasciculation of the tongue, and normal sensation. Proximal muscles are affected more than distal ones, and the lower extremities usually are weaker than the upper extremities. Evans, Drennan, and Russman proposed a functional classification to aid in planning long-term orthopaedic care: group I patients never develop the strength to sit independently and have poor head control; group II patients develop head control and can sit but are unable to walk; group III patients can pull themselves up and walk in a limited fashion, frequently with the use of orthoses; and group IV patients develop the ability to walk and run normally and to climb stairs before onset of the weakness.

Orthopaedic treatment generally is required for hip and spine problems. Fractures are frequent in these patients as well, especially nonambulators, with the femur, ankle, and humerus the most common sites. Joint contractures also can occur, especially in the upper extremities, and tend to worsen with age. Children with type I spinal muscular atrophy are markedly hypotonic and generally die as a result of the disease early in life. In these patients, orthopaedic reconstruction is not warranted; however, patients with type I spinal muscular atrophy may develop fractures that heal quickly with appropriate splinting. Many children with infantile spinal muscular atrophy (Werdnig-Hoffmann disease) are never able to walk even with braces, but most patients with the juvenile form (Kugelberg-Welander disease) are able to walk for many years. Gentle passive range-of-motion exercises and positioning instructions can be beneficial initially. Surgical release of

TABLE 35-5

Spinal Muscular Atrophy

TYPE	CLINICAL CHARACTERISTICS	PROGNOSIS
1: most severe (Werdnig-Hoffman disease)	▪ Poor head control ▪ Difficulty with swallowing and feeding ▪ Absence of deep tendon reflexes ▪ Tongue atrophy ▪ Limb and trunk hypotonia ▪ Tongue fasciculations ▪ Intercostal muscle weakness	Patients with type 1 SMA have high risk of mortality in early childhood because of pulmonary complications.
2: intermediate severity	▪ Delayed motor milestones ▪ Functional ability to maintain sitting position without support ▪ Joint contractures ▪ Intercostal muscle weakness	Patients with type 2 SMA can be expected to live into their 20s and beyond.
3: mild (Kugelberg-Welander disease)	▪ Onset at age >18 months ▪ Ambulatory ▪ Scoliosis ▪ Hand tremors ▪ Muscle fasciculations ▪ Musculoskeletal overuse syndrome ▪ Hip abductor weakness (bilateral Trendelenburg lurch) ▪ Hip extensor weakness (increased lumbar lordosis)	Patients with type 3 SMA, especially those who remain ambulatory, have life expectancy not markedly different from that of general population.

(Based on information from Mesfin A, Sponseller PD, Leet AI: Spinal muscular atrophy: manifestations and management, J Am Acad Orthop Surg 20:393, 2012.)
SMA, Spinal muscular atrophy.

contractures rarely is required. Because of the absence of movement and weight bearing, coxa valga deformity of the hip is frequent and unilateral or bilateral hip subluxation may occur (Fig. 35-29). Because many of these children are sitters, a stable and comfortable sitting position is essential. Traditionally in nonambulatory patients, proximal femoral varus derotational osteotomy (Chapter 33) has been used to produce a more stable sitting base. Efforts to maintain the reduction of the hips for good sitting balance may prevent pain and pelvic obliquity. Observation instead of surgical intervention generally is recommended because of the small number of patients having symptoms or seating problems.

Among children with spinal muscular atrophy who survive childhood, scoliosis becomes the greatest threat during adolescence. The prevalence of scoliosis is nearly 100% in children with type II spinal muscular atrophy and in children with type III muscular atrophy who become

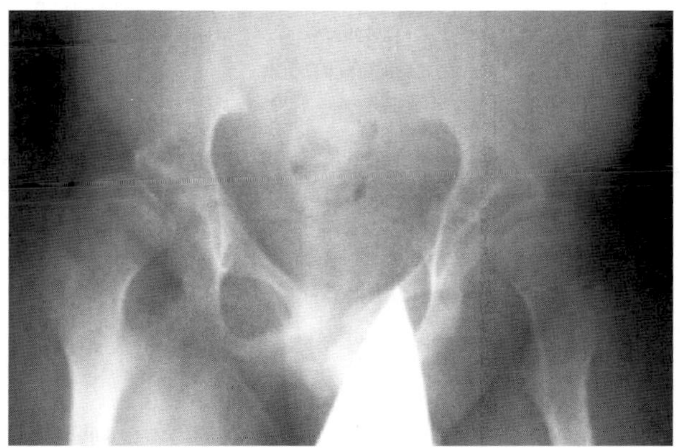

FIGURE 35-29 Coxa valga deformity and subluxation in 12-year-old child with spinal muscular atrophy.

nonambulatory. Curves typically are long and C-shaped and are most common in the thoracolumbar spine, occurring in up to 80% of patients. Scoliosis usually is progressive and severe and can limit daily function and cause cardiopulmonary problems. Bracing may be indicated during the growing years to slow curve progression, but spinal stabilization is ultimately required in almost all adolescent patients. Several authors have emphasized the importance of early surgery before the curve becomes severe and rigid. An inverse relationship between pulmonary function and scoliosis severity has been identified: for every 10-degree increase in Cobb angle, there is a 5% decrease in predicted vital capacity and a 3% decrease in peak flow. This limits the time frame during which patients with spinal muscular atrophy have sufficient lung capacity to successfully undergo spinal surgery.

The treatment of choice for most patients, especially older ones, is a long posterior fusion, using growth-friendly instrumentation. This fusion and instrumentation usually should extend to the pelvis in nonambulatory patients to prevent pelvic obliquity. Growing rod constructs have been shown to improve spine height, space available for the lungs, and control of pelvic obliquity in young patients with progressive scoliosis who are too young for definitive spinal fusion. Chandran et al. and McElroy et al. reported improvement in Cobb angles, as well as in quality of life for patients and caregivers, with few complications with the use of growing rods in patients with spinal muscular atrophy. Use of a vertical expandable prosthetic titanium rib (VEPTR; Synthes, Westchester, PA) has been reported in children with neuromuscular scoliosis, with varying results (Fig. 35-30). Livingston et al. compared the use of growing rods (9 children) with VEPTR (11 children) in spinal muscular atrophy and found that neither improved "parasol rib" deformity (collapse of the rib cage), although spinal deformity was better corrected with growing rods. At least one complication occurred in 83% of

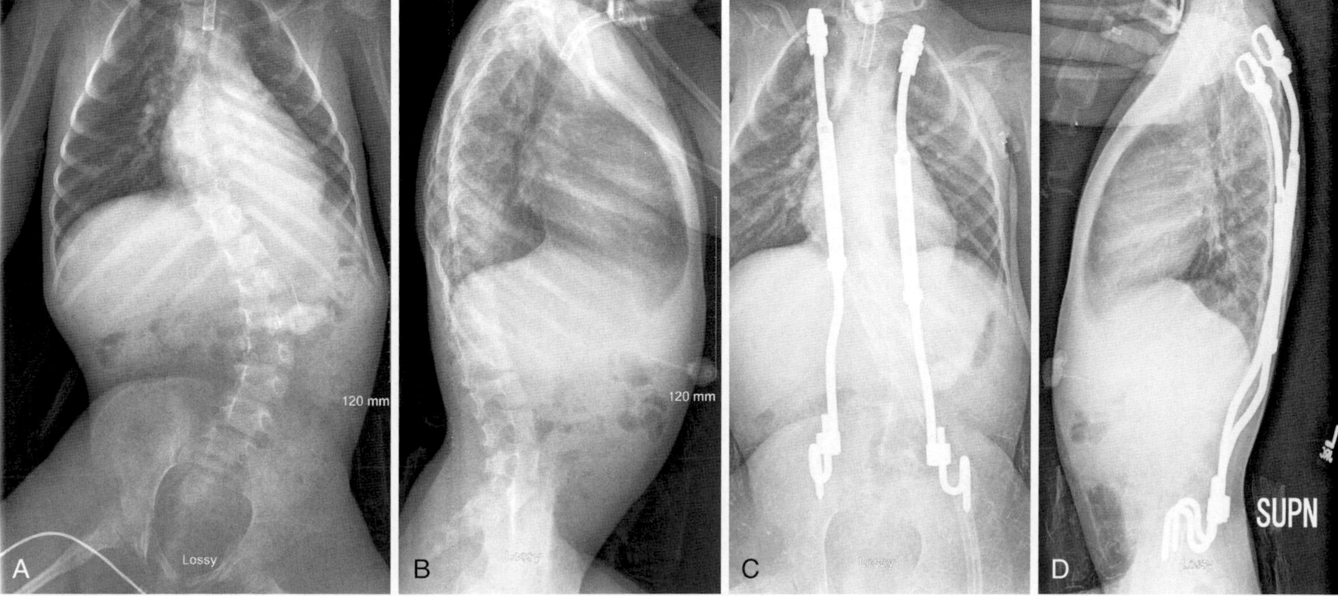

FIGURE 35-30 **A** and **B,** Spinal deformity in a young child with spinal muscular atrophy. **C** and **D,** At the age of 5 years, 2.5 years after implantation of vertical expandable prosthetic titanium rib (VEPTR).

those with VEPTR, compared with 41% of those with growing rods.

Intraoperative and postoperative complications are frequent in these patients, and thorough preoperative evaluation is mandatory. Numerous studies have found the frequency of respiratory tract infections before surgery and the vital capacity of the lungs to be good indicators of the patient's ability to tolerate surgery. Tracheostomy should be considered for any patient with frequent preoperative respiratory tract infections and a vital capacity of less than 35% of normal. Techniques of surgery for the treatment of neuromuscular scoliosis are described in Chapter 44.

REFERENCES

GENERAL

Bengtsson NE, Seto JT, Hall JK, et al: Progress and prospects of gene therapy clinical trials for the muscular dystrophies, *Hum Mol Genet* 2015 Oct 8. [Epub ahead of print].

Brooks JT, Sponseller PD: What's new in the management of neuromuscular scoliosis, *J Pediatr Orthop* 2015 Apr 13. [Epub ahead of print].

Canavese F, Sussman MD: Strategies of hip management in neuromuscular disorders: Duchenne muscular dystrophy, spinal muscular atrophy, Charcot-Marie-Tooth disease and arthrogryposis multiplex congenital, *Hip Int* 19(Suppl 6):S46, 2009.

Inal-Ince D, Savci S, Arikan H, et al: Effects of scoliosis on respiratory muscle strength in patients with neuromuscular disorders, *Spine J* 9:981, 2009.

Jirka S, Aartsma-Rus A: An update on RNA-targeting therapies for neuromuscular disorders, *Curr Opin Neurol* 28:515, 2015.

Mercuri E, Pichiecchio A, Allsop J, et al: Muscle MRI in inherited neuromuscular disorders: past, present, and future, *J Magn Reson Imaging* 25:433, 2007.

Schwend RM, Drennan JC: Cavus foot deformity in children, *J Am Acad Orthop Surg* 11:201, 2003.

Wagner S, Poirot I, Vuillerot C, Berard C: Tolerance and effectiveness on pain control of Pamidronate(r) intravenous infusions in children with neuromuscular disorders, *Ann Phys Rehabil Med* 54:348, 2011.

Yazici M, Ahser MA, Hardacker JW: The safety and efficacy of Isola-Galveston instrumentation and arthrodesis in the treatment of neuromuscular spinal deformities, *J Bone Joint Surg* 82A:524, 2000.

MUSCULAR DYSTROPHY—GENERAL

Angelini C: The role of corticosteroids in muscular dystrophy: a critical appraisal, *Muscle Nerve* 36:424, 2007.

Fishman FG, Goldstein EM, Peljovich AE: Surgical treatment of upper extremity contractures in Emery-Dreifuss muscular dystrophy, *J Pediatr Orthop B* 2015 Nov 19. [Epub ahead of print].

Griffet J, Decrocq L, Rauscent H, et al: Lower extremity surgery in muscular dystrophy, *Orthop Traumatol Surg Res* 97:634, 2011.

Rahimov F, Kunkel LM: The cell biology of disease: cellular and molecular mechanisms underlying muscular dystrophy, *J Cell Biol* 201:499, 2013.

Whitehead NP, Kim MJ, Bible KL, et al: A new therapeutic effect of simvastatin revealed by functional improvement in muscular dystrophy, *Proc Natl Acad Sci U S A* 112:12864, 2015.

Wright JG, Smith PL, Owen JL, Fehlings D: Assessing functional outcomes of children with muscular dystrophy and scoliosis: the Muscular Dystrophy Spine Questionnaire, *J Pediatr Orthop* 28:840, 2008.

DUCHENNE MUSCULAR DYSTROPHY

Abbs S, Tuffery-Giraud S, Bakker E, et al: Best Practice Guidelines on molecular diagnosis in Duchenne/Becker muscular dystrophies, *Neuromuscul Disord* 20:422, 2010.

Bos W, Westra AE, Pinxten W, et al: Risks in a trial of an innovative treatment of Duchenne muscular dystrophy, *Pediatrics* 136:1173, 2015.

Buckner JL, Bowden SA, Mahan JD: Optimizing bone health in Duchenne muscular dystrophy, *Int J Endocrinol* 2015:928385, 2015.

Bushby K, Finkel R, Birnkrant DJ, et al: Diagnosis and management of Duchenne muscular dystrophy, part 1: diagnosis and pharmacologic and psychosocial management, *Lancet Neurol* 9:77, 2010.

Cheuk DK, Wong V, Wraige E, et al: Surgery for scoliosis in Duchenne muscular dystrophy, *Cochrane Database Syst Rev* (1):CD005375, 2007.

Cheuk DK, Wong V, Wraige E, et al: Surgery for scoliosis in Duchenne muscular dystrophy, *Cochrane Database Syst Rev* (10):CD005375, 2015.

Gordon KE, Dooley JM, Sheppard KM, et al: Impact of bisphosphonates on survival for patients with Duchenne muscular dystrophy, *Pediatrics* 127:e353, 2011.

James KA, Cunniff C, Apkon SD, et al: Risk factors for first fractures among males with Duchenne or Becker muscular dystrophy, *J Pediatr Orthop* 35:640, 2015.

Karol LA: Scoliosis in patients with Duchenne muscular dystrophy, *J Bone Joint Surg* 89A(Suppl 1):155, 2007.

Kerr TP, Lin JP, Gresty MA, et al: Spinal stability is improved by inducing a lumbar lordosis in boys with Duchenne muscular dystrophy: a pilot study, *Gait Posture* 28:108, 2008.

Kim S, Campbell KA, Fox DJ, et al: Corticosteroid treatment in males with Duchenne muscular dystrophy: treatment duration and time to loss of ambulation, *J Child Neurol* 30:1275, 2015.

King WM, Ruttencutter R, Nagaraja HN, et al: Orthopedic outcomes of long-term daily corticosteroid treatment in Duchenne muscular dystrophy, *Neurology* 68:1607, 2007.

Lebel DE, Corston JA, McAdam LC, et al: Glucocorticoid treatment for the prevention of scoliosis in children with Duchenne muscular dystrophy: long-term follow-up, *J Bone Joint Surg* 95:1057, 2013.

Main M, Mercuri E, Haliloglu G, et al: Serial casting of the ankles in Duchenne muscular dystrophy: can it be an alternative to surgery? *Neuromuscul Disord* 17:277, 2007.

Manzur AY, Kuntzer T, Pike A, Swan A: Glucocorticoid corticosteroids for Duchenne muscular dystrophy, *Cochrane Database Syst Rev* (1):CD003725, 2008.

McMillan HJ, Gregas M, Darras BT, Kang PB: Serum transaminase levels in boys with Duchenne and Becker muscular dystrophy, *Pediatrics* 127:e132, 2011.

Partridge TA: Impending therapies for Duchenne muscular dystrophy, *Curr Opin Neurol* 24:415, 2011.

Shieh PB: Duchenne muscular dystrophy: clinical trials and emerging tribulations, *Curr Opin Neurol* 28:542, 2015.

Sienkiewicz D, Kulak W, Okurowska-Zawada B, et al: Duchenne muscular dystrophy: current cell therapies, *Ther Adv Neurol Disord* 8:166, 2015.

Suk KS, Lee BH, Lee HM, et al: Functional outcomes in Duchenne muscular dystrophy scoliosis: comparison of the differences between surgical and nonsurgical treatment, *J Bone Joint Surg* 96:409, 2014.

Takaso M, Nakazawa T, Imura T, et al: Two-year results for scoliosis secondary to Duchenne muscular dystrophy fused to lumbar 5 with segmental pedicle screw instrumentation, *J Orthop Sci* 15:171, 2010.

Velasco MV, Colin AA, Zurakowski D, et al: Posterior spinal fusion for scoliosis in Duchenne muscular dystrophy diminishes the rate of respiratory decline, *Spine* 32:459, 2007.

Wein N, Alfano L, Flanigan KM: Genetics and emerging treatments for Duchenne and Becker muscular dystrophy, *Pediatr Clin North Am* 62:723, 2015.

LIMB-GIRDLE DYSTROPHY

Moore SA, Shilling CJ, Westra S, et al: Limb-girdle muscular dystrophy in the United States, *J Neuropathol Exp Neurol* 65:995, 2006.

FACIOSCAPULOHUMERAL DYSTROPHY

de Greef JC, Lemmers RJ, Camano P, et al: Clinical features of facioscapulohumeral muscular dystrophy 2, *Neurology* 75:2010, 1548.

Gerevini S, Scarlato M, Maggi L, et al: Muscle MRI findings in facioscapulohumeral muscular dystrophy, *Eur Radiol* 2015 Jun 27. [Epub ahead of print].

Karceski S: Diagnosis and treatment of facioscapulohumeral muscular dystrophy: 2015 guidelines, *Neurology* 85:e41, 2015.

Lee CS, Kang SJ, Hwang CJ, et al: Early-onset facioscapulohumeral muscular dystrophy—significance of pelvic extensors in sagittal spinal imbalance, *J Pediatr Orthop B* 18:325, 2009.

Tawil R, Kissel JT, Heatwole C, et al: Evidence-based guideline summary: evaluation, diagnosis, and management of facioscapulohumeral muscular dystrophy: report of the Guideline Development, Dissemination, and Implementation Subcommittee of the American Academy of Neurology and the Practice Issues Review Panel of the American Association of Neuromuscular & Electrodiagnostic Medicine, *Neurology* 85:357, 2015.

Van Tongel A, Atoun E, Narvani A, et al: Medium to long-term outcome of thoracoscapular arthrodesis with screw fixation for fascioscapulohumeral muscular dystrophy, *J Bone Joint Surg* 95:1404, 2013.

CONGENITAL DYSTROPHY

Ho G, Cardamone M, Farrar M: Congenital and childhood myotonic dystrophy: current aspect of disease and future directions, *World J Clin Pediatr* 4:66, 2015.

Peat RA, Smith JM, Compton AG, et al: Diagnosis and etiology of congenital muscular dystrophy, *Neurology* 71:312, 2008.

Takaso M, Nakazawa T, Imura T, et al: Surgical correction of spinal deformity in patients with congenital muscular dystrophy, *J Orthop Sci* 15:493, 2010.

MYOTONIC DYSTROPHY

Canavese F, Sussman MD: Orthopaedic manifestations of congenital myotonic dystrophy during childhood and adolescence, *J Pediatr Orthop* 29:208, 2009.

Gadalla SM, Pfeiffer RM, Kristinsson SY, et al: Brain tumors in patients with myotonic dystrophy: a population-based study, *Eur J Neurol* 2015 Oct 28. [Epub ahead of print].

Johnson NE, Abbott D, Cannon-Albright LA: Relative risks for comorbidities associated with myotonic dystrophy: a population-based analysis, *Muscle Nerve* 52:659, 2015.

Johnston NE, Ekstrom AB, Campbell C, et al: Parent-reported multi-national study of the impact of congenital and childhood onset myotonic dystrophy, *Dev Med Child Neurol* 2015 Oct 28. [Epub ahead of print].

Schilling L, Forst R, Forst J, Fujak A: Orthopaedic disorders in myotonic dystrophy type 1: descriptive clinical study of 21 patients, *BMC Musculoskelet Disord* 14:338, 2013.

CHARCOT-MARIE-TOOTH DISEASE

Bamford NS, White KK, Robinett SA, et al: Neuromuscular hip dysplasia in Charcot-Marie-Tooth disease type 1A, *Dev Med Child Neurol* 51:408, 2009.

Beals TC, Nickisch F: Charcot-Marie-Tooth disease and the cavovarus foot, *Foot Ankle Clin* 13:259, 2008.

Burns J, Ryan MM, Ouvrier RA: Quality of life in children with Charcot-Marie-Tooth disease, *J Child Neurol* 25:343, 2010.

Burns J, Scheinberg A, Ryan MM, et al: Randomized trial of botulinum toxin to prevent pes cavus progression in pediatric Charcot-Marie-Tooth disease type 1A, *Muscle Nerve* 42:262, 2010.

Chan G, Bowen JR, Kumar SJ: Evaluation and treatment of hip dysplasia in Charcot-Marie-Tooth disease, *Orthop Clin North Am* 37:203, 2006.

Chung KW, Suh BC, Shy ME, et al: Different clinical and magnetic resonance imaging features between Charcot-Marie-Tooth disease type 1A and 2A, *Neuromuscul Disord* 18(6):10, 2008.

Dreher T, Wolf SI, Heitzmann D, et al: Tibialis posterior tendon transfer corrects the foot drop component of cavovarus foot deformity in Charcot-Marie-Tooth disease, *J Bone Joint Surg* 96:456, 2014.

Faldini C, Traina F, Nanni M, et al: Surgical treatment of cavus foot in Charcot-Marie-Tooth disease: a review of twenty-four cases: AAOS exhibit selection, *J Bone Joint Surg* 97:e30, 2015.

Guyton GP: Current concepts review: orthopaedic aspects of Charcot-Marie-Tooth disease, *Foot Ankle Int* 27:1003, 2006.

Hoellwarth IS, Mahan ST, Spencer SA: Painful pes planovalgus: an uncommon pediatric orthopedic presentation of Charcot-Marie-Tooth disease, *J Pediatr Orthop B* 21:428, 2012.

Karakis I, Greags M, Darras BT, et al: Clinical correlates of Charcot-Marie-Tooth disease in patients with pes cavus deformities, *Muscle Nerve* 47:488, 2013.

Karol LA, Elerson E: Scoliosis in patients with Charcot-Marie-Tooth disease, *J Bone Joint Surg* 89A:150, 2007.

Napiontek M, Pietrzak K: Joint preserving surgery versus arthrodesis in operative treatment of patients with neuromuscular polyneuropathy: questionnaire assessment, *Eur J Orthop Surg Traumatol* 25:391, 2015.

Novais EN, Bixby SD, Rennick J, et al: Hip dysplasia is more severe in Charcot-Marie-Tooth disease than in developmental dysplasia of the hip, *Clin Orthop Relat Res* 472:665, 2014.

Novais EN, Kim YJ, Carry PM, Millis MB: Periacetabular osteotomy redirects the acetabulum and improves pain in Charcot-Marie-Tooth hip dysplasia with higher complications compared with developmental dysplasia of the hip, *J Pediatr Orthop* 2015 June 3. [Epub ahead of print].

Pouwels S, de Boer A, Leufkens HG, et al: Risk of fracture in patients with Charcot-Marie-Tooth disease, *Muscle Nerve* 50:919, 2014.

Rose KJ, Raymond J, Regshauge K, et al: Serial night casting increases ankle dorsiflexion range in children and young adults with Charcot-Marie-Tooth disease: a randomised trial, *J Physiother* 56:113, 2010.

Saporta AS, Sottile SL, Miller LJ, et al: Charcot-Marie-Tooth disease subtypes and genetic testing strategies, *Ann Neurol* 69:22, 2011.

Stover MD, Podeszwa DA, De La Rocha A, Sucato DJ: Early results of the Bernese periacetabular osteotomy for symptomatic dysplasia in Charcot-Marie-Tooth disease, *Hip Int* 23(Suppl 9):S2, 2013.

VanderHave KL, Hensinger RN, King BW: Flexible cavovarus foot in children and adolescents, *Foot Ankle Clin* 18:715, 2013.

Ward CM, Dolan LA, Bennett DL, et al: Long-term results of reconstruction for treatment of a flexible cavovarus foot in Charcot-Marie-Tooth disease, *J Bone Joint Surg* 90A:2631, 2008.

Yagerman SE, Cross MB, Green DW, Scher DM: Pediatric orthopedic conditions in Charcot-Marie-Tooth disease: a literature review, *Curr Opin Pediatr* 24:50, 2012.

FRIEDREICH ATAXIA

Ashley CN, Hoang KD, Lynch DR, et al: Childhood ataxia: clinical features, pathogenesis, key unanswered questions, and future directions, *J Child Neurol* 27:1095, 2012.

Bodensteiner JB: Friedreich ataxia, *Semin Pediatr Neurol* 21:72, 2014.

La Pean A, Jeffries N, Grow C, et al: Predictors of progression in patients with Friedreich ataxia, *Mov Disord* 23:2026, 2008.

Lynch DR, Seyer L: Friedreich ataxia: new findings, new challenges, *Ann Neurol* 76:487, 2014.

Paulsen EK, Friedman LS, Myers LM, Lynch DR: Health-related quality of life in children with Friedreich ataxia, *Pediatr Neurol* 42:335, 2010.

Sival DA, Pouwels ME, Van Brederode A, et al: In children with Friedreich ataxia, muscle and ataxis parameters are associated, *Dev Med Child Neurol* 53:529, 2011.

Tsirikos AI, Smith G: Scoliosis in patients with Friedreich's ataxia, *J Bone Joint Surg* 94:684, 2012.

Tsou AY, Paulsen EK, Lagedrost SJ, et al: Mortality in Friedreich ataxia, *J Neurol Sci* 307:46, 2011.

SPINAL MUSCULAR ATROPHY

Chandran S, McCarthy J, Noonan K, et al: Early treatment of scoliosis with growing rods in children with severe spinal muscular atrophy: a preliminary report, *J Pediatr Orthop* 31:450, 2011.

Eckart M, Guenther UP, Idkowiak J, et al: The natural course of infantile spinal muscular atrophy with respiratory distress type I (SMRD1), *Pediatrics* 129:e148, 2012.

Fujak A, Kopschina C, Forst R, et al: Fractures in proximal spinal muscular atrophy, *Arch Orthop Trauma Surg* 130:775, 2010.

Fujak A, Raab W, Schuh A, et al: Natural course of scoliosis in proximal spinal muscular atrophy type II and IIIa: descriptive clinical study with retrospective data collection of 126 patients, *BMC Musculoskelet Disord* 14:283, 2013.

Funk S, Lovejoy S, Mencio G, Martus J: Rigid instrumentation for neuromuscular scoliosis improves deformity correction without increasing complications, *Spine* 41:46, 2016.

Haaker G, Fujak A: Proximal spinal muscular atrophy: current orthopedic perspective, *Appl Clin Genet* 6:113, 2013.

Halawi MJ, Lark RK, Fitch RD: Neuromuscular scoliosis: current concepts, *Orthopedics* 38:e452, 2015.

Humphrey E, Fuller HR, Morris GE: Current research on SMN protein and treatment strategies for spinal muscular atrophy, *Neuromuscul Disord* 22:193, 2012.

Kolb SJ, Kissel JT: Spinal muscular atrophy, *Neurol Clin* 33:831, 2015.

Lawton S, Hickerton C, Archibald AD, et al: A mixed methods exploration of families' experiences of the diagnosis of childhood spinal muscular atrophy, *Eur J Hum Genet* 23:575, 2015.

Lin CW, Kalb SJ, Yeh WS: Delay in diagnosis of spinal muscular atrophy: a systematic literature review, *Pediatr Neurol* 53:293, 2015.

Livingstone K, Zurakowski D, Snyder B: Growing Spine Study Group; Children's Spine Study Group: Parasol rib deformity in hypotonic neuromuscular scoliosis: a new radiographical definition and a comparison of short-term treatment outcomes with VEPTR and growing rods, *Spine* 40:E780, 2015.

McElroy MJ, Shaner AC, Crawford TO, et al: Growing rods for scoliosis in spinal muscular atrophy: structural effects, complications, and hospital stays, *Spine* 36:1305, 2011.

Mesfin A, Sponseller PD, Leet AI: Spinal muscular atrophy: manifestations and management, *J Am Acad Orthop Surg* 20:393, 2012.

Modi HN, Suh SW, Jong JY, et al: Treatment and complications in flaccid neuromuscular scoliosis (Duchenne muscular dystrophy and spinal muscular atrophy) with posterior-only pedicle screw instrumentation, *Eur Spine J* 19:384, 2010.

Sucato DJ: Spine deformity in spinal muscular atrophy, *J Bone Joint Surg* 89A(Suppl 1):148, 2007.

Tisdale S, Pellizzoni L: Disease mechanisms and therapeutic approaches in spinal muscular atrophy, *J Neurosci* 35:8691, 2015.

Tobert DG, Vitale MG: Strategies for treating scoliosis in children with spinal muscular atrophy, *Am J Orthop* 42:E99, 2013.

Vai S, Bianchi ML, Moroni I, et al: Bone and spinal muscular atrophy, *Bone* 79:116, 2015.

Wadman RI, Bosboom WM, van den Berg LH, et al: Drug treatment for spinal muscular atrophy type I, *Cochrane Database Syst Rev* (1):CD006281, 2011.

Wadman RI, Bosboom WM, van den Berg LH, et al: Drug treatment for spinal muscular atrophy types II and III, *Cochrane Database Syst Rev* (1):CD006282, 2011.

Wertz MH, Sahin M: Developing therapies for spinal muscular atrophy, *Ann N Y Acad Sci* 2015 Jul 14. [Epub ahead of print].

White KK, Song KM, Frost N, et al: VEPTR growing rods for early-onset neuromuscular scoliosis: feasible and effective, *Clin Orthop Relat Res* 469:1335, 2011.

Yuan P, Jiang L: Clinical characteristics of three subtypes of spinal muscular atrophy in children, *Brain Dev* 37:537, 2015.

Zebala LP, Bridwell KH, Baldus C, et al: Minimum 5-year radiographic results of long scoliosis fusion in juvenile spinal muscular atrophy patients: major curve progression after instrumented fusion, *J Pediatr Orthop* 31:480, 2011.

The complete list of references is available online at ***expertconsult.inkling.com****.*

PART XI

FRACTURES AND DISLOCATIONS IN CHILDREN

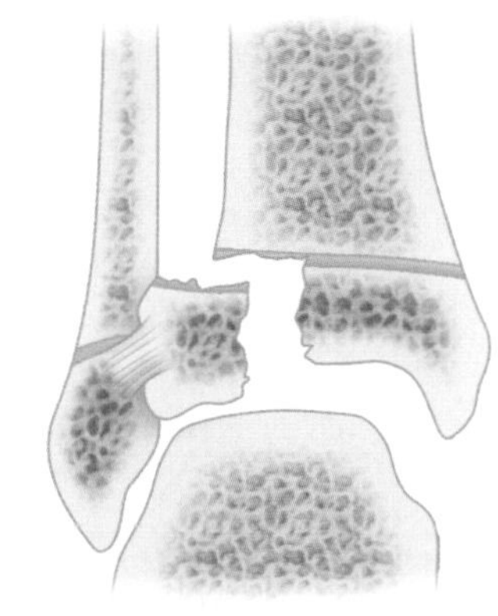

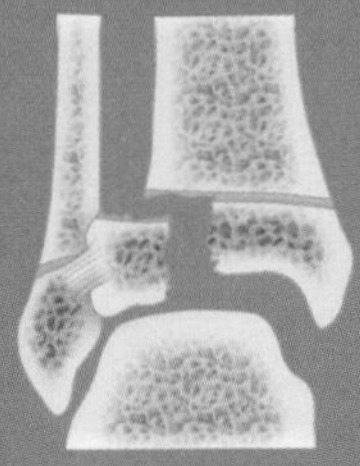

CHAPTER 36

FRACTURES AND DISLOCATIONS IN CHILDREN

Jeffery R. Sawyer, David D. Spence

GENERAL PRINCIPLES

Fractures are common in children, occurring at a rate of 12 to 30 per 1000 children every year. The risk of sustaining a fracture between birth and 16 years of age has been reported to be 42% to 64% for boys and 27% to 40% for girls. Children and adolescents, because of their unique physiologic features, such as the presence of physes, increased elasticity of bone and other connective tissue structures, as well as decreased motor control and greater head-to-body weight ratio in younger children, have different patterns of fractures than adults. Although most fractures in children heal well without long-term complications, certain fractures, especially those involving the physis and articular surface, have the potential to cause significant morbidity.

Children, unlike adults, can remodel fractures as they grow, especially those in the plane of motion of the adjacent joint. Fractures that are angulated in the coronal plane have some remodeling potential, and those that are rotationally displaced have little to none. In the upper extremity, growth is more rapid at the proximal humerus and distal radius, whereas in the lower extremity it is primarily about the knee, at the distal femur and proximal tibia. Fractures that are closer to active physes, such as proximal humeral fractures, due to rapid growth have tremendous remodeling potential compared with fractures that occur in less active physes, such as radial neck fractures where less remodeling occurs. Understanding remodeling is essential in optimizing treatment for each patient. Because of these differences, a basic understanding of skeletal growth potential and maturation is essential in caring for children with fractures.

This chapter mainly discusses fractures that require operative management. Lateral condyle and femoral neck fractures have been called "fractures of necessity" because poor outcomes are certain without operative treatment. Some fractures, such as those of the proximal humerus, rarely require surgery. Nonunion in children is rare and if present is usually caused by factors such as open fracture, soft-tissue interposition at the fracture site, pathologic lesion, or vitamin D deficiency.

GROWTH PLATE INJURIES

It has been estimated that 30% of fractures in children involve a physis and most heal without any long-term complications. It is important to have knowledge of which fractures have a low potential for causing growth disturbance, such as those in the proximal humerus, and those that have greater potential, such as those in the distal femur and tibia. Histologically, most physeal fractures occur through the proliferative zone, which is the weakest region of the physis; however, they can occur through any zone. Some physeal fractures may be related to endocrinologic changes that occur around the time of puberty.

Historically, different schemes have been used to describe and classify physeal fractures. The most widely used scheme is that proposed by Salter and Harris, which is based on the radiographic appearance of the fracture as it relates to the physis as described below (Fig. 36-1).

- Type I fractures occur through the physis only, with or without displacement.

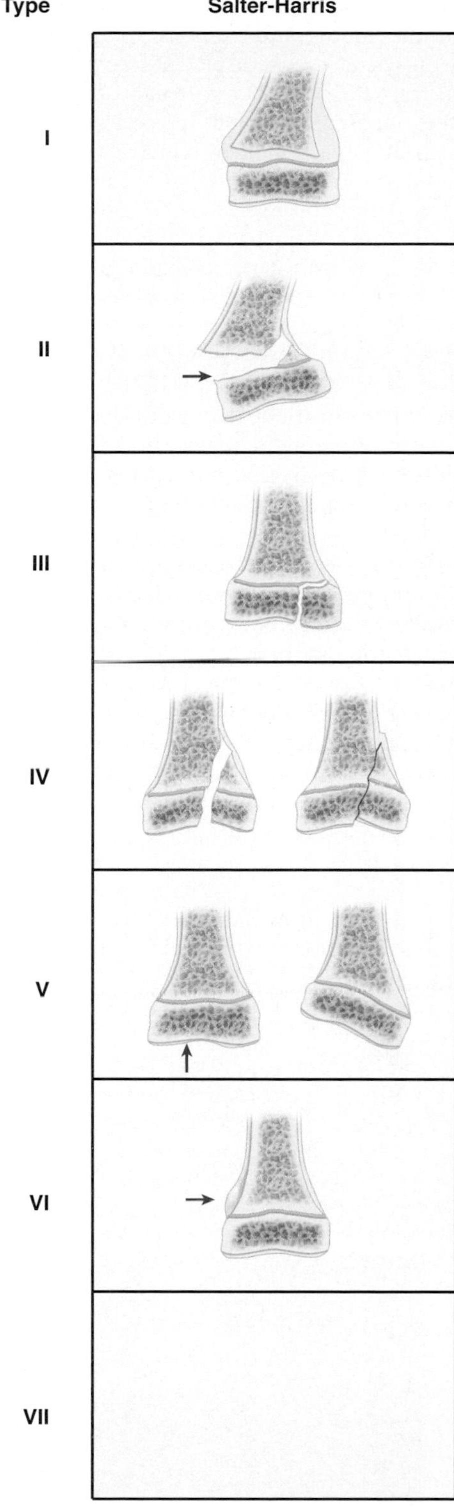

FIGURE 36-1 Classification of physeal injuries by Salter and Harris (see text).

- Type II fractures have a metaphyseal spike attached to the separated epiphysis (Thurston-Holland sign) with or without displacement.
- Type III fractures occur through the physis and epiphysis into the joint with joint incongruity when the fracture is displaced.

- Type IV fractures occur in the metaphysis and pass through the physis and epiphysis into the joint. Joint incongruity occurs with displaced fractures.
- Type V fractures, which are usually diagnosed only in retrospect, are compression or crush fractures of the physis, producing permanent damage and growth arrest.

Rang added a Type VI fracture that is caused by a shearing injury to the peripheral aspect of the physis (perichondral ring). These fractures have been classically described in lawn mower accidents when the peripheral aspect of the physis is sheared off, but they can occur with penetrating trauma and in sports as well. Type VI fractures have a high rate of angular deformity and growth arrest. Although not completely prognostic, in general, Salter-Harris type III-VI fractures have a greater risk of complications than Salter-Harris types I and II injuries. An exception might be a completely displaced Salter-Harris type I fracture that has a greater potential for growth arrest than a nondisplaced Salter-Harris type IV fracture of the distal femur.

Although many Salter-Harris types I and II fractures can be treated nonoperatively, Salter-Harris type III and IV fractures usually require operative intervention, most commonly open reduction and internal fixation because of the intraarticular nature of the fracture and the potential for posttraumatic arthritis with nonanatomic reduction. Implants crossing the physis should be avoided when possible and when used should be smooth and the smallest diameter possible, and should be removed as soon as the fracture is stable (Fig. 36-2). The treatment of specific fractures and the potential for growth arrest are discussed for each specific injury. Regardless of the injury type, parents need to be educated as to the possibility of growth disturbance and the need for long-term follow-up for any physeal fracture.

When growth arrest occurs, it can result in a shortening or angular deformity or both of the limb, depending on the size and the location of the growth arrest. Growth arrest most commonly results from a bony bar that crosses the physis. Although spontaneous correction of the bar with growth resumption has been reported, it is very rare. Central bars tend to lead to shortening, and peripheral bars tend to lead to angular deformity, but in most cases there are components of each. Certain fractures, such as distal femoral and distal tibial physeal fractures, have a higher rate of growth arrest and deformity than others. Once a bony bar occurs, the size and location of the bar can be determined using three-dimensional imaging such as computed tomography (CT) or volumetric magnetic resonance imaging (MRI). Physeal bar resection has been tried using a variety of direct and indirect methods, and the results have been unpredictable with unsuccessful outcomes occurring in 10% to 40% of patients. In general, younger patients with smaller (<30% of the physis) peripheral bars have a higher rate of success with bar resection than older patients with larger central bars. Bar resection is often combined with osteotomy to correct the resultant angular deformity as well. For large bars or those that are difficult to resect, epiphysiodesis of the remaining physis with staged angular correction and/or lengthening may be the best option.

When growth across the physis ceases symmetrically, such as with large central bars or with type V fractures, the primary problem is limb shortening. In the upper extremity, the major growth centers are the proximal humerus (arm) and distal radius and ulna (forearm). In contrast, the major growth centers in the lower extremity are the distal femur (thigh) and proximal tibia and fibula (leg) (Fig. 36-3). Using either the Mosley straight-line graph or the Paley modifiers, the amount of deformity present at skeletal maturity can be predicted. The ultimate shortening that occurs is a result of the physis involved and amount of growth remaining. The relative contribution of each physis to overall limb segment growth is shown in Figure 36-3. Shortening is much better tolerated in the upper extremity than the lower extremity, and length equalization procedures are rarely used in the upper extremity. In general, patients with a lower extremity leg-length discrepancy at maturity up to 2 cm can be treated with a shoe lift, 2 to 5 cm with contralateral epiphysiodesis, and those greater than 5 cm with limb lengthening. This can be done using various techniques described in Chapter 29.

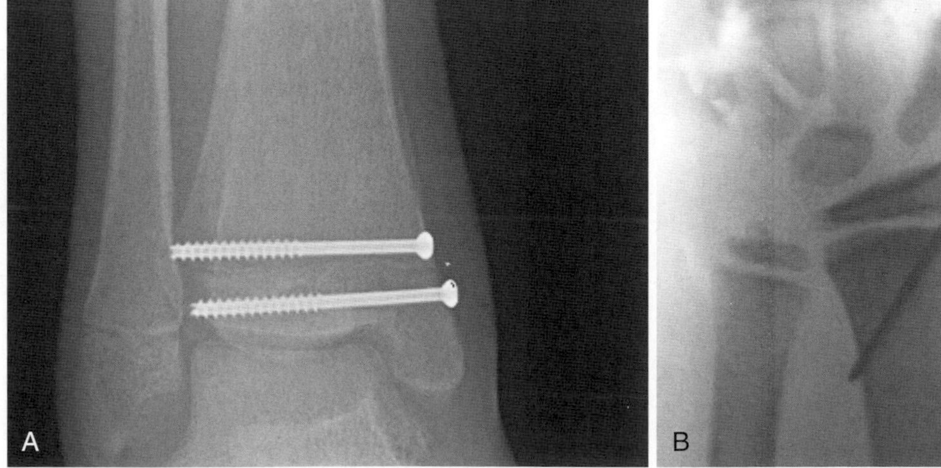

FIGURE 36-2 Fixation of physeal fracture. **A**, Correct placement of cannulated screws in metaphysis and epiphysis avoiding physis. **B**, Smooth pin crossing physis if necessary to hold reduction.

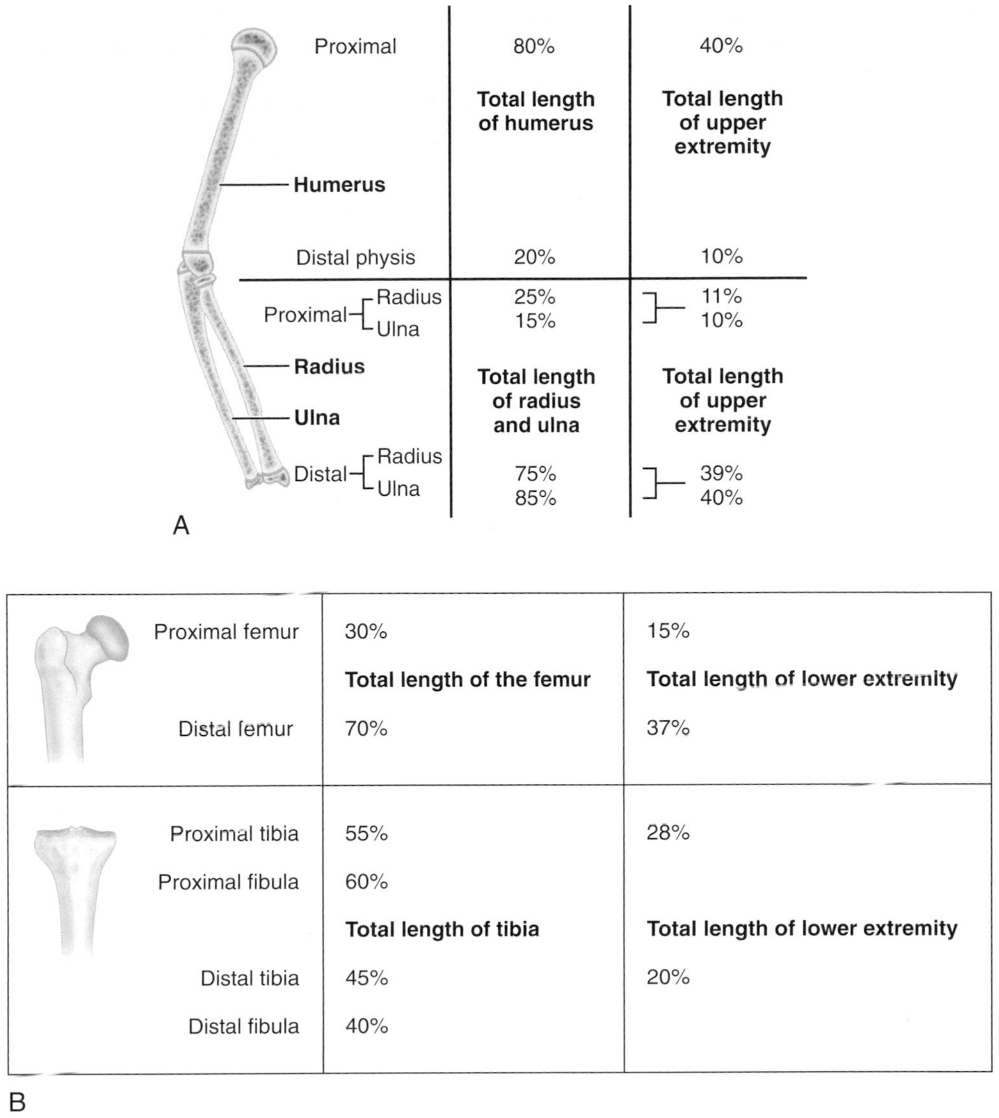

Proximal	80%	40%
Humerus	**Total length of humerus**	**Total length of upper extremity**
Distal physis	20%	10%
Proximal – Radius	25%	11%
Proximal – Ulna	15%	10%
Radius / Ulna	**Total length of radius and ulna**	**Total length of upper extremity**
Distal – Radius	75%	39%
Distal – Ulna	85%	40%

A

Proximal femur	30%	15%
	Total length of the femur	**Total length of lower extremity**
Distal femur	70%	37%
Proximal tibia	55%	28%
Proximal fibula	60%	
	Total length of tibia	**Total length of lower extremity**
Distal tibia	45%	20%
Distal fibula	40%	

B

FIGURE 36-3 **A,** Approximately 80% of the growth of humerus occurs at the proximal physis; in the ulna and radius, approximately 85% occurs at the distal physis. **B,** Approximately 70% of the growth of the femur occurs at the distal physis; in the tibia, approximately 55% occurs in the proximal physis and 60% in the proximal fibular physis, and 45% occurs at the distal tibial physis and 40% in the distal fibular physis.

OPEN FRACTURES

The general classification and principles associated with the treatment of open fractures apply to children as well. The most common open fractures in children are in the forearm and tibia followed by the hand, femur, and humerus. It is important to remember that factors such as thick active periosteum, greater periosteal bone formation potential, and lack of comorbidities lead to faster and more reliable bone healing in children than in adults. The initial management should consist of wound irrigation and debridement, antibiotics, and stabilization of the fracture. Treatment should be individualized for each patient. Timely administration of antibiotics has been shown to decrease infection rates in patients with open fractures. A survey of 181 pediatric orthopaedic surgeons showed considerable variability in treatment methods for type I open fractures in children with regard to treatment location (emergency room versus operating room), antibiotic type and duration, and irrigation solution used.

A large multicenter review of 536 children with 554 open fractures showed an overall infection rate of 3% with no difference in infection for all Gustilo and Anderson types comparing emergent (<6 hours) with delayed (>6 hours) treatment. Grade III fractures in older children and adolescents have complication rates similar to those in adults. A recent meta-analysis showed no relationship between late debridement and increased infection rates in children with open fractures as well. The treatment of specific open fractures is discussed in this chapter.

BIRTH FRACTURES

Neonates who are diagnosed with a fracture in the first week of life without any evidence of trauma are considered to have a birth fracture. The incidence is approximately 0.1/1000 live births and may be related to forced obstetric maneuvers. The most commonly fractured bones include the humerus, clavicle, and femoral shaft. Risk factors include very large or very small fetuses, breech presentation, instrumented delivery, small uterine incision (Cesarean section), twin pregnancy, prematurity and prematurity-related osteopenia, and osteogenesis imperfecta. Between 60% and 80% of patients do not have positive findings on the initial newborn examination. Prenatal ultrasound may help to identify high-risk patients, such as those with osteogenesis imperfecta before delivery.

Clinically, patients present with warmth, swelling, pain, and irritability with motion. Some children present with pseudoparalysis or failure to move a limb, which can be confused with differential diagnoses of osteomyelitis, septic arthritis, or brachial plexus palsy. Because it may take several days for some of these signs to develop, delayed diagnosis of 1 to 2 days is common. Most birth fractures do not require operative treatment, heal quickly, and remodel fully. Clavicular or humeral shaft fracture can be treated by pinning the baby's sleeve to the front of the shirt for 1 to 2 weeks until healed. Femoral shaft fractures can be treated with splinting or a Pavlik harness. Spica casting rarely is necessary. Physeal separations, especially at the distal femur and distal humerus, are rare but can occur with difficult delivery. Advanced imaging such as arthrography or ultrasound can be used to make the diagnosis. (These specific injuries are discussed later in the chapter.)

NONACCIDENTAL TRAUMA

Musculoskeletal injuries are the second most common type of injury after soft-tissue injury, occurring 10% to 70% of the time in children with nonaccidental trauma (NAT). Because of this, 30% to 50% of these children are seen by an orthopaedic surgeon. Because there is no specific test to make the diagnosis of NAT, a careful history and physical examination must be performed and appropriate use of imaging is necessary. This usually is done using a multi-disciplinary team approach. Having a high index of suspicion of NAT is essential because in up to 20% of children with NAT the diagnosis is missed on their initial medical visit. Making the diagnosis is essential because there is a high rate of reabuse and even death in children when the diagnosis is missed. It is important to be aware of risk factors for NAT and of certain injuries that are highly suggestive of this mechanism of injury. Risk factors for NAT include age younger than 2 years, fractures or injuries in different stages of healing, posterior rib fractures, and long bone fractures in young patients (Fig. 36-4). Common fractures in abused children are in the humerus, tibia, and femur. Radiographic features such as soft-tissue swelling (1 to 2 days), periosteal reaction (15 to 35 days), soft or hard callus (36 days), and bridging and remodeling (after 45 days) can be used to determine the age of the fracture. Other conditions in the differential diagnosis of NAT include metabolic bone disease and genetic conditions that can lead to bone fragility, such as osteogenesis imperfecta, rickets, renal disease, disuse osteopenia, and the use of certain medications such as corticosteroids.

Humeral shaft fractures in children younger than 3 years were at one time thought to be associated with NAT, but most are not. However, a high index of suspicion must remain for NAT in any child younger than 1 year of age with a long bone fracture. Humeral shaft fractures, although less often than clavicular fractures, can occur at birth. Risk factors include large babies, shoulder dystocia, and the use of assistive devices. These children will often present with pseudoparalysis that can be confused with a brachial plexus palsy and septic arthritis.

BOX 36-1

Standard Skeletal Survey for Suspected Child Abuse

Minimum Required Views
- Anteroposterior views of entire skeleton
- Dedicated views of hands and feet
- Lateral views of appendicular skeleton—skull and spine

Imaging Also Suggested
- Oblique views of ribs
- Oblique views of hands and feet

Optional Useful Images
- Lateral views of the joints—wrists, ankles, knees
- Orthogonal views of any fractures found

When NAT is suspected, a skeletal survey (Box 36-1) should be ordered when the child is younger than 1 year of age, when there is no history or an inconsistent history of injury, or in those in whom the fracture is attributed to NAT or domestic violence to look for secondary injuries. A skeletal survey should be performed in older children when concerns of NAT exist. Patients with buckle fractures of the distal radius and toddlers with a fracture of the tibia do not need routine skeletal survey. It should be noted that lower extremity long bone fractures in ambulatory children rarely are caused by NAT. On skeletal survey, 50% of children have one fracture, 21% will have two, 12% will have three, and 17% have more than three. Controversy exists as to which studies are optimal to include in a skeletal survey; however, rib films are essential because of the high sensitivity and specificity for NAT. Because imaging around active physes is difficult, and with improvements in plain radiographic techniques, bone scan rarely is used in the evaluation of NAT.

Certain fracture types such as spiral femoral fractures and metaphyseal corner fractures were thought to be pathognomonic for NAT. Recent studies have shown that spiral femoral fractures actually are rare in abused children and that transverse fractures are more predictive of NAT. A recent review has shown that the metaphyseal corner fracture, once thought to be pathognomonic for NAT, is very similar to fractures seen with rickets. It is important to remember that fracture morphology gives information about the direction but not the etiology of the force applied and that the presence or absence of a fracture is probably more important than its morphology.

CLAVICLE

Fractures of the clavicle are common in children and adolescents, with a peak age for clavicular fractures being 10 to 19 years of age. The majority of fractures heal well with nonoperative treatment, especially in young children. Although

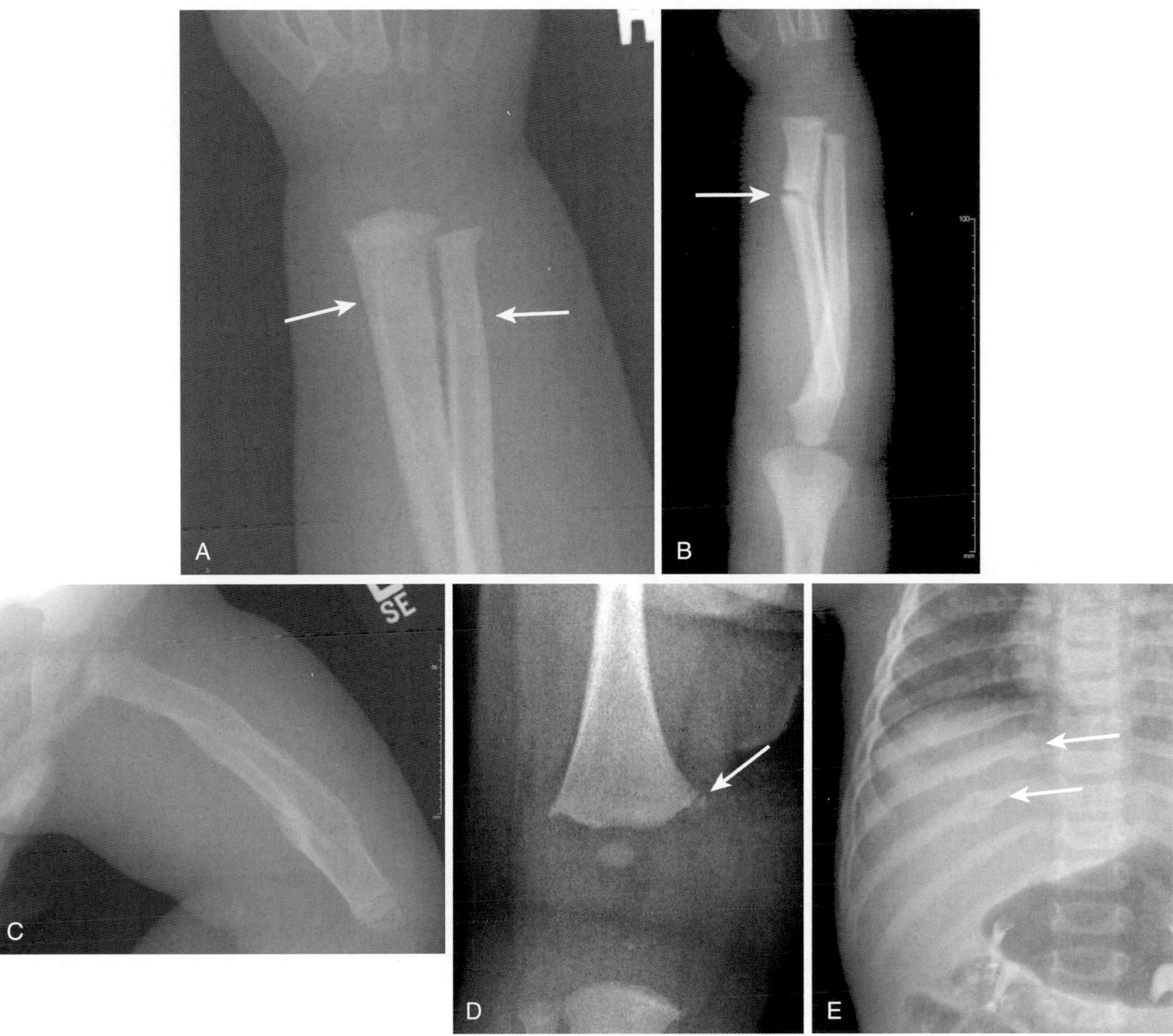

FIGURE 36-4 Child abuse. **A to C,** Six-month old child with multiple fractures at different stages of healing. **D,** Metaphyseal corner fracture. **E,** Rib fractures.

there has been a dramatic increase in the operative treatment of clavicular fractures in adults, the role of operative treatment of clavicular shaft fractures in children and adolescents remains controversial. A review of members of the Pediatric Orthopaedic Society of North America showed that the majority preferred nonoperative treatment for all fracture patterns; however, older age (16 to 19 years), evidence in the adult literature, and physician years of experience (less than 5 years) predicted operative treatment preference. Excellent clinical and radiographic outcomes have been reported for both nonoperative and operative management of these injuries. Operatively treated patients typically have a faster return to activities but also have a higher complication rate in terms of symptomatic hardware and nonunion. The rate of malunion is higher with nonoperative treatment; however, patients with established malunions have excellent functional outcome scores. Although studies have shown good outcomes with both methods of treatment, stronger evidence is needed to determine if one method is superior to the other. The indications for operative treatment are open fracture, polytrauma, floating shoulder, fractures with skin compromise, and widely displaced or shortened fractures in older adolescents. Operative treatment of these injuries is described in Chapter 57.

STERNOCLAVICULAR FRACTURES AND DISLOCATIONS

The medial clavicle is one of the last growth centers to ossify, typically between 20 and 24 years of age. Fractures of the medial clavicle are usually Salter-Harris type I or II fractures, which in most cases heal with closed management and without complications (Fig. 36-5). It can be difficult to

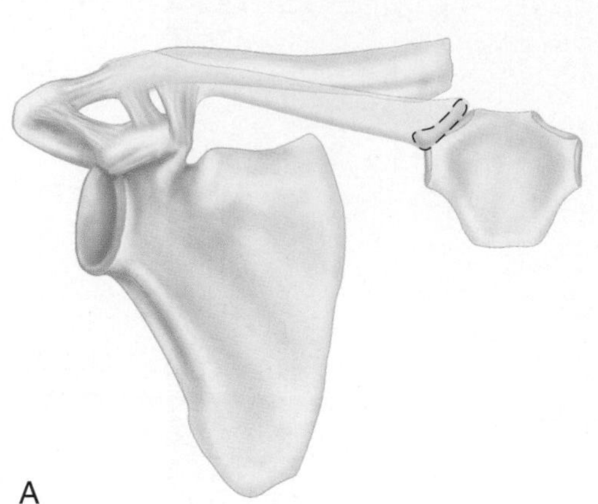

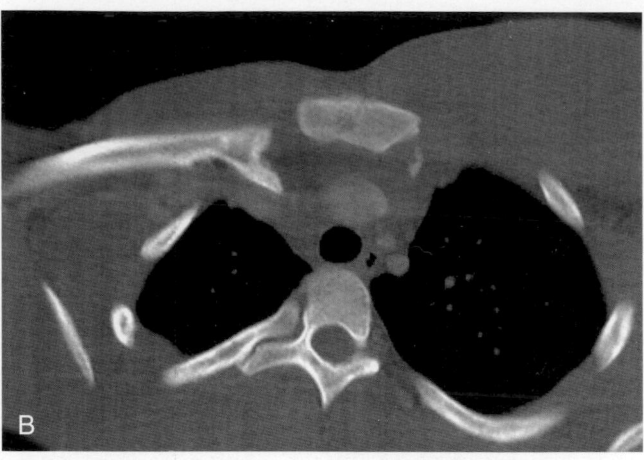

FIGURE 36-5 **A,** Injury shown is Salter-Harris type I physeal separation of medial clavicle rather than dislocation of sternoclavicular joint. **B,** CT scan showing clavicular separation.

differentiate these injuries from true sternoclavicular joint dislocations because clinically they appear similar. The use of CT scan is helpful in these situations not only to determine the fracture pattern but also to evaluate the relationship between the fracture fragments and the mediastinal structures such as the brachiocephalic vein and innominate artery with posteriorly displaced fracture dislocation. Anteriorly displaced fractures usually heal with a "bump" over the proximal clavicle but rarely are symptomatic. Up to 50% of patients with posteriorly displaced fractures may remain symptomatic, which has led some authors to recommend operative treatment of these injuries. Because the epiphyseal (proximal) fragment is small, fixation is usually achieved with FiberWire (Arthrex Inc, Naples FL) or suture repair. Care must be taken to protect the adjacent neurovascular structures and pleura. A recent meta-analysis showed that although considerable variability in the literature exists, good results can be obtained with both open and closed treatment. It also showed that early treatment is better because patients treated less than 48 hours after injury had better results than those treated later. Patients who undergo late operative treatment for chronic posterior fracture-dislocation have been shown to do well with activities of daily living but have pain when returning to the same level of athletic participation.

LATERAL (DISTAL) CLAVICULAR FRACTURES

Injuries to the distal clavicle in young children are rare. In older children and adolescents these injuries appear very similar to acromioclavicular joint injuries. These injuries are really physeal fractures in which the epiphysis and physis maintain their normal anatomic relation to the shoulder joint, whereas the distal metaphysis is displaced superiorly, away from the underlying structures. The periosteal sleeve generally is intact inferiorly, and the ligamentous structures connecting the clavicle to the coracoid usually remain attached to the periosteal sleeve (Fig. 36-6). Because the periosteal sleeve is highly osteogenic, these fractures have a tremendous potential to remodel, and most patients do well with nonoperative treatment. Operative treatment, consisting of open reduction and internal fixation, usually is reserved for adolescent patients with significant displacement and limited remodeling potential. The operative treatment of lateral clavicular injuries is discussed in Chapter 57.

ACROMIOCLAVICULAR DISLOCATIONS

There are five types of acromioclavicular injuries described in children (Fig. 36-7). Type I injury is not sufficient to completely rupture the acromioclavicular or the coracoclavicular ligaments. Type II injury damages the acromioclavicular ligaments but not the coracoclavicular ligaments; a partial periosteal sleeve (tube) tear also occurs. In type III injury the acromioclavicular ligament is completely ruptured, but the coracoclavicular ligaments are intact because they are still attached to the periosteum. The clavicle is unstable and is displaced superiorly through a rent in the periosteal sleeve (pseudodislocation). Type IV injury is identical to type III except that, in addition to being displaced superiorly, the clavicle is displaced posteriorly. Type V injury is severe; the acromioclavicular ligaments are disrupted, and, although the coracoclavicular ligaments are still attached to the periosteal sleeve, the clavicle is now unstable and its lateral end is buried in the trapezius and deltoid muscles or has pierced them and is located under the skin in the posterior aspect of the shoulder.

In many types III, IV, and V dislocations, an unrecognized fracture of the distal end of the clavicle occurs, with the acromioclavicular and coracoclavicular ligaments remaining intact and attached to the empty periosteal tube or to the most distal fragment. In children and adolescents up to age 15 years, types I, II, and III acromioclavicular separations, even with fracture of the distal third of the clavicle, can be treated by nonoperative means. In patients older than age 15 years, type III injuries may require surgery. Open reduction and internal fixation should be considered for markedly displaced types IV and V fractures (see Chapter 57).

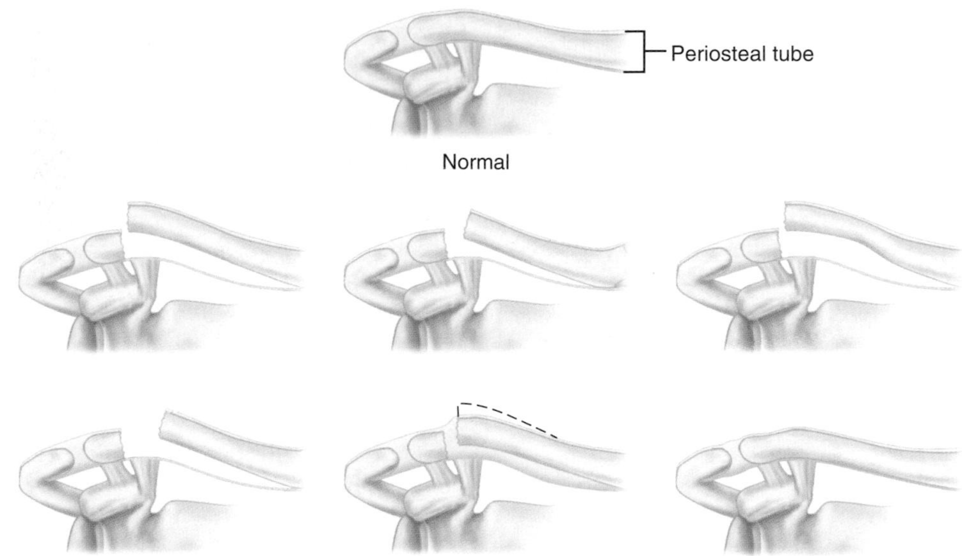

FIGURE 36-6 Distal clavicular fracture with coracoclavicular and coracoacromial ligaments still intact or at least attached to periosteal tube. Fracture in child remodels satisfactorily without surgery.

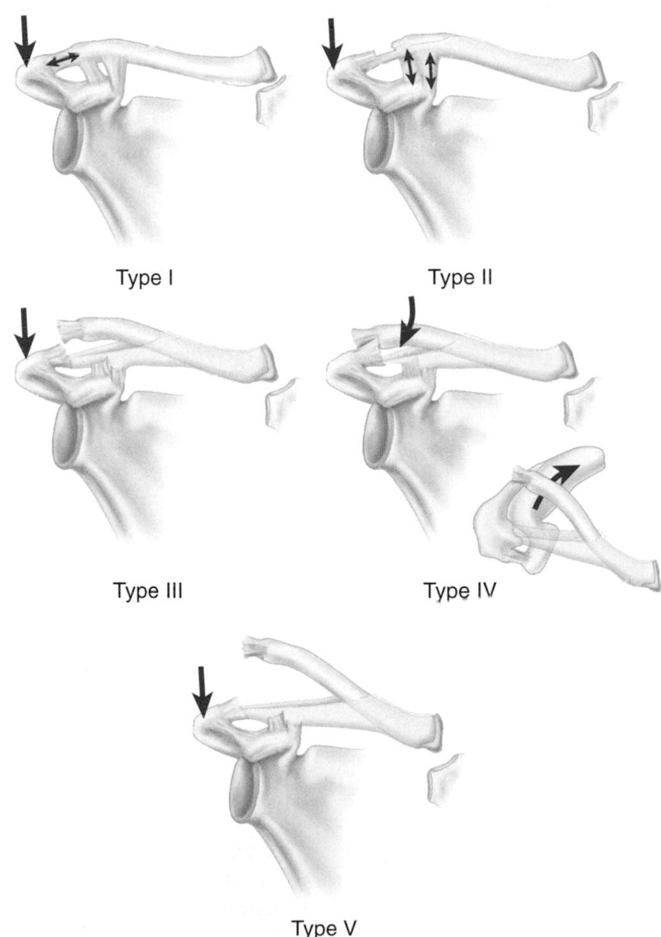

FIGURE 36-7 Five types of acromioclavicular separation occurring in children (see text). Acromioclavicular and coracoclavicular ligaments are attached to periosteal tube, although distal end of clavicle is significantly displaced in types III, IV, and V.

In types IV and V acromioclavicular dislocations, it is important to disengage the distal clavicle from the trapezius and deltoid muscles. If this is unsuccessful by closed means, surgery is indicated to remove the clavicle from the muscles and replace it in the periosteal tube. The periosteal tube should be repaired, and the deltoid-trapezius muscle fascia should be imbricated superiorly over the clavicle. If the repair is unstable, internal fixation is required, as in adults, by acromioclavicular or coracoclavicular fixation, as described in Chapter 57.

SHOULDER DISLOCATIONS

Shoulder dislocations in children are rare, and proximal humeral physeal fractures are much more common. In a review of 500 glenohumeral dislocations, only eight patients were younger than 10 years of age (1.6%). It is thought that glenohumeral dislocations in skeletally immature patients may become more common as the level of sports participation increases. A series of 14 skeletally immature patients treated with closed reduction found a redislocation rate of 21% at a mean of 5 years' follow-up. Glenohumeral dislocation has been reported when associated with a proximal humeral metaphyseal fracture. The diagnosis and management of shoulder dislocations for adolescents is similar to adults, as described in Chapter 60.

PROXIMAL HUMERAL FRACTURES

Proximal humeral fractures are relatively rare in the pediatric population, accounting for 0.5% of pediatric fractures and 4% to 7% of all epiphyseal fractures. Of the physeal fractures, the majority are Salter-Harris type II fractures and Salter-Harris types III and IV are rare. They are most often classified by the Neer-Horowitz classification as shown in Box 36-2. A systematic review of the treatment of proximal humeral fractures in children found that nonunions did not occur and malunions were exceedingly rare, regardless of the method of treatment. This is due to the rapid growth and remodeling potential of the proximal humerus, especially in young children. In children younger than 10 years, it has been shown that angulation of up to 60 degrees can remodel completely, whereas in older children and adolescents it is closer to 20 to 30 degrees. A recent cohort-matched comparison of operative and nonoperative treatment of 32 proximal humeral fractures showed no difference in complications, functional outcome, or patient satisfaction. Within the nonoperatively treated group, there was a higher rate of dissatisfaction in patients older than 12 years treated nonoperatively. They found the odds ratio of an undesirable outcome increased 3.81 for each year of age with nonoperative treatment.

CLOSED TREATMENT

Closed treatment consisting of a sling or hanging arm cast remains the primary method of treatment for these injuries given the tremendous healing and remodeling potential of the proximal humerus. Closed reduction, when necessary, can be performed with sedation and by abducting (90 degrees) and externally rotating (90 degrees) the arm relative to the shoulder. Patients can gradually increase shoulder motion as their symptoms allow. Physical therapy rarely is needed in this population.

BOX 36-2

Neer-Horowitz Classification of Humeral Physeal Fractures

I = to 5 mm of displacement
II = to one-third humeral shaft
III = to two-thirds humeral shaft
IV = more than two-thirds humeral shaft / total separation

Adapted from Neer C II, Horowitz BS: Fractures of the proximal humeral epiphyseal plate, Clin Orthop Relat Res 41:24, 1963.

OPERATIVE TREATMENT

Operative treatment usually is reserved for older children and adolescents and includes closed reduction and pinning, nailing using flexible titanium elastic intramedullary nails (TEIN), and open reduction. Indications for open reduction using the deltopectoral approach include open fracture, inability to obtain a satisfactory closed reduction, and skeletal maturity (or close to skeletal maturity) (Fig. 36-8A and B). The most common impediments to obtaining a successful closed reduction include the periosteum, biceps tendon, deltoid muscle, and comminuted bone fragments. The use of TEIN has been shown to produce good radiographic and functional results in several studies; however, implant removal is occasionally necessary because of prominence. A comparison of percutaneous pinning and TEIN found that both techniques are effective in fracture stabilization in older children. The use of TEIN was shown to have a lower complication rate than percutaneous pinning; however, TEIN use was associated with increased blood loss, operative time, and rate of reoperation for hardware removal.

CLOSED REDUCTION AND PERCUTANEOUS PINNING OF PROXIMAL HUMERUS

TECHNIQUE 36-1

- Position the patient to allow anteroposterior and axillary lateral images of the injured shoulder. Prepare and drape the patient in a sterile manner.
- Manipulate the distal fragment into slight external rotation, 90 degrees of flexion, and 70 degrees of abduction using image intensification. This brings the fragments together satisfactorily. This maneuver should push the upper part of the shaft back through the rent in the deltoid muscle and anterior periosteum and correct the anterior

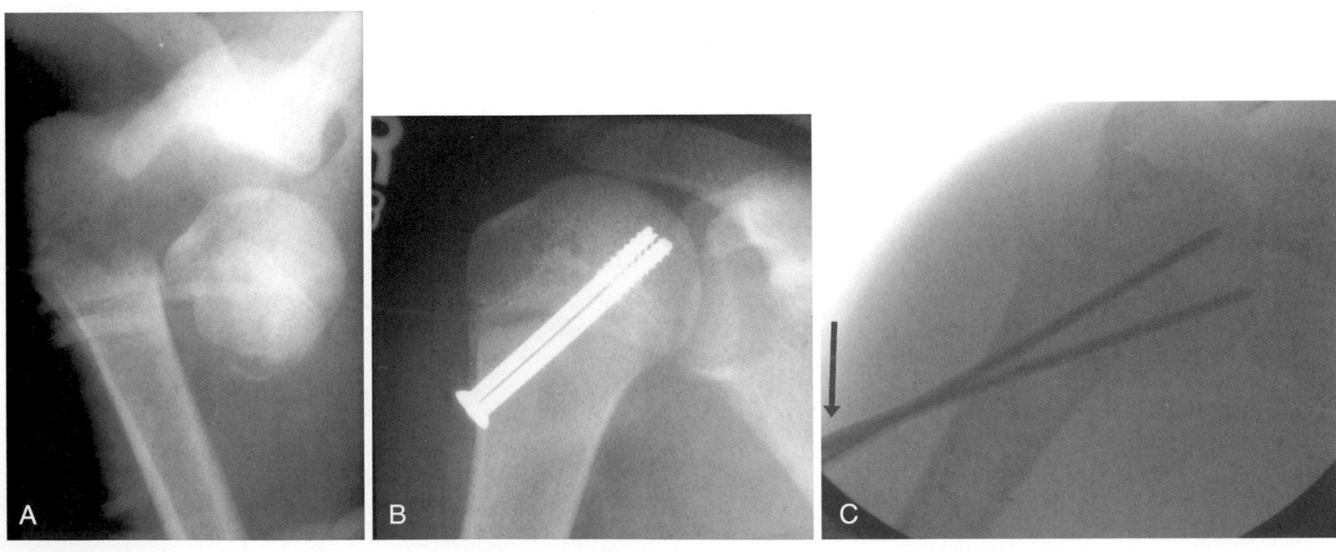

FIGURE 36-8 **A,** Irreducible dislocation-Salter-Harris type II fracture of the proximal humerus in a 15-year-old boy. **B,** After open reduction and screw fixation. **C,** Smooth Kirschner wires can also be used in younger patients.

angulation. Have an assistant support the proximal fragment to help achieve and maintain the reduction.

- Drill two terminally threaded Steinmann pins through the lateral shaft in a proximal direction into the humeral head to maintain the reduction. In older patients with large metaphyseal fragments, a cannulated screw can be used. The skin incision should be made fairly distal to accommodate the pin trajectory.
- In younger patients, smooth Kirschner wires can be used (Fig. 36-8C).

POSTOPERATIVE CARE. Patients are placed in a sling, and gentle range-of-motion exercises are started. The pins, which can be irritating to the patient, are removed in 3 to 4 weeks.

CLOSED REDUCTION AND INTRAMEDULLARY NAILING OF PROXIMAL HUMERUS

TECHNIQUE 36-2

- Position the patient to allow anteroposterior and axillary lateral images of the injured shoulder. Prepare and drape the patient in a sterile manner.
- Make a lateral incision over the supracondylar ridge. Drill two holes in the lateral cortex using a drill slightly larger than the diameter nail selected. Alternatively, one medial and one lateral hole can be drilled. If a medial nail is used, care must be taken to protect the ulnar nerve.
- Prebend the nail and pass it retrograde to the fracture site. Gently reduce the fracture using fluoroscopic guidance and pass the first nail. Repeat for the second nail either through the lateral or second medial incision.
- When the fracture reduction is adequate, cut the nails beneath the skin for later removal. If acceptable reduction after two attempts cannot be obtained, proceed with open reduction using the deltopectoral interval.

POSTOPERATIVE CARE. Place the arm in a soft dressing with sling and begin motion. Nails are typically removed in 6 months or sooner if the implant is causing symptoms.

HUMERAL SHAFT FRACTURES

Humeral shaft fractures in children are uncommon, accounting for less than 10% of all humeral fractures in children. Most occur either in children younger than 3 years or older than 12 years, and almost all of these injuries can be treated nonoperatively because of the remodeling potential of the humerus and the ability of the glenohumeral joint to accommodate for any residual malalignment. Up to 70 degrees of angulation in children younger than 5 years and 30 degrees of angulation in children ages 12 to 13 can be accepted. Less angulation in distal fractures, especially those in varus, is acceptable because of the undesirable cosmetic appearance of the arm. Closed treatment usually consists of coaptation splinting, fracture bracing, or the use of a hanging arm cast. Operative treatment, consisting of plating or the use of TEIN, has been shown to provide good results. External fixation can be used in rare conditions in which severe soft-tissue injuries are present. Indications for operative treatment include patients with polytrauma to speed mobilization and upper extremity weight bearing, a floating elbow, a pathologic lesion, and adolescents close to skeletal maturity. Radial nerve entrapment can occur, especially with distal fractures after closed reduction maneuvers. A loss of radial nerve function after closed reduction indicates potential entrapment of the nerve between the fracture fragments, and urgent nerve exploration and internal fixation are necessary. Plating techniques for children are similar to adults as discussed in Chapter 57.

CLOSED/OPEN REDUCTION AND INTRAMEDULLARY NAILING OF PROXIMAL HUMERUS

TECHNIQUE 36-3

- Position the patient to allow anteroposterior and axillary lateral images of the injured humerus. This can be done on a radiolucent table or hand table. Prepare and drape the patient in a sterile manner.
- Make a lateral incision over the supracondylar ridge. Drill two holes in the lateral cortex using a drill slightly larger than the diameter nail selected. Alternatively, one medial and one lateral hole can be drilled. If a medial nail is used, care must be taken to protect the ulnar nerve.
- Place the nail over the skin to radiographically determine where the fracture site will be on the nail. Gently bend the nail with the apex of the bow at the fracture site. Pass both nails retrograde to the fracture site. Gently reduce the fracture using fluoroscopic guidance and pass the first nail 1 to 2 cm across the fracture site. Repeat for the second nail either through the lateral or a second medial incision. Once both nails have crossed the fracture site, advance them to their final positions.
- When the fracture reduction is adequate, cut the nails beneath the skin for later removal. If acceptable reduction cannot be obtained after two attempts, proceed with open reduction.

POSTOPERATIVE CARE. Place the arm in a soft dressing with sling and begin motion. Nails typically are removed in 6 months or sooner if the implant is causing symptoms.

SUPRACONDYLAR HUMERAL FRACTURES

Supracondylar humeral fractures are the most common pediatric elbow fractures, accounting for 3% of all children's fractures. The most common age of injury is 5 to 7 years. Almost all (98%) are extension-type injuries, which usually are caused by a fall onto an outstretched hand. Flexion-type fractures, although rarer, are more difficult to reduce, have worse outcomes, and are associated with ulnar nerve injury (Fig. 36-9). Approximately 5% to 10% of children have an associated ipsilateral distal radial fracture. The most commonly used classification is that by Gartland in which type I fractures are nondisplaced, type II fractures have an intact posterior hinge, and type III fractures have complete displacement. A type IV injury has been described in which there is complete loss of the anterior and posterior periosteal hinge, making it unstable in both flexion and extension. Type IV fractures usually are the result of high-energy injury. Care must be taken when reducing a type III fracture to avoid tearing the periosteal hinge, making it a type IV injury. The diagnosis can be made in most cases using plain radiographs. Advanced imaging, such as CT, occasionally is used in an adolescent when there are concerns about a coronal split in the distal fragment or T-condylar fracture.

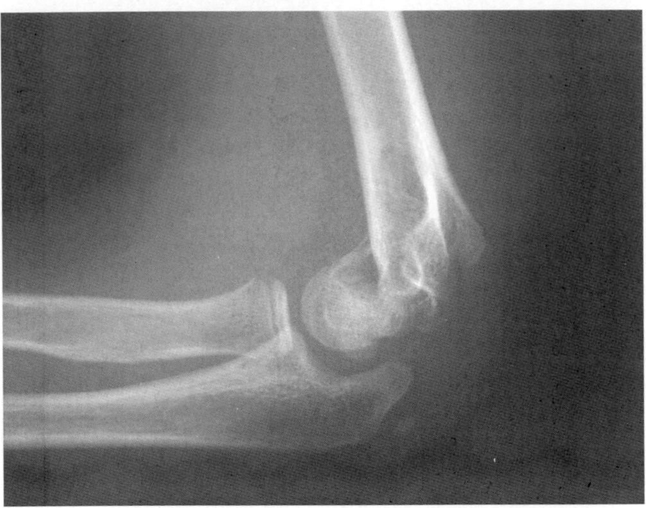

FIGURE 36-9 Flexion type supracondylar humeral fracture.

A careful neurologic examination is essential because 10% to 15% of patients have a nerve injury, with the anterior interosseous nerve being the most frequently injured in extension-type fractures. The ulnar nerve is most frequently injured in flexion-type injuries. Obese children have been shown to have a higher rate of both preoperative and postoperative nerve palsy. A loss of neurologic function after reduction is concerning for nerve entrapment at the time of reduction, and urgent open exploration of the nerve is necessary. Most nerve injuries are a result of neurapraxia and resolve within 6 to 12 weeks; electromyography is indicated if there is no return of nerve function within 3 months. A recent long-term follow-up study showed that at an average follow-up of 8 years most patients had excellent function; 100% of patients with radial nerve, 88% of patients with median nerve, and only 25% of patients with ulnar nerve injuries fully recovered.

Urgent assessment of the vascular status of the limb also is essential to minimize complications. A vascular injury, typically to the brachial artery, can occur in up to 10% to 20% of patients with a type III fracture (Fig. 36-10). Because of the rich collateral blood supply about the elbow, the hand may be well perfused even with complete disruption of the brachial artery. The vascular status of the limb can be classified as normal—pulseless but with a warm pink (perfused) hand—or pulseless—pale (nonperfused) hand. Treatment of patients with a pulseless warm hand remains controversial in terms of the need for brachial artery exploration (Fig. 36-11). A supracondylar fracture with a nonperfused hand is a surgical emergency to prevent reperfusion injury and compartment syndrome leading to Volkmann ischemic contracture.

Compartment syndrome occurs in approximately 0.1% to 0.3% of patients with supracondylar humeral fractures and is more common with concurrent fracture of the forearm or wrist.

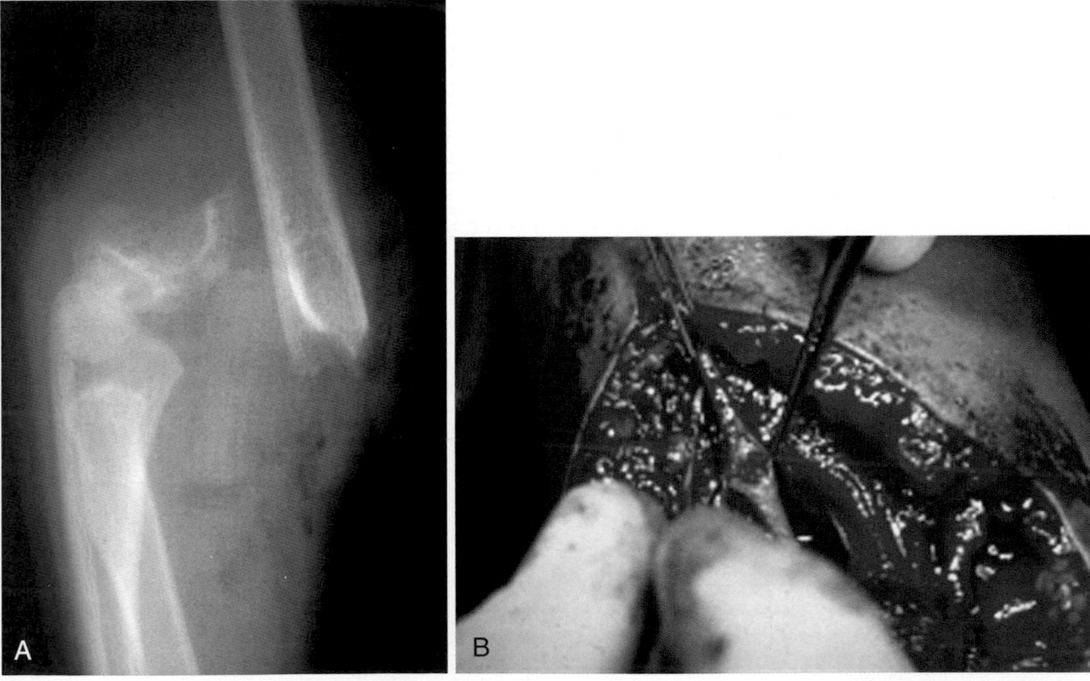

FIGURE 36-10 **A,** Type III supracondylar humeral fracture with vascular injury. **B,** Brachial artery occlusion with supracondylar humeral fracture.

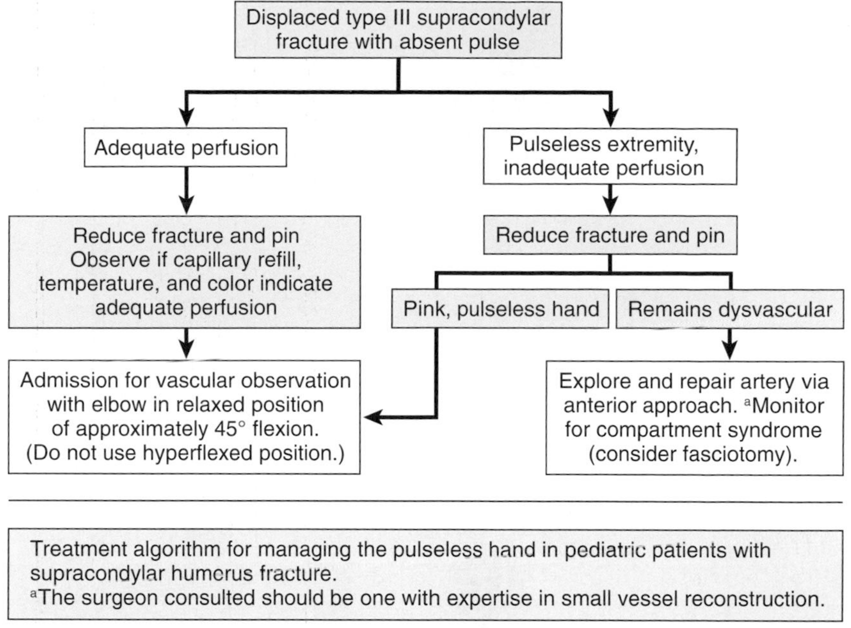

FIGURE 36-11 Management of pulseless supracondylar humeral fracture. (From: Abzug JM, Herman MJ: Management of supracondylar humerus fractures in children: current concepts, J Am Acad Orthop Surg 20:69, 2012.)

In patients with vascular compromise, urgent reduction in the operating room should be performed and the vascular status of the hand assessed. Arteriography should not be used unless the level of vascular injury is unclear in patients with polytrauma and should never delay closed reduction of a supracondylar humeral fracture. If perfusion is not restored, urgent exploration of the brachial artery with release of entrapping structures and direct repair with vein grafting if necessary should be performed by a surgeon with experience in the repair of small vessels. Prophylactic forearm and hand fasciotomies are necessary in patients with prolonged ischemia time. This is especially important in patients with concomitant nerve injuries in which the ability to detect a compartment syndrome clinically is impaired. Most patients in whom perfusion is restored (pink hand) even in the absence of a radial pulse have good long-term outcomes with observation.

Treatment of supracondylar humeral fractures is based on the Gartland type. Type I fractures are treated with long arm cast immobilization for 3 weeks followed by a brief period of protected activity. Patients with the presence of a posterior fat pad on radiographs should be presumed to have a type I fracture and treated in this fashion.

Treatment of type II injuries is somewhat controversial. Wilkins subdivided type II injuries into A and B with type IIA fractures being stable and type IIB fractures having some degree of rotation or translation making them unstable. Closed reduction and casting can be used in patients with type IIA injuries. Closed reduction and percutaneous pinning typically with two or three lateral pins has become the main form of treatment for type IIB injuries and for those in which the stability is in question. We prefer to pin most type II fractures because of concerns about the ability to maintain reduction in a splint or cast, poor patient compliance with barriers to timely follow-up, and difficulty in differentiating between type IIA and B fractures. Type III fractures are treated with closed reduction and pinning (Fig. 36-12).

Complications of percutaneous pinning occur in approximately 5% of patients, with pin migration or irritation being the most common followed by infection (1%) and elbow stiffness. The ideal pin configuration remains controversial; however, although crossed medial and lateral pins are more stable than two lateral pins in vitro, use of two or three lateral pins appears to be equal to crossed pins in vivo. A comparison study of medial crossed pins and lateral entry pins showed equal maintenance of reduction in both groups, but the crossed pin group had a 7.7% rate of iatrogenic nerve injury. This rate of iatrogenic nerve injury with crossed pins has been shown in other studies as well. If lateral pinning is used, it is important to engage both fragments and have bicortical fixation with at least two pins and at least 2 mm of pin separation at the fracture site. We prefer the use of two or three lateral pins for most type III fractures and use a medial pin for fractures that are very unstable (Figs. 36-13 and 36-14). If a medial pin is used, making a small incision and using retractors to protect the ulnar nerve, as well as avoiding pinning these fractures in maximal elbow flexion, can reduce the rate of ulnar nerve injury. It is difficult to maintain reduction of type IV fractures because of the loss of the periosteal hinges. For this reason, it may be necessary to hold the arm stable and rotate the C-arm for imaging rather than rotating the arm. The indications for open reduction, which occurs approximately 10% of the time, include irreducible fractures, open fractures, and those with suspected or confirmed neurovascular injuries. A direct anterior approach can be used in most patients with posterior displaced fracture because it provides the best access to the neurovascular structures and fracture site. Because of the muscle stripping that occurs with these injuries, the neurovascular structures are typically in a subcutaneous position (Fig. 36-15).

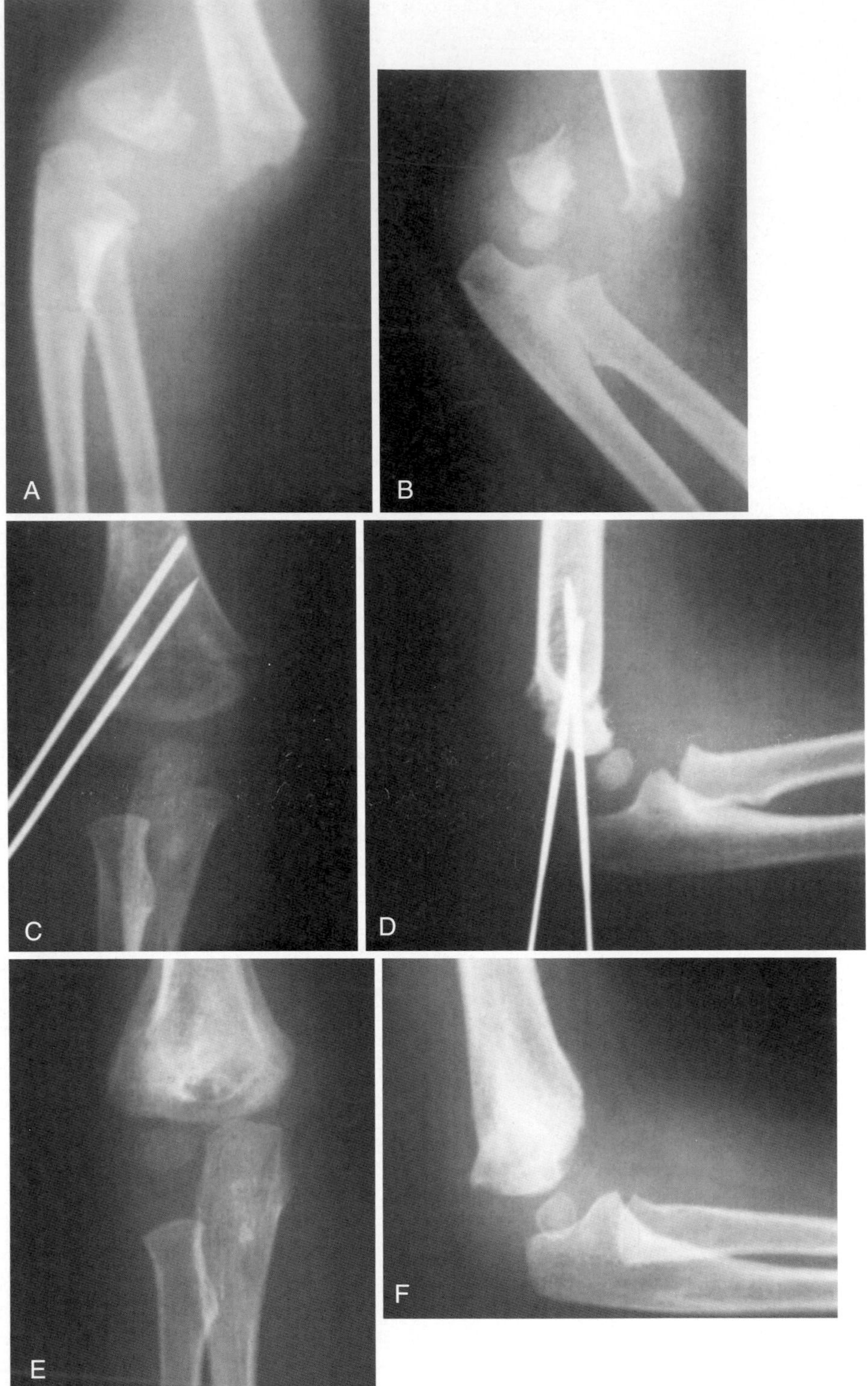

FIGURE 36-12 Fixation of supracondylar fracture. **A** and **B,** Severely displaced type III supracondylar fracture. **C** and **D,** Closed reduction and percutaneous pinning were performed. **E** and **F,** Final result.

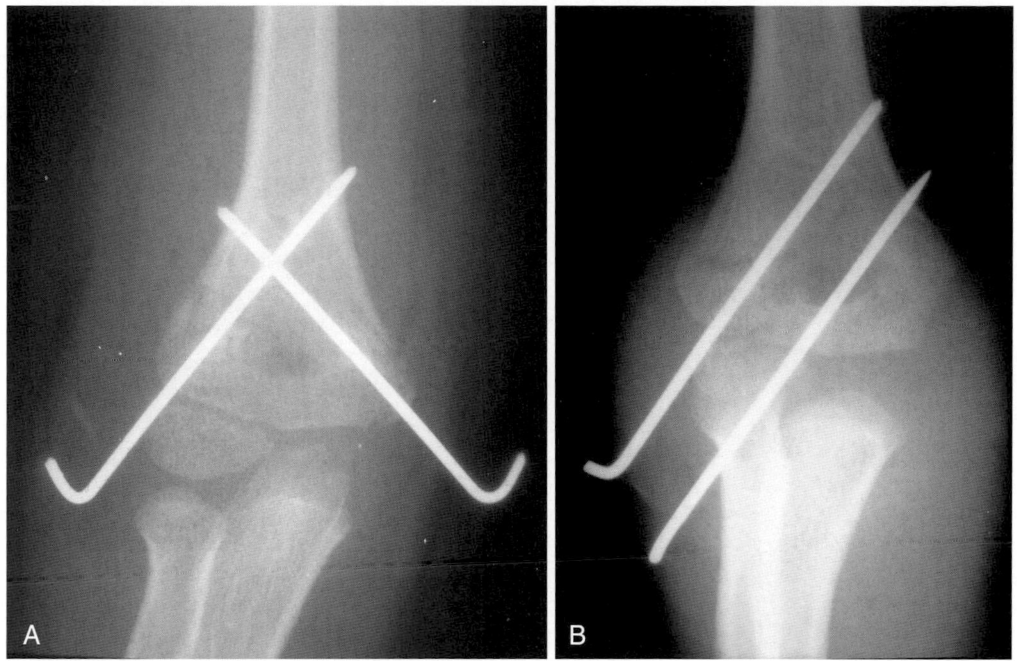

FIGURE 36-13 Fixation of supracondylar humeral fractures can be done with **(A)** two crossed pins or **(B)** two lateral pins.

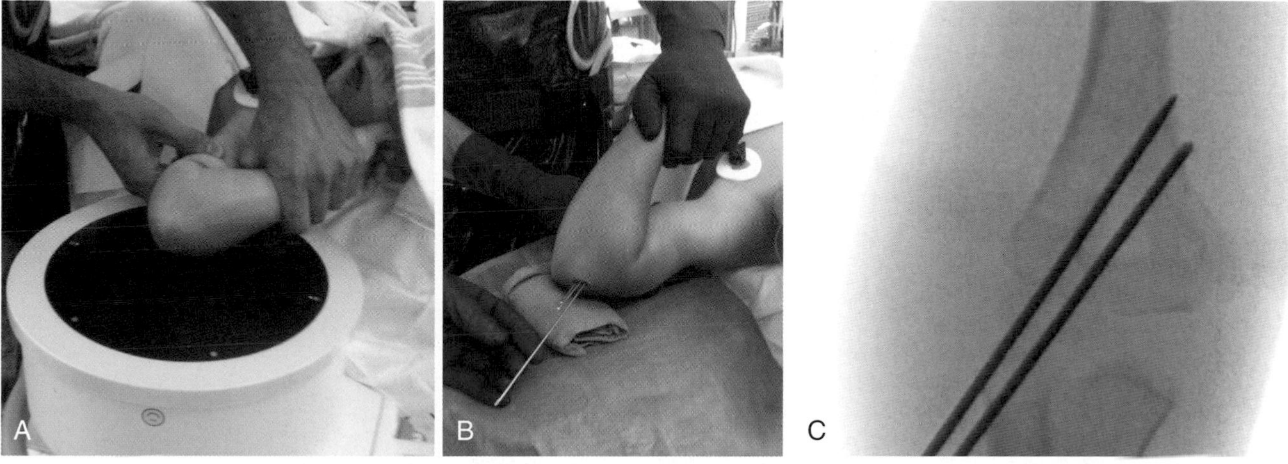

FIGURE 36-14 Pinning of supracondylar humeral fracture. **A**, Positioning of the arm on image intensifier. **B**, Confirm that the lateral pins engage the fracture fragments. **C**, Final fluoroscopic imaging. **SEE TECHNIQUE 36-4.**

CLOSED REDUCTION AND PERCUTANEOUS PINNING OF SUPRACONDYLAR FRACTURES (TWO LATERAL PINS)

TECHNIQUE 36-4

- Position the patient supine and position the elbow on an inverted image intensifier (Fig. 36-14A).
- For the more common extension type of supracondylar fracture, with countertraction on the humerus, apply traction to the forearm and examine the fracture with image intensification. With the elbow in extension, correct rotational malalignment and medial and lateral translation. Once this is corrected, maintain traction on the elbow and gently flex the elbow to 120 degrees. Use pressure on the olecranon as the elbow is flexed to correct extension of the distal fragment. Maximally flex the elbow and pronate the forearm to lock the posterior and medial soft-tissue hinges. It is important to correct rotation and translation before flexing the elbow.
- For the rarer flexion-type injury, flexing the elbow will further displace the fragment because of the disruption of the posterior periosteal hinge. In this case the elbow

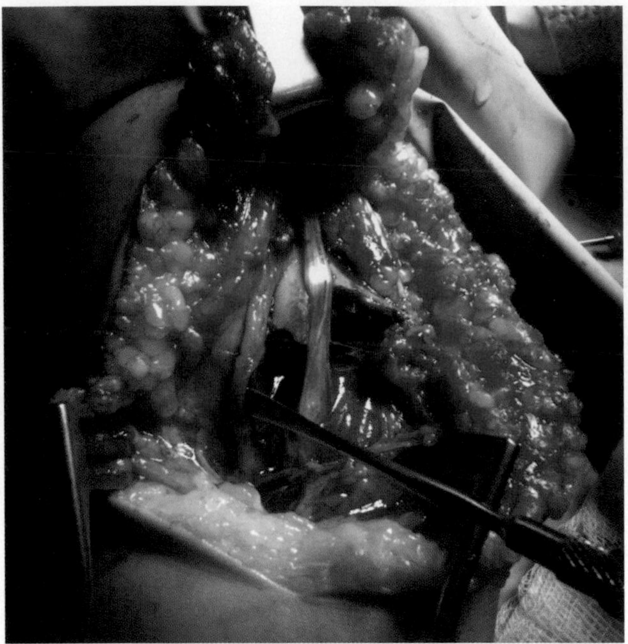

FIGURE 36-15 Neurovascular structures of the supracondylar humerus. Medial nerve and brachial artery under Freer elevator.

will need to be pinned in extension. This can be difficult, and posterior open reduction often is needed.

- Confirm the anteroposterior reduction with image intensification, aiming the beam through the forearm and rotating the humerus from medial to lateral to assess the medial and lateral column reduction. Confirm lateral reduction by externally rotating the shoulder to obtain a lateral view of the elbow.
- Maintain reduction while performing closed percutaneous pinning with image intensification to verify that the two lateral pins engage both fracture fragments (Fig. 36-14B). The pins should be divergent and not cross at the fracture site.
- If a medial pin is used, make a 1 cm incision over the medial epicondyle. Spread the soft tissues so that the epicondyle can be seen and ensure that the ulnar nerve is protected. Alternatively, a small soft-tissue drill sleeve can be used. It is not necessary to expose or explore the ulnar nerve in patients without ulnar nerve symptoms. Once the pin is placed, it can be cut outside the skin and the incision closed with absorbable suture.
- After the pins are inserted, extend the elbow as far as possible without bending the pins. With the aid of image intensification, check the stability of the reduction by rotating and stressing the elbow to determine if a third (medial or lateral) pin is necessary. Compare the carrying angle with that of the normal extremity. Cut and bend the pins outside of the skin and check final fluoroscopic images to ensure no displacement occurred during bending (Fig. 36-14C).

POSTOPERATIVE CARE. Place the patient in a well-padded posterior splint or bivalved cast with the elbow flexed at 60 degrees to relax the antecubital structures. Patients are treated in a cast for 3 to 4 weeks. The pins are then removed, and gentle range of motion is started.

See also Video 36-1.

ANTERIOR APPROACH

TECHNIQUE 36-5

- If an anterior approach is to be used, make a transverse incision over the antecubital space. This can be extended proximally and distally if necessary. The proximal extension should be performed (medial or lateral) over the proximal fragment because this is usually the site of neurovascular injury. Note that in high-energy injuries the anterior soft tissues may be stripped and the neurovascular bundle may be subcutaneous.
- Develop a plane between the biceps and brachialis tendons. Release the biceps aponeurosis while protecting the brachial artery. Retract the biceps and brachialis muscle medially and the brachioradialis laterally. Protect the radial nerve and posterior interosseous artery.
- Observe the supracondylar fragment and note its alignment with the proximal fragment. Use a small curet to remove any hematoma at the fracture site. Note any interdigitations on the ends of the bone, and by matching them reduce the fracture.
- Use two or three Steinmann pins in a manner similar to that described for percutaneous pinning. Image intensification simplifies pin placement. Cut the pins off outside the skin for easy removal later.

POSTOPERATIVE CARE. Close the incision and place the patient in a well-padded posterior splint with the elbow in 60 degrees of flexion and convert to a long arm cast to 90 degrees of flexion in 5 to 7 days. The pins are removed in 3 to 4 weeks, and gentle range-of-motion exercises are begun.

The timing of reduction for type III fractures remains controversial; however, recent studies have shown no difference in complication rates between patients treated in an urgent (less than 12 hours) or delayed (later than 12 hours) fashion. Delayed treatment requires a conscious, cooperative patient without neurovascular compromise and the ability to proceed with surgery in a timely fashion if their neurovascular examination changes with monitoring. Type II fractures can be treated safely in a delayed fashion.

Postoperatively, patients are placed either in a long arm posterior splint or a bivalved cast with the elbow in 60 degrees of flexion. Follow-up radiographs are obtained at 1 week, and the cast or splint is removed and changed to a long arm cast with the elbow in 90 degrees for an additional 2 to 3 weeks. The pins are removed in the office, and most patients regain motion without the need for physical therapy. Most children,

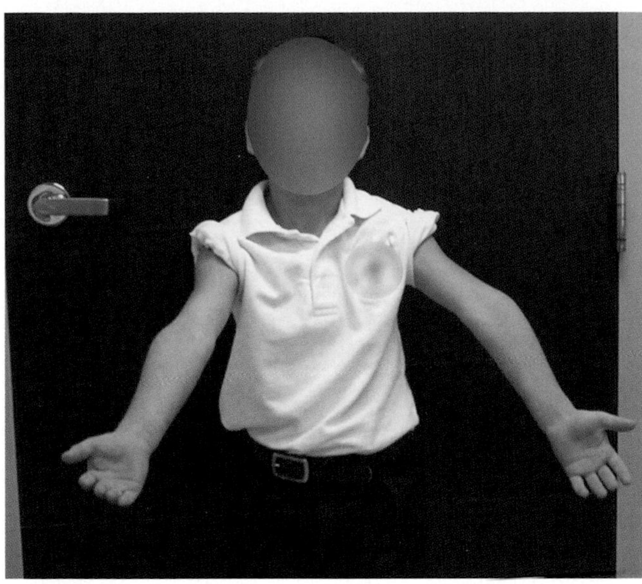

FIGURE 36-16 Cubitus varus deformity after supracondylar fracture.

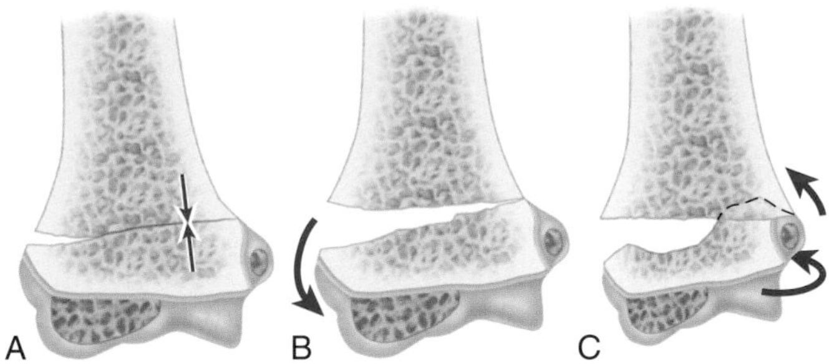

FIGURE 36-17 Mechanism of coronal tilting. **A,** Impaction of fracture medially. **B,** Tilting of fragment medially. **C,** Horizontal rotation.

unlike adults, have good mid-term and long-term functional outcomes after supracondylar humeral fracture.

Cubitus varus is the most common angular deformity that results from supracondylar fractures in children (Fig. 36-16). Cubitus valgus, although mentioned in the literature as causing tardy ulnar nerve palsy, rarely occurs and is more often caused by nonunion of lateral condylar fractures. Because the normal carrying angle increases from childhood to adulthood, an increase in valgus is not as cosmetically noticeable as a complete reversal to a varus position.

Several causes for cubitus varus have been suggested. Medial displacement and rotation of the distal fragment have been cited most often, but experimental studies showed that varus tilting of the distal fragment was the most important cause of change in the carrying angle (Fig. 36-17). Osteonecrosis and delayed growth of the trochlea, with relative overgrowth of the normal lateral side of the distal humeral epiphysis, is a rare cause of progressive cubitus varus deformity after supracondylar fracture. This progressive growth abnormality cannot be prevented by stabilization of the distal fragment because it probably is related to injury to the blood supply of the trochlea at the time of fracture.

Rotational malalignment may occur but is not a significant deformity. Malrotation of the distal humerus is compensated for to a large degree by motion of the shoulder joint. As a result, the rotational component in cubitus varus deformities is of little consequence and all that is usually necessary for correction is a lateral closing wedge osteotomy. Occasionally, a hyperextension deformity requires the addition of a flexion component.

Three basic types of osteotomies have been described: a medial opening wedge osteotomy with a bone graft, an oblique osteotomy with derotation, and a lateral closing wedge osteotomy. Uchida et al. described a three-dimensional osteotomy for correction of cubitus varus deformity in which medial and posterior tilt and rotation of the distal fragment can be corrected if necessary (Fig. 36-18).

A lateral closing wedge osteotomy is the easiest, safest, and inherently most stable osteotomy. Supracondylar osteotomy for cubitus varus should be viewed as a reconstructive procedure and not as fracture management. The fixation used can be tailored to the age of the child and degree of deformity (Fig. 36-19). A combination of screws and Kirschner wires may be needed for younger patients, whereas plate-and screw fixation is more appropriate for adolescents.

DeRosa and Graziano reported good results with a step-cut osteotomy technique fixed with a single cortical screw (Fig. 36-20). They reported no ulnar or radial nerve injuries, infections, nonunions, or hypertrophic scars, and all patients retained preoperative ranges of motion. They concluded that this osteotomy with single-screw fixation is a safe procedure that can correct multiple planes of deformity, but they emphasized the importance of careful preoperative planning and special attention to surgical detail. If a more extensive osteotomy is needed, a step-cut translation osteotomy and fixation with a Y-shaped humeral plate that allows early movement of the joint may be used (Fig. 36-21).

LATERAL CLOSING WEDGE OSTEOTOMY FOR CUBITUS VARUS

TECHNIQUE 36-6

- After standard preparation and draping and inflation of the tourniquet, approach the elbow through a lateral incision.
- With fluoroscopic guidance, insert two Kirschner wires into the lateral condyle before osteotomy and advance them just distal to the planned distal cut. Be prepared to advance these proximally after the closing wedge osteotomy has been made.
- Make a closing wedge osteotomy laterally, leaving the medial cortex intact.
- Weaken the medial cortex using drill holes. Apply a valgus stress to complete the osteotomy with the forearm in pronation and the elbow flexed.
- Close the osteotomy and advance the Kirschner wires from the lateral condyle into the medial cortex of the proximal fragment.

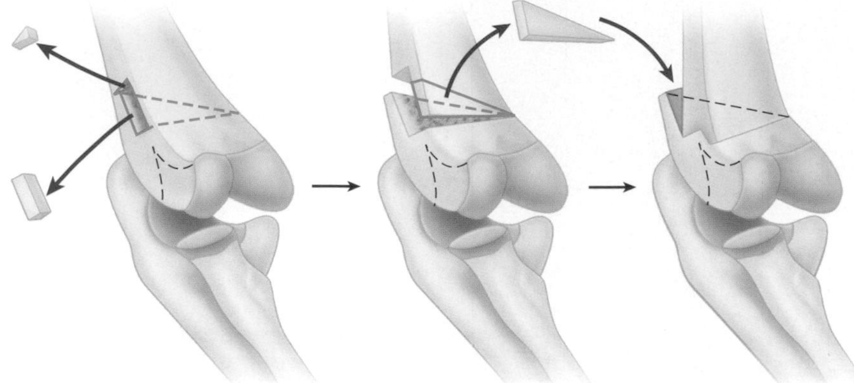

FIGURE 36-18 Three-dimensional osteotomy for correction of cubitus varus deformity. Medial and posterior tilt is corrected. After osteotomy, distal fragment is compacted with proximal fragment by adding external rotation using wedge of humeral cortex. Bone graft is added if necessary. (From Uchida Y, Ogata K, Sugioka Y: A new three-dimensional osteotomy for cubitus varus deformity after supracondylar fracture of the humerus in children, J Pediatr Orthop 11:327, 1991.)

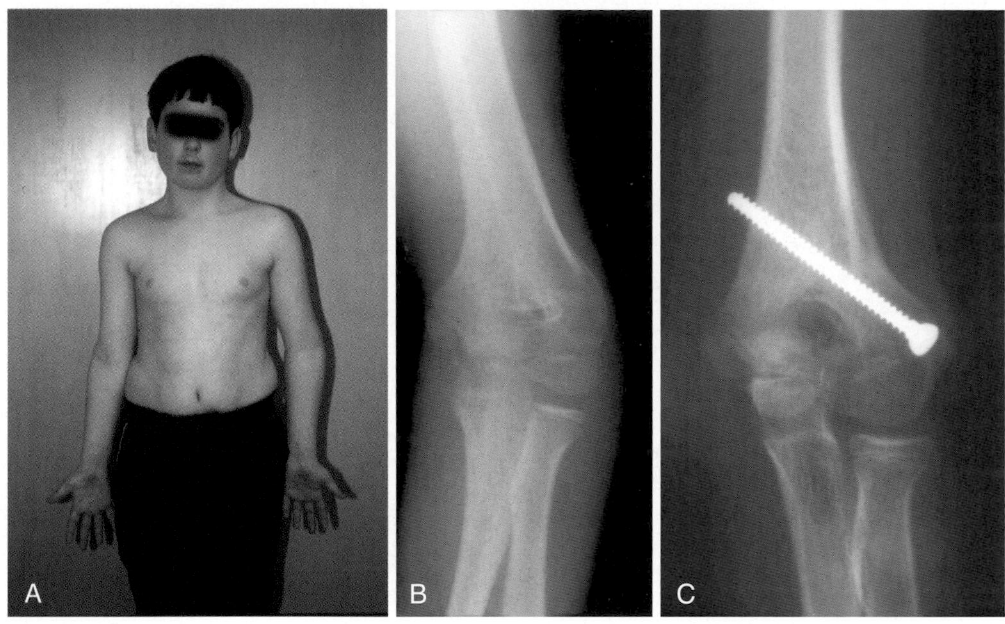

FIGURE 36-19 **A** and **B,** Cubitus varus deformity of the left elbow. **C,** After osteotomy and screw fixation.

- Leave the wires buried under the skin. A third wire can be used if necessary for stability.
- Close the wound in layers and splint the arm in 90 degrees of flexion and full pronation. A long arm cast can be applied in 5 to 7 days.

POSTOPERATIVE CARE. The wires are removed at approximately 6 weeks after surgery, and a range-of-motion exercise program is started.

LATERAL CONDYLAR FRACTURES

Fracture of the lateral condyle is the second most common (17%) pediatric elbow fracture after fracture of the supracondylar humerus, usually occurring between the ages of 4 and 6 years. The most common mechanism of injury is a fall onto an outstretched arm with the elbow in varus, which causes avulsion of the lateral humeral condyle. Alternatively, these injuries can occur, although less commonly, during a fall onto a flexed elbow. Unlike supracondylar humeral fractures, lateral condylar fractures are rarely associated with neurovascular injuries.

These injuries can be classified either anatomically or by displacement. Historically, the Milch classification was used to determine whether the fracture passed through (type I) or around (type II) the capitellum. The Milch type II fracture, which is really a Salter-Harris type II fracture, is the most common type (95%) (Fig. 36-22). More often the fractures are classified by displacement because the amount of displacement determines the method of treatment. A recent

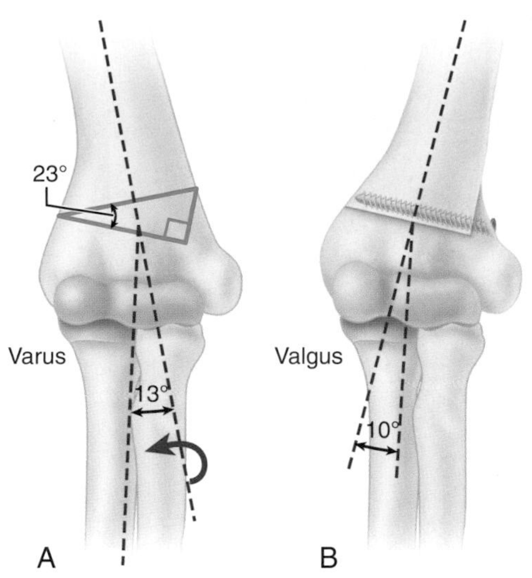

FIGURE 36-20 **A,** Osteotomy designed to correct cubitus varus deformity of 13 degrees. Distal fragment can be rotated to correct additional deformity. **B,** After wedge removal and closure, screw is used for fixation. (Redrawn from DeRosa GP, Graziano GP: A new osteotomy for cubitus varus, Clin Orthop Relat Res 236:160, 1988.) **SEE TECHNIQUE 36-6.**

displacement based classification system by Weiss et al. has been shown to be prognostic for complications. Type I fractures are displaced less than 2 mm, type II fractures are displaced more than 2 mm with an intact cartilaginous hinge, and type III fractures are displaced more than 2 mm without an intact cartilaginous hinge (Fig. 36-23). Type III fractures tend to be displaced and rotated and, in some cases, if enough trochlear stability is lost, a posterolateral subluxation of the radius and ulna can occur (Fig. 36-24). This classification also helps guide treatment, because type I fractures can be treated with a cast, type II fractures with percutaneous pinning, and type III fractures with open reduction and internal fixation.

Radiographically, it can be difficult to determine the amount of displacement because of the large amount of unossified epiphysis present. The presence of a metaphyseal fragment on the lateral radiograph is helpful in making the diagnosis (Fig. 36-25). The addition of an internal oblique radiograph also can be helpful in assessing the true amount of displacement. It can be difficult to determine the stability of the cartilaginous hinge on plain radiographs, and it may be necessary to perform stress radiographs or arthrography under anesthesia for full assessment. Advanced imaging such MRI can be used when the diagnosis is in question or to evaluate the stability of the cartilaginous hinge; however, this requires sedation to obtain satisfactory high resolution images in this age group.

Nondisplaced or minimally displaced fractures can be treated in a long arm cast for 4 to 6 weeks depending on the age of the patient. These fractures need to be watched closely because late displacement can occur. For type II fractures or fractures in which there is concern about the integrity of the cartilaginous hinge, a stress examination under anesthesia with or without arthrography may be performed. In patients with a large metaphyseal fragment, percutaneous pinning using smooth Kirschner wires or a cannulated screw is performed. Displaced fractures or those with unclear reduction require open reduction and internal fixation (Fig. 36-26). This is done through a lateral approach, taking care to avoid dissection posteriorly that may injure the blood supply to the trochlea, which enters posteriorly, and cause osteonecrosis. Fixation using smooth Kirschner wires and cannulated screws has been described with good results. Kirschner wires can be left outside the skin for short periods of time (3 to 4 weeks) with a low risk of infection. Pins can be buried under the skin for longer periods, but removal usually requires a second operative procedure.

The most common complication after fracture of the lateral condyle is loss of reduction. Therefore close follow-up is necessary for these patients. Even fractures with less than 2 mm of initial displacement can displace late.

OPEN REDUCTION AND INTERNAL FIXATION OF LATERAL CONDYLAR FRACTURE

TECHNIQUE 36-7

- Expose the elbow through a Kocher lateral approach (Fig. 1-110) and carry the dissection down to the lateral humeral condyle. In some patients, especially with type III fractures, the distal fragment is rotated and the articular cartilage is subcutaneous, and care is necessary to prevent iatrogenic articular cartilage injury. The soft-tissue dissection is between the brachioradialis and the triceps, although often the capsule is already torn. Expose the anterior surface of the joint. It is important that no dissection be performed posteriorly to prevent injury to the trochlear blood supply.
- The displacement and the size of the fragment are always greater than is apparent on radiographs because much of the fragment is cartilaginous. The fragment usually is rotated and displaced. Irrigate the joint to remove blood clots and debris, reduce the articular surface accurately, and confirm the reduction by observing the articular surface, particularly at the trochlear ridge. Because of the plastic deformation that often occurs, there may be some metaphyseal displacement, even with anatomic articular surface reduction. The fracture should be stabilized in the position of anatomic joint reduction regardless of the metaphyseal deformity.
- If a large metaphyseal fragment is present, insert two smooth Kirschner wires across it into the medial cortex of the distal humerus in a divergent fashion.
- Check the reduction and the position of the internal fixation by radiographs before closing the wound. Cut off the ends of the wires beneath the skin, but leave them long enough to allow easy removal (Fig. 36-27). Alternatively, the pins can be left outside the skin for ease of removal.
- Place the arm in a bivalved long arm cast or splint with the elbow flexed 90 degrees.

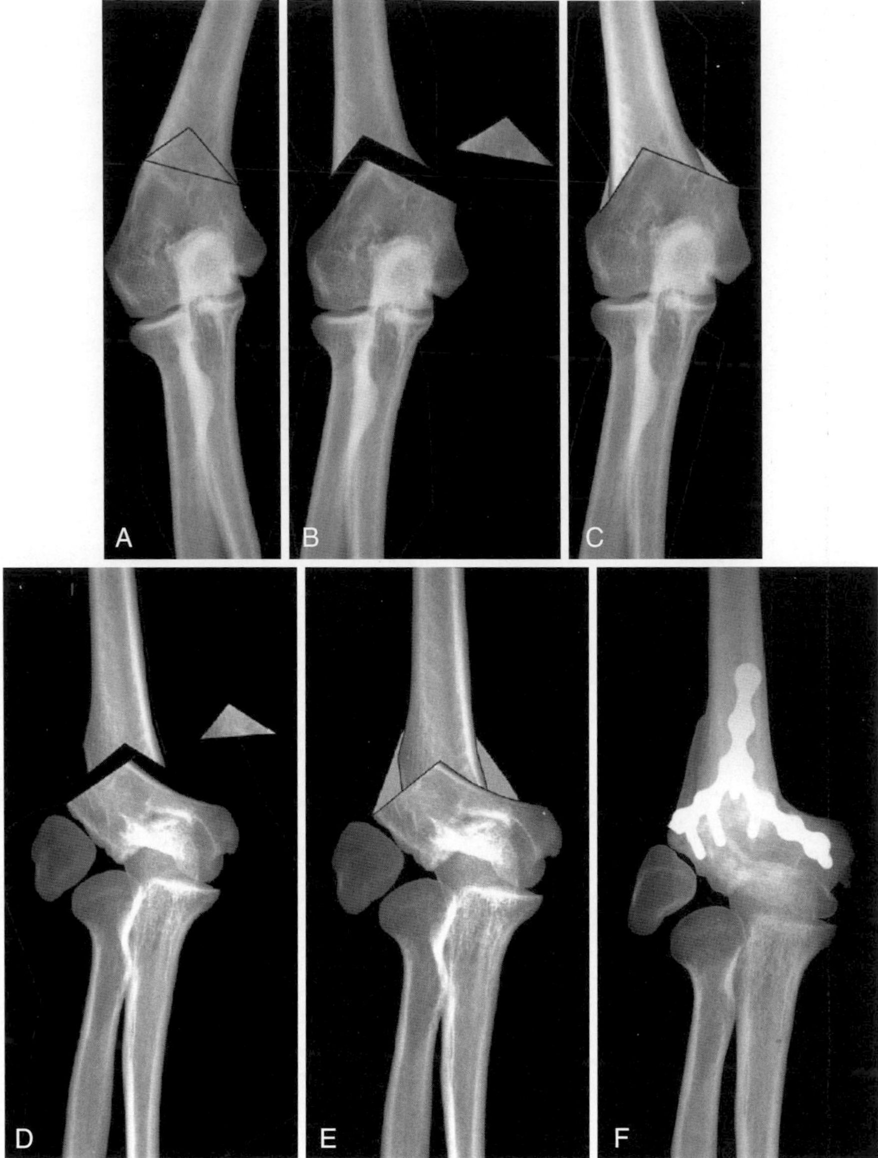

FIGURE 36-21 Step-cut translation osteotomy. **A,** After humerus-elbow-wrist angle is determined on anteroposterior radiograph, initial transverse osteotomy line is made 0.5 to 1.0 cm superior to olecranon fossa and perpendicular to axis of humerus. *Triangular area* indicates area to be resected. **B** and **C,** Cubitus varus is corrected by rotating distal fragment and translating it medially after completing initial transverse osteotomy. Triangular overlapping of proximal and distal humeral portions means that resection is indicated. For cubitus varus, degree of correction increases as location of apex moves medially. **D** and **E,** Cubitus valgus is corrected by rotating distal part of humerus medially and translating it laterally according to anatomic shape of normal elbow. **F,** Fixation of osteotomy site. (From Kim HT, Lee JS, Yoo CI: Management of cubitus varus and valgus, J Bone Joint Surg 87A:771, 2005.) **SEE TECHNIQUE 36-6.**

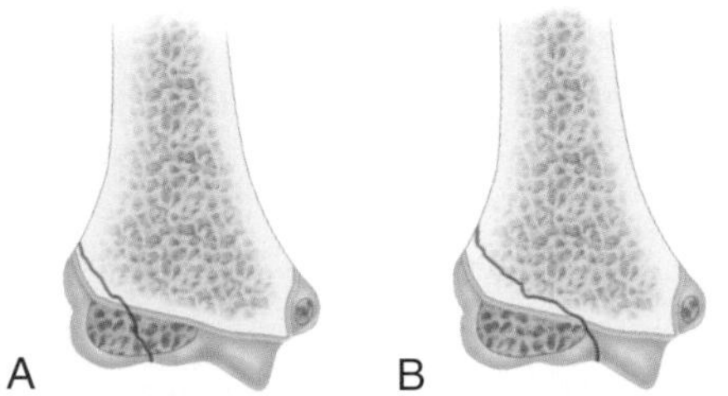

FIGURE 36-22 Lateral humeral condylar fractures. **A,** Milch type I fracture, which is Salter-Harris type IV epiphyseal fracture. **B,** Milch type II fracture, which is Salter-Harris type II epiphyseal fracture.

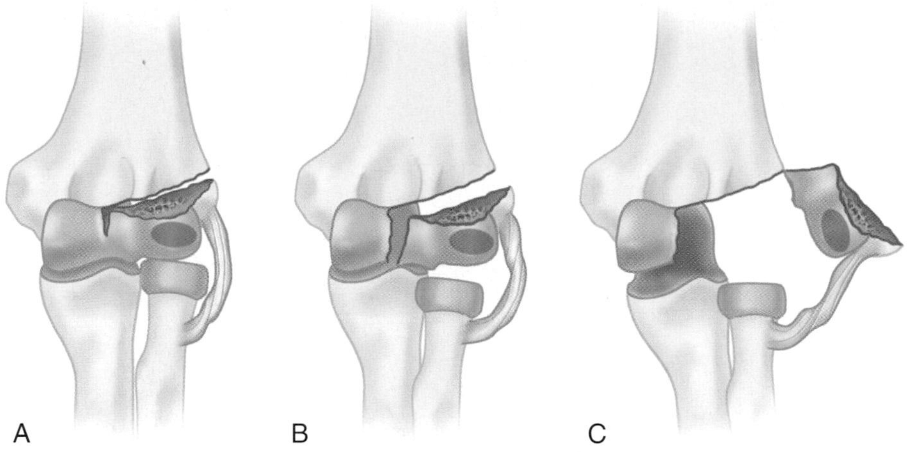

FIGURE 36-23 Weiss classification of lateral condylar fractures. **A**, Type 1 fracture, less than 2 mm displacement. **B**, Type 2 fracture, 2 mm or more displacement and congruity of the articular surface. **C**, Type 3 fracture, 2 mm or more displacement and lack of articular congruity.

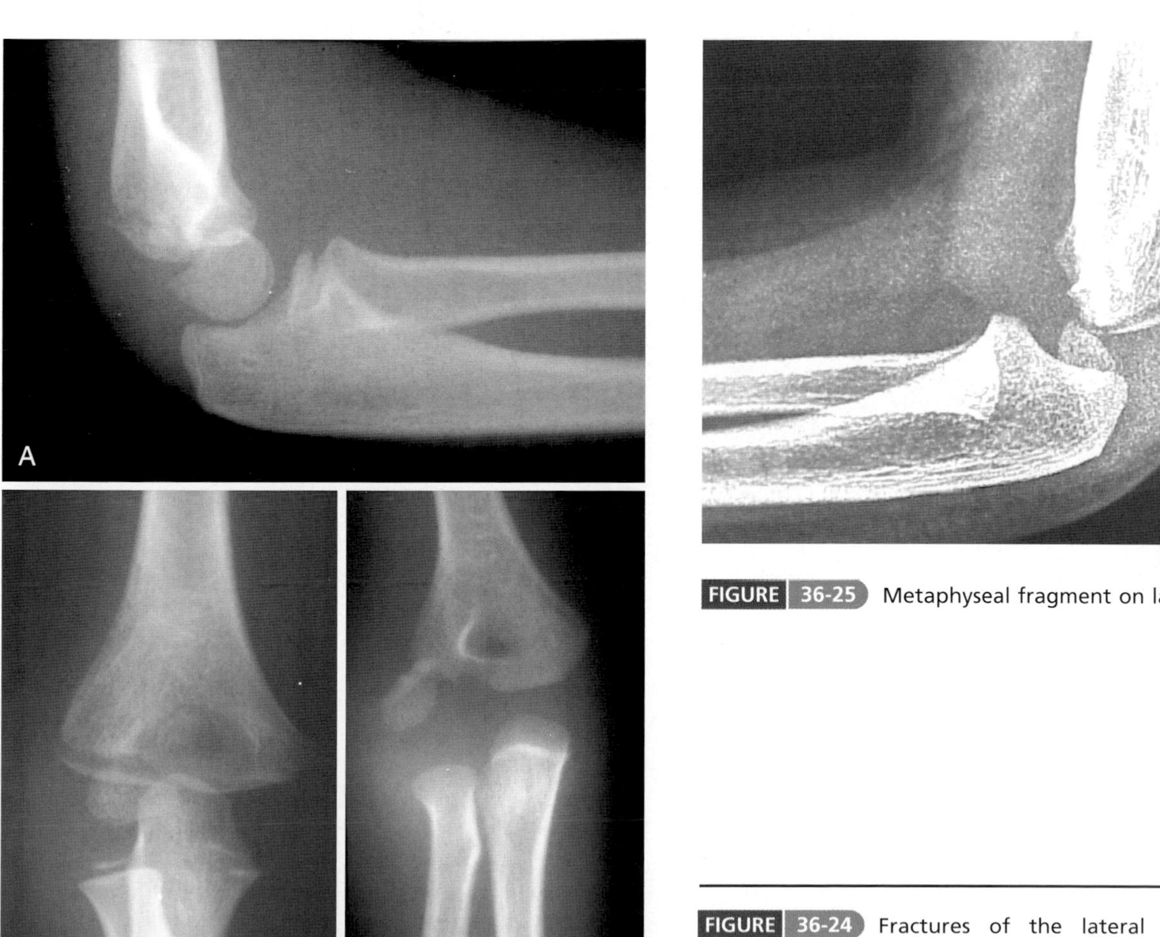

FIGURE 36-25 Metaphyseal fragment on lateral radiograph.

FIGURE 36-24 Fractures of the lateral humeral condyle. **A,** Type I, stable fracture with minimal lateral gap. **B,** Type II, fracture to epiphyseal cartilage with a lateral gap; displacement risk undefined. **C,** Type III, fracture gap as wide laterally as medially; high risk of later displacement.

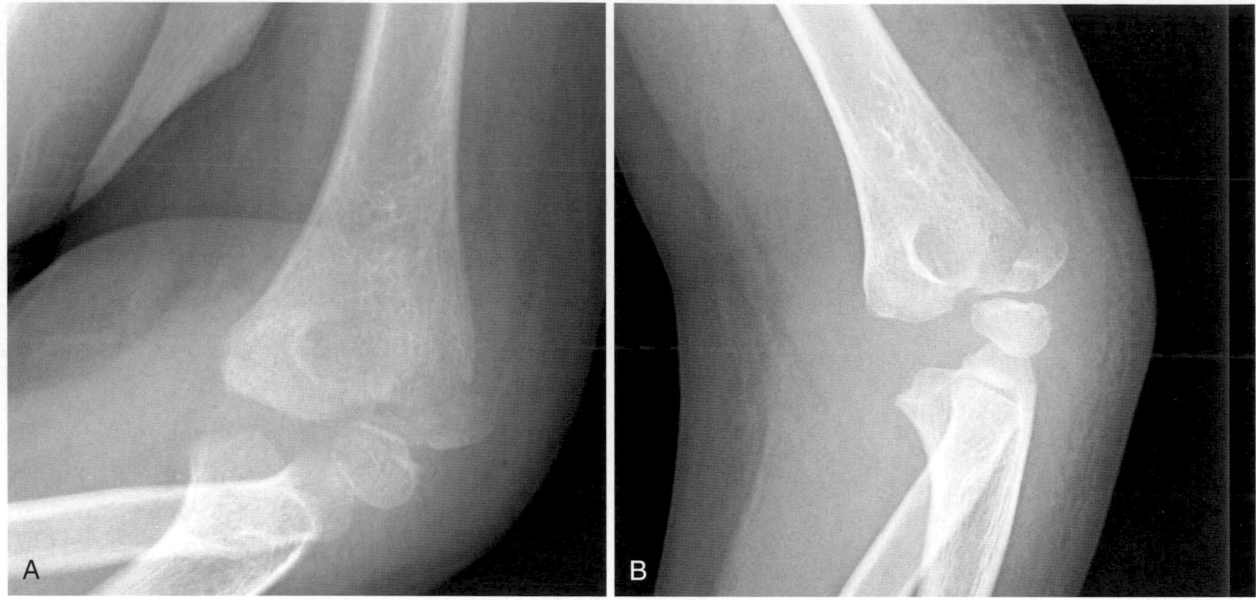

FIGURE 36-26 **A** and **B**, Radiographs showing lateral condylar fracture.

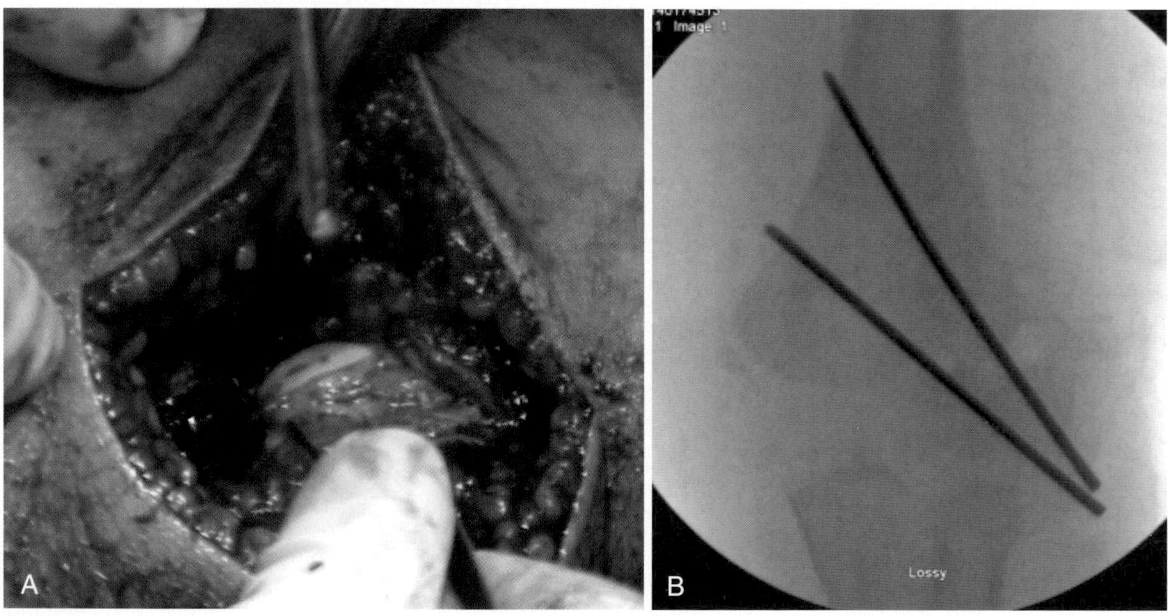

FIGURE 36-27 **A**, Open reduction and internal fixation of lateral condylar fracture shown in Figure 36-26. **B**, After open reduction and fixation with smooth wires. **SEE TECHNIQUE 36-7.**

POSTOPERATIVE CARE. Immobilization should continue 4 weeks with the arm in a cast followed in some cases by splinting. At the end of that time the pins can be removed if union is progressing. Gentle active motion of the elbow usually is resumed intermittently out of the splint. These fractures are notorious for late and delayed union, and some require immobilization with intermittent range-of-motion exercises for more than 6 weeks.

COMPLICATIONS AFTER LATERAL CONDYLAR FRACTURE

Complications from lateral condylar fractures include physeal arrest, physeal stimulation, osteonecrosis, and nonunion with resultant cubitus valgus (Fig. 36-28). Lateral condylar overgrowth, radial prominence, and variation in the carrying angle of the elbow have been attributed to transient stimulation of the lateral column of the elbow. Osteonecrosis of the capitellum (Fig. 36-29) or a small growth arrest in the central

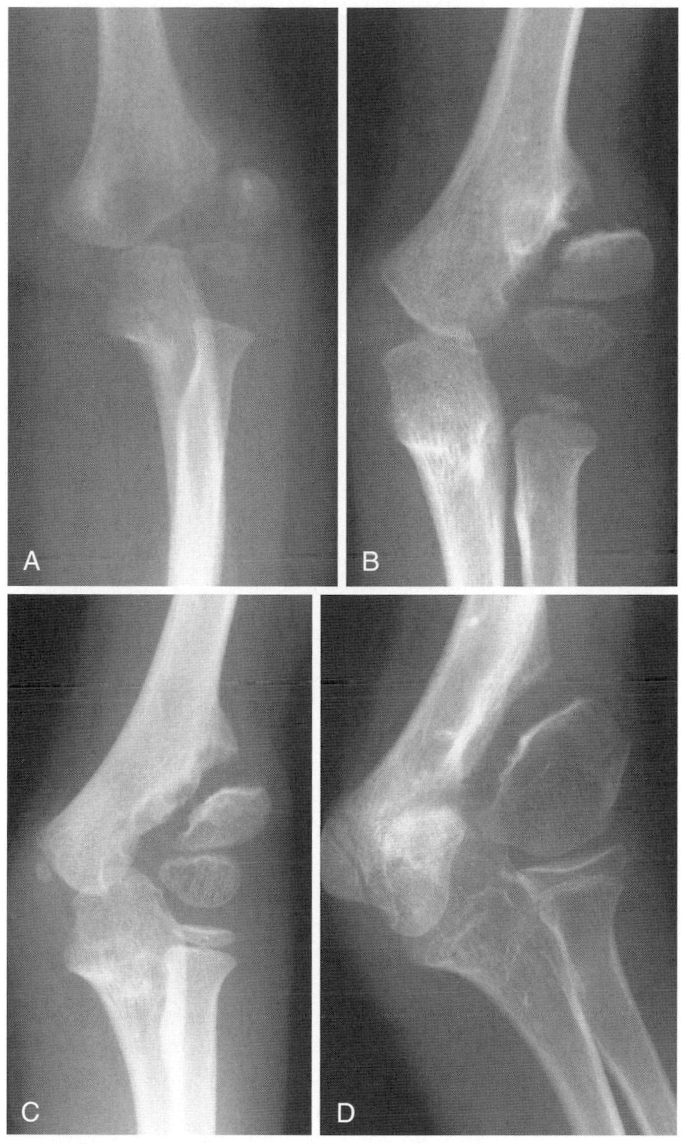

FIGURE 36-28 **A,** Fracture of lateral humeral condyle in 5-year-old boy. **B,** Established nonunion 1 year after nonoperative treatment (observation only). **C,** Apparent proximal migration of capitellum and condyle at 3 years. **D,** Severe cubitus valgus 9 years after fracture.

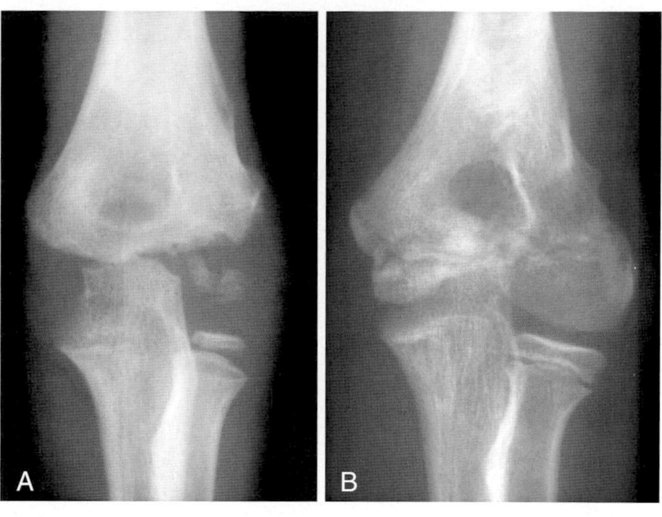

FIGURE 36-29 **A,** Fracture of the lateral humeral condyle through the ossific nucleus. **B,** Development of osteonecrosis of the capitellum.

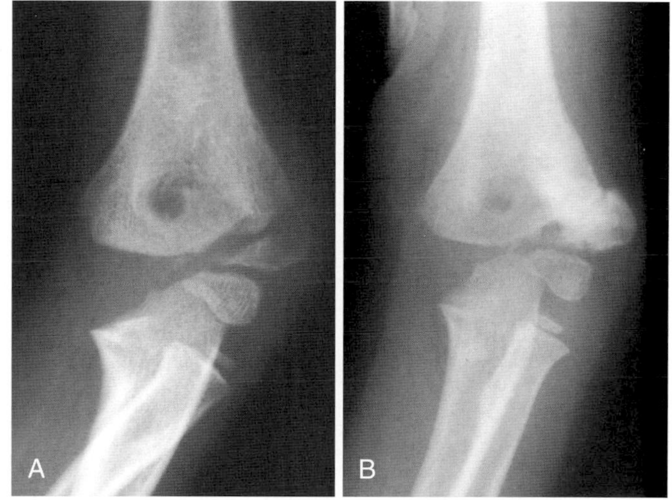

FIGURE 36-30 **A** and **B,** Nonunion of lateral condylar fracture after closed treatment.

physis occurs with "fishtail" deformity (deepening of the trochlear groove) and rare varus deformity. Because of the lack of cases, data concerning prevention, treatment, and long-term follow-up are limited.

Nonunion with resultant cubitus valgus probably is the most significant complication (Fig. 36-30). Nonunion must be differentiated from delayed union. Immobilization of the fracture even with minimal displacement for more than 6 weeks often is necessary. A delay in union may result from inadequate external immobilization or internal fixation. If union is not achieved at 12 weeks, a small wedge-shaped bone graft can be placed across the metaphyseal fragment with supplemental smooth pin or screw fixation (Fig. 36-31). If the elbow seems to be stable and is not painful and all that is present is a lucent line with no motion of the fracture fragment on stress views, observation and prolonged immobilization may be all that are necessary. If motion is present or a nonunion seems to be developing, however, early surgery is indicated. Surgery for well-established nonunions is difficult, and the goals should be to restore a more anatomic alignment of the elbow. Arthrotomy and realignment of the articular surface should be avoided because of the high risk of further elbow stiffness and osteonecrosis; osteotomy generally is a better option (Figs. 36-32 and 36-33). Rigid internal fixation should be used to promote early motion. Tardy ulnar nerve palsy can accompany lateral condyle nonunions and can be treated with ulnar nerve transposition and correction of the cubitus valgus.

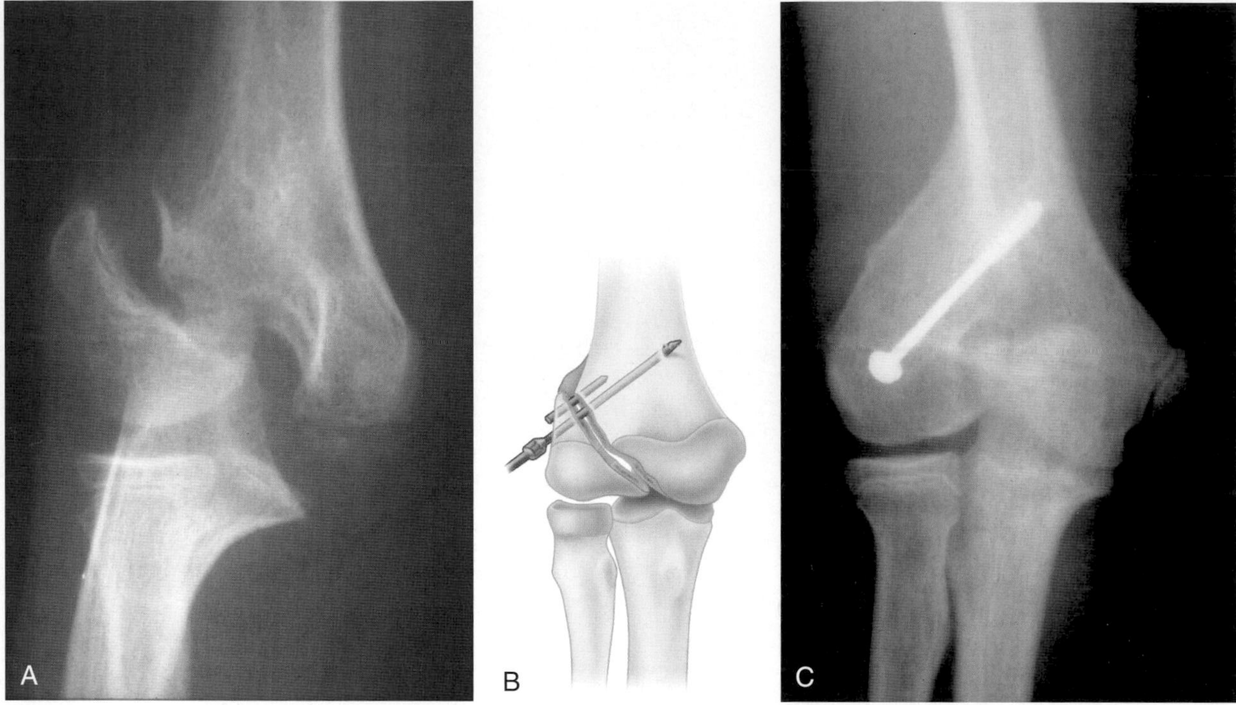

FIGURE 36-31 **A,** Nonunion of lateral condyle with distal fragment in acceptable position for bone grafting and internal fixation. **B** and **C,** Transfixed, freshened, bone-grafted nonunion; physis of condylar fragment is not violated by pin or graft.

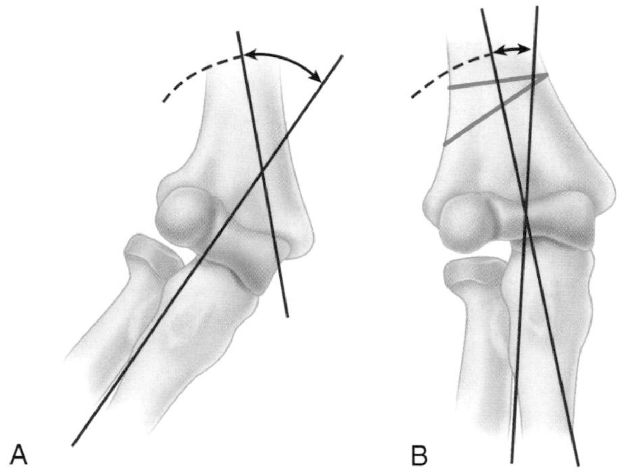

FIGURE 36-32 Correction of cubitus valgus by osteotomy. **A,** Cubitus valgus secondary to nonunion of lateral humeral condyle. **B,** Opening wedge osteotomy laterally to restore alignment.

OSTEOTOMY FOR ESTABLISHED CUBITUS VALGUS SECONDARY TO NONUNION OR GROWTH ARREST

TECHNIQUE 36-8

- Place the patient prone with the forearm supported on an arm board.
- Use a posterior muscle-splitting incision, exposing the distal humerus, but do not open the elbow joint.
- Split the fibers of the triceps muscle, retract them, and identify the ulnar nerve. When indicated for treatment of tardy ulnar nerve palsy, detach the flexor group of muscles from the medial epicondyle and transpose the nerve anteriorly. Reattach the flexor muscles.
- As a landmark, note the upper limit of the condylar fragment. Perform a simple transverse osteotomy at the level of the intersection of the forearm axis with the lateral cortex of the humerus (Fig. 36-33A and B).
- Notch the inferior surface of the proximal fragment to receive the apex of the superior surface of the distal fragment, which is moved laterally (Fig. 36-33C and D). Adduct the distal fragment until the excessive angle of abduction (valgus) has been reduced to the normal carrying angle, controlling the amount of correction by radiographs made with the extremity and the fragments in extension.
- When correction is satisfactory, fix the fragments by inserting two smooth crossed Kirschner wires, carefully flex the elbow, and immobilize it in plaster at 90 degrees.

POSTOPERATIVE CARE. The cast is left on for 4 to 6 weeks, depending on the age of the child and evidence of bony union. The wires are removed, and motion is encouraged at that time.

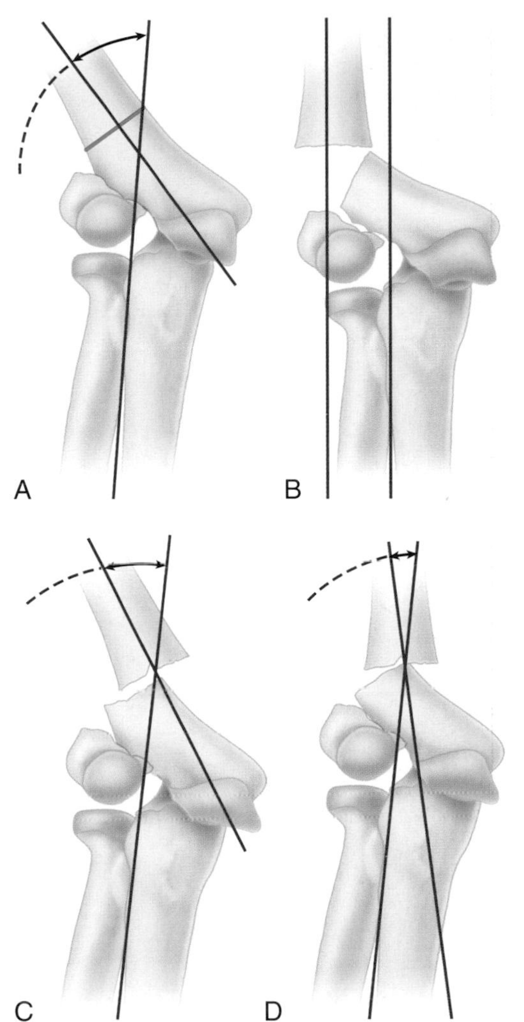

FIGURE 36-33 A and B, Milch type II significantly displaced lateral condylar fracture, in which simple osteotomy would result in unacceptable alignment. C and D, Osteotomy with lateral displacement of distal humeral fragment, aligning arm satisfactorily with forearm. **SEE TECHNIQUE 36-8.**

MEDIAL CONDYLAR FRACTURES

Fractures of the medial humeral condyle in children are rare, accounting for 1% of pediatric elbow fractures. They usually occur in slightly older children than fractures of the lateral condyle, around the ages of 3 to 8 years. They are caused by a direct fall onto the elbow or a fall onto an outstretched hand with the elbow in a varus position. Medial condylar fractures in younger children can be associated with nonaccidental trauma. Kilfoyle described three types based on displacement: type I, a greenstick or impacted fracture; type II, a fracture through the humeral condyle into the joint with little or no displacement; and type III, an epiphyseal fracture that is intraarticular and involves the medial condyle with the fragment displaced and rotated (Fig. 36-34). Type III fractures, which occur in older children, account for 25% of all medial condylar fractures. In type III fractures the flexor pronator mass, which is attached to the distal fragment, causes the distal fragment to rotate anteriorly and medially, causing the articular surface to face posteriorly and laterally. This injury often is confused with medial epicondylar fracture, which is more common but occurs in older children. Making a radiographic diagnosis can be difficult, especially in younger patients in whom the trochlea has not yet ossified, which occurs around the age of 8 years. MRI and elbow arthrography can be used to make the diagnosis in unclear cases. Medial epicondylar fractures often occur with elbow dislocations and, because of the intraarticular nature of the medial condyle, patients with medial condylar fractures, unlike those with medial epicondylar fractures, have fat pad changes evident on radiographs.

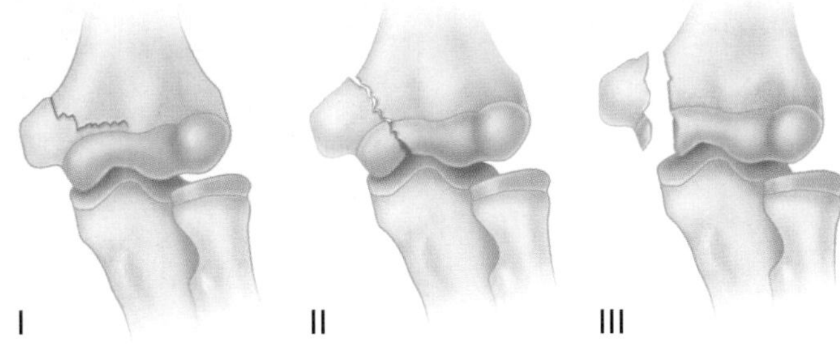

FIGURE 36-34 Three types of medial condylar fractures described by Kilfoyle: type I, impacted; type II, epiphyseal and intraarticular; and type III, displacement of entire medial condyle.

For nondisplaced fractures treatment consists of 4 to 6 weeks of cast immobilization. These fractures heal more slowly than supracondylar fractures and are more like lateral condylar fractures because of the intraarticular nature of the fracture site. The treatment for displaced fractures is open reduction and internal fixation to ensure joint congruity. This is best done through a posteromedial incision, which provides excellent exposure of the fracture site and allows for protection of the ulnar nerve. Care must be taken not to extend the dissection posteriorly to avoid injury to the trochlear blood supply. Fixation consists typically of two smooth Kirschner wires in younger children and screw or plate fixation, or both, in older children to control rotation and prevent nonunion that can occur with inadequate fracture fixation (Fig. 36-35).

COMPLICATIONS AFTER MEDIAL CONDYLAR FRACTURE

The most common complication with this fracture is failing to make the correct diagnosis (see Fig. 36-35). Once the correct diagnosis is made, nonunion is rare and usually results from inadequately stabilized fractures. Complications usually consist of nonunion with resultant cubitus varus, trochlear osteonecrosis, and loss of reduction, and the complication rate can be as high as 33%. Nonunion can be treated with revision open reduction and internal fixation and bone grafting. Many patients with osteonecrosis of the trochlea are asymptomatic and require only observation. Cubitus varus caused by growth delay or arrest of the trochlea and cubitus valgus caused by fracture-simulated overgrowth can occur with these injuries. Corrective osteotomy can be used to treat these deformities if they become painful or interfere with function.

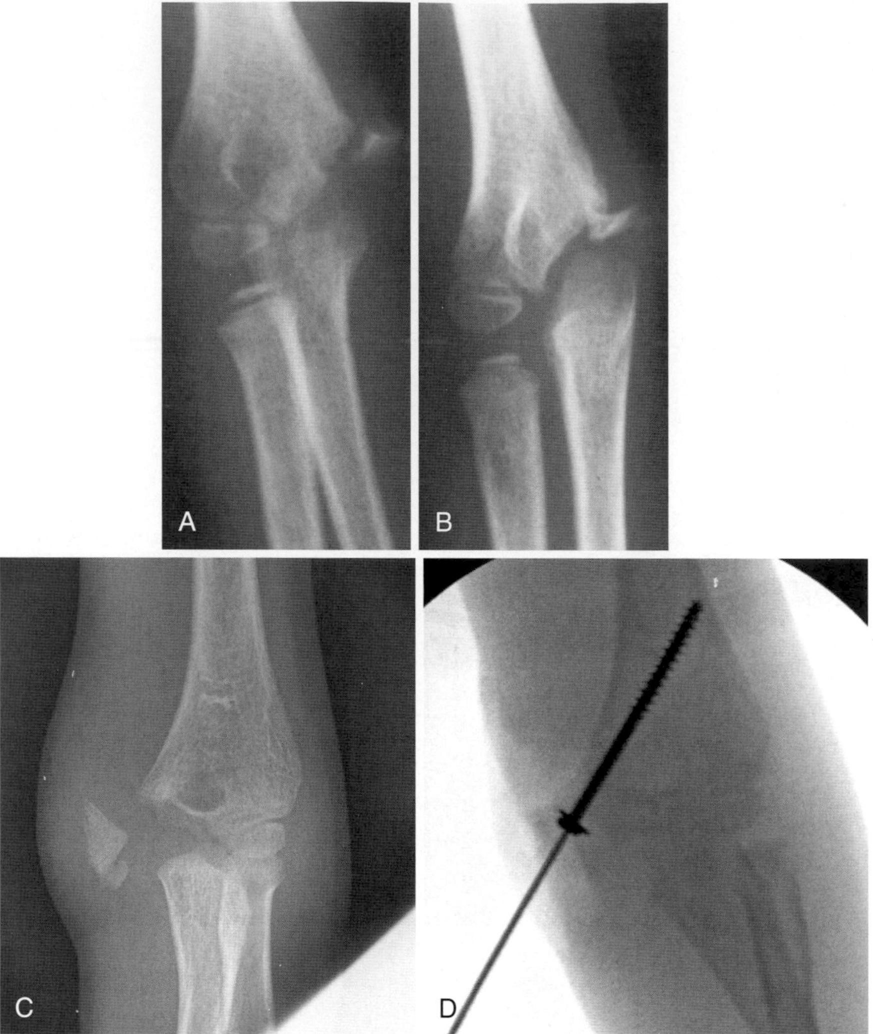

FIGURE 36-35 **A,** Fracture of medial condyle that was believed to be fracture of medial epicondyle. **B,** At 12 weeks after injury, nonunion of medial condyle. **C** and **D,** Fixation of medial condylar fracture.

OPEN REDUCTION AND INTERNAL FIXATION OF MEDIAL CONDYLAR FRACTURE

TECHNIQUE 36-9

- Begin a medial incision just distal to the medial condyle and extend it proximally parallel to the long axis of the humerus. Carry the dissection down to bone, isolating the ulnar nerve, and retract it posteriorly. The capsule usually is ruptured and need not be incised for exposure of the fracture. The capsule can be released anteriorly if more exposure desired.
- Carefully examine the detached condyle and remove all hematoma. The fragment is surprisingly large, and often a part of the capitellum is included.
- Gently reduce the fracture and hold it with a bone tenaculum without disturbing the soft-tissue attachments of the fragment. Some metaphyseal plastic deformation may occur, so it is essential to restore the normal contour of the articular surface rather than the medial column.
- Insert two smooth Kirschner wires through the condylar fragment and into the humerus in a proximal and lateral direction. Two wires are necessary to prevent rotation of the fragment. Use smooth Kirschner wires rather than screws if the child is young and cannulated screw fixation in older children. Before closing the incision, verify the position of the wires and the fragment by radiographs. Cut off the wires beneath the skin, leaving them long enough to allow easy removal.
- Close the wound and apply a splint or bivalve cast with the elbow flexed 90 degrees.

MEDIAL EPICONDYLAR FRACTURES

Medial epicondylar fractures account for approximately 10% of pediatric elbow fractures, with a peak age at occurrence of 11 to 12 years. Between 30% and 50% occur with elbow dis-

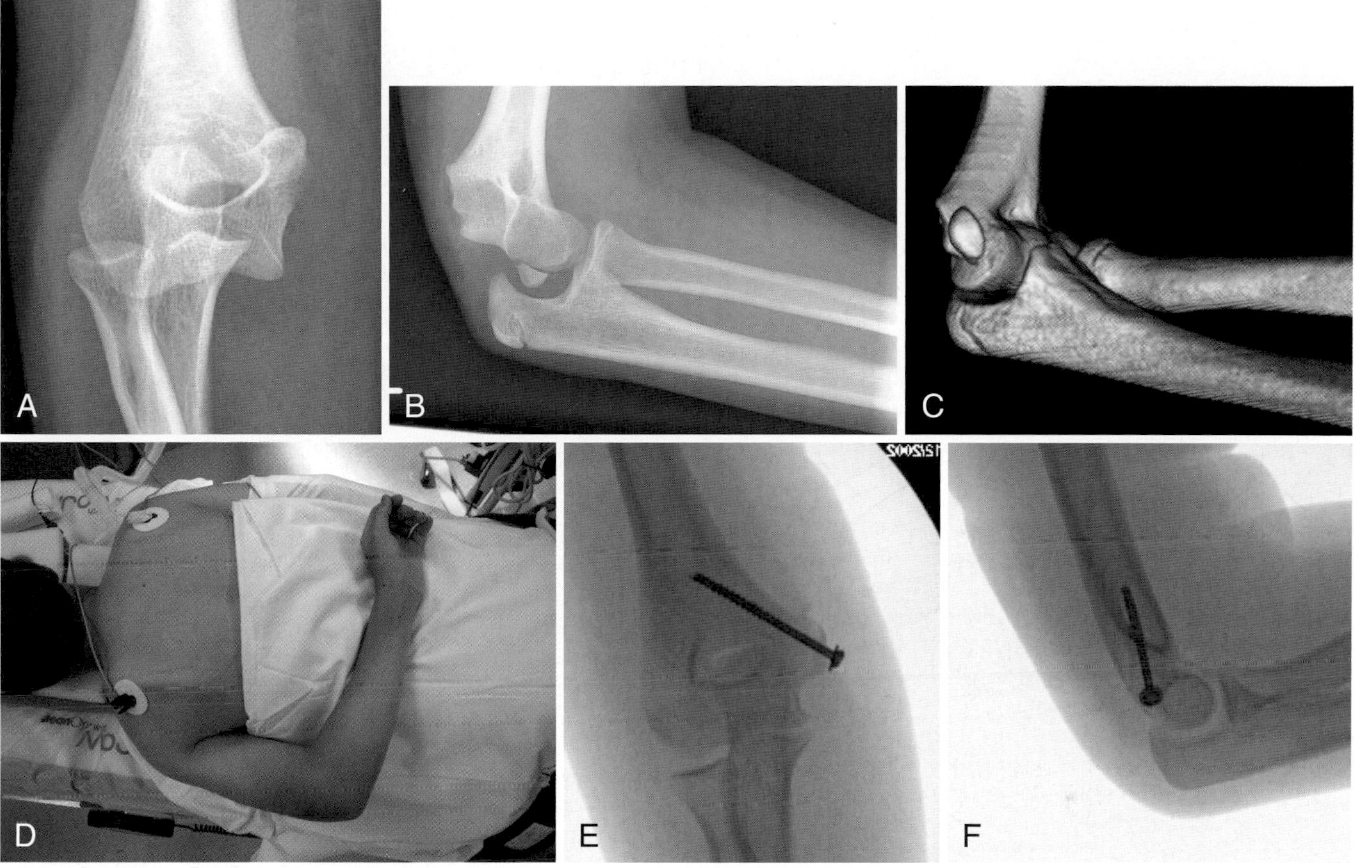

FIGURE 36-36 Anteroposterior (**A**) and lateral (**B**) radiographs of patient with an elbow dislocation and associated fracture of the medial epicondyle. **C**, Postreduction CT showing true displacement of the epicondyle. **D**, Hammerlock position allows for relaxation of forearm flexors attached to the displaced fragment. Anteroposterior (**E**) and lateral (**F**) radiographs after fixation with a cannulated screw and washer.

locations, and it is important to ensure that the medial epicondyle is not entrapped after reduction of the dislocation.

The most common mechanism of injury is an avulsion that can occur as a result of a valgus stress being placed on the extended elbow, usually after a fall. The medial epicondylar apophysis is the origin of the ulnar collateral ligament, which if under valgus stress, avulses it. It can also occur as a result of a pure avulsion by the forearm flexors and rarely with a direct blow to the elbow. In complete fractures, the avulsed apophysis displaces distally from pull of the forearm flexor mass originating on it. Radiographic and CT studies have shown that accurately measuring the true amount of displacement in all planes is difficult.

Nondisplaced fractures can be treated with 2 to 3 weeks of immobilization in a long arm cast or brace followed by gradual resumption of activity. The absolute indication for operative treatment is an entrapped intraarticular apophyseal fragment in an elbow dislocation. Other indications include fractures associated with elbow dislocations to allow early range of motion and fractures displaced more than 1 cm. A relative indication is a minimally displaced fracture in a high-demand throwing athlete. Treatment of mildly displaced fractures, less than 1 cm, remains controversial because of the difficulty in measuring true displacement, the good results being reported in small series of patients treated both operatively and nonoperatively, and the lack of comparison studies.

Surgery can be performed supine or prone in the "hammerlock position," which provides relaxation to the forearm flexor musculature, making reduction easier (Fig. 36-36). Typically a single 4.0 or 4.5-mm cannulated screw is used for fixation, and a long arm cast is worn for 2 to 3 weeks before beginning physical therapy. In comminuted fractures, smooth Kirschner wires, sutures, or both can be used to stabilize the fragments. Patients are treated with a long arm cast or brace for 2 to 3 weeks followed by physical therapy.

COMPLICATIONS AFTER MEDIAL EPICONDYLAR FRACTURE

Complications associated with medial epicondylar fractures are rare and most often associated either with missed incarcerated intraarticular fragments and elbow stiffness related to an elbow dislocation and ulnar nerve palsy. Nonunion of these fractures is rare and can be associated with long-term elbow instability leading to a tardy ulnar nerve palsy. Ulnar nerve dysesthesia is common after operative treatment especially with removal of incarcerated intraarticular fragments, which usually resolves. Ulnar nerve transposition is reserved for late palsies and not for acute ulnar nerve symptoms. Because of the subcutaneous location of the medial epicondyle, screw prominence and pain can occur and can be treated with hardware removal once satisfactory healing has occurred.

OPEN REDUCTION AND INTERNAL FIXATION FOR DISPLACED OR ENTRAPPED MEDIAL EPICONDYLE

TECHNIQUE 36-10

- Position the patient prone with a nonsterile tourniquet and place the elbow on a sterile-draped image intensifier. Mark the course of the ulnar nerve on the skin.
- Make a medial incision centered on the medial epicondyle approximately 5 cm in length.
- The ulnar nerve is posterior and should be protected for the entire procedure. For displaced fractures without entrapment, the fracture site can be viewed directly. Irrigate the fracture site thoroughly. Use a small curet to remove any remaining apophyseal cartilage on the displaced fragment to promote bony healing.
- If the fragment is entrapped within the elbow joint when the fracture site is exposed, only the bony surface of the condyle is seen; no loose fragment is visible. The medial capsule, musculotendinous origin of the long flexor muscles, and epicondyle are folded within the joint, covering the lower part of the coronoid fossa and process. With a small tenaculum, remove the epicondyle with its soft-tissue attachments from within the joint. Now consider the fragment simply as a displaced epicondylar fracture.
- Reduce the epicondyle and secure it with a screw and washer if possible, which allows for early motion. If the fracture is comminuted or the patient is very young, a smooth Kirschner wire can be used. In rare cases in which the epicondyle cannot be stabilized because of comminution, excise the fragments and attach the flexor muscles to the distal humerus using drill holes or a suture anchor(s).
- Suture the tear in the capsule and forearm muscles, close the wound, and apply a posterior splint or a bivalved cast.

POSTOPERATIVE CARE. A splint or cast is worn for 2 to 3 weeks. Alternatively, if good stability is obtained, a hinged elbow brace can be used in compliant patients to begin gentle immediate early range-of-motion exercises.

CHRONIC MEDIAL EPICONDYLE APOPHYSITIS (LITTLE LEAGUE ELBOW)

This chronic injury is related to overuse in young athletes, primarily baseball players. Excessive throwing places repetitive tension on the medial epicondylar apophysis. Overuse is a major contributor to this as the incidence is relatively low when established age-related pitch counts are followed. Patients have pain directly over the medial epicondyle, which is increased with valgus stress. Some patients have a loss of elbow extension as well. Radiographically, the apophysis is widened compared with the opposite side, and comparison views can be helpful but are not necessary to make the diagnosis.

The most important treatment is rest followed by a gradual resumption of activity. Antiinflammatory medications, splinting, and ice may be helpful for symptomatic relief. Patients, families, and coaches need to be educated about the overuse nature of this injury. Once the patient is pain free, activity can be gradually progressed, ensuring proper throwing mechanics are followed. Although this can be very debilitating in terms of sports participation, no long-term complications from this have been reported.

DISTAL HUMERAL FRACTURES

Fracture of the entire distal humeral physis, which occurs more distally than a supracondylar fracture (Fig. 36-37), most commonly occurs during a fall and most frequently in young children (mean age, 5 years). This injury has historically been underreported because making the diagnosis was difficult. With increased awareness and advanced imaging techniques such as MRI, ultrasound, and arthrography, this injury is being diagnosed with greater frequency.

The distal humeral epiphysis extends across to include the secondary ossification of the medial epicondyle until about 6 to 7 years of age in girls and 8 to 9 years in boys. Most fractures involving the entire distal humeral physis occur before the age of 6 or 7 and usually younger. The younger the child, the greater the volume of distal humerus occupied by cartilaginous epiphysis. As children mature, the volume of the epiphysis decreases, which some authors believe is protective of injury. This may explain the association between distal humeral physeal fractures and birth trauma, as well as nonaccidental trauma. In addition, the physeal line in infants is near the center of the olecranon fossa, making it prone to hyperextension injury. Malunion after these injuries is less common because of the broad surface area of the distal humerus. Because the blood supply to the medial trochlea courses through the physis, osteonecrosis of the trochlea can occur.

These fractures are classified into three groups based on the degree of ossification of the lateral condylar epiphysis. Group A fractures occur in infants up to 12 months of age,

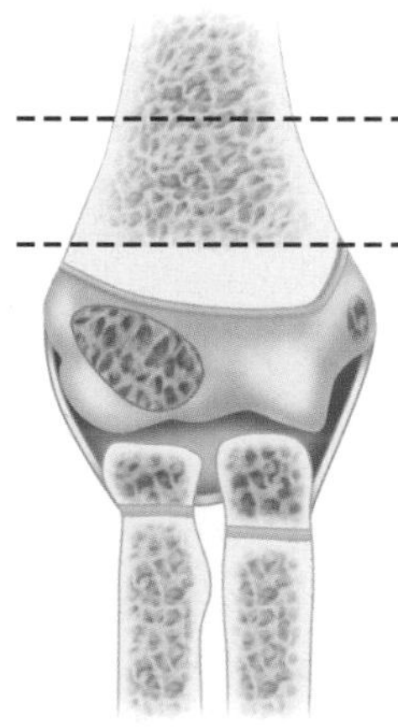

FIGURE 36-37 *Dashed horizontal lines* indicate proximal area, where supracondylar fracture occurs, and distal area, where physeal fracture-separation occurs in wider part of distal humerus in younger age group.

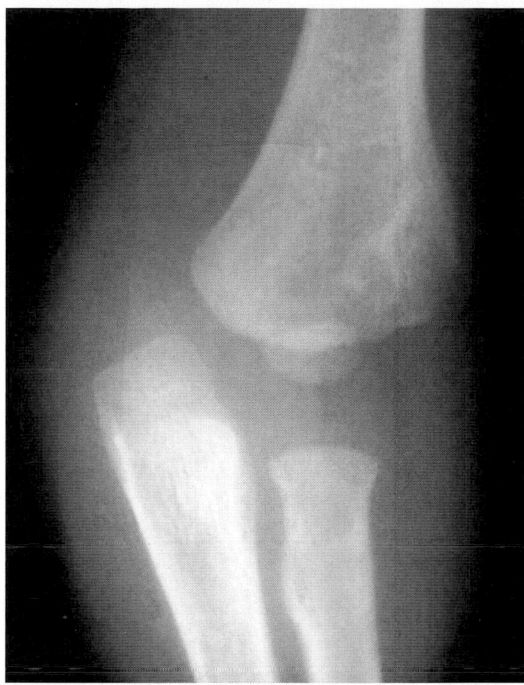

FIGURE 36-38 Transphyseal dislocation in a neonate. Note loss of normal relationship between ulna and distal humerus.

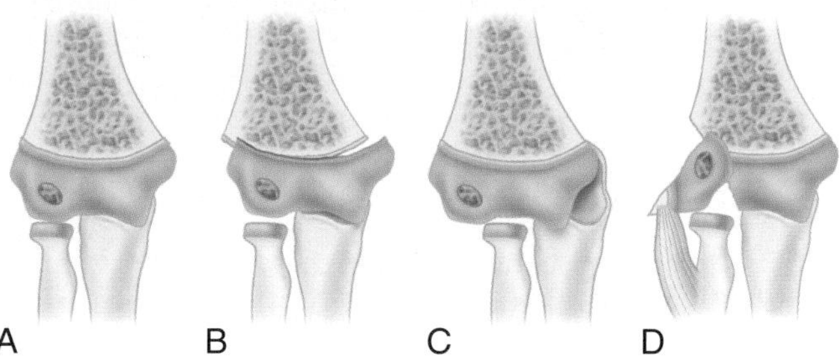

FIGURE 36-39 Elbow injuries that may be confused clinically. **A,** Normal elbow before three centers of ossification appear. **B,** Separation of entire distal humeral epiphysis. **C,** Dislocation of elbow. **D,** Lateral condylar fracture.

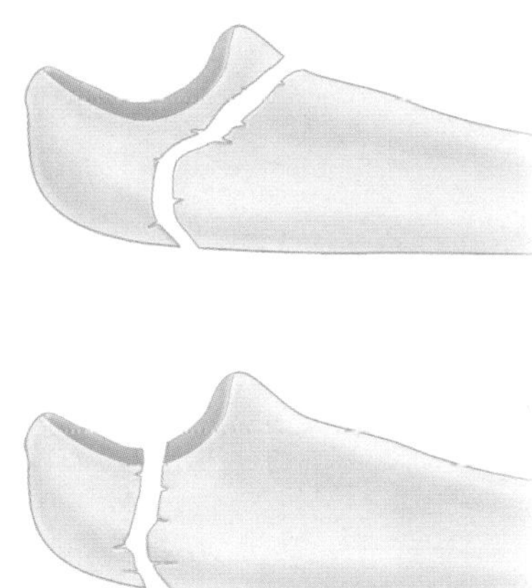

FIGURE 36-40 Two types of olecranon physeal fractures. Regardless of type, if displacement is significant, open reduction and internal fixation is probably indicated.

before the secondary ossification center of the lateral condylar epiphysis appears (and are usually Salter-Harris type I physeal injuries) (Fig. 36-38). These often are missed because the lateral condylar epiphysis lacks an ossification center. Group B fractures occur most often in children 12 months to 3 years of age in whom there is definite ossification of the lateral condyle. Group C fractures occur in older children, from 3 to 7 years of age, and result in a large metaphyseal fragment.

In an infant younger than 18 months of age whose elbow is swollen secondary to trauma or suspected trauma, a fracture involving the entire distal humeral physis should be considered. In a young infant or newborn, swelling may be minimal with little crepitus because the fracture fragments are covered in cartilage (physis) rather than bone.

Radiographic diagnosis can be difficult, especially if the ossification center of the lateral condyle is not visible. The only relationship that can be determined is that of the primary ossification centers of the distal humerus to the proximal radius and ulna (Fig. 36-39). The proximal radius and ulna maintain an anatomic relationship to each other but are displaced posteriorly and medially in relation to the distal humerus. Comparison views of the opposite uninjured elbow may be helpful to determine the presence of displacement.

Once the lateral condylar epiphysis becomes ossified, displacement of the entire distal epiphysis is much more obvious. The anatomic relationship of the lateral condylar epiphysis with the radial head is maintained, even though the distal humeral epiphysis is displaced posterior and medial in relation to the metaphysis of the humerus.

Because they have a large metaphyseal fragment, type C fractures may be confused with either a low supracondylar fracture or a fracture of the lateral condylar physis. The key diagnostic point is the smooth outline of the distal metaphysis in fractures involving the total distal physis. With supracondylar fractures, the distal portion of the distal fragment has a more irregular border.

A lateral condylar physeal fracture can be differentiated from the rare elbow dislocation in an infant can be made on radiograph. With a displaced fracture of the lateral condylar physis, the relationship between the lateral condylar epiphysis and the proximal radius usually is disrupted. If the lateral crista of the trochlea is involved, the proximal radius and ulna may be displaced posterolaterally. Elbow dislocations are rare in the peak age group for fractures of the entire distal humeral physis. With elbow dislocations, the displacement of the proximal radius and ulna is almost always posterolateral, and the relationship between the proximal radius and lateral condylar epiphysis is disrupted. Comparison views are helpful in making this diagnosis. Advanced imaging such as arthrography or MRI also can be used. Ultrasound can be helpful, especially in an infant.

TREATMENT

Treatment is first directed toward prompt recognition. Because this injury may be associated with child abuse, the parents may delay seeking treatment and ossification may already be present on the initial radiographs. These injuries, when recognized in a timely fashion, can be treated with closed reduction and percutaneous pinning (Fig. 36-40). Arthrography can be helpful to define the cartilaginous

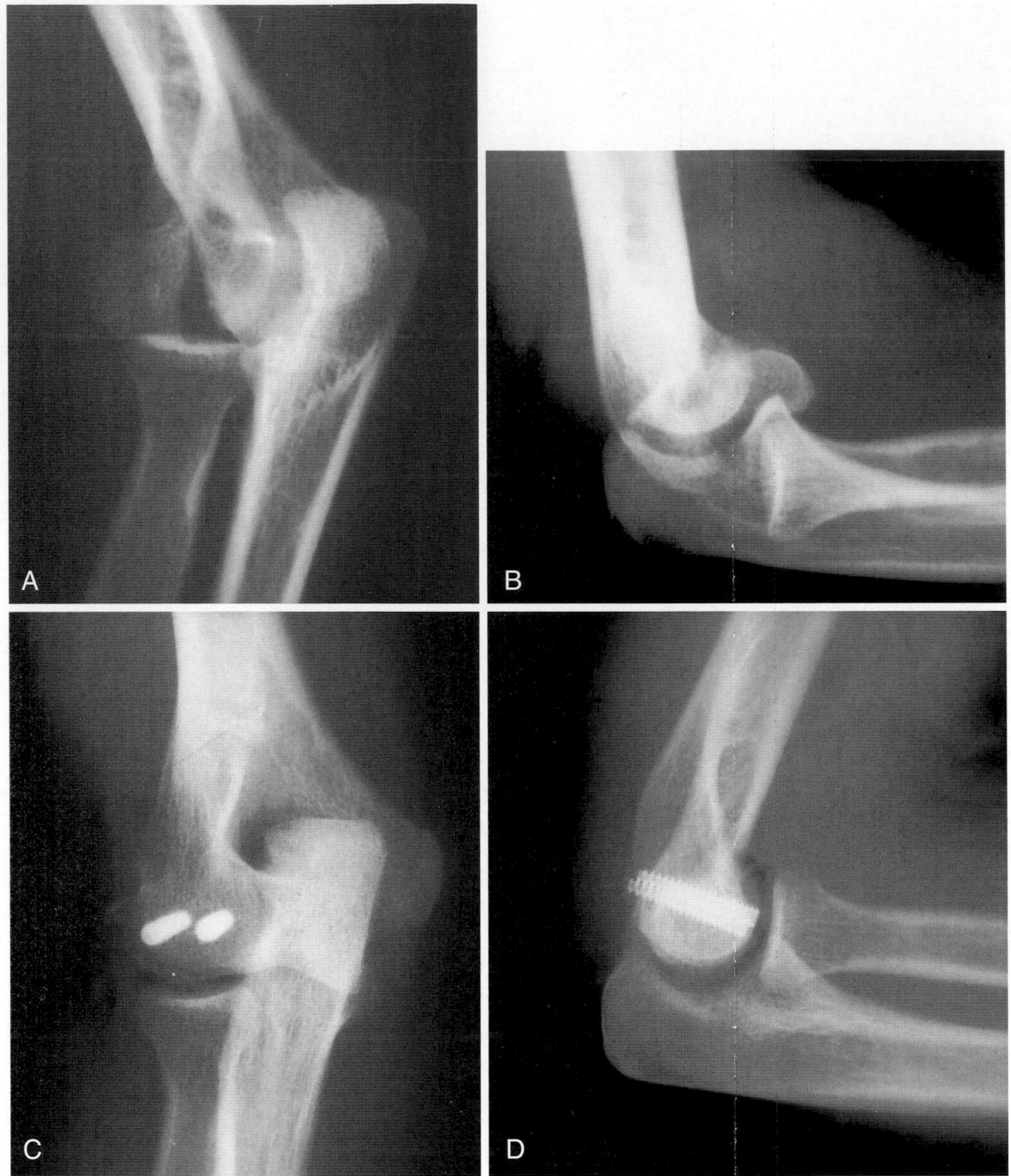

FIGURE 36-41 A and B, Capitellar fracture in an adolescent. C and D, After reduction and fixation with cannulated screws.

distal fragment. Missed untreated fractures may remodel completely without any residual deformity if the distal fragment is only medially translocated and not tilted.

CAPITELLAR FRACTURES

Fractures of the capitellum involve only the true articular surface of the lateral condyle, including in some instances the articular surface of the lateral crista of the trochlea. Generally, this fragment comes from the anterior portion of the distal articular surface that is sheared off by the radial head. Unlike in adults, these fractures are rare in children and usually occur in adolescents.

Excision of the fragment and open reduction and reattachment are the two most common forms of treatment. However, because of the intraarticular nature of the injury, closed reduction is not likely to be successful. Many small fragments can be excised through either a lateral open or arthroscopic approach. This eliminates the need for postoperative immobilization and accompanying elbow stiffness. Open reduction and internal fixation can be performed if the fragments are large enough; however, osteonecrosis of the attached fragment can occur. Compression screws have been shown to provide stable fixation (Fig. 36-41). Alternatively, a suture repair can be performed, which allows for follow-up MRI examination and eliminates the need for implant removal. Regardless of the treatment method used, patients and parents should be counseled that elbow motion will be lost after this injury.

OLECRANON FRACTURES

Isolated physeal fracture of the olecranon in children is uncommon due in part to the broad-based insertion of the triceps. When it does occur, it typically is the result of an avulsion force being applied to the olecranon with the

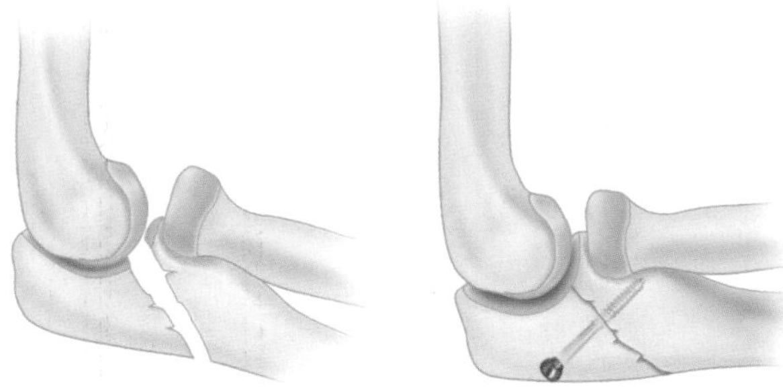

FIGURE 36-42 Metaphyseal intraarticular olecranon fracture that is unstable and requires open reduction and internal fixation, here with oblique screw.

elbow flexed. Although rare in the general population, these fractures, especially bilateral ones, are well described in children with osteogenesis imperfecta in whom refracture also is common. Apophyseal stress injuries can occur in high-level athletes, especially gymnasts and throwing athletes, and if left untreated can result in a painful nonunion. The most common fractures of the olecranon are metaphyseal, either isolated or associated with other elbow injuries. The peak age is 5 to 10 years, and olecranon fractures account for approximately 5% of pediatric elbow fractures. Isolated olecranon fractures are classified by the mechanism of injury: flexion, extension, or shear. Isolated flexion fractures most commonly occur in a fall directly onto a flexed elbow. A fall onto a hyperextended elbow is the usual mechanism of injury in supracondylar humeral fractures; however, if there is a significant varus or valgus stress applied simultaneously, a metaphyseal olecranon fracture can occur. Shear injuries, which typically produce an oblique fracture line, are rare and can occur either in flexion or extension. Associated fractures occur in 50% to 75% of children with an olecranon fracture, the most common being a proximal radial fracture and type I Monteggia injury.

Treatment for stress fractures includes time away from the causative activity followed by gradual resumption of activity. Cannulated screw fixation is used for patients with symptomatic delayed unions or nonunions. Most olecranon fractures are nondisplaced and can be treated for 3 to 4 weeks in a long arm cast with the elbow in 70 to 80 degrees of flexion. Late displacement can occur, so these fractures need to be monitored carefully. For fractures that are displaced or that had an unsatisfactory closed reduction, open reduction and internal fixation is indicated. A variety of fixation techniques, such as percutaneous pinning, tension banding, and screw and plate fixation, have been described with good outcomes (Fig. 36-42). Tension banding using bioabsorbable suture can be used in younger, smaller children to eliminate the need for implant removal. These techniques are discussed in Chapter 57. Elbow stiffness is a common complication after olecranon fracture in children, and stable fixation is essential to start early range of motion to prevent this.

RADIAL HEAD AND NECK FRACTURES

Isolated radial head fractures in children are rare because the immature radial head is cartilaginous. When they do occur, they usually are Salter-Harris type IV injuries in children 10 to 12 years of age. Patients with true radial head fractures are at increased risk of progressive radial head subluxation, osteonecrosis, and radiocapitellar arthrosis and need to be followed over the long term. Most children sustain fractures of the radial neck, which account for approximately 1% of all children's fractures and 5% of pediatric elbow fractures.

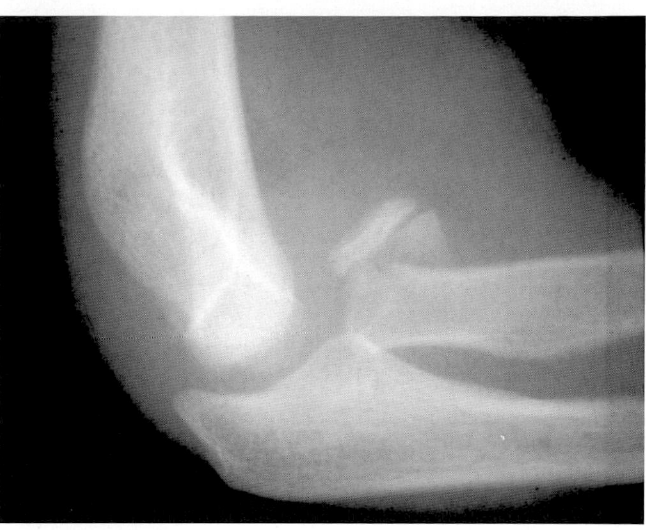

FIGURE 36-43 Displaced Salter-Harris type II fracture of the radial head and neck.

The majority of radial neck injuries occur during a fall onto an outstretched upper extremity with the elbow in a valgus position. They typically occur in the metaphysis but can extend into the proximal radial physis producing a Salter-Harris type II pattern (Fig. 36-43). Many of these fractures are angulated, with the most common direction being lateral, followed by anterior, then posterior. Radial neck fractures also can occur in conjunction with an elbow dislocation, either at the time of dislocation or during reduction (Fig. 36-44). The fracture may be completely displaced or intraarticular and may block reduction. For this reason the radial neck must be thoroughly evaluated before and after reduction of a pediatric elbow dislocation.

Making the diagnosis, especially in young children, can be difficult because of the unossified radial head. In these patients the only sign of a fracture may be a small metaphyseal fragment. A radiocapitellar view can be helpful in making the diagnosis.

Due to the remodeling potential of the proximal radius, fractures with less than 30 degrees of angulation can be treated nonoperatively as long as there is no loss of forearm rotation. Patients are placed in a long arm cast for 3 weeks and then allowed to resume range-of-motion exercises. Patients with displaced, significantly angulated or displaced fractures require reduction. This consists of a step-wise approach starting with closed reduction, progressing to percutaneous-assisted reduction, and finally open reduction and internal fixation if satisfactory reduction cannot be obtained. Because there is great potential for elbow stiffness after open reduction and internal fixation, a closed reduction with slight malalignment is preferable to an open reduction and internal fixation with anatomic alignment. The loss

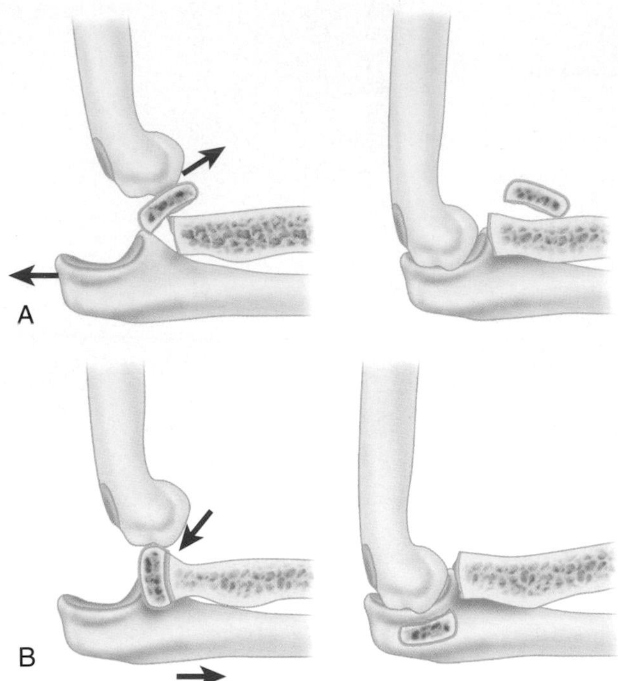

FIGURE 36-44 **A,** Fracture occurring when elbow dislocation is reduced. **B,** Fractures occurring at time of elbow dislocation.

of motion in patients with open treatment may reflect selection of most displaced fractures for open reduction and internal fixation.

Closed reduction can be performed using a variety of techniques based on the direction of displacement of the radial neck. One very useful technique is that described by Patterson. With the use of general anesthesia if needed and fluoroscopy (image intensification), an assistant stabilizes the radius distal to the fractured radial neck. With the elbow in extension and forearm rotated in the position of maximal tilt, the surgeon applies a varus stress with one hand on the elbow and lateral pressure directly over the radial head with the thumb of the other hand (Fig. 36-45). Other reduction techniques have been described with the elbow in flexion. In addition, the wrapping of the arm with an Esmarch bandage has been shown to occasionally improve fracture reduction, and this maneuver should be attempted with all radial neck reduction techniques.

A percutaneous-assisted technique is used when closed techniques have failed. The most commonly used technique involves the percutaneous manipulation of the fracture with a Kirschner wire. The wire is cut, and the blunt end is used to reduce the radial neck and head to the shaft (Fig. 36-46). The reduced radial neck can be stabilized by percutaneous pinning (Fig. 36-47). Alternatively a flexible intramedullary nail can be introduced retrograde from the distal radius using the technique described by Metaizeau. Using this technique, a flexible intramedullary nail is passed retrograde from the radial metaphysis proximally to the fracture site. Once engaged in the proximal fragment, the nail is rotated until the optimal reduction is obtained (Fig. 36-48). The fracture is then stabilized with the nail until healing has occurred.

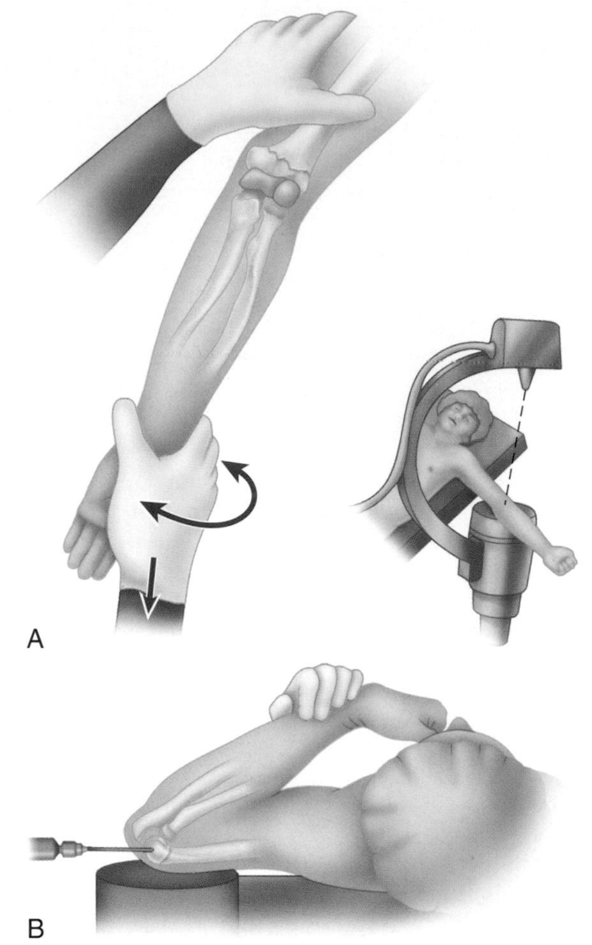

FIGURE 36-45 **A,** Rotational deformity and displacement evaluated with image intensification; anatomic correction of these deformities must be obtained before elbow is fixed. **B,** Accurate position of pins ensured by image intensification during procedure.

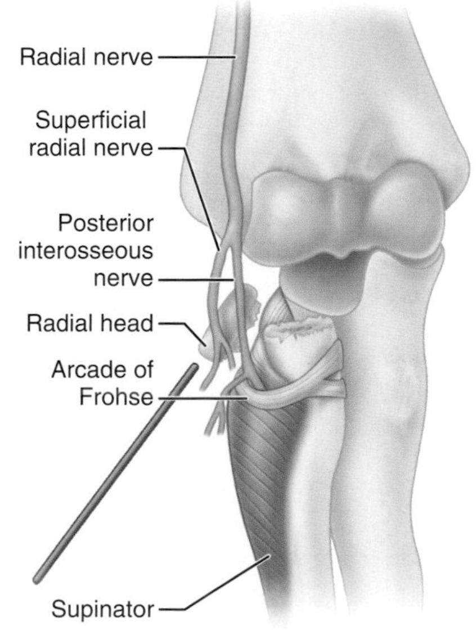

FIGURE 36-46 Radial neck fracture in relation to arcade of Frohse. During percutaneous reduction, wire should be introduced on ulnar side of radius to avoid deep branch of radial nerve.

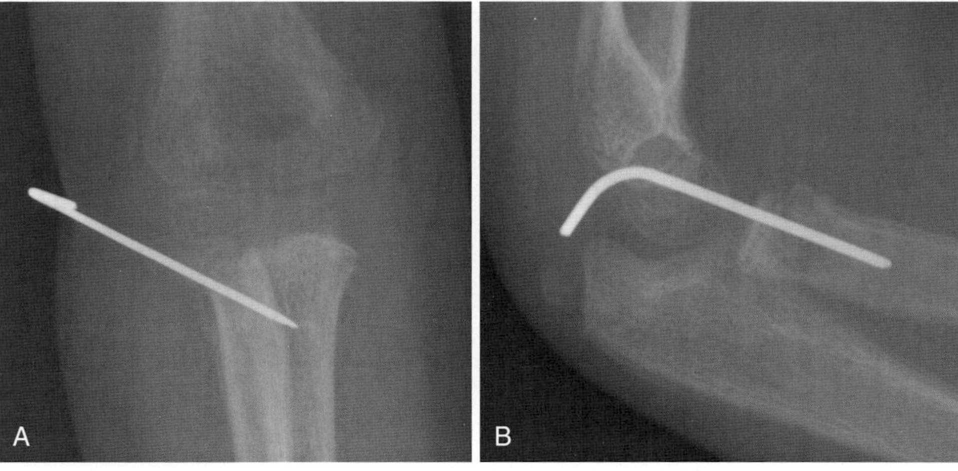

FIGURE 36-47 A and B, Anteroposterior and lateral view of radial neck pin.

In open reduction and internal fixation, most surgeons use smooth pin fixation in younger children and rigid fixation in the form of screws or plates in older children or adolescents (Fig. 36-49). Early rigid fixation allows early motion. This should be done through a lateral approach with the forearm in supination to protect the posterior interosseous nerve. Impediments to reduction such as capsular flaps or the annular ligament should be removed or repaired. Screws and plates should be placed in the "safe zone," which is the 100 degrees of circumference of the radial head that does not articulate with the proximal ulna. These techniques are described in Chapter 57.

CLOSED AND OPEN REDUCTION OF RADIAL NECK FRACTURES

TECHNIQUE 36-11

- After administering general anesthesia, place the patient supine.
- Use the manipulative technique as described by Patterson. Have an assistant hold the arm proximally, with one hand placed medially against the distal humerus, and apply straight longitudinal distal traction. Apply a varus force to the forearm and digital pressure directly over the tilted radial head to complete the reduction (Fig. 36-50). Hold the forearm in 90 degrees of flexion and in pronation. If this manipulation reduction is unsuccessful, have the assistant hold the arm with the shoulder abducted to 90 degrees and the forearm held in supination. With the use of an image intensifier and in a sterile operating field, introduce a Kirschner wire through the skin on the radial side of the elbow down to the angulated and displaced radial head and neck. Disimpact and push the radial head into anatomic position with the Kirschner wire. Remove the wire and flex the elbow to 90 degrees. The fracture can be pinned percutaneously from lateral to medial taking care to protect the posterior interosseous nerve (see Fig. 36-48).

PERCUTANEOUS REDUCTION AND PINNING

TECHNIQUE 36-12

- With the patient under general anesthesia, prepare and drape the upper limb.
- With fluoroscopy in the anteroposterior projection (Fig. 36-51A), determine the forearm rotation that exposes the maximal amount of deformity of the fracture and mark the level of the bicipital tuberosity of the proximal radius.
- Make a 1-cm dorsal skin incision at the marked level just lateral to the subcutaneous border of the ulna.
- Gently insert a periosteal elevator between the ulna and the radius, taking care not to disrupt the periosteum of the radius or ulna (Fig. 36-51B). The radial shaft usually is much more ulnarly displaced than expected, and the radial nerve is lateral to the radius at this level.
- While counter-pressure is applied against the radial head, lever the distal fragment away from the ulna (Fig. 36-51C). An assistant can aid in this maneuver by gently applying traction and rotating the forearm back and forth to disimpact the fracture fragments.
- If necessary to correct angulation, insert a percutaneous Kirschner wire into the fracture site, parallel to the radial head, and use it to lever the epiphysis perpendicular to the radial axis (Fig. 36-51D).
- Once adequate reduction has been obtained, insert an oblique Kirschner wire to provide fracture fixation.

POSTOPERATIVE CARE. A posterior splint or bivalved cast is applied and worn for 3 to 4 weeks, and the Kirschner wire is removed once fracture callus is present.

If these maneuvers are unsuccessful, reduction can be attempted using a retrograde flexible intramedullary nail.

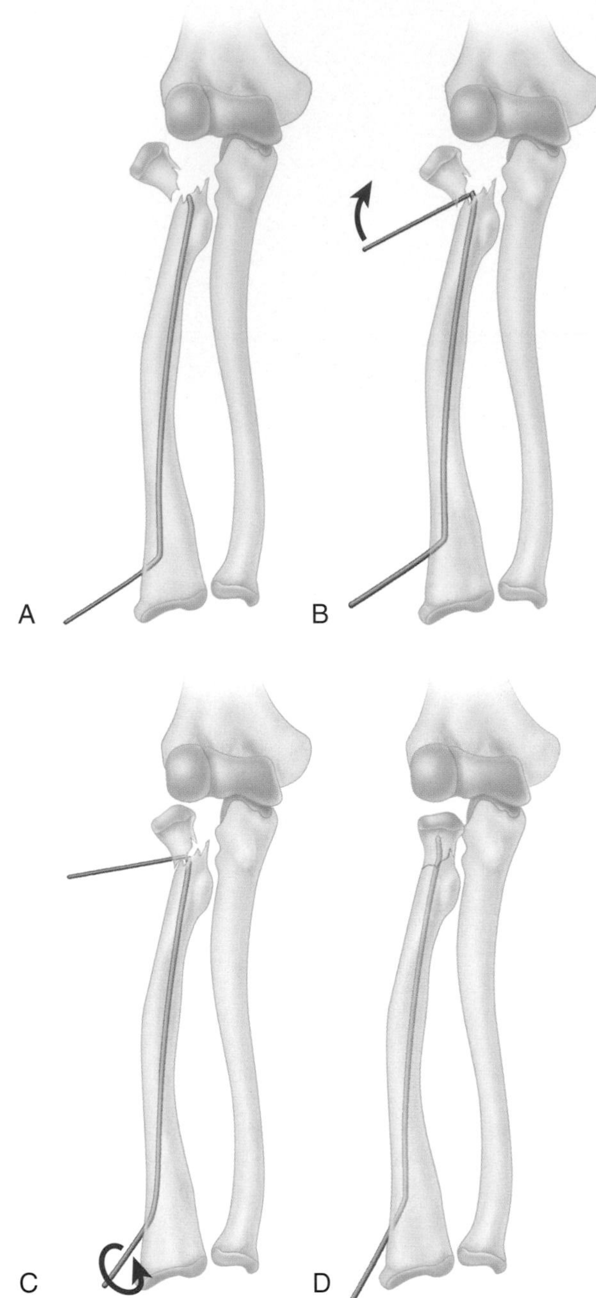

FIGURE 36-48 **A** to **D**, Reduction of radial head by leverage method and retrograde intramedullary pinning with Kirschner wire. Note slightly bent tip first pointing laterally. After it is placed in radial head, it is rotated 180 degrees along its axis. (Redrawn from Stiefel D, Meuli M, Altermatt S: Fractures of the neck of the radius in children: early experience with intramedullary pinning, J Bone Joint Surg 83B:536, 2001. Copyright British Editorial Society of Bone and Joint Surgery.) **SEE TECHNIQUE 36-11.**

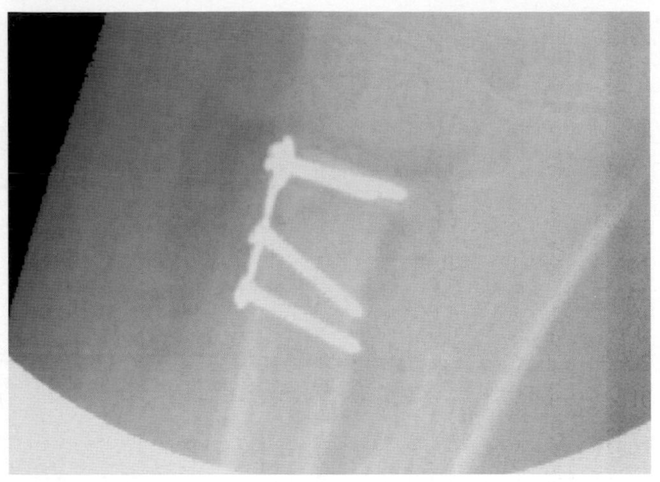

FIGURE 36-49 Open reduction and internal fixation of radial neck fracture.

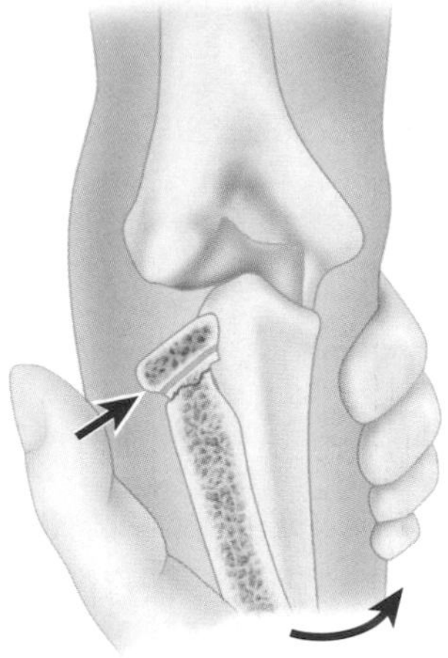

FIGURE 36-50 Mechanism of reduction of radial neck fracture. **SEE TECHNIQUE 36-11.**

CLOSED INTRAMEDULLARY NAILING

TECHNIQUE 36-13

- With the patient under general anesthesia, prepare and drape the upper limb.
- Expose the radial aspect of the distal radial metaphysis through a short radial incision 1 cm proximal to the radial physis, avoiding injury to the cutaneous branch of the radial nerve.
- Drill the cortex, starting perpendicular to the radius and then in a more proximal direction.
- Introduce the nail into the medullary canal. Advance the wire using gentle taps of the mallet to avoid perforation of the ulnar cortex of the distal radius.
- If a lateral displacement of the distal fragment remains, rotate the nail 180 degrees around its long axis so that its

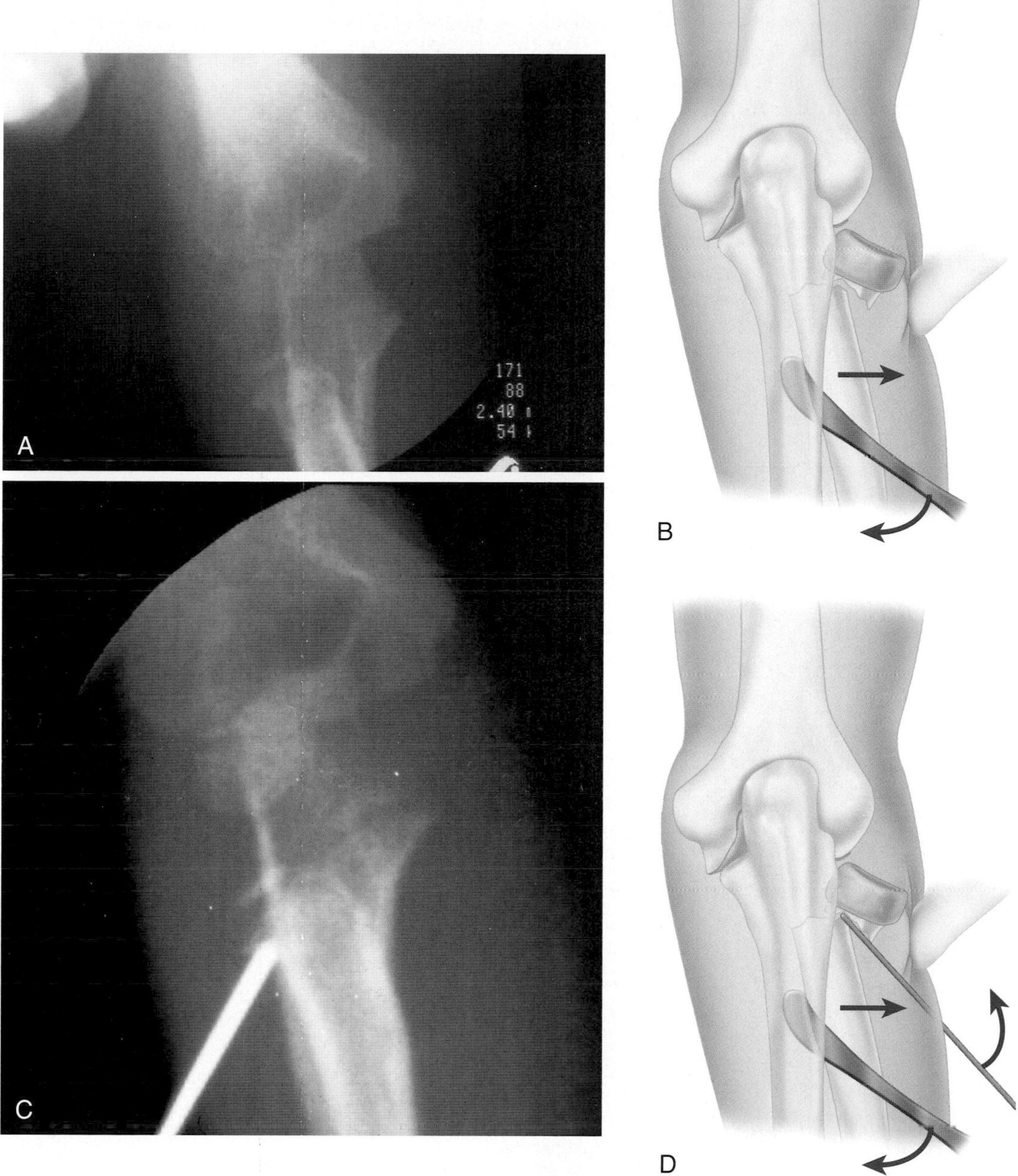

FIGURE 36-51 Wallace radial head reduction technique. **A,** Dislocated radial head fracture. **B,** Periosteal elevator is used to lever the distal fragment laterally while the thumb pushes the proximal fragment medially. **C** and **D,** Kirschner wires are used to assist the reduction if necessary. (**B** and **D**, redrawn from Erickson M, Frick S: Fractures of the proximal radius and ulna. In Beaty JH, Kasser JR, editors: Rockwood and Wilkins' fractures in children, 7th ed, Philadelphia, Wolters Kluwer, 2010.) **SEE TECHNIQUE 36-12.**

point faces inward. This produces a medial shift of the radial head and reduces it. The tension produced in the lateral intact periosteum prevents overcorrection medially.

- Cut the lower metaphyseal end of the pin and close the skin.
- When the epiphysis is impossible to reach, tilting of more than 80 degrees by external manipulation or by percutaneous pinning makes it possible to obtain at least a partial reduction, which is maintained with an intramedullary nail.

POSTOPERATIVE CARE. The arm is immobilized in a long arm cast for 2 to 3 weeks. The Kirschner wire is removed in 3 to 4 weeks once callus is present on radiographs.

COMPLICATIONS AFTER RADIAL NECK FRACTURE

Complications of treatment include loss of motion, which is most common in pronation and supination rather than flexion and extension. Malunion and nonunion can occur; however, this is rare. Patients with asymptomatic nonunions can be observed (Fig. 36-52). Radial head excision is reserved for a very select, small group of salvage cases.

CORONOID FRACTURES

Regan and Morrey classified fractures of the coronoid process as type I, a small chip fracture; type II, a fracture involving less than 50% of the process; and type III, a fracture involving more than 50% of the process (Fig. 36-53). They recommended closed treatment for types I and II fractures and open reduction and internal fixation for type III fractures if possible. Operative treatment of these injuries is more common in adolescent and adult patients. This is described in Chapter 57.

ELBOW DISLOCATIONS

Acute elbow dislocation in children is rare, accounting for approximately 5% of all children's elbow injuries. The most common type is posterior but, as in adults, dislocations can be anterior, medial, or lateral. In rare cases a proximal radioulnar joint disruption can occur (Fig 36-54). Elbow dislocations often occur in conjunction with fractures of the medial epicondyle and radial neck.

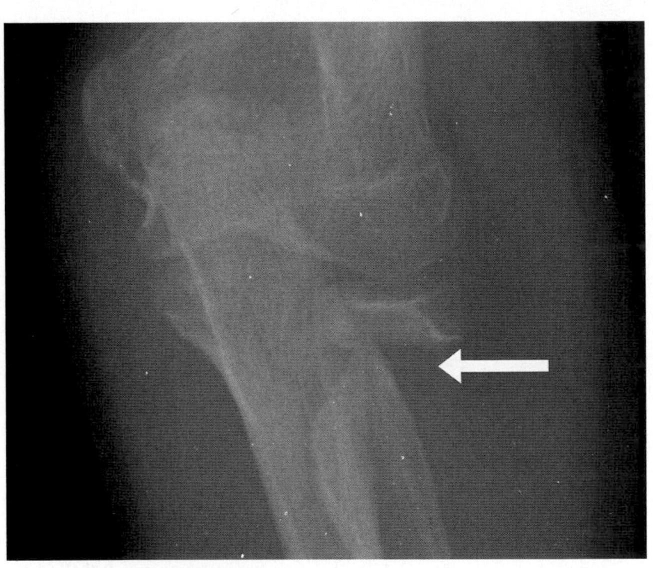

FIGURE 36-52 Radial neck nonunion.

Most patients can be treated with closed reduction, a brief period of immobilization, followed by progressive protected range of motion in a splint or brace to prevent redislocation. Indications for operative treatment include entrapped intraarticular fragments (medial epicondyle, radial neck), open fracture, or associated elbow injury that will require open reduction and internal fixation.

COMPLICATIONS AFTER ELBOW DISLOCATION

The most common complication is elbow stiffness and loss of motion, especially extension. Other rare complications include redislocation, myositis ossificans after open fractures, and neurovascular injuries. It is essential to perform a thorough neurovascular examination before and after closed or open reduction to ensure that nerve or vessel entrapment did not occur at the time of reduction.

RADIAL HEAD DISLOCATIONS (MONTEGGIA FRACTURE-DISLOCATIONS)

Monteggia fractures are relatively rare, accounting for less than 1% of all pediatric elbow dislocations, with a peak age of 4 to 10 years. Although rare, they receive considerable interest because they are often missed, resulting in poor outcomes. Radial nerve injury has been reported to occur in 10% to 20% of patients, especially those with anterior and lateral dislocations because of the proximity of the radial head to the posterior interosseous nerve.

The diagnosis of Monteggia fracture can be made with standard anteroposterior and lateral radiographs of the elbow, and it is essential that the elbow be viewed in both planes for all patients with forearm fractures. A line drawn through the center of the radial neck should extend through the central portion of the capitellum regardless of elbow position (Fig. 36-55). In rare instances when radiographs are equivocal, advanced imaging, such as CT, MRI, or ultrasound, should be used. The absence of trauma and changes such as a hypoplastic capitellum and a flattened convex radial head (Fig. 36-56) should raise suspicion for a congenital radial head dislocation, which often is bilateral.

The most commonly used classification system is that of Bado, which is based on the direction of radial head

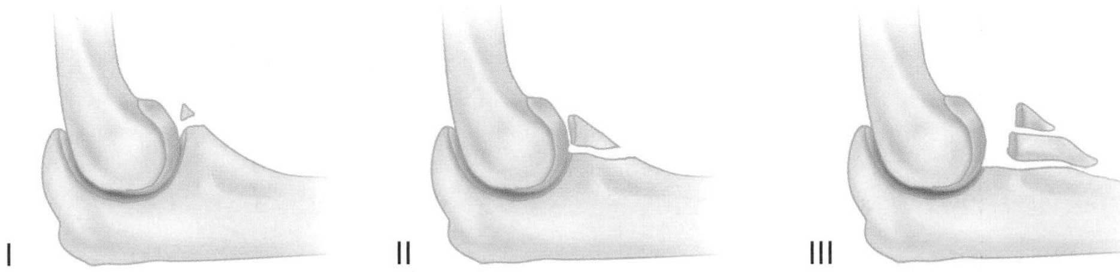

FIGURE 36-53 Classification of coronoid fractures. Type I, small fragment avulsion. Type II, involvement of less than 50% of coronoid process. Type III, involvement of more than 50% of coronoid process.

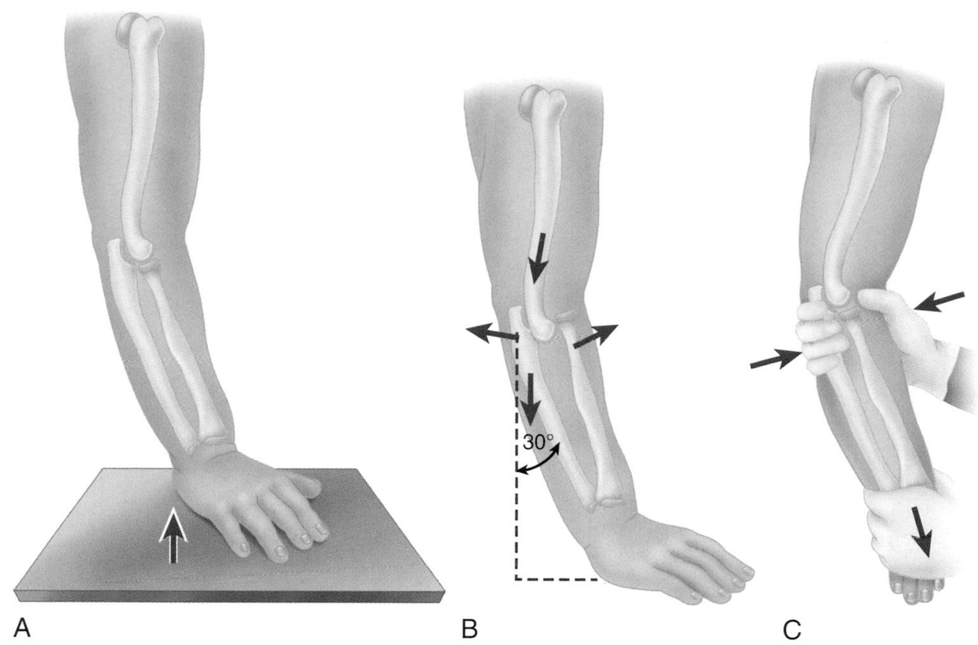

FIGURE 36-54 **A** and **B,** Mechanism of injury in a fall on outstretched hand with elbow in approximately 30 degrees of flexion. There is separation of all three articulations, with humerus acting as wedge between proximal radius and ulna **(B)**. **C,** Mechanism of reduction aims to reverse deforming forces with longitudinal traction and compression of radius and ulna together. (Redrawn from Altuntas AO, Balakumar J, Howells RJ, et al: Posterior divergent dislocation of the elbow in children and adolescents: a report of three cases and review of the literature, J Pediatr Orthop 25:317, 2005.)

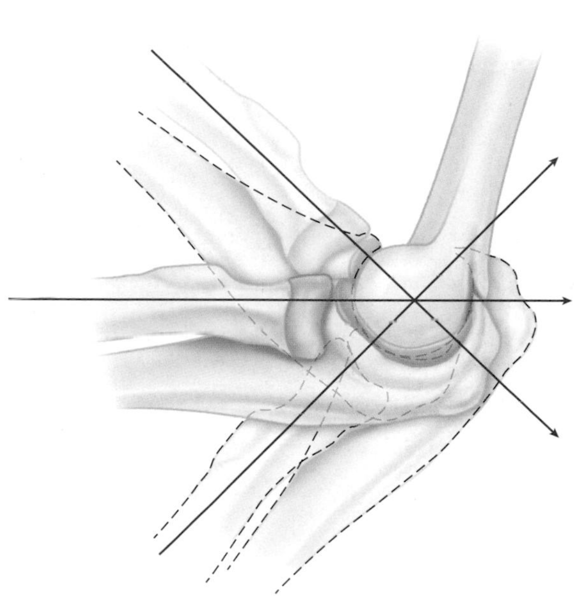

FIGURE 36-55 On the lateral radiograph, the axis of the radial head should bisect the center of the capitellum on all views, regardless of the amount of elbow flexion.

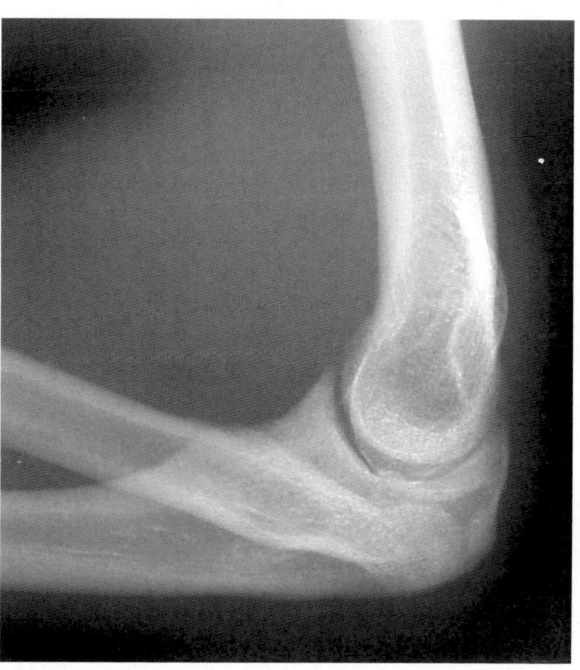

FIGURE 36-56 Congenital radial head dislocation. Note convexity of the radial head indicative of congenital rather than traumatic radial head dislocation.

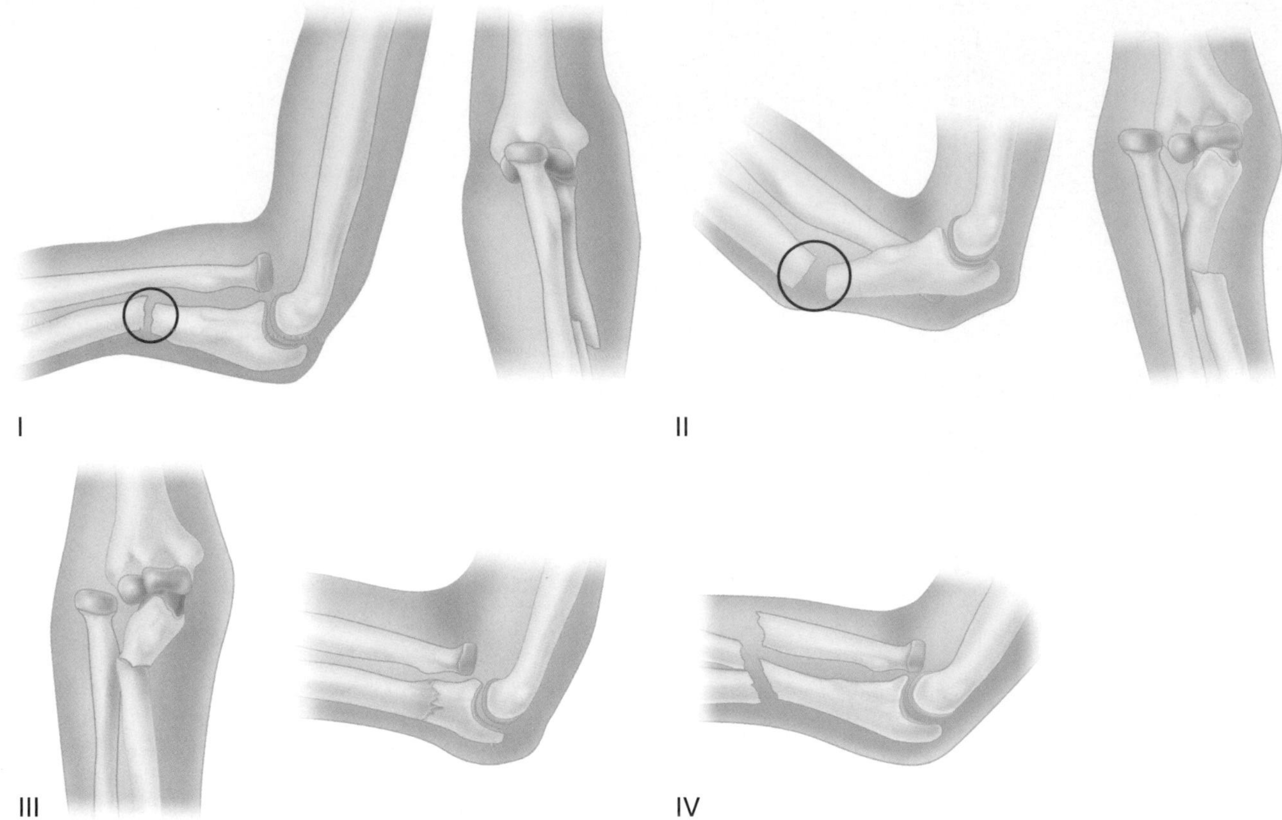

FIGURE 36-57 Types of Monteggia fractures. Type I with anterior dislocation of radial head and anterior angulation of ulnar fracture. Type II with posterior dislocation of radial head and posterior angulation of ulnar fracture. Type III with lateral dislocation of radial head and lateral angulation of ulnar fracture. Rare type IV with fractures of radial and ulnar shafts and dislocation of radial head.

dislocation (Fig. 36-57). The most common is a fracture of the proximal third of the ulna, anterior angulation of the fracture, and anterior dislocation of the radial head (type I). The second most common is a fracture of the proximal ulna, posterior angulation of the fracture, and posterior dislocation of the radial head (type II). Lateral angulation of a proximal ulnar fracture may result in a third type with lateral dislocation of the radial head (type III), and a rare fourth type may occur with a proximal both-bone fracture and anterior dislocation of the radial head (type IV) (Fig. 36-58). Although it is descriptive and straight forward, the Bado classification is not prognostic. Classification systems by Letts and Ring, based on the pattern of ulnar injury, may be more prognostic in terms of outcome given the fact that successful reduction of the ulna typically provides stability to the radiocapitellar joint (Box 36-3). In addition, there have been numerous reports of "Monteggia equivalents," including the three most common: (1) isolated radial head dislocation (see "Isolated Dislocations of Radial Head") (Fig. 36-59), (2) fracture of the proximal ulna with fracture of the radial neck, and (3) both-bone proximal third fractures with the radial fracture more proximal than the ulnar fracture (Fig. 36-60).

An isolated radial head dislocation is very rare (see Fig. 36-59). This is because many children thought to have an isolated radial head fracture have subtle plastic deformation of the ulna, which when corrected leads to stable radial head reduction (Fig. 36-61). This must be differentiated from

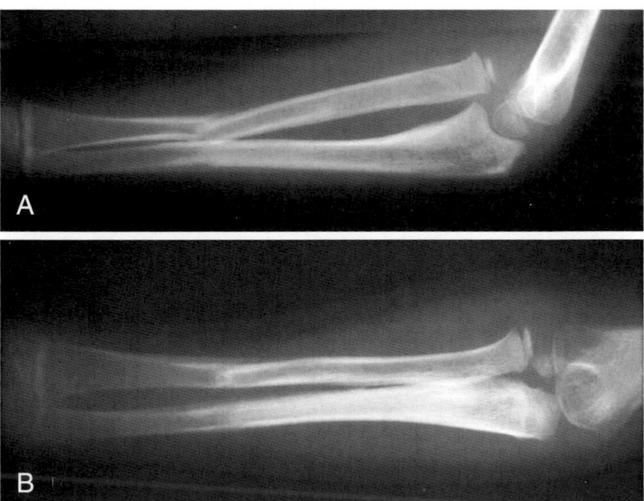

FIGURE 36-58 Type IV Monteggia fracture with fractures of radial and ulnar shafts and dislocation of radial head.

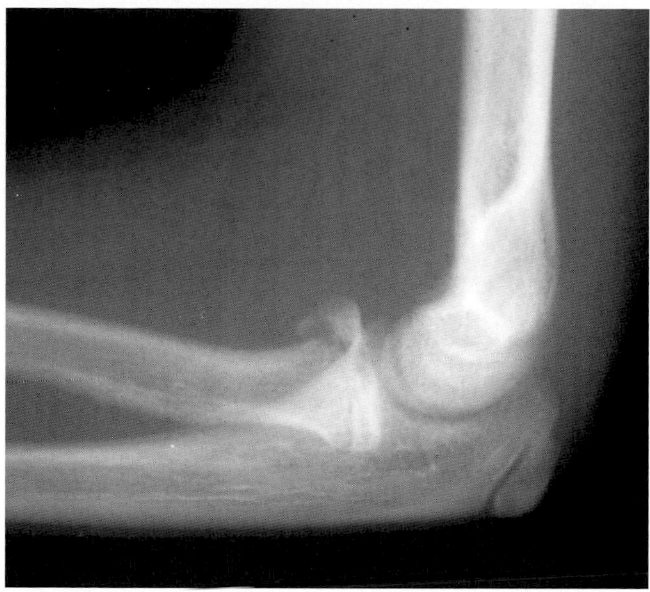

FIGURE 36-59 Fracture of the anterior third of the radial head with subsequent dislocation.

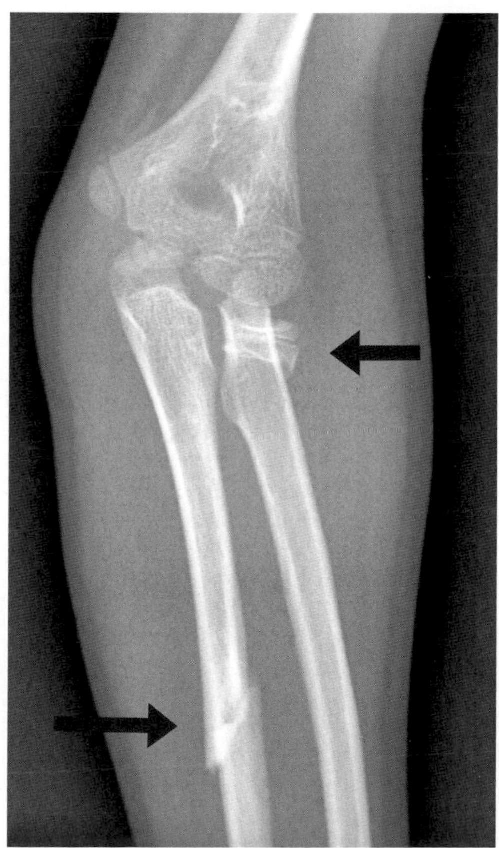

FIGURE 36-60 Monteggia variant: both-bone proximal-third fractures with radial fracture more proximal than ulnar fracture.

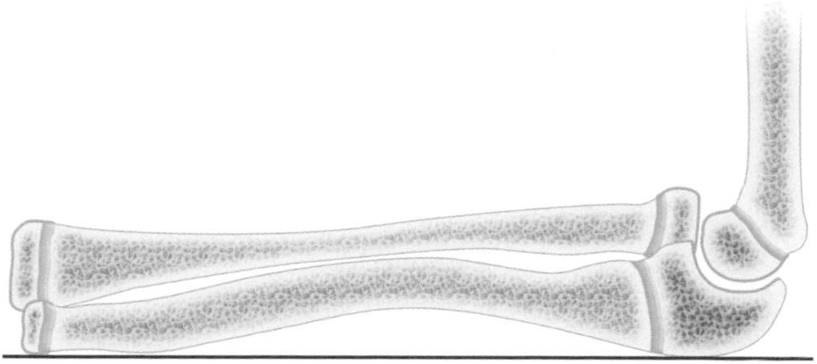

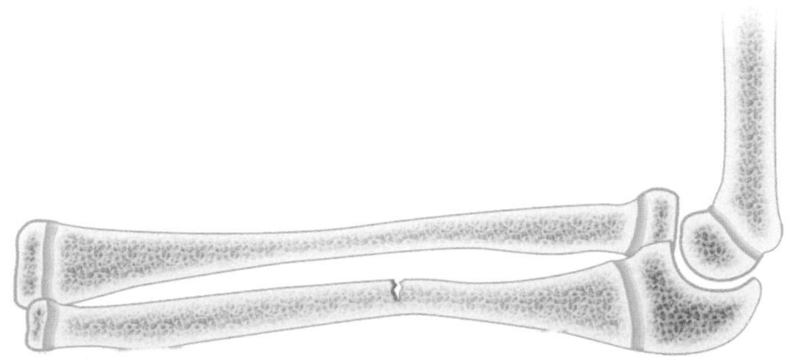

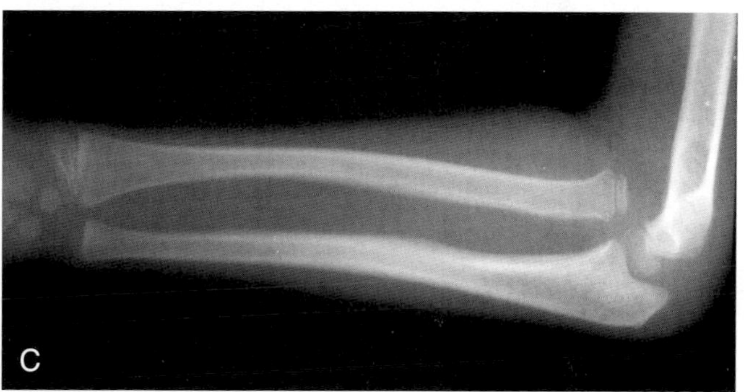

FIGURE 36-61 Plastic deformation of the ulna. **A,** Anterior bend. **B,** Anterior greenstick. **C,** Radiographic appearance.

BOX 36-3

Classification of Monteggia Fracture-Dislocations in Children According to Ulnar Injury

TYPE OF ULNAR INJURY	TREATMENT
Plastic deformation	Closed reduction of the ulnar bow and cast immobilization
Incomplete (greenstick or buckle) fracture	Closed reduction and cast immobilization
Complete transverse or short oblique fracture	Closed reduction and intramedullary Kirschner wire fixation
Long oblique or comminuted fracture	Open reduction and internal fixation with plate and screws

Modified from Ring D, Jupiter JB, Waters PM: Monteggia fractures in children, *J Am Acad Orthop Surg* 6:215, 1998.

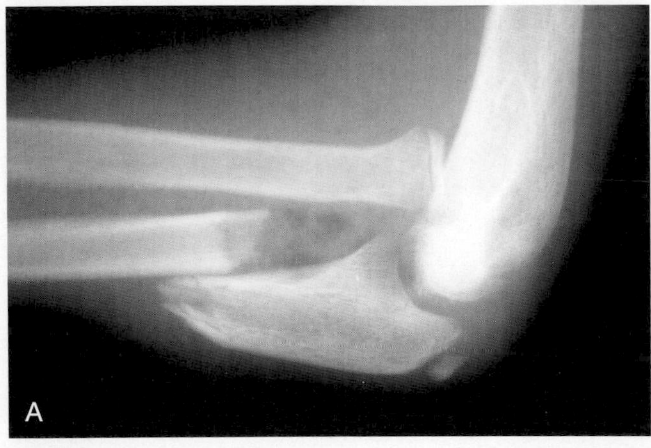

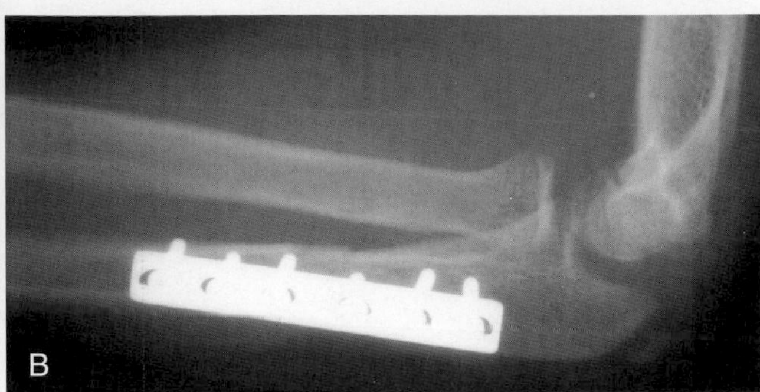

FIGURE 36-62 **A,** Monteggia fracture. **B,** After open reduction and plate fixation.

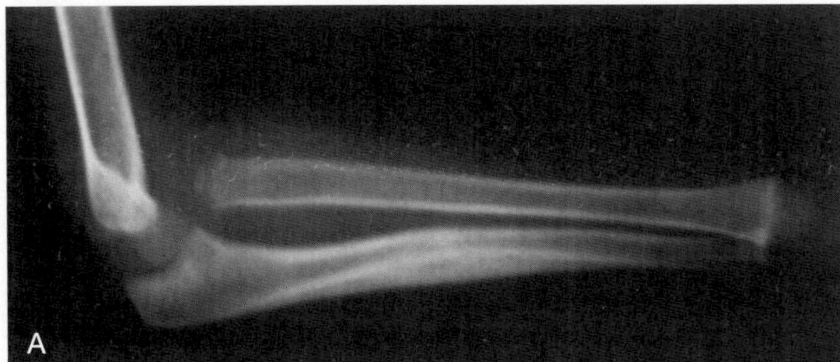

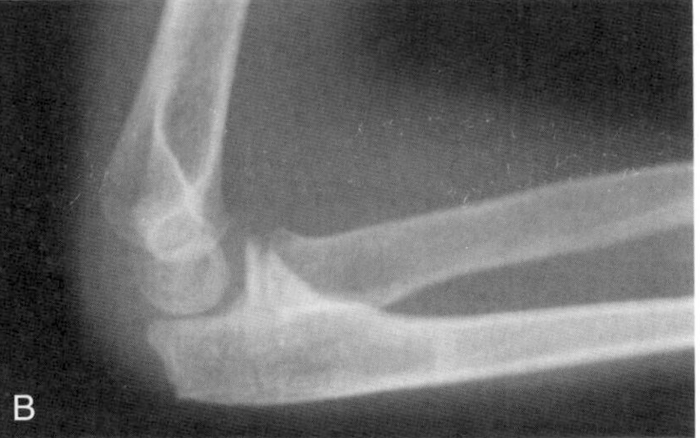

FIGURE 36-63 Malunion of ulna and anterior dislocation of radial head. **A,** Before treatment. **B,** At 3 years after surgery, showing maintenance of radial head reduction.

nursemaid's elbow in which the radiographs are completely normal.

Successful treatment of a Monteggia fracture is dependent on correcting and stabilizing the ulnar deformity, which in turn provides stability for the radiocapitellar joint. Closed reduction and cast treatment is indicated for patients with either stable or greenstick fractures of the ulna, as well as those with plastic deformation of the ulna and satisfactory reduction of the radial head. Patients should be immobilized in a long arm cast in 90 to 100 degrees of flexion and supination and followed closely radiographically for 2 to 3 weeks to ensure maintenance of radial head reduction. Operative stabilization of the ulna is necessary with either an intramedullary nail for transverse or short oblique fractures or a plate for long oblique or comminuted fracture to provide ulnar length stability (Fig. 36-62). Open reduction of the radial head combined with annular ligament reconstruction is indicated for patients with irreducible radial head dislocations caused by interposition of the annular ligament. Patients need to be followed closely postoperatively for redislocation of the radial head. Pinning of the radiocapitellar joint should be avoided when possible to prevent intraarticular pin breakage. A radiocapitellar joint unstable enough to require pinning should raise the suspicion of inadequate ulnar reduction or entrapped soft tissue.

Controversy exists as to when an acute Monteggia fracture becomes chronic. Some patients are asymptomatic while others complain of pain, decreased range of motion, or deformity. Many authors believe that, although treatment of chronic Monteggia fractures is difficult and the results unpredictable, it is better than the natural history of untreated fractures (Fig. 36-63). Generally, operative treatment is more successful in symptomatic younger patients without radial head deformity. Principles of surgical reconstruction include correction of the ulnar deformity with an ulnar osteotomy and annular ligament reconstruction. The ulnar osteotomy should be stabilized in the position of maximal stability of the radiocapitellar joint, which often creates a secondary ulnar deformity that is clinically insignificant (Fig. 36-64, Technique 36-14). Most authors recommend reconstruction of the annular ligament, either with the native ligament itself or a strip of triceps tendon or fascia as advocated by Boyd, Lloyd-Roberts, and Bell-Tawse (Fig. 36-65). Radial head resection should be avoided in younger patients because of the risk of late deformity and should only be used as a salvage procedure.

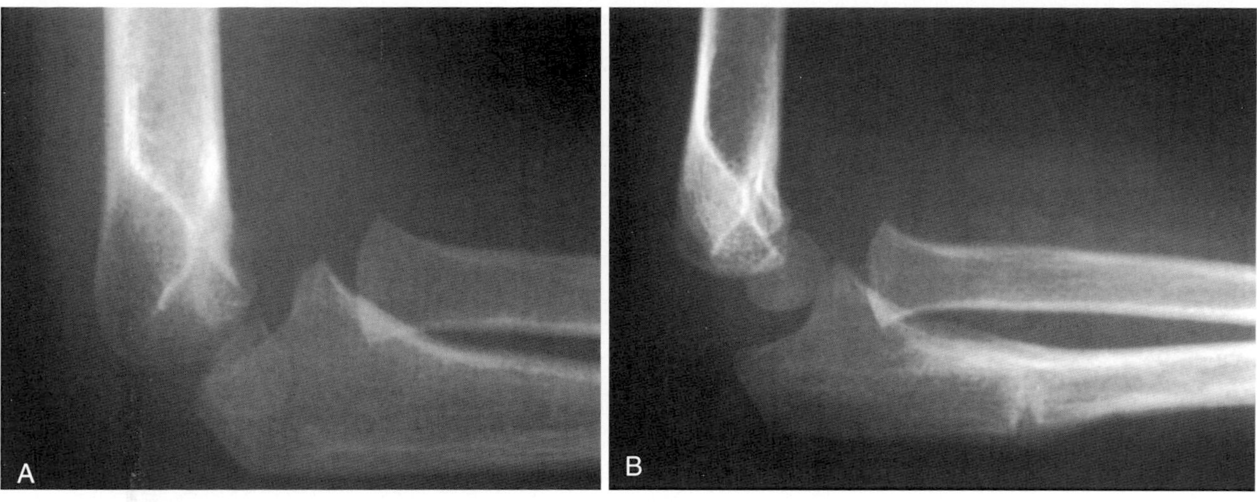

FIGURE 36-64 **A**, Deformity after Monteggia fracture. **B**, After overcorrection osteotomy (see text).

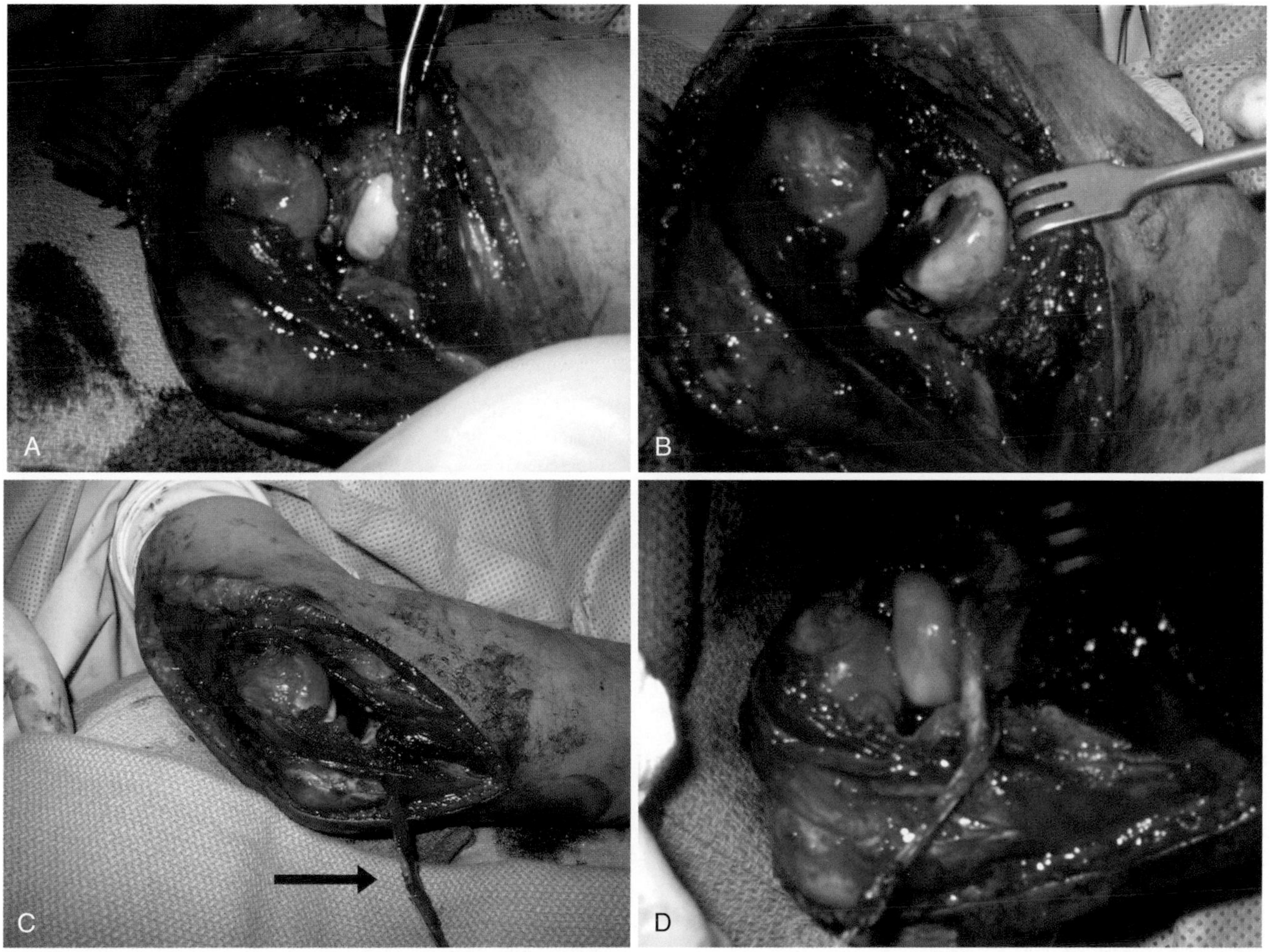

FIGURE 36-65 Lateral approach to the elbow shows incongruent radiocapitellar joint (**A**) and changes in radial head morphology (**B**). The triceps fascia has been harvested (**C**) and is used to reconstruct the annular ligament (**D**).

OVERCORRECTION OSTEOTOMY AND LIGAMENTOUS REPAIR OR RECONSTRUCTION

TECHNIQUE 36-14 *Figure 36-66*

(SHAH AND WATERS)

- Make a curvilinear incision to allow for possible triceps tendon harvesting and to perform an ulnar opening wedge osteotomy (Fig. 36-66B). Initially, open only the proximal portion.
- Identify the radial nerve between the brachialis and brachioradialis in the distal humerus. Dissect the nerve distal to its motor (posterior interosseous nerve) and sensory branches.
- Mobilize and protect the nerves throughout the remainder of the procedure.
- Expose the joint through the anconeus–extensor carpi ulnaris interval. Carry the dissection proximal and elevate the extensor-supinator mass and capsule as a single tissue plane off the distal humerus (Fig. 36-66C).
- Debride the elbow joint of synovitis and pulvinar. Pay particular attention to the proximal radioulnar joint so that it will fit anatomically into place.
- At this point, it must be determined if the native annular ligament can be used for reconstruction. Identify the central perforation in the capsular wall that separates the dislocated radial head from the joint. This is the site of opening of the original ligament. Extend the incision from the center outward to enlarge this opening. This will allow the native annular ligament to be reduced over the radial neck (Fig. 36-66D).
- Remove capsular adhesions from the radial head for reduction back into the joint. Reattach the native ligament to the ulna using the large periosteal sleeve.
- If the native ligament cannot be used, prepare to harvest the triceps fascia for ligament reconstruction.
- Attempt radial head reduction, carefully scrutinizing congruity between the radial head and capitellum. If satisfactory, proceed with ligamentous repair or reconstruction. If the radius cannot be reduced, perform an ulnar osteotomy at the site of maximal deformity, which will involve a more distal ulnar exposure (Fig. 36-66E).
- Perform periosteal dissection under fluoroscopic guidance.
- Make an opening wedge osteotomy using a laminar spreader to allow the radial head to align with the capitellum without pressure. The goal is partial overcorrection of the ulnar alignment. Alternatively, temporary anatomic pinning of the radiocapitellar joint can be done to allow opening of the ulnar osteotomy.
- Once reduced, partially fix the ulnar osteotomy proximally and distally using a plate and screws. No bone graft is necessary.
- Remove the temporary pin from the radiocapitellar joint. To ascertain radiocapitellar and radioulnar alignment, rotate the radial head, testing for a complete stable arc.
- Repair the periosteum and return attention to the ligamentous repair or reconstruction.
- If the native annular ligament can be used, repair this with mattress sutures through the ulnar periosteal tunnels. Do not tighten these sutures until all have been placed.
- If the annular ligament cannot be used, develop a 6-cm to 8-cm strip of triceps fascia from proximal to distal, elevating the periosteum from the proximal ulna to the level of the radial neck. Take care not to amputate the fascia.
- Pass the strip of tendon through the periosteum, around the radial neck, bringing it back and suturing it to itself and the ulnar periosteum. Passing and securing the tendon through the periosteum is similar to the drill holes described by Seel and Peterson.
- Repair the capsule and extensor supinator origin back to the lateral epicondylar area of the humerus.
- Before complete closure, obtain final radiographs and fluoroscopy to make sure there is a stable arc of motion in flexion and extension and pronation and supination.
- Prophylactically perform forearm fasciotomies and inspect the radial nerve before subcutaneous and skin closure.
- Apply a long arm, bivalved cast with the forearm in 60 to 90 degrees of supination and the elbow flexed 80 to 90 degrees.

POSTOPERATIVE CARE. The cast is worn for 4 to 6 weeks and then changed to a removable bivalved cast to allow active pronation and supination. Flexion and extension of the elbow are usually the first to return, with full rotary motion returning over 6 months.

GALEAZZI FRACTURES

Galeazzi fractures, or fractures of the radius with dislocation of the distal radioulnar joint (DRUJ), are rare in children. Most fractures of the distal forearm are associated with anterior displacement of the distal ulna unlike proximal forearm fractures, which are associated with posterior dislocations. True lateral radiographs are essential in making the diagnosis. Reduction of the radial fracture will reduce the DRUJ in most patients. In patients with irreducible fractures, open reduction and internal fixation of the distal radius should be performed and the DRUJ reassessed. If the DRUJ remains dislocated, then open reduction and internal fixation of the DRUJ should be performed to remove interposed structures, most commonly periosteum, extensor carpi ulnaris, or extensor digiti quinti tendon, and the triangular fibrocartilage complex (TFCC). The DRUJ may be pinned with the forearm supinated to provide additional stability.

Although this injury usually occurs in adolescents, a pediatric variant consisting of a Salter-Harris type II fracture of the distal ulna occurs before rupture of the TFCC can occur in a younger child. The treatment principles are the same as for adolescents; however, periosteal entrapment may block reduction rather than the TFCC.

NURSEMAID'S ELBOW

Nursemaid's elbow is a subluxation of the annular ligament over the radial head, most commonly occurring in children 2 to 3 years of age when longitudinal traction is placed on the

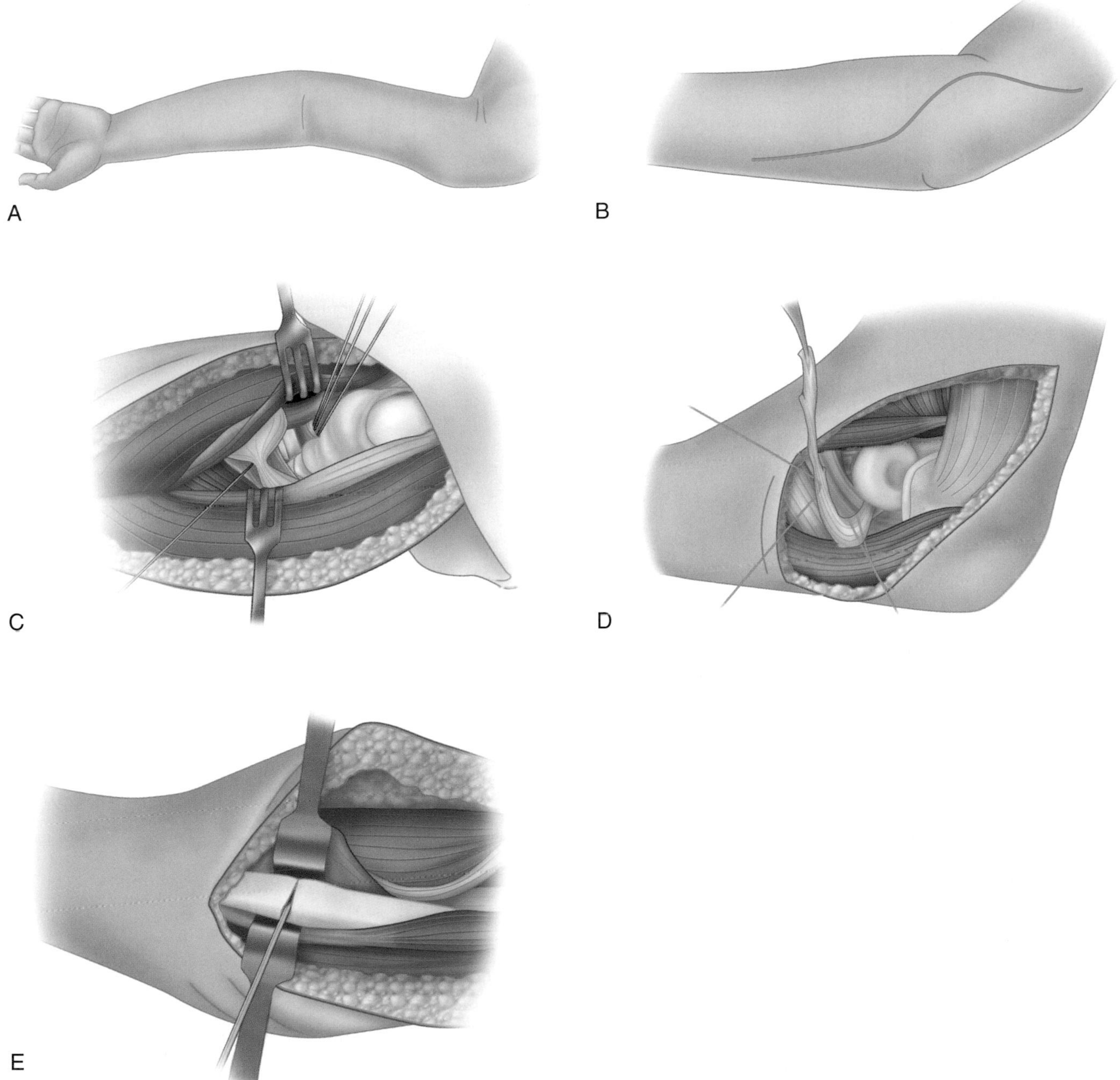

FIGURE 36-66 Reconstruction of late or chronic Monteggia fracture-dislocation. **A,** Clinical deformity of chronic Monteggia lesion with increased cubitus valgus. **B,** Extensile incision for annular ligament reconstruction and ulnar osteotomy. **C,** Exposure of radiocapitellar and radioulnar joint with elevation of extensor-supinator origin from lateral epicondyle, protection of radial nerve, and thorough joint debridement. **D,** Radial head with osteochondral change from chronic dislocation. Annular ligament has been reduced around radial neck, and sutures are in place for construction to annular ligament. **E,** Ulnar opening wedge osteotomy at site of maximal deformity. (Redrawn from Shah AS, Waters PM: Monteggia fracture-dislocations in children. In Flynn JM, Skaggs DL, Waters PM, editors: Rockwood and Wilkins' Fractures in Children, 8th edition. Philadelphia, Wolters Kluwer, 2015.) **SEE TECHNIQUE 36-14.**

upper extremity with the elbow extended and forearm supinated. Despite the well-known mechanism of injury, 30% to 40% of patients with nursemaid's elbow present without any history of a traction injury. Radiographs are normal in this condition, unlike Monteggia variants in which there is plastic deformation of the ulna. A variety of closed reduction techniques have been reported to be successful. A combination of forearm flexion and supination will reduce most pulled elbows. Immobilization with a sling has been used for several days for symptomatic relief. Recurrence is high, and parents need to be counseled to avoid traction on the child's upper limbs. Patients in which the diagnosis is unclear should be reexamined in 7 to 10 days to ensure the correct diagnosis. This usually resolves around the age of 5 years when the ligamentous structures about the elbow mature and give it more stability.

FOREARM FRACTURES

Forearm fractures are the most common fractures in children and account for up to 40% of all pediatric fractures. The forearm can be divided into three regions: proximal, middle, and distal based on unique physiologic differences such as muscle forces and growth potential. Ninety percent of the growth of the forearm occurs at the distal third, giving it tremendous remodeling capacity, unlike the proximal third where very little growth and remodeling capacity exists.

PROXIMAL THIRD FOREARM FRACTURES

Fractures of the proximal third of the forearm without radial head subluxation or dislocation are uncommon. Because of the possibility of an associated radial head dislocation, radiographs of the elbow should be obtained in any proximal forearm fracture. Many proximal fractures are unstable in flexion, making operative treatment often necessary, especially in older children and adolescents. When surgical fixation is necessary, good results can be obtained with intramedullary nailing or plate fixation. Radioulnar synostosis is rare and can occur during forearm fracture at any level but is most common in proximal third fractures. Risk factors for radioulnar synostosis include severe initial injury, displaced fractures at the same level, operative treatment, and radial head excision.

MIDDLE THIRD FOREARM FRACTURES

Diaphyseal fractures of the forearm are the third most common pediatric fracture, behind the distal radius and supracondylar humerus. The most common mechanism of injury is a fall onto an outstretched hand. Many of the fractures of the midforearm in children can be treated nonoperatively, especially in young children because of the remodeling potential. The unique physiologic characteristics of pediatric bone, including its increased elasticity, increases the potential for incomplete or greenstick fractures and plastic deformation. These fractures have no remodeling potential and reduction is necessary.

Despite increased interest in operative treatment of these injuries, closed reduction with cast application remains an essential method of treatment, especially for minimally displaced fractures in younger children. Meticulous casting technique, including an intraosseous mold, straight ulnar border, three-point molding, and close follow-up to watch for late displacement or angulation, is essential for a good outcome. The cast index, defined as the sagittal cast width divided by the coronal cast width, of less than 0.7 is predictive of successful outcome. Although this was initially described for distal radial fractures, it is a good guideline for diaphyseal fractures as well.

Indications for operative treatment include open fracture, fracture in older children, loss of reduction in a cast, malunion, floating elbow, irreducible fracture caused by soft-tissue interposition, unstable fracture pattern, shortening more than 1 cm, and refracture after cast treatment. A dramatic increase in operative treatment of diaphyseal fractures in children between the ages of 5 and 12 years has been the result of the use of intramedullary nailing. The most common procedures use stable elastic intramedullary nailing of the radius and ulna, as described by Metaizeau, or plating. Studies, including a Cochrane review and meta-analysis comparing nailing with plating, showed that there was no significant difference in outcomes between the two techniques and outcomes were good in 90% of patients. Patients with intramedullary nailing had better cosmetic results but did require a second procedure to remove the implant. The Metaizeau nailing technique involves prebending of the nails to allow for restoration of the radial bow and to facilitate optimal reduction. Most authors avoid the distal radial physis and insert the nail in the radial side of the distal radius proximal to the physis. This approach avoids nail placement in Lister's tubercle, which has been shown to have a high rate of extensor pollicis brevis tendon injury. The ulna usually is nailed antegrade either through or proximal to the proximal ulnar physis. Transphyseal nail placement is technically easier and has not been shown to cause growth arrest but is associated with a higher rate of minor implant irritation. The pins are buried below the skin, and most authors recommend a brief period of immobilization, with nail removal between 4 and 12 months after fracture when the bone is healed radiographically. Other authors have shown good results with single-bone fixation of the ulna. The advantages of this technique include decreased operative time and ease of implant removal. It is not recommended for open fractures because of the higher rate of radial malunion. Repeated attempts at closed reduction and nailing increase the risk of compartment syndrome; therefore, an open reduction should be performed after two or three unsuccessful closed attempts. The rate of delayed union primarily in the ulna using this technique is 8% to 15% and higher in boys, those with increased fracture displacement, and those who had open reduction of the ulna.

INTRAMEDULLARY FOREARM NAILING

TECHNIQUE 36-15

- Place the child supine with the affected arm on a radiolucent table and apply, but do not inflate, a pneumatic tourniquet if open reduction is required.
- Make a 5-mm longitudinal incision on the lateral (radial) side of the distal metaphysis taking care to protect the radial sensory nerve.
- Drill a hole in the bone 5 to 10 mm proximal to the metaphysis, first perpendicularly and then obliquely toward the elbow.
- Depending on the diameter of the bone, choose a titanium or stainless steel nail of the appropriate size, which is typically 2.0 mm to 3.0 mm. Introduce the nail into the radius proximally taking care not to pass it out the medial (ulnar) cortex of the radius (Fig. 36-67).
- Reduce the fracture and pass the nail into the proximal metaphysis.
- The ulna can be nailed antegrade or retrograde, although antegrade nailing is technically straightforward. To do this, mark the course of the ulnar nerve as it crosses the elbow on the skin for reference. Make a 5-mm

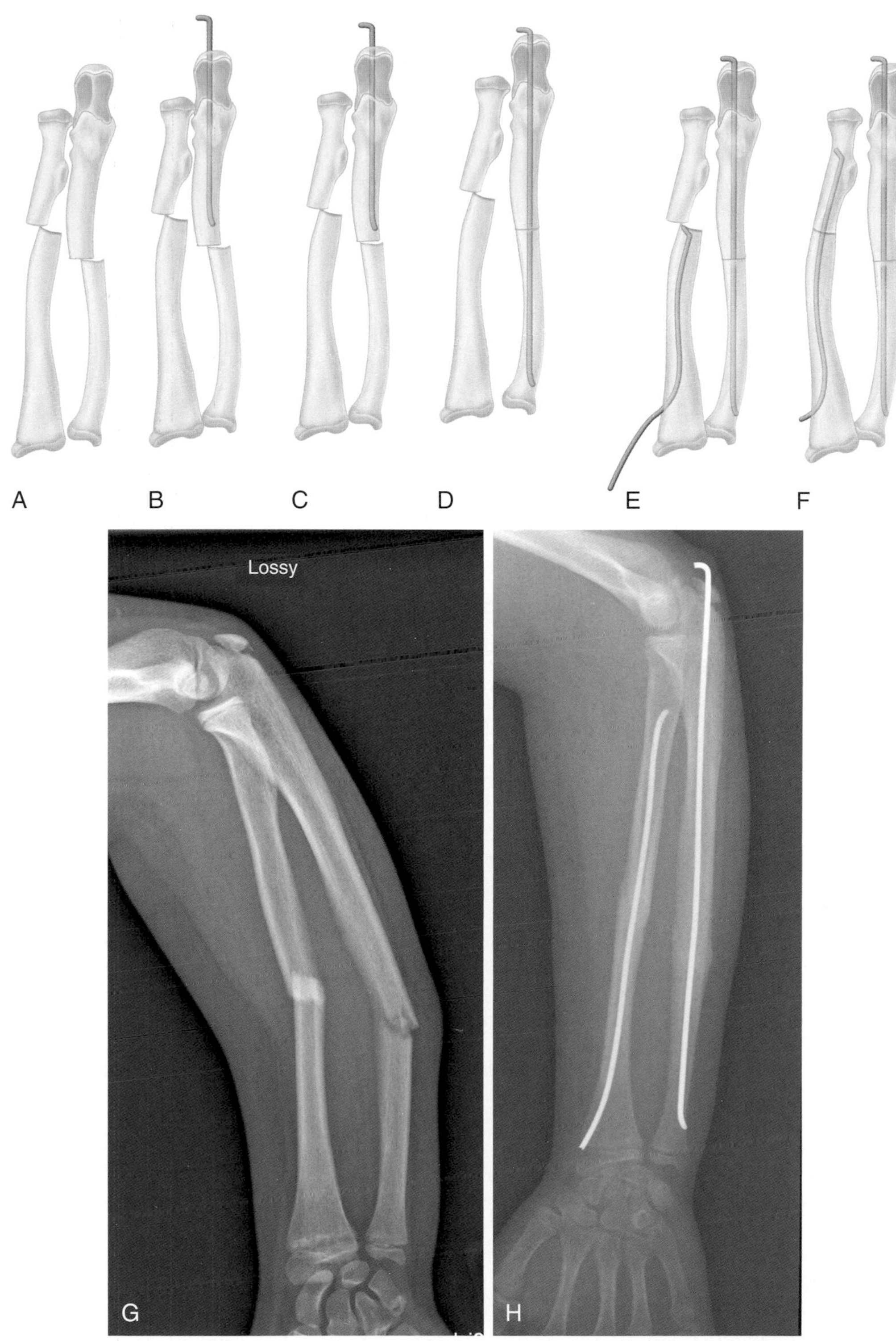

FIGURE 36-67 Intramedullary nailing of both-bone fractures of forearm. **A** and **G,** Displaced both-bone fractures. **B,** Pin is introduced into least displaced bone. **C,** Pin is advanced to fracture site. **D,** Fracture is reduced by external manipulation, and pin is advanced into proximal metaphysis. **E,** Fracture of other bone is reduced and fixed in same manner. **F** and **H,** Both pins in place. **SEE TECHNIQUE 36-15.**

longitudinal incision over the posterior olecranon and drill a small entry hole taking care to protect the ulnar nerve. Pass the nail across the fracture site in an antegrade fashion.

- Alternatively, retrograde nailing can be done in a fashion to that used for the radial nail. To do this, place a small drill hole just proximal to the distal ulnar physis. Pass the nail retrograde taking care to prevent cutout of the lateral (radial) cortex. Once the fracture is reduced and the nail is in good position, cut the nail approximately 5 mm from the entry point, irrigate, and close the soft tissues. Avoid multiple passes with the nail because this increases the risk of compartment syndrome. Open reduction should be performed if it is difficult or impossible to pass the nail in a closed fashion.
- Close all wounds. Apply a long arm, bivalved cast or splint.

POSTOPERATIVE CARE. After intramedullary nail fixation, the cast is removed after 4 to 6 weeks. The pins are removed at 6 months after fracture. Participation in sports is avoided for 2 months.

Complications reported after intramedullary nail fixation include loss of reduction after wire removal, refracture, deep infection, pin site infection, transient anterior interosseous nerve palsy, and skin ulcers over buried wires. Patients treated with intramedullary nailing for open or closed forearm fractures have been reported to have an increased incidence of compartment syndrome compared with patients treated with closed reduction and casting. Also, patients with longer operative times, increased use of intraoperative fluoroscopy, and multiple attempts at closed percutaneous pinning are at higher risk of developing compartment syndrome. Close observation and monitoring of all patients with both-bone forearm fractures is recommended, but especially of those at risk.

Plate fixation is indicated for patients with length unstable or comminuted fractures and fractures with delayed or nonunion in which the medullary canal may be inaccessible to an intramedullary nail (Chapter 57). Although plates provide better length and rotational stability, as well as restoration of the radial bow, they require longer operative time and larger incisions. Single bone plating of the radius and ulna has been reported as well, but there is a risk of malunion of the unplated bone. Refracture after plate removal is well documented in adults, but no clear data exist in children. Adolescents at or near skeletal maturity need to be counseled as to the risk of refracture after implant removal.

PLASTIC DEFORMATION AND GREENSTICK FRACTURES

Plastic deformation occurs due to the increased porosity and elasticity of a child's bone. Plastic deformation occurs as a result of microfracture along the bow. These fractures have little to no remodeling potential, especially in older children, and should be reduced to prevent cosmetic and functional complications. These can be reduced gradually under sedation either with direct manipulation or over a fulcrum. Outcomes are good as long as the injury is recognized.

Greenstick fractures are unique to children and most commonly occur in the mid-diaphysis of the radius and ulna. Fractures at the same level can be treated with closed reduction and cast application. Fractures at different levels indicate a rotational component that needs to be corrected at the time of reduction. Important features of greenstick fractures are that they have little remodeling potential and a high rate of refracture. For this reason, most authors recommend completing the greenstick fracture before casting, which allows for more abundant callus formation.

DISTAL THIRD FOREARM FRACTURES

The distal radius is the most commonly fractured bone in childhood, with a peak age of 10 years. This is typically caused by a fall onto an outstretched upper extremity. Approximately half of children with a distal radial fracture have an associated ulnar fracture. Other associated injuries, although rare, can occur and include ipsilateral scaphoid and supracondylar humeral fracture. Isolated ulnar fractures are very rare in children. The diagnosis of these injuries usually can be made with plain radiographs alone, and the elbow should be included in all imaging of distal third fractures to rule out an associated elbow injury. Advanced imaging, such as MRI and CT, is not routinely used unless the diagnosis is in question or an associated wrist injury such as scaphoid fracture is present. Ultrasound can be used to diagnose nondisplaced fractures in young children; however, it is user dependent and not readily available in all centers.

Because of its frequency, the management of distal radial fractures is one of the cornerstones of pediatric orthopaedic care. Although there has been an increase in operative treatment of these injuries, especially in older children, closed treatment is still the most common method of treatment. Because 90% of the growth of the forearm occurs distally, there is tremendous remodeling potential for these fractures, especially in young children. An age-based approach in determining acceptable alignment and need for operative treatment can be used (Table 36-1). Fundamentals of closed treatment include reduction using the periosteal hinge and a well-molded cast. It has been shown that the cast index, as described by Chess, of less than 0.7 is predictive of successful cast treatment. Buckle (torus) fractures are common, and well-designed randomized studies show that removable splint treatment is well tolerated, safe, and cost-effective for these injuries.

Physeal fractures are common, accounting for a third of all distal radial fractures. Most are Salter-Harris types I and II injuries; Salter types III to VI injuries are very rare. The risk of growth arrest is 1% to 7%. This can be treated by epiphysiodesis of the remaining physis and ulnar shortening osteotomy. Distal ulnar growth arrest is rare and can be treated with radial epiphysiodesis and ulnar lengthening osteotomy.

Closed reduction with percutaneous pinning with single or dual pins has been shown to provide good outcomes with a low complication rate. In a randomized study of percutaneous pinning compared with cast treatment, the authors found a higher rate of loss of reduction in the cast group than the pinning group. However, 38% of patients in the pinning group had mild complications related to the pin, which resolved with removal. The pins can be left outside the skin, and pin removal can be performed in the outpatient setting. The use of open reduction and internal fixation is reserved for older children who are near or at skeletal maturity.

TABLE 36-1

Recommended Acceptable Alignment Parameters for Pediatric Forearm Fracture by Age

SOURCE	AGE	ANGULATION	MALROTATION	BAYONETTE APPOSITION/DISPLACEMENT
Price (2010)	< 8 yrs	<15 deg (MS) <15 deg (DS) <10 deg (PS)	< 30 deg	100% displacement
Noonan, Price (1998)	< 9 yrs	< 15 deg	< 45 deg	<1 cm short
Tarmuzi et al. (2009)	< 10 yrs	< 20 deg		No limits
Qairul et al. (2001)	<12 yrs	< 20 deg		

From Vopat ML, Kane PM, Christino MA, et al: Treatment of diaphyseal forearm fractures in children, Orthop Rev (Pavia) 6:5325, 2014.
DS, Distal shaft; *MS*, mid-shaft; *PS*, proximal shaft.

CLOSED REDUCTION AND PERCUTANEOUS PINNING OF FRACTURES OF THE DISTAL RADIUS

TECHNIQUE 36-16

- Position the patient on the operating table with the wrist over a sterilely draped image intensifier.
- Reduce the fracture using traction and gentle manipulation, especially for a physeal fracture.
- While holding the wrist in a flexed position to stabilize the fracture, use a Kirschner wire and the image intensifier to mark the trajectory of the pin on the skin.
- Start the pin at the tip of the radial styloid and pass it proximally and ulnarly across the fracture site.
- Once the fracture is pinned, cut and bend the pin and obtain final images. It is important to leave the pin long so that it does not become buried under the skin during cast treatment.
- Place the arm in a well-padded short arm splint or bivalved cast.

POSTOPERATIVE CARE. The short arm cast is worn for 4 to 6 weeks, and the pin is then removed. Range-of-motion exercises are started, and the patient is placed in a removable splint for an additional 4 weeks.

WRIST DISLOCATIONS

Because of the proximity of the distal radial and ulnar physes to the wrist joint, wrist dislocations are extremely rare in children. When they do occur, it is usually in a skeletally mature adolescent. Treatment is similar to that in adults (Chapter 69).

SCAPHOID AND CARPAL FRACTURES

The carpal bones ossify relatively late in childhood; therefore, fractures of the carpal bones are rare and when present can be overlooked. Scaphoid fractures are the most common carpal injuries in children and adolescents with peak age of 12 to 15 years. They have become more common as more children participate in competitive sports.

The scaphoid is the largest bone in the proximal row of the carpus, and ossification begins between age 5 and 6 years and is completed between the ages of 13 and 15 years corresponding with the peak incidence of fracture. Fractures of other carpal bones generally follow their times of ossification: triquetrum, 12 to 13 years; trapezium, 13 to 14 years; trapezoid, 13 to 14 years; and hamate, 15 years. The most common mechanism of injury is a fall onto the outstretched hand with the forearm pronated. This usually produces a middle third fracture. Distal third fractures usually are caused by direct trauma or avulsion and are the most common. Proximal pole fractures are the least common.

An age-based classification that is predictive of the type of injury has been developed. Type I injuries occur in children younger than 8 years and usually are chondral. Type II injuries that occur between 8 to 11 years usually are osteochondral, and type III injuries that occur in children older than 12 years are more "adult-like" because the scaphoid is ossified. Pediatric scaphoid fractures also can be classified by location: tuberosity, transverse distal pole, avulsion of the distal pole, waist, or proximal pole. In children, fractures of the distal third of the scaphoid (transverse distal pole and tuberosity) are the most common.

The most common clinical signs of scaphoid fracture are dorsal swelling of the wrist, tenderness in the anatomic snuffbox and over the distal part of the radius, and painful dorsiflexion of the wrist or extension of the thumb. Radiographs should include anteroposterior, lateral, and scaphoid views with the wrist in ulnar deviation; however, normal radiographs do not preclude the presence of a scaphoid fracture. If a scaphoid fracture is suggested but radiographs are negative, the wrist should be immobilized and reevaluated in 2 weeks because up to 30% of patients may have positive follow-up radiographs. MRI is useful in making the diagnosis, and a normal study as early as 2 days after injury has a negative predictive value of 100%.

Fractures of the proximal pole, although rare, seem to heal uneventfully when treated by prolonged immobilization. Avulsion fractures in the distal third of the scaphoid are common in children and usually require cast immobilization only. Healing times of scaphoid fractures have been described as 3 to 4 weeks for tuberosity fractures, 4 to 16 weeks for waist fractures, 4 to 8 weeks for distal scaphoid fractures, and 3 to 6 weeks for distal avulsions. Indications for operative treatment of scaphoid fractures in pediatric patients at or near skeletal maturity are similar to those for scaphoid fractures in adults. Smooth wires rather than compression screws have been used in young children to prevent growth arrest (see Chapter 69).

A painful nonunion of the proximal scaphoid, which in children is extremely rare, may occur after a delay in treatment generally because of an incorrect diagnosis or lack of immobilization. An established nonunion in a child may be treated operatively as in an adult. A dorsal or volar approach can be used. Some authors have speculated that bipartite scaphoid may be an ununited waist fracture that has taken on the characteristics of a bipartite bone. Bipartite scaphoid usually is bilateral, asymptomatic, and not related to trauma.

Fractures of the triquetrum in children often are subtle flake avulsion or impingement fractures that require good oblique radiographs for recognition. The incidence of these fractures probably is much higher than currently known because many are misdiagnosed as wrist sprains or type I physeal injuries of the distal radius and ulna. Three weeks of cast immobilization usually is sufficient treatment.

METACARPAL FRACTURES

Fractures of the metacarpals can occur at any location; however, the most common site of metacarpal fractures in children is the metacarpal neck, usually in the small and ring fingers. The peak incidence is 15 years of age. The most common mechanisms of injury are contact sports and striking an object (e.g., boxer's fracture). Metacarpal shaft fractures usually are the result of trauma such as a direct blow.

Most fractures of the metacarpals in children can be treated closed with cast immobilization. Metacarpal shaft fractures are usually stable because of the presence of intermetacarpal ligaments and can be treated with cast immobilization. Percutaneous pinning either intramedullary or to adjacent stable metacarpals can be performed for displaced or unstable fractures. Occasionally, open reduction and internal fixation is necessary for long oblique length unstable fractures as in adults (see Chapter 67). Metacarpal neck fractures usually can be treated with closed reduction and cast immobilization. Because of the mobility of the fourth and fifth metacarpals and the excellent remodeling capacity, up to 30 to 40 degrees of residual angulation can be accepted with closed treatment. Between 10 and 20 degrees of angulation generally is thought to be acceptable in the second and third metacarpal necks. Reduction can be done using the Jones technique of flexing the metacarpophalangeal joint 90 degrees and placing a dorsally directed force on the proximal phalanx with counter pressure on the metacarpal shaft. Occasionally, a metacarpal neck fracture in a noncompliant patient or an unstable fracture requires treatment with closed reduction and percutaneous pinning.

The most important goal in treatment of these injuries is restoration of normal rotation. Normal rotation should be confirmed by the ability to flex the fingers into the palm (see Chapter 67). Even a small amount (< 10 degrees) of rotational malalignment can create overlap of the digits during flexion and cause functional limitations; corrective osteotomy to align the digit often is necessary. If troublesome malrotation persists, the fracture will not remodel and either percutaneous pinning or open reduction and internal fixation is indicated. A displaced intraarticular metacarpal head fracture, which usually is seen in older children or adolescents, may also require open reduction and internal fixation.

THUMB METACARPAL FRACTURES

Most thumb metacarpal fractures in children occur proximally near the physis rather than the distal metacarpal as in the other metacarpals (Table 36-2). As a rare variant, the thumb metacarpal may have a physis at the proximal and distal ends, and comparison views are helpful in making this diagnosis. A fracture of the thumb metacarpal base usually can be treated for 3 to 4 weeks in an abduction thumb spica cast (Fig. 36-68A). The physeal fracture that occurs most often in this area is a Salter-Harris type II injury, and it can be treated by closed reduction (Fig. 36-68B and C). Pediatric Bennett fractures can occur, however, and are Salter-Harris type III fractures (Fig. 36-68D). This fracture is intraarticular, and in a child it can result in a physeal disturbance if not treated properly. Closed reduction and percutaneous pin fixation or open reduction and internal fixation with smooth pins, as in an adult Bennett fracture is indicated (see Chapter 67) (Fig. 36-69). Occasionally, in an older adolescent, a fracture of the base of the first metacarpal that does not involve the physis (Rolando fracture) can be satisfactorily reduced and pinned percutaneously with the aid of image intensification.

TABLE 36-2

Fractures of the Thumb Metacarpal Base in Children

TYPE	DESCRIPTION	TREATMENT
A	Between physis and junction of proximal and middle thirds of bone Often transverse or slightly oblique Often some medial impaction Angulated in apex lateral direction	Closed reduction + cast Residual angulation of 20-30 degrees is acceptable depending on age of child and clinical appearance of thumb If unstable after reduction, percutaneous pinning required
B	Salter-Harris type II physeal fracture with metaphyseal fragment on medial side More common than type C	Mild angulation—no reduction, cast Moderate angulation—closed reduction + cast Severe angulation—closed reduction + percutaneous pinning; open reduction and fixation if closed reduction unsuccessful
C	Salter-Harris type II physeal fracture with metaphyseal fragment on lateral side	
D	Salter-Harris type III or IV fracture Resembles Bennett fracture in adults	Closed or open reduction and internal fixation

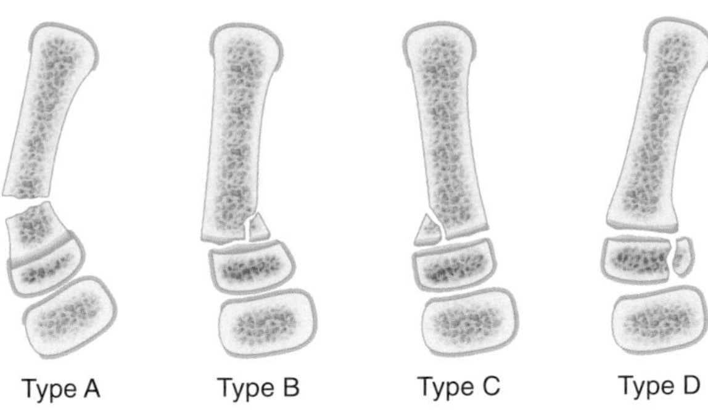

FIGURE 36-68 Classification of thumb metacarpal fractures. Type A, metaphyseal fracture. Types B and C, Salter-Harris type II physeal fractures with lateral or medial angulation. Type D, Salter-Harris type III fracture.

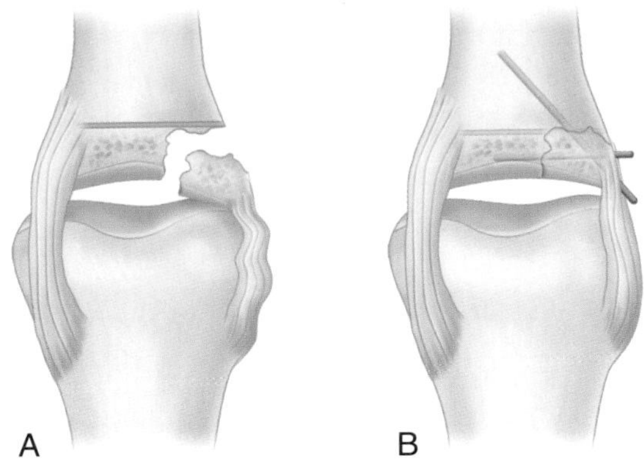

FIGURE 36-69 Example of gamekeeper thumb. **A,** Type III physeal fracture. **B,** After open reduction and internal fixation with pins.

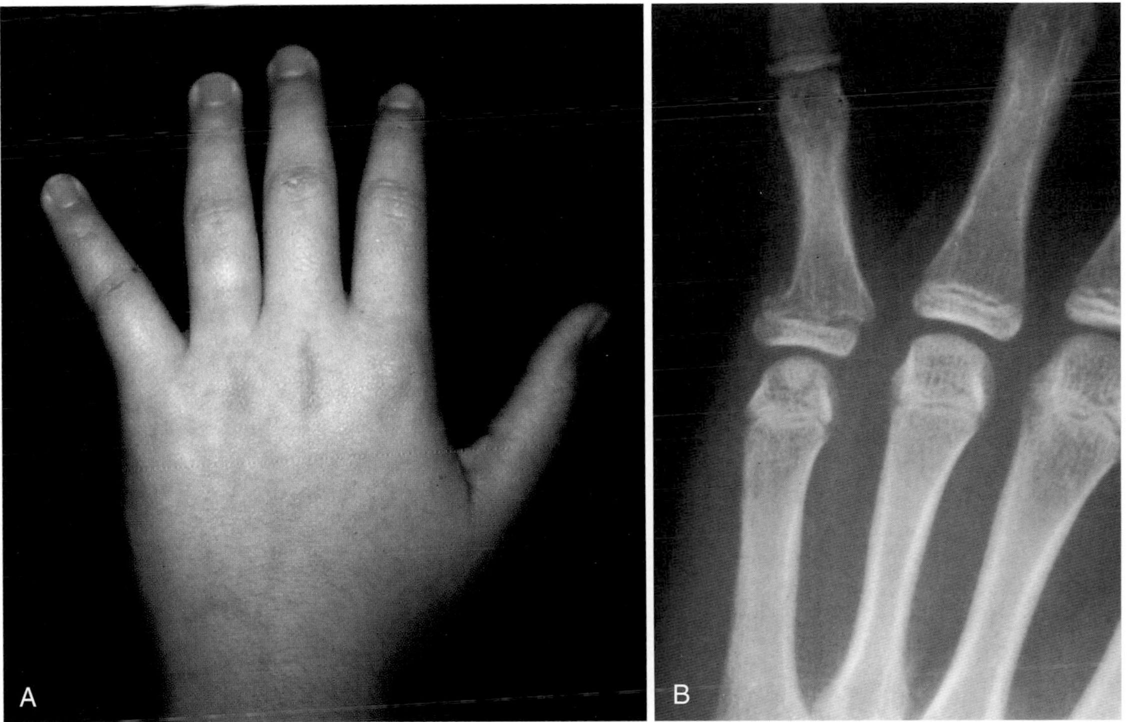

FIGURE 36-70 Extraoctave phalangeal fracture. **A,** Clinical appearance. **B,** Radiographic appearance.

PHALANGEAL FRACTURES

Phalangeal fractures are common in children, with the most common mechanism being sports activity. Up to two thirds occur in the proximal phalanx at a peak age of 12 years. They can involve the shaft, physis, neck, and condyles. The majority of proximal and middle phalangeal shaft fractures can be treated with cast immobilization for 3 to 4 weeks with closed reduction being performed for displaced fractures. Ensuring proper rotation as described previously for metacarpal fractures is essential to ensure a good outcome. Many of these fractures are physeal, and Salter-Harris type II fractures of the proximal phalanx are common. Growth arrest, however, is uncommon. Salter-Harris type III fractures of the base of the proximal or middle phalanx do occur and because of their intraarticular nature often require open reduction and internal fixation. The "extraoctave fracture," or an angulated apex radial base of the fifth proximal phalanx fracture (Fig. 36-70), can occur and is treated by placing a bolster in the fourth web space to act as fulcrum for reduction followed by casting. Irreducible fractures require open reduction and internal fixation. Fractures of the phalangeal neck and condyles usually are unstable and often require operative treatment. Nondisplaced intraarticular fractures can be treated closed with close follow-up. Open reduction and internal fixation with small diameter wires is indicated for displaced intraarticular fractures (Fig. 36-71).

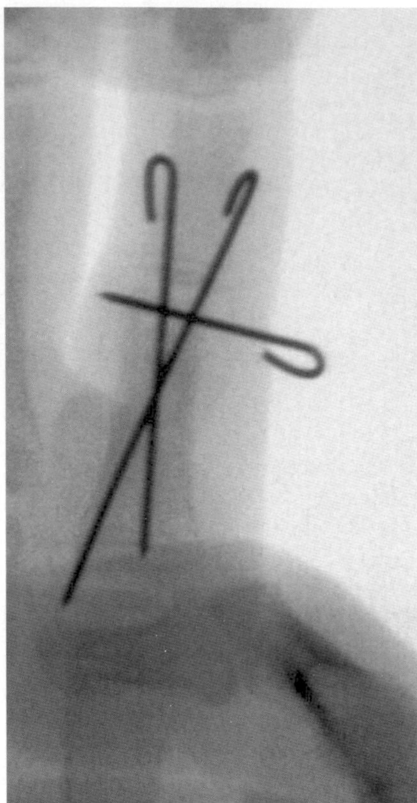

FIGURE 36-71 Pinning for phalangeal neck fracture.

OPEN REDUCTION AND INTERNAL FIXATION OF PHYSEAL FRACTURES OF PHALANGES AND METACARPALS

TECHNIQUE 36-17

- Make a straight midlateral incision (see Chapter 64) over the involved physis. After soft-tissue dissection and retraction, mobilize the neurovascular structures and lateral bands. Expose the physis, but take care not to damage it or the perichondral ring or periosteum overlying it.
- Carefully mobilize the fragments; clean out any small fragments or hematoma, and reduce the fracture anatomically. Ensure that the reduction is satisfactory at the physis and joint surface.
- With a power drill (low torque, high speed), transfix the fracture with two smooth parallel pins, preferably in the metaphysis or epiphysis. Crossed pins and pins that cross the physis generally should be avoided, but sometimes small fracture fragments cannot be adequately transfixed and held otherwise. Cut off the pins beneath the skin, but leave them long enough to be removed easily as an outpatient procedure.
- Close the soft tissues appropriately and apply a splint or cast.

POSTOPERATIVE CARE. The pins are removed at 4 weeks, and a range-of-motion exercise program is started at that time or shortly thereafter. This program should be taught to the parents and the patient and should concentrate on active range of motion only. (Passive range-of-motion exercises in a child will cause the child to withdraw or guard against any motion at all.) The parents should be warned of the possibility of growth arrest with subsequent angular deformity.

DISTAL PHALANGEAL FRACTURE

Distal phalangeal fractures can be classified as physeal or extraphyseal. Extraphyseal fractures usually are the result of crush injuries and heal uneventfully. Meticulous nailbed exploration and repair are necessary for severe injuries to prevent late nail deformity. Displaced physeal fractures are mallet finger equivalents in children because of the attachment of the flexor digitorum profundis (FDP) tendon on the distal fragment. The Seymour fracture is a Salter-Harris type I or II fracture of the distal phalanx that is associated with a nailbed injury. These injuries often are overlooked and have a high rate of infection. They usually are irreducible because of the interposed sterile matrix in the physis. Urgent irrigation and debridement are essential for a good outcome. Operative stabilization occasionally is necessary and can be done with a small smooth Kirschner wire.

COMPLICATIONS OF PHALANGEAL FRACTURES

Complications of pediatric phalangeal fractures are uncommon, but nonunion, malunion, osteonecrosis, and growth disturbance may occur. Nonunion is rare except in severe injuries in which the fracture fragments are devascularized. Malunion is more common and can result in angulation or rotational deformities and limited motion (Fig. 36-72). Although most malunions remodel satisfactorily, especially in young children, considerable deformity may require osteotomy for realignment. Waters et al. described a percutaneous technique for reduction of malunion of phalangeal neck fractures with partial bony healing (Fig. 36-73). An obliquely inserted Kirschner wire (0.9 mm to 1.6 mm, depending on the size of the child) is used to break down the callus and partially healing bone and lever the dorsally displaced and rotated condylar fragment back into the correct anatomic position. One or two percutaneous wires (0.7 mm to 1.1 mm) are used to hold the reduction. Growth disturbance can result from any injury that involves the physes but is uncommon after phalangeal fracture.

PEDIATRIC SPINE FRACTURES AND DISLOCATIONS

Spine fractures and dislocations are relatively uncommon in children, accounting for 1% to 3% of pediatric fractures; however, they are associated with a high rate of other injuries and morbidity and mortality. In older children, they are most commonly caused by motor vehicle accidents and sports. A recent review of pediatric spine fractures from a high-volume center showed that 80% of injuries occurred in older children (ages 13 to 19 years) and 60% of all patients had an associated injury, most often intrathoracic. Multiple spinal level injuries

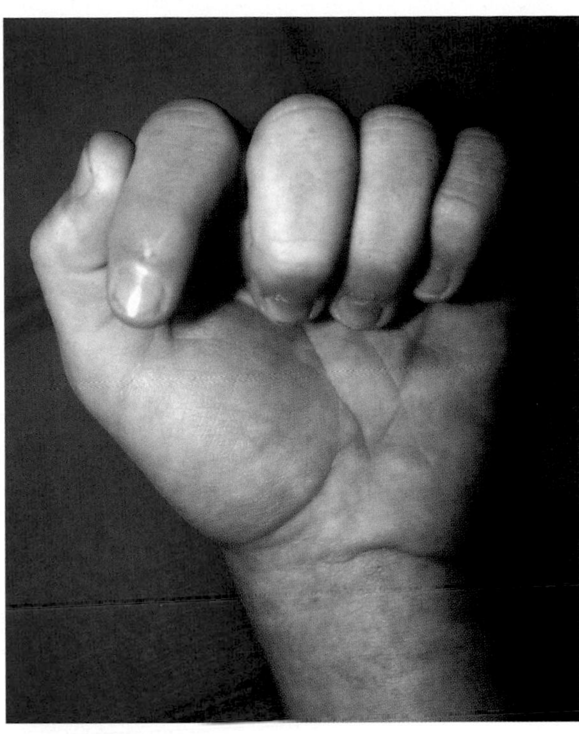

FIGURE 36-72 Malunion of phalangeal neck fracture producing malalignment of fingers.

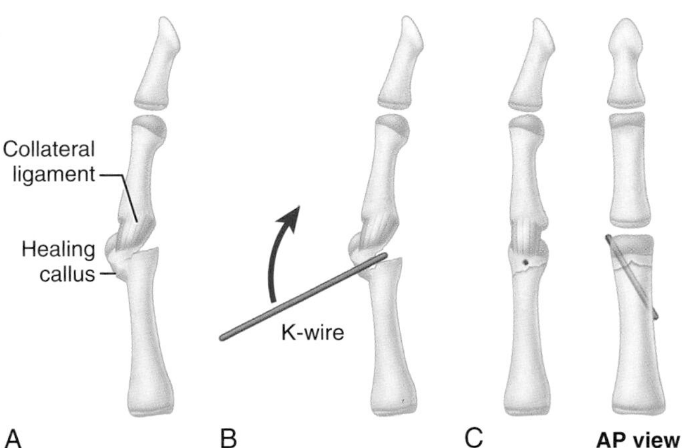

FIGURE 36-73 **A,** Percutaneous reduction of malunion of phalangeal neck fracture with partial bony healing. **B,** Kirschner wire is used to breakdown the callus and partial bony healing and lever the fragment into anatomic position. **C,** One or two percutaneous wires are used to hold the reduction.

were seen in 45% of patients, of which a third were in a different region of the spine. Therefore examination of the entire spine is essential in a child with a spine injury. Nonaccidental trauma should always be considered in young children with a cervical spine injury. Children younger than 3 years have a higher rate of spinal cord injury and mortality than older children and adolescents.

CERVICAL SPINE

Cervical spine fractures are less common in children than in adolescents or adults. They may occur at any age as a result of trauma with motor vehicle accident being the most common mechanism in a recent large series. Because of the large head-to-body weight ratio and increased ligamentous laxity in young children, upper cervical spine injuries are more common, and lower cervical spine injuries are most often seen in adolescents. The initial radiographic examination of a child with a suspected cervical spine injury consists of anteroposterior, lateral, and odontoid radiographs, which have been shown to be more sensitive than a cross-table lateral image alone. The use of CT is becoming more prevalent, especially in the adult population, but does have an increased radiation exposure. It is important to note that small children, because of their greater relative head size, need to be positioned by elevating the torso to avoid inadvertent flexion of the cervical spine. Supervised flexion-extension radiographs can be used in an awake, cooperative patient to assess cervical spine stability. The role of MRI continues to evolve; however, it is useful in detecting ligamentous injury in patients who cannot perform flexion or extension radiographs. It also is useful in detecting disc herniation and the status of the spinal cord in patients with neurologic deficits.

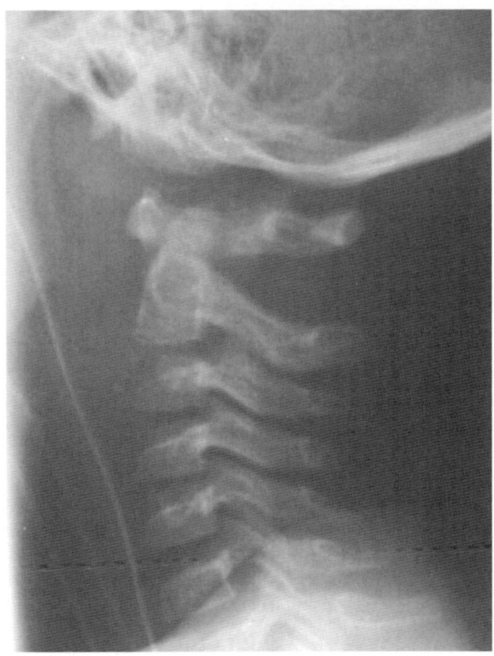

FIGURE 36-74 Atlantooccipital dislocation.

ATLANTOOCCIPITAL FRACTURES AND INSTABILITY

Occipital condyle fractures in children are extremely rare. The majority are stable and can be treated with a cervical orthosis. Atlantooccipital dislocation (AOD) was once thought to be uniformly fatal; however, with advanced trauma care more children are surviving. A recent report of 14 patients found that most were injured in automobile accidents, and complications including spinal cord and brain injury were common (Fig. 36-74). Cranial nerve injuries also can be present. At our institution over a 20-year period, we had 14 atlantooccipital dislocations that were treated with posterior occipitocervical fusion with internal fixation. All fusions united, but at the time of the most recent follow-up,

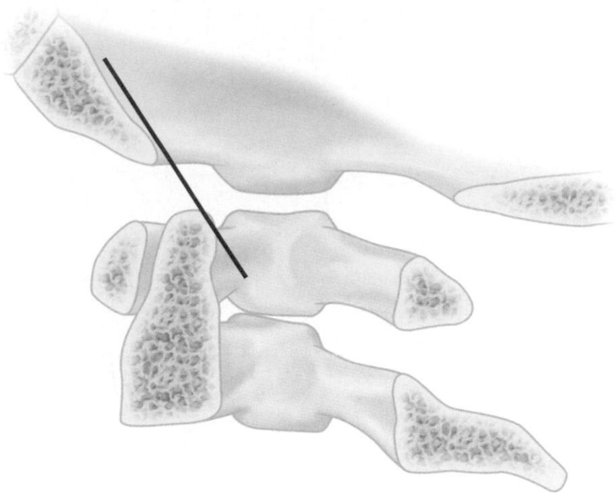

FIGURE 36-75 Wackenheim line. (Redrawn from Astur N et al: Traumatic atlanto-occipital dislocation in children, J Am Acad Orthop Surg 22:274, 2014.)

half of the patients had residual neurologic impairment. The most common postoperative complication was hydrocephalus, which should be suspected with postoperative neurologic decline.

A variety of imaging radiographic measurements has been described to aid in making the diagnosis. One helpful reproducible measurement is the Wackenheim line. The Wackenheim line drawn along the clivus should intersect tangentially the tip of the odontoid. A shift in this line either anteriorly or posteriorly from the odontoid tip is indicative of AOD (Fig. 36-75). MRI, which shows disruption of the tectorial membrane, is helpful in making this diagnosis. It is also helpful in assessing the degree of soft-tissue disruption at adjacent caudal levels. Operative stabilization, in most instances, is an occiput-to-C2 fusion using wires or screws depending on the size and anatomy of the patient. Acute hydrocephalus related to changes in cerebrospinal fluid flow is common in the early postoperative period.

UPPER CERVICAL SPINE (C1-2) INJURIES

C1 fractures are extremely uncommon in children. Often the normal synchondrosis is mistakenly identified as a fracture. Odontoid fractures are relatively common cervical spine fractures in children, with a peak incidence at 4 years. These fractures usually result from high-energy trauma such as a motor vehicle accident or fall. They typically occur through the odontoid synchondrosis at the base of the odontoid and displace anteriorly. Because of this, the diagnosis usually can be made on plain radiographs, especially the lateral view. CT with sagittal reconstruction also is helpful in confirming the diagnosis and evaluating for other associated injuries. Physician-supervised flexion-extension radiographs can be performed in an awake, cooperative patient to assess stability. Patients with more than 50% opposition of the odontoid can be treated with an extension Minerva cast or halo for 6 to 8 weeks followed by an orthosis. Many patients cannot comply with or tolerate this, and operative treatment is necessary. In patients with C1-C2 fracture, posterior fusion with instrumentation may be necessary, and a wide variety of techniques using screws or wires has been reported.

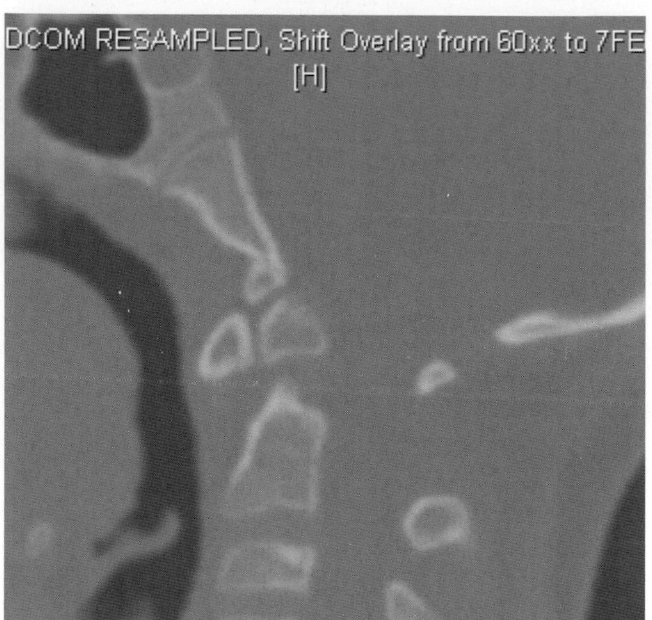

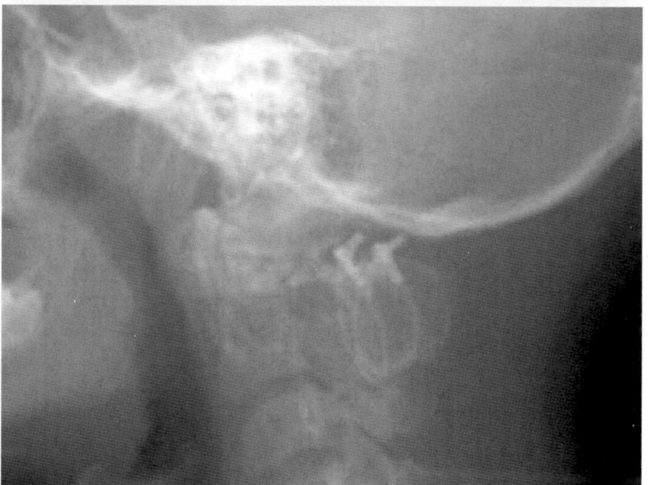

FIGURE 36-76 Os odontoideum.

An os odontoideum describes a range of deficiencies of the odontoid from complete absence to mild hypoplasia. It most commonly consists of an accessory ossicle that is separated from the body of C2, rendering it unstable (Fig. 36-76). Although most authors believe this is a congenital deformity, some have suggested this may occur as a result of a minor traumatic event to the odontoid. Presentation can range from an incidental finding to a displaced injury after a traumatic event. The diagnosis usually can be made on a lateral radiograph because the ossicle usually is smaller and more sclerotic than the normal odontoid. Supervised flexion-extension radiographs can be performed to assess the stability of the os, which correlates to the likelihood of developing neurologic symptoms from spinal cord compression. CT with sagittal reconstruction can aid in confirming the diagnosis and in operative planning. It can detect the presence of other associated cervical spine abnormalities such as a hypoplastic ring of C1. Indications for surgery include progressive or significant instability, pain, or neurologic compromise, and there is no role for nonoperative treatment in these patients. C1-C2 fusion can be performed using a variety of techniques including wiring or transarticular screw fixation depending on the surgeon's ability and patient's anatomy.

ROTATORY SUBLUXATION

Rotatory subluxation between C1 and C2 occurs most frequently after an acute upper respiratory tract infection or after low-grade trauma. It is thought that the inflammation associated with an upper respiratory tract infection increases the blood supply to the region, inducing laxity of the capsular and ligamentous structures. Patients typically present with a torticollis or "cock robin" position to their neck. Pain is common in the acute stage and is usually associated with sternocleidomastoid spasm as the child attempts to stabilize the head. In late cases the pain subsides and fixed deformity persists. Diagnosis can be made on plain films, especially the odontoid view, which shows asymmetry of the distance between the odontoid and lateral masses. CT, either dynamic or with three-dimensional reconstruction, can be used to confirm the diagnosis. Rotatory subluxation been classified by Fielding and Hawkins: type I is a unilateral facet subluxation and an intact transverse ligament, type II is a unilateral facet subluxation with transverse ligament involvement resulting in 3 mm to 5 mm of anterior displacement, type III is a bilateral facet subluxation with greater than 5 mm anterior displacement, and type IV is displacement of the atlas posteriorly rather than anteriorly. Types III and IV injuries are exceedingly rare but are associated with a high rate of neurologic injury.

Most acute subluxations can be treated nonoperatively. Patients can be placed in a soft collar and given antiinflammatory medication and diazepam for muscle spasm. If it does not resolve within a week, hospitalization and halter traction are indicated. Halo traction also can be used in severe cases. Operative treatment consisting of reduction and C1-C2 fusion is reserved for the rare acute cases that do not resolve with nonoperative treatment or those with neurologic deficits. Often it is necessary in patients with chronic subluxations to correct the head and neck deformity operatively with posterior spinal fusion and instrumentation.

LOWER CERVICAL SPINE (C3-7) INJURIES

Subaxial cervical spine injuries occur more commonly in older children and adolescents and are usually the result of high-energy injuries and sporting accidents. Both clinical and radiographic evaluation of the entire spine is necessary in these patients because of the high rate of secondary spine injuries that frequently occur at noncontiguous levels. Subaxial cervical spine injury can be a pure ligamentous disruption, facet dislocation(s), or fracture; it is similar to an adult injury. An understanding of normal developmental anatomy is helpful, as pseudosubluxation or apparent anterior translation, most commonly of C2 on C3, is a normal finding in children and adolescents. In addition, anterior wedging of the vertebral bodies is also a normal finding related to the ossification pattern of the vertebral body.

Plain radiographs are the standard initial step in the radiographic evaluation of the pediatric cervical spine. The anterior and posterior vertebral and spinolaminar lines (Fig. 36-77) are helpful in assessing the normal and pathologic anatomic relationships. CT has been shown to have improved sensitivity in making the diagnosis of cervical spine fracture

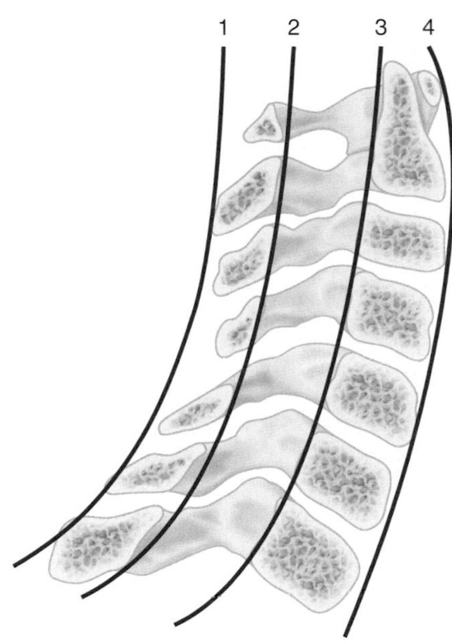

FIGURE 36-77 Spinal lines. Normal relationships in the lateral cervical spine: 1, spinous processes; 2, spinolaminar line; 3, posterior vertebral body line; 4, anterior vertebral body line. (Redrawn from Copley LA and Dormans JP: Cervical spine disorders in infants and children, J Am Acad Orthop Surg 6:204, 1998.)

but does have a higher radiation exposure. MRI is helpful in assessing the amount of ligamentous and soft-tissue disruption and detecting subtle compression fractures that may be missed on plain radiographs or CT. In a recent review at our institution, most subaxial cervical spine injuries in children and adolescents occurred at C6 and C7 and responded well to nonoperative treatment.

One unique injury in pediatric patients is spinal cord injury without radiographic abnormality (SCIWORA), first described by Pang. This condition is characterized by a spinal cord injury, either complete or incomplete, in the absence of any radiographic abnormalities. A recent meta-analysis found that in half the patients, MRI was normal, which carries a better long-term prognosis as well. It is hypothesized to be related to a severe flexion distraction injury of the cervical spine. Cadaver studies have shown that the spinal column in children due to ligamentous laxity can undergo 4 cm to 5 cm of distraction before disruption compared with 4 mm to 5 mm for the spinal cord. A stretch-related vascular mechanism has also been proposed. Delayed neurologic compromise can occur in 50% of patients, and some demonstrate transient warning signs. Recovery is unpredictable, and there is no treatment available when this occurs.

The operative techniques for treatment of these specific injuries are similar to adults and are discussed in Chapter 41.

THORACOLUMBAR SPINE

Thoracolumbar fractures are rare in young children and can be the result of nonaccidental trauma in neonates. They are more common in older children and adolescents and are usually the result of motor vehicle accidents, sports injuries, and falls. Thoracolumbar spine fractures in the absence of trauma can be associated with infection and osteopenia in

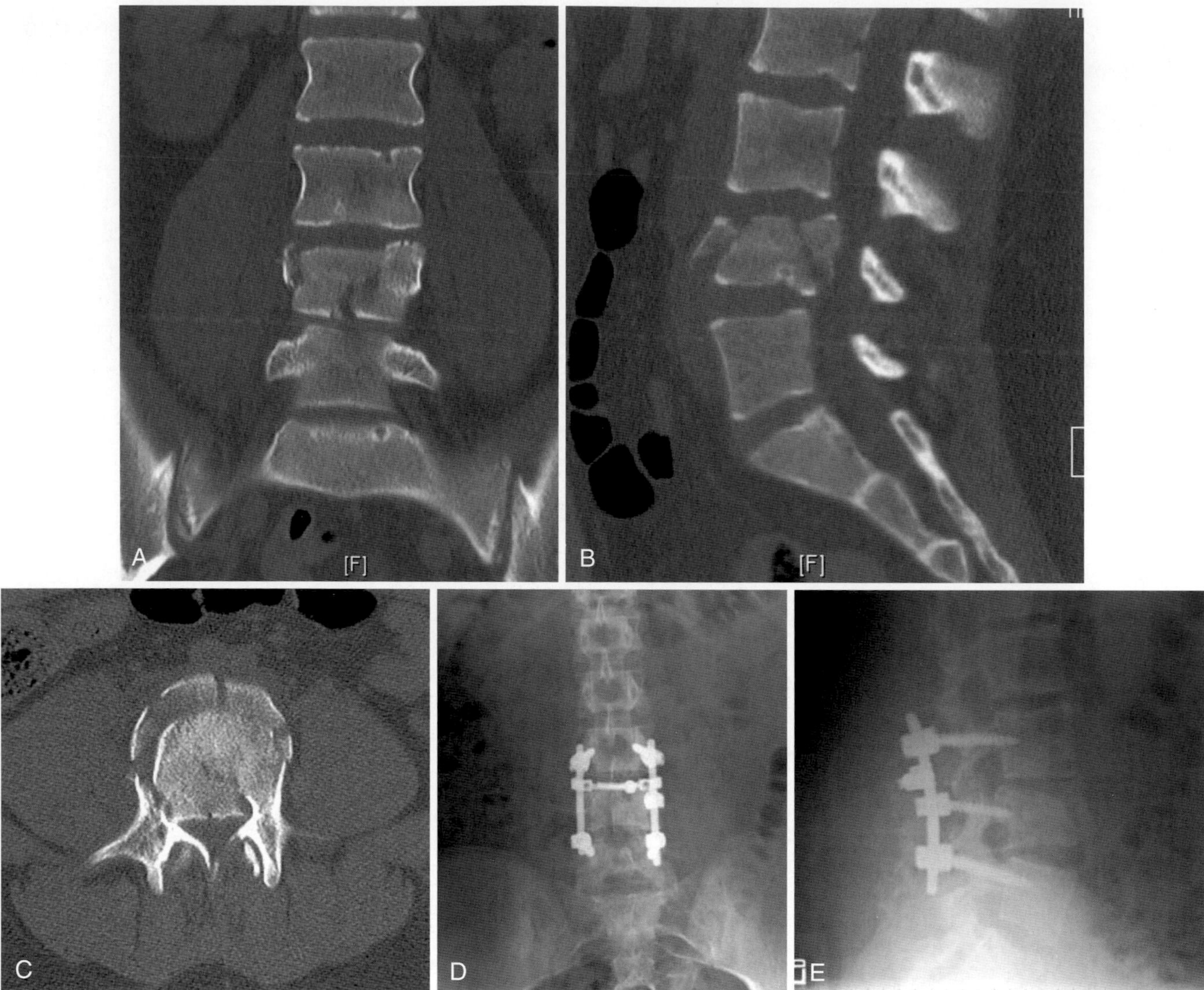

FIGURE 36-78 Burst fracture. **A,** Coronal CT). **B,** Sagittal CT. **C,** Axial MRI. **D and E,** Postoperative anteroposterior and lateral radiographs.

conditions such as juvenile osteoporosis, corticosteroid use, and certain genetic syndromes. Associated injuries, both spine and nonspine, are common and a thorough examination of the entire patient is necessary to evaluate and treat these appropriately. One such injury is the lap belt injury in which a child receives a hyperflexion injury from the lap belt causing anterior spinal compression, posterior spinal distraction, and compression of the intraabdominal structures between the lap belt and the spine. This often is diagnosed by the presence of seat belt abrasions on the patient's skin. The risk of intraabdominal injury is 42% with this injury. The role of corticosteroids in children with thoracolumbar fractures and spinal cord injuries remains controversial.

Initial radiographic evaluation should consist of anteroposterior and lateral radiographs of the entire spine and odontoid views. CT with sagittal and coronal reconstructions is helpful in making the diagnosis and evaluating spinal canal compromise (axial view) and posterior element injuries. MRI has been shown to be beneficial in assessing soft-tissue structures including the disc, spinal cord, and posterior ligamentous structures. The assessment of the posterior ligamentous structures is essential in assessing spinal stability and guiding treatment. These fractures are typically classified similarly to adult fractures based on mechanism: compression, burst, flexion distraction, and ligamentous disruption (Fig. 36-78). Treatment usually is similar to adults, which is described in Chapter 41.

The Chance, or flexion distraction, fracture commonly is seen in children and is a result of a flexion distraction force usually applied by a lap belt (Fig. 36-79). In children these can be bony, usually through the endplate, ligamentous, or both. Historically, some of these fractures, especially the isolated bony injury, were treated in braces. Several outcome studies have shown that operative treatment is superior in terms of return to function and better long-term sagittal alignment than nonoperative treatment, especially in those with abdominal injuries or significant posterior ligamentous

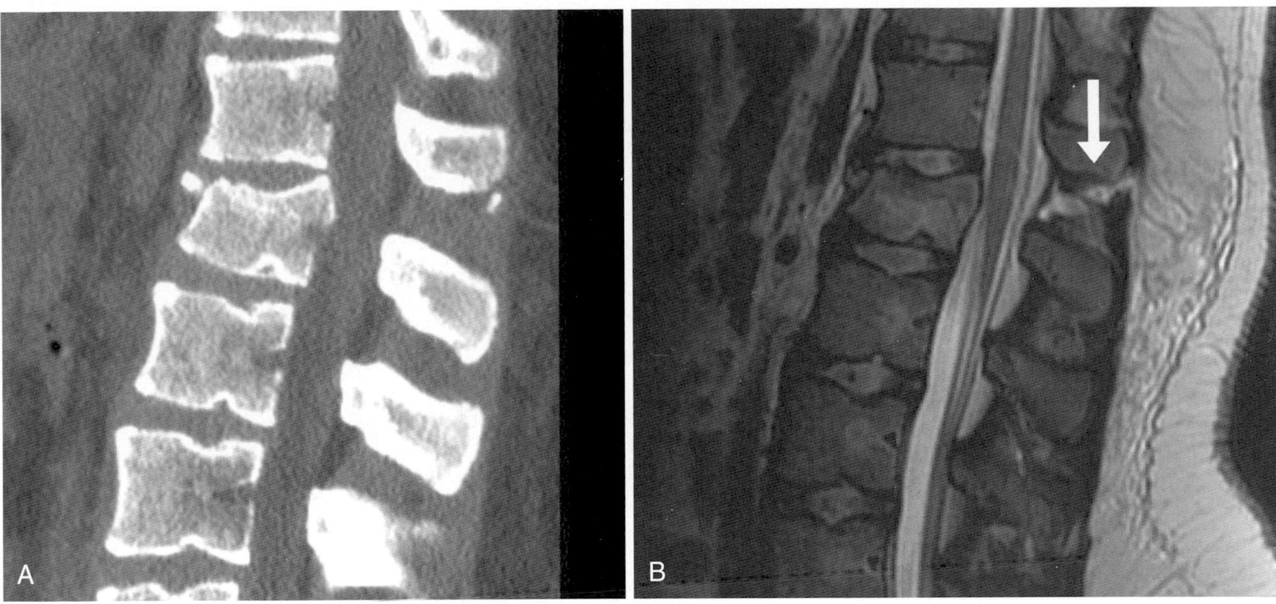

FIGURE 36-79 Chance fracture. **A**, CT. **B**, MRI.

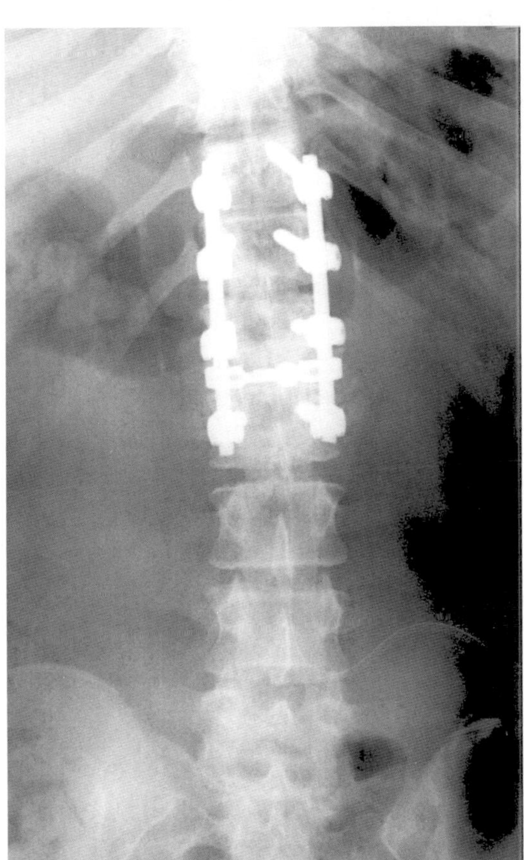

FIGURE 36-80 Chance fracture after spinal fixation.

disruption as seen on MRI (Fig. 36-80). In a multicenter study, Arkader et al. reported better clinical outcomes in patients treated operatively for Chance fractures.

Another fracture unique to pediatric patients is the endplate fracture, which is a flexion-type injury that usually occurs in an older child. A displaced fragment of a lumbar vertebral ring epiphysis in adolescents may simulate disc rupture (Fig. 36-81). The finding at surgery usually is a displaced bony fragment from the apophyseal ring, which is deficient posteriorly. This fragment can occasionally be seen on plain radiographs and can readily be seen on CT. MRI is the diagnostic imaging procedure of choice and has been reported to be able to differentiate endplate physeal fractures from herniated discs in children. In symptomatic patients, treatment consists of removal of the avulsed bony fragment.

PELVIC FRACTURES

Fractures of the pelvis in children are uncommon. Surgical fixation rarely is necessary for these fractures. Generally, the long-term results of conservative treatment are satisfactory because of the remodeling potential of the pelvis in children. However, recent literature has questioned the true remodeling potential of the immature pelvis, leading to an increase in surgical stabilization of pelvic fractures in this age group. Pelvic fractures may be associated with high-energy mechanisms, and soft-tissue injuries occurring in conjunction with pelvic fractures may be severe and require emergency treatment. Associated injuries include skull, cervical, facial, and long bone fractures; subdural hematomas, cerebral contusions, and concussions; lung contusions; hemothorax; hemopneumothorax; ruptured diaphragm; and lacerations of the spleen, liver, and kidney. Injuries that may be associated with and adjacent to pelvic fractures include damage to major blood vessels, retroperitoneal bleeding, rectal tears, and rupture or laceration of the urethra or bladder. The location and number of pelvic fractures are strongly associated with the probability of abdominal injury: 1% for isolated pubic fractures, 15% for iliac or sacral fractures, and 60% for multiple fractures of the pelvic ring. Because of these other injuries, mortality in children is high (9% to 18%). In a study of 54 patients with major pelvic fractures, 87% had associated pelvic or extrapelvic (soft-tissue) injuries; 14.8% died. Most

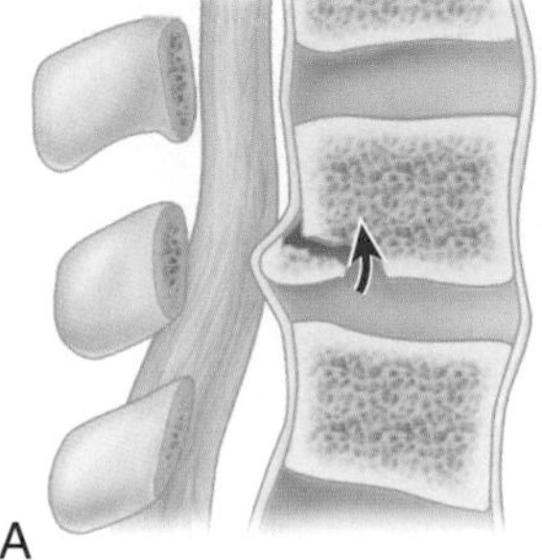

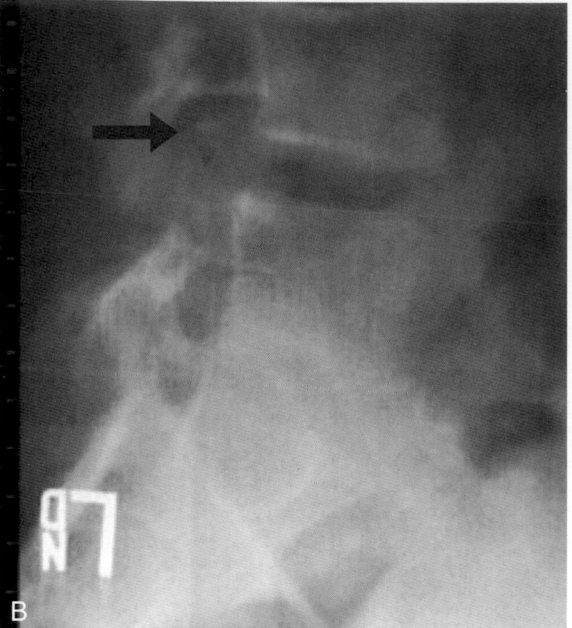

FIGURE 36-81 **A,** Posterior physeal injury that can mimic ruptured disc. **B,** Avulsion of ring apophysis has produced displaced fragment that presses on nerve root.

patients (70.4%) were treated conservatively. This suggests that the principles of management in children should not differ greatly from those in adults. Serious associated pelvic or extrapelvic injuries may pose more treatment problems than the actual pelvic fractures. The death rate from pelvic fractures alone is quite low (0% to 2.3%). Torode and Zieg reported 11 deaths in 141 patients with pelvic fractures, and 40% of patients with type IV injuries required laparotomy because of other injuries. Frequently, a child who has what radiographically appears to be a minor pelvic fracture also has had significant and possibly life-threatening soft-tissue injuries around the pelvis.

The initial evaluation of pelvic fractures usually is dictated by the mechanism of injury and associated injuries, and if a high-energy mechanism was the cause, the pediatric advanced life support protocol should be followed. This should include a thorough history, careful physical examination, laboratory tests when indicated, and appropriate imaging. If there is a high suspicion of pelvic trauma, an anteroposterior radiograph of the pelvis should be obtained. Additional radiographs, such as inlet and outlet views and Judet views of the pelvis, also may be of benefit. CT should be obtained in any patient suspected of having pelvic instability, anterior disruption, or posterior ring involvement. If a patient with a pelvic fracture becomes hemodynamically unstable, a pelvic binder should be placed. If the patient remains unstable, angiography or surgical packing should be considered based on institutional guidelines. For patients with a vertically unstable pelvis or hip joint instability, skeletal traction should be placed.

The pelvis in children differs from that in adults in that (1) more malleability is present because of the nature of the bone itself, the increased elasticity of joints, and the ability of the cartilaginous structures to absorb energy; (2) the elasticity of the joints around the pelvis is greater, which may allow for significant displacement and result in fracture of only one area rather than the traditional double break in the pelvic ring seen in adults; (3) the cartilage at the apophyses is inherently weak compared with bone, so avulsion fractures occur more frequently in children and adolescents than in adults; and (4) fractures into the triradiate cartilage can occur, causing growth arrest, which results in leg-length inequality and faulty development of the acetabulum.

In children and adolescents with pelvic fractures, isolated pubic rami and iliac wing fractures occur more often in an immature pelvis (open triradiate cartilage), whereas acetabular fractures and pubic or sacroiliac diastasis occur more often in a mature pelvis (closed triradiate cartilage). In patients with an immature pelvis, treatment of pelvic fractures should focus on associated injuries (e.g., head, abdominal) that often are the cause of mortality.

Numerous classification systems have been devised for pelvic fractures in children. The most widely used classification was proposed by Torode and Zieg and describes a four-part classification of pelvic fractures (Fig. 36-82): type I, avulsion of the bony elements of the pelvis; type II, iliac wing fractures; type III, simple ring fractures, including fractures involving the pubic rami or disruptions of the pubic symphysis; and type IV, including unstable injuries such as ring disruption fractures, hip dislocations, disruption of the sacroiliac joint, and fractures involving the acetabular portion of the pelvic ring. More recently, Shore et al. proposed a modification of the Torode and Zeig classification that subdivided type III injuries into type III-A (simple, stable anterior ring fractures) and type III-B (stable pelvic fractures involving the anterior and posterior ring). Shore et al. demonstrated that type III-B injuries were associated with increased blood product use, intensive care requirement, and length of hospital stay (Fig. 36-83).

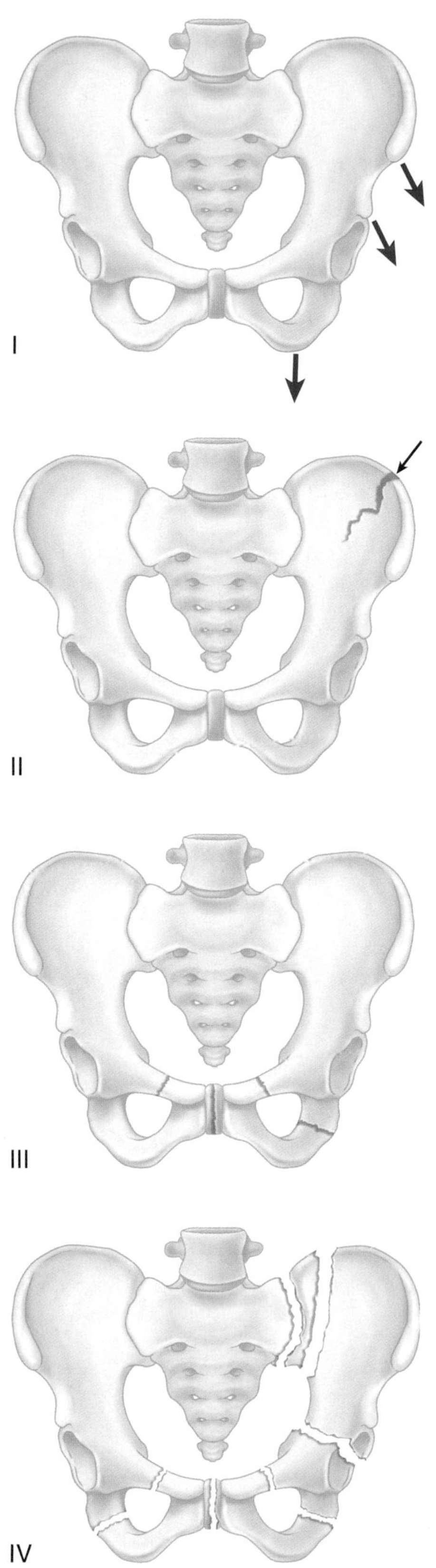

FIGURE 36-82 Torode and Zieg classification of pelvic fractures (see text).

This classification does not subdivide acetabular fractures. Quinby and Rang classified pelvic fractures into three categories: uncomplicated fractures, fractures with visceral injuries requiring surgical exploration, and fractures associated with immediate massive hemorrhage. Although this classification is useful concerning the patient's ultimate outcome, its emphasis is on associated soft-tissue injuries, rather than on the pelvic fracture itself. Moreno et al. described four types of "fracture geometry" based on radiographic appearance and used to identify patients at risk for severe hemorrhage. Adult classifications such as the AO/ASIF group and the Young and Burgess should be applied to a pelvis with a closed triradiate cartilage and emphasize fracture stability and direction of force: lateral compression, anteroposterior compression, vertical shear, and combined mechanisms (Fig. 36-84). Key and Conwell's classification of pelvic fractures in adults is based on the number of breaks in the pelvic ring. Their system, which includes acetabular fractures, also is applicable in children. We have evaluated 134 pelvic fractures in children; the percentages of the individual bones and types of fractures are given in Table 36-3. The Orthopaedic Trauma Association devised a classification scheme that consists of three main types and numerous subtypes: A, lesion sparing (or with no displacement of) posterior arch; B, incomplete disruption of posterior arch, partially stable; and C, complete disruption of posterior arch, unstable.

Comparison among studies using different systems is difficult. The most useful information is whether a fracture is stable or unstable. Most pelvic fractures in children are stable.

Three physical signs are commonly associated with pelvic fractures: (1) Destot sign, a large superficial hematoma formation beneath the inguinal ligament or in the scrotum; (2) Roux sign, a decrease in the distance of the greater trochanter to the pubic spine on the affected side in lateral compression fractures; and (3) Earle sign, a bony prominence or large hematoma and tenderness on rectal examination, indicating a significant pelvic fracture. Posterior pressure on the iliac crest causes pain at the fracture site as the pelvic ring is opened, and compression of the pelvic ring at the iliac crest from lateral to medial causes pain and possibly crepitation. Downward pressure on the symphysis pubis and posteriorly on the sacroiliac joints causes pain and motion if a break in the pelvic ring is present. Pain in the inguinal area can be elicited by flexion and extension of the hips.

As already noted most pelvic fractures in children can be treated closed, usually with protected weight bearing and activity restriction. Minor residual deformity usually is inconsequential and may remodel with growth. However, significant displacement or an unstable fracture pattern should be treated operatively. Occasionally, if the child is young and has significant diastasis of the symphysis, a spica cast alone may be used to maintain a reduced position during healing. In older children or those with unstable fracture patterns, the management of pelvic fractures should closely follow adult principles with surgical fixation that does not disrupt or alter the growth of the triradiate cartilage. If the triradiate cartilage is closed, operative techniques are the same as in adults (see Chapter 56).

AVULSION FRACTURES

Avulsion fractures occur most commonly in adolescent athletes; they occur in the anterior superior and anterior inferior

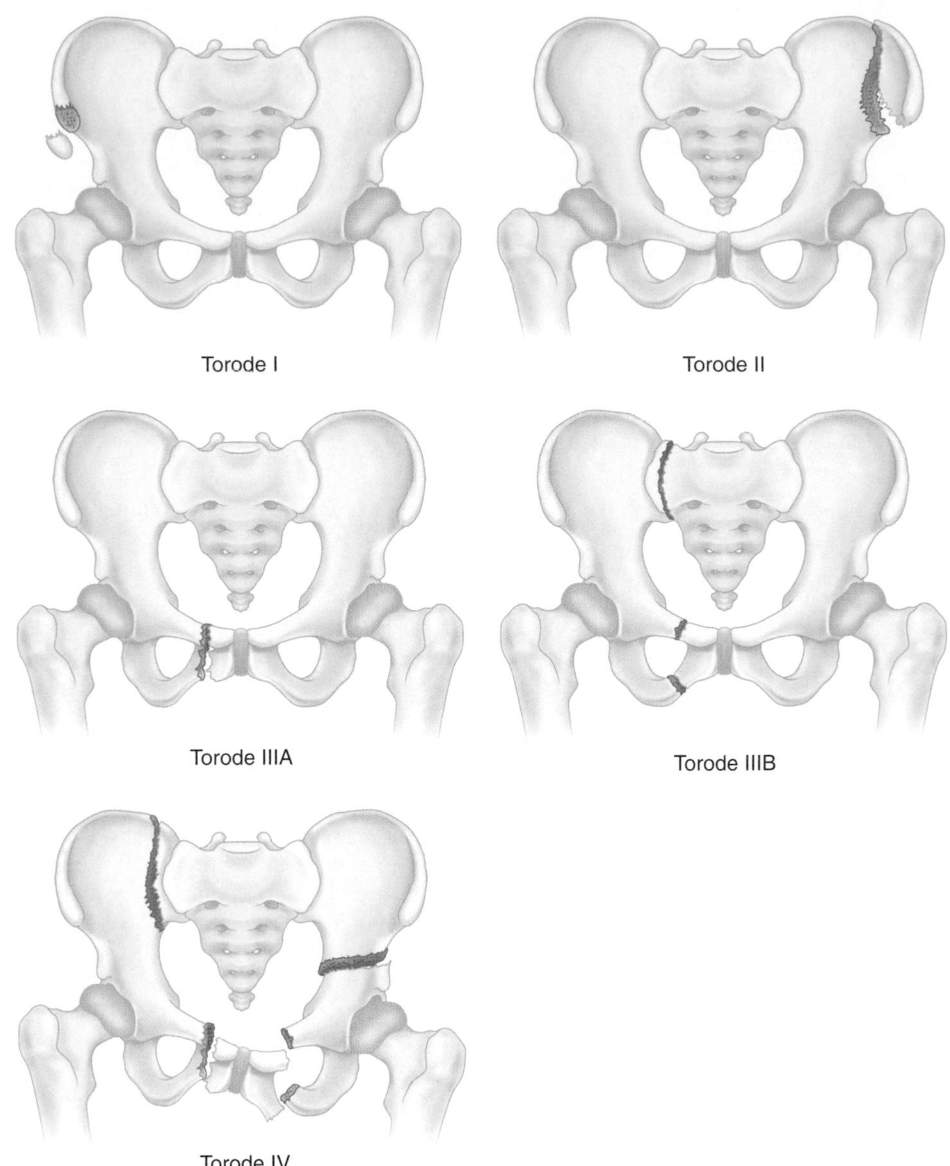

FIGURE 36-83 Shore et al. modification of Torode classification. *Torode I,* avulsion of bony elements of pelvis and separation through or adjacent to cartilaginous physis. *Torode II,* iliac wing fracture resulting from direct lateral force against pelvis causing disruption of iliac apophysis or infolding fracture of wing of ilium. *Torode IIIA,* simple stable anterior ring fracture involving pubic rami or pubic symphysis. *Torode IIIB,* stable anterior and posterior ring fracture. *Torode IV,* unstable ring disruption fracture, including ring disruptions, hip dislocations, and combined pelvic and acetabular fractures. (Redrawn from: Shore BJ, Palmer CS, Bevin C, et al: Pediatric pelvic fracture: a modification of a preexisting classification, J Pediatr Orthop 32:162, 2012.)

iliac spines and in the ischial tuberosity (Fig. 36-85) and are caused by overpull of the sartorius muscle, rectus femoris muscle, and hamstring muscles, respectively. CT scans are rarely required in this subset of pelvic injuries. Operative treatment of these injuries is rarely indicated, regardless of the amount of displacement. Rarely, excessive callus formation or myositis ossificans occurs after a displaced ischial tuberosity fracture. In two of our patients it was necessary to excise the fragment and the callus, rather than reattach the fragment. Recurrence of some excessive callus or myositis ossificans occurred, but these two patients have continued their athletic activity. Sundar and Carty described 32 avulsion fractures of the pelvis in adolescents (average age 13.8 years) seen at an average 44-month follow-up; 10 patients had disability persisting into adulthood and limitation of sports activity, and six patients continued to have persistent symptoms. Although they advocated surgical exploration and removal of ununited fragments, Sundar and Carty cautioned that operative treatment does not guarantee the return of the athlete to the same standard as before the injury. Any of these avulsion injuries, especially in the area of the ischium, can be confused with infection, myositis ossificans, and sarcoma.

TABLE 36-3

Distribution of Pelvic Fractures in Children, Campbell Clinic Series (134 Patients)

I—INDIVIDUAL BONES 66.5%				II—SINGLE BREAK 11.9%			III—DOUBLE BREAK 11.9%			IV—ACETABULUM 9.7%			
A	B	C	D	A	B	C	A	B	C	A	B	C	D
13.4%	33.6%	18%	1.5%	8.2%	3%	0.7%	3%	8.2%	0.7%	0.7%	6%	0	3%

COMPARISON WITH OTHER SERIES

	Dunn* (115 Patients)	Peltier* (186 Patients)	Reed* (84 Patients)	Hall, Klassen, Ilstrup† (204 Patients)	Campbell Clinic† (134 Patients)
I—Individual bones		10%	60.5%	24.5%	66.5%
II—Single break	70%	39%	2.5%	18.6%	11.9%
III—Double break	30%	27%	32%	31.9%	11.9%
IV—Acetabulum	Not included	24%	5%	7.8% (17.2% acetabulum and pelvis)	9.7%

Classification of Key and Conwell.
*Adult series.
†Children's series.
From Rockwood CA Jr, Wilkins KD, King RE, editors: Fractures in children, 3rd ed, Philadelphia, Lippincott, 1991.

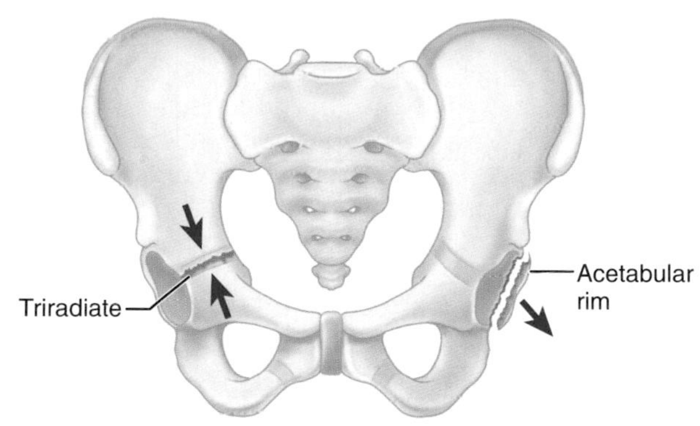

FIGURE 36-84 Small acetabular rim fracture and triradiate cartilage compression fracture.

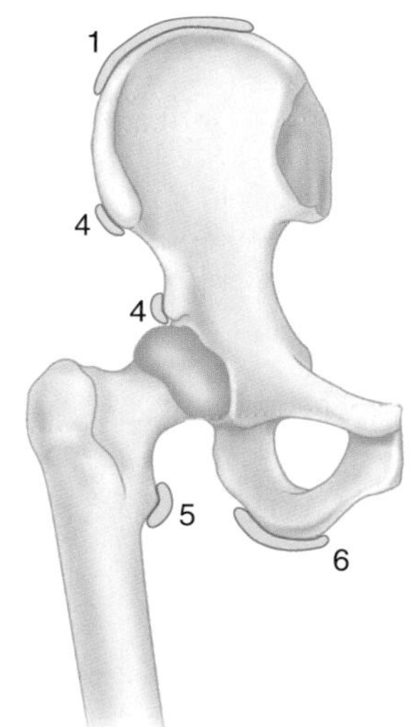

FIGURE 36-85 Distribution of 20 avulsion fractures in children reported by Fernbach and Wilkinson: iliac crest, 1; anterior superior iliac spine, 4; anterior inferior iliac spine, 4; lesser trochanter, 5; ischium or ischial apophysis, 6.

ACETABULAR FRACTURES

Acetabular fracture-dislocations in children make up 4% to 20% of pelvic fractures in the pediatric population. Damage to the triradiate cartilage in a child may cause growth arrest and a shallow, dysplastic acetabulum (Fig. 36-86). CT may help determine the extent of acetabular involvement and femoral head stability. However, in an immature pelvis, radiographs and CT may underestimate the extent of the injury; therefore MRI should be considered to evaluate the cartilaginous portion of the acetabulum, labrum, and triradiate cartilage. The Watts classification of acetabular fractures is based on the extent of acetabular involvement: (1) small fragments most often associated with dislocation of the hip (see Fig. 36-84), (2) linear fractures associated with pelvic fractures without displacement, (3) large linear fractures with hip joint instability, and (4) central fracture-dislocations.

Initial treatment should focus on a reduced hip joint. Hip reduction requires optimal sedation and muscle relaxation. Although this can be performed safely in the emergency department, many institutions prefer this maneuver to be done in the operating room to avoid femoral head displacement. It is important, however, for a dislocated hip to be reduced immediately to minimize further vascular insult to the femoral head. Hip stability should be assessed at the time of reduction, and radiographs of the contralateral hip should be obtained for comparison of joint congruency. Radiographs before reduction may reveal an occult fragment more readily than films taken after the reduction. If an incongruence is found or suspected, a CT should be performed with the possible addition of an MRI to evaluate the cause and for operative planning purposes.

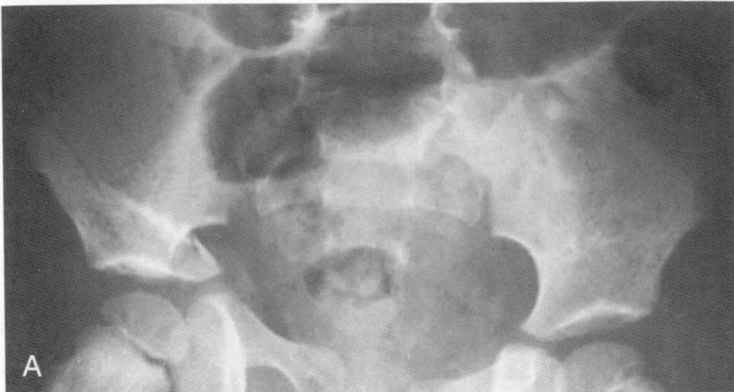

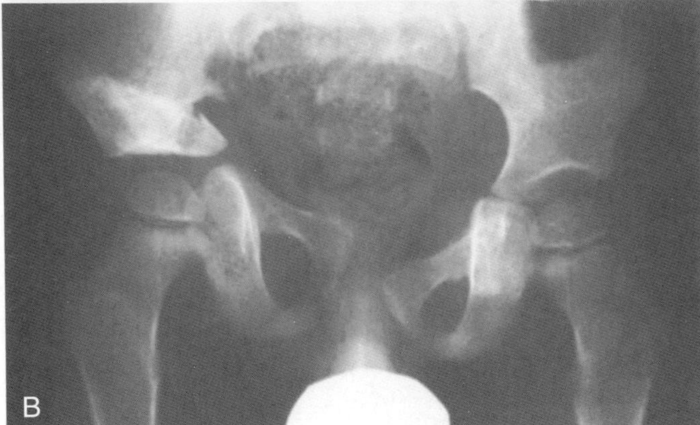

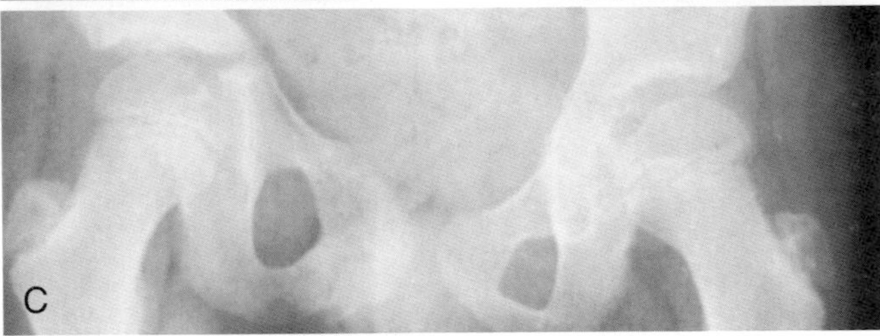

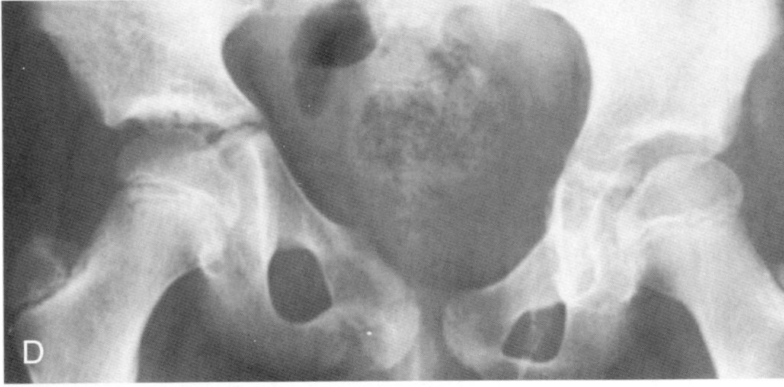

FIGURE 36-86 Premature closure of triradiate cartilage. **A,** Fracture of right ilium is visible. Fracture on left was not identified. **B,** At 4 months, fracture on right is seen again. At left, acetabulum shows increased sclerosis caused by ischial fracture into acetabulum. **C,** At 5 years, premature closure of left triradiate cartilage. **D,** At 6 years, premature closure of left triradiate cartilage and subluxation of femoral head caused by shallow acetabulum.

The treatment of many pediatric acetabular fractures is nonoperative. Stable linear fractures require only conservative treatment with a minimum of 6 to 8 weeks of non–weight bearing. Linear fractures producing hip joint instability often require a period of skeletal traction followed by definitive fixation to ensure an accurate reduction. This injury usually occurs in older children, and treatment should be the same as for adults. Central fracture-dislocations in children should be reduced promptly because the triradiate cartilage may be involved. Because injury to the triradiate cartilage is easily missed on initial radiographs, all patients with pelvic trauma should be followed clinically and radiographically for at least 1 year. Two main patterns of physeal disruption have been identified in patients with triradiate cartilage injuries: a Salter-Harris type I or II injury, which has a favorable prognosis for continued normal acetabular growth, and a Salter-Harris type V crushing injury, which has a poor prognosis because of premature closure of the triradiate physes secondary to formation of a medial osseous bridge (Fig. 36-87). In both patterns, the prognosis depends on the age of the patient at the time of injury. In young children, especially those younger than 10 years, abnormal acetabular growth can result in a shallow acetabulum. By skeletal maturity, disparate growth may increase the incongruity of the hip joint and lead to progressive subluxation. Acetabular reconstruction may be indicated for correction of the gradual subluxation of the femoral head with associated dysplasia.

HIP FRACTURES

Hip fractures include fractures of the head, neck, and intertrochanteric region of the femur and account for less than 1% of all pediatric and adolescent fractures. Different hip morphology and the presence of a physis produce hip fracture patterns that are different in children from those in adults. Complications of both the injury and treatment are frequent and should be considered during the treatment course. Late complications include osteonecrosis, coxa vara, nonunion, and premature physeal closure. Appropriate treatment of hip fractures in children is necessary to minimize these late complications. Diagnosis of a hip fracture is based on history, physical examination, and radiographs. Hip fractures in children most commonly result from a high-energy mechanism followed by pathologic fracture. As in adults, the index of suspicion for hip fracture should be high to facilitate urgent management. A standard anteroposterior radiograph of the pelvis and lateral of the hip should be obtained, as well as imaging of the entire femur. Advanced imaging may be helpful to rule out an occult injury or to evaluate the extent of the fracture.

The most widely used classification for hip fractures in the pediatric population was proposed by Delbet. This classification groups fractures according to their location: type I, transepiphyseal separations with or without dislocation of the femoral head from the acetabulum; type II, transcervical fractures, displaced and nondisplaced; type III, cervicotrochanteric fractures, displaced and nondisplaced; and type IV, intertrochanteric fractures (Fig. 36-88). The Delbet classification has proved to have prognostic value in regard to risk of osteonecrosis, healing rates, and malunion.

TYPE I, TRANSEPIPHYSEAL SEPARATIONS

Type I fractures occur when the epiphysis separates from the metaphysis. They are further subdivided into type IA, in which the epiphysis remains in the acetabulum, and type IB, in which the epiphysis is dislocated from the acetabulum. In our experience, the outcomes after type IB fractures have

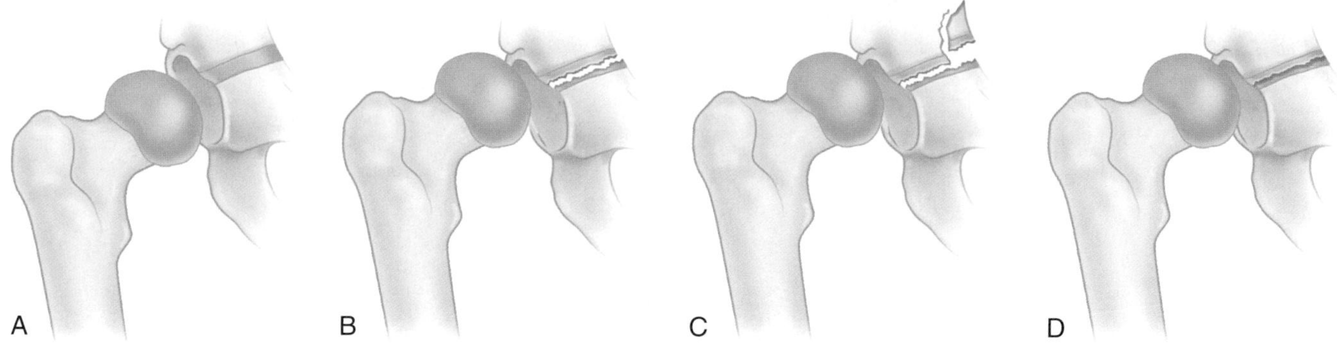

FIGURE 36-87 Types of injuries to the pelvis and triradiate cartilage. **A,** Normal hemipelvis. **B,** Salter-Harris type I fracture. **C,** Salter-Harris type II fracture. **D,** Salter-Harris type V fracture.

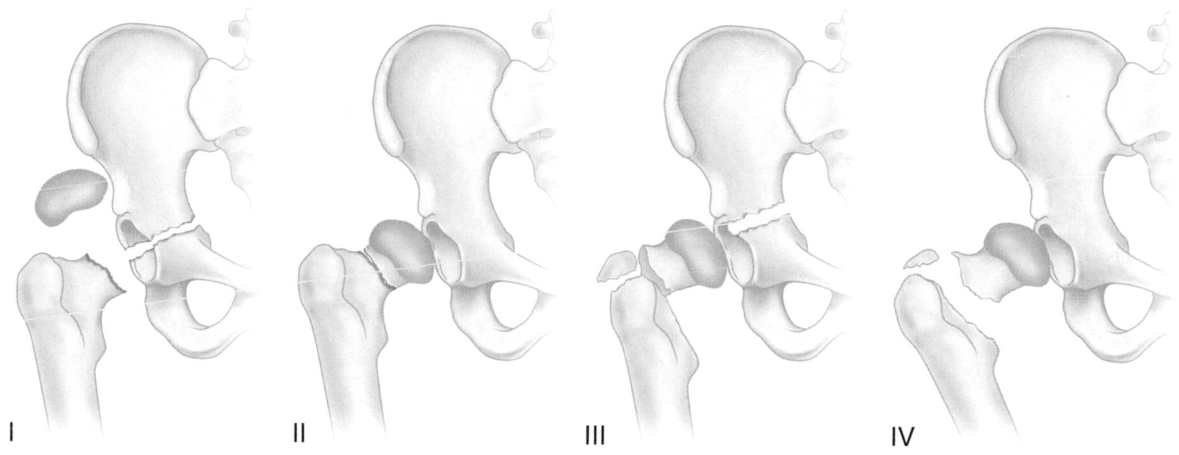

FIGURE 36-88 Delbet classification of hip fractures in children. Type I, transepiphyseal, with or without dislocation from acetabulum. Type II, transcervical. Type III, cervicotrochanteric (basicervical). Type IV, intertrochanteric.

been the worst of any of the fracture types, with an incidence of osteonecrosis of 100% in some series. Type 1A fractures may be difficult to differentiate from an unstable slipped capital femoral epiphysis (SCFE). Fractures tend to occur in younger children as the result of high-energy mechanisms, whereas SCFE is mostly seen in patients between the ages of 10 to 16 years after minor or no trauma. The presence of posterior medial callus on imaging or at the time of surgical fixation suggests that the transphyseal separation is the result of SCFE and is present in most patients with SCFE even in the absence of prodromal symptoms.

In newborns, an entity called *proximal femoral epiphysiolysis* occasionally occurs in which the physis separates probably at birth. If not considered, it may be confused with congenital dislocation or infection of the hip. Ultrasound, arthrography, or MRI is generally necessary to make the diagnosis early. At approximately 2 weeks after the separation, callus may be seen along the medial border of the femoral neck. Operative treatment with internal fixation is not needed for this separation. Clinical signs, such as pseudoparalysis of the lower extremity, and laboratory studies should aid in differentiating proximal femoral epiphysiolysis from infection.

The management of transepiphyseal separations depends on the age of the patient, displacement of the fracture, and presence of a dislocated epiphysis. All type I fractures should be managed urgently to minimize the vascular insult sustained by the injury (Figs. 36-89 and 36-90). In children younger than 2 years with a nondisplaced or minimally displaced fracture, spica cast application alone may be sufficient. If the fracture is displaced at any age and the epiphysis is located within the acetabulum, we advocate a gentle closed reduction attempt with fixation. Smooth pins are used in young patients and cannulated screws in older patients. An arthrogram may help evaluate the quality of the reduction in young patients. We routinely perform a capsulotomy to evacuate the hemarthrosis, although evidence is inconclusive that this decreases the incidence of osteonecrosis. If a gentle closed reduction does not yield a satisfactory reduction, then an open reduction should be performed through a Watson-Jones or Smith-Peterson approach (see Techniques 1-62 and 1-63), Alternatively, a surgical dislocation approach may be used; however, we have used this technique only in the setting of delayed fixation with the presence of early callus formation or in the presence of femoral head fracture. If the epiphysis is displaced from the acetabulum, a posterior approach (modified Gibson, Technique 1-68) is preferred for posterior displacement and an anterior approach (Watson-Jones or Smith-Peterson) for anterior displacement. Fixation typically

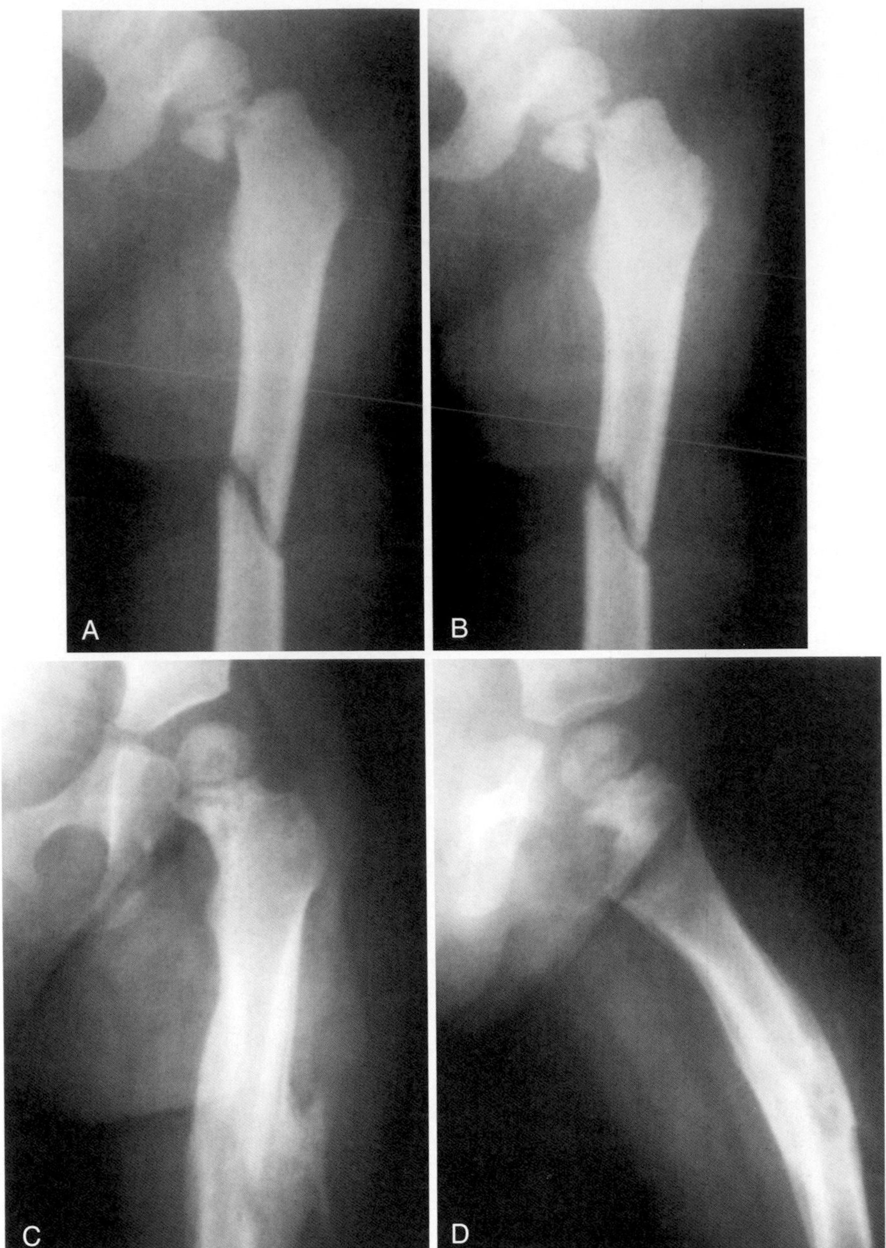

FIGURE 36-89 **A,** Type I transepiphyseal separation in 3-year-old child (with metaphyseal spike – Salter-Harris type II). **B,** Separation treated with distal femoral skeletal traction because of ipsilateral femoral fracture and to avoid crossing physis with pins in young child. **C** and **D,** At follow-up, remodeling of fracture with physis still open; patient had good range of motion.

is obtained with two or three cannulated screws. Again, smooth pins should be used in very young children to minimize the risk of premature physeal closure.

TYPE II, TRANSCERVICAL FRACTURES

Transcervical fractures are the most common hip fractures in children. Most of these are displaced, and the amount of displacement seems to be directly related to the development of osteonecrosis. We believe that displacement of the fracture is the leading variable in vascular insufficiency and that the maximal amount of displacement probably occurs at the time of injury. Capsular distention and subsequent tamponade of the vessels have been suggested to increase the incidence of osteonecrosis, and evacuation of the hematoma early by aspiration or capsular release and early internal fixation have been recommended to decrease the rate of osteonecrosis. In one report of 70 femoral neck fractures in children, however, early ORIF of type II fractures still resulted in an incidence of osteonecrosis of 35%. Type II fractures have an increased risk of varus malunion, hardware failure, and physeal arrest than more distal fractures. Internal fixation is recommended for all transcervical and basicervical fractures because of their inherent instability. A gentle closed reduction, similar to that for adult femoral neck fractures, should be done with longitudinal traction, abduction, and internal rotation, followed by fixation with pins or cannulated hip screws. Multiple closed

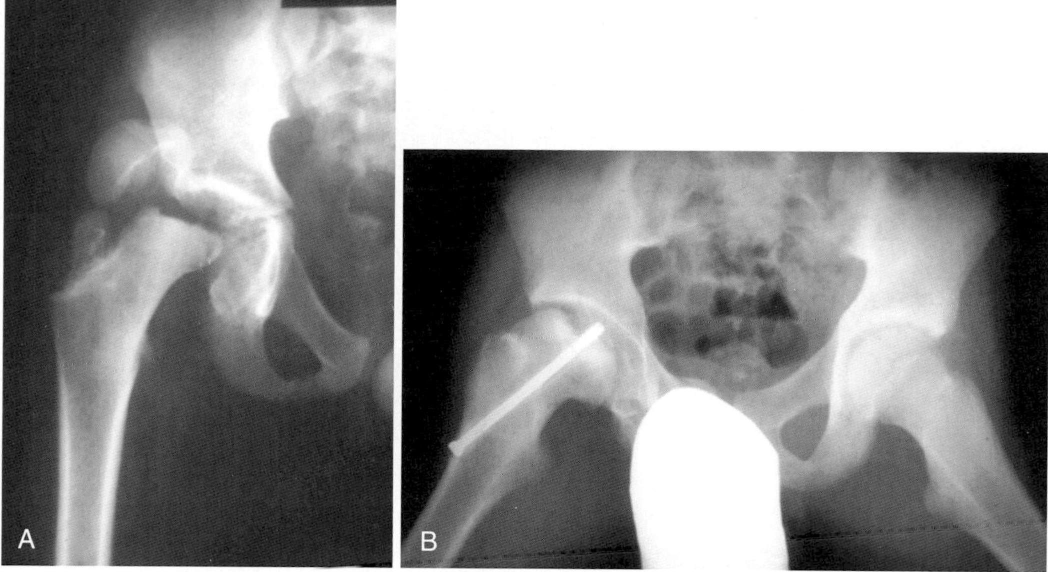

FIGURE 36-90 **A,** Type I, transepiphyseal separation with dislocation of the femoral head. **B,** Development of osteonecrosis after open reduction and fixation.

reduction attempts should be avoided. For unsatisfactory closed reductions, open reduction through an anterior Watson-Jones approach or Smith-Peterson approach is used. Percutaneous screw placement can be done with the use of an image intensifier, and a capsulotomy should be performed. The head and neck of a child's femur are extremely hard, and the use of triflanged nails or other similar devices should be avoided for fear of distraction of the fracture and possible separation of the capital femoral epiphysis. In small children, two or three pins may suffice but should be backed up with a spica cast. We routinely use two or three cannulated screws with the largest diameter that the femoral neck will accommodate. Alternatively, a pediatric or adolescent hip screw or proximal femoral locking plate may be used for basicervical fractures. Swiontkowski and Winquist recommended 4.5-mm AO cortical screws inserted short of the physis and overdrilled in the proximal fragment for a lag effect. In young children, we try to avoid crossing the physis with fixation; however, in older children or when additional stability is required, fixation is advanced across the physis. Postfixation SCFE has been reported when fixation abuts the proximal femoral physis. The priority of treatment should be achieving stable fixation instead of preservation of growth because the sequelae of failed fixation or osteonecrosis are more challenging problems than subsequent growth arrest. A spica cast with the hip in abduction is used for 6 weeks for patients with questionable fixation, young age, or questionable compliance.

TYPE III, CERVICOTROCHANTERIC FRACTURES

Type III fractures (cervicotrochanteric) are similar to fractures occurring at the base of the femoral neck in adults, although osteonecrosis after this fracture in children is more common than in adults (Fig. 36-91). A fracture in this location often allows for more stable fixation without crossing the physis; however, nonunion, malunion, premature physeal closure, and hardware failure can still occur in this subset of patients. Treatment is recommended as for type II fractures.

TYPE IV, INTERTROCHANTERIC FRACTURES

In our experience, type IV fractures (intertrochanteric) result in fewer complications than the other types. Because of the child's osteogenic potential in the trochanteric area, rapid union almost always occurs, usually within 6 to 8 weeks (Fig. 36-92). These fractures are generally extracapsular, making osteonecrosis less common, with a reported incidence of 0% to 10%.

Because intertrochanteric fractures are extracapsular, they are not treated with the same sense of urgency. However, the quality of the fracture reduction and stability of the fixation are still important to preserve the biomechanics of the hip and optimize healing. In children 3 years of age and younger, nondisplaced fractures may be treated with spica cast application alone. In the presence of displacement or age older than 3 years, internal fixation is recommended. Reduction and fixation are achieved through a lateral approach to the hip and placement of a pediatric or adolescent compressive hip screw or proximal femoral locking plate. Fixation does not need to cross the physis, and a capsulotomy does not need to be routinely performed. Stronger implants often allow for early motion without cast immobilization; however, a spica cast is recommended if noncompliance is a concern.

COMPLICATIONS

Complications after femoral neck fractures are frequent. The most serious complication of hip fractures in children is osteonecrosis. As Trueta described, the blood supply to the femoral head transitions from metaphyseal during infancy toward the lateral epiphyseal vessels during childhood with the formation of the physis, which acts as a barrier for metaphyseal blood supply. During preadolescence the artery of the ligamentum teres anastomoses to the lateral epiphyseal

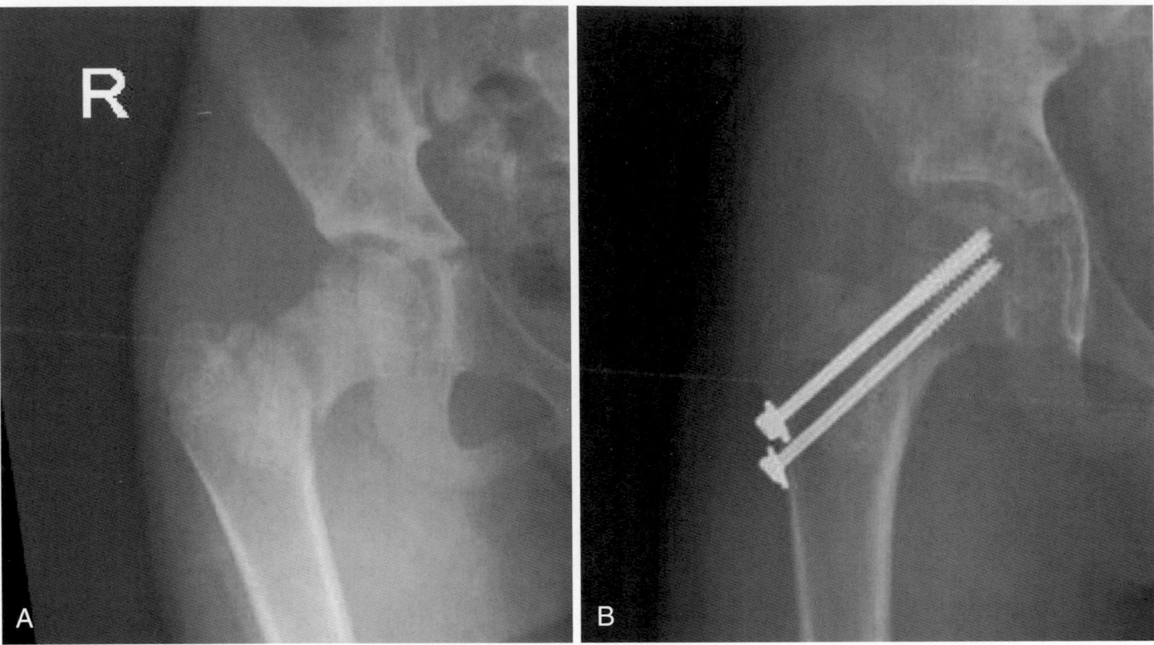

FIGURE 36-91 A, Displaced type III (cervicotrochanteric) fracture in a 6-year-old child. B, After closed reduction, capsular decompression, and fixation across the physis for additional stability.

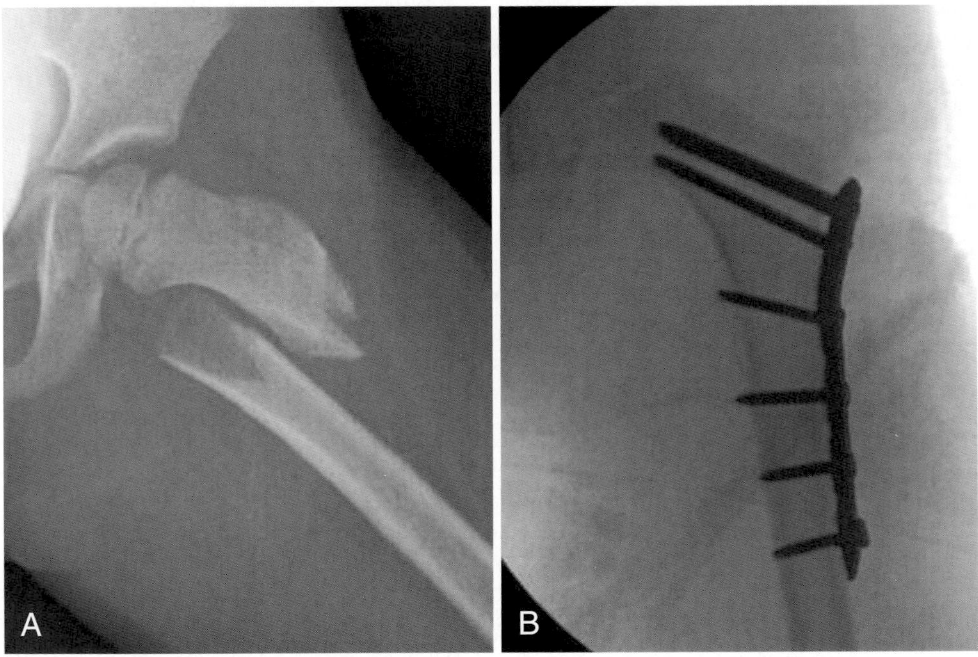

FIGURE 36-92 A, Type IV (intertrochanteric) fracture in a 5-year-old child. B, After fixation with proximal femoral locking plate.

vessels, and finally in late adolescence and into adulthood, the metaphyseal blood supply is restored. Osteonecrosis has been demonstrated to directly correlate with worse outcomes after femoral neck fractures. Spence et al. reviewed 70 femoral neck fractures at a single institution and found an overall incidence of osteonecrosis of 29%. The only independent predictors of osteonecrosis were displacement and fracture location. Yeranosian et al. reviewed 30 studies and found an overall incidence of 23%, with the fracture location and timing of reduction being the only predictors. Moon and Melhman reviewed 390 patients as part of a meta-analysis and found fracture type and patient age to be the strongest predictors of osteonecrosis, with rates of osteonecrosis of 38% for type I fractures, 28% for type II fractures, 18% for type III fractures, and 5% for type IV fractures.

Ratliff described three types of osteonecrosis: type I, whole head involvement; type II, partial head involvement; and type III, an area of osteonecrosis from the fracture line to the physis

(Fig. 36-93). Although osteonecrosis usually is diagnosed radiographically within 12 months of injury, it may not be clinically evident for several years. The prognosis and treatment options for osteonecrosis depend on the extent of the osteonecrosis, the degree of deformity and collapse, and the age at which symptoms begin (Fig. 36-94). In general, restricted weight bearing has not produced acceptable results in the treatment of osteonecrosis; reports in the literature indicate that it is successful in fewer than 25% of patients. Operative treatment options include core decompression, with or without cancellous bone grafting; nonvascularized and vascularized bone grafting (see Chapter 63); various osteotomies to rotate the necrotic segment of the femoral head out of the weight-bearing area; and even resurfacing or total hip arthroplasty in older adolescents. Some preliminary reports indicate that the addition of osteoinductive or angiogenic factors may improve the results of core decompression.

Coxa vara occurs less often when internal fixation is used. In our experience, if the neck-shaft angle is more than 120 degrees in a young child, remodeling will occur to some degree, and even if not the deformity causes little disability. If the neck-shaft angle is between 100 and 110 degrees, however, the coxa vara deformity generally does not remodel. Significant coxa vara causes a shortened extremity and an abductor or gluteal lurch and delayed degenerative joint changes. For these reasons we have routinely used a subtrochanteric valgus osteotomy for persistent coxa vara deformity and for nonunion (Fig. 36-95). A closing wedge osteotomy just distal to the greater trochanter, using a pediatric lag screw with a side plate or proximal femoral locking plate for internal fixation, is preferred. Although nonunion of the osteotomy is

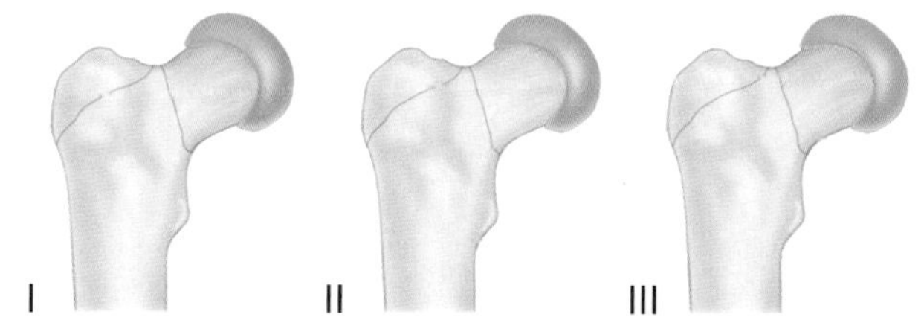

FIGURE 36-93 Three types of osteonecrosis described by Ratliff. Type I, total head involvement. Type II, segmental involvement. Type III involvement from fracture line to physis.

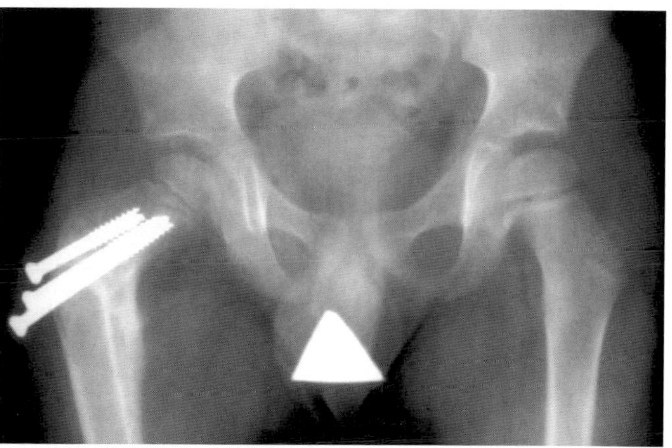

FIGURE 36-95 Coxa vara deformity after type III fracture. Fixed angle locking plates can be used to minimize the risk of coxa vara.

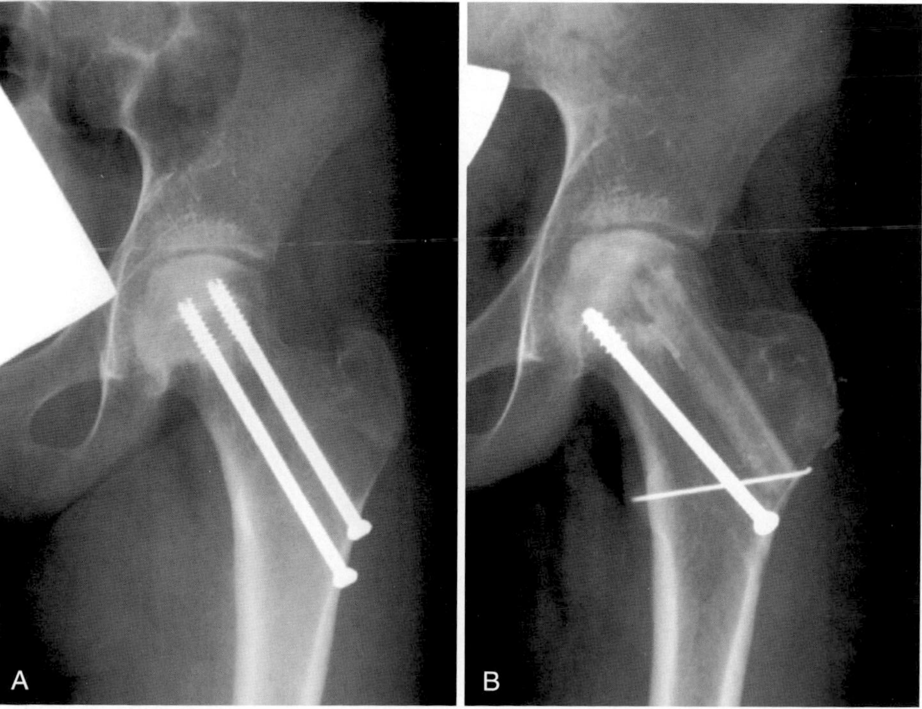

FIGURE 36-94 **A,** Osteonecrosis after type III fracture in an 11-year-old girl. The fracture was treated with urgent open reduction and internal fixation and capsular decompression. **B,** One year after vascularized fibular grafting.

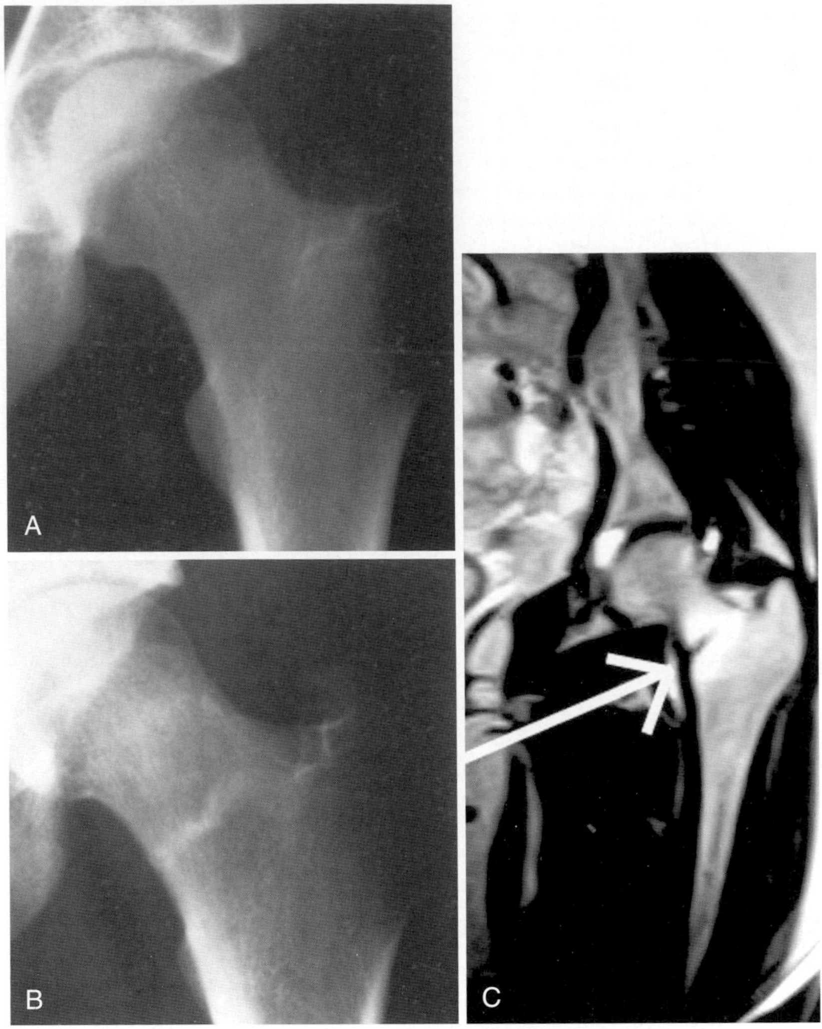

FIGURE 36-96 Stress fracture of femoral neck. **A,** Radiograph showing possible faint inferior femoral neck fracture. **B,** Radiograph made 3 weeks later revealing callus formation in inferior neck at stress fracture. **C,** MR image shows stress fracture.

rare, a one and one-half spica cast may be applied if there are concerns about the quality of the fixation or compliance of the patient.

Internal fixation also decreases the rate of nonunion, but when nonunion occurs, operative treatment should be undertaken as soon as possible. We have used a valgus subtrochanteric osteotomy to make the nonunion more horizontal and allow compressive vertical forces to aid in union. This osteotomy can be augmented, if necessary, with bone grafts. Internal fixation is routinely used across the nonunion site, with or without the use of a spica cast. A modification of the Pauwels intertrochanteric osteotomy using a 120-degree double-angle osteotomy plate has been described for the treatment of nonunion or coxa vara or both (see Technique 36-21).

Although premature physeal closure can occur, because the capital femoral physis contributes 15% of the growth of the entire lower extremity and normally closes earlier than most of the other lower extremity physes, shortening generally is less than 2 cm. The discrepancy usually is more than 2 cm only in children in whom osteonecrosis also develops. Nevertheless, we try to avoid penetrating the physis, especially in a young child. Leg-length inequality should be determined with scanograms and correlated with bone age and carefully recorded. Epiphysiodesis in the opposite extremity can be done if necessary.

Infection is uncommon after hip fractures in children. Chondrolysis after hip fractures in children has been reported, but most investigators have not found this complication.

Stress fractures of the femoral neck can occur in children, especially in adolescents. Devas noted two types: (1) a transverse type in the superior portion of the femoral neck, which may become displaced and cause severe morbidity, and (2) a compression stress fracture in the inferior portion of the femoral neck, which rarely becomes displaced, although mild varus deformity has occurred in young patients (Fig. 36-96). Internal fixation with a screw or pin is recommended for the transverse type, whereas the compression type may be treated by non–weight bearing and limitation of the child's activity; however, a stress fracture can progress to a complete fracture if proper treatment is not begun and the child is allowed to continue the same activity. The technique for closed reduction and percutaneous pin or screw fixation is described in the section on slipped capital femoral epiphysis (SCFE) (see Technique 36-23).

CLOSED REDUCTION AND INTERNAL FIXATION

TECHNIQUE 36-18

- Place the child supine on a fracture table and place the appropriately padded feet in the traction stirrups.
- Perform a gentle closed reduction by applying longitudinal traction, abduction, and internal rotation. Check the reduction with anteroposterior and lateral radiographs or with an image intensifier.
- With the use of an image intensifier, make a stab wound percutaneously or a small incision just distal to the greater trochanter and dissect through the fascia lata. Reflect the vastus lateralis anteriorly, exposing the proximal femoral shaft. Elevate the periosteum and place reverse retractors around the proximal femur to aid in exposure.
- With an image intensifier, determine the correct placement for a guide pin in the lateral shaft of the femur. Drill a guide pin across the fracture site and proximally into the femoral neck. In young children, avoid penetrating the physis, if possible. Verify the correct position of the guide pin with the image intensifier.
- Measure the exact length of the portion of the guide pin in the bone. Drill a pin or a cannulated hip screw the same length as the measured length of the guide pin parallel to or over it across the fracture site.
- Remove the guide pin and place a second pin or cannulated screw parallel to the first through the guide pin hole. Use a minimum of two pins or one 6.5-mm cannulated screw. We generally use three pins or two 6.5-mm cannulated screws, depending on the size of the child and the femoral neck. Place the pins or screws parallel and in a "cluster" formation.
- Close the incision and apply a one and one-half spica cast with the hip in the abducted position.

POSTOPERATIVE CARE. The spica cast is worn for 6 weeks. The patient progresses to weight bearing on crutches during the next 6 weeks. The pins or screws may be removed at l year when the fracture has united or when there is evidence of osteonecrosis.

OPEN REDUCTION AND INTERNAL FIXATION

TECHNIQUE 36-19

(WEBER ET AL., BOITZY)

- Place the patient supine and drape the limb so that it can be moved freely during the operation.
- Use a Watson-Jones approach to the hip joint (see Technique 1-63).
- Incise the hip joint capsule longitudinally and evacuate and flush out the hematoma, which usually is under pressure.
- Reduce the fracture with a periosteal elevator. This can be made easier by appropriate traction and internal rotation of the extremity.
- Temporarily stabilize the fracture with Kirschner wires and check the reduction in the region of the calcar. Fix the fracture permanently with cancellous screws fitted with washers. The screw threads should be in the proximal fragment only and not across the physis of the femoral head unless needed for fixation.
- Confirm the reduction radiographically and close the hip capsule.

An anterior approach, such as the Watson-Jones, can be used for displaced type II and III fractures and for type I transepiphyseal separations when the femoral head is dislocated from the acetabulum anteriorly. If the femoral head is dislocated posteriorly, a modified Gibson approach (see Technique 1-68) is used. The femoral head may be devoid of all blood supply. It should be replaced in the acetabulum, however, ensuring there are no cartilaginous or osseous fragments in the joint, and fixed to the femoral neck with cancellous screws.

POSTOPERATIVE CARE. If internal fixation is stable, touch-down weight bearing on crutches is maintained for 6 weeks. If stability is questionable, a spica cast or a long leg cast with a pelvic band should be used for 6 weeks.

VALGUS SUBTROCHANTERIC OSTEOTOMY FOR ACQUIRED COXA VARA OR NONUNION

TECHNIQUE 36-20

- Place the patient on a fracture table with an image intensifier or radiographic equipment in place to obtain anteroposterior and lateral radiographs. Prepare and drape the hip in the usual fashion. If bone grafts are to be used, prepare and drape the iliac crest also.
- Make a straight lateral longitudinal incision beginning at the greater trochanter and extending distally for 8 to 10 cm. Carry the dissection down to the lateral aspect of the femur. Elevate the periosteum and insert reverse retractors around the femur subperiosteally to expose the lateral aspect of the bone.
- Determine preoperatively the amount of valgus necessary to align the hip properly by comparing radiographs with those of the contralateral hip. We have used trigonometric functions to evaluate the effect of proximal femoral osteotomy. If a varus or a valgus osteotomy is performed in the subtrochanteric or trochanteric area, the length of the femoral head and neck fragment does not change; only the angles and the leg length change (Fig. 36-97). The amount of change in leg length can be computed by determining the change in the two angles. The change in leg length (ΔH) is equal to the length of the point from the middle of the osteotomy site to the middle of the

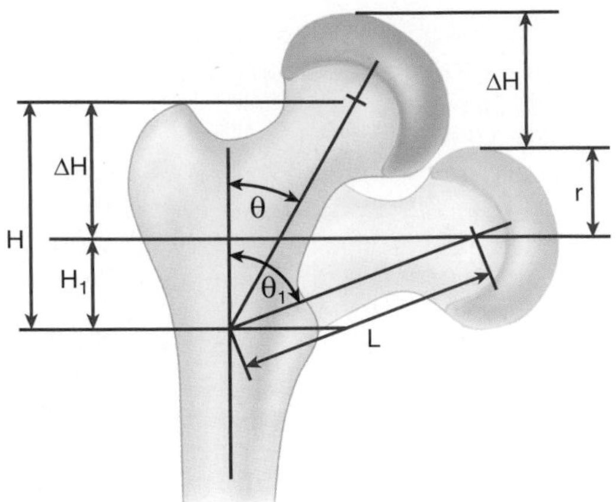

FIGURE 36-97 Illustration of constant head-neck length *L*, change in angles θ to θ_1, and ultimately change in height, ΔH. Formula is used to determine change in height; H = head-neck segment; $H_1 = L \cos \theta_1$; $\Delta H = L(\cos \theta_1 - \cos \theta)$. **SEE TECHNIQUE 36-20.**

femoral head *(L)* times the cosine of one angle minus the cosine of the new angle:

$$\Delta H = L(\cos\theta_1 - \cos\theta)$$

Going from a varus position to a valgus position increases the leg length and, conversely, going from a valgus position to a varus position decreases the leg length, or ΔH. The original angle is given for femoral head-neck segments of 2, 3, and 4 cm. The estimated increase or decrease in leg length is given for the "desired angle" obtained by a varus or valgus osteotomy.

- When the angle of correction is determined, the appropriate laterally based closing wedge osteotomy can be determined. First determine the diameter of the bone by drilling a guide pin transversely through the femur. Determine the correct size of the wedge by using a template, tangent tables (W = tangent of the angle × the diameter), or the formula $W = 0.02 \times$ diameter × angle. Outline the appropriate closing wedge osteotomy in the subtrochanteric area.
- After preparation of the osteotomy site, attention should be turned to placement of an intermediate hip compression screw or proximal femoral locking plate. Drill a hole just distal to the greater trochanter and check its placement with the image intensifier. Place an appropriate guide pin of the proper length in the femoral neck with the aid of an adjustable angle guide (Fig. 36-98A and B). If the child is young, avoid crossing the physis if possible. If the nonunion is proximal, crossing the physis may be necessary to gain union. The proximal femoral physis contributes 30% to the growth of the femur and only 15% to the entire lower extremity. Often it is preferable to obtain union of the femoral neck and manage about minor to moderate leg-length inequality afterward. Check the placement of the guide pin with image intensification.
- After the guide pin is placed, use a percutaneous direct measuring gauge to determine the lag screw length. Set the adjustable positive stop on the combination reamer for the lag screw length determined by a percutaneous direct measuring gauge. Place the reamer over the guide pin and ream until the positive stop reaches the lateral cortex (Fig. 36-98C). It is prudent to check the fluoroscopic image periodically during reaming to ensure that the guide pin is not inadvertently advancing proximally into the epiphysis.
- Set the adjustable positive stop on the lag screw tap to the same length that was reamed. Tap until the positive stop reaches the lateral cortex. Screw the appropriate intermediate compression screw over the guide pin (Fig. 36-98D and E).
- Take the plate chosen during preoperative planning and insert its barrel over the barrel guide and onto the back of the lag screw. The plate angle ultimately determines the final hip angle. Remove the barrel guide and insert a compression screw to prevent the plate from disengaging during the reduction maneuver. Use the slotted screwdriver for the pediatric compression screw or the hex screwdriver for the intermediate compression screw. If the plate obscures the osteotomy site, loosen the screw and rotate the side plate.
- Make the appropriate angled osteotomy using a power saw, remove the wedge, and align the two fragments.
- Reduce the osteotomy and secure the plate to the femur using the plate clamp. Check the rotational position of the lower extremity in extension.
- To achieve compression, insert a drill or tap guide into the distal portion of the most distal compression slot. Drill through the medial cortex. If less compression is required, follow the same steps detailed previously in the distal portion of the second or third distal slots for 2.5 mm of compression.
- Select the appropriate-length bone screw and insert it using the hex screwdriver. Use the self-holding sleeve to keep the screw from disengaging from the screwdriver (Fig. 36-98F). Finally, in the most proximal slot, the intermediate combination drill/tap guide can be angled proximally so that the drill and, ultimately, the bone screw cross the osteotomy line. Positioning the proximal bone screw in this way can provide additional stability at the osteotomy site. Insert screws into any remaining screw holes.
- The lag screw can be inserted farther to apply compression across the nonunion. To insert the lag screw for approximately 5 mm of compression, stop when the lateral cortex is midway between the two depth calibrations (Fig. 36-98G). To insert the lag screw for approximately 10 mm of compression, stop when the second depth calibration meets the lateral cortex (Fig. 36-98H).
- Close the wound in layers. Insert a suction drainage tube and apply a one and one-half spica cast with the hip in 30 to 40 degrees of abduction.
- For fixation of a nonunion, the intermediate compression hip screw should cross the nonunion site. The nonunion seems to heal better if it is made more horizontal by placing the hip in a valgus position at the subtrochanteric osteotomy site. The fibrous tissue need not be removed from the nonunion. A cancellous or cortical bone graft placed across the nonunion site may be helpful in older

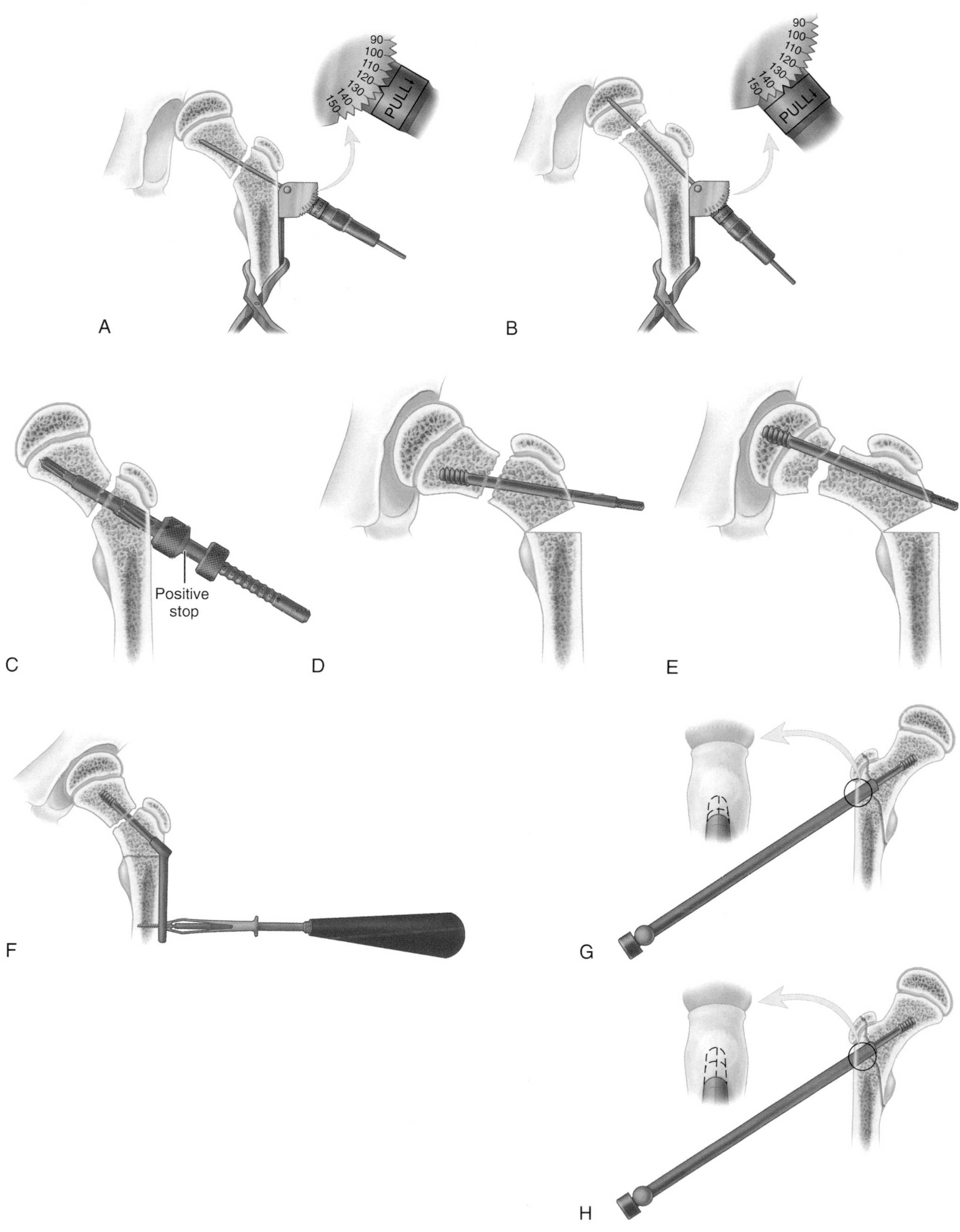

FIGURE 36-98 **A-H,** Technique for insertion of intermediate compression screw. **SEE TECHNIQUE 36-20.**

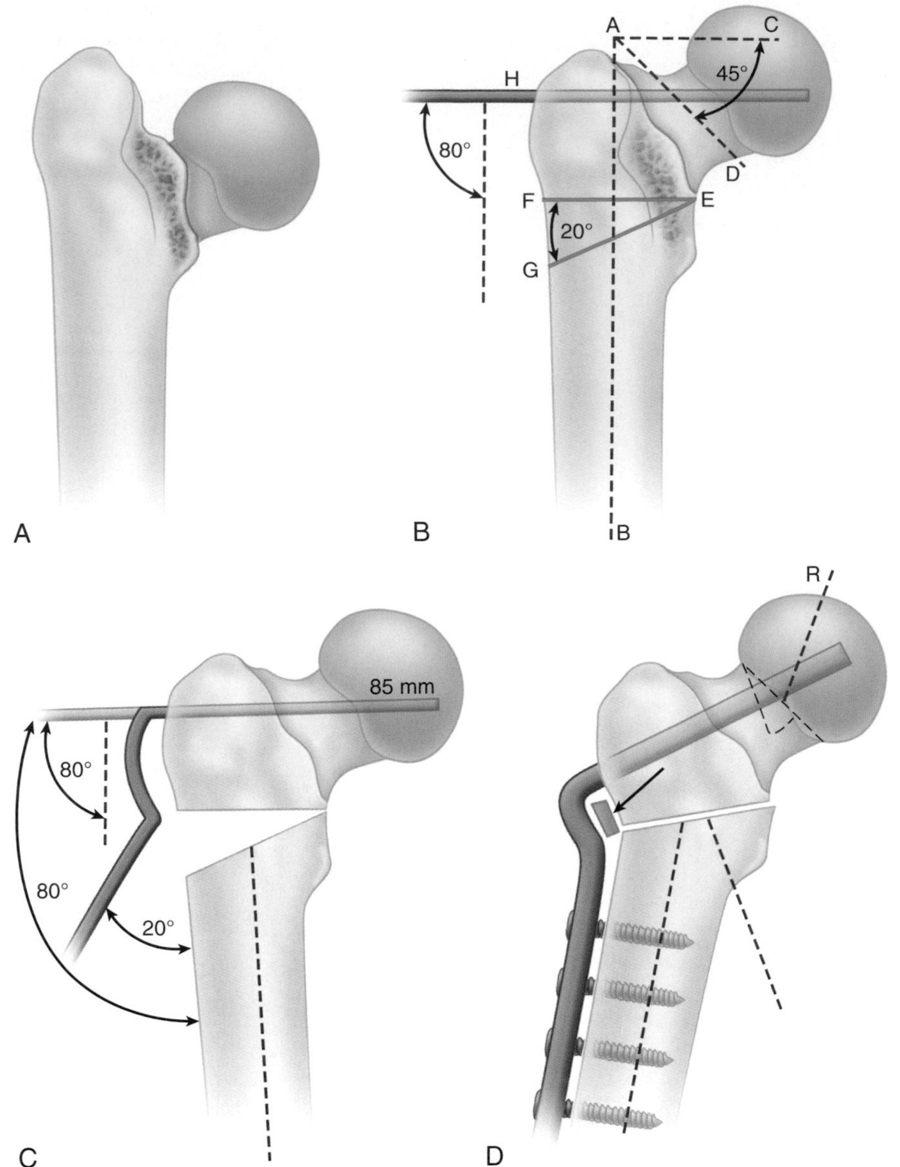

FIGURE 36-99 **A-D, Modified Pauwels intertrochanteric osteotomy for acquired coxa vara or nonunion.** (Redrawn from Magu NK, Rohilla R, Singh R, Tater R: Modified Pauwels' intertrochanteric osteotomy in neglected femoral neck fracture, Clin Orthop Relat Res 467:1064, 2009.) **SEE TECHNIQUE 36-21.**

children. The graft is inserted by drilling a hole the size of the graft up through the femoral neck adjacent and parallel to the fixation device. Care should be taken not to loosen the device. A cortical graft from the tibia or fibula can be used, but we prefer cancellous bone from the iliac crest. We have not used bone graft routinely in this procedure. In younger children with good internal fixation, making the nonunion more horizontal has been all that is necessary. A smaller version of the compression hip screw is available for younger patients.

POSTOPERATIVE CARE. The spica cast should be worn for approximately 12 weeks, depending on the age of the child. When the cast is removed, touch-down weight bearing on crutches is begun.

MODIFIED PAUWELS INTERTROCHANTERIC OSTEOTOMY FOR ACQUIRED COXA VARA OR NONUNION

TECHNIQUE 36-21

(MAGU ET AL.)

- On a tracing of a radiograph of the normal hip, determine the correct point of entry of the chisel for seating of the blade in the femoral neck, the appropriate blade length, the osteotomy line, and the appropriate intertrochanteric wedge (Fig. 36-99A and B). In a patient with open physes, make sure the blade length chosen avoids penetration of the proximal femoral physis.

- Contour a semi-tubular plate into a 120-degree double-angle plate (Fig. 36-99C).
- Attempt closed reduction through skeletal traction (if a proximal tibial pin is already in place) or manual traction.
- With image intensifier guidance, make a standard lateral approach to the hip joint and provisionally stabilize the hip with two 2-mm Kirschner wires to prevent rotation of the femoral head when the seating chisel is used to create a track for the implant blade.
- Make the two osteotomy cuts as determined on the normal hip radiograph to create a laterally based 15- to 30-degree intertrochanteric wedge of bone (Fig. 36-99B). Remove this wedge of bone to place the femoral head into a valgus position as defined by preoperative planning.
- Insert the seating chisel through the previously determined entry point, keeping the flap of the chisel parallel to the femoral shaft. Advance the chisel into the inferior half of the femoral neck for a length equal to that of the blade length of a 120-degree contoured osteotomy plate (usually 65 mm).
- Remove the chisel and insert the blade portion of the osteotomy plate into its track (Fig. 36-99C).
- Abduct the distal fragment to close the osteotomy and stabilize the plate to the femur with screws (Fig. 36-99D).

POSTOPERATIVE CARE. A hip spica cast is worn for 6 to 10 weeks, depending on the healing of the osteotomy. The cast is removed, and touch-down weight bearing on crutches is begun, followed by graduated partial and full weight bearing between 12 and 20 weeks.

TRAUMATIC HIP DISLOCATIONS

Traumatic hip dislocations in children are more common than hip fractures, although they are also rare. Trivial injury may cause a hip dislocation in young children primarily because their immature cartilage is pliable and their ligaments are lax. The reported age distribution of traumatic hip dislocations has varied among authors, with some suggesting that over half occur between the ages of 12 and 15 years, some reporting no peak age group, and some identifying two distinct groups: children 2 to 5 years old and children 11 to 15 years old. As in adults, posterior dislocations are more common than anterior ones. Factors that influence the ultimate result after dislocations of the hip are (1) the severity of the injury, (2) the interval between injury and reduction, (3) the type of treatment, (4) the period of non–weight bearing, (5) whether recurrent dislocation develops, (6) whether osteonecrosis develops, and (7) whether reduction was incomplete because of the interposition of an object in the joint. Hip dislocation with spontaneous incomplete reduction probably occurs more often than previously thought, and the diagnosis of hip subluxation may be missed initially.

Hips left unreduced for more than 24 hours usually have poor results, and osteonecrosis of the femoral head develops more frequently than in hips reduced promptly. Closed reduction often is successful if a congruous joint is obtained. Open reduction may be necessary, however, for more severe injuries or to remove any entrapped structures. Contrary to previous reports, the period of non–weight bearing does not appear to influence the development of osteonecrosis of the femoral head.

Recurrent dislocation also is more common in children than in adults because of cartilaginous pliability and ligamentous laxity. Recurrent dislocations are more frequent in children with hyperlaxity syndromes, especially Down syndrome, and may require posterior plication of the capsule and bony intervention, such as an innominate or varus osteotomy. Recurrent dislocations may be involuntary and posttraumatic and should be differentiated from voluntary dislocations, which may be habitual or nonhabitual. Additionally, Manner et al. suggested a possible association between femoroacetabular impingement (FAI) and recurrent hip dislocation, and advocated operative treatment of underlying FAI to optimize outcomes.

Osteonecrosis of the femoral head occurs after simple dislocation of the hip in an estimated 10% to 26% of adults and 8% to 10% of children (Fig. 36-100). Delays in reduction and the severity of the injury probably influence the development of osteonecrosis. Sciatic nerve palsy, heterotopic ossification, and coxa magna also have been reported as complications of hip dislocation in children.

Complete reduction may be prevented by interposition of the capsule, labrum, other soft tissue, or an osteocartilaginous fragment. An anteroposterior radiograph of the pelvis and a lateral radiograph of both hips should be made after closed reduction to compare the width of the joint spaces. If the involved joint space is wider or the Shenton line is broken, an incongruous reduction should be suspected (Fig. 36-101). If an incongruous joint is suspected, then advanced imaging with CT or MRI is obtained. If interposed structures are found, we recommend open reduction and removal of the offending material. For posterior dislocations, a posterior approach, such as a modified Gibson (see Technique 1-68) or Moore (see Technique 1-70) approach, should be used. For anterior dislocations, an anterior approach, such as the Smith-Petersen or Watson Jones (see Techniques 1-60 and 1-63) approach, is used. If the direction of dislocation cannot be determined, MRI is helpful in localizing a soft-tissue injury. A posterior approach is frequently used because this is the more common direction of dislocation. A surgical dislocation approach may be used if more extensive work is required as in the case of a femoral head fracture. At open reduction, the hip should be distracted and the acetabulum should be checked for loose bony fragments or an inverted labrum or other soft tissue. Reduction should be confirmed under direct inspection and radiographically in the operating room, ensuring that the width of the joint space has returned to normal. The technique for open reduction of an incongruous closed reduction is the same as for irreducible hip dislocation and is described in Chapter 55. For late complications, such as persistent mechanical symptoms or pain, hip arthroscopy may be useful with the most common findings being loose bodies, chondral damage, labral tears, and ligamentum teres injuries. Hip

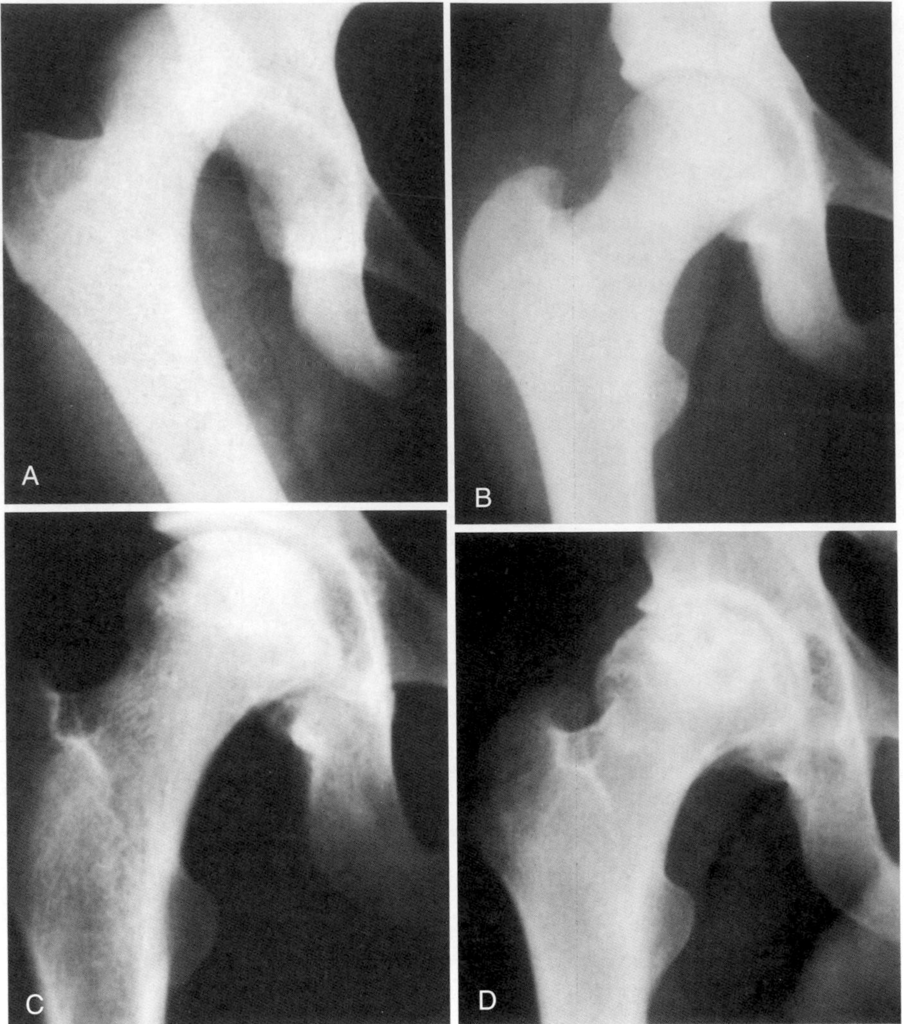

FIGURE 36-100 Osteonecrosis of femoral head after hip dislocation. **A,** Traumatic dislocation in older child. **B,** After satisfactory closed reduction. **C,** At 1 year after reduction, suggestion of early osteonecrosis. **D,** At 8 years after reduction, cystic appearance of osteonecrosis.

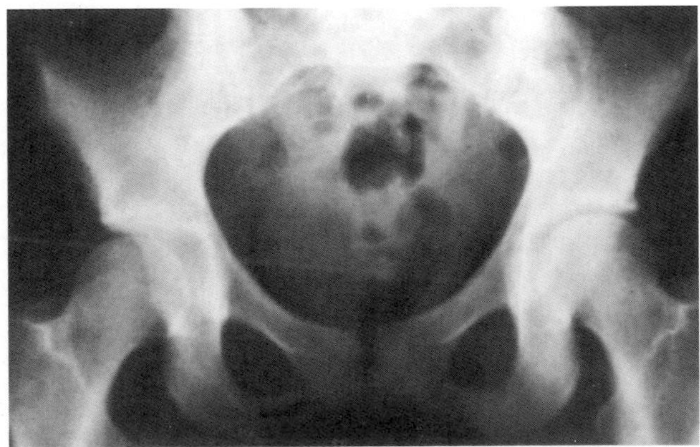

FIGURE 36-101 Incongruous reduction of hip. Radiograph of both hips after what was thought to be successful closed reduction of traumatic dislocation of the right hip in adolescent. Reduction is incongruous, however, as shown by break in Shenton line and increase in width of joint space.

arthroscopy technique and indication are discussed further in Chapter 51.

Rarely, a neglected traumatic dislocation may require open reduction in a child or adolescent. In a report of eight chronic dislocations, traction failed to obtain reduction in all eight and open reduction was required because of pain and gait disturbances. At an average follow-up of almost 8 years, six of the hips remained reduced; all had evidence of osteonecrosis. Although these results are not particularly good, they are, according to the authors, preferable to those obtained with other treatment methods or with no treatment. Other authors have recommended open reduction of neglected dislocations, even with the likelihood of osteonecrosis, because an anatomically placed femoral head maintains the stimulus for growth of the pelvis and femur, prevents deformity, and maintains limb length.

Occasionally, an ipsilateral femoral fracture occurs at the time of hip dislocation. The treatment of this combination of injuries is described in Chapter 55.

SLIPPED CAPITAL FEMORAL EPIPHYSIS

A type I transepiphyseal fracture-separation and SCFE are epiphyseal separations, but controversy over their natural histories and pathogenesis separates the two disorders. Type I transepiphyseal separations generally are caused by high-energy trauma, whereas SCFE can occur insidiously and minor trauma can cause acute separation or a chronic slip. Type I transepiphyseal separations are most common in young children, whereas SCFE occurs in a distinct older age group (age 10 to 16 years); 78% of patients with SCFE are adolescents in the rapid growth phase. SCFE occurs more frequently in obese children and is almost twice as common in boys as in girls. It occurs approximately twice as often in children of African descent than in children of European descent. The left hip is affected twice as often as the right, and bilateral involvement is reported to occur in 25% to 40% of children. When bilateral slips occur, the second slip usually occurs within 12 to 18 months of the initial slip. Patients with open triradiate cartilage are at higher risk.

Several etiologic factors have been suggested for SCFE, including local trauma, mechanical factors (especially obesity, growth spurts, and puberty), inflammatory conditions, endocrine disorders (e.g., hypothyroidism, hypopituitarism, and chronic renal disease), genetic factors, Down syndrome, and seasonal variations. Although shear forces generally are cited as causative factors, torsional forces also play a role in SCFE. Sankar et al. also demonstrated increased acetabular retroversion and overcoverage in the unaffected hip with SCFE. Moreover, in the proximal femur throughout childhood and culminating in adolescence, several pathophysiologic changes occur that increase the vulnerability of the physis, including a decrease in the neck-shaft angle, increase in the obliquity of the physis, thinning of the perichondrial ring, and change in the cellular anatomy of the physis. Liu et al. also noted that the epiphyseal tubercle may be protective at an early age until it decreases in size during adolescence. Physeal widening at this age may then allow the epiphysis to internally rotate around the tubercle. The reliable orientation of the lateral epiphyseal vessels adjacent to the tubercle might explain the low rate of osteonecrosis in chronic, stable slips. The true cause of SCFE, however, is likely multifactorial: a physis that is weakened by some underlying condition fails when it is subjected to more than normal stress, resulting in slipping of the proximal femoral epiphysis.

The clinical symptoms and radiographic signs of SCFE vary according to the type of slip, but usually include pain in the groin, hip, medial thigh, or knee and limitation of hip motion, especially internal rotation. Georgiadis and Zaltz described the medial thigh pain in SCFE as being referred by a reflex arc involving somatic sensory nerves ending at the same spinal level as opposed to being caused by irritation of the obturator nerve branches. Often when the hip is flexed the leg externally rotates in a frog-leg position because of the abnormal contact between the displaced femoral neck and the acetabular rim. SCFE should be suspected in patients age 10 to 16 years who complain of vague knee pain, which may be referred pain from the hip. Patients with chronic slips may have mild or moderate shortening of the affected extremity, the leg may be in fixed external rotation leading to an outward foot progression angle compared with the uninvolved side, and a Trendelenburg gait may be present. Unfortunately, the diagnosis is frequently delayed, which may result in more severe deformity and worse long-term outcomes. Kocher reported that delays in diagnosis occur primarily in patients with knee or distal thigh pain, patients with Medicaid coverage, and patients with stable slips.

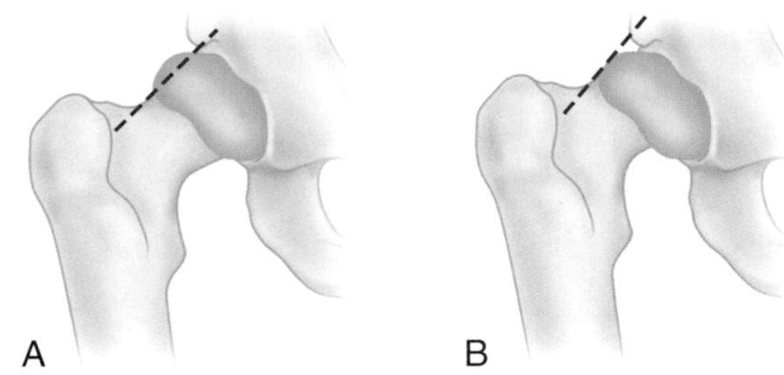

FIGURE 36-102 The Klein line: in early slips, the epiphysis is flush with or below this line. **A,** Normal hip. **B,** Slipped capital femoral epiphysis.

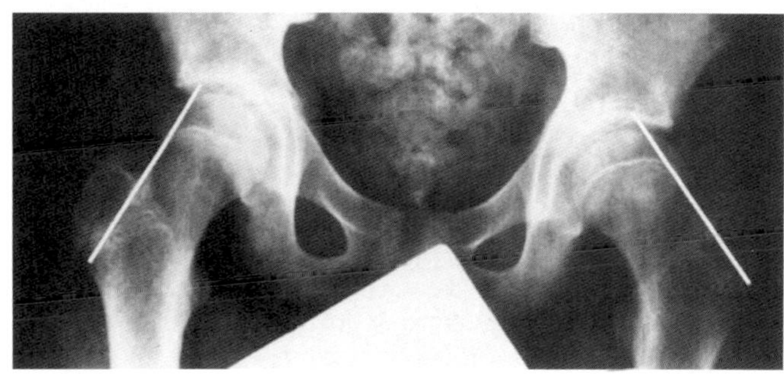

FIGURE 36-103 "Blanch" sign in slipped capital femoral epiphysis. Double density can be seen at the metaphysis of the left hip. (From Steel HH: The metaphyseal blanch sign of slipped capital femoral epiphysis, J Bone Joint Surg 68A:920, 1986.)

The diagnosis of SCFE usually is apparent from anteroposterior and frog pelvic radiographs, but special views may be helpful. The Klein line is a line along the superior aspect of the femoral neck that normally is intersected by the epiphysis. In early slips, the epiphysis is flush with or below this line (Fig. 36-102). A modification of this measurement considered a slip to have occurred if the maximal width of the epiphysis lateral to the Klein line differed 2 mm or more from the contralateral hip. This modification was reported to improve sensitivity from 40% to almost 80%. Often a double density is seen at the metaphysis on the anteroposterior radiograph as compared with the contralateral hip when the metaphysis is translated anteriorly and externally rotated relative to the epiphysis; this has been called a *metaphyseal blanch sign* (Fig. 36-103). Although not routinely used in our practice, advanced imaging may add benefit in some cases. MRI can be used for diagnosis of a subtle or "preslip" condition suggested by edema around the physis on T2-weighted images, which should be a sign that a slip is present. It also is useful in ruling out additional hip pathology or assessing femoral head perfusion. CT is helpful in determining if the physis is closed or for preoperative planning before complex osteotomies.

SCFE traditionally has been classified according to the duration of symptoms and the stability of the slip. Acute SCFE presents within 3 weeks of the onset of symptoms, whereas a chronic SCFE has a more gradual onset of symptoms of more than 3 weeks' duration. A third subset of patients may be symptomatic from a longer period and then develop more acute symptoms resulting in acute-on-chronic SCFE. Radiographs of a chronic SCFE usually show the epiphyseal displacement with evidence of bone healing or remodeling with possible secondary changes to the acetabulum and femoral neck, depending on the duration of symptoms and degree of the slip. This temporal classification of SCFE is descriptive but has little prognostic value. The most widely accepted classification of SCFE was introduced by Loder et al. and is based on the stability of the physis. A slip is classified as unstable if severe pain prevents walking, even with crutches, regardless of the duration of symptoms. With a stable slip, walking is possible, with or without crutches. Satisfactory results were obtained in 96% of stable slips compared with 47% of unstable slips. In addition, the osteonecrosis rate for the stable slips was 0% compared with 47% in the unstable group with operative intervention.

SCFE can be graded based on the severity of the slip. A preslip condition is present if there is symptomatic weakening of the physis without loss of the normal epiphyseal-metaphyseal orientation. Radiographs may demonstrate irregularity, widening, and indistinctness of the physis, and MRI demonstrates abnormal edema surrounding the physis. Mild slipping (grade I) exists when the neck is displaced less than one third of the diameter of the femoral head or when the head-shaft angle deviates from normal by 30 degrees or less on either projection as described by Southwick (Fig. 36-104). In moderate slipping (grade II), the neck is displaced between one third and one half of the diameter of the femoral head or the head-shaft angle deviates between 30 and 60 degrees from normal on either view. Severe slipping (grade III) is characterized by neck displacement of more than half the diameter of the head or deviation of the head-shaft angle of more than 60 degrees. In most large series of SCFE, 60% to 90% of slips are classified as chronic and more than half are classified as mild slips.

SCFE also can be idiopathic or atypical (associated with renal failure, radiation therapy, hypogonadism, Down syndrome, and various endocrine disorders). Children younger than 10 years old or older than 16 have been reported to be 4.2 times more likely to have atypical SFCE and 8.4 times more likely if their weight was below the 50th percentile. Slips occurring in children with underlying endocrinopathies or other risk factors may be susceptible to failure of screw fixation, progressive slipping, or contralateral slipping. When symptoms of pain continue (average 5 months) in such patients, close follow-up with radiographs or prophylactic pinning is necessary. Some authors have advocated treatment with pins that are smooth proximally and threaded distally to engage the anterolateral femoral cortex with no threads crossing the physis to allow continued growth in younger patients with renal osteodystrophy. A single cannulated 7-mm diameter screw with 10-mm threads also can be used. The screw should be placed in the center-line of the femoral head so that all screw threads are within the femoral head and not in the joint. The screw is left protruding 15 mm to 20 mm to allow further physeal growth (Fig. 36-105).

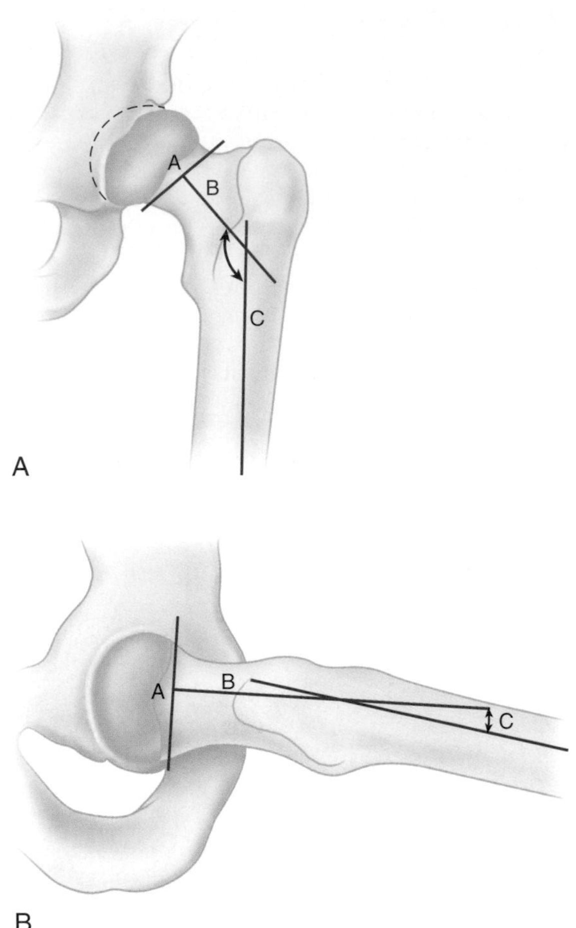

FIGURE 36-104 **A** and **B**, Measurement of head-shaft angle on anteroposterior and lateral radiographs. Line *A* connects peripheral portions of physis. Line *B* is perpendicular to line *A*, and line *C* is in long axis of femoral shaft. Intersection of lines *B* and *C* forms head-shaft angle in both views.

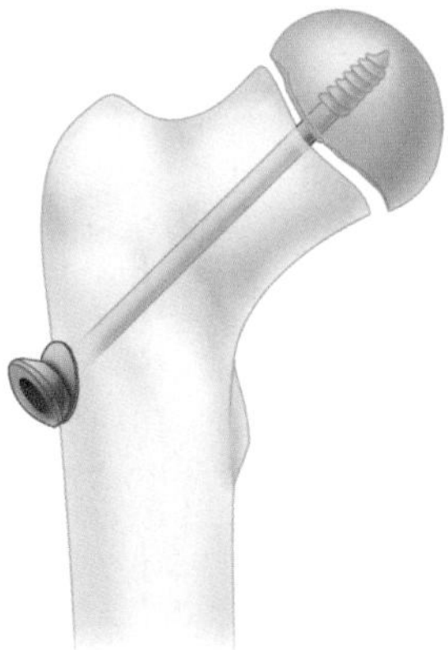

FIGURE 36-105 Principle of dynamic screw fixation. Short screw thread (10 mm) in epiphysis only, and screw and washer are left long for continued growth.

TREATMENT

The ideal treatment of SCFE would restore the biomechanics of the hip, prevent additional slipping of the epiphysis, and stimulate early physeal closure while avoiding the complications of osteonecrosis, chondrolysis, and osteoarthritis. Stabilization of the slip and closure of the physis are relatively easy to obtain by a variety of methods; however, restoration of hip biomechanics and prevention of complications has proved more difficult.

Methods of operative treatment of SCFE have included percutaneous and open *in situ* pinning, ORIF, epiphysiodesis, osteotomy, and reconstruction by arthroplasty, arthrodesis, or cheilectomy. Each technique has its proponents and opponents, and the choice of treatment must be individualized for each child, depending on age, type of slip, and severity of displacement.

IN SITU PIN OR SCREW FIXATION

Percutaneous in situ screw fixation currently is the most commonly used treatment for both stable and unstable SCFE regardless of the severity of the slip. Modern cannulated screw systems allow more accurate placement of screws and have become the implant of choice for fixation. Although earlier reports indicated that two or three pins were necessary for stability, several studies have failed to demonstrate a clinical or biomechanical advantage to multiple pins and advocate the use of a single, larger-diameter screw inserted into the center-center position of the epiphysis. Occasionally, a second screw is used at our institution if a high-grade slip is present, and a single screw does not achieve adequate stability in the unstable SCFE. Alternatively, an open procedure may be performed to restore the epiphyseal alignment and achieve stability. For unstable slips, a gentle or "incidental" reduction may be applied by simply positioning the patient in the appropriate position on the operative table, but forceful manipulation of the hip should be avoided because of the high association between a manipulative reduction and osteonecrosis.

Our techniques for determining the entry point for screw fixation and placement of the cannulated screw into the epiphysis are described in Techniques 36-22 and 36-23, respectively. Obtaining the appropriate starting point to allow passage of the screw perpendicular to the physis and into the center-center position is important; however, Merz et al. noted that a screw passed obliquely across the physis into the center-center position does not significantly alter the biomechanical stability of the construct. This may be helpful when trying to avoid screw placement that results in dynamic impingement of the screw head.

Persistent screw penetration has been the most serious disadvantage of in situ fixation. Adverse effects attributed to unrecognized implant penetration include joint sepsis, localized acetabular erosion, synovitis, postoperative hip pain, chondrolysis, and late degenerative osteoarthritis. As a practical clinical guide, placing the screw in the center of the femoral head no closer than 4 mm from the subchondral bone helps to decrease the prevalence of screw penetration (Fig. 36-106). Additionally, multiple radiographic views should be obtained to ensure persistent penetration has not occurred. Other methods such as the passage of the blunt end of the guidewire or injection of contrast dye through the cannulated screw have been described.

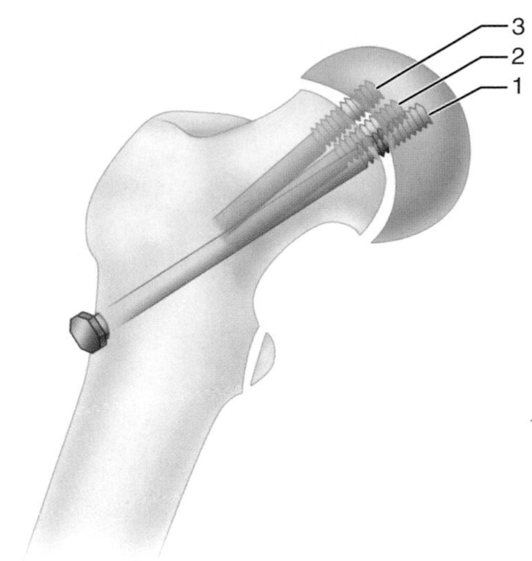

FIGURE 36-106 Screw positions in proximal femur. Position *1,* central axis of screw is located over center line of femoral head or within distance equal to one-half diameter of screw (ideal position). Position *2,* distance between axis of screw and center line of femoral head is between one half and one screw diameter. Position *3,* axis of screw is more than one screw diameter from center line. Position is given as two numbers: first for position of screw on anteroposterior radiograph and second for position as seen on lateral view. Ideal position is 1.

DETERMINING THE ENTRY POINT FOR CANNULATED SCREW FIXATION OF A SLIPPED EPIPHYSIS

TECHNIQUE 36-22

(CANALE ET AL.)

- Place the patient supine so that anteroposterior and lateral fluoroscopic views can be obtained without repositioning the patient or the extremity; a fracture table, or alternatively a radiolucent flat top table, can be used (Fig. 36-107A). The entire proximal femoral epiphysis and hip joint space should be clearly visible on both views. Prepare and drape the extremity to allow free access to the entire anterior surface of the thigh and as far medially as the pubis in the inguinal area (Fig. 36-107B). A fluoroscopic C-arm is used for an anteroposterior and an exact lateral image. On the lateral view, the femoral neck should be parallel to the femoral shaft.
- Place a guidewire on the anterior aspect of the thigh (Fig. 36-107C) so that the anteroposterior image shows it in the desired varus-valgus position (Fig. 36-107D), and mark the position of the guidewire on the anterior surface of the thigh with a marking pen.
- Place the guidewire along the lateral aspect of the thigh (Fig. 36-107E) so that it is in the correct anteroposterior position on fluoroscopic image (Fig. 36-107F), and mark the position of the wire on the skin. In SCFE, the epiphysis

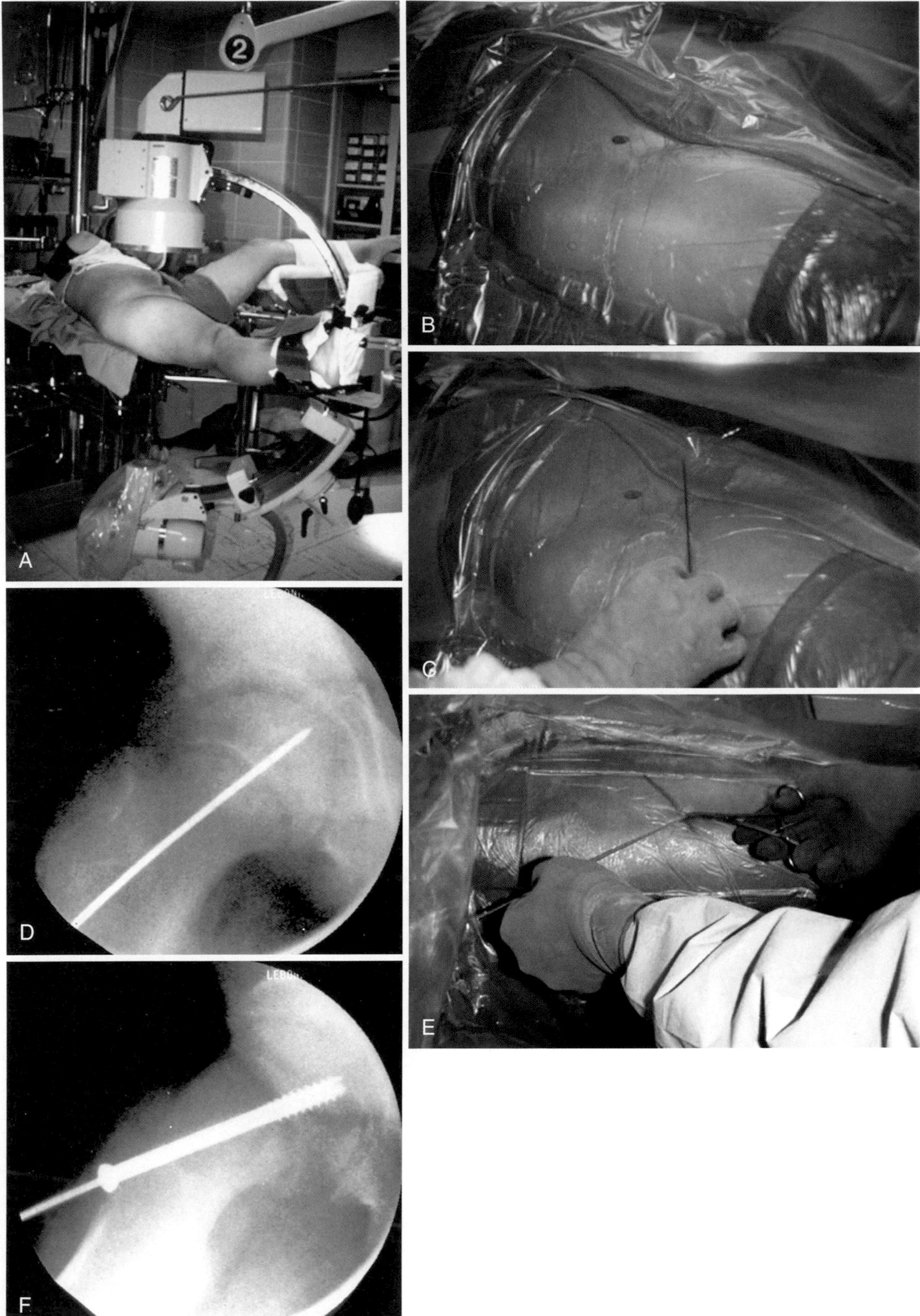

FIGURE 36-107 Technique for determining incision site for percutaneous fixation of slipped capital femoral epiphysis (see text). **A,** Positioning of patient and C-arm. **B,** Extremity is draped free to allow access to entire anterior thigh. **C,** Guidewire placed on anterior aspect of thigh. **D,** Anteroposterior image of guidewire. **E,** Guidewire placed on lateral aspect of thigh. **F,** Lateral image of guidewire. **SEE TECHNIQUE 36-22.**

is displaced posteriorly relative to the femoral neck, and this lateral guidewire angles from anterior to posterior and appears on fluoroscopic image to enter at the anterior femoral neck. The two skin lines should intersect on the anterolateral aspect of the thigh. The greater the degree of the slip (the more posterior the epiphysis), the more anterior the intersection.

- Place a guidewire, drill, or pin through a small lateral incision at the intersection of the two skin lines. Monitor proper alignment, position, and depth of insertion in the proximal femoral epiphysis on anteroposterior and lateral fluoroscopic images. Take care not to bend, kink, or notch the guidewire for fear of interosseous breakage.
- Insert the cannulated screw in the routine manner; the threads of the screw at the tip should traverse the physis (Fig. 36-107F).

DETERMINING THE ENTRY POINT FOR CANNULATED SCREW FIXATION OF A SLIPPED EPIPHYSIS

TECHNIQUE 36-23

(MORRISSY)

- Place the patient on the fracture table with the affected leg abducted 10 to 15 degrees and internally rotated as far as possible without force. This brings the femoral neck as close as possible to parallel to the floor to assist in obtaining true anterior and lateral image views. Position the image intensifier between the legs so that anteroposterior and lateral views can be obtained by moving the tube around the arc of the machine (Fig. 36-108).
- After standard preparation and draping and under image control, insert a Kirschner wire percutaneously through the anterolateral area of the thigh down to the femoral neck (Fig. 36-109), adjusting the guidewire on the anteroposterior projection to determine the axis of the femoral neck. Obtain a lateral view to determine the amount of posterior inclination necessary.
- When the starting point on the femoral neck and amount of posterior inclination have been estimated, insert the guide assembly through a small puncture wound. Advance the guide assembly to the physis and confirm placement in the central axis of the femoral head by image intensification. If the position is correct, advance the guide assembly across the plate. (If positioning is incorrect, insert a second guide assembly using the first to determine what correction in the starting point or angulation is necessary.) When the proper depth is reached (at least 0.5 cm from subchondral bone), remove the cannula and leave the guidewire in the bone.
- Determine the correct screw length by passing a guidewire of identical length along the one in the bone and measuring the difference. Advance the correct-length screw over the guide pin and remove the pin.
- Remove the leg from the traction device and move it in multiple directions, using anteroposterior and lateral views to confirm that the screw does not penetrate the joint. If two screws are deemed necessary for an acute, unstable slip, the first screw should lie in the central axis of the femoral head and the second below it, avoiding the superolateral quadrant. The second screw should stop at least 5 mm from the subchondral bone.
- Close the stab wound with a single subcuticular suture.

See also Video 36-2.

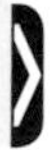

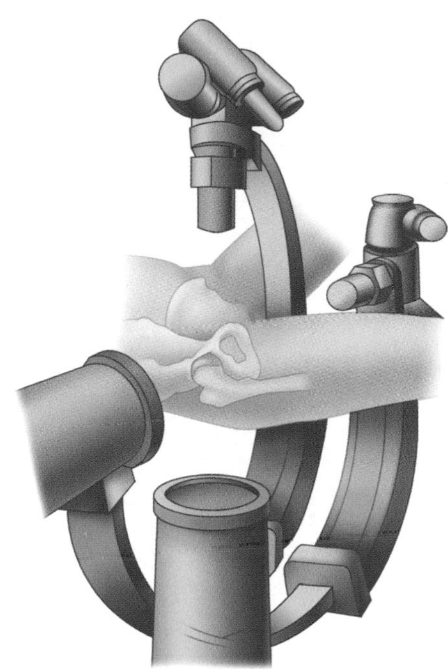

FIGURE 36-108 Percutaneous in situ fixation of slipped capital femoral epiphysis. Positioning of image intensifier to allow rotation necessary to obtain lateral and anteroposterior views. (From Morrissy RT: Slipped capital femoral epiphysis: technique of percutaneous in site fixation, J Pediatr Orthop 10:347, 1990.) **SEE TECHNIQUE 36-23.**

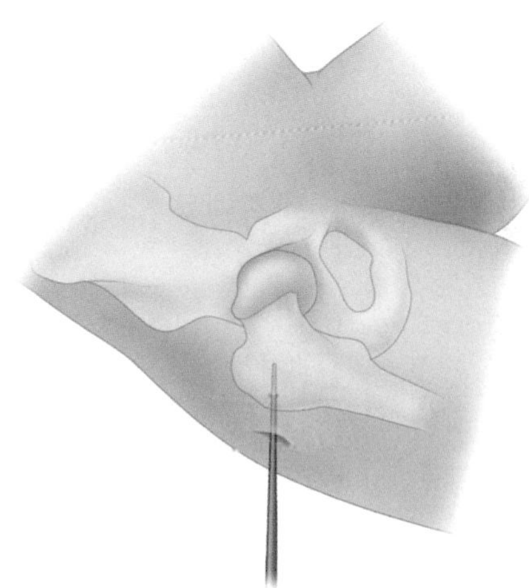

FIGURE 36-109 Kirschner wire passed percutaneously to estimated starting point on the femur. **SEE TECHNIQUE 36-23.**

POSTOPERATIVE CARE. Range-of-motion exercises are begun the day after surgery. For stable slips, patients are allowed to bear weight as tolerated with an assistive device the first day after surgery and are discharged the same day. Crutches are used until all signs of synovitis are gone and motion is free and painless (usually 2 to 3 weeks). For unstable slips, partial weight bearing is maintained with crutches for 6 to 8 weeks. All rigorous sports and other activities are limited until the physes have closed. Screw removal is not necessary, but the screws can be removed after physeal closure has been shown radiographically. The easiest method of removal is to pass a guidewire into the cannula of the screw under image control to allow the screwdriver to be guided into the head of the screw over the guidewire. However, we routinely do not remove the screws.

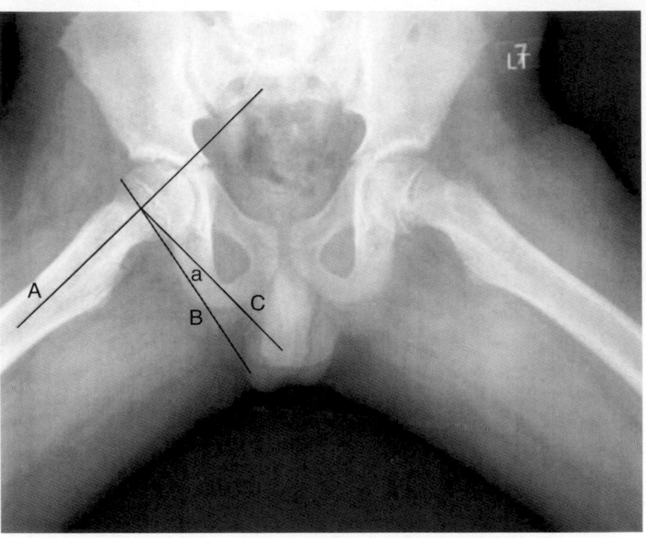

FIGURE 36-110 Posterior sloping angle of more than 12 degrees is described as predictive of the development of a contralateral slip. Line *A* is drawn along the femoral neck (diaphyseal axis). Line *B* is drawn along the plane of the physis. Line *C* is drawn perpendicular to line *A*. *a* is the posterior sloping angle. (From Park S, Hsu JE, Rendon N, et al: The utility of posterior sloping angle in predicting contralateral slipped capital femoral epiphysis, J Pediatr Orthop 30:683, 2010.)

CONTRALATERAL SLIPS

Bilateral slips are present in 20% to 30% of patients at initial presentation; the reported frequency of a subsequent, contralateral slip during the remaining growth period has ranged from 20% to 40%. Castro et al. estimated that patients with unilateral SCFE are 2335 times more likely to develop a contralateral slip than those who have never had SCFE are to have an initial slip. Even with this very high prevalence of bilateral slips, prophylactic pinning of the contralateral hip in a patient with a unilateral slip remains controversial. Because of the risks associated with prophylactic pinning of a radiographically and clinically normal hip, emphasis has been placed on trying to predict which patients with a unilateral slip will ultimately develop a second, contralateral slip.

Age appears to be one predictive factor. Females younger than 10 years of age and males younger than 12 years of age have a substantially increased incidence of contralateral SCFE, and prophylactic in situ fixation probably is indicated for these patients to prevent problems with leg-length inequality and long-term degenerative joint disease. Prophylactic fixation also may be indicated in patients with endocrine abnormalities or other processes related to their SCFE, those for whom reliable follow-up is not feasible, and those who have high risk factors for developing osteonecrosis or chondrolysis, such as obesity in younger children. A "posterior sloping" angle of more than 12 degrees (Fig. 36-110) has been described as predictive of the development of a contralateral slip. The use of a cannulated screw with a shorter threaded length that does not engage the physis has been recommended in young children to maintain stability without causing physeal closure and extremity shortening. Kocher et al. in a decision analysis found the optimal decision to be observation but advocated for contralateral fixation in patients with added risk factors or in patients in whom reliable follow-up was not feasible. Other recent studies have advocated for more routine fixation of the contralateral hip when a unilateral slip is present, especially in younger children with an open triradiate cartilage.

OPEN TECHNIQUES

Several modern open techniques for the treatment of SCFE have been developed in an attempt to improve on the high rates of complications seen with in situ fixation by addressing the acquired deformity of a slipped epiphysis and minimizing the vascular insult. The ideal treatment of a slip remains controversial but should take into account the degree of deformity, stability of the slip, risk of osteonecrosis, and an honest assessment of the skill set of the surgeon. For mild or stable slips that result in impingement or functional loss, limited open, surgical dislocation, and arthroscopic osteochondroplasty have been reported after in situ fixation with good results and are described in Chapter 6 (femoroacetabular impingement). For acute, unstable slips, some advocate an open approach to the hip through a Smith-Peterson or Watson-Jones approach with wide capsulotomy, gentle "finger" reduction, and fixation with cannulated screws. Alternatively, in moderate-grade or high-grade slips, where posterior callus formation and a contracted retinaculum may result in a block to anatomic reduction or an increase in the tension on the epiphysis vessels, a subcapital wedge resection of the femoral neck with reduction of the epiphysis may be performed with the modified Dunn technique (Technique 36-25). Ziebarth et al. reported 40 patients from two centers with moderate or severe SCFE who underwent capital realignment with the modified Dunn procedure. In their series, there were no cases of osteonecrosis at short-term follow-up, and the anatomy was restored to a slip angle of 4 to 8 degrees. The average alpha angle in their series was 40.6 degrees, and the incidence of cartilage damage, especially in stable slips, was very high. Navais et al. retrospectively compared 15 patients with severe, stable SCFE treated with the modified Dunn technique to 15 patients with severe, stable SCFE treated with in situ fixation. They found that the modified Dunn procedure resulted in better morphologic features of the femur, a higher rate of good and excellent Heyman and Herndon clinical outcome, a lower reoperation rate, and a similar occurrence of complications, which included an osteonecrosis risk of 7%. Alternatively, Sankar et al. reported 27 patients who had restoration of their capital alignment with the modified Dunn technique, but had a 15% incidence of implant failure requiring revision and 26% incidence of osteonecrosis at 22-month follow-up. Additional studies are needed to accurately assess the outcomes of this procedure for both unstable and stable slips.

Historically, several other corrective osteotomies have been described and can be divided into femoral neck and intertrochanteric osteotomies. Because moderately or severely displaced slips produce permanent irregularities in the femoral head and acetabulum, some form of realignment procedure often is indicated to restore the normal relationship of the femoral head and neck and possibly delay the onset of degenerative joint disease; however, in long-term follow-up, patients with osteotomies have been reported to have worse scores on the Iowa hip rating with each passing decade than patients without hip realignment procedures. Suggested indications for osteotomy have included problems with gait, sitting, pain, or cosmetic appearance. Often these procedures were performed more than 1 year after stabilization because of the belief that the femoral head may have the capacity to remodel. More recent data and a better understanding of SCFE-induced impingement call into question the ability of a significant deformity to remodel and raise concern that any "remodeling" may come at the cost of repetitive trauma to the labrum, chondrolabral junction, and weight-bearing acetabular cartilage. Historically, poor results with osteotomy techniques may have been partially related to a poor understanding of the blood supply to the head and intervention after irreparable damage has occurred to the articular surface.

The two basic types of corrective osteotomy are closing wedge osteotomy through the femoral neck, usually near the physis to correct the deformity, and compensatory osteotomy through the trochanteric region to produce a deformity in the opposite direction (Fig. 36-111). The advantage of osteotomy through the femoral neck is that the deformity itself is corrected, but incidences of osteonecrosis ranging from 2% to 100% and of chondrolysis from 3% to 37% have been associated with this procedure. Recent advocates of the modified Dunn procedure have proposed this technique as a viable option for patients with moderate or severe deformity; however, it does introduce a risk of osteonecrosis, and long-term results are needed before it should be widely adopted. With the exception of the modified Dunn technique, femoral neck osteotomies have been abandoned at our institution.

Trochanteric osteotomies can produce an opposite deformity to correct the coxa vara, hyperextension, and external rotation produced by a slipped epiphysis. Southwick described a biplanar osteotomy at the level of the lesser trochanter to correct the varus and hyperextension and dynamically correct the external rotation. Alternatively, the Imhaüser osteotomy can be used to primarily correct the hyperextension and secondarily to correct the varus and external rotation, as described in Technique 36-28. If the physis is not yet fused, then fixation of the physis should be achieved with a screw before the osteotomy. Trochanteric osteotomies have the advantage of low osteonecrosis rates but the disadvantage of incomplete correction of the deformity. Outcomes of trochanteric osteotomies are largely dependent on the degree of correction achieved and the extent of the underlying articular damage. Trochanteric osteotomies also have been combined at our institution with femoral neck osteochondroplasty through a surgical dislocation or limited anterior approach.

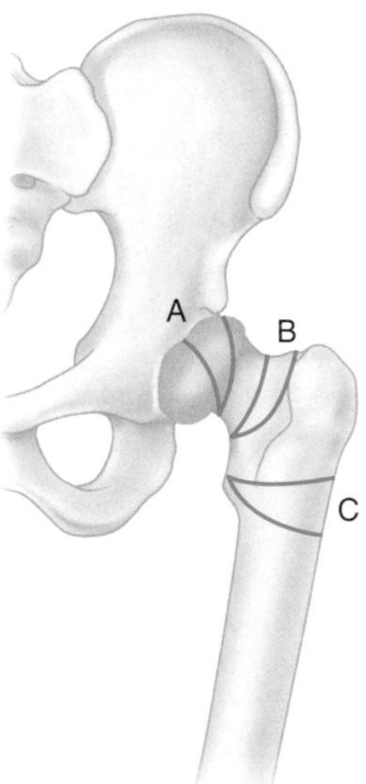

FIGURE 36-111 Osteotomies for slipped capital femoral epiphysis. *A*, Through neck near epiphysis. *B*, Through base of neck. *C*, Through trochanteric region.

POSITIONAL REDUCTION AND FIXATION FOR SCFE

TECHNIQUE 36-24

(CHEN, SCHOENECKER, DOBBS, ET AL.)

- After induction of general endotracheal anesthesia, place the patient on a fracture table with the involved extremity in gentle traction and the hip in extension, neutral rotation, and neutral abduction.
- Flex the uninvolved hip into the lithotomy position to allow an image intensifier to adequately access the pelvis. Obtain anteroposterior and lateral fluoroscopic images before making the incision. Often simple positioning results in reduction and can be determined by the remodeling of the femoral neck, particularly on the lateral view.
- If reduction is not obtained by positioning, apply minimal internal rotation (generally no more than 10 degrees) with slightly more traction; make no attempt at forceful reduction past the preacute position. This reduction reestablishes the preacute length of the retinacular vessels that supply the femoral head.
- If decompression of an intraarticular hematoma is needed, perform a capsulotomy through an anterior iliofemoral approach between the tensor fascia lata and sartorius muscles, taking care not to sacrifice the ascending branch of the lateral femoral circumflex artery.
- Once the hip joint is exposed, apply gentle flexion and internal rotation to confirm reduction under direct observation.

- Use a triangulation technique with a guidewire under fluoroscopic vision to determine the skin entry point on the anterolateral aspect of the hip.
- Advance the guidewire through the anterior aspect of the femoral neck and direct it perpendicular to the physis, slightly superiorly and anteriorly to the center of the physis.
- Place a second guidewire parallel to the first and slightly inferior and posterior to the center of the physis.
- Advance a cannulated drill over each guidewire and insert two appropriate-sized cannulated screws over the guidewires. When position of the screws is confirmed, remove the guidewires.

PERCUTANEOUS CAPSULOTOMY TO DECOMPRESS THE INTRAARTICULAR HEMATOMA

- Place long Metzenbaum scissors on the anterior femoral neck just distal to the physis under fluoroscopic confirmation.
- Use tactile confirmation to locate the generally tough hip capsule overlying the anterior femoral neck and carefully advance the scissors to perforate the capsule. Confirm this with fluoroscopy.
- Alternatively, advance a drill bit through the capsule and into the epiphysis under image intensifier guidance.

POSTOPERATIVE CARE. Patients are restricted to non–weight bearing on crutches or in a wheelchair for approximately 2 months.

SUBCAPITAL REALIGNMENT OF THE EPIPHYSIS (MODIFIED DUNN) FOR SCFE

Leunig, Slongo, and Ganz described a subcapital realignment procedure in which the femoral head is dislocated, an osteotomy of the greater trochanter is made, and the capital epiphysis is realigned and internally fixed. The rationale behind this technique is that the blood supply to the femoral head is preserved with the dislocation technique, thus avoiding osteonecrosis of the femoral head and avoiding femoroacetabular impingement by aligning the physis to the femoral neck. This is a complex procedure that should be done only by experienced hip surgeons.

TECHNIQUE 36-25

(LEUNIG, SLONGO, AND GANZ)

- Place the patient in the lateral decubitus position, with the leg draped free and placed on a sterile bag fixed to the front of the operating table.
- Make a Gibson approach (see Technique 1-68), posteriorly retracting the gluteus maximus. This approach allows exposure similar to that obtained with a Kocher-Langenbeck approach but produces a more acceptable cosmetic result.
- Retract the fascial layer between the gluteus maximus and medius along with the gluteus maximus to preserve optimal innervation and blood supply to the muscle.
- Internally rotate the leg and identify the posterior border of the gluteus medius by dissecting the overlying adipose tissue.
- Mark the level and direction of the trochanteric osteotomy with a knife, creating a line from the posterosuperior edge to the posterior border of the vastus lateralis. Place this line anterior to the trochanteric crest to avoid injury to the insertion of the external rotators. After the osteotomy, the gluteus medius, the vastus lateralis, and the long tendon of the gluteus minimus will remain attached to the trochanteric fragment. The maximal thickness of the trochanteric fragment should not exceed 1.5 cm, and the osteotomy should exit proximally just anterior to the most posterior inserting fibers of the gluteus medius to keep most of the piriformis insertion on the femur and not on the fragment.
- Expose the hip joint capsule by further dissection between the piriformis tendon and gluteus minimus, an interval that offers the best protection for the blood supply to the femoral head and allows preservation of the constant anastomosis between the inferior gluteal artery and the deep branch of the medial femoral circumflex artery.
- Flip the greater trochanteric fragment anteriorly by elevating the vastus lateralis along its posterior border to the middle of the gluteus maximus tendon insertion on the femoral shaft.
- Proximally, cut the few gluteus medius fibers remaining on the stable trochanter to allow further anterior mobilization of the trochanteric fragment.
- Flex and externally rotate the leg to increase exposure of the capsule within the gap between the piriformis and the gluteus minimus.
- Release the anterosuperior capsular insertion of the gluteus minimus muscle while preserving the long tendon of the gluteus minimus that inserts anterior on the trochanteric fragment. Up to this point in the procedure, all external rotators remain attached to the stable trochanter and protect the medial femoral circumflex artery.
- Incise the capsule close to the anterosuperior edge of the stable trochanter in a direction axial to the neck. Make a perpendicular extension along the anterior neck insertion to create a flap that can be lifted to create an inside-out capsulotomy that provides protection from cutting into cartilage and labrum.
- Extend the Z-shaped capsulotomy (for the right side) along the posterior border of the acetabulum. Direct the anteroinferior extension of the capsulotomy toward the anteroinferior border of the acetabulum. This extension must remain anterior to the lesser trochanter to avoid damage to the main branch of the medial femoral circumflex artery, which is located in the vicinity of the femur just superior and posterior to the lesser trochanter.
- Retract the anteromedial capsular flap with a small, spiked Hohmann retractor that is driven into the supra-acetabular bone just lateral to the anterior inferior iliac spine.
- Use two additional Langenbeck retractors to provide exposure for inspection of the joint for synovitis, color

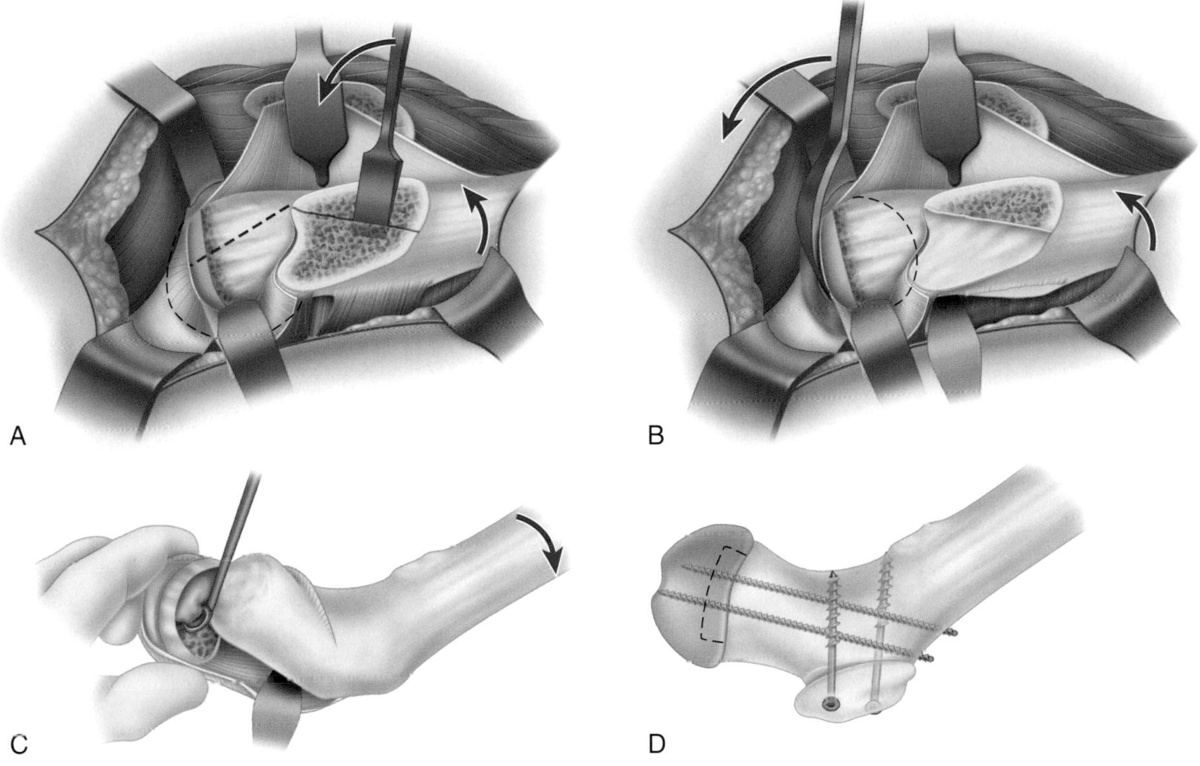

FIGURE 36-112 **A to D, Subcapital realignment of the epiphysis.** (Redrawn from Leunig M, Slongo T, Ganz R: Subcapital realignment in slipped capital femoral epiphysis: surgical hip dislocation and trimming of the stable trochanter to protect the perfusion of the epiphysis, Instr Course Lect 57:499, 2008.) **SEE TECHNIQUE 36-25.**

and quantity of synovial fluid, degree of femoral head tilt, and stability of the epiphysis on the metaphysis. If the epiphysis is mobile or stability is questionable, prophylactic pinning is recommended; however, any attempt at reducing a mobile epiphysis anatomically should be avoided at this time because there is a high risk of pathologic stretching of the retinaculum before removal of the posterior callus.

- Before surgical dislocation, drill a 2-mm hole in the femoral head to document blood perfusion. Laser Doppler flowmetry can provide dynamic control of the perfusion throughout the operation.
- Flex and externally rotate the hip and place the leg into a sterile bag over the anterior side of the table to sublux the femoral head. Use a bone hook around the femoral calcar to improve exposure of the joint.
- Document the damage pattern to the labrum and cartilage of the acetabulum and re-create the damage by the anterior metaphysis above the level of the epiphyseal contour by reducing the femoral head and moving it through flexion and internal rotation. If the epiphyseal tilt is small (<30 degrees) in a stable situation, and if trimming of the anterior metaphysis would be sufficient without creating a too thin femoral neck, full dislocation is not necessary. Create a normal offset by trimming the metaphyseal contour and pinning the epiphysis in situ.
- If slippage is more severe, dislocate the femoral head. With the head subluxed, section the round ligament with curved scissors. With manipulation of the leg and the use of special retractors on the acetabular rim and teardrop area, inspect the entire acetabulum (360 degrees).
- Rotate the leg to make visible the difference in surfaces of the femoral head and record the actual amount of epiphyseal slip. The retinaculum protecting the terminal branches of the medial femoral circumflex artery to the femoral epiphysis is clearly visible on the posterosuperior contour of the femoral neck as a somewhat mobile layer of connective tissue. Constantly moisten the femoral head cartilage during exposure.
- Reduce the femoral head into the acetabulum for creation of the soft-tissue flap consisting of the retinaculum and external rotators and containing the blood supply for the epiphysis.
- With an osteotome, carefully mobilize the area of the stable trochanter proximal to the visible physis (Fig. 36-112A) and then excise this fragment subperiosteally in an inside-out fashion.
- Incise the periosteum of the neck anterior to the visible retinaculum from the anterosuperior edge of the trochanter physis toward the femoral head. Elevate the periosteum from the posterior neck with a knife and sharp periosteal elevators, taking care to avoid suture of the anterior insertion of the retinaculum near the femoral epiphysis.
- Extend the periosteal release distally to the base of the lesser trochanter and level the remaining osseous ledge of the trochanteric base.

- In a similar manner, free the anteromedial periosteum (this is easier with the head dislocated), taking care to prevent disruption of the periosteal tube from the epiphysis (Fig. 36-112B).
- With the femoral head dislocated, use two blunt retractors to expose the femoral neck medially and laterally, avoiding any stretching of the retinaculum.
- Mobilize the epiphysis in a stepwise fashion with a curved 10-mm osteotome placed anteriorly into the physis.
- The physis is located proximal to the distal border of the epiphyseal joint cartilage. Normally, no wedge resection is necessary. With simultaneous levering with the osteotome and controlled external rotation of the leg, deliver the metaphyseal stump from the periosteal tube while the epiphysis remains in the posteromedial position. Removal of a posteromedial callus bridge in flexion-external rotation may facilitate this step.
- Spontaneous reduction of the isolated epiphysis into the acetabulum may occur at this time. Redislocation is difficult even with Kirschner wires inserted into the epiphysis. To help avoid this complication, place a small swab in the acetabulum.
- Remove visible or palpable callus formation on the posterior and posteromedial aspect of the neck. To provide a large contact area with the epiphysis, carefully round the front surface of the metaphyseal stump. Use controlled rotational maneuvers of the shaped femoral neck to allow manual fixation of the epiphysis while curettage of the remainder of the physis is performed (Fig. 36-112C). Normally, the exposed epiphyseal bone shows clear bleeding as a sign of intact perfusion.
- After removal of all callus particles, reduce the epiphysis onto the neck under visual control of the retinacular tension; reduction is easier with internal rotation of the leg. If any tension in the retinaculum occurs during this maneuver, immediately stop the reduction. Check to see that parts of the posterior soft-tissue flap are not inverted and need to be unfolded. The height of the metaphysis rarely requires reduction.
- Carefully determine the correct spatial orientation of the epiphysis. Use a palpating instrument or fluoroscopy to ensure that the border of the epiphysis has an equal distance to the neck in all planes. Visually check correct rotation relative to the location of the retinaculum and the fovea capitis. Use fluoroscopy to obtain the correct varus-valgus position.
- When the correct position is obtained, temporarily fix the epiphysis in place with a fully threaded Kirschner wire inserted in a retrograde direction through the fovea capitis, perforating the lateral cortex of the femur just distal to the vastus lateralis.
- Pull this wire back so far that its tip is level with the articular head cartilage and reduce the head into the acetabulum to allow final control of alignment with fluoroscopy. If perfect alignment of the epiphysis is achieved, insert one or two additional fully-threaded Kirschner wires from the lateral cortex of the subtrochanteric bone. Check the correct wire length visually or with fluoroscopy. The wires should be optimally distributed within the epiphysis.
- Close the periosteal tube with a few stitches, avoiding any tension. Close the capsule, also without any tension. If the tendon of the piriformis muscle is producing tension on the capsule, release it.
- Fix the trochanteric fragment with two 3.5-mm screws (Fig. 36-112D).
- Carefully close the subcutaneous adipose tissue in several layers; suction drainage usually is not necessary.

POSTOPERATIVE CARE. Continuous passive motion is used during the postoperative hospital stay. Crutches are used for toe-touch walking. Deep venous thrombosis prophylaxis with low-dose heparin is administered to obese patients only. Full weight bearing is allowed at 8 to 10 weeks, if radiographs show healing of the trochanteric osteotomy. Strengthening of the gluteus medius is begun at 6 to 8 weeks, and full muscle strength should be achieved at 10 to 12 weeks. If implant removal is required, it should not be done until at least 1 year after surgery.

COMPENSATORY BASILAR OSTEOTOMY OF THE FEMORAL NECK

A compensatory osteotomy of the base of the femoral neck that corrects the varus and retroversion components of moderate or severe chronic SCFE has been suggested to be safer than an osteotomy made near or at the physis because the line of the osteotomy is distal to the major blood supply in the posterior retinaculum. Threaded pins are used for fixation of the osteotomy and the epiphysis. Not only is the anatomic relationship of the proximal femur restored, but also further slipping is prevented.

TECHNIQUE 36-26

(KRAMER ET AL.)

- Determine preoperatively the size of wedge to be removed by measuring the degree of the slip. Determine on anteroposterior radiographs the head and neck angle. Use paper tracings of the anteroposterior and lateral radiographs and cut with scissors the wedge on the tracing paper to determine the amount of bone to be removed and the results to be obtained.
- Approach the hip laterally. Begin the skin incision 2 cm distal and lateral to the anterior superior iliac spine and curve it distally and posteriorly over the greater trochanter and then distally along the lateral surface of the femoral shaft to a point 10 cm distal to the base of the trochanter. Incise longitudinally the fascia lata. Develop the interval between the gluteus medius and tensor fasciae latae. Carry the dissection proximally to the inferior branch of the superior gluteal nerve, which innervates the latter muscle. Incise the capsule of the hip joint longitudinally along the anterosuperior surface of the femoral neck. Release widely the capsular attachment along the anterior intertrochanteric line. Reflect distally the vastus lateralis

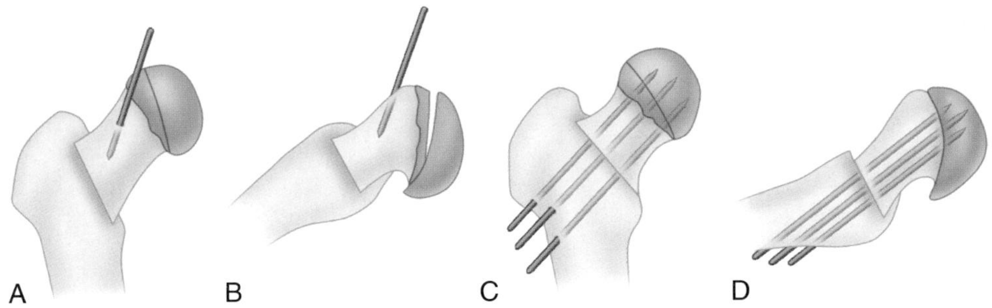

FIGURE 36-113 **A** and **B,** Widest part of wedge (at base of neck) is in line with widest part of slip, correcting varus and retroversion components, and Steinmann pin is inserted into femoral neck to control proximal fragment. If wedge is too wide anteriorly, retroversion is overly corrected. Most common mistake is to make wedge too narrow superiorly, resulting in incomplete correction of varus. **C** and **D,** Osteotomy is closed, and 5-mm threaded Steinmann pins are inserted from outer cortex of femoral shaft through femoral neck, across osteotomy site, and into femoral head. Pins fix osteotomy; because they cross the physis, they prevent any further slip. **SEE TECHNIQUE 36-26.**

to expose the base of the greater trochanter and the proximal part of the femoral shaft.

- With the capsule of the hip joint open, identify the junction between the articular cartilage of the femoral head and the callus and the junction of the callus with the normal cortex of the femoral neck. Compare the distance between these two junctions with the calculations made from the paper cutouts of the radiographs. The widest part of the wedge is in line with the widest part of the slip, in the anterior and superior aspects of the neck (Fig. 36-113A and B).
- Make the more distal osteotomy cut first, perpendicular to the femoral neck and following the anterior intertrochanteric line from proximal to distal. Extend this osteotomy cut to the posterior cortex, but leave this cortex intact. Make the second osteotomy cut with the blade of the osteotome directed obliquely so that its cutting edge stays distal to the posterior retinacular blood supply. The capsule with the blood supply reaches to the intertrochanteric line anteriorly, but posteriorly the lateral third of the neck is extracapsular. According to Kramer et al., an osteotomy made through the region of the anterior intertrochanteric line lies distal to the posterior retinacular vessels.
- Drill one or two 5-mm threaded Steinmann pins into the femoral neck proximally to ensure that the proximal portion of the femur is kept under control before completing the osteotomy (Fig. 36-113A and B). During the osteotomy, ensure that the osteotome does not fully penetrate the posterior cortex. Insert several 5-mm threaded Steinmann pins from the outer cortex of the femoral shaft through the femoral neck. Complete the osteotomy by greensticking the posterior cortex and removing the wedge of bone. Advance the threaded Steinmann pins across the osteotomy site and the physis to prevent further slipping (Fig. 36-113C and D).
- Close the capsule of the hip with interrupted sutures. Clip off the pins close to the femoral shaft and close the wound in layers. If epiphysiodesis of the greater trochanter is necessary, do it at this time.

POSTOPERATIVE CARE. Bed rest is prescribed for 2 to 3 weeks, followed by non–weight bearing. Partial weight bearing is allowed depending on the stability of the osteotomy and the weight of the patient. The threaded Steinmann pins should be removed only after the physis has fused.

EXTRACAPSULAR BASE-OF-NECK OSTEOTOMY

Extracapsular base-of-neck osteotomy has been recommended as safe and effective in preventing further slipping and improving hip range of motion in patients with severe chronic slips; however, it does not affect limb-length discrepancy. With severe slips the amount of correction of varus and posterior tilt of the femoral head is limited, and complete restoration of a normal head-shaft angle may not be possible or necessary. Removal of a wedge larger than 20 mm compromises femoral neck length and may increase greatly femoral anteversion. Also, pinning across the osteotomy site becomes more difficult when correction of more than 55 degrees of varus or valgus is attempted. These same restrictions also are applicable to intracapsular base-of-neck osteotomies and to the Southwick procedure (trochanteric osteotomy).

TECHNIQUE 36-27

(ABRAHAM ET AL.)

- Before surgery, the head-shaft angle is determined on lateral radiographs by measuring the angle formed by the epiphyseal line and the femoral shaft in the affected limb (Fig. 36-114) and comparing it with the contralateral side (or to 145 degrees). The head-shaft angle for posterior tilt or retroversion is determined on a frog-leg view and

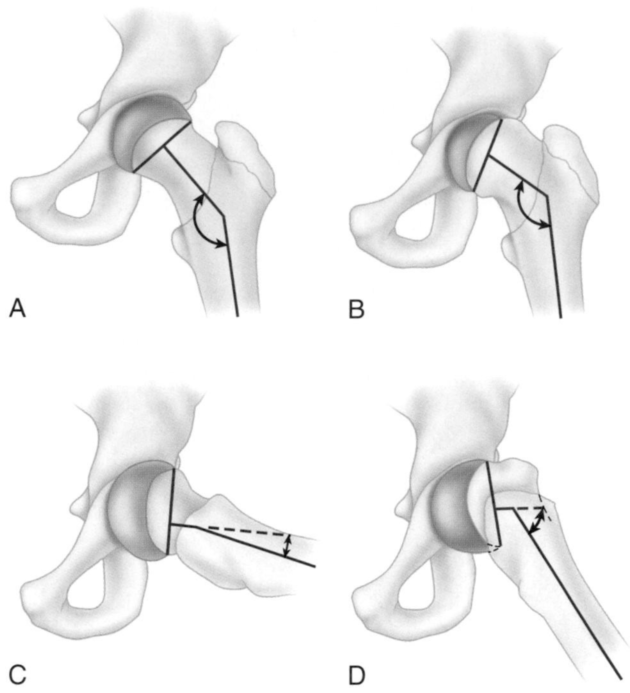

FIGURE 36-114 Extracapsular base-of-neck osteotomy: measurement of head-shaft angles on radiograph. **A,** Normal anteroposterior angle compared with slipped capital femoral epiphysis (SCFE). **B,** Moderate SCFE shows decrease in anteroposterior head-shaft angle. **C,** Normal acute angle. **D,** Severe slip shows increase in frogleg lateral head-shaft angle. (From Abraham E, Garst J, Barmada R: Treatment of moderate to severe slipped capital femoral epiphysis with extracapsular base-of-neck osteotomy, *J Pediatr Orthop* 13:294, 1993.) **SEE TECHNIQUE 36-27.**

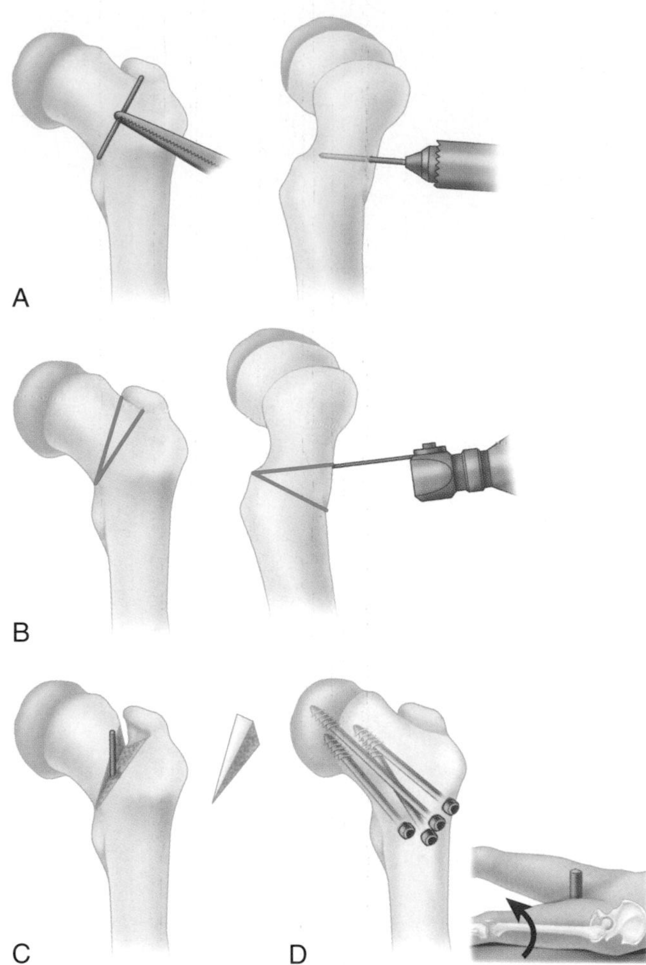

FIGURE 36-115 Extracapsular base-of-neck osteotomy (see text). **A,** Determination of proximal osteotomy cut. **B,** Osteotomy cuts. **C,** Removal of bony wedge. **D,** Fixation with cannulated screws. (From Abraham E, Garst J, Barmada R: Treatment of moderate to severe slipped capital femoral epiphysis with extracapsular base-of-neck osteotomy, *J Pediatr Orthop* 13:294, 1993.) **SEE TECHNIQUE 36-27.**

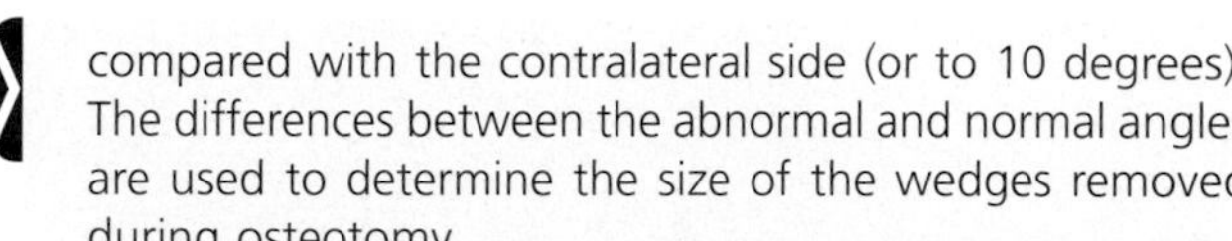

compared with the contralateral side (or to 10 degrees). The differences between the abnormal and normal angles are used to determine the size of the wedges removed during osteotomy.

- Secure the anesthetized patient on a fracture table and maximally internally rotate the involved limb by gently moving the footplate. Widely abduct the contralateral leg to make placement of fluoroscopic equipment easier. Obtain permanent anteroposterior and "shoot-through" lateral radiographs to confirm the chronicity of the slip and to outline the femoral head better. Prepare and drape the hip and patellar areas appropriately.
- Make a standard anterolateral approach and place a Charnley retractor deep to the iliotibial band. Locate the anterior joint tissue or intertrochanteric line between the gluteus medius and the vastus lateralis muscles. With a periosteal elevator, carefully elevate the anterior iliofemoral ligament. Place a narrow-tipped Hohmann retractor around the femoral neck superiorly and deep to the ischiofemoral ligament. Place another retractor deep to the iliofemoral ligament proximal to the lesser trochanter.
- Delineate a triangle on the anterior surface of the femoral neck to indicate the two-plane wedge osteotomy. Locate the proximal cut by placing a 3-cm long Kirschner wire on the anterior surface of the femur from the lesser to the greater trochanter at the base of the neck along the edge of the capsule (Fig. 36-115A). Confirm this position by fluoroscopy.
- Use a wide osteotome to mark the bone along the wire. Externally rotate the leg and drill a second Kirschner wire in the anteroposterior plane just distal to the guidewire (Fig. 36-115B). Place this wire vertical to the anterior surface of the femoral neck. Rotate the limb internally and obtain a lateral fluoroscopic view to confirm correct wire placement.
- Begin the second distal osteotomy line from the lesser trochanter to the growth plate of the greater trochanter. The angle at which this line is made from the first osteotomy line depends on the amount of correction needed. Usually a 15-mm-wide wedge, measured superiorly to the baseline of the triangle, is needed. Make the osteotomy cuts with a saw, converging them posteriorly to make a single osteotomy along the posterior cortex. Completely

remove the wedge of bone, especially superiorly, for maximal correction (Fig. 36-115C).

- While maintaining traction to prevent proximal migration of the femur, internally rotate the leg until the wedge closes completely. Abducting the leg also helps to close the osteotomy. When the patella can be internally rotated 15 degrees, adequate correction has been achieved. Remove additional bone from the metaphyseal side if necessary, but remove a maximum of 20 mm in the bony wedge.
- Fix the osteotomy with three or four cannulated screws (Fig. 36-115D). Use the first guidewire to hold the osteotomy temporarily in the desired position. Use only one screw to span the physis of the femoral head, avoiding the superolateral quadrant.
- Check alignment and screw placement on permanent radiographs before closing the wound. Usually the iliofemoral ligament and capsule are not reattached, but if they are excessively elevated from the bone, suture or staple them back to the anterior femur to preserve anterior joint stability.
- Close the wound in routine fashion and apply a sterile dressing.

POSTOPERATIVE CARE. Partial weight bearing with crutches is allowed for 6 to 8 weeks, and then full weight bearing is allowed. Weight bearing as tolerated is permitted after bilateral osteotomies.

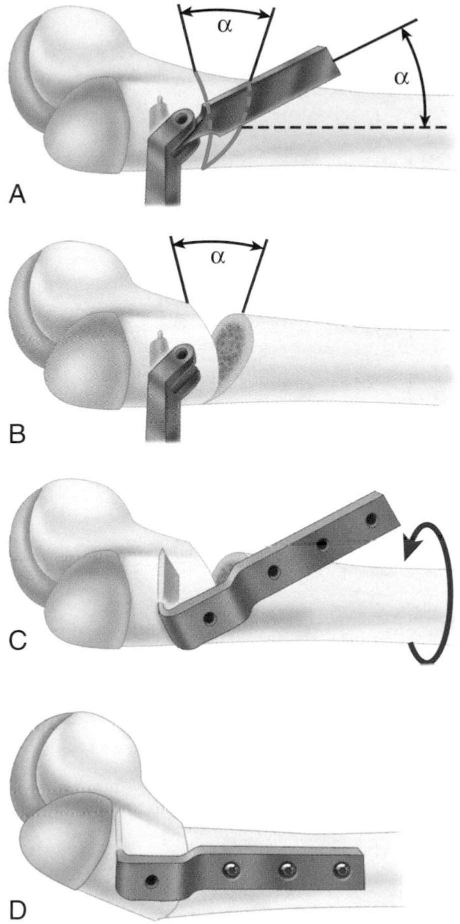

FIGURE 36-116 Intertrochanteric osteotomy (Imhäuser). **A,** Seating chisel is inserted into the neck at right angles to the shaft axis. **B,** Femoral osteotomy removes the ventral wedge. **C,** The chisel is exchanged for a blade plate, and the femur is derotated. **D,** The blade plate is fixed to the femur with screws. (Redrawn from Parsch K, Zehender H, Bühl T, Weller S: Intertrochanteric corrective osteotomy for moderate and severe chronic slipped capital femoral epiphysis, J Pediatr Orthop B 8:223, 1999.) **SEE TECHNIQUE 36-28.**

INTERTROCHANTERIC OSTEOTOMY (IMHÄUSER)

The Imhäuser osteotomy is similar to the Southwick osteotomy but is technically easier. This trochanteric osteotomy primarily corrects posterior angulation with secondary correction of external rotation and varus; thus, the osteotomy wedge is simply a closing wedge anteriorly. In theory, this reduces the varus and external rotation and allows more flexion while avoiding anterior impingement with the acetabulum. The results of intertrochanteric osteotomies have been variable, but they do appear to lessen the chance of chondrolysis and osteonecrosis that occur with osteotomies at other locations, and they do correct impending femoroacetabular impingement.

TECHNIQUE 36-28

- Through a straight lateral approach to the hip, stabilize the SCFE with a 7.3-mm cannulated, terminally threaded cancellous screw placed centrally and perpendicular to the proximal femoral physis or with Kirschner wires.
- Make the angle of insertion equal to the angle of posterior inclination of the capital epiphysis; this angle is equal to the degree of flexion of the femoral shaft that is necessary to position the epiphysis to the long axis of the femur and serves as a guide for the slotted chisel.
- Place the slotted chisel for a 90-degree angled blade plate at the base of the greater trochanter and rotate it until the anticipated anterior inclination of the side plate matches the desired degree of flexion (Fig. 36-116A). Alternatively, a proximal femoral locking plate may be used.
- Make a transverse osteotomy 2 cm distal to the chisel entry site and proximal to the lesser trochanter (Fig. 36-116B).
- Flex the distal fragment and fix it to the side plate.
- If the posterior periosteum prevents flexion of the distal fragment, release it. With increasing slip severity, increasing flexion is necessary. The flexion is accompanied by anterior translation to bring the femoral shaft in line with the proximal femoral epiphysis. This combination of movements counteracts the secondary zigzag deformity produced by a compensatory osteotomy at a site other than the primary site of deformity (the site of the slip).
- Perform an anterior capsulotomy to allow full extension of the hip after fixation of the distal fragment.
- Rotate the distal fragment medially to balance internal and external rotation of the hip and to match the

uninvolved hip as determined by preoperative examination (Fig. 36-116C).

- Fix the osteotomy with a 90-degree angled and 10-mm recessed blade plate (Fig. 36-116D).

POSTOPERATIVE CARE. A spica cast is applied with the hip in appropriate flexion, slight abduction, and internal rotation and worn for 8 to 12 weeks. Depending on the amount of healing of the osteotomy on radiograph, weight bearing is slowly increased on the operated leg. The blade plate usually is removed approximately 1 year after surgery.

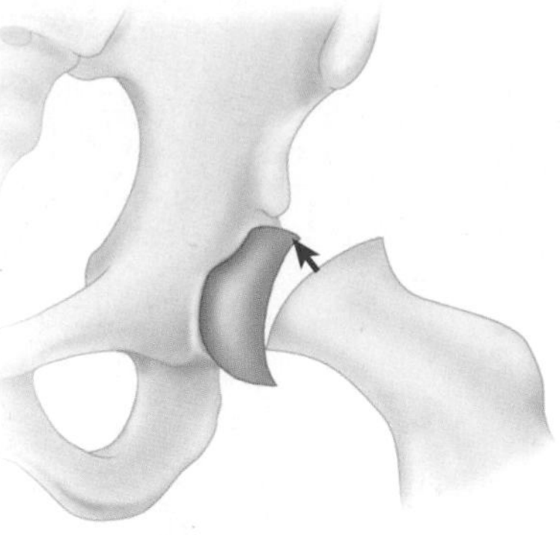

FIGURE 36-117 Anterior physeal separation.

COMPLICATIONS

OSTEONECROSIS

Osteonecrosis has been reported to occur in 10% to 40% of patients with acute unstable SCFE, although more recent reports of in situ pinning with cannulated screws generally report lower incidences (0% to 5%). Osteonecrosis is rare in chronic, stable slips and probably results from interruption of the retrograde blood supply by the original injury and is more common in acute, unstable slips. Further insult to the blood supply may result from forceful manipulations, delay in treatment in unstable slips, tamponade of the vessels, or technical errors during open procedures.

Superolateral placement of pins also has been associated with the development of osteonecrosis or at least with exacerbation of the process.

Herman et al. and Loder et al. suggested that instability may be the best predictor of osteonecrosis after acute slips, and others have confirmed that unstable slips are more likely to result in osteonecrosis than stable slips. It has been estimated that up to 50% of patients with unstable SCFE will develop osteonecrosis.

Controversy exists in the recent literature not only about the natural history of osteonecrosis after SCFE but also about treatment to alter the natural history. Although the natural history is not known for certain, treatment plans are based on these theories of cause. Those who believe that osteonecrosis occurs at the time of maximal instability recommend urgent reduction, whereas those who believe osteonecrosis is caused by a tamponade effect advocate capsulotomy, especially if manipulation is done. Hip pressures in the affected side have been shown to be double those in the unaffected side and to be higher than those of compartment syndromes after manipulation. If a significant effusion is suspected, ultrasound can be used to determine the amount of fluid and the necessity of a capsulotomy. If immediate (within 24 hours) stabilization of an acute slip cannot be accomplished because of delayed presentation, a delay of at least 7 days has been recommended by some authors to avoid the "unsafe window" during which surgical intervention may increase the risk of osteonecrosis. At our institution, however, we advocate urgent reduction, stable fixation, and routine capsulotomy for all acute, unstable slips.

Ballard and Cosgrove coined the term *physeal separation,* which is defined as the amount of separation of the anterior lip of the epiphysis from the metaphysis on a frog-leg lateral radiograph (Fig. 36-117). Of the eight hips that developed osteonecrosis in their study of 110 hips, seven had anterior physeal separation. It was concluded that anterior physeal separation is associated with a high incidence of subsequent osteonecrosis after SCFE.

CHONDROLYSIS

The diagnosis of chondrolysis requires a joint space less than 3 mm wide (normal 4 to 6 mm) and a decreased range of motion of the hip joint (Fig. 36-118). Persistent pin penetration into the joint has been the most frequently cited cause of chondrolysis, but it has been suggested that some other factor is necessary to produce chondrolysis, such as slip or an immune response.

Although fibrous ankylosis of the hip joint often occurs after chondrolysis, spontaneous partial cartilage recovery has been reported. Bed rest, traction, salicylates, nonsteroidal antiinflammatory drugs, steroids, and physical therapy have not modified the course of chondrolysis. We have had some success with intraarticular cortisone injection and operative manipulation, followed by a vigorous physical therapy program. If severe joint space narrowing persists with limitation of joint motion, arthrodesis or arthroplasty should be considered.

FEMORAL NECK FRACTURE

Femoral fractures have been reported infrequently as a complication of in situ fixation of SCFE, although several authors have reported subtrochanteric fractures. We have treated a few patients with subtrochanteric fractures through unused drill holes below screw fixation (Fig. 36-119). After trying various methods of treatment for the subtrochanteric fracture, we now recommend immediate open reduction of the fracture and internal fixation with a hip screw and a long side plate while maintaining the reduction of SCFE.

Femoral neck fracture after in situ pinning of SCFE is even less common. We have treated two patients with displaced femoral neck fractures after in situ fixation of SCFE. In both patients, treatment of the femoral neck fractures was operative and difficult and the results were less than satisfactory.

As more reports are accumulated, femoral fractures after in situ fixation of SCFE may be found to be more

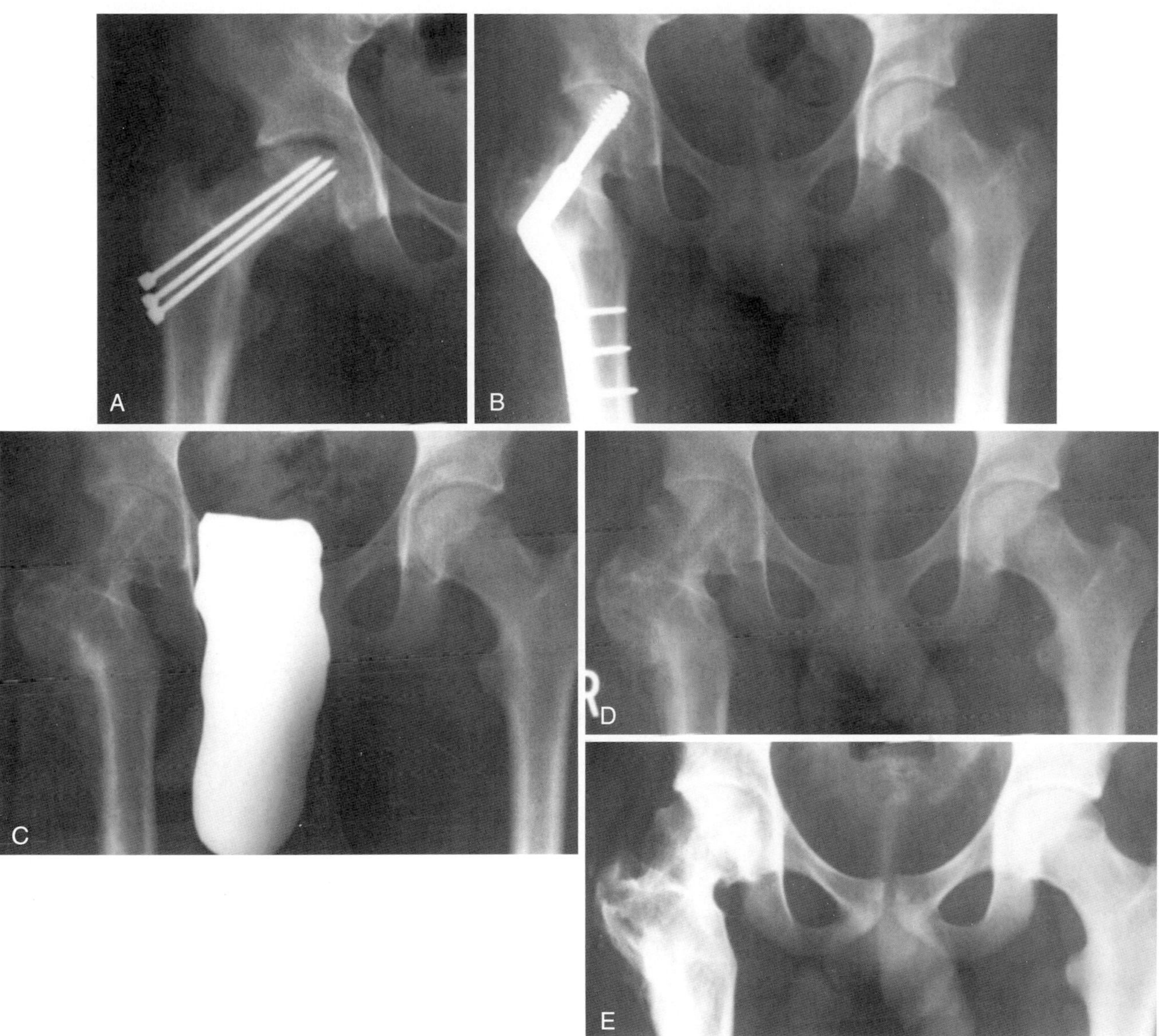

FIGURE 36-118 **A** to **E**, Chondrolysis 24 months after flexion internal rotation osteotomy for severe SCFE.

frequent than currently appreciated. The likelihood of this complication perhaps can be decreased by avoiding drilling unnecessary holes in the bone during surgery and by avoiding overzealous reaming of the femoral neck.

The necessity of pin removal after fixation of SCFE remains an area of controversy. Pin removal is not without costs and risks, and the question of whether a pin must be removed at the end of treatment remains unanswered. We currently are leaving pins and screws in place after treatment of SCFE.

CONTINUED SLIPPING

Continued slipping has occurred in patients who refused treatment, were not compliant with postoperative restrictions, and in whom stable fixation was not achieved. Progressive slipping may also occur if osteonecrosis develops and fixation is lost before physeal closure.

FEMOROACETABULAR IMPINGEMENT

Recent interest in femoroacetabular impingement (FAI), which has become a frequently reported and described entity that causes pain, decreased range of motion, and early osteoarthritis of the hip joint, has led to a better understanding of SCFE-induced impingement. These result from the anterolateral displacement of the femoral neck in relation to the femoral epiphysis producing a reduced head-neck offset, elevated alpha angle (Fig. 36-120), and cam type lesion. One study reported a high proportion (32% to 38%) of young adults with signs of clinical impingement after SCFE. Although extreme posterior angulation (slippage) obviously may cause impingement, the real question is how little angular deformity will cause impingement. This is key to in situ pinning, after which generally good early results can be expected. The literature is unclear about how much posterior angulation can be accepted during initial treatment or even

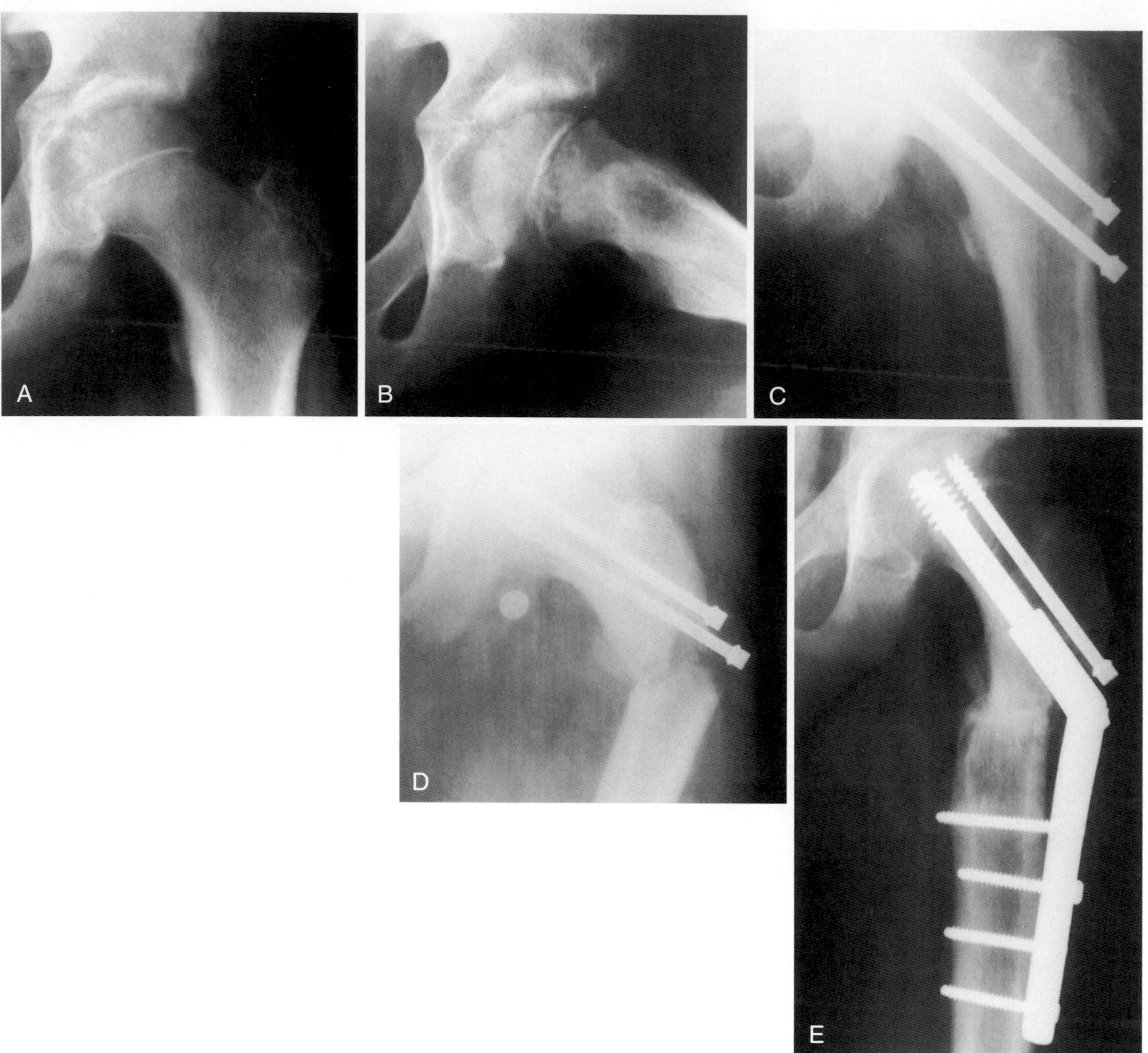

FIGURE 36-119 **A** and **B,** Slipped capital femoral epiphysis. **C,** After pin fixation, several unnecessary drill holes remain distal to last pin. **D,** After pathologic fracture through drill hole. **E,** One year after open reduction and internal fixation with compression hip screw; note evidence of union of subtrochanteric fracture. Cannulated hip screw was left in place to prevent further slipping of capital femoral epiphysis at the time of hip screw insertion.

how much angulation later will cause symptomatic FAI. According to most series, the grade of slip in adolescence cannot be used as predictor of the development of symptomatic FAI and ultimately osteoarthritis in adulthood.

The cam effect in which the femoral head or screw head abuts the acetabular labrum (Fig. 36-121) and the pincer effect in which the acetabular rim impinges on the femoral neck (Fig. 36-122) have both been described in adults who had treatment of SCFE as adolescents. FAI can be identified by arthroscopy and MRI; plain cross-table lateral radiographs dramatically demonstrate cam and pincer impingement described by Nötzli as "jamming rim" impingement (Fig. 36-123).

Femoral osteochondroplasty, valgus osteotomy, or the Imhaüser procedure (see Technique 36-28) has been recommended after in situ pinning to avoid acetabular impingement.

FEMORAL FRACTURES

Femoral fracture is a common injury. The annual rate of femoral shaft fractures in children is 20 per 100,000. With regard to age, the distribution appears to be bimodal, with peaks at 2 and 17 years. Boys have higher rates of fracture than girls at all ages. The primary mechanisms of fracture are age dependent and include falls for children younger than 6 years old, motor vehicle–pedestrian accidents for children 6 to 9 years old, and motor vehicle accidents for teenagers.

Fractures of the femur usually are classified according to location as subtrochanteric, shaft (proximal, middle, and

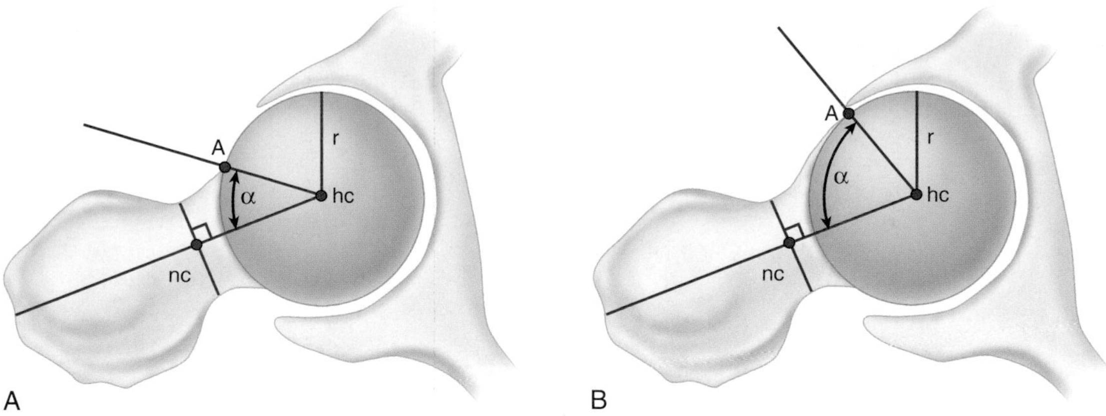

FIGURE 36-120 Anterior head-neck offset (Nötzli) angle. Point *A,* anterior point where the distance from the center of the head (*hc*) exceeds the radius (*r*) of the subchondral surface of the femoral head. α is then measured as the angle between *A-hc* and *hc-nc*, with *nc* being the center of the neck at the narrowest point. **A,** Hip in a normal individual. **B,** A typical deformation. The greater the anterior head-neck offset angle, the smaller the arc of motion required to cause cam-type impingement on the acetabular rim.

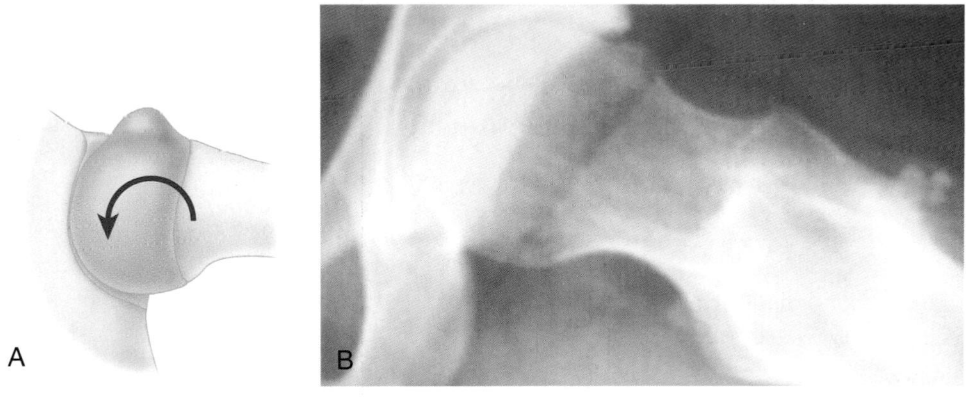

FIGURE 36-121 **A,** Cam-type impingement. **B,** Radiographic appearance.

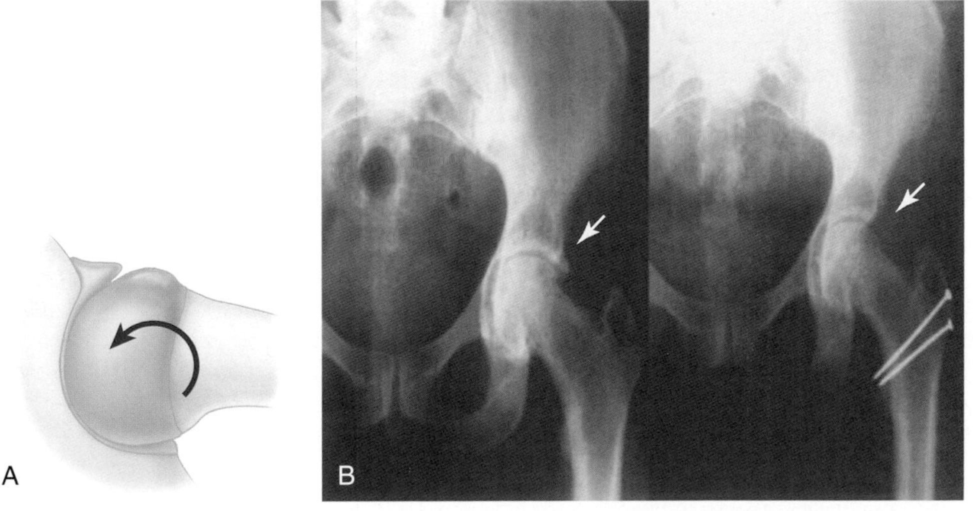

FIGURE 36-122 **A,** Pincer-type impingement. **B,** Radiographic appearance.

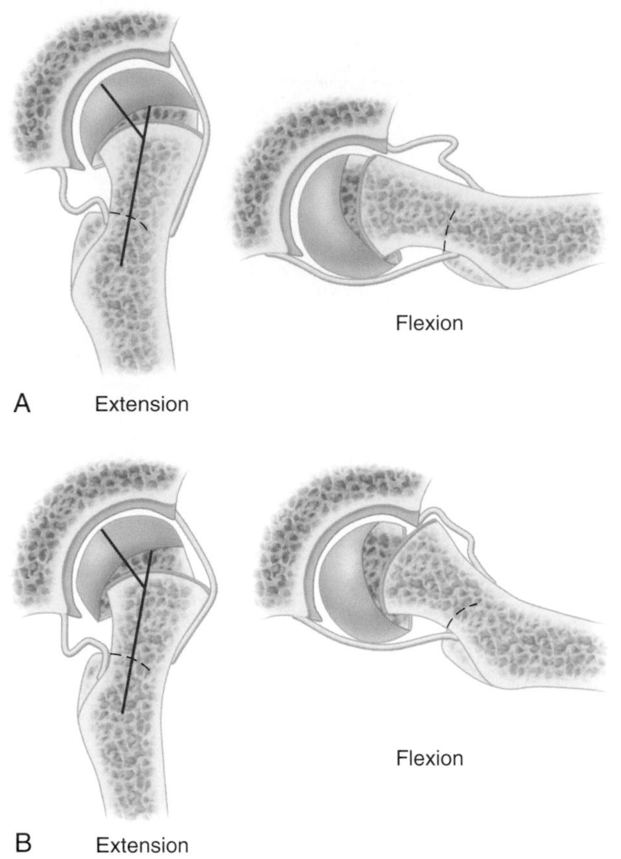

FIGURE 36-123 "Jamming rim" impingement. **A,** Mild to moderate slipped capital femoral epiphysis (SCFE) causes jamming of the femoral metaphysis against the acetabular cartilage in flexion. **B,** Severe SCFE causes impingement of the femoral neck against the acetabular rim in flexion.

distal thirds), supracondylar, and distal femoral physeal. Additionally, femoral fractures are classified by being open or closed, comminuted or noncomminuted, and by fracture pattern (transverse, spiral, or oblique). Fractures occur most commonly in the middle third of the shaft as a closed, noncomminuted, transverse fracture.

Historically, most femoral fractures in children are closed injuries and traditionally have been treated by closed methods. However, management of pediatric femoral fractures has evolved toward operative approaches because of a desire for more rapid recovery and reintegration of the patients, with the recognition that prolonged immobilization can have negative effects even in children. External fixation, submuscular plating, and intramedullary nailing all have been advocated.

Besides the usual mechanisms of injury, femoral fractures can occur at birth, can be caused by child abuse, or can be pathologic. In children younger than 1 year of age, 70% of femoral fractures are abuse related. Abuse should be suspected if any of the following are present: (1) unreasonable history; (2) inappropriate delay in coming to the hospital; (3) previous history of abuse; (4) evidence of other fractures in various stages of healing; (5) multiple acute fractures; and (6) characteristic fracture patterns. A recent study from our institution demonstrated that a transverse fracture pattern is more closely associated with abuse and should raise the index of suspicion for abuse.

In the setting of a femoral fracture, a thorough evaluation should be performed and concomitant injury ruled out. If a child sustains enough trauma to fracture the largest bone in his or her body, the child may have occult abdominal or other injuries. A careful secondary survey should be performed. Ipsilateral knee instability has been reported to occur in 4% of children with femoral fractures and may be difficult to assess at the time of injury.

FEMORAL SHAFT FRACTURES (DIAPHYSEAL FEMORAL FRACTURES)

Understanding the deforming forces applied by various structures around the femur helps in selecting the appropriate treatment of a femoral fracture. In proximal shaft and subtrochanteric fractures, the proximal fragment usually is in a position of flexion, abduction, and external rotation because of the unopposed pull of the iliopsoas, abductor, and short external rotator muscles. The adductors and extensors are intact in midshaft fractures, and the distal fragment usually is in satisfactory alignment except for some external rotation. In supracondylar fractures, the distal fragment is in a position of hyperextension because of the overpull of the gastrocnemius. The muscle imbalances are important when aligning the distal fragment to the proximal fragment whether closed or open treatment strategies are selected.

Staheli defined the ideal treatment of femoral shaft fractures in children as one that controls alignment and length, is comfortable for the child and convenient for the family, and causes the least negative psychologic impact possible. Determining the ideal treatment for each child depends on the age of the child, the location and type of fracture, the family environment, the knowledge and ability of the surgeon, and, to a lesser degree, financial considerations. Heyworth et al. reviewed femoral fractures in children 6 to 17 years old from a national database of pediatric inpatient admissions from 1997 to 2000 in about half of the United States. The frequency of operative treatment, most often consisting of internal fixation, increased significantly over this period, whereas the use of spica casting declined. This change in practice was significantly greater at pediatric hospitals than general hospitals. Sanders et al. surveyed members of the Pediatric Orthopedic Society of North America to determine their current preferences in treating femoral fractures in four age groups. For each fracture pattern, operative treatment was increasingly preferred over nonoperative treatment as patient age increased and the preferred treatments within operative and nonoperative categories changed significantly as patient age increased. There was a trend by pediatric orthopaedists to treat femoral fractures operatively in older children and nonoperatively in younger children. The consensus on treatment was that it is age dependent (Fig. 36-124).

The AAOS, after extensive review of the literature, made 14 evidence-based recommendations concerning fracture of the femur in children. Five of the recommendations with enough evidence to support a grade of recommendation (grade A or B, supported by good evidence; grade C, supported by poor evidence) are listed in Box 36-4.

Our general treatment recommendations are listed in Table 36-4.

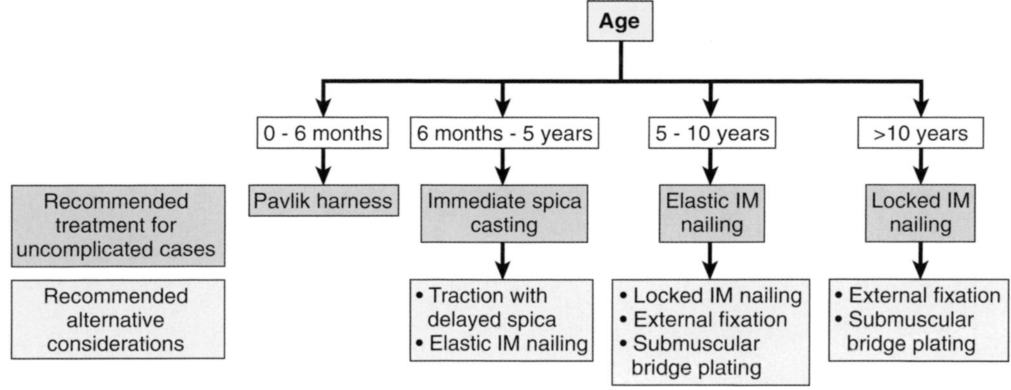

FIGURE 36-124 Algorithm for treatment of femoral fractures in children. IM, intramedullary.

BOX 36-4

Treatment Recommendations for Diaphyseal Femoral Fractures

- We recommend that children younger than 36 months with a diaphyseal femoral fracture be evaluated for child abuse (A).
- Treatment with a Pavlik harness or spica cast is an option for infants 6 months and younger with a diaphyseal femoral fracture (C).
- We suggest early spica casting or traction with delayed spica casting for children age 6 months to 5 years with a diaphyseal femoral fracture with less than 2 cm of shortening (B).
- Flexible intramedullary nailing is an option to treat diaphyseal femoral fractures in children 5 to 11 years of age (C).
- Rigid trochanteric entry nailing, submuscular plating, and flexible intramedullary nailing are treatment options for diaphyseal femoral fractures in children age 11 years to skeletal maturity, but piriformis or near piriformis entry rigid nailing is not a treatment option (C).

Several authors have evaluated the comparative economics of nonoperative and operative treatment. The charges or cost included hospital and physician charges (orthopaedists, radiologists, and anesthesiologists). Table 36-5 gives the cost or charges in different series of patients. The differences seen among series are not comparable because of many variables. On average, however, immediate or early spica casting (traction spica) cost less than prolonged traction with spica casting, intramedullary rods, or external fixation. Prolonged skeletal traction and spica casting, intramedullary rods, and external fixation frequently cost the same. The cost of reoperations for malrotation or removal of implants also was similar for the three groups.

In a very young child (birth to 6 months), a Pavlik harness can be used instead of a spica cast with cited advantages of ease of application without anesthesia; minimal hospitalization (<24 hours); easy reduction; ability to adjust the harness; minimal costs; and ease in diaper changing, nursing, and bonding. Our institution recently reported on the uses of a Pavlik harness for femoral fracture in children under 6 months of age and found excellent clinical results with minimal complication rates. Parent reliability and compliance, however, must be carefully considered before using this method of treatment.

Immediate spica casting of femoral shaft fractures in children has been recommended by several authors; best results with this method seem to be obtained in infants and young children with low-energy, length stable fracture. Although rare, a compartment syndrome secondary to spica casting also can occur. The primary problems with immediate spica casting are shortening and angulation of the fracture in high-energy femoral shaft fractures. In young children, a higher degree of angulation and shortening is accepted; these parameters become stricter with increasing age (Table 36-6).

SPICA CASTING

Early spica casting in the 90-90 position has been recommended to avoid shortening and angulation in children younger than 6 years old with a closed femoral shaft fracture stemming from low-energy trauma. Alternatively, for low-energy femoral fractures, a walking spica or single leg spica may be applied with the hip and knee flexed to 45 degrees and the cast ending above the ankle. Flynn et al. performed a prospective study comparing a walking spica with a traditional spica cast and found similar outcomes with significantly lower burden of care to the family. The walking spica group did, however, have a higher early loss of reduction requiring cast wedging in the outpatient setting.

Good results also have been reported with 90-90 skeletal traction and spica casting, although the current indication for this technique at our institution is for length-unstable fractures or concomitant injuries that prevent the patient from having a spica cast in place or from being safely sedated. If this treatment course is selected, pins for skeletal traction should be placed parallel to the axis of the knee joint (Fig. 36-125).

Adolescents do not tolerate prolonged immobilization as well as younger children, and knee pain, angulation at the fracture, and difficulty in maintaining length have been reported when 90-90 traction was used in children older than 10 years, as well as limb shortening and leg-length discrepancy, malunion, pin track infection, loss of joint motion, and

TABLE 36-4

General Treatment Guidelines in Children With Femoral Shaft Fractures

AGE	<6 MONTHS	6 MONTHS-5 YEARS	5-11 YEARS	11 YEARS-ADULT
PREFERRED TREATMENT	Pavlik harness	Early spica casting	Elastic intramedullary nail	Antegrade locked intramedullary nail
Alternate treatment because of: Head injury High velocity (comminuted) Floating knee Difficult location (proximal third and distal third) Obesity Surgical risk (multiple trauma)		Traction and spica casting	Traction and spica casting Submuscular plating Antegrade locked intramedullary nail	Submuscular plating
OPEN FRACTURES		External fixation	External fixation	External fixation

TABLE 36-5

Cost of Treatment of Femoral Shaft Fractures

SERIES	IMMEDIATE (EARLY SPICA)	TRACTION SPICA	SKELETAL INTRAMEDULLARY ROD	EXTERNAL FIXATION
Newton and Mubarak	—	$5,494	$21,093	$21,359
Clinkscales and Peterson	$5,490	$16,273	$16,056	$16,394
Stans et al.	$5,264	$15,980	$15,495	$14,478
Yandow et al.	$1,867	$11,171	—	—
Nork and Hoffinger	$22,396	$11,520	—	—
Coyte et al.	$5,970*	$7,626*	—	—

*Canadian $.

TABLE 36-6

Acceptable Angulation in Femoral Shaft Fractures

AGE	VARUS/ VALGUS (DEGREES)	ANTERIOR/ POSTERIOR (DEGREES)	SHORTENING (MM)
Birth to 2 years	30	30	15
2-5 years	15	20	20
2-10 years	10	15	15
11 years to maturity	5	10	10

From Flynn JM, Skaggs DL: Femoral shaft fractures. In Flynn JM, Skaggs DL, Waters PM (editors). Rockwood and Wilkins' Fractures in Children, 8th ed, Philadelphia, Wolters Kluwer, 2015.

muscle atrophy. As a result, internal fixation is preferred in this age group.

At our institution, if skeletal or skin traction is applied in children younger than 6 years old, longitudinal traction or traction at a 45-degree angle with up to 5 lb of weight is recommended. Overhead skin traction should not be used for femoral fractures in this age group because of the increased risk of neurovascular compromise. Neurovascular status and skin condition should be monitored carefully while the child is in traction. When length and alignment are achieved, the patient is medically stable, and appropriate callus formation is noted, a spica cast is applied. In children 6 to 10 years old, the age at which most femoral fractures occur, skeletal traction may be an option, with the application of a spica cast after 2 to 3 weeks of traction.

In older or larger children who require traction, a 5/64-inch Steinmann pin can be inserted into the distal femur or proximal tibia. If a tibial pin is used, it should be placed distal to the tibial tubercle and the proximal tibial physis to minimize the risk of growth disturbance and genu recurvatum deformity. A distal femoral traction pin may be necessary for a distal supracondylar fracture because of posterior angulation or for 90-90 degree traction in a proximal femoral fracture with anterior displacement of the proximal fragment. A femoral pin generally should not be used if intramedullary nailing is being contemplated in the course of treatment.

Peroneal nerve palsy is a rare complication of skin or skeletal traction and casting. Two of our patients younger than 2 years old developed peroneal nerve palsies after skin traction and spica casting. Spontaneous recovery occurs in most patients.

Mubarak et al. described the development of a compartment syndrome in the lower leg after application of a short leg cast used for traction to reduce femoral fractures during the application of a 90-90 spica cast. They cited as pathogenic factors traction, elevation, and pressure (Fig. 36-126). Because of the possibility of this potentially devastating complication, the use of a short leg cast for applying traction should be avoided during application of a 90-90 spica cast and alternative cast application methods should be used.

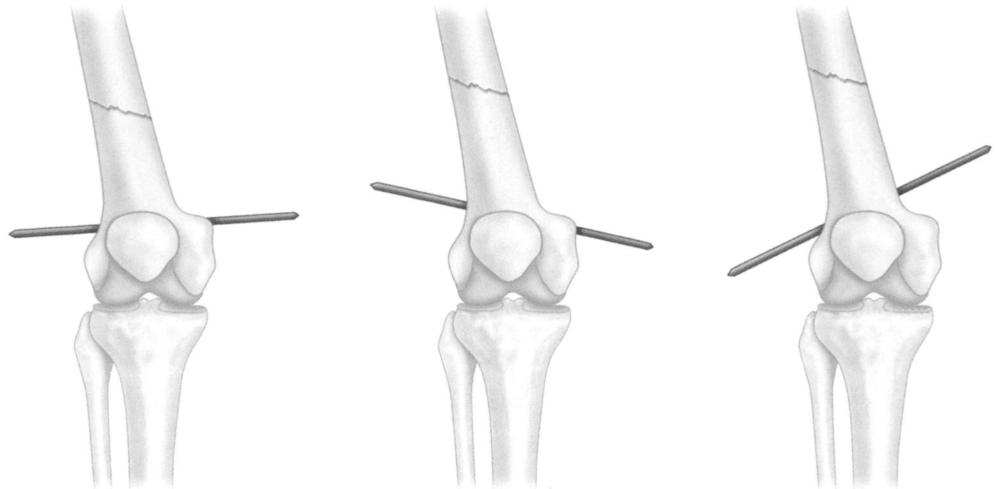

FIGURE 36-125 Position of pin in traction is either horizontal (optimal) or oblique. Oblique pins are either "to varus" or "to valgus," reflecting resultant pull of traction bow.

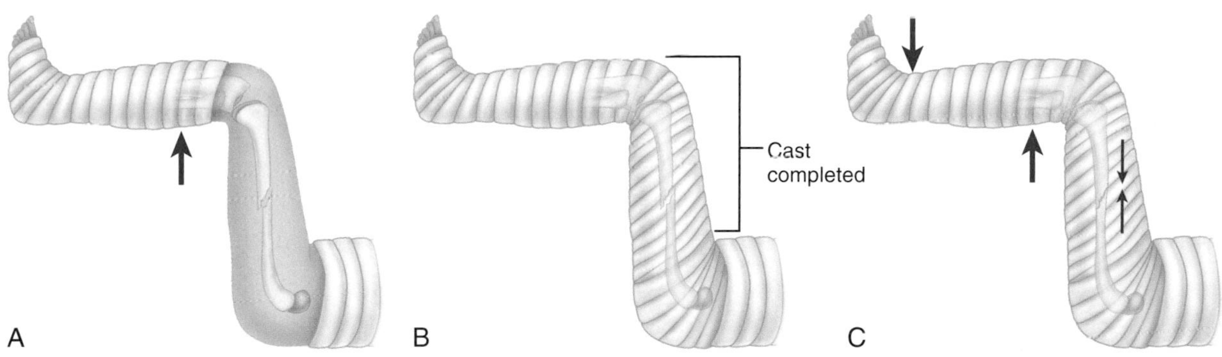

FIGURE 36-126 Pathogenic factors of traction, elevation, and pressure during the application of a short leg cast used for traction can cause compartment syndrome. **A,** Below-knee cast is applied while patient is on spica frame. **B,** Traction is applied to the short leg cast to produce distraction at the fracture site. The remainder of the cast is applied, fixing the relative distance between the leg and torso. **C,** After the child awakens from general anesthesia, there is shortening of the femur from muscular contraction, which causes the thigh and leg to slip somewhat back into the spica. This causes pressure at the corners of the cast *(arrows).* (Redrawn from Mubarak SJ, Frick S, Sink E, et al: Volkmann contracture and compartment syndromes after femur fractures in children treated with 90/90 spica casts, J Pediatr Orthop 26:567, 2006.)

SPICA CAST APPLICATION

TECHNIQUE 36-29

- After general anesthesia, remove the skeletal traction pin and sterilely clean the wound sites if traction was used.
- Apply a well-padded long leg cast with the knee flexed 45 or 90 degrees, depending on whether a traditional or walking spica is being applied. Mold the proximal part to help avoid angulation with a strong valgus mold. To avoid compartment syndrome, do not apply traction through a short leg cast to effect reduction.
- Place the child on a "spica table" or fracture table, depending on the size of the child, and check the reduction. Apply a one and one-half spica cast or full spica cast with the hip or hips flexed at 45 or 90 degrees (Fig. 36-127), with approximately 15 degrees of external rotation and 30 degrees of hip abduction. Children younger than 3 years tolerate the 90-90 degree spica cast well. This position helps prevent shortening and aids in transporting the child. (According to Flynn, automobile restraint laws in many states make it difficult or impossible to legally transport a child casted in full extension.) Knee flexion of less than 50 degrees may result in a 20% incidence of loss of reduction.
- Apply the spica to a level between the umbilicus and nipple line with a 1/4- to 1/2-inch thick towel over the thorax and under the Webril (Kendall Healthcare, Mansfield, MA), which is to be removed later to allow for chest and abdominal expansion.

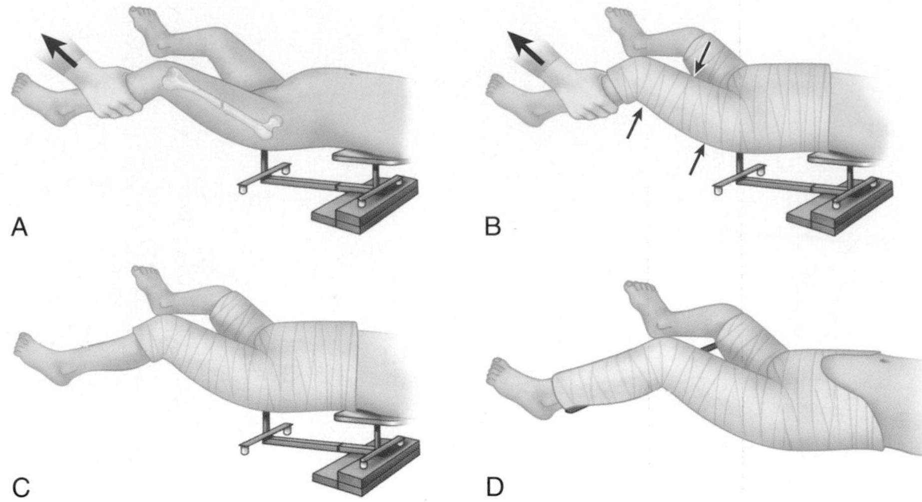

FIGURE 36-127 Technique of spica cast application. **A,** The patient is placed on a child's fracture spica table. The leg is held in about 45 degrees of flexion at the hip and knee, with traction applied to the proximal calf. **B,** The one and one-half spica cast is applied down to the proximal calf. Molding of the thigh is done during this phase. **C,** Radiographs of the femur are obtained, and any necessary wedging of the cast can be done at this time. **D,** The leg portion of the cast and the cross-bar are applied. The belly portion of the spica cast is trimmed to the umbilicus. (Redrawn from Mubarak SJ, Frick S, Sink E, et al: Volkmann contracture and compartment syndromes after femur fractures in children treated with 90/90 spica casts, J Pediatr Orthop 26:567, 2006.) **SEE TECHNIQUE 36-29.**

- Reinforce the groin, inguinal, and buttocks areas with splints to avoid breakage.
- After trimming the cast and after satisfactory radiographs are obtained, apply a wooden bar spanning the extremities and incorporate it in the cast if additional cast stability is required.

EXTERNAL FIXATION

External fixation with both monolateral and circular frames has been recommended for treatment of femoral shaft fractures in children and adolescents, with good results reported by a number of authors in patients ranging in age from 3 years to skeletal maturity. Complications, however, also have been frequent with this method of fixation. Ramseier et al., in a comparison of four fixation methods (elastic stable intramedullary nail, rigid intramedullary nail, plate, and external fixator), found that external fixation was associated with the highest number of complications. Major complications associated with external fixation of femoral fractures in children and adolescents include loss of reduction, refracture, and deep infection. The most common minor complication is pin site or pin track infection. Refracture has been reported in from 2% to 33% of patients treated with external fixation. Refracture has been suggested to occur because of the detrimental effect of prolonged rigidity imposed by the external fixator. An association has been noted between the number of cortices showing bridging callus (on anteroposterior and lateral views) at the time of fixator removal and the rate of refracture. Kesemenli et al. reported a refracture rate of only 1.8% in closed femoral fractures and a 20% rate of refracture in open fractures or in patients who had ORIF. They concluded that external fixation itself was not a risk factor for refracture. Other suggested risk factors include open fractures and bilateral fractures with the increase of time in the fixator. Factors that appear to have an inconclusive effect on refracture include fracture pattern, dynamization status, fixator type, pin size, and number of pins.

Open fractures of the femur have traditionally been stabilized with external fixation. A comparison of the results of external fixation and intramedullary nailing (both rigid and flexible nails) found that intramedullary nailing was associated with fewer complications, especially varus malunion and refracture. Infection rates appeared to be the same. Intramedullary fixation should be considered, especially for grade I open fractures. If external fixation is chosen as the method of treatment for pediatric femoral fractures, careful attention must be paid to operative technique and postoperative treatment to minimize complications.

At our institution, in a young child with polytrauma, open fracture with significant soft-tissue injury, pathologic fracture, metadiaphyseal fracture, or severe head injury, external fixation is considered as a fixation option. The technique of external fixation of fractures of the femur is described in Chapter 54.

INTRAMEDULLARY NAILING

Good results using flexible stainless steel or titanium intramedullary rods have been reported with suggested advantages of less disruption of family life, shorter hospitalization, earlier independent ambulation, and earlier return to school (Fig. 36-128). With the overall trend to more frequent internal fixation of femoral fractures, it is not surprising that the indications have expanded to include younger children. The lower age limit for flexible intramedullary nailing has not been definitively established (see AAOS Guidelines, Box

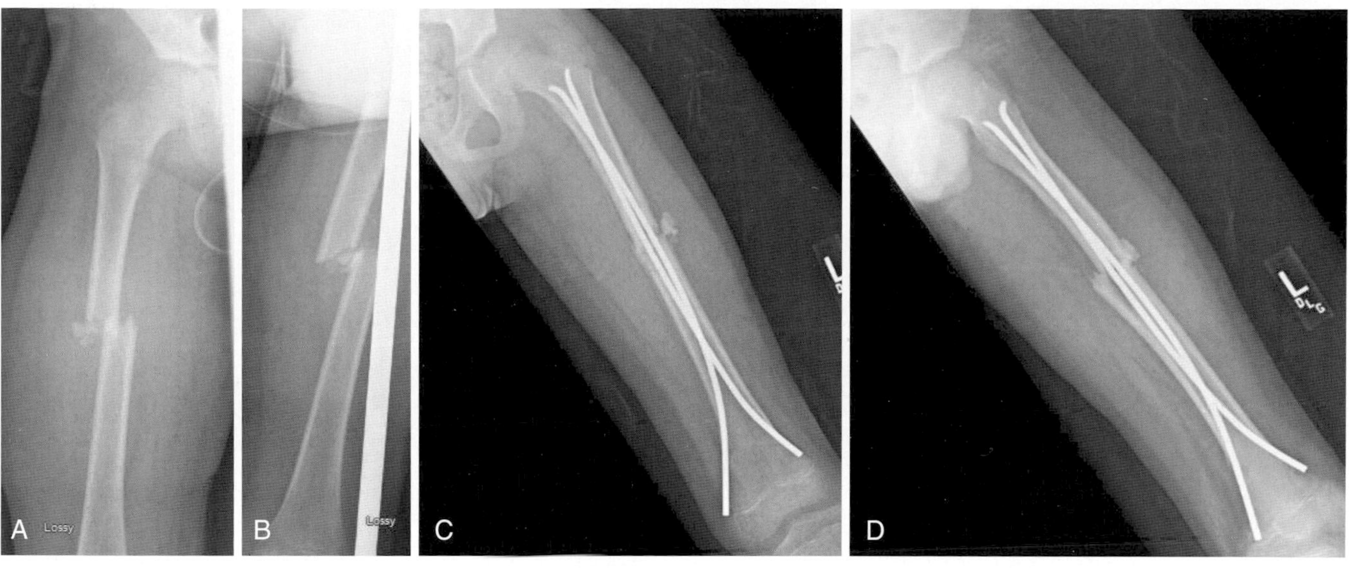

FIGURE 36-128 A and B, Femoral shaft fracture. C and D, After fixation with flexible intramedullary nails, avoiding proximal and distal physes.

36-4), but certainly there is an age at which any type of immobilization (e.g., Pavlik harness, spica cast) will produce a good result without the risk of surgical complications. Several reports have documented good results with few complications in preschool (18 months to 6 years of age) children treated with flexible intramedullary nailing. Heffernan et al. reviewed 215 patients between the ages of 2 and 6 years who were treated with either elastic nails or a spica cast and found similar complication and healing rates, with an earlier return to independent ambulation and full activities in the elastic nail group. They concluded that elastic nails were a reasonable treatment option in this age group and should be considered, especially when high-energy mechanisms are present. Long-term follow-up (at least 24 months) is recommended to monitor overgrowth, and the child's activity must be closely monitored. Malalignment and leg-length discrepancy are frequently reported complications of flexible intramedullary nailing of femoral fractures in children, but these seldom cause functional problems. Increased complication rates have been reported in unstable fractures, older patients, and overweight patients treated with titanium elastic nails. One study found that the complication rate was improved from 52% to 23% when the use of titanium elastic nailing was limited to stable fractures. Additional studies have found that the use of stainless steel nails can significantly lower the malunion rate, major complication rate, and overall cost when compared with titanium nails.

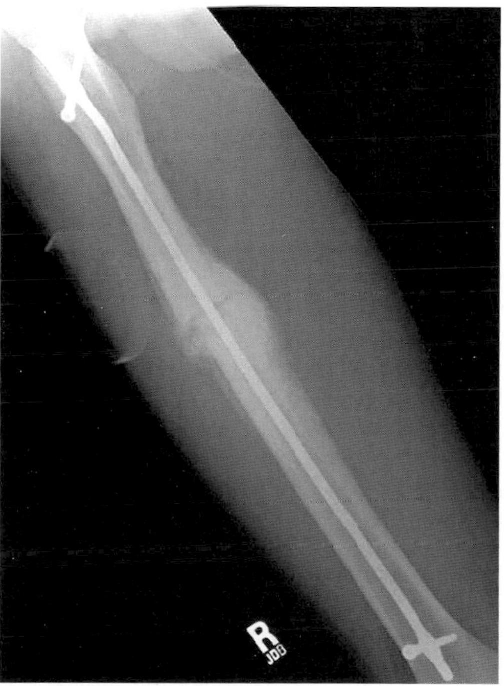

FIGURE 36-129 Flexible interlocked nailing of a femoral shaft fracture through a lateral trochanteric entry site.

A flexible interlocked intramedullary nail has been reported to reduce perioperative complications and improve outcomes, as well as reduce time to healing and time to weight bearing, by better controlling axial and rotational instability (Fig. 36-129). The nail is made of a titanium alloy that allows plastic deformation of the nail as it is introduced through a lateral trochanteric entry point into the femoral canal; the nail is locked proximally and distally with 4-mm screws. The most common complication reported with the use of this nail was trochanteric heterotopic ossification (approximately 14%); no major complications (malunion, refracture, osteonecrosis) were reported in patients with flexible locked nails, compared with 11% of patients with other fixation methods (standard flexible nails, external fixation, bridge plating, and rigid intramedullary nailing). The flexible interlocked intramedullary is recommended for fractures distal to the lesser trochanter and at least 4 cm proximal to the distal femoral physes.

Rigid intramedullary fixation of femoral shaft fractures in adolescents has been reported to result in high rates of union with short hospital stays and brief periods of immobilization that may have psychologic, social, educational, and some economic advantages over conservative treatment. In a review of our early results of intramedullary nailing of 31 femoral fractures in 30 adolescents, ranging in age from 10 to 15 years (average 12.3 years), we found that all 31 fractures united without evidence of trochanteric overgrowth, coxa valga deformity, or narrowing of the femoral neck. Two patients had bony overgrowth of more than 2cm (2.5cm and 2.8cm). Other complications included one superficial distal wound infection that resolved after intravenous antibiotic therapy and decreased sensation in the distribution of the deep peroneal nerve in one patient and in the distribution of the pudendal nerve in another; both neurologic problems resolved spontaneously. Mild heterotopic ossification over the nail proximally was found in three patients. Asymptomatic segmental osteonecrosis developed in one patient when a piriformis entry site was used and was not visible on radiographs until 15 months after fracture. A subsequent study of femoral shaft fractures in children 12 years and under treated with a rigid, locked, antegrade nailing inserted from a trochanteric entry point was conducted at our institution and demonstrated no malunion, leg-length difference, osteonecrosis, or hardware failure at final follow-up. A subsequent report by Crosby et al. on a 20-year experience with trochanteric rigid intramedullary nails in pediatric and adolescent femoral fractures demonstrated acceptable complication rates with no cases of osteonecrosis. Because of the few complications and high rate of union in our patients and other reports, we believe trochanteric rigid intramedullary nailing is the treatment of choice for femoral shaft fractures in older adolescents (12 to 16 years old) and is a reasonable option for children with risk factors for malunion, such as obesity or unstable fracture patterns.

To minimize the risk of osteonecrosis, it is important that the dissection during placement and removal not extend medial to the greater trochanter, with care to avoid extension to the capsule or the piriformis fossa. The tip of the greater trochanter in adolescents or a more lateral starting point in younger children should be used for the entry site. Only one instance of osteonecrosis has been reported when the tip of the trochanter has been used as the entry point, and no cases of osteonecrosis have been reported to our knowledge with a lateral entry point. This prevents dissection near the piriformis fossa and the origin of the lateral ascending cervical artery, which is medial to the piriformis fossa (Fig. 36-130). The proximal end of the nail should be left long (≤1cm) to make later removal easier (Fig. 36-131). Nails can be removed 9 to 18 months after radiographic union to prevent bony overgrowth over the proximal tip of the nail.

The length and diameter of the intramedullary nail may limit the use of this technique, but the development of a smaller (7 mm diameter) pediatric nail expands its application. We use a pediatric nail that has a transverse proximal interlocking screw that can be dynamized and avoids the greater trochanter and has more distal screw holes in the nail to avoid the physis (Fig. 36-132). Most small-diameter nails are solid, making passage through the fracture site a challenge. The technique of locked intramedullary nailing of the femur is described in Chapter 54.

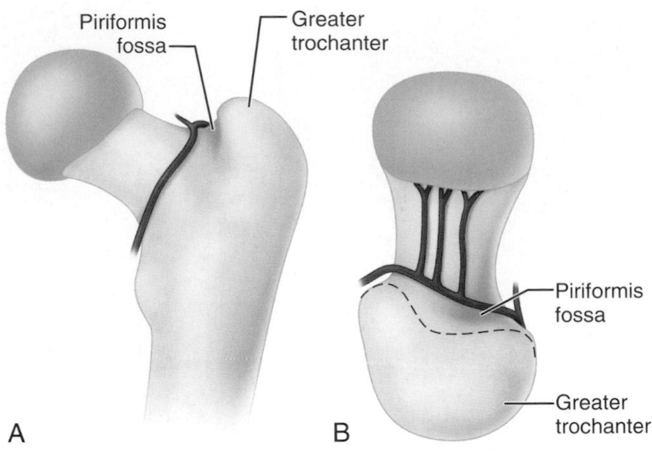

FIGURE 36-130 **A and B, Proximal femoral anatomy.** (Redrawn from Keeler KA, Dart B, Luhmann SJ, et al: Antegrade intramedullary nailing of pediatric femoral fractures using an interlocking pediatric femoral nail and a lateral trochanteric entry point, J Pediatr Orthop 29:345, 2009.)

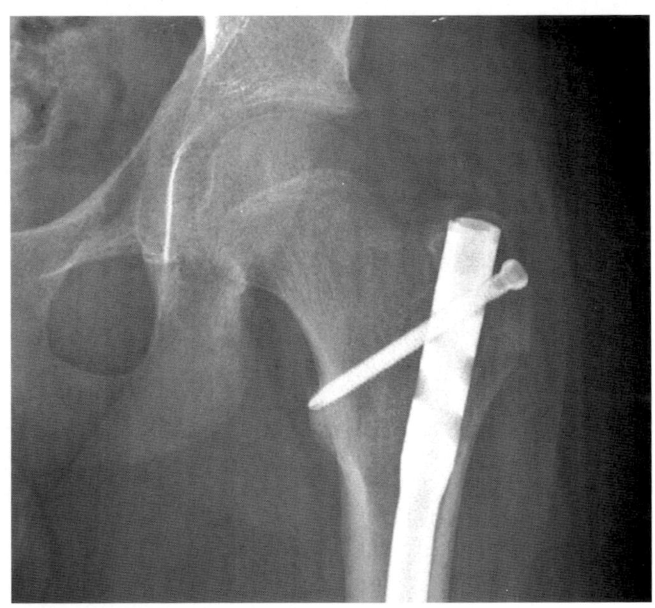

FIGURE 36-131 Proximal end of nail is left long (≤1cm) to make later removal easier.

FLEXIBLE INTRAMEDULLARY NAIL FIXATION

Biomechanical testing of flexible intramedullary nails using synthetic bone models has shown that (1) retrograde nail fixation has significantly less axial range of motion and more torsional stiffness than antegrade fixation in comminuted and transverse fracture models; (2) there is no significant difference between the mechanical properties of three different retrograde nail constructions (two C-shaped and two S-shaped and two straight flexible nails were tested), suggesting that any of the three constructs

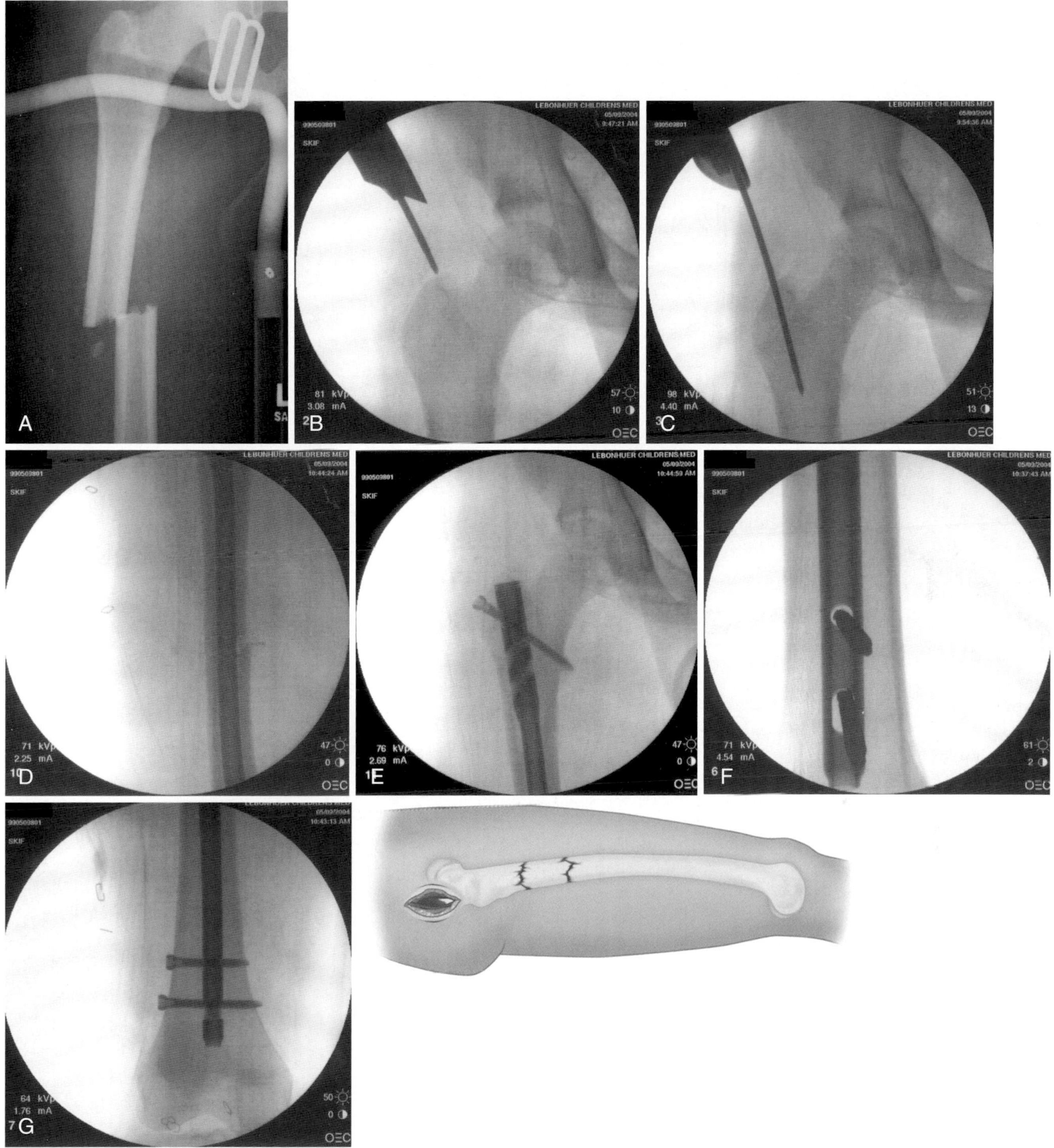

FIGURE 36-132 Pediatric TriGen intramedullary nailing. **A,** Midshaft femoral fracture in a 15-year old. **B,** Entry at tip of greater trochanter (inset shows approach). **C,** Channel reamer and guide placement. **D,** A 9-mm nail placed across fracture site. **E,** Locking of proximal screw. **F** and **G,** Concentric circle technique for distal locking.

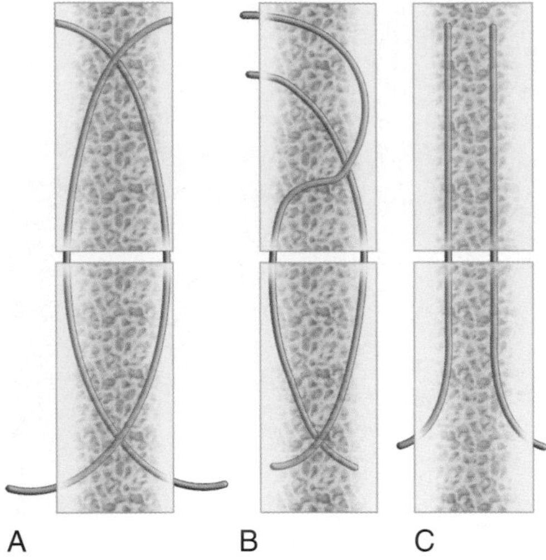

FIGURE 36-133 **A,** Midshaft diaphyseal fracture model stabilized with two C-shaped nails. **B** and **C,** Midshaft diaphyseal fracture stabilized with S-shaped and C-shaped nails **(B)** and two straight nails **(C)**.

could be used to treat femoral fractures in children; and (3) length and rotation control with two divergent flexible nails of comminuted midshaft femur fractures may be sufficient for early mobilization (Fig. 36-133). Most femoral shaft fractures in children can be stabilized using retrograde fixation. Usually, medial and lateral insertion sites are used, but a single insertion site, either medial or lateral, can be used in the distal femoral metaphysis. Two divergent C-configuration nails or one C-configuration and one S-configuration nail (bent by the surgeon at a point approximately 5cm distal to the eyelet) are routine; additional nails can be added if necessary. Special expertise is needed to stabilize subtrochanteric fractures and fractures of the distal third of the femur; antegrade insertion commonly is used for the latter. Most agree that fixation of some proximal and distal long spiral fractures may lack stability as far as rotation and angulation, and testing for stability after nailing at surgery is indicated. If instability is present, a long leg cast with a pelvic band is used short term. A prospective comparison of titanium elastic nail fixation and spica casting for treatment of femoral shaft fractures in children found that children treated with flexible nails achieved recovery milestones significantly faster than those treated with traction and spica casting. Hospital charges for the two methods were similar, and the complication rate after flexible nailing (21%) was lower than after traction and spica casting (34%).

Although mechanical studies have demonstrated equal or superior fixation with titanium nails compared with stainless steel nails, and the biomechanical properties of titanium have been suggested to be superior to those of stainless steel for intramedullary fixation, a comparison of the two devices found a malunion rate nearly four times higher with the use of titanium nails (23%) than with stainless steel nails (6%). Overall, major complications were more frequent with the titanium nails (36%) than with stainless steel nails (17%).

TECHNIQUE 36-30

- Place the patient on an orthopaedic table and reduce the fracture partially by traction guided by fluoroscopy (Fig. 36-134A and B).
- Use blunt-ended nails of quality steel (cold-hammered at 140 degrees) or titanium. The nails should be 45 cm long with diameters of 2.5, 3.0, 3.5, or 4.0 mm, depending on the child's weight and age.
- Prepare the nails preoperatively by angling them at 45 degrees about 2 cm from one end to facilitate penetration of the medullary canal and bend them into an even curve over their entire length.
- With the help of a T-handle and by rotation movements of the wrist, introduce the nails through a longitudinal drill hole made in the distal femoral metaphysis just above the physis. Use two nails, one lateral and one medial, to stabilize the fracture. Carefully impact both up the medullary canal to the fracture site. After touching the opposite internal cortex, the nails bend themselves in the direction of the long bone's axis. The nails should cross distal to the fracture site (normally 4 to 6 cm distal) (Fig. 36-134C).
- With the fracture held reduced, rotate the T-handle or manipulate the limb to direct the pins into the opposite fragment. If the first is impeded, try the second with the aid of an image intensifier. Ensure both nails are in the canal across the fracture site. When they pass the fracture level, release traction, pushing the nails farther and fixing their tips in the spongy tissue of the metaphysis, without their passing through the physis (Fig. 36-134D). Small distractions can be corrected by rotation of the pins. Avoid residual angulation by ensuring that the nails are introduced at the same level and that the tips of the nail oppose each other in both planes so that they have identical curvatures (Fig. 36-134E). Leave the distal portion of the nails slightly protruding for ease of removal (Fig. 36-134F).
- If the technique is performed correctly, the fracture is finally stabilized by two nails, each with three points of fixation. The fixation is elastic but sufficiently stable to allow automatic small position corrections by limited movements during the limb's loading.

POSTOPERATIVE CARE. Postoperatively, the limb is rested on a pillow. A knee immobilizer may give more comfort. Mobilization using crutches without weight bearing is allowed as soon as the fracture causes no pain. A spica cast can be used if rotation or angulation is evident after the procedure. At the beginning of the third week, partial weight bearing is allowed. After the appearance of calcified external callus, full weight bearing is allowed. Nails are removed when the surgeon is positive that healing has occurred, usually 6 to 12 months postoperatively.

PLATING

Plating of femoral fractures in children and adolescents has been reported by several authors, primarily for patients with severe head injury, multiple trauma, proximal or distal fractures, or length-unstable fractures (Figure 36-135). Although

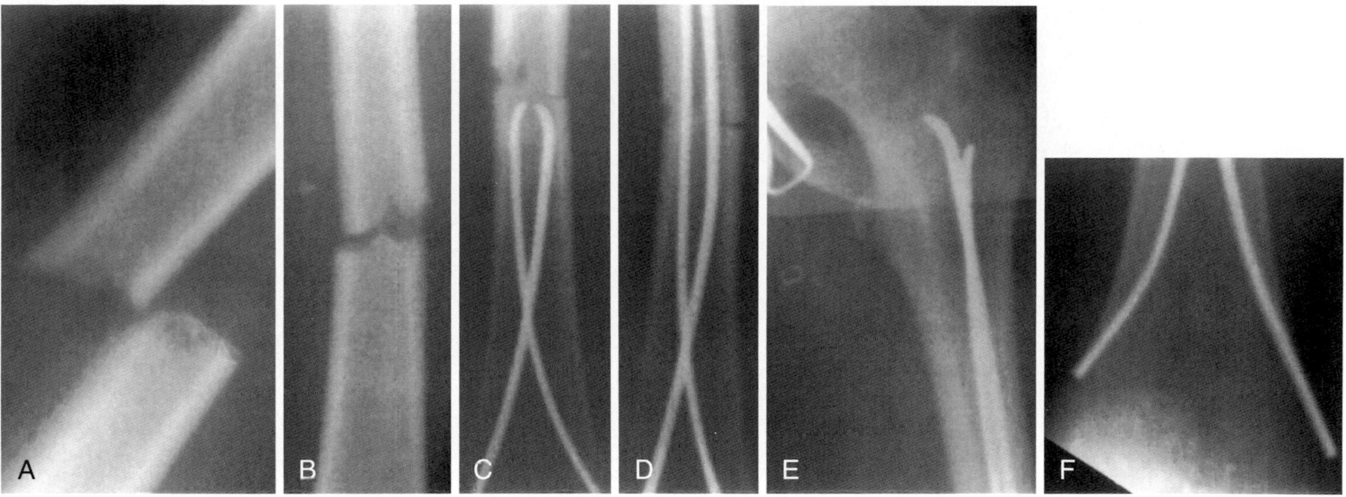

FIGURE 36-134 Flexible intramedullary nail technique. **A** and **B,** Radiographs of femoral fracture before **(A)** and after **(B)** reduction on fracture table. **C,** Both nails are placed (medial and lateral) to cross well below fracture site and stopped temporarily at fracture site for ease of passage. **D,** Both nails are driven past fracture site by manipulating distal fragment, hugging wall of intramedullary canal as necessary. **E,** Nails are driven into greater trochanteric and cervical area. **F,** Distal portions of nails are left slightly protruding for ease of removal but not too long to prevent knee motion. **SEE TECHNIQUE 36-30.**

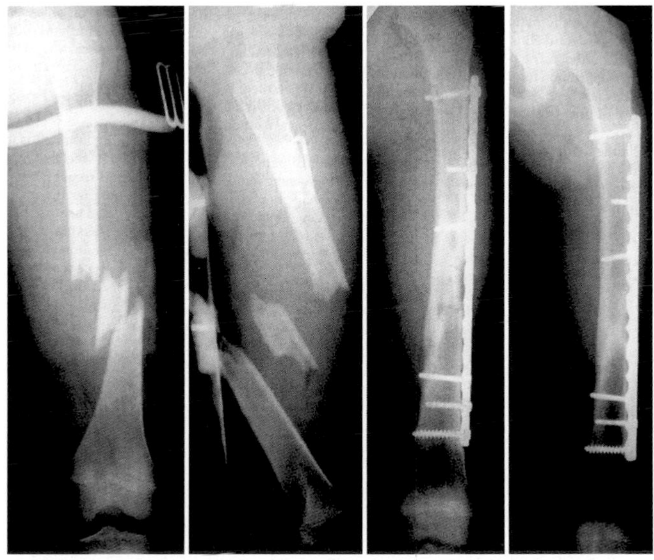

FIGURE 36-135 Submuscular bridge plating of severely comminuted segmental femoral fracture.

open plating techniques have been used in the past, a less invasive submuscular technique has been advocated by many to decrease operative time, blood loss, unsightly scars, and disruption of fracture biology. Several studies demonstrated equal or superior results of submuscular plating to elastic nails in the management of subtrochanteric, distal femoral, or length-unstable femoral fractures in regard to healing time, major or minor complication rates, and time to return to activity. Reported complications include leg-length discrepancy, refracture, hardware breakage, hypertrophic scarring, and rotational malalignment. Additionally, in a review of 85 skeletally immature diaphyseal femoral fractures treated with submuscular plate fixation, 30% of distal fractures and 12% of all fractures developed a late distal femoral valgus deformity. The authors advocated close follow-up and routine hardware removal once fracture union has occurred.

COMPLICATIONS

The most common complication after femoral shaft fractures in children is leg-length discrepancy, usually resulting from "overgrowth" of the injured femur. The exact cause of this overgrowth is unknown, but it has been attributed to age, gender, fracture type, fracture level, handedness, and amount of overriding of the fracture fragments. Age seems to be the most constant factor, but fractures in the proximal third of the femur and oblique comminuted fractures also have been associated with relatively greater growth acceleration. According to Staheli, shortening is more likely in patients older than 10 years of age and overgrowth is more likely in patients 2 to 10 years old, especially if traction has been used. Treatment with a spica cast with or without traction can result in significant shortening. This occurs when more than 2 cm of shortening is accepted and if "traction time" has not been long enough at the time of casting when excessive shortening is present at the time of initial presentation.

Although some angular deformity occurs after femoral shaft fractures in children, it usually remodels with growth. The acceptable amount of angular deformity is controversial; Table 36-6 presents our general guideline of acceptable angulation based on age. Genu recurvatum deformity of the proximal tibia has been reported after traction pin or wire placement through or near the anterior aspect of the proximal tibial physis, excessive traction, pin track infection, and prolonged cast immobilization. Occasionally, a significant angular deformity requires corrective osteotomy, but this should be delayed at least a year unless function is impaired. Torsional deformities have been reported to occur in one third to two thirds of children with femoral shaft fractures; however, most of these are mild (<10 degrees) and asymptomatic, rarely requiring treatment.

BOX 36-5

Reported Complications After Flexible Intramedullary Nail Fixation of Pediatric Femoral Fractures

- Pain or irritation at nail insertion site
- Malunion
- Loss of reduction (leading to reoperation or malunion)
- Refracture
- Neurologic deficit (transient pudendal nerve palsy, sciatic neurapraxia)
- Superficial wound infection
- Reoperation before union
  - Nail migration/skin perforation
  - Loss of reduction
  - Refracture
  - Neurologic deficit

Delayed union and nonunion of femoral shaft fractures are rare in children and occur most often after open fractures, fractures with segmental bone loss or soft tissue interposed between the fragments, and subtrochanteric fractures that have been poorly aligned with inadequate stabilization. Delayed union in a young child whose femoral fracture has been treated with casting probably should be treated by continuing cast immobilization until bridging callus forms. Rarely, bone grafting and internal fixation may be required for nonunion in an older child; an interlocking intramedullary nail usually is preferred for fixation in children older than 10 to 12 years of age. With the increased use of flexible intramedullary nails, we have noted, as expected, an increase in complications. Besides the usual complications of delayed or malunion and leg-length discrepancy, operative complications include implant failure with resulting varus deformity, protruding nails with and without skin erosion, knee stiffness, and septic arthritis. Narayanan et al. reported complications in 45 (58%) of 78 fractures treated with flexible intramedullary nailing (Box 36-5); most were minor and caused no serious sequelae.

Risk factors suggested to be associated with complications of flexible nailing include:

- Age older than 10 or 11 years and weight exceeding 49 kg
- Obesity, related to wound site complications or failure at the fracture site (40% complication rate in obese children)
- Titanium nails, compared with stainless steel nails; malunions are more frequent with flexible titanium nails
- Subtrochanteric fractures
- Comminution, more than 25% of shaft
- Open fracture
- Multiple injuries

Many of the complications associated with flexible intramedullary nailing can be prevented by careful attention to operative technique and careful follow-up.

- Pain at the insertion site can be avoided by not bending the nails at the insertion site (Fig. 36-136). Nails should be cut close to the bone, leaving less than 10 mm protruding but with enough length left to allow nail retrieval. If prominent nail migration distally occurs, it can be managed by either removing the nail at union or impacting the nail farther into the bone at reoperation.
- Malunion can be minimized by using stainless steel nails and avoiding nails that are mismatched in terms of size, determining that comminution is less than 25% of the shaft, using postoperative immobilization if necessary, and paying careful attention to the location of the fracture and final position of the nails (nails can be placed farther proximally in subtrochanteric fractures).
- Loss of reduction is a serious complication requiring reoperation and consideration of another fixation method.
- Neurologic deficits can be prevented by careful attention to traction, especially with the use of a fracture table.
- Superficial wound infections can be minimized by using perioperative antibiotics and avoiding prominent nails at the insertion site.

FRACTURES OF THE DISTAL FEMORAL PHYSIS

Fractures of the distal femoral physis are not as common as physeal injuries elsewhere, accounting for only 7% of physeal injuries of the lower extremity. At the distal femur, Salter-Harris type II physeal fractures cause more severe physeal arrests than in other parts of the skeleton. Occult Salter-Harris type V compression fractures with premature closure of the physis also occur more frequently in this location.

Salter-Harris type I fractures of the distal femoral physis rarely need operative treatment unless they are displaced. These fractures are caused more often by motor vehicle accidents or by a varus or valgus force encountered in athletic activities, and many are undisplaced (Fig. 36-137). Gentle stress radiographs may be helpful in differentiating a tear of a collateral ligament from a type I epiphyseal separation. Salter-Harris type II fractures are most common and occur in older children. Displacement usually is in the coronal plane, although it can be in the anteroposterior plane. Physeal arrest is more frequent after this fracture than after type II fractures in many other locations.

In an experimental study in rabbits, Mäkelä et al. found that destruction of 7% of the cross-sectional area of the distal femoral physis caused permanent growth disturbance and shortening of the femur. The portion of the physis beneath the metaphyseal fracture spike (Thurston-Holland sign) usually is spared. If the metaphyseal spike is medial, valgus deformity may occur because of lateral closure of the physis. If the spike is lateral, varus angulation may follow.

Salter-Harris type III fractures rarely occur. The amount of displacement is important because joint incongruity results if anatomic alignment is not restored and a bony bridge develops if the physis is not realigned exactly (Fig. 36-138A). A Salter-Harris type IV fracture is even more uncommon. It likewise requires accurate reduction. The metaphyseal spike of bone that occurs with this type of fracture is worrisome because of the increased possibility of physeal arrest from bony bridge formation (Fig. 36-138B).

When late premature physeal closure occurs, a retrospective diagnosis of a Salter-Harris type V compression injury is made. Whether this is a true compression injury, with premature closure uniformly across the distal femoral physis, was questioned by Peterson and Burkhart, who speculated whether this uniform premature physeal closure could be caused by some other mechanism, such as prolonged immobilization or an undiscovered mechanism.

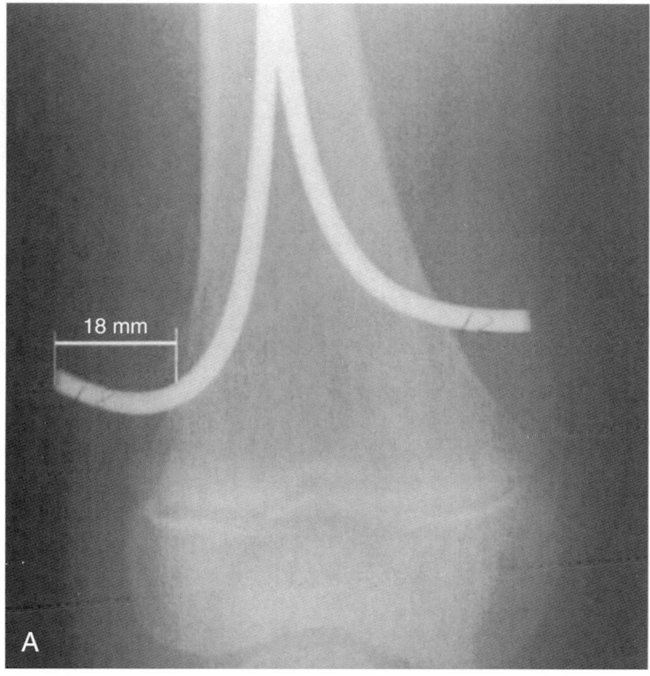

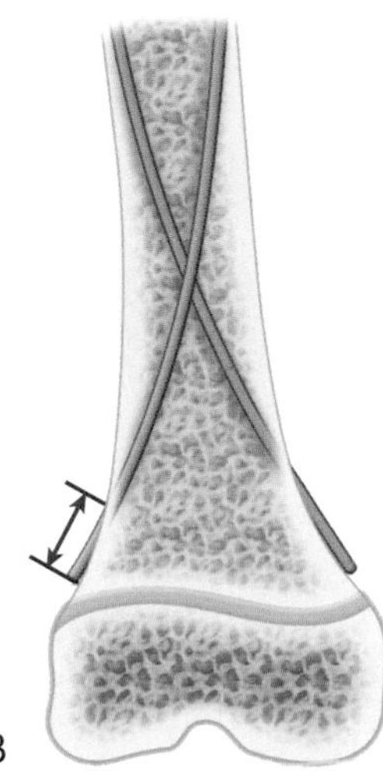

FIGURE 36-136 **A,** Bending of the nails at the insertion site can lead to postoperative irritation and pain, which may require reoperation to advance, trim, or remove the nails. **B,** Optimal position of the distal nail ends against the supracondylar flare of the metaphysis leaves the nails sufficiently out of the cortical entry site for subsequent retrieval if necessary. (From Narayanan UG, Hyman JE, Wainwright AM, et al: Complications of elastic stable intramedullary nail fixation of pediatric femoral fractures, and how to avoid them, J Pediatr Orthop 24:363, 2004.)

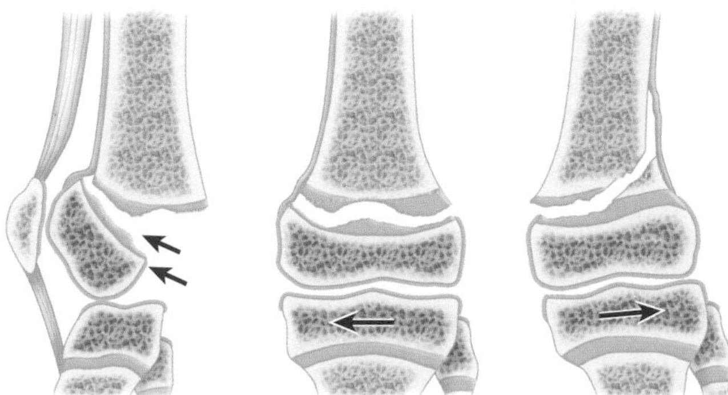

FIGURE 36-137 Various angulations of distal femoral physeal fractures, including posterior angulation, varus angulation, and valgus angulation.

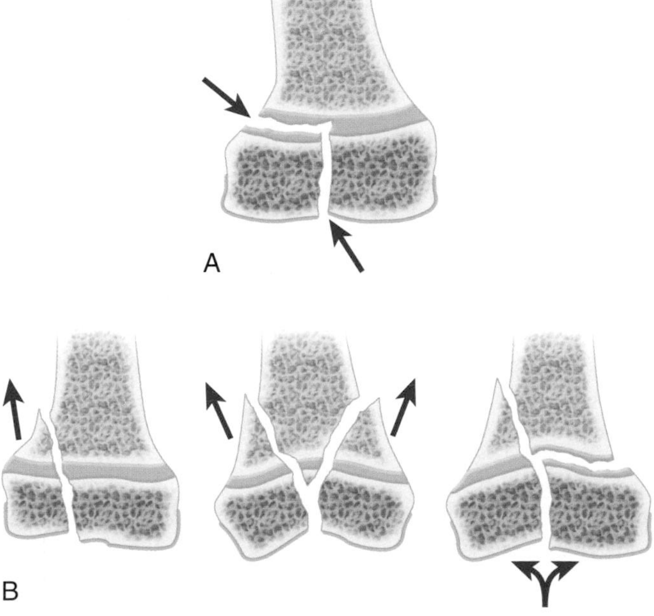

FIGURE 36-138 **A,** Salter-Harris type III distal femoral physeal fracture that requires anatomic reduction. **B,** Various types of Salter-Harris type III and IV fracture-separations, including unicondylar, bicondylar, and combination of types III and IV, which is triplane fracture.

An avulsion injury can occur at the edge of the physis, especially on the medial side. A small fragment, including a portion of the perichondrium and underlying bone, may be torn off the femur when the proximal attachment of a collateral ligament is avulsed. This uncommon injury, although assumed to be benign, can lead to localized premature physeal arrest. If physeal arrest from a bony bridge is located at the most peripheral edge of a physis, severe angular deformity can occur.

The value of the Salter-Harris classification as an indicator of the mechanism of injury and the prognosis of distal femoral physeal injuries is debatable, with some authors noting that most types I and II fractures do well, whereas others have reported unsatisfactory results and frequent

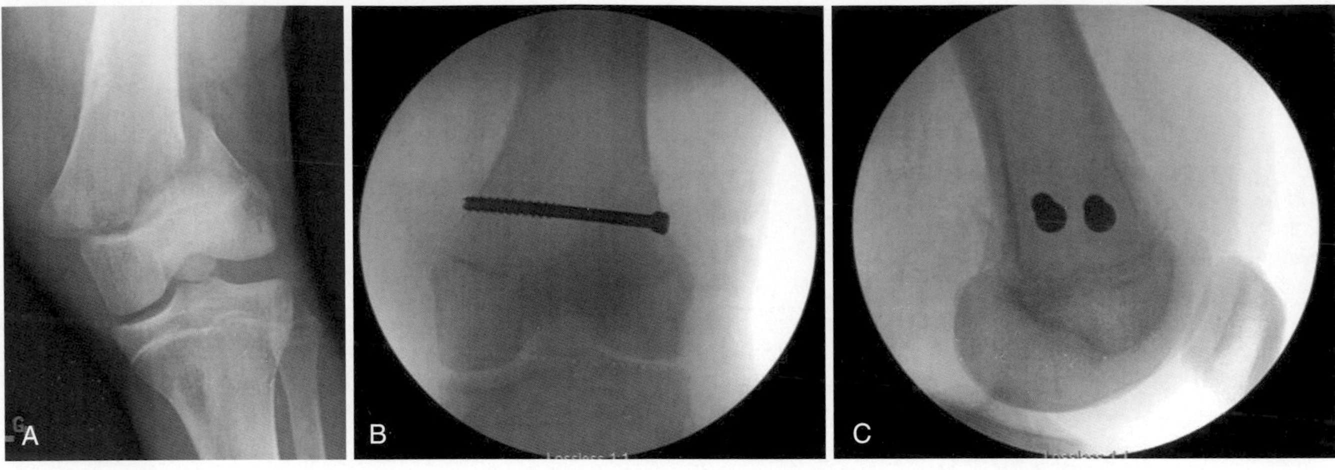

FIGURE 36-139 A, Displaced Salter-Harris type II fracture of distal femoral physis. B and C, Fixation with cannulated screws.

measurable growth disturbances in types I and II fractures. In a study of 73 patients with distal femoral physeal fractures, Arkader et al. found that both the Salter-Harris classification and displacement of the fractures were significant predictors of the final outcome.

Types I and II fractures usually are reduced with the patient under general anesthesia, and the reduction is maintained in a long leg cast with a pelvic band and pin or screw fixation in unstable fractures. These fractures are noted for redisplacement, especially if they are initially displaced anteriorly (Fig. 36-139). Closed reduction can be made easier by the use of a traction bow on a Kirschner wire in the proximal tibia. Reduction should be 90% by traction or distraction and only 10% by leverage or manipulation. Most types I and II physeal fractures do not require anatomic reduction because the fracture occurs through the zone of provisional calcification of the physis, leaving the cells responsible for growth with the ossified epiphysis, although Salter-Harris types I and II fractures in the distal femur may be an exception. If a less than anatomic reduction results, but acceptable general alignment and position are obtained, union and satisfactory growth and remodeling can be expected, especially in children younger than 10 years old in whom 20 degrees of posterior angulation would remodel. In older patients nearer skeletal maturity, only slight anteroposterior displacement and no more than 5 degrees of varus-valgus angulation are acceptable. According to Salter, it is better to accept a less than anatomic reduction with the possibility of an osteotomy later than to use forceful or repeated manipulation. In older children, a closed reduction can be done, but because of inherent instability, percutaneous cross wire fixation with the aid of image intensification may be necessary to maintain reduction (Fig. 36-140). The pins should cross the metaphysis to prevent rotation of the epiphysis. Rarely, a Salter-Harris type I or II fracture cannot be satisfactorily reduced closed because of interposition of soft tissue, and ORIF becomes necessary.

In adolescents, a large metaphyseal spike (Thurston-Holland fragment) can be stabilized with two cannulated screws. Salter-Harris type III and IV fractures require anatomic reduction. If this cannot be achieved by closed methods, ORIF is indicated. The amount of displacement that is acceptable in type III fractures has not been determined conclusively, but most authors report 2 mm or less as acceptable for closed reduction. We believe that if the surgeon thinks realistically that the amount of displacement can be decreased by performing an open reduction, this should be done. CT or MRI may be helpful when there is suspicion of injury without radiographic abnormality for evaluating articular displacement and for operative planning purposes.

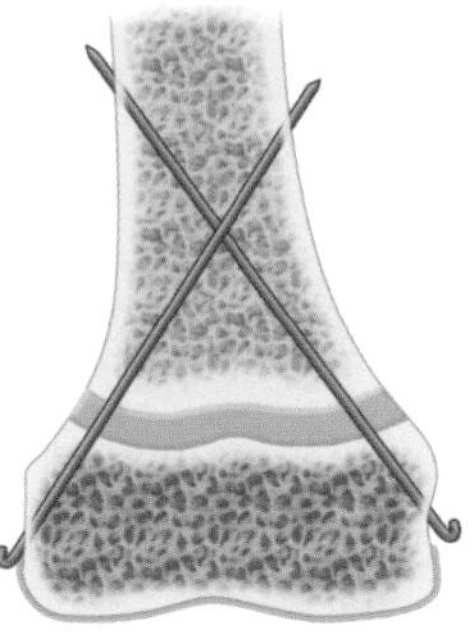

FIGURE 36-140 Cross wire fixation with aid of image intensifier. Smooth pins should be used and should penetrate the opposite cortex. **SEE TECHNIQUE 36-31.**

CLOSED OR OPEN REDUCTION

TECHNIQUE 36-31

CLOSED REDUCTION OF SALTER-HARRIS TYPES I AND II FRACTURES

- Perform closed reduction for Salter-Harris types I and II fractures.
- If the reduction is satisfactory, apply a single spica or long leg cast, depending on the direction of the original displacement.

OPEN REDUCTION OF SALTER-HARRIS TYPES I AND II FRACTURES

- If reduction cannot be maintained, insert crossed, smooth 2.4-mm (3/32-inch) Steinmann pins through the medial and lateral condyles and into the metaphysis (Fig. 36-140). If a large metaphyseal spike (Salter-Harris type II) is present after closed reduction, horizontal percutaneous pins or cannulated screws can be used.

- If the Salter-Harris type I or II fracture cannot be reduced closed, expose the epiphysis through a lateral or medial longitudinal incision, as described in Chapter 1 for intercondylar fractures.
- Reduce the separation as gently and completely as possible by manual traction and minimal leverage. If the use of instruments is necessary, avoid injury to the physis. Remove any interposed soft tissue and gently maneuver the epiphysis into position.
- After reduction is achieved, drill 2.4-mm unthreaded pins through the medial and lateral condyles so that they cross near the center of the physis and enter the metaphysis. Cut the pins off beneath the skin.
- If the pins are inserted as described and removed at 4 to 6 weeks, they are unlikely to cause any growth disturbance. If a type II or IV fracture has a large metaphyseal spike, rather than using smooth crossed pins, drill two 2.4-mm threaded pins or a cancellous screw (Fig. 36-141) through the metaphysis of the spike into the proximal metaphyseal portion of the fracture. This should provide good stability and avoids crossing the physis. If the fragment is too small, cross the physis with smooth crossed pins.

OPEN REDUCTION OF SALTER-HARRIS TYPE III FRACTURES

- If the injury is a displaced Salter-Harris type III fracture, expose the displaced condyle through an anteromedial or anterolateral incision, depending on which condyle is involved.
- An arthrotomy is necessary to ensure an anatomic reduction of the articular surface.
- Drill a large smooth pin, a cancellous screw, or a guide pin for cannulated cancellous screws into the displaced condyle to manipulate it. Gently and carefully reduce the displaced condyle into position with the pin or screw. Insert the pin or screw transversely into the intact opposite condyle without crossing the physis. Confirm the reduction by radiographs. Threaded or cancellous screws can be used across the epiphysis, as long as they do not involve, penetrate, or cross the physis.

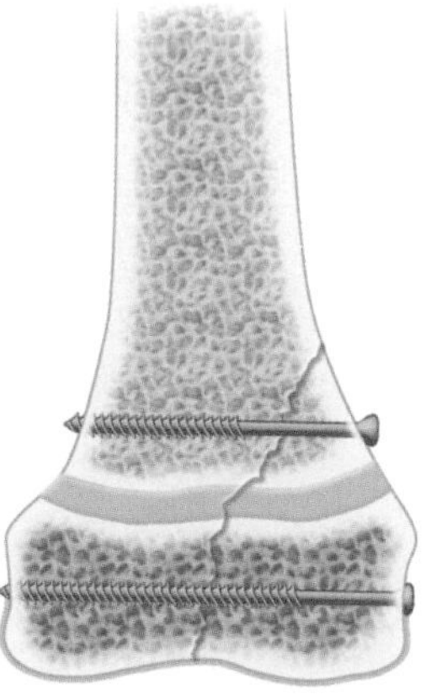

FIGURE 36-141 Salter-Harris type IV fracture metaphyseal spike is secured transversely with cancellous screws. **SEE TECHNIQUE 36-31.**

OPEN REDUCTION OF SALTER-HARRIS TYPE IV FRACTURES

- Growth disturbance occurs frequently after type IV fractures if an anatomic reduction is not achieved and fixation is not secure. Arthrotomy usually is required to ensure anatomic reduction at the articular surface.
- Approach the fracture anteromedially or anterolaterally, depending on which condyle is involved or on which side the metaphyseal spike is present.
- Reduce the articular surface and the physis precisely with smooth pins or cancellous screws. Secure the fragment to the intact condyle with transverse fixation, without crossing the physis if possible.
- If, as in type II fractures, a large displaced metaphyseal spike is present, reduce the fracture anatomically with traction and secure the metaphyseal spike to the proximal metaphyseal fragment with threaded pins, screws, or cancellous bone screws (Fig. 36-142). If the metaphyseal spike is not large enough to ensure rigid fixation, or if transverse fixation of the epiphysis cannot be secured, smooth pins can be inserted across the physis.

POSTOPERATIVE CARE. When the initial displacement is anterior, a long leg or single spica cast, depending on the stability, is applied with the knee in 45 degrees of flexion. These fractures are comparable to supracondylar fractures of the humerus in that the quadriceps and flexed knee are comparable to the triceps and flexed elbow in the maintenance of reduction. If the initial displacement is posterior, the knee should be immobilized in extension. Union usually occurs at 4 to 6 weeks. The cast and any temporary pins can be removed and an exercise program begun. Weight bearing can be permitted at 8 to 10 weeks.

COMPLICATIONS

The immediate complications of closed or open reduction include vascular impairment, peroneal nerve palsy, and recurrent displacement and angulation. Late complications include joint stiffness and physeal arrest. A recent meta-analysis that included 564 distal femoral physeal fractures found that 52% had growth disturbances, 36% in type I fractures, 58% in type II fractures, 49% in type III fractures, and 64% in type IV fractures. Leg-length discrepancies of more than 1.5cm developed in 52%. Although growth disturbance was more frequent in those treated with fixation (58%) than those without fixation (63%), clinically significant leg-length discrepancy was less frequent with fixation (27%) than without fixation (37%). Children with fractures of the distal femoral physis should be observed periodically until skeletal maturity. Epiphysiodesis of the contralateral extremity may be necessary because of premature physeal arrest with shortening or angulation or both. Angular deformity caused by bony bridge formation is common in distal femoral physeal fractures. Bony bridge resection and epiphysiodesis of the

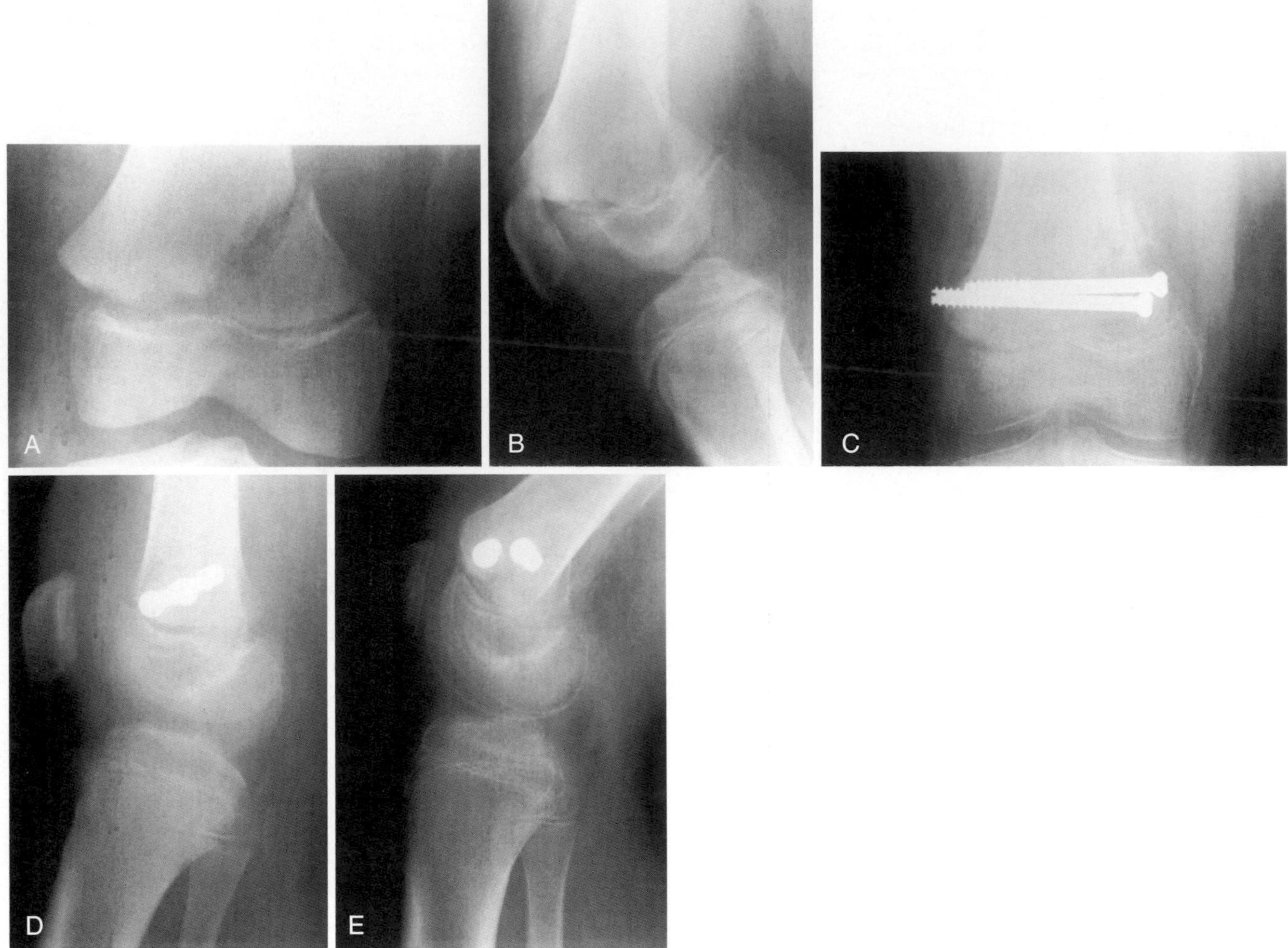

FIGURE 36-142 **A** and **B**, Salter-Harris type II fracture of distal femoral physis with small metaphyseal spike. **C** and **D**, After closed reduction and percutaneous pinning. **E**, Two weeks after surgery, loss of reduction occurred because of inadequate fixation through metaphyseal spike only. **SEE TECHNIQUE 36-31.**

opposite extremity and osteotomy may be necessary to equalize leg lengths and correct angular deformity (see Chapter 29).

KNEE FRACTURES AND DISLOCATIONS

PATELLAR DISLOCATIONS

Acute traumatic patellar dislocations usually occur in adolescents involved in athletic activities. Patients often report a twisting injury and seeing or feeling the patella dislocate and then spontaneously reduce with knee flexion. In younger children, patellofemoral dysplasia generally is an underlying cause. Less commonly, a direct blow to the medial aspect of the patella results in patellar dislocation. Factors associated with patellar dislocation include patella alta, trochlear dysplasia, hyperlaxity, an increased Q angle from torsional deformities of the femur or tibia, female sex, and a positive family history.

Diagnosis of patellar dislocation, even with spontaneous reduction, generally is easily made by clinical symptoms: diffuse tenderness and swelling around the patella, worse on the medial side; positive apprehension test with lateral translation of the patella; and hemarthrosis. Radiographs should be obtained to detect an osteochondral fracture; MRI or CT also may be valuable for evaluation of an osteochondral fracture. Stress radiographs may be needed if physeal fracture or ligament injury is suspected.

Treatment of first-time patellar dislocations usually is nonoperative, consisting of a short period of immobilization, followed by bracing and rehabilitation with return to sports activities at 6 to 12 weeks. Nonoperative management of patellar dislocations is further outlined in Chapter 60. Operative treatment is most often needed for an associated osteochondral fracture but has been recommended to reduce the risk of redislocation, which has been reported in 15% to 75% of patients. Redislocation is most frequent in young patients (<15 years of age), and the frequency decreases with increasing age.

Operative treatment is most often indicated for recurrent patellar dislocations that cause functional disability and patellar dislocations with large femoral osteochondral fractures that require fixation. Operative stabilization may

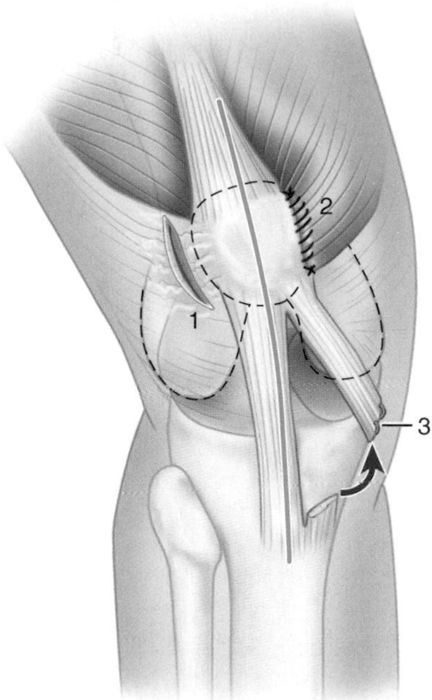

FIGURE 36-143 Schematic view of the 3-in-1 procedure. *1,* lateral release; *2,* vastus medialis muscle advancement; *3,* transfer of the medial third of the patellar tendon to the medial collateral ligament, sutured using two metal anchor sutures. (Redrawn from Oliva F, Ronga M, Longo UG, et al: The 3-in-1 procedure for recurrent dislocation of the patella in skeletally immature children and adolescents, Am J Sports Med 37:1814, 2009.) **SEE TECHNIQUE 36-33.**

occasionally be considered for high-demand athletes with a primary patellar dislocation.

Chronic recurrent subluxation or dislocation is a difficult problem. For management in a skeletally mature patient, see Chapter 45. Additional challenges are encountered in children with open physes because bony procedures at the tibial tubercle and medial patellofemoral ligament reconstruction techniques that encroach on the distal femoral physis should be avoided so as not to cause growth arrest. With this in mind, procedures have been described to correct patellar instability using soft-tissue advancement (vastus medialis), lateral release, and when needed some soft-tissue restraining procedure, such as transfer of the medial or lateral third of the patellar tendon to the medial collateral ligament (Fig. 36-143), reconstruction of the medial patellofemoral ligament, and transfer of the semitendinosus tendon through a patellar tendon (Galeazzi). Nietosvaara et al. compared operative treatment (direct repair of damaged medial structures and lateral release) to nonoperative treatment in a randomized trial involving 74 dislocations without large loose bodies in 71 patients younger than 16 years of age. Initial operative repair of the medial structures combined with lateral release did not improve the long-term outcome. Subjective results were good or excellent in 75% of those treated nonoperatively compared with 66% in those treated operatively; rates of recurrent dislocation were 71% after nonoperative treatment and 67% after operative treatment. A positive family history was identified as a risk factor for recurrence and for contralateral patellar instability.

If medial patellofemoral ligament reconstruction is selected as part of the proximal realignment, then care must be taken to avoid damage to the distal femoral physis. This can be accomplished with careful placement of the femoral tunnel distal to the physis in older adolescents or alternatively with suture or suture anchor fixation distal to the physis in younger patients. The selection of a graft is similar to that for skeletally mature patients and includes a hamstring autograft, allograft, or partial quadriceps graft. For medial patellofemoral ligament reconstruction techniques, please refer to Chapter 45.

RECONSTRUCTION OF THE PATELLOFEMORAL AND PATELLOTIBIAL LIGAMENTS WITH A SEMITENDINOSUS TENDON GRAFT

TECHNIQUE 36-32

(NIETOSVAARA ET AL.)

- Place the patient supine on a standard operating room table. After induction of general anesthesia, examine both knees, including patellofemoral tracking, before sterile preparation and draping of the limb. Apply and inflate a thigh tourniquet (pressure of 250 mm Hg).
- Through standard portals (see Chapter 51), arthroscopically examine the knee to evaluate patellar tracking, depth of the femoral trochlea, and condition of the patellofemoral joint surfaces. Remove any loose bodies.
- Make a longitudinal 4-cm skin incision medial to the tibial tubercle.
- Identify the semitendinosus and harvest its tendon with a tendon stripper, leaving the distal insertion intact.
- Place a running 2-0 Vicryl crisscross suture (Ethicon, Somerville, NJ) in the proximal end of the tendon.
- Make two additional 2-cm incisions at the inferomedial and superomedial borders of the patella.
- With a 3.2-mm cannulated drill, create a longitudinal intraosseous tunnel in the medial quadrant of the patella; enlarge the tunnel with a 4-mm drill.
- Create a subfascial tunnel between the semitendinosus insertion and the inferomedial patellar incision.
- Pass the tendon graft through this tunnel and through the patella from distal to proximal, exiting at the superomedial pole.
- From its exit at the superior aspect of the patella, tunnel the graft in a subfascial plane to the adductor tubercle and make a 3-cm incision.
- Tension the graft with the knee in 30 to 45 degrees of flexion, making sure that the patella is well seated in the trochlea. Check the tension with the knee fully extended (the graft should allow little lateral movement of the patella, only up to one-fourth of patellar width). Proper graft tension also allows congruent smooth tracking of the patella.
- Test patellar tracking and stability throughout the range of knee motion.
- Drill a 7-mm hole at the adductor tubercle and secure the graft with an absorbable 8 × 23-mm Biotenodesis screw (Arthrex, Naples, FL).

- In skeletally immature patients, do not use a Biotenodesis screw; instead, pass the graft around the adductor magnus tendon and suture it to this tendon and to itself with 0 Vicryl.
- If tightness of the lateral retinaculum does not allow congruent patellar tracking, perform a lateral retinacular release through an extended anterolateral arthroscopic portal to allow 45 degrees of rotation of the patella above the horizontal.
- In skeletally mature patients with a Q angle of more than 20 degrees, transfer the tibial tubercle 8 to 12 mm medially and fix it with two 6.5-mm lag screws.
- Release the tourniquet and close the incisions in standard manner.

POSTOPERATIVE CARE. Weight bearing and active range-of-motion exercises are allowed immediately. Patients with tibial tubercle transfer are allowed only partial weight bearing on crutches for the first 6 weeks. Return to participation in sports is allowed after 4 months.

3-IN-1 PROCEDURE FOR RECURRENT DISLOCATION OF THE PATELLA: LATERAL RELEASE, VASTUS MEDIALIS OBLIQUUS MUSCLE ADVANCEMENT, AND TRANSFER OF THE MEDIAL THIRD OF THE PATELLAR TENDON TO THE MEDIAL COLLATERAL LIGAMENT

TECHNIQUE 36-33

(OLIVA ET AL.)

- Place the patient supine on a standard operating-room table and apply a tourniquet to the thigh.
- After induction of general anesthesia, examine the knee clinically and arthroscopically.
- Make a 10-cm incision from the midpoint of the patella inferiorly to the medial aspect of the tibial tuberosity (Fig. 36-143) to expose the lateral and medial retinacula, the patellar tendon, and the superomedial aspect of the patella in the area of insertion of the vastus medialis obliquus (VMO) tendon.
- Section the lateral retinaculum proximal to the superior pole of the patella (lateral release), taking care not to breach the synovium.
- Expose the medial patellar tendon by division of the medial retinaculum and expose and release the VMO insertion.
- Prepare the medial third of the patellar tendon by detaching it as distally as possible from its tibial insertion; leave it attached to the patella proximally. Alternatively, detach the lateral third to half of the patella tendon and pass it underneath the intact medial portion.
- With the knee flexed 30 degrees, transfer the patellar tendon medially with an angle of 45 degrees with the main body of the patellar tendon. Incise the periosteum, insert two suture anchors, and suture the patellar tendon to the medial aspect of the proximal tibia and to the medial collateral ligament.
- Advance the VMO insertion 10 mm distally and laterally and secure it with continuous no. 1 Vicryl suture on the surface of the patella, which has been gently scarified with a burr.
- Close the wound in layers and apply routine dressings, bandages, and a straight-knee splint.

POSTOPERATIVE CARE. Partial weight bearing is allowed in a controlled-motion brace, progressing to full weight bearing after 2 weeks. Range of motion is slowly increased in increments with the goal of 90 degrees of flexion at 6 weeks. Gentle concentric training and proprioception training also are begun. At 8 weeks, gentle jogging in place on a "mini-tramp" is begun and progressed over the next 4 weeks. At 12 weeks, sport-specific rehabilitation is begun. Progressive return to daily activities is allowed over the next 3 months, with return to sports activities usually possible at 6 months.

PATELLAR FRACTURES

It is estimated that only 1% of all fractures occur in the patella and that only 1% of these occur in the immature skeleton, so fractures of the patella in children are rare. They usually occur in older children. Some fractures, especially osteochondral and small peripheral fractures and sleeve-type fractures, can be caused by acute dislocation of the patella, which is common in children. In adolescents, "jumper's knee" and Sinding-Larsen-Johansson syndrome occur frequently. These are avulsion injuries of the proximal and distal poles of the patella and should be considered chronic repetitive ligamentous injuries. Bipartite patella should not be confused with a patellar fracture, although it can be misleading because bipartite patella occasionally is painful in adolescent athletes. In bipartite patella, the edges of the defect usually are rounded, the condition is bilateral in approximately 50% of children, and it is almost always in the superolateral quadrant of the bone. Congenital absence of the patella or congenital hypoplasia may be seen in onychoosteodysplasia or nail-patella syndrome. Fractures of the distal pole of the patella and even transverse fractures of the patella occur often in children with cerebral palsy and spasticity of the quadriceps muscle.

A sleeve type of fracture of the distal pole of the patella has been described; often only a fleck of bone is seen on the radiograph, giving a falsely benign appearance; however, a large, cartilaginous "sleeve" is often attached to the patellar tendon that, if not replaced properly when healed and ossified, becomes malaligned and produces an abnormally elongated patella and patellar mechanism (Fig. 36-144). If this fracture occurs in conjunction with dislocation or subluxation of the patella, the elongation of the patellar mechanism makes the dislocation more unstable. MRI is helpful for evaluating the extent of the sleeve fracture and ruling out concomitant injury (Fig. 36-145).

Patellar fractures should be classified according to location, type, and amount of displacement (Fig. 36-146). A review of 67 patellar fractures in 66 children (average age of 12.4 years) at our institution determined that 19 fractures were comminuted, 18 were transverse fractures, 15 were chip fractures, 6 were vertical fractures, and 2 were sleeve fractures; 7 fractures could not be classified from the available radiographs. Treatment followed guidelines generally accepted for patellar fractures in adults, but numerous ipsilateral lower extremity fractures often dictated that treatment be determined according to the associated injury. Overall results were good in only 50% of patients. Some general trends were evident: (1) restoration of the extensor mechanism is essential, and results were less than optimal when this was not accomplished; (2) ORIF produced good results with no growth disturbance after the use of cerclage wires in patients near skeletal maturity; and (3) displaced, comminuted fractures and fractures associated with ipsilateral tibial or femoral fractures had the poorest results.

Because of the possibility of growth disturbance, and because of frequent breakage of wires in children, we routinely remove wires, pins, and screws, preferably before they break. If the fracture occurs in conjunction with an acute or recurrent dislocation of the patella, a limited lateral release and medial reefing of the retinaculum may be indicated. An osteochondral fracture of the patella or lateral femoral condyle should be suspected when acute patellar dislocation occurs.

Because in a sleeve fracture a large cartilaginous fragment usually is attached to the fleck of bone, anatomic reduction is required with displaced fractures. Malunion of the fracture may be painful and require excision of the distal fragment. If

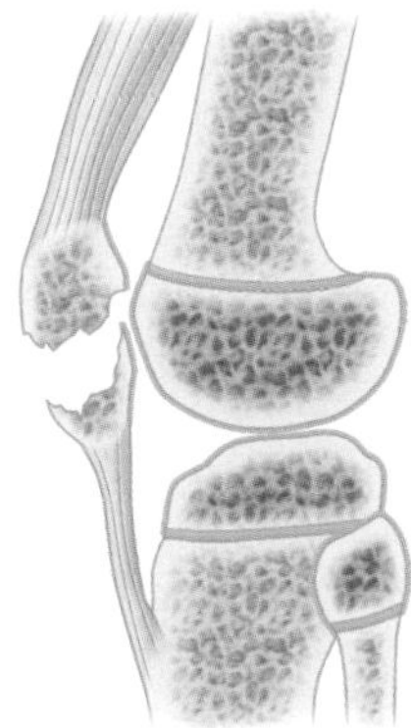

FIGURE 36-144 Substantial sleeve of avulsed cartilage when seen on radiograph appears as only "fleck" of bone and looks benign.

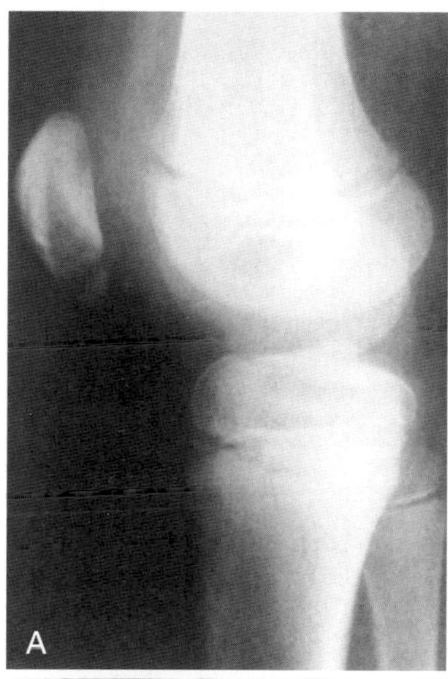

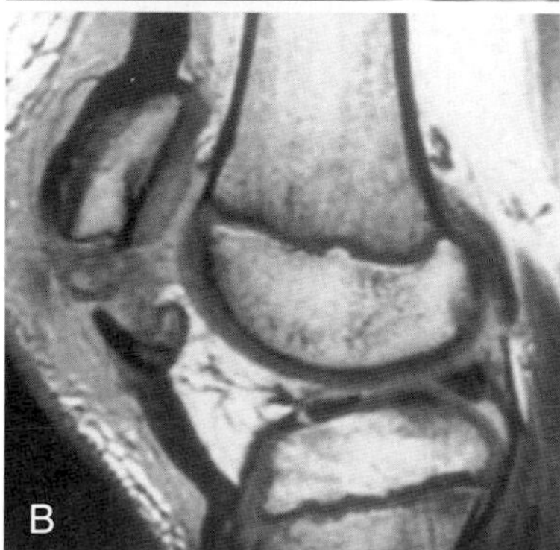

FIGURE 36-145 **A,** Apparent minor inferior pole patellar fracture. **B,** MRI reveals extent of sleeve fracture.

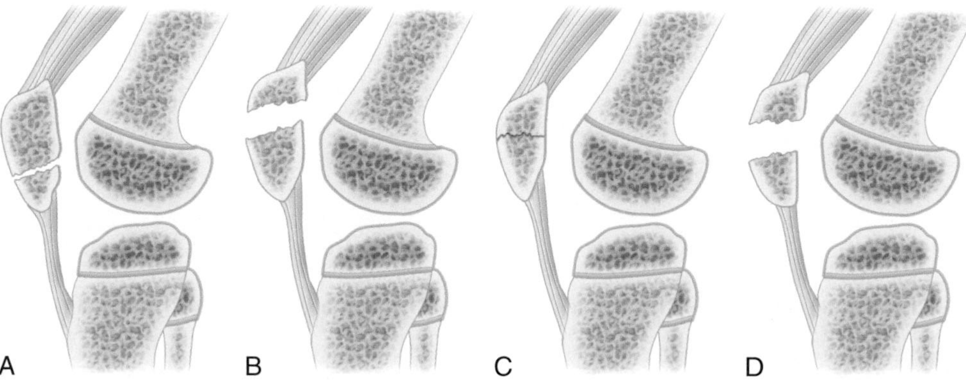

FIGURE 36-146 Types of patellar fracture. **A,** Inferior pole. **B,** Superior pole. **C,** Transverse undisplaced midsubstance. **D,** Transverse displaced midsubstance.

the sleeve fracture was caused by dislocation of the patella, healing in an elongated position may contribute to chronic recurrent dislocation.

The technique for ORIF of patellar fractures in children is the same as in adults (see Chapter 54). Because the sleeve fracture of the patella is unique to children, however, the technique of reduction and fixation is described here.

OPEN REDUCTION AND INTERNAL FIXATION OF SLEEVE FRACTURE

TECHNIQUE 36-34

(HOUGHTON AND ACKROYD)

- Place the patient supine on the operating table and prepare the leg in the usual fashion; use a tourniquet.
- Approach the inferior pole of the patella through a medial parapatellar or direct anterior incision. Expose the distal pole patellar fracture.
- Irrigate the fracture copiously with saline and with a small curet remove any clots and loose cancellous bone. Reduce the fragment with a small bone holder. Observe the fracture fragments anteriorly and try to observe the reduction posteriorly on the articular surface. If this is impossible, use a gloved finger to feel for any angulation or offset on the articular surface. Perform a tension band wiring with two Kirschner wires (see Chapter 54).
- After reduction of the fracture, place two parallel longitudinal Steinmann pins across the fracture site. Leave them protruding approximately 1/4 inch (0.5 cm) distally for easy removal. Place a tension band wire from the superior to the inferior pole of the patella, crossing itself and incorporating the parallel pins (Fig. 36-147). Tighten the wire sufficiently but not enough to overly compress and angulate the fracture fragments.
- Alternatively, a suture repair can be done through vertical tunnels in the patella in a manner similar to repair of a proximal patellar tendon rupture.
- A careful retinacular closure adds additional stability to the repair and may improve patellar tracking after healing is achieved.
- Close the wound in layers and apply an appropriate cast with the knee in slight flexion.

POSTOPERATIVE CARE. At 3 to 4 weeks, the cast is removed and range-of-motion exercises are started.

FRACTURES OF THE INTERCONDYLAR EMINENCE OF THE TIBIA

Tibial intercondylar eminence fractures account for 2% to 5% of knee injuries associated with knee effusion in children and adolescents. Tibial eminence fractures are most commonly classified according to the modified Meyers and McKeever system which describes four types: type I, little or no displacement of the fragment; type II, fragment elevated anteriorly and proximally, with some displacement but with a cartilaginous hinge posteriorly; and type III (intact fragment) and type IV (comminuted fragment), with complete displacement of the fragment (Fig. 36-148). The goal of treatment is to achieve near-anatomic reduction to restore appropriate tension of the attached anterior cruciate ligament. This has been done traditionally by closed treatment with knee extension for types I and II and by open or arthroscopic reduction and fixation for types III and IV.

The mechanism of action for tibial eminence fractures is similar to that of an anterior cruciate ligament injury, with many occurring in low-energy, noncontact activities. This injury has also been reported with higher energy mechanisms such as motor vehicle accidents, pedestrian–motor vehicle accidents, or falls from bicycles. The workup includes a careful physical examination and routine knee radiographs.

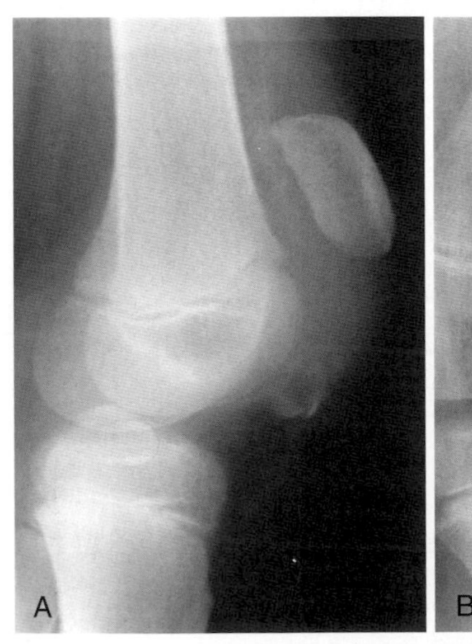

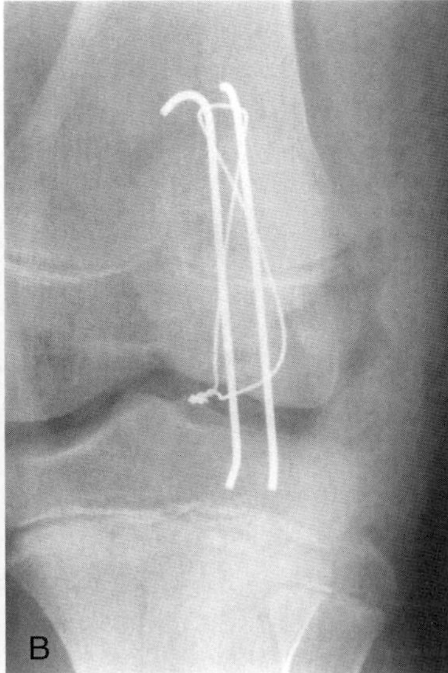

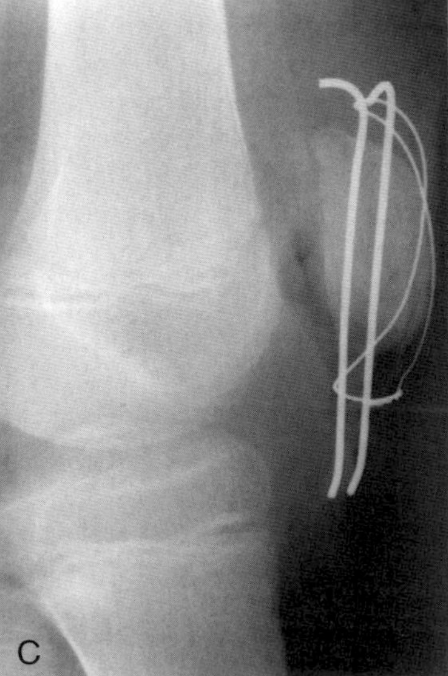

FIGURE 36-147 **A,** Patellar "sleeve" fracture. **B** and **C,** After reduction and fixation with Kirschner wires and tension band wiring. **SEE TECHNIQUE 36-34.**

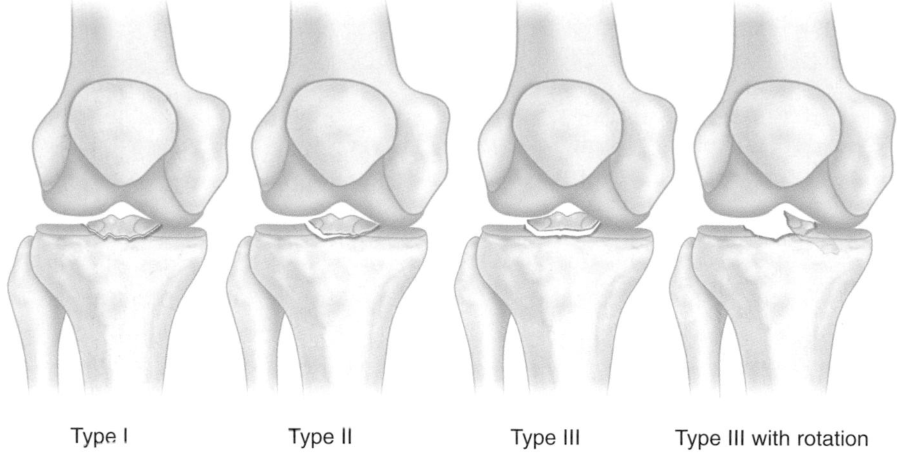

FIGURE 36-148 Meyers and McKeever classification of tibial eminence fractures.

Although the injury usually is detected with plain radiographs, CT and MRI may be used to better evaluate the extent of the injury, rule out associated injury, and for preoperative planning purposes. At our institution, we routinely use MRI to evaluate the degree of displacement, assess barriers to reduction, and evaluate associated injuries. Nonoperative management often is adequate for type I and many type II fractures if adequate reduction is achieved. If adequate reduction of the fracture is noted or restored with extension of the knee, then a cylinder or long leg cast should be applied with the knee in slight flexion. Some authors advocate the aspiration of the hemarthrosis before cast application. The fracture should be closely followed with serial radiographs. Typically, the cast can be removed by 6 weeks and the patient transitioned into a control-motion brace with progression of range of motion to full by 10 to 12 weeks.

Operative intervention is reserved for type II or III fractures that do not reduce with closed manipulation and for type IV fractures (Fig. 36-149). Kocher et al. demonstrated that meniscal or intermeniscal ligament entrapment with block to reduction is present in 26% of type II and 65% of type II fractures, necessitating open or arthroscopic reduction. Several open and arthroscopic techniques have been described for surgical repair of a displaced tibial eminence fracture. Regardless of technique, the knee should be systematically evaluated for concomitant injury, the fracture bed debrided, the fracture reduced under direct vision, and stable fixation achieved. A systematic review failed to show which of the many described techniques is superior. Whether open or arthroscopic, fixation is commonly achieved with suture fixation or screw placement. If suture fixation is selected, the suture is passed through the distal attachment of the anterior cruciate ligament and passed through drill tunnels placed in the proximal tibia and tied over a bony bridge. For screw fixation, the fragment is held reduced and a screw or bioabsorbable screw is passed across the fracture with care not to cross the physis. If additional fixation is required, some authors advocate crossing the physis with a metallic screw and then removing the screw once union has been achieved. Potential complications include nonunion, malunion, persistent laxity of the anterior cruciate ligament, loss of motion, and arthrofibrosis. Nonunion is uncommon but may be a challenge to treat, especially in very young patients in whom further growth has occurred, preventing adequate reduction of the fragment. Nonunion is more commonly encountered with nonoperative management. Malunion is a more common problem and is more commonly seen when there is a delay in diagnosis until healing has occurred. Malunion may result in a block to extension and can be treated with debridement of the elevated fragment or femoral notchplasty. A significant malunion also may result in ligamentous laxity and knee instability. If this occurs, then revision surgery or anterior cruciate ligament reconstruction should be considered. Laxity also may occur in spite of union in good position because of injury of the anterior cruciate ligament at the time of initial injury. This is encountered more frequently in types III and IV fractures, likely as a result of higher forces applied to the anterior cruciate ligament at the time of injury. Intraoperatively, the fracture bed may be gently recessed to increase the tension applied to the anterior cruciate ligament. In addition to malunion, loss of motion may occur as a result of

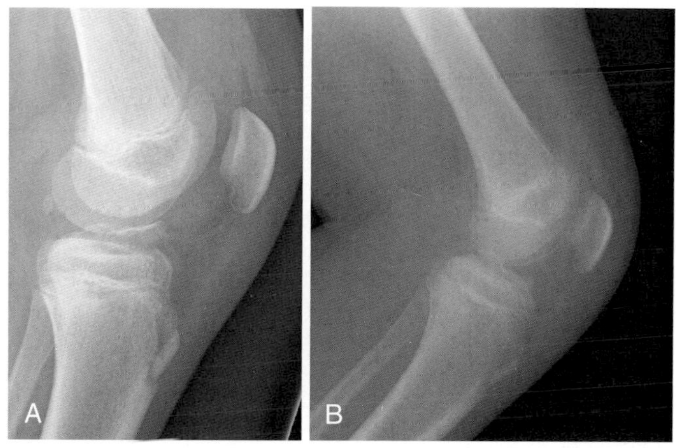

FIGURE 36-149 **A,** Type III tibial eminence fracture that could not be reduced closed. **B,** Lateral radiograph after open reduction and fixation with nonabsorbable sutures. Entrapped meniscus that prevented closed reduction was found at the time of surgery.

postoperative muscle tightness or arthrofibrosis. Patel et al. found that early posttreatment range-of-motion rehabilitation significantly improved time of return to full activity independent of age, fracture type, and operative or nonoperative management. In operatively treated fractures, arthrofibrosis occurred in 36% of knees if range of motion was initiated after 4 weeks compared with 0% in knees when early range of motion was initiated.

OPEN REDUCTION AND INTERNAL FIXATION OF TIBIAL EMINENCE FRACTURE

TECHNIQUE 36-35

- Expose the knee through the distal portion of an anteromedial parapatellar incision (see Technique 1-38). Open the capsule medially to expose the fracture fragments and the defect in the proximal tibia.
- Examine the menisci and intermeniscal ligament to ensure that they are not impeding the reduction. Place the knee in less than 30 degrees of flexion and reduce the fragment after any clots and cancellous bone have been removed from the defect.
  Alternatively, the inspection and reduction can be done with arthroscopic assistance.
- Drill two holes from distal to proximal through the tibial epiphysis. Take care to drill the holes proximal to the physis. The holes should enter the joint (1) just medial and lateral to the fracture fragments or (2) into the defect and into the fragment itself if it is large enough. Pass a 1-0 nonabsorbable suture through the most distal portion of the anterior cruciate ligament just proximal to the fracture fragment (Fig. 36-150). With suture carriers, pass the ends of the suture through the drill holes and tie them onto themselves after the reduction is satisfactory.
- Flex and extend the knee to ensure the reduction is stable. Irrigate and close the wound.

POSTOPERATIVE CARE. If stable fixation is achieved, the leg is placed in a controlled-motion brace with gradual increase in range of motion to full by 6 to 8 weeks. If a cast is used for additional stability, it should be discontinued by 4 weeks to initiate range-of-motion exercises. The patient is released to full activity only after healing has occurred and full, painless range of motion has been achieved with good strength.

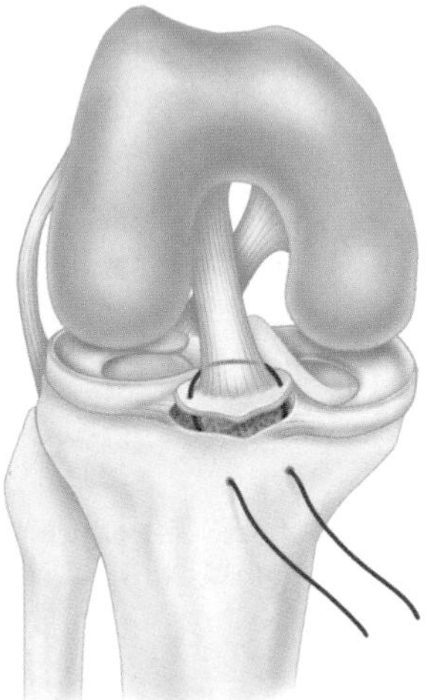

FIGURE 36-150 Repair of intercondylar eminence fracture with absorbable suture. (Redrawn from Owens BD, Crane GK, Plante T, et al: Treatment of type III tibial intercondylar eminence fractures in skeletally immature athletes, Am J Orthop 2:103, 2003.) **SEE TECHNIQUE 36-35.**

ARTHROSCOPIC REDUCTION OF TIBIAL EMINENCE FRACTURE AND INTERNAL FIXATION WITH BIOABSORBABLE NAILS

TECHNIQUE 36-36

(LILJEROS ET AL.)

- With a thigh tourniquet applied and inflated, perform standard knee arthroscopic examination through anteromedial and anterolateral portals (see Chapter 51).
- Remove the ligamentum mucosum and part of the infrapatellar fat pad to better expose the injured area.
- Remove fibrin clots and small fracture fragments from underneath the anterior tibial spine fragment and from the tibial crater.
- If the intermeniscal ligament is trapped in the fracture, interfering with reduction, free it with a probe.
- With the knee flexed to 45 degrees, reduce the fragment with a probe and temporarily fix it with a 1.6-mm AO wire introduced through a midpatellar entrance close to the medial margin of the patella (Fig. 36-151).
- Keeping as close as possible to the patella and slightly proximal to the AO wire, insert the drill guide into the joint and secure the fragment.
- Close the portals in standard fashion and apply a cast or brace with the knee in slight flexion.

POSTOPERATIVE CARE. If stable fixation is achieved, the leg is placed in a controlled-motion brace with gradual increase in range of motion to full by 6 to 8 weeks. If a cast is used for additional stability, it should be discontinued by 4 weeks to initiate range-of-motion exercises. The patient is released to full activity only after healing has occurred and full, painless range of motion has been achieved with good strength.

TIBIAL TUBEROSITY FRACTURES

Fractures of the tibial tuberosity usually occur in older children, often during jumping sports such as basketball (Fig. 36-152). These fractures were classified by Watson-Jones as

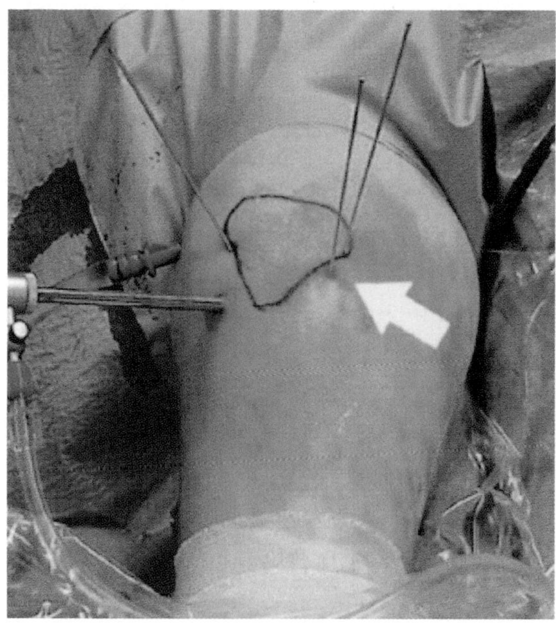

FIGURE 36-151 Arthroscopic reduction of tibial eminence fracture. (From Liljeros K, Werner S, Janarv PM: Arthroscopic fixation of anterior tibial spine fractures with bioabsorbable nails in skeletally immature patients, Am J Sports Med 37:923, 2009.) **SEE TECHNIQUE 36-36.**

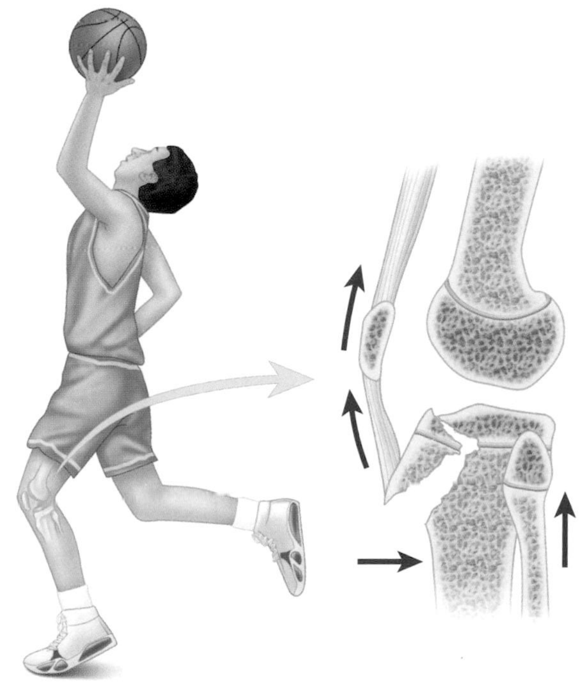

FIGURE 36-152 Mechanism of injury of flexion-avulsion injuries. These injuries are most common in adolescent boys and most often occur when attempting to push off for a jump in basketball.

type I, a small fragment that is displaced superiorly; type II, a larger fragment involving the secondary center of ossification and the proximal tibial physis, which is hinged upward; and type III, a fracture that passes proximally and posteriorly across the physis and proximal articular surface of the tibia

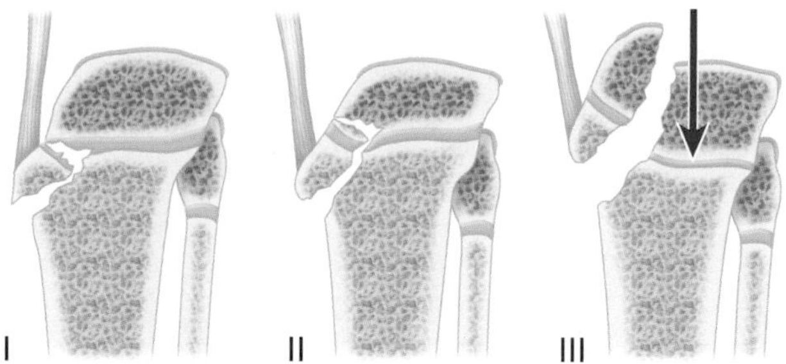

FIGURE 36-153 Types of avulsion fracture of tibial tuberosity. Type I, through secondary ossification center. Type II, at junction of primary and secondary ossification centers. Type III, across primary ossification center (Salter-Harris type III) with physis near closing posteriorly. (Redrawn from Roberts JM: Fractures and dislocations of the knee. In Rockwood CA Jr, Wilkins KE, King RE, editors: Fractures in children, Philadelphia, Lippincott, 1984.)

(Salter-Harris type III physeal fracture [Fig. 36-153]). Ogden et al. classified type III fractures further as to whether there is a rotational, comminuted, or epiphyseal component. This classification is important because type III fractures in younger children, if not anatomically reduced and held, can result in bony bridge formation, causing anterior growth arrest and hyperextension deformity; however, this complication is unlikely because these fractures usually occur in older adolescents (Fig. 36-154). Frankl described a type I-C injury as a tibial tuberosity avulsion fracture with a patellar tendon rupture from its proximal insertion. Further modifications to the classification scheme were added to include injuries to the entire proximal tibial physis. Ryu and Debenham suggested the addition of a type IV injury, in which the anterior tubercle fracture line extends completely across the tibial physis in a Salter-Harris type I pattern. Donahue et al. subdivided type IV injuries into type IV-A injuries, a strictly physeal injury, and type IV-B injuries, those with a posterior metaphyseal fragment, consistent with a Salter-Harris type II injury. Finally, a type V injury was described by Curtis and later classified by McKoy et al. with an intraarticular Salter-Harris type III extension and an associated type IV fracture, giving the fracture a Y configuration (Fig. 36-155). We have seen a number of patients, all adolescent males, with anterior tuberosity fractures combined with a posterior metaphyseal fragment (Fig. 36-156).

Differentiating between Osgood-Schlatter disease and tibial tuberosity fractures can be difficult because they both present with pain over the tibial tuberosity in jumping athletes. Osgood-Schlatter disease is a chronic traction injury at the distal attachment of the patellar tendon that results in insidious onset of inflammation along the anterior aspect of the tuberosity. A tibial tuberosity fracture, however, is an acute failure of the underlying physis. Although Osgood-Schlatter disease has been known to precede tibial tuberosity fractures, this is likely related to the strong correlation between the age and activities that result in these injuries. With Osgood-Schlatter disease, symptomatic and supportive treatment is all that is necessary, the prognosis is good, and only occasionally are symptoms prolonged by a persistent ossicle. Conversely, tibial tuberosity fractures result in an

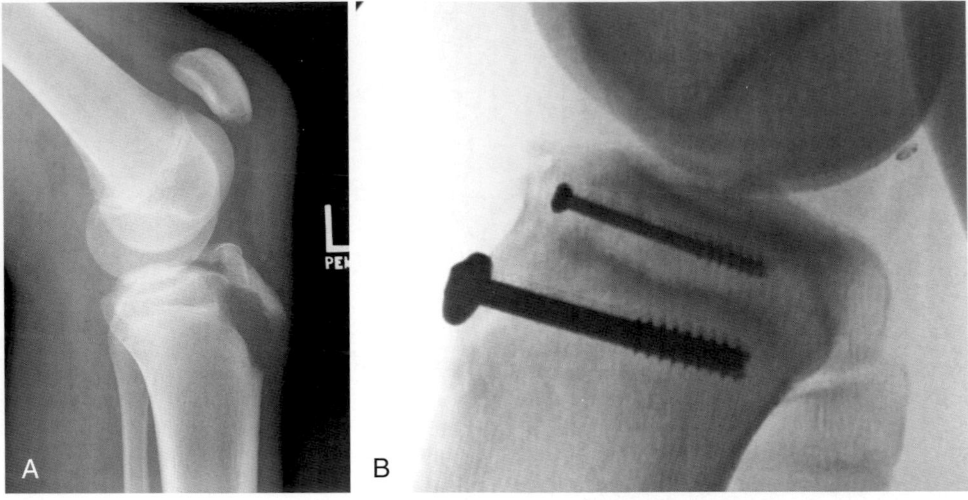

FIGURE 36-154 Tibial tuberosity fracture. **A,** Watson-Jones type III fracture (Salter-Harris type III) extending into knee joint. **B,** After open reduction and screw fixation.

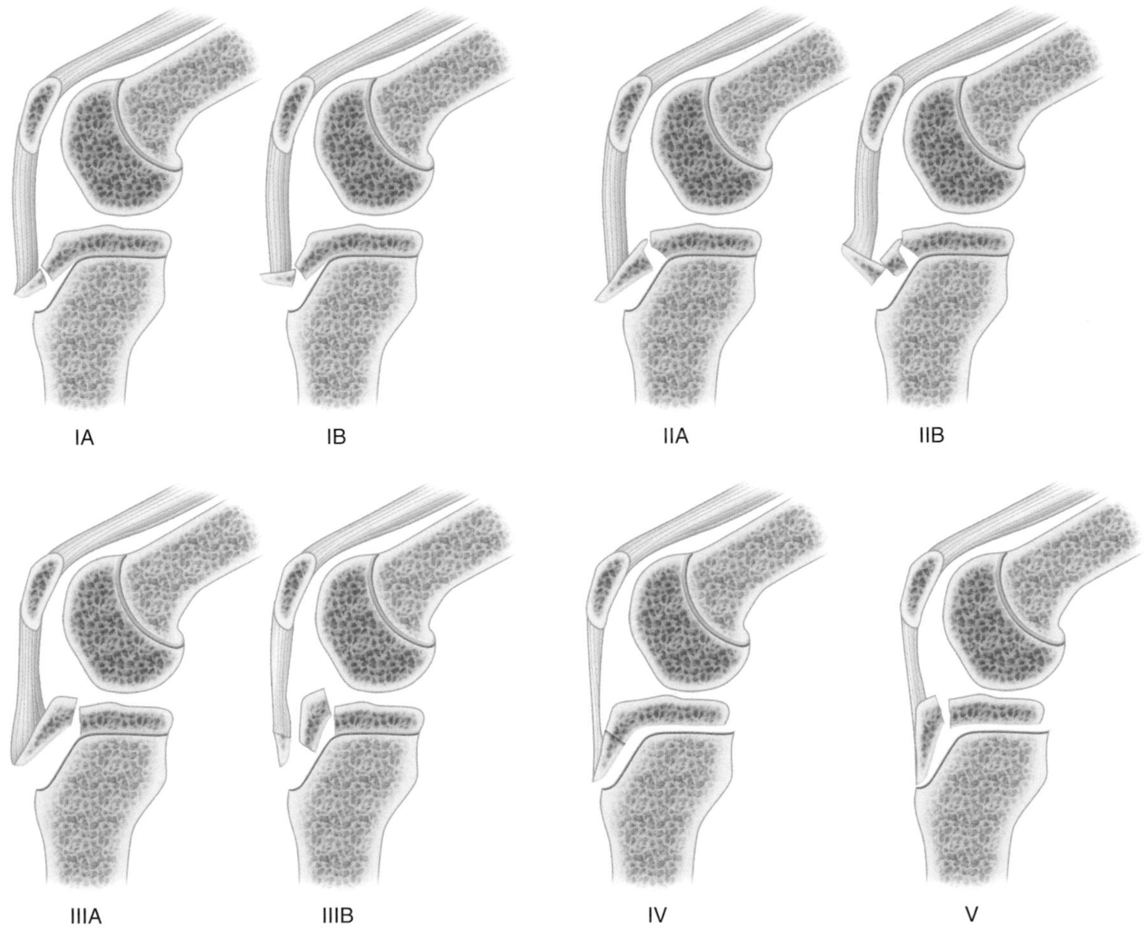

FIGURE 36-155 Classification of tibial tuberosity fractures (see text).

incompetent extensor mechanism and require urgent treatment to restore function.

Imaging workup consists of standard radiographs of the knee. Historically, the incidence of concomitant knee injury or intraarticular pathology was thought to be low because of the mechanism of action; however, several recent studies that used preoperative MRI demonstrated a higher incidence of intraarticular findings, commonly meniscal pathology and osteochondral injury, than previously reported. As a result, some authors advocate routine use of MRI as part of the

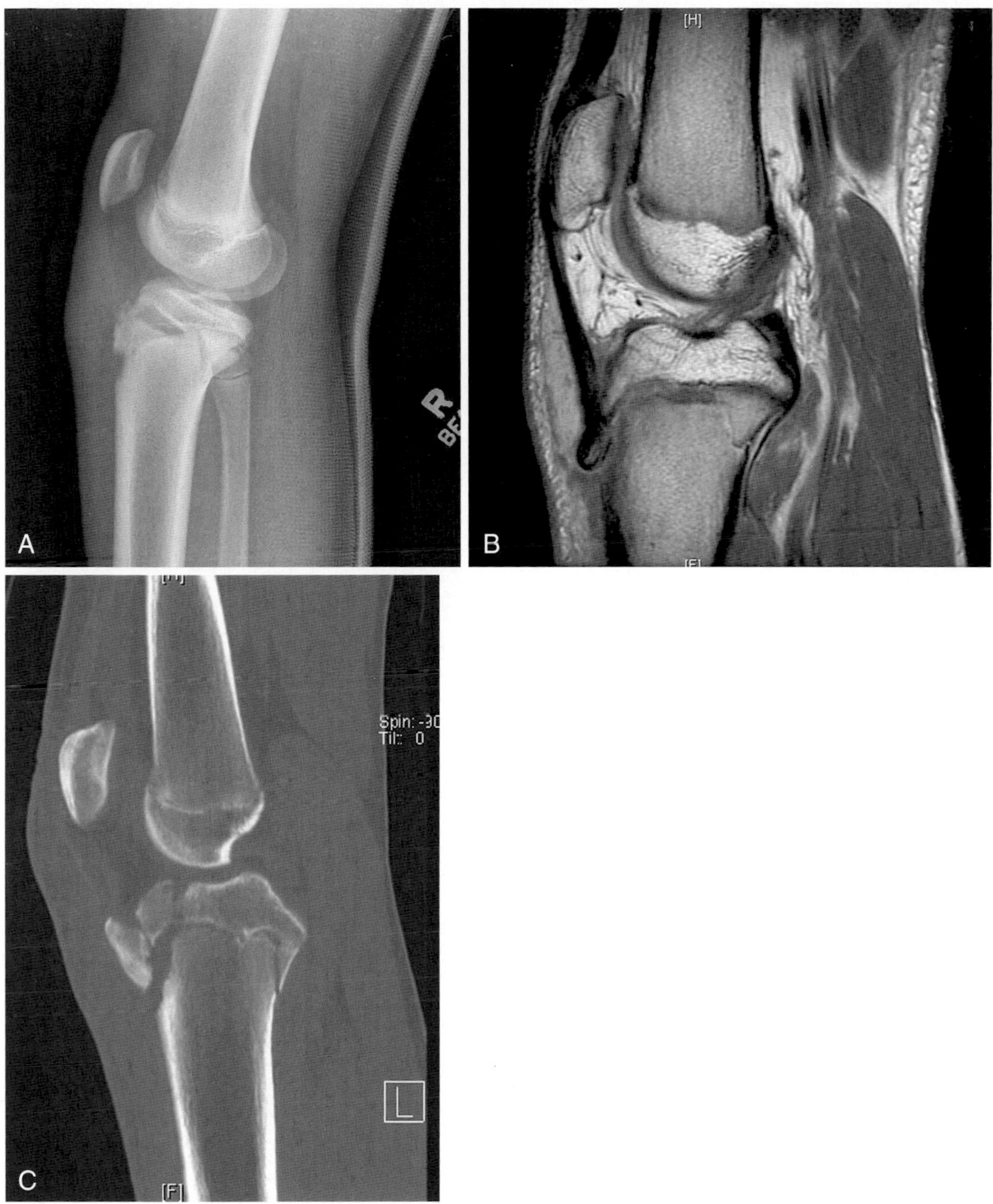

FIGURE 36-156 Anterior tibial tuberosity fracture combined with a posterior metaphyseal fracture in an adolescent male. **A,** Radiograph. **B,** MRI. **C,** CT scan.

preoperative workup, whereas others conclude that a careful inspection of the joint at time of surgery through an arthrotomy or arthroscopic assessment is sufficient.

The role of nonoperative management of tibial tuberosity fractures is limited to nondisplaced type I or type II fractures with little to no displacement. Closed treatment consists of cast immobilization in near full extension for 4 to 6 weeks followed by progressive range of motion and strengthening. Serial lateral radiographs are obtained to ensure that proximal displacement does not occur because of the pull of the quadriceps. For displacement of more than 3 mm, or for type III or greater fractures, surgical stabilization is recommended. If the fracture is reducible by closed manipulation, percutaneous fixation can be placed to maintain the reduction and allow early range of motion. If acceptable reduction is not obtained, then formal open reduction and fixation should be performed. Fixation typically is with cannulated screws; however, if the tuberosity fragment is comminuted or small, alternative methods of fixation may be used including suture, wires, suture anchors, or even plate fixation. Typically a large periosteal flap is present and, if repaired, provides addition stability to the fracture. It is hoped that with healing, fusion occurs across the traction apophysis only. We have found anterior tuberosity fractures combined with a posterior metaphyseal fragment to have a high risk of refracture after conservative treatment, and we treat these with ORIF that includes both anterior and posterior fragments (Fig. 36-157).

Complications related to tibial tuberosity fractures are uncommon. Acute compartment syndrome has been reported and often attributed to disruption of the anterior tibial recurrent vessels. We routinely admit patients with displaced

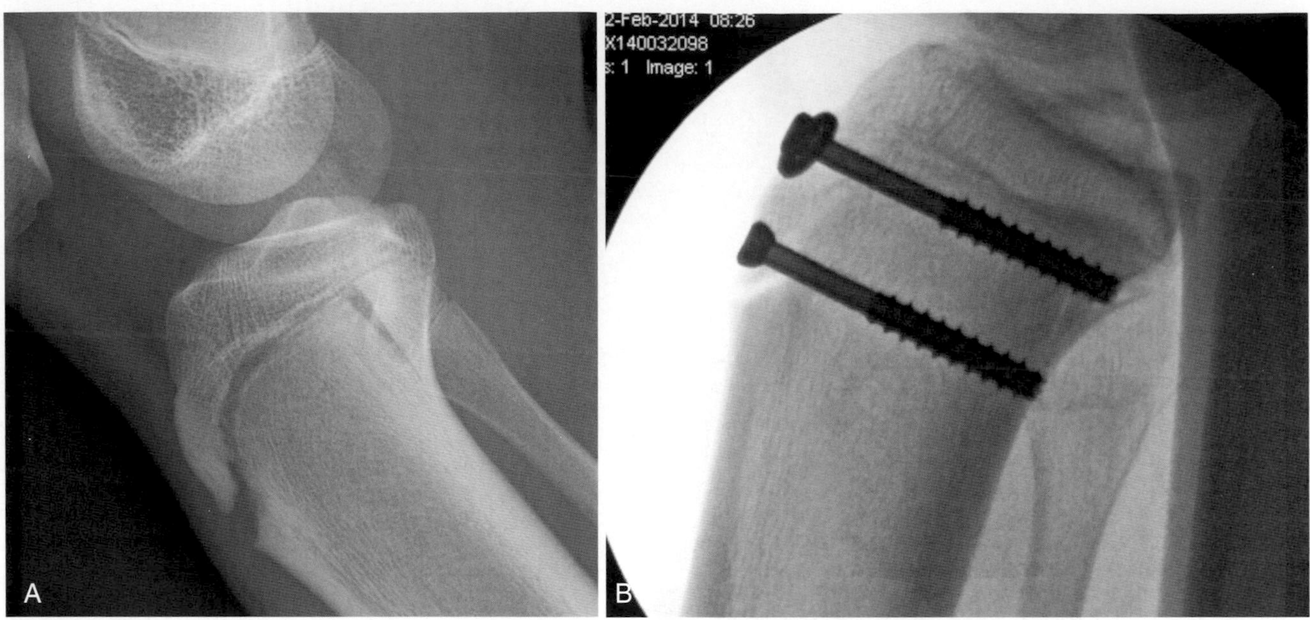

FIGURE 36-157 **A,** Anterior tibial tuberosity combined with a posterior metaphyseal fracture. **B,** Fixation with screws that includes anterior and posterior fragments.

tuberosity fractures overnight for observation regardless of treatment. Growth disturbance can occur but is rare because this fracture occurs most often toward the end of growth. If growth arrest does occur, then it may result in genu recurvatum and require surgical correction. Implant prominence is the most common complication and can be minimized by avoiding washers or using smaller, low profile implants. Our preference, however, is to use appropriate fixation to achieve a stable construct and to remove the implants once healing has occurred only if implant-related pain persists. Finally, loss of motion has been reported, but similar to tibial eminence fractures it can be minimized with stable fixation and early range of motion.

OPEN REDUCTION AND INTERNAL FIXATION

TECHNIQUE 36-37

- Make an anterior, midline incision adjacent to the tibial tuberosity and parallel to the patellar tendon. Carry the dissection laterally over the tibial tuberosity and the insertion of the patellar tendon.
- Identify any large periosteal flap, which may be avulsed medially, laterally, bilaterally, or distally. If it is frayed, resect some of it. If it is not frayed, retain it for stability.
- Expose the fracture and clean its base with a curet. Do not dissect completely free the attachments of the tibial tuberosity.
- Reduce the fracture with the knee in full extension.
- Insert guidewires for cannulated screws across the fracture. Once placed, confirm the reduction and guidewire position. If satisfactory, then place the cannulated screws in standard fashion. If the fragment is comminuted or small, then tension band, suture repair, or suture anchors may be placed to achieve fixation. Confirm the final reduction with radiographs. Suture any periosteal flap and close the wound in layers.

POSTOPERATIVE CARE. A cylinder cast or long leg cast has historically been applied with the knee in full extension for 4 to 6 weeks. If stable fixation is achieved, however, a controlled-motion brace can be used to allow for early range of motion.

OSTEOCHONDRAL FRACTURES

Osteochondral fractures of the knee occur primarily on the cartilaginous surfaces of the medial or lateral femoral condyle or the patella (Fig. 36-158). They may be caused by direct forces applied against the femur or patella or by dislocation of the patella itself (Fig. 36-159). Osteochondral fractures have been reported in over half of acute patellar dislocations, with equal numbers of capsular avulsions of the medial patellar margin and loose intraarticular fragments detached from the patella or the lateral femoral condyles (Fig. 36-160). Intraarticular fragments may be identified only after spontaneous relocation of the patella. Femoral fractures usually involve the edge of the articular surface and the middle third of the condylar arc. Usually a significant hemarthrosis follows the traumatic episode. If ligamentous instability is not present and the aspirate of the knee is sanguineous (hemarthrosis), an osteochondral fracture should be suspected, although often the fragment is not bony and cannot be seen on standard radiographs. Occasionally, just a faint density or fleck of subchondral bone can be identified. This small osseous fragment usually is part of an osteocartilaginous loose body that at surgery is surprisingly large. Additional views, such as the

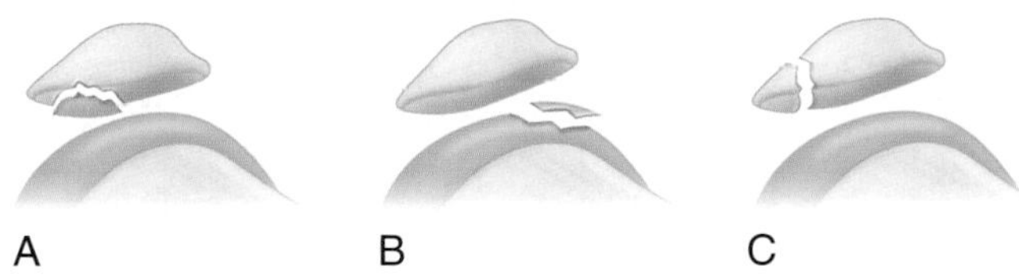

FIGURE 36-158 Three locations of osteochondral fractures caused by dislocation of patella. **A,** Inferior surface of patella. **B,** Femoral condyle. **C,** Medial surface of patella.

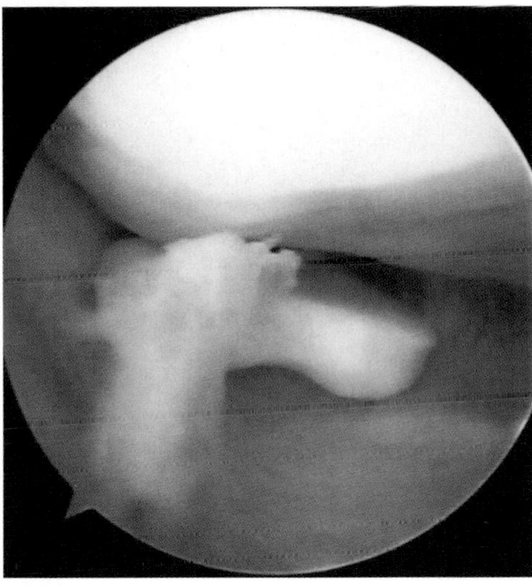

FIGURE 36-159 Osteochondral loose body from lateral femoral condyle secondary to acute patellar dislocation.

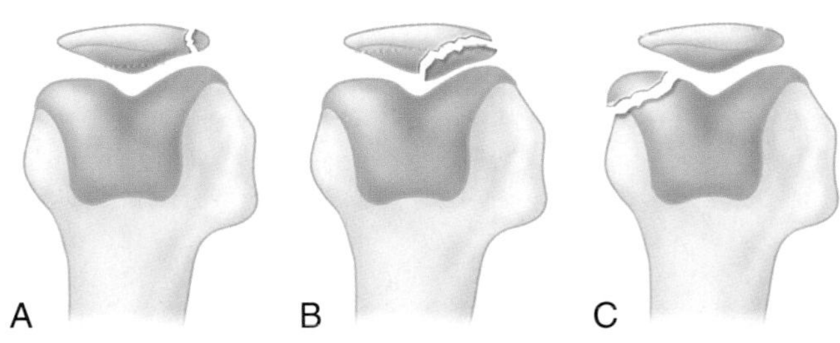

FIGURE 36-160 Most common types of osteochondral fractures in acute patellar dislocations. **A,** Medial marginal patellar avulsions. **B,** Inferomedial patellar facet. **C,** Lateral femoral condyle.

tunnel view, may improve exposure, but one study demonstrated that standard radiographs failed to identify an osteochondral fragment in 36% of children who had a loose body found at time of surgery. MRI is indicated if there is a high suspicion of osteochondral fracture. Arthroscopy is indicated to locate, identify, and remove the loose body. The defect in the patella or femur also should be identified. Small fragments or cartilaginous loose bodies can be excised, but larger fragments, particularly in weight-bearing portions of the joint, should be repaired when possible. For a more thorough discussion of osteochondral fractures, please refer to Chapter 32.

FLOATING KNEE INJURIES

Although not an injury of the knee joint, "floating knee" describes the flail knee joint segment resulting from a fracture of the shafts or adjacent metaphyses of the ipsilateral femur and tibia. This is an uncommon injury in children; it most often results from motor vehicle accidents and usually is associated with major soft-tissue damage, open fractures, and head injuries. Letts et al. proposed a five-part classification of these injuries (Fig. 36-161): type A, femoral and tibial fractures are closed diaphyseal fractures; type B, one fracture is diaphyseal, one is metaphyseal, and both are closed; type C, one fracture is diaphyseal, and the other is an epiphyseal displacement; type D, one fracture is open with major soft-tissue injury; and type E, both fractures are open with major soft-tissue injury. Their basic recommendation for treatment of these injuries is that at least one fracture (usually the tibial) must be rigidly fixed by ORIF. If mobilization of the child is essential, internal fixation of both fractures is indicated in most patients. In older children, intramedullary nailing may be more appropriate than plate fixation. Open fractures with major soft-tissue injury should be left open and stabilized with external fixation (Fig. 36-162). Outcomes of these fractures appear to be age related, with successful closed treatment of children younger than 10 years, but frequent complications and concomitant ligamentous injuries have been reported in children older than 10 years treated with reduction and fixation (intramedullary rods, plates, external fixator) of the femoral fracture. Poor results have been reported in 50% of older children because of limb-length discrepancy, angular deformity, or instability of the knee, particularly ligamentous instability.

TIBIAL AND FIBULAR FRACTURES

Fractures of the tibia and fibula are common across all age groups and represent the third most common long bone injury in children and adolescents. They are more common in males and occur from many different mechanisms. The most common location of fracture is in the distal third of the tibia followed by the middle and then proximal thirds. Many tibial and fibular fractures can be managed nonoperatively; however, these fractures require careful monitoring and management to avoid complications. Fracture patterns and potential complications vary according to location, so each anatomic site will be discussed separately. Otherwise, fractures of the tibia and fibula can be treated closed. A worrisome fracture is incomplete metaphyseal fracture of the proximal tibia. Fractures of the distal tibial and fibular physes also are of special concern because, if not treated properly, varus and valgus angulation may occur in older children and a bony bridge may form causing angular deformity in younger children.

PROXIMAL TIBIAL PHYSEAL FRACTURES

Fractures of the proximal tibial physis are uncommon fractures largely because of the anatomic stability at this location and the energy required to produce such an injury. The proximal tibial physis is partially protected by the ligamentous attachments around the knee, the fibula laterally, and the tibial tuberosity anteriorly. There also are fewer ligamentous attachments directly to the epiphysis when compared with the distal femoral epiphysis. Fractures of the epiphysis,

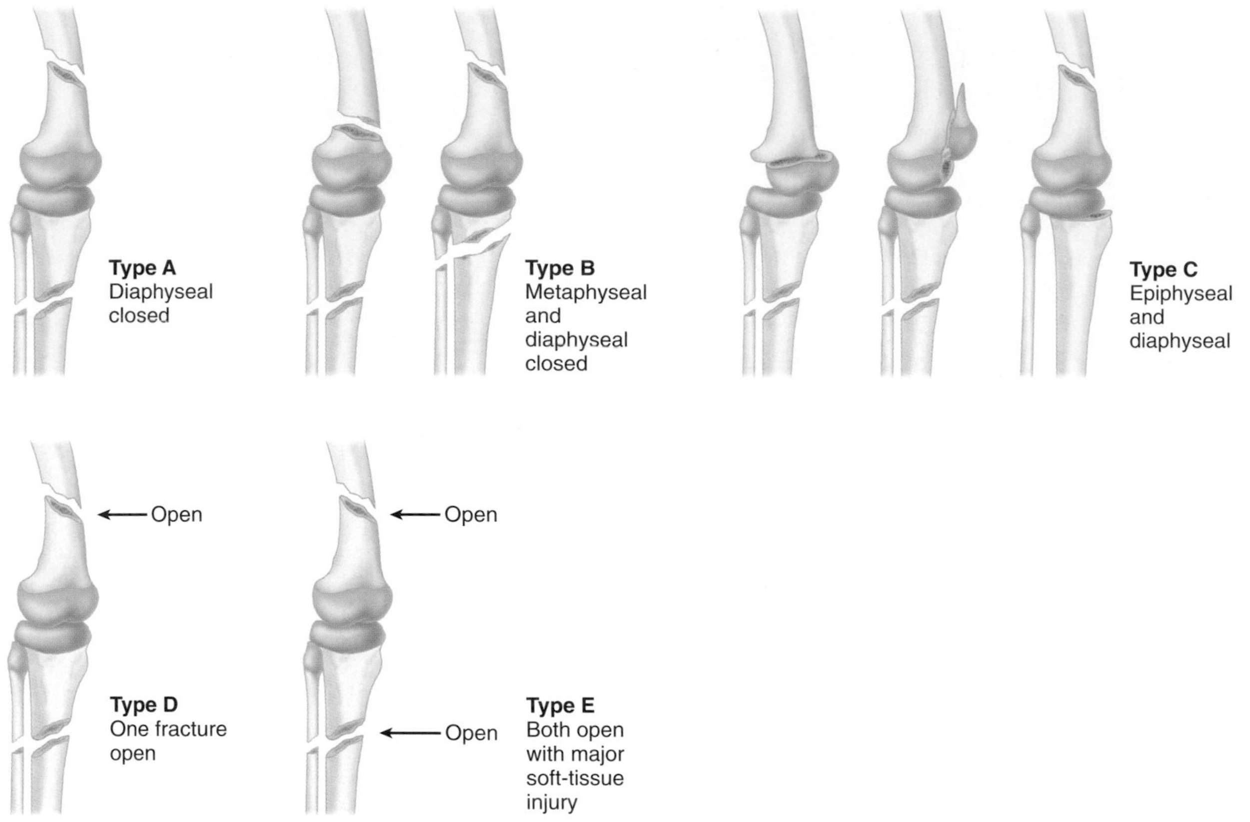

FIGURE 36-161 Classification of floating knee injuries in children (see text).

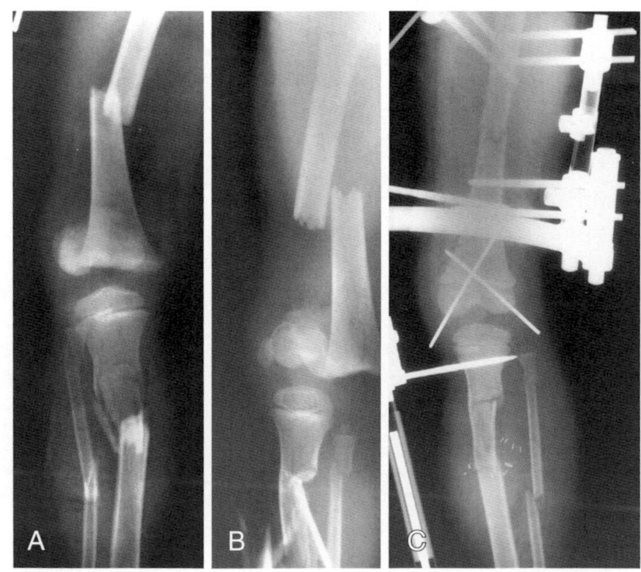

FIGURE 36-162 **A** and **B,** Severe floating knee injury with midshaft fracture of femur, Salter-Harris type I fracture of distal femoral physis, and comminuted fracture of tibial shaft. **C,** After internal fixation of distal femoral physeal fracture with crossed pins and external fixation of fractures of femoral and tibial shafts.

however, deserve special attention because of the proximity to the popliteal artery, which is tethered to the proximal tibia and may be injured when the tibial metaphysis is posteriorly displaced (Fig. 36-163). There are few dedicated studies about injuries at this location because many authors have included tibial tuberosity fractures in their series. We believe that, although there are many correlations between these two injuries, they ought to be considered separately because of some inherent differences. For type IV tibial tuberosity fractures, the proximal tibial physis also is disrupted and should be considered a true physeal injury.

Proximal tibial physeal fractures are commonly classified by the Salter-Harris classification. They can be further classified by the amount of displacement and the direction of displacement. Mubarak et al. found that by grouping fractures of the proximal tibia, including the eminence, tuberosity, and metaphyseal fractures, by direction of force and fracture pattern, there were several age-related correlations. In early childhood (ages 3 to 6 years), metaphyseal fractures were most common. In prepubescent children (ages 4 to 9 years), varus and valgus forces were the predominate mechanisms of fracture. During preadolescence (around ages 10 to 12 years), a fracture mechanism involving extension forces predominated. During adolescence (after age 13 years), the flexion-avulsion pattern consisting primarily of tibial tuberosity fracture was most common. Furthermore, tibial spine fractures occurred at age 10 years, Salter-Harris types I and II fractures at age 12 years, and Salter-Harris types III and IV

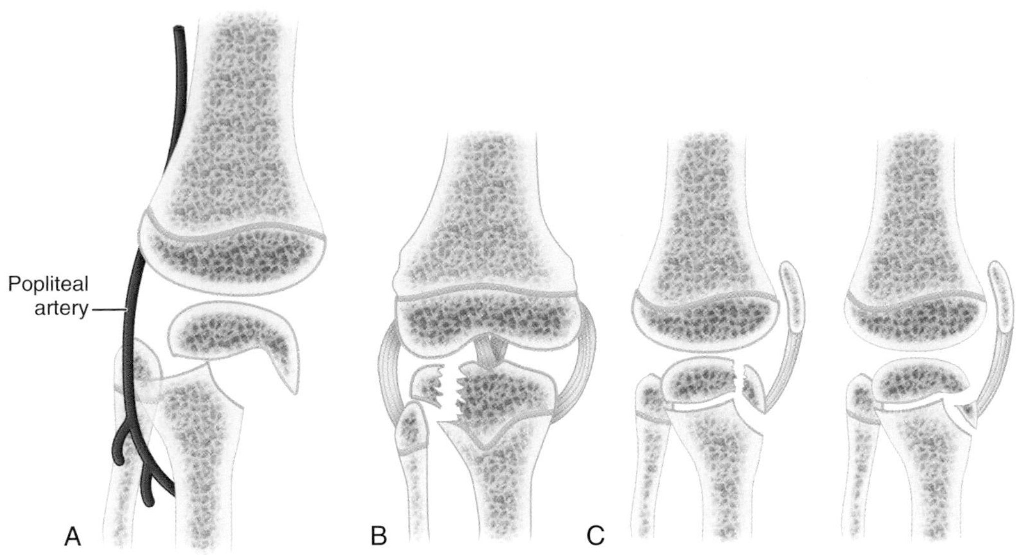

FIGURE 36-163 A, Salter-Harris types I and II fractures with posterior displacement of tibial shaft may injure popliteal artery. B, Salter-Harris type III fracture of proximal tibia. Analogous to a tibial plateau fracture. C, Fracture through tibial tuberosity and across epiphysis into knee joint similar to avulsion of epiphysis of tibial tuberosity.

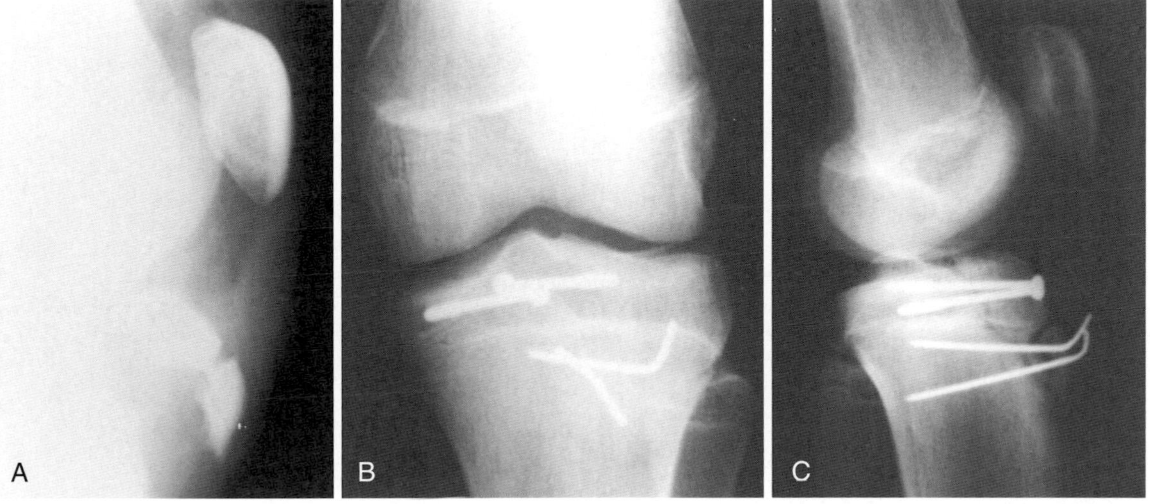

FIGURE 36-164 A, Salter-Harris type III fracture of proximal tibial physis. B and C, After open reduction and internal fixation.

physeal injuries at around age 14 years as tibial plateau equivalents.

Management of proximal tibial physeal fractures closely follows the Salter-Harris recommendations discussed earlier. Most types I and II injuries can be managed closed with cast immobilization if an adequate reduction is obtained. Gentle reduction with adequate sedation should be performed to minimize additional trauma to the physis. If the reduction is unsuccessful and there is persistent instability after reduction, vascular compromise, or impending compartment syndrome, then we prefer surgical stabilization with smooth pins across the physis or cannulated screws across the metaphyseal component. For types III or IV injuries, we accept only minimal articular displacement and have a low threshold for surgical stabilization (Fig. 36-164). Many of these fractures occur near the end of skeletal maturity and can be managed with adult techniques and implants to optimize stability and facilitate early range of motion. There is a high association between types III and IV fractures and associated intraarticular pathology. Advanced imaging with CT or MRI is helpful in determining displacement, identifying intraarticular injuries, and for preoperative planning.

Variants of Salter-Harris types III and IV fractures have been described as "triplane fractures of the proximal tibial epiphysis." These are similar to fractures that occur in the ankle in adolescent patients. Generally, these are two-part fractures that are type IV fractures and three-part fractures that are type III (Tillaux component) or type II fracture combinations. If displaced, both variants require ORIF (Fig. 36-165).

In a review of 39 proximal tibial physeal injuries at our institution, several complications occurred, including

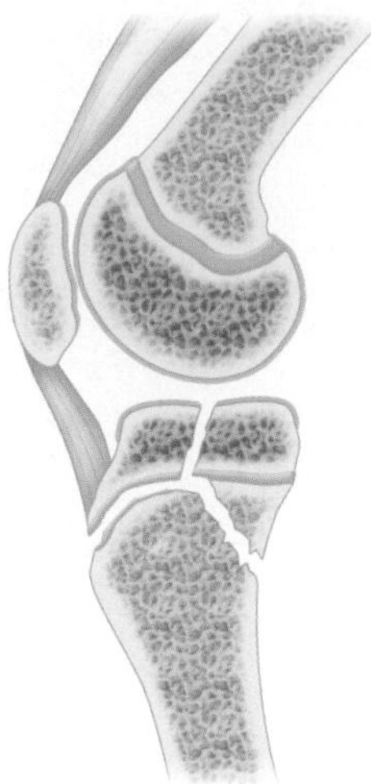

FIGURE 36-165 Sagittal view of knee depicting epiphyseal fracture pattern. Anterior and posterior fracture fragments are shown.

anterior compartment syndrome, transient and permanent peroneal nerve palsy, arterial thrombosis, angular deformity, and leg-length inequality. Any suggestion of ischemic changes, a compartment syndrome (see Chapter 48), or peroneal nerve palsy requires that immediate action be taken in the emergency department. Leg-length inequality of more than 1 inch (2.5 cm) occurred in 2 of the 39 children requiring additional treatment. Two children had joint incongruity and angular deformity.

PROXIMAL TIBIAL METAPHYSEAL FRACTURES

Fractures of the proximal tibial metaphysis occur most commonly between the ages of 3 and 8 years. The most common fracture pattern is a minimally displaced fracture created by a valgus moment to the leg from a medially directed force. Another common fracture pattern is an impaction fracture of the proximal metaphysis classically created by a trampoline injury with a young child bouncing with an older child or adult. Displaced fractures of the proximal tibial metaphysis are uncommon and are usually caused by a high-energy mechanism. Displaced fractures in this location are of concern because of their proximity to the posterior tibial artery and the possibility of damaging the vasculature of the leg.

Children with minimally displaced, low-energy fractures often present with the inability to walk. Children may describe pain in their knee or leg and have tenderness and swelling along the metaphysis. With high-energy trauma, the location of the fracture is more obvious, and careful attention should be placed on the neurovascular examination and serial compartment checks. An ankle-brachial index (ABI) test should be performed and compared with the contralateral side to rule out arterial injury if significant displacement is present.

For minimally displaced fractures, a long leg cast should be applied with the knee in slight flexion and a slight varus mold applied at the level of the fracture. For significantly angulated fractures, a reduction under sedation should be performed at the time of cast application. Displaced, high-energy fractures should be urgently reduced and surgically stabilized with age-appropriate techniques.

An uncommon but well-described complication of a proximal tibial metaphyseal fracture is a late valgus deformity. Initially described by Cozen, this phenomenon occurs in fractures of the proximal tibial metaphysis, even when nondisplaced. Radiographs often reveal a benign "greenstick" nondisplaced fracture pattern in a young child. Frequently, the fracture is treated in a straight or bent-knee cast and heals uneventfully with apparently satisfactory alignment. Later the tibia is noted to have a significant valgus angulation compared with the opposite tibia. This excess valgus may not have been preventable, and for this reason, parents should be told at the beginning of treatment about the possibility of this complication.

At what point the valgus angulation occurs and why it occurs are unknown. Numerous explanations have been advanced, however, including the following:

1. Asymmetric growth stimulation of the proximal tibial physis has been suggested. Houghton and Rooker surgically lacerated the proximal tibial periosteum medially in animals and noted a resultant valgus angulation.
2. Asymmetric growth stimulation of the medial proximal metaphysis from asymmetric vascular response has been suggested by several authors who postulated that an unbalanced vascular healing response occurs after injury to the metaphysis, causing the medial side of the tibia to outgrow the lateral side.
3. The tibial physis is stimulated more or for a longer period than the fibular physis, which may or may not have been fractured. This would cause a tethering effect, with the tibia overgrowing more medially than the fibula laterally, pulling the extremity into a valgus position.
4. Valgus angulation occurs at the time of fracture. Too often, radiographs of these fractures are taken in a cast with the knee flexed and the valgus angulation is not apparent. Radiographs of the contralateral extremity are not taken for comparison, and the amount of valgus is not appreciated. Weight bearing before solid union of the fracture also has been suggested to produce the valgus angulation.
5. Soft tissue, such as the pes anserinus, is interposed between the fragments, preventing an adequate reduction and complete healing of the fracture, which causes an exaggerated stimulation of the physis on the medial side of the tibia, resulting in overgrowth and valgus deformity (Fig. 36-166). Open reduction is recommended, especially when the fracture fragments are mildly to moderately separated medially, as is removal of the interposed material.
6. A physeal injury occurs, causing premature closure of the physis laterally, leaving the physis open medially with resultant valgus angulation.

Because the incidence, etiology, and prognosis of this deformity are unknown, prevention and treatment are controversial. The fractures usually occur between age 3 and 8 years, when the normal physiologic valgus is at its maximum. We reviewed eight children with this deformity whose ages ranged from 2 to 9 years. Similar to others, we are uncertain of the exact cause of the deformity or how to prevent it. The fracture should be treated precisely, however. First, parents should be warned before treatment is begun of the possibility of valgus deformity both during treatment and after healing has occurred. Second, a long leg cast in 5 to 10 degrees of flexion

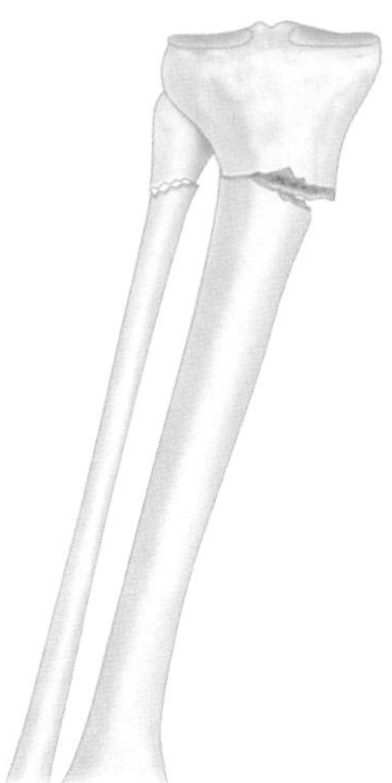

FIGURE 36-166 Opening of fracture gap medially showing that periosteum or pes anserinus could be interposed.

should be applied and radiographs of the fractured tibia and the opposite tibia should be taken frequently and compared. If any valgus angulation does occur, the cast should be wedged into a corrected position. Reduction, with the patient under general anesthesia, is recommended of any fracture with a break in the medial cortex and even minimal valgus deformity. Third, we have tried, when appropriate, to put the fractured tibia in slightly less valgus than the opposite tibia.

Of the eight children we reviewed at our institution, the deformity increased in some children 12 months after treatment. In some, the deformity improved spontaneously for 3 years after injury (Fig. 36-167). This improvement may have been caused by the normal correction of physiologic valgus seen in children 2 to 9 years old. Proximal tibial osteotomy or guided growth for significant deformity should be delayed because the deformity may correct spontaneously. Osteotomy corrects the deformity, but it also can stimulate the medial side of the tibia and cause the deformity to recur later, as noted in some of our children. Guided growth with compression of the medial physis may be the best treatment option in the rare patient who does not obtain spontaneous correction with growth.

OPEN REDUCTION AND REMOVAL OF INTERPOSED TISSUE

If interposition of soft tissue is strongly suspected or is confirmed by appropriate valgus stress radiographs with gapping of the fracture, and if the fracture is not a stress fracture, operative removal of the tissues, including the periosteum and pes anserinus, from the fracture may be necessary.

TECHNIQUE 36-38

(WEBER ET AL.)

- Place the patient supine on the operating table and prepare and drape the involved area in the usual fashion. Approach the fracture site medially through a 6-cm vertical incision.
- Carry the soft-tissue dissection down to the medial surface of the tibia and identify the fracture. Notice if the periosteum is stripped away from the medial surface of the tibia and, together with the pes anserinus, is trapped in the transverse fracture gap (Fig. 36-168A and B). Clean all debris away from the fracture, including the hematoma.
- Slide a periosteal elevator under the interposed tissues and extract them from the fracture. Hold the periosteum back with forceps (Fig. 36-168C and D) and irrigate the fracture.
- Suture the periosteum and the pes anserinus in their original positions if possible.
- Observe the fracture before closing to ensure that the gap is closed and that no further interposition of periosteum has occurred.
- Close the wound in layers and apply a long straight-leg cast.

POSTOPERATIVE CARE. Radiographs of both lower extremities in full extension should be made to ensure that no increased valgus is present in the injured tibia compared with the opposite tibia.

MIDDLE AND DISTAL TIBIAL SHAFT FRACTURES

Fractures of the shaft of the tibia, with or without associated fibular fractures, usually can be treated by closed reduction and casting. This also applies to distal tibial metaphyseal fractures. In a large series of tibial shaft fractures treated with above-knee casts, (1) initial shortening of 10 mm was compensated wholly or partially by growth acceleration; (2) mild varus deformities corrected spontaneously; (3) valgus deformity and posterior angulation persisted to some degree; and (4) rotational deformities persisted, especially internal rotation.

In general, transverse isolated fractures are less likely to displace early or late while in a cast, but spiral and oblique fractures are prone to displacement into varus or valgus for 2 to 3 weeks after injury and require careful follow-up. Fractures manipulated at 2 weeks have been found to be still mildly malleable, but fractures left for 3 weeks may not. With fractures that involve both the tibial and fibular shafts, valgus angulation is common because of the pull of the anterior and lateral compartment musculature. If the fibula is intact, the pull of the anterior compartment musculature tends to result in varus angulation as the fibula maintains the length of the lateral cortex. Posterior angulation (recurvatum) of distal tibial metaphyseal fractures can occur, especially when the ankle is held in dorsiflexion.

Spontaneous correction of angular deformity after tibial fractures has been reported to occur in boys up to age 10 years and in girls up to age 8 years; however, other reports indicate that little spontaneous correction occurs regardless of the age of the child. A summary of acceptable angulation and shortening based on age can be found in Table 36-6.

Because of the possibility of compartment syndromes, long bone fractures of the lower extremity should not be

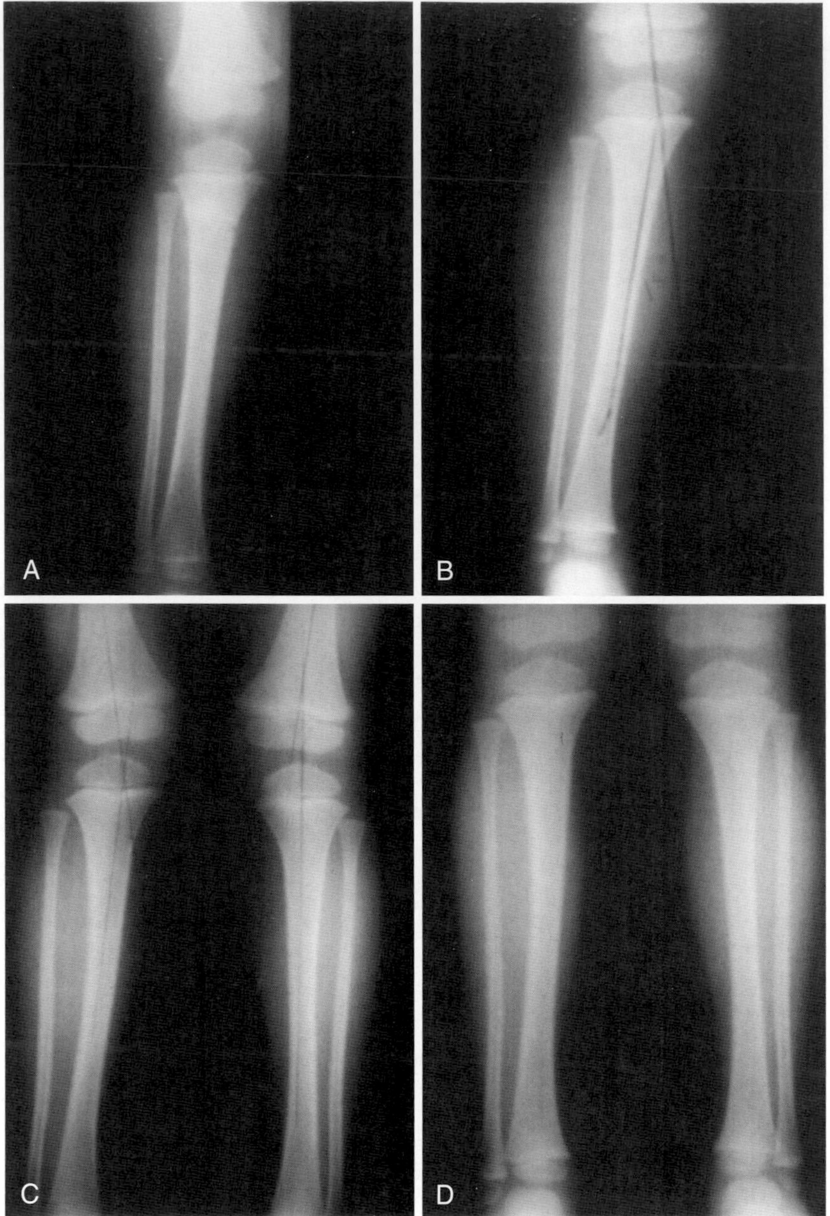

FIGURE 36-167 Spontaneous correction of valgus deformity. **A,** Proximal metaphyseal fracture at time of injury with no valgus angulation while standing. **B,** At 8 months, valgus angulation of 15 degrees is present. **C,** At 16 months, some spontaneous correction of angulation has occurred. **D,** At 2-year follow-up, valgus angulation has almost disappeared.

treated casually. A careful clinical examination should be performed and documented followed by serial examinations to monitor for signs of impending compartment syndrome. If vascular injury is suspected, an ankle-brachial index or arteriogram should be obtained at the direction of a vascular surgeon. If there is high suspicion or risk of compartment syndrome based on a thorough workup, a splint with soft-tissue dressing should be applied instead of a circular cast, and the extremity should be monitored with a suitable compartment-pressure measuring device. If compartment syndrome is anticipated or developing, surgical stabilization of the fracture should be considered and a very low threshold for compartment releases should be maintained. The treatment of impending and established compartment syndromes is described elsewhere (see Chapter 48).

Although most tibial fractures can be managed with closed treatment, there has been a trend toward expanding the indications for operative intervention of tibial fractures. The indications for operative treatment of tibial and fibular fractures in a child are:

1. Unstable fractures that cannot be adequately aligned or maintained by closed methods.
2. Open tibial fractures, which should be treated as emergencies with irrigation and debridement. If soft-tissue damage is extensive, an external fixator is used as in adults. Care should be taken not to cross the physis with pins when applying the fixator.
3. Fractures in which surgical stabilization facilitates mobilization or nursing care, such as floating knees, polytrauma, or multiple long bone injuries.

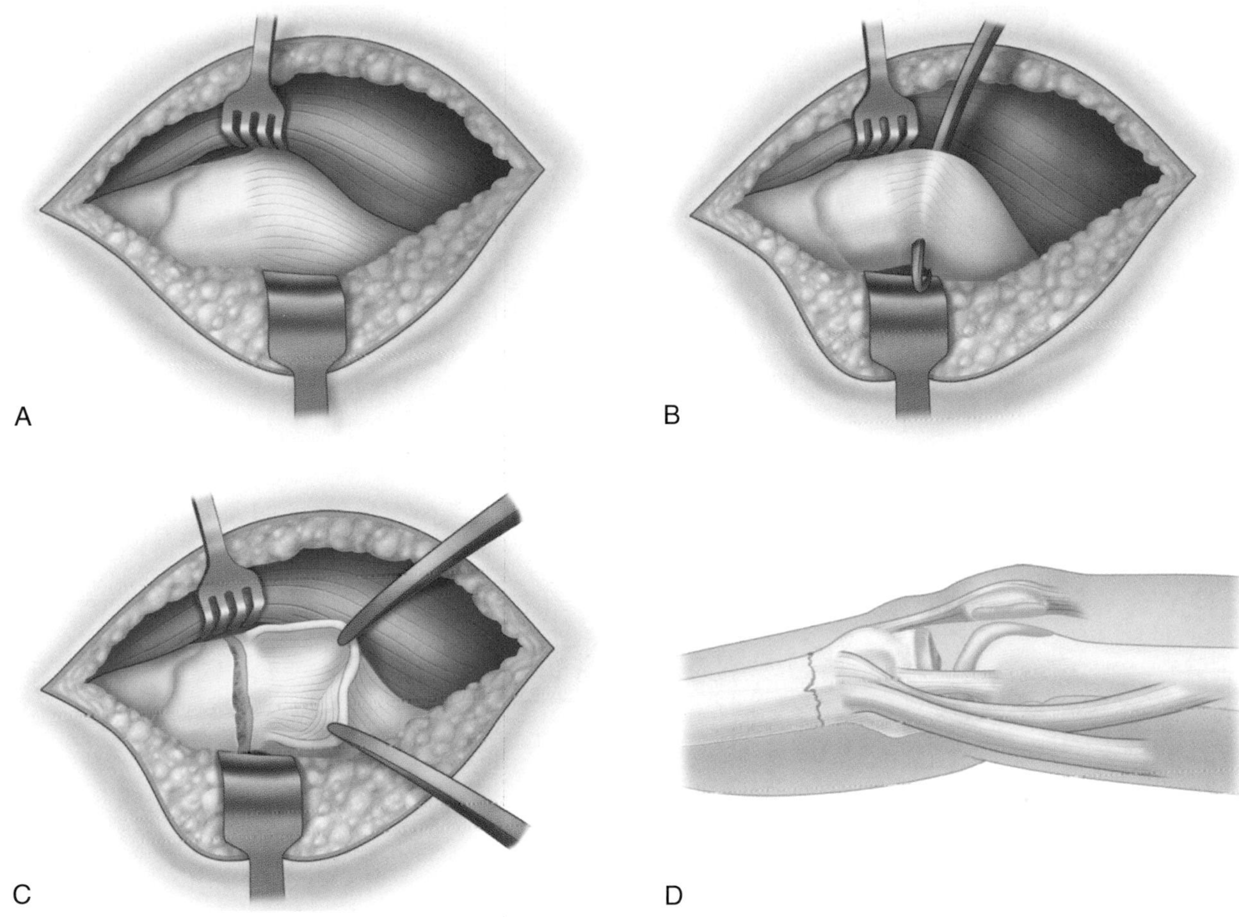

FIGURE 36-168 Weber technique for removing soft tissue from proximal metaphyseal fracture. **A,** Exposure of fracture. **B** to **D,** Removal of pes anserinus and periosteum from fracture with periosteal elevator and forceps. **SEE TECHNIQUE 36-38.**

4. Nonunions of tibial fractures, which are rare in children and are probably more serious and more difficult to manage than in adults. We have treated several children with obvious nonunions of the tibia with no other pathologic or congenital anomaly in whom internal fixation and bone grafting were required to achieve union (Fig. 36-169).

The general assumption that even grade II and III open diaphyseal fractures in children heal readily was refuted in a large series of these fractures: 55% healed primarily, 30% had delayed unions, 7.5% were classified as nonunions, and 7.5% (all with Gustilo grade IIIC fractures) required early amputation. The same factors that predispose to these complications in adults (degree of displacement, comminution, soft-tissue damage, and periosteal stripping) also contribute to delayed union and nonunion in children. Reported incidences of compartment syndrome, vascular injury, infection, and delayed union are similar to those in adults. Two complications are unique to children: late angular deformities and tibial overgrowth. Laine et al. reported eight patients with open (type IIIB or IIIC) tibial fractures who all required soft-tissue flaps and had an average bone loss of 5.4 cm. They found that with the use of a circular external fixator and the application of an algorithm based on bone loss and the ability to acutely shorten the construct, seven out of eight limbs could be salvaged, and of the seven in whom the fracture healed, all were ambulatory without assistive devices at time of final follow-up in spite of a high rate of secondary procedures.

Intramedullary nailing may be indicated because of an inability to obtain or maintain reduction in an older or larger child with an unstable fracture pattern that is at high risk of displacement or for multiple pathologic fractures in a young child, such as occur in osteogenesis imperfecta or congenital pseudarthrosis of the tibia. The ever-expanding indications for femoral intramedullary nailing in children have been extrapolated to tibial nailing, and tibial fractures in children as young as 4 years of age have been treated with flexible intramedullary nailing. A retrospective review of tibial fractures in 31 patients with open physes found shorter times to union and better functional outcomes in those treated with intramedullary nailing than in those treated with external fixation.

If intramedullary nailing is done, the proximal and distal physes should be avoided. Intramedullary nailing has been reported to be successful in stabilizing severely comminuted tibial fractures so that union is obtained without angular deformity. If possible, closed techniques of nail insertion should be used, with a small incision over the fracture if necessary for adequate reduction of the fracture. Titanium or stainless elastic intramedullary nails may be used, but the medullary canal of the tibia must be measured carefully and

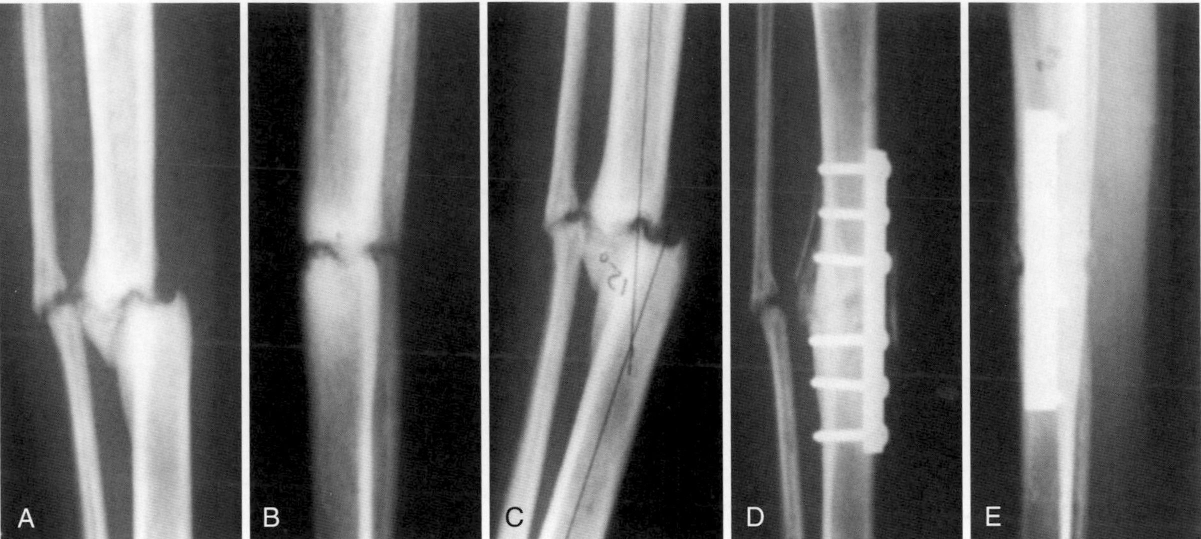

FIGURE 36-169 Nonunion of tibia and fibula in child. **A** and **B,** Nonunion before treatment. **C,** Stress radiograph showing motion at fracture. **D** and **E,** Early union after bone grafting and compression plate fixation.

the appropriate sized elastic nail selected based on the criteria described for femurs. Complications reported after intramedullary nailing of tibial fractures in children include neurovascular complications (8%), infection (8%), malunion (8%), and leg-length discrepancy (4%). In another review of tibial fractures treated with elastic intramedullary nails, delayed union occurred at a rate of 18%.

ELASTIC STABLE INTRAMEDULLARY NAILING OF TIBIAL FRACTURE

TECHNIQUE 36-39

(O'BRIEN, WEISMAN, RONCHETTI, ET AL.)

- After induction of general anesthesia and placement of a well-padded tourniquet on the proximal thigh, prepare and drape the affected leg. The tourniquet usually is not inflated.
- With the use of fluoroscopy, mark on the skin the fracture site, the proximal tibial physis, and the starting points for nail entry. The starting point for the nail entry hole is 1.5 to 2.0 cm distal to the physis.
- Make lateral longitudinal 2-cm incisions over the proximal tibial metaphysis just proximal to the starting points.
- Select two appropriately sized nails (2, 3, or 4 mm) based on the width of the medullary canal, choosing the largest possible diameter nails that will fit the medullary canal; for example, if the canal measured 6 mm, use two 3-mm nails.
- The nails come with a beveled blunt tip. Bend the very tip of the nail to 45 degrees to facilitate passage along the opposite cortex and aid in fracture reduction.
- Contour the entire length of the nail to a gentle curve such that the apex will rest at or near the fracture site after reduction. The depth of the curve should be approximately three times the diameter of the canal to achieve the optimal balance between ease of insertion and stability.
- Use a drill 0.5 cm larger than the nail in a soft-tissue sleeve to create the entry hole, confirming the entry hole with fluoroscopy in both the anteroposterior and lateral planes. Take care to avoid the tibial tubercle apophysis.
- Drill the hole in the midpoint of the anteroposterior dimension, starting perpendicular to the physis. Under fluoroscopic guidance, angle the drill caudad until it is 45 degrees from the long axis of the tibia, taking care not to drill out the far cortex or migrate toward the physis.
- Place the prebent nail on an inserter and insert it from the side opposite the distal displacement in an antegrade fashion.
- Under fluoroscopic guidance, slide the nail along the opposite cortex until the fracture is reached.
- Reduce the fracture and advance the nail across the fracture. Embed the nail in the distal tibial metaphysis without violating the cortex or the physis.
- Place the second nail from the other side in a similar fashion.
- If necessary, rotate the bent tips of the nails after passing the fracture site to effect an anatomic reduction, taking care not to distract the fracture site.
- Bend the proximal nail ends and cut them 1 cm from the cortical surface so that the nail ends will sit deep to the compartment fascia but be proud enough for easy retrieval.
- Close the wounds with an absorbable fascial and subcuticular stitch and apply a short leg cast.

POSTOPERATIVE CARE. Weight bearing is begun when evidence of bridging callus is present, usually at about 5 weeks. Nails are removed at 6 to 12 months after fracture; no immobilization is required after nail removal (Fig. 36-170).

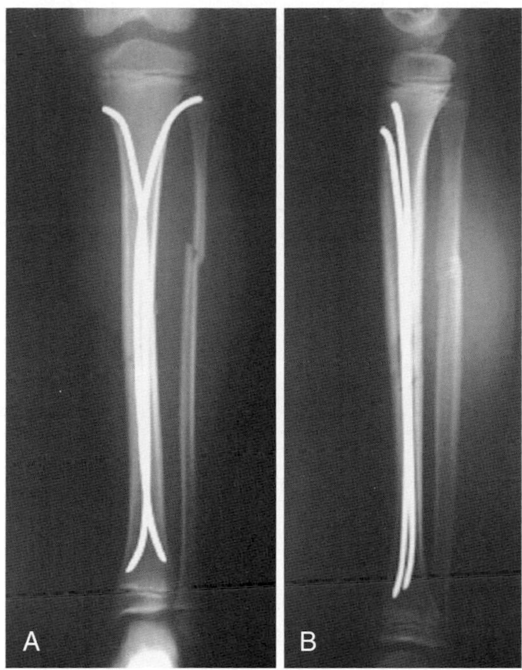

FIGURE 36-170 Grade II open fracture in 7-year-old boy. **A** and **B**, Postoperative anteroposterior and lateral radiographs of tibia and fibula. (From O'Brien T, Weisman DS, Ronchetti P, et al: Flexible titanium nailing for the treatment of the unstable pediatric tibial fracture, J Pediatr Orthop 24:601, 2004.) **SEE TECHNIQUE 36-39.**

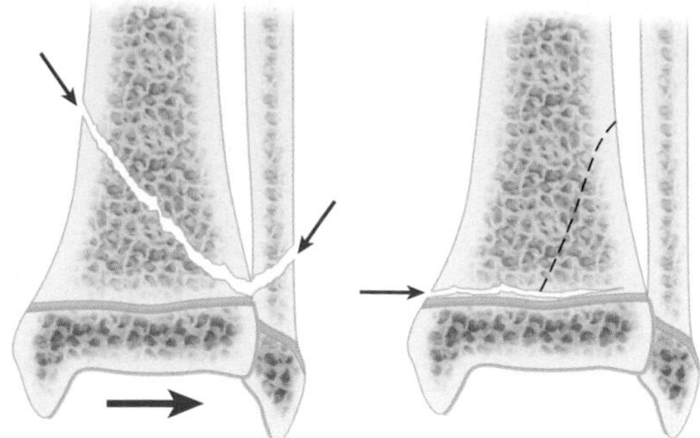

FIGURE 36-171 Salter-Harris type II physeal fractures are produced by external rotation, abduction, and plantarflexion forces.

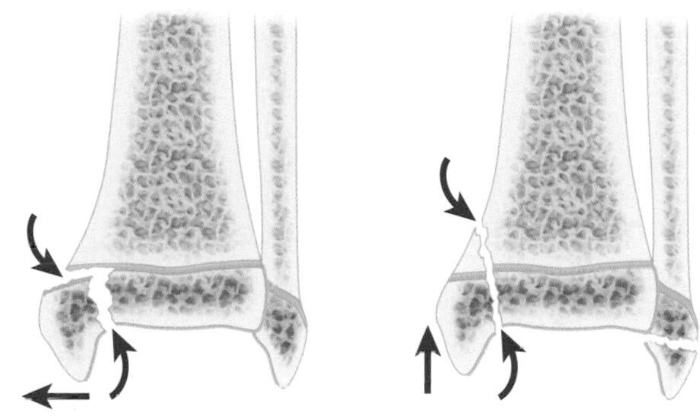

FIGURE 36-172 Salter-Harris type III and IV fractures are produced by adduction forces (supination-inversion).

DISTAL TIBIAL AND FIBULAR EPIPHYSEAL FRACTURES

Carothers and Crenshaw described the mechanism of injury of distal tibial physeal fractures using a classification of abduction, external rotation, and plantarflexion; adduction; and axial compression. Abduction, external rotation, and plantarflexion frequently produce Salter-Harris type I or II physeal fractures (Fig. 36-171); adduction produces type III or IV fractures (Fig. 36-172); and axial compression produces type V fractures. Since this original study, we have reviewed 100 ankle fractures in children. The most common were Salter-Harris type II fractures (26). Type III fractures were more common than anticipated (19), and type I fractures (9) and type IV fractures (6) were relatively rare. Also studied were six triplane and six Tillaux fractures. The remaining were distal fibular fractures, and all were Salter-Harris type I or II fractures except for one Salter-Harris type IV fracture. Most fractures of the fibular physis occur in conjunction with distal tibial fractures; Salter-Harris type III fractures usually are isolated injuries.

Fibular physeal fractures are treated for 3 to 6 weeks in a short leg cast. Salter-Harris types I and II fractures of the distal tibial physis usually are treated by closed reduction and the application of a bent-knee, long leg cast. In young children, moderate displacement after closed reduction, especially in the anteroposterior plane, can be accepted. Varus or valgus angulation in older children with type I or II fractures does not correct spontaneously, however, and excessive angulation should not be accepted (Fig. 36-173). Because the foot tolerates these positions poorly, the result is unacceptable. Two of our patients had open reduction because such a deformity could not be reduced closed. Residual gaps in the physis after closed reduction of Salter-Harris types I and II fractures may represent entrapped periosteum, which can lead to premature physeal closure. Open reduction and removal of the entrapped periosteum may be beneficial in a younger child.

In a series of 91 types I and II distal tibial physeal fractures, Rohmiller et al. reported premature physeal closure in 40%. They found a difference in the rates of premature physeal closure between fractures caused by a supination-external rotation mechanism (35%) and those caused by a pronation-abduction mechanism (54%). The most significant predictor of premature physeal closure was not initial fracture displacement but postreduction displacement. Anatomic reduction is recommended, regardless of treatment method, to decrease the risk of premature physeal closure (Fig. 36-174). In spite of treatment methods, the rate of premature physeal closure after distal tibial physeal fractures remains quite high.

Most Salter-Harris type III and IV fractures, including triplane and Tillaux fractures, require ORIF. Internal fixation methods include smooth pins or wires if the physis must be crossed, cannulated cancellous screws, and, more recently, bioabsorbable screws. Bioabsorbable screws have the advantage of not requiring second surgery for removal, but care must be taken not to damage the physis during their insertion. The amount of displacement acceptable for closed treatment has not been defined. If after a closed reduction the surgeon believes that the amount of displacement can be reduced operatively, ORIF is justified (Fig. 36-175). Surgery traditionally has been recommended for 2 to 3 mm or more

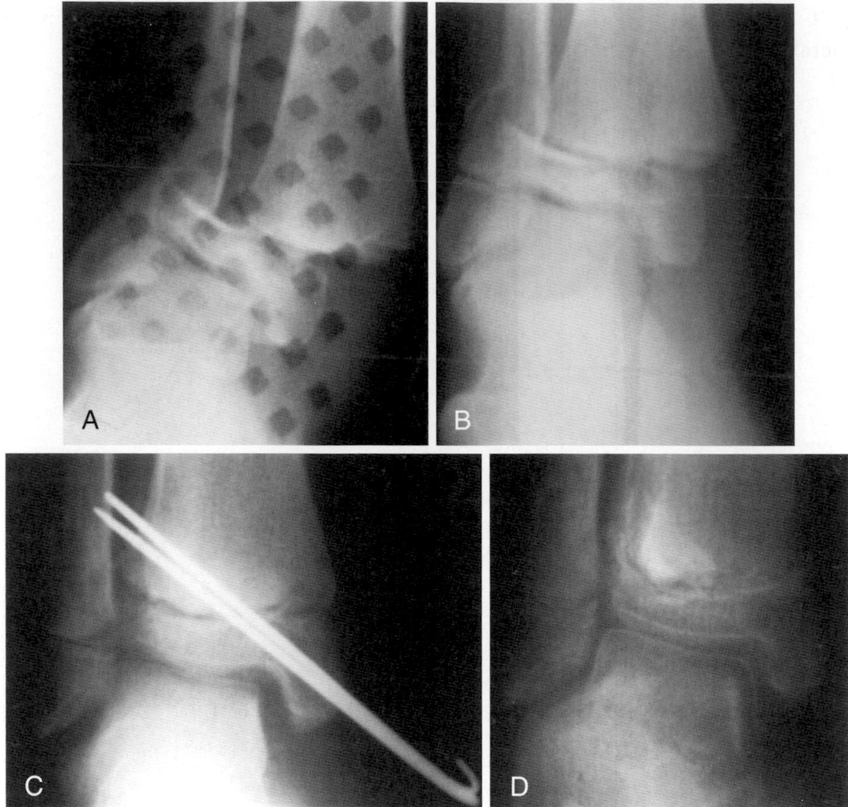

FIGURE 36-173 Open reduction of Salter-Harris type I fracture. **A,** Before treatment. **B,** After closed reduction, residual angulation is 17 degrees in this older child. **C,** After open reduction and internal fixation with smooth pins, flap of periosteum was found caught in fracture. **D,** At early follow-up, no evidence of bony bridge is seen.

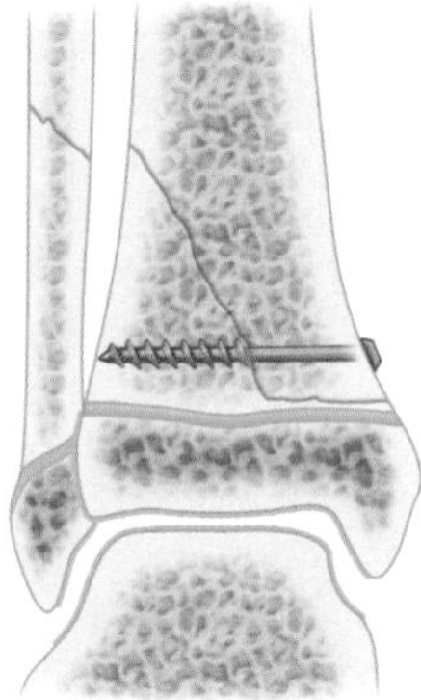

FIGURE 36-174 Cancellous screw fixing large metaphyseal spike of Salter-Harris type II fracture.

of displacement. For the most part, standards for acceptable displacement using CT techniques have not been refined or defined. The amount of displacement, the extent of comminution, and proper placement of screw fixation (at right angle to the fracture fragments) can be determined, however (Fig. 36-176).

Salter-Harris type III and IV fractures are almost always medial and occur at the plafond, with the exception of Tillaux and triplane fractures. Often a tiny triangular piece of bone is present on the metaphyseal side in a type IV fracture (Fig. 36-177). At the time of open reduction, this piece of bone can

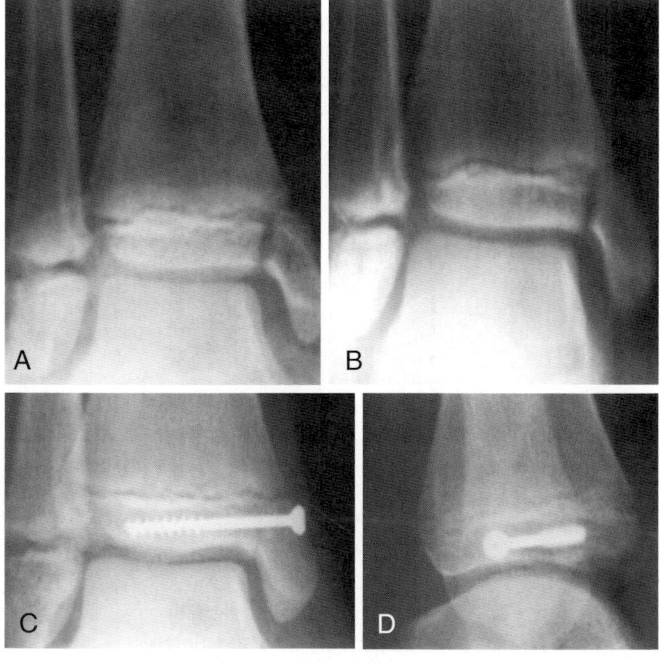

FIGURE 36-175 **A** and **B,** Anteroposterior radiographs of displaced Salter-Harris type III fracture of medial malleolus and Salter-Harris type I fracture of lateral malleolus. **C** and **D,** After open reduction and internal fixation of medial malleolar fracture with threaded screw through epiphysis.

be removed to better expose the physis and to try to prevent the formation of a peripheral bony bridge in this area. Symptomatic ossification centers in the medial malleolus should not be mistaken for Salter-Harris type III fractures.

It is best not to cross the physis with any kind of pin unless absolutely necessary for fixation to minimize the risk of a bony bridge developing where the pins cross the physis. The perichondral ring can be avulsed in this area, just as from the distal femoral physis, from a minor fracture or ligamentous or other injury and may cause peripheral growth arrest with resultant angular deformity.

Of our 100 ankle fractures, the result was poor in four type III tibial injuries and one type IV tibial injury because of varus or valgus deformity secondary to growth arrest and in one type II tibial injury because of refracture. Supramalleolar osteotomy was necessary in two injuries.

The development of a sclerotic line of growth disturbance (Park or Harris line) that appears 6 to 12 weeks after fracture has been suggested to predict the likelihood of growth arrest from the presence and displacement of the line. If the line extends across the whole width of the metaphysis in both planes, and if the line continues to grow away from the physis remaining parallel to it, growth disturbance is not likely to occur. An absence of this formation and displacement of the line may indicate abnormal growth that will result in varus or valgus angulation. Letts et al. proposed a classification of pediatric pilon fractures similar to the adult classification but amended it to include articular surface displacement of more than 5 mm and physeal displacement (Table 36-7). These type II and III fractures seem to be more severe and involve comminution of the articular surface and should be considered more complex than Salter-Harris type II, III, and IV fractures and triplane fractures.

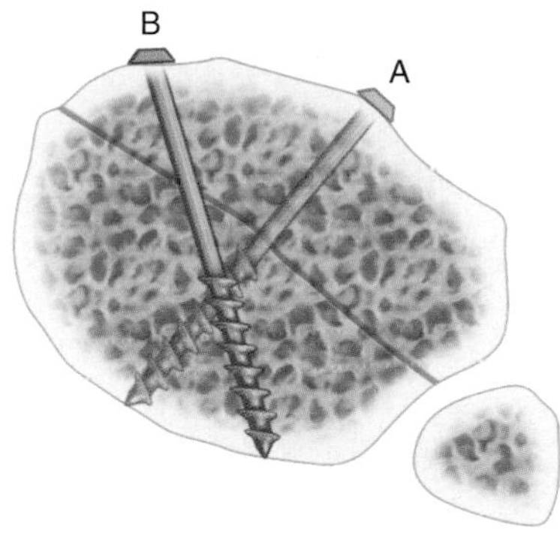

FIGURE 36-176 Distal tibial physeal fractures. Difference in entry point and direction of screw between ideal position (*A*) and observed position (*B*). (Redrawn from Cutler L, Molloy A, Dhukuram V, et al: Do CT scans aid assessment of distal tibial physeal fractures? J Bone Joint Surg 86B:239, 2004. Copyright British Editorial Society of Bone and Joint Surgery.)

High-velocity motor vehicle accidents or lawn mower injuries often produce severe open ankle fractures. These injuries may involve the distal tibial physis; a shearing fracture of the body of the talus also can be present. The result is physeal arrest and joint roughening. After an open fracture, infection can develop. External fixators can be used in the initial management until the wound is clean. Bony bridge resection and osteotomy for angular deformity may be necessary later. If infection develops or joint involvement is severe, ankle fusion may be necessary (Fig. 36-178). At the time of fusion, the physis should be preserved, and compression clamps should be used to hasten fusion. An interposed iliac bone graft can be used (see Chapter 11).

OPEN REDUCTION AND INTERNAL FIXATION

TECHNIQUE 36-40

- Place the patient supine on the operating table; prepare and drape the involved area in the usual fashion and use a tourniquet.

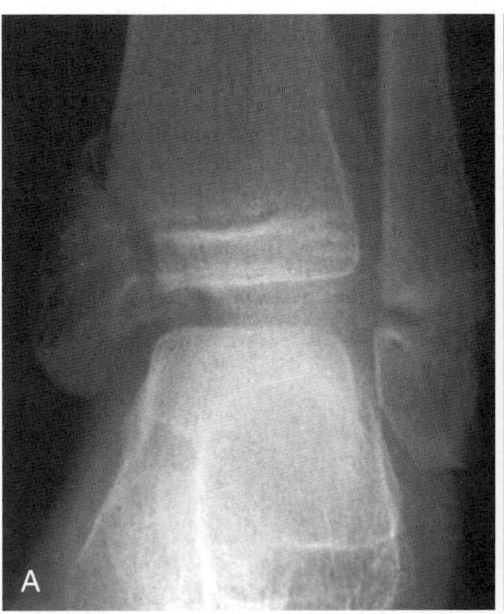

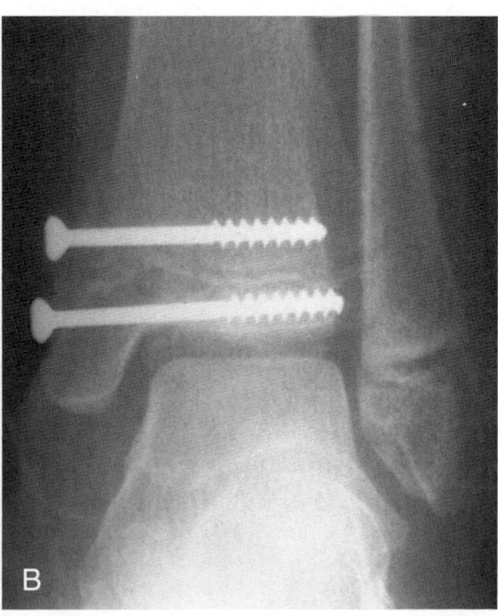

FIGURE 36-177 **A,** Salter-Harris type IV fracture of medial malleolus. **B,** After open reduction and internal fixation with threaded cancellous screws in metaphysis and epiphysis, avoiding physis.

TABLE 36-7

Pediatric Classification of Pilon Fracture

TYPE	ARTICULAR SURFACE DISPLACEMENT (mm)	PHYSEAL DISPLACEMENT (mm)	COMMINUTION	ADJACENT INJURIES
I	>5	None	None	None
II	>5	<5	2-3 fragments	None
III	>5	>5	Multiple fragments	Ipsilateral tibial shaft fracture and/or ankle dislocation

From Letts M, Davidson D, McCaffrey M: The adolescent pilon fracture: management and outcome, J Pediatr Orthop 21:20, 2001.

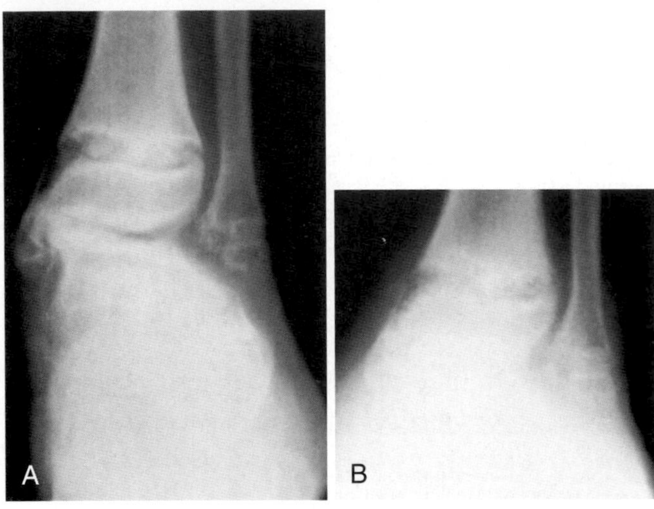

FIGURE 36-178 Severe physeal injury caused by a lawn mower. **A,** Severe injury with loss of talar dome and part of distal tibia and separation of distal tibial physis. **B,** Solid fusion with physis still open.

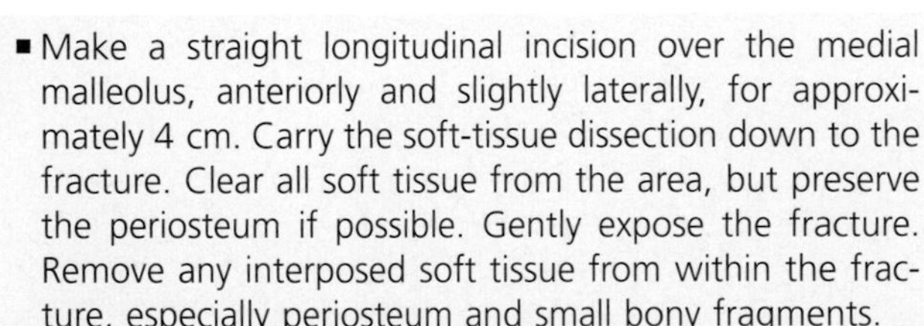

- Make a straight longitudinal incision over the medial malleolus, anteriorly and slightly laterally, for approximately 4 cm. Carry the soft-tissue dissection down to the fracture. Clear all soft tissue from the area, but preserve the periosteum if possible. Gently expose the fracture. Remove any interposed soft tissue from within the fracture, especially periosteum and small bony fragments.
- Expose the ankle joint anteriorly and, with the aid of a bone holder, reduce the fracture anatomically. If the fracture is a Salter-Harris type IV with a small metaphyseal spike, remove the spike to see the reduction better and prevent a later bony bridge at the periphery.
- Insert small, parallel, smooth Steinmann pins horizontally across the fracture. Do not cross the physis unless necessary. Use a cannulated or cancellous screw if desired, ensuring, however, that the threads do not damage the physis and the screw is horizontal across the fracture (Fig. 36-179). Check the reduction and pin or screw placement with radiographs.
- Reduce manually any fibular fracture.
- Close the wound and apply a long leg, bent-knee cast with the ankle in neutral position.

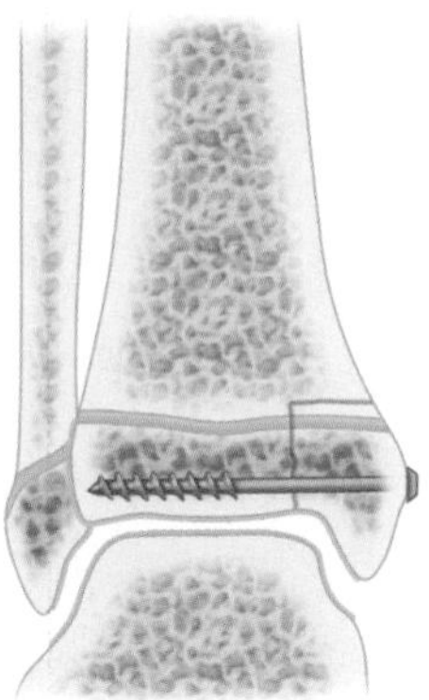

FIGURE 36-179 Salter-Harris type III or IV fracture should be fixed by horizontal pins or cancellous bone screws not involving the physis. **SEE TECHNIQUE 36-40.**

POSTOPERATIVE CARE. Weight bearing is not permitted for 4 to 6 weeks, depending on the age of the patient. A short leg, weight-bearing cast is worn for 3 weeks.

TRIPLANE FRACTURES

Triplane fractures are caused by an external rotational force and are considered a combination of Salter-Harris type II and III fractures. Marmor first coined the term *"triplane fracture of the distal part of the tibia"* in 1970 in his description of lesions consisting of three fragments: (1) the anterolateral portion of the distal tibial epiphysis; (2) the remainder of the epiphysis (anteromedial and posterior portions) with an attached posterolateral spike of the distal tibial metaphysis; and (3) the remainder of the distal tibial metaphysis and tibial shaft.

The triplane fracture has been reported to be a two-part rather than a three-part fracture. This fracture is caused by an external rotational force, and if it is a three-part fracture, it is considered a combination of Salter-Harris type II and III fractures. If it is a two-part fracture, it is a Salter-Harris type IV fracture (Figs. 36-180 and 36-181). CT or MRI evaluation has been recommended because plain radiographs alone do not show the configuration of the fracture accurately. Usually, closed reduction can be achieved by internal rotation of the foot and immobilization in a long leg cast. If a closed reduction cannot be achieved, ORIF is indicated. When adequate

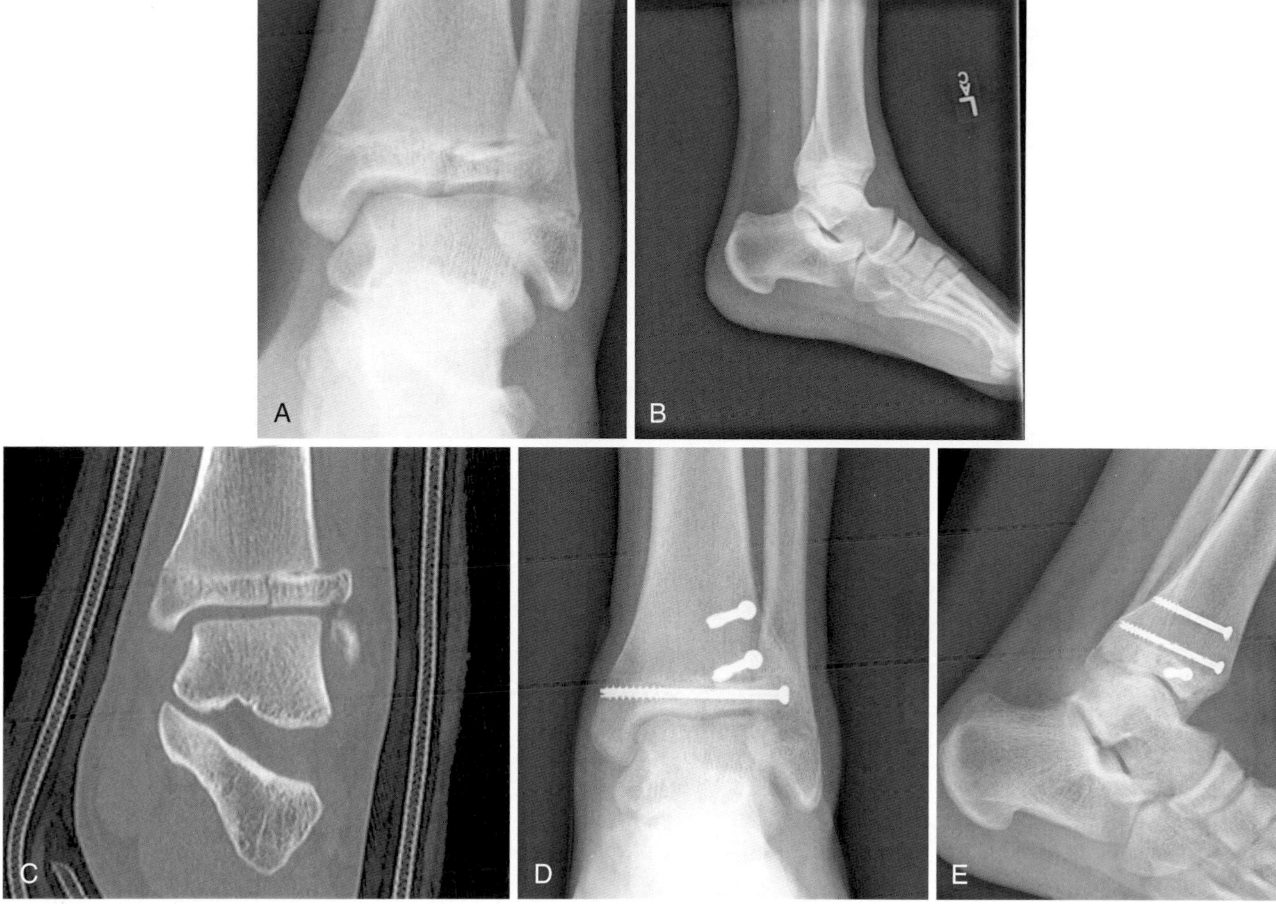

FIGURE 36-180 Distal tibial triplane fracture. **A,** Anteroposterior view showing triplane fracture. **B,** Lateral view of fracture, Salter-Harris type IV (two parts of three-part fracture, type II plus type III). **C,** Preoperative coronal CT. **D** and **E,** After open reduction and internal fixation.

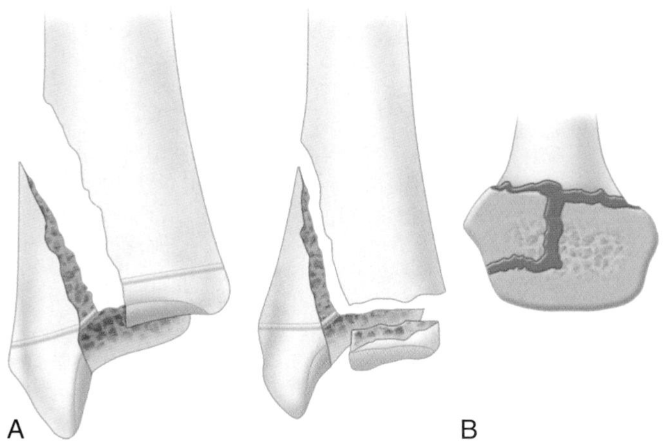

FIGURE 36-181 **A,** Example of two-fragment triplane fracture, which is Salter-Harris type IV fracture. **B,** Example of three-fragment triplane fracture, consisting of Salter-Harris type II and III fractures.

reduction (<2 mm displacement) is not achieved, degenerative changes are likely to occur. If it is a three-part fracture, open reduction of the Salter-Harris type II and type III components may be necessary and adequate exposure is required. Triplane fractures frequently occur in older children, and although physeal arrest and angular deformity can occur, they are rare.

The operative technique for triplane fractures depends on whether it is a two-part or a three-part fracture. Most two-fragment triplane fractures can be treated by closed reduction. The closed reduction should be satisfactory because this is a Salter-Harris type IV fracture with possible joint incongruity and physeal arrest. When an open reduction of this intraarticular fracture is necessary, it usually is a three-part fracture. We approach the Salter-Harris type III component laterally first. If adequate open reduction can be achieved, the Salter-Harris type II component (medially) can be treated closed; if not, both components require open reduction. The trend has been for limited incisions and cannulated screw fixation of intraarticular fragments.

TILLAUX FRACTURES

A special fracture occurring in older adolescents originally was described by Tillaux. The mechanism of injury is an external rotational force with stress placed on the anterior tibiofibular ligament, causing avulsion of the distal tibial

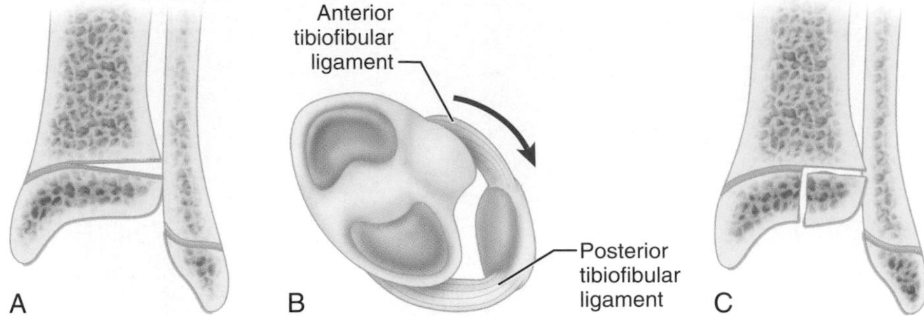

FIGURE 36-182 Mechanism of injury in Tillaux fracture. **A,** Physis in older child closing medially but still open laterally. **B,** External rotational force causes anterior tibiofibular ligament to avulse physis anterolaterally. **C,** Avulsion produces Salter-Harris type III fracture because medial part of physis is closed.

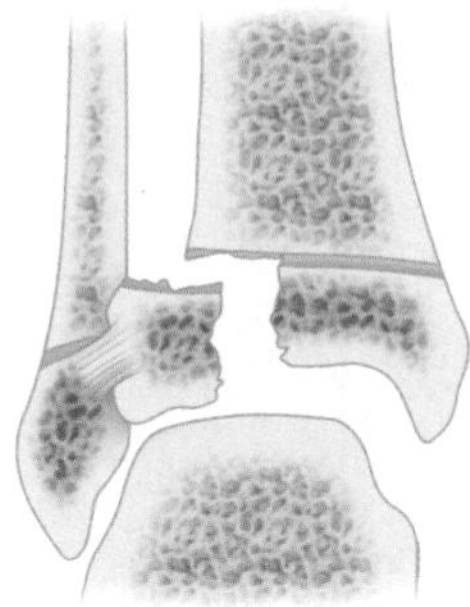

FIGURE 36-183 Tillaux fracture. See Figure 36-198 for mechanism of injury.

physis anterolaterally (Fig. 36-182). This occurs after the medial part of the physis has closed (Fig. 36-183) but before the lateral part closes. The resultant fracture through the physis runs across the epiphysis and distally into the joint, creating a Salter-Harris type III or IV fracture. If nondisplaced, these fractures can be treated conservatively with close observation to ensure a nonunion or delayed union does not occur. If there is any doubt, however, a CT is recommended to evaluate the extent of articular displacement. ORIF is indicated if the fracture is displaced (Fig. 36-184). Fracture displacement of more than 2 mm generally is considered an indication for fracture reduction and fixation.

The fracture fragment, because it is pulled off by the anterior tibiofibular ligament, is almost always anterior. Generally, Tillaux fractures occur in adolescents just before the entire physis (not just the medial part) closes, and there is little worry about using fixation across the physis as in Figure 36-185. If the child is young or there is any doubt, either smooth pins or a transverse screw across the epiphysis should be used as in see Figure 36-179.

OPEN REDUCTION AND INTERNAL FIXATION

TECHNIQUE 36-41

- Expose the type III or IV fracture anterolaterally through a 3-cm anterolateral incision.
- Gently clean and observe the fracture fragments. Take care not to disrupt the periosteum but to remove it from within the fracture.
- Use a bone holder to reduce the fracture gently. Check the reduction by examining the fragment in the ankle joint.
- Insert a small cancellous screw transversely or obliquely across the fracture but not penetrating the physis in a young child.
- Check the reduction with radiographs.
- Close the wound and apply a short leg cast.

POSTOPERATIVE CARE. Weight bearing is prohibited for 3 to 4 weeks.

FOOT AND ANKLE FRACTURES

TALAR FRACTURES

TALAR NECK FRACTURES

Fractures of the talus have three basic types: (1) fractures of the talar neck, (2) fractures of the talar body and dome, and (3) transchondral (osteochondral) fractures.

Be aware of the retrograde blood supply, which is present in a sling fashion around the talar head and neck. This blood supply enters the bone through three primary arteries: (1) artery of the tarsal sinus, (2) artery of the tarsal canal, and (3) the deltoid artery. We use the fracture classification proposed by Hawkins, which is based on the amount of disruption of the blood supply to the talus. A type I lesion is a fracture through the neck of the talus with minimal displacement and minimal damage to the blood supply of the talus, theoretically damaging only one vessel, the one entering through the talar neck. In type II lesions, the subtalar joint is subluxated or dislocated and at least two of the three sources of blood supply may be disrupted through the talar neck and entering the tarsal canal and sinus tarsi. In type III lesions, the body of the talus is dislocated from the tibia and from the calcaneus and all three of the sources of blood supply may be disrupted. The incidence of osteonecrosis is high in type III fractures.

We have described a type IV fracture that is not related to the blood supply, in which the body of the talus is dislocated or subluxated at the subtalar joint, the body of the talus

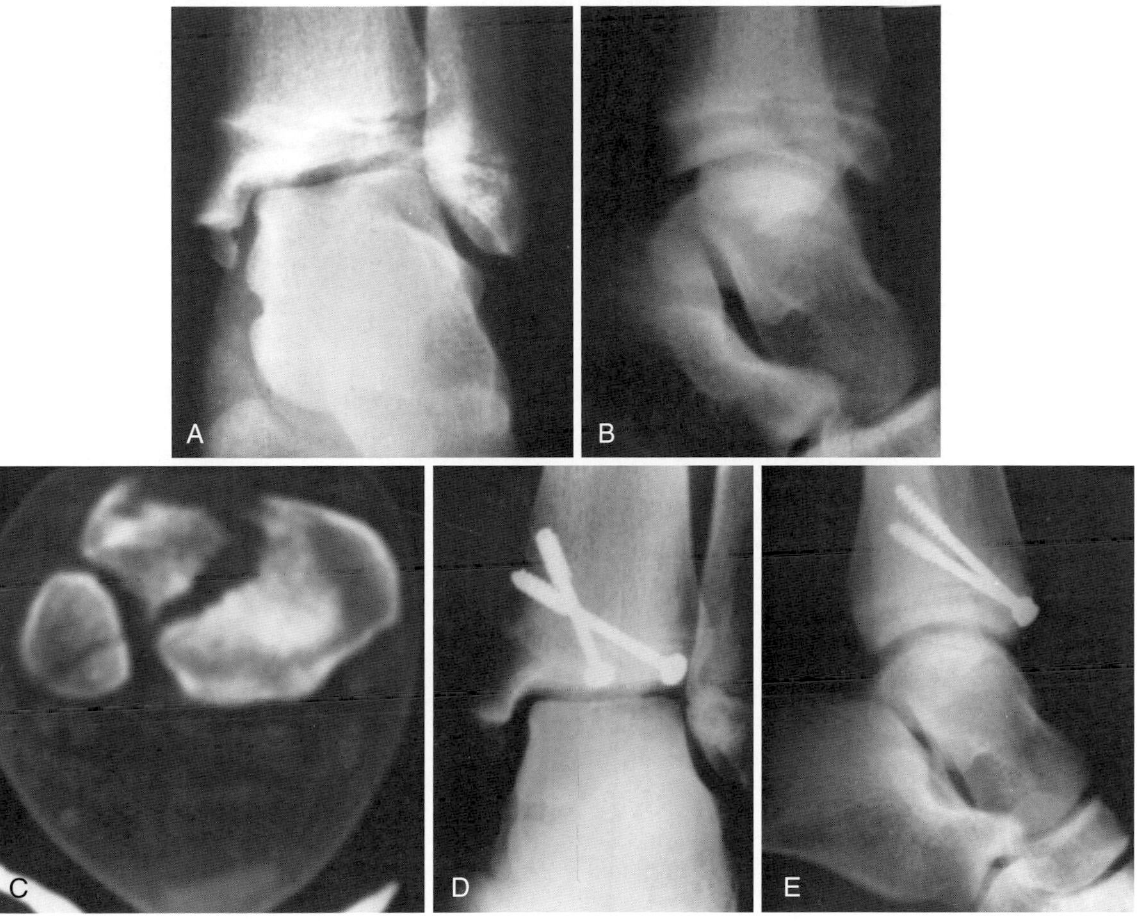

FIGURE 36-184 Tillaux fracture. **A** and **B,** Seemingly undisplaced Tillaux type of Salter-Harris type III fracture. **C,** CT scan revealing significant displacement. **D** and **E,** After satisfactory open reduction and internal fixation.

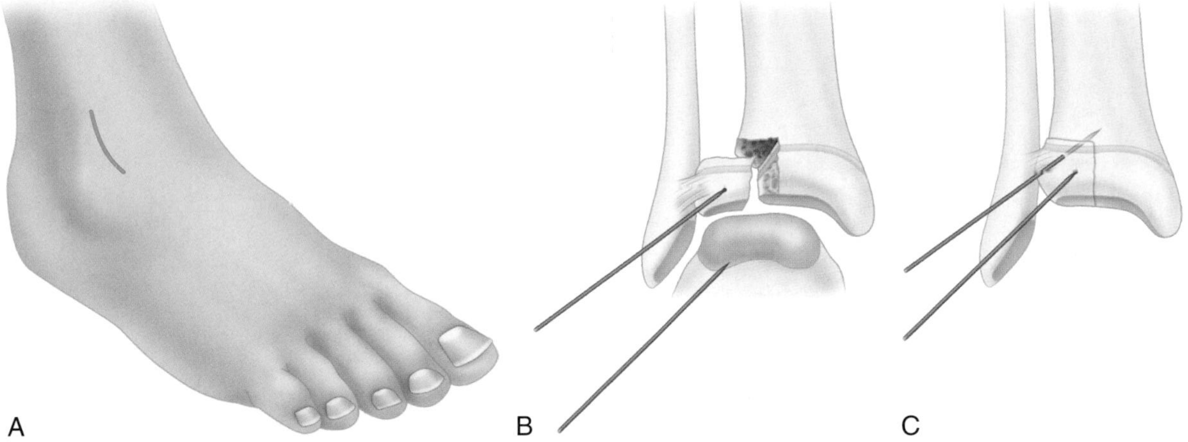

FIGURE 36-185 Percutaneous reduction and fixation of displaced Tillaux fracture. **A,** Skin incision. **B,** Steinmann pin used to reduce fracture. **C,** While fracture is held reduced with Steinmann pin, Kirschner wire is inserted in fragment and across fracture.

is dislocated at the ankle joint, the talar neck is fractured, and the head of the talus is dislocated at the talonavicular joint. Most of the fractures in our series were types I, II, or III.

We use the treatment recommended by Boyd and Knight. Closed reduction followed by non–weight bearing is the preferred treatment for type I mildly or nondisplaced fractures. If an adequate reduction cannot be obtained or maintained, ORIF is recommended. A reduction of less than 3 mm of displacement and less than 5 degrees of malalignment is considered adequate. Most of the closed reductions are done on type I fractures. In type II, III, and IV fractures, open reduction with or without internal fixation is used frequently because of the difficulty of maintaining an adequate reduction by closed methods in significantly displaced fractures. Open fractures require a thorough irrigation and debridement, and internal fixation is done only if required for stability of reduction. If the soft-tissue envelope is compromised, temporary stabilization may be achieved with a spanning external fixator until definitive fixation can be performed.

Varus malalignment is a frequent problem. A special radiographic technique is used to determine the amount of varus angulation in the anteroposterior plane. A cassette is placed directly under the foot, and the ankle is placed in maximal equinus position, the usual position after reduction of the fracture of the talar neck. This position can be maintained more easily by maximal flexion of the hip and knee. The foot is pronated 15 degrees, and the x-ray tube is directed cephalad at a 75-degree angle from the horizontal tabletop. This technique has enabled us to detect any offset or varus deformity of the head and neck of the talus.

For open reduction, an anteromedial approach is often used, retracting the neurovascular bundle laterally. Alternatively, a dual approach can be performed. Fixation is usually performed with cannulated screws from a medial to a lateral direction or small modular plates. As an alternative, cancellous lag screws can be inserted percutaneously from posterior to anterior. Techniques for talar fracture fixation are discussed further in Chapter 88.

Complications include osteonecrosis of the talar body, malunion, traumatic arthritis of the ankle and subtalar joint, and infection. Subchondral lucency present 12 weeks after injury (Hawkins line) is an indication that osteonecrosis will not occur, but this is not an absolute prognosticator. Conversely, lack of a subchondral lucency at 3 months suggests that osteonecrosis has occurred (Fig. 36-186), and advanced imaging with MRI or bone scan may confirm the diagnosis (Fig. 36-187).

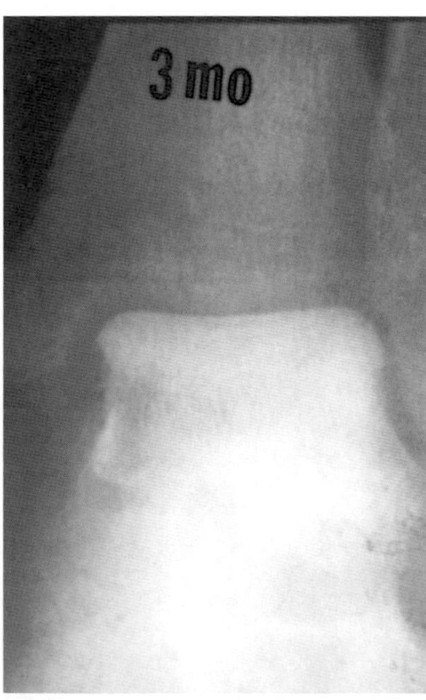

FIGURE 36-186 Hawkins line is not visible in sclerotic (latent osteonecrosis) talar dome 3 months after injury.

We evaluated a series of pediatric and adult patients for a Hawkins line to determine early if osteonecrosis was present. Osteonecrosis did not occur in any patient in whom a Hawkins line was present. A large percentage of patients in whom a Hawkins line was absent at 12 weeks developed osteonecrosis. A few patients who were immobilized for only a short time did not have a Hawkins line, however, and did not develop osteonecrosis. Not all the patients who developed osteonecrosis required operative treatment. Some did satisfactorily with patellar tendon-bearing braces. Of the 12 children, osteonecrosis developed in five, and all five healed uneventfully. The osteonecrosis process in these children was different from that in adults. They developed a sclerotic lesion in the dome and body of the talus that became a cystic lesion on radiographs; over a 2-year to 3-year period, the area resolved and all but one at long-term follow-up were asymptomatic (Fig. 36-188). Most children with osteonecrosis do not require surgery, and consequently, a prolonged period of non–weight bearing or the use of a patellar tendon-bearing, weight-relieving brace should be tried before surgery is considered. According to several reports, children younger than 12 years of age have better results and osteonecrosis has a more favorable outcome than in older children.

Malunions of talar fractures were frequent in adults; however, only 2 of the 12 children reviewed in our series had malunion. Malunion usually occurs with the distal fragment dorsiflexed or in a varus position and with the fibula rotated more anteriorly than normal. Most of our adult patients bore an excessive amount of weight on the lateral side of the foot, and many developed traumatic arthritis in the ankle and subtalar joint. The only infection in our series occurred after an open talar neck fracture. Because the talus is composed almost entirely of cancellous bone, and because fracture through the neck may seriously disrupt the blood supply, an established osteomyelitis of the talus may be resistant to treatment. Repeated sequestrectomy or attempted excision and drainage of the sinus tract are not indicated in established osteomyelitis of the talus. The results of talectomy without fusion have been poor. The preferred treatment for fractures of the talus complicated by infection is excision of the affected bone followed by arthrodesis, even in children. Operations,

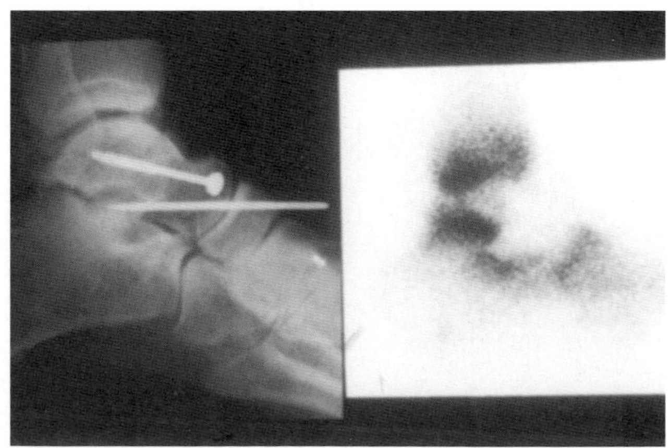

FIGURE 36-187 Bone scan 8 days after open reduction of type IV talar neck fracture with talonavicular dislocation shows decreased uptake indicating area of osteonecrosis.

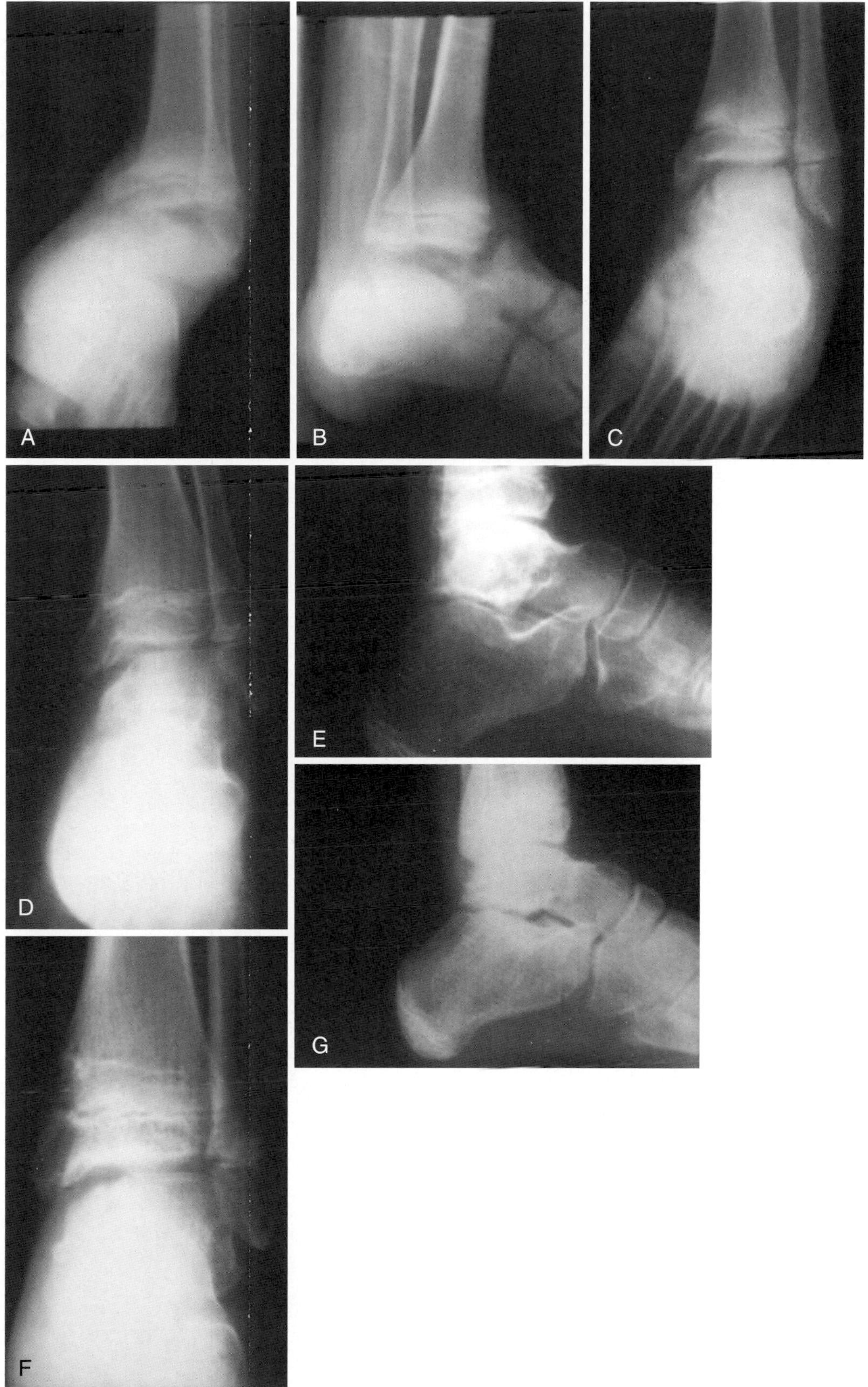

FIGURE 36-188 **A** and **B,** Type III talar neck fracture with posteromedial displacement in 9-year-old child. **C,** After closed reduction and cast immobilization. **D** and **E,** At 9 months after injury, there is evidence of healing but osteonecrosis of talus with sclerotic and cystic changes is evident. **F** and **G,** At 6 years after injury, physes are still open and some healing of osteonecrosis of talus has occurred; patient has no symptoms.

when necessary for osteonecrosis, malunion, or infection, include triple arthrodesis (see Chapter 34), ankle fusion (see Chapter 11), and talocalcaneal fusion (see Chapter 11), all of which produce better results than talectomy alone.

FRACTURES OF THE DOME AND LATERAL PROCESS OF THE TALUS

Fractures of the dome and body of the talus are rare in children but do occur in shearing injuries, especially lawn mower, bicycle spoke, and "degloving" injuries. Often severe, open shearing injuries from lawn mowers and other power equipment require excision of a portion of the talus. The wound should be irrigated, debrided, and left open; delayed closure and skin grafting, if necessary, can be performed later. The primary goal of treatment is to salvage as much length and function of the foot and ankle as possible. A large, nondisplaced, closed talar dome or body fracture can be treated satisfactorily by closed methods, especially in a child, and good results can be expected. If the fracture is significantly displaced, is intraarticular, and has cancellous bone attached to the fragment, ORIF through an anterior approach (see Technique 1-19) usually is necessary. Only rarely is osteotomy of the medial malleolus necessary for exposure. Care should be taken to avoid the physis in this area. Oblique or transverse cancellous screws inserted across the body of the talus, usually without medial malleolar osteotomy, are all that is necessary. Smaller displaced fragments often can be removed and handled in much the same manner as osteochondral fragments. A CT scan may be necessary to make the diagnosis when persistent lateral subtalar pain is present. Nondisplaced fragments can be treated closed. Large displaced fragments may need ORIF, whereas small displaced fragments can be excised to prevent subtalar arthritis (Fig. 36-189).

OSTEOCHONDRAL FRACTURES OF THE TALUS

In our experience, symptoms of osteochondral talar fractures most often begin in the second decade of life, suggesting that this is a lesion of adolescence progressing into early adulthood. We use the classification of Berndt and Harty: stage I, a small area of subchondral compression; stage II, a partially detached fragment; stage III, a completely detached fragment remaining in the crater; and stage IV, a fragment that is detached and loose in the joint (Fig. 36-190). Medial and lateral lesions appear to occur with almost equal frequency, whereas central lesions are rare.

Most lateral lesions are caused by trauma. Morphologically, lateral lesions are thin and wafer shaped and resemble osteochondral fractures. Most medial lesions are deep and morphologically cup shaped, not resembling a traumatic fracture (Fig. 36-191).

Surgery usually is required because of persistent symptoms or a loose body in the ankle joint, most often in lateral stage III or IV lesions. Stage I and II lesions generally can be treated successfully without operation. Nonoperative treatment of stage III medial lesions compares favorably with the results of operative treatment; most are asymptomatic after conservative treatment. Conversely, lateral stage III lesions generally have better results after surgical excision than after conservative treatment. We recommend operative treatment of stage III lateral lesions and all stage IV lesions; all stage I

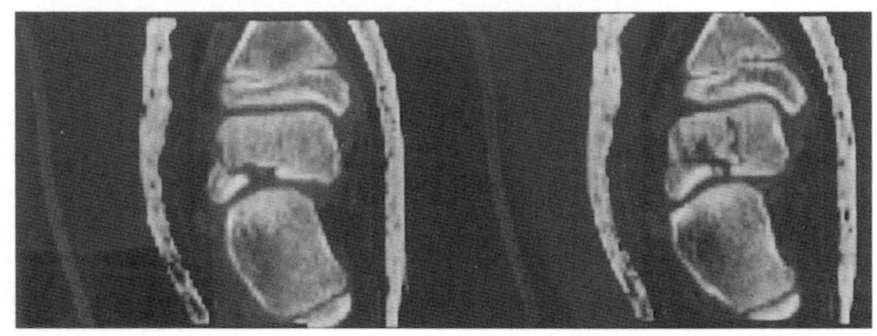

FIGURE 36-189 Coronal CT reconstruction highlighting intraarticular nature of talar lateral process fracture. (From Leibner ED, Simanovsky N, Abu-Sneinah K, et al: Fractures of the lateral process of the talus in children, J Pediatr Orthop 10B:68, 2001.)

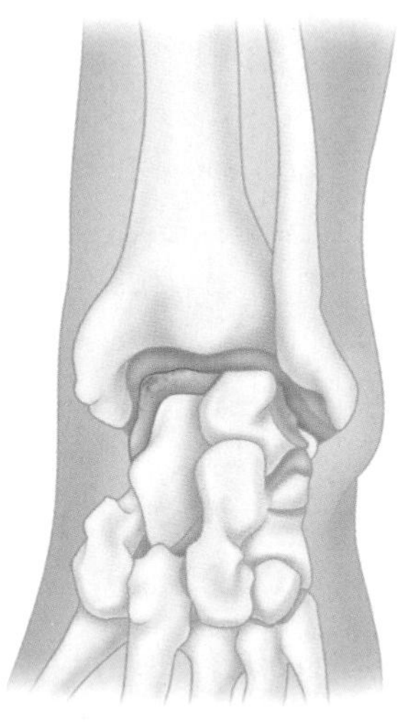

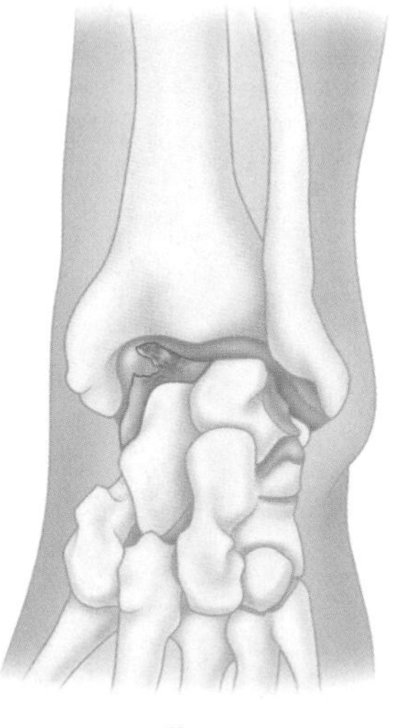

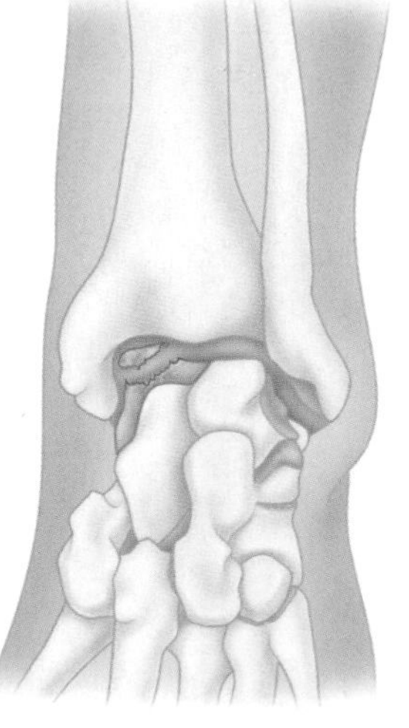

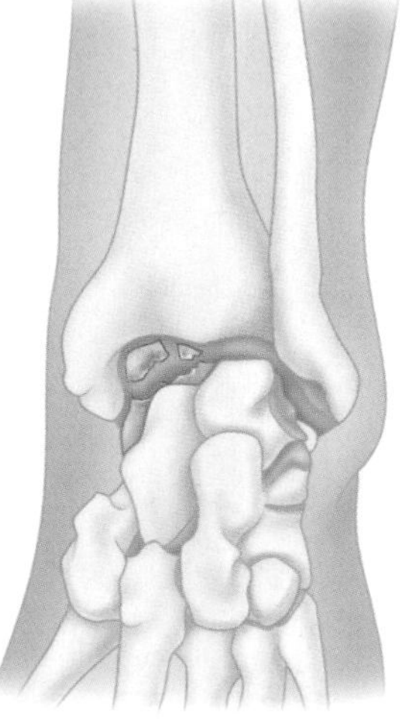

FIGURE 36-190 Four types or stages of osteochondral fractures (osteochondritis dissecans of talus). Stage I, "blister"; stage II, elevated fragment but attached; stage III, fragment detached but still in crater; stage IV, displaced fragment.

and II lesions and stage III medial lesions can be observed for healing, especially in young children and adolescents.

Histologic analysis has shown that, although morphologically the lesions were wafer shaped on the lateral side and cup shaped on the medial side, histologically they were the same. We cannot say definitely that lateral lesions are osteochondral fractures and that medial lesions are true osteochondritis dissecans. In our experience, lateral lesions have more persistent symptoms and degenerative changes than the medial lesions and require surgery more often.

Three technical operative points should be made:

1. If the osteochondral fragment appears on radiographs to be floating in its crater and riding high, with a flake of bone proximally that appears to be in the joint, the fragment probably is inverted in the crater. This means that the subchondral bone is proximal in the ankle joint and the cartilaginous portion is in the crater (Fig. 36-192). In this position, the cartilaginous fragment would not heal to the bone in the crater, and excision is indicated. This elevated, apparently "floating" fragment is pathognomonic of an inverted fragment within the crater.
2. Advanced imaging with CT is helpful in identifying the exact location and extent of the bony lesion and is important for operative planning. (Fig. 36-193).
3. Because the fibula is more posterior than the medial malleolus, osteotomy rarely is needed to reach the lateral lesions. If a CT scan shows the medial lesion to be in the middle or posterior part of the talus, however, a medial malleolar osteotomy often is necessary in skeletally mature patients. We osteotomize the medial malleolus at the plafond horizontally or obliquely. The malleolus should be predrilled to accept a cancellous screw. The malleolar fragment can be displaced with a towel clip, and the lesion is seen quite readily.

We have replaced several large fragments and held them with subchondral pins (Fig. 36-194), similar to the technique

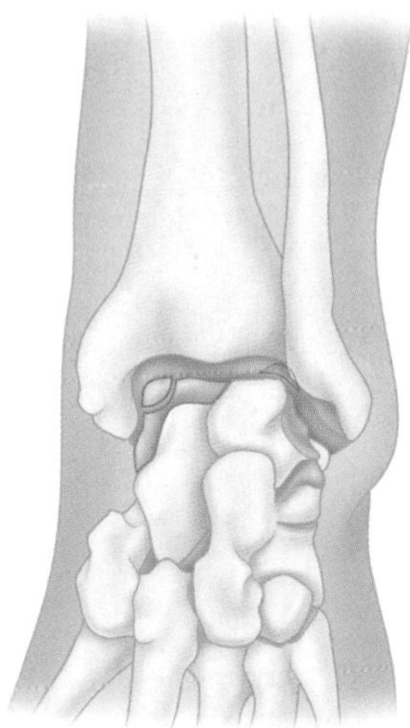

FIGURE 36-191 Morphology of medial and lateral lesions (see text).

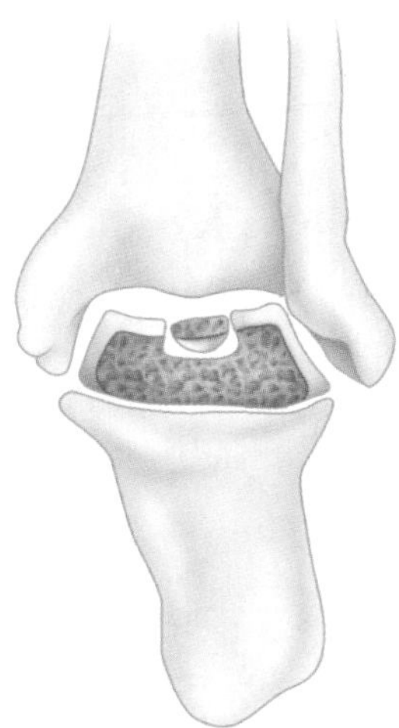

FIGURE 36-192 "Floating" fragment in reality is loose fragment turned upside down in crater.

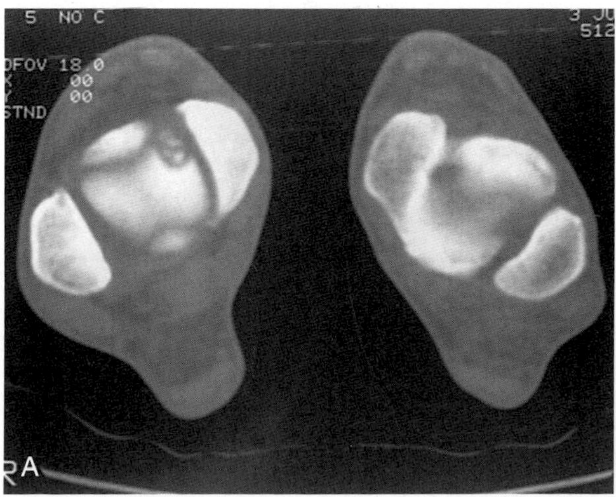

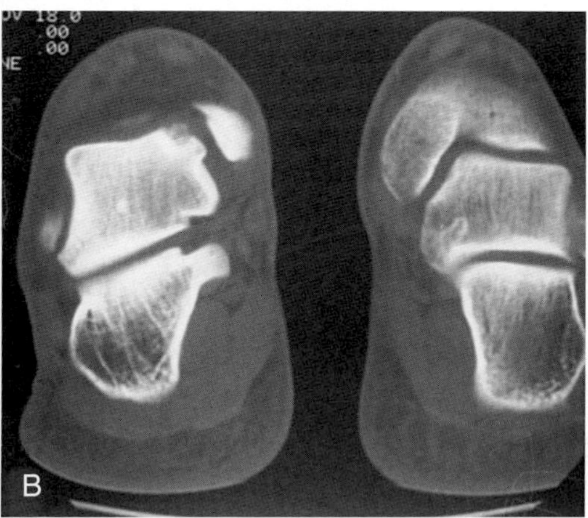

FIGURE 36-193 Osteochondral lesion in anteromedial dome of talus. **A,** CT scan in axial plane shows crater and fragments. **B,** Coronal CT scan locates lesion whether anterior, middle, or posterior, which often is difficult to determine on radiograph.

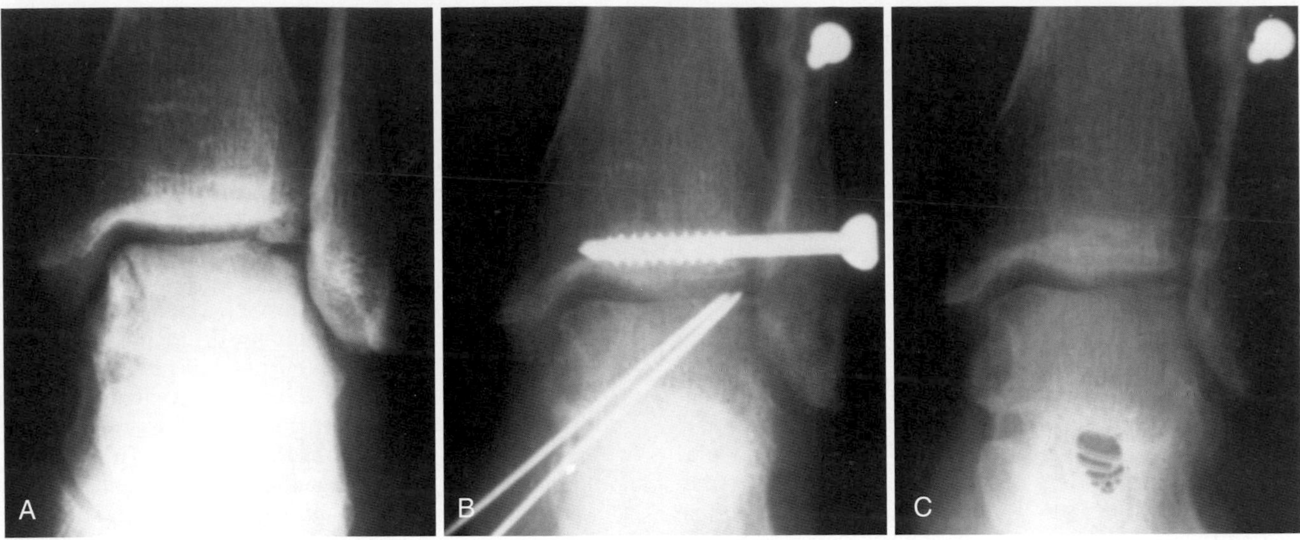

FIGURE 36-194 A, Large osteochondral fragment in lateral talus. B, After retrograde pinning of fragment; osteotomy of lateral malleolus was performed for better exposure. C, Healed lesion after removal of syndesmosis screw.

described for osteochondritis dissecans of the knee (see Chapter 32). The short-term results have been variable.

The lesions in types I, II, and III are often difficult to see at surgery and can only be palpated or "ballotted" to determine their location. Using a Keith needle or a hemostat to "ballotte" helps outline the extent of the lesion. Good results have been reported with arthroscopic excision of osteochondral lesions of the talus, but it is sometimes difficult to find and define the margins of occult lesions. With newer arthroscopy techniques and equipment, posterior and especially posteromedial lesions can be seen more easily. Often, type III lesions, if not completely detached, can be drilled, especially in children. The drilling can be done arthroscopically, percutaneously, or transmalleolarly (through the malleolus). Large fragments can be reattached, and osteochondral grafts can be inserted. Concomitant use of an image intensifier, although complex, may be of benefit. Also, computer-assisted minimally invasive treatment has been described. See the discussion of arthroscopy of the ankle joint in Chapter 50.

EXCISION OF OSTEOCHONDRAL FRAGMENT OF THE TALUS

If osteotomy of the medial malleolus is necessary, surgery on the medial side should be delayed until after closure of the physis.

TECHNIQUE 36-42

- Place the patient supine.
- Make a longitudinal incision 7 cm long over the anteromedial aspect of the ankle. Place the incision far enough medially to allow an osteotomy of the medial malleolus to be made if necessary and to allow inspection of the medial aspect of the joint. Carry the soft-tissue dissection down to the ankle joint; retract the neurovascular bundle, the anterior tibial tendon, and the common extensor tendons. Incise the capsule and expose the ankle joint. Plantarflex the foot as much as possible to try to see the lesion. If the lesion is posterior, an osteotomy usually is necessary.
- Predrill for a cancellous screw from distal to proximal through the medial malleolus into the distal tibia and remove the screw.
- Make an osteotomy obliquely across the medial malleolus at the ankle joint level perpendicular to the predrilled hole for the cancellous screw.
- With a towel clip, turn the medial malleolus distally. Evert the ankle until the medial and posterior aspects of the talar dome can be seen.
- Ballotte for any occult lesion with a Keith needle; with a small curet, remove the central necrotic area and determine the margins of the lesion. The fragment often is loose, and the subchondral bone is yellowish and hard. Remove the crater and the fragment and copiously irrigate the joint.
- With a small drill, make four or five holes in the subchondral crater for vascular ingrowth.
- Realign the medial malleolar osteotomy and insert a cancellous bone screw in the predrilled hole. Take radiographs to check for anatomic alignment of the screw and the osteotomy.
- Close the wound in layers and apply a short leg cast.

POSTOPERATIVE CARE. The patient should wear a cast or patellar tendon-bearing brace for 6 to 8 weeks, preferably non–weight bearing for a total of 8 to 12 weeks, while fibrocartilaginous tissue in the crater fills in the defect.

CALCANEAL FRACTURES

Calcaneal fractures are rare in children. They differ from calcaneal fractures in adults because (1) they occur much less frequently; (2) they do not exhibit the same fracture patterns, having less intraarticular involvement; (3) they are less serious because of the elasticity of structures in children; and (4) they remodel (Fig. 36-195). Schmidt and Weiner reported 62 calcaneal fractures in children, which they classified using a system similar to that of Essex-Lopresti (see Chapter 88). They included physeal fractures at the tuberosity and a fracture almost unique to children that involves the posterior aspect of the calcaneus with significant loss of bone that occurs in lawn mower injuries. Of the fractures, 63% were extraarticular and only 37% were intraarticular, which is the reverse of the adult fracture pattern. Displacement of the intraarticular fractures was minimal compared with adult fractures, and only two required ORIF. In several older children, the subtalar joint was obviously involved and incongruous, however, similar to the Essex-Lopresti type II fracture, with a decreased "crucial" angle and the presence of a joint compression fracture. Open fractures of the calcaneus occur more often in children than in adults, probably because of the increased incidence of lawn mower injuries.

Because displacement is uncommon in extraarticular and intraarticular fractures, most calcaneal fractures in children are expected to heal without any functional loss. The prognosis of calcaneal fractures in children is good unless a lawn mower injury results in loss of bone and soft tissue from the heel.

Harris views (ski-jump views) of the heel should be obtained, and a CT scan can be helpful because the diagnosis can be obscure secondary to minimal disturbance in the bony architecture and the high percentage of cartilage in the calcaneus of children compared with adults. Operative treatment of calcaneal fractures in children is not indicated unless subtalar joint disruption is significant. A CT scan is mandatory in preoperative operative planning. Good clinical outcomes have been reported in patients with displaced intraarticular calcaneal fractures treated with ORIF. Stress fractures of the calcaneus have been reported in children, and a bone scan may be helpful in making the diagnosis. Trott noted that cysts in the triangular space of the calcaneus become large enough for ordinary activities to produce stress or pathologic fractures.

TARSAL FRACTURES

Fractures of the tarsal bones are uncommon in children because of the flexibility of the foot. Fractures, especially of the navicular, cuboid, or cuneiform bones, usually are part of a severe injury to the foot, such as a wringer, severe compression, or lawn mower injury. The second metatarsal has been described as the cornerstone of the foot, and strong ligamentous attachments are present between the metatarsals themselves and between the cuneiforms. The most relevant anatomic features are the fixed mortise position of the base of the second metatarsal and the ligamentous attachments at this base. If there is a fracture of the base of the second metatarsal, with or without a "buckle" fracture of the cuboid, significant tarsometatarsal joint injury, although occult, has occurred. Treatment recommendations include closed reduction for gross displacement or instability, with open reduction only rarely required. Because of inherent instability, however, percutaneous Kirschner wire fixation can be used to maintain the reduction and the alignment after open or closed reduction. The wires are removed after approximately 4 weeks.

In our experience, a persistent dorsal dislocation, even in a child, produces a painful hypertrophic osseous area on the dorsum of the foot. Also, varus angulation often is present. With the patient under general anesthesia, any dislocated tarsometatarsal joints should be reduced. If this cannot be accomplished closed, ORIF of the dislocation is indicated (Fig. 36-196). Care should be taken not to violate the proximal physis of the first metatarsal.

Cuboid "nutcracker" fractures have recently been described in four children, all of whom were injured while horseback riding. The mechanism of injury is forced abduction of the forefoot, usually in combination with an axial force. Compression cuboid fractures rarely are isolated injuries, usually occurring with other midfoot fractures or dislocations. The identification of a cuboid nutcracker fracture on radiograph should prompt CT evaluation to rule out or identify other injuries. Minimally displaced isolated cuboid nutcracker fractures can be treated conservatively, but poor results are common after nonoperative treatment of displaced fractures, and operative treatment is recommended to avoid alterations in foot mechanics and function, leading to foot stiffness and pain.

OPEN REDUCTION AND INTERNAL FIXATION OF CUBOID COMPRESSION (NUTCRACKER) FRACTURE

TECHNIQUE 36-43

(CERONI ET AL.)

- Make a lateral incision along the axis from the tip of the fibula to the tip of the fifth metatarsal.
- Retract the peroneus tendons plantarly and partially elevate the extensor digitorum brevis muscle.
- Elevate the extruded lateral wall of the cuboid and inspect the fracture and adjacent joint.
- Elevate depressed fragments with a laminar spreader until the adjacent joint surfaces are congruent.
- When the shape of the cuboid is restored, fill the large corticocancellous defect with a large allograft bone block to provide stable bony support. Cut the allograft bone block overly large so that it fits into the defect with some resistance.
- This construct is stable enough that no fixation is required.
- Obtain an oblique radiograph to confirm the articular reconstruction and reestablishment of lateral column length.
- Close the wound in layers and apply a short leg cast.

POSTOPERATIVE CARE. The non–weight-bearing cast is worn for 6 weeks, followed by a walking cast for another 6 weeks. Unprotected full weight bearing is allowed at 12 weeks after surgery.

Pediatric Lisfranc fractures often are called "bunk bed" fractures because the injury occurs from a twisting force when the foot is extended, such as when a child jumps from a bunk bed. This fracture of the first tarsometatarsal area produces a subtle deformity that can be overlooked, and the

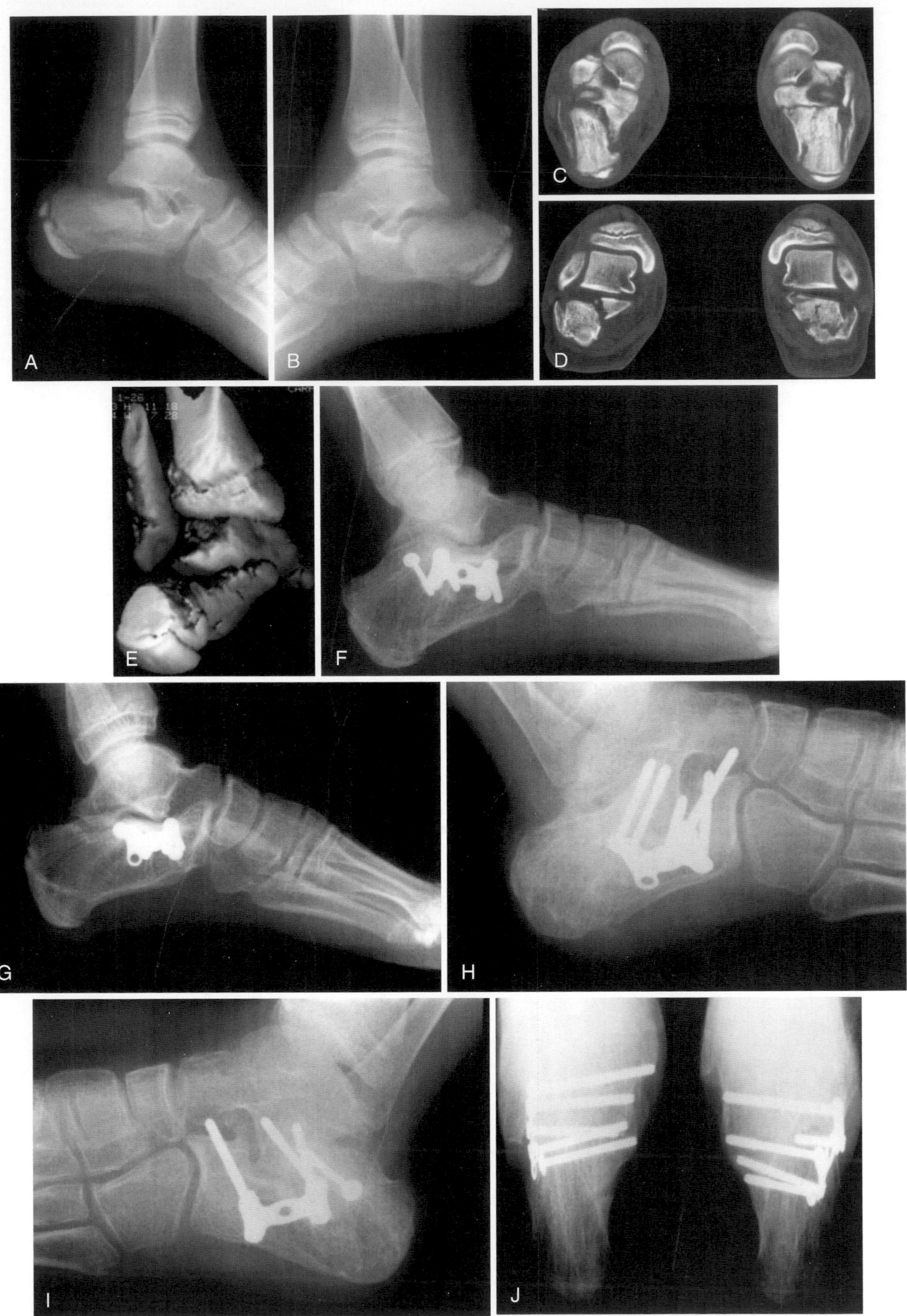

FIGURE 36-195 **A** and **B,** Lateral radiographs of bilateral severe calcaneal fractures with depression of crucial angle in child who also had T12 compression fracture resulting from a fall. **C** and **D,** CT scan at two different levels, revealing severe comminution and displacement. **E,** Three-dimensional reconstruction of lateral calcaneal fractures. **F** and **G,** Lateral radiographs after open reduction and internal fixation with contoured plates and screws. **H** to **J,** Bilateral oblique and anteroposterior radiographs at follow-up.

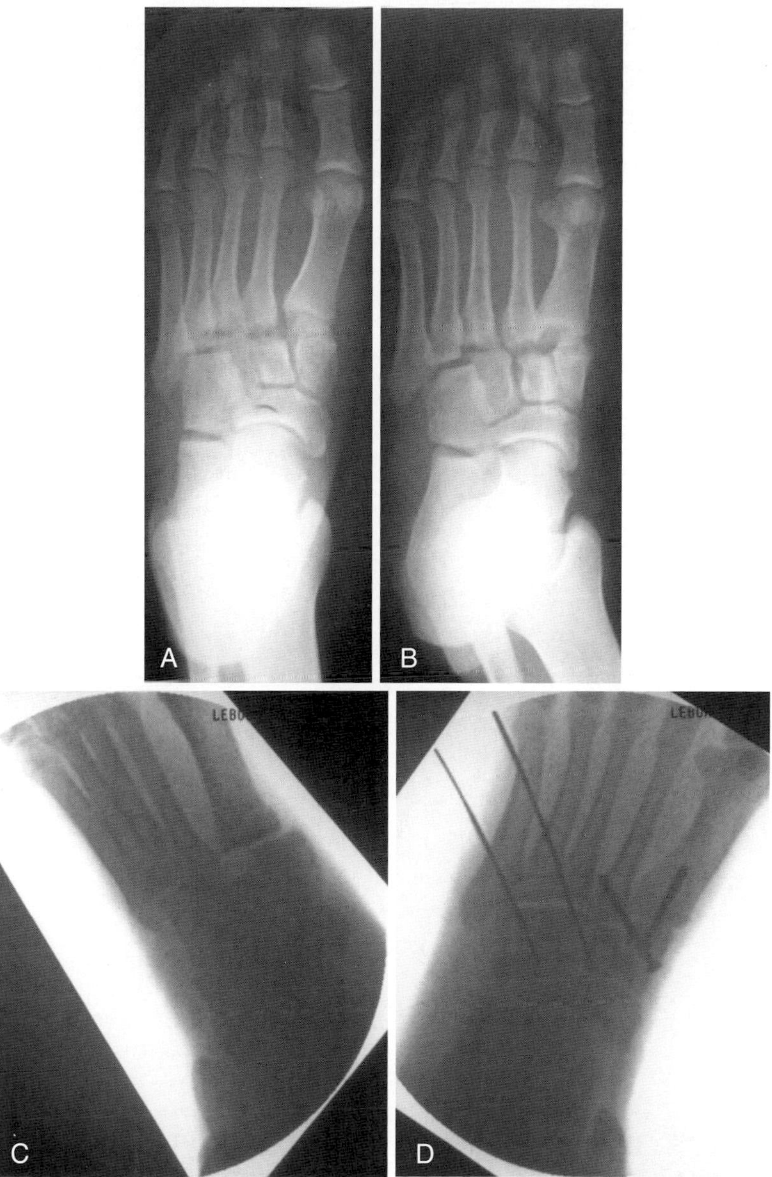

FIGURE 36-196 A, Anteroposterior radiograph appears normal. B, Oblique radiograph reveals subtle subluxation of metatarsocuneiform joint. C, At surgery, image intensification reveals extent of involvement. D, Open and percutaneous reduction and fixation of Lisfranc dislocation. Physis of first metatarsal is closed.

soft-tissue injury is more severe than is indicated by the bony injury seen on the radiographs. Often a fracture-dislocation or a fracture-subluxation of the first tarsometatarsal joint occurs or the first and second metatarsals may be involved (Fig. 36-197).

METATARSAL AND PHALANGEAL FRACTURES

Although metatarsal and phalangeal fractures in children are common, little has been written about these fractures. Perhaps this is because they usually heal uneventfully and rarely need operative treatment. Because of their strong interosseous ligaments, fractures of the proximal metatarsals usually do not become displaced significantly. Displaced fractures usually are produced by severe trauma. In addition to the fractures, the soft tissues usually are damaged considerably and swelling may be excessive. These severe injuries should be treated by elevation and observation and not by a circumferential cast. When the swelling has resolved, a displaced fracture can be reduced closed, if necessary, by longitudinal traction. For severe trauma producing multiple fractures with significant displacement, when the swelling has subsided, open reduction and smooth pin fixation are performed if necessary. This is occasionally needed in the first metatarsal of older children, where little remodeling can be expected (Fig. 36-198). Most displaced fractures of the metatarsal neck heal and usually remodel nicely in young children; however, if displacement and deformity are significant, especially in the anteroposterior plane, and multiple neck fractures are present, occasionally ORIF with longitudinal wires is necessary, especially in older children.

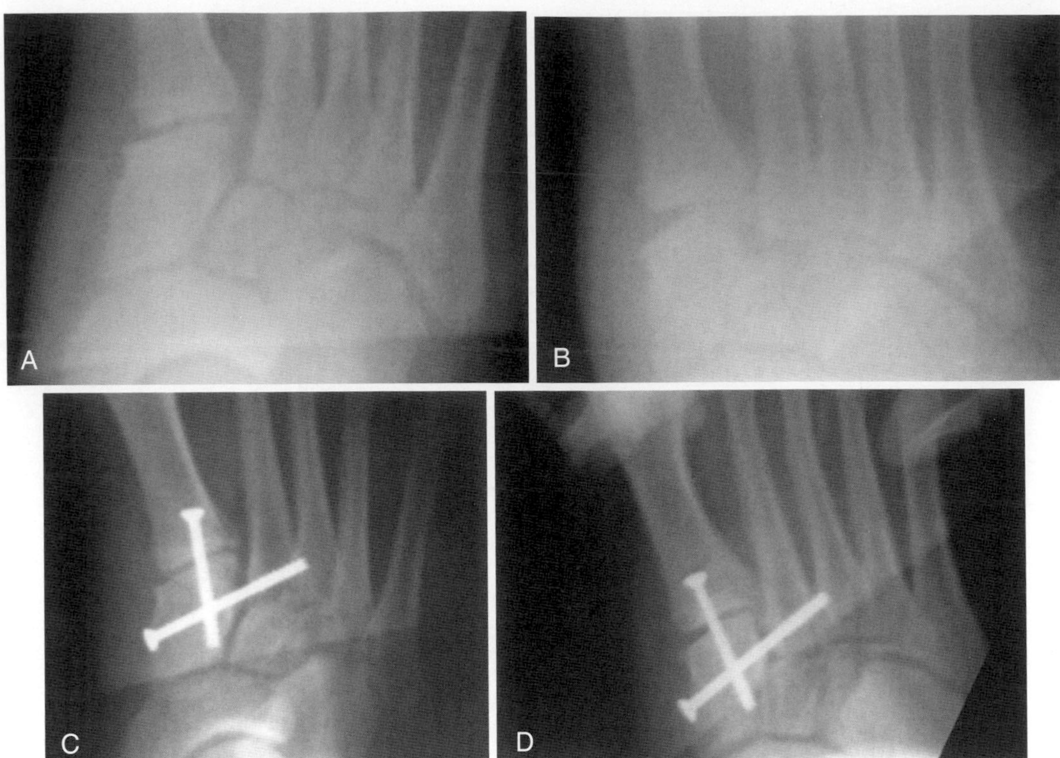

FIGURE 36-197 Anteroposterior and stress radiographs of foot with subtle Lisfranc dislocation. **A,** Radiograph appears normal. **B,** With stress into everted position, metatarsals sublux laterally. **C,** Postreduction radiograph reveals satisfactory reduction and internal fixation. **D,** Reduction maintained on eversion stress radiograph.

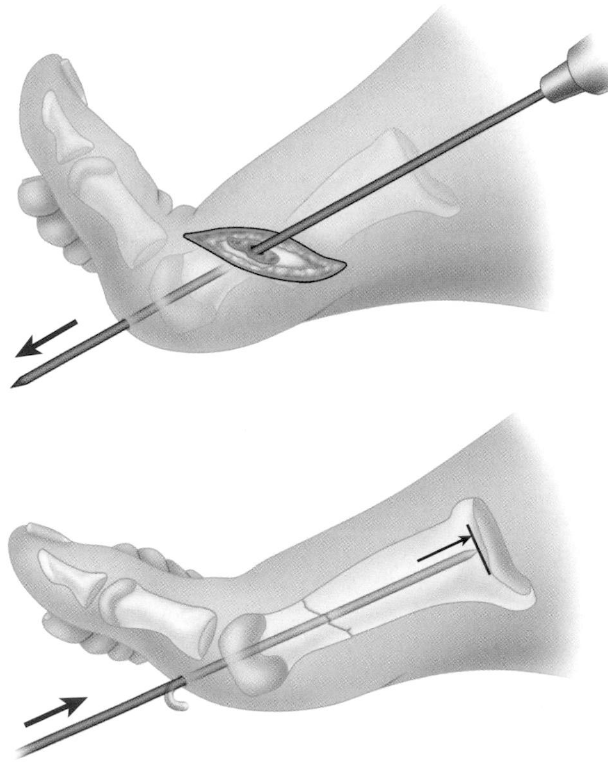

FIGURE 36-198 Method of open pinning of metatarsal shaft or neck fractures in retrograde fashion through first metatarsal head.

Stress fractures of the metatarsal shaft or neck occur in children. MRI may be helpful in diagnosis, and these fractures should be treated expectantly. We have seen a 10-year-old child with a metatarsal stress fracture, and although these fractures occur less frequently in children than in adults, they can be produced by chronic repetitive, stressful activity. Nonoperative treatment is usually appropriate combined with vitamin D supplementation. Fractures of the base of the fifth metatarsal in children and adults traditionally have been called Jones fractures, although Jones' original description from 1896 appears to be that of a diaphyseal fracture rather than an avulsion fracture of the base of the fifth metatarsal caused by overpull of the peroneus brevis muscle. Several studies have noted the uncertainty of healing of this diaphyseal fracture and recommended ORIF with a medullary screw in high-performance athletes, recreational athletes, and nonathletes with delayed union. A more recent study also suggested that fixation of Jones fractures in active adolescents should be considered to allow faster return to regular activities and prevent refracture. Avulsions of the most proximal base of the fifth metatarsal also occur in children and heal uneventfully except for some bony hypertrophy at the fracture site. This injury should be differentiated from a secondary ossification center seen on oblique views in a 10- to 13-year-old child that when painful is termed *Iselin disease* (see Chapter 32).

Fractures of the phalanges are caused primarily by hitting a hard object or compressing the toe with a heavy weight. Open fractures of the great toe distal phalanx (stubbed toe) can be worrisome. Dislocations of the phalanges usually are

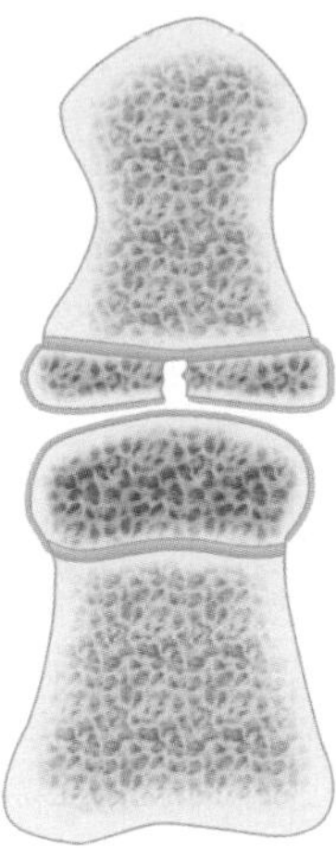

FIGURE 36-199 Fissuring (not fracture) of physis of proximal phalanx of great toe.

dorsal and can be reduced easily. Certain developmental disorders of the phalanges should not be confused with fractures. Fragmentation of the proximal epiphysis of the hallux occurs frequently (Fig. 36-199). The epiphysis may be fissured, compressed, or fragmented. Usually the physis is not fractured.

Fractures and dislocations of the phalanges should be reduced by longitudinal traction and held by "buddy" taping to the next toe. ORIF is only rarely indicated. If fracture of a phalanx is caused by a penetrating wound, as in stepping on a nail, *Pseudomonas* infection should be suspected. If the wound becomes infected, it should be irrigated and debrided and intravenous antibiotic therapy should be administered. For infected phalangeal fractures, debridement, wet dressing, intravenous administration of antibiotics, and delayed closure save some toes, especially the great toe, when impending infection or gangrene has suggested amputation. Severe open fractures occur in the forefoot and the phalanges, primarily in bicycle spoke or rotary lawn mower injuries. Treatment consists of adequate debridement of the wounds, leaving the wounds open, and delayed closure. The operative treatment of these injuries is similar to that for the digits of adults (see Chapter 88).

REFERENCES

GROWTH INJURIES, BIRTH INJURIES, AND NONACCIDENTAL TRAUMA

Anton C, Podberesky DJ: Little League shoulder: a growth plate injury, *Pediatr Radiol* 40(Suppl 1):S54, 2010.

Arkader A, Warner WC Jr, Horn BD, et al: Predicting the outcome of physeal fractures of the distal femur, *J Pediatr Orthop* 27:703, 2007.

Baldwin K, Pandya NK, Wolfgruber H, et al: Femur fractures in the pediatric population: abuse or accidental trauma? *Clin Orthop Relat Res* 469:798, 2011.

Baldwin KD, Scherl SA: Orthopaedic aspects of child abuse, *Instr Course Lect* 62:399, 2013.

Banerjee J, Asamoah FK, Singhvi D, et al: Haemoglobin level at birth is associated with short term outcomes and mortality in preterm infants, *BMC Med* 13:16, 2015.

Basha A, Amarin Z, Abu-Hassan F: Birth-associated long-bone fractures, *Int J Gynaecol Obstet* 123:127, 2013.

Clarke NM, Shelton FR, Taylor CC, et al: The incidence of fractures in children under the age of 24 months – in relation to non-accidental injury, *Injury* 43:762, 2012.

Duffy SO, Squires J, Fromkin JB, Berger RP: Use of skeletal surveys to evaluate for physical abuse: analysis of 703 consecutive skeletal surveys, *Pediatrics* 127:347, 2011.

Garrett BR, Hoffman EB, Carrara H: The effect of percutaneous pin fixation in the treatment of distal femoral physeal fractures, *J Bone Joint Surg* 93:689, 2011.

Gilbert SR, Conklin MJ: Presentation of distal humerus physeal separation, *Pediatr Emerg Care* 23:816, 2007.

Gkiokas A, Brilakis E: Spontaneous correction of partial physeal arrest: report of a case and review of the literature, *J Pediatr Orthop B* 21:369, 2012.

Harlan SR, Nixon GW, Campbell KA, et al: Follow-up skeletal surveys for nonaccidental trauma: can a more limited survey be performed? *Pediatr Radiol* 39:962, 2009.

Havranek P, Pesl T: Salter (Rang) type 6 physeal injury, *Eur J Pediatr Surg* 20:174, 2010.

Jayakumar P, Barry M, Ramachandran M: Orthopaedic aspects of paediatric non-accidental injury, *J Bone Joint Surg* 92B:189, 2010.

Jha P, Stein-Wexler R, Coulter K, et al: Optimizing bone surveys performed for suspected non-accidental trauma with attention to maximizing diagnostic yield while minimizing radiation exposure: utility of pelvic and lateral radiographs, *Pediatr Radiol* 43:668, 2013.

Kamaci S, Danisman M, Marangoz S: Neonatal physeal separation of distal humerus during cesarean section, *Am J Orthop* 43:E279, 2014.

Kang HG, Yoon SJ, Kim JR: Resection of a physeal bar under computer-assisted guidance, *J Bone Joint Surg* 92:1452, 2010.

Kaplan KM, Gruson KI, Paksima N: Bilateral humerus and corner fractures in an 18-month-old infant: a case report and review of child abuse from the resident perspective, *Bull NYU Hosp Jt Dis* 66:124, 2008.

Karmazyn B, Lewis ME, Jennings SG, et al: The prevalence of uncommon fractures on skeletal surveys performed to evaluate for suspected abuse in 930 children: should practice guidelines change? *AJR Am J Roentgenol* 197:W159, 2011.

Kemp AM, Dunstan F, Harrison S, et al: Patterns of skeletal fractures in child abuse: systematic review, *BMJ* 337:a1518, 2008.

Linder N, Linder I, Friedman E, et al: Birth trauma—risk factors and short-term neonatal outcome, *J Matern Fetal Neonatal Med* 26:1491, 2013.

Loder RT, Feinberg JR: Orthopaedic injuries in children with nonaccidental trauma: demographics and incidence from the 2000 KIDS inpatient database, *J Pediatr Orthop* 27:421, 2007.

Loraas EK, Schmale GA: Endoscopically aided physeal bar takedown and guided growth for the treatment of angular limb deformity, *J Pediatr Orthop B* 21:348, 2012.

Luri B, Koff MF, Shah P, et al: Three-dimensional magnetic resonance imaging of physeal injury: reliability and clinical utility, *J Pediatr Orthop* 34:239, 2014.

Marine MB, Corea D, Steenburg SD, et al: Is the new ACR-SPR practice guideline for addition of oblique views of the ribs to the skeletal survey for child abuse justified? *AJR Am J Roentgenol* 202:868, 2014.

Marsh JS, Polzhofer GK: Arthroscopically assisted central physeal bar resection, *J Pediatr Orthop* 26:255, 2006.

Mulpuri K, Slobogean BL, Tredwell SJ: The epidemiology of nonaccidental trauma in children, *Clin Orthop Relat Res* 469:759, 2011.

Murphy R, Kelly DM, Moisan A, Thompson NB: Transverse fractures of the femoral shaft are a better predictor of nonaccidental trauma in young children than spiral fractures are, *J Bone Joint Surg* 97A:106, 2015.

Pandya NK, Baldwin K, Kamath AF, et al: Unexplained fractures: child abuse or bone disease? A systematic review, *Clin Orthop Relat Res* 469:805, 2011.

Pandya NK, Baldwin KD, Wolfgruber H, et al: Humerus fractures in the pediatric population: an algorithm to identify abuse, *J Pediatr Orthop B* 19:535, 2010.

Pandya NK, Baldwin K, Wolfgruber H, et al: Child abuse and orthopaedic injury patterns: analysis at a level I pediatric trauma center, *J Pediatr Orthop* 29:618, 2009.

Prosser I, Lawson Z, Evans A, et al: A timetable for the radiologic features of fracture healing in young children, *AJR Am J Roentgenol* 198:1014, 2012.

Ravichandiran N, Schuh S, Bejuk M, et al: Delayed identification of pediatric abuse-related fractures, *Pediatrics* 125:60, 2010.

Sink EL, Hyman JE, Matheny T, et al: Child abuse: the role of the orthopaedic surgeon in nonaccidental trauma, *Clin Orthop Relat Res* 469:790, 2011.

Sonik A, Stein-Wexler R, Rogers KK, et al: Follow-up skeletal surveys for suspected non-accidental trauma: can a more limited survey be performed without compromising diagnostic information? *Child Abuse Negl* 34:804, 2010.

Wood JN, Fakeye O, Feudtner C, et al: Development of guidelines for skeletal survey in young children with fractures, *Pediatrics* 134:45, 2014.

Wood JN, Fakeye O, Mondestin V, et al: Development of hospital-based guidelines for skeletal survey in young children with bruises, *Pediatrics* 135:e312, 2015.

OPEN AND PATHOLOGIC FRACTURES

Bazzi AA, Brooks JT, Jain A, et al: Is nonoperative treatment of pediatric type I open fractures safe and effective? *J Child Orthop* 8:467, 2014.

Ibrahim T, Riaz M, Hegazy A, et al: Delayed surgical debridement in pediatric open fractures: a systematic review and meta-analysis, *J Child Orthop* 8:135, 2014.

Iobst CA, Spurdle C, Baitner AC, et al: A protocol for the management of pediatric type I open fractures, *J Child Orthop* 8:71, 2014.

Rapp M, Svoboda D, Wessel LM, Kaiser MM: Elastic stable intramedullary nailing (ESIN), Orthoss® and Gravitational Platelet Separation—System (GPS®): an effective method of treatment for pathologic fractures of bone cysts in children, *BMC Musculoskelet Disord* 12:45, 2011.

Wetzel RJ, Minhas SV, Patrick BC, Janicki JA: Current practice in the management of type I open fractures in children: a survey of POSNA membership, *J Pediatr Orthop* 35:762, 2015.

FRACTURES AND DISLOCATIONS INVOLVING THE CLAVICLE, PROXIMAL END OF THE HUMERUS, AND SHOULDER

Bae DS, Kocher MS, Waters PM, et al: Chronic recurrent anterior sternoclavicular joint instability: results of surgical management, *J Pediatr Orthop* 26:71, 2006.

Bae DS, Shah AS, Kalish LA, et al: Shoulder motion, strength, and functional outcomes in children with established malunion of the clavicle, *J Pediatr Orthop* 33:544, 2013.

Bahrs C, Zipplies S, Ochs BG, et al: Proximal humeral fractures in children and adolescents, *J Pediatr Orthop* 29:238, 2009.

Canavese F, Athlani L, Marengo L, et al: Evaluation of upper-extremity function following surgical treatment of displaced proximal humerus fractures in children, *J Pediatr Orthop B* 23:144, 2014.

Carry PM, Koonce R, Pan Z, Polousky JD: A survey of physician opinion: adolescent midshaft clavicle fracture treatment preferences among POSNA members, *J Pediatr Orthop* 31:44, 2011.

Chaus GW, Carry PM, Pishkenari AK, Hadley-Miller N: Operative versus nonoperative treatment of displaced proximal humeral physeal fractures: a matched cohort, *J Pediatr Orthop* 35:234, 2015.

Chee Y, Agorastides I, Garg N, et al: Treatment of severely displaced proximal humeral fractures in children with elastic stable intramedullary nailing, *J Pediatr Orthop B* 15:45, 2006.

Cordischi K, Li X, Busconi B: Intermediate outcomes after primary traumatic anterior shoulder dislocation in skeletally immature patients aged 10 to 13 years, *Orthopedics* 32:2009.

Fernandez FF, Eberhardt O, Langendörfer M, Wirth T: Treatment of severely displaced proximal humeral fractures in children with retrograde elastic stable intramedullary nailing, *Injury* 39:1453, 2008.

Goldfarb CA, Bassett GS, Sullivan S, et al: Retrosternal displacement after physeal fracture of the medial clavicle in children: treatment by open reduction and internal fixation, *J Bone Joint Surg* 83B:1168, 2001.

Hong S, Nho JH, Lee CJ, et al: Posterior shoulder dislocation with ipsilateral proximal humerus type 2 physeal fracture: case report, *J Pediatr Orthop B* 24:215, 2015.

Hutchinson PH, Bae DS, Waters PM: Intramedullary nailing versus percutaneous pin fixation of pediatric proximal humerus fractures: a comparison of complications and early radiographic results, *J Pediatr Orthop* 31:617, 2011.

Khan A, Athlani L, Rousset M, et al: Functional results of displaced proximal humerus fractures in children treated by elastic stable intramedullary nail, *Eur J Orthop Surg Traumatol* 24:164, 2014.

Mehlman CT, Yihua G, Bochang C, Zhigang W: Operative treatment of completely displaced clavicle shaft fractures in children, *J Pediatr Orthop* 29:951, 2009.

Namdari S, Ganley TJ, Baldwin K, et al: Fixation of displaced midshaft clavicle fractures in skeletally immature patients, *J Pediatr Orthop* 31:507, 2011.

Nenopoulous SP, Gigis IP, Chytas AA, et al: Outcome of distal clavicular fracture separations and dislocations in immature skeleton, *Injury* 42:376, 2011.

Pahlavan S, Bladwin KD, Pandya NK, et al: Proximal humerus fractures in the pediatric population: a systematic review, *J Child Orthop* 5:187, 2011.

Pandya NK, Behrends D, Hosalkar HS: Open reduction of proximal humerus fractures in the adolescent population, *J Child Orthop* 6:111, 2012.

Popkin CA, Levine WN, Ahmad CS: Evaluation and management of pediatric proximal humerus fractures, *J Am Acad Orthop Surg* 23:77, 2015.

Rajan RA, Hawkins MJ, Metcalfe J, et al: Elastic stable intramedullary nailing for displaced proximal humeral fractures in older children, *J Child Orthop* 2:15, 2008.

Randsborg PH, Fuglesang HF, Røtterfud JH, et al: Long-term patient-reported outcome after fractures of the clavicle in patients aged 10 to 18 years, *J Pediatr Orthop* 34:393, 2014.

Schulz J, Moor M, Roocroft J, et al: Functional and radiographic outcomes of nonoperative treatment of displaced adolescent clavicle fractures, *J Bone Joint Surg* 95A:1159, 2013.

Sykes JA, Ezetendu C, Sivitz A, et al: Posterior dislocation of sternoclavicular joint encroaching on ipsilateral vessels in 2 pediatric patients, *Pediatr Emerg Care* 27:327, 2011.

Tennent TD, Pearse EO, Eastwood DM: A new technique for stabilizing adolescent posteriorly displaced physeal medial clavicular fractures, *J Shoulder Elbow Surg* 21:1734, 2012.

Tepolt F, Carry PM, Taylor M, Hadley-Miller N: Posterior sternoclavicular joint injuries in skeletally immature patients, *Orthopedics* 37:e174, 2014.

Tepolt F, Carry PM, Heyn PC, Miller NH: Posterior sternoclavicular joint injuries in the adolescent population: a meta-analysis, *Am J Sports Med* 42:2517, 2014.

Ting BL, Bae DS, Waters PM: Chronic posterior sternoclavicular joint fracture dislocations in children and young adults: results of surgical management, *J Pediatr Orthop* 34:542, 2014.

Van Tassel D, Owens BD, Pointer L, Moriatis Wolf J: Incidence of clavicle fractures in sports: analysis of the NEISS Database, *Int J Sports Med* 35:83, 2014.

Vander Have KL, Perdue AM, Caird MS, Farley FA: Operative versus nonoperative treatment of midshaft clavicle fractures in adolescents, *J Pediatr Orthop* 30:307, 2010.

Xie F, Wang S, Jiao Q, et al: Minimally invasive treatment for severely displaced proximal humeral fractures in children using titanium elastic nails, *J Pediatr Orthop* 31:839, 2011.

SUPRACONDYLAR FRACTURES

Abbott MD, Buchler L, Loder RT, Caltoum CB: Gartland type III supracondylar humerus fractures: outcome and complications as related to operative timing and pin configuration, *J Child Orthop* 8:473, 2014.

Abzug JM, Herman MJ: Management of supracondylar humerus fractures in children: current concepts, *J Am Acad Orthop Surg* 20:69, 2012.

Altay MA, Erturk C, Altay M, et al: Ultrasonographic examination of the radial and ulnar nerves after percutaneous cross-wiring of supracondylar humerus fractures in children: a prospective, randomized controlled study, *J Pediatr Orthop B* 20:334, 2011.

Appelboam A, Reuben AD, Benger JR, et al: Elbow extension test to rule out elbow fracture: multicentre, prospective validation and observational study of diagnostic accuracy in adults and children, *BMJ* 337:a2428, 2008.

Ay S, Akinci M, Kamiloglu S, et al: Open reduction of displaced pediatric supracondylar humeral fractures through the anterior cubital approach, *J Pediatr Orthop* 25:149, 2005.

Babal JC, Mehlman CT, Klein G: Nerve injuries associated with pediatric supracondylar humeral fractures: a meta-analysis, *J Pediatr Orthop* 30:253, 2010.

Bahk MS, Srikumaran U, Ain MC, et al: Patterns of supracondylar humerus fractures, *J Pediatr Orthop* 28:493, 2008.

Bales JG, Spencer HT, Wong MA, et al: The effects of surgical delay on the outcome of pediatric supracondylar humeral fractures, *J Pediatr Orthop* 30:786, 2010.

Bashyal RK, Chu JY, Schoenecker PL, et al: Complications after pinning of supracondylar distal humerus fractures, *J Pediatr Orthop* 29:705, 2009.

Blakey CM, Biant LC, Birch R: Ischaemia and the pink, pulseless hand complicating supracondylar fractures of the humerus in childhood: long-term follow-up, *J Bone Joint Surg* 91B:1487, 2009.

Brauer CA, Lee BM, Bae DS, et al: A systematic review of medial and lateral entry pinning versus lateral entry pinning for supracondylar fractures of the humerus, *J Pediatr Orthop* 27:181, 2007.

Carmichael KD, Joyner K: Quality of reduction versus timing of surgical intervention for pediatric supracondylar humerus fractures, *Orthopedics* 29:628, 2006.

Choi PD, Melikian R, Skaggs DL: Risk factors for vascular repair and compartment syndrome in the pulseless supracondylar humerus fracture in children, *J Pediatr Orthop* 30:50, 2010.

Eberl R, Eder C, Smolle E, et al: Iatrogenic ulnar nerve injury after pin fixation and after antegrade nailing of supracondylar humeral fractures in children, *Acta Orthop* 82:606, 2011.

Fowler TP, Marsh JL: Reduction and pinning of pediatric supracondylar humerus fractures in the prone position, *J Orthop Trauma* 20:277, 2006.

Frick SL: Should you explore the brachial artery in children who have a perfused hand but no palpable radial pulse after sustaining a supracondylar humeral fracture? Commentary on articles by Amanda Weller, MD, et al: "Management of the pediatric pulseless supracondylar humeral fracture: is vascular exploration necessary?" and Brian P. Scannell, MD, et al.: "The perfused, pulseless supracondylar humeral fracture: intermediate-term follow-up of vascular status and function." *J Bone Joint Surg* 95A:e168, 2013.

Gaston RG, Cates TB, Devito D, et al: Medial and lateral pin versus lateral-entry pin fixation for type 3 supracondylar fractures in children: a prospective, surgeon-randomized study, *J Pediatr Orthop* 30:799, 2010.

Hamdi A, Poitras P, Louati H, et al: Biomechanical analysis of lateral pin placements for pediatric supracondylar humerus fractures, *J Pediatr Orthop* 30:135, 2010.

Havlas V, Trc T, Gaheer R, Schejbalova A: Manipulation of pediatric supracondylar fractures of humerus in prone position under general anesthesia, *J Pediatr Orthop* 28:660, 2008.

Howard A, Mulpuri K, Abel MF, et al: The treatment of pediatric supracondylar humerus fracture, *J Am Acad Orthop Surg* 20:320, 2012.

Isa AD, Furey A, Stone C: Functional outcome of supracondylar elbow fractures in children: a 3- to 5-year follow-up, *Can J Surg* 57:241, 2014.

Joiner ER, Skaggs DL, Arkader A, et al: Iatrogenic nerve injuries in the treatment of supracondylar humerus fractures: are we really just missing nerve injuries on preoperative examination? *J Pediatr Orthop* 34:388, 2014.

Kazimoglu C, Cetin M, Sener M, et al: Operative management of type III extension supracondylar fractures in children, *Int Orthop* 33:1089, 2009.

Kim HT, Lee JS, Yoo CI: Management of cubitus varus and valgus, *J Bone Joint Surg* 87A:771, 2005.

Kocher MS, Kasser JR, Waters PM, et al: Lateral entry compared with medial and lateral entry pin fixation for completely displaced supracondylar humeral fractures in children: a randomized clinical trial, *J Bone Joint Surg* 89A:706, 2007.

Kronner JMJR, Legakis JE, Kovacevic N, et al: An evaluation of supracondylar humerus fractures: is there a correlation between postponing treatment and the need for open surgical intervention, *J Child Orthop* 7:131, 2013.

Lacher M, Schaeffer K, Boehm R, Dietz HG: The treatment of supracondylar humeral fractures with elastic stable intramedullary nailing (ESIN) in children, *J Pediatr Orthop* 31:33, 2011.

Larson AN, Garg S, Weller A, et al: Operative treatment of type II supracondylar humerus fractures: does time to surgery affect complications, *J Pediatr Orthop* 34:382, 2014.

Lee BJ, Lee SR, Kim ST, et al: Radiographic outcomes after treatment of pediatric supracondylar humerus fractures using a treatment-based classification system, *J Orthop Trauma* 25:18, 2011.

Lee HY, Kim SJ: Treatment of displaced supracondylar fractures of the humerus in children by a pin leverage technique, *J Bone Joint Surg* 89B:646, 2007.

Lee YH, Lee SK, Kim BS, et al: Three lateral divergent or parallel pin fixations for the treatment of displaced supracondylar humerus fractures in children, *J Pediatr Orthop* 28:417, 2008.

Leitch KK, Kay RM, Femino JD, et al: Treatment of multidirectionally unstable supracondylar humeral fractures in children: a modified Gartland type-IV fracture, *J Bone Joint Surg* 88A:908, 2006.

Loizou CL, Simillis C, Hutchinson JR: A systematic review of early versus delayed treatment for type III supracondylar humeral fractures in children, *Injury* 40:245, 2009.

Luria S, Sucar A, Eylon S, et al: Vascular complications of supracondylar humeral fractures in children, *J Pediatr Orthop B* 16:133, 2007.

Mahan ST, May CD, Kocher MS: Operative management of displaced flexion supracondylar humerus fractures in children, *J Pediatr Orthop* 27:551, 2007.

Meyer CL, Kozin SH, Herman MJ, et al: Complications of pediatric supracondylar humeral fractures, *Instr Course Lect* 64:483, 2015.

Omid R, Choi PD, Skaggs DL: Supracondylar humeral fractures in children, *J Bone Joint Surg* 90A:1121, 2008.

Ramachandran M, Skaggs DL, Crawford HA, et al: Delaying treatment of supracondylar fractures in children: has the pendulum swung too far? *J Bone Joint Surg* 90B:1228, 2009.

Ramesh P, Avadhani A, Shetty AP, et al: Management of acute "'pink pulseless"' hand in pediatric supracondylar fractures of the humerus, *J Pediatr Orthop B* 20:124, 2011.

Sankar WN, Hebela NM, Skaggs DL, Flynn JM: Loss of pin fixation in displaced supracondylar humeral fractures in children: causes and prevention, *J Bone Joint Surg* 89A:713, 2007.

Seeley MA, Gagnier JJ, Srinivasan RC, et al: Obesity and its effects on pediatric supracondylar humeral fractures, *J Bone Joint Surg* 96A:e18, 2014.

Sibinski M, Sharma H, Sherlock DA: Lateral versus crossed wire fixation for displaced extension supracondylar humeral fractures in children, *Injury* 37:961, 2006.

Silva M, Pandarinath R, Garng E, et al: Inter- and intra-observer reliability of the Baumann angle of the humerus in children with supracondylar humeral fractures, *Int Orthop* 34:553, 2010.

Skaggs DL, Sankar WN, Albrektson J, et al: How safe is the operative treatment of Gartland type 2 supracondylar humerus fractures in children? *J Pediatr Orthop* 28:139, 2008.

Slobogean BL, Jackman H, Tennant S, et al: Iatrogenic ulnar nerve injury after the surgical treatment of displaced supracondylar fractures of the humerus: number needed to harm, a systematic review, *J Pediatr Orthop* 30:430, 2010.

Spencer HT, Wong M, Fong YJ, et al: Prospective longitudinal evaluation of elbow motion following pediatric supracondylar humeral fractures, *J Bone Joint Surg* 92A:904, 2010.

Srikumaran U, Tan EW, Erkula G, et al: Pin size influences sagittal alignment in percutaneously pinned pediatric supracondylar humerus fractures, *J Pediatr Orthop* 30:792, 2010.

Steinman S, Bastrom TP, Newton PO, Mubarak SJ: Beware of ulnar nerve entrapment in flexion-type supracondylar humerus fractures, *J Child Orthop* 1:177, 2007.

Valencia M, Moraleda L, Diez-Sebastian J: Long-term functional results of neurological complications of pediatric humeral supracondylar fractures, *J Pediatr Orthop* 35:606, 2015.

Walmsley PJ, Kelly MB, Robb JE, et al: Delay increases the need for open reduction of type-III supracondylar fractures of the humerus, *J Bone Joint Surg* 88B:528, 2006.

Wegmann H, Eberl R, Kraus T, et al: The impact of arterial vessel injuries associated with pediatric supracondylar humeral fractures, *J Trauma Acute Care Surg* 77:381, 2014.

Weiss JM, Kay RM, Waters P, et al: Distal humerus osteotomy for supracondylar fracture malunion in children: a study of perioperative complications, *Am J Orthop (Belle Mead NJ)* 39:22, 2010.

Weller A, Garg S, Larson AN, et al: Management of the pediatric pulseless supracondylar humeral fracture: is vascular exploration necessary? *J Bone Joint Surg* 95A:1906, 2013.

White L, Mehlman CT, Crawford AH: Perfused, pulseless, and puzzling: a systematic review of vascular injuries in pediatric supracondylar humerus fractures and results of a POSNA questionnaire, *J Pediatr Orthop* 30:328, 2010.

Woratanarat P, Angsanuntsukh C, Rattanasiri S, et al: Meta-analysis of pinning in supracondylar fracture of the humerus in children, *J Orthop Trauma* 26:48, 2011.

Yen YM, Kocher MS: Lateral entry compared with medial and lateral entry pin fixation for completely displaced supracondylar humeral fractures in children: surgical technique, *J Bone Joint Surg* 90A(Suppl 2 Pt 2):20, 2008.

Yildirim AO, Unal VS, Oken OF, et al: Timing of surgical treatment of type III supracondylar humerus fractures in pediatric patients, *J Child Orthop* 3:265, 2009.

Zamzam MM, Bakarman KA: Treatment of displaced supracondylar humeral fractures among children: crossed versus lateral pinning, *Injury* 40:625, 2009.

Zionts LE, Woodson CJ, Manjra N, Zalavras C: Time of return of elbow motion after percutaneous pinning of pediatric supracondylar humerus fractures, *Clin Orthop Relat Res* 467:2007, 2009.

LATERAL CONDYLAR FRACTURES

Beaty JH: Fractures of the lateral humeral condyle are the second most frequent elbow fracture in children, *J Orthop Trauma* 24:438, 2010.

Bernthal NM, Hoshino CM, Dichter D, et al: Recovery of elbow motion following pediatric lateral condylar fractures of the humerus, *J Bone Joint Surg* 93A:871, 2011.

Koh KH, Seo SW, Kim KM, Shim JS: Clinical and radiographic results of lateral condylar fracture of distal humerus in children, *J Pediatr Orthop* 30:425, 2010.

Lemme K, Lubicky JP, Zeni A, Riley E: Pediatric lateral condyle humeral fractures with and without associated elbow dislocations: a retrospective study, *Am J Orthop (Belle Mead NJ)* 38:453, 2009.

Song KS, Shin YW, Oh CW, et al: Closed reduction and internal fixation of completely displaced and rotated lateral condyle fractures of the humerus in children, *J Orthop Trauma* 24:434, 2010.

Weiss JM, Graves S, Yang S, et al: A new classification system predictive of complications in surgically treated pediatric humeral lateral condyle fractures, *J Pediatr Orthop* 29:602, 2009.

Yang WE, Shih CH, Lee ZL, et al: Anatomic reduction of old displaced lateral condylar fracture of the humerus in children via a posterior approach with olecranon osteotomy, *J Trauma* 64:1281, 2008.

MEDIAL EPICONDYLAR AND MEDIAL HUMERAL CONDYLAR FRACTURES

Dodds SD, Flanagin BA, Bohl DD, et al: Incarcerated medial epicondyle fracture following pediatric elbow dislocation: 11 cases, *J Hand Surg Am* 39:1739, 2014.

Edmonds EW: How displaced are "nondisplaced" fractures of the medial humeral epicondyle in children? Results of a three-dimensional computed tomography analysis, *J Bone Joint Surg* 92A:2785, 2010.

Gottschalk HP, Bastrom TP, Edmonds EW: Reliability of internal oblique elbow radiographs for measuring displacement of medial epicondyle humerus fractures: a cadaveric study, *J Pediatr Orthop* 33:26, 2013.

Haflah NH, Ibrahim S, Sapuan J, Abdullah S: An elbow dislocation in a child with missed medial epicondyle fracture and late ulnar nerve palsy, *J Pediatr Orthop B* 19:459, 2010.

Osbahr DC, Chalmers PN, Frank JS, et al: Acute avulsion fractures of the medial epicondyle while throwing in youth baseball players: a variant of Little League elbow, *J Shoulder Elbow Surg* 19:951, 2010.

Pappas N, Lawrence JT, Donegan D, et al: Intraobserver and interobserver agreement in the measurement of displaced humeral medial epicondyle fractures in children, *J Bone Joint Surg* 92A:322, 2010.

Park KB, Kwak YH: Treatment of medial epicondyle fracture without associated elbow dislocation in older children and adolescents, *Yonsei Med J* 53:1190, 2012.

Sawyer JR, Kelly DM, Beaty JH, et al: The hammerlock position for treatment of medial epicondyle fractures, *Curr Orthop Pract* 20:572, 2009.

Souder CD, Faarnsworth CL, McNeil NP, et al: The distal humerus axial view: assessment of displacement in medial epicondyle fractures, *J Pediatr Orthop* 35:449, 2015.

ELBOW JOINT FRACTURES AND DISLOCATIONS

Eberl R, Singer G, Fruhmann J, et al: Intramedullary nailing for the treatment of dislocated pediatric radial neck fractures, *Eur J Pediatr Surg* 20:250, 2010.

Elanti P, O'Farrell D: Iatrogenic radial neck fracture on closed reduction of elbow dislocation, *CJEM* 15:389, 2013.

Falciglia F, Giordano M, Aulisa AG, et al: Radial neck fractures in children: results when open reduction is indicated, *J Pediatr Orthop* 34:756, 2014.

Furushima K, Itoh Y, Iwabu S, et al: Classification of olecranon stress fractures in baseball players, *Am J Sports Med* 42:NP44, 2014.

Guitton TG, Albers RG, Ring D: Anterior olecranon fracture-dislocations of the elbow in children: a report of four cases, *J Bone Joint Surg* 91A:1487, 2009.

Heinrich SD, Butler RA: Late radial head dislocation with radial head fracture and ulnar plastic deformation, *Clin Orthop Relat Res* 460:258, 2007.

Klitscher D, Richter S, Bodenschatz K, et al: Evaluation of severely displaced radial neck fractures in children treated with elastic stable intramedullary nailing, *J Pediatr Orthop* 29:698, 2009.

Modi P, Dhammi IK, Rustagi A, Jain AK: Elbow dislocation with ipsilateral diaphyseal fractures of radius and ulna in an adult-is it type 1 or type 2 Monteggia equivalent lesion? *Chin J Traumatol* 15:303, 2012.

Paci JM, Dugas JR, Guy JA, et al: Cannulated screw fixation of refractory olecranon stress fractures with and without associated injuries allows a return to baseball, *Am J Sports Med* 41:306, 2013.

Parent S, Wedemeyer M, Mahar AT, et al: Displaced olecranon fractures in children: a biomechanical analysis of fixation methods, *J Pediatr Orthop* 28:147, 2008.

Rettig AC, Wurh TR, Mieling P: Nonunion of olecranon stress fractures in adolescent baseball pitchers: a case series of 5 athletes, *Am J Sports Med* 34:653, 2006.

Rosenbaum AJ, Leonard GR, Uhl RL, et al: Radiologic case study. Diagnosis: congenital posterior dislocation of the radial head, *Orthopedics* 37:62, 2014.

Van Zeeland NL, Bae DS, Goldfarb CA: Intra-articular radial head fracture in the skeletally immature patient: progressive radial head subluxation and rapid radiocapitellar degeneration, *J Pediatr Orthop* 31:124, 2011.

Yoon HK, Seo GW: Proximal radioulnar translocation associated with elbow dislocation and radial neck fracture in child: a case report and review of the literature, *Arch Orthop Trauma Surg* 133:1425, 2013.

FOREARM FRACTURES/MONTEGGIA FRACTURES

Abraham A, Kumar S, Chaudhry S, Ibrahim T: Surgical interventions for diaphyseal fractures of the radius and ulna in children, *Cochrane Database Syst Rev* (11):CD007907, 2011.

Altay M, Aktekin CN, Ozkurt B, et al: Intramedullary wire fixation for unstable forearm fractures in children, *Injury* 37:966, 2006.

Bader M, Sanz L, Waseem M: Forearm fractures in children: single bone fixation with elastic stable intramedullary nailing in 20 cases, *Injury* 37:923, 2006.

Baldwin K, Morrison MJ 3rd, Tomlinson LA, et al: Both bone forearm fractures in children and adolescents, which fixation strategy is superior – plates or nails? A systematic review and meta-analysis of observational studies, *J Orthop Trauma* 28:38, 2014.

Bohm ER, Bubbar V, Yong Hing K, Dzus A: Above- and below-the-elbow plaster casts for distal forearm fractures in children: a randomized controlled trial, *J Bone Joint Surg* 88A:1, 2006.

Bowman EN, Mehlman CT, Lindsell CJ, Tamai J: Nonoperative treatment of both-bone forearm shaft fractures in children: predictors of early radiographic failure, *J Pediatr Orthop* 31:23, 2011.

Carmichael KD, English C: Outcomes assessment of pediatric both-bone forearm fractures treated operatively, *Orthopedics* 30:379, 2007.

Dietz JF, Bae DS, Reigg E, et al: Single bone intramedullary fixation of the ulna in pediatric both bone forearm fractures: analysis of short-term clinical and radiographic results, *J Pediatr Orthop* 30:420, 2010.

Fernandez FF, Eberhardt O, Langendörfer M, Wirth T: Nonunion of forearm shaft fractures in children after intramedullary nailing, *J Pediatr Orthop B* 18:289, 2009.

Fernandez FF, Langendörfer M, Wirth T, Eberhardt O: Failures and complications in intramedullary nailing of children's forearm fractures, *J Child Orthop* 4:159, 2010.

Flynn JM, Jones KJ, Garner MR, Goebel J: Eleven years experience in the operative management of pediatric forearm fractures, *J Pediatr Orthop* 30:313, 2010.

Goyal T, Arora SS, Banerjee S, Kandwal P: Neglected Monteggia fracture dislocations in children: a systematic review, *J Pediatr Orthop B* 24:191, 2015.

Hammad A, Hasanin E, Lotfy W, Eladl W: Ulnar plating for the treatment of unstable fractures of the forearm in children, *Acta Orthop Belg* 73:588, 2007.

Herman MJ, Marshall ST: Forearm fractures in children and adolescents: a practical approach, *Hand Clin* 22:55, 2006.

Ho CA, Jarcis DL, Phelps JR, Wilson PL: Delayed union in internal fixation of pediatric both-bone forearm fractures, *J Pediatr Orthop B* 22:383, 2013.

Kang SB, Mangwani J, Ramachandran M, et al: Elastic intramedullary nailing of paediatric fractures of the forearm: a decade of experience in a teaching hospital in the United Kingdom, *J Bone Joint Surg* 93B:262, 2011.

Mostafa MF, El-Adl G, Enan A: Percutaneous Kirschner-wire fixation for displaced distal forearm fractures in children, *Acta Orthop Belg* 75:459, 2009.

Nakamura K, Hirachi K, Uchiyama S, et al: Long-term clinical and radiographic outcomes after open reduction for missed Monteggia fracture-dislocations in children, *J Bone Joint Surg* 91A:1394, 2009.

Paneru SR, Rijal R, Shrestha BP, et al: Randomized controlled trial comparing above- and below-elbow plaster casts for distal forearm fractures in children, *J Child Orthop* 4:233, 2010.

Price CT: Surgical management of forearm and distal radius fractures in children and adolescents, *Instr Course Lect* 57:509, 2008.

Price CT: Acceptable alignment of forearm fractures in children: open reduction indications, *J Pediatr Orthop* 30:S82, 2010.

Price CT, Knapp DR: Osteotomy for malunited forearm shaft fractures in children, *J Pediatr Orthop* 26:193, 2006.

Ramski DE, Hennrikus WP, Bae DS, et al: Pediatric Monteggia fractures: a multicenter examination of treatment strategy and early clinical and radiographic results, *J Pediatr Orthop* 35:115, 2015.

Reinhardt KR, Geldman DS, Green DW, et al: Comparison of intramedullary nailing to plating for both-bone forearm fractures in older children, *J Pediatr Orthop* 28:403, 2008.

Saul T, Ng L, Lewis RE: Point-of-care ultrasound in the diagnosis of upper extremity fracture-dislocation. A pictorial essay, *Med Ultrason* 15:230, 2013.

Sferopoulos NK: Monteggia type IV equivalent injury, *Open Orthop J* 5:198, 2011.

Shah AS, Lesniak BP, Wolter TD, et al: Stabilization of adolescent both-bone forearm fractures: a comparison of intramedullary nailing versus open reduction and internal fixation, *J Orthop Trauma* 24:440, 2010.

Sinikumpu JJ, Pokka T, Serlo W: The changing pattern of pediatric both bone forearm shaft fractures among 86,000 children from 1997 to 2009, *Eur J Pediatr Surg* 23:289, 2013.

Sood A, Kha O, Bagga T: Simultaneous Monteggia type I fracture equivalent with ipsilateral fracture of the distal radius and ulna in a child: a case report, *J Med Case Rep* 2:190, 2008.

Tan JW, Mu MZ, Liao GJ, Li JM: Pathology of the annular ligament in paediatric Monteggia fractures, *Injury* 39:451, 2008.

Tarmuzi NA, Abdullah S, Osman Z, Das S: Paediatric forearm fractures: functional outcome of conservative treatment, *Bratisl Lek Listy* 110:563, 2009.

van Geenen RC, Besselaar PP: Outcome after corrective osteotomy for malunited fractures of the forearm sustained in childhood, *J Bone Joint Surg* 89B:236, 2007.

Van Tongel A, Ackerman P, Liekens K, Berghs B: Angulated greenstick fractures of the distal forearm in children: closed reduction by pronation or supination, *Acta Orthop Belg* 77:21, 2011.

Webb WR, Galpin RD, Armstrong DG: Comparison of short and long arm plaster casts for displaced fractures in the distal third of the forearm in children, *J Bone Joint Surg* 88A:9, 2006.

HAND AND WRIST FRACTURES, DISLOCATIONS, AND FRACTURE-DISLOCATIONS

Abzug JM, Kozin SH: Seymour fractures, *J Hand Surg Am* 38:2267, 2013.

Abzug JM, Little K, Kozin SH: Physeal arrest of the distal radius, *J Am Acad Orthop Surg* 22:381, 2014.

Al-Qattan MM, Al-Qattan AM: A review of phalangeal neck fractures in children, *Injury* 46:935, 2015.

Anz AW, Bushnell BD, Bynum DK, et al: Pediatric scaphoid fractures, *J Am Acad Orthop Surg* 17:77, 2009.

Chew EM, Chong AK: Hand fractures in children: epidemiology and misdiagnosis in a tertiary referral hospital, *J Hand Surg Am* 37:1684, 2012.

Edmonds EW, Capelo RM, Stearns P, et al: Predicting initial treatment failure of fiberglass casts in pediatric distal radius fractures: utility of the second metacarpal-radius angle, *J Child Orthop* 3:375, 2009.

Faouzi HM: Scaphoid fracture associated with distal radius fracture in children: a cade report, *Chin J Traumatol* 12:187, 2009.

Gholson JJ, Bae DS, Zurakowski D, Waters PM: Scaphoid fractures in children and adolescents: contemporary injury patterns and factors influencing time to union, *J Bone Joint Surg* 93A:1210, 2011.

Huckstadt T, Klitscher D, Weltzien A, et al: Pediatric fractures of the carpal scaphoid: a retrospective clinical and radiological study, *J Pediatr Orthop* 27:447, 2007.

Krusche-Mandl I, Köttstorfer J, Thalhammer G, et al: Seymour fractures: retrospective analysis and therapeutic considerations, *J Hand Surg Am* 38:258, 2013.

Tan YW, Maffulli N: Carpal scaphoid fracture in the skeletally immature: a single centre one-year prospective study, *Acta Orthop Belg* 75:616, 2009.

Vadivelu R, Dias JJ, Burke FD, Stanton J: Hand injuries in children: a prospective study, *J Pediatr Orthop* 26:29, 2006.

SPINE FRACTURES AND DISLOCATIONS

Arkader A, Warner WC Jr, Tolo VT, et al: Pediatric Chance fractures: a multicenter perspective, *J Pediatr Orthop* 31:741, 2011.

Astur N, Sawyer JR, Klimo P Jr, et al: Traumatic atlanto-occipital dislocation in children, *J Am Acad Orthop Surg* 22:274, 2014.

Astur N, Klimo P Jr, Sawyer JR, et al: Traumatic atlanto-occipital dislocation in children: evaluation, treatment, and outcomes, *J Bone Joint Surg* 95A:e194, 2013.

Boese CK, Oppermann J, Siewe J, et al: Spinal cord injury without radiologic abnormality in children: a systematic review and meta-analysis, *J Trauma Acute Care Surg* 78:874, 2015.

de Gauzy JS, Joyve JL, Violas P, et al: Classification of Chance fracture in children using magnetic resonance imaging, *Spine* 32:E89, 2007.

Hosalkar HS, Greenbaum JN, Flynn JM, et al: Fractures of the odontoid in children with an open basilar synchondrosis, *J Bone Joint Surg* 91B:789, 2009.

Jeszensky D, Fekete TF, Lattig F, Bognár L: Intraarticular atlantooccipital fusion for the treatment of traumatic occipitocervical dislocation in a child: a new technique for selective stabilization with nine years follow-up, *Spine* 35:E421, 2010.

Knox JB, Schneider JE, Cage JM, et al: Spine trauma in a very young children: a retrospective study of 206 patients presenting to a level 1 pediatric trauma center, *J Pediatr Orthop* 34:698, 2014.

Leonard M, Sproule J, McCormack D: Paediatric spinal trauma and associated injuries, *Injury* 38:188, 2007.

Murphy RF, Davidson AR, Kelly DM, et al: Subaxial cervical spine injuries in children and adolescents, *J Pediatr Orthop* 35:136, 2015.

Rush JK, Kelly DM, Astur N, et al: Associated injuries in children and adolescents with spinal trauma, *J Pediatr Orthop* 33:393, 2013.

Vander Have KL, Caird MS, Gross S, et al: Burst fractures of the thoracic and lumbar spine in children and adolescents, *J Pediatr Orthop* 29:713, 2009.

PELVIC AND HIP FRACTURES AND DISORDERS

Abbas AA, Yoon TG, Lee JH, Hur CI: Posttraumatic avascular necrosis of the femoral head in teenagers treated by a modified transtrochanteric rotational osteotomy: a report of three cases, *J Orthop Trauma* 22:63, 2008.

Amorosa LF, Kloen P, Helfet DL: High-energy pediatric pelvic and acetabular fractures, *Orthop Clin North Am* 45:483, 2014.

Banskota AK, Speigel DA, Shrestha S, et al: Open reduction for neglected traumatic hip dislocation in children and adolescents, *J Pediatr Orthop* 27:187, 2007.

Beaty JH: Fractures of the hip in children, *Orthop Clin North Am* 37:223, 2006.

Boardman MJ, Herman MJ, Buck B, Pizzutillo PD: Hip fractures in children, *J Am Acad Orthop Surg* 17:162, 2009.

Clohisy JC, Oryhon JM, Seyler TM, et al: Function and fixation of total hip arthroplasty in patients 25 years of age or young, *Clin Orthop Relat Res* 468:3207, 2010.

Finnegan MA: CORR Insights®: delayed slipped capital femoral epiphysis after treatment of femoral neck fracture in children, *Clin Orthop Relat Res* 473:2718, 2015.

Ganz R, Horowitz K, Leunig M: Algorithm for femoral and periacetabular osteotomies in complex hip deformities, *Clin Orthop Relat Res* 468:3168, 2010.

Guimaraes JA, Mendes PH, Vallim FC, et al: Surgical treatment for unstable pelvic fractures in skeletally immature patients, *Injury* 45(Suppl 5):S40, 2014.

Herrera-Soto JA, Price CT: Traumatic hip dislocations in children and adolescents: pitfalls and complications, *J Am Acad Orthop Surg* 17:15, 2009.

Herrera-Soto JA, Price CT: Core decompression and labral support for the treatment of juvenile osteonecrosis, *J Pediatr Orthop* 31(2 Suppl):S212, 2011.

Holden CP, Holman J, Herman MJ: Pediatric pelvic fractures, *J Am Acad Orthop Surg* 15:172, 2007.

Ilizaliturri VM Jr, Gonzalez-Gutierrez B, Gonazalez-Ugalde H, Camacho-Galindo J: Hip arthroscopy after traumatic hip dislocation, *Am J Sports Med* 39(Suppl):50S, 2011.

Magu NK, Singh R, Sharma AK, Ummat V: Modified Pauwels' intertrochanteric osteotomy in neglected femoral neck fractures in children: a report of 10 cases followed for a minimum of 5 years, *J Orthop Trauma* 21:237, 2007.

Manner HM, Mast NH, Ganz R, Leunig M: Potential contribution of femoroacetabular impingement to recurrent traumatic hip dislocation, *J Pediatr Orthop B* 21:574, 2012.

Momiy JP, Clayton JL, Villalba H, et al: Pelvic fractures in children, *Am Surg* 72:962, 2006.

Neto PF, Dos Reis FB, Filho JL, et al: Nonunion of fractures of the femoral neck in children, *J Child Orthop* 2:97, 2008.

Philippon MJ, Kuppersmith DA, Wolff AB, Briggs KK: Arthroscopic findings following traumatic hip dislocation in 14 professional athletes, *Arthroscopy* 25:169, 2009.

Rao RD, Berry C, Yoganandan N, et al: Occupant and crash characteristics in thoracic and lumbar spine injuires resulting from motor vehicle collisions, *Spine J* 14:2355, 2014.

Shore BJ, Palmer CS, Bevin C, et al: Pediatric pelvic fracture: a modification of a preexisting classification, *J Pediatr Orthop* 32:162, 2012.

Shrader MW, Jacofsky DJ, Stans AA, et al: Femoral neck fractures in pediatric patients: 30 years experience at a level 1 trauma center, *Clin Orthop Relat Res* 454:169, 2007.

Spence D, DiMauro JP, Miller PE, et al: Osteonecrosis after femoral neck fractures in children and adolescents: analysis of risk factors, *J Pediatr Orthop* 36:111, 2015.

Yeranosian M, Horneff JG, Baldwin K, Hosalkar HS: Factors affecting the outcome of fractures of the femoral neck in children and adolescents: a systematic review, *Bone Joint J* 95B:135, 2013.

Zrig M, Mnif H, Koubaa M, Abid A: Traumatic hip dislocation in children, *Acta Orthop Belg* 75:328, 2009.

SLIPPED CAPITAL FEMORAL EPIPHYSIS

Anand A, Chorney GS: Patient survey of weight-bearing and physical activity after in situ pinning of slipped capital femoral epiphysis, *Am J Orthop* 36:E68, 2007.

Aronsson DD, Loder RT, Breur GJ, Weinstein SL: Slipped capital femoral epiphysis: current concepts, *J Am Acad Orthop Surg* 14:666, 2006.

Azzopardi T, Sharma S, Bennet GC: Slipped capital femoral epiphysis in children aged less than 10 years, *J Pediatr Orthop B* 19:13, 2010.

Biring GS, Hashemi-Nejad A, Catterall A: Outcomes of subcapital cuneiform osteotomy for the treatment of severe slipped capital femoral epiphysis after skeletal maturity, *J Bone Joint Surg* 88B:1379, 2006.

Castaneda P, Macias C, Rocha A, et al: Functional outcome of stable grade III slipped capital femoral epiphysis treated with in situ pinning, *J Pediatr Orthop* 29:454, 2009.

Castro FP, Bennett JT, Doulens K: Epidemiological perspective on prophylactic pinning in patients with unilateral slipped capital femoral epiphysis, *J Pediatr Orthop* 20:745, 2009.

Chen RC, Schoenecker PL, Dobbs MB, et al: Urgent reduction, fixation, and arthrotomy for unstable slipped capital femoral epiphysis, *J Pediatr Orthop* 29:687, 2009.

DeLullo JA, Thomas E, Cooney TE, et al: Femoral remodeling may influence patient outcomes in slipped capital femoral epiphysis, *Clin Orthop Relat Res* 457:163, 2007.

Diab M, Daluvoy S, Snyder BD, Kasser JR: Osteotomy does not improve early outcome after slipped capital femoral epiphysis, *J Pediatr Orthop B* 15:87, 2006.

Dodds MK, McCormack D, Mulhall KJ: Femoroacetabular impingement after slipped capital femoral epiphysis: does slip severity predict clinical symptoms? *J Pediatr Orthop* 29:535, 2009.

Fraitzl CR, Käfer W, Nelitz M, Reichel M: Radiological evidence of femoroacetabular impingement in mild slipped capital femoral epiphysis: a mean follow-up of 14.4 years after pinning in situ, *J Bone Joint Surg* 89B:1592, 2007.

Georgiadis AG, Zaltz I: Slipped capital femoral epiphysis: how to evaluate with a review and update of treatment, *Pediatr Clin North Am* 61:1119, 2014.

Goodwin RC, Mahar AT, Oswald TS, Wenger DR: Screw head impingement after in situ fixation in moderate and severe slipped capital femoral epiphysis, *J Pediatr Orthop* 27:319, 2007.

Green DW, Magekwu N, Scher DM, et al: A modification of Klein's line to improve sensitivity of the anterior-posterior radiograph in slipped capital femoral epiphysis, *J Pediatr Orthop* 29:449, 2009.

Herrera-Soto JA, Duffy MF, Birnbaum MA, Vander Have KL: Increased intracapsular pressures after unstable slipped capital femoral epiphysis, *J Pediatr Orthop* 28:723, 2008.

Ilchmann T, Parsch K: Complications at screw removal in slipped capital femoral epiphysis treated by cannulated titanium screws, *Arch Orthop Trauma Surg* 126:359, 2006.

Kalogrianitis S, Tan CK, Kemp GJ, et al: Does unstable slipped capital femoral epiphysis require urgent stabilization? *J Pediatr Orthop B* 16:6, 2007.

Kishan S, Upasani V, Mahar A, et al: Biomechanical stability of single-screw versus two-screw fixation of an unstable slipped capital femoral epiphysis model: effect of screw position in the femoral neck, *J Pediatr Orthop* 26:601, 2006.

Kocher MS, Bishop JA, Weed B, et al: Delay in diagnosis of slipped capital femoral epiphysis, *Pediatrics* 113:e322, 2004.

Leunig M, Slongo T, Ganz R: Subcapital realignment in slipped capital femoral epiphysis: surgical hip dislocation and trimming of the stable trochanter to protect the perfusion of the epiphysis, *Instr Course Lect* 57:499, 2008.

Liu RW, Armstong DG, Levine AD, et al: An anatomic study of the epiphyseal tubercle and its importance in the pathogenesis of slipped capital femoral epiphysis, *J Bone Joint Surg* 95A:e341, 2013.

Loder RT, Aronsson DD, Weinstein SL, et al: Slipped capital femoral epiphysis, *Instr Course Lect* 57:473, 2008.

Loder RT, O'Donnell PW, Didelot WP, Kayes KJ: Valgus slipped capital femoral epiphysis, *J Pediatr Orthop* 26:594, 2006.

Mamisch TC, Kim YJ, Richolt JA, et al: Femoral morphology due to impingement influences the range of motion in slipped capital femoral epiphysis, *Clin Orthop Relat Res* 467:692, 2009.

Merz MK, Amirouche F, Solitro GF, et al: Biomechanical comparison of perpendicular versus oblique in situ screw fixation of slipped capital femoral epiphysis, *J Pediatr Orthop* 35:816, 2014.

Misar A, Salama A, Freeman JV, Davies AG: Avascular necrosis in acute and acute-on-chronic slipped capital femoral epiphysis, *J Pediatr Orthop B* 16:393, 2007.

Miyanji F, Mahar A, Oka R, et al: Biomechanical comparison of fully and partially threaded screws for fixation of slipped capital femoral epiphysis, *J Pediatr Orthop* 28:49, 2008.

Palocaren T, Holmes L, Rogers K, Kumar SJ: Outcome of in situ pinning in patients with unstable slipped capital femoral epiphysis: assessment of risk factors associated with avascular necrosis, *J Pediatr Orthop* 30:31, 2010.

Parsch K, Weller S, Parsch D: Open reduction and smooth Kirschner wire fixation for unstable slipped capital femoral epiphysis, *J Pediatr Orthop* 29:1, 2009.

Riad J, Bajelidze G, Gabos PG: Bilateral slipped capital femoral epiphysis: predictive factors for contralateral slip, *J Pediatr Orthop* 27:411, 2007.

Sabharwal S, Mittal R, Zhao C: Percutaneous osteotomy for deformity correction in adolescents with severe slipped capital femoral epiphysis, *J Pediatr Orthop B* 15:396, 2006.

Sankar WN, Brighton BK, Kim YJ, et al: Acetabular morphology in slipped capital femoral epiphysis, *J Pediatr Orthop* 31:254, 2011.

Sankar WN, Novais EN, Lee C, et al: What are the risks of prophylactic pinning to prevent contralateral slipped capital femoral epiphysis? *Clin Orthop Relat Res* 471:2118, 2013.

Sankar WN, Vanderhave KL, Matheney T, et al: The modified Dunn procedure for unstable slipped capital femoral epiphysis: a multicenter perspective, *J Bone Joint Surg* 95A:585, 2013.

Segal LS, Jacobson JA, Saunders MM: Biomechanical analysis of in situ single versus double screw fixation in a nonreduced slipped capital femoral epiphysis model, *J Pediatr Orthop* 26:479, 2006.

Seller K, Raab P, Wild A, et al: Risk-benefit analysis of prophylactic pinning in slipped capital femoral epiphysis, *J Pediatr Orthop B* 10:192, 2001.

Seller K, Wild A, Westhoff B, et al: Radiological evaluation of unstable (acute) slipped capital femoral epiphysis treated by pinning with Kirschner wires, *J Pediatr Orthop B* 15:328, 2006.

Shank CF, Thiel EF, Klingele KE: Valgus slipped capital femoral epiphysis: prevalence, presentation, and treatment options, *J Pediatr Orthop* 30:140, 2010.

Spencer S, Millis MB, Kim YJ: Early results of treatment for hip impingement syndrome in slipped capital femoral epiphysis and pistol grip deformity of the femoral head-neck junction using the surgical dislocation technique, *J Pediatr Orthop* 26:281, 2006.

Tjoumakaris FP, Wallach DM, Davidson RS: Subtrochanteric osteotomy effectively treats femoroacetabular impingement after slipped capital femoral epiphysis, *Clin Orthop Relat Res* 464:230, 2007.

Upasani V, Kishan S, Oka R, et al: Biomechanical analysis of single screw fixation for slipped capital femoral epiphysis: are more threads across the physis necessary for stability, *J Pediatr Orthop* 26:474, 2006.

Witbreuk MMEH, Bolkenbaas M, Mullender MG, et al: The results of downgrading moderate and severe slipped capital femoral epiphysis by an early Imhauser femur osteotomy, *J Child Orthop* 3:405, 2009.

Woelfle JV, Fraitzl CR, Reichel H, et al: The asymptomatic contralateral hip in unilateral slipped capital femoral epiphysis: morbidity of prophylactic fixation, *J Pediatr Orthop B* 21:226, 2012.

Yildirim Y, Bautisa S, Davidson RS: Chondrolysis, osteonecrosis, and slip severity in patients with subsequent contralateral slipped capital femoral epiphysis, *J Bone Joint Surg* 90A:485, 2008.

Ziebarth K, Leunig M, Slongo T, et al: Slipped capital femoral epiphysis: relevant pathophysiological findings with open surgery, *Clin Orthop Relat Res* 471:2156, 2013.

Ziebarth K, Zilkens C, Spencer S, et al: Capital realignment for moderate and severe SCFE using a modified Dunn procedure, *Clin Orthop Relat Res* 467:704, 2009.

FEMORAL FRACTURES

Aksahin E, Celebi L, Yüksel HY, et al: Immediate incorporated hip spica casting in pediatric femoral fractures: comparison of efficacy between normal and high-risk groups, *J Pediatr Orthop* 29:39, 2009.

American Academy of Orthopaedic Surgeons: *Guideline on the treatment of pediatric diaphyseal femur fractures.* www.aaos.org/research/guidelines/PDFFguideline.asp.

Anastasopoulos J, Petratos D, Konstantoulakis C, et al: Flexible intramedullary nailing in paediatric femoral shaft fractures, *Injury* 41:578, 2010.

Arkader A, Warner WC Jr, Horn BD, et al: Predicting the outcome of physeal fractures of the distal femur, *J Pediatr Orthop* 27:703, 2007.

Baldwin K, Hsu JE, Wenger DR, Hosalkar HS: Treatment of femur fractures in school-aged children using elastic stable intramedullary nailing: a systematic review, *J Pediatr Orthop B* 20:303, 2011.

Basener CJ, Mehlman CT, DiPasquale TG: Growth disturbance after distal femoral growth plate fractures in children: a meta-analysis, *J Orthop Trauma* 23:663, 2009.

Beebe M, Kelly D, Warner WC Jr, Sawyer JR: Current controversies in the treatment of pediatric femoral shaft fractures, *Curr Orthop Pract* 20:634, 2009.

Bopst L, Reinberg O, Lutz N: Femur fracture in preschool children: experience with flexible intramedullary nailing in 72 children, *J Pediatr Orthop* 27:299, 2007.

Crosby SN, Kim EJ, Koehler DM, et al: Twenty-year experience with rigid intramedullary nailing of femoral shaft, *J Bone Joint Surg* 96A:1080, 2014.

Epps HR, Molenaar E, O'Connor DP: Immediate single-leg spica cast for pediatric femoral diaphysis fractures, *J Pediatr Orthop* 26:491, 2006.

Flynn JM, Garner MR, Jones KJ, et al: The treatment of low-energy femoral shaft fractures: a prospective study comparing the "walking spica" with the traditional spica, *J Bone Joint Surg* 93A:2196, 2011.

Garner MR, Bhat SB, Khujanazarov I, et al: Fixation of length-stable femoral shaft fractures in heavier children: flexible nails vs rigid locked nails, *J Pediatr Orthop* 31:11, 2011.

Garrett BR, Hoffman EB, Carrara H: The effect of percutaneous pin fixation in the treatment of distal femoral physeal fractures, *J Bone Joint Surg* 93B:689, 2011.

Goodwin R, Mahar AT, Oka R, et al: Biomechanical evaluation of retrograde intramedullary stabilization for femoral fractures: the effect of fracture level, *J Pediatr Orthop* 27:873, 2007.

Hedequist D, Bishop J, Hresko T: Locking plate fixation for pediatric femur fractures, *J Pediatr Orthop* 28:6, 2008.

Heffernan MJ, Gordon JE, Sabatini CS, et al: Treatment of femur fractures in young children: a multicenter comparison of flexible intramedullary nails to spica casting in young children aged 2 to 6 years, *J Pediatr Orthop* 35:126, 2015.

Heyworth BE, Hedequist DJ, Nasreddine AY, et al: Distal femoral valgus deformity following plate fixation of pediatric femoral shaft fractures, *J Bone Joint Surg* 95A:526, 2013.

Ho CA, Skaggs DL, Tang CW, Kay RM: Use of flexible intramedullary nails in pediatric femur fractures, *J Pediatr Orthop* 26:497, 2006.

Hosalkar HS, Pandya NK, Cho RH, et al: Intramedullary nailing of pediatric femoral shaft fracture, *J Am Acad Orthop Surg* 19:472, 2011.

Hui C, Joughin E, Goldstein S, et al: Femoral fractures in children younger than three years: the role of nonaccidental injury, *J Pediatr Orthop* 28:297, 2008.

Jencikove-Celerin L, Phillips JH, Werk LN, et al: Flexible interlocked nailing of pediatric femoral fractures: experience with a new flexible interlocking intramedullary nail compared with other fixation procedures, *J Pediatr Orthop* 28:864, 2008.

Keeler KA, Dart B, Luhmann SJ, et al: Antegrade intramedullary nailing of pediatric femoral fractures using an interlocking pediatric femoral nail and a lateral trochanteric entry point, *J Pediatr Orthop* 29:345, 2009.

MacNeil JA, Francis A, El-Hawary R: A systematic review of rigid, locked intramedullary nail insertion sites and avascular necrosis of the femoral head in the skeletally immature, *J Pediatr Orthop* 31:377, 2011.

Mubarak SJ, Frick S, Sink E, et al: Volkman contracture and compartment syndromes after femoral fractures in children treated with 90/90 spica casts, *J Pediatr Orthop* 26:567, 2006.

Murphy R, Kelly DM, Moisan A, et al: Transverse fractures of the femoral shaft are a better predictor of nonaccidental trauma in young children than spiral fractures are, *J Bone Joint Surg* 97A:106, 2015.

Nayeemuddin M, Higgins GA, Bache E, et al: Complication rate after operative treatment of paediatric femoral neck fractures, *J Pediatr Orthop B* 18:314, 2009.

Pombo MW, Shilt JS: The definition and treatment of pediatric subtrochanteric femur fractures with titanium elastic nails, *J Pediatr Orthop* 26:364, 2006.

Ramseier LE, Bhaskar AR, Cole WG, Howard AW: Treatment of open femur fractures in children: comparison between external fixator and intramedullary nailing, *J Pediatr Orthop* 27:749, 2007.

Ramseier LE, Janicki JA, Weir S, Narayanan UG: Femoral fractures in adolescents: a comparison of four methods of fixation, *J Bone Joint Surg* 92A:1122, 2010.

Rathjen KE, Riccio AI, De La Garza D: Stainless steel flexible intramedullary fixation of unstable femoral shaft fractures in children, *J Pediatr Orthop* 27:432, 2007.

Rush JK, Kelly DM, Sawyer JR, et al: Treatment of pediatric femur fractures with the Pavlik harness: multiyear clinical and radiographic outcomes, *J Pediatr Orthop* 33:614, 2013.

Sagan ML, Datta JC, Olney BW, et al: Residual deformity after treatment of pediatric femur fractures with flexible titanium nails, *J Pediatr Orthop* 30:638, 2010.

Simanovsky N, Porat S, Simanovsky N, Eylon S: Close reduction and intramedullary flexible titanium nails fixation of femoral shaft fractures in children under 5 years of age, *J Pediatr Orthop B* 15:293, 2006.

Sink EL, Faro F, Polousky J, et al: Decreased complications of pediatric femur fractures with a change in management, *J Pediatr Orthop* 30:633, 2010.

Sink EL, Hedequist D, Morgan SJ, Hresko T: Results and technique of unstable pediatric femoral fractures treated with submuscular bridge plating, *J Pediatr Orthop* 26:177, 2006.

Wall EJ, Jain V, Vora V, et al: Complications of titanium and stainless steel elastic nail fixation of pediatric femoral fractures, *J Bone Joint Surg* 90A:1305, 2008.

KNEE FRACTURES AND DISLOCATIONS

Ares O, Seijas R, Cugat R, et al: Treatment of fractures of the tibial tuberosity in adolescent soccer players, *Acta Orthop Belg* 77:78, 2011.

Basener CJ, Mehlman CT, DiPasquale TG: Growth disturbance after distal femoral growth plate fractures in children: a meta-analysis, *J Orthop Trauma* 23:663, 2009.

Gaffney JT: Tibia fractures in children sustained on a playground slide, *J Pediatr Orthop* 29:606, 2009.

Gans I, Baldwin KD, Ganley TJ: Treatment and management outcomes of tibial eminence fractures in pediatric patients: a systematic review, *Am J Sports Med* 42:1743, 2013.

Hung NN: Using an iliotibial tract for patellar dislocation in children, *J Child Orthop* 2:343, 2008.

Kocher MS, Micheli LJ, Gerbino P, Hresko MT: Tibial eminence fractures in children: prevalence of meniscal entrapment, *Am J Sports Med* 31:404, 2003.

Liljeros K, Werner S, Janarv PM: Arthroscopic fixation of anterior tibial spine fractures with bioabsorbable nails in skeletally immature patients, *Am J Sports Med* 37:923, 2009.

Louis ML, Guillaume JB, Launay F, et al: Surgical management of type II tibial intercondylar eminence fractures in children, *J Pediatr Orthop B* 17:231, 2008.

Mubarak SJ, Kim JR, Edmonds EW, et al: Classification of proximal tibial fractures in children, *J Child Orthop* 3:191, 2009.

Nietosvaara Y, Paukku R, Palmu S, Donell ST: Acute patellar dislocation in children and adolescents: surgical technique, *J Bone Joint Surg* 91A(Suppl 2 Pt 1):139, 2009.

Oliva F, Ronga M, Longo UG, et al: The 3-in-1 procedure for recurrent dislocation of the patella in skeletally immature children and adolescents, *Am J Sports Med* 37:1814, 2009.

Palmu S, Kallio P, Donell ST, et al: Acute patellar dislocation in children and adolescents: a randomized clinical trial, *J Bone Joint Surg* 90A:463, 2008.

Patel NM, Park MJ, Sampson NR, Ganley TJ: Tibial eminence fractures in children: earlier posttreatment mobilization results in improved outcomes, *J Pediatr Orthop* 32:139, 2012.

Rademakers MV, Kerkhoffs GM, Kager J, et al: Tibial spine fractures: a long-term follow-up study of open reduction and internal fixation, *J Orthop Trauma* 23:203, 2009.

Schmal H, Strohm PC, Niemeyer P, et al: Fractures of the patella in children and adolescents, *Acta Orthop Belg* 76:644, 2010.

Vander Have KL, Ganley TJ, Kocher MS, et al: Arthrofibrosis after surgical fixation of tibial eminence fractures in children and adolescents, *Am J Sports Med* 38:298, 2010.

Walsh SJ, Boyle MJ, Morganti V: Large osteochondral fractures of the lateral femoral condyle in the adolescent: outcome of bioabsorbable pin fixation, *J Bone Joint Surg* 90A:1473, 2008.

Wilfinger C, Castellani C, Raith J, et al: Nonoperative treatment of tibial spine fractures in children: 38 patients with a minimum follow-up of 1 year, *J Orthop Trauma* 23:519, 2009.

TIBIAL AND FIBULAR FRACTURES

Cottalorda J, Béranger V, Louahem D, et al: Salter-Harris type III and IV medial malleolar fractures. Growth arrest: is it a fate? A retrospective study of 48 cases with open reduction, *J Pediatr Orthop* 28:652, 2008.

Domzalski ME, Lipton GE, Lee D, Guille JT: Fractures of the distal tibial metaphysis in children: patterns of injury and results of treatment, *J Pediatr Orthop* 26:171, 2006.

Glass GE, Pearse M, Nanchahal J: The ortho-plastic management of Gustilo grade IIIB fractures of the tibia in children: a systematic review of the literature, *Injury* 40:876, 2009.

Gordon JE, Gregush RV, Schoenecker PL, et al: Complications after titanium elastic nailing of pediatric tibial fractures, *J Pediatr Orthop* 27:442, 2007.

Jenkins MD, Jones DL, Billings AA, et al: Early weight bearing after complete tibial shaft fractures in children, *J Pediatr Orthop B* 18:341, 2009.

Laine JC, Cherkashin A, Samchukov M, et al: The management of soft tissue and bone loss in type IIIB and IIIC pediatric open tibia fractures, *J Pediatr Orthop* 36:453, 2015.

Podeszwa DA, Wilson PL, Hollard AR, Copley LAB: Comparison of bioabsorbable versus metallic implant fixation for physeal and epiphyseal fractures of the distal tibia, *J Pediatr Orthop* 28:859, 2008.

Rohmiller MT, Gaynor TP, Pawelek J, Mubarak SJ: Salter-Harris I and II fractures of the distal tibia: does mechanism of injury relate to premature physeal closure? *J Pediatr Orthop* 26:322, 2006.

Srivastava AK, Mehlman CT, Wall EJ, Do TT: Elastic stable intramedullary nailing of tibial shaft fractures in children, *J Pediatr Orthop* 28:152, 2008.

Vallamshetla VR, De Silva U, Bache CE, Gibbons PJ: Flexible intramedullary nails for unstable fractures of the tibia in children: an eight-year experience, *J Bone Joint Surg* 88B:536, 2006.

FOOT AND ANKLE FRACTURES

Ceroni D, De Rose V, De Coulon G, Kaelin A: Cuboid nutcracker fracture due to horseback riding in children: case series and review of the literature, *J Pediatr Orthop* 27:557, 2007.

Eberl R, Singer G, Schalamon J, et al: Fractures of the talus—differences between children and adolescents, *J Trauma* 68:126, 2010.

Herrera-Soto JA, Scherb M, Duffy MF, Albright JC: Fractures of the fifth metatarsal in children and adolescents, *J Pediatr Orthop* 27:427, 2007.

Oestreich AE, Bhojwani N: Stress fractures of ankle and wrist in childhood: nature and frequency, *Pediatr Radiol* 40:1387, 2010.

Petit CJ, Lee BM, Kasser JR, Kocher MS: Operative treatment of intraarticular calcaneal fractures in the pediatric population, *J Pediatr Orthop* 27:856, 2007.

Rosenberger RE, Fink C, Bale RJ, et al: Computer-assisted minimally invasive treatment of osteochondrosis dissecans of the talus, *Oper Orthop Traumatol* 4:300, 2006.

Senaran H, Mason D, De Pellegrin M: Cuboid fractures in preschool children, *J Pediatr Orthop* 26:741, 2006.

The complete list of references is available online at expertconsult.inkling.com.

PART XII

THE SPINE

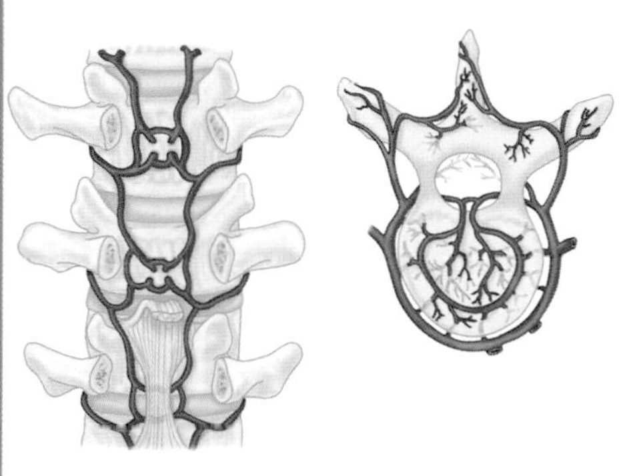

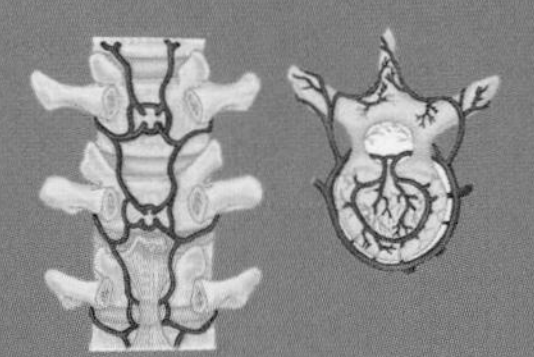

CHAPTER 37

SPINAL ANATOMY AND SURGICAL APPROACHES

Raymond J. Gardocki

ANATOMY OF VERTEBRAL COLUMN

The vertebral column comprises 33 vertebrae divided into five sections (7 cervical, 12 thoracic, 5 lumbar, 5 sacral, and 4 coccygeal) (Fig. 37-1). The sacral and coccygeal vertebrae are fused, which typically allows for 24 mobile segments. Congenital anomalies and variations in segmentation are common. The cervical and lumbar segments develop lordosis as an erect posture is acquired. The thoracic and sacral segments maintain kyphotic postures, which are found in utero, and serve as attachment points for the rib cage and pelvic girdle. In general, each mobile vertebral body increases in size when moving from cranial to caudal. A typical vertebra comprises an anterior body and a posterior arch that enclose the vertebral canal. The neural arch is composed of two pedicles laterally and two laminae posteriorly that are united to form the spinous process. To either side of the arch of the vertebral body is a transverse process and superior and inferior articular processes. The articular processes articulate with adjacent vertebrae to form synovial joints. The relative orientation of the articular processes accounts for the degree of flexion, extension, or rotation possible in each segment of the vertebral column. The spinous and transverse processes serve as levers for the numerous muscles attached to them. The length of the vertebral column averages 72 cm in men and 7 to 10 cm less in women. The vertebral canal extends throughout the length of the column and provides protection for the spinal cord, conus medullaris, and cauda equina.

ANATOMY OF SPINAL JOINTS

The individual vertebrae are connected by joints between the neural arches and between the bodies. The joints between the neural arches are the zygapophyseal joints or facet joints. They exist between the inferior articular process of one vertebra and the superior articular process of the vertebra immediately caudal. These are synovial joints with surfaces covered by articular cartilage, a synovial membrane bridging the margins of the articular cartilage, and a joint capsule enclosing them. The branches of the posterior primary rami innervate these joints.

The interbody joints contain specialized structures called *intervertebral discs.* These discs are found throughout the vertebral column except between the first and second cervical vertebrae. The discs are designed to accommodate movement, weight bearing, and shock by being strong but deformable. Each disc contains a pair of vertebral end plates with a central nucleus pulposus and a peripheral ring of anulus fibrosus sandwiched between them. They form a secondary cartilaginous joint or symphysis at each vertebral level.

The vertebral end plates are 1-mm-thick sheets of cartilage-fibrocartilage and hyaline cartilage with an increased ratio of fibrocartilage with increasing age. The nucleus pulposus is a semifluid mass of mucoid material, 70% to 90% water, with proteoglycan constituting 65% and collagen constituting 15% to 20% of the dry weight. The anulus fibrosus consists of 12 concentric lamellae, with alternating orientation of collagen fibers in successive lamellae to withstand multidirectional strain. The anulus is 60% to 70% water, with collagen constituting 50% to 60% and proteoglycan about 20% of the dry weight. With age, the proportions of proteoglycan and water decrease. The anulus and nucleus merge in a junctional zone without a strict demarcation. The discs are the largest avascular structures in the body and depend on diffusion from a specialized network of end plate blood vessels for nutrition.

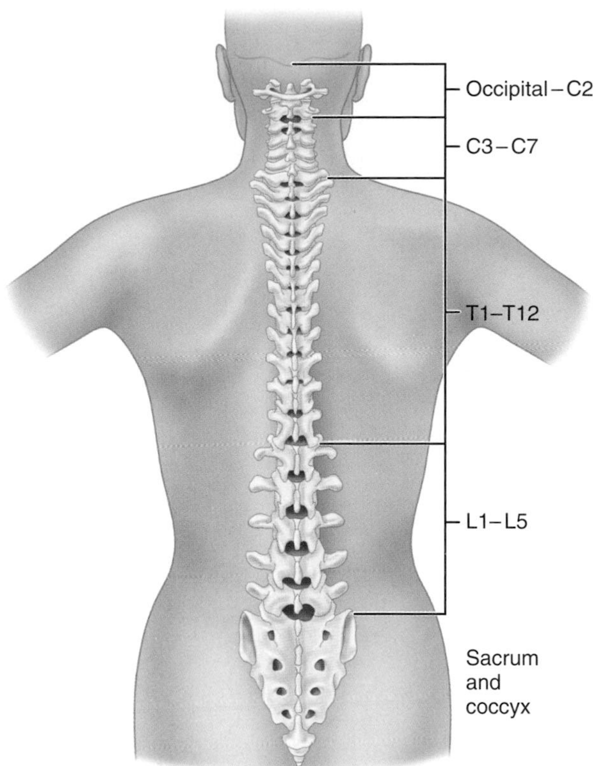

FIGURE 37-1 Vertebral column: upper cervical vertebrae (occiput to C2), lower cervical vertebrae (C3-7), thoracic vertebrae (T1-12), lumbar vertebrae (L1-5), sacrum, and coccyx.

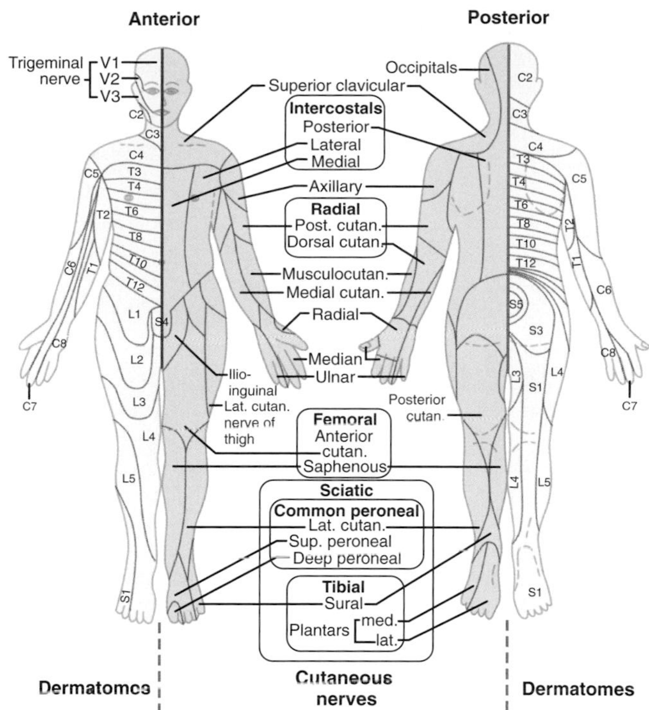

FIGURE 37-2 Dermatomal and sensory distribution. (Redrawn from Patton HD, Sundsten JW, Crill WE, et al, editors: Introduction to basic neurology, Philadelphia, 1976, WB Saunders.)

ANATOMY OF SPINAL CORD AND NERVES

The spinal cord is shorter than the vertebral column and terminates as the conus medullaris at the second lumbar vertebra in adults and the third lumbar vertebra in neonates. From the conus, a fibrous cord called the *filum terminale* extends to the dorsum of the first coccygeal segment. The spinal cord is enclosed in three protective membranes—the pia, arachnoid, and dura mater. The pia and arachnoid membranes are separated by the subarachnoid space, which contains the cerebrospinal fluid. The spinal cord has enlargements in the cervical and lumbar regions that correlate with the brachial plexus and lumbar plexus. Within the spinal cord are tracts of ascending (sensory) and descending (motor) nerve fibers. These pathways typically are arranged with cervical tracts located centrally and thoracic, lumbar, and sacral tracts located progressively peripheral. This accounts for the clinical findings of central cord syndrome and syrinx. Understanding the location of these tracts aids in understanding different spinal cord syndromes (Figs. 37-2 and 37-3; Table 37-1).

Spinal nerves exit the canal at each level. Spinal nerves C2-7 exit above the pedicle for which they are named (the C6 nerve root exits the foramen between the C5 and C6 pedicles). The C8 nerve root exits the foramen between the C7 and T1 pedicles. All spinal nerves caudal to C8 exit the foramen below the pedicle for which they are named (the L4 nerve root exits the foramen between the L4 and L5 pedicles). The final dermatomal and sensory nerve distributions are shown in Figure

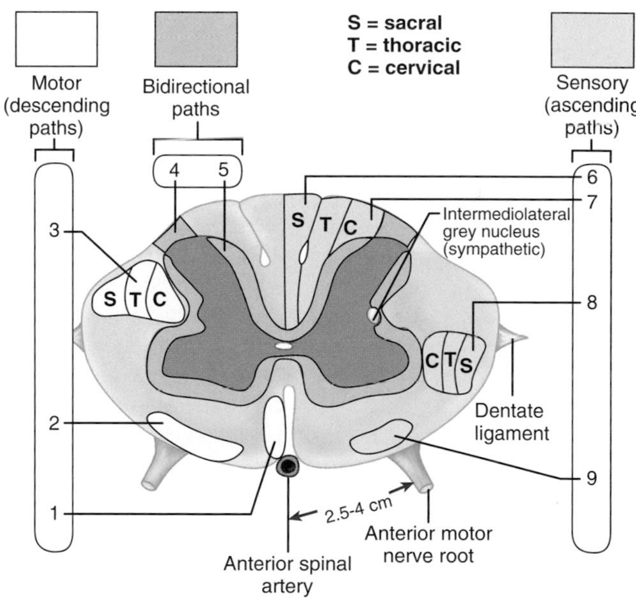

FIGURE 37-3 Schematic cross section of cervical spinal cord. (Redrawn from Patton HD, Sundsten JW, Crill WE, et al, editors: Introduction to basic neurology, Philadelphia, 1976, WB Saunders.)

37-2. Because the spinal cord is shorter than the vertebral column, the spinal nerves course more vertically as one moves caudally. Each level gives off a dorsal (sensory) root and a ventral (mostly motor) root, which combine to form the mixed spinal nerve. The dorsal root of each spinal nerve has a ganglion located near the exit zone of each foramen. This dorsal

TABLE 37-1

Ascending and Descending (Motor) Tracts

NUMBER (SEE FIG. 37-3)	PATH	FUNCTION	SIDE OF BODY
1	Anterior corticospinal tract	Skilled movement	Opposite
2	Vestibulospinal tract	Facilitates extensor muscle tone	Same
3	Lateral corticospinal (pyramidal tract)	Skilled movement	Same
4	Dorsolateral fasciculus	Pain and temperature	Bidirectional
5	Fasciculus proprius	Short spinal connections	Bidirectional
6	Fasciculus gracilis	Position/fine touch	Same
7	Fasciculus cuneatus	Position/fine touch	Same
8	Lateral spinothalamic tract	Pain and temperature	Opposite
9	Anterior spinothalamic tract	Light touch	Opposite

Modified from Patton HD, Sundsten JW, Crill WE, Swanson PD, editors: Introduction to basic neurology, Philadelphia, 1976, WB Saunders.

root ganglion is the synapse point for the ascending sensory cell bodies. This structure is sensitive to pressure and heat and can cause a dysesthetic pain response if manipulated.

ANATOMY OF CERVICAL, THORACIC, AND LUMBAR PEDICLES

Numerous studies have documented the anatomic morphology of the cervical, thoracic, and lumbar vertebrae. Advanced internal fixation techniques, including pedicle screws, have been developed and used extensively in spine surgery, not only for traumatic injuries but also for degenerative conditions. As the role for anterior and posterior spinal instrumentation continues to evolve, understanding the morphologic characteristics of the human vertebrae is crucial in avoiding complications during fixation.

Placement of screws in the cervical pedicles is controversial and carries more risk than anterior plate or lateral mass fixation. Although cervical pedicles can be suitable for screw fixation, uniformly sized cervical pedicle screws cannot be used at every level. Screw placement in the pedicles at C3, C4, and C5 requires smaller screws (<4.5 mm) and more care in placement than those of the other cervical vertebrae. CT measurements of cervical pedicle morphology found that C2 and C7 pedicles had larger mean interdiameters than all other cervical vertebrae, and that C3 had the smallest mean interdiameter. The outer pedicle width-to-height ratio increased from C2 to C7, indicating that pedicles in the upper cervical spine (C2-4) are elongated, whereas pedicles in the lower cervical spine (C6-7) are rounded. It also is crucial to know that cervical pedicles angle medially at all levels, with the most medial angulation at C5 and the least at C2 and C7. The pedicles slope upward at C2 and C3, are parallel at C4 and C5, and are angled downward at C6 and C7.

The vertebral artery from C3 to C6 is at significant risk for iatrogenic injury during pedicle screw placement. The pedicle cortex is not uniformly thick. The thinnest portion of the cortex (the lateral cortex) protects the vertebral artery, and the medial cortex toward the spinal cord is almost twice as thick as the lateral cortex. Variations in the course of the vertebral artery also place it at risk during placement of pedicle screws. At the C2 and C7-T1 levels, the vertebral artery is less at risk during pedicle screw fixation. The vertebral artery follows a more posterior and lateral course at C2, whereas at C7-T1 it is outside the transverse foramen.

Pedicle dimensions and angles change progressively from the upper thoracic spine distally. A thorough knowledge of these relationships is important when considering the use of the pedicle as a screw purchase site. A study of 2905 pedicle measurements made from T1 to L5 found that pedicles were widest at L5 and narrowest at T5 in the horizontal plane (Fig. 37-4). The widest pedicles in the sagittal plane were at T11, and the narrowest were at T1. Because of the oval shape of the pedicle, the sagittal plane width was generally larger than the horizontal plane width. The largest pedicle angle in the horizontal plane was at L5. In the sagittal plane, the pedicles angle caudad at L5 and cephalad at L3-T1. The depth to the anterior cortex was significantly longer along the pedicle axis than along a line parallel to the midline of the vertebral body at all levels except T12 and L1.

The thoracic pedicle is a convoluted, three-dimensional structure that is filled mostly with cancellous bone (62% to 79%). Panjabi et al. showed that the cortical shell is of variable density throughout its perimeter and that the lateral wall is significantly thinner than the medial wall. This seemed to be true for all levels of thoracic vertebrae.

The locations for screw insertion have been identified and described in several studies. The respective facet joint space and the middle of the transverse process are the most important reference points. An opening is made in the pedicle with a drill or hand-held curet, after which a self-tapping screw is passed through the pedicle into the vertebral body. The pedicles of the thoracic and lumbar vertebrae are tubelike bony structures that connect the anterior and posterior columns of the spine. Medial to the medial wall of the pedicle lies the dural sac. Inferior to the medial wall of the pedicle is the nerve root in the neural foramen. The lumbar roots usually are situated in the upper third of the foramen; it is more dangerous to penetrate the pedicle medially or inferiorly as opposed to laterally or superiorly.

We use three techniques for open localization of the pedicle: (1) the intersection technique, (2) the pars interarticularis technique, and (3) the mammillary process technique. It is important in preoperative planning to assess

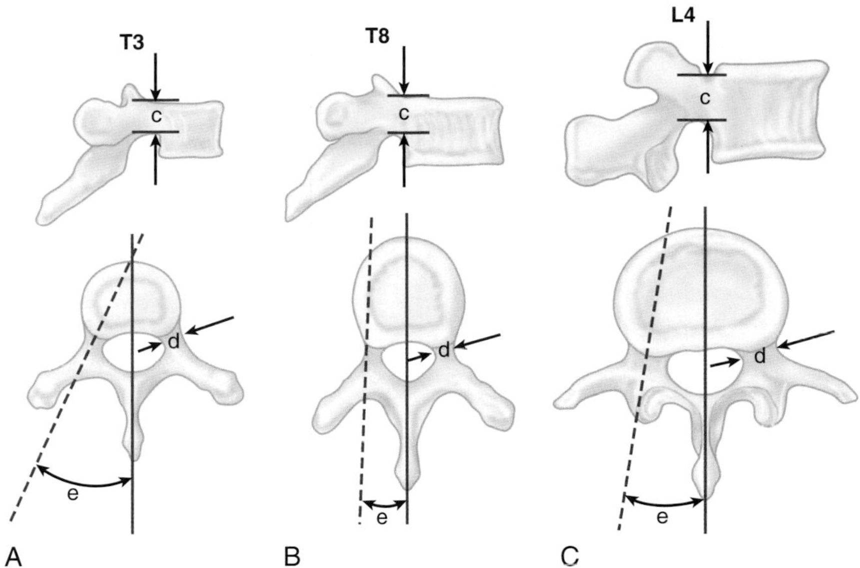

FIGURE 37-4 Pedicle dimensions of T3 **(A)**, T8 **(B)**, and L4 **(C)** vertebrae. Vertical diameter *(c)* increases from 0.7 to 1.5 cm, horizontal diameter *(d)* increases from 0.7 to 1.6 cm with minimum of 0.5 cm in T5. Direction is almost sagittal from T4 to L4. Angle *(e)* seldom extends beyond 10 degrees. More proximally, direction is more oblique: T1 = 36 degrees, T2 – 34 degrees, T3 = 23 degrees. L5 is oblique (30 degrees) but is large and easy to drill. (Redrawn from Roy-Camille R, Saillant G, Mazel CH: Plating of thoracic, thoracolumbar, and lumbar injuries with pedicle screw plates, Orthop Clin North Am 17:147, 1986.)

individual spinal anatomy with the use of high-quality anteroposterior and lateral radiographs of the lumbar and thoracic spine and axial CT or MRI at the level of the pedicle. In the lumbar spine, coaxial fluoroscopy images are a reliable guide to the true bony cortex of the pedicle. The intersection technique is perhaps the most commonly used method of localizing the pedicle. It involves dropping a line from the lateral aspect of the facet joint, which intersects a line that bisects the transverse process at a spot overlying the pedicle (Figs. 37-5 and 37-6). The pars interarticularis is the area of bone where the pedicle connects to the lamina. Because the laminae and the pars interarticularis can be identified easily at surgery, they provide landmarks by which a pedicular drill starting point can be made. The mammillary process technique is based on a small prominence of bone at the base of the transverse process. This mammillary process can be used as a starting point for transpedicular drilling. Usually the mammillary process is more lateral than the intersection technique starting point, which also is more lateral than the pars interarticularis starting point. With this in mind, different angles must be used when drilling from these sites. With the help of preoperative CT scanning or MRI at the level of the pedicle and intraoperative fluoroscopy, the angle of the pedicle to the sagittal and horizontal planes can be determined.

For percutaneous pedicle screw placement, we use fluoroscopy that is orthogonal to the target vertebral body in the anteroposterior and lateral planes and allows clear visualization of the medial wall of the pedicle and pedicle/vertebral body junction. A Jamshidi needle typically is docked on the pedicle of interest at the lamina/pedicle junction on the anteroposterior view (9 o'clock position for left pedicles and 3 o'clock position for right pedicles). For the most cephalad screw of a construct in the lumbar spine, we prefer to "cheat" the starting point a little below midline on the

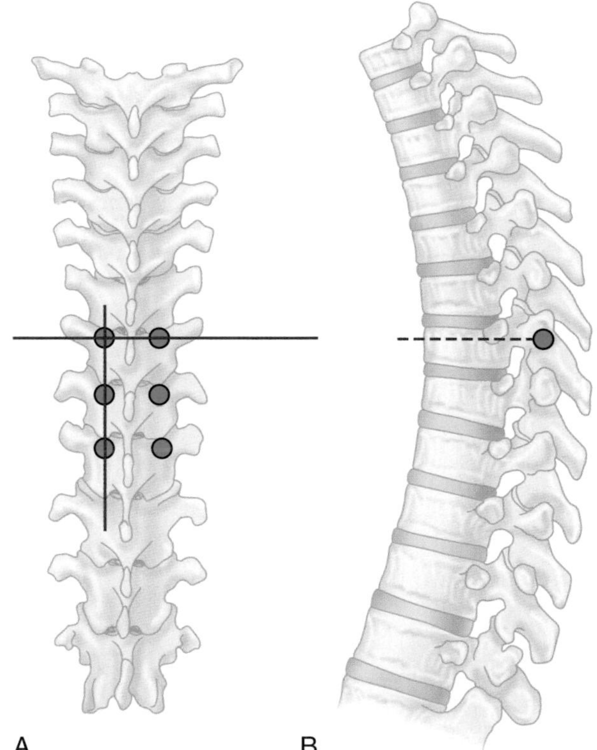

FIGURE 37-5 Pedicle entrance point in thoracic spine at intersection of lines drawn through middle of inferior articular facets and middle of insertion of transverse processes (1 mm below facet joint). **A,** Anteroposterior view. **B,** Lateral view. (Redrawn from Roy-Camille R, Saillant G, Mazel CH: Plating of thoracic, thoracolumbar, and lumbar injuries with pedicle screw plates, Orthop Clin North Am 17:147, 1986.)

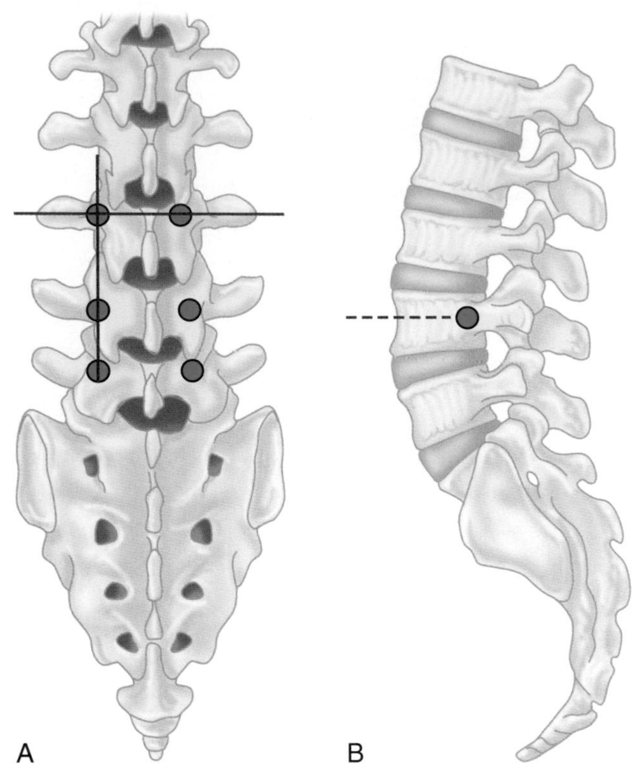

FIGURE 37-6 Pedicle entrance point in lumbar spine at intersection of two lines. On typical bony crest, it is 1 mm below articular joint. **A,** Anteroposterior view. **B,** Lateral view. (Redrawn from Roy-Camille R, Saillant G, Mazel CH: Plating of thoracic, thoracolumbar, and lumbar injuries with pedicle screw plates, Orthop Clin North Am 17:147, 1986.)

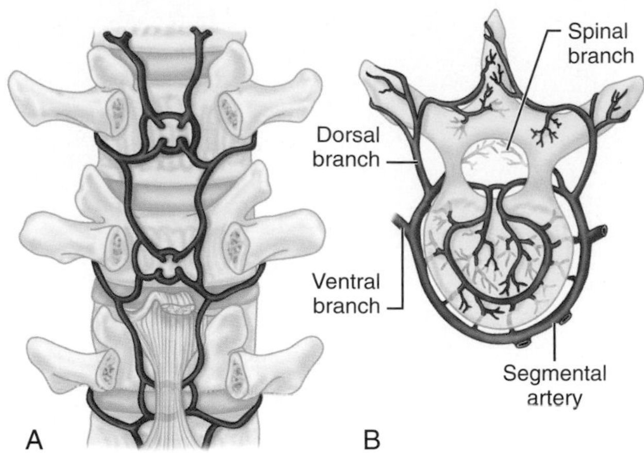

FIGURE 37-7 Vertebral blood supply. **A,** Posterior view; laminae removed to show anastomosing spinal branches of segmental arteries. **B,** Cross-sectional view; anastomosing arterial supply of vertebral body, spinal canal, and posterior elements. (Redrawn from Bullough PG, Oheneba BA: Atlas of spinal diseases, Philadelphia, 1988, JB Lippincott.)

anteroposterior view (8 o'clock for left pedicles and 4 o'clock for right pedicles) to limit encroachment of the next cephalad facet joint. Under anteroposterior imaging, the needle is then advanced down the pedicle 20 to 25 mm at a trajectory that will allow the tip of the needle to be placed at the pedicle/vertebral body junction without violating the medial wall of the pedicle. When seated, the needle should pass obliquely across the pedicle with the tip just lateral to the medial wall on the anteroposterior view and just deep to the base of the pedicle on the lateral view. This will allow passage of a guidewire into the vertebral body and placement of a cannulated percutaneous pedicle screw using a Seldinger technique. The technique of connecting rod passage depends on the hardware manufacturer.

CIRCULATION OF SPINAL CORD

The arterial supply to the spinal cord has been determined from gross anatomic dissection, latex arterial injections, and intercostal arteriography. Dommisse contributed significantly to knowledge of the blood supply, stating that the principles that govern the blood supply of the cord are constant, whereas the patterns vary with the individual. He emphasized the following factors:

1. *Dependence on three vessels.* These are the anterior median longitudinal arterial trunk and a pair of posterolateral trunks near the posterior nerve rootlets.
2. *Relative demands of gray matter and white matter.* The longitudinal arterial trunks are largest in the cervical and lumbar regions near the ganglionic enlargements and are much smaller in the thoracic region. This is because the metabolic demands of the gray matter are greater than those of the white matter, which contains fewer capillary networks.
3. *Medullary feeder (radicular) arteries of the cord.* These arteries reinforce the longitudinal arterial channels. There are 2 to 17 anteriorly and 6 to 25 posteriorly. The vertebral arteries supply 80% of the radicular arteries in the neck; arteries in the thoracic and lumbar areas arise from the aorta. The lateral sacral, the fifth lumbar, the iliolumbar, and the middle sacral arteries are important in the sacral region.
4. *Supplementary source of blood supply to the spinal cord.* The vertebral and posterior inferior cerebellar arteries are important sources of arterial supply. Sacral medullary feeders arise from the lateral sacral arteries and accompany the distal roots of the cauda equina. The flow in these vessels seems reversible and the volume adjustable in response to the metabolic demands.
5. *Segmental arteries of the spine.* At every vertebral level, a pair of segmental arteries supplies the extraspinal and intraspinal structures. The thoracic and lumbar segmental arteries arise from the aorta; the cervical segmental arteries arise from the vertebral arteries and the costocervical and thyrocervical trunks. In 60% of individuals, an additional source arises from the ascending pharyngeal branch of the external carotid artery. The lateral sacral arteries and, to a lesser extent, the fifth lumbar, iliolumbar, and middle sacral arteries supply segmental vessels in the sacral region.
5. *"Distribution point" of the segmental arteries.* The segmental arteries divide into numerous branches at the intervertebral foramen, which has been termed the *distribution point* (Fig. 37-7). A second anastomotic

network lies within the spinal canal in the loose connective tissue of the extradural space. This occurs at all levels, with the greatest concentration in the cervical and lumbar regions. The presence of the rich anastomotic channels offers alternative pathways for arterial flow, preserving spinal cord circulation after the ligation of segmental arteries.

6. *Artery of Adamkiewicz.* The artery of Adamkiewicz is the largest of the feeders of the lumbar cord; it is located on the left side, usually at the level of T9-11 (in 80% of individuals). The anterior longitudinal arterial channel of the cord rather than any single medullary feeder is crucial. The preservation of this large feeder does not ensure continued satisfactory circulation for the spinal cord. In principle, it would seem of practical value to protect and preserve each contributing artery as far as is surgically possible.
7. *Variability of patterns of supply of the spinal cord.* The variability of blood supply is a striking feature, yet there is absolute conformity with a principle of a rich supply for the cervical and lumbar cord enlargements. The supply for the thoracic cord from approximately T4 to T9 is much poorer.
8. *Direction of flow in the blood vessels of the spinal cord.* The three longitudinal arterial channels of the spinal cord can be compared with the circle of Willis at the base of the brain, but it is more extensive and more complicated, although it functions with identical principles. These channels permit reversal of flow and alterations in the volume of blood flow in response to metabolic demands. This internal arterial circle of the cord is surrounded by at least two outer arterial circles, the first of which is situated in the extradural space and the second in the extravertebral tissue planes. By virtue of the latter, the spinal cord enjoys reserve sources of blood supply through a degree of anastomosis lacking in the inner circle. The "outlet points" are limited, however, to the perforating sulcal arteries and the pial arteries of the cord.

The blood supply to the spinal cord is rich, but the spinal canal is narrowest and the blood supply is poorest at T4-9. T4-9 should be considered the critical vascular zone of the spinal cord, a zone in which interference with the circulation is most likely to result in paraplegia.

The dominance of the anterior spinal artery system has been challenged by the fact that many anterior spinal surgeries have been performed in recent years with no increase in the incidence of paralysis. This would seem to indicate that a rich anastomotic supply does exist and that it protects the spinal cord. The evidence suggests that the posterior spinal arteries may be as important as the anterior system but are as yet poorly understood. Venous drainage of the spinal cord is more difficult to define clearly than is the arterial supply (Fig. 37-8). It is well known that the venous system is highly variable. Dommisse pointed out that there are two sets of veins: veins of the spinal cord and veins that fall within the plexiform network of Batson. The veins of the spinal cord are a small component of the entire system and drain into the plexus of Batson. The Batson plexus is a large and complex venous channel extending from the base of the skull to the coccyx. It communicates directly with the superior and inferior vena cava system and the azygos system. The longitudinal venous trunks of the spinal cord are the anterior and posterior venous channels, which are the counterparts of the arterial trunks. The three components of the Batson plexus are the extradural vertebral venous plexus; the extravertebral venous plexus, which includes the segmental veins of the neck, the intercostal veins, the azygos communications in the thorax and pelvis, the lumbar veins, and the communications with the inferior vena caval system; and the veins of the bony structures of the spinal column. The venous system plays no specific role in the metabolism of the spinal cord; it communicates directly with the venous system draining the head, chest, and abdomen. This interconnection allows metastatic spread of neoplastic or infectious disease from the pelvis to the vertebral column.

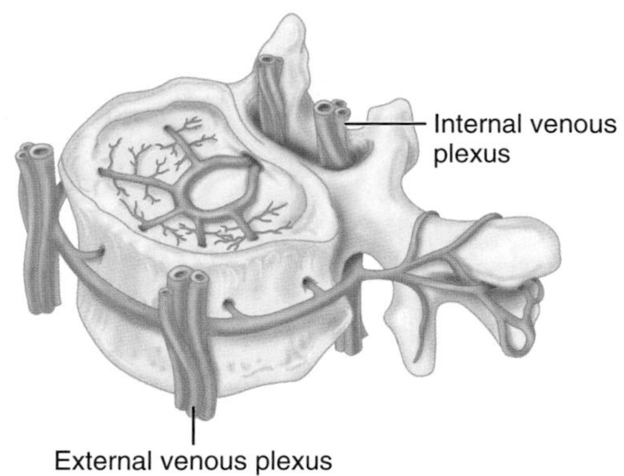

FIGURE 37-8 Venous drainage of vertebral bodies and formation of internal and external vertebral venous plexuses. (Redrawn from Bullough PG, Oheneba BA: Atlas of spinal diseases, Philadelphia, 1988, JB Lippincott.)

During anterior spinal surgery, we empirically follow these principles: (1) ligate segmental spinal arteries only as necessary to gain exposure; (2) ligate segmental spinal arteries near the aorta rather than near the vertebral foramina; (3) ligate segmental spinal arteries on one side only when possible, leaving the circulation intact on the opposite side; and (4) limit dissection in the vertebral foramina to a single level when possible so that collateral circulation is disturbed as little as possible.

SURGICAL APPROACHES

ANTERIOR APPROACHES

With the posterior approach for correction of spinal deformities well established, more attention has been placed on the anterior approach to the spinal column. Many pioneers in the field of anterior spinal surgery recognized that anterior spinal cord decompression was necessary in spinal tuberculosis and that laminectomy not only failed to relieve anterior pressure but also removed important posterior stability and produced worsening of kyphosis. Advances in major surgical procedures, including anesthesia and intensive care, have made it possible to perform spinal surgery with acceptable safety.

In general, anterior approaches to the spine are indicated for decompression of the neural elements (spinal cord, conus medullaris, cauda equina, or nerve roots) when anterior neural compression has been documented by myelography,

BOX 37-1

Relative Indications for Anterior Spinal Approaches

1. Traumatic
   a. Fractures with documented neurocompression secondary to bone or disc fragments anterior to dura
   b. Incomplete spinal cord injury (for cord recovery) with anterior extradural compression
   c. Complete spinal cord injury (for root recovery) with anterior extradural compression
   d. Late pain or paralysis after remote injuries with anterior extradural compression
   e. Herniated intervertebral disc
2. Infectious
   a. Open biopsy for diagnosis
   b. Debridement and anterior strut grafting
3. Degenerative
   a. Cervical spondylitic radiculopathy
   b. Cervical spondylitic myelopathy
   c. Thoracic disc herniation
   d. Cervical, thoracic, and lumbar interbody fusions
4. Neoplastic
   a. Extradural metastatic disease
   b. Primary vertebral body tumor
5. Deformity
   a. Kyphosis—congenital or acquired
   b. Scoliosis—congenital, acquired, or idiopathic

postmyelogram CT, or MRI. Many pathologic entities can cause significant compression of the neural elements, including traumatic, neoplastic, inflammatory, degenerative, and congenital lesions. In the lumbar spine, this indication has been expanded to include anterior interbody fusions for discogenic pain and instability.

Anterior approaches to the spine generally are made by an experienced spine surgeon, and, as a rule, it is inappropriate for surgeons who only occasionally perform spinal techniques to perform this type of surgery. In many centers, a team approach is preferred to employ the skills of an orthopaedic surgeon, neurosurgeon, thoracic surgeon, or head and neck surgeon. The orthopaedic surgeon still must have a working knowledge of the underlying viscera, fluid balance, physiology, and other elements of intensive care. Complications of anterior spine surgery are rare; however, there is a high risk of significant morbidity, and these approaches should be used with care and only in appropriate circumstances. Potential dangers include iatrogenic injury to vascular, visceral, or neurologic structures.

The exact incidence of serious complications from anterior spinal surgery is unknown. A thorough understanding of anatomic tissue planes and meticulous surgical technique are necessary to prevent serious complications. The choice of approach depends on the preference and experience of the surgeon, the patient's age and medical condition, the segment of the spine involved, the underlying pathologic process, and the presence or absence of signs of neural compression. Commonly accepted indications for anterior approaches are listed in Box 37-1.

ANTERIOR APPROACH, OCCIPUT TO C3

The anterior approach to the upper cervical spine (occiput to C3) can be transoral or retropharyngeal, depending on the pathologic process present and the experience of the surgeon.

ANTERIOR TRANSORAL APPROACH

TECHNIQUE 37-1 *Figure 37-9*

(SPETZLER)

- Position the patient supine using a Mayfield head-holding device or with skeletal traction through Gardner-Wells tongs. Monitoring of the spinal cord through somatosensory evoked potentials is recommended. The surgeon may sit directly over the patient's head.
- Pass a red rubber catheter down each nostril and suture it to the uvula. Apply traction to the catheters to pull the uvula and soft palate out of the operative field, taking care not to cause necrosis of the septal cartilage by excessive pressure.
- Insert a McGarver retractor into the open mouth and use it to retract and hold the endotracheal tube out of the way. The operating microscope is useful to improve the limited exposure.
- Prepare the oropharynx with hexachlorophene (pHisoHex) and povidone-iodine (Betadine).
- Palpate the anterior ring of C1 beneath the posterior pharynx and make an incision in the wall of the posterior pharynx from the superior aspect of C1 to the top of C3.
- Obtain hemostasis with bipolar electrocautery, taking care not to overcauterize, producing thermal necrosis of tissue and increased risk of infection.
- With a periosteal elevator, subperiosteally dissect the edges of the pharyngeal incision from the anterior ring

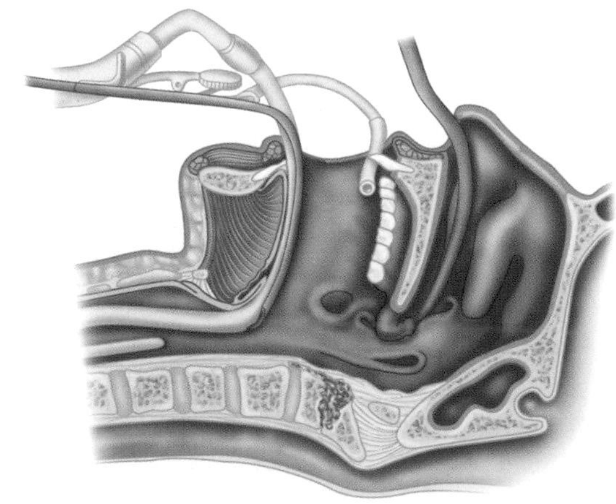

FIGURE 37-9 **Anterior transoral approach (see text).** (Redrawn from Spetzler RF: Transoral approach to the upper cervical spine. In Evarts CM, editor: *Surgery of the musculoskeletal system,* New York, 1983, Churchill Livingstone.) **SEE TECHNIQUE 37-1.**

of C1 and the anterior aspect of C2. Use traction stitches to maintain the flaps out of the way.

- Under direct vision, with the operating microscope or with magnification loupes and headlights, perform a meticulous debridement of C1 and C2 with a high-speed air drill, rongeur, or curet. When approaching the posterior longitudinal ligament, a diamond burr is safer to use in removing the last remnant of bone.
- When adequate debridement of infected bone and necrotic tissue has been accomplished, decompress the upper cervical spinal cord.
- If the cervical spine is to be fused anteriorly, harvest a corticocancellous graft from the patient's iliac crest, fashion it to fit, and insert it.
- Irrigate the operative site with antibiotic solution and close the posterior pharynx in layers.

POSTOPERATIVE CARE. An endotracheal tube is left in place overnight to maintain an adequate airway. A halo vest can be applied, or skeletal traction may be maintained before mobilization.

ANTERIOR RETROPHARYNGEAL APPROACH

The anterior retropharyngeal approach to the upper cervical spine, as described by McAfee et al., is excellent for anterior debridement of the upper cervical spine and allows placement of bone grafts for stabilization if necessary. In contrast to the transoral approach, it is entirely extramucosal and is reported to have fewer complications of wound infection and neurologic deficit.

TECHNIQUE 37-2

(MCAFEE ET AL.)

- Position the patient supine, preferably on a turning frame with skeletal traction through tongs or a halo ring. Somatosensory evoked potential monitoring of cord function is suggested during the procedure.
- Perform fiberoptic nasotracheal intubation to prevent excessive motion of the neck and to keep the oropharynx free of tubes that could depress the mandible and interfere with subsequent exposure.
- Make a right-sided transverse skin incision in the submandibular region with a vertical extension as long as required to provide adequate exposure (Fig. 37-10A). If the approach does not have to be extended below the level of the fifth cervical vertebra, there is no increased risk of damage to the recurrent laryngeal nerve.
- Carry the dissection through the platysma muscle with the enveloping superficial fascia of the neck and mobilize flaps from this area.
- Identify the marginal mandibular branch of the seventh nerve with the help of a nerve stimulator and ligate the retromandibular veins superiorly.
- Keep the dissection deep to the retromandibular vein to prevent injury to the superficial branches of the facial nerve.
- Ligate the retromandibular vein as it joins the internal jugular vein.
- Mobilize the anterior border of the sternocleidomastoid muscle by longitudinally dividing the superficial layer of the deep cervical fascia. Feel for the pulsations of the carotid artery and protect the contents of the carotid sheath.
- Resect the submandibular gland (Fig. 37-10B) and ligate the duct to prevent formation of a salivary fistula.
- Identify the digastric and stylohyoid muscles and tag and divide the tendon of the former. The facial nerve can be injured by superior retraction on the stylohyoid muscle; however, by dividing the digastric and stylohyoid muscles, the hyoid bone and hypopharynx can be mobilized medially, preventing exposure of the esophagus, hypopharynx, and nasopharynx.
- Identify the hypoglossal nerve and retract it superiorly.
- Continue dissection to the retropharyngeal space between the carotid sheath laterally and the larynx and pharynx medially. Increase exposure by ligating branches of the carotid artery and internal jugular vein, which prevent retraction of the carotid sheath laterally (Fig. 37-10C and D).
- Identify and mobilize the superior laryngeal nerve.
- Following adequate retraction of the carotid sheath laterally, divide the alar and prevertebral fascial layers longitudinally to expose the longus colli muscles. Take care to maintain the head in a neutral position and identify the midline accurately.
- Remove the longus colli muscles subperiosteally from the anterior aspect of the arch of C1 and the body of C2, avoiding injury to the vertebral arteries.
- Meticulously debride the involved osseous structures (Fig. 37-10E); if needed, perform bone grafting with autogenous iliac or fibular bone.
- Close the wound over suction drains and repair the digastric tendon. Close the platysma and skin flaps in layers.

POSTOPERATIVE CARE. The patient is maintained in skeletal traction with the head of the bed elevated to reduce swelling. Intubation is continued until pharyngeal edema has resolved, usually by 48 hours. The patient can be extubated and mobilized in a halo vest, or, if indicated, a posterior stabilization procedure can be done before mobilization.

EXTENDED MAXILLOTOMY AND SUBTOTAL MAXILLECTOMY

Cocke et al. described an extended maxillotomy and subtotal maxillectomy as an alternative to the transoral approach for exposure and removal of tumor or bone anteriorly at the base of the skull and cervical spine to C5. This procedure is technically demanding and requires a thorough knowledge of head and neck anatomy. It should be performed by a team of surgeons, including an otolaryngologist, a neurosurgeon, and an orthopaedist.

Before surgery, the size, position, and extent of the tumor or bone to be removed should be determined using the

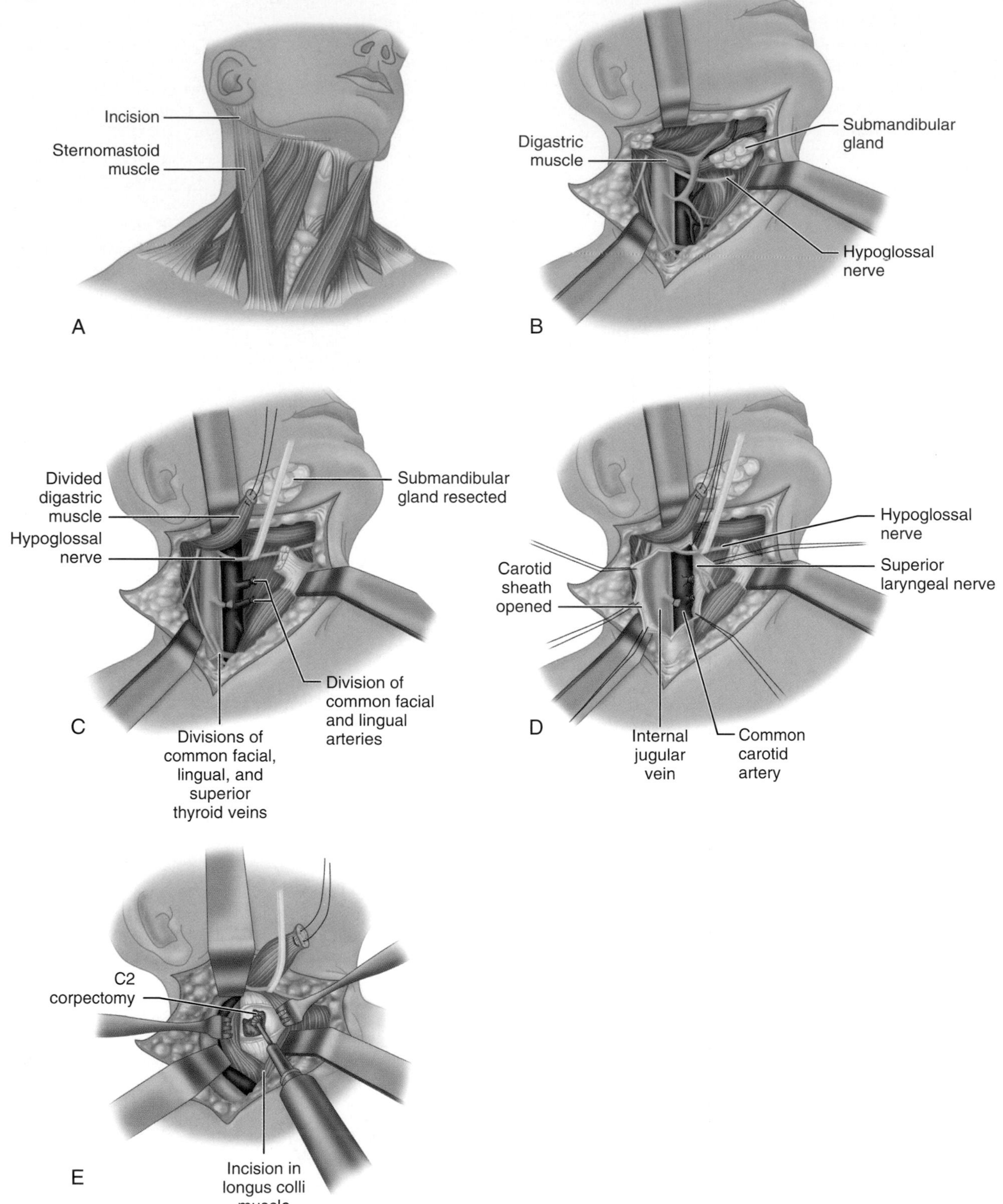

FIGURE 37-10 **A-E, Anterior retropharyngeal approach (see text).** (Redrawn from McAfee PC, Bohlman HH, Riley LH Jr, et al: The anterior retropharyngeal approach to the upper part of the cervical spine, J Bone Joint Surg 69A:1371, 1987.) **SEE TECHNIQUE 37-2**.

appropriate imaging techniques. Three to 5 days before the surgery, nasal, oral, and pharyngeal secretions are cultured to determine the proper antibiotics needed. Cephalosporin and aminoglycoside antibiotics are given before and after surgery if the floral cultures are normal and are adjusted if the flora is abnormal or resistant to these drugs.

SUBTOTAL MAXILLECTOMY

TECHNIQUE 37-3

(COCKE ET AL.)

- Position the patient on the operating table with the head elevated 25 degrees. Intubate the patient orally and move the tube to the contralateral side of the mouth.
- Perform a percutaneous endoscopic gastrostomy if the wound is to be left open or if problems are anticipated.
- Perform a tracheostomy if the exposure may be limited or if there are severe pulmonary problems. This step usually is unnecessary.
- Insert a Foley catheter and suture the eyelids closed with 6-0 nylon.
- Infiltrate the soft tissues of the upper lip, cheek, gingiva, palate, pterygoid fossa, nasopharynx, nasal septum, nasal floor, and lateral nasal wall with 1% lidocaine and 1:100,000 epinephrine.
- Pack each nasal cavity with cottonoid strips saturated with 4% cocaine and 1% phenylephrine.
- Prepare the skin with povidone-iodine and then alcohol. Drape the operative site with cloth drapes held in place with sutures or surgical clips and covered with a transparent surgical drape.
- Expose the superior maxilla through a modified Weber-Ferguson skin incision (Fig. 37-11A). Make a vertical incision through the upper lip in the philtrum from the nasolabial groove to the vermilion border. Extend the lower end to the midline and vertically in the midline through the buccal mucosa to the gingivobuccal gutter. Divide the upper lip and ligate the labial arteries. Extend the external skin incision transversely from the upper end of the lip incision in the nasolabial groove to beyond the nasal ala and superiorly along the nasofacial groove to the lower eyelid.
- Extract the central incisor tooth.
- Make a vertical midline incision through the mucoperiosteum of the anterior maxilla from the gingivobuccal

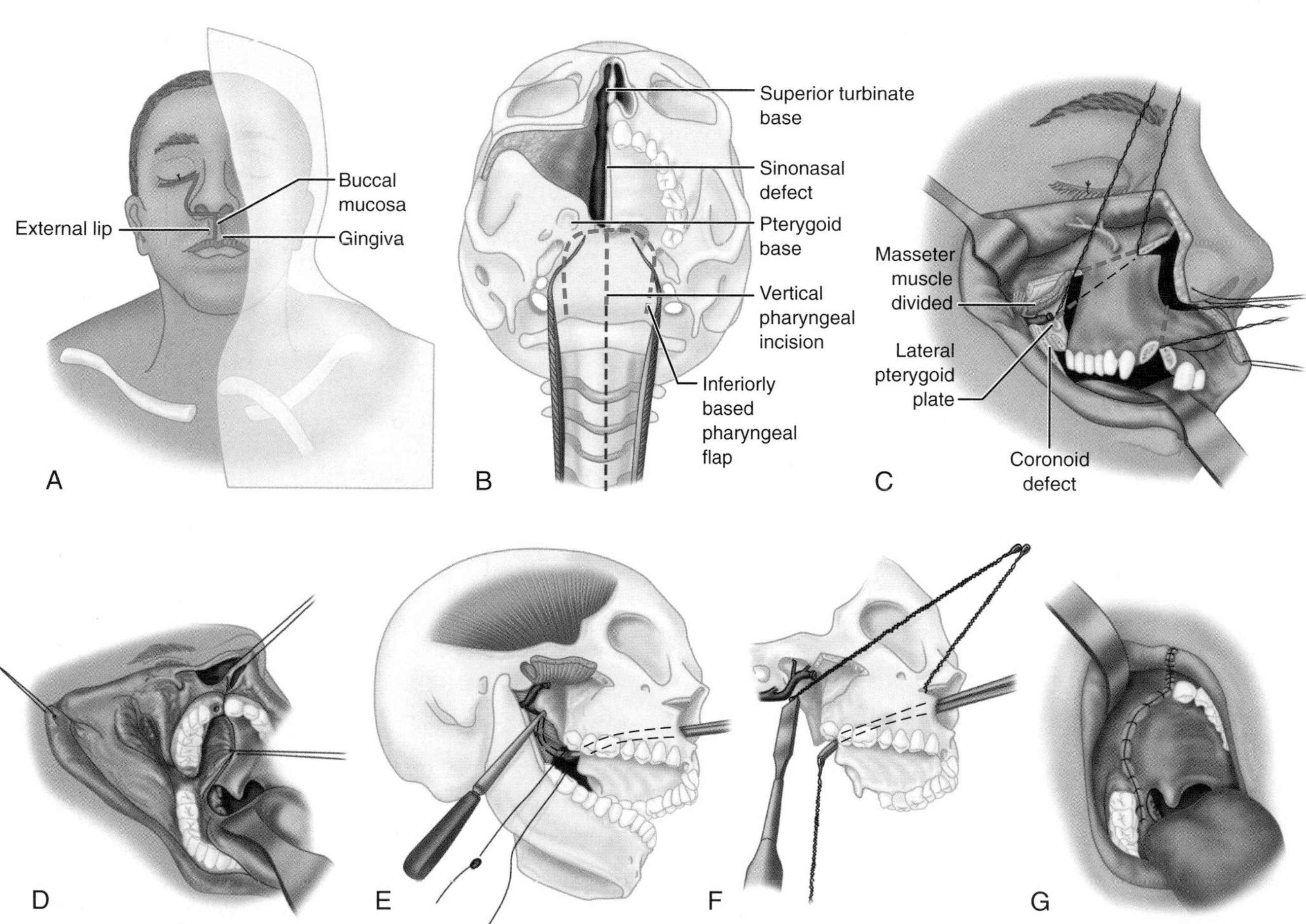

FIGURE 37-11 **A-G, Extended maxillotomy and subtotal maxillectomy (see text).** (Redrawn from Cocke EW Jr, Robertson JH, Robertson JR, et al: The extended maxillotomy and subtotal maxillectomy for excision of skull base tumors, Arch Otolaryngol Head Neck Surg 116:92, 1990.) **SEE TECHNIQUE 37-3**.

gutter to the central incisor defect and transversely through the buccal gingiva adjacent to the teeth to the retromolar region.

- Elevate the skin, subcutaneous tissues, periosteum, and mucoperiosteum of the maxilla to expose the anterior and lateral walls of the maxilla, nasal bone, piriform aperture of the nose, inferior orbital nerve, malar bone, and masseter muscle (Fig. 37-11D).
- Divide the anterior margin of the masseter muscle at its malar attachment and remove a wedge of malar bone. Use this wedge to accommodate the Gigli saw as it divides the maxilla (Fig. 37-11E and F).
- Make an incision in the lingual, hard palate mucoperiosteum adjacent to the teeth from the central incisor defect to join the retromolar incision.
- Extend the retromolar incision medial to the mandible lateral to the tonsil and to the retropharyngeal space to the level of the hyoid bone or lower pharynx, if necessary.
- Elevate the mucoperiosteum of the hard palate from the central incisor defect and alveolar ridge to and beyond the midline of the hard palate.
- Detach the soft palate with its nasal lining from the posterior margin of the hard palate.
- Divide and electrocoagulate the greater palatine vessels and nerves. Pack the palatine foramen with bone wax.
- Retract the mucoperiosteum of the hard palate, soft palate, anterior tonsillar pillar, tonsil, and pharynx medially from the prevertebral fascia. It is usually unnecessary to detach and retract the soft palate from the posterior or lateral pharyngeal walls.
- Expose the nasal cavity by detaching the nasal soft tissues from the lateral margin and base of the nasal piriform aperture (Fig. 37-11B).
- Remove a bony wedge of the ascending process of the maxilla to accommodate the upper Gigli saw (Fig. 37-11E).
- Remove the coronoid process of the mandible above the level of entrance of the inferior alveolar vessels and nerves, after dividing its temporalis muscle attachment, to expose the lateral pterygoid plate and the internal maxillary artery.
- Divide the pterygoid muscles with a Shaw knife or the cutting current of the Bovie cautery until the sharp, posterior bone edge of the lateral pterygoid plate is seen or palpated.
- Mobilize, clip, ligate, and divide the internal maxillary artery near the pterygoid plate.
- Direct the suture behind the lateral pterygoid plate into the nasopharynx and behind the posterior margin of the hard palate into the oropharynx (Fig. 37-11F).
- Pass a Kelly forceps through the nose to behind the hard palate to retrieve the medial end of the silk suture in the ligature carrier.
- Attach a Gigli saw to the lateral end of the suture and thread the saw into position to divide the upper maxilla.
- Position the upper Gigli saw (Fig. 37-11E and F) using a sharp-pointed, medium-size, curved, right-angle ligature carrier threaded with No. 2 black silk suture.
- Engage the medial arm of the saw into the ascending process wedge and its lateral arm into the malar wedge. Take care to position the saw as high as possible behind the pterygoid plate. Use a broad periosteal elevator beneath the saw on the pterygoid plate to maintain the elevated position (Fig. 37-11F).
- Position the lower Gigli saw by passing a Kelly forceps (Fig. 37-11E) through the nose into the nasopharynx behind the posterior nares of the hard palate. Engage the saw between the blades of the clamp and thread it through the nose into position for division of the hard palate (Fig. 37-11C).
- Divide the bony walls of the maxilla (Fig. 37-11C). First divide the hard palate and then the upper maxilla. Avoid entangling the saws and protect the soft tissues from injury.
- Remove the maxilla after division of its muscle attachments.
- Ligate the distal end of the internal maxillary artery.
- Place traction sutures in the soft tissues of the lip on either side of the initial lip incision and in the mucoperiosteum of the hard and soft palates. The posterior pharynx is now fully exposed.
- Infiltrate the mucous membrane covering the posterior wall of the nasopharynx, oropharynx, and the tonsillar area to the level of the hyoid bone with 1% lidocaine and epinephrine 1:100,000.
- Make a vertical midline incision through the soft tissues of the posterior wall of the nasopharynx extending from the sphenoidal sinus to the foramen magnum. Another option is to make a transverse incision from the sphenoidal sinus to the lateral nasopharyngeal wall posterior to the eustachian tube along the lateral pharyngeal wall inferiorly, posterior to the posterior tonsillar pillar behind the soft palate (Fig. 37-11B).
- Duplicate this incision on the opposite side, producing an inferiorly based pharyngeal flap (Fig. 37-11B).
- Make a more extensive exposure by extending the lateral pharyngeal wall incision through the anterior tonsillar pillar to join the retromolar incision. Extend this incision into the retropharyngeal space and retract the anterior tonsillar pillar, tonsil, and soft palate toward the midline with a traction suture. It is unnecessary to separate the soft palate completely from the pharyngeal wall.
- Extend the pharyngeal wall incision inferiorly to the level of the hyoid bone or beyond.
- Elevate, divide, and separate the superior constrictor muscle, prevertebral fascia, longus capitis muscle, and anterior longitudinal ligaments from the bony skull base and upper cervical spine ventrally.
- Expose the amount of bone to be operated on from the foramen magnum to C5. Use an operating microscope or loupe magnification for improved vision.
- Remove the offending bone with a high-speed burr, avoiding penetration of the dura.
- Close the nasopharyngeal mucous membrane and the subcutaneous tissue in one layer with interrupted sutures.
- Use a split-thickness skin or dermal graft from the thigh to resurface the buccal mucosa and any defects in the nasal surface of the hard palate.

- Use a quilting stitch to hold the graft in place without packing.
- Replace the zygoma and stabilize it with wire if it was mobilized.
- Return the maxilla to its original position and hold it in place with wire or compression plates.
- Place a nylon sack impregnated with antibiotic into the nasal cavity.
- Close the oral cavity incision with vertical interrupted mattress 3-0 polyglycolic acid sutures (Fig. 37-11G).
- Close the facial wound with 5-0 chromic and 6-0 nylon sutures.

EXTENDED MAXILLOTOMY

TECHNIQUE 37-4

- Expose the base of the skull and upper cervical spine as by the maxillectomy technique, but omit the extraction of the central incisor and the gingivolingual incision.
- Use a degloving procedure for elevation of the facial skin over the maxilla and nose to avoid facial scars.
- Divide the fibromuscular attachment of the soft palate to the pterygoid plate and hard palate, exposing the nasopharynx.
- Place the upper Gigli saw with the aid of a ligature carrier for division of the maxilla beneath the infraorbital nerve.
- Elevate the mucoperiosteum of the adjacent floor of the nose from the piriform aperture to the soft palate. Extend this elevation medially to the nasal septum and laterally to the inferior turbinate.
- Divide the bone of the nasal floor with a Stryker saw without lacerating the underlying hard palate periosteum.
- Hinge the maxilla on the hard palate, nasal mucoperiosteum, and soft palate, and rotate it medially.

POSTOPERATIVE CARE. Continuous spinal fluid drainage is maintained, and the head is elevated 45 degrees if the dura was repaired or replaced. These procedures are omitted if there was no dural tear or defect. An ice cap is used on the cheek and temple to reduce edema. Antibiotic therapy is continued until the risk of infection is minimized. Half-strength hydrogen peroxide is used for mouth irrigation to help keep the oral cavity clean. The endotracheal tube is removed when the risk of occlusion by swelling is minimized. The nasopharyngeal cavity is cleaned with saline twice daily for 2 months after pack removal. Facial sutures are removed at 4 to 6 days, and oral sutures are removed at 2 weeks.

■ ANTERIOR APPROACH, C3 TO C7

Exposure of the middle and lower cervical region of the spine is most commonly done through an anterior approach medial to the carotid sheath. A thorough knowledge of anatomic fascial planes allows a safe, direct approach to this area. The most frequent complication of the anterior approach is vocal cord paralysis caused by injury to the recurrent laryngeal nerve. Injury to the recurrent laryngeal nerve may be less common on the left side because the nerve has a more vertical course and lies in a protected position within the esophagotracheal groove. On the right the nerve leaves the main trunk of the vagus nerve and passes anterior to and under the subclavian artery, whereas on the left it passes under and posterior to the aorta at the site of origin of the ligamentum arteriosum. The nerve runs upward, having a variable relationship with the inferior thyroid artery, making the recurrent laryngeal nerve on the right side highly vulnerable to injury if the inferior thyroid vessels are not ligated as laterally as possible or if the midline structures along with the recurrent laryngeal nerve are not retracted intermittently.

The shorter, more lateral position of the right recurrent laryngeal nerve places it at risk for injury from direct trauma or from the retraction that is necessary to expose the anterior cervical vertebrae. A left-sided exposure medial to the carotid artery and internal jugular vein can be used to minimize the risk of injury. Although many spine surgeons use the right-sided approach with a low incidence of symptomatic paralysis of the recurrent laryngeal nerve, the incidence of temporary, partial, or asymptomatic paralysis may be underestimated. We believe that using the left-sided approach may reduce the risk of such injuries.

ANTERIOR APPROACH, C3 TO C7

TECHNIQUE 37-5

(SOUTHWICK AND ROBINSON)

As with other approaches to the cervical spine, skeletal traction is suggested and spinal cord monitoring can be used at the surgeon's discretion. Exposure can be carried out through either a transverse or a longitudinal incision, depending on the surgeon's preference (Fig. 37-12A). We generally use a transverse incision for one- and two-level approaches and a longitudinal incision for approaches involving three levels or more. A left-sided skin incision is preferred because of the more constant anatomy of the recurrent laryngeal nerve and the lower risk of inadvertent injury to the nerve. In general, an incision three to four fingerbreadths above the clavicle is needed to expose C3-5; an incision two to three fingerbreadths above the clavicle allows exposure of C5-7. On rare occasions, this approach can be used to access C2-3 in individuals with long, thin necks when a line drawn through the C2-3 disc space passes below the mandibular angle on lateral preoperative radiographs (Fig. 37-13).

- Center a transverse incision over the medial border of the sternocleidomastoid muscle. Infiltration of the skin and subcutaneous tissue with a 1 : 500,000 epinephrine solution assists with hemostasis.
- Incise the platysma muscle in line with the skin incision or open it vertically for more exposure.

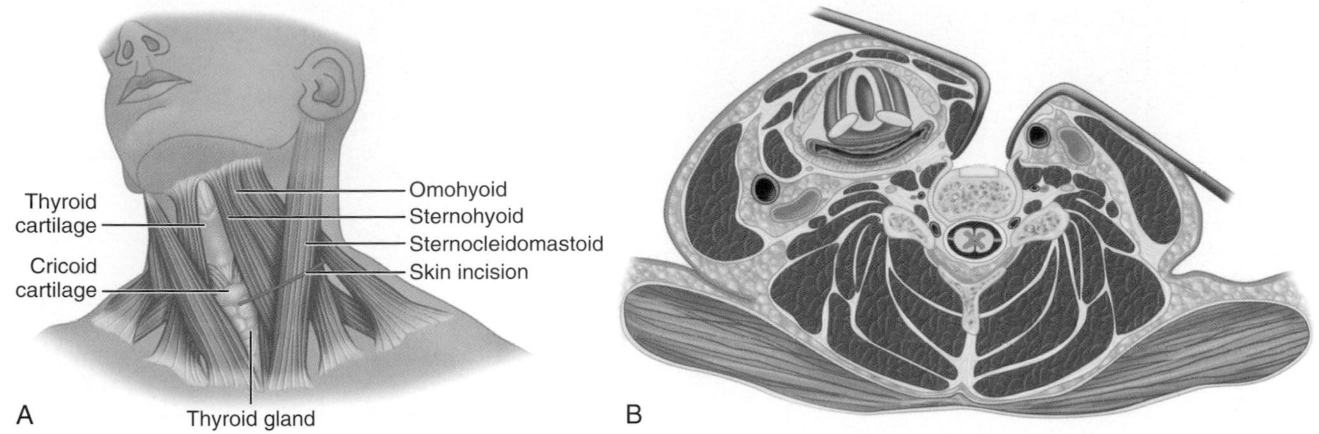

FIGURE 37-12 Anterior approach to C3-7 (see text). **A,** Incision. **B,** Thyroid gland, trachea, and esophagus have been retracted medially, and carotid sheath and its contents have been retracted laterally in opposite direction. **SEE TECHNIQUE 37-5.**

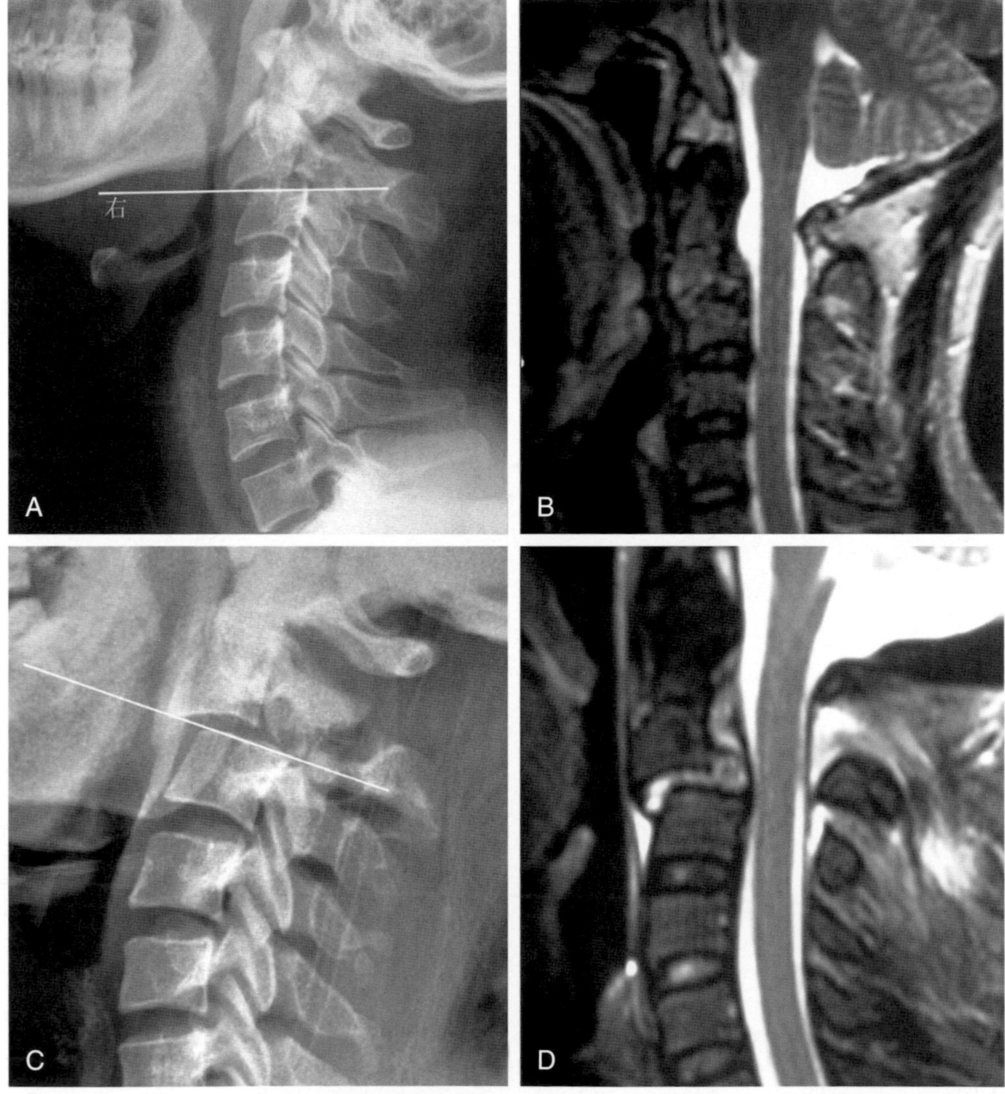

FIGURE 37-13 Lateral extension radiograph **(A)** and T2-weighted magnetic resonance image **(B).** A line based on the C3 upper endplate is drawn on a lateral extension radiograph of the cervical spine. Candidates for the subaxial anterior approach should have a mandibular angle higher than the line. Lateral extension radiograph **(C)** and T2-weighted magnetic resonance image **(D).** A large chin with a mandibular angle that extends over the line may make it difficult to reach C2 with the subaxial anterior approach. (From Zhang Y, Zhang J, Wang X, et al: Application of the cervical subaxial anterior approach at C2 in select patients, Orthopedics 36:e554, 2013.)

- Identify the anterior border of the sternocleidomastoid muscle and longitudinally incise the superficial layer of the deep cervical fascia; localize the carotid pulse by palpation.
- Carefully divide the middle layer of deep cervical fascia that encloses the omohyoid medial to the carotid sheath.
- As the sternomastoid and carotid sheath are retracted laterally, the anterior aspect of the cervical spine can be palpated. Identify the esophagus lying posterior to the trachea and retract the trachea, esophagus, and thyroid medially (Fig. 37-12B).
- Bluntly divide the deep layers of the deep cervical fascia, consisting of the pretracheal and prevertebral fascia overlying the longus colli muscles.
- Subperiosteally reflect the longus colli from the anterior aspect of the spine out laterally to the level of the uncovertebral joints. The resulting exposure is sufficient for wide debridement and bone grafting.
- Close the wound over a drain to prevent hematoma formation and possible airway obstruction.
- Approximate the platysma and skin edges in routine fashion.

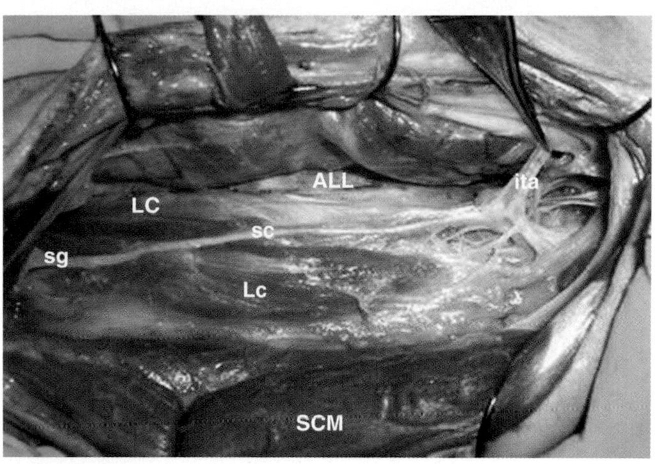

FIGURE 37-14 Anatomic dissection showing the relation of the cervical sympathetic chain *(sc)* to the longus coli muscle *(Lc)*. Also shown are the sternocleidomastoid muscle *(SMC)*, the anterior longitudinal ligament *(ALL)*, the longus capitis muscle *(LC)*, the inferior thyroidal artery *(Ita)*, and the superior ganglion of the sympathetic trunk *(sg)*. (Left side is cranial and right side is caudal.) (From Civelek E, Karasu A, Cansever T, et al: Surgical anatomy of the cervical sympathetic trunk during anterolateral approach to the cervical spine, Eur Spine J 17:991, 2008.)

ANTEROLATERAL APPROACH, C2 TO C7

Chibbaro et al. and Bruneau et al. described an anterolateral approach to the cervical spine that allows decompression of the body and roots that are affected with unilateral myelopathy and/or radiculopathy. This technique allows the removal of a wedge of cervical vertebra without the need for grafting or instrumentation. This technique also allows the direct exposure of the vertebral artery and veins by direct exposure of the vertebral foramen. It is recommended for elderly patients and smokers with unilateral anterior or lateral bony compression without instability. Cited advantages of this technique include wide decompression at a single level or multiple levels while providing direct vision of the vertebral artery and nerve roots. A disadvantage is the difficulty of the dissection with the potential injury to the vertebral artery, veins, XI cranial nerve, and the sympathetic chain, which can result in Horner syndrome (ptosis, ipsilateral miosis, and anhidrosis). In 459 procedures done since 1992, Chibbaro et al. noted no vertebral artery injury, cerebrospinal fluid leaks, dysphagia, or nerve root palsy; however, 14 patients (3%) developed Horner syndrome, which became permanent in four, and three had infections. The frequency of Horner syndrome reported in the literature is as high as 4%. The authors stressed that there is a steep learning curve with this procedure. From anatomical studies, Civelek et al. determined that the cervical sympathetic chain was on average 11.6 mm from the medial border of the longus coli muscle (Fig. 37-14). The superior ganglion was always at the level of C4, whereas the intermediate ganglion varied at its level of the cervical spine. The greatest risk to the sympathetic chain is during sectioning of the longus coli muscle transversely and dissection of the prevertebral fascia.

We have no experience with this procedure.

ANTEROLATERAL APPROACH, C2 TO C7

TECHNIQUE 37-6

(BRUNEAU ET AL., CHIBBARO ET AL.)

- Place the patient supine with the head rotated to the side opposite the incision and the neck in extension. Prepare and drape the neck as for any usual anterior cervical disc surgery.
- Identify the involved level radiographically.
- Make a longitudinal incision along the medial border of the sternocleidomastoid muscle. (At the C2-3 level the incision extends to the tip of the mastoid process superiorly and to the sternal notch for exposure of C7-T1 inferiorly.)
- Incise the platysma muscle along the plane of the skin incision.
- Open the space between the sternocleidomastoid muscle and the internal jugular vein with sharp dissection. Retract the sternocleidomastoid muscle laterally and the undissected great vessels, trachea, and esophagus medially (Fig. 37-15A).
- Identify the fatty sheath surrounding cranial nerve XI and expose the nerve from C2 to C4.
- Identify the transverse processes with a finger.
- Divide the aponeurosis of the longus coli longitudinally to identify the sympathetic chain, which lies on top of the longus coli.
- Retract the aponeurosis and the sympathetic chain laterally.

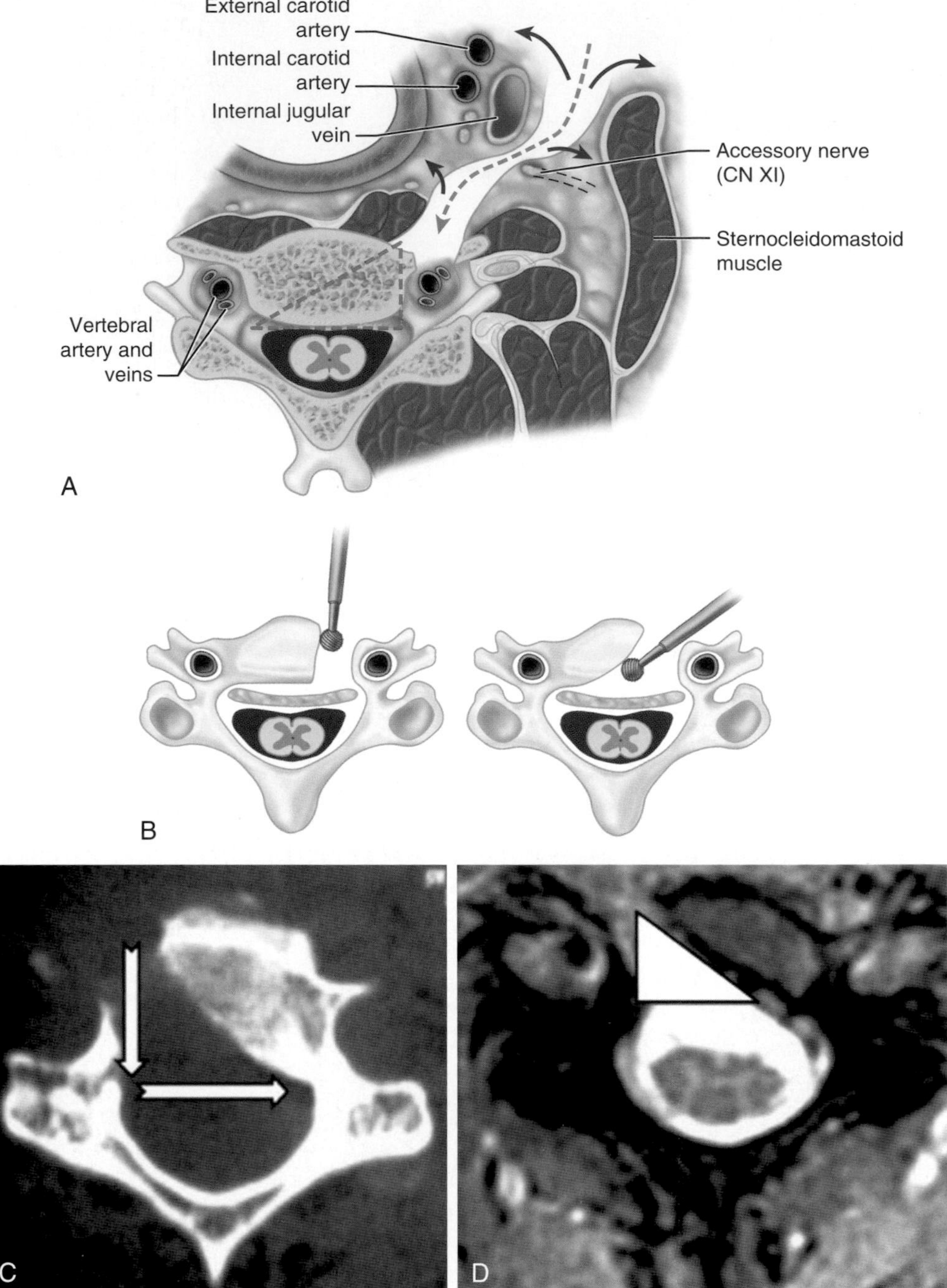

FIGURE 37-15 **A,** Anterolateral approach to the cervical spine through the interval between the sternocleidomastoid laterally and along the internal jugular vein medially with the other vascular structures including the internal carotid and external carotid. The XI cranial nerve is identified at C2 to 4 *(CN XI)*. The longus coli aponeurosis is longitudinally opened and the sympathetic chain is identified and carefully protected while exposing the uncovertebral joints and the anterior surface of the transverse process. The foramen is opened over the vertebral artery. **B,** Bony exposure through wedge-shaped lateral decompression. **C,** CT after wedge decompression. **D,** Postoperative MRI showing decompression. (From Chibbaro S, Mirone G, Bresson D, George B: Cervical spine lateral approach for myeloradiculopathy: technique and pitfalls, Surg Neurol 72:318, 2009.) **SEE TECHNIQUE 37-6**.

- Divide the longus coli longitudinally at the interval of the junction of the vertebral body and the transverse processes.
- Take care to be sure the vertebral artery is not entering at an abnormally high level such as C3, C4, or C5.
- Clear the transverse processes and the lateral aspect of the vertebral body. Confirm the level of dissection radiographically.
- Subperiosteally dissect the lateral aspect of the uncovertebral joint and medial border of the vertebral artery.
- Open the vertebral foramen laterally by removing the anterior portion of the transverse foramen with a Kerrison rongeur. This frees the cervical root from the dural root to the vertebral artery margin.
- Confirm the level of decompression again radiographically.
- Make an oblique corpectomy in the vertebra using a burr for longitudinal removal of bone from upper to lower disc spaces (Fig. 37-15B-D).
- Start with a longitudinal trench just medial to the vertebral artery and continue the bone removal medially. Preserve the posterior cortex until the wedge is completed.
- Resect the posterior cortex and the posterior longitudinal ligament to decompress the cord.
- Recheck the decompression radiographically.
- Obtain good hemostasis, irrigate the wound, and remove the retractors. The tissues will fall into place.
- Close the subcutaneous tissue and skin as desired.
- A drain can be used if necessary.
- Immobilization with a collar may be desired for soft-tissue healing.

ANTERIOR APPROACH TO CERVICOTHORACIC JUNCTION, C7 TO T1

There is no ready anterior access to the cervicothoracic junction. The rapid transition from cervical lordosis to thoracic kyphosis results in an abrupt change in the depth of the wound. Also, this is a confluent area of vital structures that are not readily retracted. The three approaches to this area are (1) the low anterior cervical approach, (2) the high transthoracic approach, and (3) the transsternal approach.

The low anterior cervical approach provides access to T1 at the inferior extent and the lower cervical spine at the superior extent of the dissection. Exposure is limited at the upper thoracic region but generally is adequate for placement of a strut graft if needed. Individual anatomic structure should be considered carefully in preoperative planning. This approach can be used if the lowest instrumented vertebra can be seen on a lateral radiograph and a line passing from the planned skin incision site to this level on the spine lies cephalad to the manubrium (Fig. 37-16).

LOW ANTERIOR CERVICAL APPROACH

TECHNIQUE 37-7

- Enter on the left side by a transverse incision placed one fingerbreadth above the clavicle.
- Extend it well across the midline, taking particular care when dissecting around the carotid sheath in the area of entry of the thoracic duct. The latter approaches the jugular vein from its lateral side, but variations are common.
- Further steps in exposure follow those of the conventional anterior cervical approach.

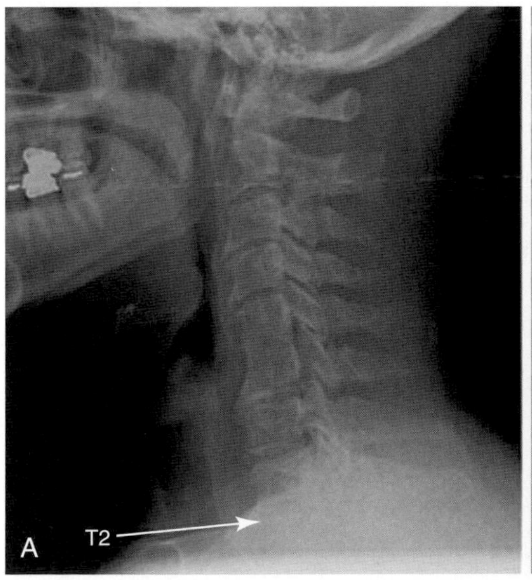

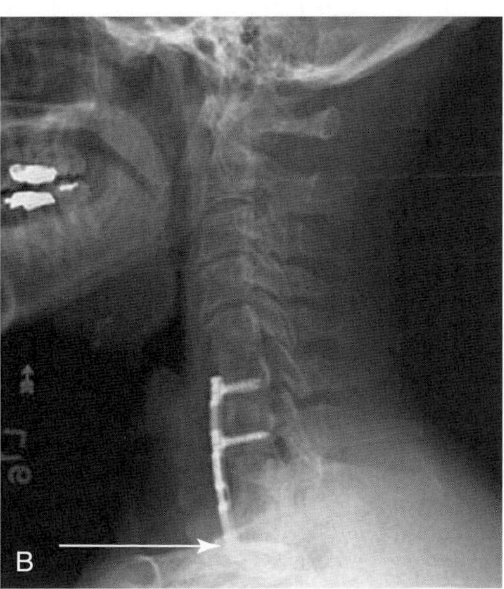

FIGURE 37-16 Criterion of Cho et al. for use of the standard Smith-Robinson approach for upper thoracic anterior fusion. **A,** On a preoperative lateral radiograph, a line drawn from the intended skin incision to the top of the manubrium (at the suprasternal notch) to the level of the disc space (T1-2) indicated that this trajectory would allow adequate exposure of the cervicothoracic junction. **B,** Fusion done through standard Smith-Robinson approach. (From Cho W, Buchowski JM, Park Y, et al: Surgical approach to the cervicothoracic junction. Can a standard Smith-Robinson approach be utilized? J Spinal Disord Tech 25:264, 2012.)

HIGH TRANSTHORACIC APPROACH

TECHNIQUE 37-8

- A kyphotic deformity of the thoracic spine tends to force the cervical spine into the chest, in which instance a high transthoracic approach is a logical choice.
- Make a periscapular incision (Fig. 37-17) and remove the second or third rib; removing the latter is necessary to provide sufficient working space in a child or if a kyphotic deformity is present. This exposes the interval between C6 and T4. Excision of the first or second rib is adequate in adults or in the absence of an exaggerated kyphosis.

For equal exposure of the thoracic and cervical spine from C4 to T4, the sternal splitting approach is recommended; it is commonly used in cardiac surgery.

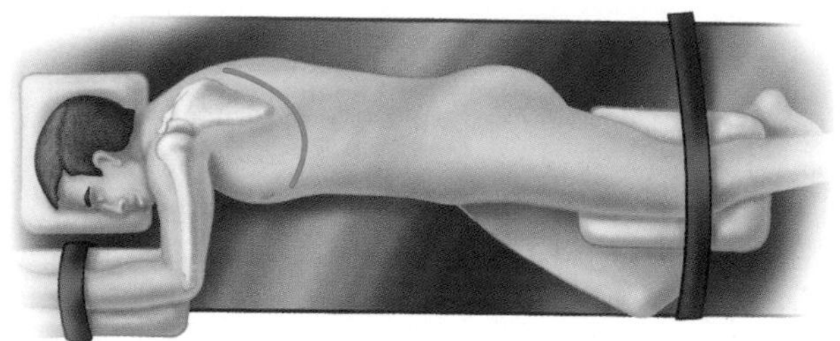

FIGURE 37-17 Patient positioning and periscapular incision for high transthoracic approach. **SEE TECHNIQUE 37-8.**

TRANSSTERNAL APPROACH

TECHNIQUE 37-9

- Make a Y-shaped or straight incision with the vertical segment passing along the midsternal area from the suprasternal notch to just below the xiphoid process (Fig. 37-18A).
- Extend the proximal end diagonally to the right and left along the base of the neck for a short distance. To avoid entering the abdominal cavity, take care to keep the dissection beneath the periosteum while exposing the distal end of the sternum. At the proximal end of the sternal notch, avoid the inferior thyroid vein.
- By blunt dissection, reflect the parietal pleura from the posterior surfaces of the sternum and costal cartilages and develop a space. Pass one finger or an instrument above and below the suprasternal space, insert a Gigli saw, and split the sternum. Spread the split sternum, and gain access to the center of the chest (Fig. 37-18B). In children, the upper portion of the exposure is posterior to the thymus and bounded by the innominate and carotid arteries and their venous counterparts.
- Develop the left side of this area bluntly.
- In patients with kyphotic deformity, the innominate vein now may be divided as it crosses the field; it may be very tense and subject to rupture. Fang et al. recommended this division. A disadvantage of ligation is that it leaves a slight postoperative enlargement of the left upper extremity that is not apparent unless carefully assessed.
- This approach provides limited access, and its success depends on accuracy in preoperative interpretation of the deformity and a high degree of surgical precision.

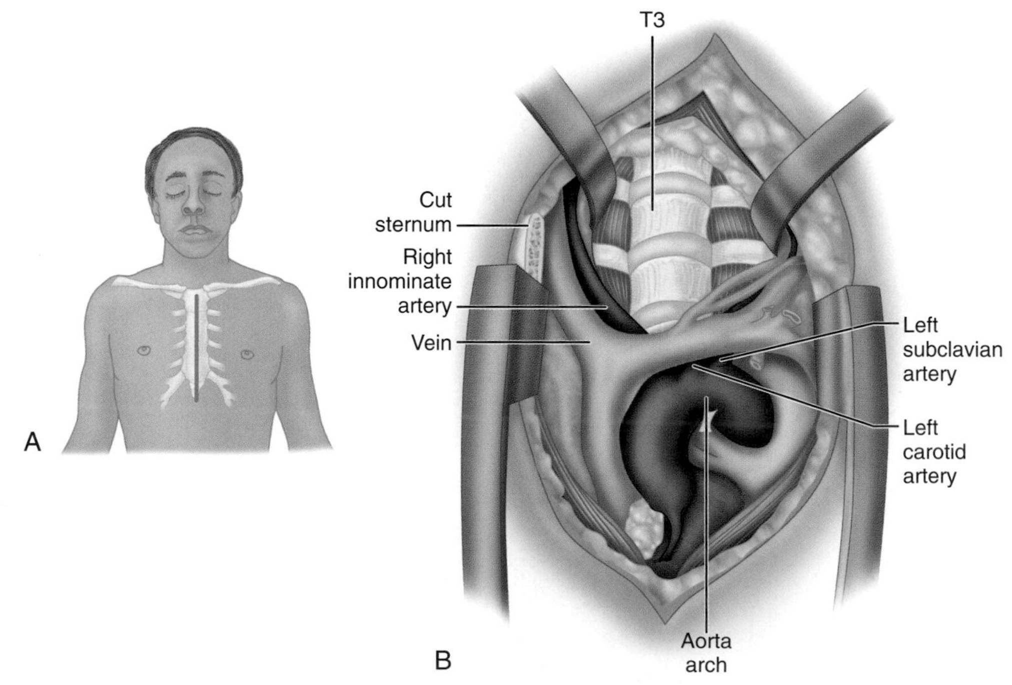

FIGURE 37-18 Transsternal approach to cervicothoracic spine (see text). **A,** Incision. **B,** Approach completed. (Redrawn from Pierce DS, Nickel VH, editors: *The total care of spinal cord injuries,* Boston, 1977, Little, Brown.) **SEE TECHNIQUE 37-9.**

MODIFIED ANTERIOR APPROACH TO CERVICOTHORACIC JUNCTION

Several authors have described an anterior approach to the cervical thoracic junction using a combined full median sternotomy and a cervical incision. Others have combined this approach with osteotomy of the clavicle or resection of the left sternoclavicular joint. The approach described by Darling et al. provides excellent exposure from C3 to T4 without the associated morbidity related to the division of the manubrium or the innominate vein. This procedure is technically simple and avoids the risk of injury to the subclavian vessels that can occur with resection of the clavicle or sternoclavicular junction.

TECHNIQUE 37-10

(DARLING ET AL.)

- Place the patient supine. If the neck is stable, place a sandbag transversely behind the shoulders to extend the neck and position the head in a head ring turned to the right. The left side is used to protect the left recurrent laryngeal nerve.
- Make an incision along the anterior border of the left sternocleidomastoid muscle to the sternal notch and continue in the midline to the level of the third costal cartilage.
- Divide the platysma in the line of the incision, retract the sternocleidomastoid laterally, and divide the omohyoid muscle.
- Retract the carotid sheath laterally, enter the prevertebral space, and develop a plane of dissection.
- Gently retract the esophagus, trachea, and adjacent recurrent laryngeal nerve to the right and elevate them away from the vertebral column.
- Incise the sternal fascia and divide the sternum in the midline from the sternal notch to the level of the second intercostal space.
- Retract the sternum laterally to the left through the synostosis between the manubrium and body of the sternum.
- Divide the strap muscles near their origin from the sternum to permit reconstruction, connecting the two portions of the incision. Do not divide the sternocleidomastoid muscle.
- Place a small chest retractor and open the partial sternotomy.
- Ligate and divide the inferior thyroid artery and middle and inferior thyroid veins. Take care not to injure the recurrent laryngeal nerve or the superior laryngeal nerve through pressure or traction.
- Dissect the thymus and mediastinal fat away from the left innominate vein.
- If exposure to T3-4 is required, divide the thymic and left innominate veins if necessary to expose the level of the aortic arch anteriorly and T4-5 posteriorly (Fig. 37-19). In completing the dissection, avoid injuring the thoracic duct as it ascends to the left of the esophagus from the level of T4 to its junction with the left internal jugular and subclavian veins.
- After spinal decompression and stabilization are completed, close the wound by approximating the manubrium with two or three heavy-gauge stainless steel wires using standard techniques.
- Reattach the strap muscles to the sternum and close the presternal fascia.
- Drain the prevertebral space with a soft Silastic drain through a separate stab wound and attach the drain to closed suction.
- Close the platysma and skin.

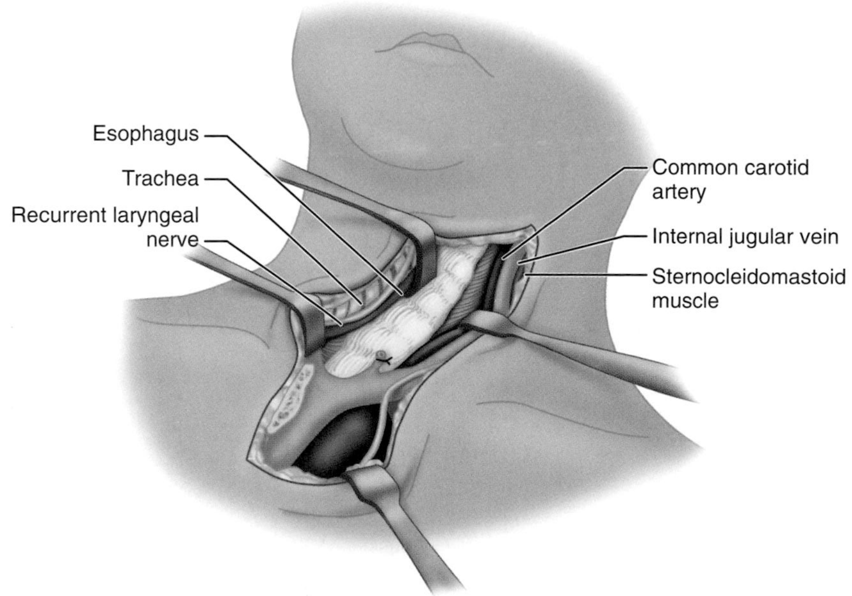

FIGURE 37-19 **Modified anterior approach to cervicothoracic junction.** (Redrawn from Darling GE, McBroom R, Perrin R: Modified anterior approach to the cervicothoracic junction, Spine 20:1519, 1995.) **SEE TECHNIQUE 37-10.**

ANTERIOR APPROACH TO THE CERVICOTHORACIC JUNCTION WITHOUT STERNOTOMY

Pointillart et al. reported that exposure of the cervicothoracic junction can be achieved with the usual anterior approach without a sternotomy. They noted that exposure of T3 and T4 may require a median manubrial resection.

TECHNIQUE 37-11

(POINTILLART ET AL.)

- Incise the skin along the medial border of the sternocleidomastoid muscle and extend it distally over the manubrium (Fig. 37-20A).
- Begin the dissection as in a standard anterior cervical approach, then extend it caudally by following the vessel-free area anterior to the vertebrae along the deep cervical fascia.
- Identify and cut the sternal ends of the sternocleidomastoid muscle and infrahyoid muscles 2 cm from their sternal insertions.
- Expose the manubrium to the medial portion of the sternoclavicular joint.
- Use finger dissection to free the posterior aspect of the manubrium for resection.
- With a high-speed drill, resect the manubrium down to the posterior cortex to allow the exposure desired (Fig. 37-20B). Excise the remaining bone with a Kerrison rongeur to complete the exposure.
- Cut the sternoclavicular ligament with scissors.
- Retract the retrosternal fat and large vessels caudally and anteriorly to expose the upper thoracic vertebra.

ANTERIOR APPROACH TO THE THORACIC SPINE

The transthoracic approach to the thoracic spine provides direct access to the vertebral bodies T2-12. The midthoracic vertebral bodies are best exposed by this approach, whereas views of the upper and lower extremes of the spine are more limited. In general, a left-sided thoracotomy incision is preferred, although some surgeons favor a right-sided thoracotomy for approaching the upper thoracic spine to avoid the subclavian and carotid arteries in the left superior mediastinum. In a left-sided thoracotomy approach the heart may be retracted anteriorly, whereas in a right-sided approach the liver may present a significant obstacle to exposure. The level of the incision should be positioned to meet the level of exposure required. Ordinarily, an intercostal space is selected at or just above the involved segment. If only one vertebral segment is involved, the rib at that level can be removed; however, if multiple levels are involved, the rib at the upper level of the proposed dissection should be removed. Because of the normal thoracic kyphosis, dissection is easier from proximal to distal. Exposure is improved by resection of a rib, and the rib provides a satisfactory bone graft, but resection is

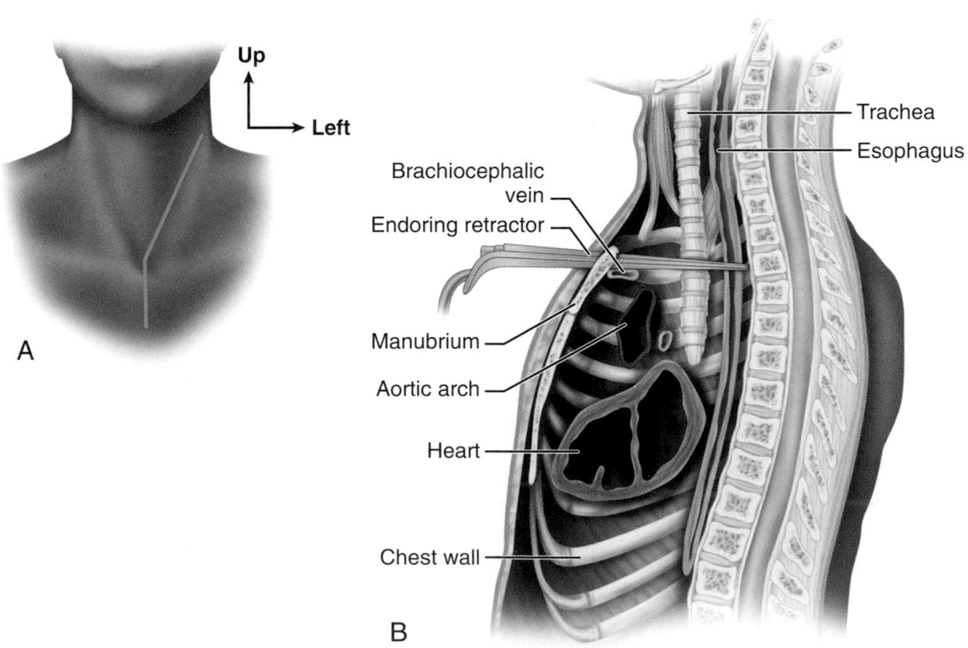

FIGURE 37-20 Anterior approach to cervicothoracic junction without sternotomy. **A,** Incision for exposure at cervicothoracic junction. **B,** Sagittal section of the chest reflecting the thoracic spine exposure possible with upper manubrium resection and retraction. (Redrawn from Pointillart V, Aurouer N, Gangnet N, Vital JM: Anterior approach to the cervicothoracic junction without sternotomy: a report of 37 cases, Spine 32:2875, 2009.) **SEE TECHNIQUE 37-11**.

unnecessary if a limited exposure is adequate for biopsy, decompression, or fusion. The transthoracic approach adds a significant operative risk and is more hazardous than the more commonly used posterior or posterolateral approaches. The increased risk of thoracotomy must be weighed against the more limited exposure provided by alternative posterior approaches.

ANTERIOR APPROACH TO THE THORACIC SPINE

TECHNIQUE 37-12

- Place the patient in the lateral decubitus position with the right side down; an inflatable beanbag is helpful in maintaining the patient's position, and the table may be flexed to increase exposure (Fig. 37-21A).
- Make an incision over the rib corresponding to the involved vertebra and expose it subperiosteally. Use electrocautery to maintain hemostasis during the exposure.
- Disarticulate the rib from the transverse process and the hemifacets of the vertebral body. Identify and preserve the intercostal nerve lying along the inferior aspect of the rib as it localizes the neural foramen leading into the spinal canal. Incise the parietal pleura and reflect it off of the spine, usually one vertebra above and one below the involved segment, to allow adequate exposure for debridement and grafting (Fig. 37-21B).
- Identify the segmental vessels that cross the midportion of each vertebral body and ligate and divide these (Fig. 37-21C).
- Carefully reflect the periosteum overlying the spine with elevators to expose the involved vertebrae.
- Use a small elevator to delineate the pedicle of the vertebrae and a Kerrison rongeur to remove the pedicle, exposing the dural sac.

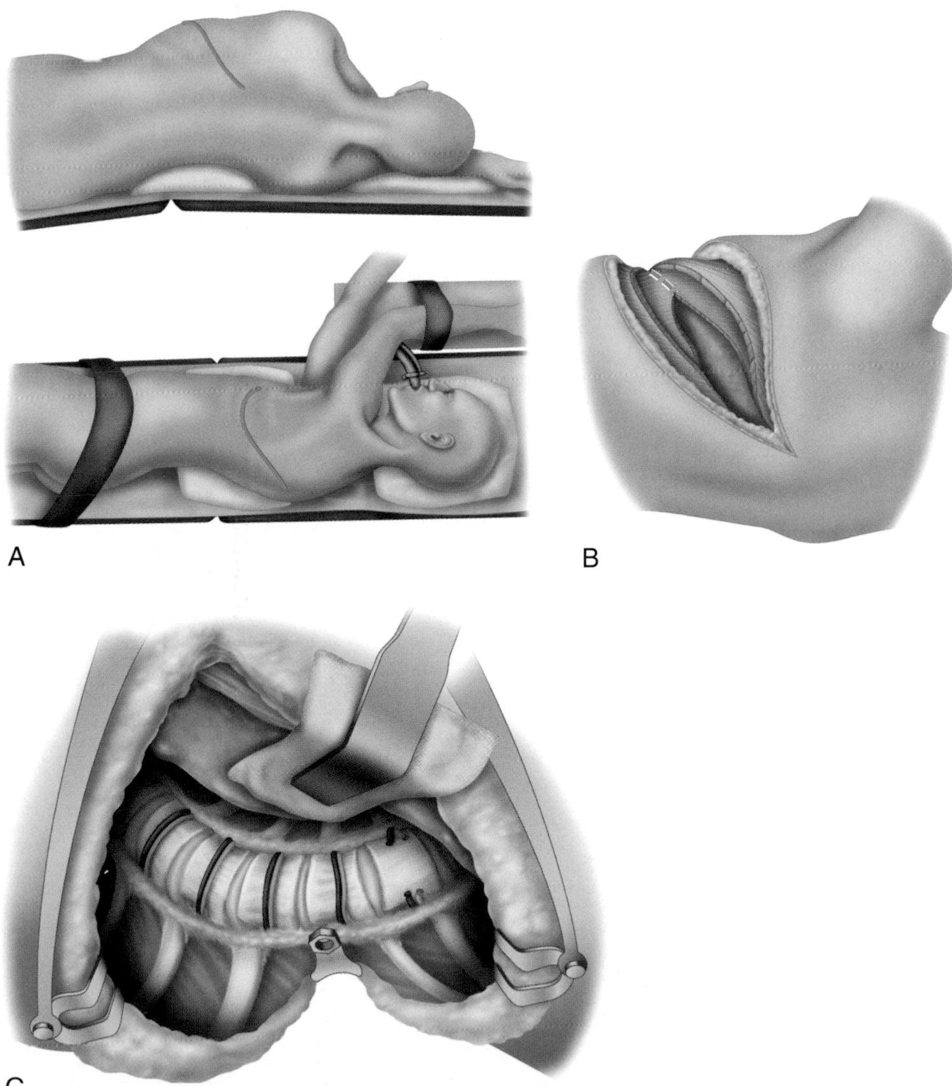

FIGURE 37-21 Transthoracic approach (see text). **A,** Positioning of patient and incision. **B,** Rib removal and division of pleura, exposing lung. **C,** Exposure of spine and division of segmental vessels over one vertebral body. **SEE TECHNIQUE 37-12.**

- Identify the disc spaces above and below the vertebrae and incise the anulus. Remove disc material using rongeurs and curets.
- An entire cross-section of the vertebral body is developed, and the anterior margin of the neural canal is identified with the posterior longitudinal ligament lying in the slight concavity on the back of the vertebral body.
- Expose sufficient segmental vessels and disc spaces to accomplish the intended procedure—usually corpectomy and strut grafting.

VIDEO-ASSISTED THORACIC SURGERY

Video-assisted thoracic surgery (VATS) has been used successfully in the anterior thoracic and thoracolumbar spine for treatment of scoliosis, kyphosis, tumors, and fractures and seems to have less morbidity than the standard thoracotomy, which can result in respiratory problems or pain after thoracotomy. Thoracoscopy has evolved rapidly and is capable of providing adequate exposure to all levels of the thoracic spine from T2 to L1; however, the learning curve is significant, and the surgical team always should include a thoracic surgeon who is competent in thoracoscopy and a spine surgeon who is well trained in endoscopic techniques.

Reported complications include intercostal neuralgia, atelectasis, excessive epidural blood loss (2500 mL), and temporary paraparesis related to operative positioning.

Although the indications for the thoracoscopic approach apparently remain the same as for open thoracotomy, some procedures require extensive internal fixation and may not be suitable for VATS. Also, patients should be informed before surgery that the thoracoscopic procedure may have to be abandoned in favor of an open procedure. Relative contraindications include preexisting pleural disease from previous surgeries.

VIDEO-ASSISTED THORACIC SURGERY

TECHNIQUE 37-13

(MACK ET AL.)

- Routine intraoperative monitoring for thoracic procedures is used, including an arterial pressure line, pulse oximeter, and end-tidal carbon dioxide measurement. Somatosensory evoked potentials should be monitored routinely for patients undergoing spinal deformity correction or corpectomy.
- Place the initial trocar in the seventh intercostal space in the posterior axillary line. Place a 10-mm, 30-degree angled rigid telescope through the 10-mm trocar. Use a 0-degree end-viewing scope and a 30-degree scope for direct vision of the intervertebral disc space to avoid impeding surgical instrumentation or obscuring the operative field. Mack et al. recommended placing the viewing port in the posterior axillary line directly over the spine and two or three access sites for working ports in the anterior axillary line to allow better access to the spine. This "reverse L" arrangement can be moved cephalad or caudad, depending on the level of the thoracic spine to be approached.
- Use the portals for placement of surgical instruments (Fig. 37-22).
- Rotate the patient anteriorly and place the patient in a Trendelenburg position for the lower thoracic spine or reverse Trendelenburg for the upper thoracic spine.
- The lung usually falls away from the operative field when completely collapsed, obviating the need for retraction instruments.
- A departure from the standard VATS approach is the positioning of the operative team. Operative procedures routinely are performed by a spine surgeon and thoracic surgeon. In contrast to other VATS procedures in which the surgeon and assistant are positioned on opposite sides of the operating table, both surgeons are positioned on the anterior side of the patient viewing a monitor on the opposite side. In addition, the camera and the viewing field are rotated 90 degrees from the standard VATS approach so that the spine is viewed horizontally.
- Perform an initial exploratory thoracoscopy to determine the correct spinal level for operative intervention.
- Count the ribs by "palpation" with a blunt grasping instrument.
- When the target level has been defined, place a 20-gauge long needle percutaneously into the disc space from the lateral aspect and confirm radiographically.
- When the correct level is ascertained, perform the specific spinal procedure.

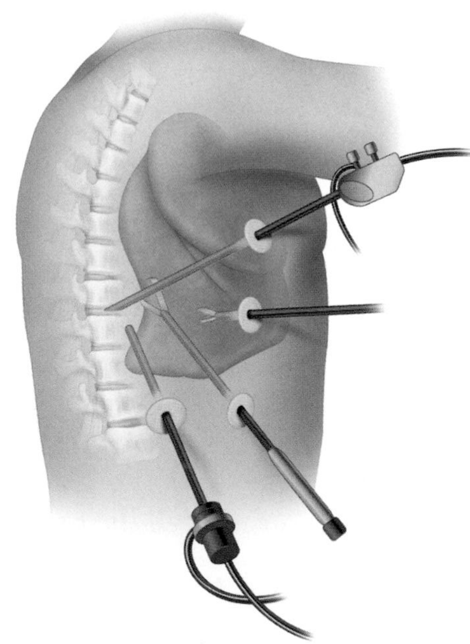

FIGURE 37-22 **Thoracoscopic instrument placement for thoracic spine procedures.** (Redrawn from Regan JJ, McAfee PC, Mack MJ, editors: Atlas of endoscopic spine surgery, St. Louis, 1995, Quality Medical Publishing.) **SEE TECHNIQUE 37-13**.

ANTERIOR APPROACH TO THE THORACOLUMBAR JUNCTION

Occasionally, it may be necessary to expose simultaneously the lower thoracic and upper lumbar vertebral bodies. Technically, this is a more difficult exposure because of the presence of the diaphragm and the increased risk involved in simultaneous exposure of the thoracic cavity and the retroperitoneal space. In most instances, thoracic lesions should be exposed through the chest, whereas lesions predominantly involving the upper lumbar spine can be exposed through an anterior retroperitoneal incision. The diaphragm is a dome-shaped organ that is muscular in the periphery and tendinous in the center. Posteriorly, it originates from the upper lumbar vertebrae through crura, the arcuate ligaments, and the 12th ribs. Anteriorly and laterally, it attaches to the cartilaginous ends of the lower six ribs and xiphoid. The diaphragm is innervated by the phrenic nerve, which descends through the thoracic cavity on the pericardium. The phrenic nerve joins the diaphragm adjacent to the fibrous pericardium, dividing into three major branches that extend peripherally in anterolateral and posterior directions. Division of these major branches may interfere with diaphragmatic function. It is best to make an incision around the periphery of the diaphragm to minimize interference with function when making a thoracoabdominal approach to the spine. We recommend a left-sided approach at the thoracolumbar junction because the vena cava on the right is less tolerant of dissection and may result in troublesome hemorrhage, and the liver may be hard to retract.

ANTERIOR APPROACH TO THE THORACOLUMBAR JUNCTION

TECHNIQUE 37-14

- Place the patient in the right lateral decubitus position and place supports beneath the buttock and shoulder.
- Make the incision curvilinear with ability to extend the cephalad or the caudal end (Fig. 37-23A).
- To gain the best access to the interval of T12-L1, resect the 10th rib, which allows exposure between T10 and L2. The only difficulty is in identifying the diaphragm as a separate structure; it tends to approximate closely the wall of the thoracic cage, allowing the edge of the lung to penetrate into the space beneath the knife as the pleura is divided (Fig. 37-23B).
- Take care in entering the abdominal cavity. Because the transversalis fascia and the peritoneum do not diverge, dissect with caution and identify the two cavities on either side of the diaphragm. To achieve confluence of the two cavities, reflect the diaphragm from the lower ribs and the crus from the side of the spine (Fig. 37-23C).
- Alternatively, incise the diaphragm 2.5 cm away from its insertion and tag it with sutures for later accurate closure.
- Incise the prevertebral fascia.
- Identify the segmental arteries and veins over the midportion of each vertebral body. Isolate these, ligate them in the midline, and expose the bone as previously described.

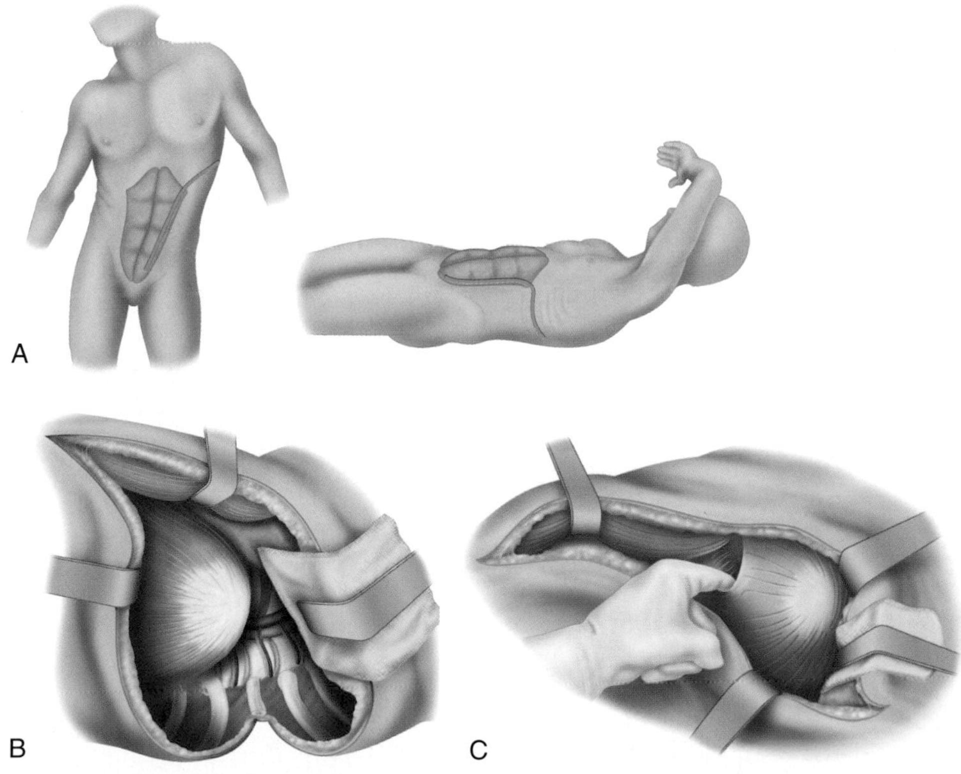

FIGURE 37-23 Thoracolumbar approach (see text). **A,** Skin incision. **B,** Transthoracic detachment of diaphragm. **C,** Retroperitoneal detachment of diaphragm. **SEE TECHNIQUE 37-14.**

MINIMALLY INVASIVE APPROACH TO THE THORACOLUMBAR JUNCTION

Although a variant of the lateral retropleural thoracotomy, the minimally invasive lateral extraceloemic (retroperitoneal/retropleural) approach can provide adequate exposure of the thoracolumbar junction to allow vertebrectomy and canal decompression from T10-L2 without the need to enter the pleural or peritoneal cavities and avoid the morbidities associated with retropleural thoracotomy. It combines the positive attributes of both the anterolateral transthoracic approach and the lateral extra-cavitary approach and is particularly useful for centrally located pathologies such as central thoracic disc herniation.

TECHNIQUE 37-15

- With the patient in a lateral decubitus position and under fluoroscopic guidance, make a 6-cm oblique incision (following the trajectory of the rib at the index level) at the midaxillary line.
- The side of the approach is chosen according to the vertebral level and the location of the abnormality, but the left-sided approach is preferred to avoid retraction of the liver and vena cava on the right.
- Dissect subperiosteally approximately 5 cm of the rib immediately overlying the target level from the underlying pleura and neurovascular bundle and remove it. Set aside the portion of resected rib for use as autograft.
- Once the parietal pleura is exposed, develop the plane between the endothoracic fascia and the pleura, taking care not to enter the pleural or peritoneal cavities (Fig. 37-24A).
- Use a sponge stick or finger dissection to bluntly mobilize the pleura anteriorly along with the diaphragm until the lateral side of the vertebral body and adjacent discs are exposed.
- If the target levels include L1, divide the medial and lateral arcuate ligaments off the costal and lumbar attachments to adequately mobilize the diaphragm. If more anterior access or exposure of L2 is needed, fully transect the crus of the diaphragm connecting the retropleural and retroperitoneal spaces.
- Retract the aorta and hemiazygos vein anteriorly. Insert sequential tubular dilators and place a tube retractor system over the largest dilator and secure it with a flexible table-mounted arm assembly (Fig. 37-24B).
- Under magnification, remove the rib head and the costovertebral ligaments at the corresponding level and complete the desired procedure with direct observation of the dura laterally and ventrally.
- If the pleural cavity is not violated there is no need for a chest tube, and postoperative mobilization can begin immediately.

ANTERIOR RETROPERITONEAL APPROACH, L1 TO L5

The anterior retroperitoneal approach to the lumbar vertebral bodies is a modification of the anterolateral approach commonly used by general surgeons for sympathectomy. It is an excellent approach that should be considered for extensive resection, debridement, or grafting at multiple levels in the lumbar spine. Depending on which portion of the lumbar spine is to be approached, the incision may be varied in placement between the 12th rib and the superior aspect of the iliac crest. The major dissection in this approach is behind the kidney in the potential space between the renal fascia and the quadratus lumborum and psoas muscles.

ANTERIOR RETROPERITONEAL APPROACH, L1 TO L5

TECHNIQUE 37-16

- Position the patient in the lateral decubitus position, generally with the right side down. The approach is made most often from the left side to avoid the liver and the inferior vena cava, which is more difficult to repair than the aorta if vascular injury occurs during the approach to the spine.
- Flex the table to increase exposure between the 12th rib and the iliac crest. Flex the hips slightly to release tension on the psoas muscle.
- Make an oblique incision over the 12th rib from the lateral border of the quadratus lumborum to the lateral border of the rectus abdominis muscle to allow exposure of the first and second lumbar vertebrae (Fig. 37-25A).
- Alternatively, place the incision several fingerbreadths below and parallel to the costal margin when exposure of the lower lumbar vertebrae (L3-5) is necessary.
- Use electrocautery to divide the subcutaneous tissue, fascia, and muscle of the external oblique, internal oblique, transversus abdominis, and transversalis fascia in line with the skin incision (Fig. 37-25B and C).
- Carefully protect the peritoneum and reflect it anteriorly by blunt dissection. If the peritoneum is entered during the approach, it must be repaired.
- Identify the psoas muscle in the retroperitoneal space and allow the ureter to fall anteriorly with the retroperitoneal fat.
- The sympathetic chain is found between the vertebral bodies and the psoas muscle laterally, whereas the genitofemoral nerve lies on the anterior aspect of the psoas muscle.
- Place a Finochietto rib retractor between the costal margin and the iliac crest to aid exposure.
- Palpate the vertebral bodies from T12 to L5 and identify and protect with a Deaver retractor the great vessels lying anterior to the spine. The lumbar segmental vessels lie in the midportion of the vertebral bodies, and the relatively avascular discs are prominent on each adjacent side of the vessels (Fig. 37-25D).
- When the appropriate involved vertebra is identified, elevate the psoas muscle bluntly off the lumbar vertebrae and retract it laterally to the level of the transverse process with a Richardson retractor. Sometimes, removal of the transverse process with a rongeur is helpful in allowing adequate retraction of the psoas muscle.

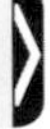

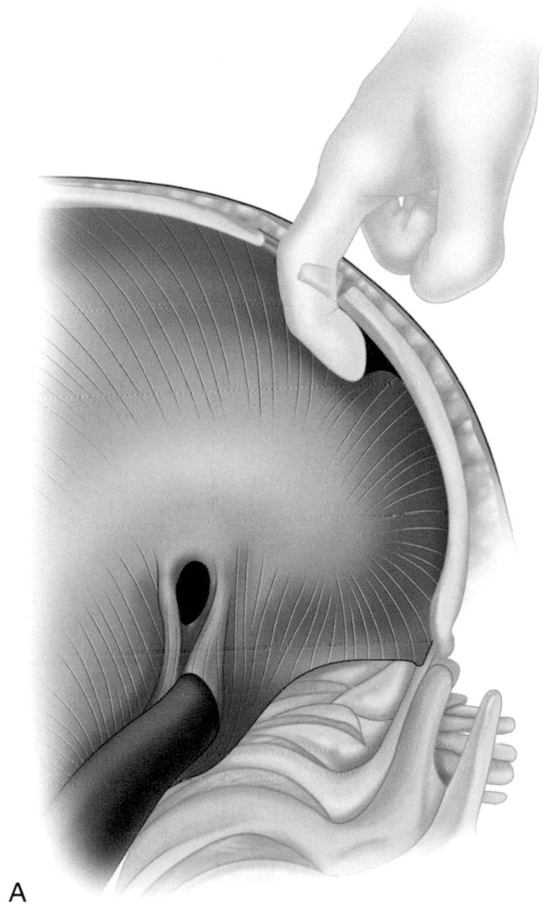

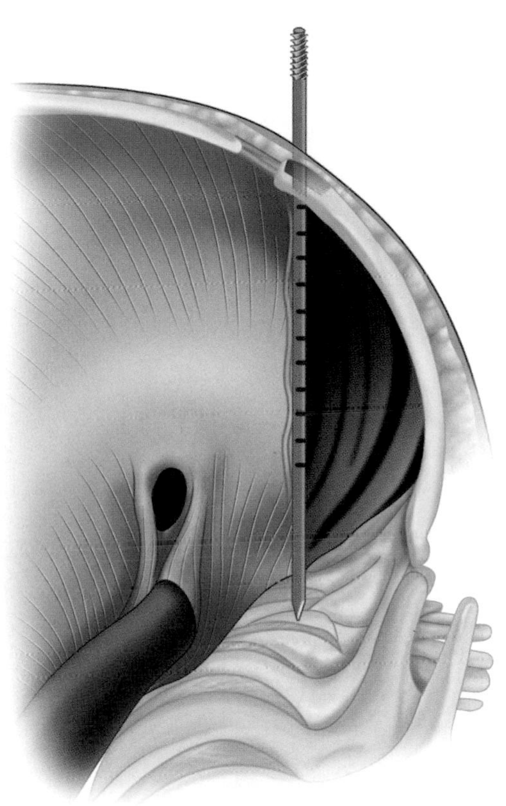

A

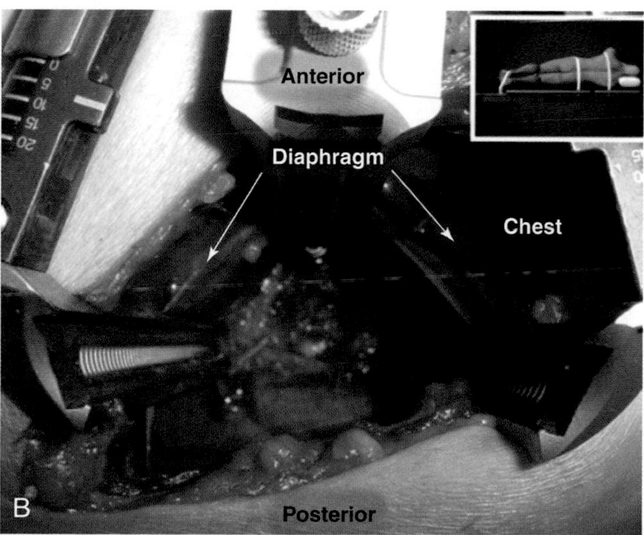

FIGURE 37-24 Minimally invasive lateral coelomic approach. **A,** Diaphragm looking from caudal to cranial demonstrating blunt dissection with the aid of a finger to develop the extracoelomic space (*left*). The diaphragm is retracted anteriorly once the costal and lumbar attachments have been mobilized (*right*). **B,** Cadaver specimen in the right lateral decubitus position (*inset*) demonstrating the view through the tubular retractor when placed in the extracoelomic space. (**A** from NuVasive, Inc. B from Dakwar E, Ahmadian A, Uribe JS: The anatomical relationship of the diaphragm to the thoracolumbar junction during minimally invasive lateral extracoelomic (retropleural/retroperitoneal) approach. Laboratory investigation, J Neurosurg Spine 16:359, 2012). **SEE TECHNIQUE 37-15.**

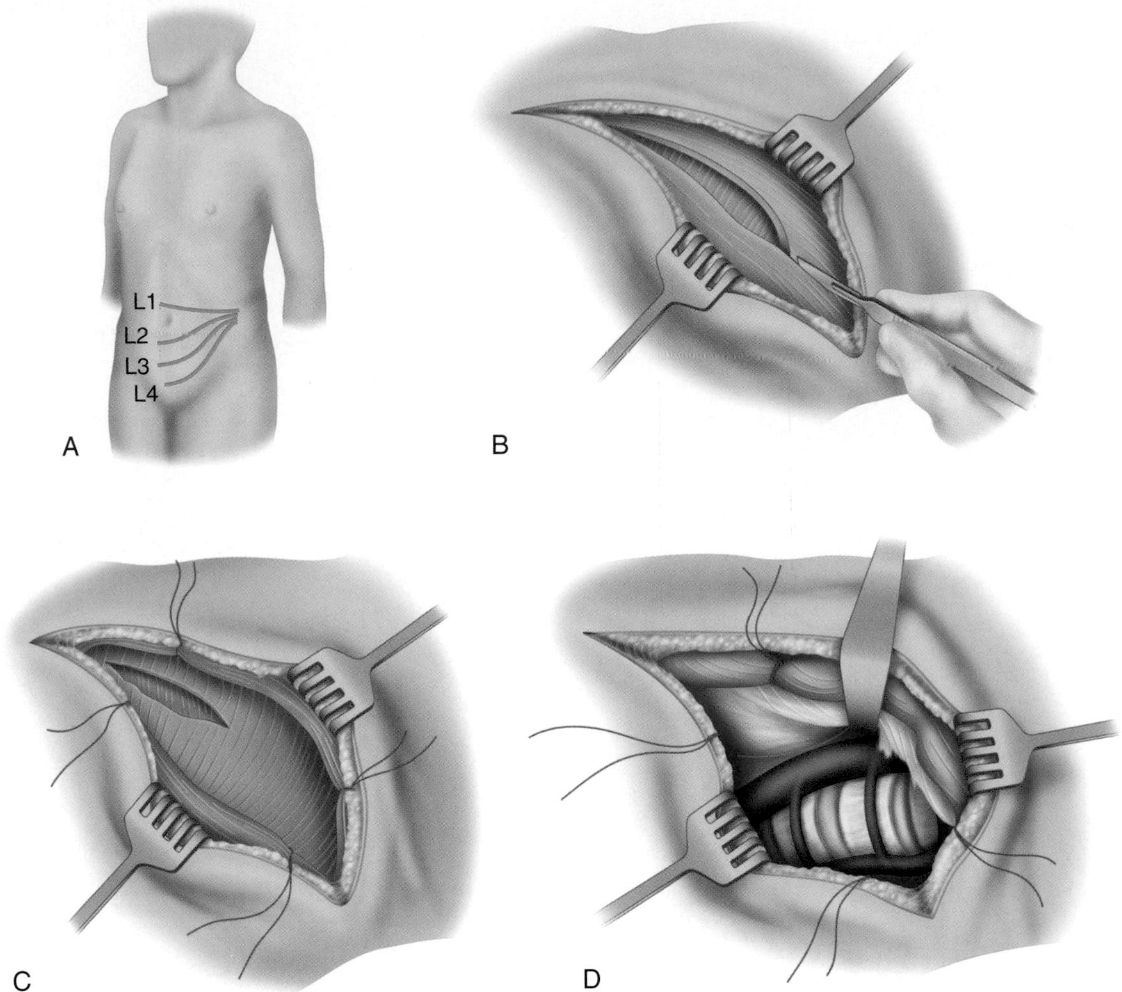

FIGURE 37-25 Anterior retroperitoneal approach (see text). **A,** Skin incisions for lumbar vertebrae. **B,** Incision of fibers of external oblique muscle. **C,** Incision into fibers of internal oblique muscle. **D,** Exposure of spine before ligation of segmental vessels. **SEE TECHNIQUE 37-16**.

- Ligate and divide the lumbar segmental vessel overlying the involved vertebra.
- Delineate the pedicle of the involved vertebra with a small elevator and locate the neural foramen with the exiting nerve root. Bipolar coagulation of vessels around the neural foramen is recommended.
- Remove the pedicle with an angled Kerrison rongeur and expose the dura.
- After completion of the spinal procedure, obtain meticulous hemostasis and close the wound in layers over a drain in the retroperitoneal space.

PERCUTANEOUS LATERAL APPROACH TO LUMBAR SPINE, L1 TO L4-5 (DLIF OR XLIF)

Ozgur et al. first described the technique of extreme lateral interbody fusion (XLIF) as a refinement of the laparoscopic lateral approach. The primary use for this approach has been the placement of an anterior lumbar interbody graft for degenerative disc disease without central canal stenosis, scoliosis, or spondylolisthesis. Park et al. analyzed the distance from a guidewire placed in 10 human cadavers using the usual lateral approach and concluded that the intrapsoas nerves are a safe distance from the radiographic center of the disc in most cases. Because of the risk of nerve injury in a small number of individuals, neural monitoring is recommended while traversing the psoas. MRI studies have been analyzed to determine the safe zones for a minimally invasive lateral approach in both normal and abnormal spines. Most levels evaluated (247) were normal, 18 were degenerative, and 19 were scoliotic. On the MR images, the overlap between the adjacent neurovascular structures and the vertebral body end plate gradually increased from L1-2 to L4-5, resulting in a very narrow safe zone at L4-5. Alteration in the anatomic location of the nerve root and the retroperitoneal vessels in patients with scoliosis further decreases this safe zone.

Knight et al. reported that 13 (22%) of 58 patients had complications after a minimally invasive direct lateral anterior lumbar fusion (DLIF) and XLIF. Approach-related complications included ipsilateral L4 nerve root injury in two

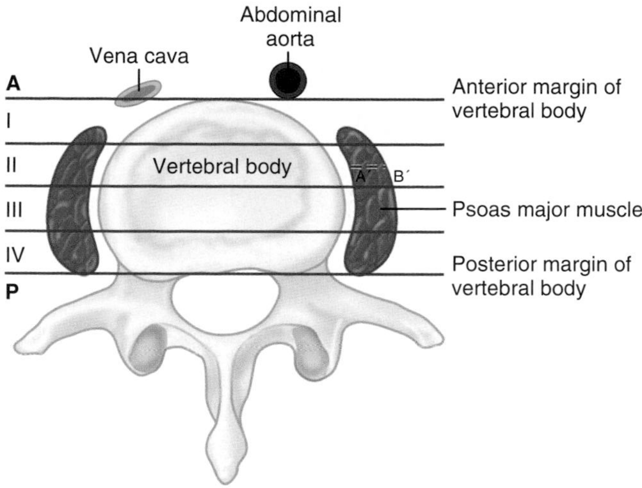

FIGURE 37-26 Zones of the lumbar vertebral body. (Redrawn from Hu WK, He SS, Zhang SC, et al: An MRI study of psoas major and abdominal large vessels with respect to the X/DLIF approach, Eur Spine J 20:557-562, 2011.)

patients, irritation of the lateral femoral cutaneous nerve in six patients, significant psoas spasm that lengthened the hospital stay in one patient, and less significant psoas irritation in five. Major complications occurred in five (8.6%) patients, including reoperation for implant subsidence in one patient and persistence of the L4 root injury at 1 year in two patients. No significant differences in complications were noted between the XLIF and DLIF procedures.

Using MR images of the lumbar spine with the vertebral body divided into four zones, each being 25% of the vertebral diameter (Fig. 37-26), Hu et al. identified the safe zones for approach using the minimally invasive lateral lumbar interbody fusion to be zones II-III at L1-2 and L2-3, zone II at L3-4, and zones I-II on the left at L4-5, and zone II on the right at L4-5 (Fig. 37-27A and B). Benglis et al. evaluated the position of the lumbar plexus in the psoas muscle of three fresh frozen human cadavers and noted that the lumbar plexus rests on the dorsal surface of the psoas muscle in a cleft created by the transverse process/vertebral body junction. The plexus progressed in a dorsal fashion from near the posterior aspect of the vertebral body at L1-2 to 0.28 of the vertebral diameter at L4-5 (Fig. 37-28). The plexus was at the greatest risk of injury at the L4-5 level.

PERCUTANEOUS LATERAL APPROACH, L1 TO L4-5

TECHNIQUE 37-17

(OZGUR ET AL.)

- After the induction of a general endotracheal anesthesia, place the patient in a right lateral decubitus position on a radiolucent operating table.
- Adjust the patient so a true 90-degree lateral image can be obtained with image intensification.
- Secure the patient in this position with taping and a bean bag or similar device.
- Adjust the table to allow maximal distance between the left rib cage and the iliac crest.
- Prepare and drape the patient for a direct lateral lumbar approach.
- Identify the midlateral position of the disc space to be entered using a Kirschner wire marker and fluoroscopic imaging (Fig. 37-29). Mark this point on the skin.
- Make a second mark posterior to the first mark at the border of the erector spinae and the abdominal oblique muscles.
- Make a 2-cm skin incision at this second mark and use blunt dissection with the index finger through the muscle layers to the retroperitoneal space; avoid entering the peritoneum (Fig. 37-30A).
- Sweep the retroperitoneal space anteriorly and palpate the psoas muscle (Fig. 37-30B).
- Turn the index finger up in a direct lateral position toward the lateral skin mark and make an incision at this mark.
- Insert the initial dilator and use the index finger to safely direct the dilator to the psoas muscle (Fig. 37-30C); confirm the position of the dilator with fluoroscopy.
- Gently separate the psoas with the initial dilator, using blunt dissection at the level determined to be in the safe zone for the level to be accessed.
- Monitor the progress of the dilator in the psoas muscle using electromyography. The stimulus necessary to elicit an electromyography response will vary with the distance from the nerve. Threshold values of more than 10 mA indicate a distance that is safe for the nerves and adequate for working.
- Take care to minimize trauma to the psoas muscle.
- Observe the progress of the dilator directly to check for nerves that may lie in the safe zone.
- Continue the dissection by spreading the midpsoas fibers laterally (Fig. 37-30D).
- Avoid the genitofemoral nerve by observing it directly until the disc is reached.
- Reconfirm placement of the initial dilator with fluoroscopy.
- Introduce subsequent dilators until the retractor can be inserted (Fig. 37-31). (This instrument varies with the system used.) Expand the retractor blades to minimize nerve pressure and maximize disc exposure.
- Confirm the final position with anteroposterior and lateral fluoroscopy before excising the disc.

ANTERIOR TRANSPERITONEAL APPROACH TO THE LUMBOSACRAL JUNCTION, L5 TO S1

Transperitoneal exposure of the lumbar spine is an alternative to the retroperitoneal approach. The advantage of the transperitoneal route is a more extensive exposure, especially at the L5-S1 level. A disadvantage is that the great vessels and hypogastric nerve plexus must be mobilized before the spine

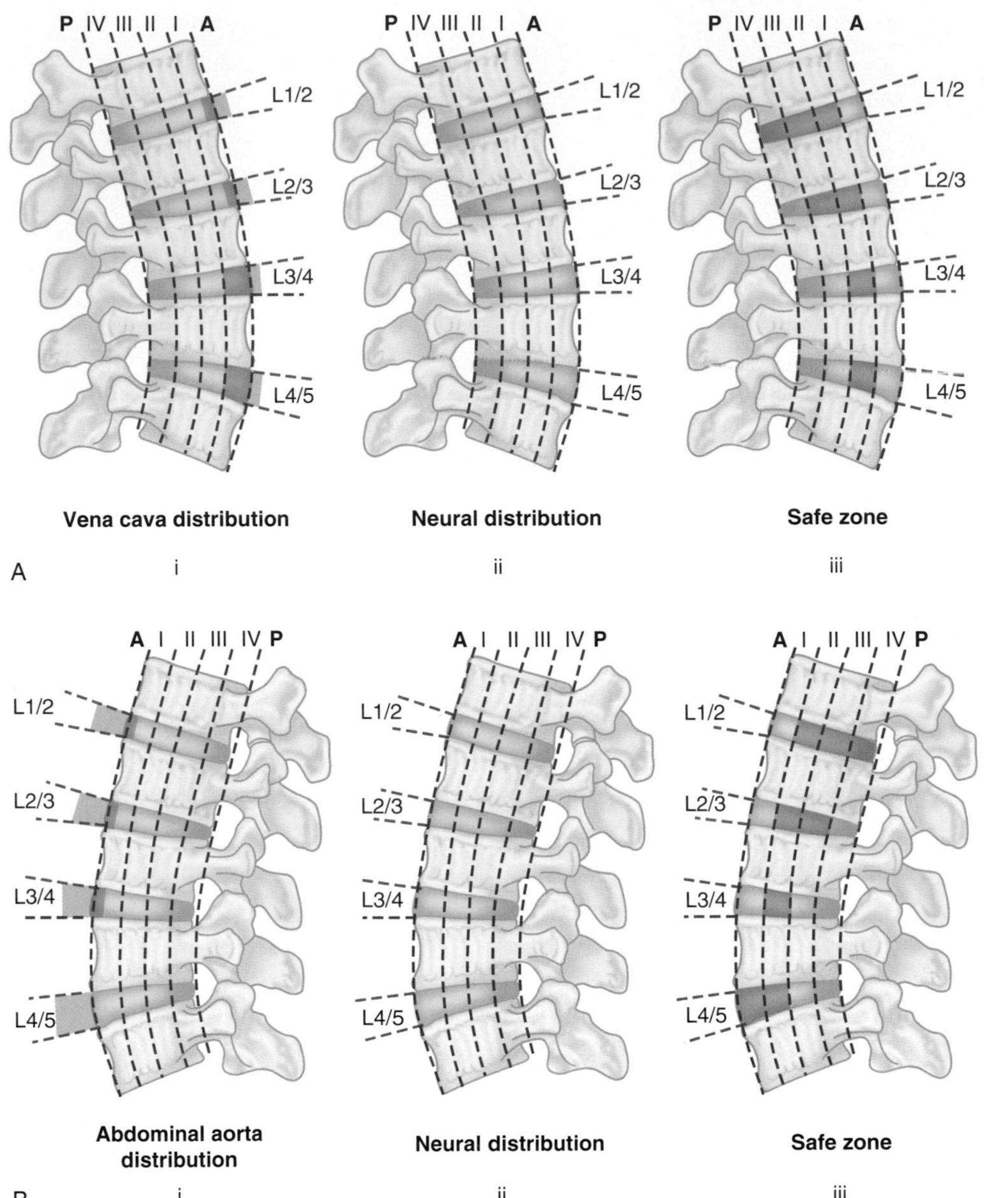

FIGURE 37-27 **A,** Right-sided XLIF approach as related to anatomic structure: *i,* vena cava distribution; *ii,* neural distribution, *iii,* safe zone. **B,** Left-sided XLIF approach associated with anatomic structures: *i,* distribution of abdominal aorta; *ii,* neural distribution; *iii,* safe zone. (From Hu WK, He SS, Zhang SC, et al: An MRI study of psoas major and abdominal large vessels with respect to the X/DLIF approach, Eur Spine J 20:557-562, 2011.)

is exposed. The superior hypogastric plexus contains the sympathetic function for the urogenital systems, and damage of this structure in men can cause complications such as retrograde ejaculation; however, damage to the superior hypogastric plexus should not produce impotence or failure of erection. Injury to the hypogastric plexus can be avoided by careful opening of the posterior peritoneum and blunt dissection of the prevertebral tissue from left to right and by opening the posterior peritoneum higher over the bifurcation of the aorta and extending the opening down over the sacral promontory. In addition, electrocautery should be kept to a minimum when dissecting within the aortic bifurcation, and until the anulus of the L5-S1 disc is clearly exposed, no transverse scalpel cuts on the front of the disc should be made.

ANTERIOR TRANSPERITONEAL APPROACH, L5 TO S1

TECHNIQUE 37-18

- Position the patient supine on the operating table and make a vertical midline or a transverse incision (Fig. 37-32A). The transverse incision is cosmetically superior and gives excellent exposure; it requires transection of the rectus abdominis sheath.
- Identify and open the sheath and transect the rectus abdominis muscle. The posterior rectus sheath, abdominal fascia, and peritoneum are conjoined in this area.

- Open the posterior rectus sheath and abdominal fascia to the peritoneum.
- Carefully open the peritoneum to avoid damage to bowel content.
- Carefully pack off the abdominal contents and identify the posterior peritoneum over the sacral promontory.
- Palpate the aorta and the common iliac vessels through the posterior peritoneum.
- Make a longitudinal incision in the posterior peritoneum in the midline around the aortic bifurcation.

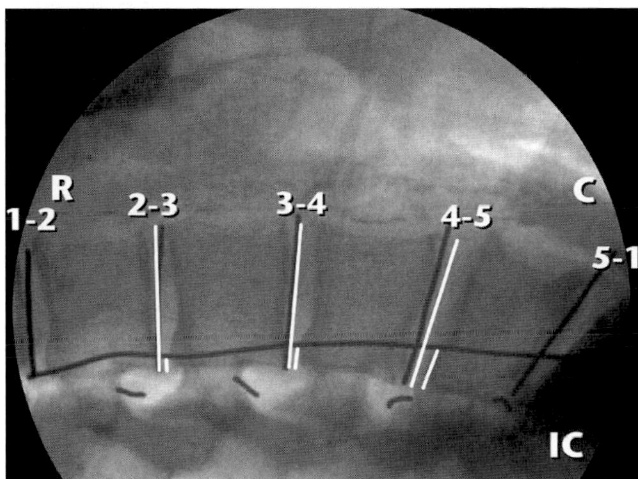

FIGURE 37-28 *White lines* show the ratio measurements: plexus to posterior end plate *(short white line)* to total length of the disc *(long white line)*. *Longitudinal dark line* is the course of the lumbar plexus as seen in the lateral view of a frozen human cadaver spine. (From Benglis DM Jr, Vanni S, Levi AD: An anatomical study of the lumbosacral plexus as related to the minimally invasive transpsoas approach to the lumbar spine, J Neurosurg Spine 10:139, 2009.)

- Extend the incision distally and to the right along the right common iliac artery to its bifurcation at the external and internal iliac arteries.
- Identify the right ureter, crossing the right iliac artery, and curve the incision medially to avoid this structure.
- Avoid the use of electrocautery anterior to the L5-S1 disc space to prevent damage to the superior hypogastric plexus.
- The left common iliac vein often lies as a flat structure across the L5-S1 disc within the aortic bifurcation. After identification of the left common iliac artery and vein, use blunt dissection to the right of the artery and hypogastric plexus and mobilize the soft tissue from left to right.
- Carefully dissect the middle sacral artery and vein from left to right (Fig. 37-32B). Longitudinal blunt dissection allows better mobilization of these vascular structures.
- If bleeding is encountered, use direct finger and sponge pressure rather than electrocautery. If electrocautery is used in this area, we recommend the bipolar rather than the unipolar machine because there is less likelihood of injuring the hypogastric plexus with a thermal burn.
- After adequate exposure of the L5-S1 disc, obtain a radiograph after inserting a 22-gauge spinal needle into the disc space. Because the L5-S1 disc and the sacrum often are angled horizontally, the body of L5 may be mistaken for the sacrum.
- Further development of the exposure proceeds as in other anterior approaches to the lumbar vertebrae.

VIDEO-ASSISTED LUMBAR SURGERY

Standard anterior approaches to the lower lumbar and lumbosacral spine include the anterior transperitoneal, anterolateral extraperitoneal, and anterior retroperitoneal approaches. As with thoracoscopy, the endoscopic technique is evolving rapidly in terms of its role in procedures involving the

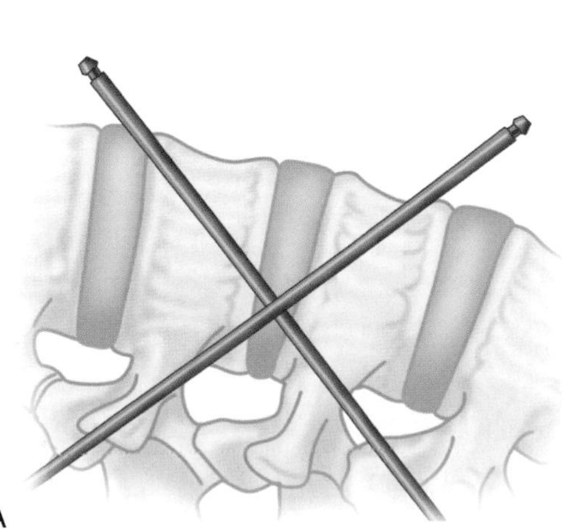

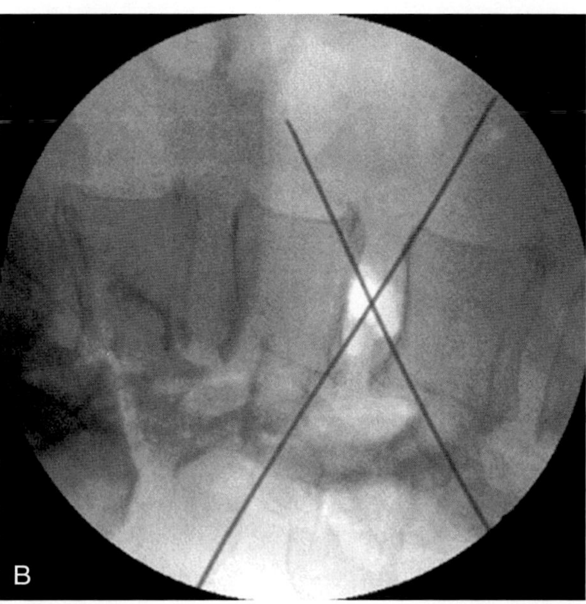

FIGURE 37-29 Percutaneous lateral approach to L1 to L4-5. **A,** Patient positioning and placement of Kirschner wires. **B,** Fluoroscopic image showing wire placement. (Redrawn from Ozgur BM, Aryan JE, Pimenta L, Taylor WR: Extreme lateral interbody fusion (XLIF): a novel surgical technique for anterior lumbar interbody fusion, Spine J 6:435, 2006.) **SEE TECHNIQUE 37-17**.

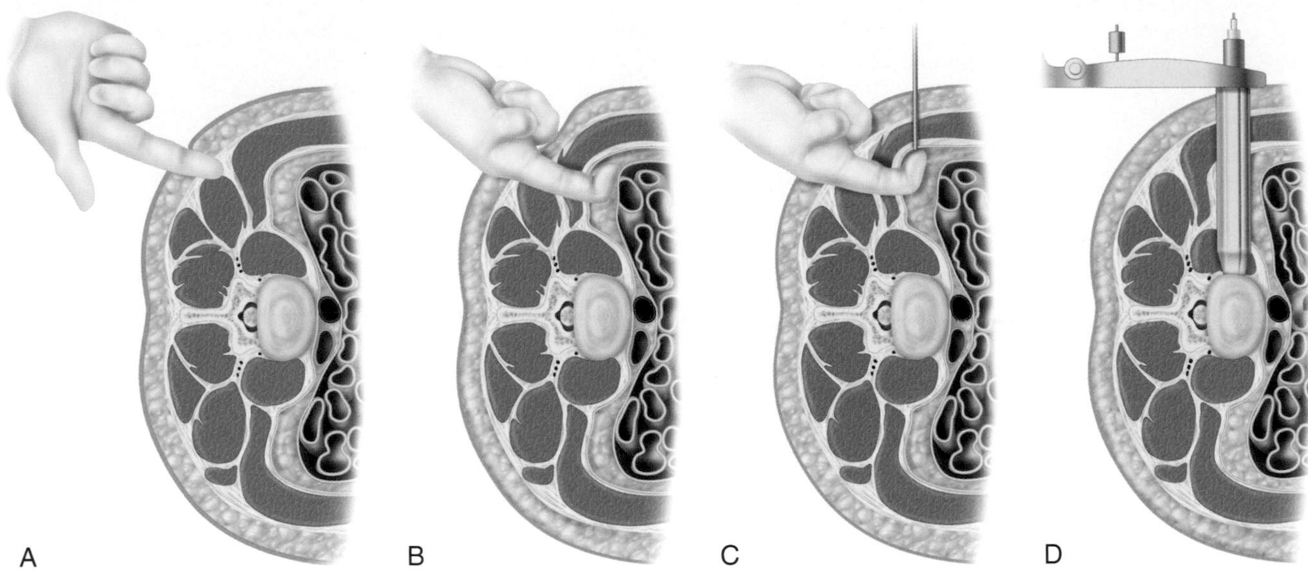

FIGURE 37-30 Percutaneous lateral approach to L1 to L4-5. **A,** Surgeon's index finger inserted into paraspinal incision site. **B,** Identification of retroperitoneal space. **C,** Guidance of the initial dilator into position. **D,** Retractor inserted into retroperitoneal space, penetrating the psoas major, positioned directly on the lateral intervertebral disc space. (Redrawn from Ozgur BM, Aryan JE, Pimenta L, Taylor WR: Extreme lateral interbody fusion (XLIF): a novel surgical technique for anterior lumbar interbody fusion, Spine J 6:435, 2006.) **SEE TECHNIQUE 37-17**.

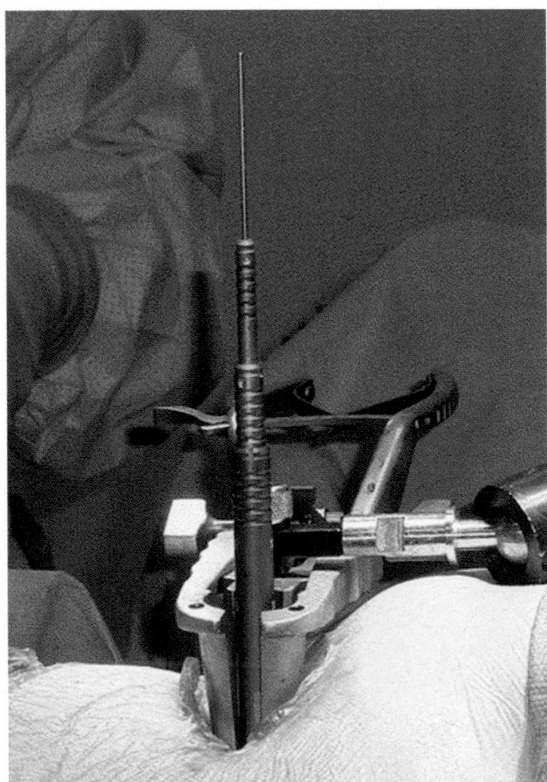

FIGURE 37-31 Operative photograph of laterally inserted dilators. With patient in lateral decubitus position, sequentially larger dilators are shown inserted, penetrating the psoas major, and resting on the desired disc space. (From Ozgur BM, Aryan JE, Pimenta L, Taylor WR: Extreme lateral interbody fusion (XLIF): a novel surgical technique for anterior lumbar interbody fusion, Spine J 6:435, 2006.) **SEE TECHNIQUE 37-17**.

anterior aspect of the lumbar spine. Transperitoneal laparoscopic approaches, which have been used for discectomy or fusion, are true endoscopic procedures that are performed with carbon dioxide insufflation and may be impeded by abdominal wall adhesions. Complications include vascular and peritoneal injuries. McAfee et al. described a minimally invasive anterior retroperitoneal approach to the lumbar spine using an endoscopic technique, and Onimus et al. described a less invasive, standard midline, extraperitoneal approach that fully preserves the abdominal innervation and is optimized with video assistance. This procedure avoids peritoneal complications, and it is anterior and midline oriented, giving direct access to the anterior aspect of the disc. Video assistance allows for a smaller incision, improved lighting, and easier presacral dissection. In addition, good exposure of the vertebral end plates is achieved, allowing a better resection and perhaps, although not reported, an improved fusion rate. In addition, surgical assistants can observe the operation despite the small incision and, if necessary, the incision can be extended cephalad or caudad if conversion to a laparotomy is necessary.

VIDEO-ASSISTED LUMBAR SURGERY

TECHNIQUE 37-19

(ONIMUS ET AL.)

- Place the patient supine and angulate the operative table to place the lumbar spine in slight extension.
- Make a 4-cm vertical incision on the midline at the umbilicus for the L4-5 approach and halfway between the

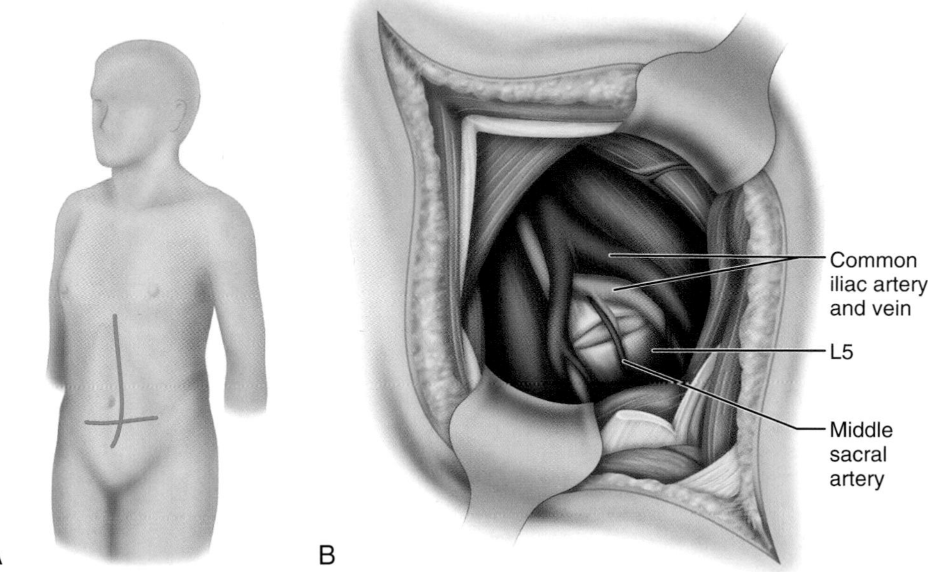

FIGURE 37-32 Transperitoneal approach to lumbar and lumbosacral spine (see text). **A**, Median longitudinal or transverse Pfannenstiel incision. **B**, Dissection of middle sacral artery and vein. **SEE TECHNIQUE 37-18.**

umbilicus and the pubic symphysis for the L5-S1 approach. In women, a more cosmetic horizontal suprapubic incision is available for the L5-S1 approach.

- After division of the linea alba, dissect on the left side between the posterior sheath of the rectus abdominis and posterior aspect of this muscle.
- Divide the posterior sheath at the lateral edge of the rectus returning to the subperitoneal fascia. The division begins at the linea arcuata. Use blunt dissection with a finger and dissecting swabs.
- The next landmark is the prominence of the psoas muscle and the iliac vessels. Reflect the ureter and peritoneum together. The lateral cleavage of the peritoneum can be increased by use of an inflatable balloon.
- Introduce a 10-mm endoscope through a lateral portal between the umbilicus and anterior superior iliac spine for exposure of L5-S1 and at the level of the umbilicus for exposure of L4-5. Introduction of the endoscope gives good exposure of the prevertebral area and allows the operation to be continued under endoscopic and direct vision.
- Expose the anterior aspect of the intervertebral disc by blunt dissection through the midline incision.
- For exposure of L5-S1, hemoclip the middle sacral vessels and divide them. Retract the common iliac vessels cranially with a specially designed retractor that is introduced through the midline incision and held in position by two Steinmann pins inserted in L5 and S1.
- For exposure of L4-5, retract the iliac vessels caudally. Divide the iliolumbar vein to allow caudal retraction of the left iliac vein.
- More acute endoscopic exposure of the vertebral plates is possible by using a 30-degree angulated arthroscope.
- Intervertebral distraction allows iliac autogenous graft insertion. The procedure can be completed with disc and vertebral plate resection.
- Close the wound on a retroperitoneal suction tube inserted through the endoscope's lateral port.

POSTOPERATIVE CARE. Standing and ambulation are allowed 2 to 3 days after surgery. A body jacket orthosis is worn for 3 months.

POSTERIOR APPROACHES

The posterior approach through a midline longitudinal incision provides access to the posterior elements of the spine at all levels, including cervical, thoracic, and lumbosacral. It is the most direct access to the spinous processes, laminae, and facets. In addition, the spinal canal can be explored and decompressed over a large area after laminectomy. Under most circumstances, the choice of approach to the spine should be dictated by the site of the primary pathologic condition. Posterior approaches to the spine rarely are indicated when the anterior spinal column is the site of an infectious process or a metastatic disease. The posterior elements usually are not involved in the pathologic process and provide stabilization for the uninvolved structures of the spinal column. Removal of the uninvolved posterior elements, as in laminectomy, may result in subluxation, dislocation, or severe angulation of the spine, causing increased compression of the neural elements and worsening of any neurologic deficit. Posterior approaches to the spine commonly are used for degenerative or traumatic spinal disorders and allow excellent exposure to perform a wide variety of fusion techniques, with or without internal stabilization. Gupta measured the distance from the midline of C1 to the vertebral artery groove in 55 adult vertebrae and found that at least 1.5 cm of the posterior arch could be safely exposed without mobilization of the vertebral artery (Fig. 37-33). With mobilization of the vertebral artery, another 10 mm of arch could be exposed in either direction.

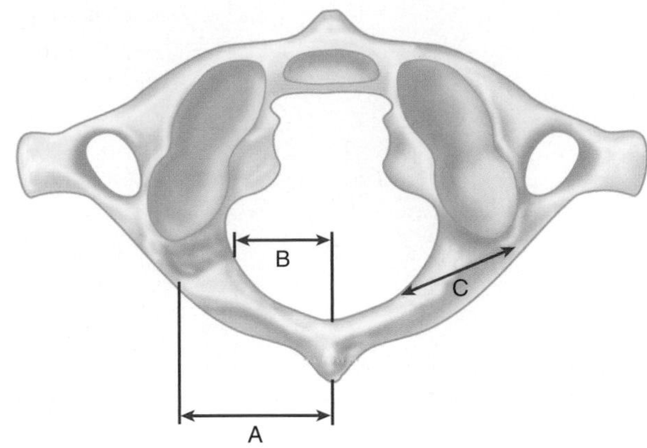

FIGURE 37-33 Distance between the posterior midline and the medial end of the vertebral artery groove at outer *(A)* and inner *(B)* cortex and the length of vertebral artery groove *(C)*. (Redrawn from Gupta T: Quantitative anatomy of vertebral artery groove on the posterior arch of atlas in relation to spinal surgical procedures, Surg Radiol Anat 30:239, 2008.)

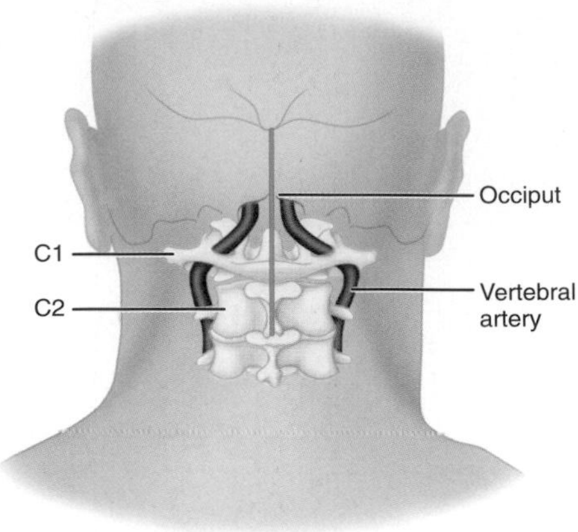

FIGURE 37-34 Posterior approach to upper cervical spine (see text). **SEE TECHNIQUE 37-20.**

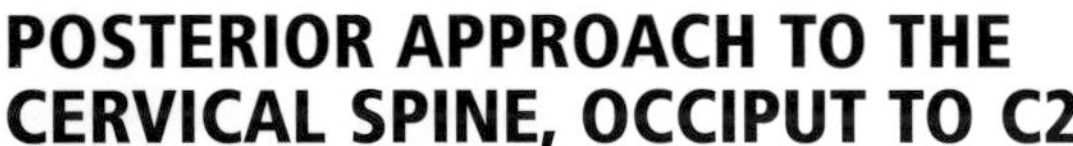

POSTERIOR APPROACH TO THE CERVICAL SPINE, OCCIPUT TO C2

TECHNIQUE 37-20

- Position the patient prone on a turning frame with skeletal traction through tongs, avoiding excessive pressure on the eyes. Alternatively, a three-point head rest can be used to provide rigid immobilization of the cervical spine during surgery.
- After routine skin preparation, attach the drapes to the neck with stay sutures or staples.
- Make a midline longitudinal skin incision from the occiput to C2 (Fig. 37-34). Infiltration of the skin and subcutaneous tissue with a dilute 1 : 500,000 epinephrine solution helps to provide hemostasis.
- Using electrocautery and elevators, expose the posterior elements subperiosteally and insert self-retaining retractors.
- It is important to deepen the incision in the midline through the thin white median raphe and avoid cutting muscle tissue. The median raphe of the cervical spine is a wandering avascular ligament and does not follow a straight midline incision. In children, do not expose any spinal levels unnecessarily to avoid spontaneous fusion at adjacent levels, including the occiput.
- When exposing the upper cervical spine, do not carry the dissection farther than 1.5 cm laterally on either side to avoid the vertebral arteries.
- When necessary, expose the occiput with elevators and insert the self-retaining retractors to expose the base of the skull and the dorsal spine of C2. The area in between contains the ring of C1; this is often deep compared with the spinous process of C2.
- While maintaining lateral retraction of the soft tissues, identify the posterior tubercle of C1 longitudinally in the midline and begin subperiosteal dissection to the bone. Often the ring of C1 is thin, and direct pressure can fracture it or cause the instrument to slip off the ring and penetrate the atlantooccipital membrane. The dura may be vulnerable on the superior and the inferior edges of the ring of C1.
- The second cervical ganglion is an important landmark on the ring of C1 laterally. It lies approximately 1.5 cm laterally on the lamina of C1 in the groove for the vertebral artery. There is little, if any, indication for dissection lateral to this groove.
- The vertebral artery may be damaged by penetration of the atlantooccipital membrane off the superior border of the ring of C1 more lateral than the usually safe 1.5 cm from the midline.
- Below C2, the lateral margins of the facet joints are the safe lateral extent of dissection.
- After exposure of the posterior occiput, the ring of C1, and the posterior elements of C2, the intended surgical procedure may be performed.
- After this, the wound is closed in layers over a drain.

POSTERIOR APPROACH TO THE CERVICAL SPINE, C3 TO C7

TECHNIQUE 37-21

- Position the patient prone on a turning frame with skeletal traction through tongs or with the head positioned in the three-point head fixation device that is attached to the table.
- The large spinous processes of C2 and C7 are prominent and can be identified by palpation. It is important to note on preoperative radiographs any posterior element deficiencies, such as an occult spina bifida, before exposure of the posterior elements.
- Make a midline skin incision over the appropriate vertebrae (Fig. 37-35) and inject the skin and subcutaneous

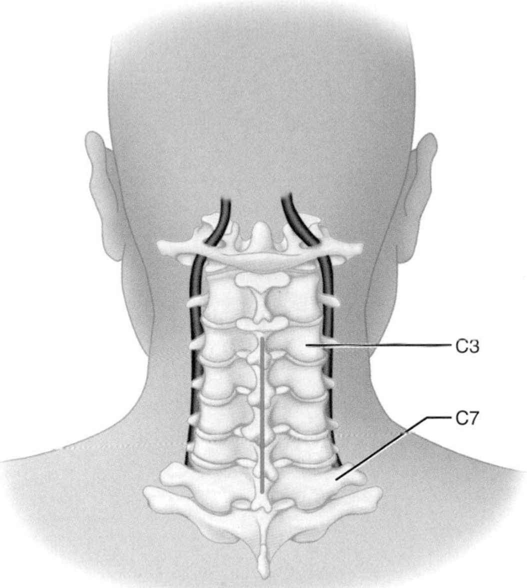

FIGURE 37-35 Posterior approach to lower cervical spine (see text). **SEE TECHNIQUE 37-21.**

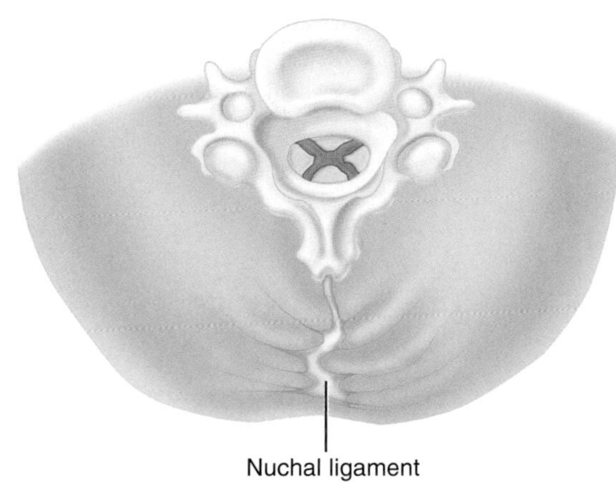

FIGURE 37-36 Posterior approach to lower cervical spine. Nuchal ligament is irregular. To maintain dry field, surgeon must stay within ligament. **SEE TECHNIQUE 37-21.**

tissues with a 1:500,000 epinephrine solution to aid in hemostasis.

- Deepen the dissection in the midline using the electrocautery knife and staying within the thin white median raphe to avoid cutting the vascular muscle tissue (Fig. 37-36). It is helpful to maintain tension on the soft tissue by inserting self-retaining retractors.
- Using electrocautery and elevators, detach the ligamentous attachments to the spinous processes and expose the posterior elements subperiosteally to the lateral edge of the facet joints, which is the extent of dissection on either side of the midline.
- After identifying the lateral edge of the facet joint, pack each level with a taped sponge to keep blood loss to a minimum.
- It is helpful to expose the spinous processes distal to proximal because the muscles can be stripped from the spinous processes in the acute angle between their insertions and the bone. If exposure in the opposite direction is attempted, the knife blade or periosteal elevator would tend to follow the direction of the fibers into the muscle and divide the vessels, increasing hemorrhage.

POSTERIOR APPROACH TO THE THORACIC SPINE, T1 TO T12

The posterior approach to the thoracic spine can be made through a standard midline longitudinal exposure with reflection of the erector spinae muscle laterally to the tips of the transverse processes. Alternatively, the thoracic vertebrae can be approached through a costotransversectomy when direct access to the transverse processes and pedicles of the thoracic spine and limited access to the vertebral bodies are indicated. Costotransversectomy should be considered for simple biopsy or local debridement. This approach does not provide the working operative area or length of exposure to the thoracic vertebral bodies that is afforded by a transthoracic approach or the midlongitudinal posterior approach.

TECHNIQUE 37-22

- Position the patient prone on a padded spinal operating frame.
- Make a long midline incision over the area to be exposed (Fig. 37-37). Infiltration of the skin, subcutaneous tissue, and erector spinae to the level of the laminae with 1:500,000 epinephrine solution helps to provide hemostasis.
- Deepen the dissection in the midline using a scalpel or the electrocautery knife through the superficial and lumbodorsal fasciae to the tips of the spinous processes.
- Expose subperiosteally the posterior elements by reflecting the erector spinae muscle laterally to the tips of the transverse processes distal to proximal, using periosteal elevators.
- Repeat the procedure until the desired number of vertebrae are exposed; where both sides of the spine require exposure, use the same technique on each side.
- Pack each segment with a taped sponge immediately after exposure to lessen bleeding.
- After satisfactory exposure of the posterior elements, obtain a radiograph to confirm proper localization of the intended level.
- After completion of the spinal procedure, close the wound in layers over a suction drain.

MINIMALLY INVASIVE APPROACHES TO THE POSTERIOR SPINE

All of the posterior approaches to the spine can be made in a minimally invasive fashion when only a limited area of dissection is needed within the lateral recess, canal, or lumbar

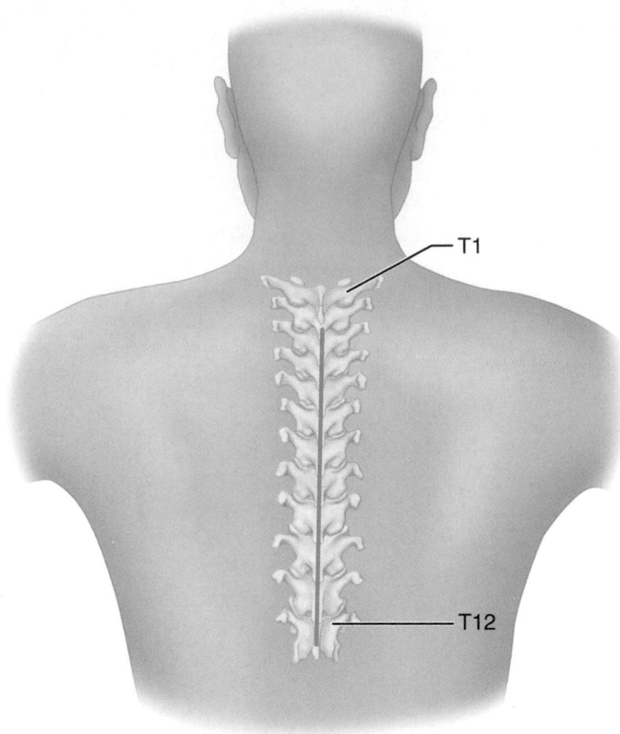

FIGURE 37-37 Posterior approach to thoracic spine (see text). **SEE TECHNIQUE 37-22.**

intervertebral foramen. The adaptation typically involves dilating through the posterior overlying fascia (thoracolumbar) and musculature, followed by inserting down to the spine a fixed or adjustable tubular retractor that is attached to a table-mounted retractor arm. The location of the incision is critical in a minimally invasive approach and depends on the exact procedure since the smaller field of view and working portal limit the surgical corridor. A 2-cm error in placement of the incision when using a 20-mm retractor is a 100% error. Planning the location of the incision based on preoperative imaging (MRI and/or CT) and fluoroscopic localization of the incision is mandatory for minimally invasive posterior approaches.

COSTOTRANSVERSECTOMY

TECHNIQUE 37-23

- Place the patient prone on a padded spinal operating frame.
- Make a straight longitudinal incision about 2.5 inches (6.3 cm) lateral to the spinous processes centered over the level of the desired vertebral dissection (Fig. 37-38A). (Alternatively, make a curved incision with its apex lateral to the midline.)
- Palpate the slight depression between the dorsal paraspinal muscle mass and the prominent posterior angle of the rib and center the incision over this groove lateral to the spinous processes.

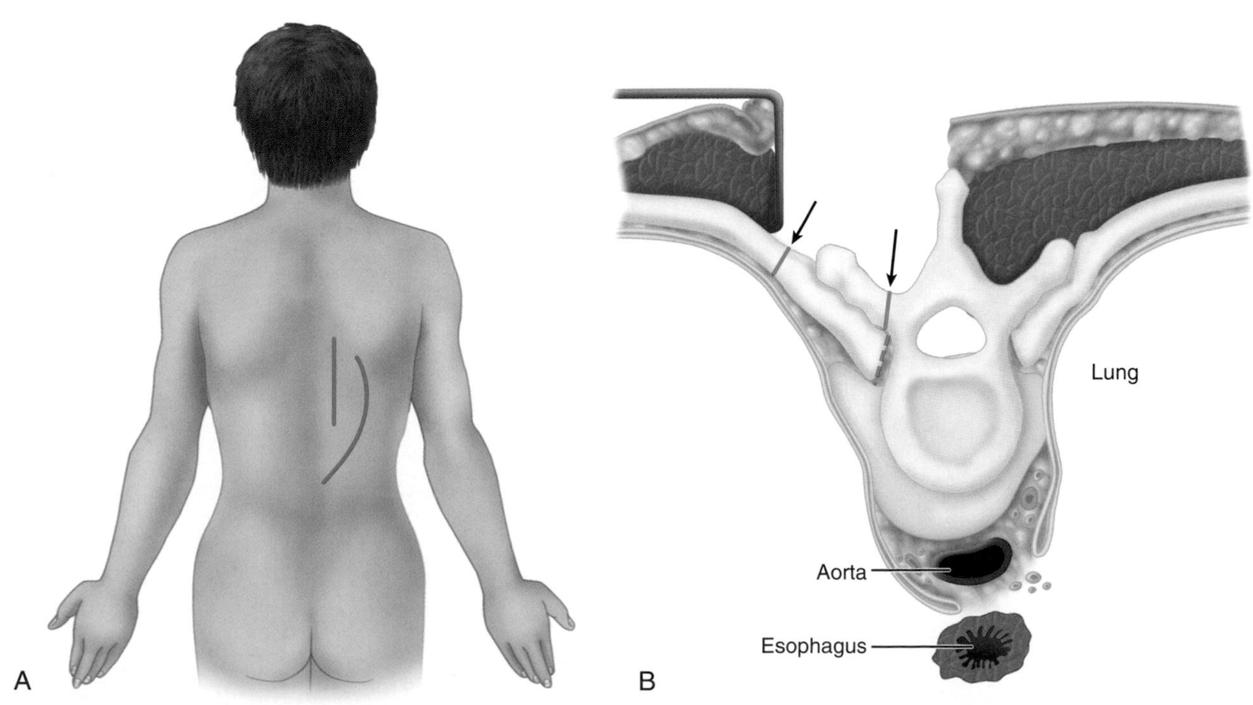

FIGURE 37-38 Costotransversectomy. **A,** Straight longitudinal incision about 2.5 inches (6.3 cm) lateral to spinous processes, centered over level of vertebral dissection. **B,** Resection of costotransverse articulation. **SEE TECHNIQUE 37-23.**

- Deepen the dissection through the subcutaneous tissues and the trapezius and latissimus dorsi muscles and the lumbodorsal fasciae, which are divided longitudinally.
- Dissect the paraspinal muscles sharply from their insertions on the ribs and transverse processes and retract them medially.
- Expose the transverse process and posterior aspects of the associated rib subperiosteally and remove a section of rib 5 to 7.5 cm long at the level of involvement. The rib generally is transected with rib cutters about 3.5 inches (~9 cm) lateral to the vertebra at its prominent posterior angle. The costotransverse ligament and joint capsule are strong and increase the inherent stability of the thoracic spine.
- Remain subperiosteal and extrapleural during this part of the exposure and protect the intercostal neurovascular bundle. Anterior to the transverse process is the vertebral pedicle, and above and below the pedicle lie the neural foramina. The nerve roots emerge from the superior portion of the foramina, giving off a dorsal and ventral ramus. The ventral ramus becomes the intercostal nerve and is joined by the intercostal vessels.
- When the pedicles, neural foramina, and neurovascular structures have been identified, proceed with dissection directly anteriorly on the pedicle to the vertebral body along a path that is relatively free of major vessels or nerves (Fig. 37-38B).
- Carefully dissect the parietal pleura with elevators anteriorly to expose the anterolateral aspect of the vertebral body, raising the sympathetic trunk and parietal pleura.
- Exposure may be increased by removal of the transverse process, pedicle, and facet joints as necessary.
- After completion of the spinal procedure, fill the wound with saline and inflate the lungs to check for air leaks.
- Close the wound in layers over a drain to prevent hematoma collection.
- Obtain a chest radiograph to document the absence of air in the pleural space, which may occur if the pleura is inadvertently entered during the exposure.

POSTERIOR APPROACH TO THE LUMBAR SPINE, L1 TO L5

The posterior approach to the lumbar spine provides access directly to the spinous processes, laminae, and facet joints at all levels. In addition, the transverse processes and pedicles can be reached through this approach. Wiltse and Spencer refined the paraspinal approach to the lumbar spine, which involves a longitudinal separation of the sacrospinalis muscle group to expose the posterolateral aspect of the lumbar spine. This approach is especially useful in removing far-lateral disc herniation, decompressing a "far out" syndrome, and inserting pedicle screws.

TECHNIQUE 37-24

- Position the patient prone or in the kneeling position on a padded spinal frame. By allowing the abdomen to hang free, intravenous pressure is decreased and blood loss is decreased as a result of collapse of the epidural venous plexus.
- Make a midline skin incision centered over the involved lumbar segment (Fig. 37-39). Infiltrating the skin and subcutaneous tissue with 1:500,000 epinephrine aids hemostasis.
- Carry the dissection down in the midline through the skin, subcutaneous tissue, and lumbodorsal fascia to the tips of the spinous processes. Use self-retaining retractors to maintain tension on soft tissues during exposure.
- Subperiosteally expose the posterior elements from distal to proximal using electrocautery and periosteal elevators to detach the muscles from the posterior elements.
- Pack each segment with a taped sponge immediately after exposure to lessen bleeding.
- If the procedure requires exposure of both sides of the spine, use the same technique on each side.
- We recommend accurate localization of the involved segment with a permanent radiograph in the operating room.
- After completion of the spinal procedure, close the wound in layers over a drain.

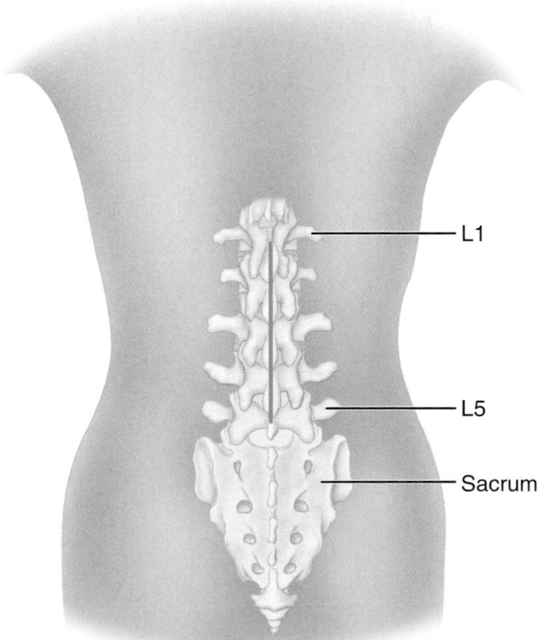

FIGURE 37-39 Posterior approach to lumbar spine (see text). **SEE TECHNIQUE 37-24.**

PARASPINAL APPROACH TO LUMBAR SPINE

TECHNIQUE 37-25

(WILTSE AND SPENCER)

- Position the patient prone or in the kneeling position on a spinal frame. By allowing the abdomen to hang free, intravenous pressure is decreased and blood loss is decreased as a result of collapse of the epidural venous plexus.
- Make a midline skin incision centered over the involved lower lumbar segment (Fig. 37-40A). Infiltration with 1 : 500,000 epinephrine helps to provide hemostasis.
- Carry dissection down to the lumbodorsal fascia and retract the skin and subcutaneous tissue laterally on either side.
- Make a fascial incision approximately 2 cm lateral to the midline (Fig. 37-40B and C).
- After the fascial layers have been divided, a natural cleavage plane is entered lying between the multifidus and longissimus muscles. Using blunt finger dissection between the muscle groups (Fig. 37-40D and E), palpate the facet joints at L4-5. Place self-retaining Gelpi retractors between the two muscle groups.
- Using electrocautery or an elevator, separate the transverse fibers of the multifidus from their heavy fascial attachments.
- Expose the lumbar transverse processes, facet joints, and laminae subperiosteally and denude them of soft tissue. Avoid carrying the dissection anterior to the transverse processes because the exiting spinal nerves lie just in front of the transverse processes and can be injured.

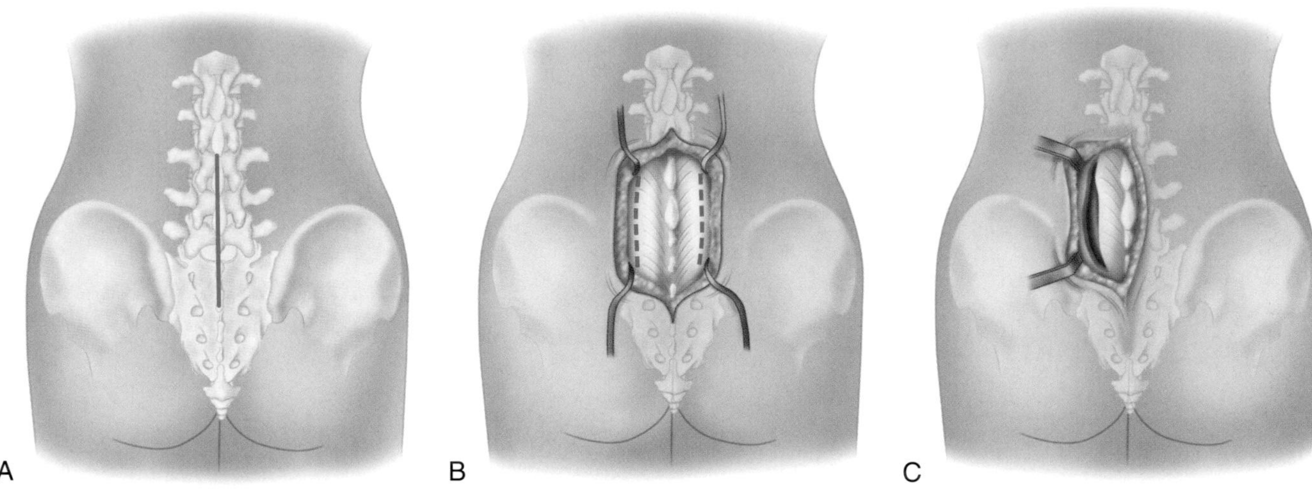

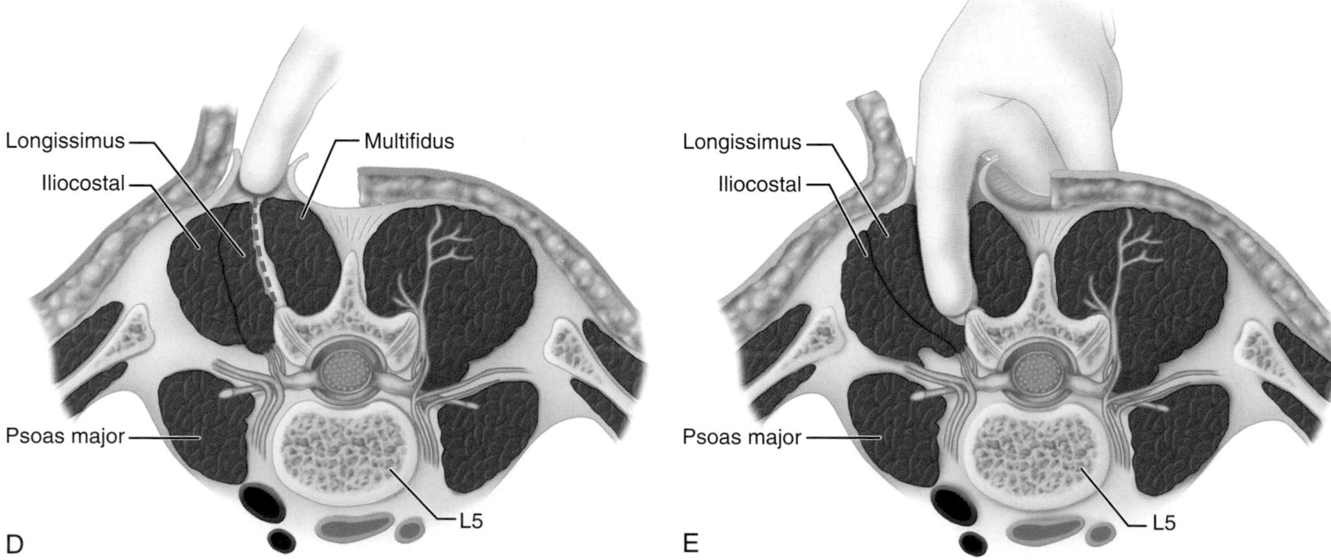

FIGURE 37-40 Paraspinal approach to lumbar spine (see text). **A,** Midline skin incision. **B** and **C,** Fascial incisions. **D** and **E,** Blunt finger dissection between muscle groups to palpate facet joints. (Redrawn from Wiltse LL, Spencer CW: New uses and refinements of the paraspinal approach of the lumbar spine, Spine 13:696, 1988.) **SEE TECHNIQUE 37-25**.

- Use bipolar cautery to control bleeding from the lumbar arteries and veins coursing above the base of the transverse processes.
- Perform unilateral or bilateral decompression and fusion of the lumbosacral spine.
- Close the wound over a suction drain and suture the skin flaps down to the fascia to remove dead space.

POSTERIOR APPROACH TO THE LUMBOSACRAL SPINE, L1 TO SACRUM

TECHNIQUE 37-26

(WAGONER)

- Make a longitudinal incision over the spinous processes of the appropriate vertebrae and incise the superficial fascia, the lumbodorsal fascia, and the supraspinous ligament longitudinally, precisely over the tips of the processes.
- With a scalpel, divide longitudinally the ligament between the two spinous processes in the most distal part of the wound.
- Insert a small, blunt periosteal elevator through this opening so that its end rests on the junction of the spinous process with the lamina of the more proximal vertebra (Fig. 37-41A). Move the handle of the elevator proximally and laterally to place under tension the muscles attached to this spinous process.
- With a scalpel moving from distal to proximal, strip the muscles subperiosteally from the lateral surface of the process.
- Place the end of the elevator in the wound so that its end rests on the junction of the spinous process with the lamina of the next most proximal vertebra and repeat the procedure as described.
- Repeat the procedure until the desired number of vertebrae have been exposed (Fig. 37-41B).
- For operations requiring exposure of both sides of the spine, use the same technique on each side.
- This approach exposes the spinous processes and medial part of the laminae.
- Increase the exposure, if desired, by further subperiosteal reflection along the laminae; expose the posterior surface of the laminae and the articular facets.
- Pack each segment with a tape sponge immediately after exposure to lessen bleeding.
- Divide the supraspinous ligament precisely over the tip of the spinous processes and denude subperiosteally the sides of the processes because this route leads through a relatively avascular field; otherwise, the arterial supply to the muscles is encountered (Fig. 37-38C).
- Blood loss can be decreased further by using electrocautery and a suction apparatus. Replace blood as it is lost.
- Expose the spinous processes from distal to proximal as just described because the muscles can then be stripped from the spinous processes in the acute angle between their insertions and the bone.

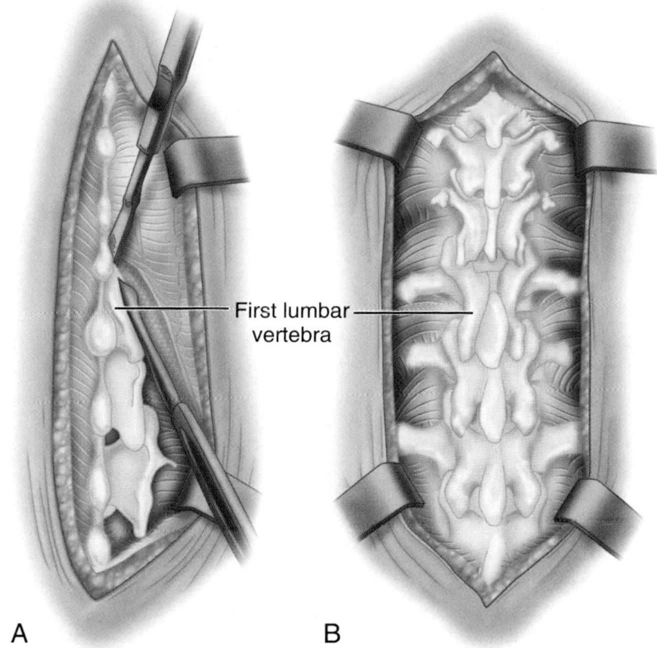

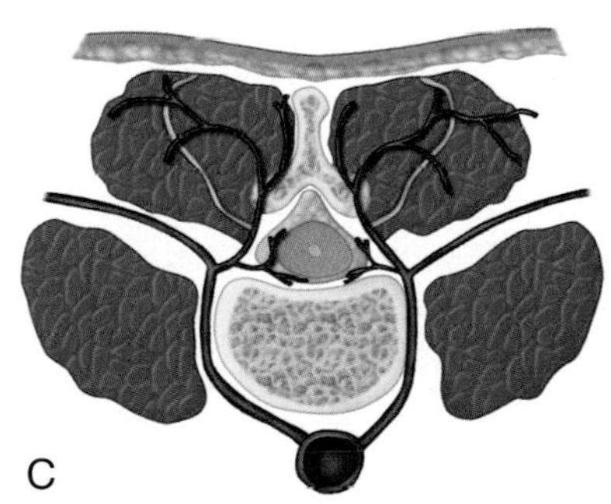

FIGURE 37-41 Approach to posterior aspect of spine. **A,** Courses of arteries supplying posterior spinal muscles, showing proximity of internal muscular branches to spinous processes. **B,** Muscle insertions are freed subperiosteally from lateral side of spinous processes and interspinous ligaments; dissection proceeds proximally, with periosteal elevator being held against bases of spinous processes. **C,** Spinous processes, laminae, and articular facets exposed. (Modified from Wagoner G: A technique for lessening hemorrhage in operations on the spine, J Bone Joint Surg 19:469, 1937.) **SEE TECHNIQUE 37-26.**

- If exposure in the opposite direction is attempted, the knife blade or periosteal elevator tends to follow the direction of the fibers into the muscle and divides the vessels, increasing hemorrhage.

POSTERIOR APPROACH TO THE SACRUM AND SACROILIAC JOINT

The posterior sacrum and sacroiliac joint are approached most commonly through a standard posterior exposure; however, the access to the sacroiliac joint is limited. Ebraheim et al. described a transosseous approach to the

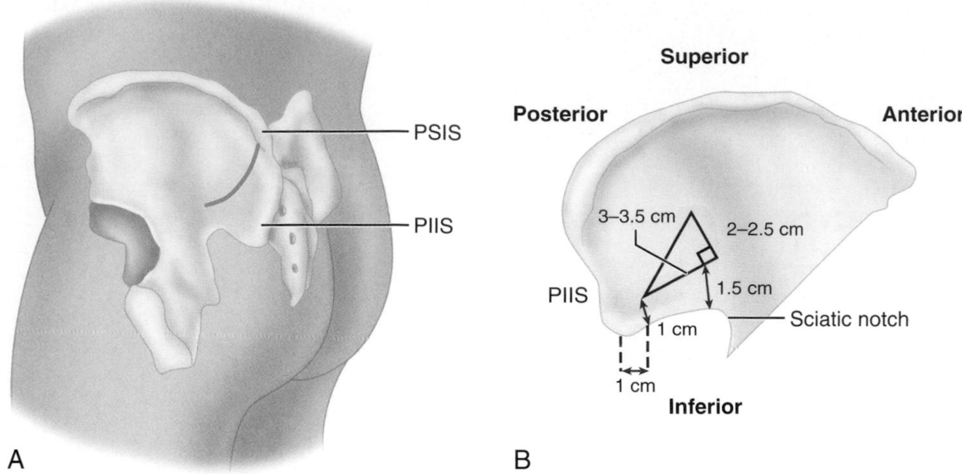

FIGURE 37-42 **Posterior approach to sacroiliac joint. A, Skin incision. B, Right triangle on outer table of posterior ilium.** ***PIIS,*** **Posterior inferior iliac spine;** ***PSIS,*** **posterior superior iliac spine.** (Redrawn from Ebraheim NA, Lu J, Biyani A, et al: Anatomic considerations for posterior approach to the sacroiliac joint, Spine 21:2709, 1996.) **SEE TECHNIQUE 37-27**.

sacroiliac joint that they suggested improves access for debridement and arthrodesis with only minimal soft-tissue dissection and iliac bone resection. Indications include trauma, infection, degenerative disease, and inflammatory processes. This approach allows direct exposure of the corresponding sacral articular surfaces.

TECHNIQUE 37-27

(EBRAHEIM ET AL.)

- Place the patient prone on padded bolsters or a spinal frame.
- Make an incision beginning at the level of the posterior superior iliac spine and extending distal to the midpoint between the posterior superior iliac spine and the posterior inferior iliac spine.
- Extend the incision laterally and distally approximately 5 cm (Fig. 37-42A).
- Divide the superficial fascia and incise the gluteus medius muscle along the line of the skin incision.
- Sharply dissect the origin of the gluteus maximus from the posterior ilium.
- Subperiosteally elevate the gluteal musculature laterally and identify the superior border of the greater sciatic notch.
- Insert one or two Steinmann pins into the ilium to assist in retracting the gluteus maximus laterally and distally. It is important not to injure the superior gluteal neurovascular bundle.
- Expose the posterior external surface of the ilium between the posterior superior iliac spine above and the superior border of the greater sciatic notch below.
- Elevate a right-angle triangular bone window from the posterior ilium using an osteotome or power saw and remove the articular cartilage from the sacrum and ilium (Fig. 37-42B). Debride the joint with curets.
- After removal of the articular cartilage, place the previously elevated bone window into its original position and carefully tamp it back into place.
- Accurate localization of the bone window in the iliac crest is important to avoid laceration to the superior gluteal artery, which may retract into the pelvis, making hemostasis difficult. Injury to the superior gluteal nerve may denervate the gluteus medius, leading to dysfunction in hip abduction. The dimensions of the right-angle triangle in the outer table of the posterior ilium are illustrated in Figure 37-42B.

REFERENCES

Adkins DE, Sandhu FA, Voyadzis JM: Minimally invasive lateral approach to the thoracolumbar junction for corpectomy, *J Clin Neurosci* 20:1289, 2013.

Baaj AA, Papadimitriou K, Amin AG, et al: Surgical anatomy of the diaphragm in the anterolateral approach to the spine: a cadaveric study, *J Spinal Disord Tech* 27:220, 2014.

Beisse R: Video-assisted techniques in the management of thoracolumbar fractures, *Orthop Clin North Am* 38:419, 2007.

Benglis DM Jr, Vanni S, Levi AD: An anatomical study of the lumbosacral plexus as related to the minimally invasive transpsoas approach to the lumbar spine: laboratory investigation, *J Neurosurg Spine* 10:139, 2009.

Cheung KMC, Mak KC, Luk KDK: Anterior approach to cervical spine, *Spine* 37:E297, 2012.

Chibbaro S, Mirone G, Bresson D, George B: Cervical spine lateral approach for myeloradiculopathy: technique and pitfalls, *Surg Neurol* 72:318, 2009.

Cho W, Buchowski JM, Park Y, et al: Surgical approach to the cervicothoracic junction. Can a standard Smith-Robinson approach be utilized? *J Spinal Disord Tech* 25:264, 2012.

Civelek E, Karasu A, Cansever T, et al: Surgical anatomy of the cervical sympathetic trunk during anterolateral approach to cervical spine, *Eur Spine J* 17:991, 2008.

Dakwar E, Ahmadian A, Uribe JS: The anatomical relationship of the diaphragm to the thoracolumbar junction during the minimally invasive lateral extracoelomic (retropleural/retroperitoneal) approach. Laboratory investigation, *J Neurosurg Spine* 16:359, 2012.

Fuentes S, Malikov S, Blondel B, et al: Cervicosternotomy as an anterior approach to the upper thoracic and cervicothoracic spinal junction, *J Neurosurg Spine* 12:160, 2010.

Gavriliu TS, Japie EM, Ghita RA, et al: Burnei's anterior transthoracic retropleural approach of the thoracic spine: a new operative technique in the treatment of spinal disorders, *J Med Life* 8:160, 2015.

Gumbs AA, Bloom ND, Bitan FD, Hanan SH: Open anterior approaches for lumbar spine procedures, *Am J Surg* 194:98, 2007.

Gupta T: Quantitative anatomy of vertebral artery groove on the posterior arch of atlas in relation to spinal surgical procedures, *Surg Radiol Anat* 30:239, 2008.

Hu WK, He SS, Zhang SC, et al: An MRI study of psoas major and abdominal large vessels with respect to the X/DLIF approach, *Eur Spine J* 20: 557–562, 2011.

Knight RQ, Schwaegler P, Hanscom D, Roh J: Direct lateral lumbar interbody fusion for degenerative conditions: early complication profile, *J Spinal Disord Tech* 22:35, 2009.

Le Huec JC, Tournier C, Aunoble S, et al: Video-assisted treatment of thoracolumbar junction fractures using a specific distractor for reduction: prospective study of 50 cases, *Eur J Spine* 19(Suppl 2):S27, 2010.

Litré CF, Duntze J, Benhima Y, et al: Anterior minimally invasive extrapleural retroperitoneal approach to the thoraco-lumbar junction of the spine, *Orthop Traumatol Surg Res* 99:94, 2013.

Ozgur BM, Aryan HE, Pimenta L, Taylor WR: Extreme lateral interbody fusion (XLIF): a novel surgical technique for anterior lumbar interbody fusion, *Spine J* 6:435, 2006.

Park DK, Lee MJ, Lin EL, et al: The relationship of intrapsoas nerves during a transpsoas approach to the lumbar spine: anatomic study, *J Spinal Disord Tech* 23:223, 2010.

Pointillart V, Aurouer N, Gangnet N, Vital JM: Anterior approach to the cervicothoracic junction without sternotomy: a report of 37 cases, *Spine* 32:2875, 2007.

Song Y, Tharin S, Divi V, et al: Anterolateral approach to the upper cervical spine: case report and operative technique, *Head Neck* 37:E115, 2015.

Zhang Y, Zhang J, Wang X, et al: Application of the cervical subaxial anterior approach at C2 in select patients, *Orthopedics* 36:e554, 2013.

The complete list of references is available online at ***expertconsult.inkling.com****.*

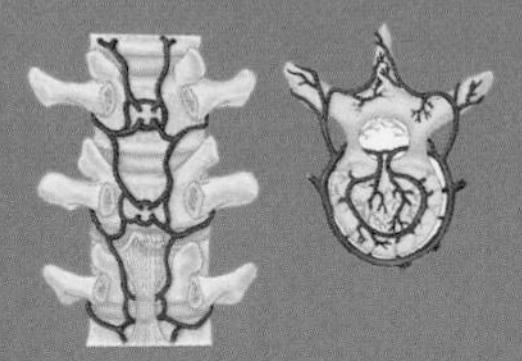

CHAPTER 38

DEGENERATIVE DISORDERS OF THE CERVICAL SPINE

Francis X. Camillo

OVERVIEW OF DISC DEGENERATION AND HERNIATION IN THE CERVICAL SPINE

In recent years, understanding of disc degeneration has undergone a significant transformation. The opportunities to improve understanding at a basic science level and a clinical level remain greater for disc disorders than for many other areas of orthopaedics. Particularly with respect to clinical applications, more effort should be made toward defining and understanding the underlying pathophysiologic processes rather than developing additional treatment options. Treatment continues to be limited not by lack of procedures but by lack of specific diagnoses with reliable natural history data that could be used to better assess and direct current and future treatment applications.

Axial spine pain, which should be distinguished from disc degeneration, is the most frequent musculoskeletal complaint. Axial spine pain—whether cervical, thoracic, or lumbar—often is attributed to disc degeneration. This degenerative process does not always cause pain, but it can lead to internal disc derangement or disc herniation. Each of these pathologic processes has unique clinical findings and treatments. The understanding of disc degeneration and the associated etiologic factors has changed markedly over the past several years. Also, efforts to make the distinction between disc degeneration and "degenerative disc disease" have made progress.

The genetic influence on disc degeneration may be attributed to a small effect from each of multiple genes or possibly a relatively large effect of a smaller number of genes. To date, several specific gene loci have been identified that are associated with disc degeneration. This association of a specific gene with degenerative disc changes has been confirmed. Other variations in the aggrecan gene, metalloproteinase-3 gene, collagen type IX, and alpha 2 and 3 gene forms also have been associated with disc pathology and symptoms. The understanding of symptoms related to disc herniations has become clearer over time than symptoms related only to disc degeneration.

Nonspecific axial pain is an international health issue of major significance and should be discriminated from pain associated with a disc herniation. Approximately 80% of individuals are affected by this symptom at some time in their lives. Impairments of the back and spine are ranked as the most frequent cause of limitation of activity in individuals younger than 45 years old by the National Center for Health Statistics (www.cdc.gov/nchs).

Nonanatomic factors, specifically work perception and psychosocial factors, are intimately intertwined with physical complaints. Compounding the diagnostic and treatment difficulties is the high incidence of significant abnormalities shown by imaging studies, which in asymptomatic matched controls is 76%. Optimal outcome primarily depends on "proper patient selection," which so far has defied satisfactory definition. Until the pathologic process is better described

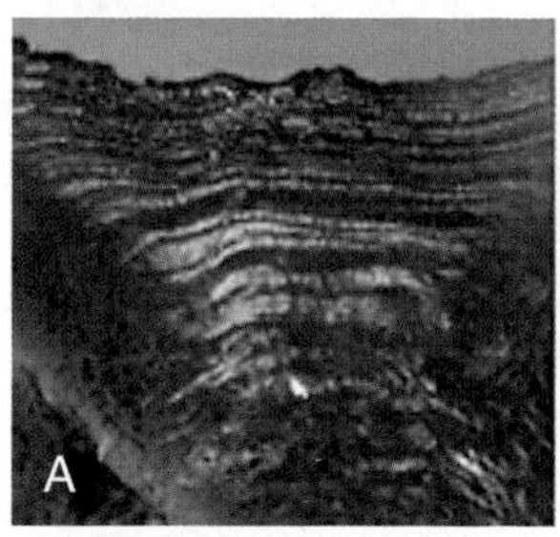

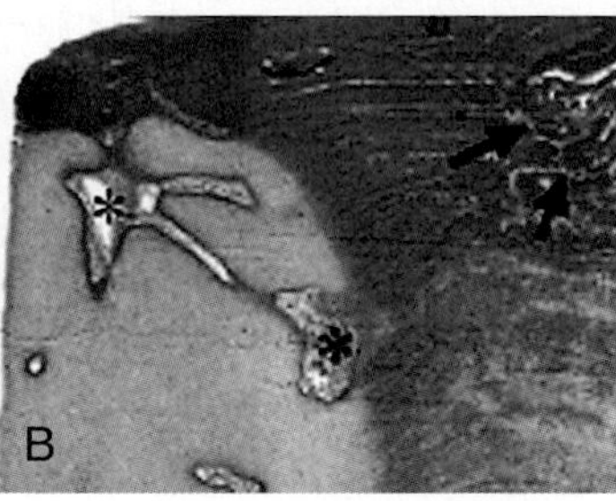

FIGURE 38-1 Histologic findings of human intervertebral discs. **A,** Specimen from 30-month-old child shows how regular concentric lamellae can be seen when specimen is viewed with polarized light. **B,** Specimen from neonate shows how outer aspect of anulus fibrosus and cartilage endplate are vascularized with blood vessels *(arrows)* and vascular channels *(asterisks)*. (**A** and **B** stained with hematoxylin and eosin; original magnification, ×10 **[A]** and ×30 **[B]**. From Roberts S, Evans H, Trivedi J, et al: Histology and pathology of the human intervertebral disc, J Bone Joint Surg 88A[Suppl 2]:10, 2006.)

and reliable criteria for the diagnosis are determined, improvement in treatment outcomes will change slowly.

DISC AND SPINE ANATOMY

The intervertebral disc has a complex structure; the nucleus pulposus has an organized matrix, which is laid down by relatively few cells. The central gelatinous nucleus is contained around the periphery by the collagenous anulus, the cartilaginous anulus, and the cartilage endplates cephalad and caudad. Collagen fibers continue from the anulus to the surrounding tissues, tying into the vertebral body along its rim and into the anterior and posterior longitudinal ligaments and the hyaline cartilage endplates superiorly and inferiorly. The cartilage endplates are secured to the osseous endplate by the calcified cartilage. Few, if any, collagen fibers cross this boundary. The anulus has a lamellar structure with interconnections between adjacent layers of collagen fibrils (Fig. 38-1).

At birth, the disc has some direct blood supply contained within the cartilaginous endplates and the anulus. These vessels recede in the first years of life, and by adulthood there is no appreciable blood supply to the disc. Over time, for reasons not well understood, the water content of the gelatinous nucleus matrix decreases with a decreased and altered proteoglycan composition. These changes lead to a more fibrous consistency of the nucleus, which ultimately fissures. Blood vessels grow into the disc through these outer fissures, with an increase in cellular proliferation and formation of cell clusters. Also, there is an increase in cell death, the mechanism of which is unknown. The cartilage endplates become thinned, with fissuring occurring with subsequent sclerosis of the subchondral endplates. The above-enumerated changes are quite similar if not identical to the changes of disc degeneration. Herniated discs have a greater number of senescent cells than nonherniated discs and have higher concentrations of matrix metalloproteinases.

The normal adult disc has a large amount of extracellular matrix and a few cells that account for about 1% by volume. These cells are of two phenotypes: anulus cells and nucleus cells. The anulus cells are more elongated and appear more like fibroblasts, whereas nucleus cells are oval and resemble chondrocytes. These two cell types behave differently and may be able to sense mechanical stresses. In culture, they respond differently to loads and produce different matrix proteins. The anulus cells produce predominantly type I collagen, whereas nucleus cells synthesize type II collagen. The characteristics of these cell types under normal and abnormal circumstances are beginning to be determined, and much is known, but this is beyond the scope of this chapter; however, this information is necessary to understand and subsequently treat disc disorders.

The cells within the disc are sustained by diffusion of nutrients into the disc through the porous central concavity of the vertebral endplate. Histologic studies have shown regions where the marrow spaces are in direct contact with the cartilage and that the central portion of the endplate is permeable to dye. Motion and weight bearing are believed to be helpful in maintaining this diffusion. The metabolic turnover of the disc is relatively high when its avascularity is considered but slow compared with other tissues. The glycosaminoglycan turnover in the disc is quite slow, requiring 500 days.

NEURAL ELEMENTS

The organization of the neural elements is strictly maintained throughout the entire neural system, even within the conus medullaris and cauda equina distally. The orientation of the nerve roots in the dural sac and at the conus medullaris follows a highly organized pattern, with the most cephalad roots lying lateral and the most caudad lying centrally. The motor roots are ventral to the sensory roots at all levels. The arachnoid mater holds the roots in these positions.

The pedicle is the key to understanding surgical spinal anatomy. The relation of the pedicle to the neural elements varies by region within the spinal column. In the cervical region, there are seven vertebrae but eight cervical roots. Accepted nomenclature allows each cervical root to exit cephalad to the pedicle of the vertebra for which it is named (e.g., the C6 nerve root exits above or cephalad to the C6 pedicle). This relationship changes in the thoracic spine because the C8 root exits between the C7 and T1 pedicles, requiring the T1 root to exit caudal or below the pedicle for which it is named. This relationship is maintained throughout the remaining more caudal segments. The naming of the disc levels is different, in that all levels where discs are present are named for the vertebral level immediately cephalad (i.e., the C6 disc is immediately caudal to the C6 vertebra, and disc pathology at that level typically would involve the C7 nerve root).

NATURAL HISTORY OF DISC DISEASE

One theory of spinal degeneration assumes that all spines degenerate and that current methods of treatment are for symptomatic relief, not for a cure. The degenerative process has been divided into three separate stages with relatively distinct findings. The first stage is dysfunction, which is seen in individuals 15 to 45 years old. It is characterized by circumferential and radial tears in the disc anulus and localized

TABLE 38-1

Spectrum of Pathologic Changes in Facet Joints and Discs and Interaction of These Changes

PHASES OF SPINAL DEGENERATION	FACET JOINTS		PATHOLOGIC RESULT		INTERVERTEBRAL DISC
Dysfunction	Synovitis	→	Dysfunction	←	Circumferential tears
	Hypermobility		↓	↖	
	Continuing degeneration	↗	Herniation	←	Radial tears
Instability	Capsular laxity	→	Instability	←	Internal disruption
	Subluxation	→	Lateral nerve entrapment	←	Disc resorption
Stabilization	Enlargement of articular processes	→	One-level stenosis	←	Osteophytes
		↘	Multilevel spondylosis and stenosis	↙	

Modified from Kirkaldy-Willis WH, editor: Managing low back pain, New York, Churchill Livingstone, 1983.

synovitis of the facet joints. The next stage is instability. This stage, found in 35- to 70-year-old patients, is characterized by internal disruption of the disc, progressive disc resorption, degeneration of the facet joints with capsular laxity, subluxation, and joint erosion. The final stage, present in patients older than 60 years, is stabilization. In this stage, the progressive development of hypertrophic bone around the disc and facet joints leads to segmental stiffening or frank ankylosis (Table 38-1).

Each spinal segment degenerates at a different rate. As one level is in the dysfunction stage, another may be entering the stabilization stage. Disc herniation in this scheme is considered a complication of disc degeneration in the dysfunction and instability stages. Spinal stenosis from degenerative arthritis in this scheme is a complication of bony overgrowth compromising neural tissue in the late instability and early stabilization stages.

In general, the literature supports an active care approach, minimizing centrally acting medications. The judicious use of epidural steroids also is supported. Nonprogressive neurologic deficits can be treated nonoperatively with expected improvement clinically. If surgery is necessary, it usually can be delayed 6 to 12 weeks to allow adequate opportunity for improvement. The important exception is a patient with cervical myelopathy, who is best treated surgically.

The natural history of degenerative disc disease is one of recurrent episodes of pain followed by periods of significant or complete relief.

Before a discussion of diagnostic studies, axial spine pain with radiation to one or more extremities must be considered. Also, understanding of certain pathophysiologic entities must be juxtaposed to other entities of which only a rudimentary understanding exists. It is doubtful if there is any other area of orthopaedics in which accurate diagnosis is as difficult or the proper treatment as challenging as in patients with persistent neck and arm or low back and leg pain. Although many patients have clear diagnoses properly arrived at by careful history and physical examination with confirmatory imaging studies, more patients with pain have absent neurologic findings other than sensory changes and have normal imaging studies or studies that do not support the clinical complaints and findings. Inability to show easily an appropriate diagnosis in a patient does not relieve the physician of the obligation to recommend treatment or to direct the patient to a setting where such treatment is available. Careful assessment of these patients to determine if they have problems that can be orthopaedically treated (operatively or nonoperatively) is imperative to avoid overtreatment and undertreatment.

Operative treatment can benefit a patient if it corrects a deformity, corrects instability, relieves neural compression, or treats a combination of these problems. Obtaining a history and completing a physical examination to determine a diagnosis that should be supported by other diagnostic studies is a useful approach; conversely, matching the diagnosis and treatment to the results of diagnostic studies, as often can be done in other subspecialties of orthopaedics (e.g., treating extremity pain based on a radiograph that shows a fracture), is more complex and difficult.

DIAGNOSTIC STUDIES

RADIOGRAPHY

The simplest and most readily available diagnostic tests for cervical pain are anteroposterior and lateral radiographs of the involved spinal region. On lateral radiographs bony abnormalities, such as subluxation, congenital narrowing, or fracture, can be identified. Soft-tissue swelling may be visible. Anteroposterior radiographs can reveal uncovertebral arthritis; potential abnormalities can be identified by looking at the relationships between pedicles and the spinous processes. Obtaining other views such as flexion and extension radiographs can reveal if instability is present. Oblique views show the foramen. These simple radiographs show a relatively high incidence of abnormal findings.

MYELOGRAPHY

The value of myelography is the ability to check all spinal regions for abnormality and to define intraspinal lesions; it may be unnecessary if clinical and CT or MRI findings are in complete agreement. The primary indications for myelography are inability to get an MRI, suspicion of an intraspinal lesion, patients with spinal instrumentation causing artifact, or questionable diagnosis resulting from conflicting clinical findings and other studies (Fig. 38-2). In addition, myelography is valuable in a previously operated spine and in patients

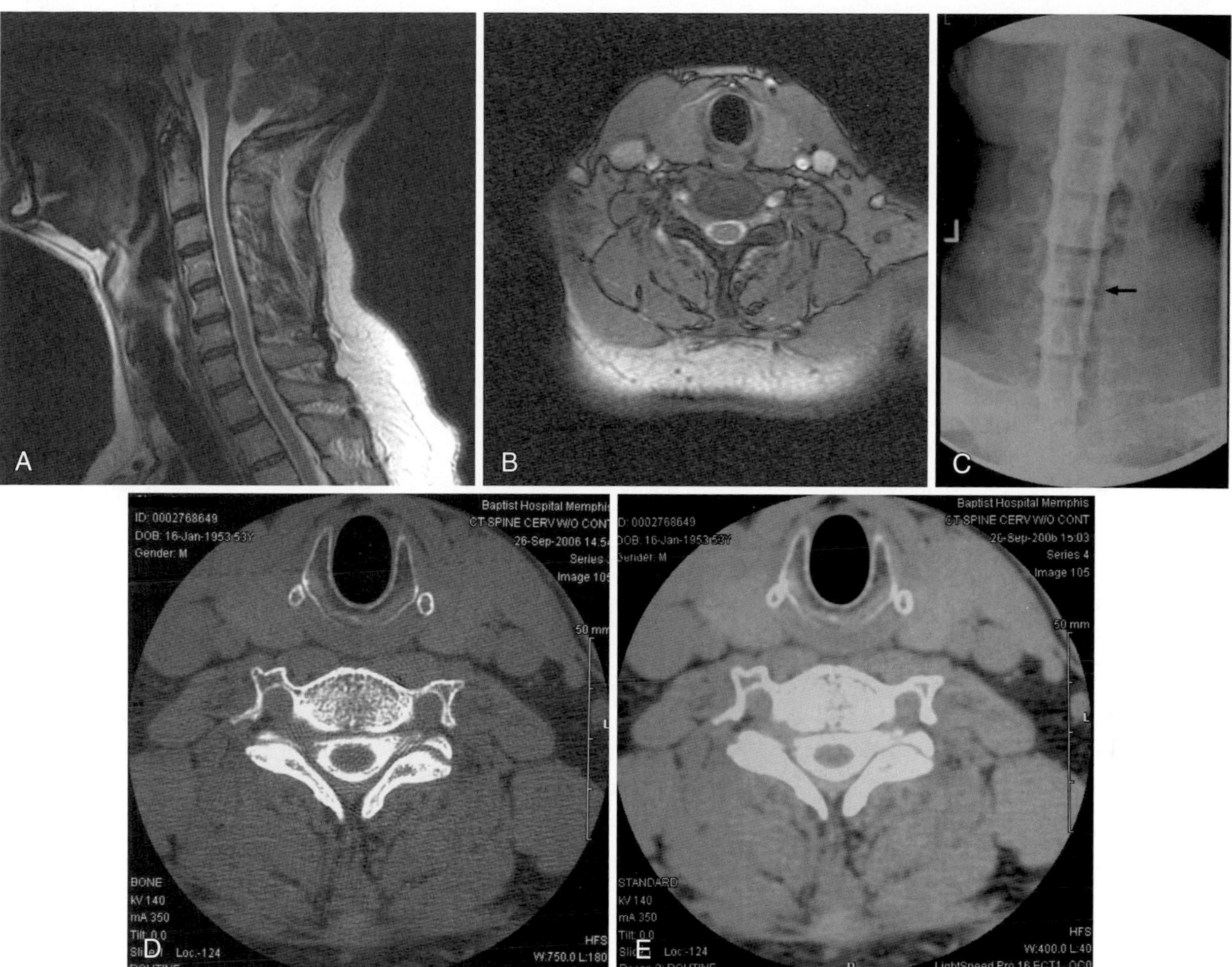

FIGURE 38-2 Forty-five-year-old patient with right C7 radiculopathy clinically. **A** and **B,** MRI was inconclusive for disc herniation. **C-E,** Postmyelogram CT clearly reveals right intraforaminal disc herniation.

with marked bony degenerative change that may be underestimated on MRI. Myelography is improved by the use of postmyelography CT in this setting and in evaluating spinal stenosis.

Several contrast agents have been used for myelography: air, oil contrast, and water-soluble (absorbable) contrast agents, including metrizamide (Amipaque), iohexol (Omnipaque), and iopamidol (Isovue-M). Because these nonionic agents are absorbable, the discomforts of removing them and the severity of the postmyelography headache have decreased.

COMPUTED TOMOGRAPHY

Most clinicians now agree that CT is an extremely useful diagnostic tool in the evaluation of spinal disease. The current technology and computer software have made possible the ability to reformat the standard axial cuts in almost any direction and magnify the images so that exact measurements of various structures can be made. Software is available to evaluate the density of a selected vertebra and compare it with vertebrae of the normal population to give a numerically reproducible estimate of vertebral density to quantitate osteopenia.

Numerous types of CT studies for the spine are available. One must be careful in ordering the study to ensure that the areas of clinical concern are included. Sagittal, axial, and coronal cuts allow a three-dimensional view of the cervical spine. Location markers allow for finer scrutiny of the area of pathology.

MAGNETIC RESONANCE IMAGING

MRI is currently the standard for advanced imaging of the spine and is superior to CT in most circumstances, in particular, identification of infections, tumors, and degenerative changes within the discs. More importantly, MRI is superior for imaging the disc and directly imaging neural structures. Also, MRI typically shows the entire region of study (i.e., cervical, thoracic, or lumbar). Of particular value is the ability to image the nerve root in the foramen, which is difficult even with postmyelography CT because the subarachnoid space and the contrast agent do not extend fully through the foramen. Despite this superiority, there are circumstances in which MRI and CT, with or without myelography, can be used in a complementary fashion.

One of the difficulties with MRI is showing anatomy that is abnormal but may be asymptomatic. MRI evidence of disc degeneration has been reported in the cervical spine in 25% of patients younger than 40 years and in 60% of patients 60 years and older. The demonstrated findings must be carefully correlated with the clinical impression. The importance of this concept cannot be overstated. The best way to obtain meaningful clinical information from MRI of the spine is to have a specific question before the study. This question is derived from a patient's history and a careful physical examination and is posed using the parameters of (1) neural compression, (2) instability, and (3) deformity. In each case, the specific location of the abnormality should be suspected before MRI and confirmed with the study. Only abnormalities in one or a combination of these categories are important, because operative techniques can treat only these problems. Failure to interpret an imaging study in this way, especially MRI, which is sensitive to anatomic abnormalities, would inevitably lead to poor clinical choices and outcomes.

OTHER DIAGNOSTIC TESTS

Numerous diagnostic tests have been used in the diagnosis of intervertebral disc disease in addition to radiography, myelography, CT, and MRI. The primary advantage of these tests is to rule out diseases other than primary disc herniation, spinal stenosis, and spinal arthritis.

Electromyography is the most notable of these tests. One advantage of electromyography is in the identification of peripheral neuropathy and diffuse neurologic involvement indicating higher or lower lesions. Electromyography and nerve conduction velocity can be helpful if a patient has a history and physical examination suggestive of radiculopathy at either the cervical or the lumbar level with inconclusive imaging studies. Paraspinal muscles in a patient with a previous posterior operation usually are abnormal and are not a reliable diagnostic finding.

Bone scans are another procedure in which positive findings usually are not indicative of intervertebral disc disease, but they can confirm neoplastic, traumatic, and arthritic problems in the spine. Various laboratory tests, such as a complete blood cell count, differential white blood cell count, C-reactive protein, biochemical profile, urinalysis, serum protein electrophoresis, and erythrocyte sedimentation rate, are extremely good screening procedures for other causes of pain in the spine. Rheumatoid screening studies, such as rheumatoid arthritis, antinuclear antibody, lupus erythematosus cell preparation, and HLA-B27, also are useful when indicated by the clinical picture.

INJECTION STUDIES

Whenever a diagnosis is in doubt, and the complaints seem real or the pathologic condition is diffuse, identification of the source of pain is problematic. The use of local anesthetics or contrast media in various specific anatomic areas can be helpful. These agents are relatively simple, safe, and minimally painful. Contrast media such as diatrizoate meglumine (Hypaque), iothalamate meglumine (Conray), iohexol (Omnipaque), iopamidol, and metrizamide (Amipaque) have been used for discography and blocks with no reported ill effects. Reports of neurologic complications with contrast media used for discography and subsequent chymopapain injection are well documented. The best choice of a contrast medium for documenting structures outside the subarachnoid space is an absorbable medium with low reactivity because it might be injected inadvertently into the subarachnoid space. Iohexol and metrizamide are the least reactive, most widely accepted, and best tolerated of the currently available contrast media. Local anesthetics, such as lidocaine (Xylocaine), tetracaine (Pontocaine), and bupivacaine (Marcaine), are used frequently epidurally and intradurally. The use of bupivacaine should be limited to low concentrations and low volumes because of reports of death after epidural anesthesia using concentrations of 0.75% or higher.

Steroids prepared for intramuscular injection also have been used frequently in the epidural space with few and usually transient complications. Spinal arachnoiditis in past years was associated with the use of epidural methylprednisolone acetate (Depo-Medrol). This complication was thought to be caused by the use of the suspending agent, polyethylene glycol, which has since been eliminated from the Depo-Medrol preparation. For epidural injections, we prefer the use of Celestone Soluspan, which is a mixture of betamethasone sodium phosphate and betamethasone acetate. Celestone Soluspan provides immediate and long-term duration of action, is highly soluble, and contains no harmful preservatives. Celestone should not be mixed with local anesthetics containing preservatives such as parabens or phenol because flocculation and clogging of the suspension can occur. If Celestone is not available, other commonly used preparations for spinal injections include methylprednisolone (Depo-Medrol) and triamcinolone acetonide (Kenalog) (Table 38-2). Isotonic saline is the only other injectable medium used frequently around the spine with no reported adverse reactions.

When discrete, well-controlled injection techniques directed at specific targets in and around the spine are used, grading the degree of pain before and after a spinal injection is helpful in determining the location of the pain generator. The patient is asked to grade the degree of pain on a 0-to-10 scale before and at various intervals after the spinal injection (Box 38-1). If a spinal injection done under fluoroscopic control results in an 80% or more decrease in the level of pain, which corresponds to the duration of action of the anesthetic agent used, we presume the target area injected to be the pain generator. Less pain reduction, 50% to 65% does not constitute a positive response.

BOX 38-1

Pain Scale and Diary

0 No pain
1 Mild pain that you are aware of but not bothered by
2 Moderate pain that you can tolerate without medication
3 Moderate pain that is discomforting and requires medication
4-5 More severe pain and you begin to feel antisocial
6 Severe pain
7-9 Intensely severe pain
10 Most severe pain (you might contemplate suicide because of it)

ACTIVITY	COMMENTS	LOCATION OF PAIN	TIME	SEVERITY OF PAIN (0-10)

TABLE 38-2

Common Corticosteroids Used in Spinal Interventions Compared With Hydrocortisone

	HYDROCORTISONE	METHYLPREDNISOLONE (DEPO-MEDROL)	TRIAMCINOLONE ACETONIDE (KENALOG)	BETAMETHASONE SODIUM PHOSPHATE AND ACETATE (CELESTONE SOLUSPAN)
Relative antiinflammatory potency	1	5	5	25
pH	5.0-7.0	7.0-8.0	4.5-6.5	6.8-7.2
Onset	Fast	Slow	Moderate	Fast
Duration of action	Short	Intermediate	Intermediate	Long
Concentration (mg/mL)	50	40-80	20	6
Relative mineralocorticoid activity	2+	0	0	0

(From el Abd O: Steroids in spine interventions. In Slipman CW, Derby D, Simeone FA, Mayer TG, editors: Interventional spine: an algorithmic approach, Philadelphia, Elsevier, 2008.)

EPIDURAL CORTISONE INJECTIONS

Epidural injections in the spine were developed to diagnose and treat spinal pain. Information obtained from epidural injections can be helpful in confirming pain generators that are responsible for a patient's discomfort. Structural abnormalities do not always cause pain, and diagnostic injections can help to correlate abnormalities seen on imaging studies with associated pain complaints. In addition, epidural injections can provide pain relief during the recovery of disc or nerve root injuries and allow patients to increase their level of physical activity. Epidural steroid injections in the treatment of disc herniation and radiculitis are performed based on the pathophysiologic mechanism of reducing inflammation; however, there is no evidence to suggest that local anesthetics with or without steroids are equally as effective as steroids alone in many settings. Because severe pain from an acute disc injury with or without radiculopathy often is time limited, therapeutic injections help to manage pain and may alleviate or decrease the need for oral analgesics.

Few serious complications occur in patients receiving epidural corticosteroid injections; however, epidural abscess, epidural hematoma, durocutaneous fistula, and Cushing syndrome have been reported as individual case reports. The most adverse immediate reaction during an epidural injection is a vasovagal reaction. Dural puncture has been estimated to occur in 0.5% to 5% of patients having cervical or lumbar epidural steroid injections. The anesthesiology literature reported a 7.5% to 75% incidence of postdural puncture (positional) headaches, with the highest estimates associated with the use of 16- and 18-gauge needles. Headache without dural puncture has been estimated to occur in 2% of patients and is attributed to air injected into the epidural space, increased intrathecal pressure from fluid around the dural sac, and possibly an undetected dural puncture. Some minor, common complaints caused by corticosteroid injected into the epidural space include nonpositional headaches, facial flushing, insomnia, low-grade fever, and transient increased back or lower extremity pain. Epidural corticosteroid injections are contraindicated in the presence of infection at the injection site, systemic infection, bleeding diathesis, uncontrolled diabetes mellitus, and congestive heart failure.

We perform epidural corticosteroid injections in a fluoroscopy suite equipped with resuscitative and monitoring equipment. Intravenous access is established in all patients with a 20-gauge angiocatheter placed in the upper extremity. Mild sedation is achieved through intravenous access. We recommend the use of fluoroscopy for diagnostic and therapeutic epidural injections for several reasons. Epidural injections performed without fluoroscopic guidance are not always made into the epidural space or the intended interspace. Even in experienced hands, needle misplacement occurs in 40% of epidural injections when done without fluoroscopic guidance. Accidental intravascular injections also can occur, and the absence of blood return with needle aspiration before injection is an unreliable indicator of this complication. In the presence of anatomic anomalies, such as a midline epidural septum or multiple separate epidural compartments, the desired flow of epidural injectants to the presumed pain generator is restricted and remains undetected without fluoroscopy. In addition, if an injection fails to relieve pain, it would be impossible without fluoroscopy to determine whether the failure was caused by a genuine poor response or by improper needle placement.

CERVICAL EPIDURAL INJECTION

Cervical epidural steroid injections have been used with some success to treat cervical spondylosis associated with acute disc disruption and radiculopathies, cervical strain syndromes with associated myofascial pain, postlaminectomy cervical pain, reflex sympathetic dystrophy, postherpetic neuralgia, acute viral brachial plexitis, and muscle contraction headaches. The best results with cervical epidural steroid injections have been in patients with acute disc herniations or well-defined radicular symptoms and in patients with limited myofascial pain. In a group of 70 patients with herniated cervical discs without myelopathy for which conservative management failed to relieve symptoms, cervical epidural steroid injections provided significant pain relief and avoided surgery in 63%. Better outcomes were noted in patients older than 50 years and those who received the injections earlier (< 100 days from diagnosis). At this time, we do not perform cervical transforaminal injections because of the

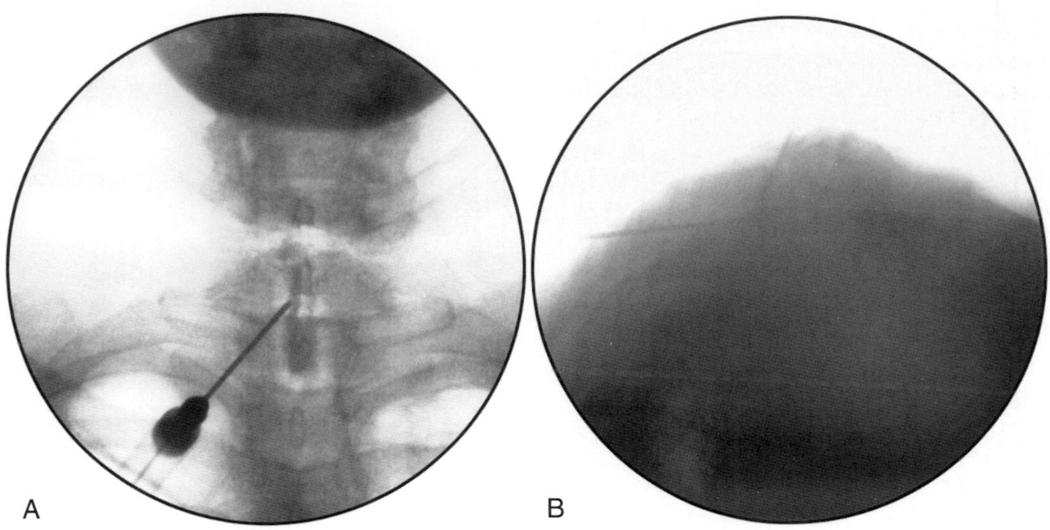

FIGURE 38-3 **A,** Posteroanterior view of cervical interlaminar epidurogram showing characteristic C7-T1 epidural contrast flow pattern. **B,** Lateral radiograph of cervical epidurogram. **SEE TECHNIQUE 38-1.**

increasing number of reports of catastrophic neurologic complications involving injury to the spinal cord and brainstem after cervical transforaminal injections. These injuries are the result of intraarterial injection into either a reinforcing radicular artery or the vertebral artery, the latter of which is the most common basis of complication. Injection into a radicular artery is an unavoidable complication but one that can be recognized by using real-time monitoring of a test dose of contrast medium. In the case of intraarterial injection, the procedure should be aborted to avoid injury to the spinal cord.

INTERLAMINAR CERVICAL EPIDURAL INJECTION

TECHNIQUE 38-1

- Place the patient prone on a pain management table. We use a low-attenuated carbon fiber tabletop that allows better imaging and permits unobstructed C-arm viewing. For optimal placement and comfort, place the patient's face in a cervical prone cutout cushion.
- Cervical epidural injections using a paramedian approach should be done routinely at the C7-T1 interspace unless previous surgery of the posterior cervical spine has been done at that level, in which case the C6-7 or T1-2 level is injected. Aseptically prepare the skin area with isopropyl alcohol and povidone-iodine several segments above and below the laminar interspace to be injected. If the patient is allergic to povidone-iodine, use chlorhexidine gluconate (Hibiclens).
- Drape the area in sterile fashion.
- Using anteroposterior fluoroscopic imaging, identify the target laminar interspace. With the use of a 27-gauge, 1/4-inch needle, anesthetize the skin so that a skin wheal is raised over the target interspace on the side of the patient's pain with 1 to 2 mL of 1% preservative-free lidocaine without epinephrine. To diminish the burning discomfort of the anesthetic, mix 3 mL of 8.4% sodium bicarbonate in a 30-mL bottle of 1% preservative-free lidocaine without epinephrine. Nick the skin with an 18-gauge hypodermic needle. Under fluoroscopic control, insert and advance a 22-gauge, 3 1/2-inch spinal needle in a vertical fashion until contact is made with the upper edge of the T1 lamina 1 to 2 mm lateral to the midline.
- Anesthetize the lamina with 1 to 2 mL of 1% preservative-free lidocaine without epinephrine. Anesthetize the soft tissues with 2 mL of 1% preservative-free lidocaine without epinephrine as the spinal needle is withdrawn.
- Insert an 18-gauge, 3 1/2-inch Tuohy epidural needle, and advance it vertically within the anesthetized soft-tissue track until contact is made with the T1 lamina under fluoroscopy.
- "Walk off" the lamina with the Tuohy needle onto the ligamentum flavum. Remove the stylet from the Tuohy needle, and attach a 10-mL syringe filled halfway with air and sterile saline. Advance the Tuohy needle into the epidural space using the loss-of-resistance technique. When loss of resistance has been achieved, aspirate to check for blood or cerebrospinal fluid (CSF). If neither blood nor CSF is evident, remove the syringe from the Tuohy needle and attach a 5-mL syringe containing 1.5 mL of nonionic contrast dye.
- Confirm epidural placement by producing an epidurogram with the nonionic contrast agent (Fig. 38-3). To confirm proper placement further, adjust the C-arm to view the area from a lateral perspective. A spot radiograph can be obtained to document placement.

- Inject a test dose of 1 to 2 mL of 1% preservative-free lidocaine without epinephrine and wait 3 minutes. If the patient does not complain of warmth, burning, or significant paresthesias or show signs of apnea, place a 10-mL syringe on the Tuohy needle and slowly inject 2 mL of 1% preservative-free lidocaine without epinephrine and 2 mL of 6 mg/mL Celestone Soluspan slowly into the epidural space. If Celestone Soluspan cannot be obtained, 40 mg/mL of triamcinolone is a good substitute.

ZYGAPOPHYSEAL (FACET) JOINT INJECTIONS

The facet joint can be a source of back or neck pain; the exact cause of the pain is unknown. Theories include meniscoid entrapment and extrapment, synovial impingement, chondromalacia facetae, capsular and synovial inflammation, and mechanical injury to the joint capsule. Osteoarthritis is another cause of facet joint pain; however, the incidence of facet joint arthropathy is equal in symptomatic and asymptomatic patients. As with other osteoarthritic joints, radiographic changes correlate poorly with pain.

Although the history and physical examination may suggest that the facet joint is the cause of spine pain, no noninvasive pathognomonic findings distinguish facet joint–mediated pain from other sources of spine pain. Fluoroscopically guided facet joint injections are commonly considered the "gold standard" for isolating or excluding the facet joint as a source of spine or extremity pain.

Clinical suspicion of facet joint pain by a spine specialist remains the major indicator for diagnostic injection, which should be done only in patients who have had pain for more than 4 weeks and only after appropriate conservative measures have failed to provide relief. Facet joint injection procedures may help to focus treatment on a specific spinal segment and provide adequate pain relief to allow progression in therapy. Either intraarticular or medial branch blocks can be used for diagnostic purposes. Although injection of cortisone into the facet joint was a popular procedure through most of the 1970s and 1980s, many investigators have found no evidence that this effectively treats low back pain caused by a facet joint. The only controlled study on the use of intraarticular corticosteroids in the cervical spine found no added benefit from intraarticular betamethasone over bupivacaine.

CERVICAL FACET JOINT

CERVICAL MEDIAL BRANCH BLOCK INJECTION

TECHNIQUE 38-2

- Place the patient prone on the pain management table. Rotate the patient's neck so that the symptomatic side is down. This allows the vertebral artery to be positioned further beneath the articular pillar, creates greater accentuation of the cervical waists, and prevents the jaw from being superimposed. Aseptically prepare and drape the side to be injected.
- Identify the target location using anteroposteriorly directed fluoroscopy. Each cervical facet joint from C3-4 to C7-T1 is supplied from the medial nerve branch above and below the joint that curves consistently around the "waist" of the articular pillar of the same numbered vertebrae (Fig. 38-4). To block the C6 facet joint nerve supply, anesthetize the C6 and C7 medial branches.
- Insert a 22- or 25-gauge, 3 1/2-inch spinal needle perpendicular to the pain management table and advance it under fluoroscopic control ventrally and medially until contact is made with periosteum. Direct the spinal needle laterally until the needle tip reaches the lateral margin of the waist of the articular pillar, and then direct the needle until it rests at the deepest point of the articular pillar's concavity under fluoroscopy.
- Remove the stylet. If there is a negative aspirate, inject 0.5 mL of 0.75% preservative-free bupivacaine.

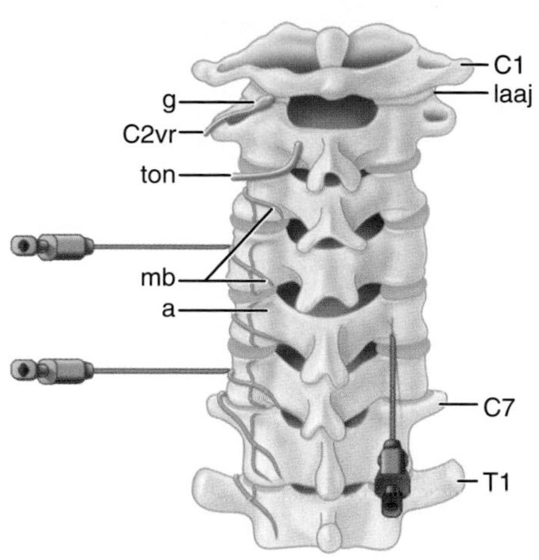

FIGURE 38-4 Proper needle placement for posterior approach to C4 and C6 medial branch blocks. Second cervical ganglion (g), third occipital nerve (ton), C2 ventral ramus (C2vr), and lateral atlantoaxial joint (laaj) are noted. a, articular facet; mb, medial branch. **SEE TECHNIQUE 38-2.**

CERVICAL DISCOGRAPHY

The approach to the cervical spine differs from the approaches used for discography of the lumbar and thoracic spine. The cervical spine is approached anteriorly rather than posteriorly. Complications associated with cervical discography because of the surrounding anatomy include injury to the trachea, esophagus, carotid artery, and jugular veins and spinal cord injury and pneumothorax. Discitis is a concern in the cervical spine; disc infection often originates from the gram-negative and anaerobic flora of the esophagus.

Traditionally, the approach to the cervical intervertebral discs has been via a paralaryngeal route that requires displacement of the trachea and esophagus away from the site of entry. A more lateral approach that is gaining popularity bypasses these structures and does not require such displacement.

CERVICAL DISCOGRAPHY

TECHNIQUE 38-3

(FALCO)

- Place the patient supine on the procedure table.
- Insert an angiocatheter into the upper extremity and begin intravenous antibiotic infusion. Alternatively, intradiscal antibiotics can be given during surgery.
- Sedate the patient, and prepare and drape the skin sterilely, including the anterolateral aspect of the neck.
- Under fluoroscopic imaging, identify the intervertebral discs with aligned endplates and sharp margins of the intervertebral discs. Approach the paralaryngeal area from the right, using a finger to displace the esophagus and trachea to the left and the carotid artery to the right. With the other hand, insert a 2- or 3 1/2-inch spinal needle over the finger through the skin and into the outer anulus of the disc. Advance the needle into the center of the disc, using anteroposterior and lateral fluoroscopic guidance.
- An alternative method is a more lateral approach to the cervical spine using a single needle. This approach may reduce the incidence of infection by passing the needle posterior to the trachea and esophagus en route to the disc space. Position the patient or the C-arm to place the cervical spine in an oblique position for optimal foraminal exposure and continue adjusting until the endplates, disc space, and uncovertebral process are in sharp focus (Fig. 38-5).
- Insert a 2- or 3 1/2-inch needle into the skin and advance it until the tip makes contact with the subjacent uncovertebral process. "Walk off" the needle just anterior to the uncovertebral process. Advance the needle into the center of the disc, using anteroposterior and lateral fluoroscopic guidance.
- After needle placement with either technique, the rest of the procedure is essentially the same as that described for thoracic or lumbar discography (Chapter 39).
- Inject either saline or a nonionic contrast dye into each disc.
- Record any pain response as none, dissimilar, similar, or exact in relationship to the patient's typical pain. Record intradiscal pressures to assist in determining if the disc is the cause of the pain.
- Perform radiography and CT of the cervical spine on completion of the study.

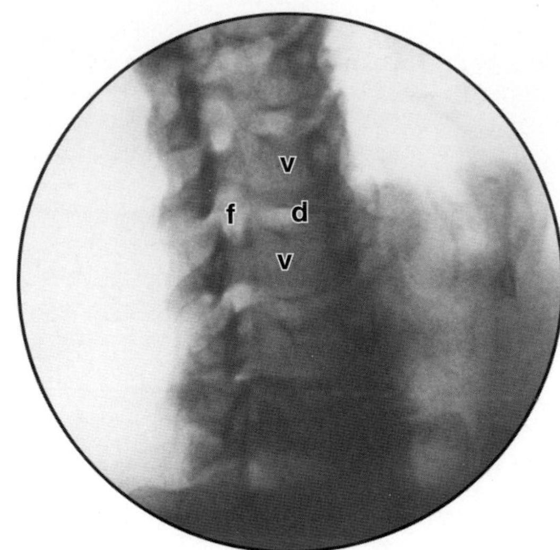

FIGURE 38-5 Foraminal position for performing cervical discography with anterolateral approach. f, foramen; v, vertebral body; d, intervertebral disc. (Courtesy of Frank J. E. Falco, MD.) **SEE TECHNIQUE 38-3.**

CERVICAL DISC DISEASE

Herniation of the cervical intervertebral disc with spinal cord compression has been identified since Key detailed the pathologic findings of two cases of cord compression by "intervertebral substance" in 1838. Cervical disc disease is slightly more common in men. Factors associated with the injury are frequent heavy lifting on the job, cigarette smoking, and frequent diving from a board. Patients with cervical disc disease also are likely to have lumbar disc disease. MRI has shown increasing cervical disc degeneration with age.

The pathophysiology of cervical disc disease is the same as degenerative disc disease in other areas of the spine. Physiologic changes in the nucleus are followed by progressive annular degeneration. Frank extrusion of nuclear material can occur as a complication of this normal degenerative process. As the disc degeneration proceeds, hypermobility of the segment can result in instability or degenerative arthritic changes or both. In contrast to those in the lumbar spine, these hypertrophic changes are predominantly at the uncovertebral joint (uncinate process) (Fig. 38-6). Hypertrophic changes eventually develop around the facet joints and vertebral bodies. Progressive stiffening of the cervical spine and loss of motion are the usual result in the end stages. Hypertrophic spurring anteriorly occasionally results in dysphagia. Increased amounts of matrix metalloproteinases, nitric oxide, prostaglandin E_2, and interleukin-6 have been identified in disc material removed from cervical disc hernias, suggesting that these products are involved in the biochemistry of disc degeneration. These substances also are implicated in pain production.

The classic approach to discs in this region has been posteriorly with laminectomy. Currently, anterior cervical discectomy with fusion is the procedure of choice when the disc is removed anteriorly to avoid disc space collapse, prevent painful and abnormal cervical motion, and speed intervertebral fusion. Foraminotomy is the procedure of choice when the disc fragment is lateral and can be removed posteriorly.

SIGNS AND SYMPTOMS

The signs and symptoms of cervical intervertebral disc disease are best separated into symptoms related to the spine itself,

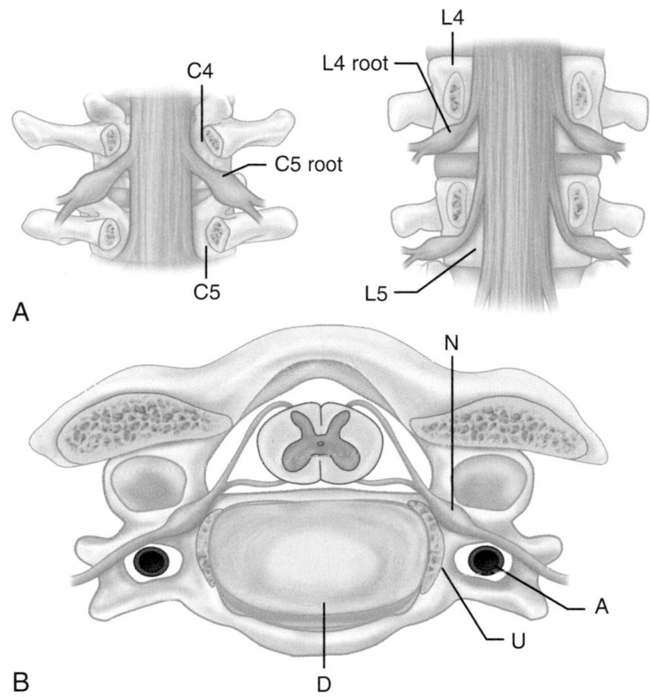

FIGURE 38-6 **A,** Comparison of points at which nerve roots emerge from cervical and lumbar spine. **B,** Cross-sectional view of cervical spine at level of disc (D). Uncinate process (U) forms ventral wall of foramen. Root (N) exits dorsal to vertebral artery (A).

symptoms related to nerve root compression, and symptoms of myelopathy. Several authors reported that when the disc is punctured anteriorly for the purpose of discography, pain is noted in the neck and shoulder. Complaints of neck pain, medial scapular pain, and shoulder pain are probably related to primary pain around the disc and spine. Anatomic studies have indicated cervical disc and ligamentous innervations. This has been inferred to be similar in the cervical spine to that of the lumbar spine with its sinu-vertebral nerve.

Symptoms of root compression usually are associated with pain radiating into the arm or chest with numbness in the fingers and motor weakness. Cervical disc disease also can mimic cardiac disease with chest and arm pain. Usually the radicular symptoms are intermittent and combined with more frequent neck and shoulder pain.

The signs of midline cervical spinal cord compression (myelopathy) are unique and varied. The pain is poorly localized and aching and may be only a minor complaint. Occasional sharp pain or generalized tingling may be described with neck extension. This is similar to the Lhermitte sign in multiple sclerosis. The pain can be in the shoulder and pelvic girdles; it is occasionally associated with a generalized feeling of weakness in the lower extremities and a feeling of instability. Global numbness in the upper extremities and difficulty with fine motor coordination are common findings. Gait disturbances and difficulty with tandem gait may be the first symptoms.

In patients with predominant cervical spondylosis, symptoms of vertebral artery compression also may be found, including dizziness, tinnitus, intermittent blurring of vision, and occasional episodes of retroocular pain. The signs of lateral root pressure from a disc or osteophytes are predominantly neurologic (Boxes 38-2 to 38-6). By evaluating multiple

BOX 38-2

C5 Nerve Root Compression

Sensory Deficit
Upper lateral arm and elbow

Motor Weakness
Deltoid
Biceps (variable)

Reflex Change
Biceps (variable)

Indicative of C4-5 disc rupture or other pathologic condition at that level.

BOX 38-3

C6 Nerve Root Compression

Sensory Deficit
Lateral forearm, thumb, and index finger

Motor Weakness
Biceps
Extensor carpi radialis longus and brevis

Reflex Change
Biceps
Brachioradialis

Indicative of C5-6 disc herniation or other local pathologic condition at that level.

BOX 38-4

C7 Nerve Root Compression

Sensory Deficit
Middle finger (variable because of overlap)

Motor Weakness
Triceps
Wrist flexors (flexor carpi radialis)
Finger extensors (variable)

Reflex Change
Triceps

Indicative of C6-7 disc rupture or other pathologic condition at that level.

BOX 38-5

C8 Nerve Root Compression

Sensory Deficit
Ring finger, little finger, and ulnar border of palm

Motor Weakness
Interossei
Finger flexors (variable)
Flexor carpi ulnaris (variable)

Reflex Change
None

Indicative of C7-T1 disc rupture or other pathologic condition at that level.

BOX 38-6

T1 Nerve Root Compression

Sensory Deficit
Medial aspect of elbow

Motor Weakness
Interossei

Reflex Change
None

Indicative of T1-2 disc rupture or other pathologic condition at that level.

motor groups, multiple levels of deep tendon reflexes, and sensory abnormalities, the level of the lesion can be localized as accurately as any other lesion in the nervous system. The multiple innervation of muscles sometimes can lead to confusion in determining the exact root involved. For this reason, MRI or other studies done for imaging confirmation of the clinical impression usually are helpful.

Rupture of the C4-5 disc with compression of the C5 nerve root should result in weakness in the deltoid and biceps muscles. The deltoid is almost entirely innervated by C5, but the biceps has dual innervation. The biceps reflex may be diminished with injury to this nerve root, although it also has a C6 component, and this must be considered. Sensory testing should show a patch on the lateral aspect of the proximal arm to be diminished (Fig. 38-7).

Rupture of the C5-6 disc with compression of the C6 root can be confused with other root levels because of dual innervation of structures. Weakness may be noted in the biceps and extensor carpi radialis longus and brevis. As mentioned earlier, the biceps is dually innervated by C5 and C6, whereas the long extensors are dually innervated by C6 and C7. The brachioradialis and biceps reflexes also may be diminished at this level. Sensory testing usually indicates a decreased sensibility over the lateral proximal forearm, thumb, and index finger.

Rupture of the C6-7 disc with compression of the C7 root frequently results in weakness of the triceps. Weakness of the wrist flexors, especially the flexor carpi radialis, also is more indicative of C7 root problems. Extensor digitorum communis weakness also can indicate C7 root involvement and may be more readily apparent because of the normal relative weakness of this muscle compared with the triceps. Weakness of the flexor carpi ulnaris usually is caused more by C8 lesions. As mentioned earlier, finger extensors also may be weakened in that they have C7 and C8 innervation. The triceps reflex may be diminished. Sensation is diminished in the middle finger. C7 sensibility varies because it is so narrow, and overlap is prominent. Definite sensibility change can be difficult to document.

Rupture between C7 and T1 with compression of the C8 nerve root results in no reflex changes. Weakness may be noted in the finger flexors and in the interossei of the hand. Sensibility is lost on the ulnar border of the palm, including the ring and little fingers. Compression of the T1 nerve root produces weakness of the interosseous muscles, decreased sensibility around the medial aspect of the elbow, and no reflex changes.

Care should be taken in the examination of the extremity when radicular problems are encountered to rule out more distal compression syndromes in the upper extremities, such as thoracic outlet syndrome, carpal tunnel syndrome, and cubital tunnel syndrome. The lower extremities should be examined with special attention to long tract signs indicating myelopathy.

Although no tests for movement of the upper extremity correspond with straight-leg raising tests in the lower extremity, the Spurling test is a maneuver that is 95% sensitive and 94% specific for diagnosing cervical nerve root pathology. A positive Spurling sign occurs when pain radiates in a dermatomal distribution ipsilaterally when the examiner turns the patient's head to the affected side while extending the neck and applying downward pressure on the head.

The shoulder abduction relief sign is another clinical sign that can be helpful in diagnosing cervical root compression syndromes. The test consists of shoulder abduction and elbow flexion with placement of the hand on the top of the head. This maneuver should relieve the arm pain caused by radicular compression. If this position is allowed to persist for 1 or 2 minutes and pain is increased, more distal compressive neuropathies such as a tardy ulnar nerve syndrome (cubital tunnel syndrome) or primary shoulder pathologic conditions often are the cause.

Cervical paraspinal spasm and limitation of neck motion are frequent findings of cervical spine disease but do not indicate a specific pathologic process. Special maneuvers involving neck motion can be helpful in the selection of conservative treatment and identification of

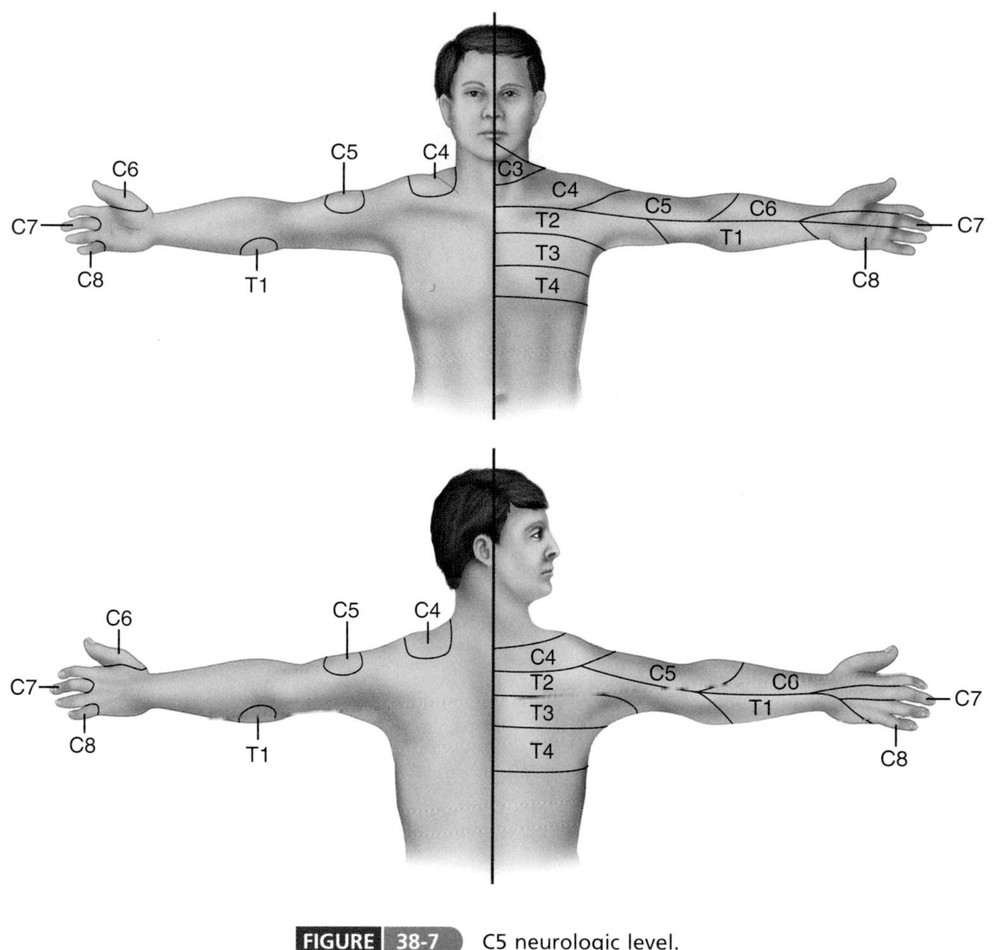

FIGURE 38-7 C5 neurologic level.

pathologic processes. The distraction test, which involves the examiner placing the hands on the occiput and jaw and distracting the cervical spine in the neutral position, can relieve root compression pain, but also can increase pain caused by ligamentous injury. Neck extension and flexion with or without traction can be helpful in selecting conservative therapies.

Patients relieved of pain with the neck extended, with or without traction, usually have hyperextension syndromes with ligamentous injury posteriorly, whereas patients relieved of pain with distraction and neck flexion are more likely to have nerve root compression caused by a soft ruptured disc or more likely hypertrophic spurs in the neural foramina. Pain usually is increased in any condition with compression. One must be careful before applying compression or distraction to ensure no cervical instability or fracture is present. One also must be careful in interpreting the distraction test to ensure the temporomandibular joint is not diseased or injured because distraction also would increase the pain in this area.

The signs of midline disc herniation are those of spinal cord compression. If the lesion is high in the cervical region, paresthesias, weakness, atrophy, and occasionally fasciculations may occur in the hands. A Hoffman sign (upper cervical spinal cord) or the inverted radial reflex also may be present when the pathology is at or above the C5/6 level. Most commonly, however, the first and most prominent symptoms are those of involvement of the corticospinal tract; less commonly, the posterior columns are affected. The primary signs are sustained clonus, hyperactive reflexes, and the Babinski reflex. Less significant findings are varying degrees of spasticity, weakness in the legs, and impairment of proprioception. Equilibrium may be grossly disturbed, but sense of pain and temperature sense rarely are lost and usually are of little localizing value.

DIFFERENTIAL DIAGNOSIS

The differential diagnosis of cervical disc disease is best separated into extrinsic and intrinsic factors. Extrinsic factors generally include disease processes extrinsic to the neck resulting in symptoms similar to primary neck problems. Included in this group are tumors of the chest; nerve compression syndromes distal to the spine; degenerative processes, such as shoulder and upper extremity arthritis; temporomandibular joint syndrome; and lesions around the shoulder, such as acute and chronic rotator cuff tears and impingement syndromes. Intrinsic problems primarily consist of lesions directly associated with the cervical spine, the most common being cervical disc degeneration with concomitant disc herniation or later development of hypertrophic arthritis. Congenital factors, such as spinal stenosis in the cervical region, also may produce symptoms. Primary and secondary tumors of the cervical spine and fractures of the cervical vertebrae also should be considered as intrinsic lesions.

Odom et al. categorized cervical disc disease into four groups: (1) unilateral soft disc protrusion with nerve root compression; (2) foraminal spur, or hard disc, with nerve root compression; (3) medial soft disc protrusion with spinal cord compression; and (4) transverse ridge or cervical spondylosis with spinal cord compression. Soft disc herniations usually affect one level, whereas hard disc herniations can affect multiple levels. Central lesions usually result in cord compression symptoms, and lateral lesions usually result in radicular symptoms.

Most of the soft disc herniations in the series of Odom et al. occurred at the C6 interspace (70%) and C5 interspace (24%). Only six occurred at the C7 interspace. Foraminal spurs also were found predominantly at the C6 interspace (48%). The C5 interspace (39%) and C7 interspace (13%) accounted for the remaining levels where foraminal spurs were found. These investigators also noted the incidence of medial soft disc protrusion with myelopathy to be rare (14 of 246 patients).

CONFIRMATORY IMAGING

Radiographic evaluation of the cervical spine frequently shows loss of normal cervical lordosis. Disc space narrowing and hypertrophic changes frequently increase with age but are not indicative of cervical disc rupture. Usually radiographs are most helpful to rule out other problems. Oblique radiographs of the cervical spine may reveal foraminal encroachment.

MRI of the cervical spine has rapidly become the major diagnostic procedure for neck, arm, and shoulder symptoms. MRI should confirm the objective clinical findings. Asymptomatic findings should be expected to increase with the age of the patient. Cervical myelography usually is indicated only after noninvasive evaluation by MRI fails to reveal the cause or level of the lesion or the patient is unable to obtain an MRI. If MRI is inconclusive, electromyography or nerve conduction velocity may be indicated to show active radiculopathy before proceeding with myelography, especially if the history and physical examination are not strongly supportive of the presence of radiculopathy.

Cervical discography is a controversial technique with limited benefits. It is not indicated in frank disc rupture, spondylosis, or spinal stenosis. The primary use is in patients with persistent neck pain without localized neurologic findings in whom standard MRI, myelography, and CT scan are inconclusive. Some investigators maintain that isolated painful discs can be identified in some patients by discography. A degenerative disc without pain on injection is not likely to be the source of the patient's complaint. Cervical discography requires considerable care and caution. It should be considered a preoperative test in patients in whom an anterior disc excision and interbody fusion are considered for primary neck and shoulder pain. Assessing the psychosocial well-being of a patient is recommended before proceeding with operative treatment. Great care is required in the technique and in the interpretation if reproducible results are desired. Cervical root blocks also have been suggested for the localization and confirmation of symptomatic root compression when used in conjunction with cervical discography. Facet joint injections also should be considered before fusion as a therapeutic and diagnostic procedure. These procedures were described earlier in this chapter.

When a component of dynamic cord compression is present, myelography remains a valuable tool, although dynamic MRI has reduced the role of myelography. Myelography is performed for ruptured cervical discs. Considerable attention must be paid to the flow of the column of contrast medium with the neck in hyperextended, neutral, and flexed positions. One cannot conclude that spinal cord compression is not present until one is certain that the cephalad flow of the medium is not obstructed with the neck acutely hyperextended. The neck should be hyperextended carefully because of the danger of further damage to the spinal cord. Cervical dynamic instability can be shown because the cephalad flow of contrast material is blocked between the lamina of the cephalad level and the disc or body of the caudal level.

NONOPERATIVE TREATMENT

As discussed earlier, most patients with symptomatic cervical disc herniations respond well to nonoperative treatment, including some patients with nonprogressive radicular weakness (between 70% and 80%). Reasonably good evidence shows that acute disc herniations decrease in size over time in the cervical region. Many conservative treatment methods for neck pain are used for multiple diagnoses. The primary purpose of the cervical spine and associated musculature is to support and mobilize the head while providing a conduit for the nervous system. The forces on the cervical spine are much smaller than on the lower spinal levels. The cervical spine is vulnerable to muscular tension forces, postural fatigue, and excessive motion. Most nonoperative treatments focus on one or more of these factors. The best primary treatment is short periods of rest, massage, ice, and antiinflammatory agents (glucocorticoids or nonsteroidal antiinflammatory) with active mobilization as soon as possible. The position of the neck for comfort is essential for relief of pain. The position of greatest relief may suggest the offending pathologic process or mechanism of injury. Patients with hyperflexion injuries usually are more comfortable with the neck in extension over a small roll under the neck. No specific position indicates lateral disc herniation, although most patients tolerate the neutral position best. Patients with spondylosis (hard disc) are most comfortable with the neck in flexion.

Cervical traction can be helpful in selected patients. Care must be exercised in instructing the patient in the proper use of traction. It should be applied to the head in the position of maximal pain relief. Traction never should be continued if it increases pain. The weights should rarely exceed 10 lb (weight of the head). The proper head halter and duration of traction sessions should be chosen to prevent irritation of the temporomandibular joint. Traction applied by a patient-controlled pneumatic force, which is more mobile than halter-type units, avoids irritation of the temporomandibular joint. Traction also should allow general relaxation of the patient. "Poor man's" traction is a simple method of evaluating the efficacy of cervical traction. It uses the weight of the unsupported head for the traction weight (about 10 lb). For extension traction, the patient is supine and the head is allowed to extend gently off the examining table or bed. For flexion, the same procedure is repeated in the prone position. The patient continues the exercise in the position that is most comfortable for 5 to 10 minutes several times daily.

The postural aspects of neck pain can be treated with more frequent changes in position and ergonomic changes in the work area to prevent fatigue and encourage good posture. Techniques to minimize or relieve tension also are helpful.

Cervical braces usually limit excessive motion. Similar to traction, they should be tailored to the most comfortable neck position. Except in cases of trauma, use of an orthosis should be limited to prevent atrophy of the musculature. They may be most helpful for patients who are very active.

Neck and shoulder exercises are most beneficial as the acute pain subsides. Isometric exercises are helpful in the acute phase. Occasionally, shoulder problems, such as adhesive capsulitis, may be found concomitantly with cervical spondylosis; complete immobilization of the painful extremity should be avoided. Physical therapy should be initiated.

OPERATIVE TREATMENT

The primary indications for operative treatment of cervical disc disease are (1) failure of nonoperative pain management; (2) increasing and significant neurologic deficit; and (3) cervical myelopathy, which predictably progresses, based on natural history studies. In most patients, the persistence of pain is the primary indication. The intensity of the persistent pain should be severe enough to interfere consistently with the patient's desired activity and greater than would reasonably be expected after operative treatment. The approach chosen should be determined by the location and type of lesion. Soft lateral discs are easily removed with the posterior approach, whereas soft central or hard discs (central or lateral) probably are best treated with an anterior approach. Any controversy that existed relative to the need for fusion with anterior discectomy essentially has been resolved with long-term follow-up studies of patients without fusion, such as that by Yamamoto et al. Osteophytes that were not removed at surgery frequently have been shown to be reabsorbed at the level of fusion. The use of a graft also prevents the collapse of the disc space and maintains adequate foraminal size.

POSTERIOR APPROACH TO THE CERVICAL SPINE

REMOVAL OF POSTEROLATERAL HERNIATIONS BY POSTERIOR APPROACH (POSTERIOR CERVICAL FORAMINOTOMY)

TECHNIQUE 38-4

- With the patient under general endotracheal anesthesia in the prone position and the head in a Mayfield positioner, flex the neck to decrease the cervical lordosis as much as possible. The upright position for surgery decreases venous bleeding, but we are reluctant to recommend its use because of concern regarding the possibility of air embolism and cerebral hypoxia in the event of a significant decline in blood pressure. Usually a slight reverse Trendelenburg position works well in posterior cervical surgery coupled with careful dissection to minimize bleeding. The shoulders are retracted inferiorly with tape if imaging of the lower cervical levels is contemplated. This imaging is needed if a microsurgical technique using tubular retractors is chosen (see Technique 38-5).
- Appropriately prepare and drape the operative field.
- Make a midline incision centered on the spinous process tip of the cephalad level involved (Fig. 38-8A) and 2 cm in length. Retract the edges of this incision and the skin withdraws in a cephalad direction so that the wound becomes properly placed.
- Divide the ligamentum nuchae longitudinally to expose the tips of the spinous processes above and below the designated area. The correct position is reasonably well ensured by palpation of the last bifid spinous process, which usually is C6. It must be verified intraoperatively, however, by a marker attached to the spinous process and documented on the lateral cervical spine radiograph.
- Dissect subperiosteally the paravertebral muscles from the laminae on the side of the lesion and retract them with a self-retaining retractor or with the help of an assistant using a hand-held retractor (Fig. 38-8B).
- With a small high-speed burr, drill away the caudal edge of the lateral portion of the lamina cephalad to the interspace. Usually minimal bone removal from the cephalad edge of the lateral portion of the caudal lamina is needed. Only a small amount of the medial portion of the facet needs to be removed in most patients. A small Kerrison rongeur (1 to 2 mm) can be used to enlarge this keyhole as needed.
- Sharply excise the ligamentum flavum with a small Kerrison rongeur and identify the nerve root, which is commonly displaced posteriorly and flattened by pressure from the underlying disc fragments (Fig. 38-8C). Removal of additional bone along the dorsal aspect of the foramen and immediately above and below the nerve root often is beneficial at this point (Fig. 38-8D).
- When the bony removal has been completed, we prefer to use the operative microscope for the remainder of the procedure. This allows more delicate work around the neural elements, while minimizing additional bone removal, and allows better hemostasis.
- The herniated nucleus pulposus most often lies slightly caudal to the center of the nerve root but occasionally is cephalad. Gently retract the nerve root superiorly to expose the extruded nuclear fragments or a distended posterior longitudinal ligament (Fig. 38-8E). The nerve root should not be retracted in a caudal direction. If additional exposure is needed, remove more bone rather than risk nerve root or spinal cord injury from traction on the root. To control troublesome venous oozing at this point, use bipolar cautery if possible. Otherwise, place tiny pledgets of cotton and thrombin-soaked absorbable gelatin sponge (Gelfoam) above and below the nerve root. Do not pack the pledgets tightly around the nerve. The nerve root can be retracted slightly in a cephalad direction to allow incision of the posterior longitudinal ligament over the herniated nucleus pulposus in a cruciate manner to permit the removal of the disc fragments (Fig. 38-8F).
- After removal of all visible loose fragments, it is imperative to search thoroughly for additional fragments laterally and medially. Ensure that the nerve root is thoroughly

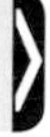

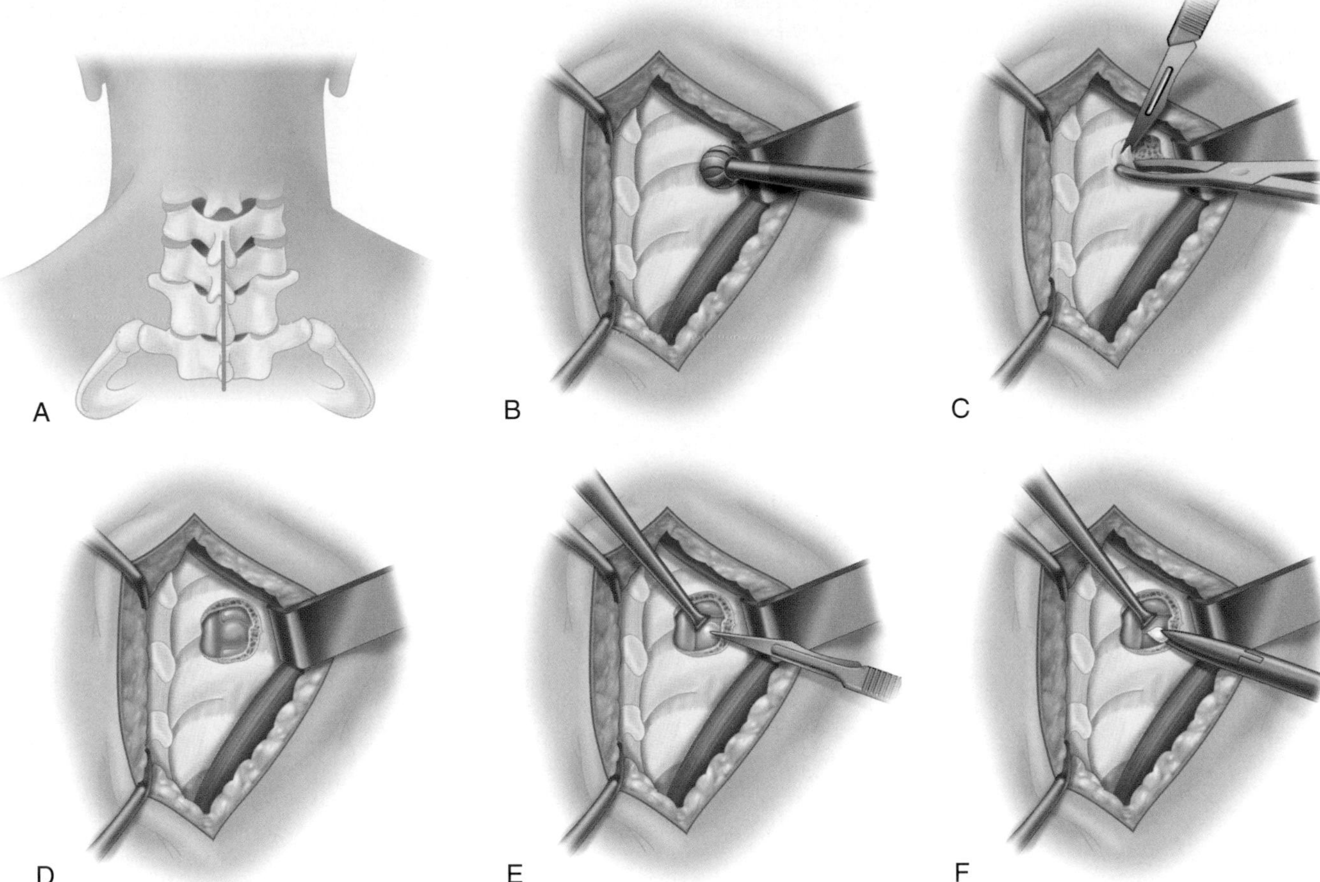

FIGURE 38-8 Technique of removal of disc between fifth and sixth cervical vertebrae. **A,** Midline incision extending from spinous process of C5 to that of C6. **B,** Paraspinal muscles have been dissected from laminae and retracted laterally. Hole is to be drilled with high-speed burr (see text). **C,** Ligamentum flavum is being dissected. **D,** Defect measuring about 1.3 cm has been made (see text) to expose nerve root and lateral aspect of dura. **E,** Nerve root has been separated from nucleus and retracted superiorly to expose herniated disc. **F,** Longitudinal ligament has been incised, and loose fragment of nucleus is being removed. **SEE TECHNIQUE 38-4.**

decompressed by inserting a probe in the intervertebral foramen. If the nerve root still seems to be tight, remove more bone from the articular facets until the nerve root is completely free. Because recurrence is so rare, do not curet the intervertebral space.

- Remove any cotton pledgets and Gelfoam after meticulous hemostasis has been achieved. Hemostasis must be complete because postoperative hemorrhage can produce cord compression and quadriplegia.
- Close the wound by suturing the fascia to the supraspinous ligament with interrupted sutures and then suturing the subcutaneous layers and skin.

POSTOPERATIVE CARE. Neurologic function is closely monitored after surgery. Discharge is permitted when the patient is ambulatory, which usually is the same day as surgery. Pain should be controlled with oral medication. Radicular pain relief usually is dramatic and prompt, although hypesthesia can persist for weeks or months. The patient is allowed to return to clerical work when comfortable and to manual labor after 6 weeks. As a rule, neither support nor physical therapy is necessary, and the patient's future activity is not restricted. Isometric neck exercises, upper extremity range-of-motion exercises, and posterior shoulder girdle exercises can be useful for patients in whom atrophy or inactivity has been considerable. A soft cervical collar can help relieve immediate postoperative pain.

MINIMALLY INVASIVE POSTERIOR APPROACHES TO THE CERVICAL SPINE

Because of the extensive subperiosteal stripping of the paraspinal musculature required for open posterior approaches, which can result in significant postoperative pain, muscle spasm, and dysfunction, less invasive procedures have been developed. Cited advantages of these "minimally invasive" techniques include shorter operative time, fewer operative risks, less blood loss, less postoperative pain, and earlier return to activity. The advent of muscle-splitting tubular retractor systems and improvements in endoscopic technology have led to the development of microendoscopic and full-endoscopic techniques for posterior cervical foraminotomy and fusion. Indications for minimally invasive posterior cervical procedures include radiculopathy caused by lateral disc herniation or foraminal stenosis, persistent or recurrent nerve root symptoms after anterior cervical discectomy, and cervical disc disease in patients for whom anterior approaches are contraindicated (e.g., those with anterior neck infection, tracheostomy, prior irradiation, previous radical neck surgery or neoplasm). Contraindications are much the same as those for open treatment and include pure axial neck pain without neurologic symptoms, gross cervical instability, symptomatic central disc herniation, and kyphotic deformity that would make posterior decompression ineffective.

MINIMALLY INVASIVE POSTERIOR CERVICAL FORAMINOTOMY WITH TUBULAR DISTRACTORS

TECHNIQUE 38-5

(GALA, O'TOOLE, VOYADZIS, AND FESSLER)

- After induction of general anesthesia, place the patient in Mayfield three-point head fixation. Progressively flex the operating table to bring the patient into a semi-sitting position so that the head is flexed but not rotated and the long axis of the cervical spine is perpendicular to the floor. The sitting position allows decreased blood accumulation in the operative field, reduces blood loss and operative times, and improves lateral fluoroscopic images because of the gravity-dependent positioning of the shoulders.
- Secure the Mayfield frame to a table-mounted cross-bar and fold the patient's arms across the lap or chest, depending on body habitus. Pad the legs, hand, and arms to prevent positional neural injury.
- Confirm the operative level on lateral fluoroscopy while holding a long Kirschner wire or Steinmann pin over the lateral side of the patient's neck.
- Mark an 18-mm longitudinal incision approximately 1.5 cm off the midline on the operative side and inject it with local anesthesia.
- Through a stab incision, advance a Kirschner wire slowly through the musculature under fluoroscopic guidance and dock it at the inferomedial edge of the rostral lateral mass of the level of interest (Fig. 38-9A). Be sure to identify and palpate bone and do not penetrate the interlaminar space where the laterally thinned ligamentum flavum may not protect against iatrogenic dural or spinal cord injury.
- Complete the incision approximately 1 cm rostral and caudal to the wire entry point and remove the wire.
- Incise the cervical fascia equal to the length of the incision with monopolar cautery or scissors so that muscle dilation can be done in a safe and controlled fashion.
- Reinsert the Kirschner wire under fluoroscopy and serially place the muscle dilators or, as an alternative, place the first dilator instead of the wire (Fig. 38-9B).
- After dilation is complete, place a 16- or 18-mm tubular retractor over the dilators and fix it over the laminofacet junction with a table-mounted flexible retractor arm (Fig. 38-9C); remove the dilators.
- Attach a 25-degree angled glass-rod endoscope to the camera, insert it, and attach it to the tube with a cylindrical plastic friction couple.
- Use monopolar cautery and pituitary rongeurs to clear the remaining soft tissue off the lateral mass and lamina, taking care to start the dissection over solid bone laterally.
- Use a small up-angled curet to gently detach the ligamentum flavum from the undersurface of the inferior edge of the lamina and use a Kerrison punch with a small footplate to begin the laminotomy (Fig. 38-9D and E).
- Subsequent steps differ little from the open procedure. Depending on the degree of facet hypertrophy, use the Kerrison punch to complete most of the laminotomy and early foraminotomy or use a drill if required. Using a fine-cutting bit and adjustable guard sleeve makes drilling around critical neural structures easier.
- After the laminotomy, remove the ligamentum flavum medially to identify the lateral edge of the dura and proximal portion of the nerve root. Doral bony resection should follow the nerve root into the foramen through a partial medial facetectomy. To maintain biomechanical integrity, preserve at least 50% of the facet.
- Carefully coagulate and incise the venous plexus overlying the nerve root.
- Use a fine-angled dissector to palpate the space ventral to the nerve root for osteophytes or disc fragments. If an osteophyte is present, use a down-angled curet to tamp the material farther ventrally into the disc space or fragment it for subsequent removal. For a soft disc herniation, use a nerve hook passed ventrally and inferiorly to the root to gently tease the fragment away from the nerve; remove it with a pituitary rongeur (Fig. 38-9F and G).
- Inspect the foramen a final time for any further signs of compression and irrigate the field with antibiotic-impregnated solution. Obtain hemostasis with bipolar cautery, bone wax, or commercial hemostatic agent.
- Remove the tube and inject local anesthetic into the fascia and muscles surrounding the incision.
- Close the wound with one or two absorbable stitches for the fascia, two or three inverted stitches for the subcutaneous layer, and a running subcuticular stitch and skin adhesive for the final skin closure.
- Place the patient supine and remove the Mayfield frame.

POSTOPERATIVE CARE. The patient is mobilized as soon as possible. No cervical collar of any type is necessary. If medically stable, patients are typically discharged after 2 to 3 hours.

Ruetten et al. described an all-endoscopic technique for posterior cervical foraminotomy using a 25-degree angle 5.9-mm arthroscope, with working canal of 3.1-mm diameter. They reported no serious complications in 91 patients, of whom only 3 had recurrence of symptoms. Postoperative pain was significantly reduced compared with a similar group of patients with open foraminotomy, and return to work was significantly quicker (19 days compared with 34 days).

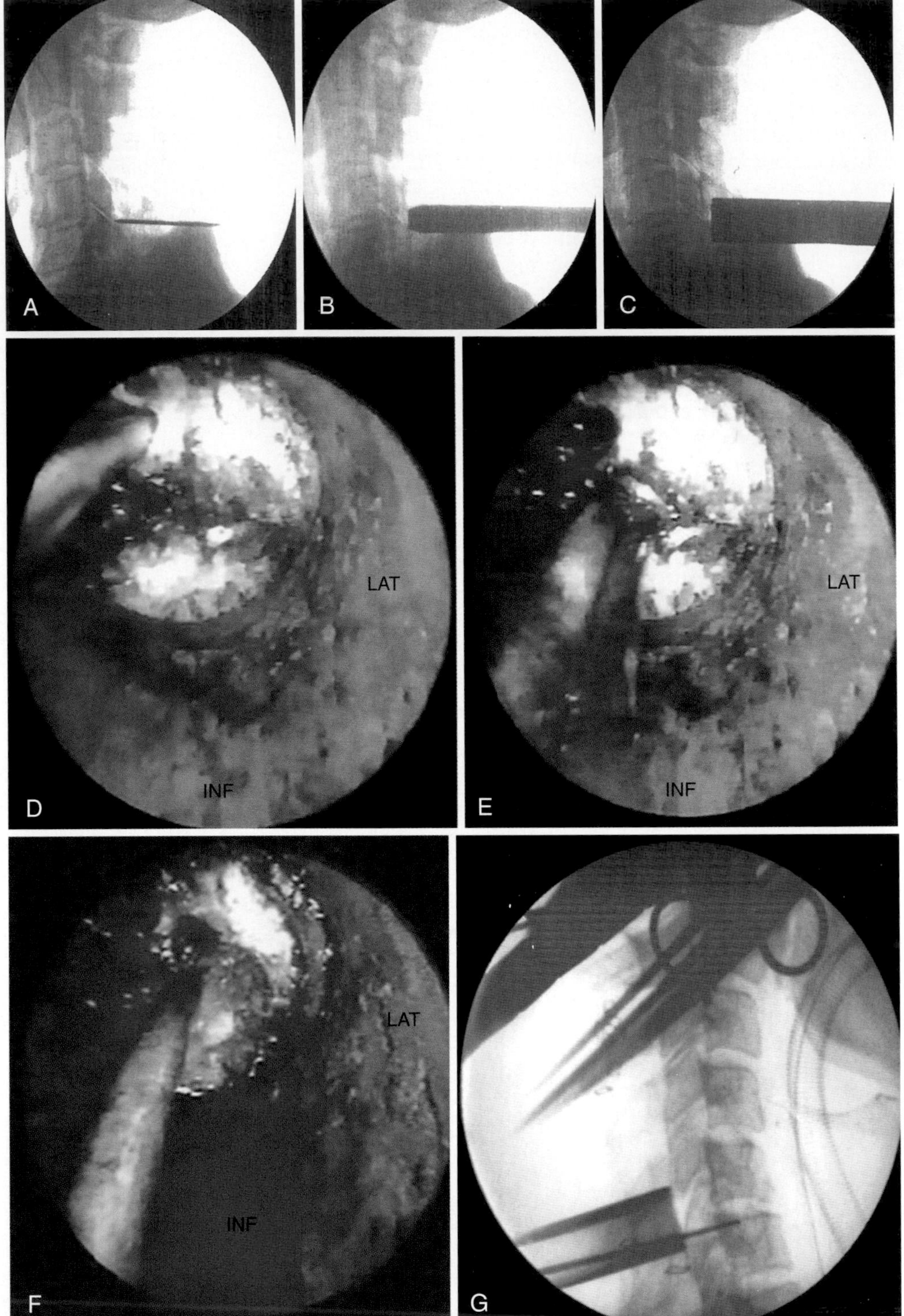

FIGURE 38-9 Minimally invasive posterior cervical foraminotomy with tubular distractors. **A,** Kirschner wire identification of area of interest. **B,** Placement of serial dilators. **C,** Placement of tubular retractor. **D** and **E,** Laminotomy and foraminotomy. **F** and **G,** Disc removal and nerve root decompression. (From Fessler RG, Khoo LT: Minimally invasive cervical microendoscopic foraminotomy: an initial clinical experience, Neurosurgery 51(Suppl 2):37, 2002.) **SEE TECHNIQUE 38-5.**

FULL-ENDOSCOPIC POSTERIOR CERVICAL FORAMINOTOMY

TECHNIQUE 38-6

(RUETTEN ET AL.)

- With the patient prone and after induction of general anesthesia, mark the line of spinal joints under radiographic control, as for a conventional open foraminotomy.
- Determine the location of the correct segment, make the skin incision, and insert a dilator into the facet joint.
- Insert the operating sheath through the dilator and remove the dilator.
- Prepare the joint segment and ligamentum flavum. Begin the foraminotomy by bone resection at the medial joint segments, resection of the lateral ligamentum flavum, and identification of the lateral edge of the dura and branching of the spinal nerve.
- Use 3-mm drills and bone punches inserted through the intraendoscopic working canal for bone resection.
- Use bipolar radiofrequency to coagulate the venous plexus.
- Depending on the particular pathology, extend the foraminotomy laterally or craniocaudally as needed. Take care to prevent excessive resection of the articular process.
- After completion of the foraminotomy, remove all instruments and close the skin. No drainage is required.

POSTOPERATIVE CARE. A soft brace is worn for 5 days.

RESULTS

In few, if any, operations in orthopaedic surgery are the results better than after the removal of a lateral herniated cervical disc. With either open or minimally invasive techniques, approximately 90% of patients have good results with relatively few complications.

ANTERIOR CERVICAL ARTHRODESIS

Anterior cervical discectomy with interbody fusion has gained wide acceptance by both orthopaedic surgeons and neurosurgeons in the management of refractory symptoms of cervical disc disease. The literature attests to a low incidence of major complications and postoperative morbidity and a high degree of success in relieving these symptoms. The fundamental difference in the many techniques is whether surgery is limited to simple discectomy and interbody fusion or whether an attempt is made to enter the spinal canal to remove osteophytes or otherwise decompress the spinal cord and nerve roots.

Extreme care must be exercised in anterior fusion of the cervical spine because of significant potential complications, including injury to the cervical viscera and neurologic and vascular injury. Reported causes of complications related to fusion by the drill and dowel method include operation of a drill without the protection of the drill guard, which allowed the drill to enter the spinal canal; displacement of a dowel bone graft into the spinal canal, either during surgery or postoperatively, which damaged the cervical cord; and the use of electrocoagulation on the posterior longitudinal ligament. The use of a tricortical iliac graft is recommended for interbody fusions.

Anterior discectomy and interbody fusion has a wide application, producing excellent results in virtually all forms of cervical disc disease and spondylosis, regardless of the objective neurologic signs. Despite subtle differences in surgical technique, the intent of the procedure is discectomy and interbody fusion with no attempt to remove osteophytes. The extent to which the posterior and posterolateral osteophytes with spondylosis contribute to the symptoms of cervical disc disease and the indications for removing them have not been completely defined. Often the discrepancy between the degree of bony spurring or other radiographic changes and the symptoms present is striking. Also, the level of neurologic involvement does not always coincide with the site of the greatest radiographic findings. Because plain radiographs cannot provide the necessary information for identifying the level or levels of neural compression, either MRI or CT myelography when indicated is strongly recommended in operative planning; both provide the detailed diagnostic information necessary. In descending order of frequency, the disc levels involved with degenerative changes are C5, C6, and C4. Correlation of the patient's symptoms with diagnostic studies is crucial because 14% of asymptomatic patients younger than 40 years of age and 28% of those older than 40 years have significant abnormalities, as shown on MRI studies. The symptoms of the degenerative processes are related to the interplay of multiple aspects of the disease process and not solely to the amount of bony spurs present. Observation of patients who have had fusions shows that a significant percentage of osteophytes but not all will be spontaneously resorbed postoperatively in the presence of a stable interbody fusion.

In our experience, simple discectomy and interbody fusion without removal of the posterior longitudinal ligament or osteophytes has been adequate in the treatment of neural compression caused by soft disc material. If the compression of neural tissue, especially the spinal cord, is caused by large osteophytes or an ossified posterior longitudinal ligament, direct decompression by removal of the compressing structures has given superior results and is recommended (Fig. 38-10). This is especially true if the T2 sequences on MRI demonstrate cord signal abnormality. In the hands of skilled surgeons, with the use of an operating microscope, a high-speed burr, small angled curets, and small Kerrison rongeurs, safe anterior excision of osteophytes and other offending structures from the spinal canal can be completed before grafting and stabilization. In selected instances, monitoring of somatosensory and motor evoked potentials is useful, primarily in patients with myelopathy or spinal cord signal abnormality, to minimize the risk of spinal cord injury from positioning or hypotension while the exposure and initial phase of decompression is being completed.

GENERAL COMPLICATIONS

For every anatomic structure present in the neck there is a possibility of a surgical error; however, poor results also occur because of poor indications and surgical technique.

The *wrong patient* may be operated on because the neck is a common target for psychogenic pain. Careful preoperative

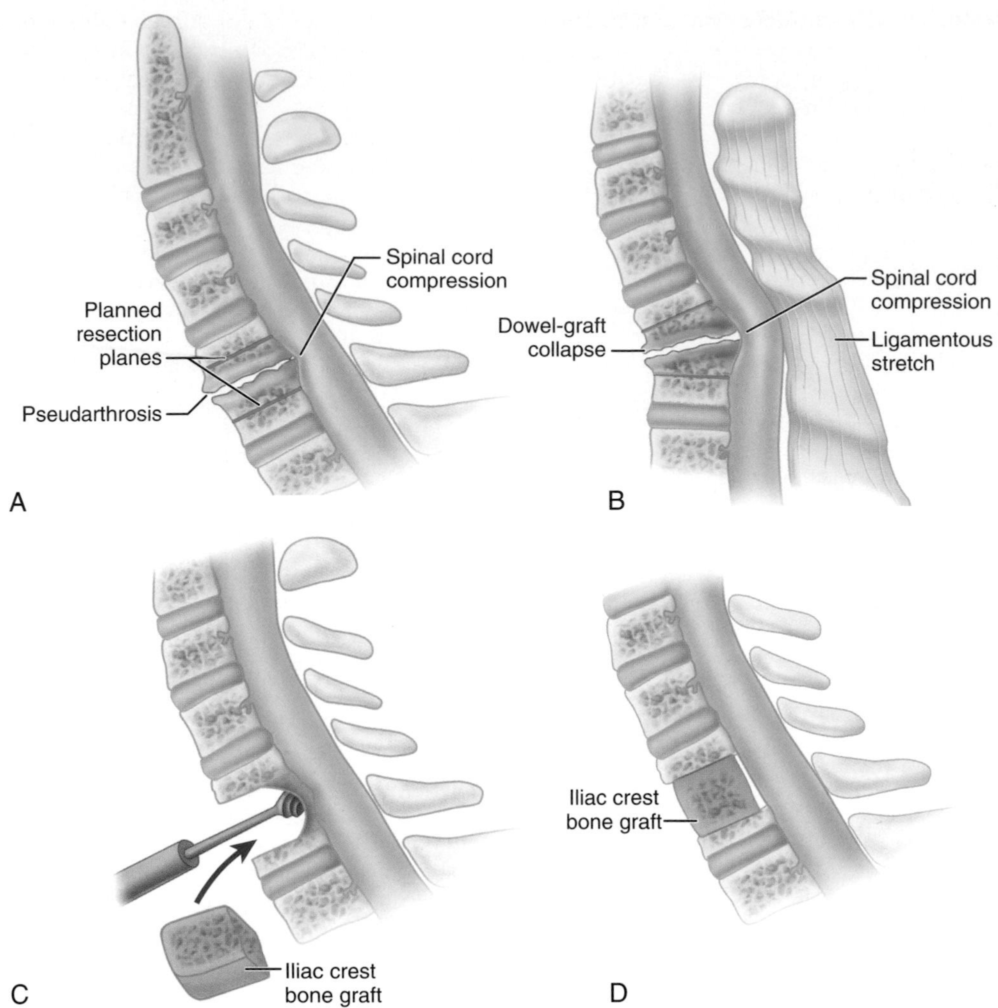

FIGURE 38-10 **A,** Typical nonunion with fibrocartilage compromising canal. **B,** Collapse of graft leads to sharp angular kyphosis, which, combined with nonunion, causes compression of cord. **C,** Decompression through anterior approach. Hemicorporectomy performed cephalad and caudad to disc space with high-speed burr to create parallel surfaces of cancellous bone. Decompression completed with angled curets. **D,** Anterior bone grafting performed with tricortical Smith-Robinson bone graft countersunk into position.

evaluation is essential to rule out a hysterical personality or a chronic anxiety state. In the absence of significant neurologic findings to localize the level of pathologic condition, great care in evaluating the patient's pain is essential. The relatively high incidence of imaging abnormalities in asymptomatic volunteers should be kept in mind. Adjunctive studies, including discography, may be of benefit. Disc degeneration may be a multifocal disease in the cervical spine; therefore, even if an examination seems to point to a single level, it is possible that within a short time other segments will become symptomatic and surgery will be of no long-term benefit. With multiple-level disc degeneration, results have not been gratifying. The best results are obtained with a single segment discectomy and fusion for definite nerve root impairment, spinal cord compression, or, less commonly, localized disc disease without root compression. Fusions of more than two segments performed for pain relief alone produce fair or poor results; improvement, not cure, is the best possible result.

The operation can be done at the *wrong level* if an incorrect vertebral count is made at surgery. Use of a localization film with a metal marker is mandatory, and the first or second cervical vertebra should always be shown on this check film. The marker needle should be directed cranially so that the tip butts the vertebra above and avoids the theca. Additionally, by placing two right-angle bends, beginning 1 cm proximal to the tip of the spinal needle, penetration of the needle beyond a depth of 1 cm is prevented.

The operation may be done in the *wrong way*; for example, the recurrent laryngeal nerve, esophagus, or pharynx can be injured by retractors. Sympathetic nervous system injuries are avoided by dissecting in the correct planes. Keeping the dissection medial to the carotid avoids the sympathetic nervous system. An approach from the left was thought to be less likely to damage the recurrent laryngeal nerve. However, this has not been proved in recent studies. One large series suggested that compression of the recurrent laryngeal nerve may well be caused by endotracheal tube position combined with tracheal retraction and may be decreased by deflating and reinflating the endotracheal tube cuff after retractor placement to allow the tube to reposition itself within the trachea. Instruments can tear the dura or compress neural tissue and must be used with extreme caution in removing the posterior disc fragments and osteophytes. Small, angled curets and Kerrison rongeurs should be sharp to prevent the need for excessive force and loss of control of the instruments. Grafts must be accurately measured and tightly fitted under compression.

The operation may be done at the *wrong time*. Timing of an operation is important; surgery should not be delayed if root conduction is significantly impaired. In patients in whom the clinical findings are purely subjective, consideration usually is given to delaying surgery until any possible litigation is settled. However, this can lead to chronic pain patterns that are difficult to eradicate. We rarely treat surgically patients who do not have objectively demonstrated neural compression or neurologic deficits. Otherwise results seem, at best, unpredictable.

POSTOPERATIVE COMPLICATIONS

All anterior surgical wounds are best drained to decrease the risks of a retropharyngeal hematoma, which can produce obstruction of the airway with its subsequent complications. A soft, closed-suction drainage system usually is inserted deep into the wound. Airway obstruction, although rare, typically occurs 12 to 36 hours postoperatively. Maximal swelling occurs 24 to 48 hours after procedure.

Extrusion of a graft is most commonly seen in the treatment of fracture-dislocations of the neck with posterior instability. This is not common in fusions for disc degeneration when posterior stability of the ligamentous structures is not impaired. At this clinic, anterior plate stabilization and cervical orthosis for 6 to 8 weeks or posterior internal fixation is a routine adjunct when posterior ligamentous stability is lost for any reason and the anterior approach for arthrodesis is necessary. At times anterior stabilization combined with external fixation with a halo vest is used. Use of the halo vest may preclude the need for posterior internal fixation.

A rectangular graft provides the best stability when compared with other graft types. Unless the graft extrudes more than 50% of its depth, or unless it causes dysphagia, revision surgery usually is not indicated. The extruded portion will be resorbed, and the graft will ossify as the arthrodesis heals. If healing time is protracted, external immobilization time should be adjusted accordingly.

Complications related to anterior instrumentation have been reported. Locking-type plate devices minimize the risk of screws backing out and esophageal or tracheal perforation. This type of device also precludes the need for bicortical drilling and thereby decreases the risk for spinal cord injury during drilling or screw placement.

Nonunion of an anterior cervical fusion is unusual. With multiple-level interbody fusions, however, the pseudarthrosis rate increases in a nonlinear fashion. For single-level fusions the literature reports a 3% to 7% nonunion rate even with autograft bone. Similar pseudarthrosis rates are noted with single-level fusions using allograft. With autogenous iliac tricortical grafts, the nonunion rate in two-level interbody fusions without anterior instrumentation ranges from 12% to 18%. However, the addition of stable internal fixation reduces this significantly. This also is true for three or more level fusions. Allograft bone should not be used for multiple-level interbody fusions without anterior plating because of a high nonunion rate. Multiple-level anterior fusions using adjunctive anterior plate fixation with allograft bone can provide satisfactory fusion rates, although the results are not as good as with autograft. When nonunions occur, typically they occur at the caudalmost segment.

If a cervical pseudarthrosis is determined to be symptomatic, usually it is best managed by posterior cervical fusion. If a significant anterior pathologic condition persists, satisfactory revision anterior surgery can be performed (see Fig. 38-10).

When anterior cervical arthrodesis is being done for traumatic disorders with resultant instability from ligamentous tears or posterior element fractures, postoperative treatment must be planned to accommodate this added factor. The postoperative care described here usually applies to arthrodesis for "stable" degenerative or other nontraumatic conditions. If cervical instability is present, or if two or more disc levels are fused, such as with corpectomy, anterior internal fixation and immobilization are routinely used.

Three basic techniques have been used for anterior cervical disc excision and fusion. The Cloward technique involves making a round hole centered at the disc space. A slightly larger, round iliac crest plug is inserted into the disc space hole. The Smith-Robinson technique involves inserting a tricortical strut of iliac crest into the disc space after removing the disc and cartilaginous endplate. The graft is inserted with the cancellous side facing the cord (posterior). This technique has been modified by fashioning the tricortical graft to be thicker in its midportion and inserting the graft with the cancellous portion facing anteriorly. The Bailey-Badgley technique involves the creation of a slot in the superior and inferior vertebral bodies. This technique is most applicable to reconstruction when one or more vertebral bodies are excised for tumor, stenosis, or other extensive pathologic conditions. This technique has been modified by using a keystone graft that increases the surface area of the graft by 30% and allows more complete locking of the graft. Biomechanically, the Smith-Robinson technique provides the greatest stability and least risk of extrusion compared with the Cloward and Bailey-Badgley types of fusions.

A left-sided approach was recommended for years to avoid recurrent laryngeal nerve injury. Recent studies, however, have shown no difference in injury rate to this nerve when comparing approaches. Approach side should be chosen based on the surgeon's comfort. Patients who have dysphagia, dysphonia, or a history of prior neck surgery on preoperative examination should undergo an evaluation of vocal cords and swallowing. If a paralyzed vocal cord is identified, the approach should be on the ipsilateral side of vocal cord paralysis.

SMITH-ROBINSON ANTERIOR CERVICAL FUSION

TECHNIQUE 38-7

(SMITH-ROBINSON ET AL.)

- Place the patient supine on the operating table with a small roll in the interscapular area.
- Apply a head halter if anterior plate fixation is to be used. Apply 5 to 10 pounds of traction to the head halter if so

desired. Otherwise, the halter is not necessary because the distraction pins and the retraction set can be used to open the disc space and allow exposure.

- Rotate the patient's head slightly to the side opposite the planned approach.
- Mark the anterior cervical skin, preferably using an existing curved skin crease, before placing the adhesive surgical field drape. The hyoid (C3), thyroid cartilage (C4-5), and cricoid cartilage (C6) are useful landmarks. The transverse-type skin incision can be used, even for three-level corpectomies if it is well placed; otherwise, an incision along the sternocleidomastoid border is useful. Throughout the exposure, meticulous hemostasis should be maintained to allow better identification of dissection planes and important anatomic structures.
- After sharply dividing the skin, sharply dissect the subcutaneous layer off the anterior fascia of the platysma to allow mobility of the wound to the desired level.
- Divide the platysma vertically near the midline by lifting it between two pairs of forceps and dividing it sharply in the cephalad and caudal directions. This allows exposure of the sternocleidomastoid border.
- Develop the interval just medial to the sternocleidomastoid to allow palpation and exposure of the carotid sheath and the overlying omohyoid muscle.
- Mobilize the omohyoid and retract caudally for access cephalad to C5 or mobilize cranially for access to C5 or caudal levels.
- Sharply divide the pretracheal fascia medial to the carotid sheath. Take care to avoid any dissection lateral to the carotid sheath that would place the sympathetic chain at risk.
- Once the pretracheal fascia has been incised, adequately develop the prevertebral space using blunt finger dissection directed medially and posteriorly.
- Place blunt hand-held retractors medially to view the paired longus colli muscles. To avoid injury to the midline structures, use bipolar cautery and small key-type elevators to subperiosteally elevate the longus colli so that self-retaining retractors can be placed deep to the medial borders of these muscles.
- Obtain a localization radiograph using a prebent spinal needle to mark the disc space before proceeding with disc excision or corpectomy.
- If the superior or inferior thyroid vessels limit exposure, ligate and divide the vessels.
- When elevating the longus colli muscles, do not extend laterally to the transverse processes to avoid the sympathetic chain and the vertebral artery. This dissection, however, must extend laterally enough to expose the anterior aspect of the uncovertebral joints bilaterally.
- Place self-retaining retractor blades deep to the longus colli bilaterally and attach to the self-retaining retractor.
- For single-level discectomy, distraction pins can be inserted. For multiple-level procedures or if screw fixation is planned, the distraction pins are best avoided because of potential microfracture at the pin sites that will compromise screw purchase.
- Once all levels are adequately exposed, use a No. 11 blade scalpel to remove the anterior anulus at each level, cutting toward the midline from each uncovertebral joint.

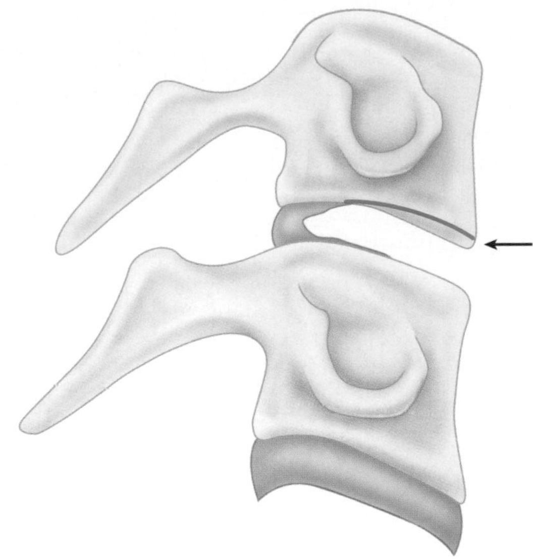

FIGURE 38-11 Diagram of bone removal with high-speed burr of anterior lip of cephalad vertebra to level matching subchondral bone at midbody level. **SEE TECHNIQUE 38-7.**

- Remove the anulus with pituitary rongeurs and curets to allow exposure of each uncinate process, which appears as a slight upward curve of the endplate of the caudal segment. This marks the safe extent of lateral dissection to avoid the vertebral artery. Remove the anterior one half to two thirds of the disc at each level in this way.
- Use an operating microscope for safe removal of the posterior disc, osteophytes, or posterior longitudinal ligament as needed.
- With a high-speed burr, remove the anterior lip of the cephalad vertebra to a level matching the subchondral bone at midbody level (Fig. 38-11). This forms a completely flat surface and enhances visibility for removing the remaining disc material and the cartilaginous endplates to the level of the posterior longitudinal ligament.
- If preoperative imaging demonstrates a soft disc fragment and this is found without violation of the posterior longitudinal ligament, further exploration of the canal is not warranted.
- If necessary, perform foraminotomy to remove uncovertebral tissue with small Kerrison rongeurs. If a defect through the posterior longitudinal ligament is found, enlarge it and explore the canal for additional fragments.
- If the surgical plan calls for complete removal of the posterior longitudinal ligament, complete all corpectomies first.
- To perform the corpectomies, use a high-speed burr to create a lateral gutter at the level of the uncinate process bilaterally that extends from one disc space to the next.
- Remove the midline bone to the same depth as the gutters and continue posteriorly until the brisk bleeding of cancellous bone gives way to cortical bone. Usually there will be significant bleeding from the posterior midpoint of the body that can be easily controlled with bipolar cautery once the cortical bone has been drilled

away. Do not use unipolar cautery in close proximity to neural tissue.

- Thin the cortical bone with the high-speed burr and remove with angled curets, or remove carefully with the burr. If necessary, remove the posterior longitudinal ligament by lifting it anteriorly with a small blunt hook and opening the epidural space with a 1-mm Kerrison rongeur. This must be done with excellent visualization and care to avoid dural injury.
- After the epidural space is entered, remove the posterior longitudinal ligament entirely if needed. If the canal is significantly compromised, carefully free it from the underlying dura with blunt dissection.
- Perform foraminotomies at this time and remove osteophytes if necessary. A small blunt probe should pass easily anterolaterally after foraminotomy. When possible, preserve the posterior longitudinal ligament to enhance construct stability.
- Carefully prepare the adjacent endplates so that all cartilage is removed, subchondral bone is preserved, the entire decompression is the width of the endplate between the uncinate processes, and the endplates are parallel to one another.
- Carefully measure the anterior to posterior dimension at each endplate. The graft depth should be 3 to 4 mm less than the shorter of the two to allow the graft to be recessed 2 mm anteriorly and not compromise the spinal canal posteriorly. Also, carefully measure the length of graft needed in the cephalad to caudal dimension. Remember to measure with and without traction being applied through the head halter so that the graft will be under proper compression. Also, make sure at this point that endplates are parallel to one another.
- Remove the disc laterally to allow visualization of the uncinate process bilaterally, which will appear as a slight upturning of the endplate and marks the safe extent of lateral decompression.
- Obtain a tricortical iliac graft using a small oscillating saw (Fig. 38-12), as described in Technique 1-8.
- During preparation of the endplate, take care to preserve the anterior cortex of the cephalad and caudal vertebrae.
- Fashion the bone graft to the appropriate depth. Position the graft with the cancellous surface directed posteriorly and bevel the cephalad and caudal posterior margins slightly to facilitate impaction. With traction applied, impact the graft into place so that the cortical portion is recessed 1 to 2 mm posterior to the anterior cortex of the vertebral bodies. There should be 2 mm of free space between the posterior margin of the graft and the spinal canal. The graft should fit snugly even when traction is being applied.
- Release traction and check the fit of the graft using a Kocher clamp to grasp it. Repeat this procedure for each additional disc space.
- Apply anterior cervical plate instrumentation if necessary with all traction released. Various systems are available and should be placed according to the manufacturer's recommendations.
- Obtain intraoperative radiographs to verify graft and hardware position.

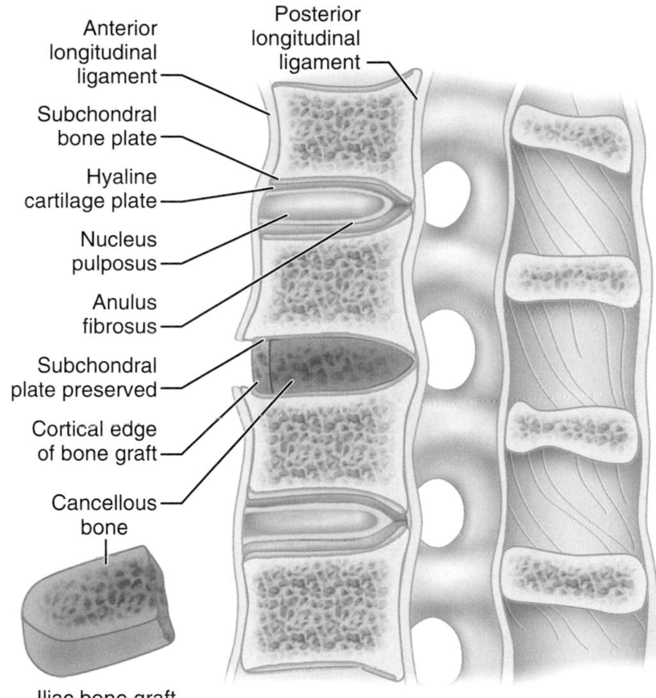

FIGURE 38-12 Technique of Robinson et al. for anterior fusion of cervical spine. **SEE TECHNIQUE 38-7.**

- Close the platysmal layer over a soft, closed-suction drain and close the skin and subcutaneous layers. Apply a thin dressing. Place the patient in a cervical orthosis before extubation.

POSTOPERATIVE CARE. The patient is allowed to be out of bed later on the day of surgery. If a drain is used, it should be removed on the first postoperative day. The cervical orthosis is continued 4 to 6 weeks for discectomy patients and 8 to 12 weeks for patients undergoing corpectomies, depending on patient compliance and radiographic appearance of the graft. Occasionally a soft collar is helpful for an additional 1 or 2 weeks. Flexion and extension lateral cervical spine radiographs should reveal no evidence of motion at the fusion site, and trabeculation should be present before discontinuation of the rigid cervical orthosis.

ANTERIOR OCCIPITOCERVICAL ARTHRODESIS BY EXTRAPHARYNGEAL EXPOSURE

Rarely, an anterior occipitocervical fusion is required for a grossly unstable cervical spine when posterior fusion is not feasible, such as in patients who have had extensive laminectomies and for rheumatoid arthritis, traumatic quadriparesis, neoplastic metastasis to the spine, and congenital abnormalities. This operation is a cranial extension of the approach described by Robinson and Smith and by Bailey

and Badgley; it permits access to the base of the occiput and the anterior aspect of all the cervical vertebrae. We have no experience with this procedure.

TECHNIQUE 38-8

(DE ANDRADE AND MACNAB)

- Maintain initial spinal stability by applying a cranial halo device with the patient on a turning frame. Keep the patient on the frame and maintain the traction throughout the operation.
- Make the exposure from the right side with an incision coursing along the anterior border of the sternocleidomastoid muscle from above the angle of the mandible to below the cricoid cartilage (Fig. 38-13A).
- Divide the platysma and deep cervical fascia in line with the incision and expose the anterior border of the sternocleidomastoid. Take care not to injure the spinal accessory nerve as it enters the anterior aspect of the sternocleidomastoid at the level of the transverse process of the atlas (Fig. 38-13B).
- Retract the sternocleidomastoid laterally and the pretracheal strap muscles anteriorly and palpate the carotid artery in its sheath. Expose the latter.
- Divide the omohyoid muscle as it crosses at the level of the cricoid cartilage (Fig. 38-13B).
- Identify the digastric muscle and hypoglossal nerve at the cranial end of the wound (Fig. 38-13B). Bluntly dissect the retropharyngeal space and enter it at the level of the thyroid cartilage.
- Divide the superior thyroid, lingual, and facial arteries and veins to gain access to the retropharyngeal space in the upper part of the wound.
- Continue blunt dissection in the retropharyngeal space and palpate the anterior arch of the atlas and the anterior tubercle in the midline. Continue above this area with the exploring finger and enter the hollow at the base of the occiput. Dissection cannot be carried farther cephalad because of the pharyngeal tubercle, to which the pharynx is attached (Fig. 38-13C).
- Insert a broad right-angled retractor under the pharynx and displace it anterosuperiorly. Use intermittent traction

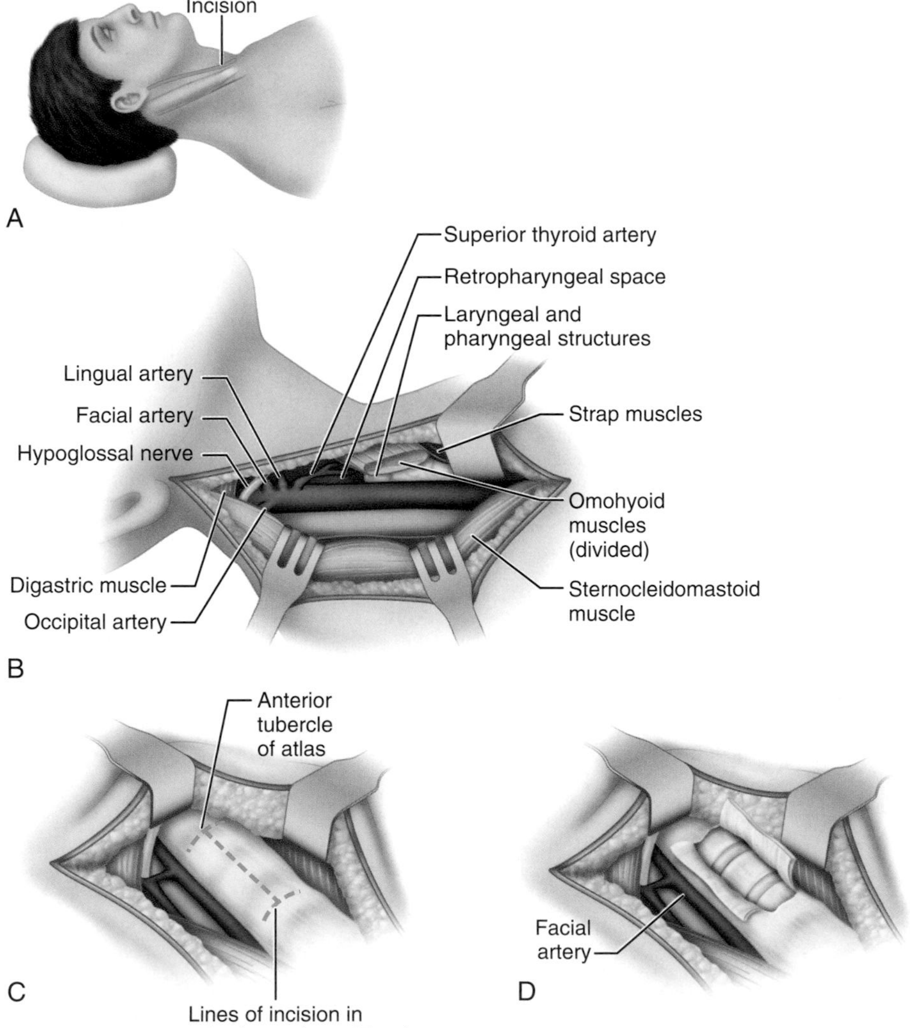

FIGURE 38-13 Technique of de Andrade and Macnab for anterior occipitocervical arthrodesis. **SEE TECHNIQUE 38-8.**

on the pharyngeal and laryngeal branches of the vagus nerve during this maneuver to minimize the risk of hoarseness. The anterior aspect of the upper cervical spine and the base of the occiput are now exposed.

- Coagulate the profuse plexus of veins under the anterior border of the longus colli. Separate the muscles from the anterior aspect of the spine by incising the anterior longitudinal ligament vertically and transversely and expose the anterior arch of C1 and the bodies of C2 and C3. The working space is approximately 4 cm because the hypoglossal nerve exits from the skull through the anterior condyloid foramen about 2 cm lateral to the midline (Fig. 38-13D).
- Roughen the anterior surface of the base of the occiput and upper cervical vertebrae with a curet.
- Obtain from the iliac crest slivers of fresh autogenous cancellous bone and place them on the anterior surface of the vertebrae to be fused. Make the slivers no thicker than 4.2 mm to prevent excessive bulging into the pharynx.
- Close the wound by suturing the platysma and skin only with a suction drain left in the retropharyngeal space for 48 hours.

POSTOPERATIVE CARE. The patient is kept on a turning frame, and traction is maintained for 6 weeks. A tracheostomy set must be kept by the bedside in case upper airway obstruction occurs. For earlier ambulation a halo vest can be applied; the halo vest is removed 16 weeks after the operation. Consolidation of the graft should occur by this time.

FIBULAR STRUT GRAFT IN CERVICAL SPINE ARTHRODESIS WITH CORPECTOMY

When performing a corpectomy, it is important to evaluate the vertebral arteries on axial images of the MRI or CT. An anomalous vertebral artery can course medially into the body, putting it at risk during removal of the vertebral body.

TECHNIQUE 38-9

(WHITECLOUD AND LAROCCA)

- Use the surgical approach of Robinson et al. (see Technique 38-7). As described in that technique, self-retaining retractors are helpful. These can be placed for cephalad and caudal retraction, as well as midline retraction achieved by placing the blades deep to the longus colli muscles that have been elevated.
- Remove a rectangular segment of the anterior longitudinal ligament and remove the anterior anulus at each disc level that is to be excised.
- Remove the anterior half to two thirds of the disc with a curet and pituitary rongeurs and identify the uncovertebral joints at each level laterally.
- With the uncovertebral joints clearly identified with the operating microscope, use a high-speed burr, small curets, and small Kerrison rongeurs to remove the remaining disc material back to the posterior longitudinal ligament at each disc level and remove the intervening vertebral bodies as described in the technique of Robinson.
- The width of the trough should be maintained at the width between the uncinate processes. The medial portion of the uncinate process can be removed, but removal should not be carried lateral to the uncinate process because this endangers the vertebral artery.
- Carry the dissection through the vertebral body until the posterior cortex is encountered. The bleeding pattern of the bone will change from a cancellous pattern to a cortical pattern at this point.
- Perform the vertebrectomy and the posterior discectomy at each level with the aid of the operating microscope or loupe magnification with the use of a headlight.
- Maintain meticulous hemostasis and use bipolar cautery on the posterior soft-tissue structures, such as the posterior longitudinal ligament.
- Apply bone wax to the cancellous surfaces laterally on the edges of the trough.
- Maintain the sides of the trough in a parasagittal plane.
- When the posterior cortex has been reached and thinned to paper thickness, use a small curet to pull the bone anteriorly, detaching it from the posterior longitudinal ligament. In this fashion, the posterior longitudinal ligament can be thinned and pathologic processes, such as ossification of the posterior longitudinal ligament where spinal cord compression occurs, can be treated.
- Remove the posterior longitudinal ligament by thinning the posterior longitudinal ligament and developing a plane just ventral to the dura. The dura can be quite attenuated in some circumstances and is easily torn. Exercise great caution during this portion of the procedure. Small curets, small Kerrison rongeurs, and micro blunt hook and micro blunt dissector are quite useful in removing the posterior longitudinal ligament and osteophytes at the posterior aspect of the uncovertebral joints.
- On completion of the decompression, use a full segment of fibula for strut graft placement.
- Place the fibular graft into prepared notches in the vertebra at both ends of the segment to be spanned.
- Notch the fibular graft at each end so that it will key into the prepared notch in each endplate. Place the endplate recess at the cephalad endplate slightly more posterior than the recess through the endplate at the caudal end to make graft insertion easier.
- Prepare the superior and inferior endplates to accept the graft by removing the cartilaginous endplate and preparing the notches. Preserve the anterior portion of the vertebral cortex to prevent graft dislodgment anteriorly.
- After the fibular graft has been cut and shaped to appropriate dimensions, increase the traction on the head and insert the graft into the superior vertebra, using an impactor to sink the inferior portion of the graft into the endplate recess, and pull distally, locking it into place. Two thirds of the graft then comes to lie posterior to the anterior aspect of the vertebral column.
- Anterior cervical plate fixation is added for stability. Take care in selecting proper plate length so that the screws will not be too close to the graft-recipient site interface.

- Check the graft position with radiographs and close the wound over soft, closed-suction drains in layers.
- Plating provides adequate stability so that only a cervical orthosis is needed after surgery. However, if screw purchase is not acceptable, halo vest immobilization should be used with the uninstrumented fibular technique or a posterior stabilizing procedure with mass screws should be considered.

POSTOPERATIVE CARE. Depending on the type of internal fixation, initial immobilization is continued with an orthosis for 6 to 8 weeks, depending on healing demonstrated on radiograph. The time required for fusion will understandably be longer with cortical bone than with a corticocancellous bone graft. Prolonged immobilization may be necessary.

POSTERIOR CERVICAL ARTHRODESIS

The techniques of posterior arthrodesis of the cervical spine are discussed in the section on fractures, dislocations, and fracture-dislocations of the cervical spine (see Chapter 41).

CERVICAL DISC ARTHROPLASTY

Currently, several different designs for cervical arthroplasty have been approved by the U.S. Food and Drug Administration (FDA) and more are in the approval process (Table 38-3). The primary argument favoring these devices is that, by avoiding anterior fusion, adjacent segment degeneration can be minimized, reducing the need for reoperation. This benefit of cervical disc arthroplasty appears to be supported by a number of randomized, controlled comparisons of arthroplasty and standard anterior cervical discectomy and fusion (ACDF) (Table 38-4). Most of these studies also noted better maintenance of motion with arthroplasty than with arthrodesis. Other studies have reported a quicker return to work (approximately 2 weeks earlier) by patients with arthroplasty. The indications for cervical disc arthroplasty appear to be similar to those for ACDF (see Chapter 41). Using the published contraindications and indications listed in the trials of four different cervical disc arthroplasty devices (Box 38-7), a review of 167 consecutive patients who had cervical spine surgery identified 95 (57%) who had absolute contraindications to this procedure. Osteopenia and concurrent lumbar degenerative disease have been reported to increase the risk of development of adjacent segment disease after cervical disc arthroplasty. Reported complications include implant migration, heterotopic ossification, and recurrent radiculopathy. Metal-on-metal disc replacements also have been found to result in a lymphocytic reaction, similar to that with metal-on-metal hip prostheses, in a few patients.

There are several additional considerations if cervical arthroplasty is to be recommended. The patient should be informed of the current expected or possible benefits and the current uncertainties involved with the procedure. Also, from an anatomic standpoint, the condition of the facets should be essentially normal because arthroplasty treats only one of the three joints at each motion segment. If there is significant disc space narrowing with facet overload and facet degeneration noted on CT, then cervical arthroplasty at this time cannot be recommended. Also, as with virtually any spine implant, the quality of the patient's bone may preclude disc replacement if osteoporosis is present. Proper implant position is crucial to the function and possible catastrophic failure of each device. The reader is referred to the specific technique guides for these parameters. Our experience with these devices is limited at this time, and their ultimate value for patient care has not been determined.

TABLE 38-3

United States Food and Drug Administration-Approved Cervical Disc Replacement Devices

Device	Manufacturer
ActivL Artificial Disc	B. Braun Aesculap Implant Systems, LLC, Center Valley, PA
Bryan Cervical Disc Medtronic	Sofamor Danek, Memphis, TN
Mobi-C Cervical Disc Prosthesis	LDR Spine USA, Inc, Austin, TX
PCM Cervical Disc	NuVasive, Inc San, Diego, CA
Prestige Cervical Disc System	Medtronic Sofamor Danek, Memphis, TN
Prodisc-C	Synthes Spine, Westchester, PA
Secure-C Artificial Cervical Disc	Globus Medical, Inc, Audubon, PA

RHEUMATOID ARTHRITIS OF THE SPINE

Rheumatoid arthritis is a systemic inflammatory disorder caused by lymphoproliferative disease within synovium, which results in cartilaginous destruction, periarticular erosions, and attenuation of ligaments and tendons. The latter along with pannus formation in the spine may cause spinal cord compression. This entity occurs twice as often in young women, with the age at diagnosis typically 30 to 50 years old. Cervical instability is the most serious and potentially lethal manifestation of rheumatoid arthritis, with radiographic changes or instability present in 19% to 88% of patients. Lumbar or thoracic pathology rarely is present in patients with rheumatoid arthritis. Risk factors for developing cervical involvement are an older age at onset, more active synovitis, higher levels of C-reactive protein, rapidly progressive erosive peripheral joint disease, and early joint subluxation. Three basic types of cervical instability are present in this disease. Atlantoaxial instability is most common, affecting 19% to 70% of patients; basilar impression or atlantoaxial impaction occurs in 38%; and subaxial subluxation occurs in 7% to 29%.

CLINICAL EVALUATION

Pain, neurologic sequelae, and instability often are the presenting symptoms. Approximately 61% of patients undergoing total joint replacement were reported to have instability in the cervical spine; 50% of these patients had no symptoms attributable to the neck preoperatively. Neck pain is reported by 40% to 88% of patients with rheumatoid arthritis of the spine, and 7% to 58% have neurologic findings. Axial neck pain usually is occipital and may be associated with

TABLE 38-4

Randomized Controlled Trials of Cervical Disc Arthroplasty

STUDY	ACDF	CDA	FOLLOW-UP	OUTCOMES
Cheng et al. (2011)	42	41	3 yr	Patients with CDA scored better in functional assessments, had more motion maintained, and had fewer complications.
Sasso et al. (2011)	221	242	4 yr	Patients with CDA had greater improvement in NDI; overall success rates: 85% with CDA, 73% with ACDF.
Garrido et al. (2011)	25	21	4 yr	CDA associated with significantly lower incidence of adjacent-level ossification.
Coric et al. (2011)	133	136	2 yr	Overall success rates: 84% with CDA, 71% with ACDF. Significantly more patients with ACDF had severe radiographic changes but no difference in reoperation rates.
Zhang et al. (2012)	60	60	2 yr	Patients with CDA had significantly better ROM; no differences in NDI or VAS for pain. Reoperation rates < 1% for CDA, 3% for ACDF.
Kelly et al. (2011)	106	103	2 yr	No difference in ROM. Significant increase in adjacent segment motion with ACDF.
Nabhan et al. (2011)	10	10	1 yr	No difference in pain relief or adjacent-segment motion.
Coric et al. (2011)	41	57	3 yr	Clinical success rates: 85% with CDA, 70% with ACDF. Angular motion improved with CDA, reduced with ACDF. Reoperation rates similar.
Jawahar et al. (2010)	34	59	3 yr	Adjacent segment degeneration equivalent. Patient satisfaction 73% with ACDF, 66% with CDA.
Heller et al. (2009)	221	242	2 yr	Significantly greater improvement in NDI score and overall success with CDA. Serious adverse events 2% with CDA, 3% with ACDF. Patients with CDA returned to work ~ 2 weeks earlier.
Cheng et al. (2009)	34	31	2 yr	Greater improvement in NDI with CDA.
Riew et al. (2008)	93	106	2 yr	Improvements in NDI, SF-36, arm/neck pain similar

ACDF, Anterior cervical discectomy and fusion; *CDA*, cervical disc arthroplasty; *NDI*, Neck Disability Index; *ROM*, range of motion; *VAS*, Visual Analog Scale.

BOX 38-7

Indications and Contraindications for Cervical Disc Replacement

Indications

- Symptomatic cervical disc disease at one or two vertebral levels between C3-T1 confirmed by imaging (MRI, CT, or myelography) showing herniated nucleus pulposus, spondylosis, or loss of disc height
- Failed ≥ 6 weeks of conservative therapy
- Between 20 and 70 years of age
- No contraindications

Contraindications

- ≥3 vertebral levels requiring treatment
- Cervical instability (translation > 3 mm and/or > 11-degree rotational difference to that or either adjacent level)
- Known allergy to implant materials (titanium, polyethylene, cobalt, chromium, and molybdenum)
- Cervical fusion adjacent to the level to be treated
- Posttraumatic vertebral body deficiency/deformity
- Facet joint degeneration
- Neck or arm pain of unknown etiology
- Axial neck pain as the solitary presenting symptom
- Severe spondylosis (bridging osteophytes, disc height loss > 50%, and absence of motion < 2 degrees)
- Osteoporosis/osteopenia
- Prior surgery at the level to be treated
- Active malignancy; history of invasive malignancy, unless treated and asymptomatic for at least 5 years
- Systemic disease (acquired immune deficiency syndrome, human immunodeficiency virus, hepatitis B or C, and insulin-dependent diabetes)
- Other metabolic bone disease (i.e., Paget disease and osteomalacia)
- Morbid obesity (body mass index [BMI] > 40 or weight > 100 lb over ideal body weight)
- Pregnant or trying to become pregnant in next 3 years
- Active local/systemic infection
- Presently on medications that can interfere with bone/soft-tissue healing (i.e., corticosteroids)
- Autoimmune spondyloarthropathies (rheumatoid arthritis)

(From Auerbach JD, Jones KJ, Fras CI, et al: The prevalence of indications and contraindications to cervical total disc replacement, Spine J 8:711, 2008.)

headaches. Myelopathic symptoms include early weakness and gait disturbance, with frequent tripping or clumsiness. Hand function may be impaired, with coordination disturbances that cause difficulty differentiating coins or buttoning clothing. Sensory changes and bowel and bladder incontinence are late myelopathic symptoms. In patients with atlantoaxial instability, vertebrobasilar insufficiency resulting from kinking of the vertebral arteries can cause vertigo, tinnitus, or visual disturbances that lead to loss of equilibrium. Neurologic evaluation in patients with rheumatoid arthritis can be difficult. Tendon ruptures, severe joint disturbances, and previous surgery can make it difficult to distinguish radicular and myelopathic symptoms from peripheral disease involvement. Any findings consistent with myelopathy should stimulate further investigation.

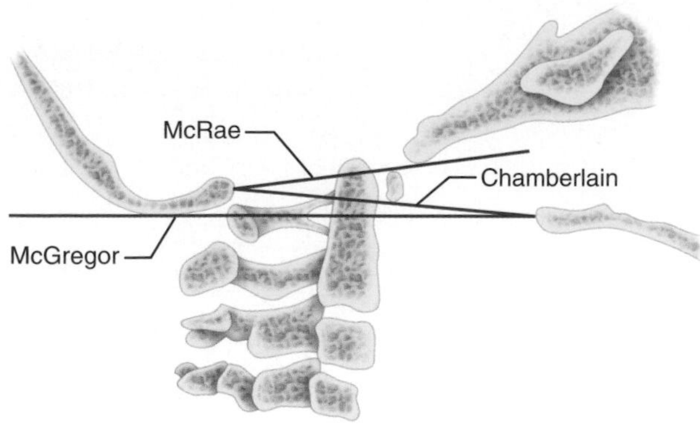

FIGURE 38-14 Drawing of base of skull and upper spine showing McGregor, McRae, and Chamberlain lines.

DIAGNOSTIC IMAGING

RADIOGRAPHY

Radiographs should include anteroposterior, lateral, odontoid, and lateral flexion and extension views. Instability and potential for neurologic sequelae are correlated best with the posterior atlantodens interval, which is determined by measuring the distance between the ventral surface of the lamina of C1 and the dorsal aspect of the odontoid; the interval should be more than 14 mm. This measurement is 97% sensitive for the presence of paralysis. In patients with preoperative paralysis caused by atlantoaxial subluxation, recovery is not expected if the spinal canal diameter is less than 10 mm. If basilar impression is coexistent, significant recovery occurs only if the space available for the cord is at least 13 mm. Therefore when patients have a posterior atlantodens interval of 14 mm or less, decompression must be considered because of the risk of paralysis from their atlantoaxial instability. Remember that the posterior atlantodens interval measured on a radiograph does not represent the actual space available for the cord because the soft tissues are not included in the measurement.

The atlantodens interval is determined by measuring the distance between the posterior edge of the anterior ring of C1 and the anterior edge of the odontoid. Normally this distance should be 3.5 mm or less in an adult. An atlantodens interval of more than 10 mm is clinically significant and suggests transverse ligament disruption; however, this measurement is not useful in predicting neurologic sequelae caused by instability, possibly because of the natural history of atlantoaxial instability. As atlantoaxial instability progresses, subsequent vertical instability develops. As this superior migration occurs, the atlantodens interval decreases. Despite significant progression of instability and potential neurologic deficit, the atlantodens interval does not increase further. Posterior subluxation is best determined by acute angulation of the cord and upper cervical spine as identified by sagittal reformatted CT, lateral air contrast tomography, or preferably MRI. Lateral subluxation implies some rotation of the atlas and is present when the lateral masses of C1 are 2 mm or more laterally than those of C2.

Atlantoaxial impaction is measured using the McGregor line (Fig. 38-14). This line is constructed from the base of the hard palate to the outer cortical table of the occiput. The tip of the odontoid is measured perpendicular to this line. Superior migration is considered present in men if the tip of the odontoid is 4.5 mm above this line. Ranawat et al. described a method of determining the degree of settling on the lateral radiograph using the minimal distance between a line drawn from the center of the anterior arch to the center of the posterior arch of the atlas and a vertical line drawn along the posterior aspect of the odontoid from the center of the pedicles of C2. They reported that the normal value was 15 mm for women and 17 mm for men, with less than 13 mm considered abnormal (Fig. 38-15). To determine vertebral settling, Redlund-Johnell and Pettersson used the minimal distance between the McGregor line and the midpoint of the inferior margin of the body of the axis on the lateral radiograph in the neutral position (Fig. 38-16). They noted the normal value to be 34 mm or more for men and 29 mm or more for women (100 patients each). In a comparative study of these two screening methods, the Redlund-Johnell method was found to be better for diagnosing basilar impression.

Subaxial subluxations produce a cascading, or "staircase," appearance of the spine. Any slippage of 4 mm or more, or 20% of the adjacent vertebral body, is considered significant. Measurement of sagittal spinal canal diameter is most useful and should be more than 13 mm. The risk of spinal cord compression and injury is higher in patients with smaller canal diameters.

COMPUTED TOMOGRAPHIC MYELOGRAPHY AND MAGNETIC RESONANCE IMAGING

Three-dimensional imaging is useful in patients who have a neurologic deficit or radiographic evidence of instability. MRI or CT myelography helps delineate the true space available for the cord. MRI is excellent for viewing soft tissues and the neural elements, but myelography followed by CT gives similar information. In addition to bony compression, pannus further decreases the space available for the cord by 3 mm or more in approximately 66% of patients. Determining the cervicomedullary angle is helpful in identifying vertical instability. A line drawn along the dorsal surface of the odontoid intersects a line drawn ventral and parallel to the medulla. This angle normally should be 135 to 175 degrees, with angles less than 135 degrees suggesting atlantoaxial impaction and correlating with the presence of myelopathy. MRI has been shown to be 100% accurate in identifying vertical settling, and it is currently the most definitive, least invasive test for cord compression. Flexion and extension MRI also has been used to determine dynamic compression

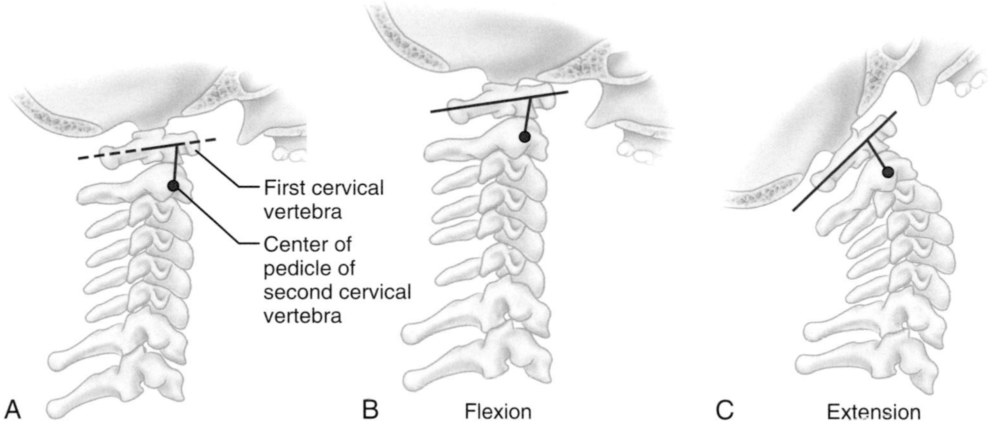

FIGURE 38-15 Ranawat et al. measurement of superior migration in rheumatoid arthritis. **A,** Diameter of ring of first cervical vertebra and distance from center of pedicle of second cervical vertebra to this diameter are measured. **B** and **C,** Measurement of superior migration is unchanged in flexion or extension of spine.

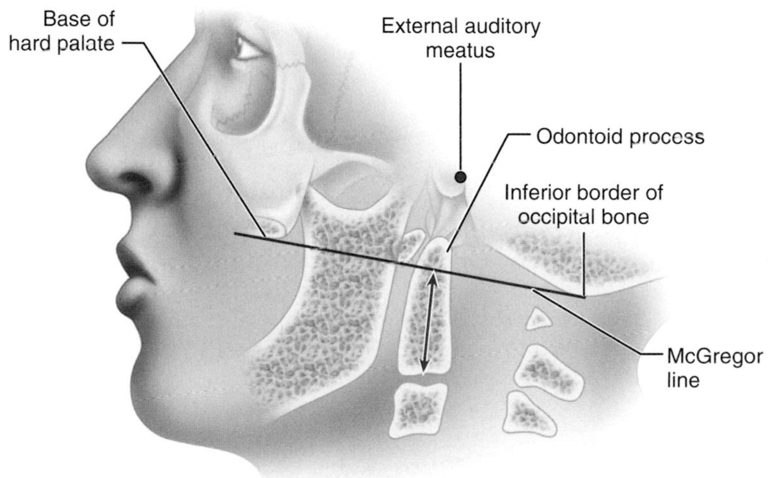

FIGURE 38-16 Redlund-Johnell determination of vertebral settling in rheumatoid arthritis. Distance is measured between McGregor line and midpoint of base of C2.

of the spinal cord. Data from anatomic studies indicate that the space available for the cord should be 14 mm at the foramen magnum, 13 mm at the atlantoaxial articulation, and 12 mm in the subaxial cervical spine.

CERVICAL INSTABILITY

Cervical disease has an early onset and is correlated with appendicular disease activity. Other factors that predict more severe spinal involvement include longer duration of disease, positive rheumatoid factor, use of steroids, and male sex. Patients with rheumatoid arthritis have a shorter life expectancy than the normal population. When cervical myelopathy is established, mortality is common if this condition remains untreated. Of 21 patients refusing surgery for cervical instability, all 21 died within 7 years of the onset of myelopathy. The incidence of sudden death from the combination of basilar impression and atlantoaxial instability is about 10%.

Atlantoaxial subluxation is the most common instability, with a reported incidence of 11% to 46% of cases at necropsy. Atlantoaxial subluxation can be anterior, posterior, or lateral, with anterior instability predominating. Posterior instability may occur in 20% and lateral instability in 7% of patients. This instability results from erosive synovitis of the atlantoaxial, atlantoodontoid, and atlantooccipital joints. Basilar impression, vertical settling, or atlantoaxial impaction is the settling of the skull onto the atlas and the atlas onto the axis as a result of erosive arthritis and bone loss. This settling can result in vertebral arterial thrombosis. According to Ranawat et al., atlantoaxial instability is present in 38% of patients with rheumatoid arthritis; however, its frequency increases with disease severity (0% in mild disease, 52% in moderate disease, and 88% in severe disease in a report by Oda et al.). Subaxial subluxations are more subtle and frequently multiple, affecting 10% to 20% of patients with rheumatoid arthritis. They are believed to result from synovitis of the facet joints and uncovertebral joints, accompanied by erosion of the ventral endplates. They may result in root compression from foraminal narrowing. Myelography, postmyelography reformatted

CT, and MRI all show root cutoff and partial or complete block. Postmyelography reformatted CT and MRI are clearly superior in identifying soft-tissue obstructions and cord compression. Absolute subluxation distances of clinical significance are unknown for this problem.

The signs and symptoms of these instability patterns include pain, stiffness, pyramidal tract involvement, vertebrobasilar insufficiency, root findings, and symptoms similar to the Lhermitte sign in multiple sclerosis. Early clinical manifestations include Hoffmann and Babinski signs and hyperreflexia.

NONOPERATIVE TREATMENT

Disease-modifying antirheumatic medications are changing the course of this disease. Early use of nonbiologic or biologic antirheumatic drugs can be beneficial in avoiding irreversible injury. The use of a combination of these medications has been shown to prevent or retard the development of anterior atlantoaxial subluxation and other cervical spine lesions in patients with an early diagnosis of rheumatoid arthritis. Patients should be under the care of a rheumatologist once the diagnosis is made.

Goals of nonoperative treatment include preventing neurologic injury, avoiding sudden death, minimizing pain, and maximizing function. Many patients, despite radiographic abnormalities, remain asymptomatic, and supportive treatment and close observation are necessary. Medical management during disease flares is important for patient comfort and should be coordinated with a rheumatologist. A cervical orthosis is helpful in some patients if pain persists. Isometric exercises help stabilize the neck without excessive motion and may help alleviate mechanical symptoms. Yearly follow-up with five-view radiographs is indicated to detect instability so that stabilization can be done before neurologic deficits develop.

OPERATIVE TREATMENT

The indications for operative treatment are neurologic impairment, instability, and pain. Fusion is recommended for patients, with or without neurological deficits, who have atlantoaxial subluxation and a posterior atlantoodontoid interval of 14 mm or less, atlantoaxial subluxation with at least 5 mm of basilar invagination, or subaxial subluxation with a sagittal spinal canal diameter of 14 mm or less. Axial imaging that shows compression of the spinal cord to a diameter of less than 6 mm also is an indication for surgery.

Atlantoaxial subluxation is best treated by posterior C1 and C2 fusion. When the subluxation is reducible, fusion may be accomplished by a posterior wiring technique (Gallie or Brooks wiring, Technique 41-7), Magerl transarticular screws (Technique 41-9), or Harms C1-2 lateral mass fixation (Technique 41-6). When the atlantoaxial subluxation is not reducible, posterior wiring techniques are contraindicated and screw fixation as described by Magerl or Harms should be used in combination with a C1 laminectomy if decompression is needed. Occipitocervical fusion also may be considered when adequate fixation cannot be achieved in C1. The need for a halo vest postoperatively should be based on the stability of the surgical fixation, bone quality, and compliance of the patient.

Preoperative planning for transarticular screws or C1 lateral mass fixation must include CT with sagittal and axial reconstructions to determine if ample lateral masses are present for fixation and to see if there are anomalies of the vertebral arteries. Stabilization alone should result in some decrease of pannus, and odontoid excision is unnecessary, unless anterior compression persists after fusion or if compression is purely bony.

In patients with basilar impression, a trial of halo or tong traction for reduction is an option, if tolerated. If reduction is accomplished, a posterior occipitocervical fusion is done. If reduction is impossible, posterior fusion is done after anterior transoral decompression or posterior decompression that includes decompression of the foramen magnum. Posterior stabilization can be obtained with wiring and cancellous struts, Luque rods, lateral mass plates, Y-plates, and newer rod-screw or rod-hook systems. The prognosis is guarded in patients with preoperative neurologic deficits, and basilar impression is associated with poorer recovery of function. As a result, aggressive treatment is indicated to prevent neurologic deficits when progressive atlantoaxial impaction is identified.

Symptomatic subaxial subluxation is best treated by surgical stabilization anteriorly or posteriorly. Anteriorly, stabilization can be achieved by discectomy or corpectomy and fusion using a cage and autograft or allograft, structural allograft, or tricortical autogenous bone graft, depending on the pathology. Posteriorly, fusion is done using wires, plates, or mass screws and rods and autogenous bone grafting. Halo traction can be used to reduce subluxations preoperatively, especially in patients with myelopathy or paraplegia. Anterior decompression and fusion are preferred for irreducible subluxations and in patients who require a decompression. Supplementation with posterior instrumentation should be considered for patients who require multilevel anterior procedures and in patients with poor bone quality.

The mortality associated with surgery for rheumatoid arthritis patients is between 5% and 10% and is higher in patients with cardiovascular disease or atlantoaxial impaction. The complication rate also is high; 25% of patients will have wound complications.

Boden and Clark developed a treatment algorithm for atlantoaxial subluxation (Fig. 38-17). The techniques for occipitocervical, atlantoaxial, and subaxial posterior cervical fusion are described in Chapter 41.

Pain is decreased after surgery in 90% to 97% of patients. Peppelman et al. reported that neurologic function improved in 95% of patients with atlantoaxial subluxations, in 76% of patients with combined atlantoaxial subluxation and atlantoaxial impaction, and in 94% of patients with subaxial subluxations. Atlantoaxial subluxations have a poor prognosis for neurologic recovery, with several studies reporting improvement of function of one Ranawat class in only 40% to 50% of patients. The severity of the preoperative neurologic deficit also influenced results.

ANKYLOSING SPONDYLITIS OF THE CERVICAL SPINE

Ankylosing spondylitis is a chronic inflammatory disease of unknown etiology. It is a seronegative spondyloarthropathy that primarily affects the axial skeleton, sacroiliac joints, and pelvis. Less commonly, involvement of peripheral joints, eyes (iritis or uveitis), heart, and lungs can occur. Inflammation of

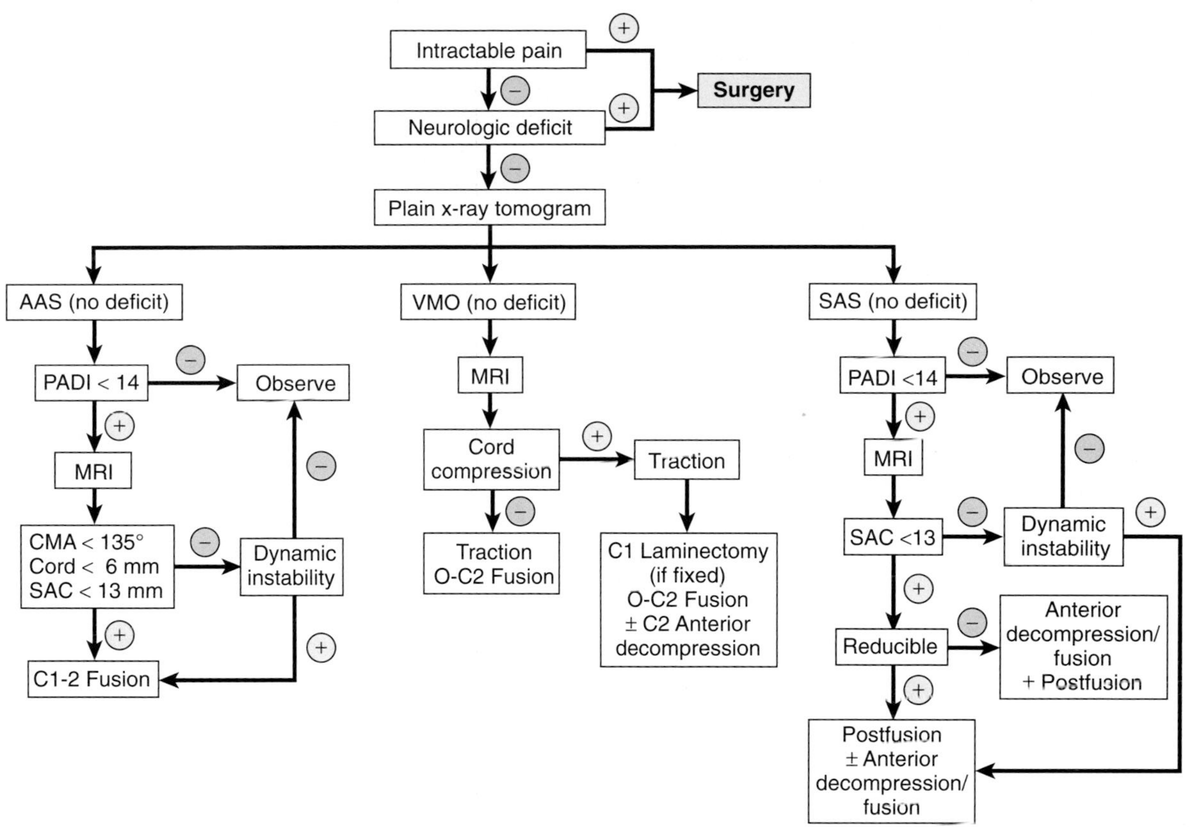

FIGURE 38-17 Algorithm for evaluation and management of rheumatoid arthritis of cervical spine. *AAS,* Atlantoaxial subluxation; *CMA,* cervicomedullary angle; *PADI,* posterior atlantodental interval; *SAC,* space available for cord; *SAS,* subaxial subluxation; *VMO,* vertical migration of odontoid. (From Boden SD, Clark CR: Rheumatoid arthritis of the cervical spine. In The Cervical Spine Research Society, Editorial Committee: The cervical spine, ed 3, Philadelphia, 1998, Lippincott-Raven.)

the spinal joints and enthesopathies cause chronic pain and stiffness and can lead to progressive ankylosis of the spine in patients with long-standing disease. Ankylosing spondylitis typically affects young adults between the ages 20 and 40 years, with a male to female ratio of 1:3. The average onset of symptoms occurs at 23 years of age; there can be an 8.5- to 11.4-year delay from initial symptoms to diagnosis. There is a known association with the HLA-B27 antigen. Eighty-eight to 96 percent of patients who have ankylosing spondylitis are HLA-B27 positive, but only 5% of the HLA-B27 population develops ankylosing spondylitis.

In the cervical spine, ankylosing spondylitis can lead to progressive deformity, causing disabling functional deficits. In addition, fused sections of the spine make it more susceptible to fracture, pseudarthrosis, or spondylodiscitis.

In the vertebral bodies, inflammatory resorption of bone at the enthesis causes periarticular osteopenia. This resorption initially is seen as a "squaring off" of the corners of the vertebral bodies. Subsequent ossification occurs in the anulus fibrosis, sparing the anterior longitudinal ligament and disc and giving the "bamboo spine" appearance on radiographs. The posterior elements are similarly affected, with ossification of the facet joints, interspinous and supraspinous ligaments, and ligamentum flavum. Atlantoaxial instability must be identified, especially in any patient having surgery for conditions associated with ankylosing spondylitis. Because of the stiff subaxial spine, instability occurs in 25% to 90% of patients with ankylosing spondylitis.

Treatment is directed at maintaining flexibility and maintaining spinal alignment with exercises and posture. Sleeping supine on a firm mattress with one pillow may help maintain sagittal alignment. Medications used in the treatment of ankylosing spondylitis fall into three categories. The first includes nonsteroidal antiinflammatory drugs that relieve pain by decreasing joint inflammation. The second group comprises disease-modifying antirheumatic drugs such as minocycline, sulfasalazine, and methotrexate. This is an unrelated group of drugs found to slow the disease process, but they do not provide a cure. Finally, tumor necrosis factor-α blockers have been shown to be effective.

Operative management in patients with ankylosing spondylitis is indicated to decrease pain and improve function. Total hip arthroplasties are the most common surgical interventions performed in this population followed by spinal osteotomies to correct sagittal imbalances.

Spinal fractures in patients with ankylosing spondylitis are always serious and frequently are life-threatening injuries. Spine osteopenia that is common in this population combined with fused segments make patients more vulnerable to fractures, especially from minor trauma. Furthermore, distorted anatomy from disc ossification, ectopic bone, and sclerosis can make the spinal fractures difficult to see on plain radiographs, and these injuries often are missed. It should be up to the treating physician to prove that the patient with ankylosis does not have a fracture after trauma. Spinal precautions and immobilization in a position accommodating the patient's

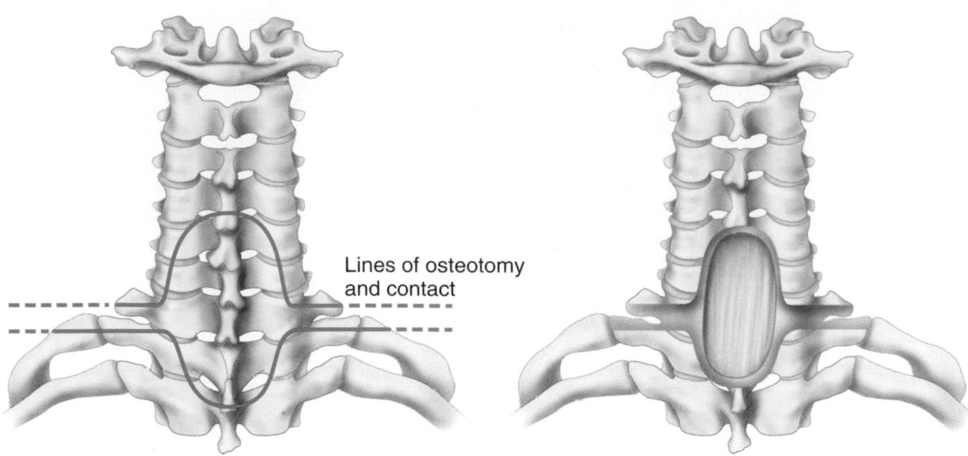

FIGURE 38-18 Extent of resection of cervical laminae for safe osteotomy. Lateral resections are beveled toward each other so that opposing surfaces are parallel and in apposition after extension osteotomy.

posture is very important. Often CT or MRI studies are needed. Fractures usually occur in the lower cervical spine, frequently are unstable, and usually are discovered late. Persistent pain may be the only finding until late neurologic loss occurs. In patients with established kyphosis, the deformity may suddenly improve. The patient's previous deformity may be unknown to individuals providing emergency care. Any perceived change in spinal alignment, even if the result of trivial trauma, should be considered a fracture in a patient with ankylosing spondylitis. The standard procedure is to immobilize the patient in the position in which he or she is found because extension may result in sudden neurologic loss. A widened anterior disc space, which may be the only obvious radiographic finding, creates an unstable configuration that is prone to translation, late neurologic loss, and slow healing. Imaging with MRI, CT, or bone scan may be helpful in making the diagnosis.

Surgical stabilization of fractures in patients with ankylosing spondylitis is associated with a high complication rate but has been shown to improve survival in this population. For stabilization of cervical fractures, combined anterior and posterior or long posterior constructs are recommended because of the poor bone quality. Anterior-only stabilization procedures are prone to failure and should be avoided. The morbidity and mortality associated with these procedures in patients with ankylosing spondylitis are very high because of the comorbidities many of these patients have.

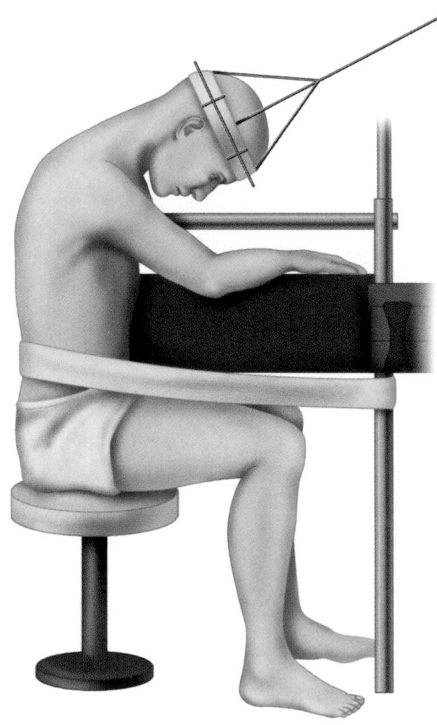

FIGURE 38-19 Position of patient for cervical osteotomy: sitting on stool with head suspended by halo and traction allows abdomen to be completely free of external pressure.

OSTEOTOMY OF THE CERVICAL SPINE

In patients with chin-on-chest deformity, often the mandible is so near the sternum that opening the mouth and chewing properly are difficult. Cervicodorsal kyphosis usually can be treated satisfactorily by lumbar osteotomy, which provides a compensatory lumbar lordosis and results in an erect posture. Cervical osteotomy may be indicated, however, (1) to elevate the chin from the sternum, improving the appearance, the ability to eat, and the ability to see ahead; (2) to prevent atlantoaxial and cervical subluxations and dislocations, which result from the weight of the head being carried forward by gravity; (3) to relieve tracheal and esophageal distortion, which causes dyspnea and dysphagia; and (4) to prevent irritation of the spinal cord tracts or excessive traction on the nerve roots, which causes neurologic disturbances.

The appropriate level for osteotomy is determined by the deformity and the degree of ossification of the anterior longitudinal ligament. Law successfully performed osteotomies at the levels of C3-4, C5-6, and C6-7, fixing the spine internally with the plates devised by Wilson and Straub for use in lumbosacral arthrodesis. Wiring of the spinal processes (see Chapter 41), or use of a halo alone, also should be effective. In the osteotomy technique described by Simmons (Fig. 38-18), decompression is done first and is extended into the neural foramina. After decompression and resection of the inferior aspect of the pedicles, extension manipulation is done. The operation is done with the patient sitting on a stool or in a dental chair and inclined forward with the arms resting on an operating table (Fig. 38-19). Overcorrection of the deformity must be avoided because otherwise the trachea and esophagus could be overstretched and become obstructed. If halo stabilization alone is used, postoperative neurologic symptoms are treated by lessening correction; if internal fixation is used for more postoperative stability, reoperation is required for adjustment of correction. The halo is worn for 3 months, and a Philadelphia collar or similar orthosis is worn an additional 6 to 8 weeks.

REFERENCES

OVERVIEW OF DISC DEGENERATION AND HERNIATION

Andersson GBJ, Howard SA, Oegema TR, et al: Directions for future research, *J Bone Joint Surg* 88A(Suppl 2):110, 2006.

Battié MC, Videman T: Lumbar disc degeneration: epidemiology and genetics, *J Bone Joint Surg* 88A(Suppl 2):3, 2006.

Hadjipavlou AG, Tzermiadianos MN, Bogduk N, Zindrick MR: The pathophysiology of disc degeneration: a critical review, *J Bone Joint Surg* 90B:1261, 2008.

Kalichman L, Hunter DJ: The genetics of intervertebral disc degeneration: familial predisposition and heritability estimation, *Joint Bone Spine* 75:383, 2008.

Poole AR: Biologic markers and disc degeneration, *J Bone Joint Surg* 88A(Suppl 2):72, 2006.

DISC AND SPINE ANATOMY

Duncan NA: Cell deformation and micromechanical environment in the intervertebral disc, *J Bone Joint Surg* 88A(Suppl 2):47, 2006.

Grunhagen T, Wilde G, Soukane DM, et al: Nutrient supply and intervertebral disc metabolism, *J Bone Joint Surg* 88A(Suppl 2):30, 2006.

Iatridis JC, MacLean JJ, Roughley PJ, et al: Effects of mechanical loading on intervertebral disc metabolism in vivo, *J Bone Joint Surg* 88A(Suppl 2):41, 2006.

Miyamoto H, Doita M, Nishida K, et al: Effects of cyclic mechanical stress on the production of inflammatory agents by nucleus pulposus and anulus fibrosus derived cells in vitro, *Spine* 31:4, 2006.

Roberts S, Trivedi J, Menage J: Histology and pathology of the human intervertebral disc, *J Bone Joint Surg* 88A(Suppl 2):10, 2006.

NATURAL HISTORY OF DISC DISEASE

Hutton MJ, Bayer JH, Powell J, Sharp DJ: Modic vertebral body changes: the natural history as assessed by consecutive magnetic resonance imaging, *Spine* 36:2304, 2011.

Lotz JC, Lurich JA: Innervation, inflammation, and hypermobility may characterize pathologic disc degeneration: review of animal model data, *J Bone Joint Surg* 88A(Suppl 2):76, 2006.

Roberts S, Evans H, Triveda J, et al: Histology and pathology of the human intervertebral disc, *J Bone Joint Surg* 88A:10, 2006.

Vernon-Roberts B, Moore RJ, Fraser RD: The natural history of age-related disc degeneration: the influence of age and pathology on cell populations in the L4-L5 disc, *Spine* 33:2767, 2008.

DIAGNOSTIC STUDIES

Haughton V: Imaging intervertebral disc degeneration, *J Bone Joint Surg* 88A(Suppl 2):15, 2006.

Shim JH, Park CK, Lee JH, et al: A comparison of angled sagittal MRI and conventional MRI in the diagnosis of herniated disc and stenosis in the cervical foramen, *Eur Spine J* 18:1109, 2009.

INJECTION STUDIES

Bogduk N: *International Spine Intervention Society practice guidelines for spinal diagnostic and treatment procedures*, San Francisco, 2004, International Spine Intervention Society.

Chen B, Rispoli L, Stitik TP, et al: Optimal needle entry angle for cervical transforaminal epidural injections, *Pain Physician* 17:139, 2014.

Cohen-Adad J, Buchbinder B, Oaklander AL: Cervical spinal cord injection of epidural corticosteroids: comprehensive longitudinal study including multiparametric magnetic resonance imaging, *Pain* 153:2292, 2012.

el Abd O: Steroids in spine interventions. In Slipman CW, Derby R, Simeone FA, Mayer TG, editors: *Interventional spine: an algorithmic approach*, Philadelphia, 2008, Elsevier.

Falco FJ, Manchikanti L, Datta S, et al: Systematic review of the therapeutic effectiveness of cervical facet joint interventions: an update, *Pain Physician* 15:E839, 2012.

Gill JS, Aner M, Jyotsna N, et al: Contralateral oblique view is superior to lateral view for interlaminar cervical and cervicothoracic epidural access, *Pain Med* 16:68, 2015.

Hoang JK, Massoglia DP, Apostol MA, et al: CT-guided cervical transforaminal steroid injections: where should the needle tip be located? *AJNR Am J Neuroradiol* 34:688, 2013.

Lin EL, Lieu V, Halevi L, et al: Cervical epidural steroid injections for symptomatic disc herniations, *J Spinal Disord Tech* 19:183, 2006.

Manchikanti L, Abdi S, Atluri S, et al: An update of comprehensive evidence-based guidelines for interventional techniques in chronic spinal pain. Part II: guidance and recommendations, *Pain Physician* 16(Suppl 2):S49, 2013.

Manchikanti L, Cash KA, Pampati V, et al: The effectiveness of fluoroscopic cervical interlaminar epidural injections in managing chronic cervical disc herniation and radiculitis: preliminary results of a randomized, double-blind, controlled trial, *Pain Physician* 13:223, 2010.

Manchikanti L, Cash KA, Pampati V, et al: A randomized, double-blind, active control trial of fluoroscopic cervical interlaminar epidural injections in chronic pain of cervical disc herniation: results of a 2-year follow-up, *Pain Physician* 16:465, 2013.

Manchikanti L, Malla Y, Cash KA, Pampati V: Do the gaps in the ligamentum flavum in the cervical spine translate into dural punctures? An analysis of 4,396 fluoroscopic interlaminar epidural injections, *Pain Physician* 18:259, 2015.

Manchikanti L, Singh V, Pampati V, et al: Comparison of the efficacy of caudal, interlaminar, and transforaminal epidural injections in managing disc herniation: is one method superior to the other? *Korean J Pain* 28:11, 2015.

Nishio I: Cervical transforaminal epidural steroid injections: a proposal for opitimizing the preprocedural evaluation with available imaging, *Reg Anesth Pain Med* 39:546, 2014.

Obernauer J, Galiano K, Gruber H, et al: Ultrasound-guided versus computed tomography-controlled facet joint injections in the middle and lower cervical spine: a prospective randomized clinical trial, *Med Ultrason* 15:10, 2013.

Pampati V, et al: Cervical epidural injections in chronic discogenic neck pain without disc herniation or radiculitis: preliminary results of a randomized, double-blind, controlled trial, *Pain Physician* 13:E265, 2010.

Park CH, Lee SH: contrast dispersion pattern and efficacy of computed tomography-guided cervical transforaminal epidural steroid injection, *Pain Physician* 17:487, 2014.

Shipley K, Riew KD, Gilula LA: Fluoroscopically guided extraforaminal cervical nerve root blocks: analysis of epidural flow of the injectate with respect to needle tip position, *Global Spine J* 4:7, 2014.

Vasudeva V, Chi J: Defining the role of epidural steroid injections in the treatment of radicular pain from degenerative cervical disk disease, *Neurosurgery* 76:N16, 2015.

Wald JT, Maus TP, Diehn FE, et al: CT-guided cervical transforaminal epidural steroid injections: technical insights, *J Neuroradiol* 41:211, 2014.

Wald JT, Maus TP, Geske JR, et al: Immediate pain response does not predict long-term outcome of CT-guided cervical transforaminal epidural steroid injections, *AJNR Am J Neuroradiol* 34:1665, 2013.

DEGENERATIVE DISC DISEASE AND INTERNAL DISC DERANGEMENT

Alvin MD, Qureshi S, Klineberg E, et al: Cervical degenerative disease: systematic review of economic analyses, *Spine* 39(22 Suppl 1):S53, 2014.

An HS, Masuda K: Relevance of in vitro and in vivo models for intervertebral disc degeneration, *J Bone Joint Surg* 88A(Suppl 2):88, 2006.

Bevevino A, Lehman RA Jr, Kang DG, et al: The effect of cervical posterior foraminotomy on segmental range of motion in the setting of total disc arthroplasty, *Spine* 39:1572, 2014.

Bono CM: Point of view. Pain and disc degeneration: a possible link derived from basic science, *Spine* 31:10, 2006.

Branch BC, Hilton DL Jr, Watts C: Minimally invasive tubular access for posterior cervical foraminotomy, *Surg Neurol Int* 6:81, 2015.

Brisby H: Pathology and possible mechanisms of nervous system response to disc degeneration, *J Bone Joint Surg* 88A(Suppl 2):68, 2006.

Brody MJ, Patel AA, Ghanayem AJ, et al: The effect of posterior decompressive procedures on segmental range of motion after cervical total disc arthroplasty, *Spine* 39:1558, 2014.

Buchowski JM, Anderson PA, Sekhon L, Riew KD: Cervical disc arthroplasty compared with arthrodesis for the treatment of myelopathy: surgical technique, *J Bone Joint Surg* 91A(Suppl 2):223, 2009.

Buerba RA, Giles E, Webb ML, et al: Increased risk of complications after anterior cervical discectomy and fusion in the elderly: an analysis of 6253 patients in the American College of Surgeons National Surgical Quality Improvement Program database, *Spine* 39:2062, 2014.

Bydon M, Mathios D, Macki M, et al: Long-term patient outcomes after posterior cervical foraminotomy: an analysis of 151 cases, *J Neurosurg Spine* 21:727, 2014.

Cardoso MJ, Mendelsohn A, Rosner MK: Cervical hybrid arthroplasty with 2 unique fusion techniques, *J Neurosurg Spine* 15:48, 2011.

Caridi JM, Pumberger M, Hughes AP: Cervical radiculopathy: a review, *HSS J* 7:265, 2011.

Cavanaugh JM, Lu Y, Chen C, et al: Pain generation in lumbar and cervical facet joints, *J Bone Joint Surg* 88A(Suppl 2):63, 2006.

Cheng L, Nie L, Li M, et al: Superiority of the BRYAN disc prosthesis for cervical myelopathy: a randomized study with 3-year followup, *Clin Orthop Relat Res* 469:3408, 2011.

Cheng L, Nie L, Zhang L, et al: Fusion versus BRYAN cervical disc in two-level cervical disc disease: a prospective, randomised study, *Int Orthop* 33:1347, 2009.

Cho W, Buchowski JM, Park Y, et al: Surgical approach to the cervicothoracic junction: can a standard Smith-Robinson approach be utilized? *J Spinal Disord Tech* 25:264, 2012.

Cho SK, Riew KD: Adjacent segment disease following cervical spine surgery, *J Am Acad Orthop Surg* 21:3, 2013.

Clark JG, Abdullah KG, Steinmetz MP, et al: Minimally invasive versus open cervical foraminotomy: a systematic review, *Global Spine J* 1:9, 2011.

Cole T, Veeravagu A, Zhang M, et al: Anterior versus posterior approach for multilevel degenerative cervical disease: a retrospective propensity score-matched study of the MarketScan database, *Spine* 40:1033, 2015.

Coric D, Nunley PD, Guyer RD, et al: Prospective, randomized multicenter study of cervical arthroplasty: 269 patients from the Kineflex-C artificial disc investigational device exemption study with a minimum 2-year follow-up, *J Neurosurg Spine* 15:348, 2011.

DeLeo JA: Basic science of pain, *J Bone Joint Surg* 88A(Suppl 2):58, 2006.

Denaro V, Papalia R, Denaro L, et al: Cervical spinal disc replacement, *J Bone Joint Surg* 91B:713, 2009.

Dohrmann G, Hsieh JC: Long-term results of anterior versus posterior operations for herniated cervical discs: analysis of 6000 patients, *Med Princ Pract* 23:70, 2014.

Evans C: Potential biologic therapies for the intervertebral disc, *J Bone Joint Surg* 88A(Suppl 2):95, 2006.

Feng H, Danfelter M, Strömqvist B, et al: Extracellular matrix in disc degeneration, *J Bone Joint Surg* 88A(Suppl 2):25, 2006.

Fineberg SJ, Ahmadinia K, Oglesby M, et al: Hospital outcomes and complications of anterior and posterior cervical fusion with bone morphogenetic protein, *Spine* 38:1304, 2013.

Garrido BJ, Wilhite J, Nakano M, et al: Adjacent-level cervical ossification after Bryan cervical disc arthroplasty compared with anterior cervical discectomy and fusion, *J Bone Joint Surg* 93:1185, 2011.

Goel VK, Panjabi MM, Patwardhan AG, et al: Test protocols for evaluation of spinal implants, *J Bone Joint Surg* 88A(Suppl 2):103, 2006.

Graham RS, Samsell BJ, Proffer A, et al: Evaluation of glycerol-reserved bone allografts in cervical spine fusion: a prospective, randomized controlled trial, *J Neurosurg Spine* 22:1, 2015.

Guyer RD, Shellock J, MacLennan B, et al: Early failure of metal-on-metal artifical disc prostheses associated with lymphocytic reaction: diagnosis and treatment experience in four cases, *Spine* 36:E492, 2011.

Heller JG, Sasso RC, Papadopoulos SM, et al: Comparison of BRYAN cervical disc arthroplasty with anterior cervical decompression and fusion: clinical and radiographic results of a randomized, controlled, clinical trial, *Spine* 34:101, 2009.

Hsu WK: Outcomes following nonoperative and operative treatment for cervical disc herniations in National Football League athletes, *Spine* 36:800, 2010.

Hsu WK: Advanced techniques in cervical spine surgery, *Instr Course Lect* 61:441, 2012.

Jacobs JJ, Hallab NJ, Urban RM, et al: Wear particles, *J Bone Joint Surg* 88A(Suppl 2):99, 2006.

Jawahar A, Cavanaugh DA, Kerr EJ 3rd, et al: Total disc arthroplasty does not affect the incidence of adjacent segment degeneration in cervical spine: results of 93 patients in three prospective randomized clinical trials, *Spine J* 10:1043, 2010.

Jeon JK, Oh CH, Chung D, et al: Prevertebral vascular esophageal consideration during percutaneous cervical disc procedures, *Spine* 39:275, 2014.

Jiang H, Zhu Z, Qiu Y, et al: Cervical disc arthroplasty versus fusion for single-level symptomatic cervical disc disease: a meta-analysis of randomized controlled trials, *Arch Orthop Trauma Surg* 132:141, 2012.

Kääpä EH, Frantsi K, Sarna S, et al: Multidisciplinary group rehabilitation versus individual physiotherapy for chronic nonspecific low back pain: a randomized trial, *Spine* 31:371, 2006.

Kelly MP, Mok JM, Frisch RF, et al: Adjacent segment motion after anterior cervical discectomy and fusion versus Prodisc-c cervical total disk arthroplasty: analysis from a randomized, controlled trial, *Spine* 36:1171, 2011.

Kim SW, Paik SH, Castro PA, et al: Analysis of factors that may influence range of motion after cervical disc arthroplasty, *Spine J* 10:683, 2010.

Larson JW, Levicoff EA, Gilbertson LG, et al: Biologic modification of animal models intervertebral disc degeneration, *J Bone Joint Surg* 88A(Suppl 2):83, 2006.

Lawrence BD, Jacobs WB, Norvell DC, et al: Anterior versus posterior approach for treatment of cervical spondylotic myelopathy: a systematic review, *Spine* 38(22 Suppl 1):S173, 2013.

Leclerc A, Chastang JF, Ozguler A, et al: Chronic back problems among persons 30 to 64 years old in France, *Spine* 31:479, 2006.

Lotz JC, Ulrich JA: Innervation, inflammation, and hypermobility may characterize pathologic disc degeneration: review of animal model data, *J Bone Joint Surg* 88A(Suppl 2):76, 2006.

Lovecchio F, Hsu WK, Smith TR, et al: Predictors of thirty-day readmission after anterior cervical fusion, *Spine* 39:127, 2014.

Lubelski D, Healy AT, Silverstein MP, et al: Reoperation rates after anterior cervical discectomy and fusion versus posterior cervical foraminotomy: a propensity-matched analysis, *Spine J* 15:1277, 2015.

Mansfield HE, Canar WJ, Gerard CS, O'Toole JE: Single-level anterior cervical discectomy and fusion versus minimally invasive posterior cervical foraminotomy for patients with cervical radiculopathy: a cost analysis, *Neurosurg Focus* 37:E9, 2014.

Maulucci CM, Ghobrial GM, Sharan AD, et al: Correlation of posterior occipitocervical angle and surgical outcomes for occipitocervical fusion, *Evid Based Spine Care J* 592:163, 2014.

McAfee PC, Geisler FH, Saiedy SS, et al: Revisability of the Charité artificial disc replacement: analysis of 688 patients enrolled in the U.S. IDE study of the Charité artificial disc, *Spine* 31:1217, 2006.

McAnany SJ, Kim JS, Overley SC, et al: A meta-analysis of cervical foraminotomy: open versus minimally invasive techniques, *Spine J* 15:849, 2015.

McAnany S, Noureldin MN, Elboghdady IM, et al: Mesenchymal stem cell allograft as a fusion adjunct in one and two level anterior cervical discectomy and fusion: a matched cohort analysis, *Spine J* 16:163, 2016.

Miller LE, Block JE: Safety and effectiveness of bone allografts in anterior cervical discectomy and fusion surgery, *Spine* 36:2045, 2011.

Nabhan A, Ishak B, Steudel WI, et al: Assessment of adjacent-segment mobility after cervical disc replacement versus fusion: RCT with 1 year's results, *Eur Spine J* 20:934, 2011.

Nanda A, Sharma M, Sonig A, et al: Surgical complications of anterior cervical diskectomy and fusion for cervical degenerative disk disease: a single surgeon's experience of 1,576 patients, *World Neurosurg* 82:1380, 2014.

Natarajan RN, Williams JR, Andersson GBJ: Modeling changes in intervertebral disc mechanics with degeneration, *J Bone Joint Surg* 88A(Suppl 2):36, 2006.

Nunley PD, Hawahar A, Kerr EJ 3rd, et al: Factors affecting the incidence of symptomatic adjacent level disease in cervical spine after total disc arthroplasty: 2-4 years follow-up of 3 prospective randomized trials, *Spine* 37:445, 2012.

Onyewu O, Manchikanti L, Falco FJ, et al: An update of the appraisal of the accuracy and utility of cervical discography in chronic neck pain, *Pain Physician* 15:E777, 2012.

O'Toole JE, Sheikh H, Eichholz KM, et al: Endoscopic posterior cervical foraminotomy and discectomy, *Neurosurg Clin N Am* 17:411, 2006.

Pahys JM, Pahys JR, Cho SK, et al: Methods to decrease postoperative infections following posterior cervical spine surgery, *J Bone Joint Surg* 95A:549, 2013.

Poole AR. Biologic markers and disc degeneration, *J Bone Joint Surg* 88A(Suppl 2):72, 2006.

Raizman NM, Yu WD, Jenkins MV, et al: Traumatic C4-C5 unilateral facet dislocation with posterior disc herniation above a prior anterior fusion, *Am J Orthop* 41:E85, 2012.

Riew KD, Buchowski JM, Sasso R, et al: Cervical disc arthroplasty compared with arthrodesis for the treatment of myelopathy, *J Bone Joint Surg* 90A:2354, 2008.

Ruetten S, Komp M, Merk H, Godolias G: Full-endoscopic cervical posterior foraminotomy for the operation of lateral disc herniations using 5.9-mm endoscopes: a prospective, randomized, controlled study, *Spine* 33:940, 2008.

Sasso RC, Anderson PA, Riew KD, Heller JG: Results of cervical arthroplasty compared with anterior discectomy and fusion: four-year clinical outcomes in a prospective, randomized controlled trial, *J Bone Joint Surg* 93A:1684, 2011.

Setton LA: Mechanobiology of the intervertebral disc and relevance to disc degeneration, *J Bone Joint Surg* 88A:52, 2006.

Shau DN, Bible JE, Samade R, et al: Utility of postoperative radiographs for cervical spine fusion: a comprehensive evaluation of operative technique, surgical indication, and duration since surgery, *Spine* 37:1994, 2012.

Singh K, Marquez-Lara A, Nandyala SV, et al: Incidence and risk factors for dysphagia after anterior cervical fusion, *Spine* 38:1820, 2013.

Skovrlj B, Gologorsky Y, Haque R, et al: Complications, outcomes, and need for fusion after minimally invasive posterior cervical foraminotomy and microdiscectomy, *Spine J* 14:2405, 2014.

Srinivasan D, La Marca F, Than KD, et al: Perioperative characteristics and complications in obese patients undergoing anterior cervical fusion surgery, *J Clin Neurosci* 21:1159, 2014.

Stadler JA 3rd, Wong AP, Graham RB, Liu JC: Complications associated with posterior approaches in minimally invasive spine decompression, *Neurosurg Clin N Am* 25:233, 2014.

Tannoury CA, An HS: Complications with the use of bone morphogenetic protein 2 (BMP-2) in spine surgery, *Spine J* 14:552, 2014.

Tortolani PJ, Cunningham BW, Eng M, et al: Prevalence of heterotopic ossification following total disc replacement: a prospective, randomized study of two hundred and seventy-six patients, *J Bone Joint Surg* 89A:82, 2007.

Tschugg A, Neururer S, Scheufler KM, et al: Comparison of posterior foraminotomy and anterior foraminotomy with fusion for treating spondylotic foraminal stenosis of the cervical spine: study protocol for a randomized controlled trial (ForaC), *Trials* 15:437, 2014.

Wang TY, Lubelski D, Abdullah KG, et al: Rates of anterior cervical discectomy and fusion after initial posterior cervical foraminotomy, *Spine J* 15:971, 2015.

White NA, Moreno DP, Brown PJ, et al: Effects of cervical arthrodesis and arthroplasty on neck response during a simulated frontal automobile collision, *Spine J* 14:2195, 2014.

Williams BJ, Smith JS, Fu KM, et al: Does BMP increase the incidence of perioperative complications in spinal fusion? A comparison of 55,862 cases of spinal fusion with and without BMP, *Spine* 36:1685, 2011.

Zhang X, Zhang X, Chen C, et al: Randomized, controlled, multicenter, clinical trial comparing BRYAN cervical disc arthroplasty with anterior cervical decompression and fusion in China, *Spine* 37:433, 2012.

Zindrick M, Harris MB, Humphreys SC, et al: Cervical disc arthroplasty, *J Am Acad Orthop Surg* 18:631, 2010.

RHEUMATOID ARTHRITIS OF THE SPINE

Joaquim AF, Ghizoni E, Tedeschi H, et al: Radiological evaluation of cervical spine involvement in rheumatoid arthritis, *Neurosurg Focus* 38:E4, 2015.

Kim HJ, Nemani VM, Riew KD, Brasington R: Cervical spine disease in rheumatoid arthritis: incidence, manifestations, and therapy, *Curr Rheumatol Rep* 17:9, 2015.

Li J, Goldstein PA: Images in anesthesiology: cranial settling: a cervical spine complication of rheumatoid arthritis, *Anesthesiology* 123:668, 2015.

Narváez J, Narváez JA, Serrallonga M, et al: Subaxial cervical spine involvement in symptomatic rheumatoid arthritis patients: comparison with cervical spondylosis, *Semin Arthritis Rheum* 45:9, 2015.

Söderman T, Olerud C, Shalabi A, et al: Static and dynamic CT imaging of the cervical spine in patients with rheumatoid arthritis, *Skeletal Radiol* 44:241, 2015.

Stein BE, Hassanzadeh H, Jain A, et al: Changing trends in cervical spine fusions in patients with rheumatoid arthritis, *Spine* 39:1178, 2014.

Wasserman BR, Moskovich R, Razi AE: Rheumatoid arthritis of the cervical spine—clinical considerations, *Bull NYU Hosp Jt Dis* 69:136, 2011.

Yurube T, Sumi M, Nishida K, et al: Incidence and aggravation of cervical spine instabilities in rheumatoid arthritis: a prospective minimum 5-year follow-up study of patients initially without cervical involvement, *Spine* 37:2136, 2012.

Yurube T, Sumi M, Nishida K, et al: Accelerated development of cervical spine instabilities in rheumatoid arthritis: a prospective minimum 5-year cohort study, *PloS ONE* 9:e88970, 2014.

Zhang T, Pope J: Cervical spine involvement in rheumatoid arthritis over time: results from a meta-analysis, *Arthritis Res Ther* 17:148, 2015.

ANKYLOSING SPONDYLITIS OF THE CERVICAL SPINE

Baraliakos X, Listing J, von der Recke A, Braun J: The natural course of radiographic progression in ankylosing spondylitis: differences between genders and appearance of characteristic radiographic features, *Curr Rheumatol Rep* 13:383, 2011.

Lin B, Zhang B, Li ZM, Li QS: Corrective surgery for deformity of the upper cervical spine due to ankylosing spondylitis, *Indian J Orthop* 48:211, 2014.

Mehdian SM, Boreham B, Hammett T: Cervical osteotomy in ankylosing spondylitis, *Eur Spine J* 21:2713, 2012.

Yang J, Huang Z, Grevitt M, et al: Precise bending rod technique a novel method for precise correction of ankylosing spondylitis kyphosis, *J Spinal Disord Tech* 2013. [Epub ahead of print].

The complete list of references is available online at ***expertconsult.inkling.com.***

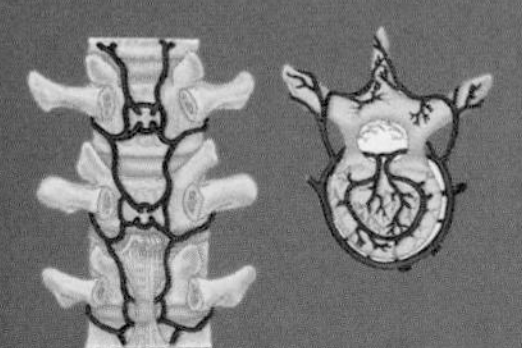

CHAPTER 39

DEGENERATIVE DISORDERS OF THE THORACIC AND LUMBAR SPINE

Raymond J. Gardocki, Ashley L. Park

OVERVIEW OF LUMBAR AND THORACIC DISC DEGENERATION AND HERNIATION

Despite an improving understanding of degenerative disc disease on the basis of its natural history and basic science, treatment results of this entity vary greatly. There is no lack of treatment options for degenerative discs; what we tend to lack is understanding of the specific cause(s) of the patient's chief complaint. Despite the fact that William Kirkaldy-Willis has described the spectrum of disc degeneration and its pathologic progression, the clinical correlation of history, physical examination, and imaging that yields a specific diagnosis remains the greatest challenge.

Over the past several decades, studies of patients with back and/or leg pain have led to improved treatment of the patients in whom a specific diagnosis was possible. This group remains the minority of patients who are evaluated for low back or leg pain. Complex psychosocial issues, depression, and secondary gain are a few of the nonanatomic problems that must be considered when evaluating these patients. In addition, the number of anatomic causes for these symptoms, whether real or perceived, has increased as understanding and diagnostic capabilities have increased.

Axial spine pain, which should be distinguished from disc degeneration, is the most frequent musculoskeletal complaint. Axial spine pain—whether cervical, thoracic, or lumbar—often is attributed to disc degeneration. This degenerative process does not always cause pain, but it can lead to internal disc derangement, disc herniation, facet arthrosis, degenerative spondylolisthesis, and stenosis that can be seen on imaging. Each of these pathologic processes has unique clinical findings and treatments. Outcomes of treatment for each of these specific pathologic entities also vary greatly despite their being from the same etiologic spectrum. The understanding of disc degeneration and the associated pathologies has changed markedly over the past several years.

The genetic influence on disc degeneration may be caused by a small effect from each of multiple genes or possibly a relatively large effect of a smaller number of genes. To date, several specific gene loci have been identified that are associated with disc degeneration. This association of a specific gene with degenerative disc changes has been confirmed. Other variations in the aggrecan gene, metalloproteinase-3 gene, collagen type IX, and alpha 2 and 3 gene forms also have been associated with disc pathology and symptoms. The understanding of symptoms and treatment success for disc herniations has surpassed those related to disc degeneration alone.

Nonspecific axial pain is an international health issue of major significance and should be discriminated from pain associated with a disc herniation. Approximately 80% of individuals are affected by this symptom at some time in their lives. Impairments of the back and spine are ranked as the most frequent cause of limitation of activity in individuals younger than 45 years old by the National Center for Health Statistics (www.cdc.gov/nchs). Physicians who treat patients with spinal disorders and spine-related complaints must distinguish the complaint of back pain, which several epidemiologic studies reveal to be relatively constant, from disability attributed to back pain. Although back pain as a presenting complaint may account for only 2% of the patients seen by a general practitioner, the cost to society and the patient in terms of lost work time, compensation, and treatment is staggering.

The total cost of low back pain in the United States is greater than $100 billion per year; one third are direct costs for care, with the remaining costs resulting from decreased productivity, lost wages, and absenteeism. Also, only about 5% of patients accounted for 75% of the costs. Typically, about 90% of patients return to work by 3 months, with most returning to work by 1 month. Patients off work for 6 months have only a 50/50 probability of ever returning to work, whereas at 1 year this probability decreases to 25%.

Nonanatomic factors, specifically work perception and psychosocial factors, are intimately intertwined with physical complaints. Compounding the diagnostic and treatment difficulties is the high incidence of significant abnormalities shown by imaging studies, which in asymptomatic matched controls is 76%. Identified risk factors for radiographically apparent disc disorders of the lumbar spine include genetic factors, age, gender, smoking, and, to a minimal degree, occupational exposure, but not socioeconomic factors. In contrast is the importance of socioeconomic factors for the development of low back pain and disability. Job dissatisfaction, physically strenuous work, psychologically stressful work, low educational attainment, and workers' compensation insurance all are associated with low back pain or disability. These data suggest that aggressive treatment between 4 weeks and 6 months is necessary for patients with low back pain. Consideration of socioeconomic factors is an important component of appropriate patient evaluation because there is an inextricable link between an individual's socioeconomic status and his or her health.

Optimal outcome primarily depends on "proper patient selection," which so far has defied satisfactory definition. Until the pathologic process is better described and reliable criteria for the diagnosis are determined, improvement in treatment outcomes will change slowly.

DISC AND SPINE ANATOMY

The anatomy of the spine and discs is discussed in detail in Chapter 37.

NEURAL ELEMENTS

The organization of the neural elements is strictly maintained throughout the entire neural system, even within the conus medullaris and cauda equina distally. The orientation of the nerve roots in the dural sac and at the conus medullaris follows a highly organized pattern, with the most cephalad roots lying lateral and the most caudad lying centrally. The motor roots are ventral to the sensory roots at all levels. The arachnoid mater holds the roots in these positions.

The pedicle is the key to understanding surgical spinal anatomy. The relation of the pedicle to the neural elements varies by region within the spinal column. In the thoracic and lumbar spine, the named root exits below the named pedicle. Discs are formally named for the vertebral bodies between which they lie (e.g., the L4-5 disc is between the L4 and L5 vertebral bodies). This allows slightly more specificity in describing the discs if there is an anatomic variant (e.g., L4-S1) and less confusion than having the vertebral body, nerve root, and disc sharing the same name. Despite being less specific, the disc often is informally named for the vertebral level immediately cephalad (e.g., the L4 disc is immediately caudal to the L4 vertebra). In the lumbar spine, lateral recess pathology, such as lateral recess stenosis or posterolateral disc herniation, typically involves the next nerve root exiting caudal to that disc; for example, an L4-5 posterolateral disc herniation would be expected to cause L5 nerve root symptoms.

At the level of the intervertebral foramen is the dorsal root ganglion (DRG). The DRG lies within the outer confines of the foramen. Distal to the ganglion, three distinct branches arise; the most prominent and important is the ventral ramus, which supplies all structures ventral to the neural canal. The second branch, the sinuvertebral nerve, is a small filamentous nerve that originates from the ventral ramus and progresses medially over the posterior aspect of the disc and vertebral bodies, innervating these structures and the posterior longitudinal ligament. The third branch is the dorsal ramus. This branch courses dorsally, piercing the intertransverse ligament near the pars interarticularis. Three branches from the dorsal ramus innervate the structures dorsal to the neural canal. The lateral and intermediate branches provide innervation to the posterior musculature and skin. The medial branch separates into three branches to innervate the facet joint at that level and the adjacent levels above and below (Fig. 39-1).

Disc innervation is through afferent axons with cell bodies within the DRG. Nociceptive signals are transmitted to the spinal cord by neurons from the DRG. Animal studies have revealed two paths between the annulus and the DRG: one from the sinuvertebral nerve and another along the paravertebral sympathetic trunk. The sinuvertebral nerve is a recurrent branch of the ventral ramus that connects back to the posterior disc at each level. The paired ganglia chains of the sympathetic trunks have axons that course through the gray rami communicantes to the spinal nerve. The disc is innervated by fibers from multiple levels. In animal models, the lateral annulus was found to be innervated by fibers coursing from the index level and two additional superior levels through the sinuvertebral nerves. Also, there was innervation through the sympathetic trunk by the DRG from the three levels even more superior than the sinuvertebral innervations. Contralateral DRG involvement also occurs through both pathways. Similar nonsegmental, multilevel innervation patterns also have been reported for the ventral disc surface. These complex multilevel innervations would help explain the pain patterns encountered clinically if similar patterns are present in humans. Also, innervations of the disc from the vertebral endplate have been shown. Intraosseous nerves follow the osseous vasculature. This endplate innervation is through a branch of the sinuvertebral nerve, the basivertebral nerve. This nerve enters the foramen, and the nerve fibers enter the vertebral margin with the vessels. The density of innervation is similar to that seen in the outer annulus, which suggests that the endplates are as important to pain generation as is the annulus.

NATURAL HISTORY OF DISC DISEASE

One theory of spinal degeneration assumes that all spines degenerate and that current methods of treatment are for

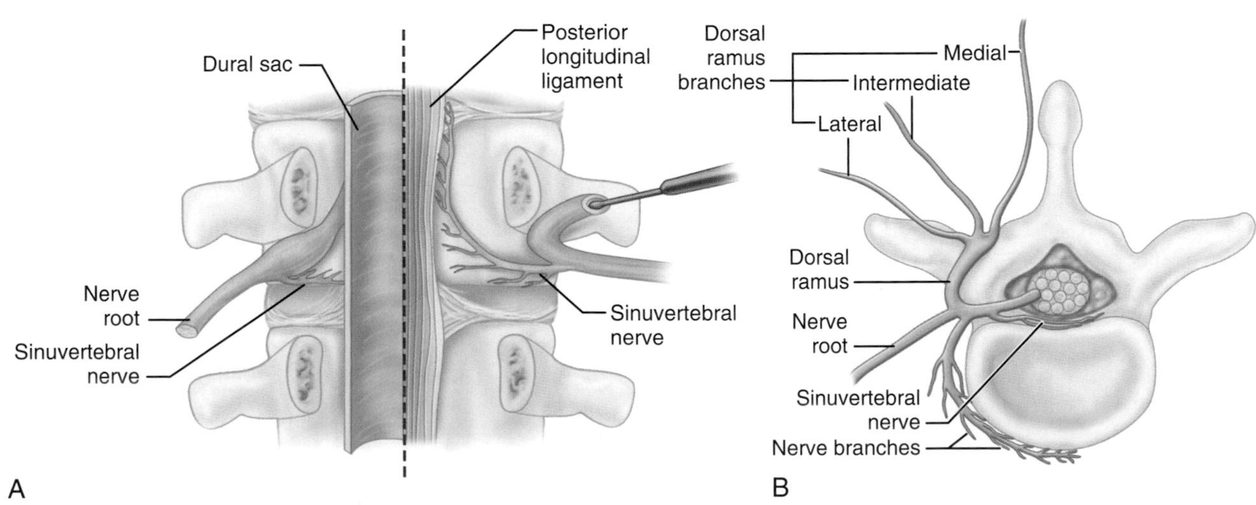

FIGURE 39-1 **A,** Dorsal view of lumbar spinal segment with lamina and facets removed. On left side, dura and root exiting at that level remain. On right side, dura has been resected and root is elevated. Sinuvertebral nerve with its course and innervation of posterior longitudinal ligament is usually obscured by nerve root and dura. **B,** Cross-sectional view of spine at level of endplate and disc. Note that sinuvertebral nerve innervates dorsal surface of disc and posterior longitudinal ligament. Additional nerve branches from ventral ramus innervate more ventral surface of disc and anterior longitudinal ligament. Dorsal ramus arises from root immediately on leaving foramen. This ramus divides into lateral, intermediate, and medial branches. Medial branch supplies primary innervation to facet joints dorsally.

symptomatic relief, not for cure. The degenerative process has been divided into three separate stages with relatively distinct findings. The first stage is dysfunction, which is seen in individuals 15 to 45 years old. It is characterized by circumferential and radial tears in the disc annulus and localized synovitis of the facet joints. The next stage is instability. This stage, found in 35- to 70-year-old individuals, is characterized by internal disruption of the disc, progressive disc resorption, and degeneration of the facet joints with capsular laxity, subluxation, and joint erosion. The final stage, present in individuals older than 60 years, is stabilization. In this stage, the progressive development of hypertrophic bone around the disc and facet joints leads to segmental stiffening or frank ankylosis (see Table 38-1).

Each spinal segment degenerates at a different rate. As one level is in the dysfunction stage, another may be entering the stabilization stage. Disc herniation in this scheme is considered a complication of disc degeneration in the dysfunction and instability stages. Spinal stenosis from degenerative arthritis in this scheme is a complication of bony overgrowth compromising neural tissue in the late instability and early stabilization stages.

Long-term follow-up studies of lumbar disc herniations have documented several principles, the foremost being that generally symptomatic lumbar disc herniation (which is only one of the consequences of disc degeneration) has a favorable outcome in most patients. The primary benefit of surgery has been noted to occur early on in the first year after surgery, but with time the statistical significance of the improvement appears to be lost. In general, the literature supports an active care approach, minimizing centrally acting medications. The judicious use of epidural steroids also is supported, but long-term results and repeated use is questionable. Nonprogressive neurologic deficits originating from the lumbar spine (except cauda equina syndrome) can be treated nonoperatively with expected clinical improvement. If surgery is necessary, it usually can be delayed 6 to 12 weeks to allow adequate opportunity for improvement. Some patients are best treated surgically, and this is discussed in the section dealing specifically with operative treatment of lumbar disc herniation.

The natural history of degenerative disc disease is one of recurrent episodes of pain followed by periods of significant or complete relief.

Before a discussion of diagnostic studies, axial spine pain with radiation to one or more extremities must be considered. Also, understanding certain pathophysiologic entities must be juxtaposed to other entities of which only a rudimentary understanding exists. It is doubtful if there is any other area of orthopaedics in which accurate diagnosis is as difficult or the proper treatment as challenging as in patients with persistent neck and arm or low back and leg pain. Although many patients have clear diagnoses properly arrived at by careful history and physical examination with confirmatory imaging studies, many patients with pain have absent neurologic findings other than sensory changes and have normal imaging studies or studies that do not support the clinical complaints and findings. Inability to easily determine an appropriate diagnosis does not relieve the physician of the obligation to recommend treatment or to direct the patient to a setting where such treatment is available. Careful assessment of these patients to determine if they have problems that can be orthopaedically treated (operatively or nonoperatively) is imperative to avoid both overtreatment and undertreatment.

Operative treatment can benefit a patient if it corrects a deformity, corrects instability, relieves neural compression, or treats a combination of these problems directly attributable to the patient's complaint. Obtaining a history and completing a physical examination to determine a diagnosis that should be supported by other diagnostic studies is fundamental; conversely, matching the diagnosis and treatment to the results of diagnostic studies, as often can be done in other subspecialties of orthopaedics (e.g., treating extremity pain based on a radiograph that shows a fracture), is more complex and difficult. The history, physical examination, and imaging studies must all confirm the same pathologic process as the source of symptoms if surgical intervention is to be reproducibly successful.

AXIAL LUMBAR PAIN

Axial lumbar pain occurs at some point in the lives of most people. Appropriate treatment for what can be at times excruciating pain generally should begin with evaluation for a significant spinal pathologic process. This pathologic process being absent, a brief (1 to 3 days) period of bed rest with institution of an antiinflammatory regimen and rapid progression to an active exercise regimen with an anticipated return to full activity should be expected and encouraged. Generally, patients treated in this manner improve significantly in 4 to 8 weeks. Diagnostic studies, including radiographs, often are not helpful because they add little information. More sophisticated imaging with CT and MRI or other studies have even less utility initially. An overdependence on the diagnosis of disc herniation can occur with early use of these diagnostic studies, which show disc herniations in 20% to 36% of normal volunteers. General imaging guidelines have been developed to help identify patients for whom radiography is indicated (Box 39-1).

Patients should understand that persistence of some pain does not indicate treatment failure, necessitating further measures; however, it is important for treating physicians to recognize that the longer a patient is limited by pain, the less likely he or she is to return to full activity.

BOX 39-1

Selective Indications for Radiography in Acute Low Back Pain

- Age > 50 years
- Significant trauma
- Neuromuscular deficits
- Unexplained weight loss (10 lb in 6 months)
- Suspicion of ankylosing spondylitis
- Drug or alcohol abuse
- History of cancer
- Use of corticosteroids
- Temperature ≥ 37.8° C (≥100° F)
- Recent visit (≤1 month) for same problem and no improvement
- Patient seeking compensation for back pain

For patients who do not respond to treatment regimens, early recognition that other issues may be involved is essential. Careful reassessment of complaints and reexamination for new information or findings and inconsistencies are necessary. Many studies of occupational back pain have revealed that depression, occupational mental stress, job satisfaction, intensity of concentration, anxiety, and marital status can be related to complaints of pain and disability. The role of these factors as causal or consequential of the symptoms remains an area of continued study; however, there is some evidence that the psychologic stresses occur before complaints of pain in some patients. Another finding that is evident from the literature is the inability of physicians to detect psychosocial factors adequately without using specific instruments designed for this purpose in patients with back pain. In one study, experienced spinal surgeons were able to identify distressed patients only 26% of the time based on patient interviews. Given the difficulty of identifying patients with psychosocial distress, being aware of the high incidence of incidental abnormal findings on imaging studies underscores the need for critical individual review of these studies by treating physicians. Severe nerve compression shown by MRI or CT correlates with symptoms of distal leg pain; however, mild-to-moderate nerve compression (Table 39-1), disc degeneration or bulging, and central stenosis do not correlate significantly with specific pain patterns.

DIAGNOSTIC STUDIES

RADIOGRAPHY

The simplest and most readily available diagnostic tests for lumbar pain are anteroposterior and lateral radiographs of the involved spinal region. These simple radiographs show a relatively high incidence of abnormal findings; however, spinal radiographs on the initial visit for acute low back pain may not contribute to patient care and are not always cost effective. Plain radiographs may be considered only after the initial therapy fails, especially in patients younger than 45 years old.

There is insignificant correlation between back pain and the radiographic findings of lumbar lordosis, transitional vertebra, disc space narrowing, disc vacuum sign, and claw spurs. In addition, the entity of disc space narrowing is extremely difficult to quantify in all but operated backs or in obviously abnormal circumstances. A study of 321 patients found that only when traction spurs or obvious disc space narrowing or both were present did the incidence of severe back and leg pain, leg weakness, and numbness increase. These positive findings had no relationship to heavy lifting, vehicular exposure, or exposure to vibrating equipment. Other studies have shown some relationship between back pain and the findings of spondylolysis, spondylolisthesis, and adult scoliosis, but these findings also can be observed in spine radiographs of asymptomatic patients.

Special radiographic views can be helpful in further defining the initial clinical radiographic impression. Oblique views are useful in defining further spondylolisthesis and spondylolysis but are of limited use in facet syndrome and hypertrophic arthritis of the lumbar spine. Lateral flexion and extension radiographs may reveal segmental instability. The interpretation of these views depends on patient cooperation, patient positioning, and reproducible technique. Lateral lumbar flexion views are valid only if done in the seated position, which maximizes lumbar kyphosis. The Ferguson view (20-degree caudocephalic anteroposterior radiograph) has been shown to be of value in the diagnosis of the "far out syndrome," that is, fifth root compression produced by a large transverse process of the fifth lumbar vertebra against the ala of the sacrum. Angled caudal views localized to areas of concern may show evidence of facet or laminar pathologic conditions.

TABLE 39-1

Classification for Spinal Nerve and Thecal Sac Deformation

SPINAL NERVE DEFORMATION IN LATERAL RECESS OR INTERVERTEBRAL FORAMEN	
0—absent	No visible disc material contacting or deforming nerve
I—minimal	Contact with disc material deforming nerve but displacement < 2 mm
II—moderate	Contact with disc material displacing ≥2 mm; nerve is still visible and not obscured by disc material
III—severe	Contact with disc material completely obscuring nerve
THECAL SAC DEFORMATION IN VERTEBRAL CANAL	
0—absent	No visible disc material contacting or deforming thecal sac
I—minimal	Disc material in contact with thecal sac
II—moderate	Disc material deforming thecal sac; anteroposterior distance of thecal sac ≥7 mm
III—severe	Disc material deforming thecal sac; anteroposterior distance of thecal sac <7 mm

(From Beattie PF, Myers SP, Stratford P, et al: Associations between patient report of symptoms and anatomical impairment visible on lumbar magnetic resonance imaging, Spine 25:819, 2000.)

MYELOGRAPHY

The value of myelography is the ability to check all spinal regions for abnormality and to define intraspinal lesions; it may be unnecessary if clinical and CT or MRI findings are in complete agreement. The primary indications for myelography are suspicion of an intraspinal lesion, patients with spinal instrumentation, or questionable diagnosis resulting from conflicting clinical findings and other studies. In addition, myelography is valuable in a previously operated spine and in patients with marked bony degenerative change that may be underestimated on MRI. Myelography is improved by the use of postmyelography CT in this setting and in evaluating spinal stenosis.

Several contrast agents have been used for myelography: air, oil contrast, and water-soluble (absorbable) contrast agents, including metrizamide (Amipaque), iohexol (Omnipaque), and iopamidol (Isovue-M). Because these nonionic agents are absorbable, the discomfort of removing them and the severity of the postmyelography headache have decreased.

Arachnoiditis is a severe complication that has been attributed occasionally to the combination of iophendylate and blood in the cerebrospinal fluid (CSF). This diagnosis usually is confirmed only by repeat myelography. Attempts at surgical neurolysis have resulted in only short-term relief and a return of symptoms within 6 to 12 months after the procedure. Time may decrease the effects of this serious problem in some patients, but progressive paralysis has been reported in rare instances. Arachnoiditis also can be caused by tuberculosis and other types of meningitis. Arachnoiditis has not been noted to be related to the use of a water-soluble contrast agent, with or without injection, in the presence of a bloody tap.

Water-soluble contrast media are now the standard agents for myelography. Their advantages include absorption by the body, enhanced definition of structures, tolerance, and the ability to vary the dosage for different contrasts. Similar to iophendylate, they are meningeal irritants, but they have not been associated with arachnoiditis. The complications of these agents include nausea, vomiting, confusion, and seizures. Rare complications include stroke, paralysis, and death. Iohexol and iopamidol have significantly lower complication rates than metrizamide. The more common complications seem to be related to patient hydration, phenothiazines, tricyclic antidepressants, and migration of contrast material into the cranial vault. Many reported complications can be prevented or minimized by using the lowest possible dose to achieve the desired degree of contrast. Adequate hydration and discontinuation of phenothiazines and tricyclic antidepressants before, during, and after the procedure also should minimize the incidence of the more common reactions. Likewise, maintenance of at least a 30-degree elevation of the patient's head until the contrast material is absorbed should help prevent reactions. Complete information about these agents and the dosages required is found in their package inserts.

Iohexol is a nonionic contrast medium approved for thoracic and lumbar myelography. The incidence of reactions to this medium is low. The most common reactions are headache (<20%), pain (8%), nausea (6%), and vomiting (3%). Serious reactions are rare and include mental disturbances and aseptic meningitis (0.01%). Good hydration is essential to minimize the common reactions. The use of phenothiazine antinauseants is contraindicated when this medium is employed. Management before and after the procedure is the same as for metrizamide.

Air contrast is used rarely and probably should be used only in situations in which myelography is mandatory and the patient is extremely allergic to iodized materials. The resolution from such a procedure is poor. Air epidurography in conjunction with CT has been suggested in patients in whom further definition between postoperative scar and recurrent disc material is required.

Myelographic technique begins with a careful explanation of the procedure to the patient before its initiation. Hydration of the patient before the procedure may minimize postmyelographic complaints. Heavy sedation rarely is needed. Proper equipment, including a fluoroscopic unit with a spot film device, image intensification, tilt table, and television monitoring, is useful. The type of needle selected also influences the risk of postdural puncture headaches, which can be severe. Smaller gauge needles (22- or 25-gauge) have been found to result in a lower incidence of postdural puncture headaches. Also, use of a Whitacre-type needle with a blunter tip and side port opening results in fewer postdural puncture headache complaints.

The most common technical complications of myelography are significant retention of contrast medium (oil contrast only), persistent headache from a dural leak, and epidural injection. These problems usually are minor. Persistent dural leaks usually are responsive to a blood patch. With the use of a water-soluble contrast medium, the persistent abnormalities caused by retained medium and epidural injection are eliminated.

MYELOGRAPHY

TECHNIQUE 39-1

- Place the patient prone on the fluoroscopic table. Use of an abdominal pillow is optional. Prepare the back in the usual surgical fashion.
- Determine needle placement by the suspected pathologic level. Placement of the needle cephalad to L2-3 is more dangerous because of the risk of damaging the conus medullaris.
- Infiltrate the selected area of injection with a local anesthetic. Use the smallest gauge needle that can be well placed. If a Whitacre-type needle is used, a 19-gauge needle may be placed through the skin, subcutaneous tissue, and fascia to form a track because this relatively blunt needle may not penetrate these structures well. Midline needle placement usually minimizes lateral nerve root irritation and epidural injection. Advance the needle with the bevel parallel to the long axis of the body. Subarachnoid placement can be enhanced by tilting the patient up to increase intraspinal pressure and minimize the epidural space.
- When the dura and arachnoid have been punctured, turn the bevel of the needle cephalad. A clear continuous flow of CSF should continue with the patient prone. Manometric studies can be done at this time if desired or indicated. Remove a volume of CSF equal to the planned injection volume for laboratory evaluation as indicated by the clinical suspicions. In most patients, a cell count, differential white blood cell count, and protein analysis are performed.
- Inject a test dose of the contrast material under fluoroscopic control to confirm a subarachnoid injection. If a mixed subdural-subarachnoid injection is suspected, change the needle depth; occasionally, a lateral radiograph may be required to confirm the proper depth. If flow is good, inject the contrast material slowly.
- Ensure continued subarachnoid injection by occasionally aspirating as the injection continues. The usual dose of iohexol for lumbar myelography in an adult is 10 to 15 mL with a concentration of 170 to 190 mg/mL. Higher concentrations of water-soluble contrast are required if higher areas of the spine are to be demonstrated. Consult the package insert of the contrast agent used. The needle can be removed if a water-soluble contrast agent (iohexol) is used.
- Allow the contrast material to flow caudally for the best views of the lumbar roots and distal sac. Make spot films in the anteroposterior, lateral, and oblique projections. A

full lumbar examination should include thoracic evaluation to about the level of T7 because lesions at the thoracic level may mimic lumbar disc disease. Take additional spot films as the contrast proceeds cranially.

- If a total or cervical myelogram is desired, allow the contrast to proceed cranially. Extend the neck and head maximally to prevent or minimize intracranial migration of the contrast medium.
- If blood is present in the initial tap, aborting the procedure if the CSF does not clear rapidly is best. It can be attempted again in several days if the patient has no symptoms related to the first tap and is well hydrated. If the proper needle position is confirmed in the anteroposterior and lateral views, and CSF flow is minimal or absent, suspect a neoplastic process. Place the needle at a higher or lower level as indicated by the circumstances. If attempts to obtain CSF continue to fail, abandon the procedure and reevaluate the clinical situation.

COMPUTED TOMOGRAPHY

CT can be a useful diagnostic tool in the evaluation of spinal disease (Fig. 39-2). The current technology and computer software have made possible the ability to reformat the standard axial cuts in almost any direction and magnify the images so that exact measurements of various structures can be made. Software is available to evaluate the density of a selected vertebra and compare it with vertebrae of the normal population to give a numerically reproducible estimate of vertebral density to quantitate osteopenia.

Numerous types of CT studies for the spine are available. One must be careful when ordering the study to ensure that the areas of clinical concern are included. The most common routine for lumbar disc herniations consists of making serial cuts through the last three lumbar intervertebral discs. If the equipment has a tilting gantry, an attempt is made to keep the axis of the cuts parallel with the discs. Frequently, the gantry cannot tilt enough, however, to allow a parallel beam through the lowest disc space. This technique does not allow demonstration of the canal at the pedicles. Another method involves making cuts through the discs without tilting the gantry. The entire canal is not shown, and the lower cuts frequently have the lower and upper endplates of adjacent vertebrae superimposed in the same view.

The most complex method consists of making multiple parallel cuts at equal intervals. This allows computer reconstruction of the images in different planes, usually sagittal and coronal. These reformatted views allow an almost three-dimensional view of the spine and most of its structures. The

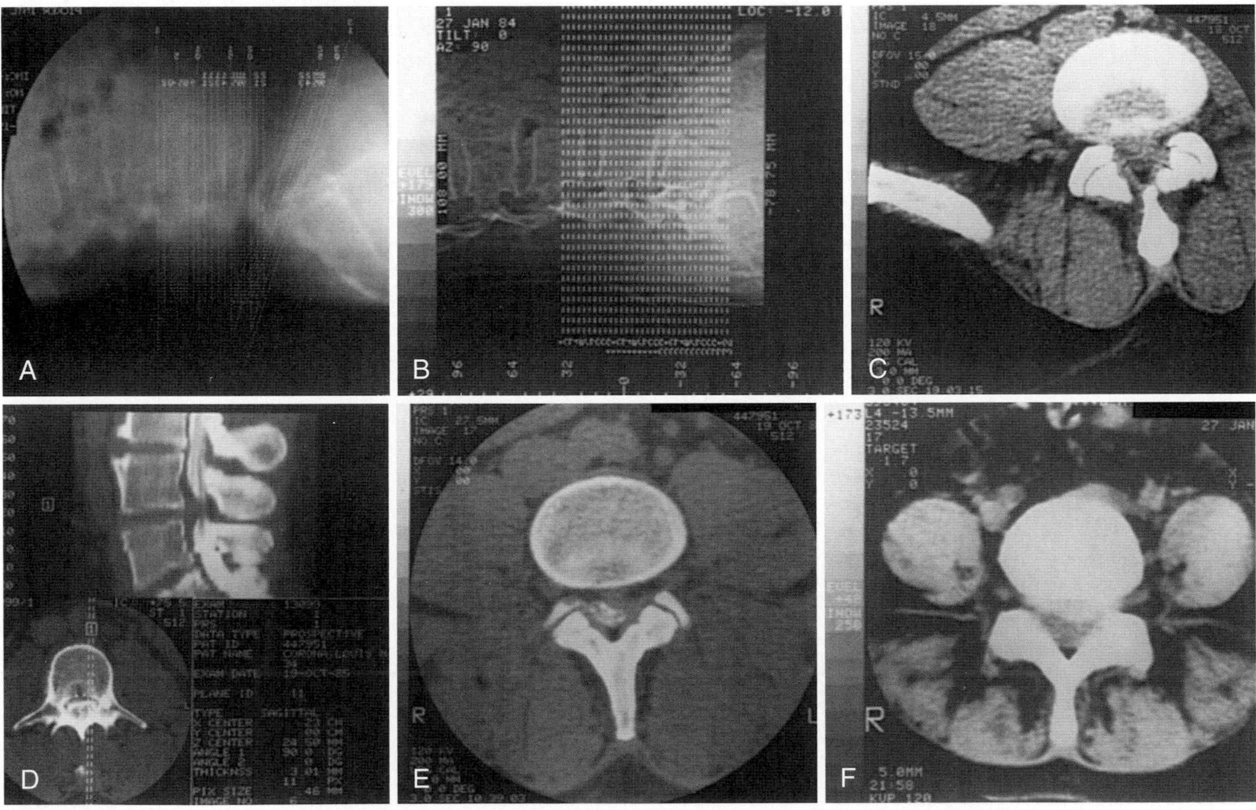

FIGURE 39-2 **A,** CT scan scout view of lumbar disc herniation at lumbar disc level showing angled gantry technique. **B,** CT scan scout view of straight gantry technique. **C,** CT scan of lumbar disc herniation at L4-5 disc level showing cross-sectional anatomy with gantry straight. **D,** CT scan of L4-5 disc herniation at lumbar disc level showing cross-sectional, sagittal, and coronal anatomy using computerized reformatted technique. **E,** CT scan of L4-5 disc herniation at lumbar disc level showing cross-sectional anatomy 2 hours after metrizamide myelography. **F,** CT scan of lumbar disc herniation at L4-5 disc level showing cross-sectional anatomy after intravenous injection for greater soft-tissue contrast.

greatest benefit of this technique is the ability to see beyond the limits of the dural sac and root sleeves. The diagnosis of foraminal encroachment by bone or disc material can be made in the face of a normal myelogram. The proper procedure can be chosen that fits all of the pathologic conditions involved.

Optimal reformatted CT should include enlarged axial and sagittal views with clear notation as to laterality and sequence of cuts. Several sections of the axial cuts should include the local soft tissue and contiguous abdominal contents. Finally, a set of images adjusted for improved bony detail should be included for evaluation of the facet joints and the lateral recesses. This study should be centered on the level of greatest clinical concern. The study can be enhanced further if done after water contrast myelography or with intravenous injection of a contrast medium. Enhancement techniques are especially useful if the spine being evaluated has been operated on previously.

This noninvasive, painless outpatient procedure can supply more information about spinal disease than was previously available with a battery of invasive and noninvasive tests usually requiring hospitalization. CT does not show intraspinal tumors or arachnoiditis and is unable to differentiate scar from recurrent disc herniation. The use of intravenous contrast medium (Fig. 39-2F) followed by CT can improve the definition between scar and disc herniation. Myelography is still required to show intraspinal tumors and to "run" the spine to detect occult or unsuspected lesions. The development of low-dose metrizamide or iohexol myelography with reformatted CT done as an outpatient procedure allows maximal information to be obtained with minimal time, risk, discomfort, and cost.

MAGNETIC RESONANCE IMAGING

MRI is currently the standard for advanced imaging of the spine and is superior to CT in most circumstances, in particular, identification of infections, tumors, and degenerative changes within the discs (Fig. 39-3). More important, MRI is superior for imaging the disc and directly images neural structures. Also, MRI typically shows the entire region of study (cervical, thoracic, or lumbar). Of particular value is the ability to image the nerve root in the foramen, which is difficult even with postmyelography CT because the subarachnoid space and the contrast agent do not extend fully through the foramen. Despite this superiority, there are circumstances in which MRI and CT, with or without myelography, can be used in a complementary fashion.

One of the difficulties with MRI is showing anatomy that is abnormal but may be asymptomatic. MRI evidence of disc degeneration has been reported in the cervical spine in 25% of patients younger than 40 years and in 60% of patients 60 years and older, and lumbar disc degeneration was found in 35% of patients 20 to 39 years old and in 100% of patients older than 50. The demonstrated findings must be carefully correlated with the clinical impression. The importance of this concept cannot be overstated. The best way to obtain meaningful clinical information from MRI of the spine is to have a specific question before the study. This question is derived from the patient's history and careful physical examination and is posed using the parameters of (1) neural compression, (2) instability, and (3) deformity. In each case the specific location of the abnormality should be suspected before MRI and confirmed with the study. Only abnormalities in one or a combination of these categories are important, and operative techniques can treat only these problems. Failure to interpret an imaging study in this way, especially MRI, which is sensitive to anatomic abnormalities, would inevitably lead to poor clinical choices and outcomes.

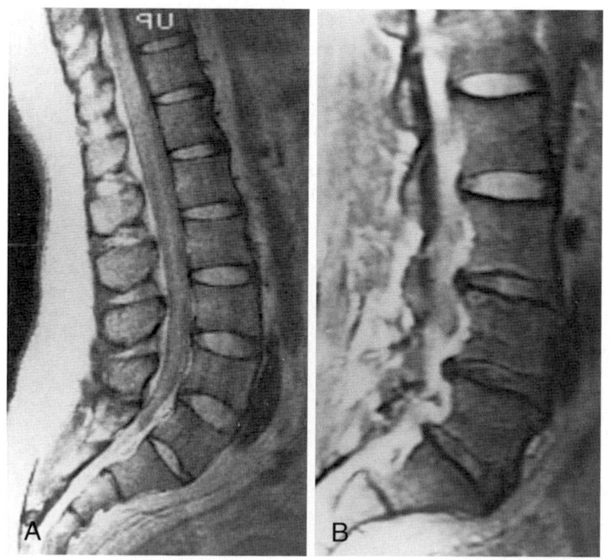

FIGURE 39-3 MRI of lumbar spine. **A,** Normal T2-weighted image. **B,** T2-weighted image showing degenerative bulging or herniated discs, or both, at L3-4, L4-5, and L5-S1.

OTHER DIAGNOSTIC TESTS

Numerous diagnostic tests have been used in the diagnosis of intervertebral disc disease in addition to radiography, myelography, CT, and MRI. The primary advantage of these tests is to rule out diseases other than primary disc herniation, spinal stenosis, and spinal arthritis.

Electromyography is the most notable of these tests. One advantage of electromyography is in the identification of peripheral neuropathy and diffuse neurologic involvement indicating higher or lower lesions. Electromyography and nerve conduction velocity can be helpful if a patient has a history and physical examination suggestive of radiculopathy at either the cervical or lumbar level with inconclusive imaging studies. Paraspinal muscles in a patient with a previous posterior operation usually are abnormal and are not a reliable diagnostic finding.

Bone scans are another procedure in which positive findings usually are not indicative of intervertebral disc disease, but they can confirm neoplastic, traumatic, and arthritic problems in the spine. Various laboratory tests, such as a complete blood cell count, differential white blood cell count, C-reactive protein, biochemical profile, urinalysis, serum protein electrophoresis, and erythrocyte sedimentation rate, are extremely good screening procedures for other causes of pain in the spine. Rheumatoid screening studies, such as those for rheumatoid arthritis, antinuclear antibody, lupus erythematosus cell preparation, and HLA-B27, also are useful when indicated by the clinical picture.

Some tests that were developed to enhance the diagnosis of intervertebral disc disease have been surpassed by more advanced technology. Lumbar venography and ultrasonographic measurement of the intervertebral canal are two examples.

INJECTION STUDIES

Whenever a diagnosis is in doubt and the complaints seem real or the pathologic condition is diffuse, identification of the source of pain is problematic. The use of local anesthetics or contrast media in various specific anatomic areas can be helpful. These agents are relatively simple, safe, and minimally painful. Contrast media such as diatrizoate meglumine (Hypaque), iothalamate meglumine (Conray), iohexol (Omnipaque), iopamidol, and metrizamide (Amipaque) have been used for discography and blocks with no reported ill effects. Reports of neurologic complications with contrast media used for discography and subsequent chymopapain injection are well documented. The best choice of a contrast medium for documenting structures outside the subarachnoid space is an absorbable medium with low reactivity, because it might be injected inadvertently into the subarachnoid space. Iohexol and metrizamide are the least reactive, most widely accepted, and best tolerated of the currently available contrast media. Local anesthetics, such as lidocaine (Xylocaine), tetracaine (Pontocaine), and bupivacaine (Marcaine), are used frequently epidurally and intradurally. The use of bupivacaine should be limited to low concentrations and low volumes because of reports of death after epidural anesthesia using concentrations of 0.75% or higher.

Steroids prepared for intramuscular injection also have been used frequently in the epidural space with few and usually transient complications. Spinal arachnoiditis in past years was associated with the use of epidural methylprednisolone acetate (Depo-Medrol). This complication was thought to be caused by the use of the suspending agent, polyethylene glycol, which has since been eliminated from the Depo-Medrol preparation. For epidural injections, we prefer the use of Celestone Soluspan, which is a mixture of betamethasone sodium phosphate and betamethasone acetate. Celestone Soluspan provides immediate and long-term duration of action, is highly soluble, and contains no harmful preservatives. Celestone should not be mixed with local anesthetics containing preservatives such as parabens or phenol because flocculation and clogging of the suspension can occur. If Celestone is not available, other commonly used preparations for spinal injections include methylprednisolone (Depo-Medrol) and triamcinolone acetonide (Kenalog) (see Table 38-2). Isotonic saline is the only other injectable medium used frequently around the spine with no reported adverse reactions. All substrates injected into the epidural space should be preservative free.

When discrete, well-controlled injection techniques directed at specific targets in and around the spine are used, grading the degree of pain before and after a spinal injection is helpful in determining the location of the pain generator. The patient is asked to grade the degree of pain on a 0-to-10 scale before and at various intervals after the spinal injection (see Box 38-1). If a spinal injection done under fluoroscopic control results in an 80% or more decrease in the level of pain, which corresponds to the duration of action of the anesthetic agent used, we presume the target area injected to be the pain generator. Less pain reduction, 50% to 65%, does not constitute a positive response.

■ EPIDURAL CORTISONE INJECTIONS

Epidural injections in the cervical, thoracic, and lumbosacral spine were developed to diagnose and treat spinal pain. Information obtained from epidural injections can be helpful in confirming pain generators that are responsible for a patient's discomfort. Structural abnormalities do not always cause pain, and diagnostic injections can help to correlate abnormalities seen on imaging studies with associated pain complaints. In addition, epidural injections can provide pain relief during the recovery of disc or nerve root injuries and allow patients to increase their level of physical activity. Because severe pain from an acute disc injury, with or without radiculopathy, often is time limited, therapeutic injections can help to manage pain and may alleviate or decrease the need for oral analgesics.

The previous literature did not reliably establish the efficacy of epidural injections because of the lack of well-controlled studies. A retrospective study comparing interlaminar to transforaminal epidural injections for symptomatic lumbar intervertebral disc herniations found that transforaminal injections resulted in better short-term pain improvement and fewer long-term operative interventions.

A number of randomized, double-blind, controlled studies have been done to evaluate the effectiveness of lumbar interlaminar injections, as well as caudal epidural injections, in the treatment of chronic discogenic pain with and without radiculitis. Overall these studies indicate that a high percentage of patients receiving the injections have significant pain relief and functional improvement. The question still remains whether there is any significant long-term benefit to these injections.

Few serious complications occur in patients receiving epidural corticosteroid injections; however, epidural abscess, epidural hematoma, durocutaneous fistula, and Cushing syndrome have been reported as individual case reports. The most adverse immediate reaction during an epidural injection is a vasovagal reaction, although this is much more common with cervical injections. Dural puncture has been estimated to occur in 0.5% to 5% of patients having cervical or lumbar epidural steroid injections. Some minor, common complaints caused by corticosteroid injected into the epidural space include nonpositional headaches, facial flushing, insomnia, low-grade fever, and transient increased back or lower extremity pain. Major adverse events can occur with epidural injections, but these are rare, their true incidence is unknown, and they have been described only in case reports. Several large series involving nearly 5000 patients with over 8000 transforaminal lumbar epidural injections reported no major adverse events and a less than 1% incidence of postinjection headache; the most frequent sequela was increased leg or back pain, which also occurred in less than 1% of patients.

Epidural corticosteroid injections are contraindicated in the presence of infection at the injection site, systemic infection, bleeding diathesis, uncontrolled diabetes mellitus, and congestive heart failure.

We perform epidural corticosteroid injections in a fluoroscopy suite equipped with resuscitative and monitoring equipment. Intravenous access is established in all patients with a 20-gauge angiocatheter placed in the upper extremity. Mild sedation is achieved through intravenous access. We recommend the use of fluoroscopy for diagnostic and therapeutic epidural injections for several reasons. Epidural injections performed without fluoroscopic guidance are not always made into the epidural space or the intended interspace. Even in experienced hands, needle misplacement occurs in 40% of caudal and 30% of lumbar epidural injections when done without fluoroscopic guidance. Accidental intravascular injections also can occur, and the absence of blood return with needle aspiration before injection is an unreliable indicator of this complication. In the presence of anatomic anomalies, such as a midline epidural septum or multiple separate epidural compartments, the desired flow of epidural injectants to the presumed pain generator is restricted and remains undetected without fluoroscopy. In addition, if an injection fails to relieve pain, it would be impossible without fluoroscopy to determine whether the failure was caused by a genuine poor response or by improper needle placement.

THORACIC EPIDURAL INJECTION

Epidural steroid injections in the thoracic spine have been shown to provide relief from thoracic radicular pain secondary to disc herniations, trauma, diabetic neuropathy, herpes zoster, and idiopathic thoracic neuralgia, although reports in the literature are few.

INTERLAMINAR THORACIC EPIDURAL INJECTION

TECHNIQUE 39-2

- A paramedian rather than a midline approach is used because of the angulation of the spinous processes.
- Place the patient prone on a pain management table. The preparation of the patient and equipment are identical to that used for interlaminar cervical epidural injections (see Technique 38-1). Aseptically prepare the skin area several segments above and below the interspace to be injected. Drape the area in sterile fashion.
- Identify the target laminar interspace using anteroposterior fluoroscopic guidance.
- Anesthetize the skin over the target interspace on the side of the patient's pain. Under fluoroscopic control, insert and advance a 22-gauge, 3½-inch spinal needle to the superior edge of the target lamina. Anesthetize the lamina and the soft tissues as the spinal needle is withdrawn.
- Mark the skin with an 18-gauge hypodermic needle and insert an 18-gauge, 3½-inch Tuohy epidural needle, and advance it at a 50- to 60-degree angle to the axis of the spine and a 15- to 30-degree angle toward the midline until contact with the lamina is made. To view the thoracic interspace better, position the C-arm so that the fluoroscopy beam is in the same plane as the Tuohy epidural needle.
- "Walk off" the lamina with the Tuohy needle into the ligamentum flavum. Remove the stylet from the Tuohy needle and, using the loss-of-resistance technique, advance it into the epidural space. When loss of resistance has been achieved, aspirate to check for blood or CSF. If neither blood nor CSF is evident, inject 1.5 mL of nonionic contrast dye to confirm epidural placement.
- To confirm proper placement further, adjust the C-arm to view the area from a lateral projection (Fig. 39-4). A spot radiograph or epidurogram can be obtained. Inject 2 mL of 1% preservative-free lidocaine without epinephrine and 2 mL of 6 mg/mL Celestone Soluspan slowly into the epidural space.

LUMBAR EPIDURAL INJECTION

Certain clinical trends are apparent with lumbar epidural steroid injections. When nerve root injury is associated with a disc herniation or lateral bony stenosis, most patients who received substantial relief of leg pain from a well-placed

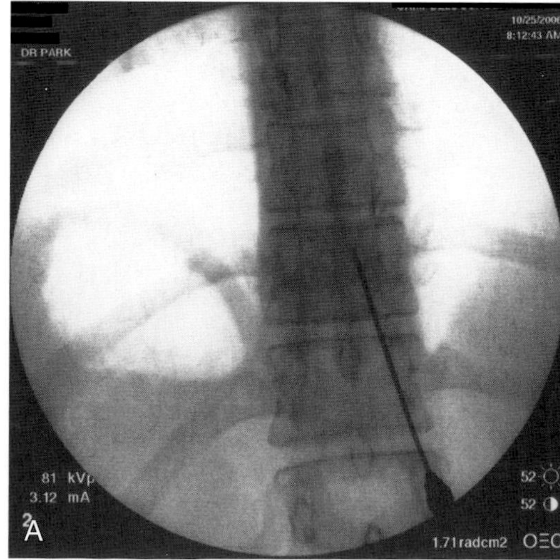

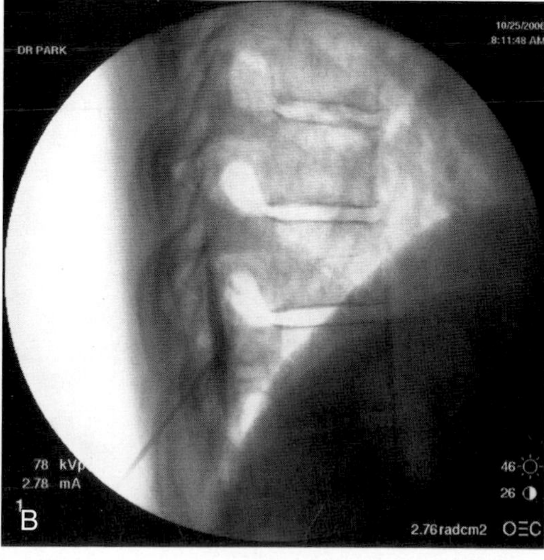

FIGURE 39-4 **A,** Posteroanterior view of thoracic interlaminar epidurogram showing characteristic contrast flow pattern. **B,** Lateral radiograph of thoracic epidurogram. **SEE TECHNIQUE 39-2.**

transforaminal injection, even if temporary, benefit from surgery for the radicular pain. Patients who do not respond and who have had radicular pain for at least 12 months are unlikely to benefit from surgery. Patients with back and leg pain of an acute nature (<3 months) respond better to epidural corticosteroids. Unless a significant reinjury results in an acute disc or nerve root injury, postsurgical patients tend to respond poorly to epidural corticosteroids.

INTERLAMINAR LUMBAR EPIDURAL INJECTION

TECHNIQUE 39-3

- Place the patient prone on a pain management table. Aseptically prepare the skin area with isopropyl alcohol and povidone-iodine several segments above and below the laminar interspace to be injected. Drape the area in a sterile fashion.
- Under anteroposterior fluoroscopy guidance, identify the target laminar interspace. Using a 27-gauge, ¼-inch needle, anesthetize the skin over the target interspace on the side of the patient's pain with 1 to 2 mL of 1% preservative-free lidocaine without epinephrine.
- Insert a 22-gauge, 3½-inch spinal needle vertically until contact is made with the upper edge of the inferior lamina at the target interspace, 1 to 2 cm lateral to the caudal tip of the inferior spinous process under fluoroscopy. Anesthetize the lamina with 2 mL of 1% preservative-free lidocaine without epinephrine. Anesthetize the soft tissue with 2 mL of 1% lidocaine as the spinal needle is withdrawn.
- Nick the skin with an 18-gauge hypodermic needle and insert a 17-gauge, 3½-inch Tuohy epidural needle and advance it vertically within the anesthetized soft-tissue track until contact with the lamina has been made under fluoroscopy.
- "Walk off" the lamina with the Tuohy needle onto the ligamentum flavum. Remove the stylet from the Tuohy needle and attach a 10-mL syringe filled halfway with air and sterile saline to the Tuohy needle. Advance the Tuohy needle into the epidural space using the loss-of-resistance technique. Avoid lateral needle placement to decrease the likelihood of encountering an epidural vein or adjacent nerve root. Remove the stylet when loss of resistance has been achieved. Aspirate to check for blood or CSF. If neither blood nor CSF is present, remove the syringe from the Tuohy needle and attach a 5-mL syringe containing 2 mL of nonionic contrast dye.
- Confirm epidural placement by producing an epidurogram with the nonionic contrast agent (Fig. 39-5). A spot radiograph can be taken to document placement.
- Remove the 5-mL syringe and place on the Tuohy needle a 10-mL syringe containing 2 mL of 1% preservative-free lidocaine and 2 mL of 6 mg/mL Celestone Soluspan. Inject the corticosteroid preparation slowly into the epidural space.

TRANSFORAMINAL LUMBAR AND SACRAL EPIDURAL INJECTION

TECHNIQUE 39-4

- Place the patient prone on a pain management table. Aseptically prepare the skin area with isopropyl alcohol and povidone-iodine several segments above and below the interspace to be injected. Drape the area in sterile fashion.
- Under anteroposterior fluoroscopic guidance, identify the target interspace. Anesthetize the soft tissues over the lateral border and midway between the two adjacent transverse processes at the target interspace.

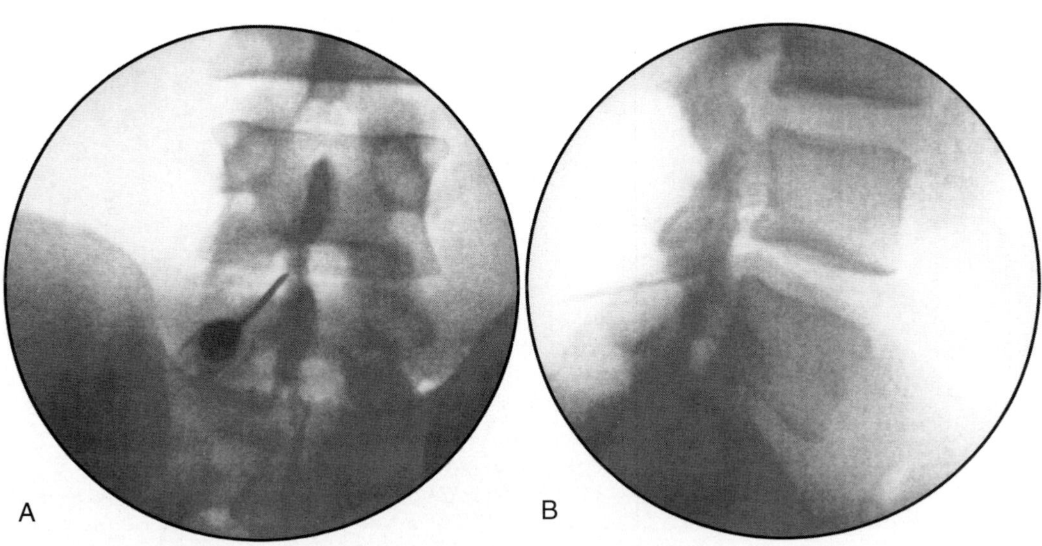

FIGURE 39-5 **A,** Posteroanterior view of lumbar interlaminar epidurogram showing characteristic contrast flow pattern. **B,** Lateral radiograph of lumbar epidurogram. **SEE TECHNIQUE 39-3.**

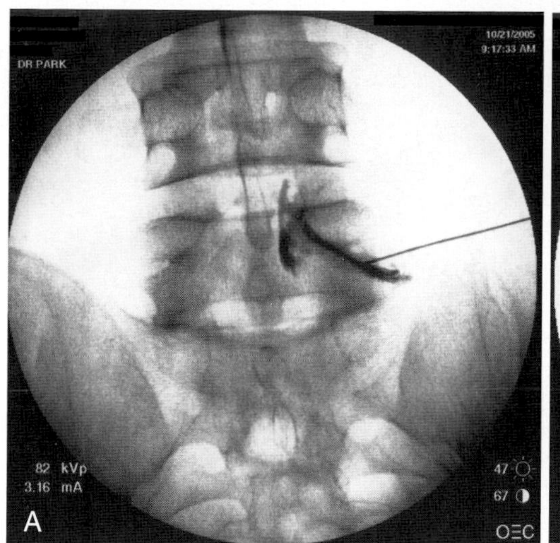

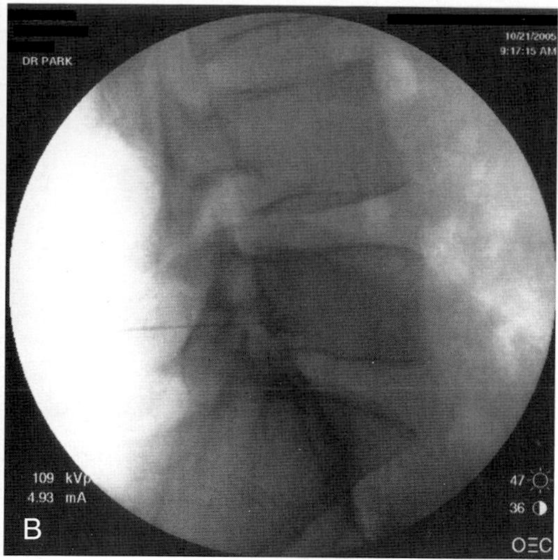

FIGURE 39-6 **A,** Right L5 selective nerve root injection contrast pattern. **B,** Lateral radiograph of L5 selective nerve block contrast flow pattern in anterior epidural space. **SEE TECHNIQUE 39-4.**

- Insert a 22-gauge, 4¾-inch spinal needle and advance it within the anesthetized soft-tissue track under fluoroscopy until contact is made with the lower edge of the superior transverse process near its junction with the superior articular process.
- Retract the spinal needle 2 to 3 mm, redirect it toward the base of the appropriate pedicle, and advance it slowly to the 6-o'clock position of the pedicle under fluoroscopy. Adjust the C-arm to a lateral projection to confirm the position and then return the C-arm to the anteroposterior view.
- Remove the stylet. Inject 1 mL of nonionic contrast agent slowly to produce a perineurosheathogram (Fig. 39-6). After an adequate dye pattern is observed, inject slowly a 2-mL volume containing 1 mL of 0.75% preservative-free bupivacaine and 1 mL of 6 mg/mL Celestone Soluspan.
- The S1 nerve root also can be injected using the transforaminal approach.
- Place the patient prone on the pain management table.
- After appropriate aseptic preparation, direct the C-arm so that the fluoroscopy beam is in a cephalocaudad and lateral-to-medial direction so that the anterior and posterior S1 foramina are aligned.
- Anesthetize the soft tissues and the dorsal aspect of the sacrum with 2 to 3 mL of 1% preservative-free lidocaine without epinephrine. Insert a 22-gauge, 3½-inch spinal needle, and advance it within the anesthetized soft-tissue track under fluoroscopy until contact is made with posterior sacral bone slightly lateral and inferior to the S1 pedicle. "Walk" the spinal needle off the sacrum into the posterior S1 foramen to the medial edge of the pedicle.
- Adjust the C-arm to a lateral projection to confirm the position and return it to the anteroposterior view.
- Remove the stylet. Inject 1 mL of nonionic contrast slowly to produce a perineurosheathogram (Fig. 39-7). After an adequate dye pattern of the S1 nerve root is obtained, insert a 2-mL volume containing 1 mL of 0.75% preservative-free bupivacaine and 1 mL of 6 mg/mL Celestone Soluspan.

CAUDAL SACRAL EPIDURAL INJECTION

TECHNIQUE 39-5

- Place the patient prone on a pain management table. Aseptically prepare the skin area from the lumbosacral junction to the coccyx with isopropyl alcohol and povidone-iodine. Drape the area in sterile fashion.
- Try to identify by palpation the sacral hiatus, which is located between the two horns of the sacral cornua. The sacral hiatus can be best observed by directing the fluoroscopic beam laterally.
- Anesthetize the soft tissues and the dorsal aspect of the sacrum with 2 to 3 mL of 1% preservative-free lidocaine without epinephrine. Keep the C-arm positioned so that the fluoroscopic beam remains lateral.
- Insert a 22-gauge, 3½-inch spinal needle between the sacral cornua at about 45 degrees, with the bevel of the spinal needle facing ventrally until contact with the sacrum is made. Using fluoroscopic guidance, redirect the spinal needle more cephalad, horizontal and parallel to the table, advancing it into the sacral canal through the sacrococcygeal ligament and into the epidural space (Fig. 39-8).
- Remove the stylet. Aspirate to check for blood or CSF. If neither blood nor CSF is evident, inject 2 mL of nonionic contrast dye to confirm placement. Move the C-arm into the anteroposterior position and look for the

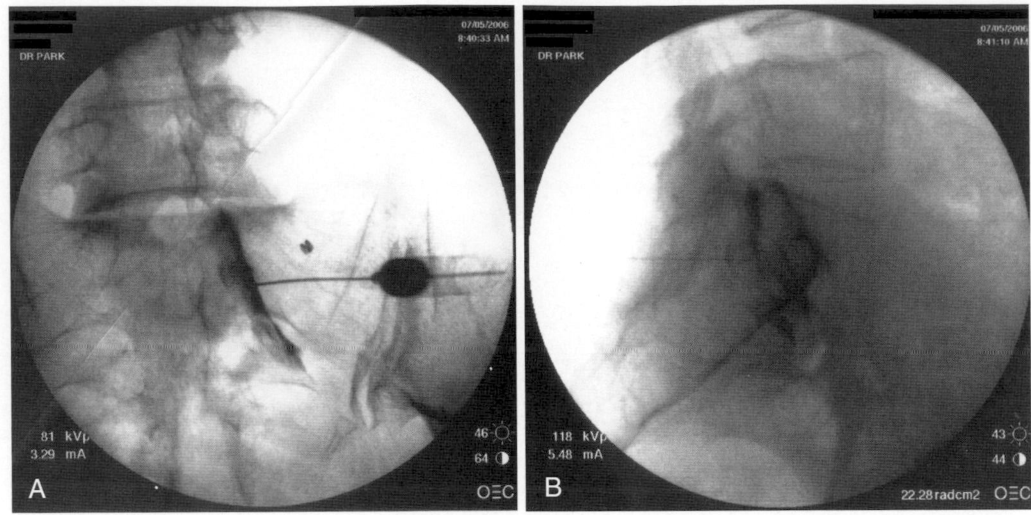

FIGURE 39-7 **A,** Right S1 selective nerve root injection contrast pattern with perineurosheathogram. **B,** Lateral radiograph of S1 contrast flow in sacral epidural space. **SEE TECHNIQUE 39-4.**

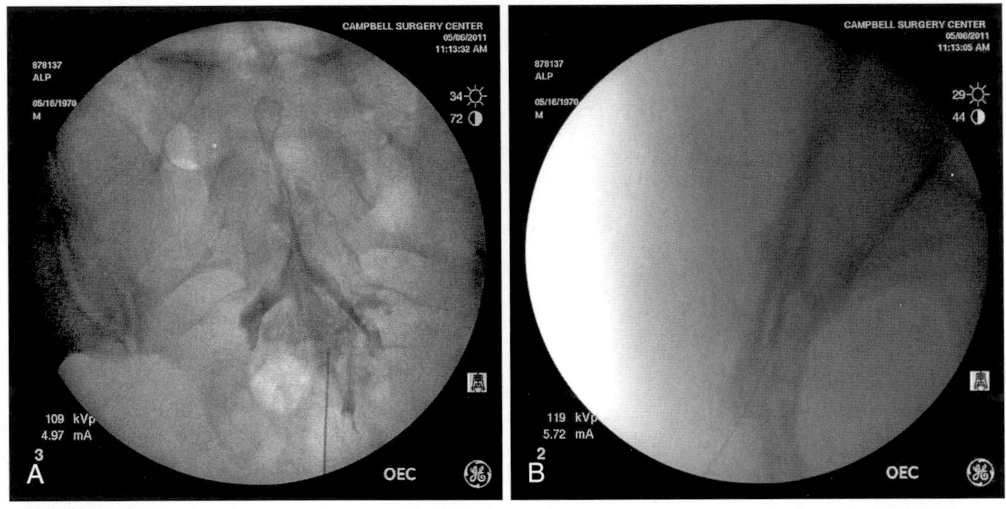

FIGURE 39-8 Fluoroscopic view (caudal approach) lumbar epidural injection. **SEE TECHNIQUE 39-5.**

characteristic "Christmas tree" pattern of epidural flow. If a vascular pattern is seen, reposition the spinal needle and confirm epidural placement with nonionic contrast dye.

- When the correct contrast pattern is obtained, slowly inject a 10-mL volume containing 3 mL of 1% preservative-free lidocaine without epinephrine, 3 mL of 6 mg/mL Celestone Soluspan, and 4 mL of sterile normal saline.

ZYGAPOPHYSEAL (FACET) JOINT INJECTIONS

The facet joint can be a source of back pain; the exact cause of the pain is unknown. Theories include meniscoid entrapment and extrapment, synovial impingement, chondromalacia facetae, capsular and synovial inflammation, and mechanical injury to the joint capsule. Osteoarthritis is another cause of facet joint pain; however, the incidence of facet joint arthropathy is equal in symptomatic and asymptomatic patients. As with other osteoarthritic joints, radiographic changes correlate poorly with pain.

Although the history and physical examination may suggest that the facet joint is the cause of spine pain, no noninvasive pathognomonic findings distinguish facet joint–mediated pain from other sources of spine pain. Fluoroscopically guided facet joint injections are commonly considered the "gold standard" for isolating or excluding the facet joint as a source of spine or extremity pain.

Clinical suspicion of facet joint pain by a spine specialist remains the major indicator for diagnostic injection, which should be done only in patients who have had pain for more than 4 weeks and only after appropriate conservative measures have failed to provide relief. Facet joint injection procedures may help to focus treatment on a specific spinal segment and provide adequate pain relief to allow progression in therapy. Either intraarticular or medial branch blocks can be used for diagnostic purposes. Although injection of cortisone into the facet joint was a popular procedure through most of the 1970s and 1980s, many investigators have found no evidence that this effectively treats low back pain caused by a facet joint. The only controlled study on the use of intraarticular corticosteroids in the cervical spine found no added benefit from intraarticular betamethasone over bupivacaine.

LUMBAR FACET JOINT

LUMBAR INTRAARTICULAR INJECTION

TECHNIQUE 39-6

- Place the patient prone on a pain management table. Aseptically prepare and drape the patient.
- Under fluoroscopic guidance, identify the target segment to be injected. Upper lumbar facet joints are oriented in the sagittal (vertical) plane and often can be seen on direct anteroposterior views, whereas the lower lumbar facet joints, especially at L5-S1, are obliquely oriented and require an ipsilateral oblique rotation of the C-arm to be seen.
- Position the C-arm under fluoroscopy until the joint silhouette first appears. Insert and advance a 22- or 25-gauge, 3½-inch spinal needle toward the target joint along the axis of the fluoroscopy beam until contact is made with the articular processes of the joint. Enter the joint cavity through the softer capsule and advance the needle only a few millimeters. Capsular penetration is perceived as a subtle change of resistance. If midpoint needle entry is difficult, redirect the spinal needle to the superior or inferior joint recesses.
- Confirm placement with less than 0.1 mL of nonionic contrast dye with a 3-mL syringe to minimize injection pressure under fluoroscopic guidance. When intraarticular placement has been verified, inject a total volume of 1 mL of injectant (local anesthetic with or without corticosteroids) into the joint.

LUMBAR MEDIAL BRANCH BLOCK INJECTION

TECHNIQUE 39-7

- Place the patient prone on a pain management table. Aseptically prepare and drape the area to be injected.
- Because there is dual innervation of each lumbar facet joint, two medial branch blocks are required. The medial branches cross the transverse processes below their origin (Fig. 39-9). The L4-5 facet joint is anesthetized by blocking the L3 medial branch at the transverse process of L4 and the L4 medial branch at the transverse process of L5.

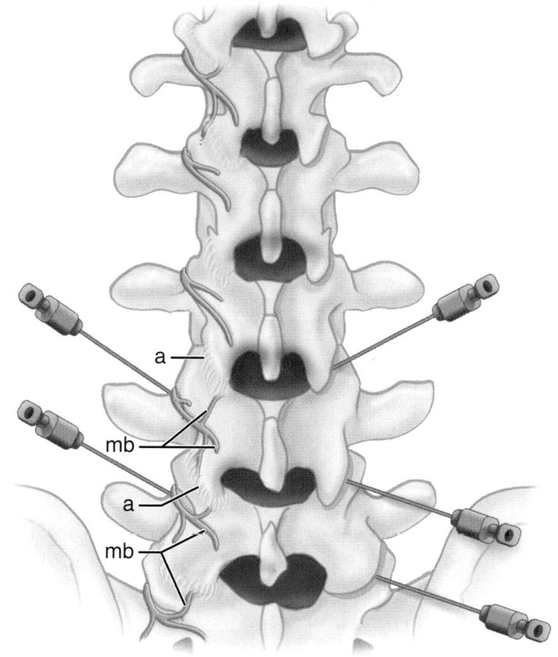

FIGURE 39-9 Posterior view of lumbar spine showing location of medial branches (mb) of dorsal rami, which innervate lumbar facet joints (a). Needle position for L3 and L4 medial branch blocks shown on left half of diagram would be used to anesthetize L4-5 facet joint. Right half of diagram shows L3-4, L4-5, and L5-S1 intraarticular facet joint injection positions. **SEE TECHNIQUE 39-7.**

In the case of the L5-S1 facet joint, anesthetize the L4 medial branch as it passes over the L5 transverse process and the L5 medial branch as it passes across the sacral ala.

- Using anteroposterior fluoroscopic imaging, identify the target transverse process. For L1 through L4 medial branch blocks, penetrate the skin using a 22- or 25-gauge, 3½-inch spinal needle lateral and superior to the target location.
- Under fluoroscopic guidance, advance the spinal needle until contact is made with the dorsal superior and medial aspects of the base of the transverse process so that the needle rests against the periosteum. To ensure optimal spinal needle placement, reposition the C-arm so that the fluoroscopy beam is ipsilateral oblique and the "Scotty dog" is seen. Position the spinal needle in the middle of the "eye" of the Scotty dog. Slowly inject (over 30 seconds) 0.5 mL of 0.75% bupivacaine.
- To inject the L5 medial branch (more correctly, the L5 dorsal ramus), position the patient prone on the pain management table with the fluoroscopic beam in the anteroposterior projection.
- Identify the sacral ala. Rotate the C-arm 15 to 20 degrees ipsilateral obliquely to maximize exposure between the junction of the sacral ala and the superior process of S1. Insert a 22- or 25-gauge, 3½-inch spinal needle directly into the osseous landmarks approximately 5 mm below

the superior junction of the sacral ala with the superior articular process of the sacrum under fluoroscopy. Rest the spinal needle on the periosteum and position the bevel of the spinal needle medial and away from the foramen to minimize flow through the L5 or S1 foramen. Slowly inject 0.5 mL of 0.75% bupivacaine.

SACROILIAC JOINT

The sacroiliac joint remains a controversial source of primary low back pain despite validated scientific studies. It often is overlooked as a source of low back pain because its anatomic location makes it difficult to examine in isolation and many provocative tests place mechanical stresses on contiguous structures. In addition, several other structures may refer pain to the sacroiliac joint.

Similar to other synovial joints, the sacroiliac joint moves; however, sacroiliac joint movement is involuntary and is caused by shear, compression, and other indirect forces. Muscles involved with secondary sacroiliac joint motion include the erectae spinae, quadratus lumborum, psoas major and minor, piriformis, latissimus dorsi, obliquus abdominis, and gluteal. Imbalances in any of these muscles as a result of central facilitation may cause them to function in a shortened state that tends to inhibit their antagonists reflexively. Theoretically, dysfunctional movement patterns may result. Postural changes and body weight also can create motion through the sacroiliac joint.

Because of the wide range of segmental innervation (L2-S2) of the sacroiliac joint, there are myriad referral zone patterns. In studies of asymptomatic subjects, the most constant referral zone was localized to a 3 × 10-cm area just inferior to the ipsilateral posterior superior iliac spine (Fig. 39-10); however, pain may be referred to the buttocks, groin, posterior thigh, calf, and foot.

Sacroiliac dysfunction, also called sacroiliac joint mechanical pain or sacroiliac joint syndrome, is the most common painful condition of this joint. The true prevalence of mediated pain from sacroiliac joint dysfunction is unknown; however, several studies indicated that it is more common than expected. Because no specific or pathognomonic historical facts or physical examination tests accurately identify the sacroiliac joint as a source of pain, diagnosis is one of exclusion. Sacroiliac joint dysfunction should be considered, however, if an injury was caused by a direct fall on the buttocks, a rear-end motor vehicle accident with the ipsilateral foot on the brake at the moment of impact, a broadside motor vehicle accident with a blow to the lateral aspect of the pelvic ring, or a fall in a hole with one leg in the hole and the other extended outside. Lumbar rotation and axial loading that can occur during ballet or ice skating is another common mechanism of injury. Although controversial, the risk of sacroiliac joint dysfunction may be increased in individuals with lumbar fusion or hip pathology. Other causes include insufficiency stress fractures; fatigue stress fractures; metabolic processes, such as deposition diseases; degenerative joint disease; infection; and inflammatory conditions, such as ankylosing spondylitis, psoriatic arthritis, and Reiter disease. The diagnosis of sacroiliac joint pain can be confirmed if symptoms are reproduced on distention of the joint capsule by provocative injection and subsequently abated with an analgesic block.

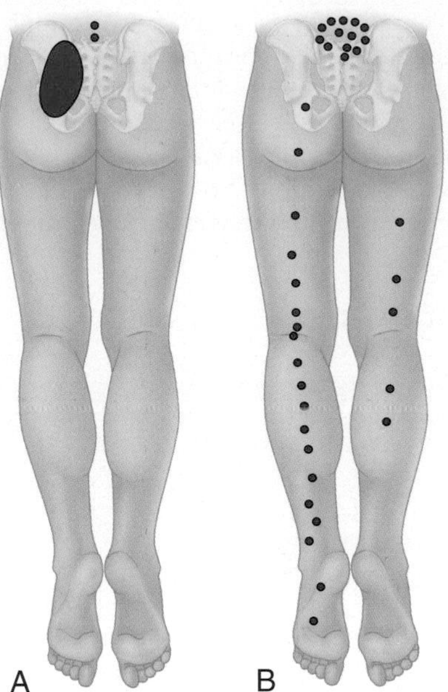

FIGURE 39-10 Pain diagram. **A,** Patient-reported pain diagram consistent with sacroiliac joint dysfunction. **B,** Patient-reported diagram inconsistent with sacroiliac joint dysfunction. (From Fortin JD, Dwyer AP, West S, et al: Sacroiliac joint: pain referral maps upon applying a new injection/arthrography technique, part I: asymptomatic volunteers, Spine 19:1475, 1994.)

SACROILIAC JOINT INJECTION

TECHNIQUE 39-8

- Place the patient prone on a pain management table. Aseptically prepare and drape the side to be injected. Rotate the C-arm until the medial (posterior) joint line is seen.
- Use a 27-gauge, ¼-inch needle to anesthetize the skin of the buttock 1 to 3 cm inferior to the lowest aspect of the joint. Using fluoroscopy, insert a 22-gauge, 3½-inch spinal needle until the needle rests 1 cm above the most posteroinferior aspect of the joint (Fig. 39-11). Rarely, a larger spinal needle is required in obese patients. Advance the spinal needle into the sacroiliac joint until capsular penetration occurs.
- Confirm intraarticular placement under fluoroscopy with 0.5 mL of nonionic contrast dye (Fig. 39-12). A spot radiograph can be taken to document placement. Inject a 2-mL volume containing 1 mL of 0.75% preservative-free bupivacaine and 1 mL of 6 mg/mL Celestone Soluspan into the joint.

DISCOGRAPHY

Discography has been used since the late 1940s for the experimental and clinical evaluation of disc disease in the cervical and lumbar regions of the spine. Since that time, discography has had a limited but important role in the evaluation of suspected disc pathology.

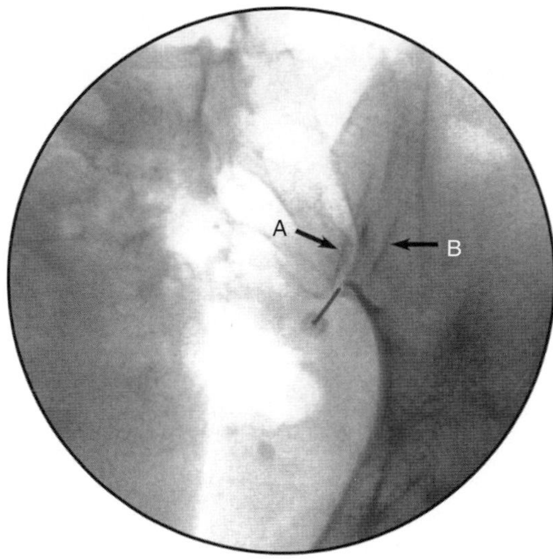

FIGURE 39-11 Sacroiliac joint injection showing medial *(A)* and lateral *(B)* joint planes (silhouettes). Entry into joint is achieved above most posteroinferior aspect of joint. **SEE TECHNIQUE 39-8.**

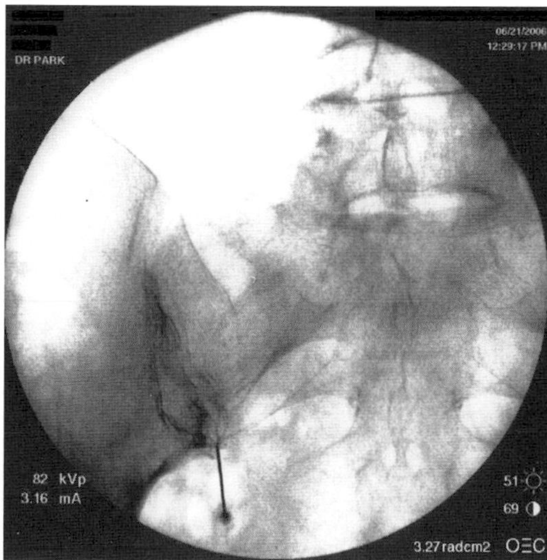

FIGURE 39-12 Left sacroiliac joint contrast pattern. **SEE TECHNIQUE 39-8.**

The clinical usefulness of the data obtained from discography is controversial. Although early studies concluded that lumbar discography was an unreliable diagnostic tool, with a 37% false-positive rate, later studies found a 0% false-positive rate for discography and concluded that, with current technique and a standardized protocol, discography was a highly reliable test.

The most important aspect of discography is provocative testing for concordant pain (i.e., pain that corresponds to a patient's usual pain) to provide information regarding the clinical significance of the disc abnormality. Although difficult to standardize, this testing distinguishes discography from other anatomic imaging techniques. If the patient is unable to distinguish customary pain from any other pain, the procedure is of no value. In patients who have a concordant response without evidence of a radial annular fissure on discography, CT should be considered because some discs that appear normal on discography show disruption on a CT scan.

Indications for lumbar discography include operative planning of spinal fusion, testing of the structural integrity of an adjacent disc to a known abnormality such as spondylolisthesis or fusion, identifying a painful disc among multiple degenerative discs, ruling out secondary internal disc disruption or suspected lateral or recurrent disc herniation, and determining the primary symptom-producing level when chemonucleolysis is being considered. Lumbar discography is most useful as a test to exclude levels from operative intervention rather than as a primary indication for operative fusion in patients with axial back pain. Thoracic discography can be a useful tool in the investigation of thoracic, chest, and upper abdominal pain. Degenerative thoracic disc disease, with or without herniation, has a highly variable clinical presentation, frequently mimicking visceral conditions and causing back or musculoskeletal pain. Discography also may be justified in medicolegal situations to establish a more definitive diagnosis even though treatment may not be planned on that disc.

Compression of the spinal cord, stenosis of the roots, bleeding disorders, allergy to the injectable material, and active infection are contraindications to diagnostic discography procedures. Although the risk of complications from discography is low, potential problems include discitis, nerve root injury, subarachnoid puncture, chemical meningitis, bleeding, and allergic reactions. In addition, in the cervical region, retropharyngeal and epidural abscess can occur. Pneumothorax is a risk in the cervical and thoracic regions.

LUMBAR DISCOGRAPHY

Lumbar discography originally was done using a transdural technique in a manner similar to myelography with a lumbar puncture. The difference between lumbar myelography and discography was that the needle used for the latter was advanced through the thecal sac. The technique later was modified, consisting of an extradural, extralaminar approach that avoided the thecal sac, and it was refined further to enable entry into the L5-S1 disc using a two-needle technique to maneuver around the iliac crest.

A patient's response during the procedure is the most important aspect of the study. Pain alone does not determine if a disc is the cause of the back pain. The concordance of the pain in regard to the quality and location are paramount in determining whether the disc is a true pain generator. A control disc is necessary to validate a positive finding on discography.

TECHNIQUE 39-9

(FALCO)

- Place the patient on a procedure or fluoroscopic table.
- Insert an angiocatheter into the upper extremity and infuse intravenous antibiotics to prevent discitis. Some physicians prefer to give antibiotics intradiscally during the procedure.

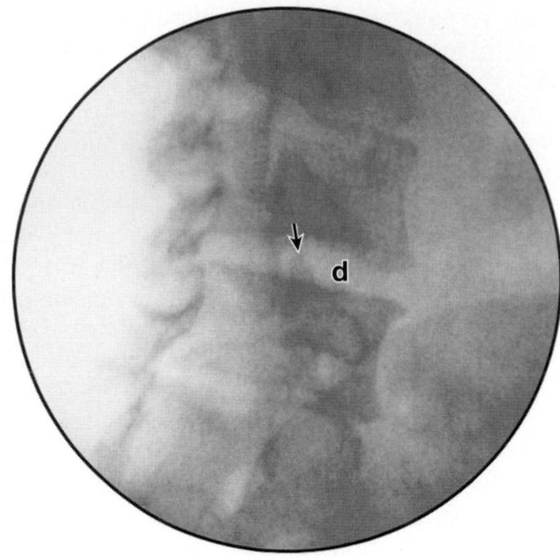

FIGURE 39-13 Lumbar spine in oblique position with superior articular process *(arrow)* dividing disc space (d) in half. (Courtesy of Frank J. E. Falco, MD.) **SEE TECHNIQUE 39-9.**

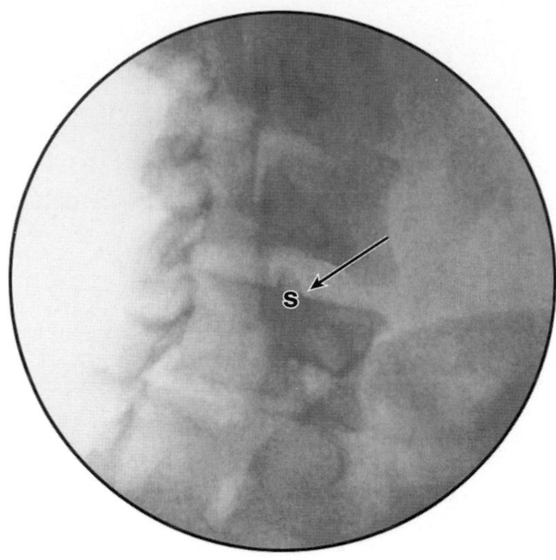

FIGURE 39-14 Disc entry point is just anterior *(arrow)* to base of superior articular process (s) and just above superior endplate of vertebral body. (Courtesy of Frank J. E. Falco, MD.) **SEE TECHNIQUE 39-9.**

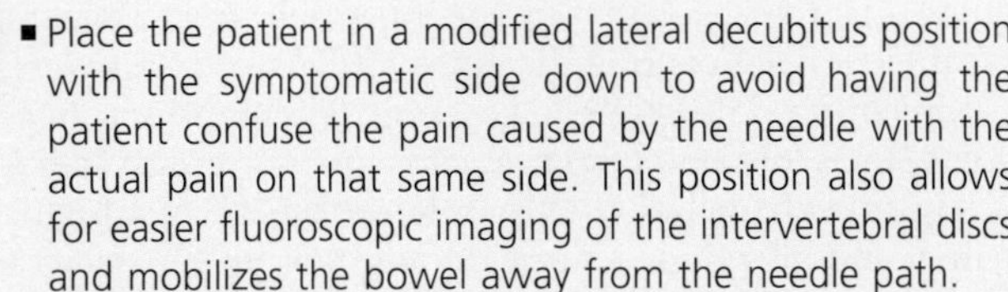

- Place the patient in a modified lateral decubitus position with the symptomatic side down to avoid having the patient confuse the pain caused by the needle with the actual pain on that same side. This position also allows for easier fluoroscopic imaging of the intervertebral discs and mobilizes the bowel away from the needle path.
- Sedate the patient with a short-acting agent. It is best to avoid analgesic agents that may alter the pain response.
- Prepare and drape the skin sterilely, including the lumbosacral region.
- Under fluoroscopic control, identify the intervertebral discs. Adjust the patient's position or the C-arm so that the lumbar spine is in an oblique position with the superior articular process dividing the intervertebral space in half (Fig. 39-13).
- Anesthetize the skin overlying the superior articular process with 1 to 2 mL of 1% lidocaine if necessary.
- Advance a single 6-inch spinal needle (or longer, depending on the patient's size) through the skin and deeper soft tissues to the outer annulus of the disc. The disc entry point is just anterior to the base of the superior articular process and just above the superior endplate of the vertebral body, which allows the needle to pass safely by the exiting nerve root (Fig. 39-14). Advance the needle into the central third of the disc, using anteroposterior and lateral fluoroscopic imaging.
- Confirm the position of the needle tip within the central third of the disc with anteroposterior and lateral fluoroscopic imaging. Inject either saline or nonionic contrast dye into each disc.
- Record any pain that the patient experiences during the injection as none, dissimilar, similar, or exact in relationship to the patient's typical low back pain. Record intradiscal pressures to assist in determining if the disc is the cause of the pain.
- Obtain radiographs of the lumbar spine on completion of the study, paying particular attention to the contrast-enhanced disc. Obtain a CT scan if necessary to assess disc anatomy further.
- An alternative method is a two-needle technique in which a 6- or 8-inch spinal needle is passed through a shorter introducer needle (typically $3\frac{1}{2}$ inches) into the disc in the same manner as a single needle. This approach may reduce the incidence of infection by allowing the procedure needle to pass into the disc space without ever penetrating the skin. The introducer needle also may assist in more accurate needle placement, reducing the risk of injuring the exiting nerve root. The two-needle approach may require more time than the single-needle technique, and the larger introducer needle could cause more pain to the patient.
- The two-needle technique often is used to enter the L5-S1 disc space with one modification. The procedure needle typically is curved (Fig. 39-15). To bypass the iliac crest, the introducer needle is advanced at an angle that places the needle tip in a position that does not line up with the L5-S1 disc space, which makes it difficult, if not impossible, for a straight procedure needle to advance into the L5-S1 disc. A curved procedure needle allows the needle tip to align with the L5-S1 disc as it is advanced toward and into the disc adjusting for malalignment.

THORACIC DISCOGRAPHY

Thoracic discography has been refined to provide a technique that is reproducible and safe. A posterolateral extralaminar approach similar to lumbar discography is used with a single-needle technique. The significant difference between thoracic and lumbar discography is the potential for complications because of the surrounding anatomy of the thoracic spine. In contrast to lumbar discography, which typically is performed in the mid to lower lumbar

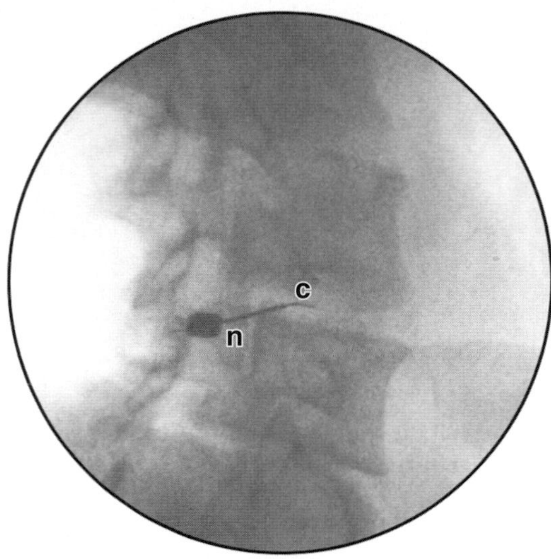

FIGURE 39-15 Curved procedure needle (c) passing through straight introducer needle (n). (Courtesy of Frank J. E. Falco, MD.) **SEE TECHNIQUE 39-9.**

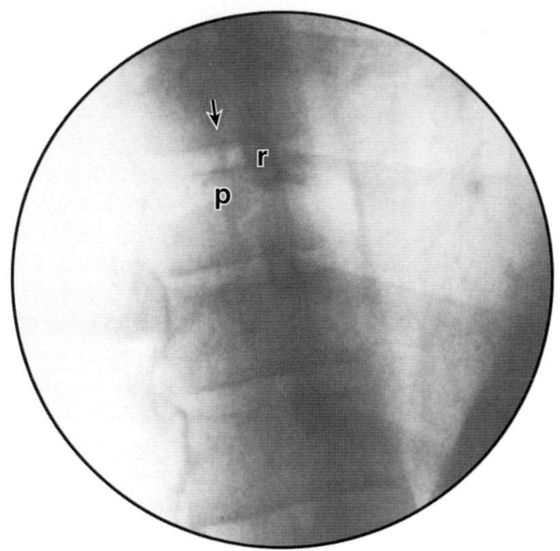

FIGURE 39-16 Oblique position with superior articular process *(arrow)* dividing thoracic intervertebral space in half. *p*, pedicle; *r*, rib head. (Courtesy of Frank J. E. Falco, MD.) **SEE TECHNIQUE 39-10.**

spine below the spinal cord and lungs, thoracic discography has the inherent risk of pneumothorax and direct spinal cord trauma; other complications include discitis and bleeding. Essentially the same protocol is used for thoracic discography as for lumbar discography.

TECHNIQUE 39-10

(FALCO)

- Place the patient in a modified lateral decubitus position on the procedure table with the symptomatic side down.
- Begin antibiotics through the intravenous catheter. Alternatively, intradiscal antibiotics may be given during the procedure.
- Sedate the patient and prepare and drape the skin in a sterile manner.
- Using fluoroscopic imaging, identify the intervertebral thoracic discs. Move the patient or adjust the C-arm obliquely to position the superior articular process so that it divides the intervertebral space in half (Fig. 39-16). At this point, the intervertebral discs and endplates, subjacent superior articular process, and adjacent rib head should be in clear view. The endplates, the superior articular process, and the rib head form a "box" (Fig. 39-17) that delineates a safe pathway into the disc, avoiding the spinal cord and lung. Keep the needle tip within the confines of this "box" while advancing it into the annulus.
- After proper positioning and exposure, anesthetize the skin overlying the superior articular process with 1 to 2 mL of 1% lidocaine if necessary.
- Advance a single 6-inch spinal needle (a shorter or longer needle can be used, depending on the patient's size) through the skin and the deeper soft tissues into the outer annulus within the "box" just anterior to the base of the superior articular process and just above the superior endplate. Continue into the central third of the disc, using anteroposterior and lateral fluoroscopic guidance.

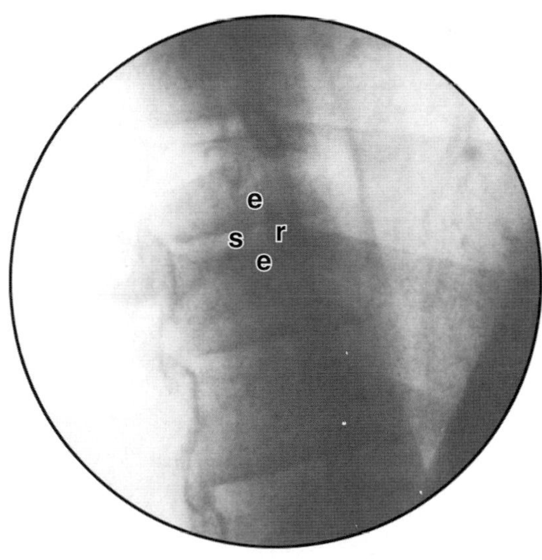

FIGURE 39-17 Thoracic endplates (e), superior articular process (s), and rib head (r) form box. (Courtesy of Frank J. E. Falco, MD.)

- Inject either saline or a nonionic contrast dye into each disc in the same manner as for lumbar discography.
- Record any pain response and analyze for reproduction of concordant pain using the same protocol as for lumbar discography.
- Obtain radiographs and CT scan of the thoracic spine on completion of the study.

THORACIC DISC DISEASE

The thoracic spine is the least common location for disc pathology. Since the 1960s, many approaches have been described and validated through clinical experience. It is apparent that posterior laminectomy has no role in the operative treatment of this problem. Other posterior approaches, such as costotransversectomy, have good indications.

Symptomatic thoracic disc herniations remain rare, with an estimated incidence of one in 1 million individuals per year. They represent 0.25% to 0.75% of the total incidence of symptomatic disc herniations. The most common age at onset is between the fourth and sixth decades. As with the other areas of the spine, the incidence of asymptomatic disc herniations is high; an estimated 37% of thoracic disc herniations are asymptomatic. Operative treatment of thoracic disc herniations is indicated in rare patients with acute disc herniation with myelopathic findings attributable to the lesion, especially progressive neurologic symptoms.

SIGNS AND SYMPTOMS

The natural history of symptomatic thoracic disc disease is similar to that in other areas, in that symptoms and function typically improve with conservative treatment and time. The clinical course can vary, however, and a high index of suspicion must be maintained to make the correct diagnosis. The differential diagnosis for the symptoms of thoracic disc herniations is fairly extensive and includes nonspinal causes occurring with the cardiopulmonary, gastrointestinal, and musculoskeletal systems. Spinal causes of similar symptoms can occur with infectious, neoplastic, degenerative, and metabolic problems within the spinal column and the spinal cord.

Two general patient populations have been documented in the literature. The smaller group of patients is younger and has a relatively short history of symptoms, often with a history of trauma. Typically, an acute soft disc herniation with either acute spinal cord compression or radiculopathy is present. Outcome generally is favorable with operative or nonoperative treatment. The larger group of patients has a longer history, often more than 6 to 12 months of symptoms, which result from chronic spinal cord or root compression. Disc degeneration, often with calcification of the disc, is the underlying process.

Pain is the most common presenting feature of thoracic disc herniations. Two patterns of pain are apparent: one is axial, and the other is bandlike radicular pain along the course of the intercostal nerve. The T10 dermatomal level is the most commonly reported distribution, regardless of the level of involvement. This is a band extending around the lower lateral thorax and caudad to the level of the umbilicus. This radicular pattern is more common with upper thoracic and lateral disc herniations. Some axial pain often occurs with this pattern as well. Associated sensory changes of paresthesias and dysesthesia in a dermatomal distribution also occur (Fig. 39-18). High thoracic discs (T2 to T5) can manifest similarly to cervical disc disease with upper arm pain, paresthesias, radiculopathy, and Horner syndrome. Myelopathy also may occur. Complaints of weakness, which may be generalized by the patient, typically involving both lower extremities occur in the form of mild paraparesis. Sustained clonus, a positive Babinski sign, and wide-based and spastic gait all are signs of myelopathy. Bowel and bladder dysfunction occur in only 15% to 20% of these patients. The neurologic evaluation of patients with thoracic disc herniations must be meticulous because there are few localizing findings. Abdominal reflexes, cremasteric reflex, dermatomal sensory evaluation, rectus abdominis contraction symmetry, lower extremity reflexes and strength and sensory examinations, and determination of long tract findings all are important.

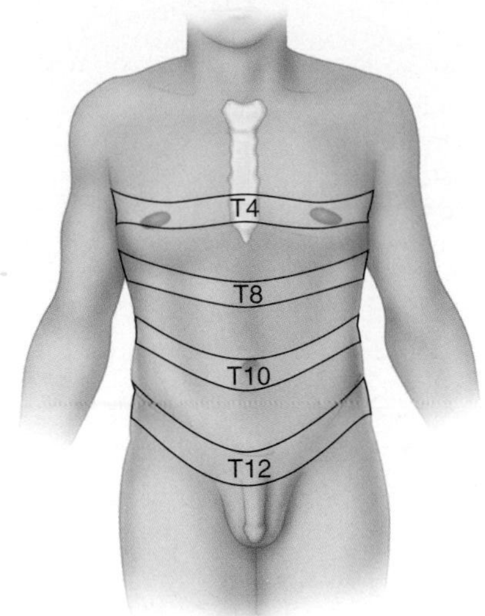

FIGURE 39-18 Sensory dermatomes of trunk region.

CONFIRMATORY IMAGING

Plain radiographs are helpful to evaluate traumatic injuries and to determine potential osseous morphologic variations that may help to localize findings, especially on intraoperative films, if these become necessary. MRI is the most important and useful imaging method to show thoracic disc herniations. In addition to the disc herniation, neoplastic or infectious pathology can be seen. The presence of intradural pathology, including disc fragments, also usually is shown on MRI. The spinal cord signal may indicate the presence of inflammation or myelomalacia as well. Despite all of these advantages, MRI may underestimate the thoracic disc herniation, which often is calcified and has low signal intensity on T1- and T2-weighted sequences.

Myelography followed by CT also can be useful in evaluating the bony anatomy and more accurately assessing the calcified portion of the herniated thoracic disc. Regardless of the imaging methods used, the appearance and presence of a thoracic disc herniation must be carefully considered and correlated with the patient's complaints and detailed examination findings.

TREATMENT RESULTS

As mentioned previously, nonoperative treatment usually is effective. A specific regimen cannot be recommended for all patients; however, the principles of short-term rest, pain relief, antiinflammatory agents, and progressive directed activity restoration seem most appropriate. These measures generally should be continued at least 6 to 12 weeks if feasible. If neurologic deficits progress or manifest as myelopathy, or if pain remains at an intolerable level, surgery should be recommended. The initial procedure recommended for this lesion was posterior thoracic laminectomy and disc excision. At least half of the lesions have been identified as being central, making the excision from this approach extremely difficult, and the results were disheartening. Most series reported fewer than half of the patients improving, with some becoming worse after posterior laminectomy and discectomy. Recent studies suggest that lateral rachiotomy (modified costotransversectomy) or an anterior transthoracic approach for discectomy produces considerably better results with no evidence of worsening after the procedure.

Video-assisted thoracic surgery (VATS) has been used in several series to remove central thoracic disc herniations successfully without the need for a thoracotomy or fusion.

OPERATIVE TREATMENT

The best operative approach for these lesions depends on the specific characteristics of the disc herniation and on the particular experience of the surgeon. Simple laminectomy has no role in the treatment of thoracic disc herniations. Posterior approaches, including costotransversectomy, transpedicular, transfacet pedicle-sparing, transdural, and lateral extracavitary approaches, all have been used successfully. Anterior approaches via thoracotomy, a transsternal approach, retropleural approach, or VATS also have been used successfully (Fig. 39-19). More recently, a number of minimally invasive posterior and anterior techniques have been developed, most using a series of muscle dilators, tubal retractors, and microscope visualization.

COSTOTRANSVERSECTOMY

Costotransversectomy is probably best suited for thoracic disc herniations that are predominantly lateral or herniations that are suspected to be extruded or sequestered. Central disc herniations are probably best approached transthoracically. Some surgeons have recommended subsequent fusion after disc removal anteriorly or laterally.

THORACIC COSTOTRANSVERSECTOMY

TECHNIQUE 39-11

- The operation usually is done with the patient under general anesthesia with a double-lumen endotracheal tube or a Carlen tube to allow lung deflation on the side of approach.
- Place the patient prone and make a long midline incision or a curved incision convex to the midline centered over the side of involvement.
- Expose the spine in the usual manner out to the ribs.
- Remove a section of rib 5.0 to 7.5 cm long at the level of involvement, avoiding damage to the intercostal nerve and artery.
- Carry the resection into the lateral side of the disc, exposing it for removal. Additional exposure can be made by laminectomy and excision of the pedicle and facet joint. Fusion is unnecessary unless more than one facet joint is removed.
- Close the wound in layers.

POSTOPERATIVE CARE. Postoperative care is similar to that for lumbar disc excision without fusion (see Technique 39-15).

THORACIC DISC EXCISION

Because of the relative age of patients with thoracic disc ruptures, special care must be taken to identify patients with pulmonary problems. In these patients, the anterior approach can be detrimental medically, making a posterolateral approach safer. Patients with midline protrusions probably are best treated with the transthoracic approach to ensure complete disc removal.

THORACIC DISCECTOMY—ANTERIOR APPROACH

TECHNIQUE 39-12

- The operation is done with the patient under general anesthesia, using a double-lumen endotracheal tube for lung deflation on the side of the approach.
- Place the patient in a lateral decubitus position. A left-sided anterior approach usually is preferred, making the operative procedure easier, if the herniation is central.
- Make a skin incision along the line of the rib that corresponds to the second thoracic vertebra above the involved intervertebral disc except for approaches to the upper five thoracic segments, where the approach is through the third rib. The skin incision is best determined by correlating preoperative imaging with intraoperative fluoroscopy.
- Cut the rib subperiosteally at its posterior and anterior ends and insert a rib retractor. Save the rib for grafting later in the procedure. One can decide on an extrapleural or transpleural approach depending on familiarity and ease. Exposure of the thoracic vertebrae should give adequate access to the front and opposite side.
- Dissect the great vessels free of the spine.
- Ligate the intersegmental vessels near the great vessels and not near the foramen. One should be able to insert the tip of a finger against the opposite side of the disc when the vascular mobilization is complete. Exposure of the intervertebral disc without disturbing more than three segmental vessels is preferable to avoid ischemic problems in the spinal cord.
- In the thoracolumbar region, strip the diaphragm from the 11th and 12th ribs. The anterior longitudinal ligament usually is sectioned to allow spreading of the intervertebral disc space.
- Remove the disc as completely as possible if fusion is planned. The use of an operating microscope or loupe magnification eases the removal of the disc near the posterior longitudinal ligament. Use curets and Kerrison rongeurs to remove the disc back to the posterior longitudinal ligament. When using this technique with fusion, removal of most of the disc is straightforward. As the posterior portion of the disc, including the herniation, is removed, however, the technique becomes more difficult. As mentioned previously, the herniation and surrounding disc usually are calcified and must be removed either piecemeal or with a high-speed drill. Careful dissection to develop a plane between tissue to be removed and the

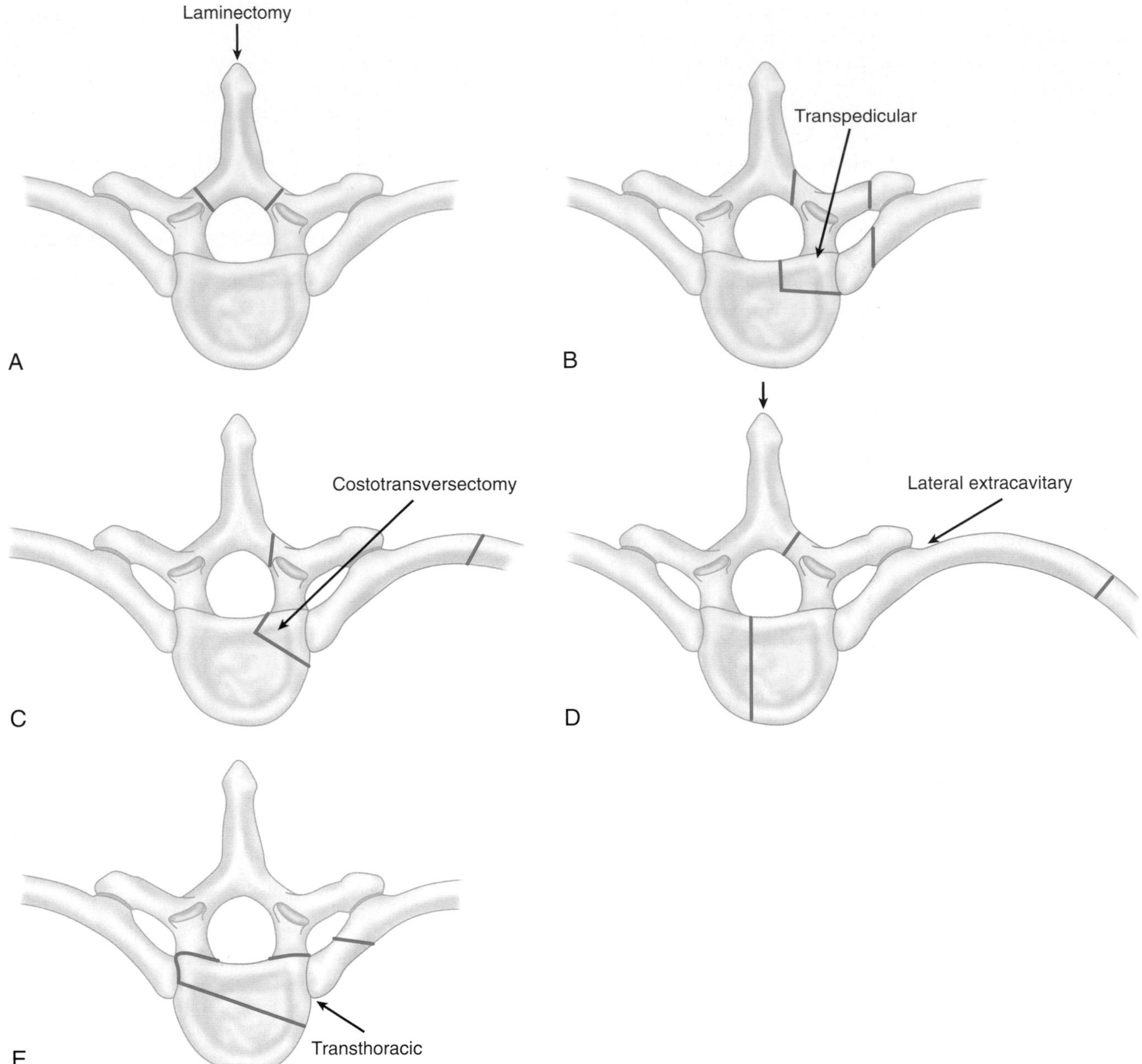

FIGURE 39-19 **A** to **E,** Exposure of thoracic disc provided by standard laminectomy **(A)**, transpedicular approach **(B)**, costotransversectomy approach **(C)**, lateral extracavitary approach **(D)**, and transthoracic approach **(E)**.

ventral dura is required. This is best done with blunt Penfield-type dissectors and small curets of various designs and orientations. Even if a drill is used, the removal of the posteriormost tissue should be done with hand instruments, not powered instruments. Expect significant bleeding from the epidural veins, which usually are congested at the level of herniation.

- After removal of the disc, strip the endplates of their cartilage.
- Make a slot on the margin of the superior endplate to accept the graft material. Preserve the subchondral bone on both sides of the disc space. Insert iliac, tibial, or rib grafts into the disc space. If multiple short rib grafts are used, they can be tied together with heavy suture material when the maximal number of grafts has been inserted. This helps maintain vertical alignment for all such grafts.
- Close the wound in the usual manner and use standard chest drainage.
- Alternatively, if fusion is not desired, a more limited resection using an operating microscope can be done.
- Also, the minimally invasive lateral extraceloemic (retroperitoneal/retropleural) approach as described in Chapter 37 can be used for herniations from T10-11 to L1-2.
- After the vascular mobilization, resect the rib head to allow observation of the pedicle and foramen caudal to

the disc space. The cephalad portion of the pedicle can be removed with a high-speed burr and Kerrison rongeurs, exposing the posterolateral aspect of the disc. This allows for careful, blunt development of the plane ventral to the dura with removal of the disc herniation and preservation of the anterior majority of the disc and limits the need for fusion. A similar technique using VATS is described in Technique 39-13.

- The transthoracic approach removing a rib two levels above the level of the lesion can be used up to T5. The transthoracic approach from T2 to T5 is best made by excision of the third or fourth rib and elevation of the scapula by sectioning of attachments of the serratus anterior and trapezius from the scapula. The approach to the T1-2 disc is best made from the neck with a sternum-splitting incision.

POSTOPERATIVE CARE. Postoperative care is the same as for a thoracotomy. The patient is allowed to walk after the chest tubes are removed. Extension in any position is prohibited. A brace or body cast that limits extension should be used if the stability of the graft is questionable. The graft usually is stable without support if only one disc space is removed. Postoperative care is the same as for anterior corpectomy and fusion if more than one disc level is removed. If no fusion is done, the patient is mobilized as pain permits without a brace.

THORACIC ENDOSCOPIC DISC EXCISION

Microsurgical and endoscopic operative techniques are highly technical, and they should be performed by a surgeon who is proficient in this technique and in the use of endoscopic equipment and with the assistance of an experienced thoracic surgeon. Ideally, the procedure should first be done on cadavers or live animals.

ENDOSCOPIC THORACIC DISCECTOMY

TECHNIQUE 39-13

(ROSENTHAL ET AL.)

- Place the patient in the left lateral decubitus position to allow a right-sided approach and displacement of the aorta and heart to the left.
- Insert four trocars in a triangular fashion along the middle axillary line converging on the disc space. Introduce a rigid endoscope with a 30-degree optic angle attached to a video camera into one of the trocars, leaving the other three as working channels.
- Deflate the lung using a Carlen tube or similar method.
- Split the parietal pleura starting at the medial part of the intervertebral space and extending up to the costovertebral process.
- Preserve and mobilize the segmental arteries and sympathetic nerve out of the operating field.
- Drill away the rib head and lateral portion of the pedicle. Remove the remaining pedicle with Kerrison rongeurs to improve exposure to the spinal canal. Removing the superior posterior portion of the vertebra caudal to the disc space allows safer removal of the disc material, which can be pulled anteriorly and inferiorly away from the spinal canal to be removed. Use endoscopic instruments for surgery in the portals.
- Remove the disc posteriorly and the posterior longitudinal ligament, restricting bone and disc removal to the posterior third of the intervertebral space and costovertebral area to maintain stability.
- Insert chest tubes in the standard fashion and set them to water suction; close the portals.

POSTOPERATIVE CARE. The patient is rapidly mobilized as tolerated by the chest tubes. Discharge is possible after the chest tubes have been removed and the patient is ambulating well.

MINIMALLY INVASIVE THORACIC DISCECTOMY

TECHNIQUE 39-14

- Place the patient in the lateral decubitus position with the affected side up.
- Localize an incision over the disc space of interest. A 5-cm portion of rib can be resected if it is overlying the disc, or the approach can sometimes be performed without rib resection.
- Using blunt finger dissection, make a retropleural approach down to the spine and dock a minimally invasive retractor system on the disc space and rib head of interest. Sometimes the pleura must be opened, but this does not change the exposure significantly because the retractor can safely retract the lung while being insufflated.
- Complete the procedure as in an open discectomy through a thoracotomy using the self-retaining retractor (many different styles are available).
- Once the procedure is finished there is no need for a chest tube if the pleura is not violated.
- Close the rib base and subcutaneous tissues in layers.

This approach can be extended down to L1-2 by mobilizing the diaphragm off the rib and transverse process attachments.

POSTOPERATIVE CARE. The patient is mobilized the day of surgery and is discharged when ambulating well.

LUMBAR DISC DISEASE

SIGNS AND SYMPTOMS

Although back pain is common from the second decade of life on, intervertebral disc disease and disc herniation are

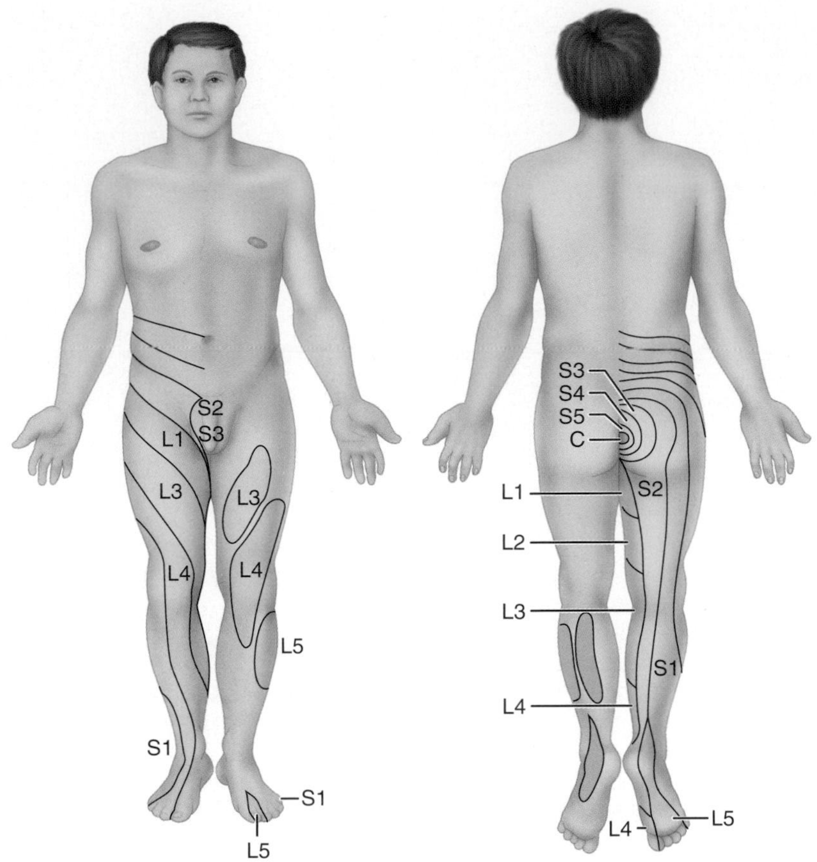

FIGURE 39-20 Diagram indicating dermatomal regions for T12-S5 nerves.

most prominent in otherwise healthy people in the third and fourth decades of life. Most people relate their back and leg pain to a traumatic incident, but close questioning frequently reveals that the patient has had intermittent episodes of back pain for many months or even years before the onset of severe leg pain. In many instances, the back pain is relatively fleeting and is relieved by rest. Heavy exertion, repetitive bending, twisting, or heavy lifting often brings on axial back pain. In other instances, an inciting event cannot be elicited. The pain usually begins in the lower back, radiating to the sacroiliac region and buttocks. The pain can radiate down the posterior thigh. Back and posterior thigh pain of this type can be elicited from many areas of the spine, including the facet joints, longitudinal ligaments, and periosteum of the vertebra. Radicular pain usually extends below the knee and follows the dermatome of the involved nerve root (Fig. 39-20).

The usual history of lumbar disc herniation is of repetitive lower back and buttock pain, relieved by a short period of rest. This pain is suddenly exacerbated, often by a flexion episode, with the appearance of leg pain. Most radicular pain from nerve root compression caused by a herniated nucleus pulposus is evidenced by leg pain equal to, or in many cases greater than, the degree of back pain. Whenever leg pain is minimal and back pain is predominant, great care should be taken before making the diagnosis of a symptomatic herniated intervertebral disc. The pain from disc herniation usually varies, increasing with activity, especially sitting. The pain can be decreased by rest, especially in the semi-Fowler position, and can be exacerbated by straining, sneezing, or coughing. Whenever the pattern of pain is bizarre or the pain is uniform in intensity, a diagnosis of symptomatic herniated disc should be viewed with some skepticism.

Other symptoms of disc herniation include weakness and paresthesias. In most patients, the weakness is intermittent, varies with activity, and is localized to the neurologic level of involvement. Paresthesias also vary and are limited to the dermatome of the involved nerve root. Whenever these complaints are generalized, the diagnosis of a simple unilateral disc herniation should be questioned.

Numbness and weakness in the involved leg and occasionally pain in the groin or testis can be associated with a high or midline lumbar disc herniation. If a fragment is large or the herniation is high, symptoms of pressure on the entire cauda equina can occur with development of cauda equina syndrome. These symptoms include numbness and weakness in both legs, rectal pain, numbness in the perineum, and paralysis of the sphincters. This diagnosis should be the primary consideration in patients who complain of sudden loss of bowel or bladder control. Whenever the diagnosis of cauda equina syndrome is caused by an acute midline herniation, evaluation and treatment should be aggressive.

The physical findings with disc disease vary because of the time intervals involved. Usually patients with acute pain show evidence of marked paraspinal spasm that is sustained during walking or motion. A scoliosis or a list in the lumbar spine may be present, and in many patients the normal lumbar lordosis is lost. As the acute episode subsides, the degree of spasm diminishes remarkably, and the loss of normal lumbar lordosis may be the only telltale sign. Point tenderness may be present over the spinous process at the level of the disc involved, and pain may extend laterally in some patients.

If there is nerve root irritation, it centers over the length of the sciatic nerve, in the sciatic notch, and more distally in the popliteal space. In addition, stretch of the sciatic nerve at the knee should reproduce buttock, thigh, and leg pain (i.e., pain distal to the knee). A Lasègue sign usually is positive on the involved side. A positive Lasègue sign or straight-leg raising should elicit buttock and leg pain distal to the knee. Occasionally, if leg pain is significant, the patient leans back from an upright sitting position and assumes the tripod position to relieve the pain. This is referred to as the "flip sign." Contralateral leg pain produced by straight-leg raising should be regarded as pathognomonic of a herniated intervertebral disc. The absence of a positive Lasègue sign should make one skeptical of the diagnosis, although older individuals may not have a positive Lasègue sign. Likewise, inappropriate findings and inconsistencies in the examination usually are nonorganic in origin (see discussion of nonspecific axial pain). If the leg pain has persisted for any length of time, atrophy of the involved limb may be present, as shown by asymmetric girth of the thigh or calf. The neurologic examination varies as determined by the level of root involvement (Boxes 39-2 to 39-4).

Unilateral disc herniation at L3-4 usually compresses the L4 root as it crosses the disc before exiting at the L4-5 intervertebral foramen below the L4 pedicle. Pain may be localized around the medial side of the leg. Numbness may be present over the anteromedial aspect of the leg. The anterior tibial muscle may be weak, as evidenced by inability to heel walk. The quadriceps and hip adductor group, both innervated from L2, L3, and L4, also may be weak and, in extended ruptures, atrophic. Reflex testing may reveal a diminished or absent patellar tendon reflex (L2, L3, and L4) or anterior tibial tendon reflex (L4). Sensory testing may show diminished sensibility over the L4 dermatome, the isolated portion of which is the medial leg (Fig. 39-20) and the autonomous zone of which is at the level of the medial malleolus.

Unilateral disc herniation at L4-5 results in compression of the L5 root. L5 root radiculopathy should produce pain in the dermatomal pattern. Numbness, when present, follows the L5 dermatome along the anterolateral aspect of the leg and the dorsum of the foot, including the great toe. The autonomous zone for this nerve is the dorsal first web of the foot and the dorsum of the third toe. Weakness may involve the extensor hallucis longus (L5), gluteus medius (L5), or extensor digitorum longus and brevis (L5). Reflex change usually is not found. A diminished posterior tibial reflex is possible but difficult to elicit.

With unilateral rupture of the disc at L5-S1, the findings of an S1 radiculopathy are noted. Pain and numbness involve the dermatome of S1. The S1 dermatome includes the lateral malleolus and the lateral and plantar surface of the foot, occasionally including the heel. There is numbness over the lateral aspect of the leg and, more important, over the lateral aspect of the foot, including the lateral three toes. The autonomous zone for this root is the dorsum of the fifth toe. Weakness may be shown in the peroneus longus and brevis (S1), gastrocnemius-soleus (S1), or gluteus maximus (S1). In general, weakness is not a usual finding in S1 radiculopathy. Occasionally, mild weakness may be shown by asymmetric fatigue with exercise of these motor groups. The ankle jerk usually is reduced or absent.

Massive extrusion of a disc involving the entire diameter of the lumbar canal or a large midline extrusion can produce pain in the back, legs, and occasionally perineum. Both legs may be paralyzed, the sphincters may be incontinent, and the ankle jerks may be absent.

BOX 39-2

L4 Root Compression*

Sensory Deficit
Posterolateral thigh, anterior knee, and medial leg

Motor Weakness
Quadriceps (variable)
Hip adductors (variable)

Anterior Tibial Weakness
Reflex change
Patellar tendon
Anterior tibial tendon (variable)

*Indicative of L3-4 disc herniation or pathologic condition localized to L4 foramen.

BOX 39-3

L5 Root Compression*

Sensory Deficit
Anterolateral leg, dorsum of the foot, and great toe

Motor Weakness
Extensor hallucis longus
Gluteus medius
Extensor digitorum longus and brevis

Reflex Change
Usually none
Posterior tibial (difficult to elicit)

*Indicative of L4-5 disc herniation or pathologic condition localized to L5 foramen.

BOX 39-4

S1 Root Compression*

Sensory Deficit
Lateral malleolus, lateral foot, heel, and web of fourth and fifth toes

Motor Weakness
Peroneus longus and brevis
Gastrocnemius-soleus complex
Gluteus maximus

Reflex Change
Achilles tendon (gastrocnemius-soleus complex)

*Indicative of L5-S1 disc herniation or pathologic condition localized to the S1 foramen.

More than 95% of the ruptures of the lumbar intervertebral discs occur at L4-5 or L5-S1. Ruptures at higher levels in many patients are not associated with a positive straight-leg raising test. In these instances, a positive femoral stretch test can be helpful. This test is done by placing the patient prone and acutely flexing the knee while placing the hand in the popliteal fossa. When this procedure results in anterior thigh pain, the result is positive and a high lesion should be suspected. In addition, these lesions may occur with a more diffuse neurologic complaint without significant localizing neurologic signs.

Often the neurologic signs associated with disc disease vary over time. If the patient has been up and walking for a period of time, the neurologic findings may be much more pronounced than if he or she has been at bed rest for several days, decreasing the pressure on the nerve root and allowing the nerve to resume its normal function. In addition, various conservative treatments can change the physical signs of disc disease.

Comparative bilateral examination of a patient with back and leg pain is essential in finding a clear-cut pattern of signs and symptoms. The evaluation commonly may change. Adverse changes in the examination may warrant more aggressive therapy, whereas improvement of the symptoms or signs should signal a resolution of the problem. Early symptoms or signs suggesting cauda equina syndrome or severe or progressive neurologic deficit should be treated aggressively from the onset.

DIFFERENTIAL DIAGNOSIS

The differential diagnosis of back and leg pain is extremely lengthy and complex. It includes diseases intrinsic to the spine and diseases involving adjacent organs but causing pain referred to the back or leg. For simplicity, lesions can be categorized as being extrinsic or intrinsic to the spine. Extrinsic lesions include diseases of the urogenital system, gastrointestinal system, vascular system, endocrine system, nervous system not localized to the spine, and extrinsic musculoskeletal system. These lesions include infections, tumors, metabolic disturbances, congenital abnormalities, and associated diseases of aging. Intrinsic lesions involve diseases that arise primarily in the spine. They include diseases of the spinal musculoskeletal system, the local hematopoietic system, and the local neurologic system. These conditions include trauma, tumors, infections, diseases of aging, and immune diseases affecting the spine or spinal nerves.

Although the predominant cause of back and leg pain in healthy individuals usually is lumbar disc disease, one must be extremely cautious to avoid a misdiagnosis, particularly given the high incidence of disc herniations present in asymptomatic patients as discussed previously. A full physical examination must be completed before making a presumptive diagnosis of herniated disc disease. Common diseases that can mimic disc disease include ankylosing spondylitis, multiple myeloma, vascular insufficiency, arthritis of the hip, osteoporosis with stress fractures, extradural tumors, peripheral neuropathy, and herpes zoster. Infrequent but reported causes of sciatica not related to disc hernia include synovial cysts, rupture of the medial head of the gastrocnemius, sacroiliac joint dysfunction, lesions in the sacrum and pelvis, and fracture of the ischial tuberosity.

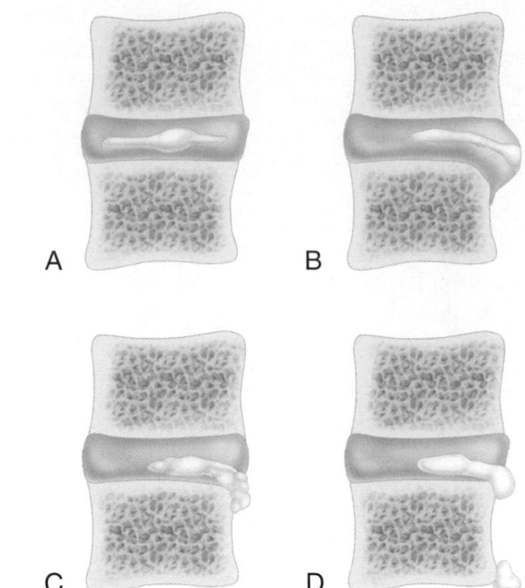

FIGURE 39-21 Types of disc herniation. **A,** Normal bulge. **B,** Protrusion. **C,** Extrusion. **D,** Sequestration.

CONFIRMATORY IMAGING

Although the diagnosis of a herniated lumbar disc should be suspected from the history and physical examination, imaging studies are necessary to rule out other causes, such as a tumor or infection. Plain radiographs are of limited use in the diagnosis because they do not show disc herniations or other intraspinal lesions, but they can show infection, tumors, or other anomalies and should be obtained, especially if surgery is planned. Currently, the most useful test for diagnosing a herniated lumbar disc is MRI (Figs. 39-21 and 39-22). Since the advent of MRI, myelography is used much less frequently, although in some situations it may help to show subtle lesions. When myelography is used, it should be followed by CT.

NONOPERATIVE TREATMENT

The number and variety of nonoperative therapies for back and leg pain are diverse and overwhelming. Treatments range from simple rest to expensive traction apparatus. All of these therapies are reported with glowing accounts of miraculous "cures"; few have been evaluated scientifically. In addition, the natural history of lumbar disc herniation is characterized by exacerbations and remissions with eventual improvement of extremity complaints in most cases, which can make any intervention appear successful to the patient. Finally, several distinct symptom complexes seem to be associated with disc disease. Few, if any, studies have isolated the response to specific and anatomically distinct diagnoses.

The simplest treatment for acute back pain is rest; generally 2 days of bed rest are better than a longer period. Biomechanical studies indicate that lying in a semi-Fowler position (i.e., on the side with the hips and knees flexed) with a pillow between the legs should relieve most pressure on the disc and nerve roots. Muscle spasm can be controlled by the application of ice, preferably with a massage over the muscles in spasm. Pain relief and antiinflammatory effect can be achieved with nonsteroidal antiinflammatory drugs (NSAIDs). Most acute exacerbations of back pain respond quickly to this

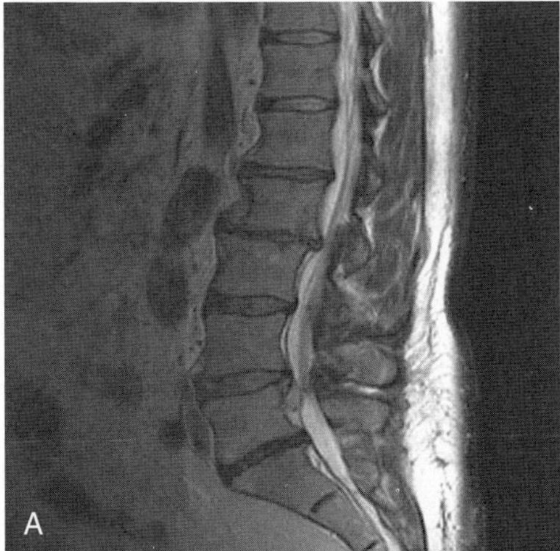

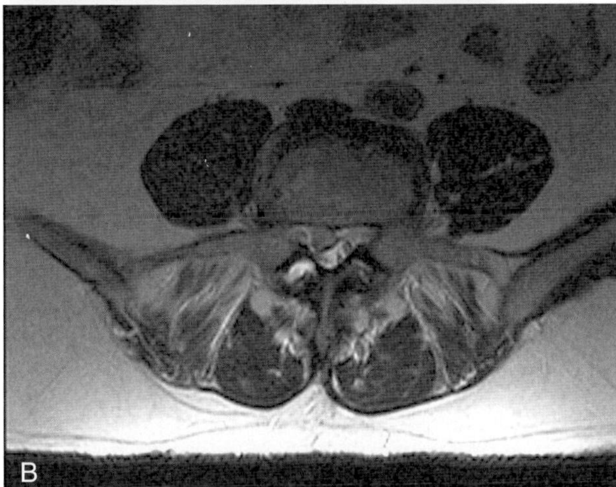

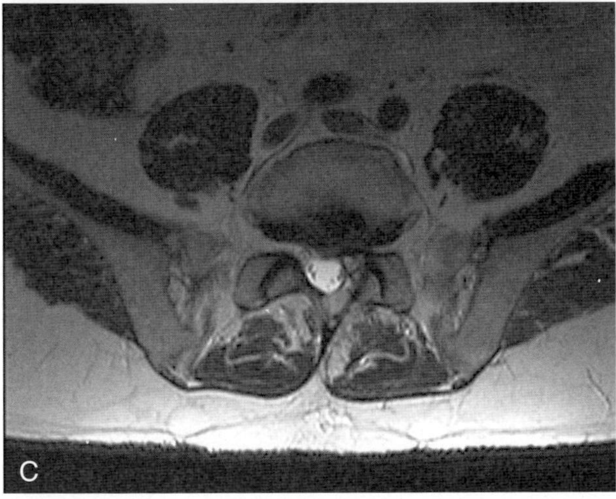

FIGURE 39-22 Sixty-one-year-old patient with right L5 radiculopathy. **A,** T2 sagittal MR image reveals sequestered L4 herniated disc fragment. **B,** T2 axial MR image shows the fragment between L5 pedicles. **C,** This patient also had asymptomatic left L5 disc extrusion.

therapy. As the pain diminishes, the patient should be encouraged to begin isometric abdominal and lower extremity exercises. Walking within the limits of comfort also is encouraged. Sitting, especially riding in a car, is discouraged. Continuation of ordinary activities within the limits permitted by pain has been shown to lead to a quicker recovery.

Education in proper posture and body mechanics is helpful in returning the patient to the usual level of activity after the acute exacerbation has improved. This education can take many forms, from individual instruction to group instruction. Back education of this type is now usually referred to as "back school." Although the concept is excellent, the quality and quantity of information provided may vary widely. The work of Bergquist-Ullman and Larsson and others indicates that patient education of this type is extremely beneficial in decreasing the amount of time lost from work initially but does little to decrease the incidence of recurrence of symptoms or length of time lost from work during recurrences. The combination of back education and combined physical therapy is superior to placebo treatment. Physical therapy can help improve activity level and physical function but should be discontinued if it aggravates the radiculopathy.

Numerous medications have been used with various results in subacute and chronic back and leg pain syndromes. The current trend seems to be moving away from the use of strong narcotics and muscle relaxants in the outpatient treatment of these syndromes. This is especially true in the instances of chronic back and leg pain where drug habituation and increased depression are frequent. Oral steroids used briefly can be beneficial as potent antiinflammatory agents. The many types of NSAIDs also are helpful when aspirin is not tolerated or is of little help. Numerous NSAIDs are available for the treatment of low back pain. When depression is prominent, mood elevators such as nortriptyline can be beneficial in reducing sleep disturbance and anxiety without increasing depression. Nortriptyline also decreases the need for narcotic medication.

Physical therapy should be used judiciously. The exercises should be fitted to the symptoms and not forced as an absolute group of activities. Patients with acute back and thigh pain eased by passive extension of the spine in the prone position can benefit from extension exercises rather than flexion exercises. Improvement in symptoms with extension indicates a good prognosis with conservative care. Patients whose pain is increased by passive extension may be improved by flexion exercises. These exercises should not be forced in the face of increased pain. This may avoid further disc extrusion. Any exercise that increases pain should be discontinued. Lower extremity exercises can increase strength and relieve stress on the back, but they also can exacerbate lower extremity arthritis. The true benefit of such treatments may be in the promotion of good posture and body mechanics rather than of strength. Numerous treatment methods have been advanced for the treatment of back pain. Some patients respond to the use of transcutaneous electrical nerve stimulation. Others do well with traction varying from skin traction in bed with 5 to 8 lb to body inversion with forces of more than 100 lb. Back braces or corsets may be helpful to other patients. Ultrasound and diathermy are other treatments used in acute back pain. The scientific efficacy of many of these treatments has not been proved.

As discussed earlier, the natural history of lumbar disc disease generally is favorable. Although low-back pain can result in significant disability, approximately 95% of patients return to their previous employment within 3 months of symptom onset. Failure to return to work within 3 months has been identified as a poor prognostic sign. Longer periods of disability equate to lower probability of returning to work: in patients with total disability lasting a year, the likelihood of returning to work is 21%, and in those with disability lasting 2 years the likelihood is less than 2%. Obesity and smoking have been shown to correlate unfavorably with low back pain and may adversely affect the progression of symptoms.

OPERATIVE TREATMENT

If nonoperative treatment for lumbar disc disease fails, the next consideration is operative treatment. Before this step is taken, the surgeon must be sure of the diagnosis. The patient must be certain that the degree of pain and impairment warrants such a step. The surgeon and the patient must realize that disc surgery is not a cure but may provide symptomatic relief. It neither stops the pathologic processes that allowed the herniation to occur nor restores the disc to a normal state. The patient still must practice good posture and body mechanics after surgery. Activities involving repetitive bending, twisting, and lifting with the spine in flexion may have to be curtailed or eliminated. If prolonged relief is to be expected, some permanent modification in the patient's lifestyle may be necessary, although often no specific limitations are applied.

The key to good results in disc surgery is appropriate patient selection. The optimal patient is one with predominant (if not only) unilateral leg pain extending below the knee that has been present for at least 6 weeks. The pain should have been decreased by rest, antiinflammatory medication, or even epidural steroids but should have returned to the initial levels after a minimum of 6 to 8 weeks of conservative care. Physical examination should reveal signs of sciatic irritation and possibly objective evidence of localizing neurologic impairment. CT, lumbar MRI, or myelography should confirm the level of involvement consistent with the patient's examination.

Operative disc removal is mandatory and urgent only in patients with cauda equina syndrome; other disc excisions should be considered elective. The elective status of surgery should allow a thorough evaluation to confirm the diagnosis, level of involvement, and physical and psychologic status of the patient. Frequently, if there is a rush to the operating room to relieve pain without proper investigation, the patient and the physician later regret the decision.

Regardless of the method chosen to treat a disc rupture surgically, the patient should be aware that the procedure is predominantly for the symptomatic relief of leg pain. Patients with predominantly back pain may not experience relief.

MICRODISCECTOMY

Most disc surgery is performed with the patient under general endotracheal anesthesia, although local anesthesia has been used with minimal complications. Patient positioning varies with the operative technique and surgeon. To position the patient in a modified kneeling position, a specialized frame or custom frame is popular. Positioning the patient in this manner allows the abdomen to hang free, minimizing epidural venous dilation and bleeding (Fig. 39-23). A headlamp allows the surgeon to direct light into the lateral recesses where a large proportion of the surgery may be required. The addition of loupe magnification also greatly improves the identification and exposure of various structures. Most surgeons also use an operative microscope to improve visibility further. The primary benefit of an operating microscope compared with loupes is the view afforded the assistant. Radiographic confirmation of the proper level is necessary. Care should be taken to protect neural structures. Epidural bleeding should be controlled with bipolar electrocautery. Any sponge, pack, or cottonoid patty placed in the wound should extend to the outside. Pituitary rongeurs should be marked at a point equal to the maximal allowable disc depth to prevent injury of viscera or great vessels.

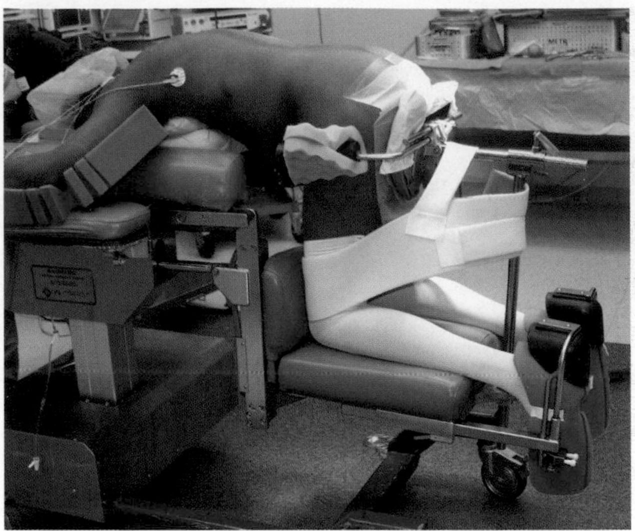

FIGURE 39-23 Knee-chest position for lumbar disc excision allows abdomen to be completely free of external pressure.

MICROSCOPIC LUMBAR DISC EXCISION

Microscopic lumbar disc excision has replaced the standard open laminectomy as the procedure of choice for herniated lumbar disc. This procedure can be done on an outpatient basis and allows better lighting, magnification, and angle of view with a much smaller exposure. Because of the limited dissection required, there is less postoperative pain and a shorter postoperative stay.

Microscopic lumbar discectomy requires an operating microscope with a 400-mm lens, a variety of small-angled Kerrison rongeurs of appropriate length, microinstruments, and preferably a combination suction/nerve root retractor. The procedure is performed with the patient prone. A specialized frame (Fig. 39-23) previously described can be used, or the patient can be positioned on chest rolls. There are several advantages to using a specialized table, such as an Andrews table: (1) it allows the belly to hang free where venous blood will pool, which results in decreased venous epidural bleeding intraoperatively; (2) the knee-chest position maximizes the lumbar kyphosis, placing the ligamentum flavum on slight tension that allows for easier removal but also opens the interlaminar space, which may provide greater canal access with less bone removal; and (3) the small footprint of the bed enables the operating microscope to be placed at the foot, which not only makes access to the ocular lens easier for both the surgeon and assistant standing on opposite sides of the table but also allows the fluoroscope to be moved into the surgical field for imaging without having to move the microscope base itself.

The microscope can be used from skin incision to closure. The initial dissection can be done under direct vision, however. A lateral radiograph is taken to confirm the level, but fluoroscopy is much quicker when used for localization. Fluoroscopy is essential for localization when using tubular retractors because the field of view is smaller, making the available margin for error in placing the skin incision less.

ENDOSCOPIC TECHNIQUES

Endoscopic techniques have been developed with the purported advantage of shortened hospital stay and faster return to activity. These techniques generally are variations of the microdiscectomy technique using an endoscope rather than the microscope and different types of retractors. This remains another alternative technique. Each system is unique, and the reader is referred to the technique guide of the various manufacturers for details. The basic principles remain the same as with microdiscectomy. Less-invasive tubular retractors also have been used in a transmuscular fashion, allowing disc excision with less soft-tissue damage because of the more precise exposure; however, better objective clinical results have not been shown with this technique.

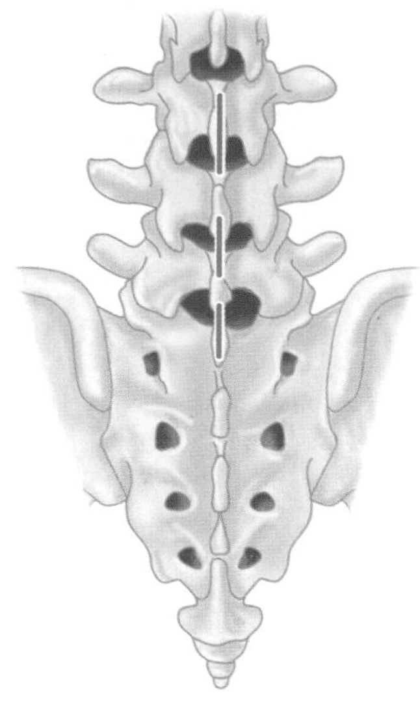

FIGURE 39-24 **Incision micro lumbar disc excision.** (From Gardocki RG: Microscopic lumbar discectomy. In Canale ST, Beaty JH, Azar FM, editors: Campbell's Core Procedures, Philadelphia, Elsevier, 2016.) **SEE TECHNIQUE 39-15.**

MICROSCOPIC LUMBAR DISCECTOMY

TECHNIQUE 39-15

APPROACH FOR USE OF MCCULLOCH RETRACTOR

- Infiltrate the operative field (paraspinous muscle, subcutaneous tissue, and skin) with 10 mL of 0.25% bupivacaine with epinephrine for preemptive analgesia and hemostasis.
- Make the incision from the midspinous process of the upper vertebra to the superior margin of the spinous process of the lower vertebra at the involved level. This usually results in a 1-inch (25 to 30 mm) skin incision. This incision may need to be moved slightly higher for higher lumbar levels (Fig. 39-24).
- Maintain meticulous hemostasis with electrocautery as the dissection is carried to the fascia.
- Incise the fascia at the midline using electrocautery. Insert a periosteal elevator in the midline incision. Using gentle lateral movements, elevate the deep fascia and muscle subperiosteally from the spinous processes and lamina on the involved side only.
- Obtain a lateral radiograph with a metal clamp attached to the spinous process to verify the level.
- With a Cobb elevator, gently sweep the remaining muscular attachments off in a lateral direction to expose the interlaminar space and the edge of each lamina. A sharp elevator makes this task easier. Meticulously cauterize all bleeding points.
- Insert the appropriate length McCulloch-type retractor into the wound with the shorter spike medial and the flat blade lateral and adjust the microscope. Shaving down the flat blades of the retractor to produce a narrower retractor can help minimize the incision size and collateral soft-tissue damage.

APPROACH FOR USE OF TUBULAR RETRACTOR

- Alternatively, the approach can be made using a tubular retractor, which further minimizes damage to the paraspinal muscles and prevents detachment of the lumbodorsal fascia from the supraspinous ligament. A curved drill is required for visualization when drilling bone through the tubular retractor because of the narrower operating corridor.
- With fluoroscopic guidance, place an 18-gauge needle through the skin and into the paraspinous muscles with a trajectory toward the target disc space, approximately the radius of the final retractor diameter away from the edge of the spinous process (e.g., 9 mm off the edge of the spinous process if the ultimate tubular retractor diameter will be 18 mm) to prevent conflict between the spinous process and tubular retractor. It is essential that the needle be orthogonal with the target disc because it will be used to define the center of the tubular approach. Typically it is best to place the needle in line with the superior endplate of the caudal vertebral body, but that depends on the type of herniation and its location.
- Infiltrate the operative field (paraspinous muscle, subcutaneous tissue, and skin) with 10 mL of 0.25% bupivacaine with epinephrine for preemptive analgesia and hemostasis.
- Make a 20-mm long incision centered on the needle stick and place the blunt end of the guidewire just through the

lumbodorsal fascia. The younger and more fit the patient, the more force necessary to pop the blunt end of the guidewire through the fascia. Do not use the sharp end of the guidewire or advance the guidewire down to bone because it is very easy to pierce the interlaminar space and dural sac with the guidewire.

- Once the guidewire is through the fascia, advance the first pencil-shaped dilator through the fascia over the guidewire and use it to gently probe for the trailing edge of the cephalad lamina, which should feel like a bump at the end of the dilator. The guidewire can be removed as soon as the lumbodorsal fascia is pierced with the first dilator.
- Sequentially dilate down to bone with enlarging tubular retractors to expose the interlaminar space. Each dilator can be used as a curet to remove soft-tissue attachments from the interlaminar space.
- Mount the final tubular retractor to a stationary arm attached to the table and obtain a final fluoroscopic image to confirm the location of the retractor orthogonal with the target disc space before bringing in the microscope and adjusting the field of view. We prefer 14 to 16 mm diameter tubular retractors for this approach, depending on the size of the patient and the level of surgical experience with this technique. Tubular retractors in the 18- to 24-mm diameter range can be used when first becoming familiar with this approach.

From this point on, the surgical technique is essentially the same for both approaches.

- Identify the ligamentum flavum and lamina. Use a curet to elevate the superficial leaf of the ligamentum flavum from the leading edge of the caudal lamina.
- Use a Kerrison rongeur to resect the superficial leaf of the ligamentum flavum to allow identification of the critical angle, which is junction of the leading edge of the caudal lamina and the medial edge of the superior articular process. Identifying the critical angle is essential in primary microlumbar discectomy because it has a constant relationship to the corresponding pedicle, traversing nerve root, and target disc. The pedicle is always just lateral to the critical angle, the traversing nerve is always just medial to the pedicle, and the disc of interest is always just cephalad to the critical angle and pedicle. It sometimes is necessary to drill the medial aspect of the inferior articular process to allow adequate visualization of the critical angle.
- Use a high-speed drill to remove the trailing edge of the cephalad lamina up to the insertion of the ligamentum flavum to allow easier and more complete removal of the ligament, keeping in mind that the ligament attaches to the lamina as you move medially. This makes initially detaching the ligament from the undersurface of the cephalad lamina with an angled curet much easier toward the midline.
- After the lateral portion of the ligamentum flavum has been detached from the caudal edge of the superior lamina and the cephalad edge of the inferior lamina with a curet, use a blunt dissector to lift the edge of the ligamentum flavum so that it can be excised with a Kerrison rongeur. Take care to orient the rongeur parallel to the nerve root as much as possible. The goal when resecting the ligamentum flavum should be removal in one piece, which prevents nibbling away at it while trying to grab and mop end with the rongeur. En bloc removal is made easier by using the rongeur to remove some bone along with the lateral edge of the ligamentum flavum from caudal to cephalad, starting at the critical angle and working up the medial edge of the superior articular process where the ligamentum flavum attaches (Fig. 39-25).
- Once the ligamentum flavum is removed, the medial wall of the corresponding pedicle should be palpable with a nerve hook or angled dissector. If not, more bone may need to be removed lateral to the critical angle. Once the medial wall of the corresponding pedicle is identified, the traversing nerve can be found just medial to it and the target disc can be found just cephalad to it.
- When the nerve root is identified, carefully mobilize the root medially. Gently dissect the nerve free from the disc fragment to avoid excessive traction on the root. Bipolar cautery for hemostasis is helpful. When mobilized, retract the root medially. If the root is difficult to mobilize, consider that a conjoined root may be present
- Make a gentle extradural exploration beneath the nerve with a 90-degree blunt hook, taking care not to tear the

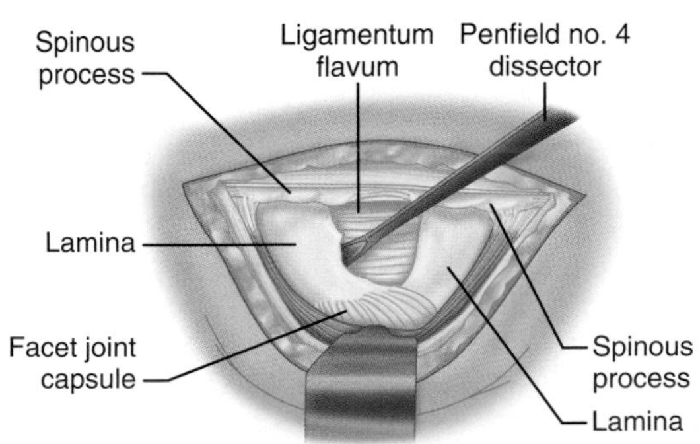

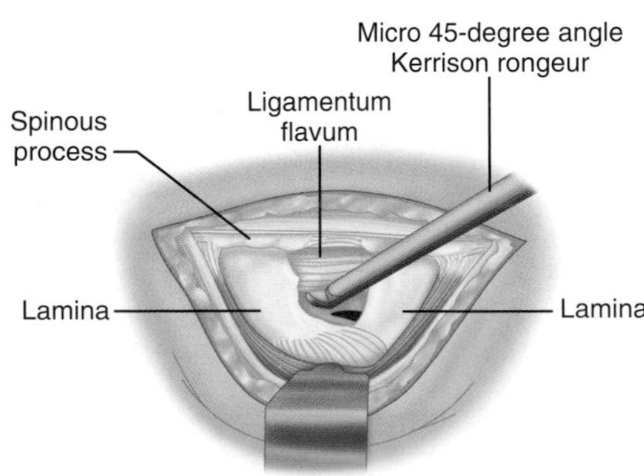

FIGURE 39-25 **Entrance to epidural space by detachment of ligamentum flavum.** (From Gardocki RG: Microscopic lumbar discectomy. In Canale ST, Beaty JH, Azar FM, editors: Campbell's Core Procedures, Philadelphia, Elsevier, 2016.) **SEE TECHNIQUE 39-15.**

dura. The small opening and magnification can make the edge of the dural sac appear to be the nerve root.

- When using bipolar cautery, ensure that only one side is in contact with the nerve root to avoid thermal injury to the nerve. Epidural fat is not removed in this procedure.
- Insert the suction/nerve root retractor with its tip turned medially under the nerve root and hold the manifold between the thumb and index finger. With the nerve root retracted, the disc is now visible as a white, fibrous, avascular structure. Under magnification, small tears may be visible in the annulus.
- Enlarge the annular tear with a Penfield no. 4 dissector and remove the disc material with the appropriate-sized pituitary rongeur. Do not insert the instrument into the disc space beyond the angle of the jaws, usually about 15 mm, to minimize the risk of anterior perforation and vascular injury. Downward pressure on the adjacent intact annulus can sometimes help express loose disc fragments from the subannular space (Fig. 39-26).
- Remove the exposed disc material. Remove additional loose disc or cartilage fragments. Inspect the root and adjacent dura for disc fragments. Forcefully irrigate the disc space using a Luer-Lok syringe and an unused no. 8 suction tip inserted into the disc space. Maintain meticulous hemostasis.
- The discectomy is complete when (1) the lateral recess is adequately decompressed; (2) the 90-degree dissection can be probed to the back of the cephalad vertebral body, the disc space, and the back of the caudal vertebral body out to the midline without any protrusions into the canal; (3) the 90-degree dissector can be spun (helicopter maneuver) beneath the traversing nerve root without any restrictions; and (4) the traversing nerve root is freely retractable both medially and laterally. It is comforting to see the dura pulsate with the heartbeat and expand and contract with respiration, but these findings alone do not indicate an adequate discectomy and decompression.
- If the expected pathologic process is not found, review preoperative imaging studies for the correct level and side. Also obtain a repeat radiograph or fluoroscopic image with a metallic marker at the disc level to verify the level. Be aware of bony anomalies that may alter the numbering of the vertebrae on imaging studies.
- Close the fascia and the skin in the usual fashion using absorbable sutures if using the McCulloch retractor. When using a tubular retraction, it can simply be removed and the skin closed subcutaneously because the lumbodorsal fascia will seal itself like Chinese finger cuffs when the paraspinous muscles contract, because the lumbodorsal fascia was only dilated between its fibers and not incised.

POSTOPERATIVE CARE. Postoperative care is similar to that after standard open disc surgery. Typically this procedure is done on an outpatient basis. Injecting the paraspinal muscles on the involved side with bupivacaine 0.25% with epinephrine at the beginning of the procedure and additional bupivacaine at the conclusion aids patient mobilization immediately postoperatively. We prefer to use a skin glue product for final skin closure without the use of dressing and allow the patient to shower the day of surgery. Activity can be allowed as tolerated once the skin incision is healed, typically in 2 weeks.

ADDITIONAL EXPOSURE TECHNIQUES

A large disc herniation or other pathologic condition, such as lateral recess stenosis or foraminal stenosis, may require a greater exposure of the nerve root. The additional pathologic condition usually can be identified before surgery. If the extent of the lesion is known before surgery, the proper approach can be planned. Additional exposure includes hemilaminectomy, total laminectomy, and facetectomy. Hemilaminectomy usually is required when identifying the root as a problem. This may occur with a conjoined root. Total laminectomy usually is reserved for patients with spinal stenoses that are central, which occur typically in cauda equina syndrome. Facetectomy usually is reserved for foraminal stenosis or severe lateral recess stenosis. If more than one facet is removed, a fusion should be considered in addition. This is especially true in the removal of facets and the disc at

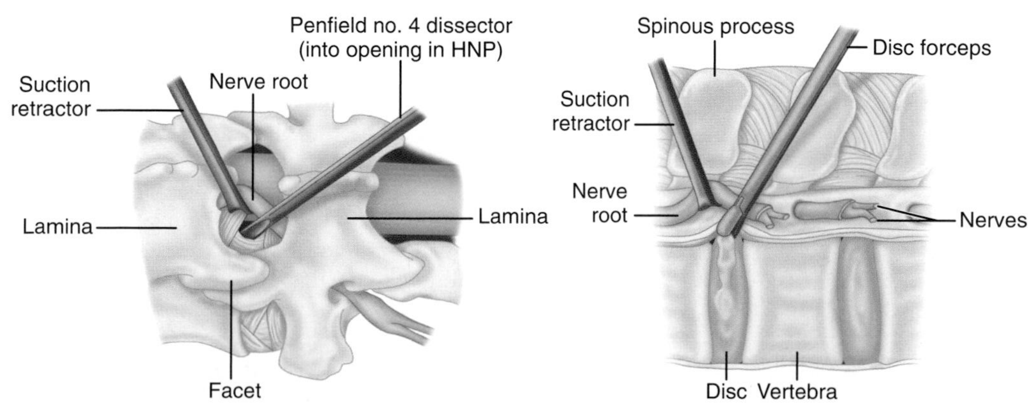

FIGURE 39-26 **Dilation of annular defect to facilitate disc fragment removal.** (From Gardocki RG: Microscopic lumbar discectomy. In Canale ST, Beaty JH, Azar FM, editors: Campbell's Core Procedures, Philadelphia, Elsevier, 2016.) **SEE TECHNIQUE 39-15.**

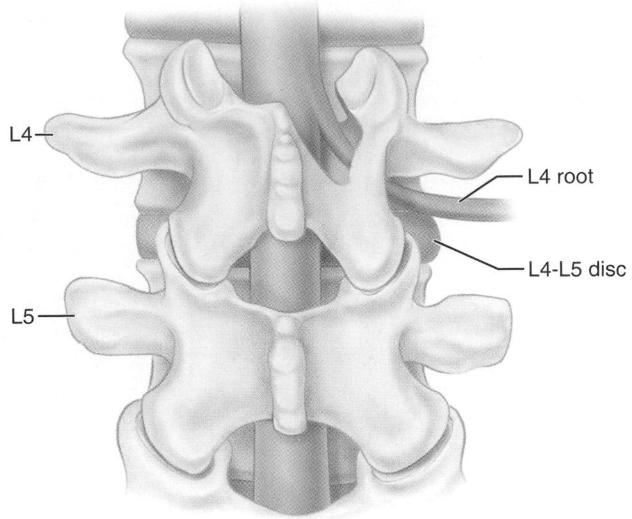

FIGURE 39-27 Lateral approach for discectomy. L4 foraminotomy allows exposure of root.

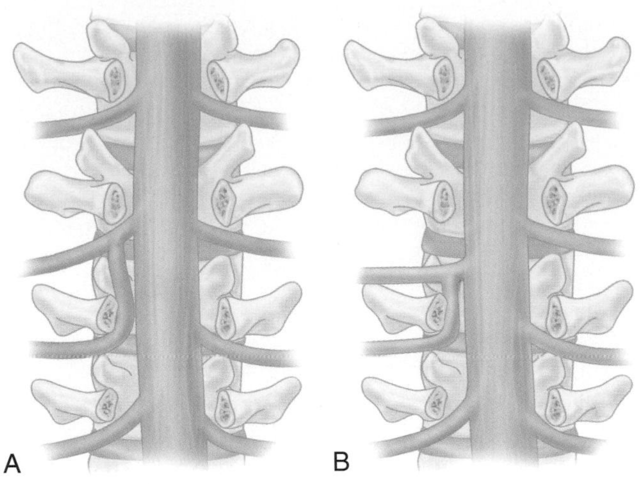

FIGURE 39-28 **A,** Type 1A conjoined nerve root. **B,** Type 1B conjoined nerve root.

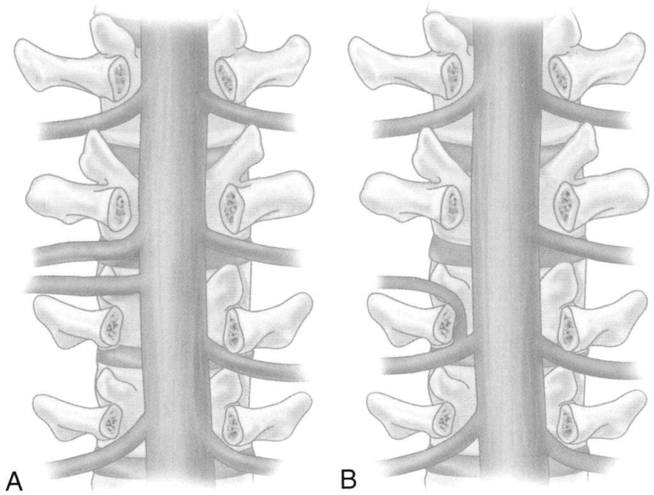

FIGURE 39-29 **A,** Type 2A conjoined nerve root. **B,** Type 2B conjoined nerve root.

the same interspace in a young, active individual with a normal disc height at that level.

Rarely, disc herniation has been reported to be intradural. An extremely large disc that cannot be dissected from the dura or the persistence of an intradural mass after dissection of the disc should alert one to this potential problem. Excision of an intradural disc requires a transdural approach, which increases the risk of complications from cerebrospinal fluid leak and intradural scarring.

A disc that is far lateral may require exposure outside the spinal canal (Fig. 39-27). This area is approached by removing the intertransverse ligament between the superior and inferior transverse processes lateral to the spinal canal. The disc hernia usually is anterior to the nerve root that is found in a mass of fat below the intertransverse ligament. A microsurgical approach is a good method for dealing with this problem. A long tubular retractor is especially useful for the far lateral approach if the tube is inserted at the proper trajectory to address the pathology in or lateral to the foramen. If the facet is not hypertrophic and the plane between the facet joint capsule and intertransverse ligament can be identified, foraminal and far lateral disc herniations can sometimes be removed without bony resection above the L5 level.

LUMBAR ROOT ANOMALIES

Several different types of nerve root anomalies are relatively common in anatomic studies but less common with imaging studies, which suggest they are underrecognized clinically. These congenital anomalies may account for a portion of the poor results from lumbar disc surgery because the abnormal and unrecognized roots may be injured. This is of even more concern with some minimally invasive techniques with less direct nerve visualization.

Conjoined nerve roots are the most common type of anomaly. Various anatomic studies show some type of conjoined root in 14% to 17% of cadavers. Clinical studies using advanced imaging, such as myelography or MRI, show conjoined roots in only 2% to 5% of patients. Conjoined roots have been classified anatomically (Figs. 39-28 to 39-31). There are three classes, the first two of which are subdivided. Type 1 occurs when two roots exit the dura with one common sheath. With type 1A anomalies, the cephalad root departs the conjoined stalk at an acute angle to exit below the appropriate pedicle, and the caudal root travels within the canal to exit also below the appropriate pedicle. If the cephalad root exits at 90 degrees from the conjoined portion, this is a type 1B anomaly. Type 2 anomalies occur when two roots exit through a single foramen. Type 2A anomalies have one vacant foramen; type 2B anomalies have a portion of one of the roots exiting via the other foramen, which may be cephalad to the foramen occupied by the two nerve roots. Type 3 anomalies occur when there is an anastomosing branch between two adjacent nerve roots. This branch crosses the disc space and can easily be injured during discectomy.

These root anomalies can cause false-positive interpretations of imaging studies and can be confused with disc bulges

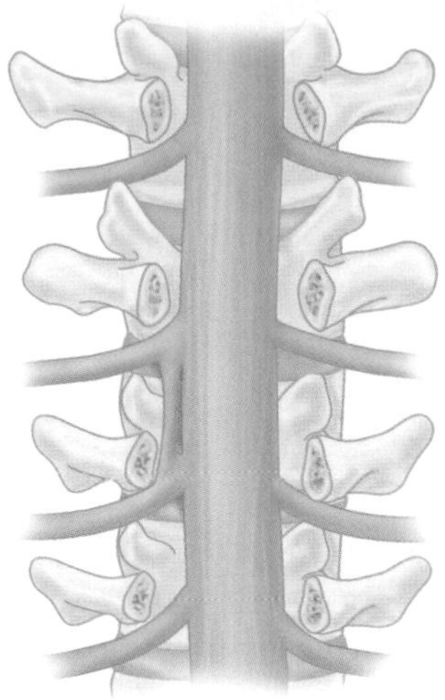

FIGURE 39-30 Type 3 conjoined nerve root.

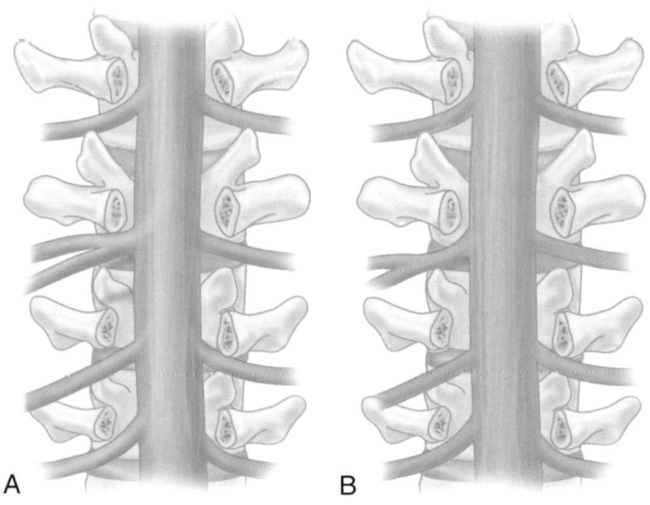

FIGURE 39-31 A and B, Furcal nerve root.

or herniations. Particularly if the herniation appears in an atypical location, such as near the pedicle, or if the signal intensity is different from disc material, a diagnosis of a conjoined root should be considered. Also, if a patient presents with a history of failed disc surgery, this diagnosis should be considered. The anomalous roots not only can be divided inadvertently but also can be injured by excessive tension because the conjoined roots usually are less mobile than normal roots. The most common location for conjoined roots involves the L5 and S1 levels. A second type of anomaly that may be as common as conjoined roots is a furcal nerve root; this refers to a bifurcation of a single nerve root. Often furcal roots are bilateral and can occur at multiple levels. Increased awareness of these anomalies is important to reduce the risk of nerve injury and to avoid surgery with an incorrect diagnosis of disc herniations. Surgical outcomes in patients with conjoined roots tend to be significantly worse than in the general population.

RESULTS OF SURGERY FOR DISC HERNIATION

Numerous retrospective and some prospective reviews of open disc surgery are available. The results of these series vary greatly with respect to patient selection, treatment method, evaluation method, length of follow-up, and conclusions. Good results range from 46% to 97%. Complications range from none to more than 10%. The reoperation rate ranges from 4% to more than 20%. A comparison between techniques also reveals similar results. There is no particular technique of discectomy that yields consistently superior results. Technical procedural differences are of minimal importance with regard to outcome.

Several points stand out in the analysis of the results of lumbar disc surgery. Patient selection seems to be crucial. Several studies noted that a low educational level is significantly correlated to poor results of surgery. Valid results of the Minnesota Multiphasic Personality Inventory (MMPI) (hysteria and hypochondriasis T-scores) appear to be good indicators of surgical outcome regardless of the degree of the pathologic condition. The duration of the current episode, the age of the patient, the presence or absence of predominant back pain, the number of previous hospitalizations, and the presence or absence of compensation for a work injury have been identified as factors affecting final outcome. In the latest report on lumbar disc herniation (2008) from the multicenter Spine Patient Outcomes Research Trial (SPORT), operative was compared with nonoperative treatment in 501 patients and additional observational cohorts (743 participants). The results were overwhelmingly in favor of surgery: patients treated operatively had far less pain, better physical function, and less disability than patients who did not have surgery. The validity of the conclusions generated by SPORT has been questioned because of the high crossover rates in the randomized intent-to-treat studies and the variability of the patient population, nonoperative treatments, and operative procedures. The finding of durability of operative results (4-year follow-up), however, is important. In a later study of patients with degenerative spondylolisthesis and spinal stenosis who had operative treatment, those with predominant leg pain had a better prognosis than those with predominant back pain.

■ COMPLICATIONS OF DISC EXCISION

The complications associated with standard disc excision and micro lumbar disc excision are similar. One large series (Table 39-2) of 2503 open disc excisions listed a postoperative mortality of 0.1%, a thromboembolism rate of 1%, a postoperative infection rate of 3.2%, and a deep disc space infection rate of 1.1%. Postoperative cauda equina lesions developed in five patients. Laceration of the major vascular structures also has been described as a rare complication of this operation. Dural tears with CSF leaks, pseudomeningocele formation, CSF fistula formation, and meningitis also are possible but are more likely after reoperation. The complications of micro lumbar disc excision seem to be less than with standard laminectomy.

In a retrospective review of 1326 patients who had spinal surgery, 51 dural tears (4%) were identified; 48 of these occurred with a posterior thoracolumbar approach. The presence of a dural tear or leak results in the potentially serious

TABLE 39-2

Complications of Lumbar Disc Surgery

COMPLICATION	INCIDENCE (%)
Cauda equina syndrome	0.2
Thrombophlebitis	1
Pulmonary embolism	0.4
Wound infection	2.2
Pyogenic spondylitis	0.07
Postoperative discitis	2 (1122 patients)
Dural tears	1.6
Nerve root injury	0.5
Cerebrospinal fluid fistula	*
Laceration of abdominal vessels	*
Injury to abdominal viscera	*

*Rare occurrence (nos. 10 and 11 not identified in Spangfort's study, but reported elsewhere).

(Modified from Spangfort EV: The lumbar disc herniation: a computer-aided analysis of 2504 operations, Acta Orthop Scand Suppl 142:1, 1972.)

problems of pseudomeningocele, CSF leak, and meningitis. Eismont, Wiesel, and Rothman suggested five basic principles in the repair of these leaks (Fig. 39-32):

1. The operative field must be unobstructed, dry, and well exposed.
2. Dural suture of a 4-0 or 6-0 gauge with a tapered or reverse cutting needle is used in a simple or a running locking stitch. If the leak is large or inaccessible, a free fat graft or fascial graft can be sutured to the dura. Fibrin glue applied to the repair also is helpful but used alone does not seal a significant leak.
3. All repairs should be tested by using the reverse Trendelenburg position and Valsalva maneuvers.
4. Paraspinous muscles and overlying fascia should be closed in two layers with nonabsorbable suture used in a watertight fashion. Drains should not be used.
5. Bed rest in the supine position should be maintained for 4 to 7 days after the repair of lumbar dural defects. A lumbar drain should be placed if the integrity of the closure is questionable.

The development of headaches on standing and a stormy postoperative period should alert one to the possibility of an undetected CSF leak. This can be confirmed by MRI.

The presence of glucose in drainage fluid is an unreliable diagnostic test. Rarely, a pseudomeningocele has been implicated as a cause of persistent pain from pressure on a nerve root by the cystic mass. In our experience, these principles are valid with the exception of maintaining bed rest. With good closure, patients can be mobilized the day after surgery. If closure is not watertight, extended bed rest with a drain may be helpful.

One of the advantages of tubular lumbar discectomy with an 18-mm or smaller diameter tube is in the treatment of small dural tears. Because the dead space is so small, these tears usually can be treated simply with fibrin glue when there is no root herniation. We follow the usual postoperative course in patients who have tubular discectomy with dural repair using fibrin glue as long as there are no postoperative headaches or symptoms of meningeal irritation. A 3-day course of acetazolamide (Diamox) is prescribed, which acts as a chemical drain by decreasing CSF production in the choroid plexus by inhibiting carbonic anhydrase. This is the same course of Diamox prescribed for acute mountain (altitude) sickness. Patients are advised to lie flat for 72 hours after surgery only if they have positional headaches.

BOX 39-5

Fibrin Glue

Ingredients

Two vials of topical thrombin, 10,000 U each
10 mL of calcium chloride
5 U of cryoprecipitate
Two 5-mL syringes
Two 22-gauge spinal needles

Instructions

1. Do not use saline that comes with thrombin.
2. Mix thrombin and calcium chloride.
3. Draw mixture into syringe.
4. Draw cryoprecipitate into second syringe.
5. Apply equal amounts to area of need.
6. Allow to set to a "Jello" consistency.

DURAL REPAIR AUGMENTED WITH FIBRIN GLUE

Dural repair can be augmented with fibrin glue. Pressure testing of a dural repair without fibrin glue reveals that the dura is able to withstand 10 mm of pressure on day 1 and 28 mm on day 7. With fibrin glue, the dura is able to withstand 28 mm on day 1 and 31 mm on day 7. Fibrin glue also can be used in areas of troublesome bleeding or difficult access for closure, such as the ventral aspect of the dura. Fibrin glue is an adjunct for closure, and every effort should be made for primary closure, even if fibrin glue is to be used. However, fibrin glue tends to be sufficient in the setting of a transmuscular approach using a tubular retractor because the amount of dead space is significantly limited and dural leaks can be tamponaded with fibrin glue alone.

TECHNIQUE 39-16

- Mix 20,000 U of topical thrombin and 10 mL of calcium chloride and draw the mixture up into a syringe.
- In another syringe, draw 5 U of cryoprecipitate, and simultaneously inject equal quantities of each onto the dural repair or tear.
- Allow the glue to set to the consistency of "Jello" (Box 39-5). Commercially available kits also are available.

■ FREE FAT GRAFTING

Fat grafting for the prevention of postoperative epidural scarring has been shown to be superior to Gelfoam in the

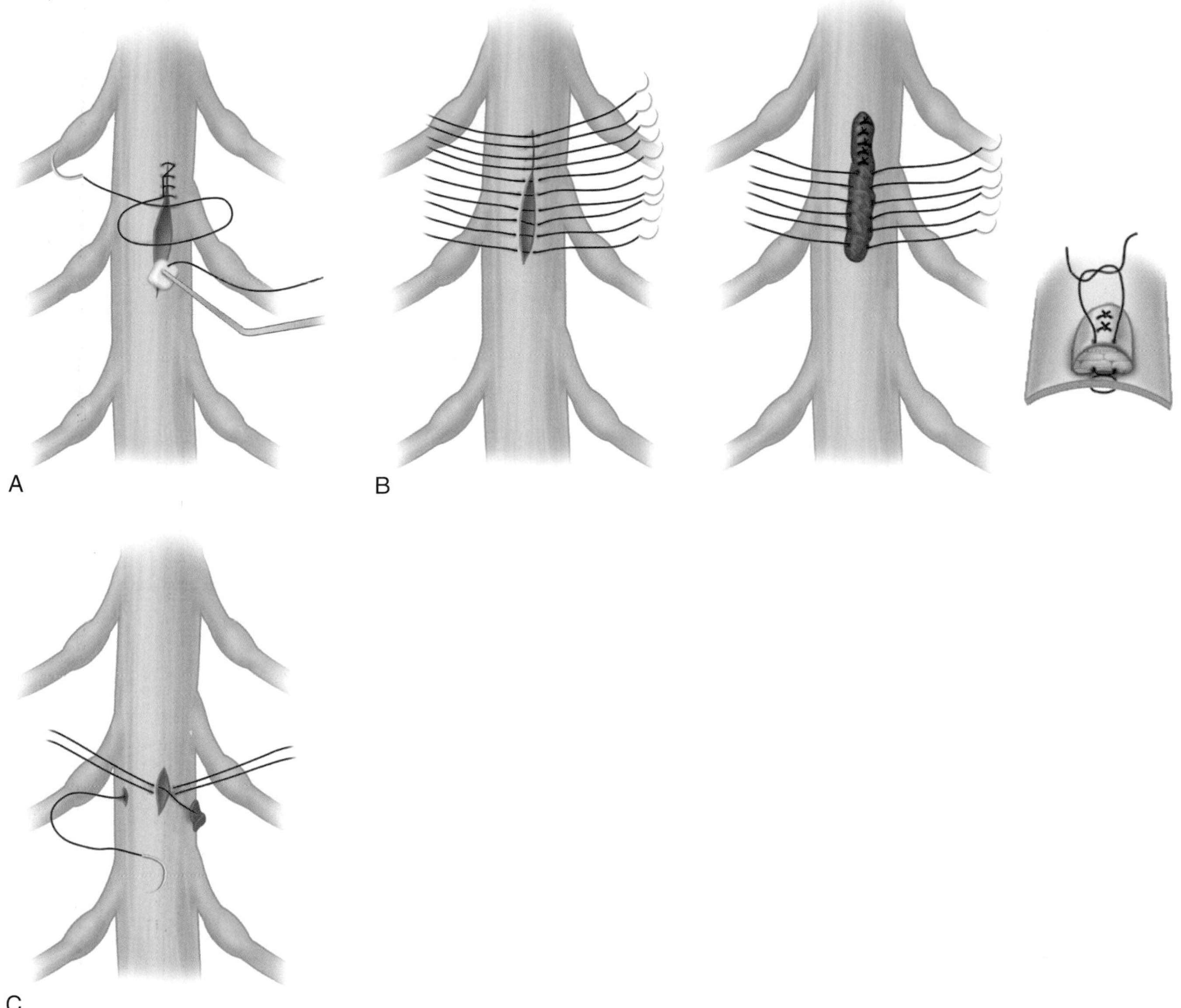

FIGURE 39-32 **A,** Dural repair using running-locking dural suture on taper or reverse-cutting, one-half-circle needle. Smaller sized suture should be used. Use of suction with sucker and small cotton pledgets is essential to protect nerve roots while operative field is kept dry of cerebrospinal fluid. **B,** Single dural stitches can be used to achieve closure, each suture end being left long. Second needle is attached to free suture end, and ends of suture are passed through piece of muscle or fat, which is tied down over repaired tear to help achieve watertight closure. Whenever dural material is inadequate to allow closure without placing excessive pressure on underlying neural tissues, free graft of fascia or fascia lata or freeze-dried dural graft should be secured to margins of dural tear using simple sutures of appropriate size. **C,** For small dural defects in relatively inaccessible areas, transdural approach can be used to pull small piece of muscle or fat into defect from inside out, sealing cerebrospinal fluid leak. Central durotomy should be large enough to expose defect from dural sac. Durotomy is closed in standard watertight fashion.

prevention of postoperative scarring. The current rationale for free fat grafting seems to be the possibility of making any reoperation easier. Neither the benefit of reduced scarring and its relationship to the prevention of postoperative pain nor the increased ease of reoperation in patients in whom fat grafting was performed has been established. Caution should be taken in applying a fat graft to a large laminar defect because this has been reported to result in an acute cauda equina syndrome in the early postoperative period. We currently reserve the use of a fat graft (or fascial grafts) for dural repairs and small laminar defects where the graft is supported by the bone. A study by Jensen et al. found that fat grafts decreased dural scarring but not radicular scar formation. The clinical outcome was not improved.

The technique of free fat grafting is straightforward. At the end of the procedure, just before the incision is closed, take a large piece of subcutaneous fat and insert it over the laminectomy defect. If the patient is thin, a separate incision over the buttock may be required to obtain sufficient fat to fill the defect.

REPEAT LUMBAR DISC SURGERY

Making the diagnosis of recurrent disc herniation is significantly more difficult than that of primary disc herniation. The clinical presentation may be identical to that of primary herniation but usually has a larger component of axial pain. Most recurrences happen in the relatively early postoperative period, primarily the first 6 months after surgery. To date, no operative technique has been shown to reduce the incidence of recurrent disc herniations, which is reported in 3% to 7% of patients. Specifically, more aggressive disc removal does not reduce this complication and may be detrimental to the function of the motion segment. MRI with intravascular contrast material has been helpful in identifying recurrent herniations. It is difficult, however, to distinguish a peridural scar from a small recurrent herniation. For patients with a history of no or minimal improvement after disc excision, the diagnostic difficulties are even greater. A possible incorrect original diagnosis, incorrect level, root anomaly, root injury, CSF leak, and infection must be considered in addition to recurrent disc herniation.

With regard to surgery for recurrent herniation, the principles of identifying and protecting the nerve root and then removing the herniation are the same as for a primary discectomy. The area of exposure generally should be larger, although usually the procedure still can be done on an outpatient basis.

REPEAT LUMBAR DISC EXCISION

TECHNIQUE 39-17

This procedure is most often used for recurrent herniation but can be used in primary disc excisions.

- After thoroughly preparing the back, identify the spinous processes of L3, L4, L5, and S1 by palpation. Inject 25 mL of 0.25% bupivacaine with epinephrine into the paraspinal muscles on the involved side.
- Make a midline incision 4 cm long, centered over the interspace where the disc herniation is located. Incise the supraspinous ligament; by subperiosteal dissection, strip the muscles from the spinous processes and laminae of these vertebrae on the side of the lesion.
- Retract the muscles with a self-retaining retractor, or with the help of an assistant, and expose one interspace at a time.
- Verify the location with a radiograph so that no mistake is made regarding the interspaces explored.
- Secure hemostasis with electrocautery, bone wax, and packs. Leave a portion of each pack completely outside the wound for ready identification.
- Identify normal tissue first. Use a curet to remove scar from the edges of the laminae carefully. Remove additional bone as necessary to expose normal dura.
- Identify the pedicles superiorly and inferiorly if there is any question of position and status of the root. Carry the dissection from the pedicles to identify each root; this may allow the development of a normal plane between the dura and scar. This requires patience, and small curets or Penfield dissectors work best. Maintain meticulous hemostasis with bipolar cautery.
- Once the lateral edge of the root is identified, it is often helpful to mobilize the root and epidural scar as a single mass off the floor of the canal using a curet, which will sometimes uncover the underlying disc herniation.
- Remove the disc herniation and explore the axilla of the root and the subligamentous space for retained fragments. Also, ensure that the nerve root is well decompressed in the lateral recess.
- Spinal fusion is not done unless an unstable spine is created by the dissection or was identified preoperatively as a correctable and symptomatic problem.
- If the initial procedure was done using the tubular retractor technique (see Technique 39-15), a tubular retractor is used for recurrent disc herniations

POSTOPERATIVE CARE. Postoperative care is the same as after disc excision (see Technique 39-15).

DISC EXCISION AND FUSION

The necessity of lumbar fusion at the same time as disc excision was first suggested by Mixter and Barr. In the first 20 years after their discovery the combination of disc excision and lumbar fusion was common. More recent data comparing disc excision alone with the combination of disc excision and fusion indicate that there is little, if any, advantage to the addition of a spinal fusion to the treatment of simple disc herniation. These studies indicate that spinal fusion increases the complication rate and lengthens recovery. The indications for lumbar fusion should be independent of the indications for disc excision for radiculopathy.

THORACIC AND LUMBAR SPINE ARTHRODESIS

Arthrodesis of the lumbosacral region is done for degenerative, traumatic, and congenital lesions. Indications for and techniques of spinal fusion and care after surgery vary from one orthopaedic center to another. Many orthopaedists prefer posterior arthrodesis, usually some modification of the intertransverse process type fusion, using a large quantity of autogenous iliac bone. Internal fixation can be used with posterior arthrodesis. Before the use of instrumentation, the current status of the implant—its risks and indications and approval by the FDA—should be reviewed carefully and completely with the patient. Posterolateral or intertransverse process fusions are used most frequently, either alone or occasionally in combination with an anterior fusion and with or without posterior internal fixation. Interbody fusions from posterior, anterior, retroperitoneal, or transperitoneal approaches are preferred by other orthopaedic surgeons.

For lumbar fusion, the best technique for a particular patient remains controversial. The decision should be based on the pathologic entity being treated, expected applicable biomechanics and healing potential of different constructs, and the surgeon's experience. With regard to the pathologic entity, consideration must be given to the spinal column and the neural elements. In this way the proper balance can be obtained between the need for possible increased instability from neural decompression and strategies to increase stability to promote fusion. After determining the optimal operative plan for a particular patient, additional controversy exists regarding the best technique to execute the plan, that is, an open technique versus a minimally invasive approach.

ANTERIOR ARTHRODESIS

TRANSTHORACIC APPROACH TO THE THORACIC SPINE

For anterior arthrodesis of the thoracic spine, a transthoracic approach provides direct access to the vertebral bodies T2 to T12. The midthoracic vertebral bodies are best exposed by this approach, whereas views of the upper and lower extremes of the spine are more limited.

TECHNIQUE 39-18

- Approach the involved vertebra as described in Chapter 37.
- Remove the disc material at the confirmed level with sharp dissection in the outer two thirds of the disc.
- Carefully remove the remaining disc material with Kerrison rongeurs and curets using magnification.
- With the disc removed and the canal free of all obstructions, prepare the endplates by removing the cartilage without penetrating the cortical bone.
- Insert tricortical bone graft, prepared structural allograft, or a bone cage as desired.
- Internal fixation may be added as necessary.
- Close the chest cavity in layers over a chest tube.

POSTOPERATIVE CARE. The patient is allowed to ambulate rapidly after the procedure. The chest tube is removed once drainage is minimal and there is no air leak. Initially a removable brace such as a Jewett brace or thoracolumbosacral orthosis can be used for ambulation. The brace can be discontinued as pain relief improves and radiographic union is noted.

Numerous indications for anterior arthrodesis of the lumbar spine are reported in the literature. At this clinic the indications include debridement of infection, tuberculosis, excision of tumors, correction of kyphosis, scoliosis, neural decompression after fracture, and to achieve stability when posterior arthrodesis is not feasible. Less frequently, we have used this technique in the treatment of spondylolisthesis or internal intervertebral disc derangements. The surgical approach used in tuberculosis by Hodgson and Stock should be applicable in most instances (see Chapter 42).

ANTERIOR DISC EXCISION AND INTERBODY FUSION OF THE LUMBAR SPINE

The rationale of management of lower back pain must be based on an accurate diagnosis. The pain syndromes in this area are many, and diagnostic pitfalls are ever present. Treatment varies according to the physical and emotional profile of the patient and the experience of the surgeon involved. Hemilaminectomy and decompression of nerve roots still constitute the most widely used surgical procedure for unremitting lower back pain. With continued instability of the anterior and posterior elements, supplemental posterior or posterolateral fusion usually proves satisfactory.

There is a group of patients for whom standard surgical procedures are unsuccessful. The following causes of persistent symptoms after disc surgery have been identified:

- Mistaken original diagnosis
- Recurrent herniation of disc material (also incomplete removal)
- Herniation of disc at another level
- Bony compression of nerve root
- Perineural adhesions
- Instability of vertebral segments
- Psychoneurosis

In this group, improved diagnostic accuracy currently can be obtained with the use of electromyography, a psychologic profile assessment, postmyelographic CT, MRI with and without gadolinium contrast, and possibly discography. Finally, differential spinal anesthesia is helpful in discriminating between the various pain types.

As a rule, failure of the usual posterior methods of fusion to relieve pain in the presence of a solid arthrodesis and in the absence of other pathology as listed earlier dictates consideration of anterior intervertebral disc excision and interbody spinal fusion. The reported outcomes of anterior interbody fusion have been variable, with success rates ranging from 36% to 90%. Although reports of long-term results are inconclusive, pain relief appears to be obtained in 80% to 90% of patients.

Suggested indications include (1) instability causing backache and sciatica, (2) spondylolisthesis of all types, (3) pain after multiple posterior explorations, and (4) failed posterior fusions. Good results have been reported with the use of three iliac wedge grafts for degenerative disease and a block graft for spondylolisthesis (Fig. 39-33).

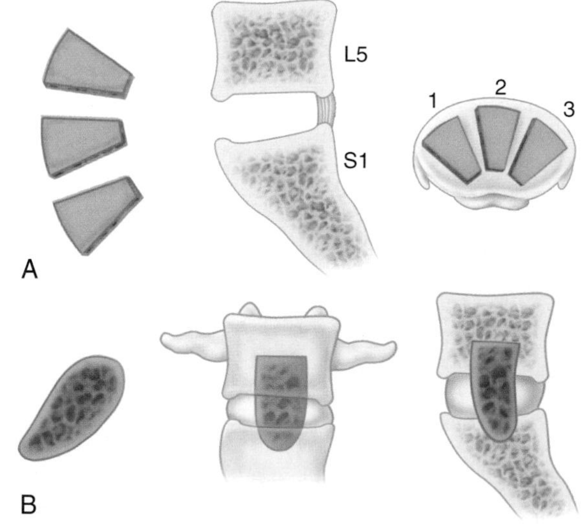

FIGURE 39-33 Freebody technique for anterior interbody fusion in lower lumbar spine. **A,** Technique for degenerative disease. **B,** Technique for spondylolisthesis.

ANTERIOR INTERBODY FUSION OF THE LUMBAR SPINE

TECHNIQUE 39-19

(GOLDNER ET AL.)

- Administer general anesthesia and place the patient in the Trendelenburg position.
- Develop the retroperitoneal approach to the vertebral bodies and identify the psoas muscle, the iliac artery and vein, and the left ureter. If more than three interspaces are to be fused, retract the ureter toward the left.
- Identify the sacral promontory by palpation.
- Inject saline solution under the prevertebral fascia over the lumbar vertebra and lift the sympathetic chain for easier dissection.
- Expose the lumbosacral disc space by retracting the left iliac artery and vein to the left.
- In exposing the fourth lumbar interspace, displace the left artery and vein and ureter to the right side.
- Elevate the anterior longitudinal ligament as a flap with the base toward the left.
- Tag the flap with sutures and retract it to give additional protection to the vessels.
- Separate the intervertebral disc and annulus from the cartilaginous endplates of the vertebrae with a thin osteotome and remove them with pituitary rongeurs and large curets.
- Clean the space thoroughly back to the posterior longitudinal ligament without removing bone, thereby keeping bleeding to a minimum until the site is ready for grafting.
- Remove the cartilaginous endplates from the vertebral bodies with an osteotome until bleeding bone is encountered.
- Cut shallow notches in the opposing surfaces of the vertebrae and measure the dimensions of the notches carefully with a caliper.
- Cut grafts from the iliac wing, making them larger than the notches for later firm impaction (Fig. 39-34).
- Hyperextend the spine, insert multiple grafts, and relieve the hyperextension.
- Bipolar electrocautery is useful in obtaining hemostasis, but take care not to coagulate the sympathetic fibers over the anterior aspect of the lumbosacral joint. Use of silver clips in this area is preferred.
- After completion of the fusion, close all layers with absorbable sutures.
- Estimate the amount of blood lost and replace it.

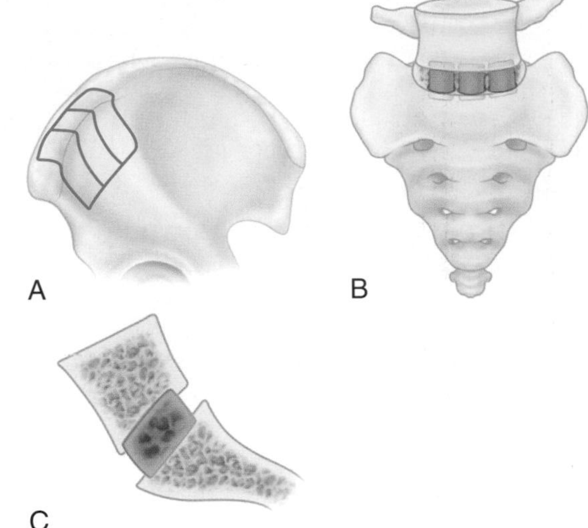

FIGURE 39-34 Technique of Goldner et al. for anterior interbody fusion of lumbosacral joint. **SEE TECHNIQUE 39-19.**

POSTOPERATIVE CARE. Nasogastric suction may be necessary for gastric decompression for about 36 hours. Attention must be paid to mobilization of the lower extremities to prevent dependency and blood pooling. Thigh-length hose for prevention of thromboembolic disease, intermittent compression boots, and low-molecular-weight heparin all are used for deep vein thrombosis prophylaxis. In-bed exercises with straight-leg raising are started on the first postoperative day and continued indefinitely. The patient is allowed to sit and walk with a low back corset used for postoperative immobilization as tolerated. Postoperative radiographs are made before discharge from the hospital to serve as a baseline for judging graft appearance. Three months later, side-bending and flexion and extension radiographs are made in the standing position to provide information about the success of arthrodesis. Radiographs are then repeated at 6 and 12 months after surgery, with the solid fusion not confirmed until 1 year after surgery. Tomograms may be useful in evaluating suspected pseudarthrosis.

We have used a retroperitoneal approach to L2, L3, L4, and L5 discs. For the L5 or lumbosacral disc, some prefer a transperitoneal approach if good anterior access is needed. The incidence of deep venous thrombosis after these approaches, especially the midline transperitoneal approach, is much higher than after ordinary spinal surgery. Suitable prophylaxis is indicated, even though it may not be successful in preventing this complication.

MINIMALLY INVASIVE ANTERIOR FUSION OF THE LUMBAR SPINE

In the fields of general surgery and thoracic surgery, the development of laparoscopic surgical techniques and VATS has allowed significant improvements to be made with respect to decreasing pain, duration of hospitalization, and recovery times for a variety of procedures (Fig. 39-35). Similarly, laparoscopic and VATS techniques have been applied to anterior spine surgery with significant improvements in these same areas. VATS is described in Technique 39-13. We have limited experience with this technique; currently it is seldom used because of the risk of catastrophic complications.

Laparoscopic transperitoneal lumbar instrumentation and fusion also has been developed, and several systems are

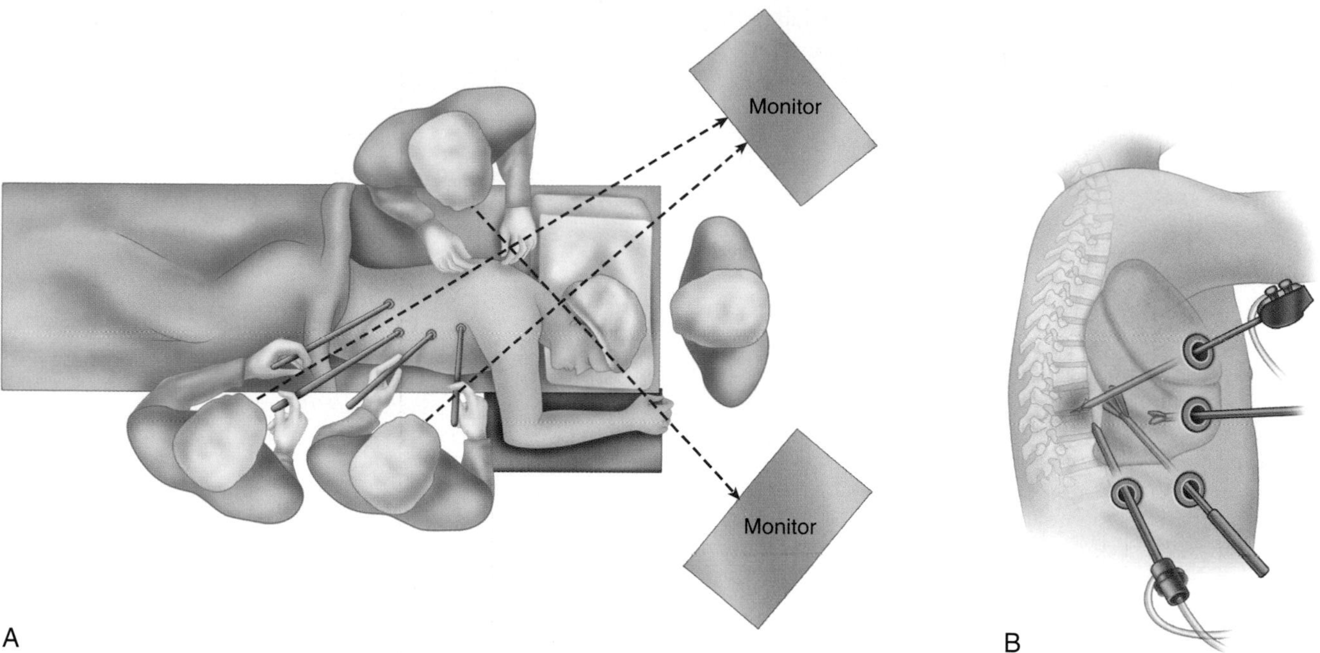

FIGURE 39-35 Video-assisted thoracic surgery is used for anterior release and interbody fusion. **A,** Patient positioned in left lateral decubitus position and portal positions marked. **B,** Portals.

currently available. These systems allow disc removal and insertion of threaded cylindrical devices, as well as trapezoidal cages packed with autogenous bone into the disc spaces, typically at the L5-S1 and the L4-L5 levels. Although these techniques provide an effective means of achieving anterior interbody fusion with maintenance of disc space distraction, they appear to require a significant learning curve. Both the VATS and laparoscopic techniques should be performed by surgeons experienced in these techniques to minimize potentially catastrophic complications. The ultimate success of the procedure depends on the proper diagnosis and patient selection. Each device has a technique guide specific to it, and the reader is referred to these guides for specific device use.

PERCUTANEOUS ANTERIOR LUMBAR ARTHRODESIS—LATERAL APPROACH TO L1 TO L4-5

Direct lateral anterior lumbar fusion and extreme lateral interbody fusion can be done through a minimally invasive direct lateral approach (see Technique 37-16); however, there is a definite learning curve for disc excision and fusion techniques done through the small access provided by the dilating retractor systems. Complications, primarily related to nerve root injury or irritation, have been reported in 22% of patients after a minimally invasive direct lateral anterior lumbar fusion and extreme lateral interbody fusion. Knowledge of "safe zones" for this approach and familiarity with the dilating retractor systems are essential for avoiding these complications.

TECHNIQUE 39-20

- After confirmation of the correct position of the retractor (see Technique 37-16) with anteroposterior and lateral fluoroscopy, center the anterior annulotomy window in the anterior half of the disc.
- Make the window opening wide enough to accommodate the implant.
- Remove the disc with standard instruments.
- Leave the posterior annulus intact.
- Release the contralateral annulus using a Cobb dissector to allow distraction of the disc space to insert the implant.
- Insert an implant that will rest on both lateral margins of the epiphyseal ring.
- Irrigate the cavity copiously.
- Carefully remove the retractor while observing the psoas muscle covering the defect and watching for bleeding.
- Close the fascial and subcutaneous layers.
- The skin can be closed with a subcuticular method.
- Supplementary posterior instrumentation must be used to maintain stability.

POSTERIOR ARTHRODESIS

Posterior arthrodeses of the lumbar and thoracic spine generally are based on the principles originated by Hibbs in 1911. In the Hibbs operation, fusion of the neural arches is induced by overlapping numerous small osseous flaps from contiguous laminae, spinous processes, and articular facets. In the thoracic spine, the arthrodesis is generally extended laterally out to the tips of the transverse processes so that the posterior cortex and cancellous bone of these portions of the vertebrae are used to widen the fusion mass. Accurate visual identification of a specific vertebral level is always difficult except when the sacrum can be exposed and thus identified. At any other level, despite the fact that identification of a given vertebra may be possible because of the anatomic peculiarities of spinous processes, laminae, and articular facets, it is always advisable to make marker radiographs at surgery. Marker films occasionally are made before surgery, using a metal marker on the skin with a scratch on the skin to identify the level. We recommend a method consisting of the radiographic identification of a marker of adequate size clamped to a spinous process within the operative field. The closer to the base of the spinous process the marker can be inserted, the more accurate and easier the identification. Cross-table lateral or anteroposterior radiographs taken on the operating table to compare with good-quality preoperative radiographs usually are sufficient for accurate identification of the vertebral level, although the quality of the portable radiographs may at times make this difficult. Patient positioning to maintain lumbar lordosis also is important.

HIBBS FUSION

With the Hibbs technique, fusion is attempted at four different points—the laminae and articular processes on each side. The procedure has been modified slightly over the years.

TECHNIQUE 39-21

(HIBBS, AS DESCRIBED BY HOWORTH)

- Incise the skin and subcutaneous tissues in the midline along the spinous processes and attach towels to the skin edges with clips or use an adhesive plastic drape. Divide the deep fascia and supraspinous ligament in line with the skin incision. With a Kirmisson or Cobb elevator, remove the supraspinous ligament from the tips of the spines.
- Strip the periosteum from the sides of the spines and the dorsal surface of the laminae with a curved elevator. Control bleeding with long thin sponge packs (Hibbs sponges).
- Incise the interspinous ligaments in the direction of their length, making a continuous longitudinal exposure.
- Elevate the muscles from the ligamentum flavum and expose the fossa distal to the lateral articulation overlying the pars interarticularis and transverse process base. Excise the fat pad in the fossa with a scalpel or curet.
- Thoroughly denude the spinous processes of periosteum and ligament with an elevator and curet, split them longitudinally and transversely with an osteotome, and remove them with the Hibbs biting forceps.
- Using a thick chisel elevator, strip away the capsules of the lateral articulations.
- Free with a curet the posterior layer (about two thirds) of the ligamentum flavum from the margins of the distal and proximal laminae in succession and peel it off the anterior layer; leave the latter to cover the dura.
- Excise the articular cartilage and cortical bone from the lateral articulations with special thin osteotomes, either straight or angled at 30, 45, or 60 degrees as required. A. D. Smith emphasized that the lateral articulations of the vertebra above the area of fusion must not be disturbed, because this may cause pain later. However, it is important to include the lateral articulations within the fusion area, because if they are not obliterated, the entire fusion is jeopardized. After curetting the lateral articulations in the fusion area, he narrowed the remaining defect by making small cuts into the articular processes parallel with the joint line so that these thin slices of bone separate slightly and fill the space. This, he believed, is preferable to packing the joint spaces with cancellous bone chips.
- Using a gouge, cut chips from the fossa below each lateral articulation and turn them into the gap left by the removal of the articular cartilage or insert a fragment of spinous process into the gap.
- Denude the fossa of cortical bone and pack it fully with chips.
- Also with a gouge, remove chips from the laminae and place them in the interlaminar space in contact with raw bone on each side. Use fragments from the spinous processes to bridge the laminae. Also use additional bone from the ilium near the posterosuperior spine or from the spinous processes beyond the fusion area.
- When large or extensive grafts are taken from the posterior ilium, postoperative pain or sensitivity of the area may be marked. Care should be taken to avoid injury to the cluneal nerves with subsequent neuroma formation. Bone from the bone bank can be used, especially if the bone available locally is scant because of spina bifida.
- The bone grafts should not extend beyond the laminae of the end vertebrae because the projecting ends of the grafts can cause irritation and pain.
- If the nucleus pulposus is to be removed, the chips are cut before exposure of the nucleus and are kept until needed. The remaining layer of the ligamentum flavum is freed as a flap with its base at the midline, is retracted for exposure of the nerve root and nucleus, and after removal of the nucleus is replaced to protect the dura.
- Suture the periosteum, ligaments, and muscles snugly over the chips with interrupted sutures. Then suture the subcutaneous tissue carefully to eliminate dead space and close the skin either with a subcuticular suture or nonabsorbable skin suture technique.

At this clinic we routinely use an adhesive plastic film material to isolate the skin surface from the wound rather than attaching towels to skin edges with clips, because clips have an unfortunate tendency to become displaced and can get lost within the wound. We routinely use modified Cobb elevators, which when sharp are efficient in stripping away the capsules of the lateral articulations. The most important single project at the time of surgery is preparing an extensive fresh cancellous bed to receive the grafts. This means denuding the facet joints, articular processes, pars interarticularis, laminae, and spinous processes. Subcuticular wound closure is used routinely to improve patient comfort.

POSTOPERATIVE CARE. We routinely use closed-wound suction for 12 to 36 hours, with removal of the suction device mandatory by 48 hours. Depending on the level of the arthrodesis, the age of the patient, and the presence or absence of internal fixation, walking is allowed in 24 to 48 hours when pain permits. For obese patients, all types of external fixation or support likely will be inadequate and limitation of activity may be the only reasonable alternative. The appropriateness of bracing remains controversial. Generally, for fusions with marked preoperative instability (e.g., burst fractures), rigid bracing is continued for 12 weeks. For fusions without marked instability (e.g., degenerative spondylolisthesis), bracing generally, if used, is less rigid and of shorter duration.

POSTEROLATERAL OR INTERTRANSVERSE FUSIONS

In 1948 Cleveland, Bosworth, and Thompson described a technique for repair of pseudarthrosis after spinal fusion in which grafts are placed posteriorly on one side over the laminae, lateral margins of the articular facets, and base of the transverse processes. Watkins described what he called a posterolateral fusion of the lumbar and lumbosacral spine in which the facets, pars interarticularis, and bases of the transverse processes are fused with chip grafts and a large graft is placed posteriorly on the transverse processes. When the lumbosacral joint is included, the grafts extend to the posterior aspect of the first sacral segment.

We, like many others, use this operation and its modifications for primary lumbar and lumbosacral fusions and in patients with pseudarthrosis, laminar defects either congenital or surgical, or spondylolisthesis with chronic pain from instability. The operation may be unilateral or bilateral but usually is bilateral, covering one or more joints depending on the stability of the area to be fused. The retraction instruments designed by McElroy and others are useful. However, one should be mindful of the ischemia caused by retractors, and they should be periodically released to allow perfusion of the paraspinal musculature. When placing the retractors, minimal retractor bulk and tension should be employed. The technique described by Watkins allows exposure for a posterolateral fusion without much need for soft-tissue retraction.

POSTEROLATERAL LUMBAR FUSION

TECHNIQUE 39-22

(WATKINS)

- Make a longitudinal skin incision along the lateral border of the paraspinal muscles, curving it medially at the distal end across the posterior crest of the ilium (Fig. 39-36A). Alternatively, a single midline skin incision can be used with bilateral fascial incisions.
- Divide the lumbodorsal fascia and establish the plane of cleavage between the border of the paraspinal muscles and the fascia overlying the transversus abdominis muscle. The tips of the transverse processes can now be palpated in the depths of the wound (Fig. 39-36B).
- Release the iliac attachment of the muscles with an osteotome, taking a thin layer of ilium. Continue the exposure of the posterior crest of the ilium by subperiosteal dissection and remove the crest almost flush with the sacroiliac joint, taking enough bone to provide one or two grafts. Removal of the iliac crest increases exposure of the spine.
- Retract the sacrospinalis muscle toward the midline and denude the transverse processes of the dorsal muscle and ligamentous attachments; expose the articular facets by excising the joint capsule.
- Remove the cartilage from the facets with an osteotome and level the area down to allow the graft to fit snugly against the facets, pars interarticularis, and base of the transverse process at each level.

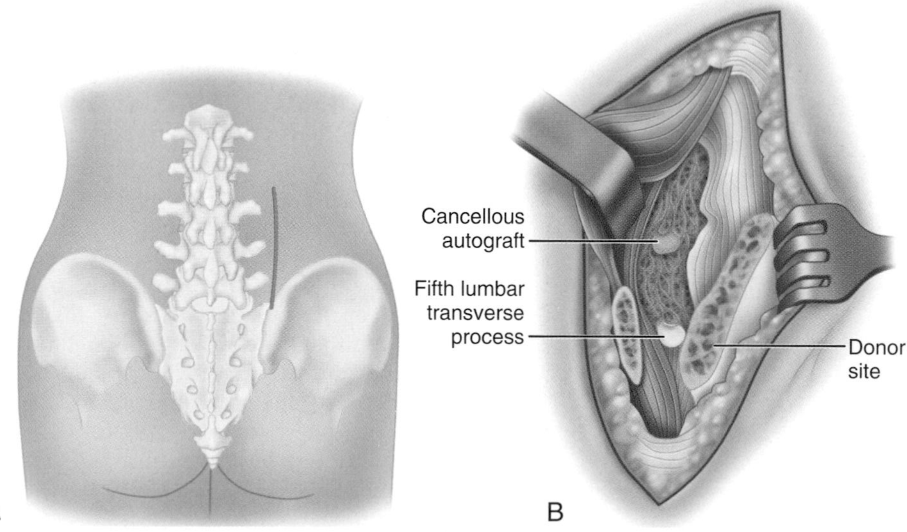

FIGURE 39-36 Watkins posterolateral fusion. **A,** Incision. **B,** Lumbothoracic fascia has been incised, paraspinal muscles have been retracted medially, and tips of transverse processes are now palpable. Split iliac crest and smaller grafts have been placed against spine. **SEE TECHNIQUE 39-22.**

- Comminute the facets with a small gouge or osteotome and turn bone chips up and down from the facet area, upper sacral area, and transverse processes.
- Split the resected iliac crest longitudinally into two grafts. Shape one to fit into the prepared bed and impact it firmly in place with its cut surface against the spine (Fig. 39-36B). Preserve the remaining graft for use on the opposite side with or without additional bone from the other iliac crest.
- Pack additional ribbons and chips of cancellous bone from the ilium about the graft.
- Allow the paraspinal muscles to fall in position over the fusion area and close the wound.

POSTOPERATIVE CARE. Postoperative care is the same as that described for posterior arthrodesis (see Technique 39-21).

Modifications of the Watkins technique include splitting of the sacrospinalis muscle longitudinally; inclusion of the laminae, as well as the articular facets and transverse processes, in the fusion (Figs. 39-37 and 39-38); and combining posterolateral fusion using a midline approach with a modified Hibbs type fusion in routine lumbar and lumbosacral fusions (Fig. 39-39). Adkins used an intertransverse or alar transverse fusion in which tibial grafts are inserted between the transverse processes of L4 and L5 and between that of L5 and the ala of the sacrum on one or both sides.

INTERTRANSVERSE LUMBAR FUSION

TECHNIQUE 39-23

(ADKINS)

- Dissect the erector spinae muscles laterally from the pedicles, exposing the transverse processes and ala of the sacrum. This is easier when the facets have been removed, but if these are intact, exposure can be obtained without disturbing them.
- Cut a groove in the upper or lower border of each transverse process with a sharp gouge or forceps. Take care not to fracture the transverse process.
- In the ala of the sacrum, first make parallel cuts in its posterosuperior border with an osteotome. Then drive a gouge across the ends of these cuts and lever the intervening bone out of the slot so made.
- For fusions of the fourth to the fifth lumbar vertebra, cut a tibial graft with V-shaped ends; insert it obliquely between the transverse processes and then rotate it into position so that it causes slight distraction of the processes and becomes firmly impacted between them.
- For the lumbosacral joint, cut the graft so that it is V-shaped at its upper end and straight but slightly oblique at its lower end. Insert one arm of the V in front of the transverse process and punch the lower end into the slot in the sacrum. If only one side is grafted, arrange the patient so that there is a slight convex curve of the spine on the operated side; thus, firm impaction occurs when the spine is straightened. Bilateral grafts are preferred. The grafts should be placed as far laterally as possible to avoid the nerve roots and to gain maximal stability.
- Alternatively, strips of iliac wing cortex no more than 2 to 3 mm thick are placed anterior to the transverse processes of L4 and L5 to bridge the gap and lie on the intertransverse fascia. Similarly, another strip is placed between the ala of the sacrum and L5 by wedging it into the space after the ala has been slotted and decorticated. Care must be taken that these grafts do not protrude too far anterior to the plane of the transverse processes. This modification does not require a tibial graft and is recommended.

POSTOPERATIVE CARE. Postoperative care is the same as that described for posterior arthrodesis (see Technique 39-21).

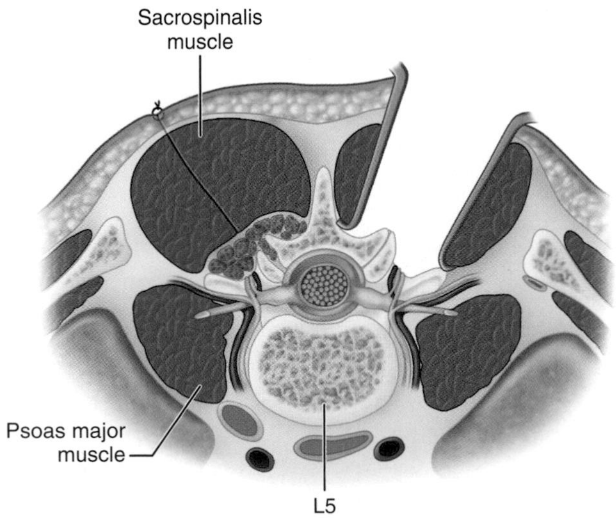

FIGURE 39-37 Technique of posterolateral fusion in which sacrospinalis muscle is split longitudinally and laminae, articular facets, and transverse processes are all included in fusion.

MINIMALLY INVASIVE TRANSFORAMINAL LUMBAR INTERBODY FUSION

A microscope and tubular retractors allow minimally invasive transforaminal lumbar interbody fusions to achieve decompression and stabilization while safely performing the procedure with less collateral damage to surrounding structures and the posterior dynamic stabilizers of the spine than with open procedures. Because the surgical corridor required is minimal, tubular retractors eliminate the need for traditional muscle-stripping techniques and preserve the form and function of the paraspinous musculature, which allows more normal physiologic function of the spine and sparing of the dynamic posterior stabilizers. Other advantages include reduced blood loss, less postoperative back pain, shorter time to ambulation, shorter hospital stay, and shorter duration of narcotic usage postoperatively compared with open approaches. Minimally invasive techniques also have been reported to result in significant reductions in total hospital costs compared with standard open techniques, and there is

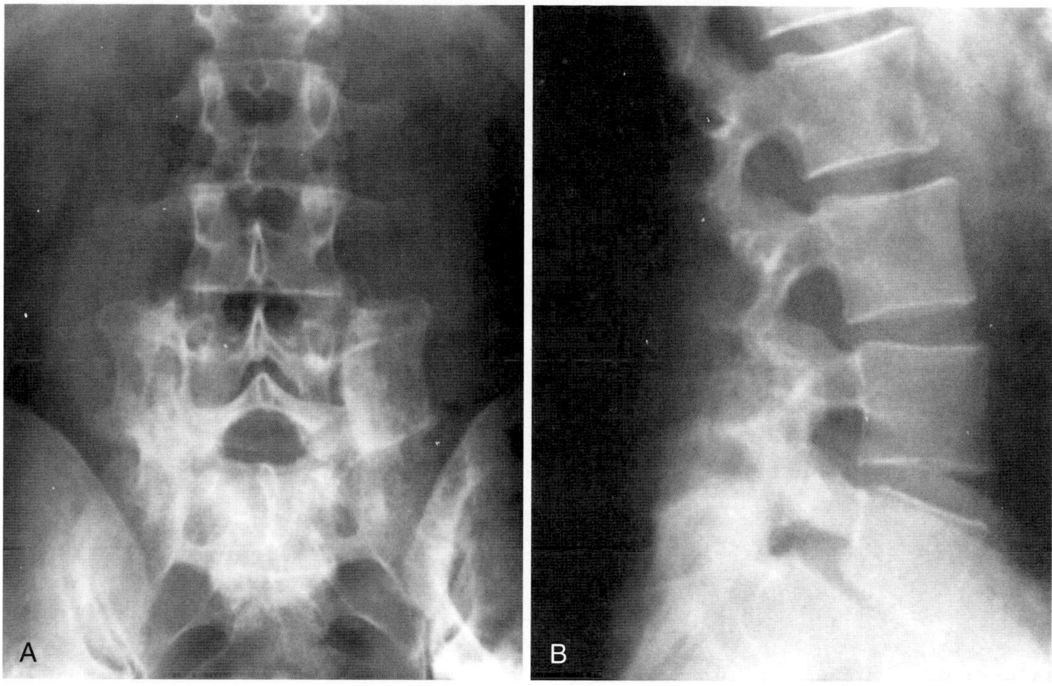

FIGURE 39-38 Bilateral posterolateral fusion for spondylolisthesis in adult. Anteroposterior **(A)** and lateral **(B)** radiographs 6 months after surgery.

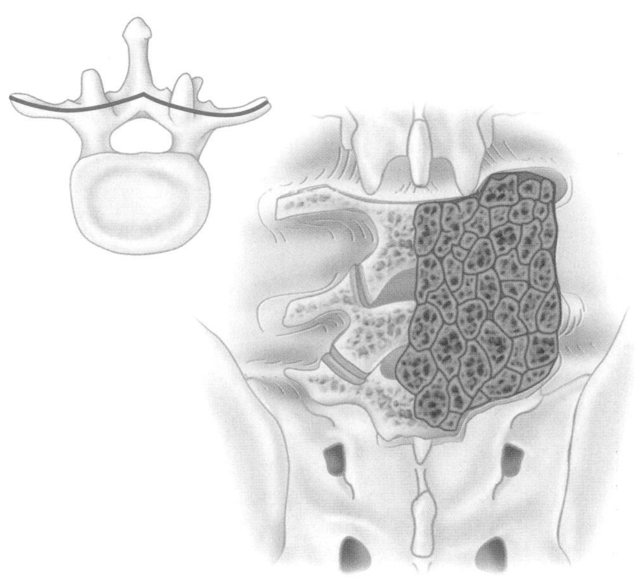

FIGURE 39-39 Slocum technique combining posterior (modified Hibbs) and posterolateral fusions. Midline incision is used. *Inset*, All bone posterior to blue line is removed.

early evidence that adjacent segment degeneration may be decreased compared with open surgery.

TECHNIQUE 39-24

(GARDOCKI)

- After induction of general endotracheal anesthesia, position the patient prone on a radiolucent table.
- Obtain lateral and anteroposterior C-arm fluoroscopic images to ensure that the pedicles can be adequately imaged.
- Insert a spinal needle into the paraspinal musculature at the interspace of interest, 40 to 60 mm lateral to the midline depending on patient depth and confirm its position with lateral fluoroscopy.
- The trajectory should approach the anterior and middle third of the disc space.
- Remove the needle and make a 20-mm vertical incision at the puncture site.
- Insert the blunt end of a guidewire through the incision and direct it toward the appropriate anatomy under fluoroscopic guidance. Advance the guidewire only through the lumbodorsal fascia, taking care not to penetrate the ligamentum flavum and to avoid inadvertent dural puncture.
- Insert the cannulated soft-tissue dilator over the guidewire with a twisting motion.
- Once the fascia is penetrated, remove the guidewire and use progressively larger dilators to create a muscle-sparing surgical corridor down to the appropriate interlaminar space while remaining orthogonal to the disc.
- Dock the appropriate-length 18- or 20-mm tubular retractor on the facet joint complex and interlaminar space.
- With the use of an operating microscope or loupe magnification, carry out a total facetectomy with a high-speed drill (preferred) or osteotomes. The osteotomy is L-shaped and should connect the interlaminar space at the base of the spinous process with the pars interarticularis just above the disc space but below the pedicle.
- Denude all removed bone of soft tissue and morcellize it for later use as interbody graft material.

- Perform a conventional discectomy by incising the annulus with a no. 15 scalpel blade lateral to the dural sac while retracting the traversing nerve root. There is no need to retract the exiting root. All cartilage should be removed from the disc space up to the outer anulus.
- Sequentially distract the disc space until the original disc space height is obtained and the normal foraminal opening is restored. This can be done with shavers, trials, or mechanical distractors depending on the system being used.
- Remove soft tissue and the cartilaginous endplate covering with scraping or curettage. Scrape medially under the midline and gradually work laterally in a sweeping motion until both caudal and cephalad endplates are cleared of soft tissue, exposing the compressed cancellous endplate of both vertebrae.
- Insert an appropriately sized graft based on the distractors or trials. The graft material can be bone, polymer, or metal. Do not place a graft that is too long because it may increase the risk of later posterior displacement.
- Countersink the graft until it is 4 to 5 mm below the posterior margin of the disc space.
- Probe the extradural space and foramina to ensure adequate decompression of the neural elements.
- Once the graft is in place, confirm positioning on anteroposterior and lateral fluoroscopic images. If positioned adequately with adequate restoration of disc height and lordosis, place bilateral percutaneous pedicle screws to allow a stable environment for fusion across the disc space.
- Use anteroposterior and lateral images of the pedicle for cannulation with an appropriately sized Jamshidi needle using a "pencil-in-cup" technique. The remaining technique varies depending on the hardware manufacturer.
- Once all hardware is adequately placed, close the incisions subcutaneously with 2-0 Vicryl and use skin glue (e.g., Dermabond or Histacryl) for final skin closure. When a 20-mm or smaller tube is used there is no need for fascial closure.

POSTOPERATIVE CARE. Patients are encouraged to walk as much as possible immediately after surgery. Bending, lifting, and twisting are restricted for a period of 3 months. All restrictions are lifted at 3 months if radiographs show appropriate progression of fusion. Hospital stay is seldom longer than 24 hours, and this procedure can sometimes be done in the outpatient setting in carefully selected patients.

INTERNAL FIXATION IN LUMBAR SPINAL FUSION

Various types of internal fixation have been used in lumbar spinal fusion. The object is to immobilize the joints during fusion and thus hasten consolidation and reduce pain and disability after surgery. Additionally, the instrumentation maintains correction of deformity and normal contours during the consolidation of the fusion mass. For many years, surgeons fixed the spinous processes of the lumbar spine with heavy wire loops, as described by Rogers for fracture-dislocation of the cervical spine.

Early methods of fixing the articular facets used bone blocks or cylindrical bone grafts to transfix the facets, particularly at the lumbosacral joint. In one bone grafting technique (McBride), soft-tissue attachments to the spinous processes and laminae were elevated, the spinous processes of L4, L5, and S1 were removed at their bases, and special trephine cutting tools were used to cut mortise bone grafts from them. The laminae were then spread forcibly with laminae distractors, and, again with the use of special trephine cutting tools, a round hole was made across each facet joint into the underlying pedicle. The bone grafts were then impacted firmly across each joint into the pedicle, and the distractors were removed. H-shaped grafts between the spinous processes also have been described for articular facet fixation.

Internal fixation (such as pedicle screws and plates) is described in Chapter 41. Again, however, before using these techniques the indications and current status of the use of these implants as approved by the FDA should be reviewed carefully with the patient. A special consent form should be signed by the patient if these devices are being used for anything other than the strictly approved indications.

TREATMENT AFTER POSTERIOR ARTHRODESIS

Opinions vary as to the proper treatment after spinal fusion. Usually the patient is placed on bed rest for a period of 12 to 24 hours; mobilization is then begun. No clear consensus exists on the duration of bed rest or the type of external support that should be used or even whether external support should be used. This depends on the pathologic condition being treated and on the location and extent of the fusion. Surgeon preference also is important in this decision and often is based more on the patient's comfort rather than immobilization for promotion of fusion, especially if instrumentation has been used for a degenerative process rather than for treatment of traumatic instability. Immobilization is continued until the patient is comfortable or until consolidation of the fusion mass occurs as seen on radiographs. Anteroposterior radiographs are made with the patient supine and in right and left bending positions, and a lateral radiograph is made with the patient in flexion and extension between 3 and 4 months postoperatively to confirm consolidation of the fusion mass. A longer period may be needed, especially in uninstrumented fusions. However, even with instrumentation the fusion mass may require a year or more to mature.

With newer, less invasive techniques, postoperative immobilization usually is not needed and patients are encouraged to gradually return to normal activities as much as possible, avoiding bending, lifting, and twisting for 3 months.

PSEUDARTHROSIS AFTER SPINAL FUSION

The possibility of pseudarthrosis after spinal arthrodesis should be remembered from the time the operation is proposed until the fusion mass is solid. A frank discussion of this problem with each patient before operation is important. The reported pseudarthrosis rate ranges from 9% to 30%. Some authors have correlated higher pseudarthrosis rates with a greater number of levels fused, but multiple studies have reported single-level pseudarthrosis rates as high as 30%. A

TABLE 39-3

Factors Affecting Fusion Rates in Lumbar Spine Surgery

	SUCCESSFUL FUSION (%)
INSTRUMENTATION TYPE	
None	84
Any	89
Semirigid	91
Rigid	88
FUSION LOCATION	
Posterolateral	85
Posterior interbody	89
Anterior interbody	86
Circumferential (360°)	91
GRAFT TYPE	
Autogenous bone alone	87
Allograft alone	86
Autogenous bone + interbody cage	90
Allograft/autogenous bone mix	86
BRACE TYPE	
None	89
Any	88
Semirigid or nonrigid	87
Rigid	88

(From Raizman NM, O'Brien JR, Poehling-Monaghan KL, Yu WD: Pseudarthrosis of the spine, J Am Acad Orthop Surg 17:494, 2009.)

critical analysis of the literature determined that instrumentation, fusion location, graft type, and brace type all affected lumbar fusion rates (Table 39-3). Careful patient selection and meticulous surgical technique in preparing the recipient site and in harvesting and preparing bone grafts are required to optimize fusion rates regardless of any other techniques that may be used.

It has been estimated that 50% of patients with pseudarthrosis have no symptoms. Persistent pain after spinal fusion with no other identifiable cause is presumed to be caused by pseudarthrosis when this condition is present. Yet, in some patients pain continues after a successful repair. Although pain can persist, repair of a pseudarthrosis is indicated when disabling pain persists; repair is contraindicated when pain is slight or absent.

The following findings are helpful in making a diagnosis of pseudarthrosis: (1) discretely localized pain and tenderness over the fusion area, (2) progression of the deformity or disease, (3) localized motion in the fusion mass, as found in biplane bending radiographs, and (4) motion in the fusion mass found on exploration. The amount of motion on flexion-extension radiographs that is consistent with solid fusion is controversial, ranging from no motion to 5 degrees of motion. When rigid instrumentation has been used, lack of motion does not necessarily indicate solid fusion; the presence of broken spinal implants does imply pseudarthrosis. Thin-cut CT scans appear to be more reliable than radiographs in evaluating fusion: a prospective study comparing imaging findings to intraoperative findings showed that CT most closely agreed with intraoperative findings compared with plain radiographs and MRI. The expense of MRI and its susceptibility to metallic artifact from instrumentation remain disadvantages to its routine use in the assessment of spinal fusion. Exploration is the only way to be absolutely certain that a fusion mass is completely solid.

Treatment of a patient with a painful pseudarthrosis involves a second attempt at fusion and may require a different approach from that used in the original fusion surgery, as well as the use of additional instrumentation, bone graft, and osteobiologic agents.

PSEUDARTHROSIS REPAIR

TECHNIQUE 39-25

(RALSTON AND THOMPSON)

- Expose the entire fusion plate subperiosteally through the old incision; if the defect is wide and filled with dense fibrous tissue, subperiosteal stripping in that area can be difficult. A narrow defect often is difficult to locate because the surface of the plate usually is irregular and the line of pseudarthrosis may be sinuous in the coronal and sagittal planes. In our experience, adherence of the overlying fibrous tissue has been the key factor that aids in identifying a pseudarthrosis. The characteristic smooth cortical surface and easily stripped fibrous "periosteum" of a solid, mature fusion mass are quite different from the adherent fibrous tissue overlying a pseudarthrosis. Meticulous inspection of the region of the facet joint is needed. Often a mature and solid fusion mass extends across the transverse processes, but motion is detectable at the facet joint, indicating the fusion mass did not incorporate to the fusion bed (i.e., the transverse processes).
- Thoroughly clean the fibrous tissue from the fusion mass in the vicinity of the pseudarthrosis. The adjacent superior and inferior borders of the fusion mass on either side of the pseudarthrosis usually will be seen to move when pressure is applied with a blunt instrument, such as a curet.
- As the defect is followed across the fusion mass, it will be found to extend into the lateral articulations on each side. Carefully explore these articulations and excise all fibrous tissue and any remaining articular cartilage down to bleeding bone.
- If the defect is wide, excise the fibrous tissue that fills it to a depth of 3 to 6 mm across the entire mass and protect the underlying spinal dura.
- Thoroughly freshen the exposed edges of the defect.
- When the defect is narrow and motion is minimal, limit the excision of the interposed soft tissue to avoid loss of fixation.
- Fashion a trough 6 mm wide and 6 mm deep on each side of the midline, extending longitudinally both well above and well below the defect.

- "Fish scale" the entire fusion mass on both sides of the defect, with the bases of the bone chips raised being away from the defect.
- Obtain both strip and chip bone grafts either from the fusion mass above or below or from the ilium, preferably the latter.
- Pack these grafts tightly into the lateral articulations, into the pseudarthrosis defect, and into the longitudinal troughs.
- Place small grafts across the pseudarthrosis line and wedge the edge of each transplant beneath the fish-scaled cortical bone chips. Use all remaining graft material to pack neatly in and about the grafts.
- Internal fixation (see Chapter 41) can be used to improve the rate of healing after pseudarthrosis repair but often is not necessary, and removal of loose hardware improves postoperative imaging capability.

DEGENERATIVE DISC DISEASE AND INTERNAL DISC DERANGEMENT

As has already been discussed, the degenerative process is fundamental to the development of disc herniations. Current research shows that genetic factors are more important than the mechanical stresses that have long been emphasized. The development of a disc herniation is only one of the pathways that the degenerative disc may follow. Alternatively, the disc may become the primary source of pain, rather than the nerve root, as is the case with herniations. This discogenic type of pain is most attributable to the internal disc derangement (IDD) that accompanies the degenerative process. Correct diagnosis and treatment of painful degenerative discs are difficult and controversial.

There are many different treatment options for this diagnosis, including fusions, disc arthroplasty, nucleoplasty, and dynamic stabilization procedures. The number of fusion operations in the United States has consistently increased since the 1970s and is significantly higher than in other developed countries. The indication for most of these procedures is IDD. Currently, only two lumbar disc replacement prostheses are approved by the FDA, but several designs are under investigation. The sole indication for these devices currently is to treat symptomatic degenerative disc disease. Likewise, the implants currently in development for nucleoplasty also are ultimately for treatment of the same process. There are multiple devices and models for "dynamic stabilization," only some of which are for the treatment of IDD. There is no shortage of treatment options. Treatment is controversial because no consensus of diagnostic criteria exists with regard to symptom type or severity, physical examination, or diagnostic imaging criteria. In addition to lack of consensus with regard to diagnosis, few prospective randomized data exist on outcomes for the numerous operative or nonoperative treatment options.

More recent research has helped considerably in understanding the anatomic basis for discogenic pain with nociceptive receptors and the innervation of the disc by the sinuvertebral nerves and basivertebral nerves being shown, as discussed earlier. Anatomic studies also are beginning to give insight into the complexities of normal disc structure and function. The understanding of pain and mechanisms that lead to inflammatory and mechanical pain is continually improving. These studies focus on the molecular structure of the matrix, the mechanical properties of the matrix, the cellular activities within the matrix, and the complexities of pain modulation (Fig. 39-40). Understanding the interplay between these processes and the complex psychosocial issues involved and instruments necessary for diagnosis allows for much more precise and rational treatment.

Current understanding of IDD defines this as a pathologic condition resulting in axial spine pain with no or minimal deformation of spinal alignment or disc contour. This is to be distinguished from measurable instability as can occur with fractures, traumatic ligamentous disruptions, degenerative listhesis, scoliosis, or other conditions. Although these conditions can be a source of pain, they are fundamentally different in that there are definite defined anatomic alterations and imaging abnormalities associated with each of these circumstances. There are no defined criteria for IDD, however.

Because there are no pathognomonic findings for IDD, the diagnosis requires a compilation of findings consistent with IDD and elimination of other diagnostic possibilities. Foremost among the consistent findings is the history. Patients usually are relatively young, in the third to sixth decades of life. Pain usually is chronic with symptoms present for several years, although the pain may have become constant or very frequent only in the previous several months. The pain is axial primarily, often with buttock and posterior thigh (sclerotomal) pain. Pain distal to the knee indicates either different or coexistent pathology. Positions and activities that increase intradiscal pressure, such as sitting or flexion, should exacerbate the symptoms. Likewise, recumbency, especially in the fetal position, often decreases the pain. This pattern of variable pain intensity is important and must be elicited carefully because the patient usually describes the pain only as constant. Pain that is constant but has little or no variation in intensity or only random fluctuations probably is not caused by IDD.

Examination reveals no weakness or reflex changes if IDD is the only diagnosis. Lumbar range of motion is mildly limited, especially in flexion, and limitation is caused by lumbosacral pain or tightness. Straight-leg raising typically causes back and buttock pain but no pain distal to the knee. There is no spasm in the paraspinal musculature, and extension usually gives some relief temporarily. The patient often has a depressed mood and should be questioned about changes or stresses at work and at home. If the patient has identified significant stresses, anger, or anxiety, the diagnosis of IDD is in question. Also, examination for Waddell signs should be included (Table 39-4), and if three or more are present, an alternative diagnosis is more likely. The examination must include the hip joints as a possible cause of buttock and thigh pain.

Imaging studies should include a lumbar spine series and dynamic films to assess deformities, measurable instability, or destructive lesions. Additional diagnostic studies should be obtained to evaluate abdominal or intrapelvic pathology that may have been suggested by the patient's history and physical examination. Additionally, MRI of the lumbar spine should

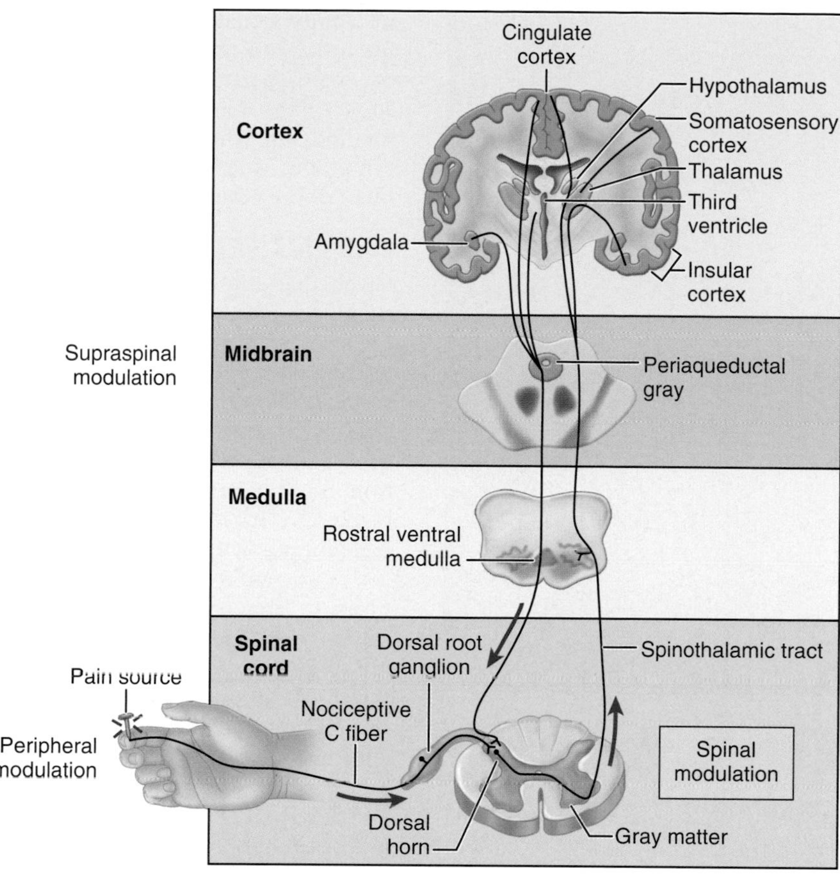

FIGURE 39-40 Main anatomic areas of pain modulation. (Redrawn from DeLeo JA: Basic science of pain, J Bone Joint Surg 88A:58, 2006.)

TABLE 39-4

Signs and Symptoms for Diagnosis of Abnormal Illness Behavior

NONORGANIC SIGNS	DESCRIPTION
Regional disturbances	Widespread region of sensory changes or weakness that is divergent from accepted neuroanatomy
Superficial/nonanatomic tenderness	Tenderness of skin to light touch (superficial) or depth tenderness felt over a widespread area not localized to one structure (nonanatomic)
Simulation	
Axial loading	Low back pain reported with pressure on the patient's head while standing
Rotation	Low back pain reported when shoulders and pelvis are rotated in the same plane as the patient stands
Distraction	
Straight-leg raising	Inconsistent limitation of straight-leg raising in supine and seated positions
Overreaction	Disproportionate verbalization, facial expression, muscle tension, collapsing, sweating during examination
NONORGANIC SYMPTOM DESCRIPTORS	
Do you get pain in your tailbone?	
Do you have numbness in your entire leg (front, side, and back of leg at the same time)?	
Do you have pain in your entire leg (front, side, and back of leg at the same time)?	
Does your whole leg ever give way?	
Have you had to go to the emergency department because of back pain?	
Has all treatment for your back made your pain worse?	

(From Fritz JM, Wainner RS, Hicks GE: The use of nonorganic signs and symptoms as a screening tool for return-to-work in patients with acute low back pain, Spine 25:1925, 2000.)

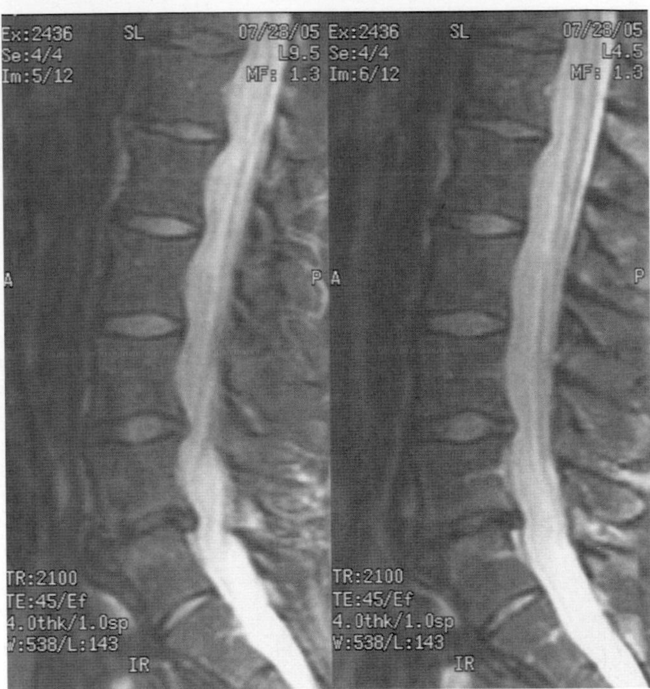

FIGURE 39-41 A 51-year-old patient with chronic axial spine pain without neurologic deficits that did not respond to nonoperative treatments.

show diminished water content in the nucleus of one or more lumbar discs (Fig. 39-41). This may or may not be associated with a loss of disc height and broad-based disc bulging. Decreased water content leads to decreased signal intensity best seen on T2-weighted sagittal images. This finding alone has no diagnostic value unless the appropriate history and physical examination also are present and there is no other discernible diagnosis.

The clinical diagnosis of IDD requires a careful and methodical assessment of many different factors. When the diagnosis is established, treatment options can be considered. Most patients can be treated without operative intervention, especially if they are educated as to the nature of the process causing their pain, specifically that it is not relentlessly progressive generally and that continued pain does not equate with progressive deterioration or disability. Often this understanding and instruction on moderate activity modification, aerobic conditioning such as walking, and core muscle strengthening allow these patients to manage their symptoms long-term without undue worry or resource consumption.

A small group of patients with persistent and debilitating symptoms may benefit from operative intervention. Before proceeding with any operative treatment, the patient should be informed that surgery leads to improvement in only 65%, leaving about 35% no better or possibly worse with respect to axial spine pain. Also, patients should understand that those who improve still have some activity limitations caused by pain or stiffness. This discussion must be very frank. For patients who still are considering surgery, a consistent and comprehensive assessment leads to the best overall outcomes. This approach is used for treating IDD, which is a diagnosis of exclusion and is separate from the treatment of measurable instability, spinal stenosis, disc herniations, spondylolisthesis, fractures, and other more objective diagnoses. The question becomes: of patients who have severe and debilitating axial spine pain that is not adequately improved with nonoperative methods and who have no objective diagnosis to explain their symptoms, which are likely to improve with surgery? Treatment of the other diagnoses is covered elsewhere.

PATIENT SELECTION PROCESS

Given that any other objective diagnosis has already been ruled out, the primary consideration in patient selection revolves around nonanatomic or psychosocial causes for disabling axial spine pain. For many years, patients with workers' compensation claims have been considered high risk for psychosocial causes of their pain, but more recent studies that independently assess this variable do not support this assertion. It has been found by several studies independently that being off work more than 8 weeks before surgery is an independent predictor of poorer outcome.

Many authors have tried to develop instruments to measure "abnormal illness behaviors." Waddell et al. defined this as "maladaptive overt illness related behavior, which is out of proportion to the underlying physical disease (including IDD) and more readily attributable to associated cognitive and affective disturbances." Waddell et al. also developed clinical tools designed to detect the presence of abnormal illness behavior by identifying physical signs or symptoms and descriptions that were nonorganic. Five nonorganic signs and seven nonorganic symptom descriptions have been identified (see Table 39-4). This group initially described these for use in patients with chronic pain and suggested that the presence of three or more was required to show abnormal illness behavior. Although these signs and symptoms cannot be used to predict return to work, the presence of multiple Waddell signs correlates with poor operative outcome and may temper the decision to offer a particular patient operative consideration.

The first formal step in patient selection for operative treatment for IDD is the MMPI. This study is done before any invasive studies to assess specifically for IDD. This instrument has been used in many studies and has been shown to be a predictor of operative outcomes, regardless of the spinal pathologic condition that is present. Riley et al. investigated the MMPI-2 and found that the results replicated the older MMPI. Patients with MMPI and MMPI-2 findings of depressed-pathologic profile and a conversion V profile reported greater dissatisfaction with operative outcomes. The MMPI is lengthy and difficult to administer in an orthopaedic clinical setting. An independent assessment by an experienced psychologist or psychiatrist who also administers the MMPI is best. By comparison, the Distress and Risk Assessment Method (DRAM) is relatively easily administered and scored and has been validated in clinical settings with regard to patients with back pain. The DRAM consists of the Modified Somatic Perception Questionnaire and the Zung Depression Index. With this simplified method, patients identified as psychologically distressed are three to four times more likely to have a poor outcome after any form of treatment.

We recommend that patients being considered for operative treatment with the working diagnosis of IDD have formal psychologic testing, which at our clinic consists of the MMPI. The current version of this test has predictive value for failure

TABLE 39-5

Classification of Nerve Fibers on the Basis of Fiber Size (Relating Fiber Size to Fiber Function and Sensitivity to Local Anesthetics)

FIBER GROUP/SUBGROUP	DIAMETER (μM)	CONDUCTION VELOCITY (m/s)	MODALITY SUBSERVED	SENSITIVITY TO LOCAL ANESTHETICS (%)
A (MYELINATED)				
A alpha	15-20	80-120	Large motor, proprioception	1
A beta	8-15	30-70	Small motor, touch, and pressure	↓*
A gamma	4-8	30-70	Muscle spindle, reflex	
A delta	3-4	10-30	Temperature, sharp pain, nociception	0.5
B (unmyelinated)	3-4	10-15	Preganglionic autonomic	0.25
C (unmyelinated)	1-2	1-2	Dull pain, temperature, nociception	0.5

*Vertical arrow indicates intermediate values in descending order.
(From Raj PP, editor: Practical management of pain, ed 3, St. Louis, 2000, Mosby.)

of operative treatment but has no predictive value for successful operative treatment. If the scoring and assessment from the psychologist administering the MMPI do not indicate the patient is at increased risk for failure, the second step in the assessment is taken.

DIFFERENTIAL SPINAL ANESTHETIC

The second formal step is the administration of a differential spinal anesthetic. This technique has been well reviewed by Raj, and the reader is referred to that work for a more complete description. Briefly, this technique, which is based anatomically on the relationship between nerve fiber size, conduction velocity, and fiber function, is shown in Table 39-5. The fiber diameter is the most critical physical dimension. The type A fibers are myelinated and subdivided into alpha, beta, gamma, and delta subtypes, each with different functions. Also, the unmyelinated B and C fibers serve different functions. The basic concept of the differential spinal is that by sequentially administering a local anesthetic agent, a predictable sequence of functional loss, beginning with sympathetic, then sensory, and finally motor blockade, is seen. The conventional technique (Table 39-6) is administered as a series of four solutions, each given in an identical fashion. The patient is questioned regarding his or her pain, and a series of observations is made by the physician to evaluate strength by dermatome, light touch, sharp and dull discrimination by dermatome, and reflexes (Table 39-7). The solutions should be referred to as "A" through "D" to avoid the term "*placebo*" in front of the patient. Also, the patient is not told ahead of time of the expected sequential changes to avoid bias. The four solutions are given as follows:

Solution A: contains no local anesthetic and serves as placebo.

Solution B: contains 0.25% procaine, which is known to represent the mean sympatholytic concentration of procaine in the subarachnoid space that is the concentration sufficient to block B fibers but usually insufficient to block A delta and C fibers

Solution C: contains 0.5% procaine, the mean sensory blocking concentration of procaine, that is, the concentration that usually is sufficient to block (in addition to B fibers) A delta and C fibers, but insufficient to block A alpha, A beta, and A gamma fibers

Solution D: contains 5% procaine and is used to provide complete blockade of all fibers

TABLE 39-6

Preparation of Solutions for Conventional Sequential Differential Spinal Blockade

SOLUTION	PREPARATION OF SOLUTION	YIELD	BLOCKADE
D	To 2 mL of 10% procaine, add 2 mL of normal saline	4 mL of 5% procaine	Motor
C	To 1 mL of 5% procaine, add 9 mL of normal saline	10 mL of 0.5% procaine	Sensory
B	To 5 mL of 0.5% procaine, add 5 mL of normal saline	10 mL of 0.25% procaine	Sympathetic
A	Draw up 10 mL of normal saline	10 mL of normal saline	

(From Raj PP, editor: Practical management of pain, ed 3, St. Louis, 2000, Mosby.)

TABLE 39-7

Observations After Each Injection

SEQUENCE	OBSERVATION
1	Blood pressure and pulse rate
2	Patient's subjective evaluation of the pain at rest
3	Reproduction of patient's pain by movement
4	Signs of sympathetic block (temperature change, psychogalvanic reflex)
5	Signs of sensory block (response to pin prick)
6	Signs of motor block (inability to move toes, feet, legs)

(From Raj PP, editor: Practical management of pain, ed 3, St. Louis, 2000, Mosby.)

Each solution is given at 5-minute intervals for appropriate patient examination with documentation of findings. The interpretation of this differential spinal anesthetic is as follows.

PSYCHOGENIC PAIN

If solution A relieves the patient's pain, the pain should tentatively be considered as "psychogenic." Between 30% and

35% of all patients with true organic pain obtain relief from an inactive agent. Relief after the normal saline solution may represent a "placebo reaction," but it also may represent a true psychogenic mechanism that is subserving the patient's pain. Clinically, these two usually can be differentiated because the placebo reaction is short lived and self-limiting, whereas pain relief provided by an inactive agent in a patient with true psychogenic pain usually is long lasting, if not permanent.

SYMPATHETIC PAIN

If the patient does not obtain relief with the placebo dose but does obtain relief from solution B, the mechanism causing pain tentatively is classified as sympathetic, provided that concomitant with the onset of pain relief there are signs of sympathetic blockade, without signs of sensory block. Although this is the mean sympatholytic dose, in some patients (who may have an increased sensitivity for A delta and C fibers) relief may be as a result of the production of hypoalgesia, analgesia, or anesthesia. The diagnosis of a sympathetic mechanism is fortunate for the patient because it may be treatable with sympathetic blocks, especially if diagnosis and treatment are started early.

SOMATIC PAIN

If 0.25% procaine (solution B) does not produce pain relief, but the 0.5% concentration (solution C) does, this usually indicates the pain is subserved by A delta and C type fibers, and the pain is classified as somatic, provided that the patient did show signs of sympathetic blockade with the previous 0.25% concentration, and the onset of pain relief is accompanied by the onset of analgesia and anesthesia. This is important because if the patient had a decreased sensitivity for B fibers, pain relief at the 0.5% concentration is from delayed sympathetic block rather than sensory block.

CENTRAL PAIN

If pain relief is not obtained by any of the preceding injections, the 5% procaine (solution D) is injected to block all fiber types. If the 5% dose gives pain relief, the mechanism is still considered somatic and it is presumed that the patient has a decreased sensitivity for A delta and C fibers. If the patient fails to obtain relief despite complete blockade, the pain is classified as "central" in origin. This is not a specific diagnosis and may indicate one of four possibilities, including (1) a central lesion, (2) psychogenic pain, (3) encephalization, or (4) malingering (see Table 39-8 for more complete information). Although this technique was used for many years, more recently, a "modified" technique has been used. This modified technique allows more rapid recovery of the patient and eliminates some ambiguities. Also, the spinal needle can be removed after a shorter time, which may reduce infection risk, and patient position can be changed more easily to re-create better the usual painful position for the patient.

MODIFIED TECHNIQUE

The modified technique requires only two solutions: normal saline and 5% procaine (Table 39-9). As with the conventional technique after informed consent (but being careful to avoid bias), a small-bore needle is placed into the subarachnoid space. At that time, 2 mL of normal saline is injected and the same observations are made. If the patient has no or only partial relief from the placebo injection, 2 mL of 5% procaine is injected, the needle is withdrawn, and the patient is placed supine. The same observations are made at 5-minute intervals, as outlined earlier (see Table 39-7).

INTERPRETATION

If the pain is relieved with the saline injection, the interpretation is the same as described earlier (i.e., consider the pain

TABLE 39-8

Diagnostic Possibilities of Central Mechanism

DIAGNOSIS	EXPLANATION/BASIS OF DIAGNOSIS
Central lesion	The patient may have a lesion in the central nervous system that is above the level of the subarachnoid sensory block. We have seen two patients who had a metastatic lesion in the precentral gyrus, which was the central origin of the patient's peripheral pain.
Psychogenic pain	The patient may have true psychogenic pain, and it is not going to respond to any level of block. This is an even more uncommon response in patients with psychogenic pain than a positive response to placebo.
Encephalization	The patient's pain may have undergone "encephalization," a poorly understood phenomenon in which persistent, severe, agonizing pain, originally of peripheral origin, becomes self-sustaining at a central level. This usually does not occur until severe pain has been endured for a prolonged period; when it has occurred, removal or blockade of the original peripheral mechanism fails to provide relief.
Malingering	The patient may be malingering. One cannot prove or disprove this with differential blocks. If a patient is involved in litigation concerning the cause of pain and anticipates financial benefit, it is unlikely that any therapeutic modality would relieve the pain. Empirically, however, we believe that a previous placebo reaction from solution A followed by no relief from solution D strongly suggests that a patient who ultimately appears to have a central mechanism is not malingering because the placebo reaction, depending as it does on a positive motivation to obtain relief, is unlikely in a malingerer. There is no way to document the validity of this theory, but it does suggest a greater motivation to obtain pain relief than to obtain financial gain.

(From Raj PP, editor: Practical management of pain, ed 3, St. Louis, 2000, Mosby.)

TABLE 39-9

Preparation of Solutions for Modified Differential Spinal Blockade

SOLUTION	PREPARATION	YIELD
D	To 1 mL of 10% procaine, add 1 mL of cerebrospinal fluid	2 mL of 5% procaine (hyperbaric)
A	Draw up 2 mL of normal saline	2 mL of normal saline

(From Raj PP, editor: Practical management of pain, ed 3, St. Louis, 2000, Mosby.)

psychogenic). If the patient does not obtain relief with the 5% procaine, the diagnosis is considered the same as when no pain relief occurs in the conventional technique (i.e., mechanism is central). If the patient obtains complete pain relief after the 5% procaine, the pain is considered organic. If the pain returns when the patient again appreciates pinprick as sharp (recovered from analgesia), the mechanism is considered somatic (i.e., subserved by A delta or C fibers or both). If pain relief persists for a prolonged time after recovery from analgesia, the mechanism is considered sympathetic.

In our experience, the primary benefit of this procedure is to distinguish patients with psychogenic or central pain mechanisms from the group with somatic pain. It is unusual to find a sympathetic etiology in this group of patients who have had extensive evaluations and trial therapies before the current evaluation was undertaken. Identification of a patient with true psychogenic or central mechanism of pain and avoiding any further operative interventions is very advantageous to a patient who is highly likely to have a poor outcome and to the conscientious surgeon who is treating this patient. If a patient has a somatic mechanism responsible for pain, the third component to the evaluation is discography.

Discography was described earlier in this chapter, and the reader is referred there for the details of the procedure (see Techniques 39-9 and 39-10). Although the technique of discography generates some controversy, the interpretation and utility of the procedure generate even more controversy. In our practice, low-pressure discography is used. To be considered positive, there must be concordant pain above a minimal threshold that is similar, if not identical, to a patient's usual axial pain. Also, there must be radiographic abnormalities with annular disruption. If the examiner determines that the patient has one or more positive discogram levels and at least one normal control level, operative treatment is offered. The type of operative treatment can be subdivided into arthrodesis or disc replacement, but even with confirmatory imaging and specific concordant discogram results, the results of surgery for axial back pain are mediocre at best.

The specific procedure that best fits each patient requires careful consideration of each available option and must involve the patient substantially in the decision-making process. With regard to arthrodesis, there are multiple options, including anterior lumbar interbody techniques, posterolateral techniques, posterior interbody techniques, and combined anterior and posterior fusion options. There are a variety of stabilization alternatives involving interbody devices, pedicle screw fixation, and combinations of these strategies. The ultimate goal in each type of surgery is a solid arthrodesis. Also, the arthrodesis may use autologous iliac bone graft, which is considered the standard, although bone morphogenetic proteins (BMPs) seem to have a role. At this time, no particular approach and no particular technique of stabilization have been shown to be superior to others, and there are several good studies that show statistical equivalency between anterior lumbar interbody fusion (ALIF), posterior lumbar interbody fusion (PLIF), and posterolateral fusion with instrumentation (Fig. 39-42). Also, there has been no superiority proved for the various minimally invasive options. Likewise, there is no study showing BMP superior to autogenous bone when used posteriorly in this setting. When used with ALIF, BMP-2 has been shown to be equal to autologous bone. Long-term questions remain, however, about use of BMP-2 in women of reproductive age. The use of BMP in anterior cervical fusions has been associated with an increased incidence of complications, especially wound infections; its use in thoracolumbar and posterior cervical fusions does not seem to be associated with more complications.

At this time, there is no commercially available prosthesis for nucleoplasty, so this remains only a potential treatment. Multiple dynamic stabilization-type devices are available. There are, however, no biomechanical or clinical data to support the use of this strategy for treatment of IDD.

THORACIC/LUMBAR DISC ARTHROPLASTY (TOTAL DISC REPLACEMENT)

A technique that has garnered great attention in the past 5 years is that of total disc replacement (TDR) (Fig. 39-43). The reason for this intense interest is the belief by many experts that this motion-preserving technique reduces adjacent motion segment degeneration, which remains problematic. There is some evidence that genetics may be more important than mechanical factors in IDD. Serious questions remain in regard to this technology, however:

1. Is motion preserved over long periods of time with TDR?
2. Does motion preservation decrease adjacent segment disease, or is this primarily determined by genetic factors?
3. What are the long-term results for TDR with issues such as wear, subsidence, or aseptic loosening?
4. What are the optimal revision strategies for TDR?

At this time, there are only three lumbar disc prostheses with FDA approval: the INMOTION, which is a modification of the Charité (Depuy Spine, Raynham, MA), the ProDisc-L (DePuy Synthes), and the activL (Aesculap, Center Valley, PA). All are approved only for single-level disc replacement. Several other lumbar disc prostheses are currently in the approval process.

The patient should be informed of the current expected or possible benefits and the current uncertainties involved with TDR. Also, from an anatomic standpoint, the condition of the facets should be essentially normal because TDR treats only one of the three joints at each motion segment. If there is significant disc space narrowing with facet overload and facet degeneration noted on CT, then TDR at this time cannot be recommended. Also, as with virtually any spine implant, the quality of the patient's bone may preclude TDR if osteoporosis is present.

The specific technique for TDR is similar to ALIF in principle. The mobilization of vascular structures needs to be

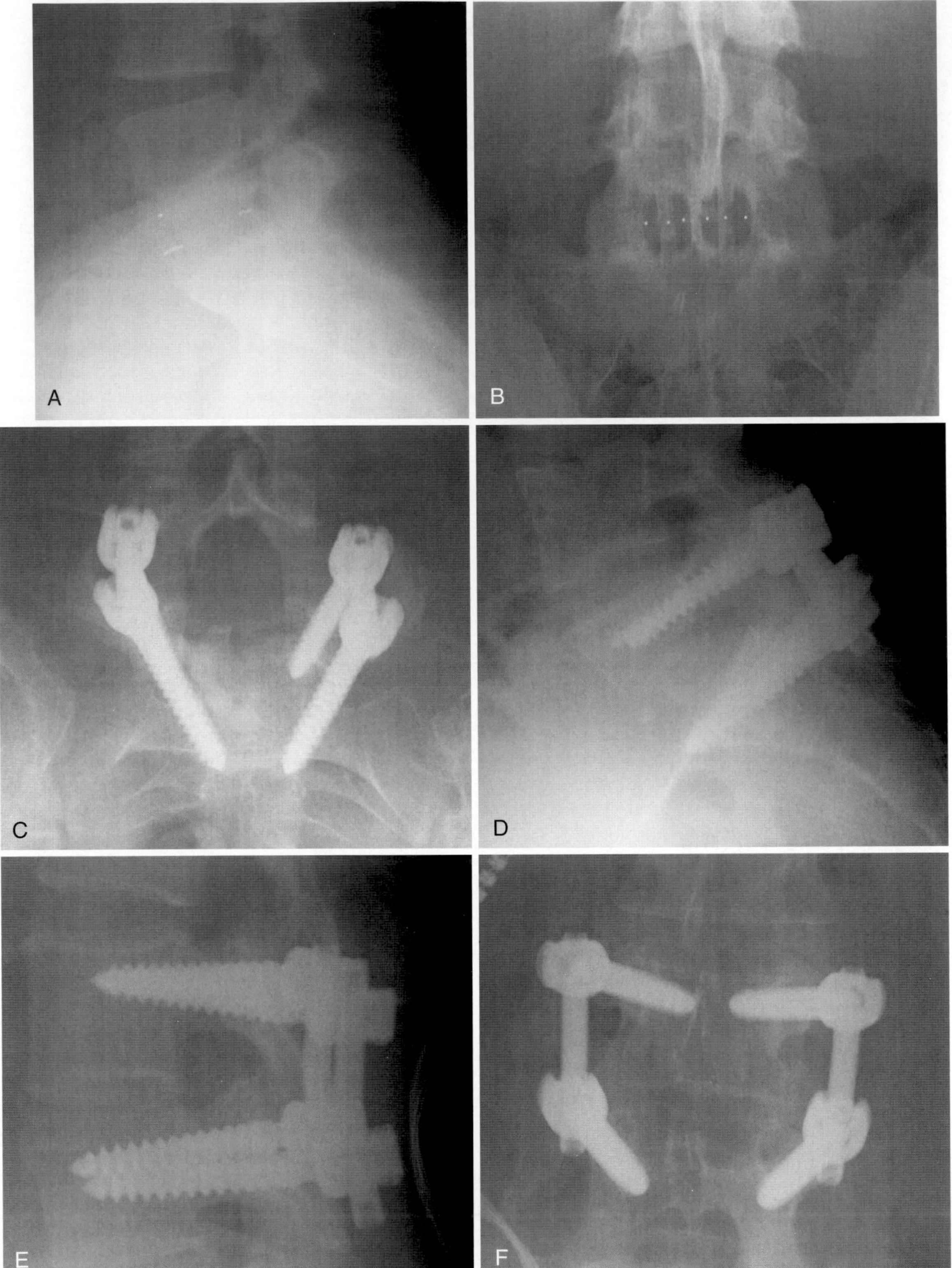

FIGURE 39-42 **A** and **B,** Solid arthrodesis after anterior lumbar antibody fusion with radiolucent threaded cages with bone morphogenetic protein type 2. **C** and **D,** Pedicle screw instrumentation with posterolateral autologous bone and transforaminal lumbar interbody fusion with allograft bone. **E** and **F,** Posterolateral fusion with autologous bone and pedicle screw instrumentation extending previous fusion.

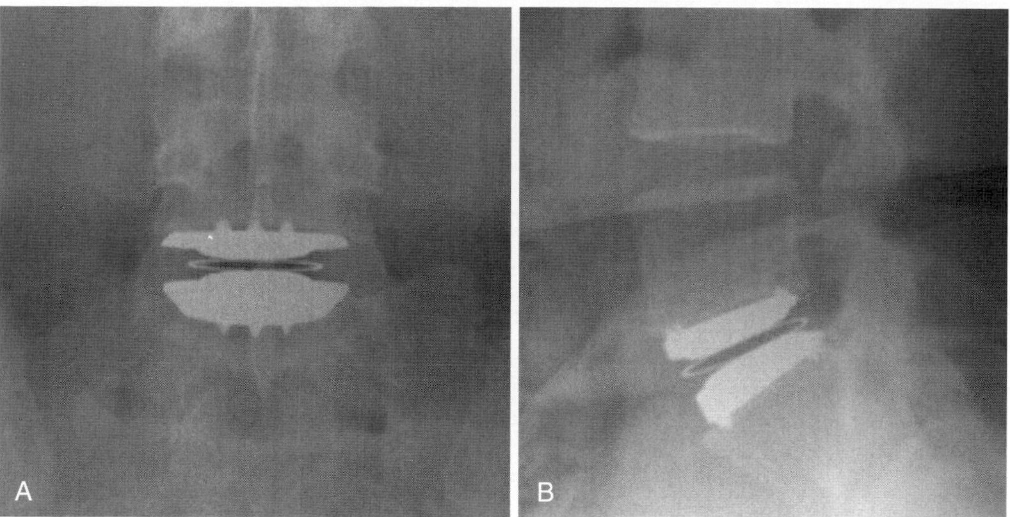

FIGURE 39-43 **A** and **B,** Anteroposterior and lateral views of patient with internal disc derangement treated with Charité total disc replacement.

slightly greater, especially at the L4 disc level. Also, proper sizing of the implant to optimize surface area of contact has been shown to reduce the risk for subsidence. Proper implant position is crucial to the function and possible catastrophic failure of each device. The reader is referred to the specific technique guides for these parameters. Our experience with these devices is limited at this time, and their ultimate value for patient care has not been determined.

FAILED SPINE SURGERY

One of the greatest problems in orthopaedic surgery and neurosurgery is the treatment of failed spine surgery. Numerous reasons for the failures have been advanced. Results from repeat surgery for disc problems seem to be best with the discovery of a new problem or identification of a previously undiagnosed or untreated problem. The best results from repeat surgery have been reported to occur in patients who have experienced 6 months or more of complete pain relief after the first procedure, when leg pain exceeds back pain, and when a definite recurrent disc can be identified. Adverse factors include scarring, previous infection, repair of pseudarthrosis, and adverse psychologic factors. Satisfactory results from reoperation have been reported to be 31% to 80%, and complications have been reported to be three to five times higher than for primary surgeries. Patients should expect improvement in the severity of symptoms rather than complete relief of pain. As the frequency of repeat back surgeries increases, the chance of a satisfactory result decreases precipitously.

The recurrence or intensification of pain in the subacute or late period after disc surgery should be treated with the usual conservative methods initially. If these methods fail to relieve the pain, the patient should be completely reevaluated. Frequently, a repeat history and physical examination give some indication of the problem. Additional testing should include psychologic testing, myelography, MRI to check for tumors or a higher disc herniation, and reformatted CT scans to check for areas of foraminal stenosis or for lateral herniation. The use of the differential spinal, root blocks, facet blocks, and discograms also can help identify the source of pain. The presence of abnormal psychologic test results or an abnormal differential spinal should serve as a modifier to any suggested treatment indicated by the other testing. Satisfactory nonoperative treatment of this problem should be attempted before additional surgery is performed. A distinct, operatively correctable, anatomic problem should be identified before surgery is contemplated. Pseudarthrosis, instability, and recurrent herniations are the diagnoses most likely to respond to further operative intervention after failed spine surgery. The operative should be tailored specifically to the anatomic problem identified.

STENOSIS OF THE THORACIC AND LUMBAR SPINE

Degenerative spinal stenosis is a progressive disorder that involves the entire spinal motion segment as described by Kirkaldy-Willis. Degeneration of the intervertebral disc results in initial relative instability and hypermobility of the facet joints. An increase in pressure on the facet joints with disc space narrowing and increasing angles of extension occurs and can lead to hypertrophy of the facet joint, particularly the superior articular process. As joint destruction progresses, the hypertrophic process ultimately may result in local ankylosis. Calcification and hypertrophy of the ligamentum flavum commonly are contributing factors. The end result anatomically is reduced spinal canal dimensions and compression of the neural elements. The resultant venous congestion and hypertension likely are responsible for the symptom-complex known as *intermittent neurogenic claudication.* Mild trauma and occupational activity do not seem to affect significantly the development of this disease, but they may exacerbate a preexisting condition.

ANATOMY

Spinal stenosis can be categorized according to the anatomic area of the spine affected, the region of each vertebral segment

TABLE 39-10

Classification of Spinal Stenosis

ANATOMIC	
ANATOMIC AREA	ANATOMIC REGION (LOCAL SEGMENT)
Cervical	Central Foraminal
Thoracic	Central Lateral recess Foraminal Extraforaminal (far-out)

PATHOLOGIC

1. Congenital
   1. Achondroplastic (dwarfism)
   2. Congenital forms of spondylolisthesis
   3. Scoliosis
   4. Kyphosis
2. Idiopathic
3. Degenerative and inflammatory
   1. Osteoarthritis
   2. Inflammatory arthritis
   3. Diffuse idiopathic skeletal hyperostosis
   4. Scoliosis
   5. Kyphosis
   6. Degenerative forms of spondylolisthesis
4. Metabolic
   1. Paget disease
   2. Fluorosis

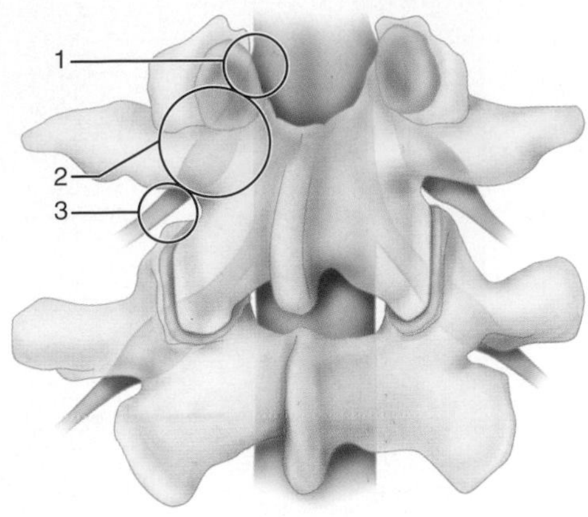

FIGURE 39-44 Zones of lateral canal as described by Lee. Entrance zone (1) is composed of cephalad and medial aspects of lateral recess, which begins at lateral aspect of thecal sac and runs obliquely down and laterally toward intervertebral foramen. Midzone (2) is located beneath pars interarticularis and just inferior to pedicle and is bound anteriorly by posterior aspect of vertebral body and posteriorly by pars; medial boundary is open to central spinal canal. Exit zone (3) is formed by intervertebral foramen.

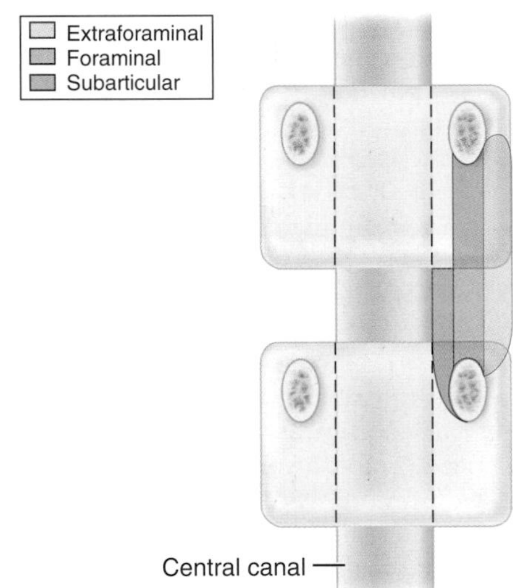

FIGURE 39-45 Central and lateral canal zones showing subarticular, foraminal, and extraforaminal divisions.

affected, and the specific pathologic entity involved (Table 39-10). Stenosis can be generalized or localized to specific anatomic areas of the cervical, thoracic, or lumbar spine. It is most common in the lumbar region, but cervical stenosis also occurs frequently. It has been rarely reported in the thoracic spine. Spinal stenosis can be localized or diffuse, affecting multiple levels, as in congenital stenosis. Degeneration of the disc occurs with disc narrowing and subsequent ligamentous redundancy, which compromises the spinal canal area. Instability may ensue. This relative hypermobility precipitates the formation of facet overgrowth and ligamentous hypertrophy. The ligamentum flavum may be markedly thickened into the lateral recess where it attaches to the facet capsule, causing nerve root compression. These phenomena occur alone or in combination to create the symptom-complex characteristic of spinal stenosis.

A description of spinal stenosis requires an understanding of the anatomy affected and the use of consistent terminology (Fig. 39-44). *Central spinal stenosis* denotes involvement of the area between the facet joints, which is occupied by the dura and its contents. Stenosis in this region usually is caused by protrusion of a disc, bulging anulus, osteophyte formation, or buckled or thickened ligamentum flavum. Symptomatic central spinal stenosis results in neurogenic claudication with generalized leg pain. Lateral to the dura is the lateral canal, which contains the nerve roots; compression in this region results in radiculopathy. The *lateral recess,* also known as "Lee's entrance zone," begins at the medial border of the superior articular process and extends to the medial border of the pedicle. This is where the nerve root exits the dura and courses distally and laterally under the superior articular facet (Fig. 39-45). The borders of the lateral recess are the pedicle laterally, the superior articular facet dorsally, the disc and posterior ligamentous complex ventrally, and the central canal medially. Facet arthritis most frequently causes stenosis in this zone, along with vertebral body spurring and disc or anulus pathology. "Lee's midzone" describes the *foraminal region,* which lies ventral to the pars. Its borders are the lateral recess medially, the posterior vertebral body and disc ventrally, the pars and intertransverse ligament dorsally, and the lateral border of the pedicle laterally.

The foramen is essentially the area between the cephalad and caudal pedicles. The dorsal root ganglion and ventral motor root occupy 30% of this space. This also is the point where the dura becomes confluent with the nerve root as epineurium. Causes of stenosis in this area are pars fracture with proliferative fibrocartilage or a lateral disc herniation. Thickening of the ligamentum flavum sometimes extends into the foramen and can be associated with a spur from the undersurface of the pars, especially if foraminal height is less than 15 mm and posterior intervertebral disc height is less than 4 mm. The *exit zone* is identified as the area lateral to the facet joint. The nerve root is present in this location and can be compressed by a "far lateral" disc, spondylolisthesis and associated subluxation, or facet arthritis.

The most common type of spinal stenosis is caused by degenerative arthritis of the spine, including Forestier disease, and is characterized by hyperostosis and spinal rigidity in elderly patients. Other processes, such as Paget disease, fluorosis, kyphosis, scoliosis, and fracture with canal narrowing, may result in spinal stenosis. Hypertrophy and ossification of the posterior longitudinal ligament, which usually are confined to the cervical spine, and diffuse idiopathic skeletal hyperostosis (DISH) syndrome also may result in an acquired form of spinal stenosis. Congenital forms caused by disorders such as achondroplasia and dysplastic spondylolisthesis are much less common.

Congenital spinal stenosis usually is central and is evident on imaging studies. Idiopathic congenital narrowing usually involves the anteroposterior dimension of the canal secondary to short pedicles; the patient otherwise is normal. In contrast, in achondroplasia the canal is narrowed in the anteroposterior plane owing to shortened pedicles and in lateral diameter because of diminished interpedicular distance. These findings occur in addition to the other characteristic features of achondroplasia.

Acquired forms of spinal stenosis usually are degenerative (Box 39-6). This process is most commonly localized to the facet joints and ligamentum flavum, with the resultant arthritic changes in the joints visible on radiographic studies. Frequently, these abnormalities are symmetric bilaterally. The L4-5 level is the most commonly involved, followed by L5-S1 and L3-4. Disc herniation and spondylolisthesis may exacerbate the narrowing further. Spondylolisthesis and spondylolysis rarely cause spinal stenosis in young patients. The combination of degenerative change, aging, and spondylolisthesis or spondylolysis in patients 50 years old or older frequently results in lateral recess or foraminal stenosis. Paget disease and fluorosis have been reported to result in central or lateral spinal stenosis. Paget disease is one form of spinal stenosis that responds well to medical treatment with calcitonin.

BOX 39-6

Types of Spinal Stenosis

Congenital

Idiopathic
Achondroplastic

Acquired

Degenerative
- Central canal
- Lateral recess, foramen
- Degenerative spondylolisthesis
- Degenerative scoliosis
- Combination of congenital and degenerative stenosis

Iatrogenic
- Postlaminectomy
- Postfusion
- Postchemonucleolysis
- Spondylolytic
- Posttraumatic

Miscellaneous
- Paget disease
- Fluorosis
- Diffuse idiopathic skeletal hyperostosis syndrome
- Hyperostotic lumbar spinal stenosis
- Oxalosis
- Pseudogout

NATURAL HISTORY

Although symptoms may arise from narrowing of the spinal canal, not all patients with narrowing develop symptoms. One study found no significant association between clinical symptoms and anteroposterior spinal canal diameter. In general, the natural history of most forms of spinal stenosis is the insidious development of symptoms. Occasionally, there can be an acute onset of symptoms precipitated by trauma or heavy activity. Many patients have significant radiographic findings with minimal complaints or physical findings. About 50% of patients treated nonoperatively report improved back and leg pain after 8 to 10 years, although functional ability after decompressive surgery has been shown in multiple studies to surpass that obtained after nonoperative treatment. A prospective, randomized study of 100 patients with symptomatic spinal stenosis treated operatively or nonoperatively found that pain relief occurred after 3 months in most patients regardless of treatment, although it took 12 months in a few patients. Results in patients treated nonoperatively deteriorated over time; however, at 4 years they were excellent or fair in 50%; 80% of patients treated operatively had good results at 4 years.

Reported studies suggest that for most patients with spinal stenosis, a stable course can be predicted, with 15% to 50% showing some improvement with nonoperative treatment. Worsening of symptoms despite adequate conservative treatment is an indication for operative treatment.

Weinstein et al. showed significantly more improvement in all primary outcomes in patients treated operatively compared with those treated nonoperatively.

CLINICAL EVALUATION

In patients with spinal stenosis, symptoms include back pain (95%), sciatica (91%), sensory disturbance in the legs (70%), motor weakness (33%), and urinary disturbance (12%). In patients with central spinal stenosis, symptoms usually are bilateral and involve the buttocks and posterior thighs in a nondermatomal distribution. With lateral recess stenosis, symptoms usually are dermatomal because they are related to a specific nerve being compressed. Patients with lateral recess stenosis may have more pain during rest and at night but more walking tolerance than patients with central stenosis.

TABLE 39-11

Differentiation of Symptoms of Vascular Claudication From Symptoms of Neurogenic Claudication

EVALUATION	VASCULAR	NEUROGENIC
Walking distance	Fixed	Variable
Palliative factors	Standing	Sitting/bending
Provocative factors	Walking	Walking/standing
Walking uphill	Painful	Painless
Bicycle test	Positive (painful)	Negative
Pulses	Absent	Present
Skin	Loss of hair; shiny	Normal
Weakness	Rarely	Occasionally
Back pain	Occasionally	Commonly
Back motion	Normal	Limited
Pain character	Cramping—distal to proximal	Numbness, aching—proximal to distal
Atrophy	Uncommon	Occasional

Differentiation of symptoms of vascular claudication from symptoms of neurogenic claudication is important (Table 39-11). Vascular symptoms typically are felt in the upper calf, are relieved after a short rest (5 minutes) while still standing, do not require sitting or bending, and worsen despite walking uphill or riding a stationary bicycle. Neurogenic claudication improves with trunk flexion, stooping, or lying but may require 20 minutes to improve. Patients often report better endurance walking uphill or up steps and tolerate riding a bicycle better than walking on a treadmill because of the flexed posture that occurs. Pushing a grocery cart also allows spinal flexion, which enhances endurance and decreases discomfort in most patients with neurogenic claudication (positive "shopping cart" sign).

Generally, physical findings with all forms of spinal stenosis are inconsistent. Distal pulses should be felt and confirmed to be strong, and internal and external rotation of the hips in extension should be full, symmetric and painless. Straight-leg raising and sciatic tension tests usually are normal. The neurologic examination usually is normal, but some abnormality may be detected if the patient is allowed to walk to the limit of pain and is then reexamined. The gait and posture after walking may reveal a positive "stoop test." This test is done by asking the patient to walk briskly. As the pain intensifies, the patient may complain of sensory symptoms followed by motor symptoms. If the patient is asked to continue to walk, he or she may assume a stooped posture and the symptoms may be eased, or if the patient sits in a chair bent forward, the same resolution of symptoms occurs.

DIAGNOSTIC IMAGING

RADIOGRAPHY

Although plain radiography cannot confirm spinal stenosis, findings such as short pedicles on the lateral view, narrowing between the pedicles on the anteroposterior view, ligament ossification, narrowing of the foramen, and hypertrophy of the posterior articular facets can be helpful hints. Leroux et al. outlined hypertrophic radiographic changes associated with hyperostosis on plain tomography and CT (Box 39-7).

BOX 39-7

Hypertrophic Radiographic Changes Associated With Hyperostosis

Plain Radiographs

Dorsal Level

1. Intervertebral osseous bridge
2. "Lobster claw"

Cervical Level

1. Exuberant osteophytosis
2. Narrow cervical canal

Lumbar Level

1. Marginal somatic osseous proliferation
2. "Candle flame"
3. "Lobster claw"
4. Intervertebral osseous bridge
5. Disc arthrosis
6. Acquired vertebral block
7. Hypertrophy of posterior articular processes
8. "Bulb" appearance of posterior articular hypertrophy
9. Anterior subluxation
10. Posterior subluxation

Lumbar Computed Tomography

1. Herniated disc
2. Disc protrusion
3. Vacuum disc sign
4. Hypertrophy of posterior articular processes
5. Osteoarthritis of apophyseal joints
6. Osseous proliferations of nonarticular aspects of superior apophyseal joint
7. Osseous proliferations of nonarticular aspects of inferior apophyseal joint
8. C/O of posterior longitudinal ligament
9. C/O of yellow ligament
10. C/O of supraspinal ligament
11. Anterior C/O of posterior articular capsule
12. Posterior C/O of posterior articular capsule
13. Anteroposterior diameter of spinal canal
14. Transverse diameters of spinal canal

(Modified from Leroux JL, Legeron P, Moulinier L, et al: Stenosis of the lumbar spinal canal in vertebral ankylosing hyperostosis, Spine 17:1213, 1992.)
C/O, Calcification or ossification or both.

The radiographic identification and confirmation of lumbar spinal stenosis have improved with the development of new imaging techniques. Initially, only central spinal stenosis was recognized, with canal narrowing to 10 mm considered absolute stenosis. This could be measured using radiographs or, preferably, myelography. Schönström, Bolender, and Spengler compared two methods of identifying central spinal stenosis: (1) anteroposterior canal measurement by CT and (2) measurement of the dural sac with myelography in patients undergoing surgery for spinal stenosis. They found no correlation between the transverse area of the bony canal in normal patients and patients with spinal stenosis. A dural sac transverse area of 100 mm^2 or less correlated with symptomatic spinal stenosis. This method allows the inclusion of soft tissue in the determination of spinal stenosis. The analysis of this area can be calculated relatively easily using standard CT software.

Currently, axial imaging has supplanted standard radiographs in the diagnosis of spinal stenosis, although radiographs are important in the initial evaluation of patients with persistent pain of more than 6 weeks' duration or of patients with "red flags" of other disease, including recent trauma, history of cancer, immunosuppression, age older than 50 years or younger than 20 years, neurologic deficit, or previous surgery. Flexion and extension views are useful to identify preexisting instability before laminectomy and may be useful in determining the need for subsequent fusion. Translation of more than 4 mm or rotation of more than 10 to 15 degrees indicates instability. A reversal of the normal trapezoidal disc geometry with widening posteriorly and narrowing anteriorly also may indicate instability.

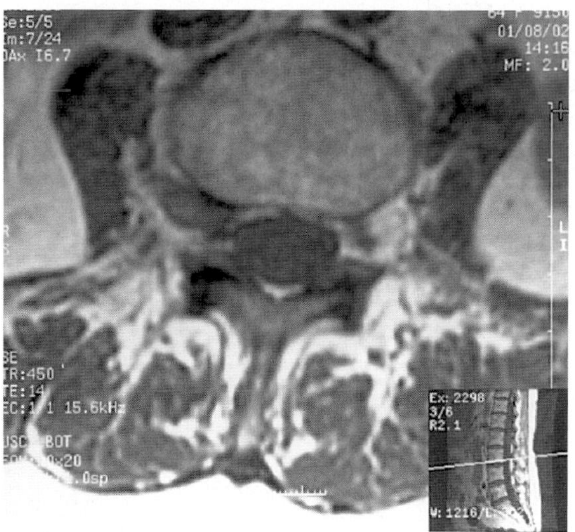

FIGURE 39-46 T1-weighted MR image showing far-lateral disc protrusion. Note obliteration of normal interval of fat between disc and root.

MAGNETIC RESONANCE IMAGING

MRI is helpful in identifying disease processes, such as tumors and infections, and is a good noninvasive study for patients with persistent lower extremity complaints after radiographic screening evaluation. MRI should be confirmatory in patients with a consistent history of neurogenic claudication or radiculopathy, but it should not be used as a screening examination because of the high rate of asymptomatic disease. Morphologic changes have been correlated with preoperative findings, such as pain and function, however, only to a limited extent. Sagittal T2-weighted MR images are a good starting point because they give a myelogram-like image. Sagittal T1-weighted images are evaluated with particular attention focused on the foramen. An absence of normal fat around the root indicates foraminal stenosis. Axial images provide a good view of the central spinal canal and its contents on T1- and T2-weighted images. Far lateral disc protrusions are identified on axial T1-weighted images by obliteration of the normal interval of fat between the disc and nerve root (Fig. 39-46). The foraminal zone is better evaluated with sagittal T1-weighted sequences, which confirm the presence of fat around the nerve root. Absolute anatomic measures also can be used, as previously discussed. Spinal deformity, including scoliosis and significant spondylolisthesis, can result in suboptimal imaging by MRI. This is secondary to the curvature of the spine in and out of the plane of the scanner on sagittal sequences and difficulty obtaining true axial cuts. Another disadvantage of MRI is the cost; nonetheless, MRI has become a useful, noninvasive diagnostic tool for the evaluation of patients with extremity complaints.

COMPUTED TOMOGRAPHIC MYELOGRAPHY

Despite the prevalence of MRI, myelography followed by CT is still accepted and widely used for operative planning in patients with spinal stenosis; it has a diagnostic accuracy of 91%. The addition of CT after a myelogram allows detection of 30% more abnormalities than with myelography alone. Because of the dynamic nature of the study, stenosis not visible on MRI with the patient recumbent may be identified on standing flexion and extension lateral views. CT after myelography characterizes the bony anatomy better than MRI, which helps the surgeon plan decompression surgery. However, imaging of the nerve roots in the foraminal region lateral to the pedicle is impossible because of the confluence of the dura with the epineurium at this point. There also is additional morbidity associated with the lumbar puncture required for myelography. Myelography followed by CT is best suited for patients with dynamic stenosis, postoperative leg pain, severe scoliosis or spondylolisthesis, metallic implants, contraindications to MRI, and lower extremity symptoms in the absence of findings on MRI.

Abnormal findings occur in 24% to 34% of asymptomatic individuals evaluated with CT myelography, just as with MRI, so clinical correlation is a must.

CT has been used to further define lateral recess stenosis and foraminal stenosis. These types of stenosis rarely are identified with myelography. The lateral recess is anatomically the area bordered laterally by the pedicle, posteriorly by the superior articular facet, and anteriorly by the posterolateral surface of the vertebral body and the adjacent intervertebral disc. The superior border of the corresponding pedicle is the narrowest portion of the lateral recess. Measurement of the recess in this area using the tomographic cross-section usually is 5 mm or greater in normal patients, but in symptomatic patients the diagnosis is confirmed if the height is 2 mm or less (Fig. 39-47). The foramen is the area of the spine bordered by the inferior edge of the pedicle cephalad, the pars interarticularis with the associated inferior articular facet and the superior articular facet from the lower segment posteriorly, the superior edge of the pedicle of the next lower vertebra caudally, and the vertebral body and disc anteriorly. This area rarely can be seen with myelography. A standard CT in the cross-sectional mode suggests narrowing if the foraminal space immediately after the pedicle cut is present for only one or two more cuts (provided that the cuts are close together). The best way to appreciate foraminal narrowing is to reformat the lumbar scan, which can create sagittal views through the pedicles and structures situated laterally.

Wiltse et al. described a far-out compression of the root that occurs predominantly in spondylolisthesis when the root is compressed by a large L5 transverse process subluxed below the root and pressing the root against the ala of the sacrum. This diagnosis is best confirmed with a reformatted CT scan with coronal cuts (Fig. 39-48).

Some studies have attempted to correlate clinical outcomes with pathologic findings on myelography and CT. A retrospective review found that patients who had a block on myelogram had a better chance of obtaining a good outcome. Another study confirmed postoperative stenosis in 64% of 191 patients at 4-year follow-up. Slight differences were noted in the Oswestry questionnaire between patients with and without stenosis but not in walking distances, and instability was present in 21% without demonstrable clinical effect. The degree of decompression on CT myelography did not correlate at all with outcomes, and regardless of the number of levels that had decompression, the results were similar. Nonetheless, decompression of all symptomatic levels with evidence of compression is recommended to enhance neural circulation and function and to avoid reoperation for recurrent spinal stenosis.

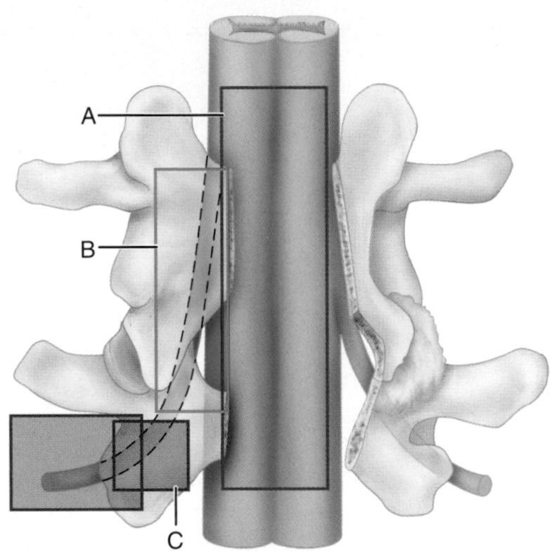

FIGURE 39-47 Three-dimensional illustration of segmental stenoses. *A,* Anatomic. *B,* Segmental. *C,* Pathologic.

OTHER DIAGNOSTIC STUDIES

Electrodiagnostic studies should be used if the diagnosis of neuropathy is uncertain, especially in patients with diabetes mellitus. Needle electromyographic study was shown to have a lower false-positive rate than MRI in asymptomatic patients. The diagnostic use of such studies, including somatosensory evoked potentials, is limited by the lack of prospective studies to determine sensitivity or specificity. Vascular Doppler examinations are useful to identify inflow problems into the lower extremities and should be accompanied by a vascular surgery consultation when indicated. Differential diagnosis also can be aided by the use of exercise testing. Tenhula et al. described a bicycle-treadmill test that stresses the patient in an upright position on an exercise treadmill and subsequently in a seated position on an exercise bicycle that allows spinal flexion. Earlier onset of leg symptoms with level walking and delayed onset of symptoms with inclined treadmill walking were significantly associated with stenosis. Exercise treadmill testing also is useful to help determine baseline function for quantitative evaluation of functional status after surgery. This study showed significant postoperative improvement in

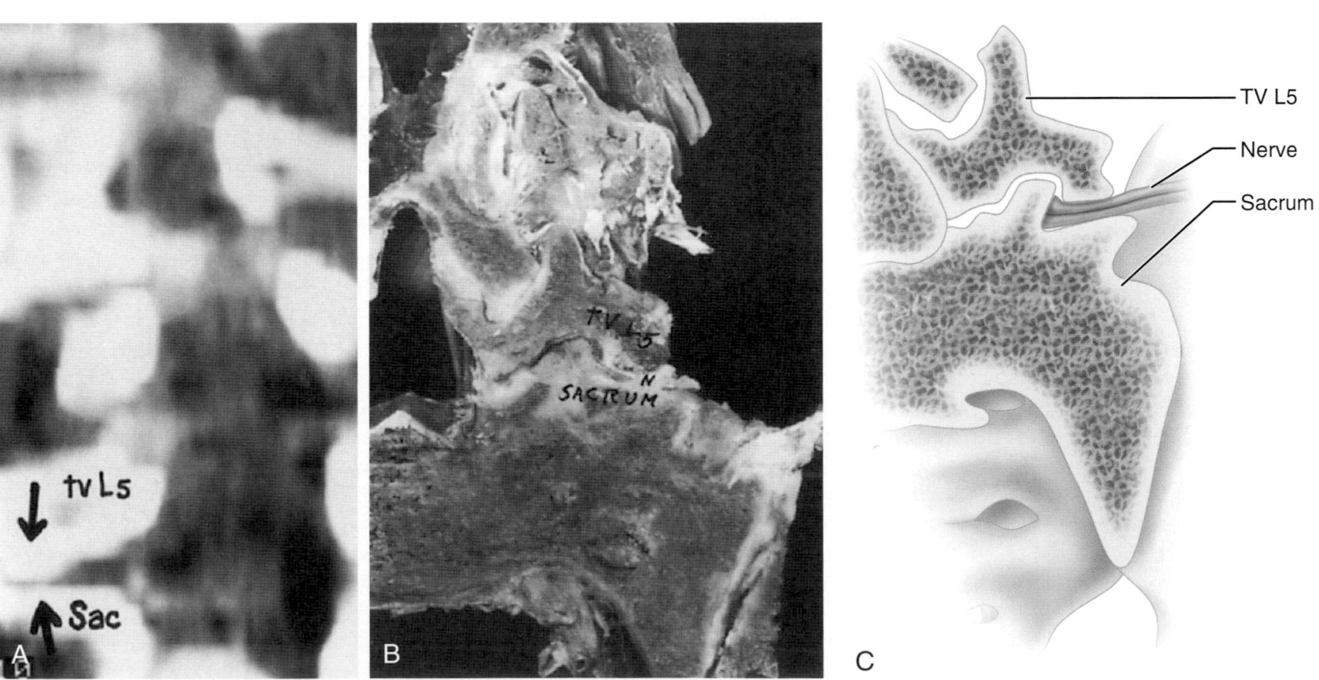

FIGURE 39-48 **A,** Coronal view of CT scan showing impingement of transverse process of L5 on sacrum. **B,** Coronal section showing right transverse process. **C,** Drawing of coronal section. (From Wiltse LL, Guyer RD, Spencer CW, et al: Alar transverse process impingement of the L5 spinal nerve: the far-out syndrome, Spine 9:31, 1984.)

treadmill walking and bicycling duration (88% preoperatively and 9% postoperatively for walking; 41% preoperatively and 17% postoperatively for bicycling), lower visual analogue scale pain scores, and a later onset of pain.

NONOPERATIVE TREATMENT

Symptoms of spinal stenosis usually respond favorably to nonoperative management (satisfactory results in 69% at 3 years according to Simotas et al.). Despite symptoms of back pain, radiculopathy, or neurogenic claudication, conservative management is successful in most patients. Patients with radicular type pain respond well to nonoperative treatment, but those with scoliosis tend to have worse results. Conservative measures should include rest not exceeding 2 days, pain management with antiinflammatory medications or acetaminophen, and participation in a trunk-stabilization exercise program, along with good aerobic fitness. Other methods should be reserved for patients who are limited by pain and should be used to maximize participation in the exercise program. Traction has no proven benefit in the adult lumbar spine. For a patient with unremitting symptoms of radiculopathy or neurogenic claudication, epidural steroid injections may be useful in alleviating symptoms to allow better participation in physical therapy. Epidural steroids can give significant symptomatic relief, although no scientific study has documented long-term efficacy.

Manchikanti et al. reported significant pain relief in 76% of 25 patients who had percutaneous adhesiolysis with injection of lidocaine, hypertonic sodium chloride solution, and nonparticulate betamethasone. If spinal stenosis is present with coexistent degenerative arthritis in the hips or knees, some permanent limitation in activity may be necessary regardless of treatment.

■ EPIDURAL STEROID INJECTION

Spinal stenosis and the resultant mechanical compression of neural elements can cause structural and chemical injury to the nerve roots. Edema and venous congestion of the nerve roots can lead to further compression and ischemic neuritis. This may result in the leakage of neurotoxins, such as phospholipase and leukotriene B, which can lead to increased inflammation and edema. Steroids are potent antiinflammatory medications and result in a decrease in leukocyte migration, the inhibition of cytokines, and membrane stabilization. These actions coupled with their ability to reduce edema provide the rationale for the use of epidural steroid injections in spinal stenosis. Epidural steroid injections have been used in the treatment of spinal stenosis for many years, and no validated long-term outcomes have been reported to substantiate their use. Significant improvement in pain scores, however, has been reported at 3 months. Patients with a healthier emotional status and those with a higher body mass index reportedly experience more pain relief. A prospective, randomized study found caudal epidural injections (lidocaine 0.5%) with or without steroids to be effective in approximately 60% of patients in the short term.

The technique of placement—caudal, translaminar, or transforaminal—also is debated, as is whether fluoroscopy should be used. Lee et al. reported improvement in 87.5% of 216 patients using fluoroscopically guided caudal epidural steroid injection; however, they included minimal improvement in these results. Although one study reported no difference between interlaminar and transforaminal injection, Lee et al. noted that bilateral transforaminal epidural injection allowed delivery of a higher concentration of injectate. Using anatomic landmarks for caudal injections, Stitz et al. reported accurate placement in 65% to 74% of patients, with intravascular placement in 4%. Accurate placement of translaminar injections seems to be equally difficult, with successful placement reported in 70%.

Spinal canal dimension has not been shown to be predictive of success or failure of epidural steroid injection. Complications are infrequent but can occur and include hypercorticism, epidural hematoma, temporary paralysis, retinal hemorrhage, epidural abscess, chemical meningitis, and intracranial air. A 5% incidence of dural puncture has been reported, and, if it occurs, subarachnoid injection of steroids or local anesthetic should be avoided to prevent mechanical or chemical nerve root irritation. Headaches occur in 1% to 5% of patients and are related to dural puncture or the use of the caudal injection route. In patients with headaches associated with caudal injections, the cause has not been determined because dural puncture should not occur at this level, because the dural sleeve has terminated at midsacrum.

The ideal candidate for epidural steroid injection seems to be a patient who has acute radicular symptoms or neurogenic claudication unresponsive to traditional analgesics and rest, with significant impairment in activities of daily living. We have used this technique successfully in our treatment algorithm for neurogenic claudication and radiculopathy both as a diagnostic and therapeutic procedure. The authors prefer transforaminal injections because they allow more ventral placement of injectate in the foramen and lateral recess.

OPERATIVE TREATMENT

The primary indication for surgery in patients with spinal stenosis is increasing pain that is resistant to conservative measures. Because the primary complaint often is back pain and some leg pain, pain relief after surgery may not be complete. Operative intervention should be expected to give good relief of claudicatory leg pain with variable response to back pain. Most series report a 64% to 91% rate of improvement, with 42% in patients with diabetes, but most patients still have some minor complaints, usually referable to the preexisting degenerative arthritis of the spine. Neurologic findings, if present, improve inconsistently after surgery. Pearson et al. noted that patients whose predominant complaint was leg pain improved significantly more with operative treatment than those whose predominant complaint was low back pain. Both, however, improved significantly with operative treatment compared with conservative treatment. Reoperation rates vary from 6% to 23%. Prognostic factors include better results with a disc herniation, stenosis at a single level, weakness of less than 6 weeks' duration, monoradiculopathy, and age younger than 65 years. Depression, psychiatric disease, cardiovascular disease, higher body mass index, scoliosis, and disorders affecting ambulation have been associated with a poorer prognosis. Reversal of neurologic consequences of spinal stenosis seems to be a relative indication for surgery unless the symptoms are acute.

Radiographic findings alone are never an indication for surgery. Factors predicting outcome vary, and correlation of

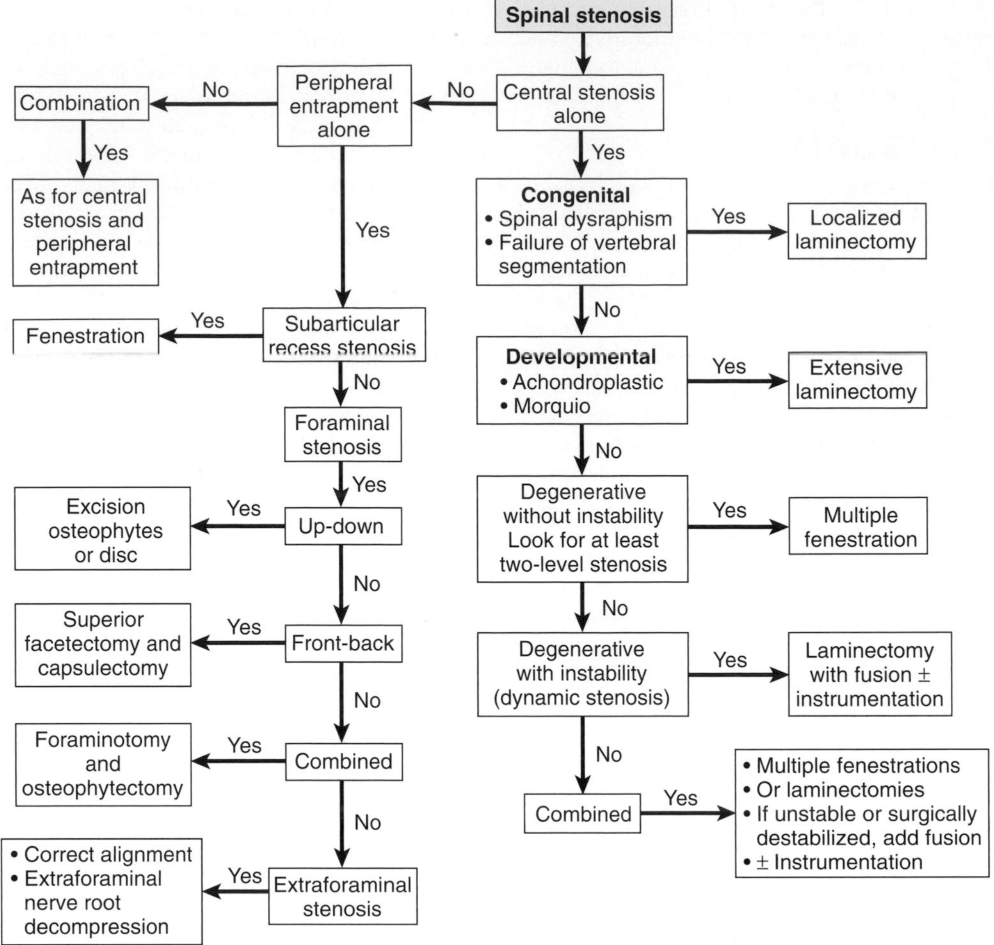

FIGURE 39-49 Algorithm for treatment of spinal stenosis. (From Hadjipavlou AG, Simmons JW, Pope MH: An algorithmic approach to the investigation, treatment, and complications of surgery for low back pain, Semin Spine Surg 10:193, 1998.)

imaging with symptoms seems to be the best guarantee of improvement after surgery. Localized lesions on radiograph without general involvement respond best. Ganz reported a 96% success rate in patients whose preoperative symptoms were relieved by postural change.

A patient's inability to tolerate the restricted lifestyle necessitated by the disease and the failure of a good conservative treatment regimen should be the primary determining factors for surgery in a well-informed patient. The patient should understand the potential for the operation to fail to relieve pain or to worsen it, especially in regard to the axial component of the symptoms. In addition to the general risks of spinal surgery, the severity of symptoms and lifestyle modifications should be considered. Lumbar spinal stenosis does not result in paralysis, only decreased ambulatory capacity, and conservative management is warranted indefinitely in a patient with good function and manageable symptoms. Delaying surgical treatment for a trial of nonoperative treatment has not been shown to affect outcome; however, one study reported less favorable results in patients who had symptoms for more than 33 months.

Cervical and thoracic spinal stenoses are associated with painless paralysis in the form of cervical and thoracic myelopathy and require closer attention and follow-up.

PRINCIPLES OF SPINAL STENOSIS SURGERY

Decompression by laminectomy or a fenestration procedure is the treatment of choice for lumbar spinal stenosis (Fig. 39-49). Fusion is required if excessive bony resection compromises stability or if isthmic or degenerative spondylolisthesis, scoliosis, or kyphosis is present. Other important indications for fusion include adjacent segment degeneration after prior fusion and recurrent stenosis or herniated disc after decompression. Laminectomy may be preferable in older patients with severe, multilevel stenosis, whereas fenestration procedures, consisting of bilateral laminotomies and partial facetectomies that preserve the midline structures, are an alternative in younger patients with intact discs. This is an especially attractive procedure when performed through a minimally invasive approach because injury to the dynamic spinal stabilizers is minimized. In one recent study, fewer complications and less postoperative instability were reported after bilateral laminotomies than after laminectomy.

Whenever possible, the source of pain should be localized with selective root blocks preoperatively to allow a more focal decompression. At surgery, specific attention should be directed to the symptomatic area, which may result in less extensive decompression than would normally be done with the pain source unconfirmed. If radical decompression of only one root is necessary, additional stabilization by fusion with or without instrumentation is usually unnecessary. The removal of more than one complete facet joint may require instrumented fusion. It is advisable to prepare the patient for fusion in case the findings at surgery require a more radical approach than anticipated. When both an ipsilateral lateral recess decompression and foraminal decompressions are necessary, a TLIF can be used without risking subsequent instability at the level. Positioning the patient with the abdomen hanging free minimizes bleeding. If fusion is likely, the hips should remain extended to prevent positional kyphosis. The authors do not recommend the use of a kyphosing frame when a fusion is performed. As in disc surgery, a microscope or magnifying loupes and a headlamp are helpful. The microscope allows for a smaller incision with less damage while maintaining binocular vision and depth perception caused by the smaller interocular distance of the microscope. When proceeding with the decompression, care should be taken to watch for adhesions that can result in dural tears, even if no previous surgery has been done. Frequently, the narrowing in the lateral recess and foramen is so great that a Kerrison rongeur cannot be used without damaging the root. Alternatively, dissection in the lateral recess and foramen may require a small, sharp osteotome or a high-speed burr, which allows the surgeon to thin the bone sufficiently to allow removal with angled curets. In contrast to disc surgery, for decompression the lateral recess is best seen from the opposite side of the table. During open procedures, the operating surgeon may find it necessary to switch sides during the operation to view the pathology and nerve roots better. Blunt probes with increasing diameters also are useful for determining adequate foraminal enlargement. Disc herniation should be treated at the same time as the spinal stenosis. A good approach is to start the decompression at a point of lesser stenosis and work toward the area of most severe stenosis. This often frees the neural structures enough to make the final decompression simpler and decreases the risk of damage to dura or nerve roots. This approach is especially useful when a minimally invasive undercutting laminoplasty technique is used to operatively treat spinal stenosis.

■ ADJACENT SEGMENT DEGENERATION

Adjacent disc degeneration and stenosis, or the transition syndrome, deserves special mention. It is known that disc degeneration occurs adjacent to a fusion in 35% to 45% of patients because of the ensuing hypermobility of the unfused joint, usually above the fusion mass. Adjacent segment stenosis below the fusion mass, although less frequent, always occurred along with stenosis above the fusion in a study by Lehmann et al.

Adjacent segment breakdown may cause symptoms that require surgery in 30% of patients. Pathology, including spinal stenosis, herniated nucleus pulposus, and instability, may require treatment years after successful surgery. Breakdown is possible one or two levels above lumbosacral fusions and above or below thoracolumbar and "floating" lumbar fusions. Schlegel et al. reported 58 patients who developed spinal stenosis, disc herniation, or instability at a segment adjacent to a previously asymptomatic fusion that was done an average of 13.1 years earlier, although 70% had good or excellent results. These clinical findings have been substantiated by subsequent biomechanical studies that confirmed kinematic changes in segments adjacent to spinal fusions. Simple malalignment that occurs during patient positioning when the hips are not extended may result in hypolordosis and increase the load across implants and increase posterior shear and laminar strain at adjacent levels. These changes may help to explain the cause of adjacent segment breakdown. Posterior lumbar interbody fusion (PLIF) also resulted in adjacent segment changes in all patients, but this did not affect results at 5 years in the series of Miyakoshi et al. In a study comparing patients with spondylolytic spondylolisthesis, degenerative spondylolisthesis, and spinal stenosis, Yu et al. found no significant differences in superior adjacent segment degeneration, instability, or clinical outcome after partial or total laminectomy and single-level PLIF.

Rigidity of instrumentation has been hypothesized to correlate with motion at adjacent segments. Studies have fueled interest in less rigid and dynamic stabilization constructs. In a prospective study with 4-year radiographic follow-up comparing rigid, semirigid, and dynamic instrumentation devices, Korovessis et al. found no differences in adjacent segment degeneration among the three groups. It is undetermined whether more rigid fusion increases the likelihood of adjacent segment changes. There is some evidence that maintaining the function of the posterior dynamic stabilizing paraspinous musculature, including the multifidus, may lead to decreased rates of adjacent segment degeneration after lumber fusion.

Fusion is more difficult as the number of levels fused increases, with L4-5 being the most frequent site of pseudarthrosis. The addition of a second level of fusion should be avoided if possible, and fusing a degenerative disc as a prophylactic measure does not seem to be supported by the data available. The actual source of transition syndromes is unknown; however, postoperative hypolordosis and rigidity of the fused segment probably contribute to the problem along with disruption of the posterior dynamic muscular stabilizers damaged during open posterior approaches. Surgery should attempt to maintain normal segmental lordosis and global sagittal balance, in addition to fusing the fewest segments possible while minimizing collateral damage to the paraspinous musculature and lumbodorsal fascia.

Complications are relatively infrequent after decompression for spinal stenosis and occur more often in patients with multiple comorbid conditions, especially diabetes. Comorbidities also contribute to poorer patient satisfaction and increased operative complications. Previous reports have cited increased morbidity and mortality associated with stenosis surgery in the elderly, although one study found that advanced age did not decrease patient satisfaction or return to activities, and there was no increase in morbidity associated with surgery for stenosis in the elderly.

Deep venous thrombosis also must be considered in patients after decompression. The incidence of this complication varies but is likely higher than reported. Pulmonary emboli are exceedingly rare, however. Prophylaxis is best limited to pneumatic compression devices of the foot or calf and early ambulation because the risk of epidural hematoma from pharmacologic agents is greater than the risk of a significant pulmonary event or deep venous thrombosis. Reoperation is necessary in 9% to 23% of patients with spinal stenosis.

DECOMPRESSION

There are no universal indicators of outcome after decompression. The number of levels requiring decompression have not been shown to affect the surgical results. Factors associated with poorer outcomes have included questionable radiographic confirmation of stenosis, female sex, litigation, previous failed surgery, and the presence of spondylolisthesis. A patient's self-assessment of health may be the best predictor of satisfaction. Cardiac comorbidity also may be predictive. Yukawa et al. found that the severity of central canal narrowing at a single level did not affect postoperative improvement in either functional ability, as determined by treadmill and bicycle testing, or patient self-assessment. Patients with multilevel stenosis had similar improvements in postoperative assessment scores.

Jönsson reported successful results after operative treatment in 62% to 67% of patients, although they noted deterioration at 5 years, with 18% requiring reoperation. Patients with a 6-mm or less anteroposterior canal diameter preoperatively had better results. Patients with hip arthritis, diabetes mellitus, previous surgery, vertebral fracture, or a postoperative complication had worse results. Although most are satisfied with the results of decompression, continued severe back pain and the inability to walk a distance have been reported. The Maine Lumbar Spine Group found that long-term (8 to 10 years) results were better after operative than nonoperative treatment. However, approximately half of the patients reported improvement in their back pain, leg pain, or both and were satisfied with their current status regardless of whether they were treated operatively or nonoperatively.

The cost of spinal stenosis surgery (decompressive laminectomy) at 2 years compared favorably with other treatment modalities in one Spine Patient Outcomes Research Trial (SPORT) study.

Progressive instability after decompression does not predict poor results. It appears that normal walking, sensory deficits, and ability to perform activities of daily living improved despite instability. Some further anterolisthesis is tolerated well after decompression, and it is appropriate to observe these patients for further symptoms before recommending fusion because 30% of patients develop anterolisthesis after decompression.

MIDLINE DECOMPRESSION (NEURAL ARCH RESECTION)

TECHNIQUE 39-26

- Perform the procedure with the patient under general endotracheal anesthesia. Position the patient prone using the frame of choice.
- Make the incision in the midline centered over the level of stenosis. Localizing radiographs should be taken to verify the level of surgery. Carry the incision in the midline to the fascia.
- Strip the fascia and muscle subperiosteally from the spinous processes and laminae to the facet joints to expose the pars interarticularis. Avoid damaging facet joints that are not involved in the bony dissection.
- Identify and remove the spinous processes of the levels to be decompressed. Clear the soft tissue with a sharp curet.
- Remove the lamina with a Kerrison rongeur or high-speed burr up to the insertion of the ligamentum flavum. If the lamina is extremely thick, a high-speed drill with a diamond or side-cutting burr can be used to thin the outer cortex to allow easier removal of the inner portion with a Kerrison rongeur. The lamina may be removed with impunity up to the insertion of the ligamentum flavum. Once the ligamentum insertion is identified, the ligamentum can be detached from the lamina with a curet. Take special care in removal of the lamina after the ligamentum flavum is released. The neural structures will be found compressed, and the usual space for instrument insertion may be unavailable. Remove the lamina until the pedicles can be felt. It can be helpful to begin the lateral recess decompression with the high-speed burr before removal of the ligamentum flavum to avoid having to place a rongeur into an already stenotic canal.
- Using the pedicle as a guide, identify the nerve root and trace it out to the foramen.
- With a chisel or rongeur, carefully remove the medial portion of the superior facet that forms the upper portion of the lateral recess (Fig. 39-50). Check the foramen for patency with an angled dural elevator or graduated probes. If there is further restriction, carry the dissection laterally and open the foramen; do not remove more than half of the pars. Undercutting into the foramen is especially helpful in this regard.

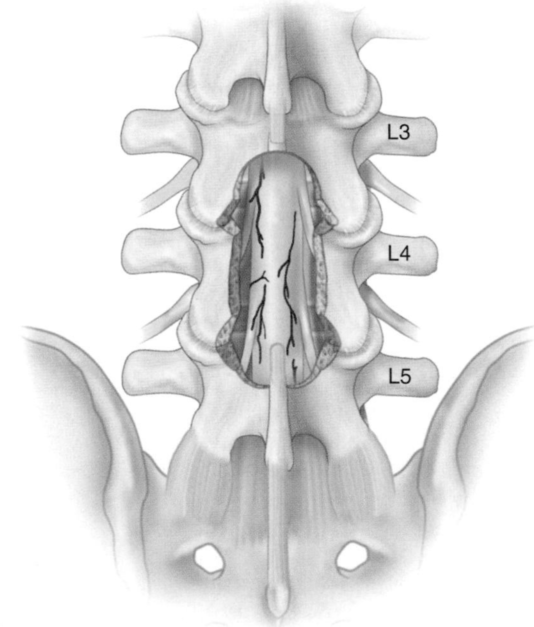

FIGURE 39-50 Typical midline decompression for spinal stenosis. Note medial facetectomy and foraminotomy with preservation of the pars. Decompression is from inferior border of L3 pedicle to superior border of L5 pedicle, exposing both lateral borders of dura in lateral recess. **SEE TECHNIQUE 39-26.**

- Inspect the disc and remove gross herniations unilaterally, but try to avoid bilateral annulotomy because this compromises stability. Usually the disc is bulging, and the anulus is firm. Remove the anulus and bony ridge ventrally if it is kinking the nerve. This procedure involves some risk of nerve injury and requires a bloodless field. If safety is a concern, a complete facetectomy may be better.
- Complete the dissection at all symptomatic levels. Decompression should be from the caudal aspect of the most proximal pedicle to the cephalad aspect of the most distal pedicle, allowing observation of the lateral margins of the dura in the lateral recesses. This can be done with preservation of the proximal portion of the lamina and the intervening ligamentum flavum at the level above and below. Many failed decompressions are the result of inadequate decompression of the foraminal region, so probing the foramen is mandatory to determine if the decompression is adequate.
- If no obstructions are noted and all areas have been decompressed adequately, ensure hemostasis with bipolar cautery and the temporary use of thrombin-soaked absorbable gelatin sponge (Gelfoam). Inspect for cerebrospinal fluid leakage. If desired, take a large fat graft from the incision or buttock and place it over the laminectomy defect. A ⅛-inch diameter drain can be placed deep in the wound, exiting through a separate stab incision. Close the wound in layers.

LESS-INVASIVE DECOMPRESSION

The consequences of bone and ligament removal must be considered when performing decompression for spinal stenosis. Removal of the spinous processes, laminae, variable portions of the facets and pars, supraspinous and interspinous ligaments, ligamentum flavum, and portions of facet capsules is routine during these operative procedures. Denervation of the paraspinal musculature occurs with wide exposures, which results in altered muscle function. A minimally invasive technique allows decompression of the significant compressing anatomy while preserving paraspinal muscles, the spinous processes, and intervening supraspinous and interspinous ligaments. Results with full-endoscopic techniques have been shown to be equal to those of conventional procedures, with the advantages of fewer complications. Although Kelleher et al. noted that minimally invasive decompression is effective in most patients, including those with degenerative spondylolisthesis; patients with scoliosis, especially with listhesis, have a significantly higher revision rate, and this must be considered when making treatment decisions.

SPINOUS PROCESS OSTEOTOMY (DECOMPRESSION)

Weiner et al. reported a 47% improvement in the Low Back Outcome Score and a 66% improvement in average pain level in 46 of 50 patients evaluated 9 months after surgery. Spinous process osteotomy was done at one to four levels; the only complications were dural tears in four patients. Although three patients died of unrelated causes, 38 of the 46 remaining patients were satisfied or very satisfied with their operative results. On reexploration or postoperative CT scans, spinous processes usually united with the remaining lamina in patients with short decompressions, although nonunion did not correlate with poor results. Complete laminectomy may be necessary if adequate decompression is impossible through the limited laminotomy in patients with severe involvement.

SPINOUS PROCESS OSTEOTOMY (DECOMPRESSION)

TECHNIQUE 39-27

(WEINER ET AL.)

- Patient positioning and localization of spinal levels are as described in Technique 39-26.
- Make a midline incision to expose the dorsolumbar fascia. Make a paramedian incision in the fascia, preserving the supraspinous and interspinous ligaments with subperiosteal dissection of the paraspinal muscles from the spinous process and laminae. Avoid lifting the multifidus muscles beyond the medial aspect of the facet joint to preserve their innervation.
- With a curved osteotome, free each spinous process from the lamina at its base. Release only the levels shown to be affected on preoperative imaging.
- When the spinous process is freed, retract it to one side with the paraspinal muscles beneath the retractor and the other blade of the retractor beneath the multifidus muscles to expose the midline (Fig. 39-51A). Resect approximately half of the cephalad lamina and one fourth of the caudal lamina along with the underlying ligamentum flavum.
- Using a loupe or microscope for magnification, undercut the lateral recess and open the foraminal zone (Fig. 39-51B). Complete laminectomy is recommended for severe stenosis or congenital stenosis involving all anatomic zones (central, lateral recess, and foraminal zones).
- Close the incision in routine fashion, allowing the spinous process to return to its normal position with suture of the fascia (Fig. 39-51C).

MICRODECOMPRESSION

Microdecompression can be done in patients without disc herniations or instability, including degenerative spondylolisthesis with a risk of worsening instability. This is a technically demanding procedure and is not recommended for patients with severe stenosis or congenital stenosis, which require complete laminectomy. McCulloch reported that decompressions were done at one to five levels without intraoperative complications in 30 patients treated for neurogenic claudication unresponsive to nonoperative measures. One superficial wound infection occurred. Of the 30 patients, 26 were very satisfied or fairly satisfied with their results; all but one stated that they would recommend the procedure to a friend with a similar problem. Good to

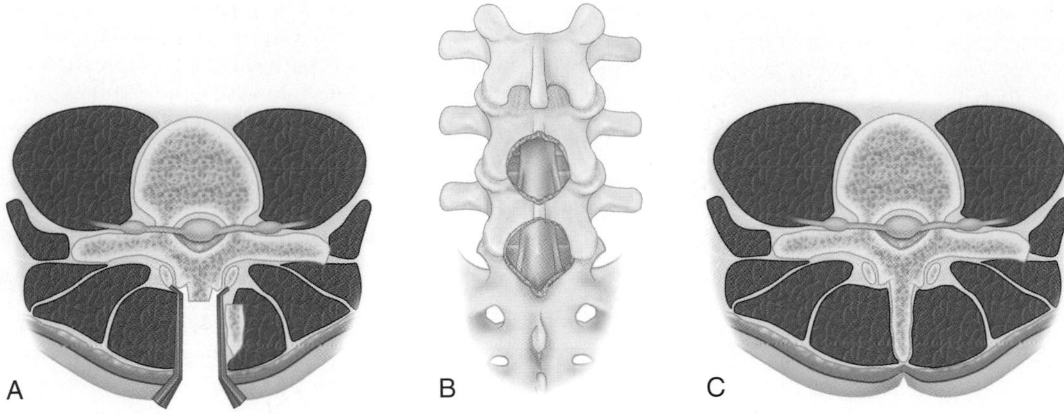

FIGURE 39-51 Spinous process osteotomy described by Weiner et al. **A,** Muscle is taken down on only one side and only to medial facet border. **B,** Decompression is performed under microscopic magnification. **C,** After closure, spine returns to normal position. **SEE TECHNIQUE 39-27.**

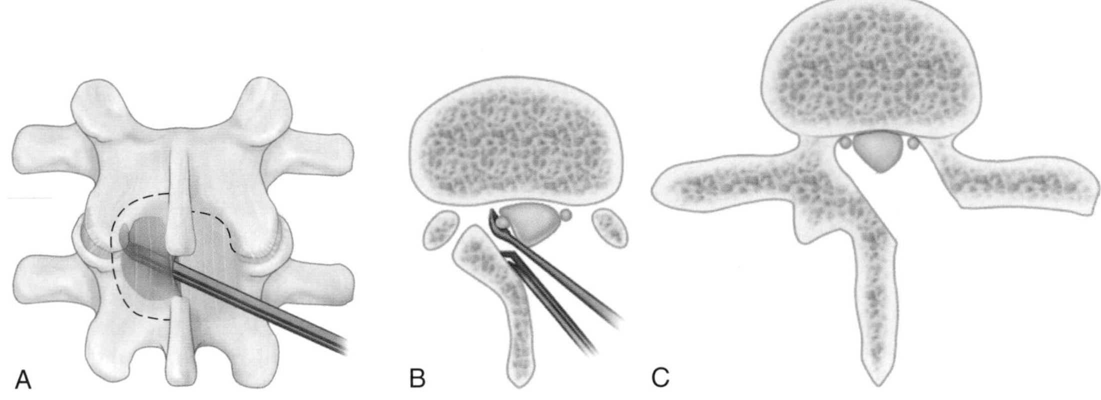

FIGURE 39-52 Microdecompression. **A,** Muscle is taken down on only one side, and ipsilateral decompressive hemilaminotomy is done; contralateral side is accessed under midline structures. **B,** Sac and root are gently retracted for contralateral decompression. **C,** End result is complete decompression with preservation of paraspinal musculature and interspinous and supraspinous ligaments, limited dead space, and excellent cosmetic result. **SEE TECHNIQUE 39-28.**

excellent results also have been reported (Orpen et al.) in 82 of 100 patients using a slightly modified microdecompression technique that allows decompression on both sides of the spine through a unilateral, hemilaminectomy approach.

TECHNIQUE 39-28

(MCCULLOCH)

- Place the patient in a kneeling position to increase interlaminar distance and identify the operative level on standard radiographs.
- Make a midline incision centered over the affected levels documented on preoperative imaging studies. Make a paramedian fascial incision on the most symptomatic side 1 cm from the midline.
- Elevate the multifidus muscles subperiosteally from the spinous process and laminae, but do not retract them beyond the medial aspect of the facet joint. Obtain unilateral interlaminar exposure and maintain it with a discectomy retractor.
- Under microscopic magnification, perform laminotomy cephalad until the origin of the ligamentum flavum is encountered. Use undercutting to preserve as much dorsal bone as possible; angle the microscope to accomplish this.
- In a similar fashion, resect the proximal one fourth of the caudal lamina, completing removal of the ligamentum flavum from origin to insertion. Angling of the microscope into the lateral recess allows further decompression of the cephalad and caudal nerve roots and lateral dura.
- When decompression is completed on one side, angle the microscope toward the midline for contralateral decompression (Fig. 39-52A). Rotation of the operative table allows better viewing of the contralateral structures (Fig. 39-52B).
- Use a no. 4 Penfield elevator or similar instrument to release adhesions between the dura and opposite ligamentum flavum, which is resected in a similar fashion.
- Remove the bone at the base of the spinous processes of the cephalad and caudal levels to provide adequate vision

of the opposite side (Fig. 39-52C). Some removal of the deepest portions of the interspinous ligament also is necessary to view the structures across the midline adequately.

- For surgeons comfortable with advanced minimally invasive techniques, the same laminoplasty procedure can be performed through a fixed tubular retractor using a transmuscular approach with less damage to the paraspinous musculature. This minimizes the need to dissect the multifidus attachment from the spinous process and lamina. Maintaining the dynamic stabilizers may lead to decreased rates of adjacent segment instability.

POSTOPERATIVE CARE. There are no special considerations after a simple decompression. The patient should be examined carefully for the first few days for new neurologic changes that may indicate the formation of an epidural hematoma. The patient is encouraged to walk on the first day. Sutures are removed at 14 days if nonabsorbable sutures have been used. We prefer the use of absorbable subcutaneous sutures with a glue-type product for the final skin closure. The same limitations as after disc surgery apply to decompressions without fusion. For patients engaged in heavy manual labor, a permanent job change may be required. Return to work also is similar to return after disc surgery.

DECOMPRESSION WITH FUSION

The indications for spinal fusion with decompression for spinal stenosis are becoming more clearly defined. Preoperative and intraoperative factors must be carefully considered when decompression and fusion surgery are contemplated. Serious thought should be given to performing arthrodesis in addition to decompression in patients with preoperative degenerative spondylolisthesis, scoliosis, kyphosis, stenosis at a previously decompressed level, or stenosis adjacent to a previously fused lumbar segment. The finding of a synovial facet joint cyst radiographically or intraoperatively is important because these have been associated with development or progression of slipping postoperatively. Because cysts reflect derangement of the facet joint, fusion should be considered after decompression and excision of synovial cysts in patients with spinal stenosis with or without preoperative instability.

The prevalence of postoperative problems related to instability varies, possibly because of the great variations in the extent of the operative decompression, but the likelihood of iatrogenic instability remains low if established principles of decompression are followed. White and Wiltse noted subluxation after decompression in 66% of patients with degenerative spondylolisthesis. They suggested that a fusion be done in conjunction with decompression in (1) patients younger than 60 years old with instability caused by the loss of an articular process on one side, (2) patients younger than 55 years old with a midline decompression for degenerative spondylolisthesis that preserves the facets, and (3) patients younger than 50 years old with isthmic spondylolisthesis. The complete removal of one facet, or more than 50% resection of both facets, may result in instability. In addition, generalized spinal stenosis that requires extensive decompression with the loss of multiple articular processes may require fusion. When complete bilateral facetectomies are necessary, the addition of a lateral fusion may be difficult and the bone graft may impinge on the exposed nerve roots. In this instance, an anterior interbody fusion is warranted to prevent postoperative instability. Posterior segmental instrumentation for posterior spinal fusion has decreased the high incidence of pseudarthrosis after long lumbar fusions.

The complications of this procedure are similar to the complications of disc surgery; however, the risk of nerve root damage and dural laceration is greater. The rates of infection, thrombophlebitis, and pulmonary embolism also are slightly higher. When a facet has been partially resected, later facet or pars fracture may account for a recurrence of symptoms, although the most important cause of failure to relieve symptoms has been found to be inadequate decompression. Bone regrowth has been noted in 88% of patients after total laminectomy and in all patients with associated spondylolisthesis.

INTERSPINOUS DISTRACTION

A distraction technique recently has been described as an alternative to decompression surgery. A spacer is inserted into the interspinous space as far anteriorly and as close to the posterior aspect of the lamina as possible. This procedure requires no ligamentous or bony resection, and the spinal canal is not breached, eliminating the risk of neural damage. Symptomatic benefit has been reported in 54% at 1 year in one study and in 78% at 4.2 years in another for degenerative spinal stenosis. Verhoof et al., however, did not recommend its use for the treatment of spinal stenosis in the presence of degenerative spondylolisthesis because of the unacceptably high failure rate. Fifty-eight percent of their patients required decompression and posterolateral fusion within 24 months. Long-term follow-up data are still lacking.

ANKYLOSING SPONDYLITIS

Ankylosing spondylitis is a chronic inflammatory disease of unknown etiology. It is a seronegative spondyloarthropathy that primarily affects the axial skeleton, sacroiliac joints, and pelvis. Less commonly, involvement of peripheral joints, eyes (iritis or uveitis), heart, and lungs can occur. Inflammation of the spinal joints and enthesopathies cause chronic pain and stiffness and can lead to progressive ankylosis of the spine in patients with long-standing disease. Ankylosing spondylitis typically affects young adults between the ages 20 and 40 years, with a male to female ratio of 1:3. The average onset of symptoms occurs at 23 years of age; there can be an 8.5- to 11.4-year delay from initial symptoms to diagnosis. There is a known association with the HLA-B27 antigen. Between 88% and 96% of patients who have ankylosing spondylitis are HLA-B27 positive, but only 5% of the HLA-B27 population develops ankylosing spondylitis.

Initially, morning stiffness is the primary symptom. Other early symptoms usually are chronic pain and stiffness in the middle and lower spine, as well as buttock pain from the sacroiliac joint. The symptoms are nonspecific for ankylosing spondylitis. As the disease progresses, ankylosis of the sacroiliac joints and spine can occur. Ankylosis usually progresses from caudal to cephalad. After ankylosis, however, pain symptoms often improve. Other symptoms may be related to hip arthritis, which occasionally progresses to spontaneous arthrodesis. Pulmonary cavitary lesions with fibrosis occur, as do aortic insufficiency and conduction defects. Amyloid deposition can cause renal failure. Uveitis requires special ophthalmologic care and follow-up to prevent permanent vision changes. Breathing may be restricted because of fusion of the costochondral and costovertebral articulations.

In the spine, ankylosis can lead to a loss of lumbar spinal lordosis and progressive kyphosis of the cervical and thoracic spine. This combined with hip flexion deformities can result in a loss of sagittal balance and disabling functional deficits, such as an inability to look above the horizon or to lie in bed. Furthermore, fused sections of the spine make it more susceptible to fracture, pseudarthrosis, or spondylodiscitis.

Radiographs initially show fusion of the sacroiliac joints, which characteristically occurs bilaterally. In the vertebral bodies, inflammatory resorption of bone at the enthesis causes periarticular osteopenia. This resorption initially is seen as a "squaring off" of the corners of the vertebral bodies. Subsequent ossification occurs in the anulus fibrosis, sparing the anterior longitudinal ligament and disc and giving the "bamboo spine" appearance on radiographs. The posterior elements are similarly affected, with ossification of the facet joints, interspinous and supraspinous ligaments, and ligamentum flavum. Atlantoaxial instability must be identified, especially in any patient having surgery for conditions associated with ankylosing spondylitis. Because of the stiff subaxial spine, instability occurs in 25% to 90% of patients with ankylosing spondylitis.

Treatment is directed at maintaining flexibility with stretching of the hip flexors and hamstrings and maintaining spinal alignment with exercises and posture. Sleeping supine on a firm mattress with one pillow may help maintain sagittal alignment and prevent hip flexion contractures. Medications used in the treatment of ankylosing spondylitis fall into three categories. The first includes nonsteroidal antiinflammatory drugs that relieve pain by decreasing joint inflammation. The second group comprises disease-modifying antirheumatic drugs such as minocycline, sulfasalazine, and methotrexate. This is an unrelated group of drugs found to slow the disease process, but they do not provide a cure. Finally, tumor necrosis factor-α blockers have been shown to be effective.

Operative management in patients with ankylosing spondylitis is indicated to decrease pain and improve function. Total hip arthroplasties are the most common surgical interventions performed in this population followed by spinal osteotomies to correct sagittal imbalances.

Spinal fractures in patients with ankylosing spondylitis are always serious and frequently are life-threatening injuries. Spine osteopenia that is common in this population combined with fused segments make patients more vulnerable to fractures, especially from minor trauma. Furthermore, distorted anatomy from disc ossification, ectopic bone, and sclerosis can make the spinal fractures difficult to see on plain radiographs, and these injuries often are missed. It should be up to the treating physician to prove that the patient with ankylosis does not have a fracture after trauma. Spinal precautions and immobilization in a position accommodating the patient's posture is very important. Often CT or MRI studies are needed. Fractures usually occur in the lower cervical spine, frequently are unstable, and usually are discovered late. Persistent pain may be the only finding until late neurologic loss occurs. In patients with established kyphosis, the deformity may suddenly improve. The patient's previous deformity may be unknown to individuals providing emergency care. Any perceived change in spinal alignment, even if the result of trivial trauma, should be considered a fracture in a patient with ankylosing spondylitis. The standard procedure is to immobilize the patient in the position in which he or she is found because extension may result in sudden neurologic loss. A widened anterior disc space, which may be the only obvious radiographic finding, creates an unstable configuration that is prone to translation, late neurologic loss, and slow healing. Imaging with MRI, CT, or bone scan may be helpful in making the diagnosis.

Surgical stabilization of fractures in patients with ankylosing spondylitis can be challenging. For cervical fractures, anterior and posterior or long posterior constructs are recommended because of the poor bone quality. Thoracolumbar fractures can be stabilized with a long posterior construct across the fractured level. More recently, percutaneous techniques of long-segment stabilization are being used. The morbidity and mortality associated with these procedures in patients with ankylosing spondylitis are very high because of the comorbidities many of these patients have.

OSTEOTOMY OF THE LUMBAR SPINE

Smith-Petersen, Larson, and Aufranc in 1945 described an osteotomy of the spine to correct the flexion deformity that often develops in ankylosing spondylitis and sometimes in rheumatoid arthritis. Since then, others have reported similar procedures. The technique described by Smith-Petersen et al. is done in one stage. Others have described surgery done in two stages, consisting of division of the anterior longitudinal ligament under direct vision instead of allowing it to rupture when the deformity is corrected by gentle manipulation, as in the method of Smith-Petersen et al.

If the flexion deformity is severe, the patient's field of vision is limited to a small area near the feet and walking is extremely difficult. This is evident by looking at the chin-brow to vertical angle (Fig. 39-53). Respiration becomes almost completely diaphragmatic. Gastrointestinal symptoms resulting from pressure of the costal margin on the contents of the upper abdomen are common; dysphagia or choking may occur. In addition to improvement in function, the improvement in appearance made by correcting the deformity is important to the patient. If extreme, the deformity should be corrected in two or more stages because of contracture of soft tissues and the danger of damaging the aorta, the inferior vena cava, and the major nerves to the lower extremities. According to Law, 25 to 45 degrees of correction usually can be obtained, resulting in marked improvement functionally and cosmetically. Initially, mortality was about 10% with operative treatment; however, a later series reported no deaths or serious complications.

The safest and most efficient position for this procedure is with the patient lying on his or her side. This lateral position has several advantages: (1) it is easier to place the grossly deformed patient on the table; (2) the danger of injuring the ankylosed cervical spine by pressure of the forehead against the table is eliminated; (3) the anesthesia is easier to manage because maintaining a clear airway and free respiratory exchange is less difficult; and (4) the operation is easier because any blood would flow out from the depth of the wound rather than into it. Adams described hyperextending the spine with an ingenious three-point pressure apparatus, and Simmons described surgery with the patient on his or her side and under local anesthesia. When the osteotomy is complete, the patient is turned prone, carefully fracturing the anterior longitudinal ligament with the patient briefly under nitrous oxide and fentanyl anesthesia.

The osteotomy usually is made at the upper lumbar level because the spinal canal here is large, and the osteotomy is distal to the end of the cord. A lumbar lordosis is created to compensate for the thoracic kyphosis; motion of the spine is not increased. Osteotomy methods include resection of the spinous processes from the laminae to the pedicles, simple wedge resection of the spinous processes into the neural foramina (Fig. 39-54A and B), chevron excision of the laminae and spinous processes (Fig. 39-54C and D), and combined anterior opening wedge osteotomy after posterior resection of the spinous processes and laminae.

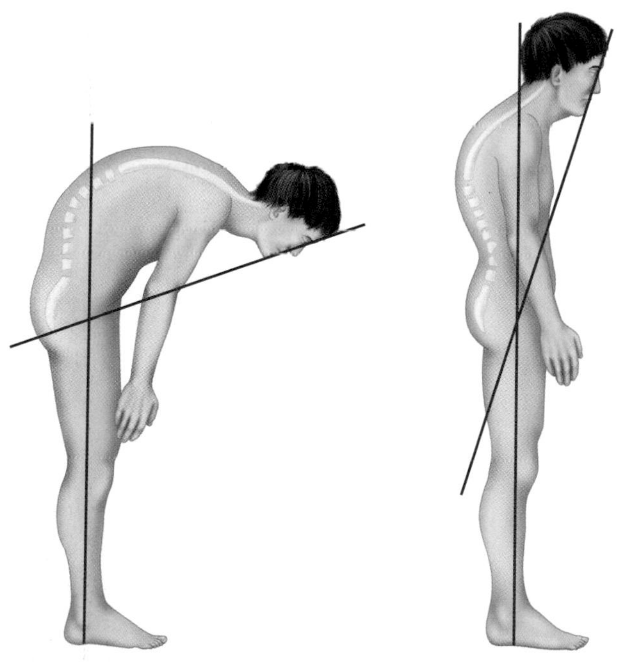

FIGURE 39-53 Chin-brow to vertical angle is measured from brow to chin to vertical while patient stands with hips and knees extended and neck in fixed or neutral position.

An average correction from 80 to 44 degrees has been reported after upper lumbar osteotomy, with correction maintained by internal fixation. Manual osteoclasis worked best in patients with calcified ligaments. Complications from this procedure include hypertension, gastrointestinal problems, neurologic defects, urinary tract infections, psychologic problems, dural tears with leakage, retrograde ejaculation, and, rarely, rupture of the aorta.

Spinal osteotomy is a demanding procedure for which proper training and experience are mandatory. The surgeon should be familiar with the several options available.

SMITH-PETERSEN OSTEOTOMY

The Smith-Petersen osteotomy is an excellent option for correction of smaller degrees of spinal deformity. Bone is removed through the pars and facet joints (Fig. 39-54C and D). If a previous fusion has been done, care should be taken to thin the fusion mass gradually until the ligamentum flavum or dura is exposed. Symmetric resection is necessary to prevent creating a coronal deformity. Removal of the underlying ligament also is helpful in preventing buckling of the dura or iatrogenic spinal stenosis. Approximately 10 degrees of correction can be obtained with each 10 mm of resection. Excessive resection should be avoided because it may result in foraminal stenosis. In patients with degenerative discs, decreased flexibility may limit the amount of correction that can be obtained. The osteotomy is closed with compression or with in situ rod contouring, and bone graft is applied.

PEDICLE SUBTRACTION OSTEOTOMY

Pedicle subtraction osteotomy (Fig. 39-54A and B) is best suited for patients who have significant sagittal imbalance of 4 cm or more and immobile or fused discs. Pedicle subtraction osteotomy is inherently safer than the Smith-Petersen osteotomy because it avoids multiple osteotomies. Typically, 30 degrees or more of correction can be obtained with a single posterior osteotomy, preferably at the level of the deformity. If the deformity is at the spinal cord level, pedicle subtraction osteotomy can be used, but manipulation of the cord must be avoided. Thomasen and Thiranont and Netrawichien described the use of this osteotomy after laminectomy and pedicle resection. In their technique, compression instrumentation was used, along with simultaneous flexion of the

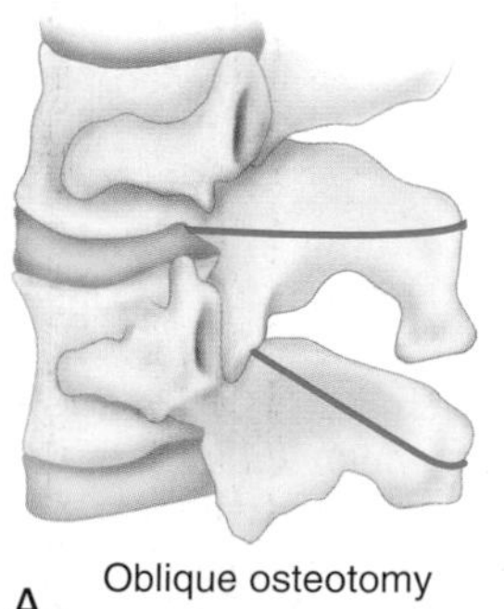

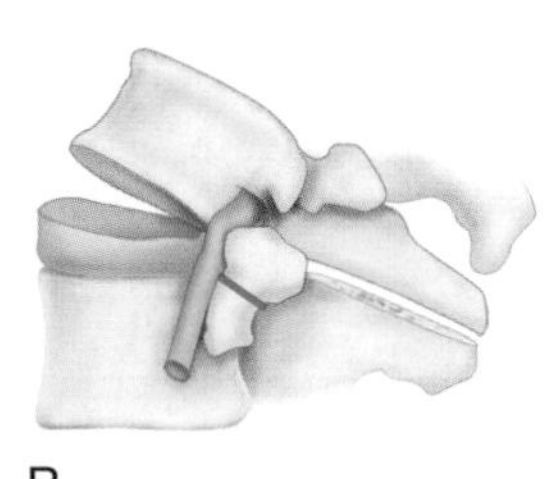

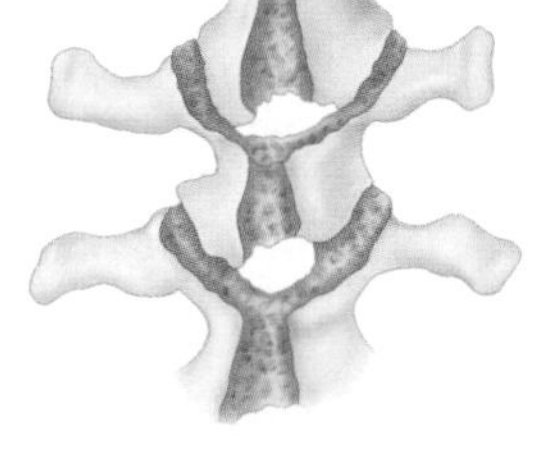

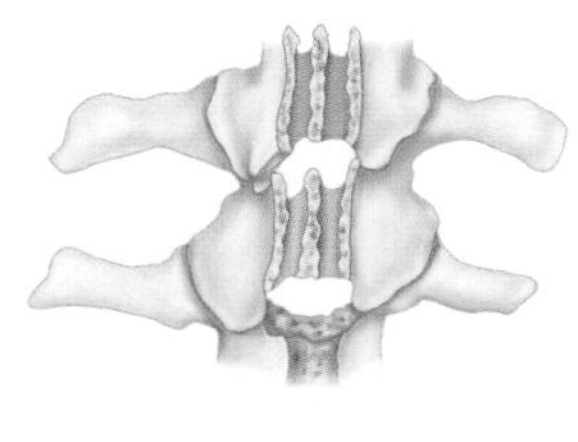

FIGURE 39-54 Methods of high lumbar spinal osteotomy. **A** and **B**, Simple wedge resection of spinous processes into neural foramina. **C** and **D**, Chevron excision of laminae and spinous processes.

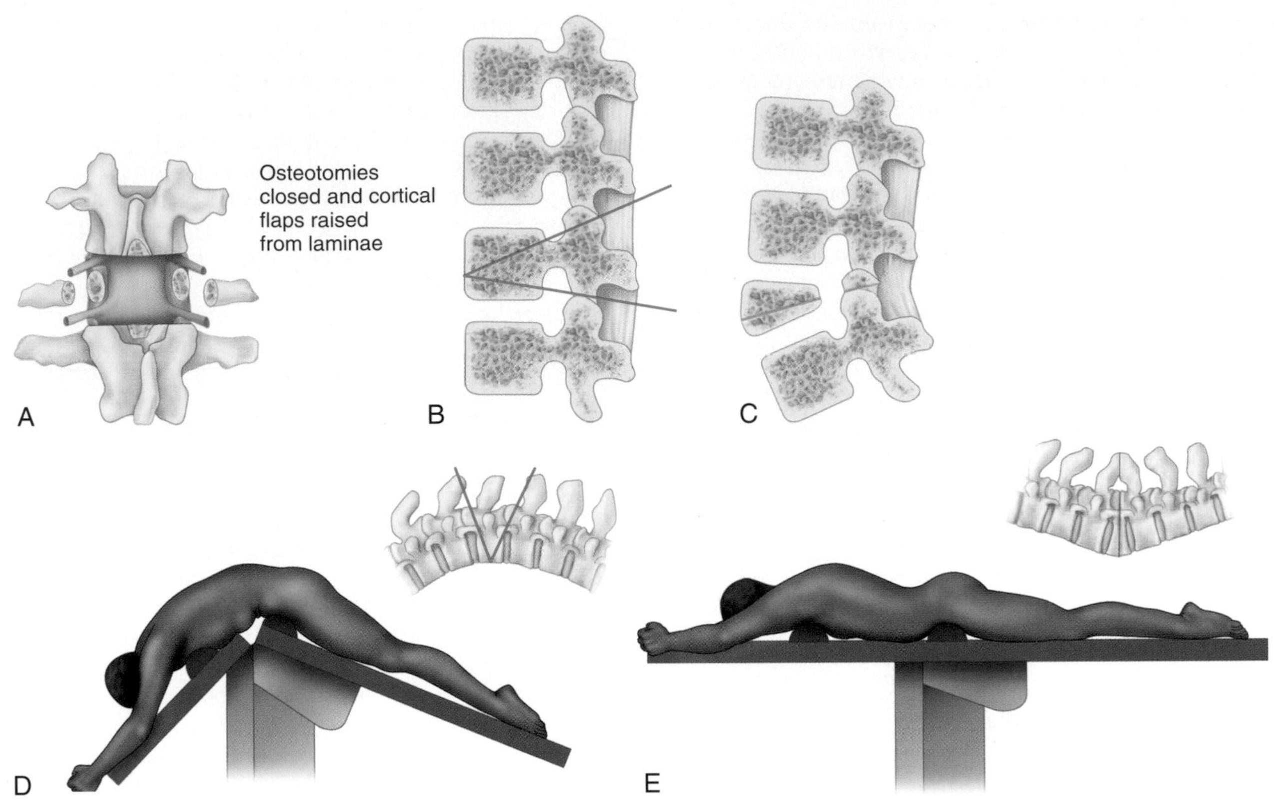

FIGURE 39-55 **A,** Total laminectomy. **B,** Rather than osteotomy with opening of disc in front, Thomasen used resection of posterior wedge and resection of pedicles **(C)**. Patient's position on operating table before **(D)** and after **(E)** reduction of osteotomy. Osteotomy gap is closed when table is brought from flexed to straight position.

head and foot of the operating table (Fig. 39-55). Care must be taken to avoid compression of the dura or creation of a coronal deformity. A wake-up test is done after correction and cancellous bone grafting have been completed.

EGGSHELL OSTEOTOMY

The eggshell osteotomy requires anterior and posterior approaches and usually is reserved for severe sagittal or coronal imbalance of more than 10 cm from the midline (Fig. 39-56). This is a spinal shortening procedure with anterior decancellization followed by removal of posterior elements, instrumentation, deformity correction, and fusion.

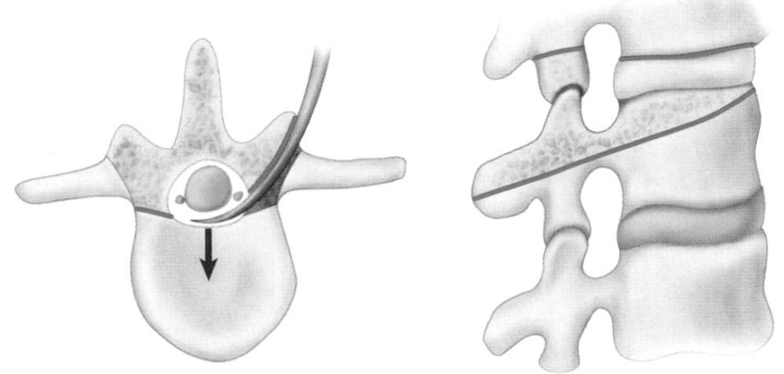

FIGURE 39-56 Heinig eggshell procedure. After posterior elements have been removed and pedicles have been collapsed outward, long, sharp curet is used to collapse "eggshell."

ADULT SPINAL DEFORMITY

Although nearly 60% of the adult population has some form of spinal deformity, only approximately 6% are symptomatic. Most patients with symptoms from their spinal deformity are 70 years of age or older, and most report pain and impaired health-related quality of life. Approximately 60% of patients with late-onset degenerative scoliosis are female. Degenerative curves tend to be short segment, usually lumbar, and less severe than the curves in idiopathic scoliosis. Symptoms of spinal stenosis are more common in patients with degenerative scoliosis. The goal of treatment of degenerative scoliosis is to relieve back pain and the symptoms of spinal stenosis, whereas the treatment goals for adult idiopathic scoliosis usually are pain control and deformity correction. Treatment of adult idiopathic and degenerative scoliosis requires a different approach from that used for typical adolescent idiopathic scoliosis, is more challenging, and is more likely to have complications such as dural tears, nonunion, implant breakage, and wound infection. Adult spinal deformity curves tend to be more rigid than those in adolescents, and surgery is further complicated by the prevalence of medical comorbidities and osteopenia in these older patients.

INCIDENCE AND PROGRESSION OF DEFORMITY

Adult idiopathic scoliosis is defined as a coronal deformity of more than 10 degrees with associated structural changes in a patient older than 20 years at time of diagnosis, most commonly in patients in their late 30s. Women are affected much more frequently than men, similar to the incidence of adolescent scoliosis. Studies have shown a prevalence of 2% to 4% for curves of more than 10 degrees. According to Weinstein and Ponseti, thoracic curves of more than 50 degrees progress approximately 1 degree per year up to 75 degrees, when progression slows to about 0.3 degrees per year, finally stopping at about 90 degrees. Lumbar curves progress at a rate of 0.4 degrees per year after reaching only 30 degrees; a more aggressive approach is warranted for lumbar curves, especially after progression is documented. Predictors of lumbar curve progression include L5 above the intercristal line, apical rotation of more than 30%, an unbalanced or decompensated curve, a thoracic curve of more than 50 degrees, and a thoracolumbar or lumbar curve of more than 30 degrees. Sixty-eight percent of adult curves progress more than 5 degrees over time.

Patients with idiopathic scoliosis rarely develop significant pulmonary complications, even with curves exceeding 100 degrees. In the absence of overt thoracic lordosis, surgery generally is not warranted to maintain or improve pulmonary function in adults.

Degenerative scoliosis develops in patients with previously straight spines after age 40 years, typically affecting the lumbar spine with an associated lumbar hypolordosis, lateral olisthesis, and spinal stenosis. Men and women are affected more equally than patients with idiopathic curves, with 60% to 70% of those affected being women. Degenerative scoliosis occurs in 6% to 30% of the elderly population, with most curves being minor, affecting fewer segments (two to five segments) than in adult idiopathic scoliosis (seven to 11 segments), with an equal distribution of right and left lumbar curves. Rotary subluxation varies and seems to be worse after decompression surgery without fusion. Curves can be progressive, but the natural history has not been elucidated conclusively. Progression of 1 to 6 degrees a year has been reported. Symptoms of spinal stenosis occur most often in degenerative curves that have defects in the convexity and concavity, possibly because significant degenerative changes preceded the development of the scoliosis. As a result, treatment of degenerative scoliosis often is necessary to relieve spinal stenosis by decompression, with instrumented fusion to prevent instability and further progression of deformity.

CLASSIFICATION

In general, adult scoliosis can be broadly divided into two categories: deformity due to progression of untreated or inadequately treated adolescent idiopathic scoliosis (AIS) or de novo scoliosis, which is primary degenerative scoliosis that results from asymmetric disc and facet joint degeneration. Deformity as a result of progression of AIS typically manifests as long, gradually progressive thoracic or thoracolumbar curves, whereas de novo deformity presents as sharp lumbar or thoracolumbar curves with an apex at L2-3 or L3-4. A third type of adult spinal deformity can be caused by an adjacent idiopathic curve or metabolic bone disease. More recently, the Scoliosis Research Society (SRS)-Schwab classification system has been developed. This system takes into account the coronal curve type, pelvic parameters, and sagittal balance (Fig. 39-57). It has been validated in a number of studies and has shown excellent interobserver and intraobserver reliability.

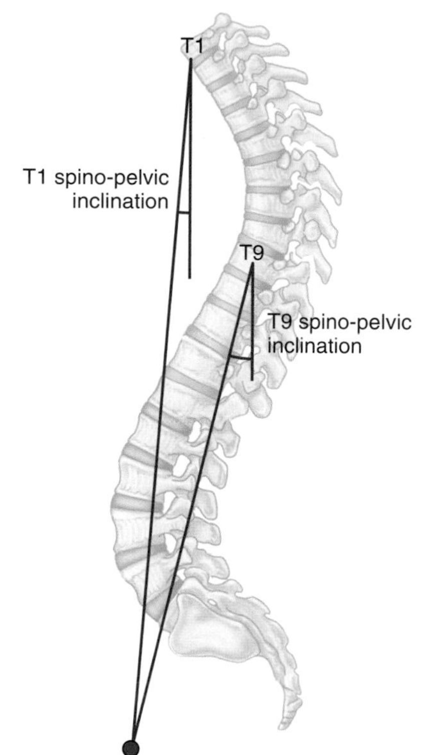

FIGURE 39-57 Measurement of the T1 spinopelvic inclination angle.

SAGITTAL AND CORONAL BALANCE

In the treatment of adult spinal deformities, whether idiopathic or degenerative in origin, it is important to understand the normal sagittal relationships. In a normal spine, the primary curvature is kyphosis of the thoracic spine, which develops first in infants. Subsequent to upright posture, the secondary lordotic curvatures in the cervical and lumbar spine develop between 5 and 15 years old. Curves in men and women are similar at the cessation of growth, although the curves develop more quickly in women.

Sagittal balance is the alignment that is necessary to center the head over the pelvis or hips in the sagittal and coronal planes. A plumb line dropped from the center of the C7 vertebral body is referred to as the *sagittal vertical axis.* On the standing lateral long-cassette view, the plumb line normally falls through or behind the sacrum. Normal values for the sagittal vertical axis in adults are from +48 mm to −48 mm, with negative values indicating a position behind the sacral promontory. An alternative means of measuring sagittal balance is the T1 spinopelvic inclination angle (T1SPI), which is measured as the angle between a vertical plumb line from T1 and a line drawn from T1 to the center of the bicoxofemoral axis (Fig. 39-57). The advantage of using T1SPI over the sagittal vertical axis is that it is not vulnerable to radiographic calibration errors. Another method of assessing sagittal balance is the T1 pelvic angle (TPA). Similar to the T1SPI, TPA is the angle formed by a line drawn from the center of T1 to the bicoxofemoral axis and then to the center

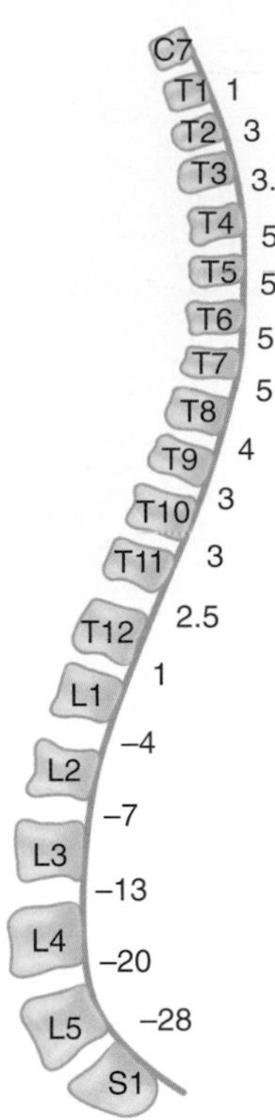

FIGURE 39-58 Bernhardt and Bridwell segmental sagittal measures of thoracic and lumbar spine. Note contribution of L4-5 and L5-S1 discs to overall lumbar lordosis (67%).

of the S1 endplate. The two distinct advantages of TPA are that it does not require radiographic calibration and it integrates both T1SPI and pelvic tilt, both of which have been shown to correlate with outcome scores.

Coronal balance is quantified globally by the amount of offset between the C7 plumb line and the center-sacral vertical line (CSVL) and the offset between the apical vertebra from the CSVL. Any translation of the coronal vertical axis to either side of the midline is considered decompensation.

Sagittal and coronal vertical axes are used to evaluate and estimate global balance. Global balance is the result of segmental alignment of the functional spinal unit and regional alignment of the cervical, thoracic, and lumbar segments. Bernhardt and Bridwell measured 102 radiographs of normal spines to determine normal sagittal plane alignment (Fig. 39-58). By convention, kyphosis is represented as a positive measurement and lordosis is represented as a negative value. In a normal adult spine, there is a small amount of kyphosis segmentally at each end of the thoracic kyphosis, reaching a maximum at the apical region (T6-7) of about +5 degrees. Apical discs or vertebrae are identified in the sagittal plane as those that are parallel to the floor. Considered independently, the thoracolumbar junction is a transition zone of force transmission and alignment. In this region, a shift occurs from the thoracic kyphosis to lumbar lordosis. The first lordotic disc is typically at L1-2, and normal thoracolumbar alignment as measured from the cephalad T12 endplate to the caudal L2 endplate is 0 to −10 degrees. The lumbar spine is a region of lordosis, reaching a maximal segmental lordosis at L4-5 and L5-S1. The sagittal apex of the lumbar spine usually is L3. Greater than 60% of lumbar lordosis is created by the discs at L4-5 and L5-S1, which contribute −20 degrees and −28 degrees to the regional lordotic measurement.

Because most lordosis is present in the distal lumbar spine, it is important to maintain normal segmental and regional interrelationships so that global balance is preserved. As a rule of thumb, on a lateral radiograph taken with the patient facing the surgeon's right, there is a "sagittal clock," as described by Bridwell. In a normal, standing patient, the apical L3 disc or endplate points at the 3-o'clock position, L4 points at the 4-o'clock position, and L5 points at the 5-o'clock position. If this regional alignment is maintained, the likelihood of a postoperative flatback deformity is minimized.

Achieving appropriate sagittal balance in adult spinal deformity correction is essential. The relationship between balanced sagittal vertical axis (SVA) and health-related quality of life scores has been well established in the literature. Sagittal malalignment results in compensatory pelvic retroversion (increased pelvic tilt), which helps the patient maintain an upright posture; however, pelvic retroversion has been shown to increase energy expenditure and negatively affect ambulation. Some patients are limited in their ability to compensate with pelvic retroversion because of hip flexion contractures or stiffness. Schwab et al. listed as goals of surgical correction (1) SVA less than 50 mm, (2) T1SPI less than 0 degrees, (3) pelvic incidence-lumbar lordosis mismatch less than 9 degrees, and (4) pelvic tilt less than 20 degrees.

SPINOPELVIC ALIGNMENT

Recent research has established the importance of spinopelvic parameters—pelvic incidence, pelvic tilt, and sacral slope—in the evaluation of adult patients with spinal deformity (Fig. 39-59). Pelvic incidence is defined as the angle between a line perpendicular to the center of the sacral endplate and a line drawn from the center of the sacral endplate to the center of the bicoxofemoral axis (Fig. 39-59A). It is important to understand that pelvic incidence is a fixed morphologic parameter that does not change after skeletal maturity. Pelvic incidence can be considered the "take-off" degree of the lumbar spine; the higher this angle, the more lumbar lordosis required to maintain an upright posture. Average pelvic incidence in adults is 52 ± 10 degrees. Pelvic tilt, on the other hand, is a variable angle that represents the amount of compensatory pelvic retroversion the patient is using to maintain an upright posture (Fig. 39-59B). It is defined as the angle between a vertical reference line through the bicoxofemoral axis and a line from the center of the bicoxofemoral axis to the center of the sacral endplate. A pelvic tilt of less than 20 degrees is considered normal, and values of more than 30 degrees are considered markedly increased. Finally, sacral slope is defined by the angle between a horizontal reference line and a line parallel to the superior sacral endplate (Fig. 39-59C).

CLINICAL EVALUATION

Back pain occurs in 60% to 80% of patients with idiopathic scoliosis, which is similar to the occurrence in the general population. Pain is the chief presenting complaint in 25% to 80% of patients with adult idiopathic curvatures. This can include mechanical back pain, buttock pain, and, occasionally, radiculopathy or neurogenic claudication. Neurogenic claudication occurs in 13% as a result of degenerative changes

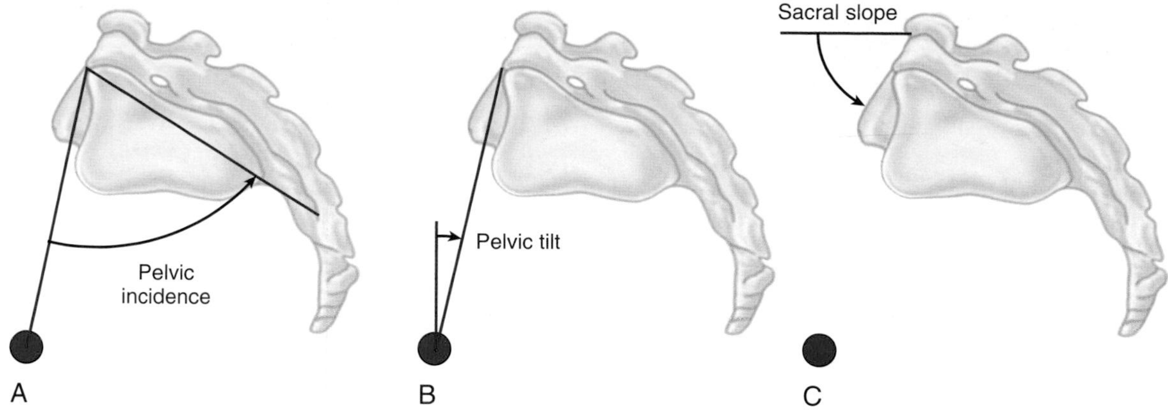

FIGURE 39-59 Measurement of pelvic incidence **(A)**, pelvic tilt **(B)**, and sacral slope **(C)**.

within or, more commonly, distal to the lumbar curve. Radiculopathy occurs in only 4%, with entrapment of nerve roots within the foramina of the concavity. In contrast to degenerative scoliosis, most adult patients with idiopathic scoliosis have more mechanical symptoms than neurologic complaints. Patients may relate symptoms of curve progression, such as a progressive lean or list to one side, changes in waistline symmetry, hip prominence, protuberant or flaccid abdomen, hemline changes, or a loss in height in the absence of fracture. Neurologic symptoms may include radiculopathy or neurogenic claudication, which usually is a result of degenerative changes in the distal fractional curve. Diminished pulmonary function in patients with curves of more than 60 degrees or cor pulmonale in patients with curves of more than 100 degrees occasionally is caused by the scoliosis and should be evaluated carefully to rule out other causes. Predictors of pain include curves of more than 45 degrees, lumbar curves, and thoracolumbar and lumbar curves of more than 45 degrees with apical rotation and coronal decompensation.

Physical examination findings usually are negative except for the spinal deformity. The skin should be examined for evidence of pathologic lesions and hair patches that suggest underlying intraspinal anomalies. If spinal cord anomalies exist, atrophy may be evident in the lower extremities or intrinsic atrophy of the foot may be present with pes cavus and clawing of the toes. Reflexes should be documented, as should the results of a comprehensive neurologic examination.

The deformity should be evaluated by looking for structural features of the rib and lumbar paraspinal prominence on forward bending while also recording flexibility. This test also helps to determine which curve is primary because more rotation and subsequent prominence is found in the more structural primary curve. If rib prominence exceeds 3 cm, thoracoplasty should be considered if surgery is performed. Trunk shift is identified by dropping an imaginary line perpendicular to the floor from the lateral ribs. This line should symmetrically intersect the pelvis. Plumb lines should be dropped to evaluate for coronal decompensation and to help in estimating sagittal balance. Special attention should be paid to the left shoulder because instrumentation of a curve with a structural upper thoracic curve must include this segment to avoid a high left shoulder postoperatively. Waistline asymmetry should be noted, and any limb-length inequality must be considered. Equalizing limb length with ¼-inch blocks sometimes is helpful if limb-length discrepancy is more than 1 inch. Placing the patient prone on the examination table often gives information regarding curve flexibility and the extent of deformity that will be found during intraoperative positioning. Some surgeons find traction and bending films useful to evaluate curve flexibility.

In degenerative scoliosis, symptoms of neurogenic claudication are present in 71% to 90% of patients and usually cause them to seek medical attention, with deformity incidentally noted. These symptoms often do not improve with forward bending, and to obtain relief patients support the trunk with the arms or assume a supine position. This is in contrast to the usual patient with spinal stenosis and neurogenic claudication. Radiculopathy from facet overgrowth, foraminal stenosis within the concavity of curvature, or nerve root tension along the curve convexity can occur, although neurologic deficits are rare, and back pain is ubiquitous. Primary treatment is directed at decompression of spinal stenosis, with fusion or instrumentation indicated based on the potential for increased instability.

Physical findings are nonspecific in most patients. Motion usually is preserved, but patients guard against hyperextension. Symptoms may be reproduced by this maneuver in the presence of spinal stenosis. Neurologic examination rarely identifies significant motor, sensory, or reflex deficits; however, any abnormal findings should be documented. Evaluation of distal pulses is necessary to help rule out peripheral vascular disease and vascular claudication. Bilateral absence of Achilles tendon reflexes may be an indicator of peripheral neuropathy. Flattening of the lumbar spine represents degenerative change, and a lumbar prominence on forward bending accentuates the convexity of a coronal deformity. Sagittal and coronal balance should be estimated clinically. When contemplating any decompressive or stabilizing procedure, correction of the entire degenerative scoliotic segment must be considered because of sagittal or coronal decompensation.

ANATOMY AND BIOMECHANICS

Adult scoliosis shares most of the anatomic features of idiopathic adolescent scoliosis. Unique to adult patients with scoliosis are the diminished elasticity of the ligamentous structures and the narrowing of disc spaces that combine to stiffen primary and secondary or compensatory curves. Osteopenia also must be considered in older patients, especially in patients with risk factors for osteoporosis, such as glucoid use, postmenopausal status, and a personal or family history of fragility fractures.

The biomechanics of the bone-implant interface must be considered if long instrumentation constructs are used, especially when extended to the sacrum. Because of the long lever arm produced in long deformity constructs and the relatively poor fixation obtained in the sacrum, S1 screws have a high likelihood of biomechanical failure if not protected. To obtain purchase anterior to the biomechanical pivot point at the anterior sacrum, many surgeons choose iliac instrumentation. The two most commonly used modern instrumentation options for protecting the S1 screws are iliac screws and S2-alar-iliac (SAI) screws. Iliac screws provide strong fixation and ease of insertion with the potential risk of hardware prominence and the theoretical technical difficulty of rod alignment with the S1 screws. SAI screws somewhat mitigate the hardware prominence and rod alignment issues of traditional iliac screws. Fixation can be augmented with a load-sharing structural interbody fusion device. The most significant biomechanical increase in posterior instrumentation strength is with the addition of the iliac screws. The superiority of any of these techniques has not been established, and the surgeon's experience and preference determine the choice.

Finally, osteoporosis is a significant consideration in the treatment of these patients. Although there is no cause-and-effect relationship between bone density and degenerative scoliosis, these patients usually are older and more predisposed to osteoporosis. Compression fractures and compromised operative fixation may complicate the treatment of patients with concomitant disease. Attention should be paid to the optimization of bone metabolism and bone density before any major spinal deformity surgery. If indicated, supplementary vitamin D and calcium should be started before surgery and continued afterward throughout the phases of bone healing.

DIAGNOSTIC IMAGING

RADIOGRAPHY

For both idiopathic and degenerative scoliosis, standing radiographs on 36-inch cassettes must be obtained and scrutinized for coronal and, more important, sagittal balance. It is critical for this to be conducted in a standardized fashion. Patients should be instructed to stand in a neutral upright position with the hips and knees comfortably extended and the fingers on the clavicles (shoulders at 45 degrees of forward elevation). Lateral bending radiographs over a foam fulcrum are ideal for assessing flexibility, although standard maximal effort bending films often suffice. Often, simple prone radiographs give a good estimate of sagittal and coronal alignment that can be found intraoperatively. For sagittal deformities, appropriate fulcrum bending films can be obtained to determine flexibility. Push prone views, as described by Kleinmann et al. and Vedantam et al., are useful in determining the response of the lowest instrumented vertebra to instrumentation. With degenerative scoliosis, degenerative disc changes and flattening of the normal lumbar lordosis are present. With both degenerative and idiopathic scoliosis, rotary subluxation may be evident in some patients, with lateral olisthesis of varying degrees.

COMPUTED TOMOGRAPHIC MYELOGRAPHY AND MAGNETIC RESONANCE IMAGING

By providing information regarding central, lateral recess, and foraminal stenosis, MRI is very useful in the preoperative evaluation of adult patients with spinal deformity. In addition, disc hydration and excessive facet degeneration are useful pieces of information provided by T2-weighted sequences that may influence whether surgery stops at or includes a lower degenerative segment. The degree of desiccation of the L5-S1 disc should prompt extra consideration to end at the adjacent disc above or include the degenerative segment. Adjacent segment pathology is common, and in older patients it may be prudent to include such diseased discs.

CT myelogram can be used instead of MRI in patients with contraindications (such as a pacemaker); however, it is an invasive procedure and should not be used routinely. Non-myelogram CT scans can be useful in patients with extreme deformity or prior surgery. Finally, DICOM images from CT scans can be used by 3D printers to create life-size, three-dimensional models, which occasionally can be useful for surgical planning in severe deformities.

NONOPERATIVE TREATMENT

Recent studies have called into question the value of nonoperative care in adult scoliosis, given the high cost and lack of improvement in outcome measures. However, given the potential morbidity of surgical treatment, we believe that attempting traditional methods of nonoperative treatment of back and leg pain are appropriate in patients with adult scoliosis. Orthoses may be helpful for the relief of axial degenerative symptoms. Intermittent use of a soft thoracolumbosacral orthosis (TLSO) is better tolerated than use of a rigid TLSO by older, often endomorphic, patients. The orthosis should be worn during symptomatic periods and kept to a minimum otherwise. Correction of deformity or prevention of progression of these curves is impossible, and an orthosis is used only for the management of symptoms; the patient should be aware of the treatment goals. Physical therapy should be continued in addition to bracing, with the ultimate goal of paraspinal strengthening and subsequent core stabilization that allow the brace to be discarded. Cognitive behavioral therapy is another key aspect of the patient with chronic pain that should not be overlooked.

OPERATIVE TREATMENT

When adequate nonoperative treatment has failed in a patient with unremitting symptoms or radiographic progression, surgery should be considered. Curves of more than 50 degrees with documented progression, loss of pulmonary function (believed to be caused by the scoliosis when curves exceed 60 degrees), progressive neurologic changes, and significant coronal or sagittal decompensation are relative indications for surgery. Cosmetic considerations are a genuine concern for patients as well and may play a small role in operative decision-making. The goal of surgery is to maintain a balanced spine, with the head centered over the pelvis, while fusing the minimum number of segments possible.

Although improvement radiographically and clinically can be expected with operative treatment, the overall incidence of complications has been reported to be from 13% to 40% and the incidence of pseudarthrosis is 13% to 17%. Several authors have noted that although elderly patients have the greatest risk of complications, they show greater improvement in pain and disability compared with younger patients. Revision rates are relatively low.

A spinal implant should be used that allows segmental placement of screws and allows iliac fixation. If fusion of the lumbosacral joint is anticipated, interbody fusion has traditionally been obtained with allograft or fusion cages that are cut to maintain the normal segmental lordotic disc alignment. The use of cell-saver autotransfusion is encouraged. Spinal cord monitoring should include somatosensory and transcranial motor evoked potentials. If useful data are obtained and maintained with somatosensory and motor evoked potentials, wake-up testing is unnecessary until the conclusion of the surgery. If pedicle screws are used below T8, pedicle screw stimulation can be useful to confirm proper placement. Although we find free-hand pedicle screw technique to be safe and to reduce patient and surgical team radiation exposure, some surgeons may not be comfortable with this. Fluoroscopy or computer-aided navigation enhances the use of anatomic landmarks and is helpful for some surgeons, especially in the setting of deformity and prior fusion. Regardless, this surgery is complex and has an extended recuperation period, with a significant risk of complications, which the patient must understand when operative treatment is chosen.

DECOMPRESSION IN DEGENERATIVE SCOLIOSIS

Decompression alone is a viable option for a patient with symptomatic spinal stenosis and minimal kyphosis, a neutral sagittal vertical axis, and no instability on dynamic imaging. Attempts should be made to avoid destabilizing the spine during decompression, and fusion should be done if more than 50% of either facets or an entire facet is resected. Degenerative scoliosis should be considered the coronal variant of spondylolisthesis; if the ligamentous structures are violated and facet and disc resections are necessary, fusion should be considered. Decompression alone is inadequate if claudicatory leg symptoms originate from foraminal stenosis within the concavity of a degenerative curve. Transfeldt et al. found a higher complication rate in patients with full curve fusion and less improvement in the Oswestry Disability Index than in patients with decompression alone.

POSTERIOR INSTRUMENTATION AND FUSION

IDIOPATHIC SCOLIOSIS

Patients with flexible idiopathic curves of less than 70 degrees and no significant kyphosis or decompensation are candidates for posterior instrumentation and fusion alone. This can be done with numerous instrumentation systems and techniques (see Chapter 44). The ideal candidate for a posterior procedure has a smaller, flexible curve; hypokyphosis; and a flexible compensatory lumbar curve. Posterior procedures also are an appropriate choice for a King type V or Lenke subclass 2 or 4 structural upper thoracic curve. Similar correction clinically and radiographically has been reported with posterior-only approaches compared with combined anterior and posterior procedures, with the advantages of decreased blood loss, anesthesia, and operative time.

Standard posterior approaches are used, and instrumentation may include hooks, wires, or screws for curve correction. The current trend involves the use of all-pedicle screw constructs for deformity correction because of the segmental fixation that is obtained and the three-column control that is provided by a pedicle screw placed into the vertebral body. With this fixation, derotation may be possible to some extent during the correction maneuver. Another benefit of the use of pedicle screws is the extraspinal placement of implants, which avoids the space-occupying phenomenon created by hooks or wires placed within the spinal canal. Finally, the cortical fixation of a screw through the pedicle is superior biomechanically to hook fixation, which makes this technique appealing for an osteoporotic adult spine. These benefits are not without risks, however, and the primary concern is pedicle screw malposition that affects the great vessels or the spinal cord, dura, or nerve roots. When done by surgeons with proper training, pedicle screw placement so far has been safe and effective for the treatment of adult scoliosis; however, it is wise to discuss procedures in detail with patients before surgery and to explain the inherent risks involved.

Selection of fusion levels is similar to that in adolescent scoliosis patients. The goal of surgery is a balanced spine with the head centered over the pelvis in the sagittal and coronal planes. Fusion should be from stable vertebra to stable vertebra, unless pedicle screw instrumentation is used, and fusion can safely be stopped short of the stable vertebra. For curves with features similar to King types II and V curves without severe kyphosis, pedicle screw fixation seems ideal. This technique allows fusion of the curve from end vertebra to end vertebra, which can save one to three fusion levels distally in some patients compared with typical hook constructs. In adults, flexibility of the compensatory curve must be considered more than in adolescents with scoliosis because overcorrection of the thoracic curve in a spine with a relatively inflexible lumbar curve results in decompensation and an unsatisfactory result. It is prudent to apply only a conservative amount of correction that can be accommodated by the compensatory curve so that normal balance is restored and further progression is halted. The amount of correction that can be obtained is estimated from preoperative bending films.

Avoiding a flatback deformity during posterior distraction is mandatory because this deformity is much easier to prevent than to treat. Nonetheless, because of pseudarthrosis, implant failure, transition syndromes, adjacent level fracture, patient positioning, and other technical reasons, flatback deformity can occur in some patients under the best of circumstances. Concave distraction of the lumbar spine, especially beyond L2, should be avoided because this maneuver is kyphogenic. Segmental instrumentation allows differential correction along the same rod, which is helpful in preventing flatback deformity and shoulder decompensation. Avoiding distraction, or even applying some convex compression, along with precontouring the rods into lordosis helps to maintain normal lumbar alignment.

DEGENERATIVE SCOLIOSIS

In a patient with a flexible spine and mild-to-moderate scoliosis, symptomatic spinal stenosis is treated with traditional decompression. Occasionally, facetectomy or partial pedicle resection is necessary to decompress symptomatic nerve roots. In this situation, posterior intertransverse fusion is recommended. If laxity is present, instrumentation should extend from neutral and stable vertebrae at each end of the construct. Ending the instrumented fusion at a level of kyphosis potentiates adjacent segment changes and may result in a proximal junctional kyphosis, which remains a particularly vexing problem for deformity surgeons. Rotary subluxation also can occur after decompression alone in the presence of unstable degenerative scoliosis. The fusion should end at a neutrally rotated, level, and stable end vertebra and should restore sagittal and coronal balance. Care should be taken to avoid stopping instrumentation and fusion at any apical segments or at the apex of a kyphosis or scoliosis because this creates deformity later.

ANTERIOR SPINAL INSTRUMENTATION AND FUSION

Deformity correction through an anterior approach is described in Chapter 44, but it warrants mention here because anterior instrumentation and fusion with third-generation implants have given excellent deformity correction in adults and have not caused significant problems with kyphosis as did the early Zielke and Dwyer implants. With single-rod or double-rod implant systems and structural grafts, anterior deformity correction is a viable alternative for lumbar and thoracolumbar curves because it allows short segment correction of flexible curves. Primary thoracic curves with flexible and compensatory lumbar curves in adults also can be treated effectively with anterior fusion. Correction must be appropriate, however, for the ability of the lumbar curve to compensate; overcorrection in adults results in more decompensation than in the flexible spines of children with scoliosis. Also, as in pediatric deformities, strict attention must be paid to the upper thoracic spinal segment from T1 or T2 to T6 to prevent shoulder asymmetry owing to a structural upper thoracic curve. An upper thoracic curve is a relative contraindication for anterior spinal instrumentation and fusion unless measures are taken to allow persistent tilt of the cephalad end vertebra, which would allow the upper thoracic curve to remain balanced. Anterior interbody fusion, either from a direct anterior or far lateral approach, can be especially helpful in restoring lordosis and indirectly decompressing foraminal stenosis in degenerative scoliosis but usually requires additional posterior stabilization.

POSTOPERATIVE MANAGEMENT

Patients are commonly monitored overnight in the intensive care unit with frequent neurologic evaluations and observation to prevent complications associated with fluid shifts, which occur after such long procedures. Sitting is encouraged the day after surgery, and formal physical therapy is initiated. Walking as tolerated is encouraged with assistance until independent ambulation is achieved. With modern pedicle screw constructs, a thoracolumbar orthosis generally is not necessary. The Foley catheter is removed when the patient is able to get to a bedside commode with minimal assistance. Antibiotics can be discontinued when drains are pulled or at 24 hours postoperatively, depending on surgeon preference, and oral narcotic analgesics usually are well tolerated by the third day after surgery. Pneumatic leg compression devices are used as prophylaxis against deep vein thrombosis because of the possible risk of epidural hematoma associated with pharmacologic agents. These are discontinued when the patient is fully independent with ambulation. Nonsteroidal antiinflammatory medications are avoided for 3 months postoperatively because of their potential inhibitory effect on fusion.

COMBINED ANTERIOR AND POSTERIOR FUSIONS

For a rigid curve of more than 70 degrees or a curve that is decompensated sagittally or coronally, or for instrumentation that crosses the lumbosacral joint, a combined approach can be more powerful. For severe rigid thoracic deformities of more than 100 degrees, which often are associated with translation of the trunk of more than 4 to 6 cm anterior or lateral to the pelvis, Boachie-Adjei and Bradford showed that vertebrectomy, as a combined or staged procedure, was effective in achieving spinal balance. It is preferable to complete combined procedures, if possible, under a single anesthesia because this results in fewer complications and a shorter hospitalization; however, if any portion of the procedure is unexpectedly long, blood loss is excessive, or a patient is unable to tolerate continuation of the procedure, it is prudent to postpone the second stage of the procedure. Parenteral nutrition between stages is recommended because patients often develop a postoperative ileus and do not tolerate enteral nutrition.

When a combined procedure is used, the first stage usually includes anterior release, discectomy, and fusion of the primary curve. If instrumentation is extended to the lumbosacral joint, interbody fusion is advisable at L4-5 and L5-S1, with structural grafting of these discs to maintain lordosis, improve fusion rates, and decrease stresses on the posterior implants. Morselized bone graft is placed in the thoracic disc spaces and usually consists of the rib excised for the exposure. Supplemental bone graft can be obtained from the inner table of the anterior iliac crest if the rib is small or osteoporotic. Instrumentation may or may not be necessary during the anterior portion of the procedure and is placed at the surgeon's discretion.

After anterior release and fusion, posterior instrumentation and fusion are done, with segmental fixation from stable vertebra to stable vertebra. Care is taken to avoid ending an instrumentation construct at the apex of a curve in either the coronal or the sagittal plane because of the risk of later decompensation. It also is prudent to include any disc level with severe degenerative changes, especially in degenerative deformities.

Boachie-Adjei and Cunningham reported the use of a hybrid approach consisting of limited anterior and overlapping posterior instrumentation for adult thoracolumbar and lumbar scoliosis. They noted 59% and 68% correction in thoracolumbar and lumbar curves, respectively.

PEDICLE SUBTRACTION OSTEOTOMY

This is a very useful technique for correction of sagittal imbalance when performed below the level of the conus. It can achieve greater correction than Smith-Petersen type osteotomies alone and may be necessary in the setting of sagittal imbalance in a previously fused spine.

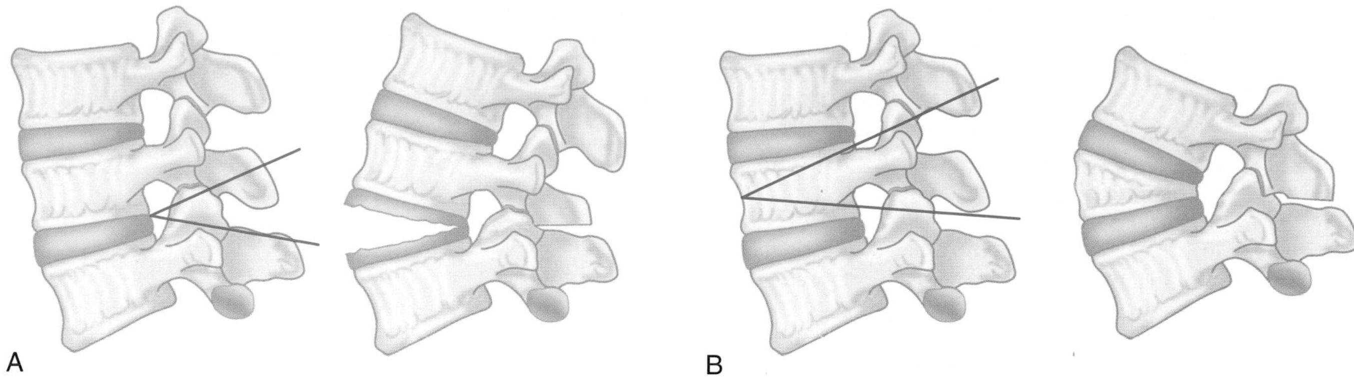

FIGURE 39-60 **A,** Smith-Petersen osteotomy. **B,** Pedicle subtraction osteotomy. **SEE TECHNIQUE 39-29.**

TECHNIQUE 39-29

(BRIDWELL ET AL.)

- Pedicle screws should be placed as the first step. We prefer using a freehand technique whenever possible to reduce radiation exposure to the operative team and patient.
- Extend the central laminectomy to include all posterior elements, using Leksell and Kerrison rongeurs and osteotomes as much as possible to save bone graft material. This posterior element resection is, in essence, a Smith-Petersen osteotomy above and below the pedicles that are to be resected (Fig. 39-60A).
- Use an osteotome to create the transverse process osteotomy.
- Resect the pedicle itself with a Leksell rongeur, high speed burr, or both.
- Carefully dissect along the vertebral wall with a small Cobb or Penfield elevator to avoid injuring the segmental vessels. Place specialized spoon retractors along the lateral aspect of the vertebral body.
- To make the osteotomy, a decancellation or sharp osteotomy technique can be used. Using an osteotome provides better control of the geometry of the osteotomy, thereby affording more precise and greater correction. Commercial osteotomy guides can guide the amount of resection required to achieve the desired angular correction. It is critical during this step to avoid iatrogenic injury, via stretch or direct sharp injury, to the dural sac and nerve roots. This is best accomplished with a nerve root retractor and a no. 4 Penfield.
- Before the osteotomy is completed, a temporary rod can be placed to allow for controlled closure.
- Once the posterior vertebral wall is sufficiently thinned, use specialized impactors to impact the posterior body wall into the defect. It is critical to ensure that the dural sac is free of adhesions at this point.
- With a high-speed drill, resect the lateral vertebral wall, taking care to avoid injury to the nerve roots and dural sac. Alternatively, a thin Leksell rongeur can be used.
- Close the osteotomy by applying compression or cantilever bending maneuvers to the spine. During this process, it is critical to make sure that the decompression is wide enough above and below to avoid injury or iatrogenic stenosis to the dural sac.

OTHER TECHNIQUES

The newest generation of implants can be used to treat most deformities, allowing instrumentation of all thoracic levels down to the sacrum and pelvis. Approaches and techniques generally have remained the same, however. Pedicle screw instrumentation has been used in all levels in the treatment of spinal deformities, with excellent clinical and radiographic results. For lumbar curves, pedicle screw instrumentation is applied to the convexity and compressed to create lordosis; for typical thoracic curves, the pedicle screws are applied to the concavity of the deformity and distracted to restore kyphosis. Any compensatory curves must be treated appropriately with compression where lordosis is required and with distraction where kyphosis is desired. Upper thoracic curves are controlled by compression of the convexity because most of these curves also are kyphotic.

Computer-navigation devices can be a helpful technique in the placement of pedicle screws; however, given the additional setup time required and the safety and ease of freehand techniques, we typically reserve navigation for placement of pedicle screws across a fusion mass that has lost all anatomic landmarks. This technique initially was used with CT and MRI but more recently has been used with fluoroscopy. Fluoroscopy has the advantage of "real-time" images that are not dependent on patient position and are not subject to as much error from motion as are CT and MRI. These technologies can confirm anatomic relationships and, although expensive, are being used more frequently. Scheufler et al. reported that intraoperative biplanar fluoroscopy and CT-guided navigation significantly facilitated correction and instrumentation while reducing radiation exposure to the surgeon in less-invasive decompression and fusion procedures.

For skilled endoscopic spinal surgeons, video-assisted thoracoscopic surgery provides excellent visualization through relatively small incisions with the potential to decrease blood loss, postoperative pain, periscapular winging, and pulmonary dysfunction. The learning curve is very steep, however, with initial procedures taking a good deal longer than a typical thoracotomy. This technique requires double lumen intubation and places increased demands on the anesthesia staff. Although video-assisted thoracoscopic surgery continues to develop, the options for its use in anterior instrumentation are still limited. In adult patients with spinal deformity, in whom osteoporosis and osteopenia are prevalent, structural grafts may be more difficult to place endoscopically, limiting the application of video-assisted thoracoscopic surgery.

Direct lateral or far lateral approaches to the interbody space in the lumbar spine are especially useful for degenerative scoliosis. These techniques allow for complete disc resection with a bony bed for fusion, excellent correction of coronal deformities, and very good indirect decompression of foraminal stenosis caused by degenerative changes and scoliotic foraminal compression. These are not typically done as stand-alone procedures and deformity corrections benefit from the addition of posterior pedicle screw instrumentation, which can be done posteriorly if the posterior fusion is omitted.

Anand et al. reported that minimally invasive multilevel percutaneous correction and fusion through a direct lateral transpsoas approach allowed multisegment correction with less blood loss and morbidity than an open approach. Reported complications of combined transpsoas extreme lateral interbody fusion and posterior pedicle screw instrumentation have included intraoperative bowel injury, motor radiculopathy, and postoperative thigh paresthesias or dysesthesias. The rate of major complications after a far lateral approach in one study, however, compared favorably to that of other procedures (12%). For these reasons, we commonly perform multilevel lateral interbody fusion and/or anterior interbody fusion as the first stage of adult deformity fusion surgery.

ILIAC FIXATION

Modern instrumentation techniques for correction of spinal deformity in adult patients often include iliac fixation. These large (> 8.0 mm diameter) and very long (> 80 mm) screws obtain purchase anterior to the lumbosacral pivot point. This creates a more rigid construct and unloads the S1 screws, which, even with tricortical purchase, can be prone to loosening and even fracture. Iliac fixation should be considered when fusion constructs extend proximally to L3 or beyond and when there is insufficient sacral fixation, significant sagittal or coronal imbalance that requires correction, L5 or S1 defects from tumor or infection, or an L5-S1 pseudarthrosis.

Although many iliac fixation techniques have been developed, currently the two most popular choices are iliac screws and S2-alar-iliac screws (S2AI). Traditional iliac screws involve placing a screw from the posterior superior iliac spine (PSIS) toward the anterior superior iliac spine (ASIS). This screw can be safely placed freehand or with the use of intraoperative fluoroscopy. However, there are two distinct disadvantages of this technique: (1) symptomatic screw prominence and (2) difficulty with aligning the iliac screw tulip with the S1 tulip without the use of an offset connector. Alternatively, the S2AI screw obviates both of these issues by starting more medially and distally, between the S1 and S2 foramen, extending through the SI joint, and obtaining purchase in the ilium. Early experience with the S2AI screws suggest they cause fewer symptomatic hardware issues requiring removal. Adult deformity surgeons should be able to place both types of iliac fixation in case anatomic or hardware issues preclude one option.

BOX 39-8

Classification of Coccydynia

Based on Etiology
- Idiopathic
- Traumatic

Based on Pathology
- Degeneration of the sacrococcygeal and intercoccygeal disc and joints
- Morphology of the coccyx: types II, III, IV, presence of a bony spicule and coccygeal retroversion
- Mobility of the coccyx: hypermobile or posterior subluxation
- Referred pain: lumbar pathology or arachnoiditis of the sacral nerve roots, spasm of the pelvic floor muscles, inflammation of the pericoccygeal soft tissues
- Other: neoplasm, crystal deposits, infection, somatization or neurosis

Based on Coccygeal Morphology
- Type I—curved gently forward
- Type II—marked curve with apex pointing straight forward
- Type III—angled forward sharply between the first and second or second and third segments
- Type IV—anteriorly subluxed at the level of the sacrococcygeal joint or first or second intercoccygeal joint
- Type V—coccygeal retroversion with spicule
- Type VI—scoliotic deformity

(Modified from Nathan ST, Fisher BE, Roberts CS: Coccydynia: a review of pathoanatomy, aetiology, treatment and outcome, J Bone Joint Surg 92B:1622, 2010. Copyright British Editorial Society of Bone and Joint Surgery.)

COCCYGEAL PAIN

Pain in the region of the coccyx is referred to as coccydynia or coccygodynia. Although the literature indicates that this is a rare disorder, physicians in our group who specialize in spine care evaluate and treat several cases of coccygeal pain every year.

The most common causes of coccydynia that we have observed in our practice are a single direct axial trauma, such as falling directly on the coccyx, and a subtle form of cumulative trauma that occurs as a result of long periods of sitting awkwardly. As with other musculoskeletal disorders, however, other causes need to be considered (Box 39-8). In the absence of any obvious pathologic changes involving the coccyx, coccygeal pain is classified as idiopathic and may actually be the result of spasticity or abnormalities affecting the musculature of the pelvic floor.

Body mass index appears to correlate with different coccygeal configurations (Table 39-12) and different coccygeal lesions. Obese patients have mainly posterior subluxation, normal-weight patients have mainly a hypermobile or

TABLE 39-12

Frequency of Different Coccygeal Lesions Correlated With Patient Body Mass Index (BMI)

	POSTERIOR LUXATION	ANTERIOR LUXATION	HYPERMOBILITY	SPICULE	NORMAL COCCYX
Obese patients BMI > 27.4	51%	4%	27%	2%	16%
Normal-weight patients BMI 19.5 to ≤ 27.4	15%	6%	30%	16%	33%
Thin patients BMI < 19.5	4%	4%	15%	29%	48%

(Modified from Maigne JY, Doursounian L, Chatellier G: Causes and mechanisms of common coccydynia: role of body mass index and coccygeal trauma, Spine (Phila Pa) 25:3072, 2000.)

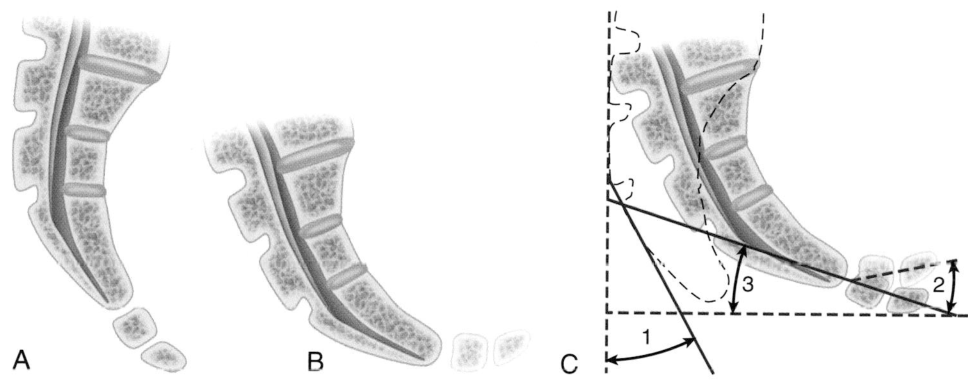

FIGURE 39-61 Evaluation of coccygeal mobility. **A,** Standing radiograph. **B,** Sitting radiograph shows flexion of the coccyx. **C,** Superimposition of sitting radiograph on standing radiograph, matching the sacrum by pivoting the sitting film through an angle representing sagittal pelvic rotation (angle 1 = angle of rotation). Coccygeal mobility is indicated by angle 2 (angle of mobility). Angle 3 is the angle at which the coccyx strikes the seat surface (angle of incidence).

radiographically normal coccyx, and thin patients have mainly anterior subluxation and spicules.

The most common presenting complaint is pain in and around the coccyx without significant low-back pain or radiation or referral of pain. Typically, the pain is associated with sitting and is exacerbated when rising from a seated position. Palpation in the region of the coccyx may reveal localized tenderness and swelling. Although coccydynia is a clinical diagnosis, imaging studies are helpful in the evaluation. Radiographs obtained with the patient sitting and standing are most useful because they allow measurement of the sagittal rotation of the pelvis and the coccygeal angle of incidence (Fig. 39-61). Advanced imaging studies, such as MRI and technetium-99 m bone scans, may demonstrate inflammation of the sacrococcygeal area, indicating coccygeal hypermobility, and are helpful to rule out some forms of underlying pathology such as chordoma.

Nonsurgical methods such as NSAIDs and use of a donut cushion remain the standard initial treatment for coccydynia and are successful in approximately 90% of patients. When these methods fail to relieve pain, we have had success in reducing or eliminating coccygeal pain with the injection of a local anesthetic and corticosteroids under fluoroscopic guidance. Although there is no clear consensus in the literature regarding the exact site of injection, we generally target the vestigial disc at the point of maximal tenderness over the coccyx.

COCCYGEAL INJECTION

TECHNIQUE 39-30

- Place the patient prone on a pain management table, with the legs slightly abducted and the feet "pigeon-toed" in.
- Aseptically prepare the skin area from the lumbosacral junction to the coccyx with isopropyl alcohol and povidone-iodine. Drape the area in sterile fashion.
- Adjust the C-arm to an anteroposterior projection to visualize the coccyx. Insert a 22-gauge, 3.5-inch spinal needle with the bevel facing ventrally in the midline.
- A lateral fluoroscopic image can be used to confirm the depth of the needle. Great care must be taken to prevent overinsertion because of the proximity of the rectum to the ventral surface of the coccyx.
- The needle should be inserted down to the point of maximal tenderness on the coccyx, which will radiographically correlate with a vestigial disc segment. The goal is to dock the needle on the painful vestigial disc in the midline.
- Once the needle is docked, remove the stylet and aspirate to check for blood. If blood is not evident, inject 0.5 mL

of nonionic contract dye to confirm placement. When the correct contrast pattern is obtained, slowly inject a 5-mL volume consisting of 2 mL of 1 : 1 preservative-free lidocaine without epinephrine and 3 mL of 6 mg/mL Celestone Soluspan.

Excision of the mobile segment or total coccygectomy may be indicated for patients in whom conservative management fails, especially those with radiographic evidence of hypermobility or subluxation; success rates ranging from 60% to 91% have been reported in this group of patients. Outcomes of surgery are not as good in patients with normal coccygeal mobility. Excision is considered only if the patient gets relief of the coccygeal pain that corresponds to the duration of the local anesthetic at a minimum. If the local anesthetic yield no relief, then resection of the coccyx is unlikely to as well.

REFERENCES

OVERVIEW OF DISC DEGENERATION AND HERNIATION

Andersson GBJ, Howard SA, Oegema TR, et al: Directions for future research, *J Bone Joint Surg* 88A(Suppl 2):110, 2006.

Battié MC, Videman T: Lumbar disc degeneration: epidemiology and genetics, *J Bone Joint Surg* 88A(Suppl 2):3, 2006.

Bogduk N: Degenerative joint disease of the spine, *Radiol Clin North Am* 50:613, 2012.

Hadjipavlou AG, Tzermiadianos MN, Bogduk N, Zindrick MR: The pathophysiology of disc degeneration: a critical review, *J Bone Joint Surg* 90B:1261, 2008.

Hestbaek L, Leboeuf-Yde C, Kyvik KO, et al: The course of low back pain from adolescence to adulthood: eight-year follow-up of 9600 twins, *Spine* 31:468, 2006.

Hughes SP, Freemont AJ, Hukins DW, et al: The pathogenesis of degeneration of the intervertebral disc and emerging therapies in the management of back pain, *J Bone Joint Surg* 94A:1298, 2012.

Kadow T, Sowa G, Vo N, Kang JD: Molecular basis of intervertebral disc degeneration and herniations: what are the important translational questions?, *Clin Orthop Relat Res* 473:2015, 1903.

Kalichman L, Hunter DJ: The genetics of intervertebral disc degeneration: familial predisposition and heritability estimation, *Joint Bone Spine* 75:383, 2008.

Katz JN: Lumbar disc disorders and low-back pain: socioeconomic factors and consequences, *J Bone Joint Surg* 88A(Suppl 2):21, 2006.

Menezes-Reis R, Bonugli GP, Dalto VF, et al: The association between lumbar spine sagittal alignment and L4-L5 disc degeneration among asymptomatic young adults, *Spine* 2016. [Epub ahead of print].

Poole AR: Biologic markers and disc degeneration, *J Bone Joint Surg* 88A(Suppl 2):72, 2006.

Schroeder JE, Dettori JR, Brodt ED, Kaplan L: Disc degeneration after disc herniation: are we accelerating the process?, *Evid Based Spine Care J* 3:33, 2012.

Wasiak R, Kim JY, Pransky G: Work disability and costs caused by recurrence of low back pain: longer and more costly than in first episodes, *Spine* 31:219, 2006.

Weber KT, Jacobsen TD, Maidhof R, et al: Developments in intervertebral disc disease research: pathophysiology, mechanobiology, and therapeutics, *Curr Ev Musculoskelet Med* 8:18, 2015.

DISC AND SPINE ANATOMY

Abuzayed B, Tuna Y, Gazioglu N: Thorascopic anatomy and approaches of the anterior thoracic spine: cadaver study, *Surg Radiol Anat* 34:539, 2012.

Duncan NA: Cell deformation and micromechanical environment in the intervertebral disc, *J Bone Joint Surg* 88A(Suppl 2):47, 2006.

Grunhagen T, Wilde G, Soukane DM, et al: Nutrient supply and intervertebral disc metabolism, *J Bone Joint Surg* 88A(Suppl 2):30, 2006.

Iatridis JC, MacLean JJ, Roughley PJ, et al: Effects of mechanical loading on intervertebral disc metabolism in vivo, *J Bone Joint Surg* 88A(Suppl 2):41, 2006.

Miyamoto H, Doita M, Nishida K, et al: Effects of cyclic mechanical stress on the production of inflammatory agents by nucleus pulposus and anulus fibrosus derived cells in vitro, *Spine* 31:4, 2006.

Morimoto T, Snonhata M, Kitajima M, et al: The termination level of the conus medullaris and lumbosacral transitional vertebrae, *J Orthop Sci* 18:878, 2013.

Pattappa G, Li Z, Peroglio M, et al: Diversity of intervertebral disc cells: phenotype and function, *J Anat* 221:480, 2012.

Roberts S, Trivedi J, Menage J: Histology and pathology of the human intervertebral disc, *J Bone Joint Surg* 88A(Suppl 2):10, 2006.

Teske W, Boudelal R, Zirke S, et al: Anatomical study of preganglionic spinal nerve and disc relation at different lumbar levels: special aspect for microscopoic spine surgery, *Technol Health Care* 23:343, 2015.

Zhong W, Driscoll SJ, Wu M, et al: In vivo morphological features of human lumbar discs, *Medicine (Baltimore)* 93:e333, 2014.

NATURAL HISTORY OF DISC DISEASE

Cribb GL, Jaffray DC, Cassar-Pullicino VN: Observations on the natural history of massive lumbar disc herniation, *J Bone Joint Surg* 89B:782, 2007.

Hutton MJ, Bayer JH, Powell J, Sharp DJ: Modic vertebral body changes: the natural history as assessed by consecutive magnetic resonance imaging, *Spine* 36:2304, 2011.

Kjaer P, Tunset A, Boyle E, Jensen TS: Progression of lumbar disc herniations over an eight-year period in a group of adult Danes from the general population—a longitudinal MRI study using quantitative measures, *BMC Musculoskelet Disord* 17:26, 2015.

Lotz JC: Lurich JA: Innervation, inflammation, and hypermobility may characterize pathologic disc degeneration: review of animal model data, *J Bone Joint Surg* 88A(Suppl 2):76, 2006.

Rahme R, Moussa R, Bou-Nassif R, et al: What happens to Modic changes following lumbar discectomy? Analysis of a cohort of 41 patients with a 3- to 5-year follow-up period, *J Neurosurg Spine* 13:562, 2010.

Roberts S, Evans H, Triveda J, et al: Histology and pathology of the human intervertebral disc, *J Bone Joint Surg* 88A:10, 2006.

Sharma A, Parsons M, Pilgram T: Temporal interactions of degenerative changes in individual components of the lumbar interbertebral discs: a sequential magnetic resonance imaging study in patients less than 40 years of age, *Spine* 36:2011, 1794.

Vernon-Roberts B, Moore RJ, Fraser RD: The natural history of age-related disc degeneration: the influence of age and pathology on cell populations in the L4-L5 disc, *Spine* 33:2767, 2008.

Weiner BK, Vilendecic M, Ledic D, et al: Endplate changes following discectomy: natural history and associations between imaging and clinical data, *Eur Spine J* 24:2449, 2015.

DIAGNOSTIC STUDIES

Eck JC, Sharan A, Resnick DK, et al: Guideline update for the performance of fusion procedures for degenerative disease of the lumbar. Part 6: discography for patient selection, *J Neurosurg Spine* 21:37, 2014.

Haughton V: Imaging intervertebral disc degeneration, *J Bone Joint Surg* 88A(Suppl 2):15, 2006.

Reeves RS, Furman MB: Discography's role in low back pain management, *Pain Manag* 2:151, 2012.

Shim JH, Park CK, Lee JH, et al: A comparison of angled sagittal MRI and conventional MRI in the diagnosis of herniated disc and stenosis in the cervical foramen, *Eur Spine J* 18:1109, 2009.

Singh V, Manchikanti L, Onyewu O, et al: An update of the appraisal of the accuracy of thoracic discography as a diagnostic test for chronic spinal pain, *Pain Physician* 15:E757, 2012.

Yu Y, Liu W, Song D, et al: Diagnosis of discogenic low back pain in patients with probable symptoms but negative discography, *Arch Orthop Trauma Surg* 132:627, 2012.

Willems P: Decision making in surgical treatment of chronic low back pain: the performance of prognostic tests to select patients for lumbar pinal fusion, *Acta Orthop Suppl* 84:1, 2013.

INJECTION STUDIES

Ackerman WE 3rd, Ahmad M: The efficacy of lumbar epidural steroid injections in patients with lumbar disc herniations, *Anesth Analg* 104:1217, 2007.

Benyamin RM, Wang VC, Vallejo R, et al: A systematic evaluation of thoracic interlaminar epidural injections, *Pain Physician* 15:E497, 2012.

Bydon M, Macki M, De la Garza-Ramos R, et al: The cost-effectiveness of CT-guided sacroiliac joint injections: a measure of QALY gained, *Neurol Res* 36:915, 2014.

el Abd O: Steroids in spine interventions. In Slipman CW, Derby R, Simeone FA, Mayer TG, editors: *Interventional spine: an algorithmic approach*, Philadelphia, 2008, Elsevier.

Falco FJ, Manchikanti L, Datta S, et al: An update of the effectiveness of therapeutic lumbar facet joint interventions, *Pain Physician* 15:E909, 2012.

Fekete T, Woernle C, Mannion AF, et al: The effect of epidural steroid injection on postoperative outcome in patients from the lumbar spinal stenosis outcome study, *Spine* 40:1303, 2015.

Fotladou A, Wojcik A, Shaju A: Management of low back pain with facet joint injections and nerve root blocks under computed tomography guidance. A prospective study, *Skeletal Radiol* 41:1081, 2012.

Gerszten PC, Smuck M, Rathmell JP, et al: Plasma disc decompression compared with fluoroscopy-guided transforaminal epidural steroid injections for symptomatic contained lumbar disc herniation: a prospective, randomized, controlled trial, *J Neurosurg Spine* 12:357, 2010.

Hwang SY, Lee JW, Lee GY, Kang HS: Lumbar facet joint injection: feasibility as an alternative method in high-risk patients, *Eur Radiol* 23:3153, 2013.

Iversen T, Solberg TK, Romner B, et al: Effect of caudal epidural steroid or saline injection in chronic lumbar radiculopathy: multicentre, blinded, randomised controlled trial, *BMJ* 343:d5278, 2011.

Kaufmann TJ, Geske JR, Murthy NS, et al: Clinical effectiveness of single lumbar transforaminal epidural steroid injections, *Pain Med* 14:1126, 2013.

Lee JH, An JH, Lee SH: Comparison of the effectiveness of interlaminar and bilateral transforaminal epidural steroid injections in treatment of patients with lumbosacral disc herniation and spinal stenosis, *Clin J Pain* 25:206, 2009.

Manchikanti L, Benyamin RM, Falco Fj, et al: Do epidural injections provide short- and long-term relief for lumbar disc herniation? A systematic review, *Clin Orthop Relat Res* 473:2015, 1940.

Manchikanti L, Cash KA, McManus CD, et al: Preliminary results of a randomized, double-blind, controlled trial of fluoroscopic lumbar interlaminar epidural injections in managing chronic lumbar discogenic pain without disc herniation or radiculitis, *Pain Physician* 13:E279, 2010.

Manchikanti L, Kaye AD, Manchikanti K, et al: Efficacy of epidural injections in the treatment of lumbar central spinal stenosis: a systematic review, *Anesth Pain Med* 5:e23139, 2015.

Manchikanti L, Malla Y, Wargo BW, et al: A prospective evaluation of complications of 10,000 fluoroscopically directed epidural injections, *Pain Physician* 15:131, 2012.

Manchikanti L, Singh V, Cash KA, et al: Preliminary results of a randomized, equivalence trial of fluoroscopic caudal epidural injections in managing chronic low back pain, part 2: disc herniation and radiculitis, *Pain Physician* 11:801, 2008.

Manchikanti L, Singh V, Falco FJ, et al: Evaluation of the effectiveness of lumbar interlaminar epidural injections in managing chronic pain of lumbar disc herniation or radiculitis: a randomized, double-blind, controlled trial, *Pain Physician* 13:343, 2010.

Mandel S, Schilling J, Peterson E, et al: A retrospective analysis of vertebral body fractures following epidural steroid injections, *J Bone Joint Surg* 95A:961, 2013.

McCormick Z, Cushman D, Casey E, et al: Factors associated with pain reduction after transforaminal epidural steroid injection for lumbosacral radicular pain, *Arch Phys Med Rehabil* 95:2350, 2014.

Quraishi NA: Transforaminal injection of corticosteroids for lumbar radiculopathy: systemtic review and meta-analysis, *Eur Spine J* 21:214, 2012.

Rados I, Sakic K, Fingler M, Kapural L: Efficacy of interlaminar vs transforaminal epidural steroid injection for the treatment of chronic unilateral radicular pain: prospective, randomized study, *Pain Med* 12:1316, 2011.

Ribeiro LH, Furtado RN, Konai MS, et al: Effect of facet joint injection versus systematic steroids in low back pain: a randomized controlled trial, *Spine* 38:2013, 1995.

Schaufele MK, Hatch L, Jones W: Interlaminar versus transforaminal epidural injections for the treatment of symptomatic lumbar intervertebral disc herniations, *Pain Physician* 9:361, 2006.

Schütz U, Cakir B, Dreinhöfer K, et al: Diagnostic value of lumbar facet joint injection: a prospective triple cross-over study, *PLoS ONE* 6:e27991, 2011.

Zou YC, Li YK, Yu CF, et al: A cadaveric study on sacroiliac joint injection, *Int Surg* 100:320, 2015.

THORACIC DISC DISEASE

Arnold PM, Johnson PL, Anderson KK: Surgical management of multiple thoracic disc herniations via a transfacet approach: a report of 15 cases, *J Neurosurg Spine* 15:76, 2011.

Arts MP, Bartels RH: Anterior or posterior approach of thoracic disc herniation? A comparative cohort of mini-transthoracic versus transpedicular discectomies, *Spine J* 14:2014, 1654.

Ayhan S, Nelson C, Gok B, et al: Transthoracic surgical treatment for centrally located thoracic disc herniations presenting with myelopathy: a 5-year institutional experience, *J Spinal Disord Tech* 23:79, 2010.

Bartels RH, Peul WC: Mini-thoracotomy or thoracoscopic treatment for medially located thoracic herniated disc?, *Spine* 32:E581, 2007.

Chandra SP, Ramdurg SR, Kurwale N, et al: Extended costotransversectomy to achieve circumferential fusion for pathologies causing thoracic instability, *Spine J* 14:2094, 2014.

Choi KY, Eun SS, Lee SH, Lee HY: Percutaneous endoscopic thoracic discectomy: transforaminal approach, *Minim Invasive Neurosurg* 53:25, 2010.

Coppes MH, Bakker NA, Metzemaekers JD, Groen RJ: Posterior transdural disectomy: a new approach for the removal of a central thoracic disc herniation, *Eur Spine J* 21:623, 2011.

Cornips EM, Janssen ML, Beuls EA: Thoracic disc herniation and acute myelopathy: clinical presentation, neuroimaging findings, surgical considerations, and outcome, *J Neurosurg Spine* 14:520, 2011.

Danielsson AJ, Romberg K, Nachemson AL: Spinal range of motion, muscle endurance, and back pain and function at least 20 years after fusion or brace treatment for adolescent idiopathic scoliosis: a case-control study, *Spine* 31:275, 2006.

Elhadi AM, Zehri AH, Zaidi HA, et al: Surgical efficacy of minimally invasive thoracic discectomy, *J Clin Neurosci* 22:2015, 1708.

Khoo LT, Smith ZA, Asgarzadie F, et al: Minimally invasive extracavitary approach for thoracic discectomy and interbody fusion: 1-year-clinical and radiographic outcomes in 13 patients compared with a cohort of traditional anterior transthoracic approaches, *J Neurosurg Spine* 14:250, 2011.

Lubelski D, Abdullah KG, Steinmetz MP, et al: Lateral extracavitary, costotransversectomy, and transthoracic thoracotomy approaches to the thoracic spine: review of techniques and complications, *J Spinal Disord Tech* 26:222, 2013.

Oppenlander ME, Clark JC, Kalyvas J, Dickman CA: Indications and techniques for spinal instrumentation in thoracic disk surgery, *Clin Spine Surg* 29:E99, 2016.

Sheikh H, Samartzis D, Perez-Cruet MJ: Techniques for the operative management of thoracic disc herniation: minimally invasive thoracic microdiscectomy, *Orthop Clin North Am* 38:351, 2007.

Snyder LA, Smith ZA, Dahdaleh NS, Fessler RG: Minimally invasive treatment of thoracic disc herniations, *Neurosurg Clin N Am* 25:271, 2014.

Wait SD, Fox DJ, Kenny KJ, Dickman CA: Thoracoscopic resection of symptomatic herniated discs: clinical results in 121 patients, *Spine* 37:35, 2012.

Watanabe K, Yabuki S, Konno S, Kikuchi S: Complications of endoscopic spinal surgery: a retrospective study of thoracoscopy and retroperitoneoscopy, *J Orthop Sci* 12:42, 2007.

Yamasaki R, Okuda S, Maeno T, et al: Surgical outcomes of posterior thoracic interbody fusion for thoracic disc herniations, *Eur Spine J* 22:2496, 2013.

Yanni DS, Connery C, Perin NI: Video-assisted thoracoscopic surgery combined with a tubular retractor system for minimally invasive thoracic discectomy, *Neurosurgery* 68(1 Suppl Operative):138, 2011.

Yoshihara H: Surgical treatment for thoracic disc herniation: an update, *Spine* 39:E406, 2014.

Yoshihara H, Yoneoka D: Comparison of in-hospital morbidity and mortality rates between anterior and nonanterior approach procedures for thoracic disc herniation, *Spine* 39:E728, 2014.

LUMBAR DISC DISEASE

ETIOLOGY, DIAGNOSIS, AND CONSERVATIVE TREATMENT

Bass EC, Nau WH, Diederich CJ, et al: Intradiscal thermal therapy does not simulate biologic remodeling in an in vivo sheep model, *Spine* 31:139, 2006.

Battié MC, Videman T: Lumbar disc degeneration: epidemiology and genetics, *J Bone Joint Surg* 88A(Suppl 2):3, 2006.

Battié MC, Videman T, Kaprio J, et al: The Twin Spine Study: contributions to a changing view of disc degeneration, *Spine J* 9:47, 2009.

Carragee EJ, Don AS, Hurwitz EL, et al: ISSLS Prize Winner: Does discography cause accelerated progression of degeneration changes in the lumbar disc: a ten-year matched cohort study, *Spine* 34(2338):2009, 2009.

Daffner SD, Hymanson HJ, Wang JC: Cost and use of conservative management of lumbar disc herniation before surgical discectomy, *Spine J* 10:463, 2010.

de Schepper EI, Damen J, van Meurs JB, et al: The association between lumbar disc degeneration and low back pain: the influence of age, gender, and individual radiographic features, *Spine* 35:531, 2010.

Finckh A, Zufferey P, Schurch M-A, et al: Short-term efficacy of intravenous pulse glucocorticoids in acute discogenic sciatica: a randomized controlled trial, *Spine* 31:377, 2006.

Golinvaux NS, Bohl DD, Basques BA, et al: Comparison of the lumbar disc herniation patients randomized in SPORT to 6,846 discectomy patients from NSQIP: demographic, perioperative variables, and complications correlate well, *Spine J* 15:685, 2015.

Hahne AJ, Ford JJ, McMeeken JM: Conservative management of lumbar disc herniation with associated radiculopathy: a systematic review, *Spine* 35:E488, 2010.

Jegede KA, Ndu A, Grauer JN: Contemporary management of symptomatic lumbar disc herniations, *Orthop Clin North Am* 41:217, 2010.

Jiang H, Deng Y, Wang T, et al: Interleukin-23 may contribute to the pathogenesis of lumbar disc herniation through the IL-23/IL-17 pathway, *J Orthop Surg Res* 11:12, 2016.

Katz JN: Lumbar disc disorders and low back pain: socioeconomic factors and consequences, *J Bone Joint Surg* 88A(Suppl 2):21, 2006.

Kerr D, Zhao W, Lurie JD: What are the long-term predictors of outcomes for lumbar disc herniation? A randomized and observational study, *Clin Orthop Relat Res* 473:2015, 1920.

Kido T, Okuyama K, Chiga M, et al: Clinical diagnosis of upper lumbar disc herniation: pain and/or numbness distribution are more useful for appropriate level diagnosis, *J Orthop Sci* 2016. [Epub ahead of print].

Kim SW, Yeom JS, Park SK, et al: Inter- and intra-observer reliability of MRI for lumbar lateral disc herniation, *Clin Orthop Surg* 1:34, 2009.

Lee BH, Kim TH, Park MS, et al: Comparison of effects of nonoperative treatment and decompression surgery on risk of patients with lumbar spinal stenosis falling: evaluation with functional mobility tests, *J Bone Joint Surg* 96A:e110, 2014.

Li Y, Fredrickson V, Resnick DK: How should we grade lumbar disc herniation and nerve root compression? A systematic review, *Clin Orthop Relat Res* 473:2015, 1896.

Madigan L, Vaccaro AR, Spector LR, Milam RA: Management of symptomatic lumbar degenerative disk disease, *J Am Acad Orthop Surg* 17:102, 2009.

Malik KM, Cohen SP, Walega DR, Benzon HT: Diagnostic criteria and treatment of discogenic pain: a systematic review of recent clinical literature, *Spine J* 13:2013, 1675.

Oktay AB, Albayrak NB, Akgul YS: Computer aided diagnosis of degenerative intervertebral disc diseases from lumbar MR images, *Comput Med Imaging Graph* 38:613, 2014.

Pearson A, Blood E, Luire J, et al: Predominant leg pain associated with better surgical outcomes in degenerative spondylolisthesis and spinal stenosis. Results from the Spine Patient Outcomes Research Trial (SPORT), *Spine* 36:219, 2011.

Pneumaticos SG, Reitman CA, Lindsey RW: Diskography in the evaluation of low back pain, *J Am Acad Orthop Surg* 14:46, 2006.

Rabinovitch DL, Peliowski A, Furlan AD: Influence of lumbar epidural injection volume on poain relief for radicular leg pain and/or low back spine, *Spine J* 9:509, 2009.

Siemionow K, An H, Masuda K, et al: The effects of age, gender, ethnicity, and spinal level on the rate of intervertebral disc degeneration: a review of 1712 intervertebral discs, *Spine* 36:1333, 2011.

Smeets RJEM, Sittink H, Hidding A, et al: Do patients with chronic low back pain have a lower level of aerobic fitness than healthy controls: are pain, disability, fear of injury, working status, or level of leisure time activity associated with the difference in aerobic fitness level?, *Spine* 31:90, 2006.

van der Windt DA, Simons E, Riphagen II, et al: Physical examination for lumbar radiculopathy due to disc herniation in patients with low-back pain, *Cochrane Database Syst Rev* (2):CD007431, 2010.

Wade KR, Robertson PA, Thambyah A, Broom ND: How healthy discs herniate: a biomechanical and microstructural study investigating the combined effects of compression rate and flexion, *Spine* 39:1018, 2014.

Weinstein JN, Lurie JD, Tosteson TD, et al: Surgical versus nonoperative treatment for lumbar disc herniation: four-year results for the Spine Patient Outcomes Research Trial (SPORT), *Spine* 33:2789, 2008.

Weinstein JN, Lurie JD, Tosteson TD, et al: Surgical compared with nonoperative treatment for lumbar degenerative spondylolisthesis: four-year results in the Spine Patient Outcomes Research Trial (SPORT) randomized and observational cohorts, *J Bone Joint Surg* 91A:1295, 2009.

Weinstein JN, Tosteson TD, Lurie JD, et al: Surgical versus nonoperative treatment for lumbar spinal stenosis: four-year results for the Spine Patient Outcomes Research Trial (SPORT), *Spine* 35:1329, 2010.

Yu PF, Jiang FD, Liu JT, Jiang H: Outcomes of conservative treatment for ruptured lumbar disc herniation, *Acta Orthop Belg* 79:726, 2013.

OPERATIVE TREATMENT

Aichmair A, Du JY, Shue J, et al: Microdiscectomy for the treatment of lumbar disc herniation: an evaluation of reoperations and long-term outcomes, *Evid Based Spine Care J* 5:77, 2014.

Awad JN, Moskovich R: Lumbar disc herniations: surgical versus nonsurgical treatment, *Clin Orthop Relat Res* 443:183, 2006.

Banagan K, Gelb D, Poelstra K, Ludwig S: Anatomic mapping of lumbar nerve roots during a direct lateral transpsoas approach to the spine: a cadaveric study, *Spine* 36:E687, 2011.

Bydon M, De la Garza-Ramos R, et al: Impact of smoking on compications and pseudarthrosis rates after single- and 2-level posterolateral fusion of the lumbar spine, *Spine* 39:2014, 1765.

Dafford EE, Anerson PA: Comparison of dural repair techniques, *Spine J* 15:1099, 2015.

Dohrmann GJ, Mansour N: Long-term results of various operations for lumbar disc herniation: analysis of over 39,000 patients, *Med Princ Pract* 24:285, 2015.

Fakouri B, Shetty NR, White TC: Is sequestrectomy a viable alternative to microdiscectomy? A systematic review of the literature, *Clin Orthop Relat Res* 473:2015, 1957.

Fakouri B, Stovell MG, Allom R: A comparative study of lumbar microdiscectomy in obese and non-obese patients, *J Spinal Disord Tech* 28:E352, 2015.

Feng H, Danfelter M, Stromquist B, et al: Extracellular matrix in disc degeneration, *J Bone Joint Surg* 88A(Suppl 2):25, 2006.

Fischer CR, Ducoffe AR, Errico TJ: Posterior lumbar fusion: choice of approach and adjunct techniques, *J Am Acad Orthop Surg* 22:503, 2014.

Gotfryd A, Avanzi O: A systematic review of randomised clinical trials using posterior discectomy to treat lumbar disc herniations, *Int Orthop* 33:11, 2009.

Guerin P, El Fegoun AB, Obeid I, et al: Incidental durotomy during spine surgery: incidence, management and complications. A retrospective review, *Injury* 43:397, 2012.

Houten JK, Alexandre LC, Nasser R, Wollowick AL: Nerve injury during the transpsoas approach for lumbar fusion, *J Neurosurg Spine* 15:280, 2011.

Hsu WK, McCarthy KJ, Savage JW, et al: The Professional Athlete Spine Initiative: outcomes after lumbar disc herniation in 342 elite professional athletes, *Spine J* 11:180, 2011.

Kamper SJ, Ostelo RW, Rubinstein SM, et al: Minimally invasive surgery for lumbar disc herniation: a systematic review and meta-analysis, *Eur Spine J* 23:1021, 2014.

Kelly MP, Mok JM, Berven S: Dynamic constructs for spinal fusion: an evidence-based review, *Orthop Clin North Am* 41:203, 2010.

Kerr D, Zhao W, Lurie JD: What are long term predictors of outcomes for lumbar disc herniation? A randomized and observational study, *Clin Orthop Relat Res* 473:2015, 1920.

Lau D, Han SJ, Lee JG, et al: Minimally invasive compared to open microdiscectomy for lumbar disc herniation, *J Clin Neurosci* 18:81, 2011.

Li X, Hu Z, Cui J, et al: Percutaneous endoscopic lumbar discectomy for recurrent lumbar disc herniation, *Int J Surg* 27:8, 2016.

Lindley EM, McCullough MA, Burger EL, et al: Complications of axial lumbar interbody fusion, *J Neurosurg Spine* 15:273, 2011.

Lurie JD, Faucett SC, Hanscom B, et al: Lumbar discectomy outcomes vary by herniation level in the Spine Patient Outcomes Research Trial, *J Bone Joint Surg* 90A:2008, 1811.

Lurie JD, Tosteson TD, Tosteson AN, et al: Surgical versus nonoperative treatment for lumbar disc herniation: eight-year results for the spine patient outcomes research trial, *Spine* 39:3, 2014.

Osterman H, Seitsalo S, Karppinen J, Malmivaara A: Effectiveness of microdiscectomy for lumbar disc herniation: a randomized controlled trial with 2 years of follow-up, *Spine* 31:2409, 2006.

Overley SC, McAnany SJ, Andelman S, et al: Return to play in elite athletes after lumbar microdiscectomy: a meta-analysis, *Spine* 41:713, 2016.

Phan K, Rao PJ, Kam AC, Mobbs RJ: Minimally invasive versus open transforaminal lumbar interbody fusion for treatment of degenerative lumbar disease: systematic review and meta-analysis, *Eur Spine J* 24:1017, 2015.

Ran J, Hu Y, Zheng Z, et al: Comparison of discectomy versus sequestrectomy in lumbar disc herniation: a meta-analysis of comparative studies, *PLoS ONE* 10:e0121816, 2015.

Ruetten S, Komp M, Merk H, Godolias G: Use of newly developed instruments and endoscopes: full-endoscopic resection of lumbar disc herniations via the interlaminar and lateral transforaminal approach, *J Neurosurg Spine* 6:521, 2007.

Sidhu GS, Henkelman E, Vaccaro AR, et al: Minimally invasive versus open posterior lumbar interbody fusion: a systematic review, *Clin Orthop Relat Res* 472:2014, 1792.

Soliman J, Harvey A, Howes G, et al: Limited microdiscectomy for lumbar disk herniation: a retrospective long-term outcome analysis, *J Spinal Disord Tech* 27:E8, 2014.

Strömqvist F, Strömqvist B, Jönsson B, et al: Outcome of surgical treatment of lumbar disc herniation in young individuals, *Bone Joint J* 97B:2015, 1675.

Talia AJ, Wong ML, Lau HC, Kaye AH: Comparison of the different surgical approaches for lumbar interbody fusion, *J Clin Neurosci* 22:243, 2015.

Wang K, Hong X, Zhou BY, et al: Evaluation of transforaminal endoscopic lumbar discectomy in the treatment of lumbar disc herniation, *Int Orthop* 39:2015, 1599.

Weistroffer JK, Hsu WK: Return-to-play rates in National Football League linemen after treatment for lumbar disk herniation, *Am J Sports Med* 39:632, 2011.

Wong AP, Smith ZA, Nixon AT, et al: Intraoperative and perioperative complications in minimally invasive transforaminal lumbar interbody fusion: a review of 513 patients, *J Neurosurg Spine* 22:487, 2015.

DEGENERATIVE DISC DISEASE AND INTERNAL DISC DERANGEMENT

An HS, Masuda K: Relevance of in vitro and in vivo models for intervertebral disc degeneration, *J Bone Joint Surg* 88A(Suppl 2):88, 2006.

Bono CM: Point of view. Pain and disc degeneration: a possible link derived from basic science, *Spine* 31:10, 2006.

Brisby H: Pathology and possible mechanisms of nervous system response to disc degeneration, *J Bone Joint Surg* 88A(Suppl 2):68, 2006.

Buttermann GR, Mullin WJ: Two-level circumferential lumbar fusion comparing midline and paraspinal posterior approach: 5-year interim outcomes of a randomized, blinded, prospsective study, *J Spinal Disord Tech* 28:E534, 2015.

DeLeo JA: Basic science of pain, *J Bone Joint Surg* 88A(Suppl 2):58, 2006.

Evans C: Potential biologic therapies for the intervertebral disc, *J Bone Joint Surg* 88A(Suppl 2):95, 2006.

Feng H, Danfelter M, Strömqvist B, et al: Extracellular matrix in disc degeneration, *J Bone Joint Surg* 88A(Suppl 2):25, 2006.

Goel VK, Panjabi MM, Patwardhan AG, et al: Test protocols for evaluation of spinal implants, *J Bone Joint Surg* 88A(Suppl 2):103, 2006.

Guyer RD, Shellock J, MacLennan B, et al: Early failure of metal-on-metal artifical disc prostheses associated with lymphocytic reaction: diagnosis and treatment experience in four cases, *Spine* 36:E492, 2011.

Jacobs JJ, Hallab NJ, Urban RM, et al: Wear particles, *J Bone Joint Surg* 88A(Suppl 2):99, 2006.

Kääpä EH, Frantsi K, Sarna S, et al: Multidisciplinary group rehabilitation versus individual physiotherapy for chronic nonspecific low back pain: a randomized trial, *Spine* 31:371, 2006.

Lao LF, Zhong GB, Li QY, Liu ZD: Kinetic magnetic resonance analysis of spinal degeneration: a systematic review, *Orthop Surg* 6:294, 2014.

Larson JW, Levicoff EA, Gilbertson LG, et al: Biologic modification of animal models intervertebral disc degeneration, *J Bone Joint Surg* 88A(Suppl 2):83, 2006.

Leclerc A, Chastang JF, Ozguler A, et al: Chronic back problems among persons 30 to 64 years old in France, *Spine* 31:479, 2006.

Lee JC, Cha JG, Yoo JH, et al: Radiographic grading of facet degeration, is it reliable? – a comparison of MR or CT grading with histologic grading in lumbar fusion candidates, *Spine J* 12:507, 2012.

Lotz JC, Ulrich JA: Innervation, inflammation, and hypermobility may characterize pathologic disc degeneration: review of animal model data, *J Bone Joint Surg* 88A(Suppl 2):76, 2006.

McAfee PC, Geisler FH, Saiedy SS, et al: Revisability of the Charité artificial disc replacement: analysis of 688 patients enrolled in the U.S. IDE study of the Charité artificial disc, *Spine* 31:1217, 2006.

Natarajan RN, Williams JR, Andersson GBJ: Modeling changes in intervertebral disc mechanics with degeneration, *J Bone Joint Surg* 88A(Suppl 2):36, 2006.

Phan K, Rao PJ, Kam AC, Mobbs RJ: Minimally invasive versus open transforaminal lumbar interbody fusion for treatment of degenerative lumbar disease: systematic review and meta-analysis, *Eur Spine J* 24:1017, 2015.

Poole AR: Biologic markers and disc degeneration, *J Bone Joint Surg* 88A(Suppl 2):72, 2006.

Regan JJ, McAfee PC, Blumenthal SL, et al: Evaluation of surgical volume and the early experience with lumbar total disc replacement as part of the investigational device exemption study of the Charité artificial disc, *Spine* 31:2270, 2006.

Setton LA: Mechanobiology of the intervertebral disc and relevance to disc degeneration, *J Bone Joint Surg* 88A(S2):52, 2006.

Tortolani PJ, Cunningham BW, Eng M, et al: Prevalence of heterotopic ossification following total disc replacement: a prospective, randomized study of two hundred and seventy-six patients, *J Bone Joint Surg* 89A:82, 2007.

Williams BJ, Smith JS, Fu KM, et al: Does BMP increase the incidence of perioperative complications in spinal fusion? A comparison of 55,862 cases of spinal fusion with and without BMP, *Spine* 36:2011, 1685.

FAILED SPINE SURGERY

Adogwa O, Parker SL, Shau D, et al: Long-term outcomes of revision fusion for lumbar pseudarthrosis, *J Neurosurg Spine* 15:393, 2011.

Alanay A, Vyas R, Shamie AN, et al: Safety and efficacy of implant removal for patients with recurrent back pain after a failed degenerative lumbar spine surgery, *J Spinal Disord Tech* 20:271, 2007.

Ambrossi GL, McGirt MJ, Sciubba DM, et al: Recurrent lumbar disc herniation after single-level lumbar discectomy: incidence and health care cost analysis, *Neurosurgery* 65:574, 2009.

Bordoni B, Marelli F: Failed back surgery syndrome: review and new hypotheses, *J Pain Res* 9:17, 2016.

Brau SA, Delamarter RB, Kropf MA, et al: Access strategies for revision in anterior lumbar surgery, *Spine* 33:2008, 1662.

Bronson WH, Koehler SM, Qureshi SA, Hecht AC: The importance of pain radiography in the evaluation of radiculopathy after failed diskectomy, *Orthopedics* 33:358, 2010.

Chan CW, Peng P: Failed back syndrome, *Pain Med* 12:577, 2011.

Choi KC, Ahn Y, Kang BU, et al: Failed anterior lumbar interbody fusion due to incomplete foraminal decompression, *Acta Neurochir (Wien)* 153:567, 2011.

Choudhary RK, Ahmed HA: Primary and revision lumbar discectomy, *J Bone Joint Surg* 86B:621, 2004.

Chun DS, Baker KC, Hsu WK: Lumbar pseudarthrosis: a review of current diagnosis and treatment, *Neurosurg Focus* 39:E10, 2015.

Czerwein JK Jr, Thakur N, Migliori SJ, et al: Complications of anterior lumbar surgery, *J Am Acad Orthop Surg* 19:251, 2011.

Dede O, Thuillier D, Pekmezci M, et al: Revision surgery for lumbar pseudarthrosis, *Spine J* 15:977, 2015.

Dickson DD, Lenke LG, Bridwell KH, Koester LA: Risk factors for and assessment of symptomatic pseudarthrosis after lumbar pedicle subtraction osteotomy in adult spinal deformity, *Spine* 39:1190, 2014.

Diwan AD, Parvartaneni H, Cammisa F: Failed degenerative lumbar spine surgery, *Orthop Clin North Am* 34:309, 2003.

Eichholz KM, Ryken TC: Complications of revision spinal surgery, *Neurosurg Focus* 14:E1, 2003.

Farjoodi P, Skolasky RL, Riley LH 3rd: The effects of hospital and surgeon volume on postoperative complications after lumbar spine surgery, *Spine* 36:2069, 2011.

Glenn JS, Yaker J, Guyer RD, Ohnmeiss DD: Anterior discectomy and total disc replacement for three patients with multiple recurrent lumbar disc herniations, *Spine J* 11:e1, 2011.

Guo JJ, Yang H, Tang T: Long-term outcomes of the revision open lumbar discectomy by fenestration: a follow-up study of more than 10 years, *Int Orthop* 33:1341, 2009.

Hazard RG: Failed back surgery syndrome: surgical and nonsurgical approaches, *Clin Orthop Relat Res* 443:228, 2006.

Kostuik JP: Complications and surgical revision for failed disc arthroplasty, *Spine J* 4(6 Suppl):289S, 2004.

Lee SH, Kang BU, Ahy Y, et al: Operative failure of percutaneous endoscopic lumbar discectomy: a radiologic analysis of 55 cases, *Spine* 31:E285, 2006.

Liu G, Buchowski JM, Bunmaprasert T, et al: Revision surgery following cervical laminoplasty: etiology and treatment strategies, *Spine* 34:2760, 2009.

McCunniff PT, Young ES, Ahmadinia K, et al: Smoking is associated with increased blood loss and transfusion use after lumbar spinal surgery, *Clin Orthop Relat Res* 474:1019, 2016.

Mobbs RJ, Phan K, Thayaparan GK, Rao PJ: Anterior lumbar interbody fusion as a salvage technique for pseudarthrosis following posterior lumbar fusion surgery, *Global Spine J* 6:14, 2016.

Morgan-Hough CV, Jones PW, Eisenstein SM: Primary and revision lumbar discectomy: a 16-year review from one centre, *J Bone Joint Surg* 85B:871, 2003.

Papadopoulos EC, Girardi FP, Sandhu HS, et al: Outcome of revision discectomies following recurrent lumbar disc herniation, *Spine* 31:1473, 2006.

Patel AA, Brodke DS, Pimenta L, et al: Revision strategies in lumbar total disc arthroplasty, *Spine* 33:1276, 2008.

Rabb CH: Failed back syndrome and epidural fibrosis, *Spine J* 10:454, 2010.

Rasizman NM, O'Brien JR, Poehling-Monaghan KL, Yu WD: Pseudarthrosis of the spine, *J Am Acad Orthop Surg* 17:494, 2009.

Ruetten S, Komp M, Merk H, Godolias G: Recurrent lumbar disc herniation after conventional discectomy: a prospective, randomized study comparing full-endoscopic interlaminar and transforaminal versus microsurgical revision, *J Spinal Disord Tech* 22:122, 2009.

Schwender JD, Casnellie MT, Perra JH, et al: Perioperative complications in revision anterior lumbar spine surgery: incidence and risk factors, *Spine* 34:87, 2009.

Selznick LA, Shamji MF, Isaacs RE: Minimally invasive interbody fusion for revision lumbar surgery: technical feasibility and safety, *J Spinal Disord Tech* 22:207, 2009.

Smith JS, Ogden AT, Shafizadeh S, Fessier RG: Clinical outcomes after microendoscopic discectomy for recurrent lumbar disc herniation, *J Spinal Disord Tech* 23:30, 2010.

Suk KS, Lee HM, Moon SH, Kim NH: Recurrent lumbar disc herniation: results of operative management, *Spine* 26:672, 2001.

Tormenti MJ, Maserati MB, Bonfield CM, et al: Perioperative surgical complications of transforaminal lumbar interbody fusion: a single-center experience, *J Neurosurg Spine* 2011. [Epub ahead of print].

Turunen V, Nyyssönen T, Miettinen H, et al: Lumbar instrumented posterolateral fusion in spondylolisthetic and failed back patients: a long-term follow-up study spanning 11-13 years, *Eur Spine J* 21:2140, 2012.

Vargas-Soto HA, Mehbod A, Mullaney KJ, et al: Salvage procedures for pseudarthrosis after transforaminal lumbar interbody fusion (TLIF)—anterior-only versus anterior-posterior surgery: a clinical and radiological outcome study, *J Surg Orthop Adv* 18:200, 2009.

Wang MY, Green BA: Laminoplasty for the treatment of failed anterior cervical spine surgery, *Neurosurg Focus* 15:E7, 2003.

SPINAL STENOSIS

Aalto TJ, Malmivaara A, Kovacs F, et al: Preoperative predictors for postoperative clinical outcome in lumbar spinal stenosis: systematic review, *Spine* 31:E648, 2006.

Ammendolia C, Stuber KJ, Rok E, et al: Nonoperative treatment for lumbar spinal stenosis with neurogenic claudication, *Cochrane Database Syst Rev* (8):CD010712, 2013.

Athiviraham A, Wali ZA, Yen D: Predictive factors influencing clinical outcome with operative management of lumbar spinal stenosis, *Spine* J11:613, 2011.

Athiviraham A, Yen D: Is spinal stenosis better treated surgically or nonsurgically?, *Clin Orthop Relat Res* 458:90, 2007.

Atlas SJ, Delitto A: Spinal stenosis: surgical versus nonsurgical treatment, *Clin Orthop Relat Res* 443:198, 2006.

Ben-Galim P, Reitman CA: The distended facet sign: an indicator of position-dependent spinal stenosis and degenerative spondylolisthesis, *Spine J* 7:245, 2007.

Briggs VG, Li W, Kaplan MS, et al: Injection treatment and back pain associated with degenerative lumbar spinal stenosis in older adults, *Pain Physician* 13:E347, 2010.

Celik SE, Celik S, Göksu K, et al: Microdecompressive laminotomy with a 5-year follow-up period for severe lumbar spinal stenosis, *J Spinal Disord Tech* 23:229, 2010.

Chiodo A, Haig AJ, Yamakawa KS, et al: Needle EMG has a lower false positive rate than MRI in asymptomatic older adults being evaluated for lumbar spinal stenosis, *Clin Neurophysiol* 118:751, 2007.

Daffner SD, Wang JC: The pathophysiology and nonsurgical treatment of lumbar spinal stenosis, *Instr Course Lect* 58:657, 2009.

Dean CL, Gabriel JP, Cassinelli EH, et al: Degenerative spondylolisthesis of the cervical spine: analysis of 58 patients treated with anterior cervical decompression and fusion, *Spine* J9:439, 2009.

Englund J: Lumbar spinal stenosis, *Curr Sports Med Rep* 6:50, 2007.

Försth P, Michaëlsson K, Sandén B: Does fusion improve the outcome after decompressive surgery for lumbar spinal stenosis? A two-year follow-up study involving 5390 patients, *Bone Joint J* 95B:960, 2013.

Geisser ME, Haig AJ, Tong HC, et al: Spinal canal size and clinical symptoms among persons diagnosed with lumbar spinal stenosis, *Clin J Pain* 23:780, 2007.

Genevay S, Atlas SJ: Lumbar spinal stenosis, *Best Pract Res Clin Rheumatol* 24:253, 2010.

Harrast MA: Epidural steroid injections for lumbar spinal stenosis, *Curr Rev Musculoskelet Med* 1:32, 2008.

Harrop JS, Hilibrand A, Mihalovich KE, et al: Cost-effectiveness of surgical treatment for degenerative spondylolisthesis and spinal stenosis, *Spine* 39(22 Suppl 1):S75, 2014.

He B, Yan L, Xu Z, et al: Treatment strategies for the surgical complications of thoracic spinal stenosis: a retrospective analysis of two hundred and eighty three cases, *Int Orthop* 38:117, 2014.

Hong SW, Choi KY, Ahn Y, et al: A comparison of unilateral and bilateral laminotomies for decompression of L4-L5 spinal stenosis, *Spine* 36:E172, 2011.

Hsieh MK, Chen LH, Niu CC, et al: Combined anterior lumbar interbody fusion and instrumented posterolateral fusion for degenerative lumbar scoliosis: indication and surgical outcomes, *BMC Surg* 15:26, 2015.

Issack PS, Cunningham ME, Pumberger M, et al: Degenerative lumbar spinal stenosis: evaluation and management, *J Am Acad Orthop Surg* 20:527, 2012.

Jalil Y, Carvalho C, Becker R: Long-term clinical and radiological postoperative outcomes after an interspinous microdecompression of degenerative lumbar spinal stenosis, *Spine* 39:368, 2014.

Kaptan H, Kasimcan O, Cakiroglu K, et al: Lumbar spinal stenosis in elderly patients, *Ann NY Acad Sci* 1100:173, 2007.

Kelleher MO, Timlin M, Persaud O, Rampersaud YR: Success and failure of minimally invasive decompression for focal lumbar spinal stenosis in patients with and without deformity, *Spine* 35:E981, 2010.

Kikuike K, Miyamoto K, Hosoe H, Shimizu K: One-staged combined cervical and lumbar decompression for patients with tandem spinal stenosis on cervical and lumbar spine: analyses of clinical outcomes with minimum 3 years follow-up, *J Spinal Disord Tech* 22:593, 2009.

Komp M, Hahn P, Merk H, et al: Bilateral operation of lumbar degenerative central spinal stenosis in full-endoscopic interlaminar technique with unilateral approach: prospective 2-year results of 74 patients, *J Spinal Disord Tech* 24:281, 2011.

Kondrashov DG, Hannibal M, Hsu KY, Zucherman JF: Interspinous process decompression with the X-STOP device for lumbar spinal stenosis: a 4-year follow-up study, *J Spinal Disord Tech* 19:323, 2006.

Kovacs FM, Urrútia G, Alarcón JD: Surgery versus conservative treatment for symptomatic lumbar spinal stenosis: a systematic review of randomized controlled trials, *Spine* 36:E1335, 2011.

Lad SP, Babu R, Ugiliweneza B, et al: Surgery for spinal stenosis: long-term reoperation rates, health care cost, and impact of instrumentation, *Spine* 39:978, 2014.

Lee JH, An JH, Lee SH: Comparison of the effectiveness of interlaminar and bilateral transforaminal epidural steroid injections in treatment of patients with lumbosacral disc herniation and spinal stenosis, *Clin J Pain* 25:206, 2009.

Lee JW, Myung JS, Park KW, et al: Fluoroscopically guided caudal epidural steroid injection for management of degenerative lumbar spinal stenosis: short- and long-term results, *Skeletal Radiol* 39:691, 2010.

Lee JY, Whang PG, Lee JY, et al: Lumbar spinal stenosis, *Instr Course Lect* 62:383, 2013.

Leonardi MA, Zanetti M, Min K: Extent of decompression and incidence of postoperative epidural hematoma among different techniques of spinal decompression in degenerative lumbar spinal stenosis, *J Spinal Disord Tech* 26:407, 2013.

Li C, He Q, Tang Y, Ruan D: The fate of adjacent segments with pre-existing degeneration after lumbar posterolateral fusion: the influence of degenerative grading, *Eur Spine J* 24:2468, 2015.

Lieberman I: Surgery reduced pain and disability in lumbar spinal stenosis better than nonoperative treatment, *J Bone Joint Surg* 89A:2007, 1872.

Malmivaara A, Slätis P, Heliövaara M, et al: Surgical or nonoperative treatment for lumbar spinal stenosis? A randomized controlled trial, *Spine* 32:1, 2007.

Manchikanti L, Cash KA, McManus CD, et al: Preliminary results of a randomized, equivalence trial of fluoroscopic caudal epidural injections in managing chronic low back pain: Part 4—spinal stenosis, *Pain Physician* 11:833, 2008.

Manchikanti L, Cash KA, McManus CD, et al: The preliminary results of a comparative effectiveness evaluation of adhesiolysis and caudal epidural injections in managing chronic low back pain secondary to spinal stenosis: a randomized, conrolled trial, *Pain Physician* 12:E341, 2009.

Manchikanti L, Dunbar EE: Correlation of spinal canal dimensions to efficacy of epidural steroid injection in spinal stenosis, *J Spinal Disord Tech* 20:546, 2007.

Meyer F, Börm W, Thomé C: Degenerative cervical spinal stenosis: current strategies in diagnosis and treatment, *Dtsch Arztebl Int* 105:366, 2008.

Minamide A, Yoshida M, Maio K: The natural clinical course of lumbar spinal stenosis: a longitudinal cohort study over a minimum of 10 years, *J Orthop Sci* 18:693, 2013.

Miyamoto H, Sumi M, Uno K, et al: Clinical outcome of nonoperative treatment for lumbar spinal stenosis, and predictive factors relating to prognosis, in a 5-year minimum follow-up, *J Spinal Disord Tech* 21:563, 2008.

Nemani VM, Aichmair A, Taher F, et al: Rate of revision surgery after stand-alone lateral lumbar interbody fusion for lumbar spinal stenosis, *Spine* 39:E326, 2014.

Ng LC, Tafazal S, Sell P: The effect of duration of symptoms on standard outcome measures in the surgical treatment of spinal stenosis, *Eur Spine J* 16:199, 2007.

Orpen NM, Corner JA, Shetty RR, Marshall R: Micro-decompression for lumbar spinal stenosis: the early outcome using a modified surgical technique, *J Bone Joint Surg* 92B:550, 2010.

Parker SL, Godil SS, Mendenhall SK, et al: Two-year comprehensive medical management of degenerative lumbar spine disease (lumbar spondylolisthesis, stenosis, or disc herniation): a value analysis of cost, pain, disability, and quality of life: clinical article, *J Neurosurg Spine* 21:143, 2014.

Pearson A, Blood E, Lurie J, et al: Predominant leg pain is associated with better surgical outcomes in degenerative spondylolisthesis and spinal stenosis: results from the Spine Patient Outcomes Research Trial (SPORT), *Spine* 36:219, 2011.

Pearson A, Blood E, Lurie J, et al: Degenerative spondylolisthesis versus spinal stenosis: does a slip matter? Comparison of baseline characteristics and outcomes (SPORTS), *Spine* 35:298, 2010.

Pearson A, Lurie J, Tosteson T, et al: Who should have surgery for spinal stenosis? Treatment effect predictors in SPORT, *Spine* 37:2012, 1791.

Podichetty VK, Spears J, Isaacs RE, et al: Complications associated with minimally invasive decompression for lumbar spinal stenosis, *J Spinal Disord Tech* 19:161, 2006.

Resnick DK, Watters WC 3rd, Mummaneni PV, et al: Guideline update for the performance of fusion procedures for degenerative disease of the lumbar spine. Part 10: lumbar fusion for stenosis without spondylolisthesis, *J Neurosurg Spine* 21:62, 2014.

Resnick DK, Watters WC 3rd, Mummaneni PV, et al: Guideline update for the performance of fusion procedures for degenerative disease of the lumbar spine. Part 9: lumbar fusion for stenosis with spondylolisthesis, *J Neurosurg Spine* 21:54, 2014.

Sangwan SS, Kundu ZS, Walecha P, et al: Degenerative lumbar spinal stenosis—results of expansive laminoplasty, *Int Orthop* 32:805, 2008.

Sasai K, Umeda M, Maruyama T, et al: Microsurgical bilateral decompression via a unilateral approach for lumbar spinal canal stenosis including degenerative spondylolisthesis, *J Neurosurg Spine* 9:554, 2008.

Sekiguchi M, Wakita T, Otani K, et al: Lumbar spinal stenosis-specific symptom scale: validity and responsiveness, *Spine* 39:E1388, 2014.

Siddiqui M, Karadimas E, Nicol M, et al: Effects of X-STOP device on sagittal lumbar spine kinematics in spinal stenosis, *J Spinal Disord Tech* 19:328, 2006.

Siddiqui M, Smith FW, Wardlaw D: One-ear results of X-Stop interspinous implant for the treatment of lumbar spinal stenosis, *Spine* 32:1345, 2007.

Sigmundsson FG, Jönsson B, Strömqvist B: Preoperative pain pattern predicts surgical outcome more than type of surgery in patients with central spinal stenosis without concomitant spondylolisthesis: a register study of 9051 patients, *Spine* 39:E199, 2014.

Sigmundsson FG, Jönsson B, Strömqvist B: Outcome of decompression with and without fusion in spinal stenosis with degenerative spondylolisthesis in relation to preoperative pain pattern—a register study of 1,624 patients, *Spine J* 15:638, 2015.

Sigmundsson FG, Kang XP, Jönsson B, Strömqvist B: Correlation between disability and MRI findings in lumbar spinal stenosis: a prospective study of 109 patients operated on by decompression, *Acta Orthop* 82:204, 2011.

Slätis P, Malimivaara A, Heliövaara M, et al: Long-term results of surgery for lumbar spinal stenosis: a randomised controlled trial, *Eur Spine J* 20:1174, 2011.

Smith CC, Booker T, Schaufele MK, Weiss P: Interlaminar versus transforaminal epidural steroid injections for the treatment of symptomatic lumbar spinal stenosis, *Pain Med* 11:2010, 1511.

Spengler DM: Surgery reduced pain at two years but did not differ from nonsurgical treatment for physical function in lumbar spinal stenosis, *J Bone Joint Surg* 90A:2553, 2008.

Takahashi N, Kikuci S, Yabuki S, et al: Diagnostic value of the lumbar-extension-loading test in patients with lumbar spinal stenosis: a cross-sectional study, *BMC Musculoskeletal Disord* 15:529, 2014.

Tosteson AN, Luri JD, Tosteson TD, et al: Surgical treatment of spinal stenosis with and without degenerative spondylolisthesis: cost-effectiveness after 2 years, *Ann Intern Med* 149:845, 2008.

Trouillier H, Birkenmaier C, Rauch A, et al: Posterior lumbar interbody fusion (PLIF) with cages and local bone graft in the treatment of spinal stenosis, *Acta Orthop Belg* 72:460, 2006.

Watters WC 3rd, Baisden J, Gilbert TJ: Degenerative lumbar spinal stenosis: an evidence-based clinical guideline for the diagnosis and treatment of degenerative lumbar spinal stenosis, *Spine J* 8:305, 2008.

Weinstein JN, Tosteson TD, Luri JD, et al: Surgical versus nonsurgical therapy for lumbar spinal stenosis, *N Engl J Med* 358:794, 2008.

Zhang L, Chen R, Xie P, et al: Diagnostic value of the nerve root sedimentation sign, a radiological sign using magnetic resonance imaging, for detecting lumbar spinal stenosis: a meta-analysis, *Skeletal Radiol* 44:519, 2015.

ADULT IDIOPATHIC AND DEGENERATIVE SCOLIOSIS

Anand N, Baron EM, Thaiyananthan G, et al: Minimally invasive multilevel percutaneous correction and fusion for adult lumbar degenerative scoliosis: a technique and feasibility study, *J Spinal Disord Tech* 21:259, 2008.

Bach K, Ahmadian A, Deukmedjian A, Uribe JS: Minimally invasive surgical techniques in adult degenerative spinal deformity: a systematic review, *Clin Orthop Relat Res* 472:2014, 1749.

Berven SH, Hohenstein NA, Savage JW, Tribus CB: Does the outcome of adult deformity surgery justify the complications in the elderly (above 70 y of age) patients?, *J Spinal Disord Tech* 28:271, 2015.

Boachie-Adjei O, Charles G, Cunningham ME: Partially overlapping limited anterior and posterior instrumentation for adult thoracolumbar and lumbar scoliosis: a description of novel spinal instrumentation, "the hybrid technique, *HSS J* 1:93, 2007.

Bridwell KH, Glassman S, Horton W, et al: Does treatment (nonoperative and operative) improve the two-year quality of life in patients with adult symptomatic lumbar scoliosis: a prospective multicenter evidence-based medicine study, *Spine* 34:3171, 2009.

Crawford CH 3rd, Glassman SD: Surgical treatment of lumbar spinal stenosis associated with adult scoliosis, *Instr Course Lect* 58:669, 2009.

Deviren V, Metz LN: Anterior instrumented arthrodesis for adult idiopathic scoliosis, *Neurosurg Clin North Am* 18:273, 2007.

Fu L, Chang MS, Crandall DG, Revella J: Does obesity affect surgical outcomes in degenerative scoliosis?, *Spine* 39:2049, 2014.

Good CR, Lenke LG, Bridwell KH, et al: Can posterior-only surgery provide similar radiographic and clinical results as combined anterior (throacotomy/ thoracoabdominal)/ posterior approaches for adult scoliosis?, *Spine* 35:210, 2010.

Graham RB, Sugrue PA, Koski TR: Adult degenerative scoliosis, *Clin Spine Surg* 29:95, 2016.

Ha KY, Jang WH, Kim YH, Park DC: Clinical relevance of the SRS-Schwab classification for degenerative lumbar scoliosis, *Spine* 41:E282, 2016.

Hallager DW, Hansen LV, Dragsted CR, et al: A comprehensive analysis of the SRS-Schwab Adult Spinal Deformity Classification and confounding variables—a prospective, non-US cross-sectional study in 292 patients, *Spine* 41:E589, 2016.

Hassanzadeh H, Jain A, El Dafrawy MH, et al: Clinical results and functional outcomes of primary and revision spinal deformity surgery in adults, *J Bone Joint Surg* 95A:1413, 2013.

Hong JY, Suh SW, Modi HN, et al: Correlation of pelvic orientation with adult scoliosis, *J Spinal Disord Tech* 23:461, 2010.

Isaacs RE, Hyde J, Goodrich JA, et al: A prospective, nonrandomized, multicenter evaluation of extreme lateral interbody fusion for the treatment of adult degenerative scoliosis: perioperative outcomes and complications, *Spine* 35:S322, 2010.

Kim YB, Lenke LG, Kim YJ, et al: Surgical treatment of adult scoliosis: is anterior apical release and fusion necessary for the lumbar curve?, *Spine* 33:1125, 2008.

Lehman RA Jr, Kang DG, Lenke LG, et al: Pulmonary function following adult spinal deformity surgery: minimum two-year follow-up, *J Bone Joint Surg* 97A:32, 2015.

Li G, Passias P, Kozanek M, et al: Adult scoliosis in patients over sixty-five years of age: outcomes of operative versus nonoperative treatment at a minimum two-year follow-up, *Spine* 34:2165, 2009.

Li M, Shen Y, Gao ZL, et al: Surgical treatment of adult idiopathic scoliosis: long-term clinical radiographic outcomes, *Orthopedics* 34:180, 2011.

Liu S, Diebo BG, Henry JK, et al: The benefit of nonoperative treatment for adult spinal deformity: identifying predictors for reaching a minimal clinically important difference, *Spine J* 16:210, 2016.

Manoharan SR, Baker DK, Pasara SM, et al: Thirty-day readmissions following adult spinal deformity surgery: an analysis of the national surgical quality improvement program (NSQIP) database, *Spine J* 2016. [Epub ahead of print].

Passias PG, Soroceanu A, Yang S, et al: Predictors of revision surgical procedure excluding wound complications in adults spinal deformity and impact on patient-reported outcomes and satisfaction: a two-year follow-up, *J Bone Joint Surg* 98A:536, 2016.

Pichelmann MA, Lenke LG, Bridwell KH, et al: Revision rates following primary adult spinal deformity surgery: six hundred forty-three consecutive patients followed-up to twenty-two years postoperative, *Spine* 35:219, 2010.

Riouallon G, Bouyer B, Wolff S: Risk of revision surgery for adult idiopathic scoliosis: a survival analysis of 517 cases over 25 years, *Eur Spine J* 2016. [Epub ahead of print].

Rose PS, Lenke LG, Bridwell KH, et al: Pedicle screw instrumentation for adult idiopathic scoliosis: an improvement over hook/hybrid fixation, *Spine* 34:852, 2009.

Sansur CA, Smith JS, Coe JD, et al: Scoliosis research society morbidity and mortality of adult scoliosis surgery, *Spine* 36:E593, 2011.

Scheer JK, Khanna R, Lopez AJ, et al: The concave versus convex approach for minimally invasive lateral lumbar interbody fusion for thoracolumbar degenerative scoliosis, *J Clin Neurosurg* 22:2015, 1588.

Scheer JK, Mundis GM, Klineberg E, et al: Post-operative recovery following adult spinal deformity surgery: comparative analysis of age in 149 patients during 1-year follow up, *Spine* 40:2015, 1505.

Scheufler KM, Cyron D, Dohmen H, Eckardt A: Less invasive surgical correction of adult degenerative scoliosis, part 1: technique and radiographic results, *Neurosurgery* 67:697, 2010.

Scheufler KM, Cyron D, Dohmen H, Eckardt A: Less invasive surgical correction of adult degenerative scoliosis, part II: complications and clinical outcome, *Neurosurgery* 67:2010, 1609.

Shaw R, Skovrlj B, Cho SK: Association between age and complications in adult scoliosis surgery: an analysis of the Scoliosis Research Society Morbidity and Mortality database, *Spine* 41:508, 2016.

Smith JS, Klineberg E, Lafage V, et al: Prospective multicenter assessment of perioperative and minimum 2-year postoperative complication rates associated with adult spinal deformity surgery, *J Neurosurg Spine* 26:1–14, 2016.

Smith JS, Lafage V, Shaffrey CI, et al: Outcomes of operative and nonoperative treatment for adult spinal deformity: a prospective, multicenter, propensity-matched cohort assessment with minimum 2-year follow-up, *Neurosurgery* 78:851, 2016.

Smith JS, Shaffrey CI, Glassman SD, et al: Risk-benefit assessment of surgery for adult scoliosis: an analysis based on patient age, *Spine* 36:2011.

Soroceanu A, Burton DC, Diebo BG, et al: Impact of obesity on complications, infection, and patient-reported outcomes in adult spinal deformity surgery, *J Neurosurg Spine* 2015. [Epub ahead of print].

Soroceanu A, Diebo BG, Burton D, et al: Radiographical and implant-related complications in adult spinal deformity surgery: incidence, patient risk factors, and impact on health-related quality of life, *Spine* 40:1414, 2015.

Swamy G, Berven SH, Bradford DS: The selection of L5 versus S1 in long fusions for adult idiopathic scoliosis, *Neurosurg Clin North Am* 18:281, 2007.

Tormenti MJ, Maserati MB, Bonfield CM, et al: Complications and radiographic correction in adult scoliosis following combined transpsoas extreme lateral interbody fusion and posterior pedicle screw instrumentation, *Neurosurg Focus* 28:E7, 2010.

Transfeldt EE, Topp R, Mehbod AA, Winter RB: Surgical outcomes of decompression, decompression with limited fusion, and decompression with full curve fusion for degenerative scoliosis with radiculopathy, *Spine* 35:2010, 1872.

Verla T, Adogwa O, Toche U, et al: Impact of increasing age on outcomes of spinal fusion in adult idiopathic scoliosis, *World Neurosurg* 87:591, 2016.

Wang G, Hu J, Liu X, Cao Y: Surgical treatments for degenerative lumbar scoliosis: a meta analysis, *Eur Spine J* 24:2015, 1792.

Weistroffer JK, Perra JH, Lonstein JE, et al: Complications in long fusions to the sacrum for adult scoliosis: minimum five-year analysis of fifty patients, *Spine* 33:1478, 2008.

Wollowick AL, Kang DG, Lehman RA Jr: Timing of surgical staging in adults spinal deformity surgery: is later better?, *Spine J* 13:2013, 1723.

Worley N, Marascalchi B, Jalai CM, et al: Predictors of inpatient morbidity and mortality in adult spinal deformity surgery, *Eur Spine J* 25:819, 2016.

Yadla S, Maltenfort MG, Ratliff JK, Harrop JS: Adult scoliosis surgery out comes: a systematic review, *Neurosurg Focus* 28:E3, 2010.

Yagi M, Boachie-Adjei O, King AB: Characterization of osteopenia/osteoporosis in adult scoliosis. Does bone density affect surgical outcome?, *Spine* 36:2011, 1652.

Zhu F, Bao H, Liu Z, et al: Unanticipated revision surgery in adult spinal deformity: an experience with 815 cases at one institution, *Spine* 39(26 Spec No.):B36, 2014.

ANKYLOSING SPONDYLITIS

Arun R, Dabke HV, Mehdian H: Comparison of three types of lumbar osteotomy for ankylosing spondylitis: a case series and evolution of a safe technique for instrumented fusion, *Eur Spine J* 20:2252, 2011.

Baraliakos X, Listing J, von der Recke A, Braun J: The natural course of radiographic progression in ankylosing spondylitis: differences between genders and appearance of characteristic radiographic features, *Curr Rheum Rep* 13:383, 2011.

Park YS, Him HS, Baek SW: Spinal osteotomy in ankylosing spondylitis: radiological, clinical, and psychological results, *Spine J* 14:2014, 1921.

Park YS, Kim HS, Baek SW, Oh JH: Preoperative computer-based simulations for the correction of kyphotic deformities in ankylosing spondylitis patients, *Spine J* 14:2420, 2014.

Ravinsky RA, Ouellet JA, Brodt ED, Dettori JR: Vertebral osteotomies in ankylosing spondylitis—comparison of outcomes following closing wedge osteotomy versus opening wedge osteotomy: a systematic review, *Evid Based Spine Care J* 4:18, 2013.

Zhang W, Zheng M: Operative strategy for different types of thoracolumbar stress fractures in ankylosing spondylitis, *J Spinal Disord Tech* 27:423, 2014.

Zheng GQ, Song K, Zhang YG, et al: Two-level spinal osteotomy for severe thoracolumbar kyphosis in ankylosing spondylitis: experience with 48 patients, *Spine* 39:1055, 2014.

COCCYGEAL PAIN

Balain B, Eisenstein SM, Alo GO, et al: Coccygectomy for coccydynia: case series and review of literature, *Spine* 31:414, 2006.

Haddad B, Prasad V, Khan W, et al: Favourable outcomes of coccygectomy for refractory coccygodynia, *Ann R Coll Surg Engl* 96:136, 2014.

Hanley EN, Ode G, Jackson BJ, Seymour R: Coccygectomy for patients with chronic coccydynia: a prospective, observational study of 98 patients, *Bone Joint J* 98B:526, 2016.

Karadimas EJ, Trypsiannis G, Giannoudis PV: Surgical treatment of coccygodynia: an analytic review of the literature, *Eur Spine J* 20:698, 2011.

Kerr EE, Benson D, Schrot RJ: Coccygectomy for chronic refractory coccygodynia: clinical case series and literature review, *J Neurosurg Spine* 14:654, 2011.

Lirette LS, Chaiban G, Tolba R, Eissa H: Coccydynia: an overview of the anatomy, etiology, and treatment of coccyx pain, *Oschsner J* 14:84, 2014.

Maigne J, Pigeau I, Aguer N, et al: Chronic coccydynia in adolescents: a series of 53 patients, *Eur J Phys Rehabi Med* 47:245, 2011.

Maigne JY, Doursounian L, Chatellier G: Causes and mechanisms of common coccydynia: role of body mass index and coccygeal trauma, *Spine* 25:3072, 2000.

Maigne JY, Lagauche D, Doursounian L: Instability of the coccyx in coccydynia, *J Bone Joint Surg* 92B:1038, 2000.

Mitra R, Cheung L, Perry P: Efficacy of fluoroscopically guided steroid injections in the management of coccydynia, *Pain Physician* 10:775, 2007.

Nathan ST, Fisher BE, Roberts CS: Coccydynia: a review of pathoanatomy, aetiology, treatment and outcome, *J Bone Joint Surg* 92B:2010, 1622.

Patel R, Appannagari A, Whang PG: Coccydynia, *Curr Rev Musculoskelet Med* 1:223, 2008.

Perkins R, Schofferman J, Reynolds J: Coccygectomy for severe refractory sacrococcygeal joint pain, *J Spine Disord Tech* 16:100, 2003.

Ramieri A, Domenicucci M, Cellocco P, et al: Acute traumatic instability of the coccyx: results in 28 consecutive coccygectomies, *Eur Spine J* 22(Suppl 6):S939, 2013.

Richette P, Maigne JY, Bardin T: Coccydynia related to calcium crystal deposition, *Spine* 33:E620, 2008.

Trollegaard AM, Aarby NS, Hellberg S: Coccygectomy: an effective treatment option for chronic coccydynia: retrospective results in 41 consecutive patients, *J Bone Joint Surg* 92B:242, 2010.

Woon JT, Stringer MD: Clinical anatomy of the coccyx: a systematic review, *Clin Anat* 25:158, 2012.

Woon JT, Stringer MD: CT morphology of the normal human adult coccyx, *Anat Sci Int* 89:126, 2014.

The complete list of references is available online at ***expertconsult.inkling.com****.*

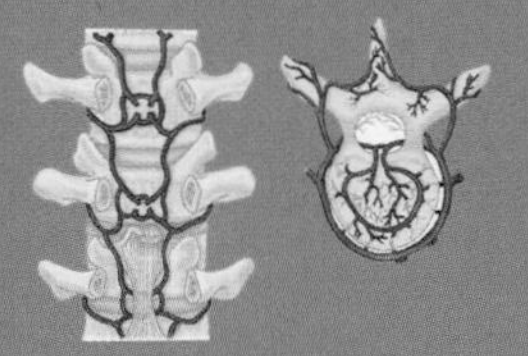

CHAPTER 40

SPONDYLOLISTHESIS

Keith D. Williams

GENERAL INFORMATION

Spondylolisthesis is a descriptive term derived from the Greek spondylo (spine) and olisthesis (slip) and was first described by Herbinaux, an obstetrician, in 1782. The varied etiologies of spondylolisthesis have been classified by Wiltse. The common feature of the various types is anterior translation of the cephalad vertebra relative to the adjacent caudal segment. The biomechanical force causing this translation is the anteriorly directed vector created by the contraction of the posteriorly located erector spinae muscles, coupled with the force of gravity acting on the upper body mass through the lordotic lumbar spine and lumbosacral junction, which explains why this deformity is not seen in children before they are ambulatory. For spondylolisthesis to occur there must be a failure of anatomic structure(s) that normally resist this anteriorly directed force. These structures include the facets, annulus fibrosus, posterior bony arch, and pedicles. Symptoms of spondylolisthesis include axial pain, neurogenic claudication, radiculopathy, and even cauda equina syndrome. In addition, the deformity associated with spondylolisthesis can range from not clinically apparent to severe with significant sagittal imbalance and associated truncal shortening.

ETIOLOGY

Wiltse initially described five different etiologies of spondylolisthesis and later added iatrogenic instability as a sixth type. The most common types are dysplastic, isthmic, and degenerative. In a radiographic study over a 25-year period, Fredrickson et al. found that 92% of children with spondylolysis also had dysplastic features of the lumbar spine, specifically spina bifida occulta, which persisted into adulthood in 70%.

Congenital malformations of the posterior elements, especially elongation of the pars interarticularis and spina bifida occulta, can significantly compromise the ability of the posterior bony elements to resist the anteriorly directed forces applied to the spine can have this consequence. Even though these anomalies are present at birth the spondylolisthesis does not occur until after the child is able to ambulate, which causes the anteriorly directed force to be generated. As the forces increase with growth, the annulus is unable to restrain the caudal-ventral force, which leads to the development of the spondylolisthesis. As the anterior translation occurs progressively, severe spinal stenosis can result with variable neurologic sequelae.

Fracture of the pars interarticularis results in an isthmic type of spondylolisthesis. Development of a pars interarticularis stress fracture is the most common reason for a spondylolysis. Less commonly, fatigue fracture with healing and resultant elongation of the pars or acute traumatic pars fracture can result in an isthmic spondylolisthesis. The incidence of spondylolysis is 0% at birth and increases to 7% by age 18. Most people with spondylolysis will develop a grade 1 slip over time. Longitudinal studies to evaluate the risk factors for developing a high-grade (greater than 50%) slip have identified several radiographic factors of importance, including disc degeneration, high slip angle, and increased pelvic incidence. It remains unclear which, if any, of these findings may actually cause slip progression and which may result from it.

Degenerative spondylolisthesis occurs as a result of the degenerative cascade as described by Kirkaldy-Willis. The loss of disc height allows the cephalad vertebra to translate anteriorly. The associated hypertrophic facet and ligamentous changes result in spinal stenosis centrally and in the lateral recess more so than in other types of spondylolisthesis (Fig. 40-1).

CLASSIFICATION

Two classification systems are most commonly used to describe spondylolisthesis. The Wiltse classification describes

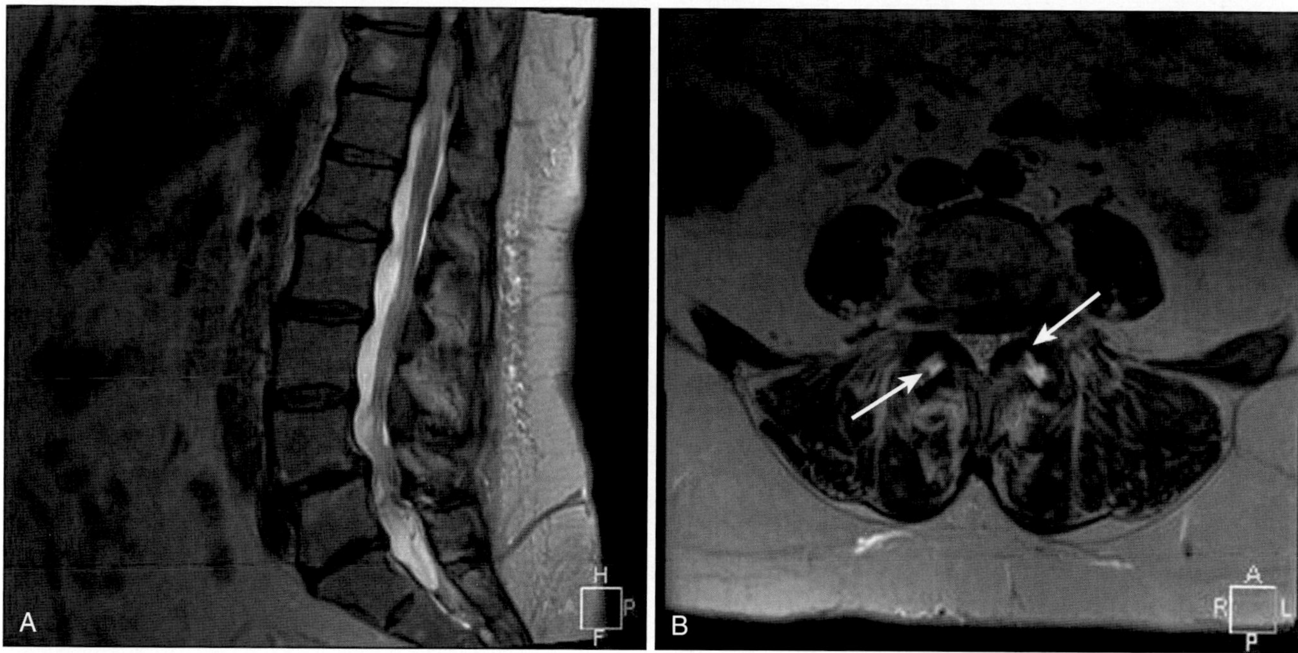

FIGURE 40-1 Degenerative spondylolisthesis with spinal stenosis. **A,** Sagittal CT. **B,** On axial view, note hypertrophic facet and ligamentum flavum (*right arrow*) and facet effusions (*left arrow*) indicating dynamic instability.

BOX 40-1

Classification of Spondylolisthesis (Wiltse et al.)

Type I, dysplastic—Congenital abnormalities of the upper sacral facets or inferior facets of the fifth lumbar vertebra that allow slipping of L5 to S1. No pars interarticularis defect is present in this type.

Type II, isthmic—Defect in pars interarticularis allows forward slipping of L5 on S1. Three types of isthmic spondylolistheses are recognized:

- Stress fracture of pars interarticularis (lytic)
- Elongated but intact pars interarticularis
- Acute fracture of pars interarticularis

Type III, degenerative—Intersegmental instability of long duration with subsequent remodeling of the articular processes at the level of involvement

Type IV, traumatic—Fractures in the area of the bony hook other than the pars interarticularis, such as the pedicle, lamina, or facet

Type V, pathologic—Generalized or localized bone disease and structural weakness of the bone, such as osteogenesis imperfecta

six types of spondylolisthesis based on the location of the deficiency of the posterior elements that allows the listhesis to occur (Box 40-1). The other classification system in common usage was developed by Marchetti and Bartolozzi and divides spondylolisthesis types into dysplastic and acquired types. In addition to classification systems based primarily on etiology, Meyerding devised a widely used grading system based on the amount of translation at the affected level that provides an easily determined metric for the severity of the slip. This grading system divides the superior endplate of the caudal vertebra into four equal portions. This allows for five possible grades, based on the position of the posterior wall of the cephalad vertebral body relative to the four segments of the superior endplate below (Table 40-1 and Fig. 40-2).

WILTSE CLASSIFICATION

TYPE 1 DYSPLASTIC

Malformation or dysplasia of the posterior elements, particularly the pars or inferior facet of the cephalad vertebra or the superior facet of the caudal vertebra (or both), results in a loss of the normal buttressing effect to resist the anterior and caudally directed forces on the L5 vertebra as a result of gravity and contraction of the erector spinae muscles. This dysplasia most often occurs at the lumbopelvic junction and affects the geometry of the sacrum and L5. In addition congenital defects such as spina bifida or elongation of the pars can result in instability and resultant progressive slippage.

TYPE 2 ISTHMIC

The hallmark of this type is a defect in the pars interarticularis. This defect can be lytic, the result of a stress fracture (most common), attributed to bone remodeling of microfractures resulting in an elongated pars, or an acute pars fracture. Isthmic spondylolisthesis often occurs in children, adolescents, and young adults, but can occur into the fifth decade. Because of the cortical nature of the bone of the pars fracture healing potential is relatively poor.

TYPE 3 DEGENERATIVE

Degenerative spondylolisthesis is the most common type. It results from segmental instability as a result of disc degeneration and facet remodeling and thus occurs later in life.

Patients with degenerative spondylolisthesis are more likely to have a dynamic component to their deformity, meaning the amount of translation is affected by their body position. This type of listhesis is most common at the L4-L5 level, usually in women over 50 years of age, particularly those of African descent. For patients with a dynamic component, it is important to obtain upright films, because the spondylolisthesis may not be visible on supine imaging such as MRI.

TYPE 4 TRAUMATIC

This is an uncommon type of spondylolisthesis. Unlike the isthmic type, the fracture is not through the pars. Rather, it is through any other part of the posterior elements, usually involving the pedicles or facets. These tend to be high-energy injuries.

TYPE 5 PATHOLOGIC

This also is an uncommon etiology involving a pathologic process that affects the posterior arch, such as infection or Paget disease, leading to instability at the affected segment.

TABLE 40-1

Meyerding Classification of Spondylolisthesis

GRADE	DISPLACEMENT*
I	0-25%
II	26-50%
III	51-75%
IV	76-100%
V (spondyloptosis)	> 100%

*As measured on lateral radiograph, distance from the posterior edge of the superior vertebral body to the posterior edge of the adjacent inferior vertebral body; distance is reported as a percentage of the total superior vertebral body length.

TYPE 6 IATROGENIC

This type was added after the original description of the classification. Iatrogenic spondylolisthesis occurs when there has been surgical treatment at the involved segment and the instability is the result of the surgical intervention. Most commonly this is as a result of transection of the pars with facetectomy or excessive pars thinning and subsequent fracture of the pars leading to instability.

MARCHETTI-BARTOLOZZI CLASSIFICATION

Marchetti and Bartolozzi subclassified the dysplastic type of spondylolisthesis into high dysplasia and low dysplasia types (Box 40-2). In the low dysplasia type, the S1 endplate and the L5 vertebral body maintain a normal anatomic shape. In the high dysplasia type, the S1 endplate becomes rounded and takes on a more trapezoidal shape of the L5 vertebral body. This system was first described in 1982 with a subsequent revision in 1994. The purpose of the classification is to determine what factors may predict progression of the spondylolisthesis and thereby direct treatment. This classification divides the presumed etiologies of spondylolisthesis into two categories: developmental, in which there is a morphologic abnormality of the anatomy, or acquired, in which the anatomy is normal and the deformity results from trauma, degeneration, or pathologic causes.

DEVELOPMENTAL SPONDYLOLISTHESIS

The cardinal feature of this group is that there is some degree of dysplasia of the posterior elements present. This category is further divided into low dysplasia and high dysplasia based on the severity of the anomalies present, as indicated by the degree of kyphosis at the affected level and the slip angle.

Developmental high dysplastic spondylolisthesis is characterized by major deficiencies of the posterior arches, intervertebral discs, upper endplate of S1 (which often is rounded) and the body of L5, which is trapezoidal. The pars is often

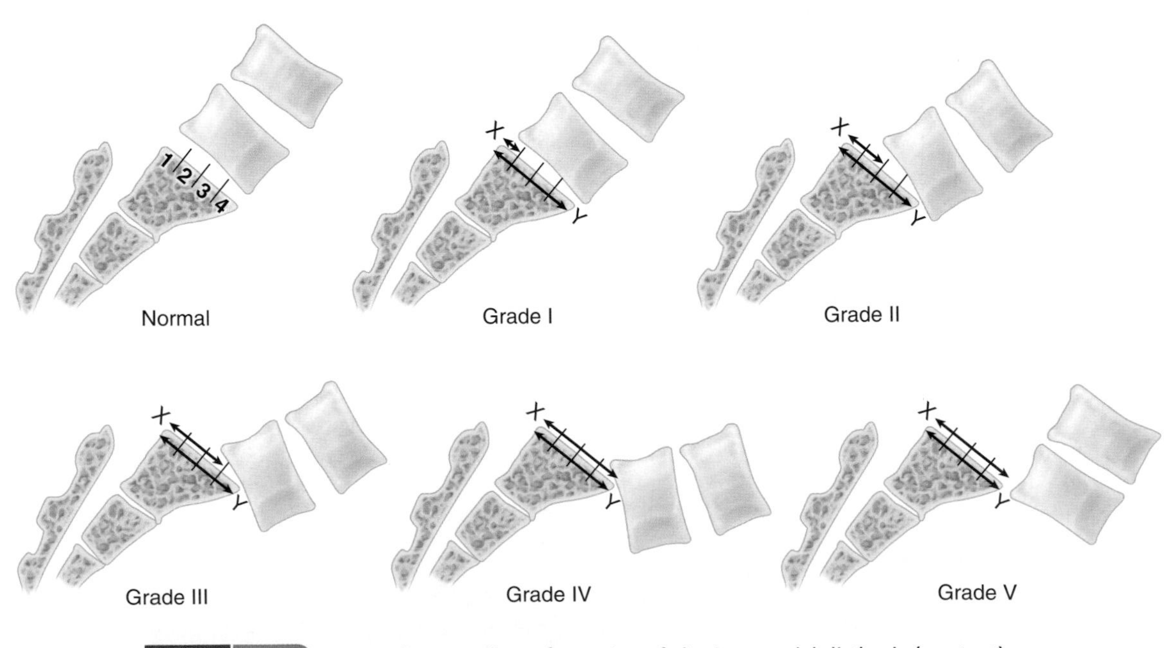

FIGURE 40-2 Meyerding grading of severity of slip in spondylolisthesis (see text).

BOX 40-2

Classification of Spondylolisthesis (Marchetti and Bartolozzi)

Developmental
High dysplastic
With lysis
With elongation
Low dysplastic
With lysis
With elongation

Acquired
Traumatic
Acute fracture
Stress fracture
Post surgery
Direct surgery
Indirect surgery
Pathologic
Local pathology
Systemic pathology
Degenerative
Primary
Secondary

From deWald RL: Spondylolisthesis. In Bridwell KH, DeWald RL, editors: The textbook of spinal surgery, ed 3, Philadelphia, 2011, Lippincott Williams & Wilkins.

elongated or lytic. In adolescents, the L5-S1 level is most commonly affected. Patients with this type of spondylolisthesis often have progression of the spondylolisthesis before adulthood. The risk of progression is directly proportional to the severity of dysplasia.

In *developmental low dysplastic spondylolisthesis*, the L4 and L5 bodies remain rectangular and the S1 endplate remains flat. Also there is no hyperlordosis and verticalization of the sacrum. Progression is less common and when present is a small increase in translation and not an increase in kyphosis and slip angle.

ACQUIRED TRAUMATIC SPONDYLOLISTHESIS

This type is rare and results from significant trauma with fracture of the pars or other portions of the posterior elements.

ACQUIRED POSTSURGICAL SPONDYLOLISTHESIS

This type is subdivided into direct and indirect types. In the direct type, the instability is at the level of surgical intervention because of fracture or bony resection such as facetectomy. The indirect type occurs at a level adjacent to prior surgery such as a fusion.

ACQUIRED PATHOLOGIC SPONDYLOLISTHESIS

This type results from pathologic processes affecting the integrity of the posterior elements such as infection or Paget disease.

ACQUIRED DEGENERATIVE SPONDYLOLISTHESIS

This occurs as a result of degenerative changes in the disc and facets without any disruption of the pars and occurs without a history of prior surgery.

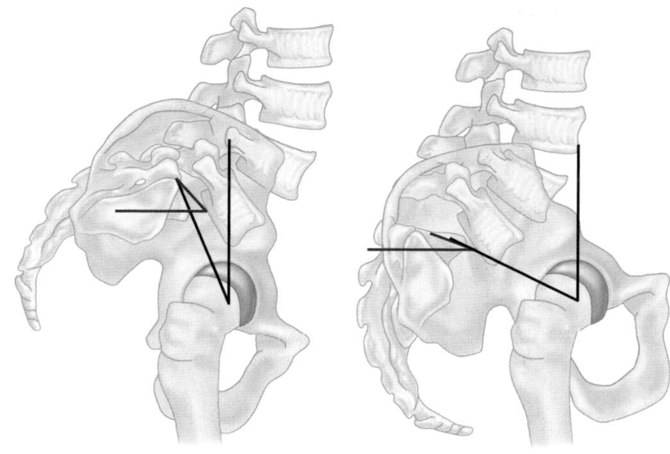

FIGURE 40-3 **Balanced and unbalanced pelvis as described by Hresko et al. Balanced pelvis has a high sacral slope (*red lines*) and low pelvic tilt (*black lines*). Unbalanced pelvis has a low sacral slop and high pelvic tilt.** (Redrawn from Tebet MA: Current concepts on the sagittal balance and classification of spondylolysis and spondylolisthesis, Rev Bras Orthop 49:3, 2014.)

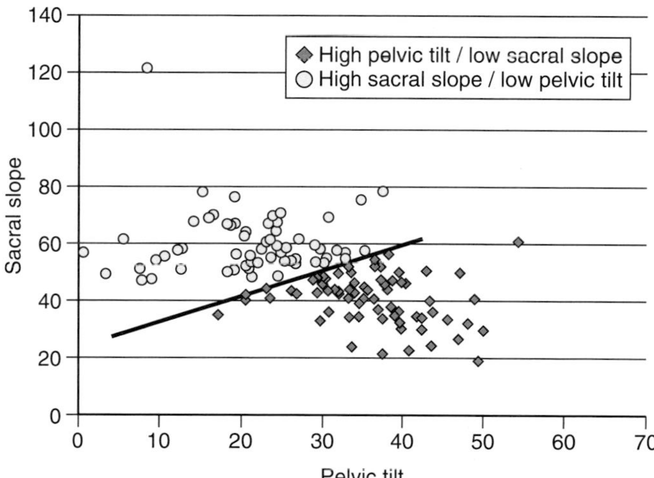

FIGURE 40-4 **Nomogram defining groups based on relation between pelvic tilt and sacral slope.** (From Hresko MT, Labelle H, Roussouly P, Berthonnaud E: Classification of high-grade spondylolistheses based on pelvic version and spine balance. Possible rational for reduction, Spine 32:2208, 2007.)

The classification of Marchetti and Bartolozzi is most useful in evaluating patients who have developmental, high dysplastic spondylolisthesis. In this group, the relationship between pelvic incidence, sacral slope, and pelvic tilt is most relevant. The pelvis is either "balanced " or "unbalanced" (Fig. 40-3), and Hresko et al. developed a nomogram (Fig. 40-4) to help define each group based on the relation between pelvic tilt and sacral slope.

RADIOGRAPHIC PELVIC PARAMETERS

The relationship between spinopelvic alignment and spondylolisthesis has been an area of intense evaluation in recent years. This is true for dysplastic spondylolisthesis as well as other types of spondylolisthesis. Ferrero et al. compared 654 patients with degenerative spondylolisthesis with 709 asymptomatic matched volunteers and concluded that those with degenerative spondylolisthesis had increased pelvic incidence and that there were several subgroups based on C7 tilt, emphasizing the need to evaluate overall spinopelvic balance in patients with degenerative spondylolisthesis.

LUMBOSACRAL DYSPLASIA

The primary areas of posterior dysplasia include the facet joints, pars interarticularis, and spina bifida occulta. These dysplastic posterior changes lead to an inability of the L5 vertebra to resist the anterior and ventral forces created by the upright posture on the lordotic spine. This increases the anterior column stresses and can lead to growth related abnormalities and bone remodeling abnormalities that combine to cause anterior column dysplasia that can exacerbate the posterior deficiencies. As a result of these changes a progressive deformity consisting of kyphosis at the lumbosacral junction and translation of L5 on the rounded S1 endplate can occur, resulting in an unbalanced spinopelvic alignment. Evaluation of sacral "doming" is important because this has been identified as a risk factor for slip progression. The Spinal Deformity Study Group (SDSG) index (Fig. 40-5) has excellent intraobserver and interobserver reliability. An SDSG index of 25% has been suggested to be the threshold of significant sacral deformity.

As the L5 disc becomes more vertical on the standing lateral radiograph, the ability of the dysplastic posterior elements to resist the shear stresses progressively decreases. To correct the inability of the dysplastic L5 posterior elements to resist this shear force at the lumbosacral junction, the posterior tension band needs to be restored and anterior column support needs to be reestablished.

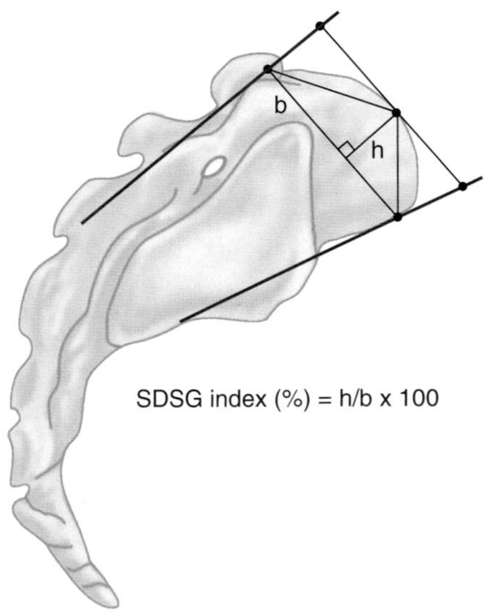

FIGURE 40-5 Spinal Deformity Study Group (SDSG) index for assessment of sacral doming. (Redrawn from Berthonnaud E, Dimnet J, Labelle H, et al: Spondylolisthesis. In O'Brien MF, Kuklo TR, Blanke KM, et al, editors: Spinal Deformity Study Group radiographic measurement manual. Memphis TN: Medtronic Sofamor Danek, 2004.)

SPINOPELVIC ALIGNMENT

In recent years numerous studies have demonstrated that spinopelvic alignment is important to maintain an energy-efficient posture. An understanding of the relationship between sacropelvic morphology and spinopelvic balance is particularly important in evaluating developmental dysplastic spondylolisthesis in adolescents and young adults. As understanding of this relationship improves, the ability to determine optimal treatment regimens should also increase. Patients with developmental dysplastic spondylolisthesis have abnormal sacropelvic morphology, which can result in abnormal sacropelvic orientation.

One of the most important radiographic parameters is *pelvic incidence* (PI). Other parameters remain under evaluation, as does the optimal method to measure each parameter. Pelvic incidence is significantly increased in patients with degenerative spondylolisthesis and dysplastic spondylolisthesis, and the relative increase in pelvic incidence correlates directly with the severity of the slip. Pelvic incidence is defined as the angle between a line perpendicular to the sacral endplate at its midpoint extending caudally and a line joining the midpoint of the sacral endplate to the hip axis (Fig. 40-6). It is important to understand that pelvic incidence is a morphologic measurement, meaning it is determined by the individual anatomy and it is not affected by the position of the sacropelvis in space. The pelvic incidence does increase slightly with growth before stabilizing in adulthood. Patients with spondylolisthesis have higher than normal values and the higher the grade of the spondylolisthesis the higher the pelvic incidence. Huang et al. found, however, that pelvic incidence does not predict the probability of spondylolisthesis progression.

Two other important radiographic parameters are the *sacral slope* (SS) and *pelvic tilt* (PT) (Fig. 40-7). Both of these measurements are determined by pelvic orientation on a standing lateral radiograph; their values are dependent on the position of the sacropelvis in space. Sacral slope is the angle formed by a line parallel to the sacral endplate and a horizontal line, and pelvic tilt is the angle formed by a vertical line passing through the hip axis and a line from the hip axis to the mid-point of the sacral endplate. The equation SS+PT=PI is true for a given individual in the standing position. Labelle et al. concluded that because pelvic incidence is a constant anatomic pelvic variable specific to each individual and strongly determines sacral slope, pelvic tilt, and LL, which are position-dependent variables, this study suggests that pelvic anatomy has a direct influence on the development of a spondylolisthesis

The *slip angle* is a measure of the local kyphosis at the L5-S1 level (Fig. 40-8A). It is defined as the angle formed between a line perpendicular to the posterior aspect of the upper sacrum and a line parallel to the L5 inferior endplate. The slip angle has been found to have some predictive value for slip progression when it is larger than 30 degrees.

The *lumbosacral angle* is defined as the angle formed by the intersection of a line perpendicular to the upper sacrum and a line parallel to the upper endplate of the L5 vertebra (Fig. 40-8B and C). It has been found to have some predictive value for progression when it is larger than 10 degrees.

NATURAL HISTORY

The few natural history studies that are available provide limited information in light of our current understanding of

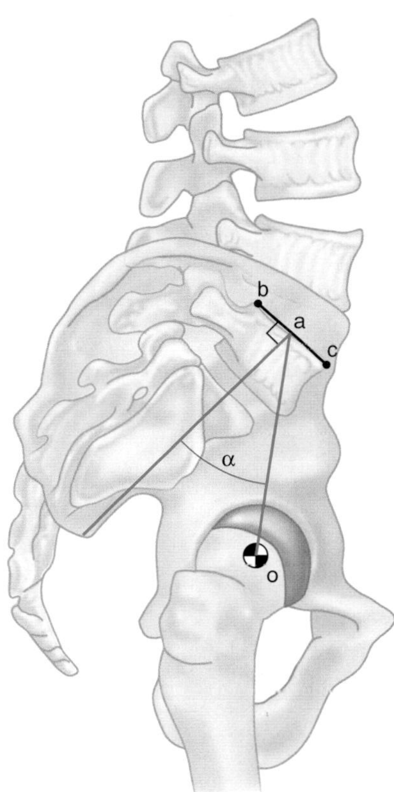

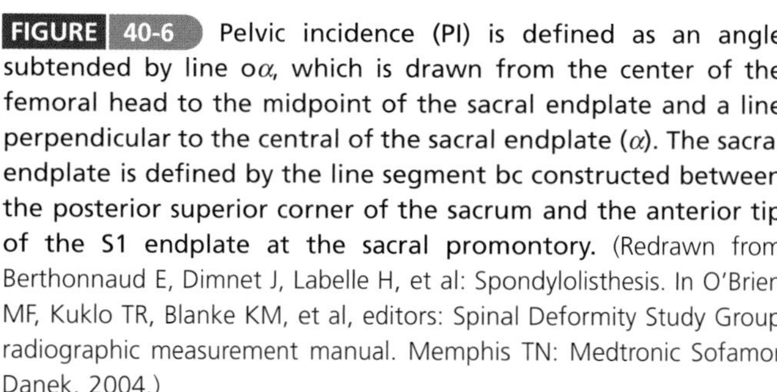

FIGURE 40-6 Pelvic incidence (PI) is defined as an angle subtended by line oα, which is drawn from the center of the femoral head to the midpoint of the sacral endplate and a line perpendicular to the central of the sacral endplate (α). The sacral endplate is defined by the line segment bc constructed between the posterior superior corner of the sacrum and the anterior tip of the S1 endplate at the sacral promontory. (Redrawn from Berthonnaud E, Dimnet J, Labelle H, et al: Spondylolisthesis. In O'Brien MF, Kuklo TR, Blanke KM, et al, editors: Spinal Deformity Study Group radiographic measurement manual. Memphis TN: Medtronic Sofamor Danek, 2004.)

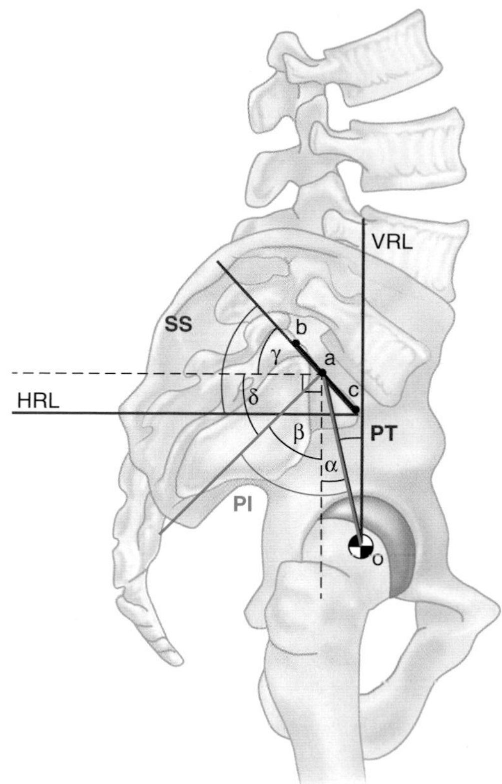

FIGURE 40-7 Mathematical relationship between pelvic incidence (PI), sacral slope (SS), and pelvic tilt (PT). *HRL*, Horizontal reference line; *VRL*, vertical reference line. (Redrawn from Berthonnaud E, Dimnet J, Labelle H, et al: Spondylolisthesis. In O'Brien MF, Kuklo TR, Blanke KM, et al, editors: Spinal Deformity Study Group radiographic measurement manual. Memphis TN: Medtronic Sofamor Danek, 2004.)

the different types of spondylolisthesis. It is clear that the natural history of developmental spondylolisthesis is different from that of acquired spondylolisthesis because of a lytic defect in an otherwise normal pars, and degenerative spondylolisthesis is different from both of these. Also, the association of spondylolysis and spondylolisthesis with clinically relevant low back pain is not clear. A recent systematic review by Andrade et al. failed to establish this link and suggested careful evaluation of the cause of low back pain even in patients with isthmic spondylolisthesis.

With *spondylolytic spondylolisthesis* there appears to be a familial association: approximately 26% of those with isthmic spondylolisthesis have a first-degree relative who also had an isthmic spondylolisthesis. A long-term follow-up study (45 years) by Beutler et al. found the risk of progression to be very small, and no children with a unilateral lytic defect had a slip that progressed. Clinically there was no difference between the general population and those with a grade I or II slip. Most children (approximately 90%) with a lytic defect have been found to have spina bifida occulta, suggesting a dysplastic etiology. The incidence of lytic defects increases with age, from 4.4% at age 6 to 6.0% in adults. Risk factors for progression remain unclear. Some authors have found that females, those with higher grade slips (> 50%) at the time of diagnosis, and those diagnosed before adolescent growth have a greater probability of progression.

Developmental spondylolisthesis with dysplasia is more likely to progress than the spondylolytic type. Dysplasia of the anterior sacrum correlates best with progression in the dysplastic group. Long-term follow-up of Meyerding types III and IV spondylolisthesis treated both operatively and nonoperatively found that most patients had done relatively well. None had severe neurologic sequelae, and only 45% had even mild neurologic symptoms. At 18-year follow-up, 36% of patients treated nonoperatively were asymptomatic. Yue et al. studied 27 patients with spondyloptosis and found pars defects in 89% and also spina bifida occulta in 89%. All of these patients had an abnormality of the proximal sacrum with rounding, suggesting that a physeal injury contributed to the deformity of the sacral endplate.

Degenerative spondylolisthesis usually occurs at the L4-5 level, primarily affects females over the age of 50, and is more frequent in people of African descent. Slip progression has been found to occur in about 30% of patients, but there

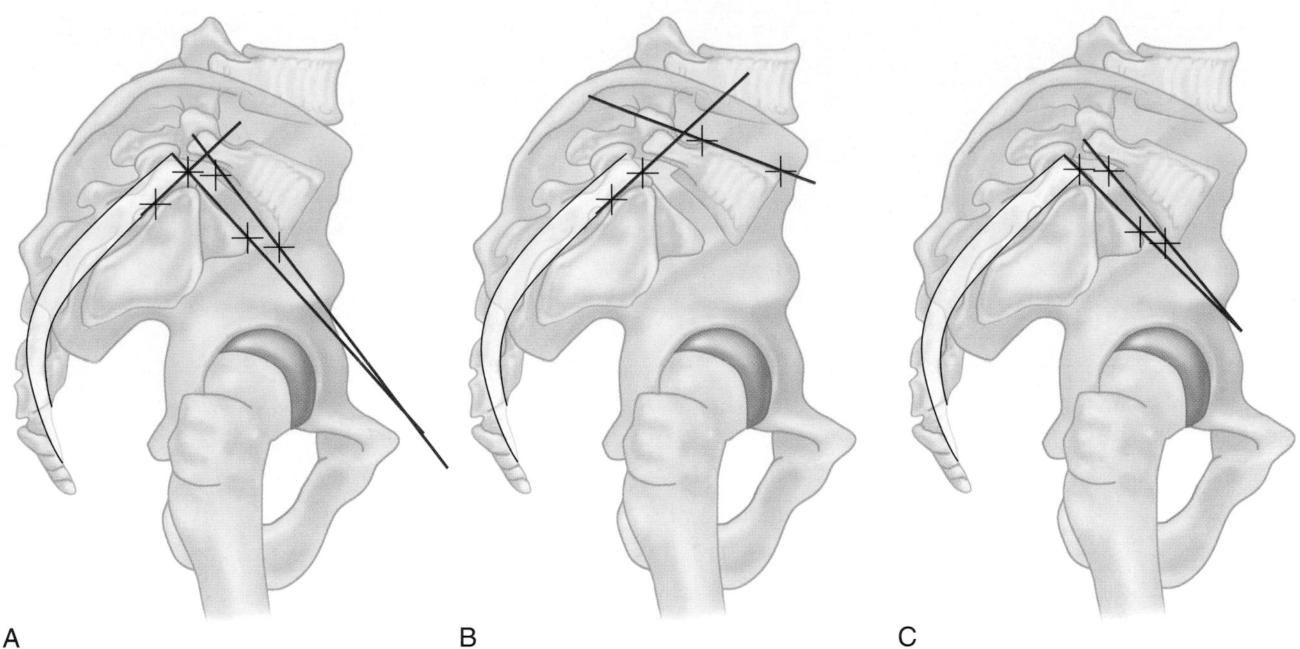

FIGURE 40-8 **A, Slip angle. B, Lumbosacral angle (Dubousset). C, Lumbosacral angle (Spinal Deformity Study Group).** (Redrawn from Glavas P, Mac-Thiong JM, Parent S, et al: Assessment of lumbosacral kyphosis in spondylolisthesis: a computer-assisted reliability study of six measurement techniques, Eur Spine J 18:212, 2009.)

usually is only mild progression. If neurologic symptoms are present, operative treatment is superior to nonoperative treatment. Matsunaga et al. found that 76% of patients without neurologic symptoms remained stable over long-term follow-up (10 to 18 years). A more recent study of 200 individuals by Enyo et al. found a baseline incidence of degenerative spondylolisthesis of 10% in those between the ages of 40 and 75 years. When the same group was radiographically re-examined 15 years later, the incidence had increased to 22.5%, with 14% of the previously normal population having developed a new degenerative spondylolisthesis. Factors associated with risk of progression were L4-5 degenerative spondylolisthesis present before age 60, female sex, and facet sagittalization.

SPONDYLOLYSIS

PATIENT PRESENTATION

Spondylolysis without any spondylolisthesis is present in 2% to 5% of the population, but only a portion become symptomatic. An even smaller portion potentially require surgical treatment. Typically the patient is an athletically active teenager with back pain and sometimes with leg pain as well. Some patients participate in organized sports year round. Often the back pain is presumed to be muscular in origin, which can delay the diagnosis substantially. Examination reveals localized pain, most commonly in the midline at the lumbosacral junction. Palpation with the patient prone to relax the extensor musculature is helpful to determine the level of involvement. For those with leg pain, nerve tension signs are present but somewhat muted relative to patients with radiculopathy caused by disc herniation.

DIAGNOSTIC EVALUATION

The radiographic evaluation includes upright lumbar radiographs including oblique views if suspicion is high for spondylolysis (Fig. 40-9). Additionally a bone scan with single photon emission computed tomography (SPECT) is ordered (Fig. 40-10). If the SPECT scan is positive, a high-resolution CT scan of the involved level should be obtained to definitively confirm the spondylolysis (Fig. 40-11). This is necessary to distinguish an area of stress reaction from a lytic defect because treatment is different. For patients with a positive SPECT scan but without a spondylolysis, 4 to 6 weeks of avoidance of sports or other high-intensity exercise usually is sufficient to allow symptom resolution. For patients with a positive SPECT scan and a pars defect visible on CT scan, 6 weeks in a rigid orthosis while upright usually is sufficient to resolve symptoms. Bony union occurs in only 25% of patients even with the use of an orthosis. There is no high-level evidence in the literature supporting the use of a rigid orthosis. In both those with healed fractures and those with fibrous unions a program of trunk and pelvic stabilization is initiated with a gradual return to full activities. Patients are allowed to return to full activity based on clinical outcome, not necessarily radiographic evidence of bony healing. Patients who remain symptomatic longer than 3 months with this treatment regimen require either more significant activity modifications or consideration for operative treatment depending on the severity of symptoms.

EVALUATION FOR OPERATIVE TREATMENT

For patients being considered for operative treatment, upright lateral flexion/extension radiographs are obtained. We prefer seated films, although others prefer standing lateral bending radiographs. This is necessary to detect the presence of a

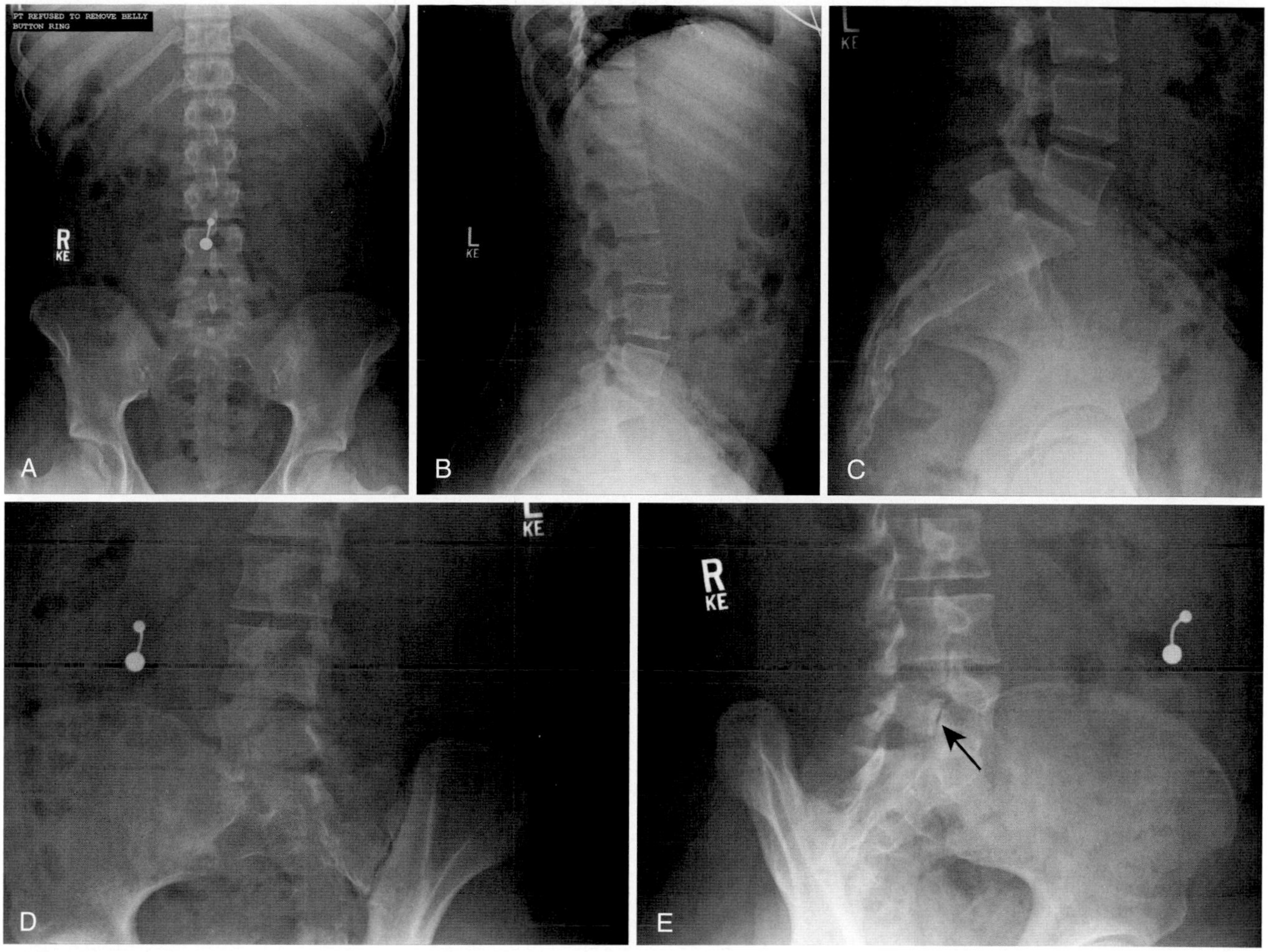

FIGURE 40-9 Upright radiographic views for evaluation of suspected spondylolysis. **A**, Anteroposterior. **B**, Lateral. **C**, Spot lateral. **D** and **E**, Bilateral oblique (arrow shows pars defect).

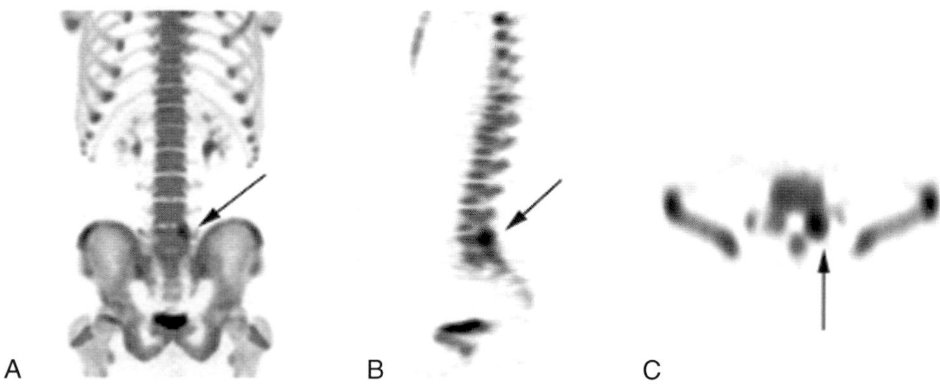

FIGURE 40-10 Coronal (**A**), sagittal (**B**), and axial (**C**) SPECT scans show increased activity in the region of the pars interarticularis in an adolescent athlete. (From spondylolysis in young athletes, Physiopedia, www.physiopedia.com/Spondylolysis_in_Young_Athletes#Diagnosis.)

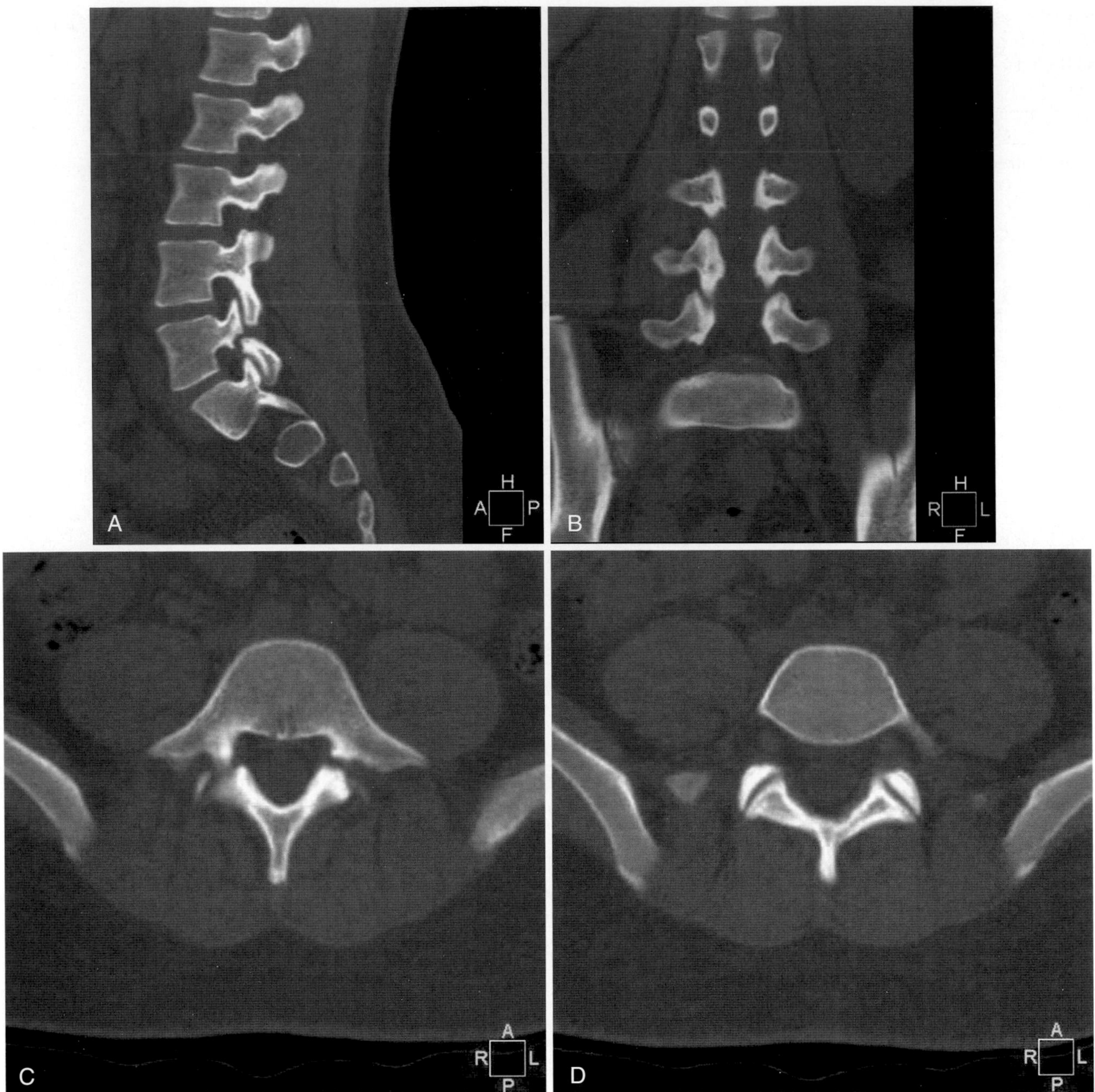

FIGURE 40-11 Sagittal **(A)**, coronal **(B)**, and axial **(C and D)** CT scans confirm spondylolysis.

significant spondylolisthesis, which may not be evident even on an upright standing lateral radiograph. To be a candidate for repair of the pars interarticularis several radiographic criteria must be met: (1) absence of spondylolisthesis, (2) absence of degenerative change at the involved disc level (best determined by MRI), (3) absence of degenerative facet changes (best determined by high resolution CT scan), and (4) absence of dysplastic changes such as spina bifida occulta, elongation of the pars interarticularis, or dysplastic facet morphology, which are all contraindications for direct pars repair (best evaluated by CT scan). In addition to these radiographic evaluations, it sometimes is helpful to use a diagnostic pars injection with a very small volume of local anesthetic. Typically, we use this when more than one level of spondylolysis is present or in other circumstances when the etiology of symptoms is not completely clear.

OPERATIVE TREATMENT

The original papers on posterior spinal fusion by Albee and Hibbs independently described the procedure for the treatment of spondylolysis and spondylolisthesis over 100 years ago. Later came descriptions of posterolateral fusions and still later the use of autogenous iliac bone graft for fusion. Buck described direct osteosynthesis of the pars fracture with a screw technique in 1970. Subsequently several different techniques have been described that use pedicle screw fixation at the involved level and various rod or hook constructs. Each construct is intended to allow compression across the lytic defect. No one technique has been shown to be superior. It is likely that the bone grafting method and technique are the most critical aspect of the procedure. We have used iliac crest bone graft in this setting, which can be harvested with minimal morbidity or risk of complication in this group of young patients.

REPAIR OF PARS INTERARTICULARIS DEFECT

TECHNIQUE 40-1

PATIENT POSITIONING

- Position the patient prone on a Jackson table after induction of anesthesia. Proper positioning is important to avoid complications.
- Make sure the chest pad is just above the nipple line with the hip pads centered at the anterior superior iliac spine.
- Support the face without pressure on the eyes and align the cervical spine in neutral to a flexed position.
- Cervical extension can be caused by some commercially available pillows for the Jackson frame and should be avoided.
- Place the hips in extension or in only slight flexion and flex the knees using pillows to decrease nerve tension.
- Confirm pedal pulses to ensure the femoral artery is not compressed by the anterior superior iliac spine pad.
- Position the upper extremities with the elbows at the level of the shoulders, placing the arm forward about 30 degrees and the elbow flexed less than 90 degrees to minimize ulnar nerve tension. Ensure that the elbows are well padded, as are all bony prominences. Administer prophylactic antibiotics and, after sterile preparation and draping are completed, complete the intraoperative "Time Out."

EXPOSURE AND GRAFT HARVEST

- Localize the involved level radiographically and make a midline incision overlying this location.
- Carry dissection down to the fascia and obtain a localization image with a clamp affixed to the spinous process, which is then marked with a rongeur confirming the level.
- Use Cobb elevators and electrocautery to expose the entire spinous process of the lytic level and the caudal portion of the spinous process cephalad to the lytic level.
- Expose the lamina at each level, taking care to avoid injury to the facet capsule.
- Expose the L4-5 facet capsule and lateral superior articular mass of L5 for repair of an L5 pars defect because the pedicle screw will be placed at the L5 level.
- Meticulously expose the pars at the involved level and expose the entire lamina of the lytic level bilaterally.
- Carefully curet the fibrocartilage out of the lytic defect to expose bone on both sides of the defect.
- Expose the base of the transverse process at the involved level.
- Use an awl to penetrate the cortex and advance a pedicle probe into the vertebral body, using fluoroscopy to assist in screw hole preparation.
- Take a slightly cranial orientation with the probe to move the ultimate position of the screw head away from the facet.
- Make a separate incision overlying the posterior superior iliac spine and carry dissection down to the fascia, which is divided along the lateral margin of the posterior superior iliac spine.
- Carefully elevate the fascia as a single layer to expose the iliac crest. There is no need to expose the outer table.
- Use an osteotome to reflect the cortex of the crest and expose the cancellous bone of the ilium.
- Use a narrow gouge to harvest multiples strips of cancellous bone. After harvesting the available bone, repair the fascia well and close the wound in layers.

PEDICLE SCREW INSERTION

- Use a high-speed burr to decorticate the base of the transverse process, lateral superior articular mass, and the pars interarticularis. Carefully place the strips of cancellous bone onto the decorticated surfaces.
- Place a polyaxial pedicle screw at the appropriate level (e.g., L5). The screw chosen usually is a smaller diameter than would be chosen for a fusion as the stresses are less and a smaller diameter screw is less likely to impinge on the facet capsule.
- Repeat pedicle screw placement on the contralateral side.
- With the defect grafted and both screws in place, use a sterile intubating stylet as a template to form a "V" shape with the caudal aspect of the L5 spinous process at the apex of the "V" and the upper ends engaging each of the pedicle screws (Fig. 40-12). Tubular benders will likely be needed to get the desired amount of rod contouring.
- Leave the rod long until after contouring is complete, because it is difficult to contour a short rod to the degree necessary. Cut the rod and place it caudal to the L5 spinous process at its base and apply compression to the rod and secure it with set screws. Torque the set screws to the manufacturer's specifications.
- Close the lumbodorsal fascia to bone to restore the normal resting length of the paraspinal musculature and close the subcutaneous and subcuticular layers.

POSTOPERATIVE CARE. Postoperatively the patient receives analgesics and muscle relaxants and begins mobilization immediately. Typically these patients are independent and able to be discharged home within 2 days.

ADULT ISTHMIC SPONDYLOLISTHESIS

Patients with isthmic spondylolisthesis are the second largest group of patients with spondylolisthesis presenting to the spine surgeon. Only degenerative spondylolisthesis is more common. Most patients with isthmic spondylolisthesis (some

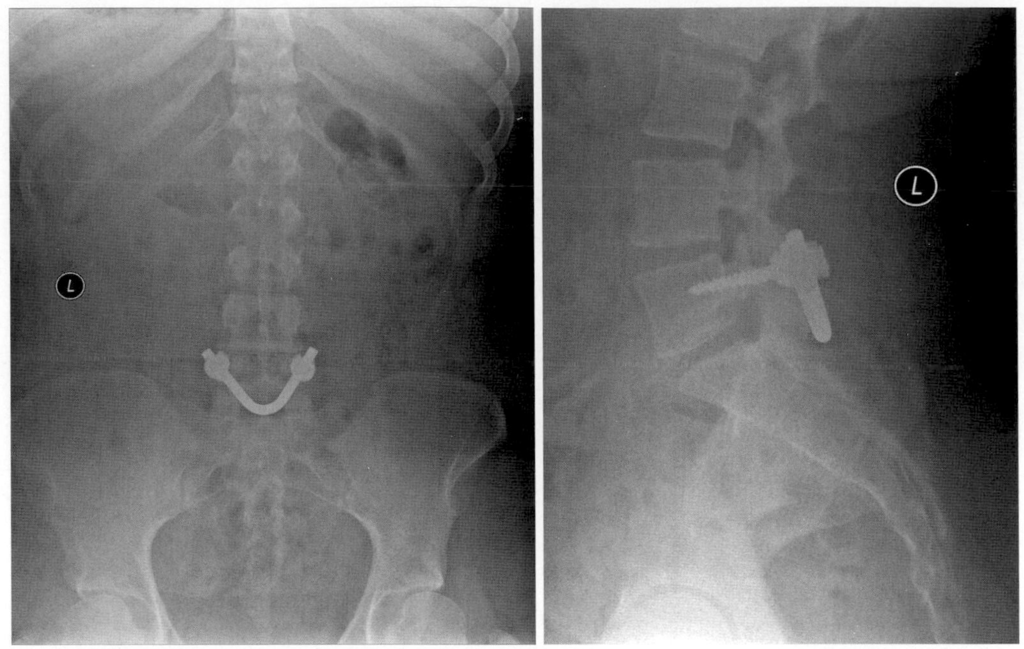

FIGURE 40-12 In situ posterolateral instrumented fusion. **SEE TECHNIQUE 40-2.**

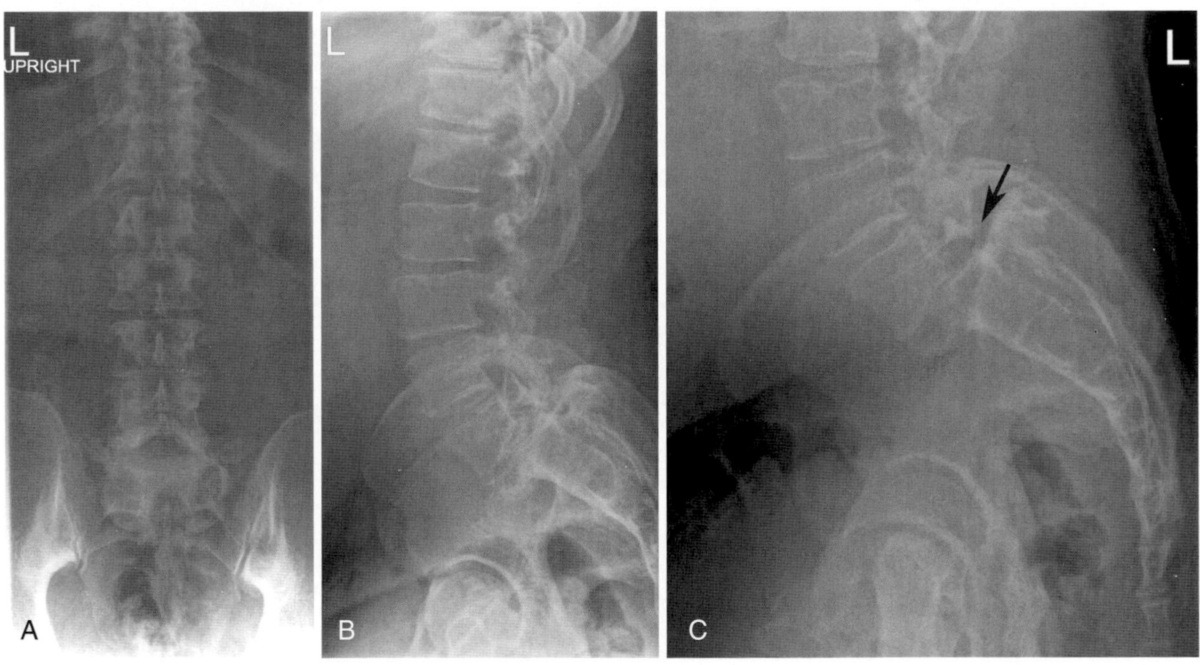

FIGURE 40-13 Initial radiographic evaluation of isthmic spondylolisthesis. **A,** Standing anteroposterior view. **B,** Standing lateral view. **C,** Spot view at L5-S1 level (arrow shows pars defect).

prefer the term "lytic acquired spondylolisthesis") present with low-grade deformities (less than a 50% slip); 90% to 95% involve the L5-S1 level, with 5% to 8% at L4-L5, and very few at the more cephalic levels. Low-grade slips are much more common than those of more than 50% by a ratio of 10:1; however, the severity can range from spondylolysis (no slip) all the way to grade V. Fortunately, most cases of low-grade isthmic spondylolisthesis are not associated with significant kyphosis or spinal imbalance. The typical presentation is a patient with axial low-back pain that tends to be mechanical and radicular pain in an L5 distribution. Initial radiographic evaluation should consist of standing anteroposterior and lateral views, as well as a spot view at the L5-S1 level (Fig. 40-13). The spondylolisthesis generally is easily diagnosed, and upright lateral flexion/extension films are useful to diagnose dynamic instability, which is common at the L4-L5 level but not at the L5-S1 level. The radiographic assessment must also include an evaluation of the regional and, if needed, global spinal balance. If significant imbalance is present, the treatment plan must correct this if surgery is indicated.

PATHOPHYSIOLOGY

The simple presence of an isthmic spondylolisthesis is not sufficient to identify the cause of the patient's symptoms because 7% of the population has spondylolysis, with or without spondylolisthesis, and most are asymptomatic. From retrospective long-term studies it has been found that about 80% of acquired lytic defects occur between the ages of 5 and 10 years, with the remaining 20% of fractures occurring before the age of 20 years. In most patients, spondylolisthesis is asymptomatic. Determining whether spondylolisthesis is the source of back pain requires a careful evaluation of the complaints. Mechanical back pain can originate from the pars defect but also from the disc, which often is more degenerative than would be expected for the patient's age because of the abnormal stresses applied to the disc as a result of the lack of stability. Radicular complaints involving the L5 root can be generated by several different pathologic processes. As the disc degenerates and loses height, the foraminal cross-sectional area is diminished, leaving less space available for the nerve root. The annulus remains attached to the inferior endplate of the cephalad vertebra and, as this vertebra translates anteriorly, the annulus becomes located posterior to the vertebra (pseudoherniation) and occupies space within the foramen. In addition, the pseudarthrosis that forms at the pars defect consists of cartilage, bone, and fibrous tissue, all of which occupy space within the foramen. Thus, the cross-sectional area of the foramen is decreased in a cephalocaudal direction by the loss of disc height and the pseudoherniation and in an anterior to posterior direction by the fibrocartilaginous tissue of the pseudarthrosis. If there is translational instability at the involved level, this can cause traction on the nerve root and produce radicular symptoms as well. In addition to these possibilities at the L5-S1 level, the L5 root can be compromised by lateral recess stenosis at the L4-5 level or less commonly by a disc herniation at the L4 disc level. Determination of the patient's primary complaint (mechanical back pain or radicular pain) will have a significant impact on the type of surgery that will be most appropriate if conservative treatment is not successful.

NONOPERATIVE TREATMENT

For many patients in the 5-to-10-year age group the initial fracture event causes minimal or no pain. For older adolescents and young adults, there is more often an acute episode of low back pain that may be associated with a specific occurrence. Typically, with the initial presentation, there is no or minimal translation present. The initial management of patients with spondylolysis is covered in the section on pars repair (p. 1737). If the patient has a spondylolisthesis of more than 1 to 2 mm at presentation, an orthosis is not recommended because fracture healing is unlikely with significant displacement. In the absence of significant neurologic deficits, patients are initially treated with a brief period of rest, anti-inflammatory medications, and muscle relaxers. Narcotics are used very sparingly, if at all, and the patient is mobilized as early as possible. Once the acute symptoms begin to subside, a program of low-impact aerobic exercise, trunk stabilization avoiding extension, and hamstring stretching is instituted. This often is successful in allowing the patient to return to full activity over a period of 8 to 12 weeks. Even with good resolution of mechanical symptoms, the patient needs to understand that trunk stabilization exercises will be necessary indefinitely to manage the expected episodic back pain.

Patients with a lytic defect of the pars have abnormal load sharing. Normally 20% of the axial load of the lumbar spine is transmitted through the posterior column, with 80% transmitted anteriorly. When a pars fracture is present, no load is carried posteriorly and all the load is transferred to the anterior column, which leads to premature disc degeneration and potentially episodic back pain; however, with proper exercise and relatively minor activity modifications, most patients can be managed nonoperatively throughout their lives.

Neurologic symptoms are less common in younger patients and often develop as the patient enters the third to fourth decades. The presence of significant neurologic deficits is an indication that operative treatment may soon become necessary because the chronic changes causing the neurologic symptoms will not resolve, although they often can be mitigated in the short-to-intermediate (months) term, but generally not the long term. For patients with significant neurologic symptoms or more than 6 months of persistent back pain not adequately controlled with the above treatment regimen, operative treatment is recommended.

It is important to realize that adult patients with low-grade isthmic spondylolisthesis and progressive complaints of lower back and hip pain may well have hip or knee pathology contributing to their symptoms. Before embarking on operative management of the spinal pathology, evaluation of these two areas is worthwhile. If the patient has significant degenerative changes of the hip, an intra-articular hip injection can be confirmatory as to whether the hip is the primary pathology. In patients with significant hip or knee degeneration, correction of these problems usually is recommended before spinal surgery. The mechanical lumbar complaints often improve with improvement in gait and aerobic activities made possible by pain reduction. When neurologic symptoms predominate, spinal surgery generally should be done first.

OPERATIVE TREATMENT

■ SURGICAL OPTIONS

Patients with isthmic spondylolisthesis can be appropriately managed using a number of techniques; however, some surgical procedures generally should not be considered in this patient group. Because patients with spondylolisthesis have instability at the involved segment, by definition, a total laminectomy (Gill procedure) in isolation is contraindicated. For similar reasons, techniques intended to achieve "dynamic fusion" are not appropriate in this group of patients. Inserting a posterior device designed to apply a distractive force at the level of an isthmic spondylolisthesis is contraindicated because distraction cannot be applied through the lytic defect. Pars repair can be a good procedure in the right patient population (see Technique 40-1); however, adult patients with isthmic spondylolisthesis-related symptoms generally are not good candidates because of the associated disc degeneration and facet arthrosis that are almost always present in this older group of patients.

EVALUATION FOR OPERATIVE TREATMENT

To appropriately plan operative treatment, additional imaging is needed. Standing lateral and posteroanterior scoliosis radiographs should be obtained to adequately assess the patient's global balance. These images should include the skull and both proximal femurs so the hip axis can be determined. The slip angle is not likely to be significantly positive in patients with low-grade acquired lytic spondylolisthesis; however, when it is positive (kyphotic), anterior column support generally will be needed. Usually the sacral endplate morphology is relatively normal, indicating that the sacral buttress is maintained. The sacral table angle can be used to assess the sacral buttress (Fig. 40-14). Each L5 transverse processes should have at least 2 cm^2 of surface area. Given the high incidence of dysplastic changes in this group of patients, we normally obtain a high-resolution CT scan to evaluate pedicle morphology, adequacy of the L5 transverse process, sacral morphology, facet arthritis at adjacent levels, and the bony foraminal dimensions. If the patient has significant radicular symptoms, an MRI usually is obtained to determine the specific location and etiology of the nerve root symptoms, which usually are caused by nerve compression but traction on the nerve root caused by instability also is possible. Although a pseudoherniation is common and can be readily seen on the MRI and may explain L5 root symptoms, the L4 disc must also be assessed. Occasionally, a patient may have an L4 disc herniation causing the L5 root symptoms, and this generally can be managed more simply with a microdiscectomy at the L4 level rather than operative stabilization at the L5-S1 level if the patient has only mild axial back-pain complaints. Also the health of the adjacent disc levels can be assessed on MRI, which will influence how many levels may need to be fused and the method of fusion. Some authors have recommended provocative discography to evaluate adjacent levels, but we have not found this to be reliable. We have found that a pars injection with a small volume of long-acting local anesthetic is helpful as a diagnostic tool when evaluating patients with extensive degenerative changes at multiple levels in addition to isthmic spondylolisthesis.

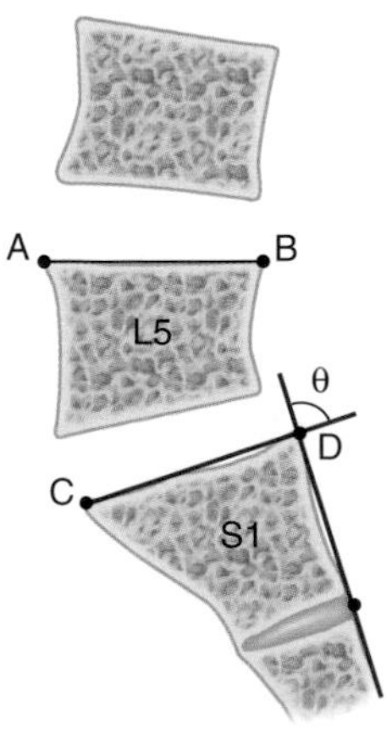

FIGURE 40-14 The sacral table angle is measured between a line along the sacral endplate and a line drawn along the posterior aspect of the S1 vertebral body.

OUTCOMES OF OPERATIVE TREATMENT

An appropriate individualized treatment plan should be based on the patient's specific symptoms. Do they have only mechanical back pain? Do they have predominantly nerve root symptomatology? Do they have significant components of both? For patients with primarily mechanical lumbar pain, stabilization without decompression (direct or indirect) can be appropriate. If they have significant neurologic deficits, direct decompression is optimal, but indirect decompression often is adequate if there are neurologic symptoms without deficits, but this depends on the pathology demonstrated on imaging. The first randomized study to demonstrate improved outcomes of operative treatment compared with nonoperative treatment in this patient group was that of Möller and Hedlund. Their findings were recently confirmed in a systematic review by Schulte et al. For patients with appropriate operative intervention, a good-to-excellent outcome (based on patient-reported outcomes) can be expected in about 85%. The primary determinant of good outcomes is the success of achieving a fusion. Kwon and Albert showed in their literature review that using rigid pedicle screw constructs improves fusion rates in patients with acquired lytic spondylolisthesis. They found a 90% fusion rate with the use of rigid pedicle screw instrumentation and a 77% fusion rate in uninstrumented cases. In children, a posterolateral uninstrumented fusion has been more successful than in adults.

Open posterior fusions can be done using a midline approach or the muscle-splitting approach described by Wiltse and Spencer (see Technique 37-25), which uses the intermuscular plane between the multifidus and longissimus muscles. The latter approach is considered by most to have the advantage of being less traumatic to the musculature and producing less "fusion disease" attributable to muscle fibrosis postoperatively. The muscle-splitting approach is not recommended if a direct decompression is planned. Current minimally invasive techniques are an extension of this concept and are less traumatic to the soft tissues; however, so far it remains unclear if they will prove superior with respect to fusion rates and clinical outcomes. For patients requiring direct decompression and interbody support, we prefer a midline exposure extending out to the tip of the transverse processes bilaterally. Steps are taken to minimize the muscle ischemia associated with this approach in an effort to minimize the potential for persistent pain related to "fusion disease."

Another finding by Kwon and Albert was that patients who had a laminectomy had a slightly lower fusion rate and slightly lower outcome scores than those without laminectomy, but neither of these reached statistical significance. These authors did find a statistically significant difference in fusion rates between circumferential fusions (anterior lumbar interbody or combined posterior lumbar interbody fusion or transforaminal lumbar interbody fusion with posterior spinal fusion) and either anterior only or posterior only fusions. Patients with an interbody fusion and a posterior fusion had the highest fusion rate (98%) compared with anterior only (75%) or posterior only fusion (83%). Clinical success rates were similar: 86% for circumferential fusion, 79% for anterior fusion only, and 75% for posterior only fusion. An economic evaluation by Bydon et al. found that adding an interbody device increased the cost per quality-adjusted life-year (QALY) compared with a posterolateral fusion alone initially; however, when the costs of reoperations were factored in, the addition of interbody fusion resulted in a modest cost savings compared with posterolateral fusion alone. Lee et al. found that complication rates and fusion rates were similar in adult patients with posterolateral fusion alone and those with posterolateral interbody fusion for isthmic spondylolisthesis.

OPERATIVE PLANNING

After clinical and imaging evaluations are complete, specific surgical procedures can be recommended based on the findings. For patients without significant neurologic complaints and with good spinal alignment, instrumented posterolateral fusion can be recommended if there is sufficient surface area for fusion. In many patients, the L5 transverse process is hypoplastic and may be inadequate (less than 2 cm^2 of surface area). For patients with inadequate area for posterolateral fusion, a posterior-only approach with circumferential fusion (posterior or transforaminal lumbar interbody fusion) or an anterior lumbar interbody fusion with posterior supplemental fixation provides a good alternative. An uninstrumented posterior-only fusion rarely is recommended in this patient population.

For patients with nerve root symptoms, direct or indirect decompression is a necessary part of the procedure. Indirect decompression is accomplished through realignment and reestablishment of the disc height using an interbody spacer device including allograft bone. Currently, a variety of devices are available for this purpose, including femoral cortical allografts, polyetheretherketone (PEEK) cages, titanium mesh cages, expandable cages, and carbon fiber devices. These devices are used in conjunction with autograft bone, allograft bone, and bone morphogenetic proteins (BMP) in an off-label application. A recent randomized, controlled, multicenter trial showed that BMP-7 (OP-1) with a collagen carrier was not as effective as autologous iliac crest bone for obtaining fusion. Because of the higher fusion rate with autologous iliac crest grafts (74%) than with BMP (54%), these authors did not recommend the use of BMP in instrumented posterior lumbar fusion procedures.

Indirect reduction can be accomplished with a transforaminal lumbar interbody fusion combined with an instrumented posterolateral fusion. For patients who need a direct decompression in addition to the realignment and reduction, we generally prefer a posterior lumbar interbody fusion coupled with an instrumented posterolateral fusion.

IN SITU POSTEROLATERAL INSTRUMENTED FUSION: WILTSE AND SPENCER APPROACH

TECHNIQUE 40-2

- After induction of anesthesia, position the patient as described in Technique 40-1. Montgomery et al. demonstrated that proper positioning allows some reduction of the spondylolisthesis.
- Apply pneumatic compression devices and initiate neuromonitoring (see Chapter 44) if it is used.
- Administer prophylactic antibiotics and tranexamic acid if it will be used. After sterile preparation and draping are completed, complete the intraoperative "Time Out."
- Make a midline skin incision at the L5-S1 level down to the fascia and carry dissection laterally superficial to the fascia on both sides about 4 cm for the length of the skin incision (see Technique 37-25).
- On each side of the midline make a 4 cm to 5 cm long fascial incision 3 cm off the midline at the approximate interval between the multifidus and longissimus muscles, curving the incisions slightly medially at the inferior end.
- Use blunt dissection to develop the plane down to the L5-S1 facet joint.
- Expose the L5 transverse process and the sacral ala subperiosteally.
- Verify the correct level radiographically with a towel clip applied to the transverse process. Once the correct level is confirmed, make a generous facetectomy.
- Prepare the pedicle screw holes at the L5 level and the S1 level bilaterally, using fluoroscopy to assist in pedicle location and orientation.
- Prepare the S1 screw holes for a bicortical technique for enhanced screw purchase. Penetrate the sacral cortex medially at the promontory just caudal to the endplate.
- Sound each screw hole to ensure there are no cortical breaches and place a cottonoid for hemostasis.
- Bone removal often is required to allow placement of the L5 screw, which also enlarges the area for bone graft incorporation.
- Place polyaxial pedicle screws bilaterally at L5 and S1 after thorough decortication and placement of bone graft under direct vision. Generally, a separate autologous iliac graft is harvested or local autograft is combined with allograft cancellous bone soaked in antibiotic solution at least 30 minutes before implantation. Some have recommended off-label use of BMP or demineralized bone matrix to augment local autograft.
- Contour the rods and affix them with the set screws, which are torqued according to the manufacturer's recommendation (Fig. 40-14).
- Thoroughly irrigate the wound throughout the procedure and again before closure. Note that if BMP is used irrigation should not be done after BMP has been placed into the wound.
- Administer a second dose of tranexamic acid before wound closure.
- Close the fascial wounds with interrupted sutures and place two subcutaneous drains. Minimize dead space by tacking the subcutaneous layer to the fascia bilaterally. Complete subcutaneous and subcuticular closure.
- This procedure can be done through a midline fascial incision (see Technique 37-24) rather than the Wiltse and Spencer approach (see Technique 37-25). If a midline incision is used, close the fascia over a drain and to the spinous processes to maintain proper muscle resting length in the lordotic spine.

POSTOPERATIVE CARE. The patient is mobilized without a brace beginning the morning after surgery. Parenteral and oral analgesics and muscle relaxers are given to facilitate rest and mobilization. Generally patients are independent with activity and can be discharged the third or fourth postoperative day.

POSTERIOR INSTRUMENTED FUSION WITH INTERBODY FUSION (PLIF AND TLIF)

This is the procedure we most commonly use for adult patients with low-grade isthmic spondylolisthesis. It is preferred because of the ability to restore normal lumbosacral alignment parameters when necessary and restore disc height. Posterior and transforaminal lumbar interbody fusion techniques are very similar and are described together. Each is combined with a posterolateral fusion to achieve a circumferential arthrodesis. A posterior lumbar interbody fusion (PLIF) is preferred because a complete laminectomy (Gill procedure) usually is done for direct decompression in these patients.

TECHNIQUE 40-3

- Position the patient as described in Technique 40-1 and complete sterile preparation and draping, followed by the intraoperative "Time Out."
- Make a midline incision centered at the L5-S1 level (Fig. 40-15A).
- Release the fascia and obtain a localization image with a clamp on the spinous process to confirm the operative level. Use a rongeur to mark the spinous process that had the clamp applied as a reference.
- Carry subperiosteal dissection laterally over the lamina at the L4, L5, and S1 levels.
- Remove the joint capsule at the L5-S1 level bilaterally, but preserve the capsule at the L4-5 facet.
- Expose the transverse process of L5 and the sacral ala bilaterally and prepare pedicle screw holes at the L5 level and the S1 level bilaterally, using fluoroscopy to assist in pedicle location and orientation.
- Prepare the S1 screw holes for a bicortical technique for enhanced screw purchase. Penetrate the sacral cortex medially at the promontory just caudal to the endplate. Sound each screw hole to ensure there are no cortical breaches and place a cottonoid for hemostasis.
- Remove the posterior elements of the L5 vertebra (Gill fragment) piecemeal or en bloc. For en bloc removal, detach the ligamentum flavum from the caudal and cephalad margins using small angled curettes. As the fragment is mobilized, advance the curet down to the pseudarthrosis site to release the fibrocartilaginous tissue around the L5 nerve root. Careful dissection is necessary here as the nerve root usually is already quite compressed and aggressive curetting may damage the root (Fig. 40-16).
- Once the lamina has been removed, remove additional fibrocartilage from around the nerve root with a Kerrison rongeur. The exiting L5 root should be visible all the way to the lateral aspect of the foramen. The operating microscope is very helpful during this dissection.
- Through the S1 foraminotomy identify the traversing S1 root. Remove the ligamentum attached to the L4 lamina to adequately decompress the L5 root in the L4-5 lateral recess as well. Removal of the osteophyte from the medial aspect of the L5 facet may also be needed.
- After the decompression is completed, decorticate the transverse processes and sacral alae and pack the lateral gutter with a sponge for hemostasis.
- Insert the pedicle screws to allow distraction (if necessary) across the disc space to facilitate disc removal and reduction of the spondylolisthesis. Standard polyaxial screws and rod reduction tools usually can be used at L5 if the amount of translation desired is less than 1.5 cm. If more translation is needed, reduction screws with extended threaded portions are quite helpful.

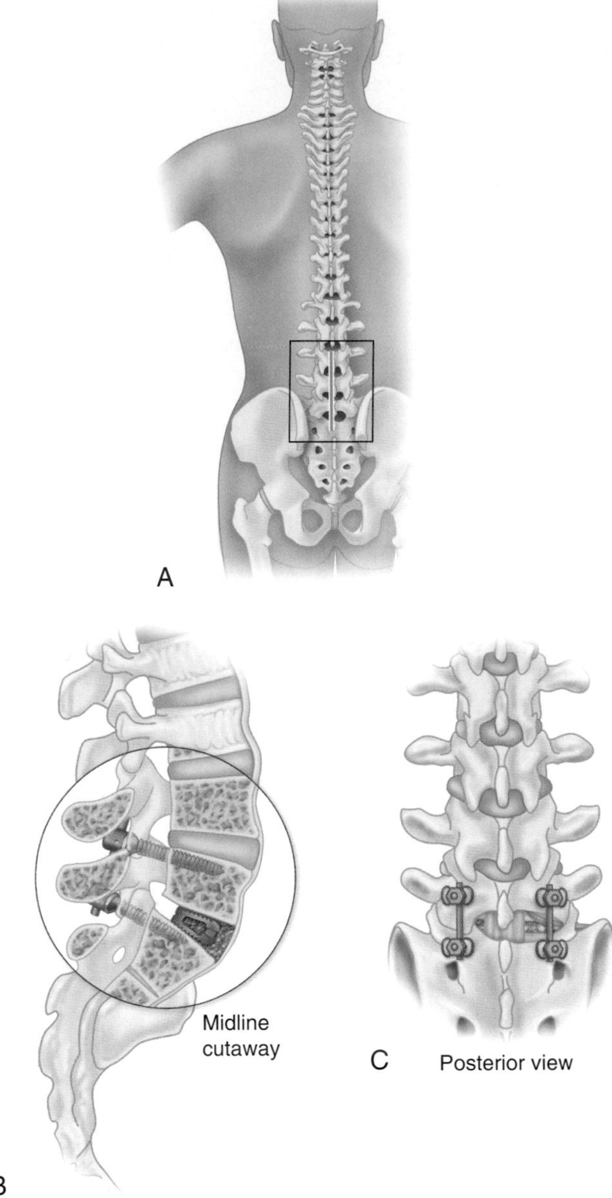

FIGURE 40-15 Posterior instrumented fusion with interbody fusion. **A**, Incision. **B**, Polyaxial screws inserted at S1 and expandable cage device placed. **C**, Rods inserted. **SEE TECHNIQUE 40-3.**

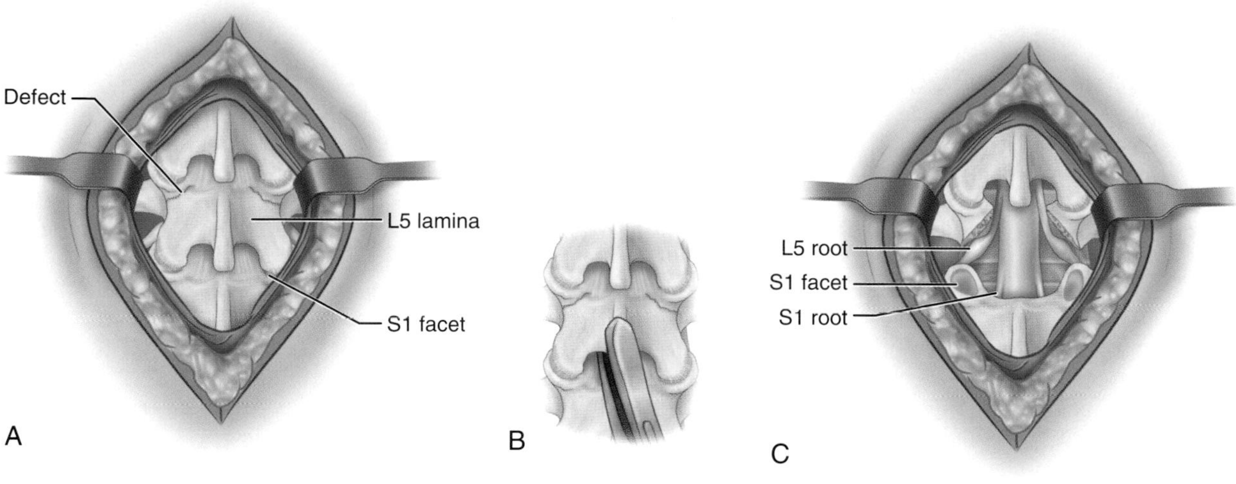

FIGURE 40-16 Gill-Manning-White laminectomy for decompression. **SEE TECHNIQUE 40-3.**

- Insert standard polyaxial screws at the S1 level (Fig. 40-15B). Typically with sufficient decompression, the pedicles can be directly inspected for cortical breaches at the L5 and S1 locations. If neuromonitoring is used, screw resistance can be determined. We use an impedance of 10mA as a threshold for a safe screw. Neuromonitoring is most useful to detect deficits caused by tension during reduction of the spondylolisthesis.
- Cut a working rod and contour it to allow rod placement. Secure this working rod to the S1 screw and then gradually reduce it into the L5 screw while maintaining a distractive force between the two screws (Fig. 40-15C). Reduce the rods bilaterally in a gradual alternating fashion, taking care not to apply so much force that the L5 screw pulls out. Monitor the translation of the L5 vertebra fluoroscopically.
- Release of the posterior annulus and disc space preparation is the next phase of the procedure. Often there is a leash of epidural veins in the axilla of the L5 nerve root that cross the disc. Coagulate these vessels with bipolar cautery, if possible, before annulotomy. They can be difficult to control otherwise, but Gelfoam and thrombin usually are effective.
- Make a wide annulotomy by retracting the thecal sac medially. This can be done bilaterally if two cages are planned or unilaterally if one of the elongated designs is to be used. In either case, the posterior osteophyte extending from L5 may need to be removed with an osteotome to adequately open the annulotomy and access the disc space.
- Use intervertebral reamers/sizers and curets to prepare the endplates, with fluoroscopic monitoring of instrument position within the disc space to avoid anterior annulus violation and potential vascular injury.
- As the discectomy and annulotomy proceed, gradually reduce the L5 vertebra until reduction is satisfactory. Loosen the contralateral set screw somewhat to allow this reduction to occur.
- Once the endplates are prepared and the reduction is satisfactory, thoroughly irrigate the disc space to remove any residual soft tissue.
- Pack allograft cancellous bone against the anterior annulus and morsellized local autograft bone in behind this. Submerge the allograft cancellous bone in antibiotic irrigation solution at the beginning of the case and maintain it there until implantation. This has decreased postoperative deep wound infections associated with allograft bone usage. Take care to leave adequate space to allow placement of the interbody device no more posteriorly than midbody so lordosis can be achieved.
- The goals of cage placement are to restore disc height and improve alignment with sufficient lordosis through the segment. Biomechanically, coverage of 35% of the endplate is desirable for stability. This can be achieved with two or more smaller devices, such as mesh cages packed with bone, or a larger footprint single device. We prefer a single expandable cage device packed with local autograft placed just anterior to the midbody. The subchondral bone is strongest around the perimeter of the endplate and weakest centrally, increasing the risk of cage subsidence if the device is too small or only centrally located.
- Once the device is transversely positioned, expand it to the predetermined desired height.
- Release the distraction from the working rods, which may need to be cut or exchanged because they likely will be too long and may impinge on the L4-5 facet joint.
- Remove the sponge and place bone graft in the lateral gutter.
- Place the final rods and apply mild compression for lordosis, being mindful of the L5 foramina dimensions.
- Torque the set screws to specifications of the manufacturer.
- Irrigate the wound throughout the procedure and thoroughly at the conclusion of the instrumentation. If BMP has been used, irrigation should not be done after it is placed into the wound.

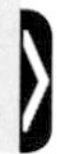

- Place a fluted drain (because of the exposed dura) and close the fascia to the remaining spinous processes with interrupted sutures to restore the normal resting length of the muscle. Close the subcutaneous and subcuticular layers individually. Administer a second dose of tranexamic acid as wound closure begins.

The procedure for a transforaminal lumbar interbody fusion (TLIF) is very similar to the PLIF as just described when done through a midline approach. When indirect decompression through the spinal implants is sufficient, TLIF may be preferred and can be done without the need for the Gill laminectomy. The discectomy and annulus removal are not as complete with this approach and the ability to translate the vertebra is more limited. Indirect decompression can be accomplished through a Wiltse approach or with minimally invasive techniques in patients with less severe pathology.

POSTOPERATIVE CARE. The patient is mobilized without a brace beginning the morning after surgery. Parenteral and oral analgesics and muscle relaxers are given to facilitate rest and mobilization. Generally patients are independent with activity and can be discharged the third or fourth postoperative day with open techniques and somewhat sooner with minimally invasive methods.

ANTERIOR LUMBAR INTERBODY FUSION

There are certain advantages to anterior lumbar interbody fusions, particularly for high-grade spondylolisthesis, because of the soft-tissue release than can be obtained to allow reduction; however, this usually is not the first choice for treatment of low-grade isthmic spondylolisthesis. The two general circumstances in which this technique is most commonly used are (1) patients appropriate for posterolateral in situ fusion with prohibitively small transverse processes and (2) as a salvage procedure in patients who had an in situ posterolateral fusion but developed a nonunion. In the first instance, supplemental posterior instrumentation normally is used, as well as the anterior surgery, to restore the posterior tension band. In the second case, the anterior procedure should be done before the previously placed posterior instrumentation has failed. This procedure is best done by an experienced spine surgeon. The risks of the approach need to be clearly discussed with the patient, particularly the risk of retrograde ejaculation in young male patients, as well as other risks.

TECHNIQUE 40-4

- Position the patient supine on a radiolucent table, such as the OSI flat top. After induction of anesthesia, fold the patient's arms across the chest on pillows and secure them in place. Place a pillow behind the knees to flex the hips and knees slightly.
- Apply pneumatic compressive devices and affix an O_2 saturation monitor to the left great toe.
- Place a bolster under the patient at the lumbosacral junction; this can be an inflatable pressure bag or rolled towels.
- Sterilely prepare and drape the infraumbilical area and administer prophylactic antibiotics. Complete the intraoperative "Time Out."
- Image the operative level fluoroscopically and determine the level of the incision.
- Make a low transverse incision down to the rectus sheath. Open the rectus sheath and mobilize the left rectus muscle toward the midline.
- Open the posterior sheath distal to the arcuate line and enter the preperitoneal space. Mobilize the peritoneal contents to the patient's right.
- After the ureter has been positively identified, set up a table-mounted retractor with several retractor blades.
- Identify the aortic bifurcation and carefully expose the anterior spine. Usually the aortic bifurcation is located at the L4 disc level, but this is variable and a fluoroscopic lateral view is used to definitively confirm the level.
- When the L5 disc level is located caudal to the bifurcation, divide the middle lumbar vessels and mobilize the left iliac vein and artery to the left.
- The dissection at the level of the disc space should be done gently and without the use of electrocautery, only bipolar cautery. The oxygen sensor on the hallux allows monitoring of the level of retraction on the artery.
- Once the disc is sufficiently exposed, make a wide annulotomy and carry out the disc excision with curets and Kerrison rongeurs.
- Use lateral image intensifier views as the posterior disc preparation is completed, which can be taken back all the way to the posterior longitudinal ligament. The most common error is inadequate posterior release.
- If the sacrum is rounded, use an osteotome to reshape it to provide a flat surface for the interbody device. A variety of cage devices are available, including titanium cages and mesh cylinders, PEEK devices with fixation capabilities, femoral allograft bone, and carbon fiber implants. The commercially available systems have trial sizes with varying degrees of lordosis to determine the optimal size and footprint. Usually by this point the spondylolisthesis has been substantially if not completely reduced.
- To obtain a fusion, harvest autograft bone or use BMP to fill the chamber within the implant. Take care if BMP is placed posteriorly and the annulus has been violated because bone can form in the canal or BMP-induced radiculitis may affect the nerve root.
- Once the interbody device is implanted (Fig. 40-17), close the wound in the usual fashion.

This same technique can be used at the L4 disc level or L3. Exposure at the L4 level is often difficult and usually requires sacrifice of the iliolumbar vein, which ascends from the left common iliac vein and must be identified and divided before the vein can be sufficiently mobilized. Excess traction on the iliac veins also can lead to deep venous thrombosis in the postoperative period.

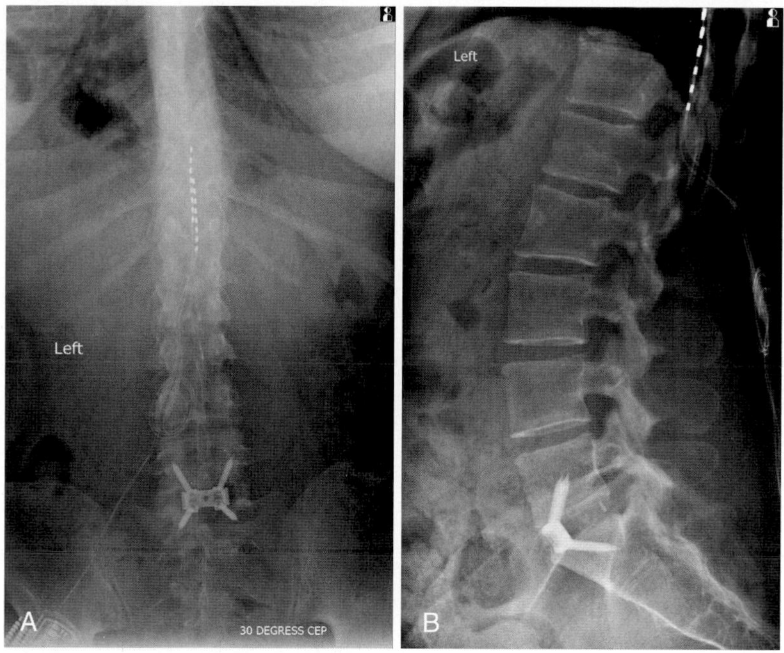

FIGURE 40-17 Ferguson (**A**) and lateral spot view (**B**) of anterior lumbar interbody fusion.

POSTOPERATIVE CARE. The patient is allowed a clear liquid diet the next day and mobilization is started on the first postoperative day, usually without a brace. Patients usually can be discharged home the second or third postoperative day. If aggressive disc space mobilization was needed, these patients usually complain of significant lumbar pain when ambulation is initiated.

DEGENERATIVE SPONDYLOLISTHESIS

Degenerative spondylolisthesis is the most common form seen in adults. It is more homogeneous with respect to pathoanatomy than the acquired lytic type because there usually is no contributory dysplasia. Degenerative spondylolisthesis is most frequent in women over the age of 50 years, especially those of African descent, and typically occurs at the L4-5 level (Fig. 40-18). It is believed to result from the degenerative cascade, as described by Kirkaldy-Willis. The L4-5 level is affected six times more often than other levels, and spondylolisthesis is four times more likely above a sacralized L5 segment. Degenerative spondylolisthesis is present in 10% of women over 60 years of age, many of whom are asymptomatic. Diabetes has been present in a disproportionate number of study patients, and Imada et al. found that patients who had undergone oophorectomy had a three times greater rate of degenerative spondylolisthesis than did patients who had not undergone oophorectomy.

PATHOPHYSIOLOGY

Degenerative spondylolisthesis is differentiated from isthmic spondylolisthesis by the presence of an intact pars (see Fig. 40-18). Because the arch is intact and moves forward with the L4 vertebral body, progressive spinal stenosis occurs in addition to facet degenerative changes. The true deformity of degenerative spondylolisthesis does not seem to be pure translation, but rather a rotary deformity that may distort the dura and its contents and exaggerate the appearance of spinal stenosis. Existing theories to explain the development of degenerative spondylolisthesis include the primary occurrence of sagittal facets and disc degeneration, with secondary facet changes accounting for anterolisthesis. The sagittal facet theory suggests a predilection for slippage because of facet orientation that does not resist anterior translation forces and, over time, results in degenerative spondylolisthesis. The disc degenerative theory proposes that the disc narrows first, and subsequent overloading of the facets results in accelerated arthritic changes, secondary remodeling, and anterolisthesis. Facet arthritic changes seem to be more severe than disc space narrowing, with the most advanced anterolisthesis present when disc narrowing is more pronounced. A continuum seems to exist as degeneration progresses. In addition, facets that are aligned in a more sagittal orientation provide less stability at the involved level, but whether these changes result from chronic instability or from a primary anatomic variant is debatable. Boden et al. showed that sagittal facet angles of more than 45 degrees at L4-5 predicted a 25 times greater likelihood of degenerative spondylolisthesis. Despite the increased frequency of degenerative spondylolisthesis in women, there seems to be no sex-specific difference in facet orientation, which calls into question the theory that sagittal facet joints are a primary cause of degenerative spondylolisthesis. Sagittal facet orientation has been correlated with disc space narrowing, suggesting that disc narrowing increases loading of the facet, resulting in secondary facet changes. Regardless of the exact nature of the first inciting event, this instability causes facet arthritis, disc degeneration, and ligamentous hypertrophy, which all contribute to produce symptoms. Facet orientation may be part of the

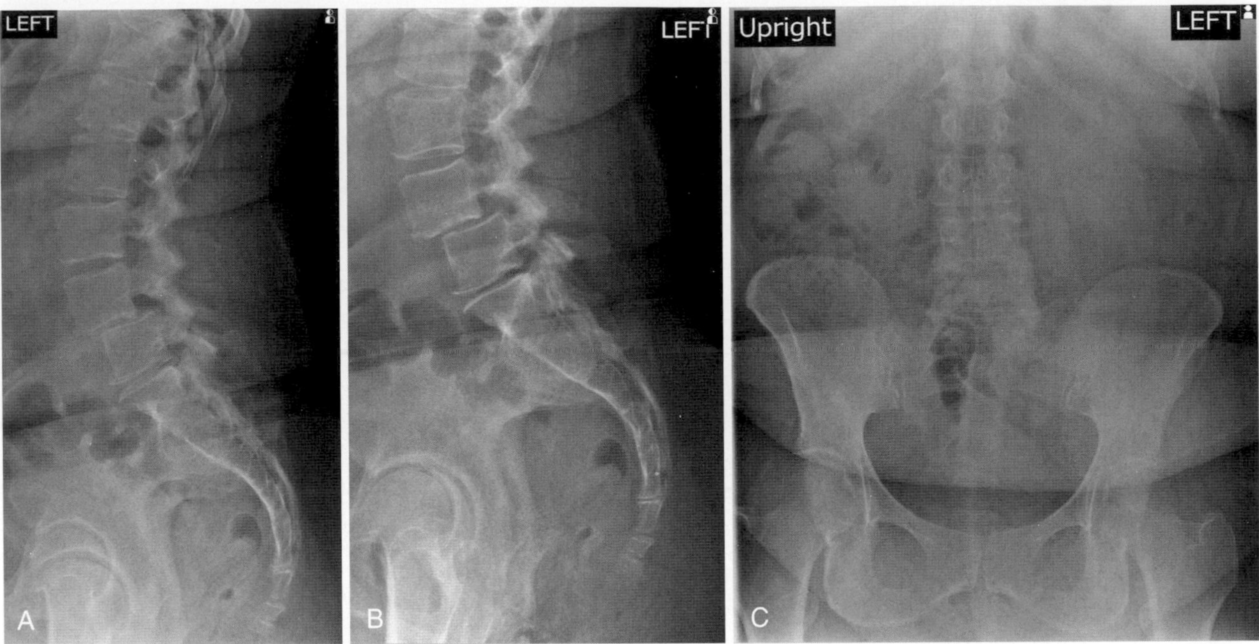

FIGURE 40-18 Degenerative spondylolisthesis at L4-5. Degenerative spondylolisthesis can be differentiated from isthmic spondylolisthesis by the presence of an intact pars (see Fig. 40-9).

consideration of potential instability when evaluating a patient for surgery, especially decompression alone. Most of the literature describing natural history concerns spinal stenosis rather than degenerative spondylolisthesis. Matsunaga et al. reported that in 145 patients examined annually for a minimum of 10 years, progressive spondylolisthesis occurred in 34% and further disc space narrowing continued in the patients without further slip. Patients with disc space narrowing, spur formation, and ligamentous ossification did not develop an increased amount of slip. There was no correlation between radiographic findings and a patient's clinical picture. Low back pain improved in patients with continued disc space narrowing, which may imply autostabilization. Of the 145 patients, 76% remained without neurologic deficits; however, 83% of patients with neurologic symptoms, including claudication and vesicorectal disorder, experienced a deterioration in their disorder and had a poor prognosis. This finding is in agreement with an earlier study by Matsunaga et al., which showed that, over 60 to 176 months, progressive slipping occurred in 30% of patients without significant effect on clinical outcome.

NONOPERATIVE TREATMENT

The symptoms attributed to degenerative spondylolisthesis tend to be stable over time or progress rather slowly. The typical complaints related to degenerative spondylolisthesis include lower back pain and lower extremity pain and weakness that are claudicatory in nature, meaning they progress in severity and distribution with ambulation and standing. The neurologic symptoms are related to spinal stenosis, which may exist not only at the level of the spondylolisthesis but at other degenerative levels. The back pain may respond to physical therapy for core strengthening with avoidance of extension exercises, although there is no clear optimal regimen. Aerobic conditioning also has a role in reducing symptoms and maintaining cardiac fitness. Activities such as stationary bike, swimming, elliptical machines, and walking as tolerated are all reasonable to try. Antiinflammatory drugs also are helpful for some patients. All of these measures must be used over the long term because of the chronic nature of this problem. Most patients remain stable with regard to symptoms over long periods, with intermittent periods of exacerbation. For those patients with worsening symptoms, 12 weeks of directed treatment is reasonable before recommending operative intervention unless the patient develops a progressive neurologic deficit. Patients with neurologic symptoms, particularly radiculopathy, may benefit from epidural steroid injections, although the benefit may only be temporary. No literature exists to support the use of a series of two or three epidural steroid injections unless symptoms improve partially after the first injection. If the first injection is done without fluoroscopy and is ineffective, a second injection can be done with fluoroscopy to ensure proper placement and diffusion. Further injections are not warranted if there is not a favorable response after a single well-placed injection. There is some evidence that response to injections can be used to diagnostically confirm the anatomic origin of the symptoms (when done under fluoroscopy) and that the short-term response to injections may correlate well with operative outcomes. If epidural steroid injection is successful, physical therapy should be instituted.

OPERATIVE TREATMENT AND OUTCOMES

The decision to consider operative treatment is based on the degree of disability and the severity of pain experienced by the patient. If the symptoms significantly limit the patient's necessary activities or those the patient enjoys, even after a reasonable trial of nonoperative care, operative treatment

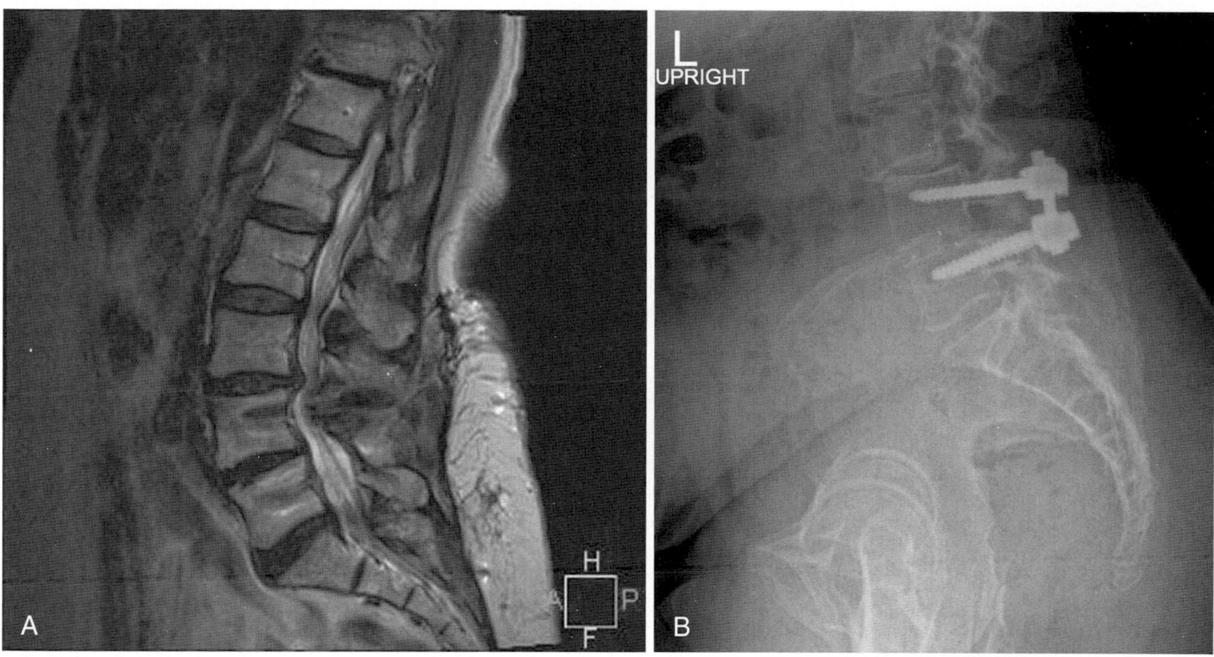

FIGURE 40-19 Evaluation of instability in degenerative spondylolisthesis. **A,** L3-4 spondylolisthesis appears reduced on supine MRI. **B,** L3-4 spondylolisthesis is visible on standing lateral radiographic spot view.

should be considered. Only 10% to 15% of patients with degenerative spondylolisthesis require surgery. In general, patients complaining primarily of neurogenic claudication or radiculopathy tend to have more improvement than those experiencing primarily axial low back pain. This is because many of the patients with primarily axial pain have degenerative levels other than the spondylolisthetic level contributing to their symptoms. The Spine Patient Outcome Research Trial (SPORT) study demonstrated a significant benefit for patients with degenerative spondylolisthesis treated with decompression and fusion (type of fusion was not controlled) at the 2-year and 4-year time frame compared with nonoperatively treated patients. This prospective, randomized, multicenter study has provided the highest level of evidence to date supporting the benefit of operative treatment in this group of patients. In a study by Golinvaux et al., the SPORT findings were determined to be generalizable to a larger group of patients in the National Surgical Quality Improvement Program (NSQIP) database. Additional economic studies have found the cost per QALY for operative treatment of degenerative spondylolisthesis to be $64,000 per QALY at 4 years, which is substantially less than the cost at 2 years. Multiple studies have found patient satisfaction rates of 85% to 90% in the operatively treated patients, with successful fusion being a key factor. In addition, Schulte et al. found "good" evidence in a literature review that operative treatment for degenerative spondylolisthesis is superior to nonoperative treatment in appropriately selected patients.

OPERATIVE PLANNING

There should be an awareness that other pathologies can mimic or overlap the signs and symptoms of degenerative spondylolisthesis and the associated spinal stenosis. Primary among these conditions are vascular claudication, degenerative hip arthritis, and peripheral neuropathy. If the history and physical examination findings are inconsistent with degenerative spondylolisthesis, evaluation for these problems should be considered.

Once the decision to recommend operative treatment has been made, a determination as to what type of operation is most appropriate for an individual patient also must be made. This determination is based on the patient's primary complaints and imaging findings. Standing lateral and anteroposterior radiographs are imperative because 15% of deformities spontaneously reduce on supine imaging such as an MRI (Fig. 40-19). Instability is considered to be present when 4 mm of translation or 10 degrees of sagittal rotation greater than the adjacent level is identified. Disc space narrowing indicates degenerative changes. Upright flexion-extension lateral views may reveal translational motion, indicating a more unstable motion segment. The Ferguson anteroposterior view shows any significant degenerative changes in the lumbosacral joint and allows a better view of the transverse processes of L5. Hypoplastic transverse processes also should prompt consideration for interbody fusion because of the paucity of bony substrate for fusion, especially for lumbosacral fusions. Dynamically unstable spondylolisthesis also may benefit from interbody fusions that improve stability through annular tension and decrease shear stress on posterior instrumentation by sharing load through the disc space. The presence of retrolisthesis or lateral listhesis also should be noted. In addition to plain radiographs, advanced neuroimaging is necessary to appropriately evaluate these patients. MRI generally is satisfactory, but a significant subset of patients cannot have an MRI because of the presence of a pacemaker or cardiac stents for example. In this case, lumbar myelography and post-myelogram high-resolution CT scans are quite satisfactory and often demonstrate the bony pathology better than MRI. Post-myelogram CT scans do not show pathology as well in the middle and lateral foramen because the subarachnoid space is not present out to the dorsal root ganglion and, thus, there is no contrast present in this area. Intraforaminal stenosis is relatively common, affecting the L4 nerve root, which is compressed against the inferior aspect of the L4 pedicle by annulus from a pseudoherniation. The most severe stenosis usually is located at the level of the spondylolisthesis, but the entire course of each symptomatic nerve root must be thoroughly assessed. Usually the L5 root is compressed in the L4-5 lateral recess, but there may be other pathology, such as a synovial cyst or disc herniation, affecting the same root or a different root level. The presence of a facet effusion more than 2 mm in width is highly suggestive of instability at that level and should prompt close inspection of the upright dynamic radiographs.

The most common procedure performed for degenerative spondylolisthesis is bilateral decompression and fusion. We typically use a posterior interbody technique with instrumentation. A meta-analysis evaluating patients with degenerative spondylolisthesis treated with decompression alone or decompression with posterolateral fusion, with or without instrumentation, found similar fusion rates (93% and 86%) and satisfaction rates (86% and 90%) with or without instrumentation. The nonfused group had a 69% satisfaction rate and 31% had slip progression. Other studies have found that patients with a solid fusion have better clinical outcomes than those who develop nonunions. Instrumentation and interbody stabilization both have been found to improve fusion rates but also to increase cost and potential risk.

The operative procedure chosen should aim to correct the identified sources of symptoms, not radiographic abnormalities. Fusion generally is recommended at the level of the spondylolisthesis but usually is not necessary at other levels requiring only decompression. Many patients with degenerative spondylolisthesis at the L4-5 level have some degenerative disc changes at the L5-S1 disc level as well. There remains some controversy of how best to manage the L5 degenerative disc changes in the absence of instability at that level. Choi et al. in a retrospective study found that the presence of L5 disc degeneration which was not treated at the time of L4-5 anterior fusion with posterior instrumentation did not affect the clinical or radiographic outcome. Although fusion for axial pain attributable only to degenerative change is very controversial and not well supported in the literature, fusion in the setting of instability is much more accepted and there is substantial literature support. The fusion can be done posterolaterally, with or without instrumentation. Fusions with interbody implants (either PLIF or TLIF) are commonly used to treat patients with degenerative spondylolisthesis. Less commonly, anterior fusions are appropriate in this patient population. There is, however, also evidence to support decompression alone for the treatment of degenerative spondylolisthesis. Decompression alone can be the most appropriate procedure in some elderly patients or those with significant comorbidities who may not tolerate the added morbidity of a fusion, especially with instrumentation.

The procedure we use most often for degenerative spondylolisthesis is posterior decompression and fusion with interbody support combined with a posterolateral instrumented fusion. The primary advantage of this approach is that it allows optimal decompression and has a higher fusion rate than posterolateral instrumented fusion or interbody fusion alone. Higher fusion rates in general correlate with better patient outcomes. One potential drawback of this approach is that biomechanically the interbody fusion increases the stiffness of the fused segment and this may increase the rate of adjacent segment degeneration. Minimally invasive posterior decompression and fusion techniques are described in Chapter 29.

LUMBAR DECOMPRESSION

TECHNIQUE 40-5

- Position the patient, prepare and drape the operative area, and administer prophylactic antibiotics as described in Technique 40-1. Keeping the hips relatively extended is important to simulate the anatomy in the standing position to allow adequate assessment of the decompression. If a frame is used that flexes the lumbar spine to open the inter-laminar space, this must be taken into account to avoid an inadequate decompression.
- Make a midline incision centered at the level to be decompressed.
- Carry dissection down to the fascia and obtain a localization image with a clamp affixed to the spinous process to confirm the level. Mark this spinous process with a rongeur.
- Use Cobb elevators and electrocautery to subperiosteally expose the spinous processes and laminae of the levels to be decompressed bilaterally, taking care to preserve the facet capsule at each level.
- Expose the pars interarticularis so it is fully visible to avoid inadvertent excessive thinning of the pars, predisposing to pars fracture in the postoperative period.
- For a complete laminectomy, use a rongeur to remove the entire spinous process of the involved level and the caudal 1/3 of the cephalad level. For L4-5 decompression this would mean removal of the caudal portion of L3 and the entire spinous process of L4. This will allow adequate access to the L4 and the L5 nerve roots.
- Once the bone at the base of the spinous process has been thinned with the rongeur or with the use of a high-speed burr, identify the midline cleft in the ligamentum flavum.
- Use a small curet to detach the ligamentum flavum from the caudal margin of the cephalad (L4) level. Use of the operating microscope is very helpful.
- Remove the thinned lamina with a Kerrison rongeur proceeding from caudal to cephalad to have better protection of the dura by the ligamentum flavum.
- Carry the decompression up to the caudal margin of the L3 lamina, focusing initially on the central canal stenosis.
- Once the central decompression is complete, turn attention to the lateral recess and foraminal stenosis as demonstrated by the imaging studies. It generally is easier for the surgeon to work on the side of the patient opposite the side on which he or she is standing.
- With the dura gently retracted with a Penfield #4 dissector, undercut the medial portion of the L3 inferior facet

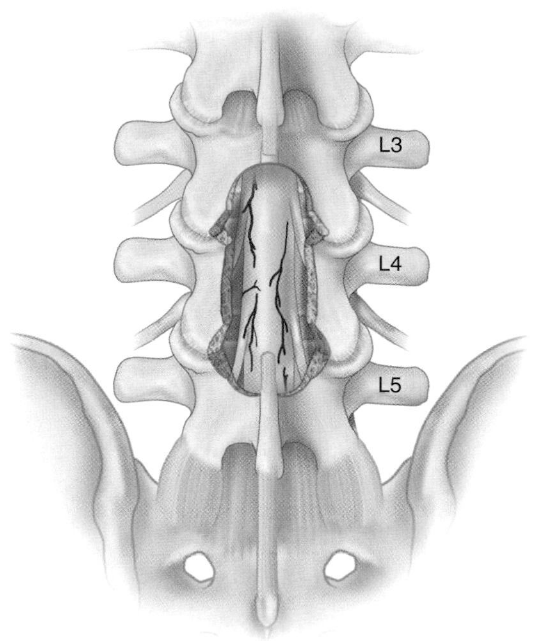

FIGURE 40-20 Typical midline decompression for spinal stenosis. Note medial facetectomy and foraminotomy with preservation of the pars. Decompression is from inferior border of L3 pedicle to superior border of L5 pedicle, exposing both lateral borders of dura in lateral recess.

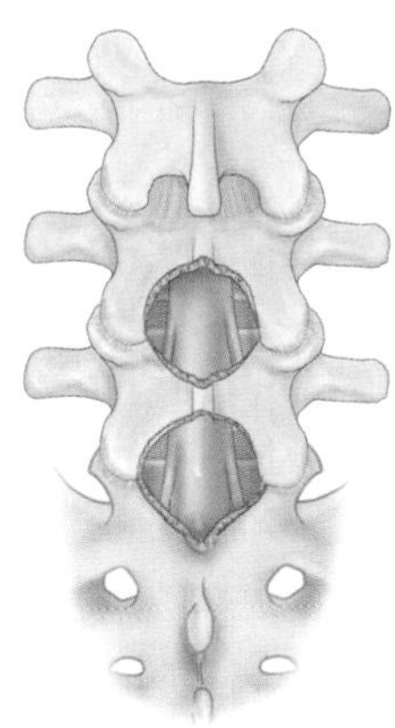

FIGURE 40-21 Decompression completed under microscopic magnification. **SEE TECHNIQUE 40-5.**

with a Kerrison rongeur. Identify the L4 nerve root and follow it into the foramen.

- Complete the foraminotomy such that a Murphy ball hook can pass easily between the root and the inferior aspect of the pedicle (ensuring an adequate cephalocaudal dimension) and posterior to the root ventral to the L4 pars (ensuring an adequate anteroposterior dimension) (Fig. 40-20).
- Pay careful attention to the amount of bony removal from the L4 pars so as not to risk fracture.
- After the L3 medial facetectomy and L4 foraminotomy are complete, decompress the L5 root in the L4-5 lateral recess. Again, gently retract the dura and remove the osteophyte extending from the medial aspect of the L5 superior articular mass and ligamentum flavum. Remove the bone to the level of the medial aspect of the L5 pedicle, which marks the lateral extent of the canal. Complete the foraminotomy at the L5 level as described above for the L4 root.
- At this point the decompression is complete. If it was necessary to perform a complete facetectomy or if extensive bone removal was needed to adequately decompress the L4 nerve root, a fusion should be added.
- An alternative technique is a laminoforaminotomy (Fig. 40-21), which can be unilateral or bilateral.
- After achieving thorough hemostasis, irrigate the wound and close it over a fluted drain because of the exposed dura. Close the fascia to the spinous process where possible to better restore the normal resting length of the paraspinal musculature. Close the subcutaneous and subcuticular layers.

POSTOPERATIVE CARE. Patients are started on oral analgesics and scheduled muscle relaxers. Mobilization is started either the evening of surgery or the next morning. Most patients are independent with mobility and can be discharged home the same day or at least by the second postoperative day.

LUMBAR DECOMPRESSION AND POSTEROLATERAL FUSION WITH OR WITHOUT INSTRUMENTATION

TECHNIQUE 40-6

- Position the patient, prepare and drape the operative area, and carry out preoperative tasks as described in Technique 40-1.
- Make a midline incision centered at the level to be decompressed.
- Carry dissection down to the fascia and obtain a localization image with a clamp affixed to the spinous process to confirm the level. Mark this spinous process with a rongeur.
- Use Cobb elevators and electrocautery to subperiosteally expose the spinous processes and laminae of the levels to be decompressed bilaterally, taking care to preserve the facet capsule at the cephalad level (L3-4) level that is not to be fused.
- Use a Cobb elevator to sweep the musculature off the capsule and carry the exposure down the lateral aspect of the superior articular mass onto the transverse process which is fully exposed.
- At the caudal facet (L4-5) level, remove the capsule and expose the transverse process.

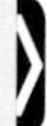

- Expose the intertransverse membrane, taking care not to violate this membrane to avoid a hematoma or nerve injury.
- Completely expose the transverse processes.
- At this point, prepare the screw holes in the following manner if pedicle screw instrumentation is to be used. Use a bone awl to penetrate the cortex at the junction of the transverse process and the superior articular mass. Advance a pedicle probe into the pedicle. Use a sound to ensure there are no cortical breaches, although after the laminectomy the pedicles can be inspected visually as well. After the screw holes are prepared, place cottonoids for hemostasis while the decompression is completed.
- Complete the laminectomy and foraminotomy as described in Technique 40-5 and proceed with fusion.
- Decorticate the transverse process of L4 and L5, the lateral surface of the articular mass and the pars with a high-speed drill, and carefully pack bone graft into the lateral gutter.
- In addition, decorticate the L4-5 facet joint and pack it with bone.
- If instrumentation is to be used, insert the screws at each level after the bone graft is placed. Otherwise the screws make decortication and graft placement more difficult.
- Cut the rods and secure them with set screws which are tightened to the manufacturer's recommended torque. Take care to make sure the rods do not impinge on the cephalad joint.
- After achieving thorough hemostasis, irrigate the wound and close it over a fluted drain because of the exposed dura. Close the fascia to the spinous process where possible to better restore the normal resting length of the paraspinal musculature. Close the subcutaneous and subcuticular layers.

POSTOPERATIVE CARE. Patients are started on oral analgesics and scheduled muscle relaxers. A single dose of 5 mg of epidural preservative-free morphine gives excellent postoperative pain relief, but does require close monitoring for respiratory depression postoperatively. Mobilization is started the next morning. Most patients are independent with mobility and can be discharged home by the third postoperative day.

LUMBAR DECOMPRESSION AND COMBINED POSTEROLATERAL AND INTERBODY FUSION (TLIF OR PLIF)

The preferred procedure for treating degenerative spondylolisthesis is posterolateral fusion combined with TLIF.

TECHNIQUE 40-7

- Patient positioning, approach, decompression, and placement of screw holes are as described in Technique 40-6.
- Place the interbody device from the side with the most severe nerve root compression and patient complaints. Thin the inferior facet on the selected side with a rongeur and keep the bone for later use.
- Use a small curet to detach the ligamentum flavum from the caudal lamina and remove the remaining inferior facet (of L4) and pars unilaterally with a Kerrison rongeur; preserve the bone for later use.
- Using the operating microscope, identify the exiting L4 root and decompress it to the lateral aspect of the foramen.
- Use a large rongeur to remove the cephalad 50% of the L5 superior articular mass to allow the desired trajectory for insertion of the interbody device.
- Decompress the L5 nerve root to the medial border of the L5 pedicle and into the L5 foramen so that a Murphy ball hook will pass cephalad and posterior to the L5 root, indicating satisfactory decompression.
- Contralateral decompression is done at this point if desired. In some patients the indirect decompression from the interbody device placement will be sufficient.
- Next, prepare the disc space. Coagulate the epidural veins crossing the disc space with bipolar cautery. Once they begin to bleed they are harder to control.
- Incise the annulus in the axilla of the L4 nerve root, retracting the thecal sac slightly medially and the L4 root laterally.
- Introduce disc reamer distractors into the disc space, monitoring the depth of penetration on lateral fluoroscopic views.
- Use ring and cup curets to scrape the endplates after the desired implant height is determined with the reamer distractor.
- Complete careful disc removal to prepare the disc space and to mobilize the segment.
- Once the endplates are prepared, thoroughly irrigate the disc space to remove any residual soft tissue.
- Pack allograft cancellous bone against the anterior annulus and morsellized local autograft bone behind this. This allograft cancellous bone is submerged in antibiotic irrigation solution at the beginning of the case and maintained there until implantation. This has decreased deep wound infections post operatively associated with allograft bone usage.
- Take care to leave adequate space to allow placement of the interbody device no more posteriorly than midbody so lordosis can be achieved. The goals of cage placement are to restore disc height and improve alignment with sufficient lordosis through the segment. Biomechanically coverage of 35% of the endplate is desirable for stability. We prefer a single expandable cage device packed with local autograft placed just anterior to the midbody. The subchondral bone is strongest around the perimeter of the endplate and weakest centrally, increasing the risk of cage subsidence if the device is too small or only centrally located.
- Once the device is transversely positioned, expand it to the predetermined desired height.
- To proceed with the fusion, decorticate the transverse process of L4 and L5, the lateral surface of the articular mass, and the pars opposite the TLIF with a high-speed drill, and carefully pack bone graft into the lateral gutter.

- Decorticate the remaining L4-5 facet joint and pack with bone.
- Insert pedicle screws at each level after the bone graft is placed. Otherwise the screws make decortication and graft placement more difficult.
- Cut the rods and secure them with set screws which are tightened to the manufacturer's recommended torque. Take care to make sure the rods do not impinge on the cephalad joint.
- After achieving thorough hemostasis, irrigate the wound and close it over a fluted drain because of the exposed dura. Close the fascia to the spinous process where possible to better restore the normal resting length of the paraspinal musculature. Close the subcutaneous and subcuticular layers. Administer a second dose of tranexamic acid as wound closure begins.

POSTOPERATIVE CARE. Postoperative management is the same as after Technique 40-6.

ANTERIOR LUMBAR INTERBODY FUSION

There is relatively little role for this procedure as a first choice in treating degenerative spondylolisthesis because of the need for direct decompression in almost all of these patients. For patients with previous adequate decompression and persistent instability or failed posterolateral fusion anterior lumbar interbody fusion (ALIF) can be a reasonable option (see Technique 40-4).

PERIOPERATIVE MANAGEMENT AND COMPLICATIONS

PREOPERATIVE MANAGEMENT

The best way to manage complications is to avoid them wherever possible. This begins with an understanding of the risks associated with a particular surgical technique and the particular needs and pathology of a given patient. Having a candid preoperative discussion with the patient and his or her family about the specific and relative risks of different treatment options is an important step in limiting the risks of complications that are most unacceptable to that patient. A detailed description of potential procedures should be provided to the patient in lay terms. Additionally, printed material or a list of web sites, such as those sponsored by the American Academy of Orthopaedic Surgeons, the Scoliosis Research Society, and the Pediatric Orthopaedic Society of North America, with reliable patient information is helpful. The surgeon should discuss any planned "off label" uses of implants and disclose any financial benefit from industry that may be derived from the procedure. In this way, the patient can make an informed decision as to his or her choice of procedure.

The surgeon also should carefully evaluate the patient and document any medical conditions or circumstances that may increase the risk of complications. A careful neurologic examination to detect even subtle abnormalities which may indicate a greater risk of nerve root injury during or after surgery should be documented. If the patient has a history of diabetes, prior deep vein thrombosis (DVT), previous surgical infection, or osteoporosis, or is a current nicotine user, this should be documented and addressed preoperatively to enhance postoperative results. In adult patients, particularly those with degenerative spondylolisthesis, assessment of vitamin D levels preoperatively and correction where indicated are warranted. Baseline information should be obtained from the patient using the patient-reported outcome instrument to be used at follow-up.

INTRAOPERATIVE MANAGEMENT

The surgical treatment of spondylolisthesis is complex, ranging from a single-level in situ fusion without instrumentation to a combined anterior and posterior procedure involving direct deformity correction and instrumentation. Intraoperatively, the surgeon can affect the risk of infection, excessive hemorrhage, DVT, neurologic deficits both in and out of the surgical field, and development of pseudarthrosis by the choices that are made and techniques used.

Some actions should be routine, such as careful patient positioning to decrease neurologic risk, administration of prophylactic antibiotics, administration of agents to decrease excessive bleeding, use of appropriate neuromonitoring in selected cases. The use of careful and precise surgical techniques also is important, including careful soft-tissue management, particularly in patients with significant dysplasia; bone graft bed preparation; type of bone graft selected; choice of implants; accurate instrumentation placement; and careful manipulations of the spine with the instrumentation.

POSTOPERATIVE MANAGEMENT

After the surgery is completed, the avoidance of complications is primarily accomplished by completing appropriate prophylactic antibiotic therapy, using mechanical DVT prophylaxis, and carefully monitoring the patient's neurologic status. Patient positioning and use of external spine support also may be appropriate in some circumstances. If use of an orthosis is planned, having it available preoperatively facilitates immediate mobilization, although if significant deformity correction is planned, fitting is best done postoperatively

SPECIFIC COMPLICATIONS

The list of possible complications and the management of each is beyond the scope of this chapter. The most common complications following surgery for spondylolisthesis (of any etiology) are pseudarthrosis, instrumentation failure, neurologic deficits, vascular injury, and infection.

PSEUDARTHROSIS

The most frequent serious complication following surgery for spondylolisthesis in most series is pseudarthrosis, although infection is more common in some series. The development of pseudarthrosis is linked to other complications, such as progression of deformity and instrumentation failure as well. Eliminating nicotine use and correcting vitamin D deficiency preoperatively have been shown to reduce the risk of pseudarthrosis in spinal fusion in general although not clearly in fusion for spondylolisthesis. Much of the spondylolisthesis literature deals with children and adolescents, and these issues are likely most relevant to older patients with degenerative spondylolisthesis. For large slip angles with sagittal imbalance and high-grade translational deformities, several studies have shown that correcting the segmental kyphosis appears to reduce the risk of pseudarthrosis more than reducing the translation. Careful preparation of the fusion bed (posteriorly and anteriorly) is important. The transverse processes should each have a surface area of at least 2 cm^2, and decorticating the pars (when present) and the lateral superior articular mass is necessary. There is good evidence that having adequate anterior column support is an important factor to reduce the risk of pseudarthrosis, and usually this is accomplished with the use of an anteriorly placed graft but this is not universally required.

The diagnosis of pseudarthrosis often is difficult unless there is obvious and rapid loss of fixation or progression of deformity, both of which necessitate early surgical correction. Persistent complaints of back pain beyond 4 to 6 months, return of pain after initial resolution of back pain, worsening or new neurologic complaints, or persistent gait abnormality should prompt consideration of the diagnosis of pseudarthrosis. Evaluation involves standing plain radiographs, upright dynamic radiographs, and usually CT scans to try to detect the nonunion (Fig. 40-22). Generally, a pseudarthrosis is not diagnosed until a year after surgery because of the slow nature of fusion consolidation and incorporation. Findings such as a persistent lucent line at the fusion site (best seen on sagittal and coronal CT reconstructions) and visible motion on dynamic radiographs are most diagnostic. Findings such as broken hardware or lucencies around screws are suggestive but not always conclusive evidence of nonunion. In addition, it is important to realize that the mere presence of a pseudarthrosis, even when diagnostically not in doubt, is not an indication for revision surgery. If symptoms warrant revision surgery, a careful assessment of the potential reason for failure

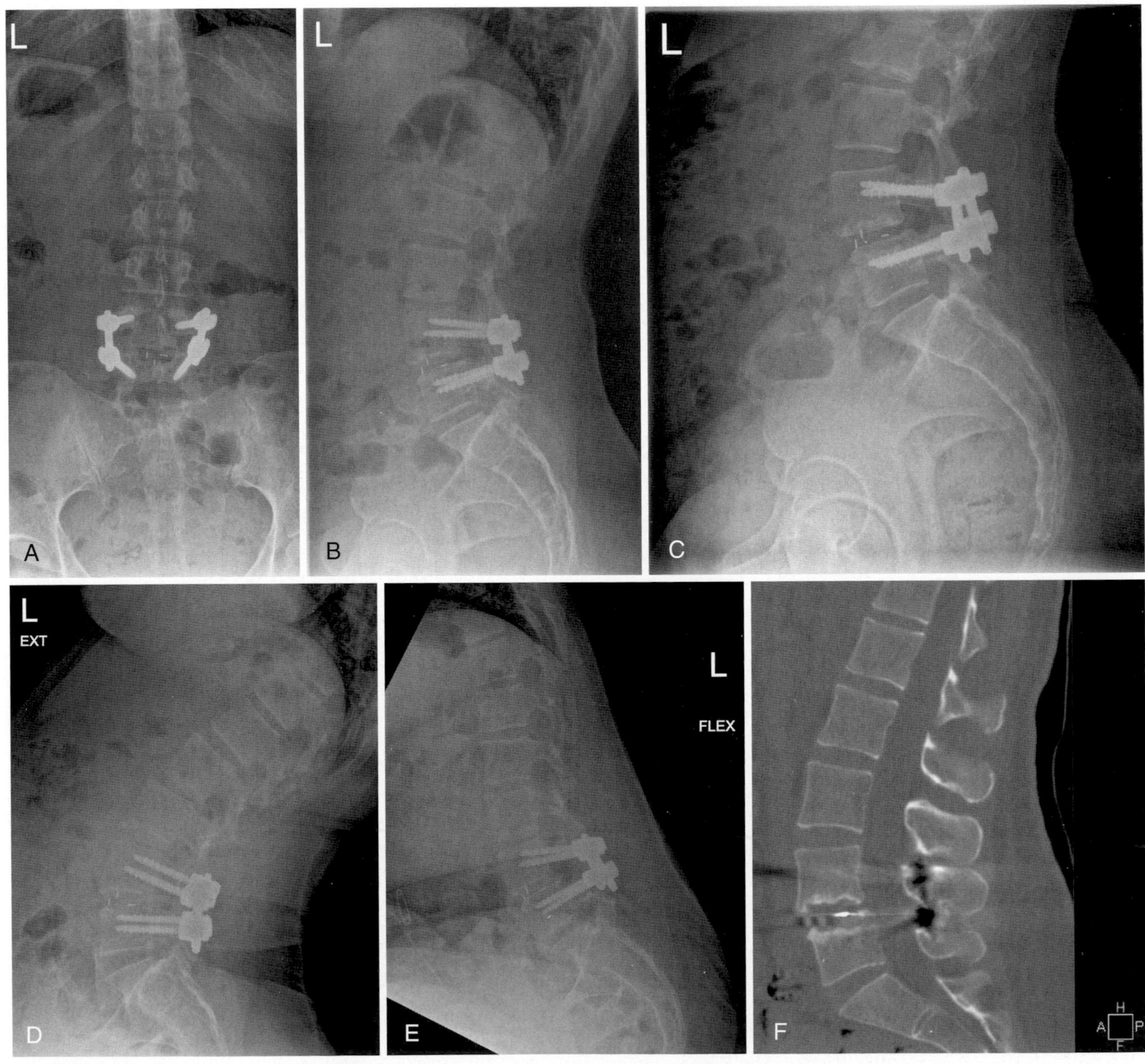

FIGURE 40-22 Pseudarthrosis at L4-5. **A** to **C**, Plain radiographs. **D** and **E**, Upright dynamic radiographs. **F**, CT scan.

of the index procedure is important. Making the effort to determine if the failure is, for example, host-related, is a biomechanical failure caused by the construct chosen, or resulted from poor execution of an appropriate construct is warranted to avoid the same outcome.

NEUROLOGIC DEFICITS

The avoidance of neurologic deficits begins with patient positioning. Taking care to pad all bony prominences, particularly the ulnar nerve at the elbow and the peroneal nerve at the knee, avoids palsies at these sites indirectly related to the surgery. In addition, keeping the knees flexed can decrease tension, particularly on the L5 root which is most at risk. The selective use of neuromonitoring, including motor evoked potentials, electromyography, somatosensory evoked potentials, impedance testing of pedicle screws, and even direct nerve stimulation of the L5 root, can all be useful techniques. Any intraoperative change in neuromonitoring parameters should be promptly evaluated. Technical issues and those related to anesthesia should be assessed, and if no clear cause is evident, the surgeon should suspect an actual neurologic injury. The anatomy and applied forces should be evaluated, and distractive or translational forces should be decreased until there is no tension on any of the neural structures. Caution should be used when applying corrective forces, particularly if the maneuver will cause tension on the L5 root. A cadaver study demonstrated that in spondylolisthesis reduction only 21% of the nerve strain occurs with the first 50% of the reduction and 79% of the measured nerve strain occurs when the final 50% of the reduction is accomplished.

Neurologic deficits also can occur from dissection around compromised neural structures. Decompression of the L5 root in particular should be cautiously undertaken to remove the fibrocartilaginous tissue in the foramen. If a developmental dysplastic spondylolisthesis is being reduced, careful dissection to release the nerve all the way out to the ala is necessary.

Malpositioned hardware is another potential cause for neurologic deficits. The anatomy can be quite abnormal with dysplastic type deformities, and careful preoperative planning and intraoperative fluoroscopy, and potentially image guided navigation, can be helpful in achieving proper and safe implant placement.

With anterior exposures of the lower lumbar spine, there is a small risk of retrograde ejaculation attributed to autonomic nerve injury. If this approach is selected, some patients may want to use a sperm bank preoperatively. Intraoperatively, limiting the use of electrocautery and gently dissecting only the area needed to access the disc space reduces this risk.

Cauda equina syndrome can occur in the immediate postoperative period. This may be attributed to a hematoma, which should be immediately decompressed, and if the segment was not instrumented initially, it should be at that time.

VASCULAR COMPLICATIONS

Preoperative positioning is important to decrease the risk of certain vascular complications. Postoperative blindness is a rare (1/60,000 to 1/100,000) postanesthetic complication that occurs more often in spine surgery than in other types of orthopaedic surgery, particularly if the patient is prone. It seems to be related to hypotension with ischemia in the distribution of the central retinal artery. There is some evidence that external pressure on the globe in the prone position may contribute, but the evidence is unclear. In any case attention to the eyes in a prone patient is warranted.

Pressure can also be placed on the femoral artery by the pad at the level of the anterior superior iliac spine of a prone patient. Verifying the presence of the pedal pulses once the patient is prone will mitigate this risk.

Direct vascular injury can occur with anterior or posterior spinal surgery. With anterior surgery, exposing and gaining control of the vascular injury are more direct. Vascular injury occurring from a posterior procedure may not be immediately apparent if it is a venous or a small arterial injury. After a short period of time, the patient may show signs of hypovolemia, and attention should move to vascular repair.

Postoperative vascular complications occur primarily in the form of DVT and very early pulmonary embolism. In patients undergoing postoperative venography without mechanical prophylaxis, some studies have reported a DVT rate of 10% to 15%, but this is decreased in similar studies using mechanical prophylaxis to 0.3% to 2%. However, in a study by Yoshioka et al., patients undergoing posterior single-level interbody fusion had a 10% rate of DVT even with mechanical prophylaxis.

INFECTION

An infection in a patient with spinal instrumentation in place is always a serious concern. Postoperative infections can manifest in the first few days following surgery or months later. Several factors are associated with infections, such as blood loss and operative time, which are likely surrogates for the complexity of the procedure. If a patient develops a pseudarthrosis, the possibility of infection should be considered and appropriately evaluated. In the immediate postoperative period, the presence of increasing pain, fever, wound drainage, wound erythema, or elevated C-reactive protein levels should raise suspicion of infection. The incidence of infection in the literature in instrumented lumbar spinal fusions is as high as 21%. In our experience, the infection rate for one- and two-level lumbar fusions with instrumentation should be less than 1% to 2%. The most common organisms include *Staphylococcus,* both coagulase negative and positive, including methicillin-resistant *Staphylococcus aureus* (MRSA), *Escherichia coli*, *Pseudomonas*, and *Enterobacter*. In the presence of wound drainage, it is prudent presume infection and to wash out the wound to determine if the infection is deep to the fascia or not. Appropriate antibiotic therapy should be administered. Factors shown to increase infection risk include smoking, diabetes, and obesity.

REFERENCES

Abdu WA, Lurie JD, Spratt KF, et al: Degenerative spondylolisthesis: does fusion method influence outcome? Four-year results of the spine patient outcomes research trial, *Spine* 34:2351, 2009.

Ahmad S, Hamad A, Bhalla A, et al: The outcome of decompression alone for lumbar spinal stenosis with degenerative spondylolisthesis, *Eur Spine J* 2016. [Epub ahead of print].

Andrade NS, Ashton CM, Wray NP, et al: Systematic review of observational studies reveals no association between low back pain and lumbar spondylolysis with or without isthmic spondylolisthesis, *Eur Spine J* 24:1289, 2015.

Bydon M, Macki M, Abt NB, et al: The cost-effectiveness of interbody fusions versus posterolateral fusions in 137 patients with lumbar spondylolisthesis, *Spine J* 15:492, 2015.

Choi KC, Shim HK, Kim JS, Lee SH: Does pre-existing L5-S1 degeneration affect outcomes after isolated L4-5 fusion for spondylolisthesis?, *J Orthop Surg Res* 10:39, 2015.

Delawi D, Jacobs W, van Susante JL, et al: OP-1 compared with iliac crest autograft in instrumented posterolateral fusion: a randomized, multicenter non-inferiority trial, *J Bone Joint Surg* 98:441, 2016.

Don AS, Roberson PA: Facet joint orientation in spondylolysis and isthmic spondylolisthesis, *J Spinal Disord Tech* 21:112, 2008.

Enyo Y, Yoshimura N, Yamada H, et al: Radiographic natural course of lumbar degenerative spondylolisthesis and its risk factors related to the progression and onset in a 15-year community-based cohort study: the Miyama study, *J Orthop Sci* 20:978, 2015.

Fernández-Fairen M, Sala P, Ramírez H, Gil J: A prospective randomized study of unilateral versus bilateral instrumented posterolateral lumbar fusion in degenerative spondylolisthesis, *Spine* 32:395, 2007.

Ferrero E, Ould-Slimane M, Gille O, et al: Sagittal spinopelvic alignment in 654 degenerative spondylolisthesis, *Eur Spine J* 24:1219, 2015.

Gavaskar AS, Achimuthu R: Transfacetal fusion for low-grade degenerative spondylolisthesis of the lumbar spine: results of a prospective single center study, *J Spinal Disord Tech* 23:162, 2010.

Ghogawala Z, Dziura J, Butler WE, et al: Laminectomy plus fusion versus laminectomy alone for lumbar spondylolisthesis, *N Engl J Med* 374:1424, 2016.

Glavas P, Mac-Thiong JM, Parent S, et al: Assessment of lumbosacral kyphosis in spondylolisthesis: a computer-assisted reliability study of six measurement techniques, *Eur Spine J* 18:212, 2009.

Golinvaux NS, Basques BA, Bohl DD, et al: Comparison of 368 patients undergoing surgery for lumbar degenerative spondylolisthesis from the SPORT trial with 955 from the NSQIP database, *Spine* 40:342, 2015.

Gottschalk MB, Premkumar A, Sweeney K, et al: Posterolateral lumbar arthrodesis with and without interbody arthrodesis for L4-L5 degenerative spondylolisthesis, *Spine* 40:917, 2015.

Ha KY, Na KH, Shin JH, Kim KW: Comparison of posterolateral fusion with and without additional posterior lumbar interbody fusion for degenerative lumbar spondylolisthesis, *J Spinal Disord Tech* 21:229, 2008.

Helenius I, Lamberg T, Osterman K, et al: Posterolateral, anterior, or circumferential fusion in situ for high-grade spondylolisthesis in young patients: a long-term evaluation using the Scoliosis Research Society questionnaire, *Spine* 31:190, 2006.

Hong SW, Lee HY, Kim KH, Lee SH: Interspinous ligamentoplasty in the treatment of degenerative spondylolisthesis: midterm clinical results, *J Neurosurg Spine* 13:27, 2010.

Hresko MT, Labelle H, Roussouly P, et al: Classification of high-grade spondylolisthesis based on pelvic version and spine balance: possible rationale for reduction, *Spine* 32:2208, 2007.

Huang KY, Lin RM, Lee YL, Li JD: Factors affecting disability and physical function in degenerative lumbar spondylolisthesis of L4–5: evaluation with axially loaded MRI, *Eur Spine J* 18:1851, 2009.

Kaner T, Dalbayrak S, Oktenoglu T, et al: Comparison of posterior dynamic and posterior rigid transpedicular stabilization with fusion to treat degenerative spondylolisthesis, *Orthopedics* 12:33, 2010.

Kim KT, Lee SH, Lee YH: Clinical outcomes of 3 fusion methods through the posterior approach in the lumbar spine, *Spine* 31:1351, 2006.

Kim KH, Lee SH, Shim CS, et al: Adjacent segment disease after interbody fusion and pedicle screw fixations for isolated L4-L5 spondylolisthesis: a minimum five-year follow-up, *Spine* 35:625, 2010.

Lee GW, Lee SM, Ahn MW, et al: Comparison of posterolateral lumbar fusion and posterior lumbar interbody fusion for patients younger than 60 years with isthmic spondylolisthesis, *Spine* 39:E1475, 2014.

Liao JC, Chen WJ, Chen LH, et al: Surgical outcomes of degenerative spondylolisthesis with L5-S1 disc degeneration: comparison between lumbar floating fusion and lumbosacral fusion at a minimum five-year follow-up, *Spine* 36:1600, 2011.

Macki M, Bydon M, Weingart R, et al: Posterolateral fusion with interbody for lumbar spondylolisthesis is associated with less repeat surgery than posterolateral fusion alone, *Clin Neurol Neurosurg* 138:117, 2015.

Mac-Thiong JM, Labelle H: A proposal for a surgical classification of pediatric lumbosacral spondylolisthesis based on current literature, *Eur Spine J* 15:1425, 2006.

Mac-Thiong J-M, Labelle H, Berthonnaud É, et al: Sagittal spinopelvic balance in normal children and adolescents, *Eur Spine J* 16:227, 2007.

Martin CR, Gruszczynski AT, Braunsfurth HA, et al: The surgical management of degenerative lumbar spondylolisthesis: a systematic review, *Spine* 32:1791, 2007.

McAnany SJ, Baird EO, Qureshi SA, et al: Posterolateral fusion versus interbody fusion for degenerative spondylolisthesis: a systematic review and meta-analysis, *Spine* 2016. [Epub ahead of print].

McGuire KJ, Khaleel MA, Rihn JA, et al: The effect of high obesity on outcomes of treatment for lumbar spinal conditions: subgroup analysis of the spine patient outcomes research trial, *Spine* 39:1975, 2014.

Mehta VA, Amin A, Omeis I, et al: Implications of spinoplevic alignment for the spine surgeon, *Neurosurgery* 76(Suppl 1):S42, 2015.

Musacchio MJ, Lauryssen C, Davis RJ, et al: Evaluation of decompression and interlaminar stabilization compared with decompression and fusion for the treatment of lumbar spinal stenosis: 5-year follow-up of a prospective, randomized, controlled trial, *Int J Spine Surg* 10:6, 2016.

Okuyam AK, Kido T, Unoki E, Chiba M: PLIF with a titanium cage and excised facet joint bone for degenerative spondylolisthesis—in augmentation with a pedicle screw, *J Spinal Disord Tech* 20:53, 2007.

Park Y, Ha JW: Comparison of one-level posterior lumbar interbody fusion performed with a minimally invasive approach or a traditional open approach, *Spine* 32:537, 2007.

Pateder DB, Benzel E: Noninstrumented facet fusion in patients undergoing lumbar laminectomy for degenerative spondylolisthesis, *J Surg Orthop Adv* 19:153, 2010.

Pearson AM, Lurie JD, Blood EA, et al: Spine patient outcomes research trial: radiographic predictors of clinical outcomes after operative or nonoperative treatment of degenerative spondylolisthesis, *Spine* 33:2759, 2008.

Poussa M, Remes V, Lamberg T, et al: Treatment of severe spondylolisthesis in adolescence with reduction or fusion in situ: long-term clinical, radiologic, and functional outcome, *Spine* 31:583, 2006.

Rihn JA, Hilibrand AS, Zhao W, et al: Effectiveness of surgery for lumbar stenosis and degenerative spondylolisthesis in the octogenarian population: analysis of the Spine Patient Outcomes Research Trial (SPORT) data, *J Bone Joint Surg* 97:177, 2015.

Sailhan F, Gollogly S, Roussouly P, et al: The radiographic results and neurologic complications of instrumented reduction and fusion of high-grade spondylolisthesis without decompression of the neural elements: a retrospective review of 44 patients, *Spine* 31:161, 2006.

Sansur CA, Reames DL, Smith JS, et al: Morbidity and mortality in the surgical treatment of 10,242 adults with spondylolisthesis, *J Neurosurg Spine* 13:589, 2010.

Sato S, Yagi M, Machida M, et al: Reoperation rate and risk factors of elective spinal surgery for degenerative spondylolisthesis: minimum 5-year follow-up, *Spine J* 15:1536, 2015.

Schaeren S, Broger I, Jeanneret B: Minimum four-year follow-up of spinal stenosis with degenerative spondylolisthesis treated with decompression and dynamic stabilization, *Spine* 33:E636, 2008.

Schulte TL, Ringel F, Quante M, et al: Surgery for adult spondylolisthesis: a systematic review of the evidence, *Eur Spine J* 25:2359, 2016.

Sigmundsson FG, Jönsson B, Strömqvist B: Outcome of decompression with and without fusion in spinal stenosis with degenerative spondylolisthesis in relation to preoperative pain pattern: a register study of 1,624 patients, *Spine J* 15:638, 2015.

Transfeldt EE, Mehbod AA: Evidence-based medicine analysis of isthmic spondylolisthesis treatment including reduction versus fusion in situ for high-grade slips, *Spine* 32(Suppl):S126, 2007.

Tsutsumimoto T, Shimogata M, Ohta H, Misawa H: Mini-open versus conventional open posterior lumbar interbody fusion for the treatment of lumbar degenerative spondylolisthesis: comparison of paraspinal muscle damage and slip reduction, *Spine* 34:1923, 2009.

Tsutsumimoto T, Shimogata M, Yoshimura Y, Misawa H: Union versus nonunion after posterolateral lumbar fusion: a comparison of long-term surgical outcomes in patients with degenerative lumbar spondylolisthesis, *Eur Spine J* 17:1107, 2008.

Verhoof OJ, Bron JL, Wapstra FH, van Royen BJ: High failure rate of the interspinous distraction device (X-stop) for the treatment of lumbar spinal stenosis caused by degenerative spondylolisthesis, *Eur Spine J* 17:188, 2008.

Wang Z, Parent S, Mac-Thiong J-M, et al: Influence of sacropelvic morphology in developmental spondylolisthesis, *Spine* 33:2185, 2008.

Weinstein JN, Lurie JD, Tosteson TD, et al: Surgical versus nonsurgical treatment for lumbar degenerative spondylolisthesis, *N Engl J Med* 356:2257, 2007.

Weinstein JN, Lurie JD, Tosteson TD, et al: Surgical compared with nonoperative treatment for lumbar degenerative spondylolisthesis: four-year results in the Spine Patient Outcomes Research Trial (SPORT) randomized and observational cohorts, *J Bone Joint Surg* 91A:1295, 2009.

Wu CH, Kao YH, Yang SC, et al: Supplementary pedicle screw fixation in spinal fusion for degenerative spondylolisthesis in patients aged 65 and over: outcome after a minimum of 2 years follow-up in 82 patients, *Acta Orthop* 79:67, 2008.

Yan DL, Pei FX, Li J, Soo CL: Comparative study of PLIF and TLIF treatment in adult degenerative spondylolisthesis, *Eur Spine J* 17:1311, 2008.

Yoshioka K, Murakami H, Demura S, et al: Prevalence and risk factors for development of venous thromboembolism after degenerative spinal surgery, *Spine* 40:E301, 2015.

Yu CH, Lee JE, Yang JJ, et al: Adjacent segment degeneration after single-level PLIF: comparison between spondylolytic spondylolisthesis, degenerative spondylolisthesis and spinal stenosis, *Asian Spine J* 5:82, 2011.

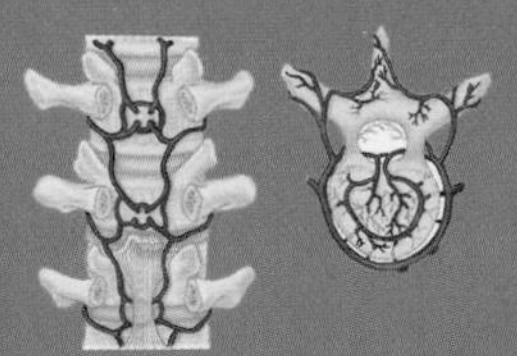

CHAPTER 41

FRACTURES, DISLOCATIONS, AND FRACTURE-DISLOCATIONS OF THE SPINE

Keith D. Williams

Many factors make assessing and treating patients with injuries to the spinal column and spinal cord demanding. The most critical responsibilities are early recognition of the injuries, prevention of neurologic deterioration, optimization of initial medical management, correct interpretation of all the diagnostic evaluations, and delivery of the most appropriate definitive care.

The cervical spine is functionally the most important region of the spine. The complex anatomy, spinal biomechanics, and the common traumatic mechanisms involved make the cervical spine also the most difficult to assess. Careful evaluation of each region is necessary. No definitive level I or II evidence studies exist to guide clinicians through much of this process, and errors can have devastating consequences for patients. The process is made even more difficult by coexisting injuries and comorbidities that often are present in severely traumatized patients who are at risk for a significant spinal injury. An orderly and thoughtful approach that is based on the best available evidence gives patients the highest probability for an optimal outcome.

The scope of the problem is demonstrated by information from the National Spinal Cord Injury Statistical Center in Birmingham, Alabama (www.nscisc.uab.edu/). The estimated annual incidence of spinal cord injury is approximately 12,500 new cases per year. Significant spinal column injuries are about twice as common as those causing spinal cord injury. Additionally, an estimated 240,000 to 337,000 people in the United States are living with the sequelae of spinal cord injury. The most common causes of these injuries are motor vehicle accidents (38%), falls (30%), violence (14%, primarily gunshot wounds), and sports mishaps (9%). Over the past few decades the average age at the time of injury has increased from 28.7 to 40.7 years, and the causes have shifted slightly toward falls and away from motor vehicle accidents and violence. Most patients with spinal cord injuries are men (80.7%). African-Americans are overrepresented based on general population trends and represent 24% of all spinal cord injuries, although 63% of patients are Caucasian. The most common neurologic category since 2005 has been incomplete tetraplegia (45%), followed by incomplete paraplegia (21%), complete paraplegia (20%), and, least commonly, complete tetraplegia (14%). Complete injuries have decreased slightly in recent years.

INITIAL MANAGEMENT OF SPINAL INJURY

Evaluation and management of the patient begin at the scene of the injury, and proper transport of the patient is very important. A retrospective review has shown that as many as 26% of spinal cord injuries occurred during transport or the early stages of evaluation at the primary medical facility. The deterioration was attributed primarily to poor immobilization and improper initial handling of the patients. Standardized protocols among emergency medical personnel have improved the safety of transport, but some controversy still remains. Total spine immobilization is recommended for all patients with a potential spinal injury. A hard collar with supports beside the head on an appropriately sized spine board for the age of the patient is used. This allows the patient to be moved and tilted as needed for transport. A 2- to 3-cm occipital pad is used in adults to avoid relative extension. In children, a spine board with an occipital recess is used to avoid relative flexion. Several studies have questioned whether all patients with potential injury need this form of immobilization because of the risk of pressure sores from the backboard. Also, studies have revealed that intracranial pressure can be elevated by as much as 25 mm Hg by the use of a rigid cervical collar. The clinical importance of this in a patient with a head injury has not been determined. At the present time, this type of immobilization with the head taped to the board and the torso secured remains the most accepted method for patient transport. This recommendation is based on level III evidence, and it is unlikely there will be better evidence developed because of ethical limitations and practical issues of moving injured patients. The patient should be moved from a spine board and have the cervical spine cleared as soon as is safely possible. This is best done after the patient reaches a facility able to fully assess and treat all injuries that are present.

INITIAL SPINE ASSESSMENT

After the ABC (airway, breathing, and circulation) of the Advanced Trauma Life Support (ATLS) protocol has been completed, a thorough orthopaedic history should be obtained and full physical examination should be done. Important information includes the injury mechanism, preinjury functional level of the patient, patient report of weakness or sensory changes, signs of blunt head trauma, spine tenderness, spinal step offs, and interspinous widening. Findings of flaccidity in the extremities, incontinence, or penile erection may indicate spinal cord injury. A detailed neurologic examination, which includes motor function, sensory function, and rectal tone, recorded on the American Spinal Injury Association (ASIA) form and an assessment of mental status are part of this examination. The diagnostic imaging of a patient is inextricably linked to the neurologic examination. The initial spinal assessment of a trauma patient is to determine if the patient has a spinal cord injury. If an injury is found, all initial CT imaging, including that of the spine, is completed as rapidly as possible and treatment initiated. If a patient does not have a spinal cord injury, it should be determined if he or she meets the criteria to be considered asymptomatic with respect to the cervical spine. If the patient is found to be asymptomatic, then the cervical spine can be cleared clinically without the need for radiography. There are five specific criteria described in the National Emergency X-Radiography Utilization Study (NEXUS) that must be fulfilled to classify a patient as asymptomatic. This study, which by design and execution provides level I evidence, is derived from 21 institutions and 34,069 patients. The purpose of the study was to develop a decision rule that would reduce the number of radiographic examinations in trauma patients without missing significant injuries. The five specific criteria are noted in Table 41-1.

Using these criteria, one third of the trauma patients evaluated in the 21 community emergency departments or level 1 trauma centers were found to be asymptomatic (range 14% to 58%). The determination of a patient's level of alertness is the first step in the workup specifically for a spinal injury, which should begin immediately after the ABCs have been evaluated. If the patient is asymptomatic by the criteria

TABLE 41-1

Criteria for Patients to Be Considered Asymptomatic

CRITERION	COMMENT
No posterior midline cervical spine tenderness	Midline posterior tenderness is deemed to be present if the patient reports pain on palpation of the posterior midline neck from the nuchal ridge to the prominence of the T1 vertebra, or if the patient evinces pain with direct palpation of any cervical spinous process.
No evidence of intoxication	Patients should be considered intoxicated if they have either of the following: a recent history provided by the patient or an observer of intoxication or intoxicant ingestion or evidence of intoxication on physical examination such as an odor of alcohol, slurred speech, ataxia, dysmetria, or other cerebellar findings or any behavior consistent with intoxication. Patients also may be considered to be intoxicated if tests of body fluids are positive for alcohol above 0.08 mg/dL or other drugs that affect the level of alertness.
A normal level of alertness	An altered level of alertness can include any of the following: a Glasgow Coma Scale score of 14 or less; disorientation to person, place, time, or events; inability to remember three objects at 5 minutes; a delayed or inappropriate response to external stimuli; or other findings.
No focal neurologic deficit	A focal neurologic deficit is any focal neurologic finding on motor or sensory examination.
No painful distracting injuries	No precise definition of painful distracting injury is possible. This category includes any condition thought by the clinician to be producing pain sufficient to distract the patient from a second cervical injury. Such injuries may include, but are not limited to, any long-bone fracture; visceral injury requiring surgical consultation; large laceration; degloving injury; crush injury; large burns; or any other injury causing acute functional impairment. Physicians may also classify any injury as distracting if it is thought to have the potential to impair the patient's ability to appreciate other injuries.

Adapted from Stiell IG, Clement CM, McKnight RD: The Canadian C-spine rule versus the NEXUS low-risk criteria in patients with trauma, N Engl J Med 349:2510, 2003.

of the NEXUS trial, no radiographs of the cervical spine are needed and the cervical spine may be "cleared" on clinical grounds, which significantly expedites care. Patients who are not alert or who do not meet the NEXUS trial criteria for other reasons require radiographic evaluation. The patient's motor and sensory examination should be documented thoroughly; the ASIA form is the accepted instrument that best serves this important function. For patients who are found to have a neurologic deficit, serial neurologic examinations are recorded using this form, which has proven to be useful in detecting clinical deterioration and guiding decisions on additional imaging or other interventions that may become necessary. For patients with neurologic deficits, ASIA forms are completed every 4 to 6 hours usually for the first 24 hours after arrival, but this varies based on the patient's course. If a patient is found to have a cervical spinal cord injury, then medical management and imaging workup will need to address this injury as the first priority in all but the most critically injured patients. In some patients immediate reduction of fractures or dislocations may be most appropriate, whereas other patients may benefit from MRI before proceeding with treatment.

Controversy persists about the optimal diagnostic imaging protocol for trauma patients as it relates to the spine. There are several objectives for which there is general consensus among trauma surgeons and spine surgeons. First is the detection of any significant spinal injury that places the patient at risk for neurologic deterioration. This may be an osseous injury, a soft-tissue injury, including posterior ligament complex injuries and other important injuries such as disc disruptions, or a combination of the two. Second, make a determination that there is no significant injury as early as possible to allow discontinuation of cervical immobilization and lifting of spine precautions. This will help avoid the recognized morbidities of immobilization and to facilitate other aspects of the patient's care. Rose et al. found that patients meeting the NEXUS criteria who had a "distracting injury" were correctly assessed on clinical grounds alone with 99% sensitivity and 99% negative predictive value. They concluded that the number of CT scans in this cohort of patients could be reduced by 61% and suggested that radiographic evaluation is unnecessary for safe clearance of the asymptomatic cervical spine in awake and alert blunt trauma patients with "distracting injuries." Additionally, the imaging should assess for associated injuries, including vertebral artery injuries in the cervical region or visceral injuries involving the chest, abdomen, and pelvic areas when evaluating the thoracic, lumbar, and sacral spine regions. The initial evaluation of the spine (thoracic to sacrum) is best done using multidetector computed tomography (MDCT) with both sagittal and coronal reformatted images (Fig. 41-1).

SPINE PRECAUTIONS

The topic of spinal precautions often is mentioned but rarely described in publications regarding trauma to the spine. Specific practices are likely inconsistent among institutions. The following protocol is derived from our experience. Spinal immobilization has already been described as it pertains to transport of an injured patient, but, as mentioned, one of the goals of the initial assessment is to be able to remove the patient from the backboard quickly once hemodynamic stability has been obtained and CT evaluation completed. Even if a significant spinal injury at any level is found, the patient can be moved to a bed but maintained with a cervical collar in place on a pillow as needed to avoid cervical extension. Patients with ankylosing spondylitis may require several pillows to keep them more upright because of their rigid cervicothoracic kyphosis (see Chapter 38). If a patient is to be placed in cervical traction, the crossmember for the traction pulley is fixed to the bed frame such that the traction vector maintains neutral alignment and adjusts if the bed position is altered. With this level of precaution, a patient can be placed head up using the reverse Trendelenburg function of the bed. If the cervical CT is negative for injury and cervical immobilization is to be continued pending further evaluation, then the patient is allowed to be fully upright in a properly fitted rigid cervical orthosis until spinal clearance is possible unless other injuries prevent this. Prasarn et al. demonstrated in a cadaver study that a kinetic bed caused less cervical displacement through an injured segment than the traditional log roll maneuver.

Patients with unstable thoracic or lumbar injuries, such as fracture-dislocation or other injuries that will be treated with internal stabilization, are maintained flat in bed (using the reverse-Trendelenburg position to elevate the head) and log-rolled side-back-side every 2 hours while awake until the spine is stabilized. For patients with spinal cord injuries in whom operative stabilization will be delayed more than 24 to 48 hours a Roto-Rest (KCI, San Antonio, TX) type bed is preferred (also used in patients with cervical injuries). Once the thoracolumbar fracture is stabilized, or for those patients being treated in an orthosis, elevating the head of the bed 0 to 30 degrees is allowed without donning the orthosis. The orthosis is required when the head of the bed is above 30 degrees.

Keeping the head of the bed elevated is strongly encouraged if blood pressure, intracranial pressure, and other vital parameters permit, to reduce the risk of aspiration and to assist with pulmonary toilet. Once spinal stability is achieved, continued frequent turning of the patient or the use of a therapeutic air mattress is preferred as long as mobility is severely limited for any reason.

DIAGNOSTIC IMAGING

Injuries that involve the thoracic, lumbar, or sacral regions of the spine generally can be diagnosed using CT, which has been established as the diagnostic imaging modality of choice in these areas. It usually is obtained as part of the primary workup by the trauma surgeons or the physicians in the emergency department. Additional evaluation with MRI in these areas or use of other modalities typically is not necessary, although there are circumstances in which this is appropriate. Because these CT studies are obtained routinely for other reasons, the specific indications for radiographic evaluations of these areas have not been extensively studied. Additional attention is given to this topic in later sections dealing specifically with injuries to these areas.

Patients who have cervical spine symptoms require imaging evaluation, and the recommendations for this process have changed in recent years. The standard radiographic evaluation of the cervical spine for trauma patients until relatively recently has been anteroposterior, lateral, and open-mouth odontoid views. This three-view protocol has proven reliable when technically adequate images are

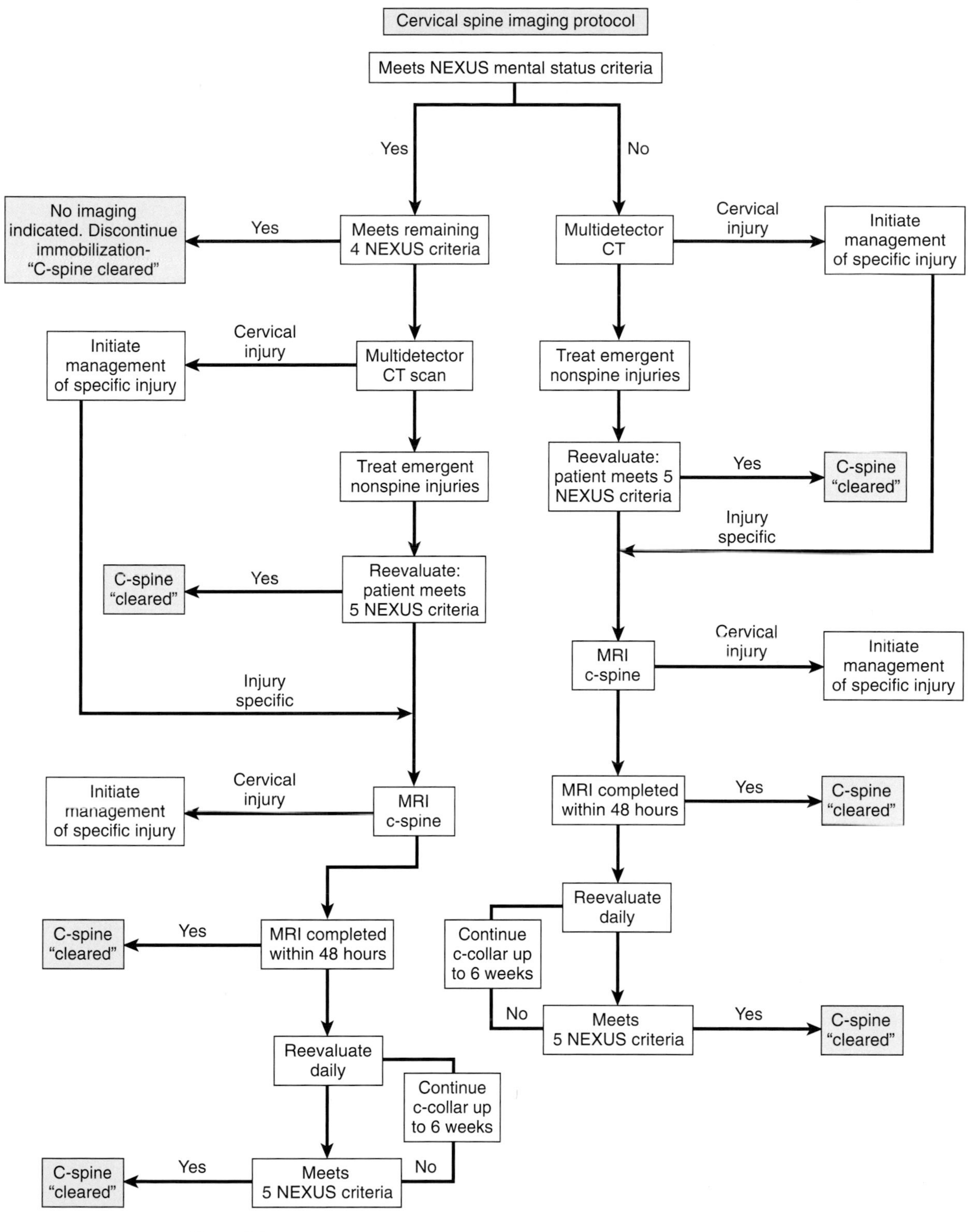

FIGURE 41-1 Cervical spine imaging in patients without spinal cord injury.

obtained, but has been documented to fail in demonstrating a small number of significant cervical injuries. Because the incidence of cervical injury in trauma patients is between 2% and 6%, a very high sensitivity is required to optimally evaluate symptomatic patients. In a series of 32,117 patients, Davis found 34 missed injuries. As has also been documented in numerous other studies, the most common reason the injury was missed in Davis' series was failure to obtain adequate radiographs of the injured level (23 patients). Eight patients in the series had incorrect readings of adequate films, and only one patient was documented to have adequate radiographs that did not demonstrate the injury even in retrospect. Most studies on this topic have found that the occipitocervical junction and the cervicothoracic junction are the areas where injuries are most likely to be missed. Several studies have provided level I evidence that the negative predictive value of an adequate three-view series is from 93% to 98%; however, in these same studies the sensitivity was only 62% to 84%. Assuming a series of 100 patients, 6% of whom have cervical injury, five of six cervical injuries could be detected as abnormal on a three-view radiographic series and one truly injured patient would not be distinguished radiographically from the 94 correctly identified true negative series. This deficiency of plain radiographs is not improved with the addition of oblique films for a five-view series.

With greater availability of multidetector computed tomography (MDCT) there has been a transition to using this modality for the primary evaluation of the cervical spine in trauma patients based on level II and III evidence. Combining the cervical CT scan with the head-chest, abdomen, and pelvic scan, which often is ordered for these patients, has resulted in a lower cost than if the cervical study is done separately. Also, because the patient is already in the scanner and the scan times are much faster with MDCT compared with conventional CT, it actually takes less time to obtain an MDCT than it would for a three-view series of plain radiographs. When the relatively high proportions of technically inadequate studies that require CT are factored in, the MDCT has been found to be cost effective relative to plain radiographs. Despite these advantages, the higher radiation dose to the patient remains a concern with MDCT. Although comparisons between MDCT with coronal plane and sagittal plane reconstructions and plain radiographs have found higher sensitivity in detecting injuries with MDCT, several studies comparing autopsy findings with injuries noted on CT before death found that not all injuries present at autopsy were demonstrated by CT. Molina et al. found significant injuries in a small number of patients that were not demonstrated on the CT images. This indicates that CT may not be the "gold standard" by which to judge all other diagnostic imaging techniques. The role of MRI in the evaluation of the cervical spine in symptomatic patients to supplement MDCT continues to develop as the deficiencies of MDCT are better understood. The high cost, limited availability, and restricted monitoring and access to the patient imposed by MRI continue to limit its use. Despite these shortcomings, a significant number of studies demonstrate improved diagnostic sensitivity with the use of MRI. Sarani et al. retrospectively found injuries on MRI in 42 of 164 (26%) trauma patients. All 164 patients had negative CT scans, and treatment was altered in 74% of these patients either with surgery or continuation of immobilization. In the subset of patients who could not be examined because of altered mental status, Sarani et al. found injuries on MRI in 5 of 46 (11%) patients who had negative CT scans, and 80% of these patients required surgery. Pourtaheri et al. found in a subset of patients with cervical fractures and altered mental status that MRI was very useful; MRI found additional injuries in 48% that changed treatment for 39%. This treatment change was from nonoperative to operative treatment 24% of the time. The clearest indication for MRI in a trauma patient is for the evaluation of an unexplained neurologic deficit at any spinal level. MRI has a higher sensitivity for detecting soft-tissue injuries, which are not well demonstrated on CT. MRI can detect a missed spinal column injury or neural compressive pathologic processes, such as disc fragments, epidural hematoma, or the presence of significant canal stenosis from other causes. For patients with a demonstrated injury and neurologic deficit at a corresponding level, MRI usually offers little additional information for that injury. However, noncontiguous injuries occur in up to 15% of patients. Because of this high rate of additional injuries, patients with cervical injuries demonstrated on MDCT at our institution are evaluated with MRI to assess for soft-tissue injuries. This practice has resulted in alteration of the treatment plan for a significant percentage of patients when additional injuries are detected. Using MRI to assist in the "clearance" of the cervical spine remains controversial at this time. Although many of these additional injuries are significant and do alter treatment, some of the injuries are not clinically significant, so specific indications for obtaining MRI need to be defined. Determining which MRI findings correlate with clinical instability also needs to be better defined. If a patient has abnormal findings on CT suggesting soft-tissue injury, such as soft-tissue density anterior to the midbody of C3 greater than 5 mm, a widened disc space (>1 to 2 mm) at one level relative to adjacent disc levels particularly if there is an anterior osteophyte avulsion at that level (Fig. 41-2), or excessive widening of the interspinous distance posteriorly, MRI should be obtained. An additional confounding issue is the timing of the MRI. Because MRI is most effective for evaluating soft-tissue injury, either by showing discontinuity of anatomic structures such as the ligamentum flavum and annulus fibrosus or hemorrhage and edema associated with tissue disruption, the timing of the study is very important. If the MRI is obtained within the first 48 hours after injury, the sensitivity for hemorrhage and edema is optimal. The ability of MRI to identify injury after 48 hours is dependent on the direct demonstration of tissue disruption or subluxation of the spine. Emery et al. found that MRI done an average of 11 days from injury failed to demonstrate known soft-tissue injuries in 2 of 19 patients. Evaluation of the available literature revealed level III evidence to support the "clearance" of the cervical spine in a symptomatic patient if CT and MRI done within 48 hours of injury are found to be normal. Our process is to obtain an MRI in the obtunded patient within this 48-hour window if the patient is stable enough to undergo the study. A patient is not considered obtunded if the mental status is altered because of the presence of substances that will only transiently impair the patient. In this case the patient has CT examination and remains in a rigid orthosis with repeat examinations until the impairment has resolved and a determination is made to either "clear" the cervical spine on clinical grounds or proceed with MRI within 48 hours. If the condition of the patient does not allow the MRI to be completed within 48 hours and the patient remains obtunded, an MRI is obtained as soon as the patient can safely undergo the study and any identified injuries are treated. However, if the delayed MRI does not directly demonstrate an injury, the patient is kept in a rigid orthosis for up to 6 weeks as treatment for presumed soft-tissue injury or until his or her mental status improves and he or she can be cleared on clinical grounds by meeting the NEXUS criteria. This protocol has been effective in avoiding neurologic deterioration because of missed injuries. Although there has been occasional morbidity such as decubitus ulcers attributable to the orthosis, this is very rare. Skin breakdown on the posterior scalp above the orthosis results from improper fit of the orthosis, not keeping the patient upright, and not turning the patient adequately. No more serious morbidities from immobilization have occurred, although nursing care, especially tracheostomy care, is

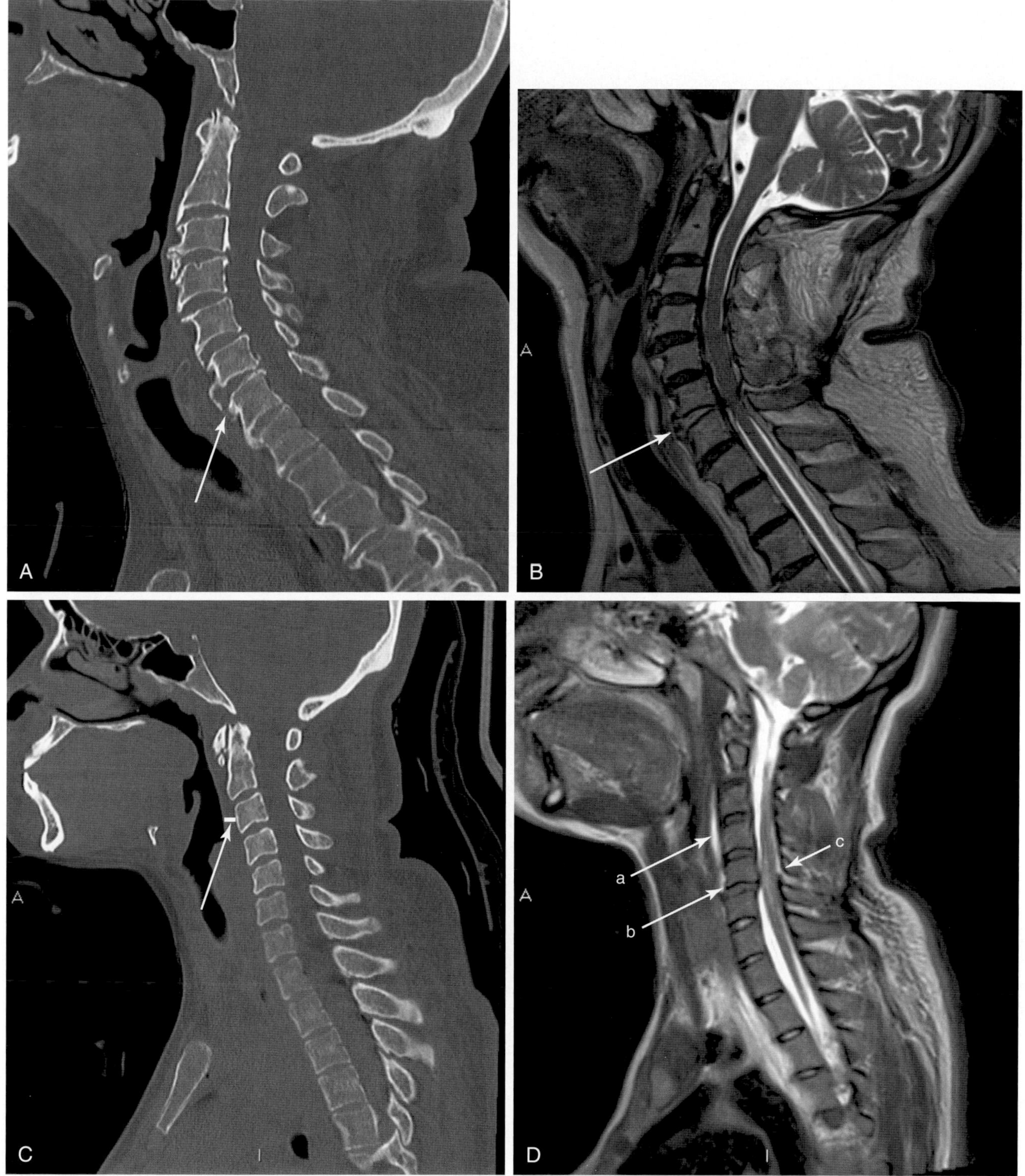

FIGURE 41-2 **A,** Disruption of C6 osteophyte suggesting disruption through the disc *(arrow).* **B,** Increased signal through C6 disc indicates disruption of disc *(arrow).* **C,** Retropharyngeal soft tissue more than 5 mm on midsagittal image *(arrow).* **D,** *Arrow a* indicates hemorrhage causing widening of soft-tissue density at C3 level. *Arrow b* indicates anterior annulus disruption. *Arrow c* indicates disruption of ligamentum flavum. Also note cord edema and swelling.

Continued

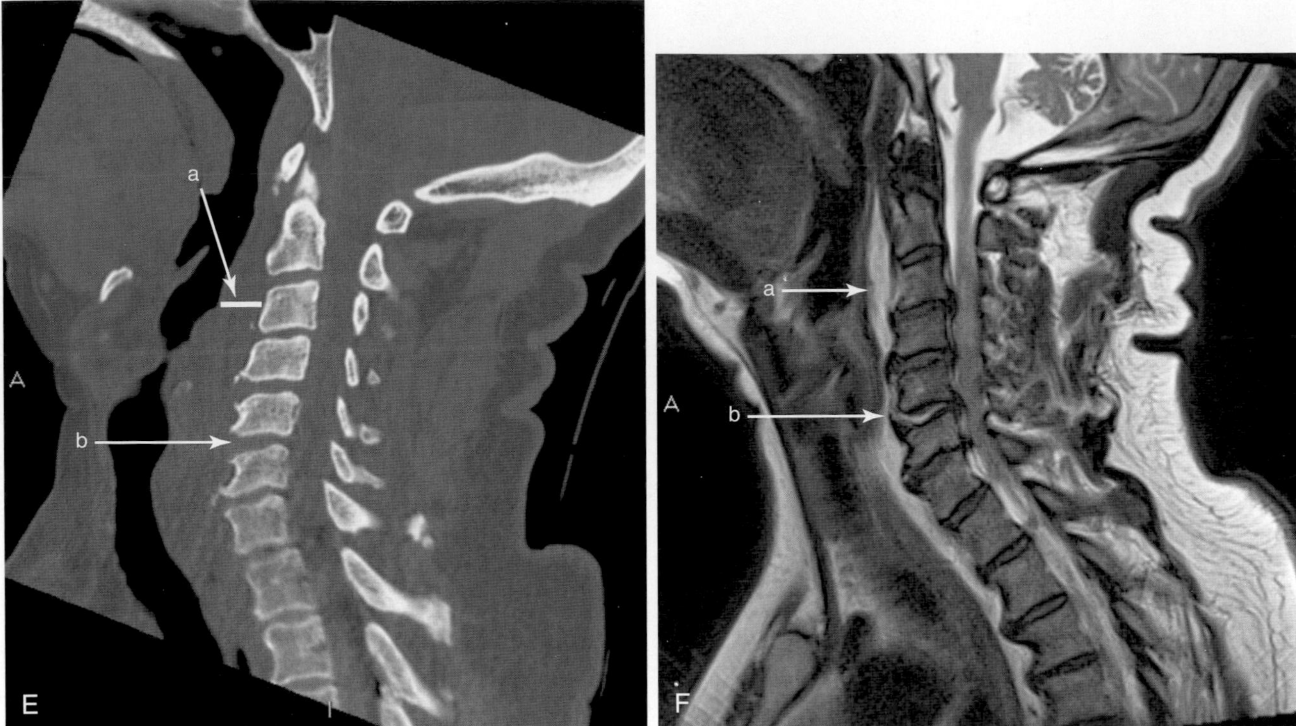

FIGURE 41-2, cont'd E, *Arrow a* indicates more than 5 mm of soft-tissue density at C3 level. *Arrow b* indicates subtle angulation through C5 disc level. F, *Arrow a* indicates hemorrhage at C3 level. *Arrow b* indicates disruption through anterior annulus and through the disc space.

somewhat more difficult. Thus, the primary indications for cervical MRI are unexplained neurologic deficit, identified cervical injury, CT findings suggestive of soft-tissue injury, or a patient with altered mental status after intoxicants are metabolized. When possible, MRI is performed within 48 hours.

ADDITIONAL IMAGING

It is unusual for additional imaging to be required beyond that described. We have not found dynamic studies to be useful acutely to evaluate the cervical spine. There is a high rate of inadequate studies for a variety of reasons, foremost of which is inadequate range of motion. In obtunded patients, there have been reports of major neurologic injury caused by obtaining dynamic images. If a nonobtunded patient has adequate motion for flexion and extension lateral radiographs, typically clearance can be done on clinical grounds using the NEXUS criteria without further imaging.

On rare occasions a patient may have findings on MDCT suggestive but not definitive of a soft-tissue injury. Typically, an MRI study would be obtained, but in certain patients this is contraindicated (e.g., if the patient has a pacemaker). In these instances a "stretch test" as described by White, Southwick, and Panjabi is done to more completely assess the stability of the spine. This test allows measurement of the displacement within a motion segment under controlled conditions to identify soft-tissue injuries. Gardner-Wells tongs are applied before this test is performed. A head halter can be used but is less desirable because of the amount of weight that potentially may be used. The possible end points for the test are a change in neurologic status, an increase of 1.7 mm between adjacent vertebrae at any level, an angulatory change of 7.5 degrees at any disc level, or reaching one third of body weight or 65 lb, whichever is less. A prerequisite to performing a "stretch test" is that the patient must be alert and able to provide a consistent feedback for neurologic examination (Box 41-1). Resuscitation should be complete, and the patient should be hemodynamically stable. Head CT should confirm no fracture near the planned cranial pin sites.

BOX 41-1

End Points for Stretch Test

- Change in neurologic status
- Increase of 1.7 mm between adjacent vertebrae at any level
- Angulatory change of 7.5 degrees at any disc level
- Reaching one third of body weight or weight limit for tongs, whichever is less

APPLICATION OF GARDNER-WELLS TONGS

TECHNIQUE 41-1

- Stabilize the patient's neck with a rigid cervical orthosis. A small bolster may be needed under the occiput or shoulders to maintain neutral cervical alignment.

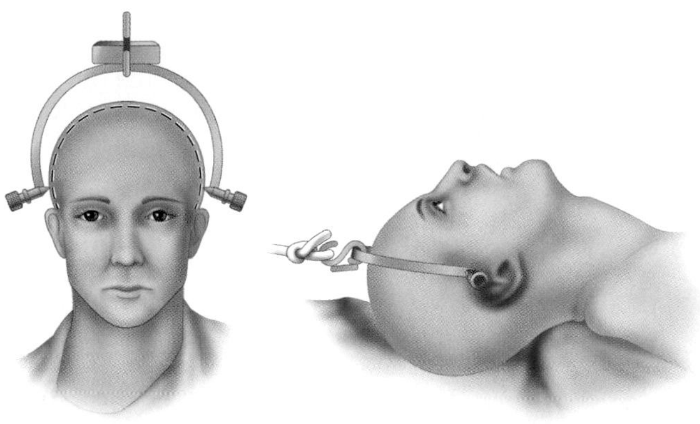

FIGURE 41-3 Gardner-Wells tongs placed just above ears, below greatest diameter of skull. **SEE TECHNIQUE 41-1.**

- Identify a point 1 to 2 cm above the top of the ear and 0 to 2 cm posterior to the auditory meatus bilaterally. Pull the hair back over this area. If necessary, remove a small amount of hair to expose the skin.
- If slight extension is desired, place the pins in line with the auditory meatus but no farther forward to avoid injury to the temporal artery. Placing the pins more posteriorly will result in slight flexion. Flexion or extension also can be accomplished by adjusting the level of the traction pulley or by placing a bolster under the shoulders as needed.
- Clean the pin sites with an antiseptic soap and antiseptic solution.
- Infiltrate the pin sites with 1% or 2% lidocaine down to the periosteum.
- Check the tongs to ensure that the central pin is recessed, the pin points are not damaged, and the S hook is in place to attach the weight.
- Gently place the tongs over the patient's head and advance the pins toward the skin. Put the pins in a symmetric position.
- To avoid rotation, center the tongs by observing the patient's nose in the middle of the tongs.
- Advance the pins until the central pin protrudes by 1 mm. This will occur on one side only. Tighten the locking nuts securely after the pins are seated.
- The tongs are now set and traction can be applied. The other restraints can be removed. No dressing is needed.
- Place the pulley for the traction rope at a level to achieve in-line traction for the cervical spine (Fig. 41-3).

STRETCH TEST

This test must always be done with direct supervision by the attending orthopaedic surgeon.

TECHNIQUE 41-2

- Apply traction through secured cranial skeletal traction. Use of a head halter may be considered only if a small amount of weight is expected to be used. If a head halter is used, place a small piece of gauze sponge between the molars for patient comfort. Carefully place a rolled towel or sheet under the patient's head or neck as needed to maintain neutral alignment.
- Place the radiographic film as close as possible to the patient's neck, position the x-ray tube 72 inches from the film, and make a lateral exposure. This will serve as the baseline image.
- Begin with 10 lb of weight and increase traction in 3- to 5-lb increments. Complete a full neurologic examination and obtain a lateral radiograph before adding the next weight increment.
- The test is considered positive and should be discontinued and traction removed if any neurologic changes occur or if any abnormal separation or angulation occurs. The radiographic criterion is an increase of 1.7 mm between adjacent vertebrae or a change of 7.5 degrees at an intervertebral disc level relative to the baseline image that was obtained.
- By completing a neurologic examination and allowing the radiographic image to be processed, an adequate time of at least 5 minutes elapses between weight increases to overcome any muscle spasm that may occur.
- Be certain to compare measurements on each new radiograph to the baseline image, *not* the previous image.
- The test is considered negative for instability if traction equal to one third of body weight or 65 lb is reached without radiographic or neurologic change.

NEUROLOGIC ASSESSMENT

To properly direct the diagnostic imaging necessary for a patient, the neurologic examination findings play a key role. Assessment of mental status using the Glasgow Coma Scale (GCS) (Table 41-2) determines the level of consciousness. If the GCS score is not 15, then imaging will be required as outlined earlier. Clearly document the motor and sensory examination, including the function of the rectal sphincter and the presence of perianal sensation. We have used the ASIA form provided on the ASIA website (www.asia-spinalinjury.org/publications/59544_sc_Exam_Sheet_r4.pdf). Using the ASIA form, sensation is recorded for light touch and pinprick in 28 dermatomal distributions on each side of the body (Fig. 41-4). Pinprick testing is done using a sterile needle rather than a pinwheel. A score of 2 (normal), 1 (altered), or 0 (absent) is determined for each dermatome, and specific "key" areas are identified on the diagram within each dermatome as optimal test locations. In addition, the presence of sensation for deep anal pressure is made to help determine if a spinal cord injury is complete or incomplete. Important dermatomal landmarks are the nipple line (T4), xiphoid process (T7), umbilicus (T10), inguinal region (T12, L1), and perianal region (S4 and S5). Motor function is scored 0/5 to 5/5 in each of 10 specific myotomes per side (Table 41-3). Also, the presence or absence of voluntary anal sphincter contraction is recorded. In some

TABLE 41-2

Glasgow Coma Scale

	POINTS
EYES OPEN	
Spontaneous	4
To sound	3
To pain	2
Never	1
BEST VERBAL RESPONSE	
Oriented	5
Confused conversation	4
Inappropriate words	3
Incomprehensible words	2
None	1
BEST MOTOR RESPONSE	
Obeys commands	6
Localizes pain	5
Flexion withdrawal	4
Abnormal	3
Extension	2
None	1

From Teasdale G, Jennett B: Assessment and prognosis of coma after head injury, Acta Neurochir 34:45, 1976.

TABLE 41-3

Key Muscle Groups Used in ASIA Motor Source Evaluation of Spinal Cord Injury

LEVEL	MUSCLE GROUP
C5	Elbow flexors (biceps, brachialis)
C6	Wrist extensors (extensor carpi radialis longus and brevis)
C7	Elbow extensors (triceps)
C8	Finger flexors (flexor digitorum profundus to the middle finger)
T1	Small finger abductors (abductor digiti minimi)
L2	Hip flexors (iliopsoas)
L3	Knee extensors (quadriceps)
L4	Ankle dorsiflexors (tibialis anterior)
L5	Long toe extensors (extensor hallucis longus)
S1	Ankle plantar flexors (gastrocnemius, soleus)

From Beaty JH, editor: Orthopaedic knowledge update, home study syllabus 6, Rosemont, IL, 1999, American Academy of Orthopaedic Surgeons, p 654.

circumstances, the designation of "NT" for not testable or 5*/5 (weakness as expected, considered normal strength because of inhibiting factors such as fractures) are most appropriate. Before making a definitive determination of injury type the patient must be out of spinal shock. This usually occurs within 24 to 48 hours but can take substantially longer and is indicated by the return of the bulbocavernosus reflex and anal wink (Figs. 41-5 and 41-6). On page 2 of the ASIA document, the requirements for each motor grade are given along with the definitions of the ASIA Impairment Scale and a flow chart to properly interpret it. Using the ASIA Impairment Scale, a determination is made to classify the spinal cord–injured patient. The level of injury is named by the most caudal myotome and dermatome level with *both* normal motor *and* sensory function. Type A patients are motor complete and sensory complete, with no motor or sensory function more than three segments caudal to the named injury level. Function within the zone of partial preservation should be recorded because a change by even a single level can be very significant, especially in the cervical region. Type B patients are motor complete but sensory incomplete (incomplete sensory loss but complete motor loss with *no* motor function more than three segments caudal to the named injury level); sensory sparing may be only light touch, pinprick in the perianal segments, or deep anal pressure. Type C patients have either voluntary sphincter contraction *or* voluntary motor function more than three segments below the named injury level with sacral sensory sparing. This motor sparing can be in non-key myotomes according to the standard at this time. More than half of functioning key myotomes are graded *less* than 3/5. Type D patients have *at least* half of functioning key myotomes greater than or equal to grade 3/5. Type E patients have a spinal cord injury that improves to normal. This type is not used to describe a patient without a spinal cord injury initially. This examination should allow the clinician to distinguish spinal cord injuries from isolated nerve root or nerve plexus type injuries.

The initial neurologic examination should be completed as soon as possible after the arrival of the patient to establish the correct baseline for the patient to which all subsequent examinations will be compared. It is our practice to complete serial neurologic assessments on patients with spinal cord injuries or unstable spinal column injuries every 4 to 6 hours for at least the first 24 hours and continue less frequent reassessments thereafter based on the patient's clinical course. This regimen is derived from experience in a busy level I trauma center but is not evidence based, and it is unlikely that evidence-based practices could be used to examine how frequently optimal evaluations should be done. In addition to the motor and sensory examinations, it is important to include examination of the deep tendon reflexes. Acute spinal cord injury results in flaccid paralysis and areflexia. The presence of pathologic reflexes such as a Babinski or Hoffmann reflex or clonus indicates a more chronic process, which may be acutely worsened by trauma such as a central cord injury in the setting of chronic cervical stenosis. The purpose for serial examinations is to detect any neurologic change and institute management changes to improve the patient's ultimate neurologic outcome. Deterioration of neurologic function can be caused by intracranial processes such as hemorrhage, metabolic processes such as acidosis, or spinal pathologic processes. Bony malalignment causing spinal cord compression, hypotension, expanding epidural hematoma, spinal cord infarction, inadequate immobilization, or improper movement of a patient are some of the reasons for deterioration that must be considered by the orthopaedic surgeon in collaboration with other consultants so treatment can be adjusted appropriately. Likewise, if a patient is noted to improve, management may need to be altered as well with regard to planning of spinal stabilization or nonoperative spinal interventions.

Patient Name ____________________

Examiner Name ____________________ Date/Time of Exam____________________

ASIA AMERICAN SPINAL INJURY ASSOCIATION

STANDARD NEUROLOGIC CLASSFICATION OF SPINAL CORD INJURY

ISCoS

MOTOR

KEY MUSCLES (scoring on reverse side)

	R	L	
C5			Elbow flexors
C6			Wrist extensors
C7			Elbow extensors
C8			Finger flexsors (distal phalanx of middle finger)
T1			Finger abductors (little finger)

UPPER LIMB TOTAL (MAXIMUM) ☐ + ☐ = ☐ (25) (25) (50)

Comments:

	R	L	
L2			Hip flexors
L3			Knee extensors
L4			Ankle dorsiflexors
L5			Long toe extensors
S1			Ankle plantar flexors

Voluntary anal contraction (Yes/No) ☐

LOWER LIMB TOTAL (MAXIMUM) ☐ + ☐ = ☐ (25) (25) (50)

	LIGHT TOUCH R	LIGHT TOUCH L	PIN PRICK R	PIN PRICK L
C2				
C3				
C4				
C5				
C6				
C7				
C8				
T1				
T2				
T3				
T4				
T5				
T6				
T7				
T8				
T9				
T10				
T11				
T12				
L1				
L2				
L3				
L4				
L5				
S1				
S2				
S3				
S4-5				
TOTALS (MAXIMUM)	(50)	(50)	(50)	(50)

☐ Any anal sensation (Yes/No)

☐ + ☐ = ☐ PIN PRICK SCORE (max: 112)

☐ + ☐ = ☐ LIGHT TOUCH SCORE (max: 112)

SENSORY

KEY SENSORY POINTS

0 = absent
1 = impaired
2 = normal
NT = not testable

NEUROLOGIC LEVEL (The most caudal segment with normal function)		R	L	COMPLETE OR INCOMPLETE? (Incomplete = Any sensory or motor function in S4-S5)	☐	ZONE OF PARTIAL PRESERVATION (Caudal extent of partially innervated segments)		R	L
	SENSORY	☐	☐	ASIA IMPAIRMENT SCALE	☐		SENSORY	☐	☐
	MOTOR	☐	☐				MOTOR	☐	☐

REV 03/06

A

MUSCLE GRADING

0 Total paralysis

1 Palpable or visible contraction

2 Active movement, full range of motion, gravity eliminated

3 Active movement, full range of motion, against gravity

4 Active movement, full range of motion, against gravity and provides some resistance

5 Active movement, full range of motion, against gravity and provides normal resistance

5* Muscle able to exert, in examiner's judgment, sufficient resistance to be considered normal if identifiable inhibiting factors were not present

NT not testable. Patient unable to reliably exert effort or muscle unavailable for testing due to factors such as immobilization, pain on effort, or contracture.

ASIA IMPAIRMENT SCALE

☐ **A = Complete:** No motor or sensory function is preserved in the sacral segments S4-S5.

☐ **B = Incomplete:** Sensory but not motor function is preserved below the neurologic level and includes the sacral segments S4-S5.

☐ **C = Incomplete:** Motor function is preserved below the neurologic level, and more than half of key muscles below the neurologic level have a muscle grade less than 3.

☐ **D = Incomplete:** Motor function is preserved below the neurologic level, and at least half of key muscles below the neurologic level have a muscle grade of 3 or more.

☐ **E = Normal:** Motor and sensory function are normal.

CLINICAL SYNDROMES (OPTIONAL)

☐ Central Cord
☐ Brown-Séquard
☐ Anterior Cord
☐ Conus Medullaris
☐ Cauda Equina

STEPS IN CLASSIFICATION

The following order is recommended in determining the classification of individuals with SCI.

1. Determine sensory levels for right and left sides.
2. Determine motor levels for right and left sides.
   Note: in regions where there is no myotome to test, the motor level is presumed to be the same as the sensory level.
3. Determine the single neurologic level.
   This is the lowest segment where motor and sensory function is normal on both sides, and is the most caudad of the sensory and motor levels determined in steps 1 and 2.
4. Determine whether the injury is Complete or Incomplete (sacral sparing). After spinal shock resolved:
   If voluntary and contraction = **No** *AND all S4-5 sensory scores =* **0** *AND any anal sensation =* **No**, *then injury is COMPLETE. Otherwise injury is incomplete.*
5. Determine ASIA Impairment Scale (AIS) Grade:

Is injury Complete? If **YES**, AIS=A Record ZPP (For ZPP record lowest dermatome or myotome on each side with some (non-zero score) preservation)

NO ↓

Is injury motor Incomplete? If **NO**, AIS=B (Yes=voluntary anal contraction OR motor function more than three levels below the motor level on a given side.)

YES ↓

Are at least half of the key muscles below the (single) neurologic level graded 3 or better?

NO ↓ AIS=C

YES ↓ AIS=D

If sensation and motor function is normal in all segments, AIS=E
Note: AIS E is used in follow up testing when an individual with a documented SCI has recovered normal function. If at initial testing no deficits are found, the individual is neurologically intact; the ASIA Impairment Scale does not apply.

B

FIGURE 41-4 **A,** Standard neurologic classification of spinal cord injury from the American Spinal Injury Association (ASIA). **B,** Muscle grading and ASIA impairment scale.

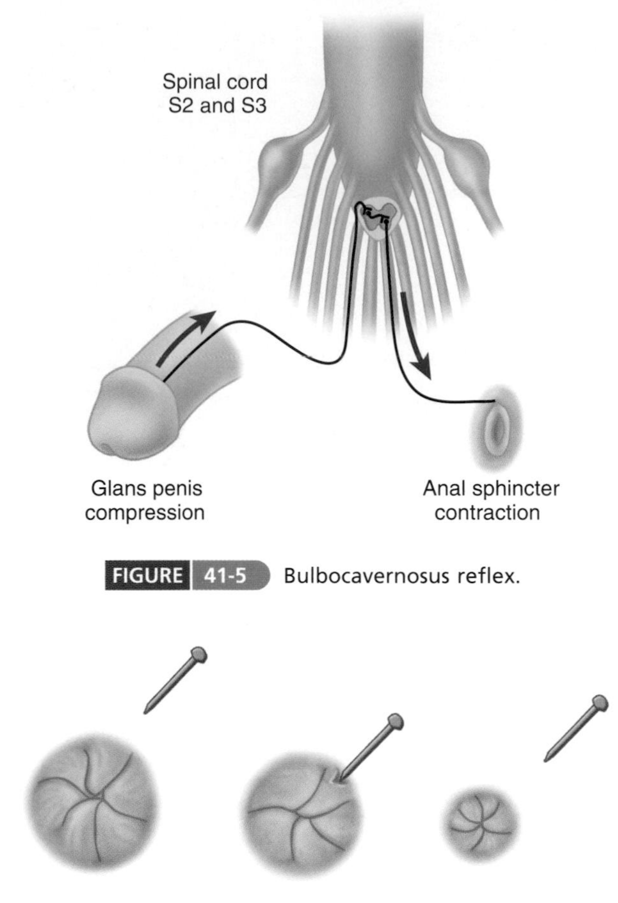

FIGURE 41-5 Bulbocavernosus reflex.

FIGURE 41-6 Anal wink. Contracture of external sphincter caused by pin prick.

SPINAL CORD INJURY

NEUROGENIC AND SPINAL SHOCK

Neurogenic shock refers to hemodynamic instability that occurs with rostral cord injuries related to the loss of sympathetic tone to the peripheral vasculature and heart, the consequences of which are bradycardia, hypotension, and hypothermia caused by absent thermoregulation. The combination of hypotension and bradycardia should alert the clinician to this cause of shock rather than hemorrhagic shock, which may coexist, particularly in patients with other injuries. Aggressive treatment of hypotension of any cause is a priority in patients with spinal cord injury. *Spinal shock* refers to a temporary dysfunction of the spinal cord, with a loss of reflexes and sensorimotor function caudal to the level of injury. It is manifested by absence of anal wink and bulbocavernosus reflexes and by flaccid paralysis. It is a temporary phenomenon and recovers usually in 24 to 48 hours even in severe injuries but can persist for weeks or rarely months. There is no specific treatment for spinal shock.

For patients with a spinal cord injury, rapid diagnosis and institution of measures to minimize secondary spinal cord injury may be the most important interventions possible to improve ultimate neurologic and functional recovery. The controversy concerning the timing of surgery is centered on the concept of minimizing the secondary injury. Numerous studies such as the Surgical Timing in Acute Spinal Cord Injury Study (STACIS) have attempted to determine the optimal timing of surgical decompression and stabilization. At present, this remains somewhat of an open question, but evidence is mounting in favor of early decompression to enhance neurologic outcomes. Often this decompression is most rapidly accomplished by placing the patient in skeletal traction. This maneuver can be done much more quickly than operative treatment in most circumstances. In addition, multiple studies provide level III evidence that earlier decompression and stabilization are associated with shorter hospital stays and lower overall treatment costs for these patients. In a clinical study with direct measurements of spinal cord pressure and spinal cord perfusion, Werndle et al. found that spinal realignment and stabilization did not lead to improved spinal cord perfusion. This was attributed to spinal cord swelling within the inelastic dura mater.

The secondary injury cascade refers to the additional neurologic injury that results from cord ischemia, leading to electrolyte shifts with cell membrane alterations and accumulation of neurotransmitters and inflammatory mediators including free radicals that further injure neural tissue. A detailed discussion of these mechanisms is beyond the scope of this text; however, it must be recognized that proper medical management of a patient with a spinal cord injury is an important component in the overall care. The secondary mechanisms follow the initial or primary mechanical injury caused by compression, distraction, shear, or laceration of the spinal cord. The secondary injury cascade occurs over a period of hours to days, depending on the severity of injury and other injuries that may be present. Based on a number of animal models and level III evidence, it appears that the injury caused by ischemia of the spinal cord is the central feature of this secondary injury process. Avoiding or minimizing ischemia of the spinal cord appears to improve neurologic outcome. Spinal cord ischemia results in changes locally, with loss of autoregulation of spinal cord blood flow and changes to the systemic vasculature. These systemic alterations include cardiac rhythm irregularities, bradycardia, decreased mean arterial pressure, decreased cardiac output, and decreased peripheral vascular resistance. All of these abnormalities have the effect of a positive feedback loop to worsen the cord ischemia and thus worsen hemodynamic parameters. All of these hemodynamic parameters tend to be worse with more severe and more rostral injuries. Respiratory insufficiency or failure often accompanies spinal cord injury because of weakness of the respiratory muscles resulting in hypoxemia, which, in turn, worsens the spinal cord ischemia. Early detection and treatment of cardiopulmonary dysfunction does reduce the morbidity and mortality caused by these mechanisms. The goal for optimal blood pressure management is a mean arterial pressure of 85 to 90 mm Hg with maintenance of 100% oxygen saturation. This is based on clinical observations and level III evidence, which remains the best guidance available to date. To properly treat these patients, arterial lines and central venous access or even Swan-Ganz catheters may be needed. Initially, hypotension should be treated as hemorrhagic in origin and fluid resuscitation should be with a balanced solution (e.g., lactated Ringer solution). After adequate crystalloid volume replacement, blood transfusion may be needed. If hypotension has not responded after fluid resuscitation and transfusion with normal central venous pressure, pressor agents should be administered to maintain the mean arterial pressure in the desired range. Agents such as dobutamine, dopamine, or norepinephrine, with both α- and β-agonist properties, are preferred over pure α agonists such as phenylephrine that can lead to reflex bradycardia. The duration of pressure support to maintain the median arterial pressure has been somewhat arbitrarily stated to be 7 days, but there is no evidence to support either a longer or shorter period of time. Supplemental oxygen should be administered and ventilator settings adjusted to keep oxygenation at or near 100% during this period as well.

IMMEDIATE SPINAL REDUCTION

The primary objective for rapid cervical reduction and stabilization is to improve spinal cord blood flow and thus minimize the harmful effects of ischemia. In animal models, rapidly relieving spinal cord compression has been shown to be beneficial. The short period of time from injury to decompression determined in these studies to be optimal has not been clinically achievable. One intervention that can be accomplished in some patients to relieve spinal cord compression and improve cord blood flow is to reduce fractures and dislocations using skeletal traction. If the injury is recognized and the patient is emergently taken to the radiology suite, often the reduction can be achieved within the first 1 to 2 hours after the patient arrives at the hospital. To be effective this must be done absolutely as soon as possible even if the initial workup has not been completed. However, limited evidence exists as to how beneficial this may be, and there is some risk from other undetected injuries in this setting. Closed reduction usually can be accomplished significantly faster than can be achieved by operative means, and completion of the evaluation in a hemodynamically stable patient can usually safely follow the reduction. Closed reduction is not always possible and is not appropriate to attempt, for example, in patients with distraction type injuries at other levels, in obtunded patients, in patients with certain cranial fractures, or if the patient becomes hemodynamically unstable.

A great deal of controversy exists regarding timing of cervical reductions and the need for cervical MRI, particularly in the context of a patient with unilateral or bilateral facet fractures or dislocations. The controversy has been centered on whether there is a need to obtain prereduction MRI to determine if there is a disc herniation. The value of this information compared with the risk of the increased time to reduction has not been established. Consideration must be given to several pieces of information when treating these patients. The first is that dislocation of the spine with spinal cord compression is definitely associated with neurologic injury. Rizzolo et al. reported that in 55% of patients with facet injuries, disc herniations or disruptions occurred and that often the disc material displaced into the canal. The importance of this is not clear as it relates to spinal reduction. Vaccaro et al. documented by MRI that more disc herniations were present after reduction than before reduction, but disc displacement did not correlate with neurologic deterioration in a small series of patients. Grauer et al. noted the significant variability of using MRI in the setting of cervical dislocations among spine surgeons based on their primary specialty. The second important fact is that only rarely has closed spinal reduction been associated with neurologic worsening if the patient is awake and alert at the time of reduction. Although there is no level I evidence on this topic, it appears that the important issue is whether the patient is awake and alert at the time of reduction, not the presence of a disc injury. Many clinical series that were reported over a period of decades found only 11 of 1200 awake patients (<1%) who developed permanent neurologic worsening after closed reduction. At least two were root level injuries. Additionally, one or two patients had transient worsening that returned to baseline. Reduction was accomplished in 80% of patients, which should allow for better spinal cord perfusion. Thus, the risk of causing additional harm in an awake and alert patient with a cervical facet fracture or dislocation and a significant neurologic deficit is very low. In an awake and alert patient with a cervical fracture or dislocation with a significant neurologic deficit, we recommend expeditious reduction without obtaining an MRI.

Significant neurologic injury in our protocol has been determined to mean less than grade 3/5 in more than one half of the key myotomes caudal to the level of injury (ASIA Impairment Scale A, B, or C). By using this regimen, most awake and alert patients have reductions before obtaining an MRI. These patients do have MRI after reduction but before definitive treatment to assist in surgical planning. For the rare patient with a bilateral facet injury, or more likely a unilateral facet injury, and more than half of the key myotomes caudal to the injury level grade 3/5 or higher, an MRI is obtained before reduction even if the patient is awake and alert. The rationale is that if a patient's neurologic function is grade 3/5 or higher initially, there is more potential for harm with immediate reduction and less benefit. If during the process of reduction worsening of neurologic deficit occurs, the attempt at reduction is terminated. Immediate MRI is obtained, and operative treatment is undertaken, depending on the pathologic process present. If the patient is obtunded, closed reduction cannot be undertaken safely and immediate reduction is not attempted. For patients in whom closed reduction is attempted but not successful, MRI is completed to help guide the surgical approach.

■ CLOSED REDUCTION TECHNIQUE

After placement of cranial tongs, the technique used is the same as that described for the stretch test (see Technique 41-2) and should be supervised by the attending surgeon. The end points are the same as well with respect to all the motion segments without the fracture or dislocation and with the addition of achieving a reduction at the injured level. The injured segment should not be distracted more than 1.7 mm relative to the adjacent uninjured level during the reduction. Once a reduction is accomplished, the traction is reduced to 10 to 15 lb and the patient's diagnostic evaluation is completed. The patient is maintained in traction with the head of bed elevated to 30 degrees until definitive stabilization is accomplished unless other injuries make it necessary to alter this position. As noted previously, a small bolster may be needed under the patient's head or shoulders to achieve a neutral alignment in traction. Closed reduction should be successful in approximately 80% of patients. Further treatment after successful or failed reduction is discussed in the section regarding subaxial injuries.

SPINAL CORD INJURY TREATMENT

At this time there remains no effective treatment to reverse spinal cord injury that has been established by level I evidence. Many patients do improve neurologically, and in some the improvement is very dramatic. The measures that have been established to date are those detailed earlier that reduce the secondary injury. These include rapid realignment of the spine when appropriate, maintaining mean arterial pressure at 85 to 90 mm Hg, and maintaining 100% oxygen saturation. The use of maintaining a mean arterial pressure (MAP) in the range of 85 to 90 mm Hg continues to be evaluated. Hawryluk et al. evaluated minute-by-minute data on 100 patients with spinal cord injuries and found a correlation between maintaining a MAP of 85 to 90 mm Hg and better neurologic outcomes; intermittent lapses below the target range negatively affected outcomes. Also, the effect appeared most important during the first 3 days after injury. An extensive literature review of cervical spinal cord injuries by the Congress of Neurological Surgeons also recommends maintaining MAP between 85 and 90 mm Hg during the first 7 days after injury. There has been extensive research into various interventions to discover any possible clinical benefit that may aid patients with spinal cord injury. One such intervention that initially gained clinical acceptance was the use of high-dose methylprednisolone using the National Acute Spinal Cord Injury Study (NASCIS) II and then the NASCIS III protocols. Subsequent evaluations of these studies found significant flaws in the data analysis, and the claimed benefits of corticosteroid use have not been realized. These protocols are generally not recommended as treatment options to patients because significant complications are associated with these very high corticosteroid doses, which outweigh any benefit. However, the diagnosis of a severe spinal cord injury is devastating to patients, and they are informed of these protocols if they meet the inclusion criteria. If after careful counseling on the potentially harmful consequences that are associated with the protocol a patient chooses this therapy, it is administered and the informed consent is thoroughly documented.

SPINAL CORD SYNDROMES

When evaluating patients with spinal cord injuries, incomplete injuries must be distinguished from those that are complete because treatment decisions are based on this determination. If a complete spinal cord injury exists, the patient may regain some function within the zone of partial preservation but needs to understand that functional recovery at a more caudal level is not to be expected. This determination cannot be made until spinal shock has resolved and a reliable detailed neurologic examination is possible. In the case of an incomplete spinal cord injury, there are several recognized syndromes. If the injury can be categorized as one of these syndromes, prognostic information can be provided to the patient in general terms, but determination of specific functional recovery remains impossible at this time. There are, however, some generalizations that help inform the patient: (1) the greater the sparing of motor and sensory function is caudal to the injury, the greater is the expected recovery; (2) the earlier that recovery appears and the more rapidly it progresses, the greater is the expected recovery; and (3) recovery can occur over 12 to 15 months, but once progress ceases further recovery should not be expected. The most recognized syndromes are central cord syndrome, Brown-Séquard syndrome, anterior cord syndrome, posterior cord syndrome, conus medullaris syndrome, and cauda equina syndrome. There are some injuries that do not fit well into these described syndromes, and prognostic information cannot be given for these mixed syndromes.

Central cord syndrome is the most common. It consists of injury to the central area of the spinal cord, including gray and white matter (Fig. 41-7B). The centrally located upper extremity motor neurons in the corticospinal tracts are the most severely affected, and the lower extremity tracts are affected to a lesser extent. Generally, patients have a tetraparesis involving the upper extremities to a greater degree than the lower extremities with greater dysfunction distally in the extremities than proximally. Sensory sparing varies, but usually sacral pinprick sensation is preserved. These patients frequently show early partial recovery and may have preexisting cord compression and may not have spinal instability. Prognosis varies, but more than 50% of patients have return of bowel and bladder control, become ambulatory, and have improved hand function (Table 41-4). This syndrome usually results from a hyperextension injury in an older individual with preexisting osteoarthritis of the spine. The spinal cord is pinched between the vertebral body anteriorly and the buckling ligamentum flavum and lamina posteriorly (Fig. 41-7A). It also may occur in younger patients with flexion injuries.

Brown-Séquard syndrome is an injury to either side of the spinal cord (Fig. 41-7C) and usually is the result of a unilateral laminar or pedicle fracture, penetrating injury, or rotational injury resulting in a subluxation. It is characterized by motor weakness on the side of the lesion and the contralateral loss of pain and temperature sensation. Prognosis for recovery is good, with significant neurologic improvement often occurring. Pollard and Apple noted that only central cord and Brown-Séquard syndromes were statistically associated with improved recovery at 2 years after injury.

Anterior cord syndrome usually is caused by a hyperflexion injury in which bone or disc fragments compress the anterior spinal artery and cord. It is characterized by complete motor loss and loss of pain and temperature discrimination below the level of injury. The posterior columns are spared to varying degrees (Fig. 41-7D), resulting in preservation of deep touch, position sense, and vibratory sensation.

TABLE 41-4

Function Attained After Central Cord Lesion

	ADMISSION (%)	PRESENT AT DISCHARGE (%)	FOLLOW-UP (%)
Ambulation	33.3	77	59
Hand function	26	42	56
Bladder function	17	—	53
Bowel function	9.5	—	53

Chronic sequelae of central cord damage: (1) increased spasticity and pyramidal tract involvement; (2) incidence of 23.8%; and (3) prognosis poor with progressive neurologic loss.

From Bosch A, Stauffer ES, Nickel VL: Incomplete traumatic quadriplegia: a ten-year review, JAMA 216:473, 1971.

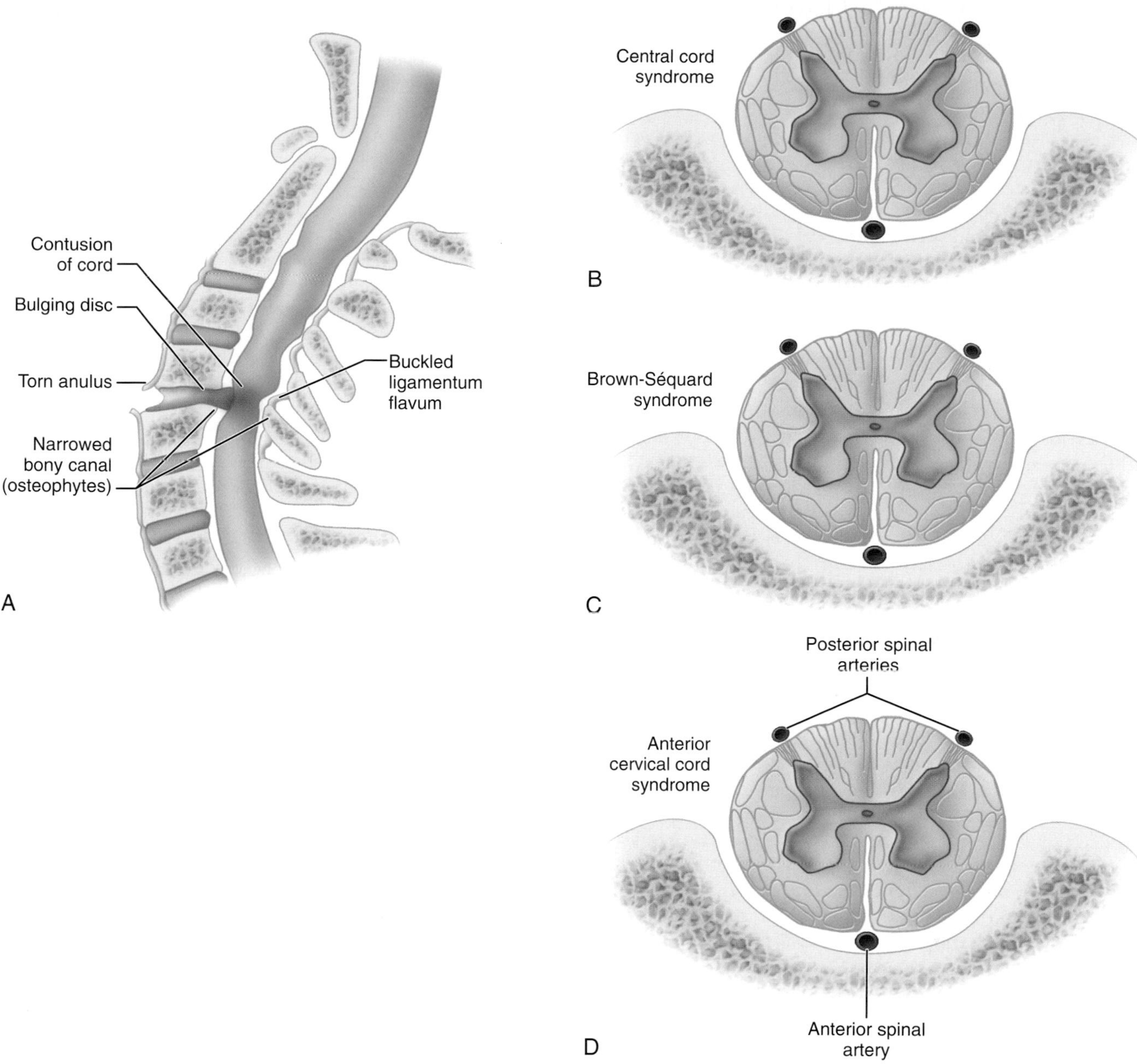

FIGURE 41-7 Spinal cord lesions. **A** and **B,** Central cord syndrome: spinal cord is pinned between vertebral body and buckling ligamentum flavum. **C,** Brown-Séquard syndrome. **D,** Anterior cervical cord syndrome.

Prognosis for significant recovery in this injury is poor. Posterior cord syndrome involves the dorsal columns of the spinal cord and produces loss of proprioception and vibratory sense while preserving other sensory and motor functions. This syndrome is rare and usually is caused by an extension injury.

Conus medullaris syndrome, or injury of the sacral cord (conus) and lumbar nerve roots within the spinal canal, usually results in areflexic bladder, bowel, and lower extremities. Most of these injuries occur between T11 and L2 and result in flaccid paralysis in the lower extremities and loss of all bladder and perianal muscle control. The irreversible nature of this injury to the sacral segments is evidenced by the persistent absence of the bulbocavernosus reflex and the perianal wink. Motor function in the lower extremities between L1 and L4 may be present if nerve root sparing occurs.

Cauda equina syndrome, or injury between the conus and the lumbosacral nerve roots within the spinal canal, also can result in an areflexic bladder, bowel, and lower limbs. With a complete cauda equina injury, all peripheral nerves to the bowel, bladder, perianal area, and lower extremities are lost and the bulbocavernosus reflex, anal wink, and all reflex activity in the lower extremities are absent, indicating absence of any function in the cauda equina. The cauda equina injuries are lower motor neuron injuries, and there is a possibility of return of function of the nerve rootlets if they have not been completely transected or destroyed. Most often, cauda equina syndrome manifests as a neurologically incomplete lesion.

CERVICAL SPINE INJURIES

HALO VEST IMMOBILIZATION AND CERVICAL ORTHOSES

Cervical immobilization is a mainstay of treatment for many cervical injuries. There is extensive clinical experience covered in the orthopaedic literature over many years regarding cervical immobilization. This literature base is mostly level III and level IV evidence studies. Unfortunately, controlled randomized prospectively collected data on specific means of immobilization for specific injuries are not available. It is unlikely such data will become available given the difficulty of devising an ethical study that could appropriately collect this information.

The first modern halo vest was developed at Ranchos Los Amigos and described by Perry and Nickels in 1959. Numerous modifications have been made to the halo vest, and other orthoses for the cervical spine have been developed. These orthoses generally have been designed to serve one of two purposes: immobilization during extrication and transport procedures or adjunctive or definitive treatment for unstable cervical injuries. The adjunctive role is either as temporary immobilization preoperatively or to provide immobilization after surgical stabilization. The goals of stable fixation and early mobilization are appropriate with spinal injuries, but often a short period of external support is recommended after surgery.

Extrication-type collars are not appropriate for treatment because they are too restrictive and would cause skin breakdown with prolonged use. They should be exchanged or removed if immobilization is not needed after initial assessment of the patient. The most commonly used types of orthoses for the cervical spine include a soft collar, a two-piece "rigid" collar, a Sternal Occipital Mandibular Immobilizer (SOMI), a Minerva (similar to a SOMI with some forehead control), and a halo vest. Several authors have compared the relative ability of these devices to limit motion in the cervical spine. Studies comparing limitation of motion in normal volunteers using devices of the same basic type usually have not found statistically significant differences between devices within the same class. These studies generally have shown progressively more limitation of motion by the orthosis type in the sequence they are listed above. These studies usually measure global motion of the cervical region and are limited in that the study participants do not have cervical injuries and as such their spinal biomechanics may be different than patients. Other authors have used cadaver models to assess the effectiveness of different orthoses in limiting motion after instability is created at a specific cervical level. Richter et al. studied an odontoid fracture model and found the halo vest to be more effective than a two-piece collar or a Minerva type brace. In another cadaver study, Horodyski et al. found that a two-piece rigid collar did not limit motion effectively after severe C5-C6 instability was created. Other studies have found atypical motion, such as "snaking," at individual levels that is caused by orthoses, especially the more restrictive types, during activities of daily living. Further studies are needed to evaluate the effect of these devices with mastication, swallowing, and oral hygiene, although these devices have been shown to affect these activities.

The halo vest has been studied more than other types of braces, and several findings have been determined. The halo vest is the most effective brace for limiting motion within the cervical spine. This appears true for the craniocervical junction, subaxial region, and cervicothoracic junction. Motion is allowed to a greater extent in the junctional areas than in the midcervical region in the halo vest. However, it is clear that motion remains throughout the cervical spine even with a halo vest properly applied. Despite this persistent motion, the halo vest has proven effective in the management of many types of cervical injuries, especially bony injuries involving the craniocervical junction. As surgical methods have improved, the halo vest has remained useful in part because for many upper cervical injuries normal motion can be preserved after fracture union. This region is responsible for a large portion of the normal cervical spine, and this motion is often permanently sacrificed with operative stabilization.

The use of halo vest immobilization does have significant associated complications. Recently, several studies have examined the morbidity and mortality associated with immobilization in a halo vest in elderly blunt trauma victims; however, no high-quality studies have prospectively evaluated this subgroup of patients. Retrospective studies in the trauma literature have noted an increased mortality rate in elderly trauma patients with cervical fractures treated with immobilization with a halo vest compared with those treated operatively or with a collar.

In institutions with higher death rates in patients with cervical spine injuries, higher rates of respiratory complications and deep vein thrombosis also were noted, suggesting that this group may not have been mobilized as well as the other subgroups evaluated. In a more thorough but still retrospective evaluation, Bransford et al. did not find an increased death rate associated with use of a halo vest. This study, which was a retrospective review of all patients at a level I trauma center for 8 years, evaluated treatment outcomes, complications, injury type, and patient age. Successful treatment was reported in 85% of patients treated with halo vest immobilization, although 11% of patients had the time in a halo vest shortened because of complications such as pin site infections. Treatment success was defined as healing of the injury in satisfactory alignment without additional intervention or secondary neurologic deterioration. The adverse events encountered in this study included death, pin site problems, pulmonary deterioration, skin breakdown, dysphagia, neurologic deterioration, and other miscellaneous complications. Twenty-two of 311 patients died after halo vest immobilization was initiated, and 19 of these deaths were within 21 days of starting halo vest immobilization. Review by a seven-member panel as to the cause of death, contributing comorbidities, and specifically whether the halo vest immobilization was a contributing cause of death was done in each case. It was determined that all 22 patients died for reasons that were not attributable to halo vest immobilization. The most common region treated with halo vest immobilization was the occiput to C2, especially odontoid fractures, although about a third of patients had subaxial injuries. Also, there were a significant proportion of study patients with more than one injury.

Complications of halo vest immobilization are frequent, with some studies having complication rates as high as 59%, although most studies identify complications in about 35% of patients. The most common type of complications involve pin site infection or loosening, which account for about 40% of all complications. Most pin site infections respond well to oral antibiotics if started early. Local pin cleaning daily and close follow-up of these patients allow early detection of these problems. Occasionally, infections are more serious and require pin site change or early discontinuation of halo vest immobilization. The most serious infections, which rarely occur, can lead to intracranial abscess requiring debridement and possibly result in death. Other less common pin-related complications include dural penetration, loosening without infection, or even skull fracture at or near the pin site. Another common complication of halo vest immobilization is failure to maintain adequate fracture reduction and spinal alignment. Rates of persistent instability with halo vest immobilization are 30% to 35% in most series. Most of these complications are detected in the first 7 to 10 days if radiographic imaging at the time halo vest immobilization is started is compared with imaging obtained after mobilization has been accomplished. Conversion to an alternative treatment may be necessary if alignment is not maintained because of the increased probability of nonunion. Nonunion detected after adequate halo vest immobilization for 12 to 16 weeks also may require surgical stabilization. Neurologic deterioration secondary to persistent instability also is a concern, although this is not common with halo vest immobilization. More serious complications, such as pneumonia or respiratory insufficiency, can occur but most often are related to inadequate mobilization of the patient. If a determination is made that adequate stability will not be attained with halo vest immobilization to allow mobilization to the full extent that the patient's other injuries would allow, then other treatment should be undertaken if possible. In this way, most of the serious complications can be avoided. Most of the later but less serious complications related to the pins are avoided by using care in applying the halo vest immobilization and by having appropriate follow-up.

HALO VEST APPLICATION

There are a variety of halo vest designs available. We typically have used a graphite horseshoe ring and four titanium pins. In patients younger than the age of 10 years, either six or eight pins may be used (see Chapter 43). Proper sizing and location of the ring are important to reduce pin loosening or ring migration. The ring selected should be the smallest diameter that can be placed below the equator of the cranium and allow at least 1 cm of clearance circumferentially. A larger ring that is farther from the bone will increase motion at the pin-bone interface, as occurs with other external fixation components when placed farther from the bone. Planned pin locations also must be carefully evaluated on CT for possible fracture.

TECHNIQUE 41-3

- Select the smallest ring that allows at least 1 cm skin clearance when placed below the largest diameter of the skull.
- The anterior pins should be above the lateral third of the eyebrow. This position avoids the supraorbital and supratrochlear nerves and the temporalis muscle. The posterior pins usually are slightly lower than the anterior pins and posterior to the ear (Fig. 41-8).
- Position the posterior piece of the vest under the patient so that the shoulder strap is properly located.
- Shave hair if needed and cleanse each pin site with antiseptic solution three times.
- Using the ring positioning pins, set the ring position and have an assistant hold the ring in this position.
- Place a needle through the pin location in the ring to be used and inject 0.5 mL of local anesthetic subperiosteally. Avoid raising a large skin wheal when injecting because this leads to traction on the skin after pin placement.
- Have the patient gently close his eyes and maintain this during ring placement to make sure the upper lids can be closed after placement of the pins.
- Place each pin down to the skin surface.
- Tighten by hand one opposing pair of pins (e.g., right anterior with left posterior) one full turn and then tighten the other pair; repeat until all pins are as tight as possible by hand. This avoids translating the ring in one direction while tightening the pins.
- Using a torque-limiting screwdriver set at 8 in/lb, tighten the pins in a figure-of-eight sequence one full rotation each until all four are at 8 in/lb. Lower torque will increase pin loosening, and higher torque increases the risk of skull penetration.
- Securely tighten the locking nut on each pin.
- Apply the anterior vest piece and secure the shoulder and abdominal straps.
- Engage the four supports from the vest into the ring and adjust the position to allow unrestricted movement of the xiphoid hinge if necessary. Tighten all set screws to the manufacturer's suggested torque.
- Radiographically verify that the fracture reduction and spinal alignment are acceptable.
- In 24 hours, retighten the pins to 8 in/lb of torque.
- Begin daily pin cleaning with H_2O_2 or povidone-iodine solution.

POSTOPERATIVE CARE. Daily pin cleaning is continued and, depending on how active the patient is, the superstructure of the halo vest is tightened every 2 to 4 weeks. The patient is mobilized as completely as the noncervical injuries will allow, and the cervical spine is imaged to verify that fracture reduction and overall alignment are stable. After the period of halo vest immobilization is completed and the pins are removed, the pin sites should be cleaned. Manually mobilizing the skin to prevent scar tethering to the periosteum allows for more normal facial expression and less noticeable scars.

RADIOGRAPHIC EVALUATION PROTOCOL

The helical CT scan is the imaging modality of choice for the diagnosis of cervical fractures and dislocations. Axial images, sagittal reconstructions, and coronal plane reconstructions each provide optimal visualization for particular injuries.

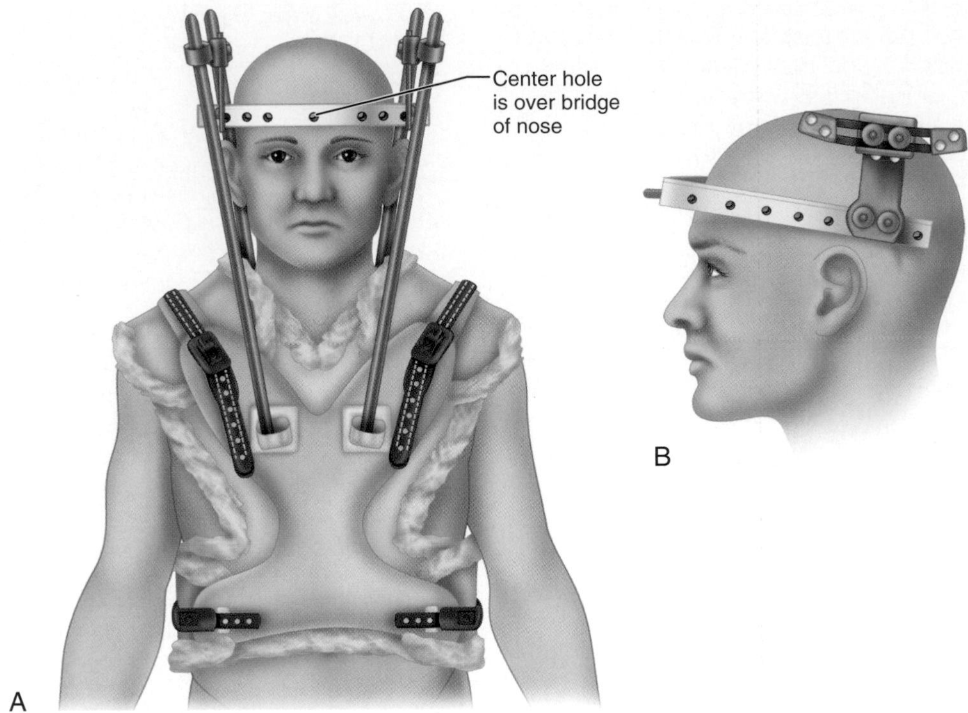

FIGURE 41-8 When applying halo ring, pin sites should be 1 cm above lateral one third of eyebrows and same distance above tops of ears in occipital area (mastoid area). **SEE TECHNIQUE 41-3.**

Having a systematic and methodical routine for viewing these series is required to detect injuries. Beginning with the sagittal reconstructions, three images are of particular value. These are the midline image and each of the parasagittal plane images through the occipital condyle-C1 joint and the facet joints on each side. These parasagittal images should be evaluated specifically for (1) congruity of the occipital condyle-C1 joint, which should be concentric and should not be more than 2 mm wide laterally; (2) intact isthmus at the C2 level; and (3) a normal relationship at each facet joint and intact lateral masses. The midline image should be evaluated specifically for (1) relation of the Wackenheim line to the dens (normally tangential to the posterior aspect of the dens); (2) widening of the atlantodens interval (normal < 3 mm; abnormal > 5 mm); (3) soft-tissue swelling at the C3 midbody (normal < 5 mm); (4) bony integrity of the dens; (5) anterior vertebral body alignment; (6) posterior vertebral body alignment; (7) alignment of the spinolaminar line; and (8) assessment for excess angulation or widening of each disc space.

The coronal reconstructions are best for evaluating the occiput-C1 joints, the C1-C2 joints, and the bony integrity of the dens.

The continuity of the posterior bony arch at each cervical level and the occiput is best determined on the axial images. Fractures involving the body, pedicle, foramen transversarium, lateral mass, lamina, and spinous process can be seen at individual levels (Fig. 41-9).

OCCIPITOCERVICAL DISSOCIATION INJURY PATTERNS

Injuries to the craniocervical junction can occur at a variety of locations. Atlantooccipital dislocations, C1-C2 dislocations, or combinations of fractures and dislocations involving the occiput, atlas, and the axis can disrupt the tectorial membrane, alar and apical ligaments, transverse atlantal ligament, and joint capsules at occiput-C1 or C1-C2. Some injuries such as fracture of the occipital condyle or isolated joint capsule injuries may be stable. However, these injuries may occur as components of a more complex injury with occipital cervical instability, which can be fatal if not treated. Often these injuries result in fatalities before the patient is transported. The diagnosis of craniocervical junction injuries requires awareness of and suspicion for the expected injury patterns. The presence of cranial nerve (CN) VI, CN X, or CN XII palsies, subarachnoid hemorrhage at the craniovertebral junction, or soft-tissue swelling anterior to the upper cervical spine should increase suspicion of a craniovertebral injury. More severe deficits, including monoparesis, hemiparesis, quadriparesis, apnea, or other high cord symptoms, also have been reported with these injuries. Careful evaluation of the CT images, particularly the reconstruction images, is needed because these injuries often are dislocations and only the relative position of one bony structure to another may be abnormal without the presence of a fracture. Atlantooccipital dislocation has become recognized more frequently as awareness of the injury has increased and initial patient care has improved. The best method for the diagnosis of atlantooccipital dislocation has not been definitively determined. Older methods based on lateral radiographs such as the Power's ratio (basion to posterior arch distance/opisthion to anterior arch distance) and the basion atlas interval/basion dens interval (BAI-BDI) have been described (Fig. 41-10). The BAI/BDI method as described by Harris et al. is the most reliable method using lateral radiographs. With the use of

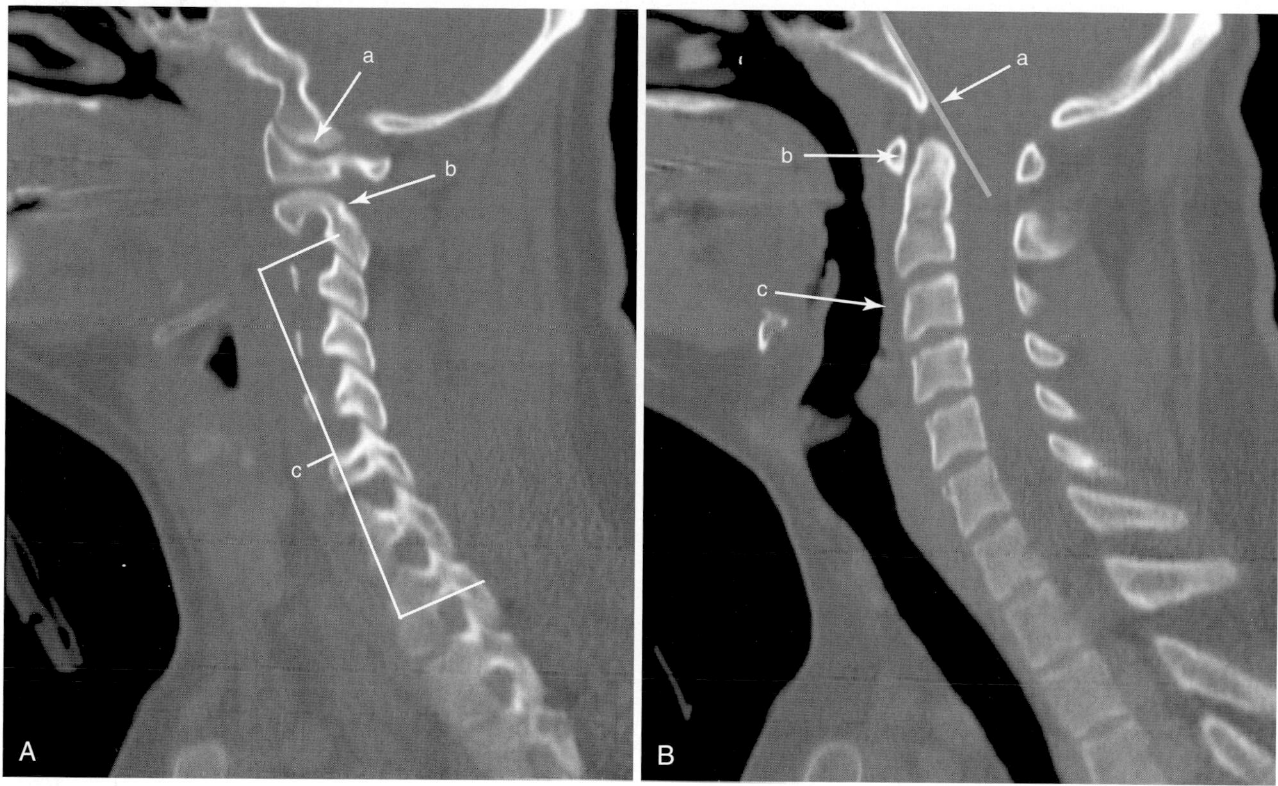

FIGURE 41-9 **A,** *Arrow a* indicates normal occiput-C1 joint congruity. *Arrow b* indicates intact C2 isthmus. *Bracket c* indicates normal facet relationships throughout the cervical spine. **B,** *Arrow a* indicates Wackenheim line with normal relationship between clivus and posterior dens. *Arrow b* indicates atlantodens interval, which is normal in width. *Arrow c* indicates normal soft-tissue density width less than 5 mm at C3 midbody.

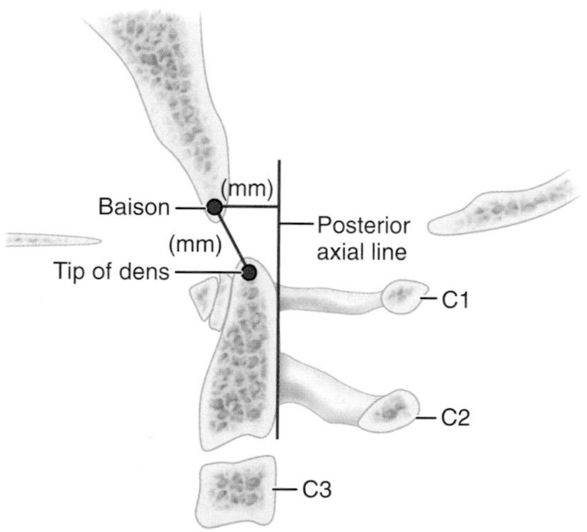

FIGURE 41-10 Measurement technique for the basion dens interval and basion-axial interval described by Harris et al.

helical CT scans, more detailed analysis of the bony relationships is possible. The method that we have used to diagnose the presence of atlantooccipital dislocation is to evaluate each of the occipital condyle-C1 joints for congruity and concentricity. If both joints are normal, there is no atlantooccipital dislocation. In addition, the relationship of the Wackenheim line to the dens is evaluated. If this relationship also is normal, there is no distraction injury between C1 and C2. The most commonly used classification system for atlantooccipital dislocation is the Traynelis system, which is described by direction of displacement, but it lacks treatment guidance. The Traynelis classification includes type I (anterior); type II (longitudinal); type III (posterior); and "other," which includes lateral or multidirectional displacement. Review of the literature revealed that patients with occipitocervical displacement who were not initially diagnosed had neurologic worsening 73% of the time before the diagnosis was recognized and about half did not improve even to their baseline neurologic examination after treatment. Ten percent of patients placed in traction had neurologic worsening in a small number of reported cases. Also, patients treated definitively with external immobilization excluding traction had a 40% rate of neurologic worsening that necessitated stabilization. Another 27% who did not worsen neurologically failed to achieve stability even after up to 22 weeks of immobilization. Patients treated with halo vest immobilization temporarily while awaiting operative stabilization had 0% neurologic worsening preoperatively. This evidence is level III but has led us to recommend operative stabilization for all patients with occipitocervical dislocations. Initial management is in a halo vest to provide provisional stabilization until the patient can undergo posterior occipitocervical fusion. Traction is not used under usual circumstances. Typically, fusion is from the occiput to C2 or C3, with multiple points of skull fixation and C1 lateral mass screws, C2 isthmus screws, and, when needed, C3 or lower lateral mass screws with autologous bone grafting. Some injuries to individual craniocervical structures without dislocation can be treated without operative stabilization.

OCCIPITOCERVICAL FUSION USING MODULAR PLATE AND ROD CONSTRUCT, SEGMENTAL FIXATION WITH OCCIPITAL PLATING, C1 LATERAL MASS SCREW, C2 ISTHMIC (PARS) SCREWS, AND LATERAL MASS FIXATION

The preferred method of occiput to cervical fusion uses a modular plate and rod system that incorporates multiple skull fixation points and multiple fixation points to the upper cervical spine. If the injury is soft tissue only at the occiput-C1 level, the construct usually can stop at the C2 level. If fixation is compromised by injury at the C1 or C2 level, fixation should be extended caudally to C3 or lower depending on the injury pattern.

The awake patient is moved to the turning frame and placed supine. General anesthesia is initiated as is neuromonitoring for appropriate patients. Typically, the patient will be in a halo vest on arrival to the operating room. A Mayfield head positioner is directly attached to the halo ring, and the anterior vest and supports are removed. If the patient is not in a halo vest, the Mayfield pinion head holder is used. After turning the bed, the posterior portion of the vest is removed. Fluoroscopic images are obtained to verify reduction of the injury and to make sure the position of the head is satisfactory for fusion. A position of slight occipitocervical flexion is preferred to allow the patient to potentially ambulate and perform daily activities with less difficulty (Fig. 41-11).

TECHNIQUE 41-4

- Shave the head several centimeters above the inion (posterior occipital protuberance).
- Prepare and drape the posterior head and neck, as well as the posterior iliac crest donor site.
- Score the skin sharply from the inion to the planned caudal level and inject dilute epinephrine solution (1 mg in 500 mL normal saline) through the score incision into the dermis and paraspinal musculature.
- Complete the skin incision sharply and then use electrocautery to dissect to the skull and spinous processes to at least the C3 level (if construct is planned to C2 level).
- Using Cobb elevators and electrocautery, subperiosteally expose the occiput from the inion to the foramen magnum.
- Expose the posterior ring of C1 laterally a distance of 15 mm from the midline or to the vertebral artery sulcus, whichever is less. Take care to keep the electrocautery on the ring of C1 and do not cauterize the atlantooccipital membrane, which is thin.
- Expose the bifid portion of the C2 spinous process and elevate the muscular attachments subperiosteally so that at closure the two sides can be sutured through bone to the spinous process of C2.
- Expose the spinous process, laminae, and entire lateral mass bilaterally at each level as needed, preserving the facet capsule at levels not to be included in the fusion.
- The C2 spinal nerve (greater occipital nerve) crosses posterior to the C2 isthmus in a dense venous plexus. Using bipolar cautery and a Penfield No. 4 elevator, gently mobilize this plexus cephalad, beginning at the upper lateral margin of the C2 lamina until the medial border of the C2 isthmus is visible. Expect bleeding during this step and control it with bipolar cautery, Gelfoam or Surgicel, and cottonoids.
- In a similar fashion, expose only the caudal edge of the ring of C1 laterally to a point even with the C2 isthmus and mobilize the venous plexus and C2 nerve caudally to allow exposure of the C1 lateral mass inferior to the posterior ring and vertebral artery.
- Using an image intensifier, verify that cervical alignment and injury reduction are satisfactory.
- The C1 screw is placed as described by Harms and Melcher. Using a hand drill placed just caudal to the ring of C1 and 3 to 4 mm lateral to the medial edge of the lateral mass, advance the drill at an angle of 10 degrees medially and slightly cephalad to a point just posterior to the anterior margin of the dens on a lateral image intensifier view. This allows for unicortical screw placement and lowers the risk of injury to the internal carotid artery and hypoglossal nerve anterior to the C1 lateral mass.
- Place a polyaxial screw with a 10-mm smooth shank extension to the drilled depth.
- Place the C2 isthmic screw in a method similar to that described by Magerl and Seeman (see Technique 41-9). Place a Penfield No. 4 elevator to palpate and if possible view the isthmus medial cortex and determine the line of entry points on the inferior facet of C2 that will allow the medially directed drill to enter the isthmus. Using the lateral image intensifier view, select the point on this line that will orient the drill up the center of the isthmus. Use a high-speed burr to penetrate only the cortex at that point. Typically, the drill will be directed 25 degrees medially and 20 to 30 degrees cephalad, but anatomy varies considerably and careful review of the CT scan is required. Direct the hand drill up the isthmus under fluoroscopic control to a point at the posterior margin of the C2 foramen transversarium as seen on the lateral image intensifier view.
- Place the appropriate length polyaxial screw to stop at the posterior foramen transversarium. In our experience this provides excellent fixation without placing the vertebral artery at risk by crossing the foramen transversarium into the C2 body.
- If additional lateral mass screws are to be used, they are placed using Anderson's modification of the technique of Magerl. Identify the four boundaries of the lateral mass and determine the geometric center of the rectangle defined by these boundaries. Penetrate the cortex 1 mm medial to the center point using a high-speed burr. Using this starting point, orient the hand drill laterally and cephalad by resting the drill sleeve at the margin of the tip of the spinous process of the next most caudal level (C4

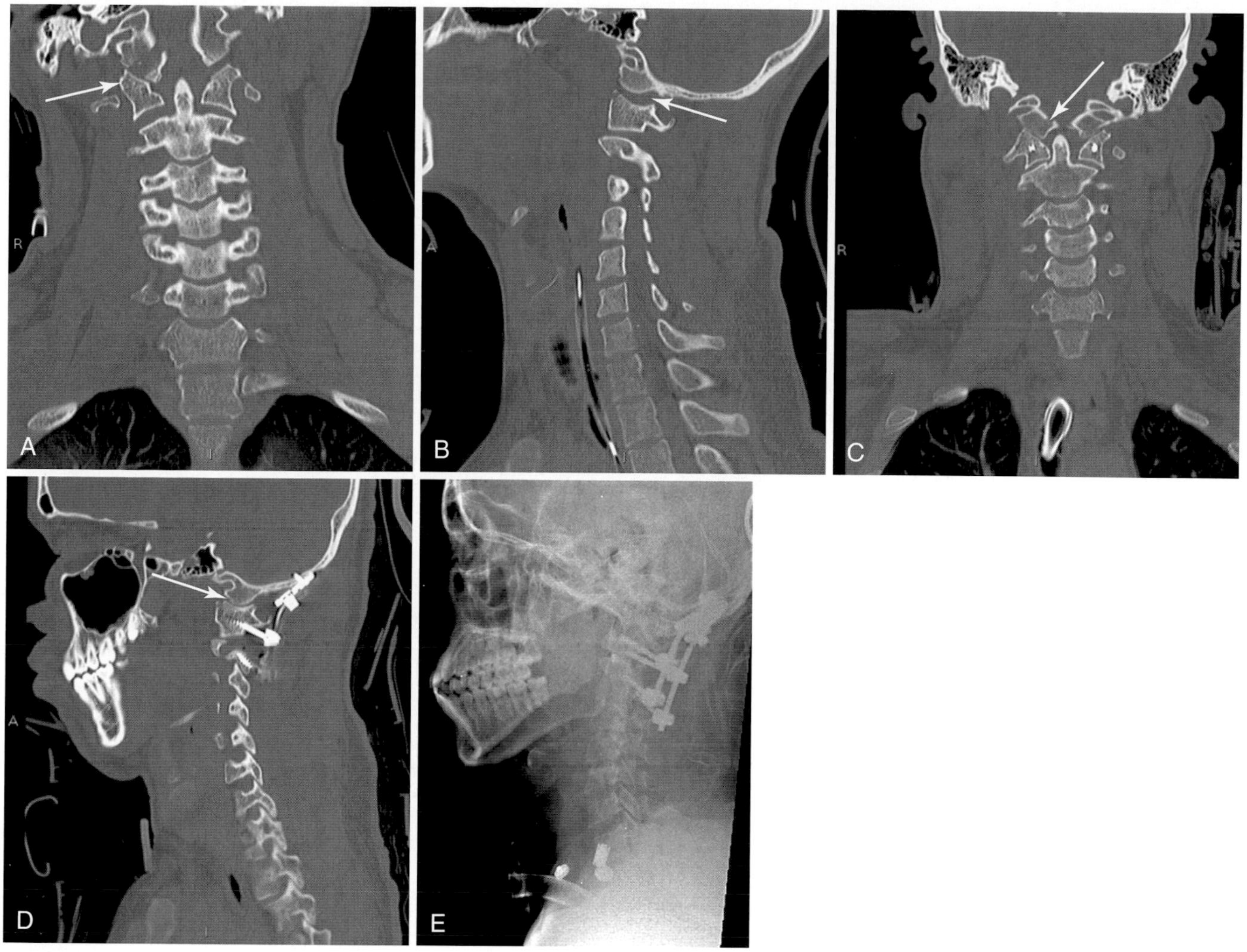

FIGURE 41-11 **A,** *Arrow* indicates fracture of right occipital condyle in patient with occipital-cervical dissociation injury. **B,** *Arrow* indicates widened and incongruous occipital condyle-C1 joint. **C,** *Arrow* indicates the right occipital condyle fracture has been reduced. *Arrow* indicates the left occipital condyle-C1 joint is congruous. **D,** Anatomic alignment with fixation to the skull, C1 lateral mass, and C2 isthmus. **E,** Lateral radiograph of occipitocervical plate-rod construct. **SEE TECHNIQUE 41-4.**

spinous process for a C3 screw). Incrementally advance the drill until the far cortex is breached and the appropriate length screw is placed bicortically. Unicortical 14-mm screws have been shown to provide satisfactory fixation and can be used if desired.

- After placement of these screws, the rod position at the skull can be determined. Some modular systems allow for either a single midline plate or two unilateral plates to be used. The occipital bone is thicker along the midline ridge, and screw purchase is enhanced if this bone can be used. However, if the midline plate does not align well with the screws as placed, bilateral plates are preferred. If two plates will be used, contour and place them to engage the thickest bone possible.
- For each occipital screw placed through the plate, use a hand drill for bicortical screw placement in the thinner lateral bone, which often is only 5 to 6 mm thick. Unicortical screws can be placed in the thicker midline bone.
- After affixing the plate component to the occiput, contour, cut, and connect the rod to the cervical screws and plate on each side. If two plates are used, it is often easier to attach the contoured rod to the plate. Engage the rod into the cervical screws and then place the screws through the plate after it is in position.
- Tighten all connections securely.
- Harvest iliac bone graft as described in Technique 1-8.
- Decorticate the occipital bone and the posterior elements of the exposed levels using a high-speed burr.
- Carefully place morselized autologous bone graft over the decorticated areas. Avoid packing the bone over the atlantooccipital membrane because compression here may result in apnea from brainstem compression. For this reason, final hemostasis should be meticulous.
- Check final alignment and reduction.
- Close the fascial layer over a drain back to bone when possible with particular attention to the C2 level.
- Close the wound in layers with a subcuticular skin closure.

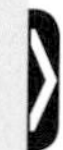

ALTERNATIVE C2 PEDICLE SCREW TECHNIQUE

A C2 pedicle screw is placed using a very similar technique to that described earlier for the isthmic screw. The primary difference is that the pedicle screw is longer and passes into the C2 body. In so doing, the course of the vertebral artery is traversed and therefore the artery is at higher risk for injury. The other difference is that with pedicle screws the trajectory is less medially oriented. Careful preoperative planning is needed because at least 8% to 10% of patients do not have anatomy that allows safe pedicle screw placement. This is especially true in women. The biomechanical advantage of the longer pedicle screw does not seem clinically important, and in general little is gained for the patient for the added risk. The isthmic screw technique is our preferred method. Several studies recently evaluated the safety and accuracy of C2 pedicle screw placement using either intraoperative CT or navigation systems, both of which were found to improve screw placement.

POSTOPERATIVE CARE. The patient is maintained in a cervical collar for 8 to 12 weeks postoperatively until healing of the fusion has progressed satisfactorily. The drain is removed on the first postoperative day.

OCCIPITOCERVICAL FUSION USING WIRES AND BONE GRAFT

TECHNIQUE 41-5

(WERTHEIM AND BOHLMAN)

- The initial positioning, induction of anesthesia, preparation, neuromonitoring, and exposure are as described in Technique 41-4.
- Use a high-speed burr to penetrate the cortex on each side of the midline ridge of bone that extends from the inion to the foramen magnum (Fig. 41-12A). Use a towel clip to form a connection between the two openings in the cortex. Take care not to penetrate the inner cortex of the occipital bone.
- Make a hole through the base of the spinous process of C2 using a towel clip or bone tenaculum.
- Pass a 20-gauge wire through, around, and back through the hole in the spinous process of C2 to encircle the caudal portion of the C2 process and a second wire through the channel in the occipital bone in similar fashion.

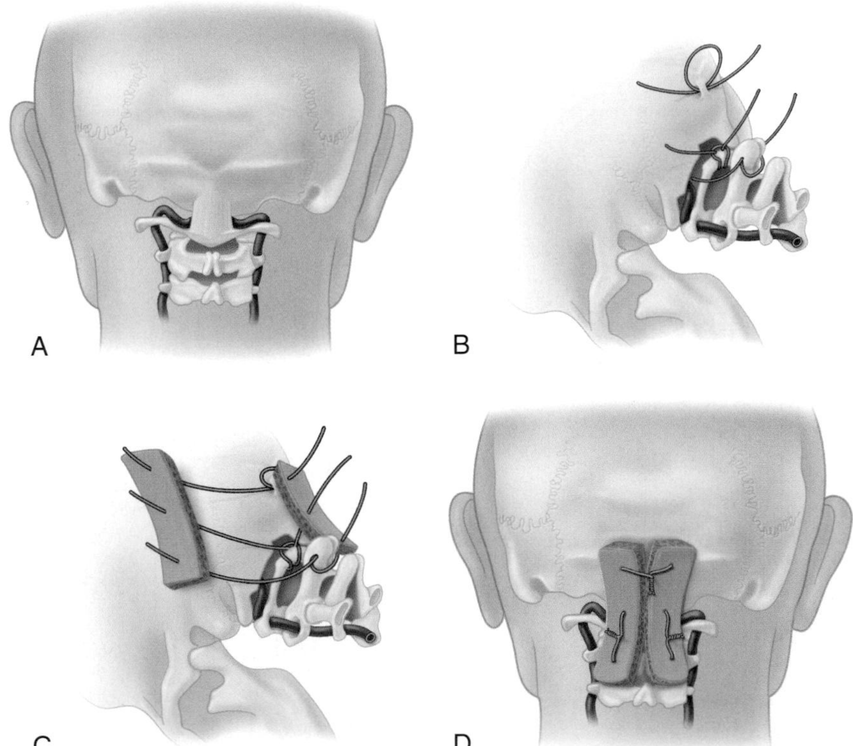

FIGURE 41-12 Wertheim and Bohlman method of occipitocervical fusion. **A,** Burr is used to create ridge in external occipital protuberance, and hole is made in ridge. **B,** Wires are passed through outer table of occiput, under arch of atlas, and through spinous process of axis. **C,** Grafts are placed on wires. **D,** Wires are tightened to secure grafts in place. **SEE TECHNIQUE 41-5.**

- Use a small angled curet to dissect the ventral side of the C1 lamina bilaterally to allow for midline sublaminar wire passage.
- Cut a 24-inch length of 20-gauge wire and bend it tightly back on itself at its midpoint. Contour the loop of wire into a "C" shape.
- Pass the loop of 20-gauge wire from caudal to rostral sublaminarly at the C1 level. Flatten the curve in the wire as needed to minimize intrusion of the wire into the spinal canal. A small blunt hook passed from the rostral side can be used to engage the loop of wire and pull the wire so that intrusion of the wire is minimized as it is advanced rostrally (Fig. 41-12B).
- Pass the free ends of the sublaminar wire through the looped portion and tighten the wire around the C1 lamina in the midline.
- Measure the distance from the occipital wire to the wire through the C2 spinous process and harvest a corticocancellous bone graft from the ilium outer table that can be divided into two 1.5-cm wide grafts that are long enough to span this distance with all wires passing through the graft.
- Decorticate the occiput and the laminae at C1 and C2 with a high-speed burr.
- Drill through each slab of bone graft to allow the wire to come through at each level (Fig. 41-12C).
- Tighten the occipital wire ends in the midline until the luster of the wire dulls slightly and turn down the cut end of the wires between the two grafts.
- Tighten the C1 and C2 wires together over the bone graft in a similar way. The grafts should be very secure (Fig. 41-12D).
- Close the fascial layer over a drain back to bone where possible with particular attention to the C2 level.
- Close the remaining wound in layers and the skin with a subcuticular closure. Reapply the halo vest.

POSTOPERATIVE CARE. Halo vest immobilization is continued until graft consolidation, which usually occurs in 12 to 16 weeks. The drain is removed on the first postoperative day.

OCCIPITAL CONDYLE FRACTURES

Fractures of the occipital condyle are recognized more often now with increased use of screening CT with reformatted images (Fig. 41-13). They occur in association with traumatic brain injuries in over half the cases, and frequently patients have additional cervical fractures. Dysfunction of cranial nerves is uncommon, but involvement of CN VI, CN IX, CN X, CN XI, and CN XII has been reported. Cranial nerve palsies most often are reported when fractures of the occipital condyle are untreated. These fractures do occur as isolated injuries but are most significant when they occur as part of a more severe craniocervical injury, such as occipital cervical dislocation. The occipital condyles articulate with the C1 lateral masses and are attached to the dens by the paired alar ligaments. The alar ligaments function to limit rotation of the occiput and atlas with respect to C2. The mechanisms for fractures of the occipital condyle usually are axial loading and lateral bending. Anderson and Montesano described the classification that is most commonly used: type I, impaction; type II, basilar skull fracture; and type III, avulsion fracture. Type I and type II fractures are stable and can be treated with a rigid orthosis or halo vest for 8 to 12 weeks. Type III fractures are potentially unstable, especially if displaced more than

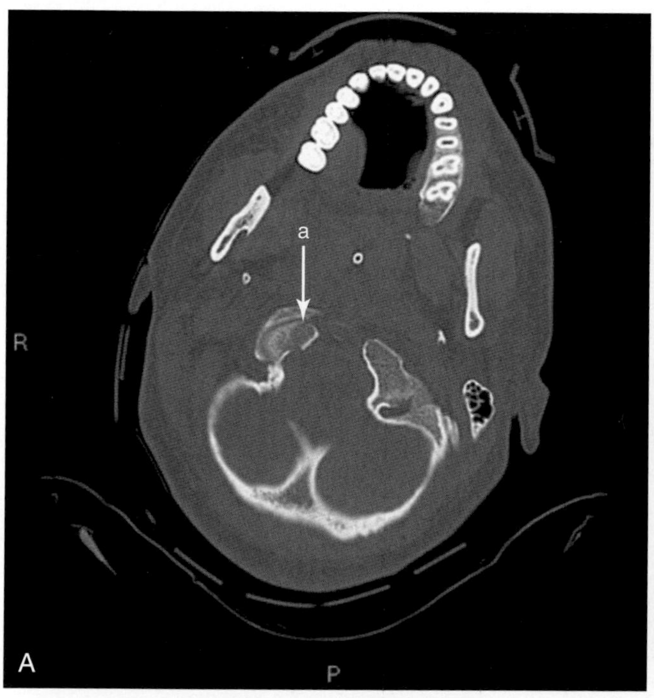

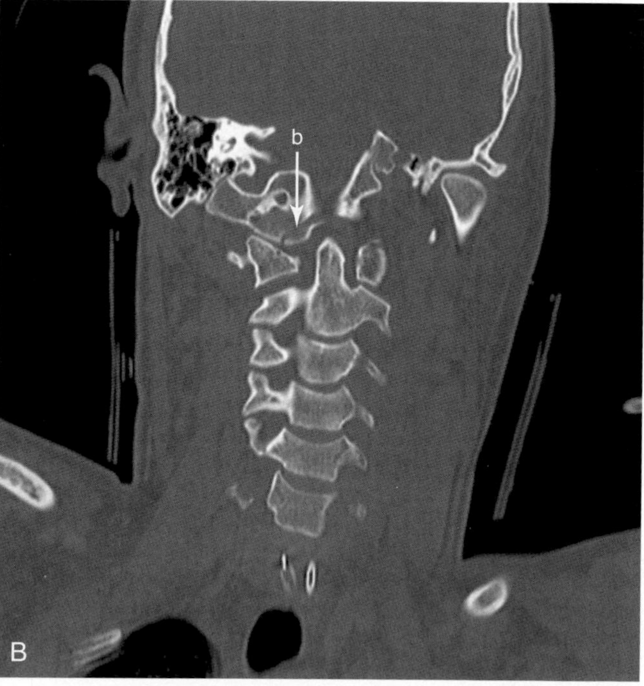

FIGURE 41-13 A and B, Right occipital condyle fracture *(arrows)*.

2 mm, because of the avulsion of the alar ligament that may be bilateral, and 12 weeks of immobilization in a halo vest is recommended. If instability persists after a period of adequate immobilization, occiput to C2 fusion may be indicated. Surgical treatment rarely is needed.

TRANSVERSE ATLANTAL LIGAMENT RUPTURE

Rupture of the transverse atlantal ligament or cruciform ligament usually occurs from a force applied to the back of the head, such as occurs in a fall. Thus, injuries involving the transverse atlantal ligament can be a purely ligamentous midsubstance tear of the ligament or can occur as the result of an avulsion of the insertion into the C1 lateral mass. Dickman et al. classified these injuries as type I, disruptions of the substance of the ligament, and type II, fractures and avulsions involving the tubercle insertion of the transverse atlantal ligament on the lateral mass of C1. Treatment is based on classification type. According to Dickman et al., type I injuries are incapable of healing without internal fixation and they should be treated with early surgery. Type II injuries, which render the transverse ligament physiologically incompetent even if the ligament substance is not torn, should be treated initially with a rigid cervical orthosis. Dickman et al. had a 74% success rate with nonoperative treatment of type II injuries, reserving surgery for patients who had a nonunion and persistent instability after 3 to 4 months of immobilization. Conversely, 26% of type II injuries in this study failed to heal after immobilization, suggesting that close follow-up is needed to determine which patients require delayed operative intervention. Usually the anterior subluxation of the ring of C1 can be detected on flexion films and the instability can be reduced in extension (Fig. 41-14). Lateral views should be checked carefully for retropharyngeal swelling, which suggests an acute injury, and for small flecks of bone avulsed off the lateral masses of C1, which may indicate avulsion of the ligament. The primary indication of this injury is instability at C1-2 on flexion and extension films. Anterior widening of the atlantodens interval of more than 3 mm on the midsagittal CT reconstruction or on a flexion view suggests that the transverse ligament is incompetent. MRI has become the standard imaging modality to evaluate the integrity of the transverse atlantal ligament. Flexion and extension views should be made under the supervision of the physician, and the patient must be monitored closely for alterations in neurologic or respiratory function. As described by Dickman et al., midsubstance injury of the transverse atlantal ligament will not heal with immobilization, and operative treatment is indicated. Posterior C1-C2 fusion using the fixation technique described by Harms and Seeman and autologous bone graft is preferred. This technique is more rigid than wiring and has the advantage over wiring methods in that it can be used in the presence of fractures of the posterior ring of C1. An alternative fixation method is the Gallie method of wiring that creates a posteriorly directed force on C1 to reduce any atlantodens interval widening (Fig. 41-14C). An intact dens will prevent overreduction of C1. A Brooks-Jenkins bone block technique should not be used because it cannot maintain the reduction as well. In 12 patients with ruptures of the transverse ligament, Levine and Edwards found an average loss of correction of 4 mm after bone block techniques and 1 mm after Gallie wiring.

POSTERIOR C1-C2 FUSION TECHNIQUES

The preferred method for C1-C2 fusion for most injuries is to use a polyaxial screw placed in the C1 lateral mass and an

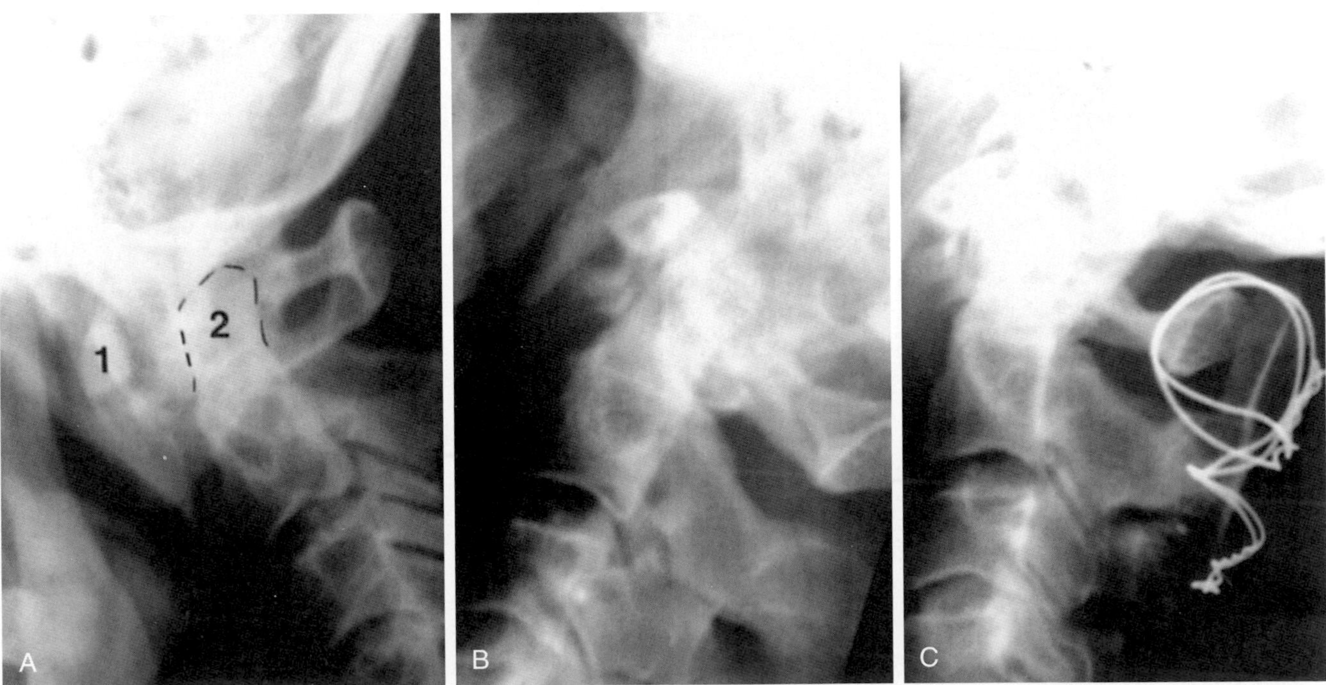

FIGURE 41-14 Patient sustained severe blow to back of head, resulting in instability of C1-2 complex because of torn transverse ligament. **A** and **B**, Note widening of atlantodens interval in flexion **(A)** and reduction in extension **(B)**. **C**, After Gallie wiring.

isthmic screw placed at C2 with autologous iliac bone graft. This is a stable construct and can be used in the presence of a posterior ring fracture of C1. Wiring techniques are less rigid but have proven effective for many years when done properly and in the appropriate setting. The Gallie technique creates a posteriorly directed force on C1 and can be used with transverse atlantal ligament injuries and other injuries that require a posterior force vector to maintain the reduction. The Gallie technique does not resist rotational forces well because the fixation is midline. The awake patient is moved to the turning frame bed in the supine position, and general anesthesia is initiated. The Mayfield pinion head holder is applied to avoid pressure on the eyes, and the patient is turned to the prone position.

POSTERIOR C1-C2 FUSION USING ROD AND SCREW CONSTRUCT WITH C1 LATERAL MASS SCREWS

TECHNIQUE 41-6

(HARMS)

- Shave the head to the level of the inion (posterior occipital protuberance).
- Prepare and drape the posterior head and neck, as well as the posterior iliac crest donor site.
- Score the skin sharply from foramen magnum to the C3 level and inject dilute epinephrine solution (1 mg in 500 mL normal saline) through the score incision into the dermis and paraspinal musculature.
- Complete the skin incision sharply and then use electrocautery to dissect to the skull and spinous processes to the C3 level.
- Using Cobb elevators and electrocautery subperiosteally, expose the occiput just above the foramen magnum bilaterally.
- Expose the posterior ring of C1 laterally a distance of 15 mm from the midline or to the vertebral artery sulcus, whichever is less. Take care to keep the electrocautery on the ring of C1 and do not cauterize the atlantooccipital membrane, which is thin.
- Expose the bifid portion of the C2 spinous process and elevate the muscular attachments subperiosteally so that at closure the two sides can be sutured through bone to the spinous process of C2.
- Expose the C2 spinous process, laminae, and entire lateral mass bilaterally, preserving the facet capsule at C2-C3.
- The C2 spinal nerve (greater occipital nerve) crosses posterior to the C2 isthmus in a dense venous plexus. Using bipolar cautery and a Penfield No. 4 elevator, gently mobilize this plexus cephalad beginning at the upper lateral margin of the C2 lamina until the medial border of the C2 isthmus is visible. Expect bleeding during this step, which can be significant and can be controlled with Gelfoam or Surgicel and cottonoids. Some authors advocate sacrificing the nerve, but in our experience this is unnecessary.
- In similar fashion, expose only the caudal edge of the ring of C1 laterally to a point even with the C2 isthmus and then mobilize the venous plexus and C2 nerve caudally to allow exposure of the C1 lateral mass inferior to the posterior ring and vertebral artery.
- Using an image intensifier, verify that injury reduction is satisfactory.
- The C1 screw is placed as described by Goel and by Harms and Melcher. Using a hand drill placed just caudal to the ring of C1 and 3 to 4 mm lateral to the medial edge of the lateral mass, advance the drill at an angle of 10 degrees medially and slightly cephalad to a point just posterior to the anterior margin of the dens on a lateral image intensifier view. This allows for unicortical screw placement and lowers the risk of injury to the internal carotid artery and hypoglossal nerve anterior to the C1 lateral mass.
- Place a polyaxial screw with a 10-mm smooth shank extension to the drilled depth.
- The C2 isthmic screw is placed in a method similar to that described by Magerl. Place a Penfield No. 4 elevator to allow a view of the isthmus medial cortex and determine the line of entry points on the inferior facet of C2 that will allow the medially directed drill to enter the isthmus. Using the lateral image intensifier view, select the point on this line that will orient the drill up the center of the isthmus. A high-speed burr is used to penetrate only the cortex at that point. Typically, the drill will be directed 25 degrees medially and 20 to 30 degrees cephalad, but anatomy varies considerably and careful review of the CT scan is required. Direct the hand drill up the isthmus under fluoroscopic control to a point at the posterior margin of the C2 foramen transversarium as seen on the lateral image intensifier view (see Technique 41-4).
- Place the appropriate length polyaxial screw to stop at the posterior foramen transversarium. In our experience, this gives excellent fixation without placing the vertebral artery at risk by crossing the foramen transversarium into the C2 body.
- Cut and contour the rod as desired. Place the rod and tighten the blocker screws securely.
- Harvest iliac bone graft as described in Technique 1-8.
- Decorticate the laminae of C1 and C2 using a high-speed burr.
- Carefully place morselized autologous bone graft over the decorticated areas. Avoid packing the bone over the atlantooccipital membrane because compression here may result in apnea from brainstem compression. For this same reason, final hemostasis should be meticulous.
- Check final alignment and reduction.
- Close the fascial layer over a drain, securely incorporating bone at the C2 spinous process level.
- Close the wound in layers with a subcuticular skin closure.

POSTOPERATIVE CARE. The patient is maintained in a rigid cervical orthosis for 8 to 12 weeks. The patient's clinical course and flexion and extension radiographs are used to verify stability and fusion progression. The drain is removed on the first postoperative day.

POSTERIOR C1-C2 FUSION USING THE MODIFIED GALLIE POSTERIOR WIRING TECHNIQUE

TECHNIQUE 41-7

(GALLIE, MODIFIED)

- Patient positioning, administration of anesthesia, preparation, and exposure are as described in Technique 41-6.
- After exposing the C2 spinous process, laminae, and entire lateral mass bilaterally, and preserving the facet capsule at C2-C3, use a small angled curet to dissect the ventral side of the C1 lamina to allow for midline sublaminar wire passage.
- Cut a 24-inch length of 20-gauge wire and bend it tightly back onto itself at its midpoint. Contour the loop of wire into a "C" shape.
- Pass the loop of 20-gauge wire from caudal to rostral sublaminarly at the C1 level. Flatten the curve in the wire as needed to minimize intrusion of the wire into the spinal canal. A small blunt hook passed from the rostral side can be used to engage the loop of wire and pull the wire so that intrusion of the wire is minimized as it is advanced rostrally. Alternatively, pass a suture to tie to the wire and use this to pull the wire rostrally.
- Pass the free ends of the sublaminar wire through the looped portion and tighten the wire around the C1 lamina in the midline at the rostral margin of the C1 ring.
- Make a hole through the base of the spinous process of C2 using a towel clip or bone tenaculum.
- Harvest a corticocancellous bone graft and notch it on one side to fit over the rostral edge of the C2 spinous process. Decorticate the C1 and C2 laminae and place the graft as an onlay type graft.
- Place one of the free ends of the wire over the graft and through the C2 spinous process and tighten to the other free wire end until the wire luster begins to change (Fig. 41-15).
- Check final alignment and reduction.
- Close the fascial layer securely over a drain, incorporating bone at the C2 spinous process level.
- Close the wound in layers with a subcuticular skin closure.

POSTOPERATIVE CARE. The patient is maintained is a halo vest for 10 to 12 weeks. The patient's clinical course and flexion and extension radiographs are used to verify stability and fusion progression. The drain is removed on the first postoperative day.

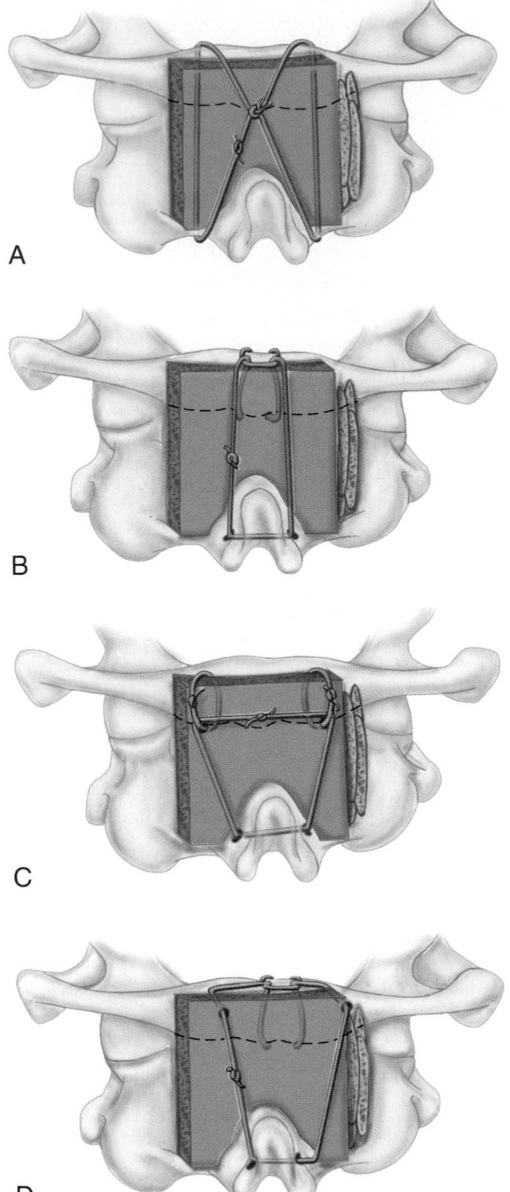

FIGURE 41-15 Modified Gallie method of using wires to hold graft in place. **A,** Wire passes under lamina of atlas and axis and is tied over graft. **B,** Wire passes under lamina of atlas and through spine of axis and is tied over graft. **C,** Wire passes through holes drilled in lamina of atlas and through spine of axis; holes are drilled through graft. **D,** Wire passes under lamina of atlas and through spine of axis; holes are drilled through graft. **SEE TECHNIQUE 41-7.**

ATLAS FRACTURES

The first description of a C1 fracture was by Cooper in 1822, and Jefferson published his case review adding four new cases in 1920. This paper contained his classification system, which has subsequently been revised by multiple authors, but his description of a burst fracture of the ring of C1 continues to carry the label of a "Jefferson fracture" (Fig. 41-16). Spence et al. published their work in 1970 on injuries to the transverse ligament in association with C1 fractures in 10 cadaver specimens. They found that if the total lateral displacement of the lateral masses was 6.9 mm or more then the transverse ligament was likely incompetent. This determination based on plain radiographs is referred to as the rule of Spence. Later, this was revised to 8.1 mm to account for magnification on plain radiographs. Dickman et al. studied 39 patients with injuries to the transverse atlantal ligament with plain radiographs, thin-cut CT, and high-resolution MRI. MRI was found to be very sensitive in detecting rupture of the transverse ligament, and their classification of these injuries was

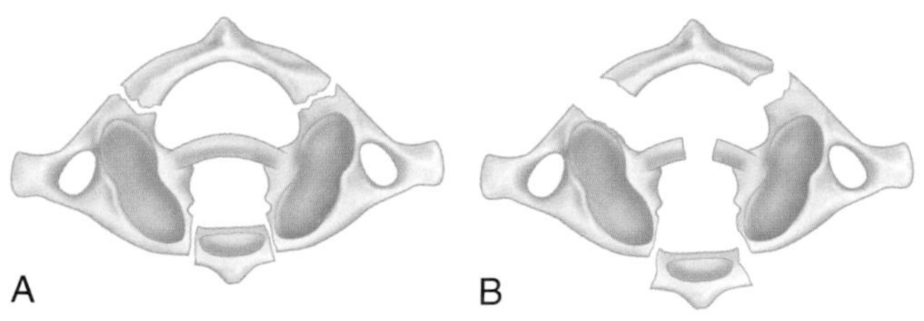

FIGURE 41-16 **A,** Axial view of stable Jefferson fracture (transverse ligament intact). **B,** Axial view of unstable Jefferson fracture (transverse ligament ruptured).

described previously. These authors found that applying the rule of Spence would have missed 61% of the transverse ligament injuries.

Biomechanical studies by Panjabi et al. and Oda et al. have shown that axial loading is the primary force that leads to C1 fractures. Because the C1 lateral masses are wedge shaped, axial loading creates a hoop stress and bone failure occurs at the weakest points that are just anterior and posterior to the lateral masses. Less force is required if the head is in extension when force is applied. Even when the transverse atlantal ligament is injured, the alar ligaments, joint capsules, and tectorial membrane are spared with axial-loading injuries. This is an important difference for transverse atlantal ligament injuries associated with C1 fractures and those associated with more complex injuries of the craniocervical junction. Landells and Van Peteghem modified Jefferson's classification into three fracture types, which is useful for treatment. Type I injuries include isolated anterior or posterior arch fractures, type II injuries involve the anterior and posterior portion of the ring, and type III injuries involve the lateral mass with or without a fracture of the ring.

TREATMENT

Treatment of atlas fractures is determined primarily by the presence or absence of associated cervical injuries. Fractures at other cervical levels occur in 30% to 70% patients with C1 fractures. By far, odontoid fractures and C2 isthmic (hangman) fractures are the most common injuries associated with C1 fractures. Landells and Van Peteghem found that type I injuries were the most common and were not associated with neurologic injuries. Our treatment regimen for isolated C1 fractures is to use a rigid collar for nondisplaced type I fractures and type III fractures of the lateral mass if the ring is not disrupted. For type I fractures with displacement, type II fractures, and type III fractures that disrupt the ring, a halo vest is used for external immobilization. Immobilization is maintained for 6 to 8 weeks if the ring is intact (some type III) and for 10 to 12 weeks if the ring is disrupted. It is rare to operatively stabilize isolated atlas fractures even if the transverse atlantal ligament is disrupted. Stability after immobilization is demonstrated on flexion-extension radiographs if the atlantodens interval is maintained at less than 3 mm. If this distance is greater than 5 mm, posterior C1-C2 fusion is recommended. The techniques are the same as described earlier for transverse atlantal ligament injuries, with some authors recommending the use of a crosslink with the screw and rod method to help maintain the C1 reduction. Appropriate external immobilization has been shown in many level III and IV studies to result in stable unions in a high percentage of patients, but outcome measures for range of motion and persistent pain have not been widely studied. Ruf et al. described a transoral technique for primary fracture stabilization without fusion, but the indication for this technique remains to be determined at this time given reliable outcomes with immobilization.

Treatment of atlas fractures that occur with ligamentous injuries or other fractures is based primarily on the concomitant injuries. The additional fractures increase the level of instability, but external immobilization with a halo vest for 12 to 16 weeks has proven sufficient in the vast majority of cases that usually involve the axis. If the halo vest does not maintain alignment sufficiently when the patient is mobilized, operative stabilization is indicated. Traction can be used to reduce the lateral mass displacement before halo vest treatment, but the halo cannot maintain the distractive force, and 3 weeks of traction may be needed to allow healing adequate to prevent loss of reduction once halo vest immobilization is initiated. Patients with disruption of the transverse atlantal ligament can have unstable injuries regardless of the type of C1 fracture; however, this injury is different from transverse atlantal ligament injuries associated with flexion or distractive mechanisms. Transverse atlantal ligament injuries from axial load mechanisms have been shown to have preservation of the joint capsules and alar ligaments. This explains why lateral mass displacement reduces with traction and why external immobilization can be successful in achieving stability when transverse atlantal ligament injuries are present by MRI in association with Jefferson fractures. The characterization of C1 fractures as "unstable" based on the presence of transverse atlantal ligament disruption is based on an oversimplification of the anatomy and may not be an adequate criterion for operative intervention.

For the rare patient who requires operative stabilization as primary treatment or after failed immobilization, posterior C1-C2 fusion is done (see Technique 41-6).

AXIS FRACTURES

The most common fractures of the axis are those involving the odontoid process. The remaining fractures are those involving the isthmus (hangman), which are the next most common fracture patterns of the axis body. Although any of these fracture types can occur with concomitant cervical injuries, they frequently occur as isolated fractures and are discussed separately. Odontoid fractures are especially common in the elderly, and in this patient group the most common mechanism is a low-energy fall.

ODONTOID FRACTURES

The classification of odontoid fractures described by Anderson and D'Alonzo in 1974 remains the most widely used system. Their scheme has three fracture types: type I, avulsion of the tip of the odontoid; type II, fracture through the base or waist of the odontoid process; and type III, originally described as fractures of the body below the base of the odontoid (Fig. 41-17). Additional fracture characteristics have been studied in numerous publications, including degree of initial fracture displacement, angulation through the fracture, patient age, fracture orientation, and smoking history of the patient. With respect to treatment outcomes, the primary factors that have been shown to be significant are fracture

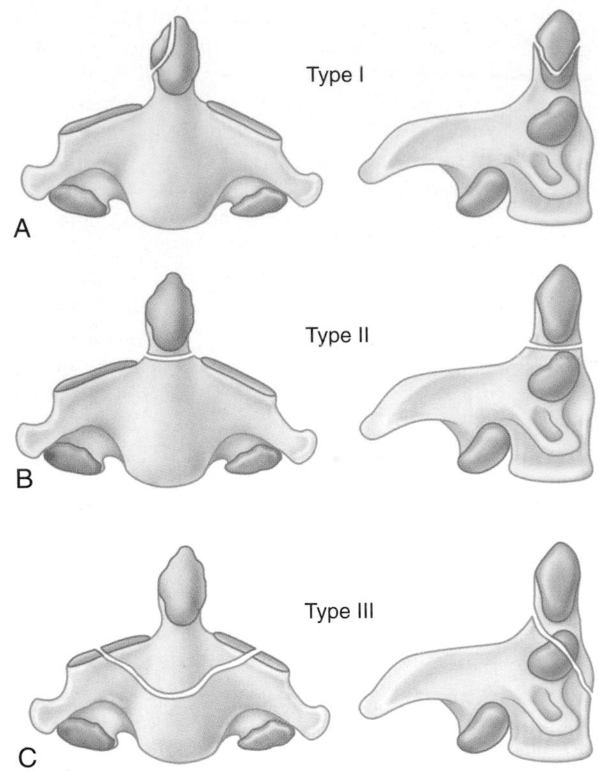

FIGURE 41-17 A-C, Three types of odontoid process fractures as seen in anteroposterior and lateral planes. Type I is oblique fracture through upper part of odontoid process. Type II is fracture at junction of odontoid process and body of second cervical vertebra. Type III is fracture through upper body of vertebra.

type, initial fracture displacement of 6 mm, and age (progressively worse outcomes are noted when patients are stratified by age).

TREATMENT

Many methods of treatment have been described for odontoid fractures, including no treatment, traction and a collar, rigid immobilization, anterior primary osteosynthesis, and posterior fusion of the C1-C2 joint. A multicenter review that included patients who did not receive treatment found that none of these patients went on to fracture union. Older literature described delayed myelopathy and death in patients with a history of untreated or nonunited odontoid fractures, indicating the importance of achieving fracture union. No level I evidence is available to make treatment recommendations; however, there is level III evidence on which treatment options can be based. Julien et al. found that type I and III fractures can be treated with rigid external immobilization such as a halo vest. One hundred percent union rates were reported for type I fractures, 65% for type II fractures, and 84% for type III fractures. Greene et al. noted an 80% union rate in type II fractures with immobilization, although in a small number the immobilization was extended beyond 13 weeks. The higher rate of success with immobilization in Greene et al.'s study may be because of early surgical treatment in 20 patients who had greater than 6 mm of displacement or more comminuted fractures that were not stable after initial halo placement. Again, this study found 100% union rates for type I fractures and 98.5% union rates for type III fractures treated with immobilization. Type III fractures treated with collars had substantially lower healing rates of 50% to 65% compared with union rates using halo vest immobilization. Collar immobilization has been found effective in type I fractures in several small series because this pattern is very infrequent.

Our treatment regimen has been to use rigid immobilization for isolated type I and type III fractures. Most often halo vest immobilization is used, but rigid collars are an option especially for the rare type I fractures. For treatment of type II fractures that are minimally displaced, immobilization is recommended because it preserves motion at the highly mobile C1-C2 joint. If anatomic reduction is achieved and there is no loss of reduction after mobilization, fracture healing with preservation of motion can be expected in 80%. All patients treated with halo vest immobilization should be aggressively mobilized and made ambulatory if at all possible, especially elderly patients. Mortality rates as high as 42% have been reported in patients with halo vest immobilization who are nonambulatory and not mobilized. Schoenfeld et al. found that the mortality was the same at various time points whether patients were treated in a collar or with halo vest immobilization, suggesting that factors other than simply treatment with halo vest immobilization result in the high mortality rates seen in elderly patients. In their study, patients with type II fractures treated operatively had lower mortality than those treated nonoperatively. Schoenfeld et al. did find a progressively higher mortality in both the operative and nonoperative treatment groups with age, and the benefits of surgery were in those age 74 years and younger. Wood et al. also found that operative benefits were greater in those under the age of 75 years. They also found that aspiration pneumonia was the most common cause of death in both operatively (55%) and nonoperatively (64%) treated patients. Vaccaro et al. showed in a level II study that neither operatively or nonoperatively treated geriatric patients returned to their preinjury functional levels. The surgically treated patients had a smaller loss than those treated nonoperatively, but the study was not randomized. We generally reserve operative treatment for type II fractures in patients in whom anatomic reduction cannot be achieved in traction or is not maintained with immobilization. Stabilization also is recommended if initial fracture translation is 6 mm or more and in patients who are not expected to be able to mobilize because of other injuries and comorbidities. Several studies have noted a trend toward operative treatment of type II fractures in the elderly in particular. This recommendation is based on level III evidence. In these patients, posterior C1-C2 fusion or anterior primary osteosynthesis may be recommended. The primary advantage of anterior fracture fixation is maintenance of motion at C1-C2, which accounts for 50% of cervical rotation, and expected acute fracture union rates of 80% to 95%. Posterior fusion of C1-C2 sacrifices this motion but can reliably achieve stability in 85% to 98% of patients and is preferred by some authors. Anterior screw fixation is not appropriate for nonunions which are treated with posterior fusion. Ni et al. described a technique of posterior instrumentation without fusion as a salvage method when anterior osteosynthesis is not possible; instrumentation is removed once fracture healing is complete. The Neck Disability Index

(NDI) scores were improved, as was range of motion after hardware removal. The C1 screw was placed using the Resnick modification for screw entry point.

ANTERIOR ODONTOID SCREW FIXATION

Anterior screw fixation can be accomplished with a single-screw or two-screw technique. Comparable union rates of 81% and 85% for the single-screw and two-screw techniques, respectively, have been reported. More important than the number of screws used is the orientation of the fracture and proper technique to achieve a lag effect. Fractures that are transverse or oblique from anterosuperior to posteroinferior are best suited for this technique because the compression from the screw(s) will be applied perpendicular to the fracture line. This technique is challenging because obtaining an anatomic reduction requires visualization on anteroposterior and lateral dual image intensifiers that are both draped into the operative field simultaneously (Fig. 41-18).

TECHNIQUE 41-8

(ETTER)

- After general endotracheal anesthesia has been induced and the patient has been positioned supine on the operating table, reduce displaced fractures in traction with either a head halter, Gardner-Wells tongs, or a halo ring.
- Anatomic reduction must be obtained before internal fixation with the cannulated screw system.
- Insert a large nasogastric tube to allow localization of the esophagus and to prevent perforation.
- Use a padded occipital ring attached to the operating table to stabilize the patient's head. The head and neck must be positioned to allow maximal access to the anterior cervical spine. A large vertical mandibular-sternal distance is required because of the size of the instrumentation and the steep inferior angle of approach necessary for screw placement. With traction applied even posteriorly displaced fractures will usually reduce in maximal cervical extension. This position improves access to the C2 level. High-resolution fluoroscopic image intensification in the anteroposterior and lateral planes is necessary for insertion of the screws. Place cotton sponges in the mouth to maximally open the jaw for an adequate open-mouth view (Fig. 41-18A).
- Before beginning the surgical procedure, confirm a free working path for the instrumentation by placing a long Kirschner wire along the side of the neck in the direction of the intended screw placement and confirm safe trajectory on the lateral image intensifier view. If clearance of the sternum is inadequate, modify the patient's position (Fig. 41-18B to D).
- Prepare and drape the operative field in a sterile fashion, with sterile draping of both the image intensifiers.
- Make an anteromedial approach to the cervical spine through a transverse skin incision 6 to 7 cm long at the level of the C5-6 disc space as determined using the Kirschner wire.
- Because of the steep angle of inclination required relative to the anterior plane of the neck, undermine the skin deep to the subcutaneous adipose layer and split the platysma muscle longitudinally in line with its fibers 2 to 3 cm lateral to the midline.
- Bluntly dissect the pretrachial fascia and develop an interval between the carotid sheath laterally and the strap muscles overlying the trachea and esophagus medially.
- Bluntly develop the prevertebral space anteriorly along the front of the cervical spine until the anteroinferior margin of the C2 body is reached.
- Place a radiolucent retractor on the anterior body of C2, gently retracting the trachea and esophagus to allow direct visualization of the C2 disc. Delineate the C2-3 intervertebral disc space and vertically incise the anterior longitudinal ligament at this level, confirming the desired entry point on the anteroposterior view for the screw(s). Ligation of the superior thyroid artery may be necessary for exposure of the C2-3 level.
- Identify with lateral image intensification the entry site through the C2 endplate and *not* through the body at the anterior margin just proximal to the endplate (Fig. 41-18E).
- Using a long drill sleeve, insert one or two 1.2-mm Kirschner wires. If one screw is planned it should be placed midline on the anteroposterior view. If using two screws, the guidewires should converge slightly but remain separated enough to allow both to fully penetrate the tip of the odontoid. On the lateral view, wire entry is at the anterior edge of the endplate and oriented to exit just posterior to the tip of the odontoid. Check advancement of the wire frequently to confirm proper trajectory. Redirecting these wires after incorrect placement is difficult.
- Verify penetration of the dens cortex and appropriate wire alignment by image intensification in two planes.
- Measure directly the guidewire insertion depth. Insert the cannulated drill bit for the cannulated 3.5-mm screw over each guidewire and drill the length of the wire to penetrate the tip of the odontoid. Monitor frequently on image intensifier views to avoid advancing the guidewire toward the brainstem. Also make certain the drill is perfectly aligned in both planes with the wire to avoid wire fracture attributed to binding within the bone.
- Insert self-tapping 3.5-mm screws of appropriate length over each guidewire and advance them with the cannulated screwdriver until the opposing apical cortical bone is secured again, using image intensifier views to make sure not to advance the wire as the screw advances, which occurs easily after drilling (Fig. 41-18F).
- The screw heads tend to encroach on the anterior margin of the C2-3 intervertebral disc, frequently requiring removal of a small amount of annulus to create a recess. Ideally, the screw heads are recessed into the disc space just inferior to the endplate.
- Always use tissue protection guards during drilling to avoid damage to soft-tissue structures.
- Close the platysma and remaining layers over a fluted style drain, which is removed the following day.

POSTOPERATIVE CARE. The patient is observed closely for respiratory status in the intensive care unit for the first

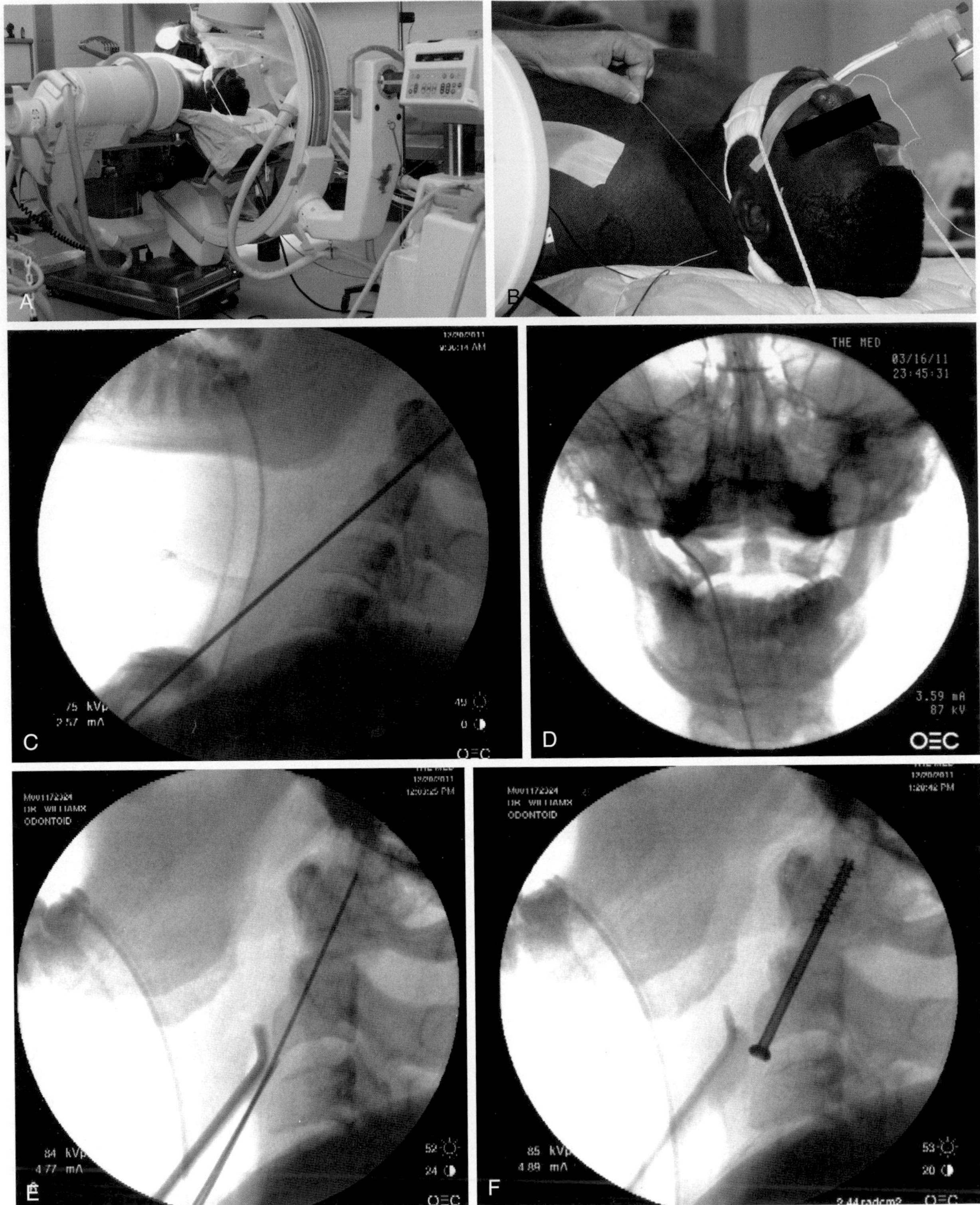

FIGURE 41-18 Odontoid fracture. **A,** Patient positioned with traction applied and image intensifiers for open-mouth and lateral images in position. **B,** Wire held in place while lateral view is obtained to indicate level of incision placement. **C,** Image with wire held in place. **D,** Open-mouth view. **E,** Lateral view after placement of first guidewire. **F,** Bicortical screw placement. **SEE TECHNIQUE 41-8.**

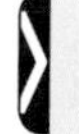

24 hours after surgery. A rigid cervical orthosis is applied and is worn for 6 to 8 weeks. The orthosis may be removed for eating. Clinical and radiographic evaluations are performed at 6, 12, and 24 weeks.

POSTERIOR STABILIZATION

The criteria for posterior stabilization are the same as for anterior fixation and are based primarily on retrospective series. Posterior fixation using one of several techniques generally offers biomechanical advantages over anterior fixation but does not allow for preservation of motion at the C1-C2 joint, which is a significant morbidity. Posterior C1-C2 fusion using the rod and screw technique popularized by Harms (see Technique 41-6) is the method usually preferred, using C2 isthmic screws rather than C2 pedicle screws in most cases. Other techniques have been described and are of use in treating odontoid fractures. Other techniques that can be useful are C1-C2 transarticular screw fixation and C1-C2 translaminar screw fixation. C1-C2 transarticular screw fixation as described by Magerl and Seemann preceded the Harms method and provides more rigid fixation than traditional posterior wiring methods, such as the Gallie or Brooks-Jenkins method. Transarticular screw placement is technically difficult, and there are clearly some patients who cannot be treated with this method because of anatomic constraints that are present in as many as 23% of patients. A properly placed transarticular screw passes through the C2 isthmus and crosses the C1-C2 facet joint and into the anterior portion of the C1 lateral mass (Fig. 41-19). Careful review of the C2 anatomy is required because in some people the vertebral artery is too medial to allow screw placement or the isthmus is too small to accept the screw. Other structures at risk include the internal carotid artery and hypoglossal nerve, which typically lie less than 3 mm anterior to the C1 lateral mass and can be injured if the screw is too long. Additionally, the patient's body habitus can make the necessary approach angle difficult if there is excessive cervicothoracic kyphosis.

POSTERIOR FUSION OF C1-C2

The Harms method (see Technique 41-6) usually is preferred because anatomic limitations are uncommon at C1 and the C2 isthmic screw orientation can vary to accommodate the patient's anatomy.

POSTERIOR C1-C2 TRANSARTICULAR SCREWS

TECHNIQUE 41-9

(MAGERL AND SEEMANN)

- Careful preoperative planning is needed to assess safety of screw placement.
- Patient preparation, positioning, and administration of anesthesia are as described in Technique 41-6.
- Use lateral image intensification to check the reduction of the C1-C2 complex.
- Perform midline posterior cervical exposure in the routine fashion from C2 to C3. The exposure should be to the lateral edge of the C2 lateral mass.
- Expose the medial wall of the isthmus up to the C1-C2 joint. If possible, curet or burr the joint. The area around the greater occipital nerve is highly vascular.
- Place intraarticular bone graft.
- Identify the landmarks for the entry portal of the transarticular screw at the lower medial edge of the inferior articular process of C2 (Fig. 41-20A). Determine the proper trajectory of the screw and make a stab incision in the skin if needed to attain the correct trajectory, which may be at C7.
- Using a 2-mm bit, incrementally drill through the isthmus near its posteromedial surface, exiting from the articular surface of C2 at the posterior aspect of the superior articular surface and entering the lateral mass of the atlas. If the isthmus is oriented too medially, the exiting drill will miss the C1 lateral mass or the drill will exit the isthmus laterally and risk injuring the vertebral artery. The drill bit should just perforate the anterior cortex of the lateral mass of C1 (Fig. 41-20B).
- Determine the appropriate screw length (Fig. 41-20C). Use a 3.5-mm cortical tap to cut threads in the drill hole and insert the appropriate 3.5-mm cortical screw across the C1-2 joint. Typically, screws are 34 to 43 mm in length. Take care not to extend more than 1 mm anterior to the C1 lateral mass. Cannulated screws can be used.
- After placing the C1-2 transarticular screws, perform a traditional posterior C1-2 fusion using either the Gallie or the Brooks technique if intraarticular grafting was not possible (Fig. 41-20D).
- Close the wound in layers over a drain, taking care to reattach the fascia to bone at the C2 level. Use a subcuticular skin closure.

POSTOPERATIVE CARE. Because this technique provides excellent rotational stability, postoperative immobilization with a halo vest usually is unnecessary. A cervical collar may be worn for 8 to 12 weeks. The drain is removed on the first postoperative day.

POSTERIOR C1-C2 FUSION WITH C2 TRANSLAMINAR SCREWS

This technique was described in 2004 as an alternative technique with less risk for vertebral artery injury, although there are other risks such as dural or spinal cord injuries. When the procedure is done properly, these are small risks. The technique employs two screws inserted through the base of the C2 spinous process and contained within the lamina on the contralateral side. The screws must be placed with one slightly more caudal on one side and directed cephalad at a steeper angle than the other screw. The translaminar screws are then connected to the C1 lateral mass screws. Biomechanically, this method has equivalence to the Harms technique for C1-C2 fusion but not for occiput-C2 fusion. If the construct is to extend below C2, rod contouring can be problematic because the translaminar screws are not aligned with the lateral mass screws.

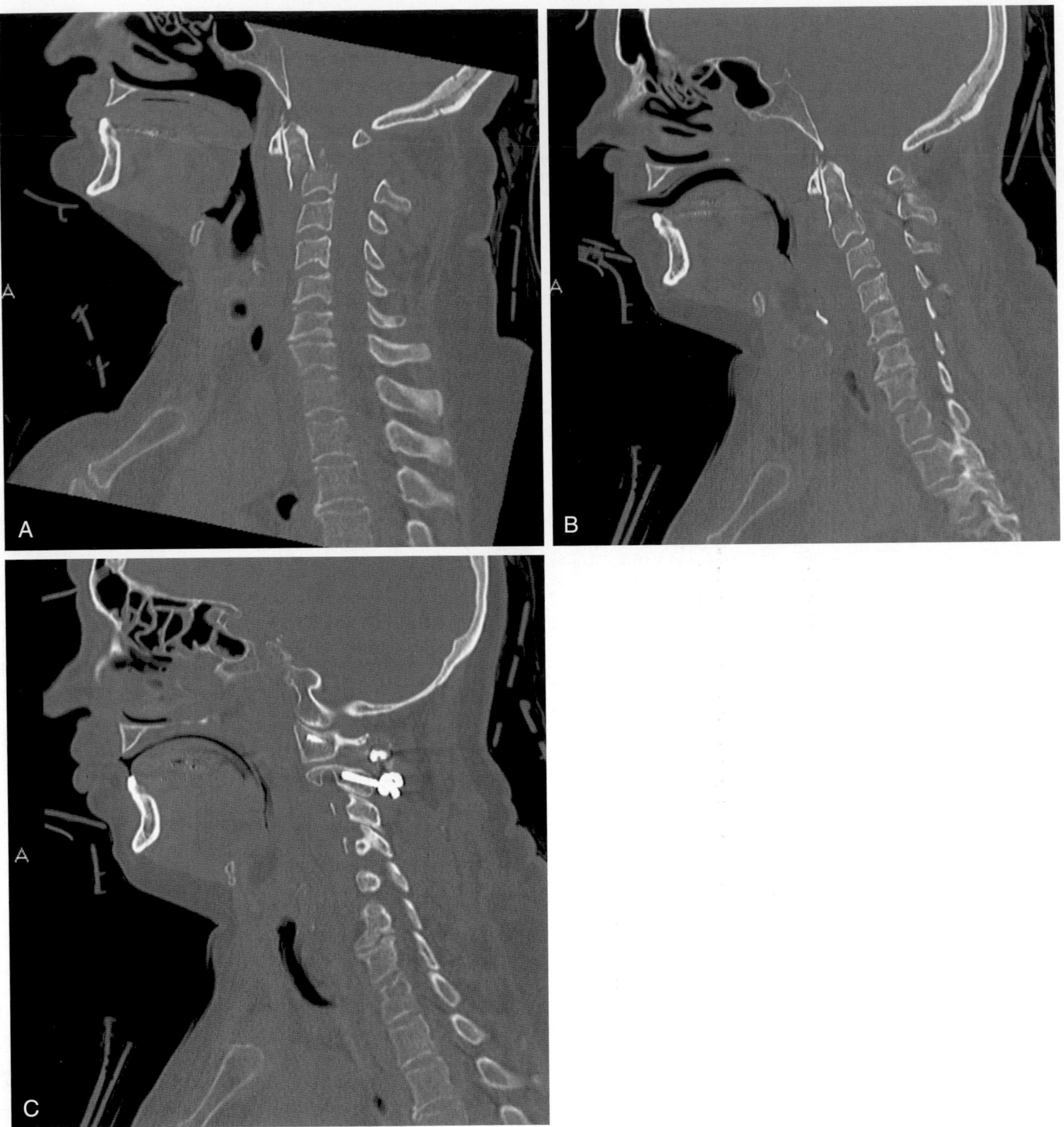

FIGURE 41-19 **A,** Anterior displaced odontoid fracture. **B,** Anatomic reduction achieved. **C,** C1 lateral mass screw and C2 isthmus screw in good position.

Generally, this method is used if anatomic constraints preclude C2 isthmic screw placement with known vertebral artery injuries preoperatively.

TECHNIQUE 41-10

(WRIGHT)

- Patient preparation, positioning, and administration of anesthesia are as described in Technique 41-6.
- Use lateral image intensification to check the reduction of the C1-2 complex.
- Perform posterior midline exposure of the cervical spine from the occiput to C2.
- Place the C1 lateral mass screws as described in Technique 41-6.
- Fully expose the caudal edge of the C2 lamina at the midline and extend it laterally.
- Use an angled curet to detach the ligamentum flavum from the ventral surface and the cephalad and caudal margin of C2 so that a Penfield No. 4 dissector or other blunt instrument can be used to palpate the anterior C2 lamina during screw placement.

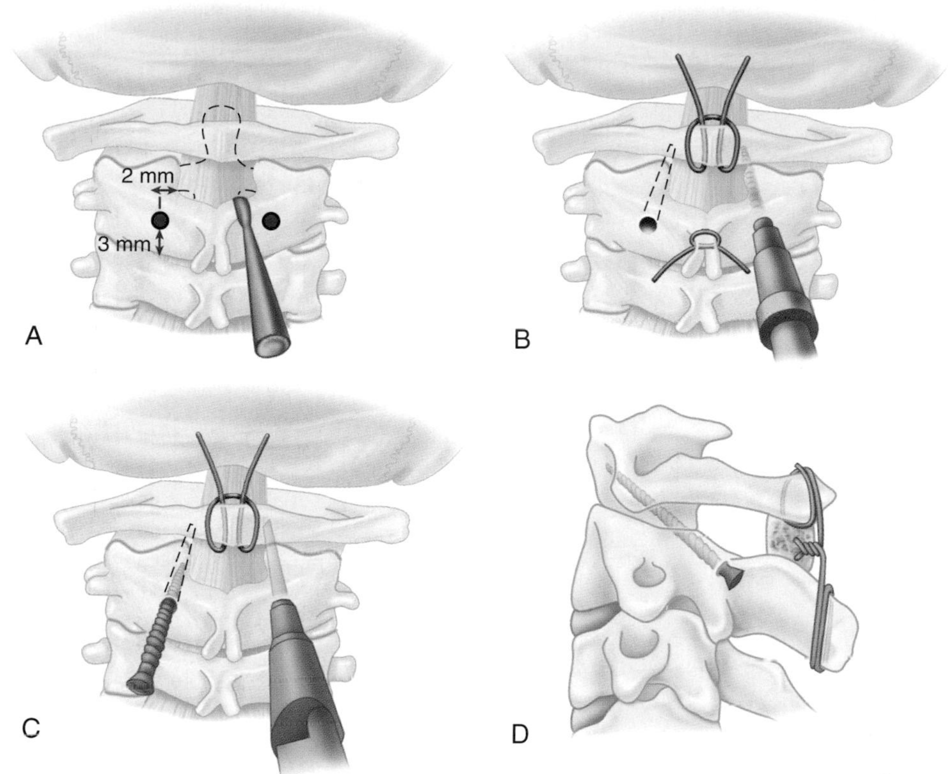

FIGURE 41-20 C1-2 transarticular screw fixation (Magerl and Seemann). **A,** Landmarks for entry point of transarticular screw. **B,** Wires are brought around arch of C1 and spinous process of C2 to manipulate these two vertebrae. Screw holes are drilled through isthmus near its posterior and medial surface of C2 and outer lateral mass of atlas. **C,** Measuring screw length and tapping with 3.5-mm cortical tap. **D,** Proper screw placement for C1-2 fusion. **SEE TECHNIQUE 41-9.**

- With a Penfield No. 4 dissector or blunt hook ventral to the lamina, use the drill to penetrate the cortex at the base of the C2 spinous process at the location determined preoperatively to allow room for both screws. Using the Penfield dissector as a guide, maintain the drill posterior to the canal and advance it laterally into the C2 inferior articular mass. The drill should not penetrate the posterior or anterior cortex as it is advanced. Screw lengths usually are 25 to 35 mm.
- Place the contralateral screw similarly.
- Contour the rod to engage the C1 lateral mass screws and secure the connections.
- Perform a traditional posterior C1-2 fusion using either the Gallie or the Brooks technique. Alternatively, morselized bone graft can be used.
- Close the wound in layers over a drain, taking care to reattach the fascia to bone at the C2 level. Use a subcuticular skin closure.

POSTOPERATIVE CARE. Postoperative immobilization with a halo vest usually is unnecessary. A cervical collar may be worn for 8 to 12 weeks. The drain is removed on the first postoperative day.

POSTERIOR C1-C2 WIRING

Wiring techniques are seldom used as the primary method of stabilization, but they remain useful for adjunctive stabilization and to maintain corticocancellous grafts in position. The Brooks and Jenkins method provides a bone block between the arch of C1 and the C2 lamina. The wires are located laterally and provide more rotational stability than is provided by the midline Gallie wiring.

TECHNIQUE 41-11

(BROOKS AND JENKINS)

- Patient preparation, positioning, and administration of anesthesia are as described in Technique 41-6.
- Expose the C1-2 level through a midline incision.
- Use a small-angled curet to clear the ventral surface of the C1 and C2 lamina.
- Using an aneurysm needle, pass a No. 2 Mersilene suture on each side of the midline in a cephalad to caudal direction, first under the arch of the atlas and then under the lamina of the axis (Fig. 41-21A). These sutures serve as guides to introduce two doubled 20-gauge stainless steel

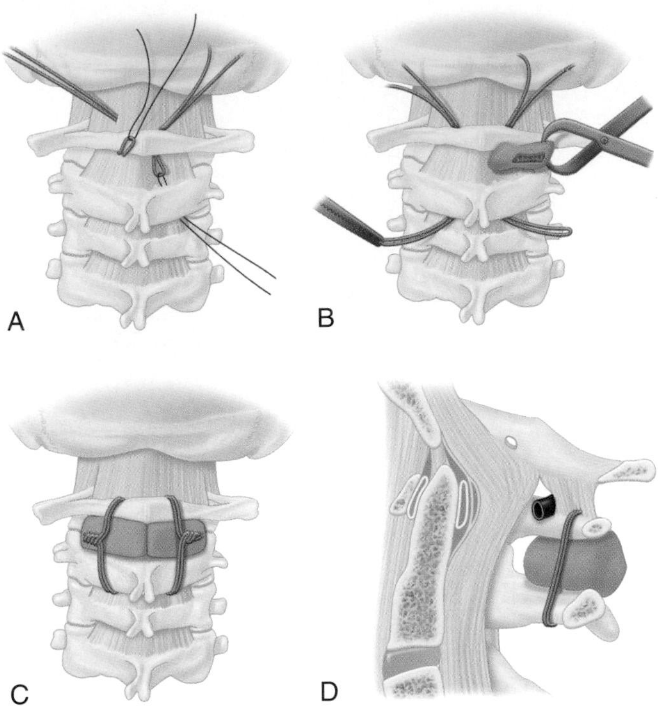

FIGURE 41-21 Brooks and Jenkins technique of atlantoaxial fusion. **A,** Insertion of wires under atlas and axis. **B,** Wires in place with graft being inserted. **C** and **D,** Bone grafts secured by wires (anteroposterior and lateral views). **SEE TECHNIQUE 41-11.**

wires into place. Alternatively, braided cables can be passed in place of the wires to increase flexibility and strength significantly. The suture is tied to the wire or cable, which is then pulled, using the suture to maintain tension on the wire or cable to minimize canal intrusion as it is passed.

- Obtain a full-thickness rectangular bone graft approximately 1.5 × 4.0 cm from the iliac crest. Divide the graft in half along the short axis. Bevel the grafts to fit snugly into the interval between the arch of the atlas and each lamina of the axis with the cancellous portion of the graft in contact with the ring of C1 and the lamina of C2 (Fig. 41-21B).
- While holding the grafts in position on each side of the midline and maintaining the width of the interlaminar space, tighten the doubled wires over them and twist and tie the wires to secure the grafts (Fig. 41-21C and D).
- Irrigate and close the wound in layers over suction drain.

POSTOPERATIVE CARE. When used as a primary fusion method, halo vest immobilization is continued for 10 to 12 weeks. If wiring is adjunctive, immobilization is based on the primary stabilization method.

TRAUMATIC SPONDYLOLISTHESIS OF THE AXIS (HANGMAN FRACTURE)

Fractures of the posterior elements of the axis through the isthmic portion or pars interarticularis are relatively common. The term *hangman fracture* was coined by Schneider in 1965, although the mechanism for the typical injury is quite different from that occurring with a judicial hanging. The usual mechanism causing this fracture pattern is hyperextension and axial loading, although some injury patterns involve flexion as well. Effendi et al. classified the injury into three types based on the apparent mechanism of injury and the radiographic characteristics. Type I injury is caused by hyperextension and is minimally displaced (0 to 2 mm of translation of the C2 body relative to C3) with no kyphosis through the disc space. Type II injury is caused by hyperextension and axial loading followed by flexion. The fracture line is relatively vertical in orientation with at least 3 mm of translation through the C2 disc. Levine and Edwards modified the Effendi type II fracture to include a flexion-distraction injury that has a relatively horizontal fracture line and significant kyphosis through the C2 disc with posterior annulus disruption but minimal translation of C2 on C3 (Fig. 41-22). Type III fractures are flexion-compression injuries, and in addition to the traumatic spondylolisthesis, dislocation of the C2-C3 facet joints occurs. One additional fracture pattern of note, reported by Starr and Eismont, occurs when the fracture extends into the posterior body of the axis on one or both sides. This variant is important because it is associated with a higher rate of neurologic injury (Fig. 41-23).

TREATMENT

Treatment of traumatic spondylolisthesis of the axis is based on fracture type, and immobilization of the fracture usually is adequate. Francis et al. reported that 95 of 123 patients healed satisfactorily with immobilization. In most series, operative treatment was performed for patients with radiographic instability despite appropriate external bracing, for patients with type III injuries, and for patients demonstrating instability after immobilization.

Type I injuries generally do not have associated ligamentous injuries, given the mechanism, and can be treated with a rigid collar. Type II and IIa injuries must be distinguished from one another because treatment is quite different. Type II injury usually can be reduced with traction if necessary, and then the patient is placed in a halo vest for 12 weeks. The patient with a type IIa fracture should not be placed in traction because of the posterior discal disruption, which allows for overdistraction and potential neurologic injury. Type IIa injuries should be reduced with gentle manual extension and slight compression, and the patient is maintained in a halo vest for 12 weeks. Type III fracture-dislocations require open reduction of the dislocation because the arch fragment cannot be controlled with traction because of the fracture. In some patients, direct stabilization of the fracture with a C2 pedicle screws placed as described earlier is possible as definitive treatment. More commonly, these screws are combined with C3 lateral mass screws and a rod construct to accomplish fusion at the C2-C3 level. If the C2 level cannot be stabilized with screw placement, a C1-C3 fusion with lateral mass screws at each level is recommended. Anterior C2-C3 stabilization is an option. The Starr and Eismont variant is treated in traction initially and then halo vest immobilization for 12 weeks. If reduction cannot be maintained, posterior fusion using C2 isthmic or pedicle screws and C3 lateral mass screws with a rod construct is most appropriate. This posterior fixation is biomechanically more stable than anterior C2-C3

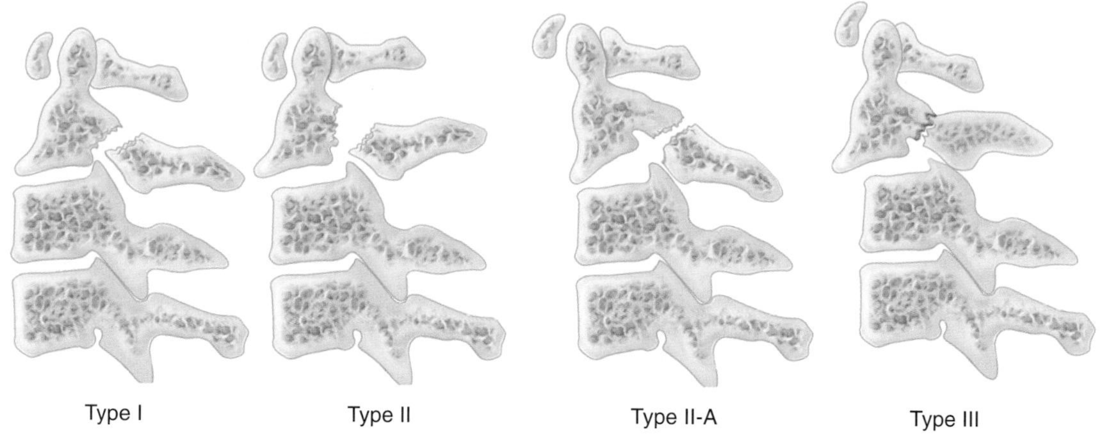

FIGURE 41-22 Hangman fracture (see text).

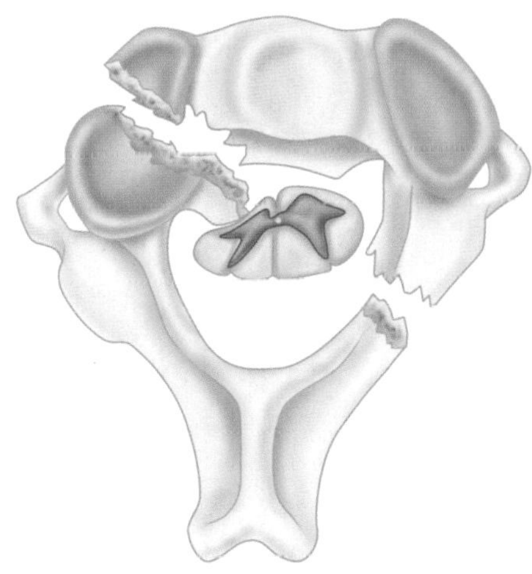

FIGURE 41-23 Atypical hangman fracture with cord impingement described by Starr and Eismont.

stabilization. Placement of this instrumentation is described in Technique 41-6.

SUBAXIAL CERVICAL SPINE INJURY (C3-T1)

■ CLASSIFICATION

Although the axis is the individual vertebra most commonly injured, the subaxial region of the cervical spine accounts for about 65% of all cervical spine injuries and most cervical spinal cord injuries. Despite the relatively high incidence of subaxial injuries (C3-T1), the optimal management often is not clear from existing medical literature. There are several reasons for this, including development of improved surgical methods and options with improved outcomes and lower morbidities. Also, no ideal classification system exists that allows reproducible and valid characterization of specific injuries that are required to compare treatments and outcomes. There have been many efforts to classify these injuries, and improvements continue to be made. Central to any classification is the concept of spinal stability, which classically has been defined by White and Panjabi as "the ability of the spine under physiologic loads to maintain an association between vertebral segments in such a way that there is neither damage nor subsequent irritation of the spinal cord or nerve roots, and, in addition, there is no development of incapacitating deformity or pain because of structural changes." The ability to make a determination of current and future stability is dependent on a complete understanding of spinal biomechanics and the ability to definitively determine the presence of injury to all the various anatomic components of the spinal column. Acute instability is caused by bone or soft-tissue injury that places the neural elements at risk of injury with any subsequent loading or deformity. Chronic instability is the result of progressive deformity that may cause neurologic deterioration, prevent recovery of injured neural tissue, or cause increasing pain or decreasing function.

In a series of cadaver studies, White and Panjabi systematically cut the various supporting structures and noted the resulting instabilities of the spine. The supporting structures of the subaxial spine can be divided into two groups: anterior and posterior (Fig. 41-24). A motion segment is made up of two adjacent vertebrae and the intervening soft tissues. If a motion segment has all the anterior elements and one posterior element, or all the posterior elements and one anterior element, it remains stable under physiologic loads. White, Southwick, and Panjabi developed a checklist for the diagnosis of clinical instability of the subaxial cervical spine (Box 41-2). This checklist includes radiographic criteria to consider in determination of clinical instability. These criteria include sagittal translation of 3.5 mm on a lateral view (Fig. 41-25). An additional criterion is more than 11 degrees of angulation of one vertebra relative to another on a lateral radiograph (Fig. 41-26).

This body of information and imaging capabilities continue to improve. The classification system described by Allen and Ferguson remains the most widely used, although several alternative systems have been described. The Allen and Ferguson system is based on a mechanistic description of the injury based on the radiographic appearance of the cervical spine. These authors reviewed 165 subaxial injuries and categorized them into six common patterns and then further subdivided each pattern into stages of severity of osseous and ligamentous injury (Table 41-5).

The terminology of this system has become familiar to spine surgeons and is accepted to describe injuries, but precise

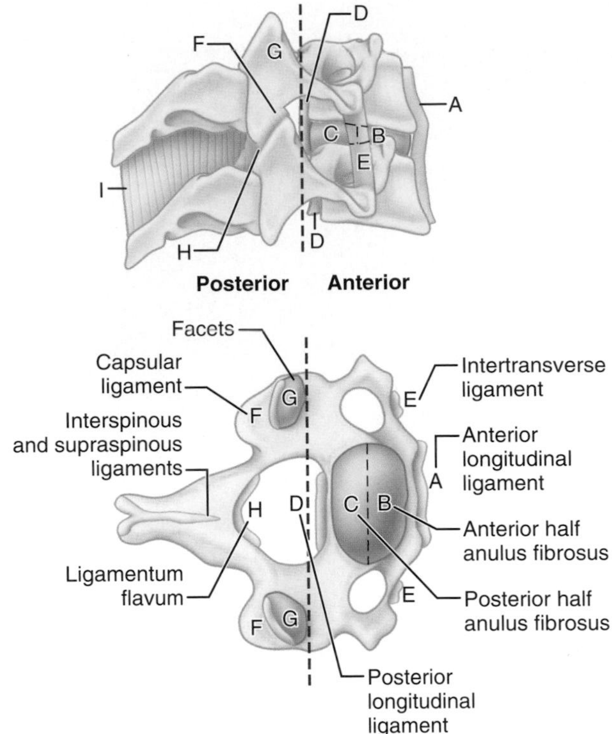

FIGURE 41-24 Important anterior and posterior supporting structures of spine.

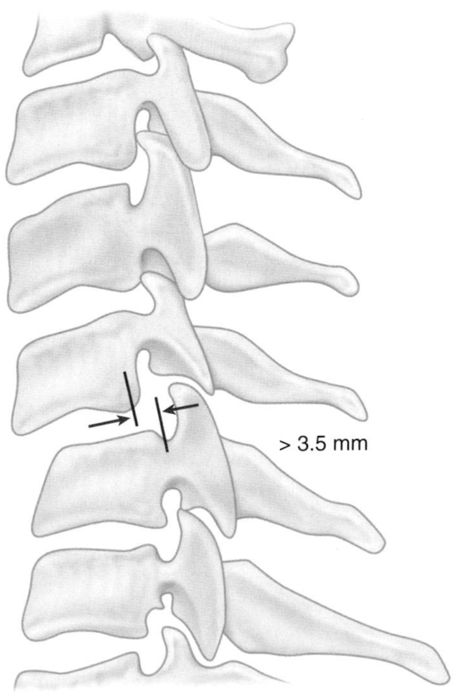

FIGURE 41-25 **Sagittal plane translation of more than 3.5 mm suggests clinical instability.** (Redrawn from White AA, Johnson RM, Panjabi MM: Biomechanical analysis of clinical stability in the cervical spine, Clin Orthop Relat Res 109:85, 1975.)

BOX 41-2

Checklist for Diagnosis of Clinical Instability in Lower Cervical Spine*

Element	Point Value
Anterior elements destroyed or unable to function	2
Posterior elements destroyed or unable to function	2
Relative sagittal plane translation >3.5 mm	2
Relative sagittal plane rotation >11 degrees	2
Positive stretch test	2
Medullary (cord) damage	2
Root damage	1
Abnormal disc narrowing	1
Dangerous loading anticipated	1

*Total of 5 or more = unstable

From White AA, Southwick WO, Panjabi MM: Clinical instability in the lower cervical spine: a review of past and current concepts, Spine 1:15, 1976.

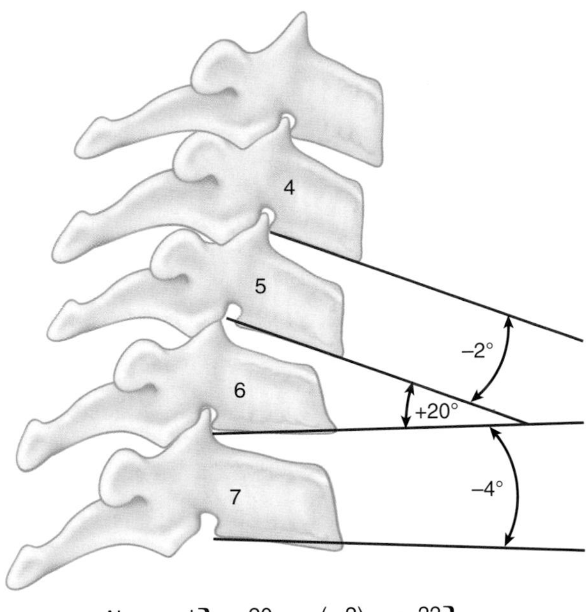

FIGURE 41-26 **Significant sagittal plane rotation (>11 degrees) suggests instability.** (Redrawn from White AA, Johnson RM, Panjabi MM: Biomechanical analysis of clinical stability in the cervical spine, Clin Orthop Relat Res 109:85, 1975.)

definitions of each stage are lacking. An alternative classification system was proposed by Moore et al. and subsequently modified by Vaccaro et al. and presented as the Subaxial Injury Classification (SLIC) scoring system. This particular system has three categories that are scored and summed. The authors proposed that the numerical value obtained can then be used to determine whether nonoperative or operative treatment should be performed. The categories that are scored are morphology, discoligamentous complex integrity, and neurologic status of the patient. An increasing score within

TABLE 41-5

Allen and Ferguson Classification of Subaxial Cervical Spine Fractures

	COMPRESSIVE FLEXION—FIVE STAGES
Compressive flexion stage 1	Blunting of the anterosuperior vertebral margin to a rounded contour, with no evidence of failure of the posterior ligamentous complex
Compressive flexion stage 2	In addition to the changes seen in stage 1, obliquity of the anterior vertebral body with loss of some anterior height of the centrum. The anteroinferior vertebral body has a "beak" appearance, concavity of the inferior endplate may be increased, and the vertebral body may have a vertical fracture.
Compressive flexion stage 3	In addition to the characteristics of a stage 2 injury, fracture line passing obliquely from the anterior surface of the vertebra through the centrum and extending through the inferior subchondral plate and a fracture of the beak.
Compressive flexion stage 4	Deformation of the centrum and fracture of the beak with mild (<3 mm) displacement of the inferoposterior vertebral margin into the spinal canal
Compressive flexion stage 5	Bony injuries as in stage 3 but with more than 3 mm of displacement of the posterior portion of the vertebral body posteriorly into the spinal canal. The vertebral arch remains intact, the articular facets are separated, and the interspinous process space is increased at the level of injury, suggesting a posterior ligamentous disruption in a tension mode.
	VERTICAL COMPRESSION—THREE STAGES
Vertical compression stage 1	Fracture of the superior or inferior endplate with a "cupping" deformity. Failure of the endplate is central rather than anterior, and posterior ligamentous failure is not evident.
Vertical compression stage 2	Fracture of both vertebral endplates with cupping deformities. Fracture lines through the centrum may be present, but displacement is minimal.
Vertical compression stage 3	Progression of the vertebral body damage described in stage 2. The centrum is fragmented, and the displacement is peripheral in multiple directions. Most commonly, the centrum fails, with significant impaction and fragmentation. The posterior aspect of the vertebral body is fractured and may be displaced into the spinal canal. The vertebral arch may be intact with no evidence of ligamentous failure, or it may be comminuted with significant failure of the posterior ligamentous complex; the ligamentous disruption is between the fractured vertebra and the one below it.
	DISTRACTIVE FLEXION—FOUR STAGES
Distractive flexion stage 1	Failure of the posterior ligamentous complex, as evidenced by facet subluxation in flexion, with abnormal divergence of the spinous process.
Distractive flexion stage 2	Unilateral facet dislocation (the degree of posterior ligamentous failure ranges from partial failure sufficient only to permit the abnormal displacement to complete failure of the anterior and posterior ligamentous complexes, which is uncommon). Subluxation of the facet on the side opposite the dislocation suggests severe ligamentous injury. In addition, a small fleck of bone may be displaced from the posterior surface of the articular process, which is displaced anteriorly. Widening of the uncovertebral joint on the side of the dislocation and displacement of the tip of the spinous process toward the side of the dislocation may be seen. Beatson serially divided the posterior interspinous ligaments, facet capsule, posterior longitudinal ligament, annulus fibrosus, and anterior longitudinal ligament and found that unilateral facet dislocation can occur with rupture of only the posterior interspinous ligament and the facet capsule.
Distractive flexion stage 3	Bilateral facet dislocations, with approximately 50% anterior subluxation of the vertebral body. Blunting of the anterosuperior margin of the inferior vertebra to a rounded corner may or may not be present. Beatson showed that rupture of the interspinous ligament, the capsules of both facet joints, the posterior longitudinal ligament, and the annulus fibrosus of the intervertebral disc was necessary to create this lesion.
Distractive flexion stage 4	Full vertebral body width displacement anteriorly or a grossly unstable motion segment, giving the appearance of a "floating" vertebra
	COMPRESSIVE EXTENSION—FIVE STAGES
Compressive extension stage 1	Unilateral vertebral arch fracture with or without anterior rotatory vertebral displacement. Posterior element failure may consist of a linear fracture through the articular process, impaction of the articular process, and ipsilateral pedicle and lamina fractures, resulting in the "transverse facet" appearance on anteroposterior radiographs, or a combination of ipsilateral pedicle and articular process fractures.

Continued

TABLE 41-5

Allen and Ferguson Classification of Subaxial Cervical Spine Fractures—cont'd

Compressive extension stage 2	Bilaminar fractures without evidence of other tissue failure. Typically, the laminar fractures occur at multiple contiguous levels.
Compressive extension stage 3	Bilateral vertebral arch fractures with fracture of the articular processes, pedicles, lamina, or some bilateral combination, without vertebral body displacement
Compressive extension stage 4	Bilateral vertebral arch fractures with partial vertebral body width displacement anteriorly
Compressive extension stage 5	Bilateral vertebral arch fracture with full vertebral body width displacement anteriorly. The posterior portion of the vertebral arch of the fractured vertebra does not displace, and the anterior portion of the arch remains with the centrum. Ligament failure occurs at two levels: posteriorly between the fractured vertebra and the one above it and anteriorly between the fractured vertebra and the one below it. Characteristically, the anterosuperior portion of the vertebra below is sheared off by the anteriorly displaced centrum.
DISTRACTIVE EXTENSION—TWO STAGES	
Distractive extension stage 1	Either failure of the anterior ligamentous complex or a transverse fracture of the centrum. The injury usually is ligamentous, and there may be a fracture of the adjacent anterior vertebral margin. The radiographic clue to this injury is abnormal widening of the disc space.
Distractive extension stage 2	Evidence of failure of the posterior ligamentous complex, with displacement of the upper vertebral body posteriorly into the spinal canal, in addition to the changes seen in stage 1 injuries. Because displacement of this type tends to reduce spontaneously when the head is placed in a neutral position, radiographic evidence of the displacement may be minimal, rarely greater than 3 mm on initial films with the patient supine.
LATERAL FLEXION—TWO STAGES	
Lateral flexion stage 1	Asymmetric compression fracture of the centrum and ipsilateral vertebral arch fracture, without displacement of the arch on the anteroposterior view. Compression of the articular process or comminution of the corner of the vertebral arch may be present.
Lateral flexion stage 2	Lateral asymmetric compression of the centrum and either ipsilateral displaced vertebral arch fracture or ligamentous failure on the contralateral side with separation of the articular processes. Ipsilateral and compressive and contralateral disruptive vertebral arch injuries may be present.

each category is intended to reflect increasingly severe injury (Table 41-6). The primary improvement of this severity scoring system is the reincorporation of the neurologic status of the patient, which is integral to the determination of spinal stability. This severity score was compared with the Allen and Ferguson system among a group of experienced spine surgeons, and the two systems had similar reliability for treatment recommendations. With continued improvements in imaging, particularly of the soft-tissue components of the spine, determination of the optimal classification of or treatment for a particular injury can be decided with certainty.

TREATMENT

Until there is a validated classification system that substantially improves on the available systems, spine surgeons will continue to use the best information available coupled with experience to determine treatments. A systematic approach as discussed earlier in this chapter is necessary when determining treatment. After the imaging has been obtained and any emergent closed reduction attempt completed, a decision for definitive treatment is necessary.

Most cervical injuries do not disrupt the structural integrity of the spine sufficiently to require operative intervention. Evaluating individual injuries based on the three-column biomechanical model has been the basis for our treatment rationale in each region of the spine. The anterior column consists of the anterior longitudinal ligament and the anterior half of the vertebral body and disc, the middle column consists of the posterior half of the body and disc and the posterior longitudinal ligament, and the posterior column includes the pedicles and all posterior osseous and ligamentous structures. The controlling principle is that single-column injuries without neurologic deficit will, in general, be stable without progressive deformity, neurologic injury, or postinjury pain. This has been consistent with our practice experience, and these patients do well with immobilization. In contrast, injuries that involve three columns are considered unstable even when there is no neurologic deficit (rare) and typically require operative stabilization. This, of course, leaves the two-column injuries, which are considered unstable. These tend to be treated operatively, but some of these injuries can be treated with immobilization. In our experience, immobilization has a low morbidity when the patient is able to mobilize immediately. In patients with two-column injuries, the neurologic status often is the determining factor as to whether operative treatment is recommended. Patients with incomplete injuries or complete injuries generally are treated operatively, whereas those with normal results of examination or possibly isolated root injuries may be treated with immobilization. Other injuries, comorbidities, congenital anomalies, and degenerative conditions can influence the treatment decision.

TABLE 41-6

Subaxial Injury Classification (SLIC) Scale

	POINTS
MORPHOLOGY	
No abnormality	0
Compression + burst	1+1 = 2
Distraction (e.g., facet perch, hyperextension)	3
Rotation or translation (e.g., facet dislocation, unstable teardrop, or advanced stage flexion compression injury)	4
DISCOLIGAMENTOUS COMPLEX	
Intact	0
Indeterminate (e.g., isolated interspinous widening, magnetic resonance imaging signal change only)	1
Disrupted (e.g., widening of anterior disc space, facet perch, or dislocation)	2
NEUROLOGIC STATUS	
Intact	0
Root injury	1
Compete cord injury	2
Incomplete cord injury	3
Continuous cord compression (neuro-modifier in the setting of a neurologic deficit)	+1

From Dorak M, Fisher CG, Fehlings MG, et al: The surgical approach to subaxial cervical spine injuries, Spine 32:2620, 2007.

The goals of stabilization are to realign the spine, prevent further loss of neurologic function, enhance neurologic recovery, restore biomechanical integrity to the spine, and promote early functional recovery. Operative treatment for subaxial spine injuries can be from an anterior, posterior, or combined (360-degree) approach. There are a variety of acceptable treatment options that can achieve these goals in a given patient. The simplest and most direct strategy is to base the approach on the area of greatest structural injury. Injuries that require reconstruction of the anterior column support generally are approached anteriorly, and posterior injuries requiring direct reduction of dislocations are approached posteriorly.

The primary advantages of anterior surgery include decompression of the neural elements and restoration of the axial load-bearing support function with use of a strut graft and anterior plating, particularly over one to two motion segments. Maintaining the patient supine during surgery also is an advantage if the patient has significant pulmonary dysfunction from blunt trauma or infection. Wound complications are infrequent with anterior surgery, although dysphagia has been recognized more frequently in recent years. Access to any level from the C2 disc to the C7 disc is possible in most patients but can be quite challenging in obese patients or those with short necks. Adequate decompression often can be accomplished with a discectomy. In a trauma setting, this is preferred to a corpectomy, which is inherently less stable. At times, such as with a burst fracture, a corpectomy is needed, and adequate stability is achieved with careful fitting and placement of the strut graft or cage and use of unicortical screws and a locking type plate. The dynamic type plates are of questionable benefit in degenerative indications but really do not have a place in the management of trauma patients because of the greater level of instability. Preservation of intact endplates and careful sizing of the strut graft without overdistracting the facets posteriorly also are critical to achieving enough stability to allow primary bone healing at the graft-host interface. There are multiple series in the literature demonstrating good outcomes with this type of anterior-only construct even with posterior ligamentous injuries. Postoperative immobilization in an orthosis generally is adequate with satisfactory plating. If fixation is compromised because of the injury pattern or bone quality, consideration should be given to posterior fixation or halo vest immobilization that may be advantageous for the patient rather than additional surgery. Anterior reconstruction and plating has been shown by Johnson et al. to have a high failure rate if the endplates are not intact, especially if there are associated facet fractures at the level treated with discectomy and reconstruction. Corpectomies at more than two levels are rare for trauma indications but if needed should be supplemented with posterior instrumentation. Combined approaches rarely are needed for a good outcome except as discussed.

Posterior fixation with current segmental fixation systems allows treatment of the most unstable injuries, even those that extend across the craniocervical or cervicothoracic junctions. These constructs use rods with lateral mass fixation from C3-C6 and pedicle screw placement at C2, C7 and in the upper thoracic region. Pedicle screws can be placed at C7 and are biomechanically superior to C7 lateral mass screws. Pedicle screws are technically more difficult to place than lateral mass screws at C3 to C6 and usually offer no significant benefit. When necessary, fixation can be extended above C3 as has already been discussed. Because posterior fixation restores the posterior tension band and segmental fixation is possible, these constructs are stiffer than anterior constructs in flexion and torsion, so fusion rates are superior for multilevel fusions treated posteriorly than for similar length anterior constructs. Decompression done posteriorly is not associated with quite the same level of neurologic improvement in some studies, probably because of less effective restoration of blood flow to the anterior cord as was shown by Brodke et al. If posterior decompression is done, it should always be accompanied by stabilization and fusion in the setting of trauma. Because of the more extensive dissection required posteriorly, there has been a higher incidence of wound infection and greater blood loss relative to anterior procedures. However, for limited posterior approaches, such as for direct reduction of facet dislocations and fusion, wound-related complications are rare. Patients who are designated as poor hosts are more likely to be osteoporotic, and, in general, posterior methods are preferred because segmental fixation is possible.

EXTENSION INJURIES

An extension injury is the result of hyperextension of the cervical spine (Fig. 41-27). Often the patient is older and had a relatively low-energy mechanism of injury such as a same level fall. The injury occurs in part from a loss of motion in

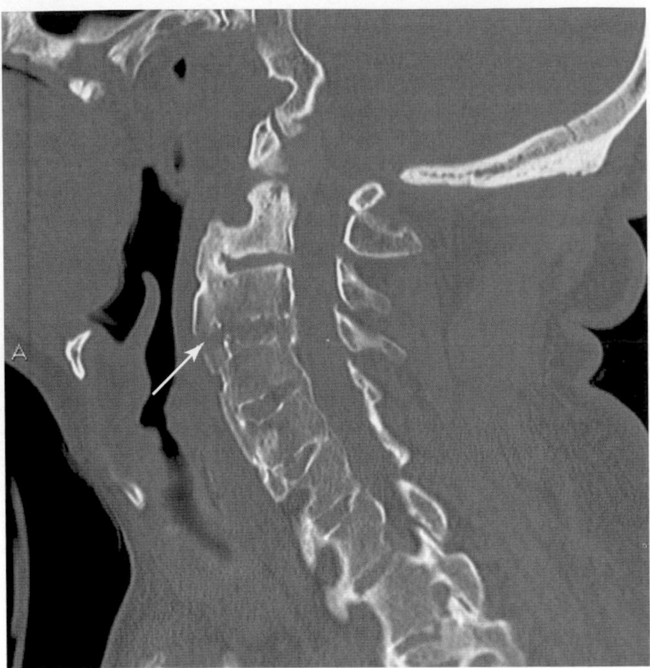

FIGURE 41-27 Extension fracture through C3 disc level in a patient with diffuse idiopathic skeletal hyperostosis.

the cervical spine, which is unable to dissipate the energy without failure. The patient may have diffuse idiopathic skeletal hyperostosis (DISH) or ankylosing spondylitis that predisposes to this injury pattern. Patients with ankylosing spondylitis actually have a fracture through the disc space and are treated somewhat differently (see later section). Patients with an incomplete disc disruption usually can be treated with immobilization. Patients with an annulus disruption that extends through the anterior and posterior margins of the annulus fibrosus are treated with anterior discectomy and fusion with bone graft and an anterior locking plate.

■ BURST FRACTURES

This injury is exemplified by shortening of the vertebral body, with comminution and retropulsion of the vertebral body into the canal (Fig. 41-28). These injuries are usually treated with corpectomy and anterior reconstruction with a tricortical iliac bone graft, fibular allograft, or cylindrical mesh cage packed with the resected vertebral body and anterior plating. The endplates are prepared to maintain intact subchondral bone as a secure footing for the chosen strut type. Usually, these patients are relatively young and do not have preexisting disease of the posterior longitudinal ligament, which is not injured by axial loading. The posterior longitudinal ligament should be preserved and will provide a counterforce for the implanted strut unless decompression cannot be satisfactorily accomplished without posterior longitudinal ligament resection. An anterior locking plate is then applied.

■ FACET DISLOCATIONS

Facet dislocations should be distinguished from facet fractures with subluxation. Bilateral facet dislocations are severe pure soft-tissue injuries with disruption of the facet capsules, which are the most important posterior ligamentous stabilizers. Additional injury occurs to the interspinous ligaments and posterior longitudinal ligament, and the posterior disc is disrupted with possible herniation. Anterior translation of up to 50% of the vertebral body dimension occurs. The algorithm for imaging and reduction should be followed. After failed or successful closed reduction, MRI is obtained. If there is a significant disc herniation present, anterior cervical discectomy with fusion and bone graft is done. If reduction was accomplished preoperatively or at the time of discectomy and fusion, an anterior locking plate is applied. This construct is stable with a reduced facet dislocation that has no bony injury. If reduction cannot be accomplished at the time of discectomy, the graft is placed and the anterior wound is closed, followed by open posterior reduction and fusion with instrumentation. If the closed reduction fails and MRI demonstrates no significant disc herniation, open posterior reduction with stabilization is the treatment of choice. Open reduction in an anesthetized patient is associated with a higher rate of spinal cord injury than closed reduction in an awake patient, as previously discussed. Unilateral facet dislocations usually have only about 25% translation, but the management scheme is similar. In some patients with unilateral facet dislocations with successful closed reduction, consideration to closed treatment is reasonable if there is no persistent neural compression, but close radiographic follow-up is essential because subluxation can recur even weeks later.

■ FACET FRACTURE WITH SUBLUXATION

When there is a facet fracture associated with subluxation, this injury usually will reduce easily with traction but will not remain reduced because of the osseous injury. If there is no fracture of either endplate, anterior discectomy with fusion, bone grafting, and anterior locking plate application is an option but should be undertaken with caution. This construct is subject to shear forces because of the incompetent facet(s), and displacement can occur. Although neurologic worsening is unusual, it has certainly been reported. Loss of fixation will require revision. Careful follow-up is recommended, and the patient must be compliant with orthosis usage. Alternatively, posterior instrumentation and fusion provide more stability and will maintain alignment more consistently, but an additional level of fusion generally is needed because fixation usually is not possible at the fractured level.

■ FRACTURE-DISLOCATIONS

These are the most severe injuries usually with soft-tissue and osseous injuries, translational displacement in one or more planes, and associated spinal cord injury. Closed reduction must be undertaken with caution to avoid overdistracting the injured segment and potentially worsening the spinal cord injury. In this injury group, combined anterior and posterior surgery often is the more conservative approach, although a combined approach is not always needed. The principle of treating the most severely injured area first is followed to reestablish spinal alignment and decompress the spinal cord. This usually is accomplished anteriorly first, and if necessary posterior supplemental stabilization and fusion are added at a second stage and may be delayed depending on the overall condition of the patient (Fig. 41-29).

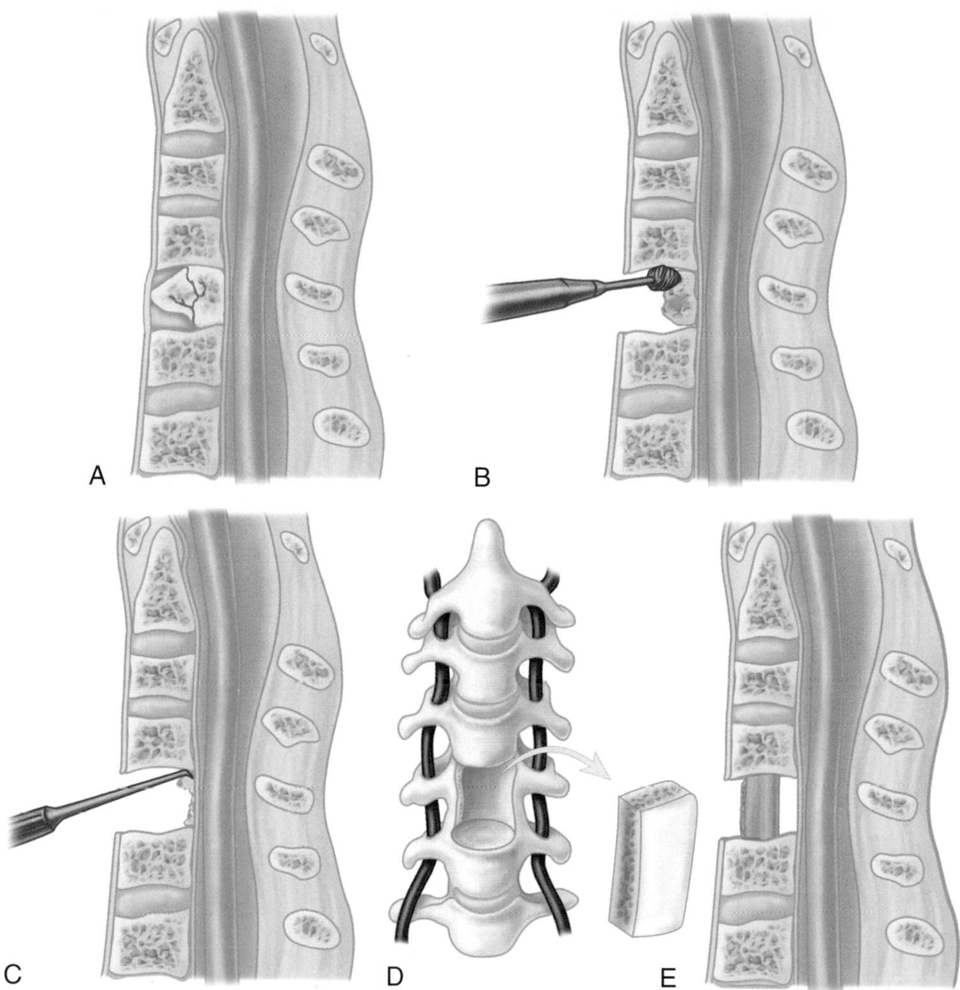

FIGURE 41-28 **A,** Typical burst fracture at C5 with retropulsed bone and disc fragments in spinal canal compressing neural elements. **B,** Disc material above and below fractured vertebra has been removed, and high-speed power burr is used to remove bone back to level of posterior longitudinal ligament. **C,** Residual posterior vertebral margin is removed with small curet to decompress neural elements. **D,** Extent of anterior cervical corpectomy. **E,** Placement of tricortical iliac crest graft after adequate cervical decompression. **SEE TECHNIQUE 41-12.**

ANTERIOR CERVICAL DISCECTOMY AND FUSION WITH LOCKING PLATE

TECHNIQUE 41-12

- If the patient is already in traction, maintain traction and alignment. Coordinate with the anesthesiologist for an awake intubation or manually maintain head position and use a GlideScope (Veriathon Inc., Bothell, WA). If the patient has a spinal cord injury, maintain a mean arterial pressure of 85 to 90 mm Hg during the procedure.
- Expose the spine through either a transverse or a longitudinal incision, depending on the surgeon's preference. We usually prefer a left-sided transverse incision (Fig. 41-30) because of the more constant anatomy of the recurrent laryngeal nerve and the lower risk of inadvertent injury.
- Make a 3-cm incision at the cricoid level for the C5 disc or adjust accordingly. A transverse incision can be used even for an extensile exposure. Locate the skin incision with the midpoint on the lateral border of the trachea on the side of the approach.
- Incise the skin and dissect through the subcutaneous layer to the platysma. Sharply dissect the fat off the platysma fascia at least 10 mm in all directions from the incision.
- Incise the platysma muscle vertically in line with its fibers.
- In the lateral portion of the wound, identify the medial border of the sternocleidomastoid muscle and bluntly develop the plane to the carotid sheath. At the C5 disc level it will be covered by the omohyoid muscle.
- Sweep the omohyoid superiorly or inferiorly (at the C5 disc level) as needed and sharply incise the pretracheal fascia along the medial border of the carotid sheath.
- With blunt finger dissection, develop the plane of the prevertebral space. Use a Kitner dissector to better define

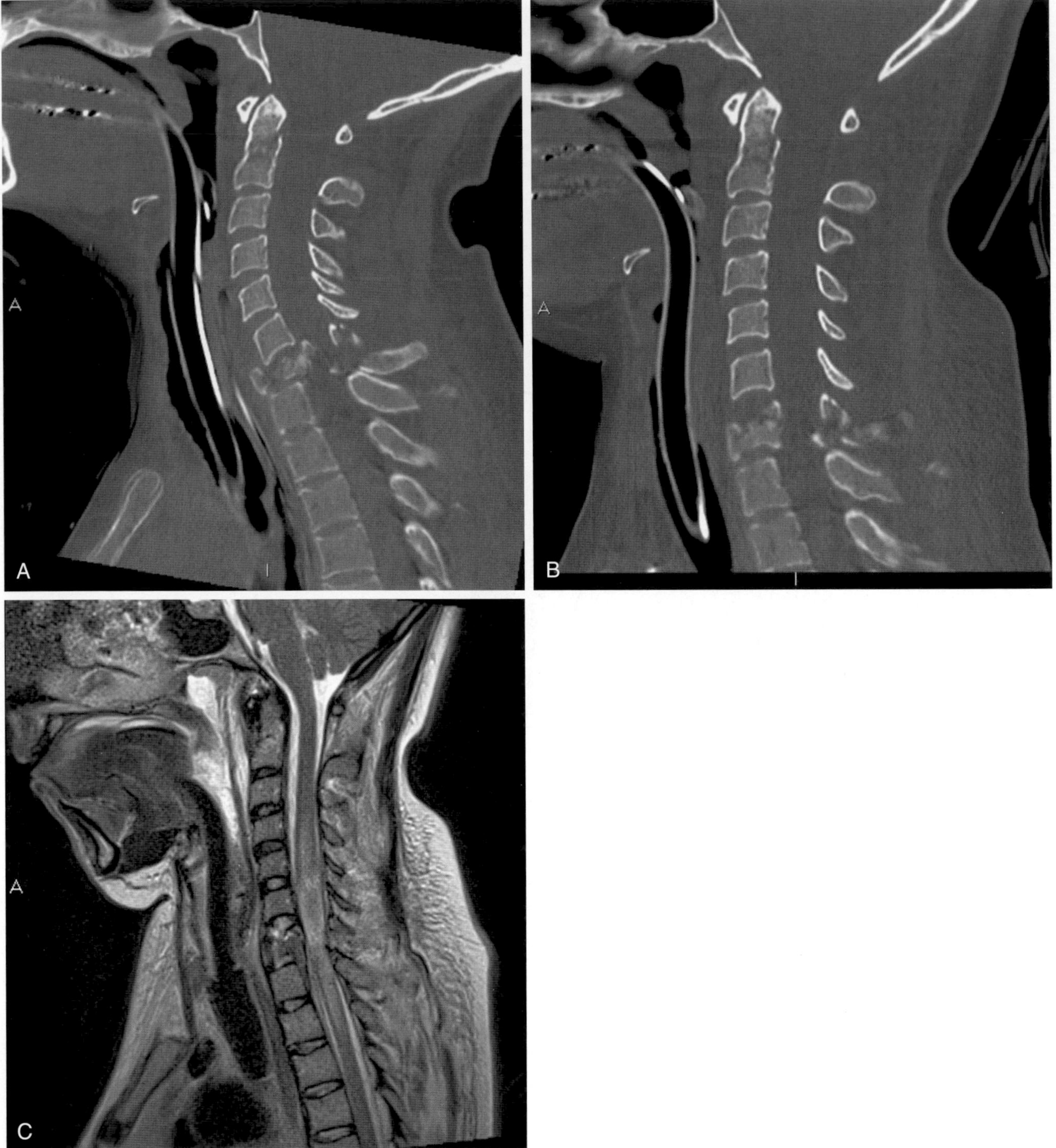

FIGURE 41-29 **A,** Fracture-dislocation involving C6 and C7 levels. Note C2 fracture. **B,** Alignment has been improved with skeletal traction. **C,** MR image after traction reveals severe spinal cord swelling and increased signal.

the anterior spine that is visible between the longus colli muscles.

- Radiographically identify the injured level with a metallic marker within the injured disc or bone and permanently store the image.
- Using blunt retractors, mobilize the trachea and esophagus just enough to safely elevate the longus colli muscles bilaterally from the midbody of the superior end vertebra to the midbody of the inferior end vertebra but avoid unnecessary exposure that may lead to adjacent segment degeneration.
- Place a self-retaining retractor with the blade deep to the medial border of the longus colli on each side of the spine at the affected level.

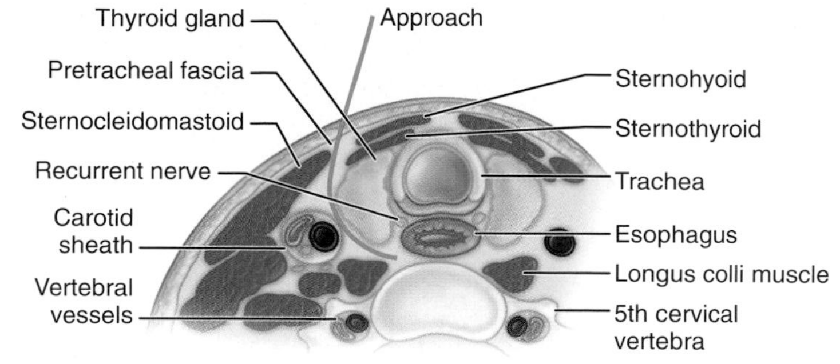

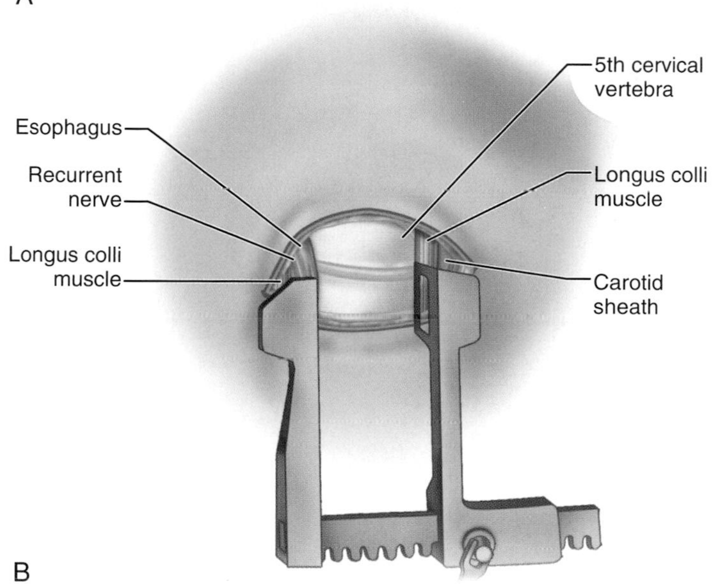

FIGURE 41-30 **A,** Anterior approach to middle and lower cervical spine through left-sided transverse incision is carried medially to carotid sheath and laterally to trachea and esophagus. **B,** Deep dissection to middle and lower cervical spine. Thorough knowledge of anatomic fascial planes is mandatory to gain adequate exposure of the anterior aspect of the cervical spine. **SEE TECHNIQUES 41-12 AND 41-13.**

- Incise the injured disc widely to the level of the uncinate process bilaterally. Use curets to remove most of the disc and clearly view the uncinate process bilaterally.
- Under the operating microscope, use a high-speed burr to remove the anteriormost portion of the inferior body of the cephalad vertebra. This bone removal is only to the level of the highest point of the concavity of the inferior endplate. This allows the endplate to be flat, and it forms a right angle with the anterior and posterior body walls and preserves the subchondral bone (Fig. 41-28). Remove any anterior osteophyte as well. With this anterior bone resection, visibility is enhanced and the posterior disc material, posterior longitudinal ligament, and posterior osteophytes can be removed as needed. If the foramina are tight, perform foraminotomies. Contour the superior endplate of the inferior vertebra with a burr, preserving the subchondral bone and creating a flat surface with an equal interval between the adjacent endplates left to right and front to back.
- Carefully measure the height of the disc space both with traction applied and without traction. Do not size the graft to maintain the traction interval if there is more than 1 mm difference between the measurements. The graft size should allow stable fit without being excessively tight.
- Either harvest tricortical iliac graft or select a composite corticocancellous allograft product. The graft typically is 12 to 13 mm in anterior to posterior dimension so it can be countersunk 2 mm and not intrude into the canal. Tamp the graft into place and verify radiographically or by direct vision that the posterior graft does not enter the canal. With traction removed the graft should be stable enough to resist being pulled easily from the disc space.
- Select the shortest locking plate possible to avoid impingement injury to the adjacent discs. The prepared endplates should be just visible through the screw holes of the plate when it is properly positioned (Fig. 41-31).
- Drill and place unicortical screws most commonly 14 mm in length. Make sure screws are placed at the correct angle to optimize locking of the screw and plate. Engage the anti-backout mechanism of the plate after placing all four screws.

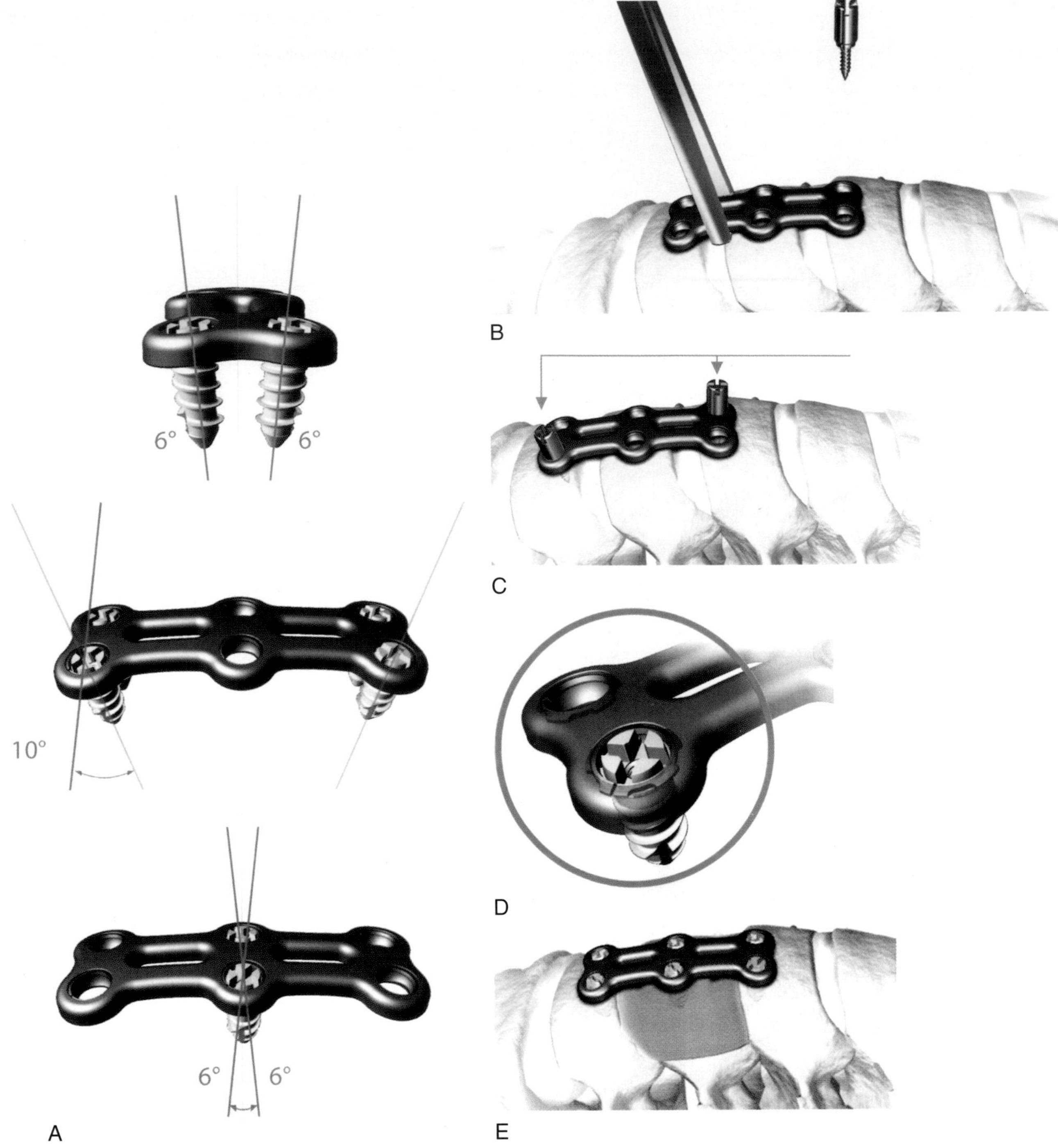

FIGURE 41-31 Anterior cervical discectomy and plating. **SEE TECHNIQUE 41-12.**

- Achieve meticulous hemostasis and close the platysma over a fluted style drain; close the remaining layers.

See also Video 41-1.

POSTOPERATIVE CARE. A rigid orthosis is worn for 4 to 6 weeks until there is radiographic evidence of healing at the graft interfaces. Flexion and extension radiographs are obtained to verify stability and to determine if the orthosis can be discontinued.

ANTERIOR CERVICAL CORPECTOMY AND FUSION, WITH ANTERIOR LOCKING PLATE

TECHNIQUE 41-13

- Preparation, positioning, and exposure are as described in Technique 41-12 with the exception being that a 4-cm incision is made at the cricoid level for C5 (Fig. 41-30).

- Incise the disc widely to the level of the uncinate process bilaterally above and below the fractured vertebra. Use curets to remove most of the disc and clearly view the uncinate process bilaterally at each level. If a metal cage or fibular allograft is to be used, remove the injured body piecemeal and save it to fill the cage or graft. If structural autograft will be used, remove the body with a high-speed burr. This is our preferred method.
- Under the operating microscope, use a high-speed burr to make a vertical groove on each side of the body to be removed that begins above the uncinate process of the normal vertebra caudally to the uncinate process of the injured segment. These grooves define the area of bone to be removed. Using the burr, remove all the bone between the two grooves, deepening each groove as needed. This can be done very rapidly until the cancellous bone of the body gives way to cortical bone, indicating the posterior cortex has been reached. By staying medial to the uncinate the vertebral artery can be avoided, although rarely a tortuous artery can erode medial to the uncinate, and this should be detected on the CT during preoperative planning. Remove the posterior cortex with the burr as well.
- Remove the posterior longitudinal ligament and posterior osteophytes as needed and perform foraminotomies as needed. Normally, the corpectomy defect is at least 17 mm in width. Remove the anterior portion of the cephalad end vertebra to leave a flat surface with preservation of the subchondral bone. Similarly, contour the superior endplate of the caudal end vertebra. The two endplates should each be flat and parallel to one another.
- Carefully measure the distance between the endplates with and without traction applied. When there is little to no movement when traction is discontinued, very careful sizing of the graft is required to avoid graft subsidence or displacement.
- Obtain an appropriate length autograft, fibular allograft, or cage filled with local bone.
- Reapply traction and increase slightly if needed to insert the strut and carefully tamp the strut into place. Because of the inclination of the endplates the graft will be more posterior at the caudal end than it is rostrally when it is resting squarely on each endplate. Verify radiographically or by direct vision that the strut does not extend into the canal. With traction removed, the strut should be stable enough to resist being pulled easily from the corpectomy defect.
- Select the shortest locking plate possible to avoid impingement injury to the adjacent discs. The prepared endplates should be just visible through the screw holes of the plate when it is properly positioned. Drill and place unicortical screws most commonly 14 mm in length. Make sure screws are placed at the correct angle to optimize locking of the screw and plate. Engage the anti-backout mechanism of the plate after placing all four screws. Screws are not placed into the strut.
- Achieve meticulous hemostasis and close the platysma over a fluted drain; close the remaining layers.

POSTOPERATIVE CARE. A rigid orthosis is worn for 6 to 8 weeks depending on the stability of the final construct and radiographic evidence of graft incorporation. Flexion and extension radiographs are obtained to verify stability and discontinue the orthosis.

POSTERIOR SUBAXIAL FIXATION AND FUSION

The instrumentation systems for posterior fixation are polyaxial screws that can be placed in the lateral mass with unicortical or bicortical purchase, or they can be placed in the pedicle. Lateral mass fixation has been shown to be effective and safe and is the preferred method in most instances. The primary exception is the lateral mass of C7, which is smaller, and where fixation is biomechanically inferior to other levels. If the construct is to be continued into the thoracic region, which is typically the case if C7 is included in the fusion, then C7 fixation usually is not included because there is insufficient space for the screw head of the T1 screw and a C7 screw on the rod. If C7 fixation is desirable, pedicle screw placement usually is preferred over lateral mass fixation at this level. The technique for lateral mass screw placement is that of Magerl, as modified by Anderson.

TECHNIQUE 41-14

(MAGERL)

- If the patient is already in traction, maintain traction and alignment. Coordinate with the anesthesiologist for an awake intubation or manually maintain head position and use a GlideScope. If the patient has a spinal cord injury, maintain a mean arterial pressure of 85 to 90 mm Hg throughout the procedure. Use a turning frame such as the Jackson table to position the patient prone.
- Radiographically verify injury reduction; if pedicle screws are to be used, make sure imaging can adequately be accomplished before preparation and draping.
- Incise the skin over the area of exposure. Infiltrate the subcutaneous tissue and muscle with 1 mg epinephrine in 500 mL normal saline.
- Expose the posterior cervical spine subperiosteally to the lateral border of the facet joints after verifying levels.
- If an unreduced dislocation is present, use a Penfield No. 4 dissector or Freer elevator to gently unlock the joint(s). Make a hole in the base of the spinous process of each of the involved vertebrae. Using a tenaculum through each spinous process, carefully distract and posteriorly translate the dislocated vertebra to reduce both facets while an assistant simultaneously uses a Penfield No. 4 dissector to guide the inferior facet into the reduced position. If this cannot be accomplished, remove a small amount of bone from the superior margin of the inferior facet and repeat the process. Postreduction stability is decreased as more bone is resected.
- Remove any facet capsules in the area to be fused and identify the boundaries of the lateral mass, which consist of the superior joint line, the inferior joint line, the lateral

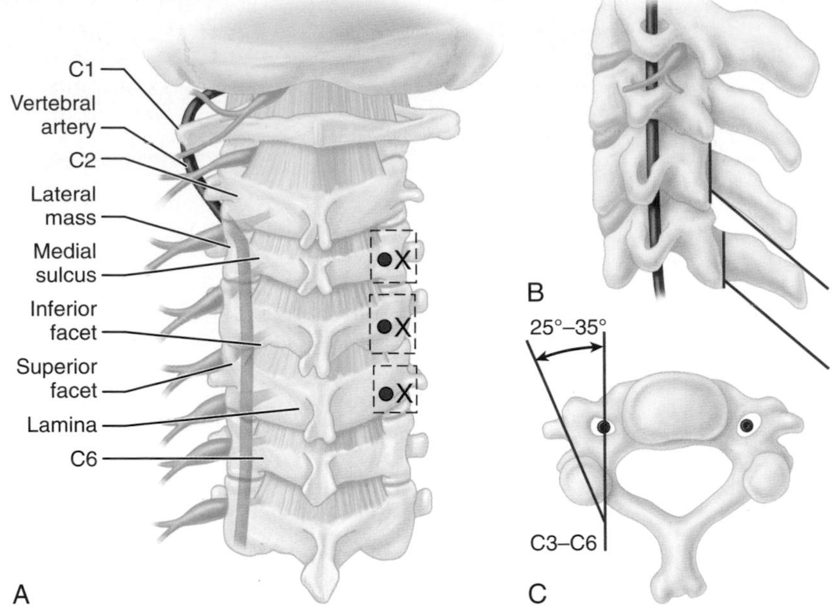

FIGURE 41-32 Posterior cervical plating. **A,** Landmarks used for identifying center of lateral mass and point for drilling. **B,** Relationship of facet joints, nerve root, and drill angle. **C,** Superior view of cervical vertebra showing relationship of drill angle, foramen transversarium, and vertebral artery. **SEE TECHNIQUE 41-14.**

border, and the medial sulcus at the junction with the lamina (Fig. 41-32A).

- If a laminectomy or laminoplasty is planned, do not perform it until the screw holes are completed so the bony landmarks can be used.
- Select an entry portal 1 mm medial to the center of the lateral mass and penetrate only the cortex with a burr.
- Drilling of the lateral mass should be directed 25 to 35 degrees laterally and 25 degrees cephalad (parallel to the plane of the facet joint) for C3 to C6 (Fig. 41-32B). This trajectory can reliably be accomplished by placing the drill guide against the midpoint of the posterior tip (remove large osteophytes if present) of the spinous process of the vertebra caudal to the level being drilled. Use a hand drill set to a depth of 14 mm that will provide unicortical fixation in most patients.
- If bicortical fixation is planned, use a drill of preset length and drill in 2-mm increments. Use a ball-tipped wire to sound the drill hole after each advance of the drill and feel the far cortex. Ideally, the drill will exit just lateral to the vertebral artery, but the artery is at risk if the drill is too medially directed.
- If a cervical pedicle screw is to be placed, carefully review the CT preoperatively to measure the size and orientation of the pedicle. The entry point into the pedicle as described by Abumi and Kaneda is just lateral to the center point of the lateral mass. Penetrate the cortex and advance a probe into the pedicle. The direction of the probe is 30 to 40 degrees medially relative to the sagittal plane, which also has been found to be 90 degrees relative to the ipsilateral lamina. With regard to orientation in the cephalad to caudal direction, this varies by level and usually is slightly caudal at the C7 level and can be identified using image intensification. Ludwig et al. recommended making a laminoforaminotomy and directly palpating the superomedial pedicle to help orient the probe.
- If a thoracic pedicle screw is to be placed, the technique described for all thoracic pedicle screws is used (see Technique 41-15).
- Place each screw. Decorticate the lateral mass and lamina and burr each joint. Cut and contour the rod and secure the rod to the screws with the blockers.
- Pack the bone graft into place.
- Close the wound in layers over a drain.

POSTOPERATIVE CARE. A rigid orthosis is used for 6 weeks and is removed if reduction has been maintained and flexion and extension films indicate there is no motion at the stabilized level(s).

ANKYLOSING SPONDYLITIS

Patients with ankylosing spondylitis form a subgroup of patients who merit special consideration with regard to spinal injuries in general and cervical spine injuries in particular. These patients can present with injury from high-energy mechanisms, but often there is a relatively low-energy mechanism such as a same-level fall. If there is no neurologic deficit, a high level of clinical suspicion must be maintained to avoid potentially serious harm to the patient. The injury mechanism is most often extension such as a blow to the face or head while falling. Because of the ossification of the outer portions of the disc, the spine is unable to absorb the energy imparted and a fracture occurs. The radiographic findings can be very subtle and often require CT or MRI to be appreciated. These fractures are most common in the C5 to T1 region, and noncontiguous injuries are reported in 10% of patients. Patients with a history of ankylosing spondylitis or those who have a characteristic kyphotic deformity at the cervicothoracic junction should be supported to maintain the kyphosis during the evaluation process and should not be laid flat. If a fracture is identified, these patients almost always require operative treatment with posterior segmental fixation over relatively long spans because osteoporotic bone typically coexists with ankylosing spondylitis. Before stabilization, the patient should be moved as infrequently as possible to minimize risk of neurologic worsening. A rigid collar is not adequate for immobilization, and halo vest immobilization should be instituted early as a temporary measure. Halo vest immobilization also is helpful when moving the patient for surgery. Turning the patient into the prone position requires planning and considerable care. These patients are at risk for significant epidural bleeding; a decline in neurologic function requires immediate investigation and early decompression to optimize outcomes. Careful assessment of the entire spine is necessary because of the high incidence of noncontiguous injuries.

VERTEBRAL ARTERY INJURIES

Considerable controversy remains regarding the optimal screening criteria and treatment of vertebral artery injuries associated with cervical fractures more than 50 years after the first description of this relationship by Carpenter. There have been numerous studies with prospectively collected data primarily to establish the incidence and evaluate treatment options. Based on a literature review, Fassett et al. found a 0.5% incidence of vertebral artery injuries in trauma patients; however, 70% had associated cervical fractures. The fractures most commonly associated with vertebral artery injury are those involving the foramen transversarium, the C1 to C3 levels, and displaced fractures or dislocations. The injury patterns associated with vascular artery injury have been further characterized by Lebl et al., who showed an association of vascular artery injury with foramen transversarium fractures displaced >1 mm, basilar skull fractures, ankylosing spondylitis, diffuse idiopathic skeletal hyperostosis, occipitocervical dislocations, and facet subluxations and dislocations. The clinical presentation of vertebral artery injury is highly variable. Patients can remain asymptomatic or develop signs of posterior circulation stroke with a reported mortality in some series as high as 33%, although in the study of Lebl et al. mortality was 4.8%. Foramen transversarium fractures at the level of entry of the vertebral artery are probably more significant than other levels, and although this usually is C6, in 5% of people the artery enters the C7 foramen transversarium. To date, the most reliable diagnostic method has been catheter cerebral angiography, although CT angiography and MR angiography continue to improve. Diagnostic associated complications do occur, which in some series include an iatrogenic stroke incidence of 1%. Treatment is anticoagulation with heparin acutely and may be maintained for 3 to 6 months; in some series, observation is recommended. Because no level I evidence guides treatment, careful coordinated treatment for each individual patient is indicated because it is not yet clear if current treatment improves patient outcomes.

Another important aspect of vertebral artery injury is the influence it may have on operative planning with regard to the cervical spine. Because the vertebral artery is at risk with certain instrumentation techniques, the presence of a vertebral artery injury must be factored into the treatment plan, as well as the effects of anticoagulation therapy if this is instituted.

THORACIC AND LUMBAR INJURIES

Thoracolumbar injuries usually are the result of high-energy trauma, and often associated visceral injuries are present in patients who have sustained significant injuries in this region. As was discussed for cervical injuries, patients with a suspected thoracolumbar injury need rapid evaluation in the trauma assessment area. This should follow the ATLS protocol with a secondary survey that includes inspection and palpation of the entire spine, noting skin condition, tenderness, stepoffs, mental status, motor and sensory examination in the extremities, and a rectal examination for tone and the presence or absence of spinal reflexes. The ASIA form is used to record the neurologic findings. The radiographic assessment should be completed as expeditiously as possible to allow the spine to be cleared and to remove the patient from the spine board or, if injury is present, to identify the injury so prompt treatment can be undertaken. To this end, CT has become the standard method for evaluation of the thoracic and lumbar regions. CT of the chest, abdomen, and pelvis with contrast enhancement is routinely obtained in the same population at risk for thoracic or lumbar spine fractures to assess for visceral injury. Several authors have shown that CT of the chest, abdomen, and pelvis has superior specificity and sensitivity for detecting injuries compared with plain radiographs. Additionally, CT of the chest, abdomen, and pelvis allows completion of the evaluation more quickly and with fewer transfers of the patient. Hauser et al. found that neither CT of the chest, abdomen, and pelvis nor plain radiographs failed to demonstrate any unstable thoracic or lumbar injuries in the 222 patients studied. Identification of additional injuries considered minor by CT of the chest, abdomen, and pelvis compared with plain radiographs was shown to change treatment with respect to pain management and how patients were mobilized. These minor injuries included spinous process and transverse process fractures without displacement.

CLASSIFICATION

The classification of thoracic and lumbar spine injuries is still evolving more than 80 years after the first published report of Böhler. The classification of these injuries remains difficult in part because the goals of classification, anatomic structures to consider, and definitions have not been agreed upon by the community of spine surgeons. Thus, some systems have been developed to direct treatment, whereas others are not intended for this purpose. Terminology, particularly relating to "stability" of the spine, does not have a universally agreed upon definition, which introduces conflicting meanings in different schemes (Box 41-3). Nicoll et al. were the first to focus on patient outcomes and found that anatomic reduction was not crucial to good outcomes in a population of miners who were

BOX 41-3

Factors Related to Spinal Instability

Neurologic Function
- Degree of neurologic deficit
- Potential for additional neurologic injury

Structural Disruption
- Severity of overall structural damage
- Comminution of the vertebral body
- Degree of canal compromise
- Disruption of spinal ligaments
- Disruption of the facet joints, lamina, and pedicles
- Disruption of the intervertebral disc
- Presence of multiple contiguous injuries
- Effect of previous destabilizing procedures

Deformity
- Severity of deformity (kyphosis or scoliosis)
- Buckling of the spinal column (loss of height)
- Potential for progression of deformity
- Redisplacement after reduction
- Potential for late collapse

Anticipated Function
- Loss of stiffness
- Expected future physical exertion
- Potential for developing chronic pain
- Potential impact on future employment

From Mirza SK, Mirza MJ, Chapman JR, Anderson PA: Classifications of thoracic and lumbar fractures: rationale and supporting data, J Am Acad Orthop Surg 10:364, 2002.

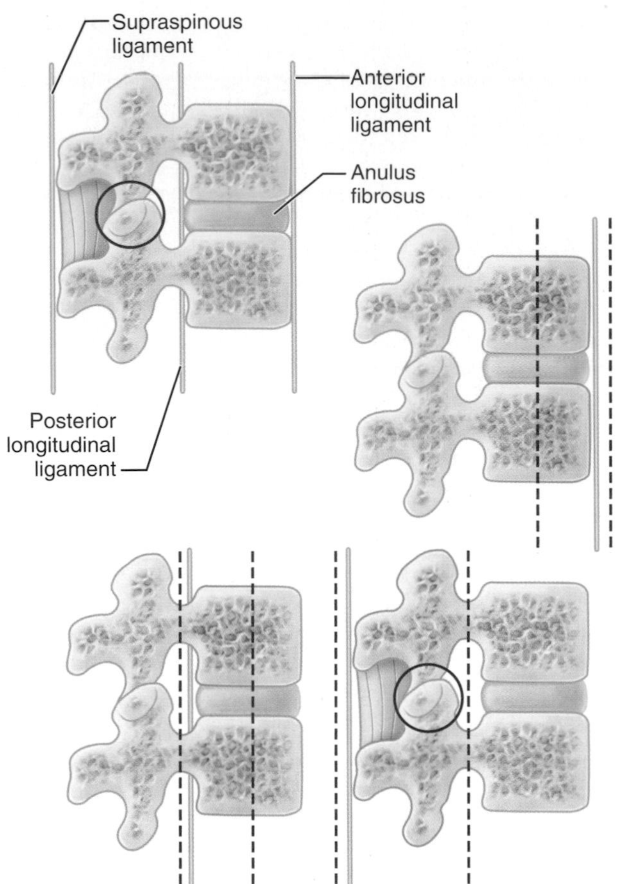

FIGURE 41-33 Three-column classification of spinal instability. Illustrations of anterior, middle, and posterior columns (see text).

the basis of their studies. They also classified fractures as stable or unstable based on the probability of increasing deformity and spinal cord injury. Other systems use "instability" as a surrogate term for neurologic injury and consider injuries unstable if a neurologic injury is present without considering the fracture pattern. To classify fractures it is necessary to image the spine, but imaging has changed significantly in the past several years; CT is now the modality of choice in most centers. The use of MRI remains controversial and has a limited role in the thoracic and lumbar regions. There have been some reports indicating MRI can accurately image the ligamentous structures, but to date these have not been corroborated by large multicenter studies. Classification systems have followed treatment options that have become more diverse as instrumentation for posterior segmental fixation, anterior reconstruction and fixation, intraosseous techniques, and minimally invasive systems have been used in the trauma setting.

Most of the various classification systems currently in use are either based on a presumed mechanism of injury with specific injury patterns recognized or they are based on fracture morphology. The Denis classification, based on a three-column model of the spine (Fig. 41-33), is an example of a mechanistic system that remains in widespread use. The AO system (Fig. 41-34) is based on fracture morphology with more severe injuries progressing from type A to type C with subtypes 1 to 3 within each type of injury. These subtypes are further subdivided into 53 possible patterns. In 2005, a collaborative effort of the Spine Trauma Study Group produced the Thoracolumbar Injury Severity Score (TLISS) system. This system incorporates the neurologic examination of the patient in a more direct way than previous systems and uses this information with the fracture morphology and the integrity of the posterior ligamentous complex to derive a numeric score for a given injury. The numeric value is then used to guide treatment options, and these treatment options are based on consensus opinions. This system was subsequently modified to become the Thoracolumbar Injury Classification and Severity Score (TLICS) by the original author in an effort to improve the reliability of classifying injuries (Table 41-7). There have been numerous articles evaluating the reliability of various classification systems and comparing one system to another or comparing the results of the same surgeons classifying the same cases at different time points. Generally, these studies have not shown one classification system to be superior to another. The TLICS system is appealing because it incorporates the neurologic function of the patient, which is the single most important determinant of functional outcome for a patient with spine injury. Although the reliability of the system has been found to be equivalent to other systems, the validity of the criteria has not been demonstrated, which also is the case for the other classifications. Also, the treatment recommendations are level IV evidence as consensus opinion.

Denis developed the three-column model as an extension of the work of several other authors based on his review of

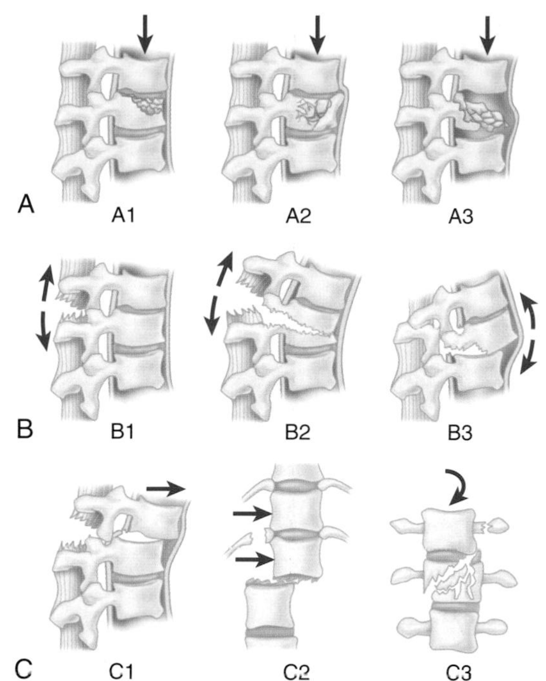

FIGURE 41-34 AO/Magerl classification of spinal injuries. **A,** Compression injuries: A1, impaction; A2, split; A3, burst. **B,** Distraction injuries: B1, posterior ligamentous; B2, posterior osseous; B3, anterior through disc. **C,** Torsion injuries: C1, type A with torsion; C2, type B with torsion; C3, torsion shear.

TABLE 41-7

Thoracolumbar Injury Classification and Severity Score

	POINTS
FRACTURE MECHANISM	
Compression fracture	1
Burst fracture	1
Translation/rotation	3
Distraction	4
NEUROLOGIC INVOLVEMENT	
Intact	0
Nerve root	2
Cord, conus medullaris, incomplete	3
Cord, conus medullaris, complete	2
Cauda equina	3
POSTERIOR LIGAMENTOUS COMPLEX INTEGRITY	
Intact	0
Injury suspected/indeterminate	2
Injured	3

Score of ≤ 3: nonoperative treatment; score of ≥ 5: operative treatment; score of 4: either nonoperative or operative treatment, depending on qualifiers such as comorbid medical conditions and other injuries.

From Vaccaro AR, Zeiller SC, Hulbert RJ, et al: The thoracolumbar injury severity score: a proposed treatment algorithm, J Spinal Disord Tech 18:209, 2005.

412 thoracolumbar injuries, only 53 of which had CT scans. His goal was to highlight the injury patterns resulting from specific injury mechanisms, and this system did not consider treatment or functional outcomes that have become increasingly important to demonstrate. Denis introduced the abstract idea of the "middle column," which is not a distinct anatomic structure but rather the posterior half of the vertebral body, posterior half of the intervertebral disc, and the posterior longitudinal ligament. The mode of failure of the middle column was used to determine the injury type and the risk of neurologic injury. His description did not include a definition of stability. Injuries were designated as minor (e.g., transverse process, pars interarticularis, spinous process) or as major. The major injuries were divided into four categories based on the presumed mechanism of compression, burst, seat belt (Chance injury), or fracture-dislocation. In a CT study of 100 consecutive patients with potentially unstable fractures and fracture-dislocations, McAfee et al. determined the mechanisms of failure of the middle osteoligamentous complex and developed a new system based on these mechanisms. McAfee et al. categorized the failure of the middle osteoligamentous complex into one of three modes: axial compression, axial distraction, or translation. We have found their simplified system useful in classifying injuries of the thoracolumbar spine.

Wedge compression fractures cause isolated failure of the anterior column and result from forward flexion. They rarely are associated with neurologic deficit except when multiple adjacent vertebral levels are affected.

In stable burst fractures, the anterior and middle columns fail because of a compressive load, with no loss of integrity of the posterior elements.

In unstable burst fractures, the anterior and middle columns fail in compression and the posterior column is disrupted. The posterior column can fail in compression, lateral flexion, or rotation. There is a tendency for posttraumatic kyphosis and progressive neural symptoms because of instability. If the anterior and middle columns fail in compression, the posterior column cannot fail in distraction.

Chance fractures are horizontally oriented distraction injuries of the vertebral bodies caused by flexion around an axis anterior to the anterior longitudinal ligament. The entire vertebra is pulled apart by a strong tensile force.

In flexion compression injuries, the flexion axis is posterior to the anterior longitudinal ligament. The anterior column fails in compression, whereas the middle and posterior columns fail in tension. This injury is unstable because the ligamentum flavum, interspinous ligaments, and supraspinous ligaments usually are disrupted.

Translational injuries are characterized by malalignment of the neural canal, which has been totally disrupted. Usually all three columns have failed in shear. At the affected level, one part of the spinal canal has been displaced in the transverse plane.

TREATMENT

The treatment of fractures that involve the thoracic and lumbar spine remains controversial for several reasons. The first is the determination of which injuries are truly best treated operatively and which are best treated nonoperatively; the second is the optimal approach for patients who will be treated operatively; and the third is whether operative treatment should include a direct decompression or if indirect decompression is sufficient. The optimal nonoperative treatment likewise is not settled with respect to whether a postural reduction should be performed, whether initial casting or a thoracolumbosacral orthosis (TLSO) should be used for the duration, or whether treatment should include a period of recumbency or if mobilization should be started quickly. To date, there are only two randomized controlled trials comparing operative with nonoperative treatment of thoracolumbar fractures. In the study of Wood et al. of 53 patients, there were no significant radiographic or functional outcome advantages to operative treatment. In addition, patients treated operatively had a much higher cost of care and higher complication rate than those treated nonoperatively. In a second study, however, Siebenga et al. did report outcome advantages of short-segment posterior fixation compared with nonoperative treatment. A larger series of patients was reported more recently with a novel methodology based on surgeon equipoise as an inclusion criteria to limit bias without the severe limitations of a prospective randomized controlled study. This study, by Stadhouder et al., retrospectively compared 190 patients treated at two different centers either operatively or nonoperatively for thoracolumbar injuries regardless of neurologic status, with the 190 patients selected from 636 total patients on the basis of discordant treatment recommendations from the two centers. The follow-up averaged 6.2 years with a 2-year minimum. Functional outcomes with respect to pain and return to work were determined for 137 of these patients. The authors concluded that with regard to functional recovery and return to work there was no significant difference in the two groups. The operative group had more patients with neurologic deficits and showed a trend toward more neurologic improvement, but this did not reach statistical significance. A systematic literature review by Bakhsheshian et al. confirmed these earlier findings in that functional outcomes after nonoperative treatment were equal to those after operative treatment in patients without neurologic deficits. They also noted that the optimal conservative management method has not been determined. In a review of 5748 patients, Verlaan et al. found that the admission ASIA score is the best predictor of neurologic recovery and that neurologic recovery is not predicted by operative or nonoperative care. To date, no clear benefit for neurologic recovery has been noted after operative treatment. Multiple studies have demonstrated that neurologic recovery does occur in patients with thoracolumbar fractures treated nonoperatively. Typically, incomplete injuries (ASIA B-D) will improve one grade with either form of treatment; several studies, including that of Wood et al., showed no benefit to surgery with respect to correcting spinal canal stenosis caused by retropulsion of bony fragments. Daniels et al., in a retrospective series of 24,098 patients with thoracolumbar injuries from 25 U.S. hospitals, found that 91.7% of patients had no neurologic injury. Nine percent of patients without a neurologic injury were treated operatively compared with 61.4% of patients who had a neurologic deficit. The type of hospital setting where treatment was rendered was a significant determinant of whether a patient received operative or nonoperative care. Patients, with or without neurologic injury, treated at an urban teaching hospital or a high-volume hospital were more likely to have surgery than at a nonteaching hospital. These numbers were significantly different. Numerous relatively small series have described percutaneous instrumentation, often in neurologically intact patients who have been found to do well with nonoperative treatment, and do not contain relevant patient-reported outcomes. The technique appears to be safe, but clinical benefit remains to be determined. Several reports have indicated that patients with instrumented thoracolumbar fractures without fusion have similar kyphosis progression over long-term follow-up as patients with instrumentation and fusion.

The issues of approach and the need for decompression often are linked. Although there is no definitive literature proving the benefits of operative decompression in thoracolumbar fractures, most spine surgeons would not recommend allowing persistent neural compression in the presence of a neurologic deficit. This is based on numerous animal studies dating back several decades that have shown a correlation between neurologic recovery and decompression of neural tissue, which allows for restoration of regional blood flow. Also, a study done by Bohlman et al. demonstrated neurologic recovery occurring after a recovery plateau was reached when a late decompression was done. There is no absolute value for canal compromise that has been found to correlate with neurologic deficit. Panjabi et al. demonstrated with a dynamic injury model that the canal encroachment at the time of injury was 85% greater than was evident on static postinjury images. This explains why there is no correlation between canal compromise on static postinjury imaging studies and neurologic deficit. Direct decompression is not indicated if the patient has no neurologic deficit even with significant canal encroachment at presentation, because this is not related to the development of a subsequent deficit. An indirect decompression often is accomplished during operative stabilization for thoracolumbar injuries. The approach that affords the best opportunity for decompression is selected when a direct decompression is deemed warranted because fixation options have become more versatile, and stable fixation usually is possible with either anterior or posterior fixation, and rarely combined fixation is necessary depending on which anatomic structures are injured.

In our practice, the treatment of thoracic and lumbar fractures is determined primarily by the neurologic status of a patient, a determination of spinal column functional integrity based on which specific structures are injured, and the type and magnitude of deformity present. Most patients with thoracic or lumbar injuries do not have neurologic compromise, and most of these patients are treated nonoperatively. A relatively small portion of these patients have injury patterns that necessitate operative treatment. Progressive neurologic deficit is one circumstance that results in a change to operative treatment. This occurs infrequently; in most studies the incidence is between 0 and 2% of patients, which is consistent with our experience. Patients who develop significant worsening of their deformity with global imbalance in the sagittal or coronal plane rather than regional deformity are treated operatively. There is poor correlation between regional kyphosis at the injured level and functional outcome, although injury to the posterior ligamentous complex is considered structurally important. To detect changes in overall alignment, upright radiographs are obtained after the patient has begun to mobilize.

Patients who have spinal cord, conus medullaris, or cauda equina injuries are most often treated operatively. Short-segment posterior instrumentation is the most common construct used, but specific construct design is dictated by the injury pattern and the neurology of the patient. Anatomic fracture reduction, although desirable, has not been the primary treatment objective. The acceptable limits of residual deformity in the sagittal and coronal planes before functional outcome is compromised have not been determined. In his original series of patients, Nicoll et al. found that of the 50 patients who returned to full function, working as miners for at least 2 years, 24 (48%) had some residual deformity. What is not clear is whether these same patients would have reached functional recovery more quickly and with less difficulty had the deformity not been present.

Nonoperative treatment consists of a TLSO for most patients with injuries at or caudal to T7 to help control lateral bending, although Jewett-type braces also are used fairly frequently if lateral bending is less of a concern and if dictated by body habitus. Injuries that are rostral to T7 are difficult to brace, especially if there are rib fractures at the injured level. Comorbidities, concomitant injuries, and anticipated activity level of the patient are some of the individual factors considered when determining whether brace treatment is a reasonable option for a particular patient. Brace treatment is initiated as soon as possible to begin mobilization, and a postural reduction usually is not done. After the patient has mobilized sufficiently, upright radiographs centered at the injury level are reviewed to confirm adequate maintenance of alignment and full-length radiographs are obtained as soon as feasible. The orthosis is worn at all times when the patient is upright beyond 30 degrees from horizontal for 12 weeks or longer if clinical progress is not as rapid as expected.

COMPRESSION FRACTURES

Compression fractures are characterized by loss of vertebral height anteriorly, with no loss of posterior vertebral height and no posterior ligamentous or bony injury. MRI is not routinely indicated unless ligamentous injury is suspected because of more than 25 degrees of segmental kyphosis. Compression fracture treatment is with a TLSO for 12 weeks with medical management of pain, which is significant, and graduated return to activity. The most severe pain usually improves after 3 to 6 weeks. Upright radiographs must be reviewed after mobilization to verify that there is no worsening of deformity. If the patient has a posterior ligamentous injury and an anterior body fracture, operative treatment is an option. Short-segment posterior tension band reconstruction that can be percutaneously placed has shown promise in this setting, but longer-term study is needed. Intraosseous procedures such as kyphoplasty should be reserved for low-energy pathologic fractures. Higher-energy fractures can have fracture lines not visible on CT scan that may extend through the posterior cortex, allowing ingress of bone cement into the spinal canal.

BURST FRACTURES

The key features of this injury are posterior vertebral body cortex fracture with retropulsion of bone into the canal and widening of the interpedicular distance relative to the adjacent levels. Multiple studies have shown that there is no reliable correlation between degree of canal compromise and neurologic function, so the percentage of canal compromise is not used as a stand-alone indication for surgery. It is very uncommon for a patient to develop a neurologic deficit with proper immobilization for a burst fracture even in the setting of severe canal compromise. Fractures of the laminae that are nondisplaced and vertically oriented do not significantly affect the ability of the spine to bear axial load forces, and the mere presence of such a fracture line does not require operative intervention. Such fractures can, however, entrap nerve rootlets, and if neurologic deficits necessitate decompression, then stabilization will be necessary after decompression. If the patient has a neurologic deficit involving more than a single root level, operative decompression and stabilization are recommended. The decompression can be indirect using distraction and ligamentotaxis through the intact posterior longitudinal ligament or a direct decompression that can be done either anteriorly or posteriorly. If there is a horizontally oriented injury posteriorly in the pars interarticularis, laminae, or a facet disruption, this would suggest a distraction force and not an axial load injury, and the posterior longitudinal ligament may be disrupted, so ligamentotaxis should not be employed. For patients without neurologic deficit who are treated operatively, posterior indirect reduction is used. The terms *stable burst* and *unstable burst* are ambiguous and in our opinion should be avoided in favor of a structural assessment of each specific portion of vertebrae. This allows an overall assessment of the structural integrity of the spine and forms the most logical basis for treatment. If operative treatment is chosen, it also can help direct the anatomic approach and the extent of stabilization that is needed. If operative stabilization is undertaken, short-segment constructs to preserve motion segments are desirable, particularly in the mid and lower lumbar levels. The load-bearing fracture classification of McCormack et al. is helpful in determining if a short construct is likely to fail based on fracture characteristics (Fig. 41-35). For injuries that cannot be stabilized using short constructs, a longer construct can be used in the thoracic spine without sacrificing clinically important motion. In the lumbar spine, anterior decompression and reconstruction usually allow preservation of motion segments and rarely need supplemental posterior stabilization at the same levels. The patient's neurologic status and coexisting injuries must be considered in operative planning. Achieving adequate stability to allow fracture and fusion healing to progress to definitive stability is the objective. For patients requiring the most complete decompression of the spinal cord, direct anterior decompression is favored.

DISTRACTION INJURIES

The cardinal feature of this type of injury is lengthening of the posterior spine that extends into the middle portion or possibly all the way through the anteriormost portion of the spine. It is important to distinguish between flexion-distraction injuries and flexion-compression injuries. Both injuries have posterior lengthening, indicating injury to the posterior osteoligamentous complex. The difference is where the instantaneous center of rotation is located at the time of injury. Flexion-distraction injuries are best represented by the "Chance" injury, described in 1948. This injury classically is located in the upper lumbar spine in people involved in motor vehicle collisions who were using two-point restraints across the lap. Upon impact, the lumbar spine flexes around

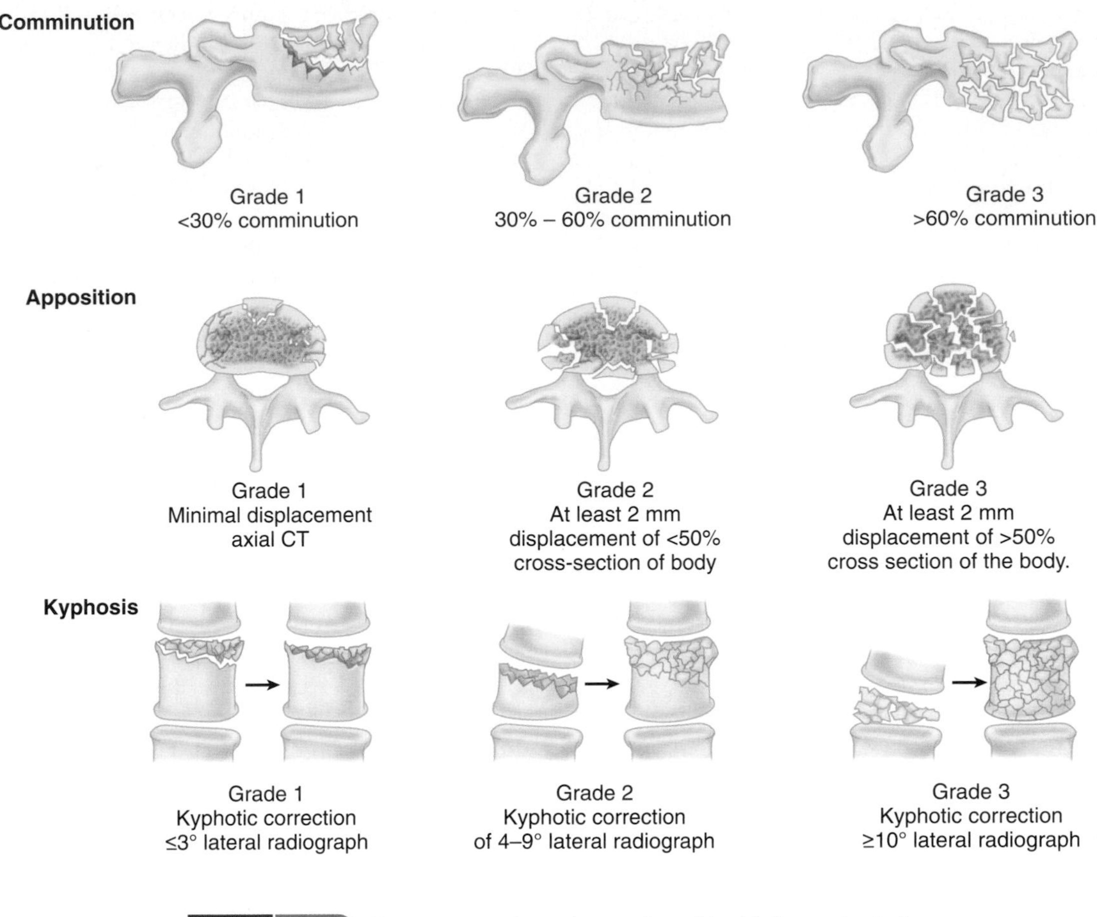

FIGURE 41-35 Fracture severity values assigned by McCormack et al.

the lap belt, and the injury occurs as the osseous structures, ligamentous structures, or both fail in tension around the center of rotation created by the seat belt, compressing the abdominal contents against the anterior spine. Because the rotation occurs around a point anterior to the spine, the lengthening occurs even though the anterior longitudinal ligament that fails in tension, so there is no structure left intact. It is important to recognize this if operative treatment is to be undertaken. Posterior compression constructs are used to stabilize these injuries, and distraction should be avoided because there is no intact structure to prevent excessive lengthening of the spine and neural elements. Flexion-compression injuries occur when the center of rotation is located within the spine such that posterior structures fail in tension and anterior structures fail in compression. Compression is a failure mode for bone but not for ligamentous structures, so in this instance the anterior longitudinal ligament is preserved and can be used as a hinge point during operative stabilization. Operative stabilization can be achieved posteriorly, using careful and monitored distraction and a rod with slightly overcontoured lordosis. This allows better correction of the kyphosis that is present with this type of injury than a compression construct. Because the posterior bone injury occurs in distraction and there is minimal comminution once reduction is achieved, the injuries are able to withstand some axial loading, so short constructs generally are sufficient. Distraction injuries often are associated with neurologic deficits, and these injuries are treated operatively with short constructs and removal of the torn ligamentum flavum that can enfold into the canal, especially if a compression construct is used. If the injury is a true Chance bone injury with no neurologic deficit, satisfactory reduction can be obtained with a hyperextension TLSO for 12 weeks.

EXTENSION INJURIES

Extension injuries are identified by anterior spinal lengthening and most commonly occur in the thoracic spine. Unlike the cervical extension injuries, which can be purely ligamentous or fractures, the injuries in the thoracic and lumbar regions are almost always fractures in patients with ankylosing spondylitis or disseminated idiopathic skeletal hyperostosis. For patients with a minimal neurologic deficit on presentation, the early recognition of this injury pattern is crucial to avoid iatrogenic injury associated with moving the patient for further evaluation or treatment of other injuries. These injuries are very unstable, and translation, usually retrolisthesis, can cause spinal cord injury. It is critical to avoid placing the patient in a horizontal supine position. Early stabilization with a long posterior construct using segmental fixation is the recommended treatment. In addition to neurologic deficits from translation of the spinal column, patients are at risk for development of epidural hematomas. If a patient has neurologic worsening, emergent MRI is indicated to assess the spinal canal alignment and for a hematoma. During the evaluation, the patient is supported in his or her native kyphosis.

FRACTURE-DISLOCATIONS

The pathognomonic feature for this type of injury is translational displacement in the axial plane. The displacement may be most evident on either the sagittal or the coronal reconstruction but may not be well demonstrated on the axial images unless two vertebral bodies happen to be imaged on the same axial slice. There also can be a rotational component (either flexion or extension) present; some injuries have distraction as a major component, but the translational displacement identifies the fracture-dislocation. This injury pattern is the most severe and is usually associated with a significant neurologic injury. These injuries are unstable in shear and require long constructs with segmental fixation. Fracture reduction and proper spinal alignment are more important goals in these injuries than decompression because many have complete neurologic injuries that will not be improved by decompression. Achieving final stability is dependent on achieving a solid fusion.

DECOMPRESSION

The role of surgical decompression is controversial. There are regional differences in cord blood flow and differences in susceptibility to neural injury by anatomic region, progressing from spinal cord to conus medullaris and cauda equina. The spinal canal in the thoracic area is small, and the cord blood supply is sparse; significant neurologic injury is common with severe fractures and dislocations in the thoracic spine. Fractures or fracture-dislocations in the lumbar region may result in marked displacement and still cause little or no neurologic deficit. Not only is the canal larger in this area, but also the spinal cord ends at approximately the first lumbar vertebra, and the cauda equina is less vulnerable than the cord to injury. Wilcox et al. in an in vitro dynamic model showed that maximal compression of the cord and narrowing of the spinal canal occur at the time of impact; both improved after recoil of the spine. The degree of final narrowing of the canal was poorly related to the CT obtained after injury. Krompinger et al. reported that late CT analysis of patients with burst fractures treated conservatively showed significant resolution of bony canal compromise. This finding also was demonstrated by Wood et al. The remodeling process seems to be age and time dependent and follows expected principles of bone remodeling to applied stress. Fontijne et al. showed that remodeling and reconstitution of the spinal canal occurs within the first 12 months after injury (50% of normal diameter at injury and 75% at 1-year follow-up). These authors concluded that conservative management of thoracolumbar burst fractures is followed by a marked degree of spontaneous redevelopment of the deformed spinal canal, which supports conservative management of thoracolumbar burst fractures in selected patients. Neurologic deficits have not developed in these patients. The treatment of thoracic and lumbar burst fractures must be individualized, and canal compromise from retropulsed bone fragments is not in itself an absolute indication for surgical decompression.

Canal compromise without residual neural tissue, which is not correlated with neural injury, must be distinguished from residual neural compression, which does correlate with neural injury. Compression of the neural elements by retropulsed bone fragments can be relieved indirectly by the application of distractive forces through posterior instrumentation or directly by exploration of the spinal canal through a posterolateral or anterior approach. There is no universal agreement as to indications for each of these. The indirect approach to decompression of the spinal canal using ligamentotaxis is a technique that uses the posterior instrumentation and a distraction force applied to the intact posterior longitudinal ligament to reduce the retropulsed bone from the spinal canal by tensioning the posterior longitudinal ligament. Numerous authors have documented excellent results with this technique, and it is a familiar technique to most orthopaedic surgeons. Problems with this technique occur if surgery is delayed for more than 10 to 14 days because indirect reduction of the spinal canal cannot be achieved after fracture healing begins. In addition, severely comminuted fractures with multiple pieces of bone pushed into the spinal canal may not be completely reduced by distraction instrumentation. If the reverse cortical sign is present, the posterior longitudinal ligament is likely not intact and ligamentotaxis will not occur.

The posterolateral technique for decompression of the spinal canal is effective at the thoracolumbar junction and in the lumbar spine. This procedure involves hemilaminectomy and removal of a pedicle with a high-speed burr to allow posterolateral decompression of the dura along its anterior aspect (Fig. 41-36). In the thoracic spine, where less room is available for the cord, this technique involves increased risk to the neural elements. The anterior approach allows direct decompression of the thecal sac but is a less familiar approach to many surgeons. Visceral and vascular structures may be injured, and this approach carries the greatest risk of potential morbidity. In addition, anterior decompression and placement of a strut graft or cage provides modest immediate stability to the fracture if the anterior longitudinal ligament is preserved. To have adequate stability, anterior fixation is needed if anterior decompression is done. The role of anterior internal fixation devices has evolved in recent years, and these devices have proven to be safe and beneficial in achieving spinal stabilization. The need for additional posterior stabilization procedures has been eliminated in some patients. When anterior decompression and strut grafting or cage placement are performed in the presence of posterior instability, posterior instrumentation and fusion can be done to improve stability. This combined posterior and anterior fixation allows for shorter constructs.

At this time, we favor early posterior instrumentation with indirect or posterolateral direct decompression in most patients requiring operative treatment. If significant residual neural compression (not mere canal compromise) exists postoperatively in a patient with an incomplete spinal cord injury, an anterior decompression and reconstruction are done if no significant clinical improvement over a reasonable period of time is noted. Posterior decompression must be carefully considered in all patients with posterior vertical laminar fractures because of the increased frequency of dural tears with exposed nerve roots and the possibility of severe posttraumatic arachnoiditis. Careful neurologic examination is required to detect some deficits; however, in severely injured or obtunded patients, reliable neurologic examination may not be possible. Ozturk et al. found dural tears in 25% of 25 patients with thoracic and lumbar burst fractures in

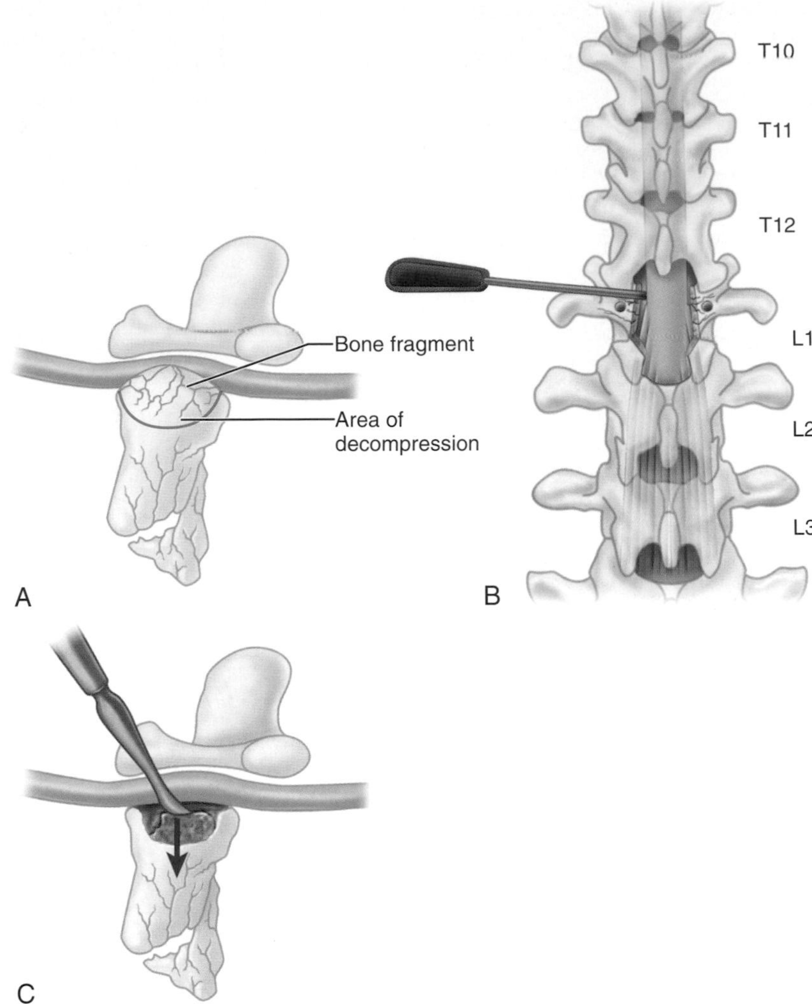

FIGURE 41-36 Posterolateral decompression technique. **A,** L1 burst fracture. **B,** Pedicle, transverse process, and lateral portions of T12-L1 facet are removed after L1 root has been isolated. **C,** After fragments have been undercut, they are reduced into vertebral body.

conjunction with vertical lamina fractures. They were more common at L2 to L4. For patients with severe but incomplete spinal cord injuries at the T12 to L3 levels, anterior decompression and reconstruction is the favored treatment. A minimally invasive approach is used when possible.

Postoperatively, a CT scan of the spine with sagittal reconstruction is obtained through the injured segment to evaluate further the adequacy of spinal cord decompression. In a retrospective review of 49 nonparaplegic patients who sustained an acute, unstable, thoracolumbar burst fracture, Danisa et al. concluded that patients treated with posterior surgery had a statistically significant lower operative time and blood loss. They noted no significant intergroup differences between those treated with anterior decompression and fusion, posterior decompression and fusion, and combined anteroposterior surgery when considering postoperative kyphotic correction, neurologic function, pain assessment, or the ability to return to work. Posterior surgery was found to be as effective as anterior or anteroposterior surgery when treating unstable thoracolumbar burst fractures. Of the three procedures, posterior surgery takes the least time, causes the least blood loss, and is the least expensive.

POSTERIOR STABILIZATION

THORACIC AND LUMBAR SEGMENTAL FIXATION WITH PEDICLE SCREWS

Pedicle screw and rod constructs have continued to increase in use for both thoracic and lumbar fractures over the past decade. By using segmental fixation, rod contouring, and compression and distraction forces as indicated on an individual rod, excellent fracture reduction is possible. Most current systems offer a variety of screw size options and a choice of rod material for the surgeon to tailor stabilization to the specific patient need. Minimally invasive techniques currently are not quite as versatile but do allow for corrective force application such as compression or distraction. The role of minimally invasive stabilization is not well established, and at this time we rarely use these techniques. We believe spinal implants should be used only by experienced spinal surgeons who have a thorough knowledge of spinal anatomy to reduce the incidence of complications, including pedicle fracture, dural tear, nerve root injury, spinal cord injury, and vascular injuries. Image intensification is routinely used to assist in screw placement; image-guided navigation has not been found useful except in unusual cases.

TECHNIQUE 41-15

- A fully radiolucent table is used. Position the patient to allow for postural reduction when placed prone using a four-post frame or chest rolls placed transversely or longitudinally, depending on the extent of postural support desired. If the patient is neurologically intact or incomplete, neuromonitoring is used if the spinal canal dimensions will be manipulated (e.g. distraction for ligamentotaxis and indirect fracture reduction) during the operation.
- Obtain images of the spine to confirm the degree of postural spinal reduction after positioning and determine the limits of the incision.
- Prepare and drape the thoracolumbar spine to be instrumented and the iliac crest if desired.
- Harvest morselized cancellous bone graft from the iliac crest.
- Make a score incision from one spinous process above the area to be instrumented to one spinous process below the area to be instrumented.
- Infiltrate the incision, subcutaneous tissue, and muscle with epinephrine solution (1 mg in 500mL of saline) and then complete the incision sharply.
- Continue the dissection with electrocautery to the fascia. Delineate the fascia for later closure. Continue the dissection through the fascia and subperiosteally expose the necessary levels.
- Use electrocautery to release the muscle from the bone carefully at the level of the fracture. Watch for evidence of a cerebrospinal fluid leak or the presence of free nerve roots.
- Continue to widen the dissection to the tips of the transverse processes in the thoracic and lumbar spine.
- Use image intensification to identify the upper level to be instrumented.

THORACIC PEDICLE SCREW PLACEMENT

- Obtain a true anteroposterior view of the vertebra. On this view the superior endplate should appear as a sharply defined line with the superiormost portion of the pedicle just rostral to the endplate. The pedicles should be symmetric with one another, and the tip of the spinous process should be superimposed in the midline of the vertebra. It is critical to adjust the image until such a view is acquired.
- Position a burr near the superior medial base of the transverse process such that it is superimposed at the 2-o'clock position on the right pedicle or the 10-o'clock position on the left pedicle on the anteroposterior view. Use the burr to penetrate the cortex in this location. Use this as the starting point for a pedicle probe.
- Advance the pedicle probe, monitoring the anteroposterior image and directing the probe medially such that it crosses from the lateral cortex of the pedicle to the medial cortex of the pedicle as it penetrates deeper into the pedicle. The trajectory of the probe should be chosen such that the tip of probe rests at the medial border of the pedicle image after advancing to a depth of 18 mm. This will allow the probe to traverse the length of the pedicle and enter the posterior vertebral body in most patients before becoming medial to the medial margin of the pedicle. This can be confirmed on lateral image intensifier views if the anatomy is atypical. As the probe is advanced, direct it slightly caudally.
- With the probe confirmed in the vertebral body, advance it to the desired depth. It is not necessary to advance into the anterior third of the body.
- Use a small ball-tipped probe to sound the pedicle for cortical breaches in all four quadrants and to confirm the vertebral body was not penetrated anteriorly.
- Place the largest diameter screw that the pedicle will accept. This can be determined from the anteroposterior view of the pedicle. The most narrow pedicles are typically at the T4 to T6 levels. If the bone is very dense or the screw is very large in relation to the pedicle, a tap is used before screw placement.
- If the pedicle is too narrow to accept even the smallest diameter screw, this same technique will allow for safe screw placement with a "in-out-in" path of the pedicle probe. It will enter the bone and then exit the bone into the costovertebral joint and reenter through the lateral pedicle wall to enter the vertebral body. This allows for safe screw placement, although screw purchase is less than with an intact pedicle.
- Most commonly, polyaxial screws are used, although monoaxial screws are occasionally used if more rigidity is needed.
- Place all thoracic screws in a similar fashion (Fig. 41-37). *Details of rod placement follow lumbar screw technique.*

LUMBAR PEDICLE SCREW PLACEMENT

- In the upper lumbar segments the same technique described for the thoracic spine is useful because these pedicles can be quite narrow, especially at L1 and L2. For the lower levels with larger pedicles, we usually prefer to place the lumbar screws using a lateral image of the vertebra being instrumented to help guide screw placement.
- Obtain a true lateral view of the vertebra as indicated by sharply defined endplates with perfectly superimposed pedicles. Adjust the image intensifier until this image is obtained.
- Place the burr just posterior to the junction of the transverse process and the superior articular mass in line with the bisector of the pedicle on the lateral image intensifier view. Penetrate the cortex at this location, which is near the junction of the pars interarticularis and the superior articular mass. Decorticating the transverse process before screw insertion improves the effectiveness of decortication and enhances the fusion bed.
- Use the cortical opening as the starting point and advance a pedicle probe into the pedicle. The probe is advanced anteriorly and medially simultaneously. Direct the probe more medially at the lower lumbar levels (usually 20 to 30 degrees at L5 and 0 to 10 degrees at the L1 level). The cephalad to caudal orientation is guided by the image

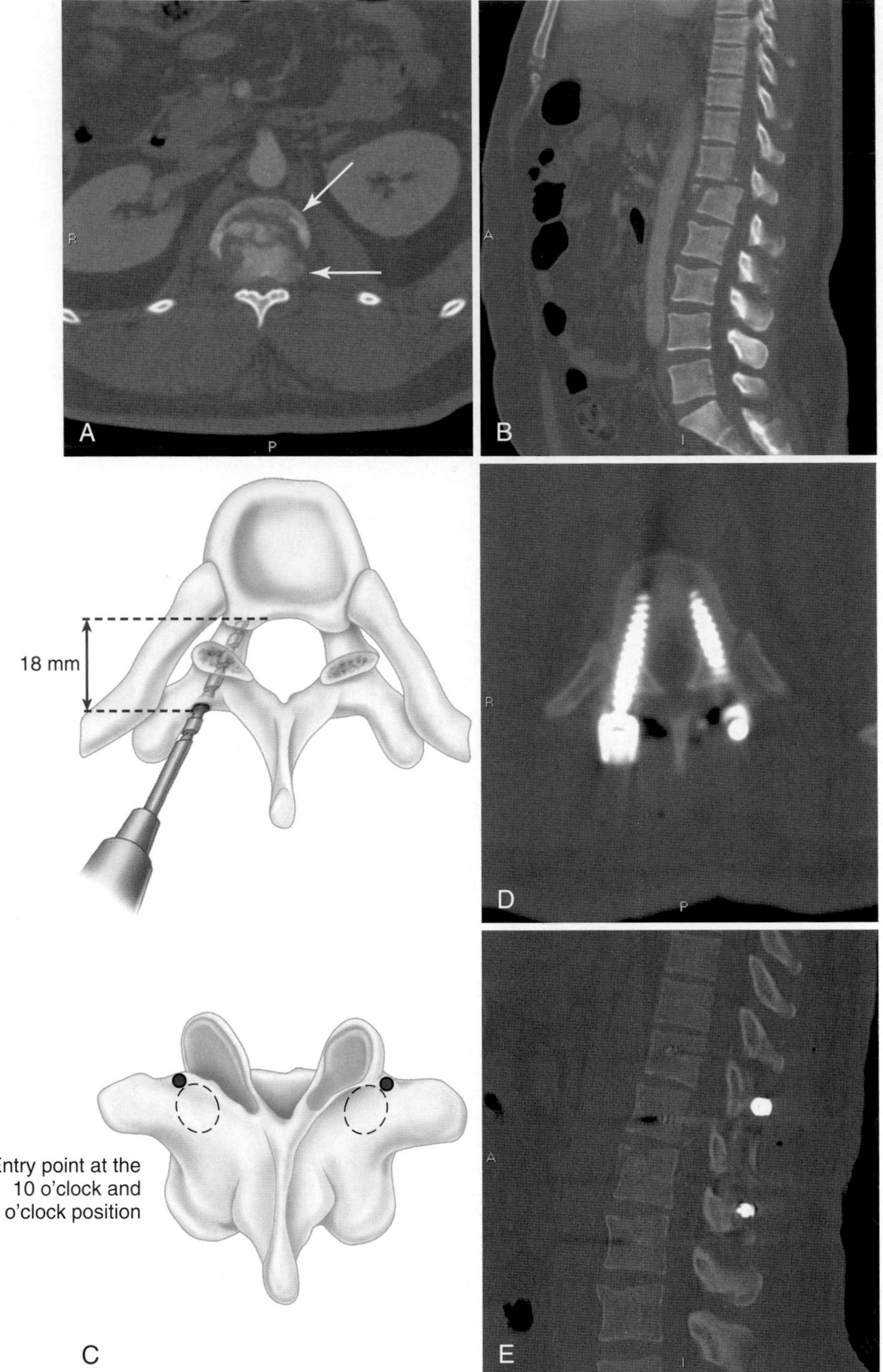

FIGURE 41-37 Axial (**A**) and sagittal (**B**) reformatted images in patient with T12-L1 fracture-dislocation. **C,** Pedicles are drilled to a depth of 18 mm from entry points at the 10-o'clock and 2-o'clock positions. **D** and **E,** Pedicle screws in place with restoration of anatomic alignment. **SEE TECHNIQUE 37-15.**

intensifier view. Advance the probe to the anterior third of the body.

- Use a small ball-tipped probe to sound the pedicle in all four quadrants and to palpate the vertebral body laterally and anteriorly to make sure there are no cortical breaches.
- The largest diameter screw the pedicle will accept (up to a 6.5-mm screw) is typically placed. Larger screws can be placed but little is usually gained, and the larger screws are more likely to cause pedicle fracture and loss of screw purchase. Polyaxial screws are most commonly used, but monoaxial screws can be useful when short constructs

with a single level of fixation above or below the fracture is used. Using a tap will lower the risk of pedicle fracture in sclerotic bone.
- Place the screw after placing the bone graft onto the decorticated surface.
- Adjust the image intensifier to obtain an "end on" view of the screw to verify radiographically that the screw is within the pedicle.
- Place the remaining screws in the same fashion.

ROD PLACEMENT

- Direct decompression, if needed, is completed before rod placement. Costotransversectomy is not used as frequently as transpedicular decompression, but both are useful techniques.
- Cut the rod, allowing some excess length if distraction will be applied.
- Contour the rod to assist in achieving reduction. This usually means undercontouring the kyphosis to help reduce the kyphotic deformity as the rod is reduced into the screw "tulip."
- Reduce the rod to the screws, using multiple reduction instruments if needed to avoid excessive pull on any individual screw, and insert the blockers into the screw "tulip" loosely at each level.
- Apply distraction or compression as the injury dictates and complete in situ rod contouring if necessary to reduce the fracture. Apply final tightening to the blockers and place crosslinks if necessary.
- Confirm adequacy of the reduction on anteroposterior and lateral views.
- Decorticate the posterior elements and transverse processes at each instrumented level and place the bone graft onto the decorticated surface. In the lumbar spine, decortication and graft placement are best done before screw placement. Cancellous allograft can be used if additional bone is needed.
- Close the fascia over a drain with suture passed through the spinous processes.
- Close remaining layers using a subcuticular skin closure for fewer wound problems.

POSTOPERATIVE CARE. Postoperatively a CT scan can be obtained to verify screw position and to determine if there is any residual neural compression in a patient with a neurologic deficit. The patient is mobilized on the first postoperative day with an orthosis unless other injuries preclude this. The orthosis is continued 8 to 12 weeks, depending on resolution of pain and radiographic follow-up for evidence of healing and maintenance of spinal alignment.

ANTERIOR STABILIZATION

Anterior reconstruction can provide satisfactory stability without necessarily requiring a posterior procedure. Sasso et al. reviewed a series of 40 patients with three-column injuries who were treated with anterior reconstruction and found that 91% of those with incomplete neurologic deficits improved one modified Frankel grade and 95% of patients had satisfactory healing with maintenance of alignment. The study was retrospective but included multiple surgeons and two sites.

The approach for anterior reconstruction varies considerably by level of injury (T4 to L3), and many centers have a joint approach using either a cardiovascular surgeon or general surgeon along with a spine surgeon. The primary advantages of an anterior reconstruction are direct decompression and restoration of the axial load-bearing portion of the spine with a strut device. With restoration of some load bearing through the anterior spine, shorter constructs are possible that can allow preservation of more normal motion segments in some clinical settings. Correction of kyphosis also is enhanced with a direct anterior approach. The anterior construct can consist of bone graft or a metallic cage that may be adjustable with respect to length in conjunction with a plate or rod device with screw fixation. Additionally, with a direct anterior decompression of the spinal canal, it is possible to completely remove retropulsed fragments of bone or disc material. The morbidity of the standard thoracotomy and retroperitoneal approaches prohibits their use in many patients, making these advantages less attractive relative to the more common posterior approach. However, with advances in retractor systems and fixation devices so that adjunctive posterior fixation is not necessary, a larger proportion of injuries can now be operatively treated anteriorly. Also, the dimensions of the implants have decreased somewhat, allowing for safer implantation of the devices. Even with these advances, injuries with posterior ligamentous complex disruption should be considered very carefully before recommending anterior-only stabilization. Injuries with translational displacement usually are treated with posterior constructs. Anterior fixation devices consist of a plate or paired rods secured to the spine with bone screws or bolts that have a threaded portion extending through the plate and accepting a nut to capture the plate. Most systems have two fixation points at each vertebral level to better resist flexion. Construct stability is most dependent on the fit of the strut (bone or cage), followed by the integrity of the endplates the strut is in contact with, native bone quality, and the inherent fixation device properties that can be decreased with technical errors in placement.

ANTERIOR PLATING

TECHNIQUE 41-16

- After induction of anesthesia, place the patient in a right lateral decubitus position, with appropriate padding to allow for a left-sided thoracic or retroperitoneal approach. Only rarely is a right-sided approach indicated. Secure the patient to the table to prevent him or her from rolling forward or backward during the procedure, which if undetected can lead to increased risk for neurologic or vascular injury. It is important that the patient remain in a true lateral position so screw trajectory can be correctly determined (Fig. 41-38A). Neuromonitoring generally is used when anterior thoracic or lumbar decompression is planned.
- Complete routine skin preparation including the iliac crest if this will be used as a graft.

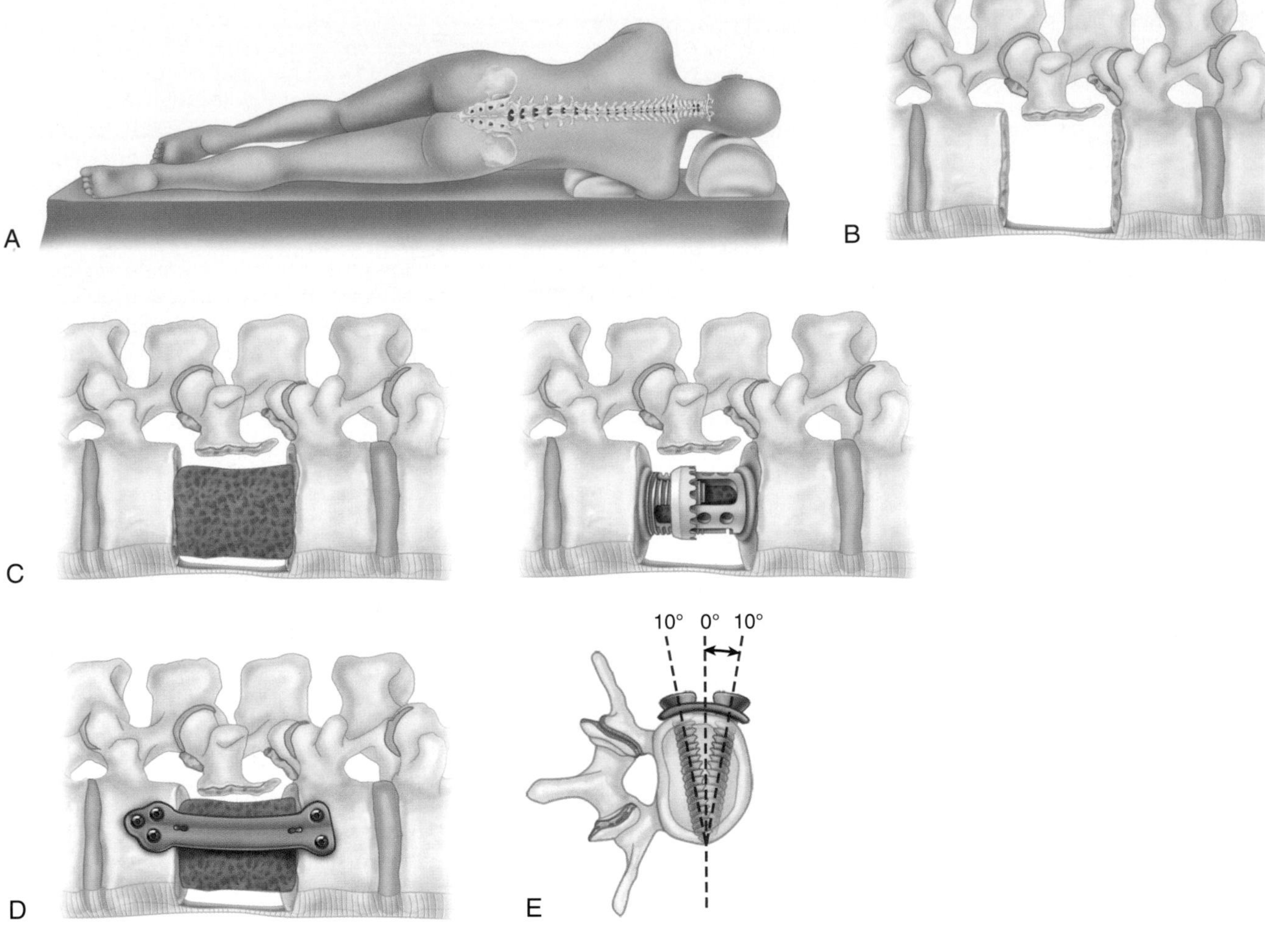

FIGURE 41-38 Anterior stabilization technique. **SEE TECHNIQUE 41-16.**

- Use the image intensifier to locate the intended incision directly lateral to the injured segment. In the thoracic spine this is typically through the rib that is two levels above the injured level. For lumbar injuries a retroperitoneal approach through the 10th or 11th rib usually is used.
- Make an incision overlying the rib and dissect down to the rib periosteum with electrocautery. Elevate the periosteum circumferentially around the rib and elevate the neurovascular bundle from the inferior rib margin. Resect the portion of the rib necessary for access to the spine. Make sure to remove enough rib posteriorly. The rib can be used along with the resected vertebral body for bone graft and should be maintained.
- For a transthoracic approach (T4 to T10), enter the pleural space and retract the lung with a wet laparotomy sponge. Shape a malleable retractor to maintain the operative field. Some prefer to deflate the lung and use a double-lumen endotracheal tube, but we have not routinely found this to be necessary to maintain the lung out of the field. Identify the aorta by palpation and ligate the segmental vessels 1 cm from the aorta. Divide between ligatures at the injured level and at the level above and below the injured level. Vascular clips can be used to supplement the ligatures. Ligating the artery of Adamkiewicz, which has a variable location, is an inherent risk of this procedure.
- For a retroperitoneal approach (T11 to L3), maintain the pleura intact if possible and enter the retroperitoneal space, dissecting bluntly down to the iliopsoas. Use a wet laparotomy sponge and a malleable retractor to maintain the operative field. Ligate the segmental arteries at the injured level and the level above and below 1 cm from the aorta. Divide between ligatures with supplemental vascular clips if needed. The artery of Adamkiewicz can be as low as L2. The crus of the diaphragm is taken down as needed, depending on the level of injury. Elevate the iliopsoas from the spine from the anterior margin, taking care to avoid the genitofemoral nerve and ureter.
- Incise the discs above and below the injured segment and remove most of the disc, leaving the anteriormost disc and anterior longitudinal ligament intact. Protect the aorta from sharp instruments with a malleable retractor placed gently between the aorta and the anterior spine.

- Using the space created by removing the discs, remove the vertebral body in its midportion, again leaving the anterior longitudinal ligament and anteriormost bone in place. An osteotome is useful to remove the posterior bone, which is preserved for graft. During bone removal ensure that the patient position has not changed to avoid inadvertent entry into the spinal canal (Fig. 41-38B).
- After creating a cavity in the midportion of the body, remove the posterior bone by progressively thinning the remaining bone and pulling it into the created defect across the canal to the level of the far pedicle medial wall to achieve a satisfactory decompression. If decompression of the posterior cortex is begun on the far side of the canal, troublesome bulging of the dura into the space created by removing the vertebral body is minimized and the surgeon's view is less obstructed.
- Take care throughout not to violate the endplates of the intact vertebra that will support the strut.
- Meticulously clean the two endplates of all cartilage and soft tissue. A surgical assistant should apply firm, anteriorly directed pressure over the spine to correct kyphosis. Measure the corpectomy defect for length of the strut in the corrected position. Additional anterior distraction with a lamina spreader can be applied but must not injure the endplates. Release of the anterior longitudinal ligament seldom is necessary in acute injuries.
- Obtain a bone graft or cage device of the desired length. Fill allograft humeral shaft or a metallic cage with the available bone from the operative field. With kyphosis correction maintained, impact the strut into place. The strut should be secure once it is in position, but avoid excessive length because it increases the risk of mechanical failure through subsidence. Image intensification views are used to verify spinal alignment and satisfactory placement of the strut (Fig. 41-38C and D).
- Determine the appropriate plate length and position the plate.
- Determine the transverse dimension of the intact vertebra so appropriate-length screws or bolts can be used for bicortical fixation, depending on the device used.
- Identify the entry points of screws as shown (Fig. 41-38E).
- Place the first screw in the posterior position of the caudal vertebra. Take care when determining placement of this screw to drill and place the screw parallel to the end plate and directed away from the spinal canal.
- Place the adjacent screw, again parallel to the endplate and angled slightly posteriorly.
- Place the screws at the cephalad level similarly. Some devices allow for additional compression to be applied if desired.
- Once all screws are secured, obtain hemostasis and close the wound in a routine manner over suction drains or chest tube as appropriate.

POSTOPERATIVE CARE. The patient is kept at bed rest until the chest tube is removed. The patient is then mobilized in a TLSO that is worn at all times when the spine is more vertical than 30 degrees from the horizontal plane. The TLSO is used for 12 to 16 weeks, depending on the clinical course.

SACRAL FRACTURES AND SPINOPELVIC DISSOCIATION INJURIES

The sacrum plays a central role in the stability of both the pelvis and the spinal column. The complex of ligaments that invest the sacrum anteriorly and posteriorly, the ligaments of the pelvic floor, and the osseous structure of the sacrum and pelvis all contribute to lumbopelvic stability and help prevent injury to the neurovascular structures in the region. The important neurologic structures at risk with sacral injuries include not only the L5 and S1 roots but also the lower sacral roots and autonomic nerves that are important for continence of the bowel and bladder and sexual function. Injuries to the sacrum are frequently missed at presentation because these patients often are involved in high-energy trauma and present with multiple injuries and may be hemodynamically unstable on arrival to the treating facility. Denis reported a large series of patients with sacral fractures, and 30% were identified late. This indicates how important a careful examination and a high index of suspicion are for detection of these injuries. As discussed earlier, the ATLS protocol should be followed for trauma patients, including palpation and inspection of the spine and posterior pelvis. Soft-tissue injuries are common in patients with sacral fractures, including Morel-Lavallée lesions that can significantly complicate the ultimate care for the patient. The neurologic evaluation must include a rectal examination to assess rectal tone and maximal contraction of the anal sphincter. The ASIA neurologic examination form should be completed to document possible L5 or S1 root injuries. The usual presence of a Foley catheter prevents assessment of bladder continence. Likewise, there is no clinical examination to detect injury to the anterior rami of S2 to S5, which contribute to the parasympathetic system and are important for sexual function and normal bladder and rectal function. Injuries to the sacrum also can damage the sympathetic ganglia of the inferior hypogastric plexus that are medial to the S2 to S4 foramina anteriorly. The L5 nerve is at risk at the anterior junction of the ala and the sacral promontory, and the S1 nerve root can be injured within the foramen. Extremity motor and sensory testing and rectal examination with pinprick and light touch examination in the perianal concentric dermatomes should be done to evaluate S2 to S5 function, as well as eliciting the anal wink and bulbocavernosus and cremasteric reflexes.

Plain radiographs have not proven sensitive in demonstrating injuries to the sacrum and lumbosacral region. CT of the chest, abdomen, and pelvis is the imaging modality of choice to screen for injuries to the pelvis and sacrum. If injuries are identified, a dedicated CT scan of the pelvis with 2-mm slices and sagittal and coronal reformatted images should be obtained. When there are associated neurologic injuries with displaced fractures, MRI also may be of value, but the best indications for MRI presently have not been fully delineated.

CLASSIFICATION

A discussion of all pelvic fractures is beyond the scope of this section; only the relatively rare injuries with subluxation or dislocation of the L5-S1 joint and fractures of the sacrum that are associated with lumbopelvic instability are covered.

Multiple classification schemes have been devised for these injuries over the past several decades, but there is no single system that encompasses sacral and lumbopelvic injuries. Denis et al. categorized 236 sacral fractures into three types based on three zones (Fig. 41-39). Zone 1 fractures are lateral to the neuroforamina and were the most common in the series, accounting for 50% of injuries with a 6% incidence of L5 and S1 injuries. Zone 2 injuries are through the neuroforamina and accounted for 34% of the injuries, and 28% of these patients had neurologic deficits unilaterally at the L5, S1, or S2 levels. Some zone 2 injuries have a shear component that increases the instability of the injury and increases the risk of nonunion. Zone 3 injuries are medial to the foramen and involve the spinal canal, comprising the remaining 16% of injuries. Sixty percent of patients have neurologic symptoms that involve bowel and bladder dysfunction, and 76% have sexual dysfunction. Roy-Camille et al. and Strange-Vognsen and Lebech subclassified the Denis zone 3 injuries that have a transverse component that connects the zone 3 fracture to another fracture on the contralateral side in zone 1 or 2 (Fig. 41-40). Isler developed a classification to describe injuries at the lumbosacral joint level with increasing probability of lumbosacral subluxation progressing from type 1 to type 3 injuries (Fig. 41-41).

TREATMENT

Many sacral fractures can be treated nonoperatively as well as some pelvic fractures, and a more complete discussion of these injuries is presented in other chapters. Fractures of the sacrum that are displaced and unstable or are associated with pelvic instability or spinal instability require operative treatment. Disruptions of the sacroiliac joint and some vertically unstable sacral fractures can be treated with percutaneous iliosacral screws. The best trajectory is horizontal with purchase in the S1 body. For Denis zone 2 injuries, compression should be avoided to reduce risk of injury to the L5 root, which is at risk of being iatrogenically compressed within the fracture. If compression is not achieved, fracture stability is compromised.

Injuries with subluxation or dislocation at the lumbosacral joint or that involve spinopelvic dissociation can be treated with lumbosacral or lumbopelvic fixation constructs. Nonoperative treatment of these injuries generally is not recommended because of the high nonunion rates, severe chronic pain, and neurologic worsening that can occur and can be very difficult to treat late (Table 41-8).

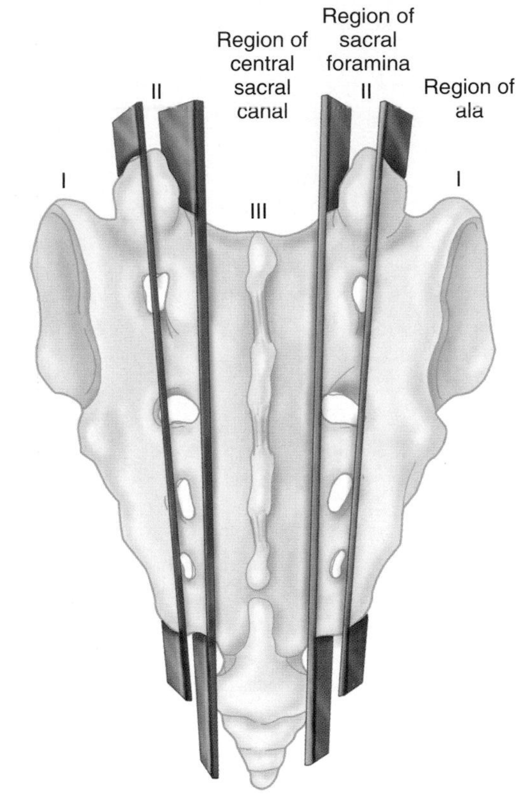

FIGURE 41-39 Three zones of sacrum described by Denis et al.: region of ala, region of sacral foramina, and region of central sacral canal.

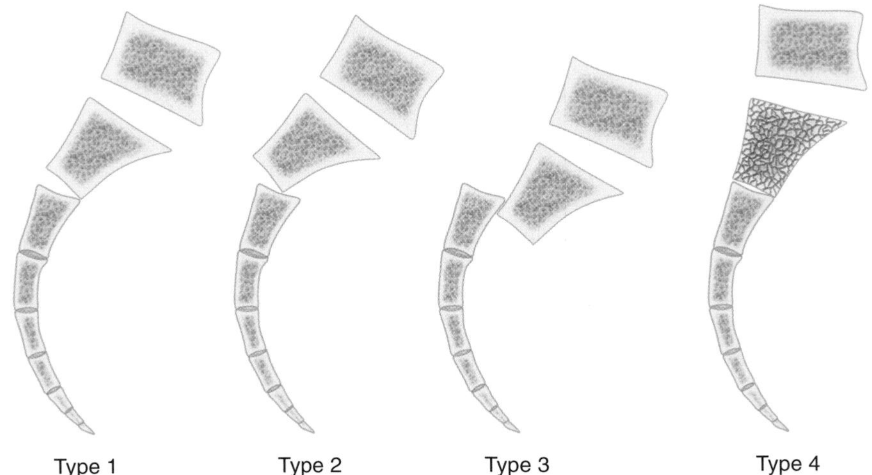

FIGURE 41-40 Roy-Camille and Strange-Vognsen and Lebech subclassifications of Denis zone 3 fractures. Type 1, angulation with no translation; type 2, angulation and translation; type 3, complete displacement of cephalad and caudal sacrum; type 4, segmental comminution. (Reproduced from Vaccaro AR, Kim DH, Brodke DS, et al: Diagnosis and management of sacral spine fractures, Instr Course Lect 53:375, 2004).

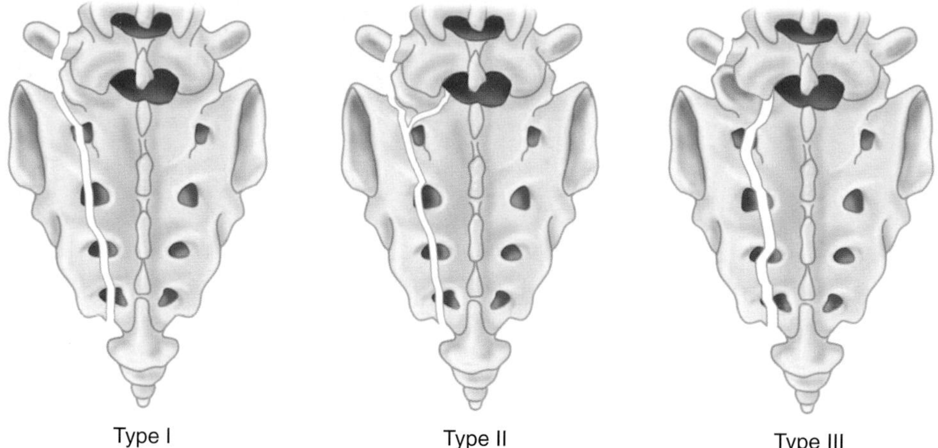

FIGURE 41-41 Isler classification for fractures of sacrum and lumbosacral junction. Type I, injury lateral to L5-S1 facet joint affecting pelvic ring stability; type II, injury through L5-S1 facet joint associated with displacement and neurologic symptoms; type III, injury involving spinal canal that is unstable. (From Vaccaro AR, Kim DH, Brodke DS, et al: Diagnosis and management of sacral spine fractures, Instr Course Lect 53:375, 2004.)

TABLE 41-8

Gibbons Classification of Cauda Equina Impairment

TYPE	NEUROLOGIC DEFICIT
1	None
2	Paresthesias only
3	Lower extremity motor deficit
4	Bowel/bladder dysfunction

From Shildhauer TA, Bellabarba C, Nork SE, et al: Decompression and lumbopelvic fixation for sacral fracture-dislocations with spino-pelvic dissociation, J Orthop Trauma 20:447, 2006.

The operative approach we use to stabilize these injuries is similar to that described by Schildhauer et al. The goals of treatment are to decompress the sacral nerves, restore stability, and improve alignment. Lindahl et al. reviewed 36 cases to determine factors associated with neurologic recovery and late pain. The severity of translation through the fracture correlated with neurologic recovery, and the quality of reduction correlated with pelvic pain. The patients are initially resuscitated and stabilized with respect to other injuries, and definitive spinopelvic fixation is completed as soon as the patient is able to tolerate the surgery. Ruatti et al. described a reduction maneuver that is done closed and as early as possible, even if definitive stabilization will be delayed. The technique involves strong and rapidly applied traction through femoral traction and countertraction applied to the torso with extension of the lumbosacral spine over a bolster. The average time to surgery reported by Schildhauer et al. was 6 days. If the patient has anterior pelvic instability, this is reconstructed first. Posterior stabilization is then done when the soft tissues are thought to be satisfactory. This stabilization is done through a midline approach, using pedicle screw fixation in the lower lumbar and S1 segments if possible and iliac screws. Because of the large forces being neutralized by the pedicle screws, we have used at least four points of fixation in the lumbar spine, and this was also the recommendation by Schildhauer et al. Typically, the construct begins at L4 with bilateral screws at this level and the L5 level. The S1 pedicles often are fractured and not available for screw placement, but if they are intact, L4 can be left out of the construct. Fusion is done across all instrumented spine levels. The sacroiliac joints are not fused. Iliac fixation consists of iliac screws inserted at the posterior superior iliac spine and directed through the sciatic buttress toward the anterior superior iliac spine and, when possible, iliosacral screws are placed. We have typically used a single iliac screw on each side (8.5 mm × 100 to 120 mm) and supplemented with iliosacral screws if reduction allows. Schildhauer et al. recommended two iliac screws per side or one iliosacral screw and one iliac screw per side. In either case, biomechanical data are not available. The prominence of the implants is an issue to consider because of the high wound complication rate. When placing the iliac screws, every effort is made not to elevate soft tissue unnecessarily, and the posterior superior iliac spine is instrumented using the "teardrop" view on image intensification with very minimal direct visualization. The iliac screw is started on the ventral portion of the posterior superior iliac spine near the sacroiliac joint to minimize the prominence of the screw head (Fig. 41-42). This also helps in connecting the rod. This usually can be done without a separate connecting rod and minimizes the hardware profile. A wide decompression of the sacral nerve roots is completed with removed bone used for bone grafting at the L4 to S1 segments. Dural lacerations are directly repaired when possible and patched with dural graft and fibrin glue if primary closure cannot be obtained. Reduction often is difficult, and using Schanz pins inserted into the S1 body to assist in disimpacting the fracture and restoring length is helpful, as is the use of a femoral distractor attached to a Schanz pin in the L5 pedicle and a pin in the ilium. Once reduction is achieved, bilateral rods are contoured and secured to the screws. Contouring the rods before determining the site for the iliac screws is very helpful. After placing the rods bilaterally, they are compressed toward one another and a crosslink is applied (Fig. 41-43). Another reduction technique described by Starantzis involves a temporary rod

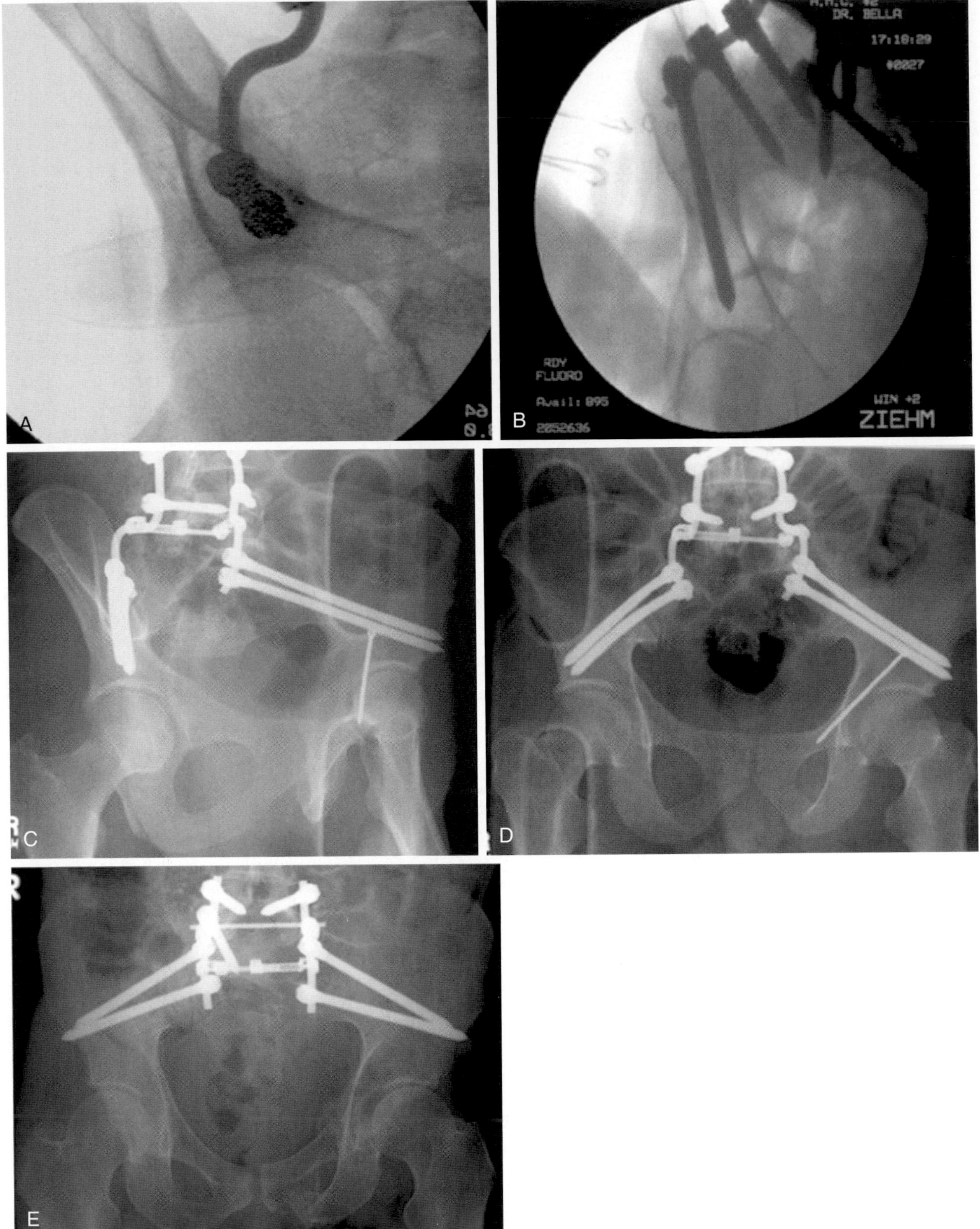

FIGURE 41-42 Obturator-outlet and obturator inlet views and iliac oblique intraoperative views guide accurate screw insertion. **A,** Bone corridor between posterior superior iliac spine and anterior inferior iliac spine, in which iliac screws are ideally placed, projects as teardrop on combination obturator-outlet oblique image. **B,** Screw is extraosseous if it extends beyond cortical boundary of radiographic teardrop. Intraosseous screw placement between inner and outer tables of ilium can also be guided and confirmed with obturator-inlet oblique view. **C,** Iliac oblique image ensures accurate screw length and appropriate location above greater sciatic notch. **D,** Two iliac screws positioned parallel or more cephalad (**E**) can be used for placement of second iliac screw, yielding triangular configuration. (From Shildhauer TA, Bellabara C, Nork SE, et al: Decompression and lumbopelvic fixation for sacral fracture-dislocations with spino-pelvic dissociation, J Orthop Trauma 20:447, 2006.)

on one side from L4 to the pelvis with a reduction screw placed at L4. A rod reduction tool is placed at L4, and distraction is applied to the reduction tower (persuader) until length has been restored. With the fracture out to length, the rod is reduced into the L4 screw and provisionally fixed. Fixation does allow mobilization without bracing, but persistent pain, neurologic dysfunction in the lower extremities, sexual dysfunction, and incontinence often remain problematic, and treatment recommendations must be individualized (Fig. 41-44).

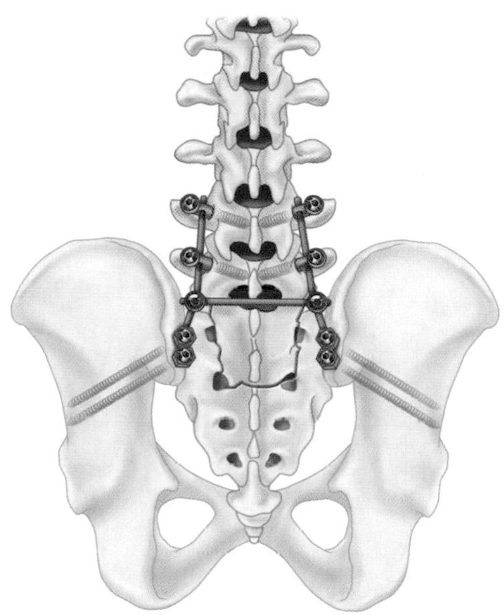

FIGURE 41-43 Lumbopelvic fixation for sacral fracture with spinopelvic dissociation.

For injuries that involve lumbosacral subluxation or dislocation without pelvic ring or vertical sacral fracture, stabilization is accomplished with pedicle screw fixation at L4 and L5 on the cephalic side of the injury and S1 and S2 fixation on the caudal side of the injury. Bone grafting is used posteriorly. If S1 fixation is not possible because of the injury pattern, fixation to the pelvis is used without fusion of the sacroiliac joint.

LUMBOPELVIC FIXATION (TRIANGULAR OSTEOSYNTHESIS)

TECHNIQUE 41-17

(SHILDHAUER)

- Bowel preparation is completed preoperatively. After induction of anesthesia, position the patient prone on a radiolucent four-poster frame that can accommodate an anterior pelvic fixator if needed, such as a Jackson frame. Somatosensory evoked potentials and electromyographic monitoring are initiated. Use image intensification to obtain a lateral view of the sacrum.
- After routine skin preparation and draping, make a midline incision extending caudally far enough to allow adequate decompression, without unnecessary skin tension.

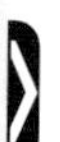

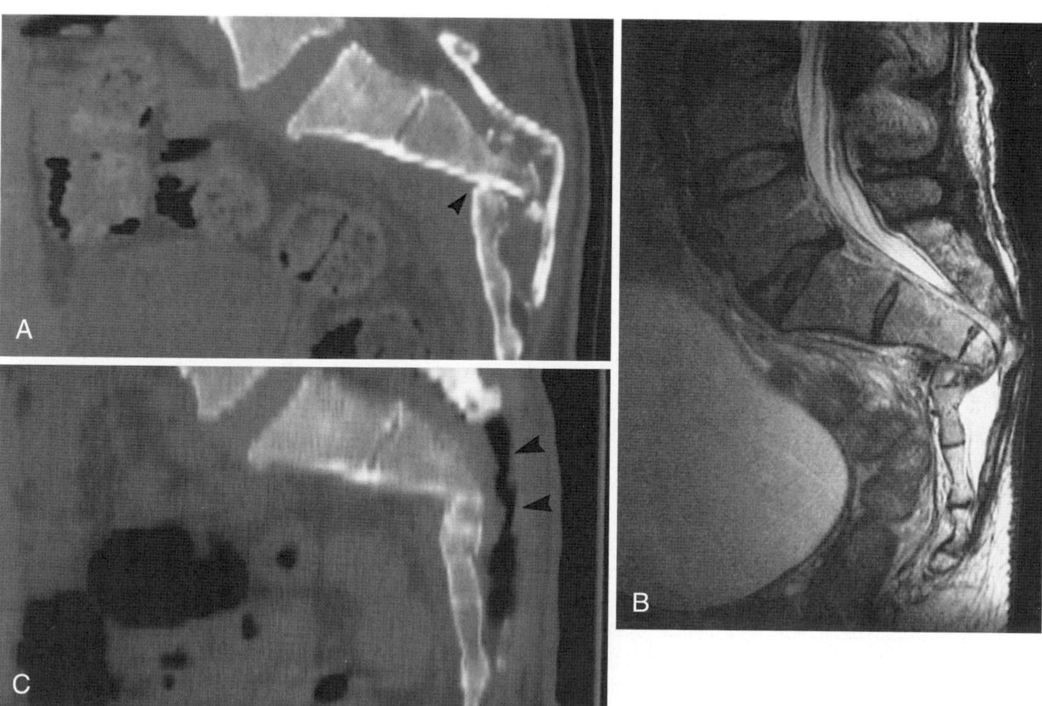

FIGURE 41-44 **A,** Sagittal CT scan of transverse fracture through S3 resulting in transection of sacral nerve roots *(arrowhead).* **B,** MR image of sacral fracture resulting in complete canal compromise. **C,** Postoperative CT scan shows decompression of sacral spinal canal after laminectomy *(arrowheads).*

- Divide tissue down to fascia with electrocautery and carefully elevate the soft tissue subperiosteally to expose the necessary lumbar segments and sacrum. Expose the transverse processes at each lumbar level and the intertransverse ligament. Subperiosteally expose the sacral ala at least 1.5 cm lateral to the lateral face of the sacral facet. Expose the posterior sacrum caudally to the fracture site and laterally as wide as the spinal canal. The posterior superior iliac spine will overhang this area, but it is not necessary to elevate the soft tissue from the sacroiliac joint and the posterior superior iliac spine, and this tissue should be left attached to the maximal extent possible. Only a small area of the ventral portion of the posterior superior iliac spine must be visible.
- Using Kerrison rongeurs and small curets, unroof the spinal canal and expect the nerves to be compressed or impaled by the bone. Repair the dural injury if possible. Mobilize the sacral roots and push the ventral bone anteriorly if needed to relieve tension on the roots.
- Reducing the fracture is difficult. Place a Schanz pin in the posterior body of S1 between the S1 and S2 foramen to manipulate the spine in relation to the pelvis. Femoral traction and a femoral distractor between the spine and ilium can be used. If reduction can be adequately achieved, iliosacral screws can sometimes be placed as transfixation screws, taking care not to compress through the vertical foramina fractures. Individual anatomy and incomplete reduction may preclude safe placement of iliosacral screws.
- Correction of the angulation and some shortening through the fracture site improve the decompression.
- Decorticate the sacral ala and transverse processes and pack the lateral gutter for hemostasis. Decortication after pedicle screw placement is less effective and may limit fusion.
- Obtain a true lateral view of the vertebra, as indicated by sharply defined endplates with perfectly superimposed pedicles. Adjust the image intensifier until this image is obtained.
- Place the bur just posterior to the junction of the transverse process and the superior articular mass in line with the bisector of the pedicle on the lateral image intensifier view. Penetrate the cortex at this location, which will also be near the junction of the pars interarticularis and the superior articular mass.
- Use the cortical opening as the starting point and advance a pedicle awl into the pedicle. Advance the awl anteriorly and medially simultaneously. The pedicle awl must be advanced carefully owing to the mobility of the spine. If S1 screws will be placed, bicortical purchase is optimal with screws exiting the anterior promontory just caudal to the S1 endplate. The S1 screws should be medialized so the screw tips are at or near the midline.
- Use a small ball-tipped probe to sound the pedicle in all four quadrants and to palpate the vertebral body laterally and anteriorly to make sure there are no cortical breaches. The probe should exit anteriorly at S1.
- The largest-diameter screw that the pedicle will accept (up to a 6.5 mm) is typically placed. Larger screws can be placed, but little is usually gained, and the larger screws are more likely to cause pedicle fracture and loss of screw purchase. Polyaxial screws are used. Using a tap for the anterior S1 cortex will lower the risk of pedicle fracture in sclerotic bone. Place the bone graft onto the decorticated surface before screw insertion.
- Adjust the image intensifier to obtain an "end on" view of the screw to verify radiographically that the screw is within the pedicle.
- Place the remaining screws in the same fashion.
- Contour rods so they will be adjacent to the posterior superior iliac spine when connected to the lumbar screws. Adjust the image intensifier for the "teardrop" view after verifying that a true lateral view of the pelvis with superimposition of the sciatic notches can be obtained (Fig. 41-42). Select the entry point into the posterior superior iliac spine on the teardrop view and advance the straight pedicle awl or 3.2-mm drill to a depth of 100 to 140 mm remaining within the confines of the teardrop. Sound the hole for cortical defects and place a large caliber screw. We have used a single 8.5-mm screw even if iliosacral screws cannot be placed. Schildhauer et al. recommends two iliac screws that may need to be somewhat smaller depending on the teardrop size.
- Confirm that the iliac screws are intraosseous bilaterally, using obturator-outlet oblique and obturator-inlet oblique views, and confirm their length on the iliac oblique views.
- Secure the rods to the screws.
- Compress the rods toward one another and crosslink at the lumbosacral level to minimize hardware prominence.
- Decorticate the facet joints and pack with additional bone.
- Carefully close the fascia back to bone where possible over a suction drain.
- Close the thin subcutaneous layer and then the skin with subcuticular suture.

POSTOPERATIVE CARE. The patient is maintained off the wound as much as possible for the first several days. The drain is removed on the first postoperative day usually, and mobilization without a brace is allowed. Full weight bearing is allowed unless precluded by pelvic or other injuries.

REFERENCES

GENERAL

Aarabi B, Alexander M, Mirvis ST, et al: Predictors of outcome in acute traumatic central cord syndrome due to spinal stenosis, *J Neurosurg Spine* 14:122, 2011.

Aarabi B, Hadley MN, Dhall SS, et al: Management of acute traumatic central cord syndrome (ATCCS), *Neurosurgery* 72(Suppl 2):195, 2013.

American Spinal Injury Association (ASIA): www.asia-spinalinjury.org/publications/index.html. 2006.

Bono CM, Heggeness M, Mich C, et al: Commentary North American Spine Society. Newly released vertebroplasty randomized controlled trials: a tale of two trials, *Spine J* 10:238, 2010.

Carreon LY, Dimar JR: Early versus late stabilization of spine injuries: a systematic review, *Spine* 36:E727, 2011.

Cooper K, Glenn CA, Martin M, et al: Risk factors for surgical site infection after instrumented fixation in spine trauma, *J Clin Neurosci* 23:123, 2016.

Daly MC, Patel MS, Bhatia NN, Bederman SS: The influence of insurance status on the surgical treatment of acute spinal fractures, *Spine* 41:E37, 2016.

Dhall SS, Hadley MN, Aarabi B, et al: Nutritional support after spinal cord injury, *Neurosurgery* 72(Suppl 2):255, 2013.

Dinar JR, Carreon LY, Riina J, et al: Early versus late stabilization of the spine in the polytrauma patient, *Spine* 21S:S187, 2010.

Fehlings MG, Rabin D, Sears W, et al: Current practice in the timing of surgical intervention in spinal cord injury, *Spine* 35:S166, 2010.

Fehlings MG, Wilson JR: Timing of surgical intervention of spinal trauma: what does the evidence indicate? *Spine* 35:S159, 2010.

Harris MB, Sethi RK: The initial assessment and management of the multiple-trauma patient with an associated spine injury, *Spine* 31:59, 2006.

Hawryluk G, Whetstone W, Saigal R, et al: Mean arterial blood pressure correlated with neurological recovery after human spinal cord injury: analysis of high frequency of physiologic data, *J Neurotrauma* 32:1958, 2015.

Huang P, Anissipour A, McGee W, Lemak L: Return-to-play recommendations after cervical, thoracic, and lumbar spine injuries: a comprehensive review, *Sports Health* 8:19, 2016.

Hurlbert RJ, Hadley MN, Walters BC, et al: Pharmacological therapy for acute spinal cord injury, *Neurosurgery* 72(Suppl 2):93, 2013.

Kallmes DF, Comstock BA, Heagerty PJ, et al: A randomized trial of vertebroplasty for osteoporotic spinal fractures, *N Engl J Med* 361:569, 2009.

Kerwin AJ, Riffen MM, Tepas JJ, et al: Best practice determination of timing of spinal fracture fixation as defined by analysis of the National Trauma Data Bank, *J Trauma* 65:824, 2008.

Lenehan B, Fisher CG, Vaccaro A, et al: The urgency of surgical decompression in acute central cord injuries with spondylolis and without instability, *Spine* 35:S180, 2010.

Levi AD, Hurlbert J, Anderson P, et al: Neurologic deterioration secondary to unrecognized spinal instability following trauma—a multicenter study, *Spine* 31:451, 2006.

Mac-Thiong JM, Feldman DE, Thompson C, et al: Does timing of surgery affect hospitalization costs and length of stay for acute care following a traumatic spinal cord injury? *J Neurotrauma* 29:2816, 2012.

Molina DK, Nichols JJ, Dimalo VJ: The sensitivity of computed tomography (CT) scans in detecting trauma: are CT scans reliable enough for courtroom testimony? *J Trauma* 63:625, 2007.

Pakzad H, Roffey DM, Knight H, et al: Delay in operative stabilization of spine fractures in multitrauma patients without neurologic injuries: effects on outcomes, *J Can Chir* 54:270, 2011.

Ploumis A, Ponnappan RK, Bessey JT, et al: Thromboprophylaxis in spinal trauma surgery: consensus among spine trauma surgeons, *Spine J* 9:530, 2009.

Ploumis A, Ponnappan RK, Sarbello J, et al: Thromboprophylaxis in traumatic and elective spinal surgery: analysis of questionnaire response and current practice of spine trauma surgeons, *Spine* 35:323, 2010.

Rechtine GR: Nonoperative management and treatment of spinal injuries, *Spine* 31:S22, 2006.

Samuel AM, Grant RA, Bohl DD, et al: Delayed surgery after acute traumatic central cord syndrome is associated with reduced mortality, *Spine* 40:349, 2015.

Schoenfeld AJ, Lehman RA, Hsu JR: Evaluation and management of combat-related spinal injuries: a review based on recent experiences, *Spine J* 12:817, 2012.

Rozzelle CJ, Aarabi B, Dhall SS, et al: Spinal cord injury without radiographic abnormality (SCIWORA), *Neurosurgery* 72(Suppl 2):227, 2013.

van Middendorp JJ, Audigé L, Hanson B, et al: What should an ideal spinal injury classification system consist of? A methodological review and conceptual proposal for future classifications, *Eur Spine J* 19:1238, 2010.

Werndle MC, Saadoun S, Phang I, et al: Monitoring of spinal cord perfusion pressure in acute spinal cord injury: initial findings of the Injured Spinal Cord Pressure Evaluation Study, *Crit Care Med* 42:646, 2014.

Wupperman R, Davis R, Obremskey WT: Level of evidence in spine compared to other orthopedic journals, *Spine* 32:388, 2007.

CERVICAL SPINE

Aarabi B, Koltz M, Ibrahimi D: Hyperextension cervical spine injuries and traumatic central cord syndrome, *Neurosurg Focus* 25:E9, 2008.

Aarabi B, Mirvis S, Shanmuganathan K, et al: Comparative effectiveness of surgical versus nonoperative management of unilateral, nondisplaced, subaxial cervical spine facet fractures without evidence of spinal cord injury, *J Neurosurg Spine* 20:270, 2014.

Aarabi B, Walters BC, Dhall SS, et al: Subaxial cervical spine injury classification systems, *Neurosurgery* 72(Suppl 2):170, 2013.

Anderson PA, Moore TA, Davis KW, et al: Cervical spine injury severity score, *J Bone Joint Surg* 89A:1057, 2007.

Aryan HE, Newman B, Nottmeier EW, et al: Stabilization of the atlantoaxial complex via C-1 lateral mass and C-2 pedicle screw fixation in a multicenter clinical experience of 102 patients: modification of the Harms and Goel techniques, *J Neurosurg Spine* 8:222, 2008.

Bailitz J, Starr F, Beecroft M, et al: CT should replace three-view radiographs as the initial screening test in patients at high, moderate, and low risk for blunt cervical spine injury: a prospective comparison, *J Trauma* 66:1605, 2009.

Bayley E, Zia Z, Kerslake R, Boszczyk BM: The ipsilateral lamina-pedicle angle: can it be used to guide pedicle screw placement in the sub-axial cervical spine? *Eur Spine J* 19:458, 2010.

Bayley E, Zia Z, Kerslake R, et al: Lamina-guided lateral mass screw placement in the sub-axial cervical spine, *Eur Spine J* 19:660, 2010.

Beaty N, Slavin J, Diaz C, et al: Cervical spine injury from gunshot wounds, *J Neurosurg Spine* 21:442, 2014.

Bellabarba C, Mirza SK, West A, et al: Diagnosis and treatment of craniocervical dislocation in a series of 17 consecutive survivors during an 8-year period, *J Neurosurg Spine* 4:429, 2006.

Bliuc D, Nguyen ND, Milch VE, et al: Mortality risk associated with low-trauma osteoporotic fracture and subsequent fracture in men and women, *JAMA* 301:513, 2009.

Bono CM, Vaccaro AR, Fehlings M, et al: Measurement techniques for lower cervical spine injuries. Consensus statement of the Spine Trauma Study Group, *Spine* 31:603, 2006.

Bono CM, Vaccaro AR, Fehlings M, et al: Measurement techniques for upper cervical spine injuries, *Spine* 32:593, 2007.

Bransford R, Falicov A, Nguyen Q, Chapman J: Unilateral C-1 lateral mass sagittal split fracture: an unstable Jefferson fracture variant, *J Neurosurg Spine* 10:466, 2009.

Bransford RJ, Lee MJ, Reis A: Posterior fixation of the upper cervical spine: contemporary techniques, *J Am Acad Orthop Surg* 19:63, 2011.

Bransford RJ, Stevens DW, Uyeji S, et al: Halo vest treatment of cervical spine injuries: a success and survivorship analysis, *Spine* 34:1561, 2009.

Chin KR, Auerbach JD, Adams SB, et al: Mastication causing segmental spinal motion in common cervical orthoses, *Spine* 31:430, 2006.

Chittiboina P, Wylen E, Ogden A, et al: Traumatic spondylolisthesis of the axis: a biomechanical comparison of clinically relevant anterior and posterior fusion techniques, *J Neurosurg Spine* 11:379, 2009.

Como JJ, Diaz JJ, Dunham M, et al: Practice management guidelines for identification of cervical spine injuries following trauma: update from the Eastern Association for Surgery of Trauma Practice management Guidelines Committee, *J Trauma* 67:651, 2009.

Daentzer D, Flörkemeier T: Conservative treatment of upper cervical spine injuries with the halo vest: an appropriate option for all patients independent of their age? *J Neurosurg Spine* 10:543, 2009.

Daffner RH, Hackney DB, Dalinka MK, et al: *Suspected spine trauma*, Reston, VA, 2007, American College of Radiology.

Daniels AH, Arthur M, Hart RA: Variability in rates of arthrodesis procedures for patients with cervical spine injuries with and without associated spinal cord injury, *J Bone Joint Surg* 89A:317, 2007.

De Iure F, Donthineni R, Boriani S: Outcomes of C1 and C2 posterior screw fixation for upper cervical spine fusion, *Eur Spin J* 18:S2, 2009.

Denaro V, Di Martino A: Current concepts in cervical spine surgery. Editorial comment, *Clin Orthop Relat Res* 469:631, 2011.

Derger T, Place H, Piper C, et al: Analysis of cervical angiograms in cervical spine trauma patients, does it make a difference? *J Spinal Disord Tech* 2014 Aug 1 [Epub ahead of print].

Dhall SS, Hadley MN, Aarabi B, et al: Deep venous thrombosis and thromboembolism in patients with cervical spinal cord injuries, *Neurosurgery* 72(Suppl 2):244, 2013.

DiPaola CP, Conrad BP, Horodyski M, et al: Cervical spin motion generated with manual versus Jackson table turning methods in a cadaveric C1-C2 global instability model, *Spine* 34:2912, 2009.

Duane TM, Dechert T, Wolfe LG, et al: Clinical examination and its reliability in identifying cervical spine fractures, *J Trauma* 62:1405, 2007.

Duggal N, Chamberlain RH, Perez-Garza LE, et al: Hangman's fracture: a biomechanical comparison of stabilization techniques, *Spine* 32:182, 2007.

Dunham CM, Brocker BP, Collier BD, Gemmel DJ: Risks associated with magnetic resonance imaging and cervical collar in comatose, blunt trauma patients with negative comprehensive cervical spine computed tomography and no apparent spinal deficit, *Crit Care* 12:R89, 2008.

Dvorak MF, Fisher CG, Aarabi B, et al: Clinical outcomes of 90 isolated unilateral facet fractures, subluxations and dislocations treated surgically and nonoperatively, *Spine* 32:3007, 2007.

Dvorak MF, Fisher CG, Fehlings MG, et al: The surgical approach to subaxial cervical spine injuries: an evidence based algorithm based on the SLIC classification system, *Spine* 32:2620, 2007.

Fassett DR, Dailey AT, Vaccaro AR: Vertebral artery injuries associated with cervical spine injuries: a review of the literature, *J Spinal Disord Tech* 21:252, 2008.

Fehlings MG, Vaccaro A, Wilson JR, et al: Early versus delayed decompression for traumatic cervical spinal cord injury: results of the Surgical Timing in Acute Spinal Cord Injury Study (STASCIS), *PLoS ONE* 7:e32037, 2012.

Gabriel JP, Muzumdar AM, Khalil S, Ingalhalikar A: A novel crossed rod configuration incorporating translaminar screws for occipitocervical internal fixation: an in vitro biomechanical study, *Spine J* 11:30, 2011.

Gebauer G, Osterman M, Harrop J, Vaccaro A: Spinal cord injury results from injury missed on CT scan: the danger of relying on CT alone for collar removal, *Clin Orthop Relat Res* 470:1652, 2012.

Gelb DE, Aarabi B, Dhall SS, et al: Treatment of subaxial cervical spinal injuries, *Neurosurgery* 72(Suppl 2):187, 2013.

Gelb DE, Hadley MN, Bizhan A, et al: Initial closed reduction of cervical spinal fracture-dislocation injuries, *Neurosurgery* 72(Suppl 2):73, 2013.

Goode T, Young A, Wilson SP, et al: Evaluation of cervical spine fracture in the elderly: can we trust our physical examination? *Am Surg* 80:182, 2014.

Grauer JN, Vaccaro AR, Lee JY, et al: The timing and influence of MRI on the management of patients with cervical facet dislocations remains highly variable, *J Spinal Disord Tech* 22:96, 2009.

Griffith B, Kelly M, Vallee M, et al: Screening cervical spine CT in the emergency department, phase 2: a prospective assessment of use, *AJNR Am J Neuroradiol* 34:809, 2013.

Hadley MN, Walters BC, Bizhan A, et al: Clinical assessment following acute cervical spinal cord injury, *Neurosurgery* 72(Suppl 2):40, 2013.

Harrigan MR, Hadley MN, Dhall SS, et al: Management of vertebral artery injuries following non-penetrating cervical trauma, *Neurosurgery* 72(Suppl 2):234, 2013.

Harris TJ, Blackmore CC, Mirza SK, Jurkovich GJ: Clearing the cervical spine in obtunded patients, *Spine* 33:1547, 2008.

Harshavardhana NS, Dabke HV: Risk factors for vertebral artery injuries in cervical spine trauma, *Orthop Rev (Pavia)* 6:5429, 2014.

Haus BM, Harris MB: Case report. Nonoperative treatment of an unstable Jefferson fracture using a cervical collar, *Clin Orthop Relat Res* 466:1257, 2008.

Helgeson MD, Lehman RA, Sasso RC, et al: Biomechanical analysis of occipitocervical stability afforded by three fixation techniques, *Spine J* 11:245, 2011.

Hohl JB, Lee JY, Horton JA, Rihn JA: A novel classification system for traumatic central cord syndrome: the central cord injury scale (CCIS), *Spine* 35:E238, 2010.

Hong JT, Sung JH, Son BC, et al: Significance of laminar screw fixation in the subaxial cervical spine, *Spine* 33:1739, 2008.

Horodyski M, DiPaola CP, Conrad BP, Rechtine GR 2nd: Cervical collars are insufficient for immobilizing an unstable cervical spine injury, *J Emerg Med* 41:513, 2011.

Humphry S, Clarke A, Hutton M, Chan D: Erect radiographs to assess clinical instability in patients with blunt cervical spine trauma, *J Bone Joint Surg* 94A:e174, 2012.

Ivancic PC, Beauchman NN, Tweardy L: Effect of halo-vest components on stabilizing the injured cervical spine, *Spine* 34:167, 2009.

Joaquim AF, Ghizoni E, Tedeschi H, et al: Upper cervical injuries—a rational approach to guide surgical management, *J Spinal Cord Med* 37:139, 2014.

Kadwar E, Uribe JS, Padhya TA, Vale FL: Management of delayed esophageal perforations after anterior cervical spinal surgery, *J Neurosurg* 11:320, 2009.

Kakarla UK, Chang SW, Theodore N, Sonntag VKH: Atlas fractures, *Neurosurgery* 66:A60, 2010.

Kalantar BS, Hipp JA, Reitman CA, et al: Diagnosis of unstable cervical spine injuries: laboratory support for the use of axial traction to diagnose cervical spine instability, *J Trauma* 69:889, 2010.

Karimi MT, kamali M, Fatoye F: Evaluation of the efficiency of cervical orthoses on cervical fracture: a review of literature, *J Craniovertebr Junction Spine* 7:13, 2016.

Kasimatis GB, Panagiotopoulos E, Gliatis J, et al: Complications of anterior surgery in cervical spine trauma: an overview, *Clin Neurol Neurosurg* 111:18, 2009.

Kast E, Mohr K, Richter HP, Borm W: Complications of transpedicular screw fixation in the cervical spine, *Eur Spine J* 15:327, 2006.

Khan SN, Erickson G, Sena MJ, Gupta MC: use of flexion and extension radiographs of the cervical spine to rule out acute instability in patients with negative computed tomography scans, *J Orthop Trauma* 25:51, 2011.

Khanna P, Chau C, Dublin A, et al: The value of cervical magnetic resonance imaging in the evaluation of the obtunded or comatose patient with cervical trauma, no other abnormal neurologic findings, and a normal cervical computed tomography, *J Trauma* 72:699, 2012.

Koech F, Ackland HM, Varma DK, et al: Nonoperative management of type II odontoid fractures in the elderly, *Spine* 33:2881, 2008.

Lebl DR, Bono CM, Velmahos G, et al: Vertebral artery injury associated with blunt cervical spine trauma: a multivariate regression analysis, *Spine* 38:1352, 2013.

Leonard R, Belafsky P: Dysphagia following C-spine surgery with anterior instrumentation: evidence from fluoroscopic swallow studies, *Spine* 36:2217, 2011.

Levi AD, Hurlbert RJ, Anderson P, et al: Neurologic deterioration secondary to unrecognized spinal instability following trauma—a multicenter study, *Spine* 31:451, 2006.

Li F, Chen Q, Xu K: The treatment of concomitant odontoid fracture and lower cervical spine injuries, *Spine* 33:E693, 2008.

Li Z, Li F, Hou S, et al: Anterior discectomy/corpectomy and fusion with internal fixation for the treatment of unstable hangman's fractures: a retrospective study of 38 cases, *J Neurosurg Spine* 22:387, 2015.

Lockwood MM, Smith GA, Tanenbaum J, et al: Screening via CT angiogram after traumatic cervical spine fractures: narrowing imaging to improve cost effectiveness. Experience of a Level 1 trauma center, *J Neurosurg Spine* 24:490, 2016.

Longo UG, Denaro L, Campi S, et al: Upper cervical spine injuries: indications and limits of the conservative management in halo vest. A systematic review of efficacy and safety, *Injury* 41:1127, 2010.

Machino M, Yukawa Y, Ito K, et al: Can magnetic resonance imaging reflect the prognosis in patients of cervical spinal cord injury without radiographic abnormality? *Spine* 36:E1568, 2011.

Malham GM, Ackland HM, Jones R, et al: Occipital condyle fractures: incidence and clinical follow-up at a level 1 trauma centre, *Emerg Radiol* 16:291, 2009.

Malik SA, Murphy M, Connolly P, O'Bryne J: Evaluation of morbidity, mortality and outcome following cervical spine injuires in elderly patients, *Eur Spine J* 17:585, 2008.

Martinez-Pérez R, Paredes I, Cepeda S, et al: Spinal cord injury after blunt cervical spine trauma: correlation of soft-tissue damage and extension of lesion, *AJNR Am J Neuroradiol* 35:1029, 2014.

Maserati MB, Stephens B, Zohny Z, et al: Occipital condyle fractures: clinical decision rule and surgical management, *J Neurosurg Spine* 11:388, 2009.

Miller CP, Brubacher JW, Biswas D, et al: The incidence of non-contiguous spinal fractures and other traumatic injuries associated with cervical spine fractures, *Spine* 36:1532, 2011.

Moore TA, Vaccaro AR, Anderson PA: Classification of lower cervical spinal injuries, *Spine* 31:S37, 2006.

Mueller CA, Peters I, Podlogar M, et al: Vertebral artery injuries following cervical spine trauma: a prospective observational study, *Eur Spine J* 20:2202, 2011.

Nadeau M, McLchlin SD, Bailey SI, et al: A biomechanical assessment of soft-tissue damage in the cervical spine following a unilateral facet injury, *J Bone Joint Surg* 94A:e156, 2012.

Ni B, Guo Q, Lu X, et al: Posterior reduction and temporary fixation for odontoid fracture. A salvage maneuver to anterior screw fixation, *Spine* 40:E168, 2015.

Pang D, Nemzek WR, Zovickian J: Atlanto-occipital dislocation, part 1: normal occipital condyle-C1 interval in 89 children, *Neurosurgery* 61:514, 2007.

Pang D, Nemzek WR, Zovickian J: Atlanto-occipital dislocation, part 2: the clinical use of (occipital) condyle-C1 interval, comparison with other diagnostic methods, and the manifestation, management, and outcome of atlanto-occipital dislocation in children, *Neurosurgery* 61:995, 2007.

Park J, Scheer JK , Lim TJ, et al: Biomechanical analysis of Goel technique for C1-2 fusion: laboratory investigation, *J Neurosurg Spine* 14:639, 2011.

Park SH, Sung JK, Lee SH, et al: High anterior cervical approach to the upper cervical spine, *Surg Neurol* 68:519, 2007.

Paxinos O, Ghanayem AJ, Zindrick MR, et al: Anterior cervical discectomy and fusion with a locked pate and wedged graft effectively stabilizes flexion-distraction stage 3 injury in the lower cervical spine: a biomechanical study, *Spine* 34:E9, 2008.

Pimentel L, Diegelmann L: Evaluation and management of acute cervical spine trauma, *Emerg Med Clin North Am* 28:719, 2010.

Pourtaheri S, Emami A, Sinha K, et al: The role of magnetic resonance imaging in acute cervical spine fractures, *Spine J* 14:2546, 2014.

Prasarn ML, Horodyski MB, Behrend C, et al: Is it safe to use a kinetic therapy bed for care of patients with cervical spine injuries? *Injury* 46:388, 2015.

Rayes M, Mittal M, Rengachary SS, Mittal S: Hangman's fracture: a historical and biomechanical perspective: historical vignette, *J Neurosurg* 14:198, 2011.

Reinhold M, Magerl F, Rieger M, et al: Cervical pedicle screw placement: feasibility and accuracy of two new insertion techniques based on morphometric data, *Eur Spine J* 16:47, 2007.

Rose MK, Rosal LM, Gonzalez RP, et al: Clinical clearance of the cervical spine in patients with distracting injuries: it is time to dispel the myth, *J Trauma Acute Care Surg* 73:498, 2012.

Rozzell CJ, Aarabi B, Dhall SS, et al: Os odontoideum, *Neurosurgery* 72(Suppl 2):159, 2013.

Rozzelle CJ, Aarabi B, Dhall SS, et al: Management of pediatric cervical spine and spinal cord injuries, *Neurosurgery* 72(Suppl 2):205, 2013.

Ryken TC, Aarabi B, Dhall SS, et al: Management of isolated fractures of the atlas in adults, *Neurosurgery* 72(Suppl 2):127, 2013.

Ryken TC, Hadley MN, Aarabi B, et al: Management of acute combination fractures of the atlas and axis in adults, *Neurosurgery* 72(Suppl 2):151, 2013.

Ryken TC, Hadley MN, Aarabi B, et al: Management of isolated fractures of the axis in adults, *Neurosurgery* 72(Suppl 2):132, 2013.

Ryken TC, Hadley MN, Walters BC, et al: Radiographic assessment, *Neurosurgery* 72(Suppl 2):54, 2013.

Ryken TC, Hurlbert RJ, Hadley MN, et al: The acute cardiopulmonary management of patients with cervical spinal cord injuries, *Neurosurgery* 72(Suppl 2):84, 2013.

Sarani B, Waring S, Sonnad S, Schwab W: Magnetic resonance imaging is a useful adjunct in the evaluation of the cervical spine of injured patients, *J Trauma* 63:637, 2007.

Schoenfeld AJ, Bono CM, Reichmann WM, et al: Type II odontoid fractures of the cervical spine: do treatment type and medical comorbidities affect mortality in elderly patients? *Spine* 36:879, 2011.

Sciubba DM, McLoughlin GS, Gokaslan ZL, et al: Are computed tomography scans adequate in assessing cervical spine pain following blunt trauma? *Emerg Med J* 24:803, 2007.

Sciubba DM, Petteys RJ: Evaluation of blunt cervical spine injury, *South Med J* 102:823, 2009.

Shaneyfelt TM, Centor RM: Reassessment of clinical practice guidelines: go gently into that good night, *JAMA* 301:868, 2009.

Shin JJ, Kim SJ, Kim TH, et al: Optimal use of the halo-vest orthosis for upper cervical spine injuries, *Yonsei Med J* 51:648, 2010.

Singh PK, Garg K, Sawarkar D, et al: Computed tomography-guided C2 pedicle screw placement for treatment of unstable hangman fractures, *Spine* 39:E1058, 2014.

Smith HE, Vaccaro AR, Maltenfort M, et al: Trends in surgical management for type II odontoid fracture: 20 years of experience at a regional spinal cord injury center, *Orthopedics* 31:650, 2008.

Sokolowski MJ, Jackson AP, Haak MH, et al: Acute outcomes of cervical spine injuries in the elderly: atlantoaxial vs subaxial injuries, *J Spinal Cord Med* 30:238, 2007.

Song KJ, Kim GH, Lee KB: The efficacy of the modified classification system of soft-tissue injury in extension injury of the lower cervical spine, *Spine* 33:E488, 2008.

Spector LR, Kim DH, Affonso J, et al: Use of computed tomography to predict failure of nonoperative treatment of unilateral facet fractures of the cervical spine, *Spine* 31:2827, 2006.

Stelfox HT, Velmahos GC, Gettings E, et al: Computed tomography for early and safe discontinuation of cervical spine immobilization in obtunded multiply injured patients, *J Trauma* 63:630, 2007.

Tan J, Sun G, Qian L, et al: C1 lateral mass-C2 pedicle screws and crosslink compression fixation for unstable atlas fracture, *Spine* 34:2505, 2009.

Tessitore E, Momjian A, Payer M: Posterior reduction and fixation of an unstable Jefferson fracture with C1 lateral mass screws, C2 isthmus screws, and crosslink fixation: technical case report, *Op Neurosurg* 63:ONSE100, 2008.

Theodore N, Aarabi B, Dhall S, et al: Occipital condyle fractures, *Neurosurgery* 72(Suppl 2):106, 2013.

Theodore N, Aarabi B, Dhall S, et al: The diagnosis and management of traumatic atlanto-occipital dislocation injuries, *Neurosurgery* 72(Suppl 2):114, 2013.

Theodore N, Aarabi B, Dhall SS, et al: Transportation of patients with acute traumatic cervical spine injuries, *Neurosurgery* 72(Suppl 2):35, 2013.

Theodore N, Hadley MN, Bizhan A, et al: Prehospital cervical spinal immobilization after trauma, *Neurosurgery* 72(Suppl 2):22, 2013.

Tsutsumi S, Ueta T, Shiba K, et al: Effects of the second national acute spinal cord injury study of high-dose methylprednisolone therapy on acute cervical spinal cord injury—results in spinal injuries center, *Spine* 31:2992, 2006.

Umerani MS, Abbas A, Sharif S: Clinical outcome in patients with early versus delayed decompression in cervical spine trauma, *Asian Spine J* 8:427, 2014.

Vaccaro AR, Hulbert RJ, Patel AA, et al: The subaxial cervical spine injury classification system. A novel approach to recognize the importance of morphology, neurology, and integrity of the disco-ligamentous complex, *Spine* 32:2365, 2007.

Vaccaro AR, Kepler CK, Kopjar B, et al: Functional and quality-of-life outcomes in geriatric patients with type-II dens fracture, *J Bone Joint Surg* 95A:729, 2013.

Walters BC: Methodology of the guidelines for the management of acute cervical spine and spinal cord injuries, *Neurosurgery* 72(Suppl 2):17, 2013.

Woods BI, Hohl JB, Braly B, et al: Mortality in elderly patients following operative and nonoperative management of odontoid fractures, *J Spinal Disord Tech* 27:321, 2014.

Wu AM, Wang XY, Chi YL, et al: Management of acute combination atlas-axis fractures with percutaneous triple anterior screw fixation in elderly patients, *Orthop Traumatol Surg Res* 98:894, 2012.

Wu JC, Huang WC, Chen YC, et al: Stabilization of subaxial cervical spines by lateral mass screw fixation with modified Magerl's technique, *Surg Neurol* 70:S1:25, 2008.

Xiao ZM, Zhan XL, Gong DF, et al: C2 pedicle screw and plate combined with C1 titanium cable fixation for the treatment of atlantoaxial instability not suitable for placement of C1 screw, *J Spinal Disord Tech* 21:514, 2008.

Zakrison TL, Williams BH: Cervical spine evaluation in the bluntly injured patient, *Int J Surg* 2016 Jan 28 [Epub ahead of print].

Zehnder SW, Lenarz CJ, Place HM: Teachability and reliability of a new classification system for lower cervical spinal injuries, *Spine* 34:2039, 2009.

Zhao L, Xu R, Liu J, et al: Comparison of two techniques for transarticular screw implantation in the subaxial cervical spine, *J Spinal Disord Tech* 24:125, 2011.

THORACIC AND LUMBAR SPINE AND SACRUM

Aebi M: Classification of thoracolumbar fractures and dislocations, *Eur Spine J* 19:S2, 2010.

Bakhsheshian J, Dahdaleh NS, Fakurnejad S, et al: Evidence-based management of traumatic thoracolumbar burst fractures: a systematic review of nonoperative management, *Neurosurg Focus* 37:E1, 2014.

Bederman SS, Hassan JM, Shah KN, et al: Fixation techniques for complex traumatic transverse sacral fractures, *Spine* 38:E1028, 2013.

Bellabarba C, Fisher C, Chapman JR, et al: Does early fracture fixation of thoracolumbar spine fractures decrease morbidity or mortality? *Spine* 35:S138, 2010.

Bellabarba C, Schildhauer TA, Vaccaro AR, Chapman JR: Complications associated with surgical stabilization of high-grade sacral fracture dislocations with spino-pelvic instability, *Spine* 31:S80, 2006.

Bernstein MP, Mirvis SE, Shanmuganathan K: Chance-type fractures of the thoracolumbar spine: imaging analysis in 53 patients, *Am J Radiol* 187:859, 2006.

Bono CM, Heggeness M, Mick C, et al: North American Spine Society newly released vertebroplasty randomized controlled trials: a tale of two trials, *Spine J* 10:238, 2010.

Bono CM, Vaccaro AR, Hurlbert RJ, et al: Validating a newly proposed classification system for thoracolumbar spine trauma: looking to the future of the thoracolumbar injury classification and severity score, *J Orthop Trauma* 20:567, 2006.

Bransford R, Bellabarba C, Thompson JH, et al: The safety of fluoroscopically-assisted thoracic pedicle screw instrumentation for spine trauma, *J Trauma* 60:1047, 2006.

Cauley JA, Hochberg MC, Lui LY, et al: Long-term risk of incident vertebral fractures, *JAMA* 298:2761, 2007.

Chou PH, MA HL, Wang ST, et al: Fusion may not be a necessary procedure for surgically treated burst fractures of the thoracolumbar and lumbar spines. A follow-up of at least ten years, *J Bone Joint Surg* 96A:1724, 2014.

Dai LY, Jiang LS, Jiang SD: Conservative treatment of thoracolumbar burst fractures: a long-term follow-up results with special reference to the load sharing classification, *Spine* 33:2536, 2008.

Daniels AH, Arthur M, Hart RA: Variability in rates of arthrodesis for patients with thoracolumbar spine fractures with and without associated neurologic injury, *Spine* 32:2334, 2007.

Dekutoski MB, Hayes ML, Utter AP, et al: Pathologic correlation of posterior ligamentous injury with MRI, *Orthopedics* 33:00, 2010.

Dhall SS, Wadhwa R, Yang MY, et al: Traumatic thoracolumbar spinal injury: an algorithm for minimally invasive surgical management, *Neurosurg Focus* 37:E9, 2014.

D'Oro A, Spoonamore MJ, Cohen JR, et al: Effects of fusion and conservative treatment on disc degeneration and rates of subsequent surgery after thoracolumbar fracture, *J Neurosurg Spine* 24:476, 2016.

Elgafy H, Bellabarba C: Three-column ligamentous extension injury of the thoracic spine: a case report and review of the literature, *Spine* 32:E785, 2007.

Gnanenthiran SR, Adie S, Harris IA: Nonoperative versus operative treatment for thoracolumbar burst fractures without neurologic deficit: a meta-analysis, *Clin Orthop Relat Res* 470:567, 2012.

Grossbach AJ, Dahdaleh NS, Abel TJ, et al: Flexion-distraction injuries of the thoracolumbar spine: open fusion versus percutaneous pedicle screw fixation, *Neurosurg Focus* E2, 2013.

Hak DJ, Baran S, Stahel P: Sacral fractures: current strategies in diagnosis and management, *Orthopedics* 32:752, 2009.

Harris MB, Shi LL, Vacarro AR, et al: Nonsurgical treatment of thoracolumbar spinal fractures, *Instr Course Lect* 58:629, 2009.

Harrop JS, Vaccaro AR, Hurlbert RJ, et al: Intrarater and interrater reliability and validity in the assessment of the mechanism of injury and integrity of the posterior ligamentous complex: a novel injury severity scoring system for thoracolumbar injuries, *J Neurosurg Spine* 4:118, 2006.

He S, Zhang H, Zhao Q, et al: Posterior approach in treating sacral fracture combied with lumbopelvic dissociation, *Orthopedics* 37:e1027, 2014.

Hulme PA, Krebs J, Ferguson SJ, et al: Vertebroplasty and kyphoplasty: a systematic review of 69 clinical studies, *Spine* 31:1983, 2006.

Inaba K, Munera F, McKennely M, et al: Visceral torso computed tomography for clearance of the thoracolumbar spine in trauma: a review of the literature, *J Trauma* 60:915, 2006.

Inaba K, Nosanov L, Menaker J, et al: Prospective derivation of a clinical decision rule for thoracolumbar spine evaluation after blunt trauma: an American Association for the Surgery of Trauma Multi-Institutional Trials Group study, *J Trauma* 78:459, 2015.

Jaffray DC, Eisenstein SM, Balain B, et al: Early mobilisation of thoracolumbar burst fractures without neurology: a natural history observation, *Bone Joint J* 98B:97, 2016.

Joaquim AF, Fernandes YB, Cavalcante RAC, et al: Evaluation of the thoracolumbar injury classification system in thoracic and lumbar spinal trauma, *Spine* 36:33, 2011.

Kakaria UK, Little AS, Chang SW, et al: Placement of percutaneous thoracic pedicle screws using NeuroNavigation, *World Neurosurg* 74:606, 2010.

Keynan O, Fisher CG, Vaccaro A, et al: Radiographic measurement parameters in thoracolumbar fractures: a systematic review and consensus statement of the spine trauma study group, *Spine* 31:E156, 2006.

Kingwell SP, Noonan VK, Fisher CG, et al: Relationship of neural axis level of injury to motor recovery and health-related quality of life in patients with a thoracolumbar spinal injury, *J Bone Joint Surg* 92A:1591, 2010.

Korovessis P, Hadjipavlou A, Repantis T: Minimally invasive short posterior instrumentation plus balloon kyphoplasty with calcium phosphate for burst and severe compression lumbar fractures, *Spine* 33:658, 2008.

Korovessis P, Repantis T, Petsinis G, et al: Direct reduction of thoracolumbar burst fractures by means of balloon kyphoplasty with calcium phosphate and stabilization with pedicle-screw instrumentation and fusion, *Spine* 33:E100, 2008.

Kose KC, Inanmaz ME, Isik C, et al: Shsort segment pedicle screw instrumentation with an index level screw and cantilevered hyperlordotic reduction in the treatment of type-A fractures of the thoracolumbar spine, *Bone Joint J* 96B:541, 2014.

Koshimune K, Itao Y, Sugimoto Y, Kikuchi T: Minimally invasive spinopelvic fixation for unstable bilateral sacral fractures, *Clin Spine Surg* 29:124, 2016.

Lee JY, Vaccaro AR, Schweitzer KM, et al: Assessment of injury to the thoracolumbar posterior ligamentous complex in the setting of normal-appearing plain radiography, *Spine J* 7:422, 2007.

Lenarz CJ, Place H, Lenke LG, et al: Comparative reliability of 3 thoracolumbar fracture classification systems, *J Spinal Disord Tech* 22:422, 2009.

Lindahl J, Mäkinen TJ, Koskinen SK, Söderlund T: Factors associated with outcome of spinopelvic dissociation treated with lumbopelvic fixation, *Injury* 45:1914, 2014.

McAnany SJ, Overley SC, Kim JS, et al: Open versus minimally invasive fixation techniques for thoracolumbar trauma: a meta-analysis, *Global Spine J* 6:186, 2016.

McHenry TP, Mirza SK, Wang JJ, et al: Risk factors for respiratory failure following operative stabilization of thoracic and lumbar spine fractures, *J Bone Joint Surg* 88A:997, 2006.

Mehta S, Auerbach JD, Born CT, Chin KR: Sacral fractures, *J Am Acad Orthop Surg* 14:656, 2006.

Meves R, Avanzi O: Correlation among canal compromise, neurologic deficit, and injury severity in thoracolumbar burst fractures, *Spine* 31:2137, 2006.

Min KS, Zamorano DP, Wahba GM, et al: Comparison of two-transsacral-screw fixation versus triangular osteosynthesis for transforaminal sacral fractures, *Orthopedics* 37:e754, 2014.

Ozturk C, Ersozlu S, Aydinli U: Importance of greenstick lamina fractures in low lumbar burst fractures, *Int Orthop* 30:295, 2006.

Patel AA, Dailey A, Brodke DS, et al: Thoracolumbar spine trauma classification: the Thorcolumbar Injury Classification and Severity Score system and case examples, *J Neurosurg Spine* 10:201, 2009.

Patel AA, Vaccaro AR, Albert TJ, et al: The adoption of a new classification system: time-dependent variation in interobserver reliability of the thoracolumbar injury severity score classification system, *Spine* 32:E105, 2007.

Pflugmacher R, Agarwal A, Kandziora F, Klostermann CK: Balloon kyphoplasty combined with posterior instrumentation for the treatment of burst fractures of the spine—1-year results, *J Orthop Trauma* 23:126, 2009.

Rihn JA, Anderson DT, Sasso RC, et al: Emergency evaluation, imaging, and classification of thoracolumbar injuries, *Instr Course Lect* 58:619, 2009.

Ruatti S, Kerschbaumer G, Gay E, et al: Technique for reduction and percutaneous fixation of U- and H-shaped sacral fractures, *Orthop Traumatol Surg Res* 99:625, 2013.

Sagi HC, Militano U, Caron T, Lindvall E: A comprehensive analysis with minimum 1-year follow-up of vertically unstable transforaminal sacral fractures treated with triangular osteosynthesis, *J Orthop Trauma* 23:313, 2009.

Saiki K, Hirabayashi S, Sakai H, Inokuchi K: Traumatic anterior lumbosacral dislocation caused by hyperextension mechanism in preexisting L5 spondylolysis: a case report and review of literature, *J Spinal Disord Tech* 19:455, 2006.

Sasani M, Özer F: Single-stage posterior corpectomy and expandable cage placement for treatment of thoracic or lumbar burst fractures, *Spine* 34:E33, 2008.

Scheer JK, Bakhsheshian J, Fakurnejad S, et al: Evidence-based medicine of traumatic thoracolumbar burst fractures: a systematic review of operative management across 20 years, *Global Spine J* 5:73, 2015.

Schildhauer TA, Bellabarba C, Nork SE, et al: Decompression and lumbopelvic fixation for sacral fracture-dislocations with spino-pelvic dissociation, *J Orthop Trauma* 20:447, 2006.

Schweitzer KM, Vaccaro AR, Lee JY, et al: Confusion regarding mechanisms of injury in the setting of thoracolumbar spinal trauma: a survey of the Spine Trauma Study Group (STSG), *J Spinal Disord Tech* 19:528, 2006.

Sethi MK, Schoenfeld AJ, Bono CM, Harris MB: The evolution of thoracolumbar injury classification systems, *Spine J* 9:780, 2009.

Siebenga J, Leferink VJ, Segers MJ, et al: Treatment of traumatic thoracolumbar spine fractures: a multicenter prospective randomized study of operative versus nonsurgical treatment, *Spine* 31:2881, 2006.

Sixta S, Moore FO, Ditillo MF, et al: Screening for thoracolumbar spinal injuries in blunt trauma: an Eastern Association for the Surgery of Trauma practice management guideline, *J Trauma Acute Care Surg* 73:S326, 2012.

Skaggs DL, Avramis I, Myung K, Weiss J: Sacral facet fractures in elite athletes, *Spine* 37:E514, 2012.

Stadhouder A, Buskens E, de Klerk LW, et al: Traumatic thoracic and lumbar spinal fractures: operative or nonoperative treatment. Comparison of two treatment strategies by means of surgeon equipoise, *Spine* 33:1006, 2008.

Stadhouder A, Öner FC, Wilson KW, et al: Surgeon equipoise as an inclusion criterion for the evaluation of nonoperative versus operative treatment of thoracolumbar spinal injuries, *Spine J* 8:975, 2008.

Starantzis KA, Mirzashahi B, Behrbalk E, et al: Open reduction and posterior instrumentation of type 3 high transverse sacral fracture-dislocation, *J Neurosurg Spine* 21:286, 2014.

Taylor RS, Fritzell P, Taylor RJ: Balloon kyphoplasty in the management of vertebral compression fractures: an updated systematic review and meta-analysis, *Eur Spine J* 16:1085, 2007.

Taylor RS, Taylor RJ, Fritzell P: Balloon kyphoplasty and vertebroplasty for vertebral compression fractures: a comparative systematic review of efficacy and safety, *Spine* 31:2747, 2006.

Tötterman A, Glott T, Madsen JE, Roise O: Unstable sacral fractures: associated injuries and morbidity at 1 year, *Spine* 31:E628, 2006.

Tsou PM, Wang J, Khoo L, et al: A thoracic and lumbar spine injury severity classification based on neurologic function grade, spinal canal deformity, and spinal biomechanical stability, *Spine J* 6:636, 2006.

Vaccaro AR, Lee JY, Schweitzer KM, et al: Assessment of injury to the posterior ligamentous complex in thoracolumbar spine trauma, *Spine J* 6:524, 2006.

Vaccaro AR, Lim MR, Hurlbert J, et al: Surgical decision making for unstable thoracolumbar spine injuries: results of a consensus panel review by the spine trauma study group, *J Spinal Disord Tech* 19:1, 2006.

Vaccaro AR, Rihn JA, Saravanja D, et al: Injury of the posterior ligamentous complex of the thoracolumbar spine: a prospective evaluation of the diagnostic accuracy of magnetic resonance imaging, *Spine* 34:E841, 2009.

Vaccaro AR, Schroeder GD, Kepler CK, et al: The surgical algorithm for the AOSpine thoracolumbar spine injury classification system, *Eur Spine J* 25:1087, 2016.

Vanek P, Bradac O, Konopkova R, et al: Treatment of thoracolumbar trauma by short-segment percutaneous transpedicular screw instrumentation: prospective comparative study with a minimum 2-year follow-up, *J Neurosurg Spine* 20:150, 2014.

Wang XY, Dai LY, Xu HZ, Chi YL: The load-sharing classification of thoracolumbar fractures: an in vitro biomechanical validation, *Spine* 32:1214, 2007.

Whang PG, Vaccaro AR, Poelstra KA, et al: The influence of fracture mechanism and morphology on the reliability and validity of two novel thoracolumbar injury classification systems, *Spine* 32:791, 2007.

Yi L, Jingping B, Gele J, et al: Operative versus non-operative treatment for thoracolumbar burst fractures without neurological deficit (review), *Cochrane Database Syst Rev* 8(4):CD005079, 2006.

Zdeblick TA: *Z-plate anterior thoracolumbar instrumentation: surgical technique*, Memphis, TN, 2006, Danek Medical.

The complete list of references is available online at ***expertconsult.inkling.com****.*

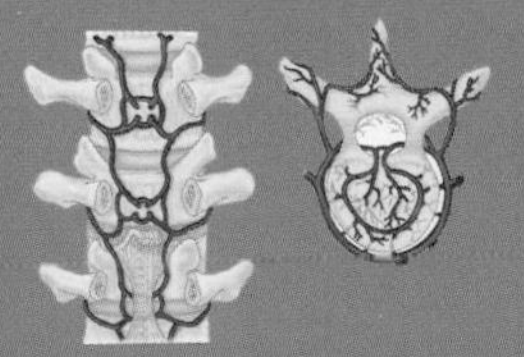

CHAPTER 42

INFECTIONS AND TUMORS OF THE SPINE

Francis X. Camillo

INFECTIONS OF THE SPINE

Spinal infections are relatively rare, accounting for only 2% to 4% of all osteomyelitis infections. Unfortunately, delays in diagnosis and treatment are common due to the manner in which these infections present. Symptoms may be vague, and there are no pathognomonic clinical signs or definitive laboratory tests or to make the diagnosis. Spinal infections can be categorized into different groups based on location of infection, mode of transmission, and infecting pathogen. The location can be in the vertebral body, disc space, paraspinal region, or epidural space. Transmission of the infection can occur by hematogenous seeding, contiguous spread, or by direct inoculation. Pathogens can be gram positive, with *Staphylococcus aureus* being the most common, gram negative, fungal, or acid fast.

SPINAL ANATOMY

Knowledge of the structure and composition of the spinal elements is essential to understanding spinal infections. The intervertebral disc previously was identified as the most commonly infected spinal element, but more recent evidence points to the metaphyses and cartilaginous end plates as the starting areas for bloodborne infections. The disc space now is considered the primary starting area only for infections that result from direct inoculation.

The nucleus pulposus is avascular, receiving nutrients through diffusion across the end plates. Coventry et al., in a microscopic study, found that in adults older than 30 years of age the intervertebral disc receives its nutrition from tissue fluids rather than from a direct blood supply. They noted multiple holes in the end plates of the vertebral bodies. These holes allow for the transport of nutrients through the end plates into the central portion of the disc.

The microvasculature of the vertebral end plates contains vessels oriented obliquely in the cartilage toward the intervertebral disc. These were found to originate from the circumferential vessels fed from the arterial plexus outside the perichondrium and from nearby metaphyseal marrow vessels. The cartilaginous end plate, which is highly vascular, seems to be the anatomic area in which the arterial supply ends.

PYOGENIC VERTEBRAL OSTEOMYELITIS AND DISCITIS

Pyogenic vertebral osteomyelitis and discitis represent 2% to 7% of all cases of pyogenic osteomyelitis. There is a bimodal age distribution with a small peak in childhood and then a larger spike in adulthood around the age of 50. Males are affected more frequently than females. Pyogenic osteomyelitis and discitis are most common in the lumbar spine (50% to 60%), followed by thoracic (30% to 40%) and cervical spine (10%). Seventeen percent of infected patients present with neurologic deficits. Infections higher in the spine are more likely to present with paralysis. The most common organism reported is *S. aureus* (65%). Drug abusers have been noted to more likely have *Pseudomonas aeruginosa* infections. Paralysis has been found to be the most common complication of *S. aureus* infection.

Pyogenic vertebral osteomyelitis and discitis usually result from the hematogenous spread of pyogenic bacteria. The bacteria may originate from an infection in the urinary tract, respiratory tract, soft tissue, or elsewhere. Although it was previously thought that infection spread through the vertebral veins known as Batson venous plexus, this has been disproven. The arterial spread of infection originates in the end plate of the vertebra. The highly vascular end plate is an area with high volume and slow blood flow—an environment that provides conditions conducive for microorganism seeding and growth. Bloodborne organisms sludging in these low-flow anastomoses can lead to a local suppurative infection. This infection can cause tissue necrosis, bony collapse, and spread of the infection into the adjacent intervertebral disc spaces, the epidural space, or into paravertebral structures.

The course of the infection varies with the infecting organism and the patient's immune status. The infection itself may create a malnourished condition that compromises the immune system.

Paralysis from spinal infection may occur early or late. Early onset of paralysis frequently suggests epidural extension of an abscess. Late paralysis may be caused by the development of significant kyphosis, vertebral collapse with retropulsion of bone and debris, or late abscess formation in more indolent infections. Four factors that indicate an increased predisposition to paralysis in pyogenic and fungal vertebral osteomyelitis include age; a higher vertebral level of infection (cervical); the presence of debilitating disease, such as diabetes mellitus, rheumatoid arthritis, or chronic steroid usage; and S. *aureus* infections. Paralysis from tuberculosis is not related to those factors.

CLINICAL PRESENTATION

The most common presenting symptom of spinal infection is back pain or neck pain (85% in one study). No pathognomonic features of the pain occur with vertebral osteomyelitis or discitis, which can lead to a delay in diagnosis. Pain is worse at night and can occur with changes in position, ambulation, and other forms of activity. The intensity of the pain varies from mild to extreme. Constitutional symptoms include anorexia, malaise, night sweats, intermittent fever, and weight loss. Spinal deformity may be a late presentation of the disease. Paralysis is a serious complication but rarely is the presenting complaint. A history of an immune-suppressing disease or a recent infection, or both, is common.

Temperature elevation, if present, usually is minimal. Localized tenderness over the involved area is the most common physical sign. Sustained paraspinal spasm also is indicative of the acute process. Limitation of motion of the involved spinal segments because of pain is frequent. Torticollis may result from infection in the cervical spine, and bizarre posturing and physical positions that could be considered psychogenic in origin are frequent. Other possible findings include the Kernig sign (severe stiffness of the hamstring) and generalized weakness. Clinical findings in elderly and immunosuppressed individuals may be minimal.

Because of the depth of the spine, abscess formation is difficult to identify unless it points superficially. Frequently, these areas of abscess pointing are some distance from the primary process. A paraspinal abscess commonly presents as a swelling in the groin below the Poupart ligament (inguinal ligament) because of extension along the psoas muscle. Straight leg raising examination usually is not helpful because it may be negative or may elicit back or rarely leg pain.

The development of neurologic signs should suggest the possibility of neural compression from abscess formation, bone collapse, or direct neural infection. Neurologic findings rarely are radicular and more frequently involve multiple nerve groups. As might be expected, neurologic symptoms become more frequent at higher spinal levels; they are most frequent with infections in the cervical and thoracic areas and are least common with infections in the thoracolumbar region. In our experience, when neurologic symptoms appear, they progress rapidly unless active decompression or drainage is undertaken.

LABORATORY STUDIES

The erythrocyte sedimentation rate (ESR) is used to help identify and clinically monitor osteomyelitic disc space infection. The ESR is not diagnostic and indicates only an inflammatory process, as do most of the radiographic findings. The ESR is elevated in 71% to 97% of children with vertebral osteomyelitis. In 37% of adults with osteomyelitis, the rate is greater than 100 mm/h, and in 67%, rates greater than 50 mm/h are noted. The ESR normally is elevated after surgery (approximately 25 mm/h), peaking at 5 days but may stay elevated for 4 weeks. Persistent elevation of the ESR 4 weeks after surgery, with associated clinical findings, indicates a persistent infection.

C-reactive protein (CRP) has proven to be a more sensitive marker for early detection of postoperative spine infections when compared with ESR. CRP levels tend to peak within the first 2 postoperative days and then decline rapidly. A continued elevation of the CRP in the immediate postoperative period (4 to 7 days) or a second rise is a strong indicator of an infection. Thelander and Larsson compared the CRP with the ESR as an indicator of infection after surgery on the spine, including microscopic and conventional disc excision and anterior and posterior spinal fusion. They noted in all patients that results of both tests were elevated initially after the surgery, but in all the patients the CRP value had returned to normal by 14 days whereas the ESR took much longer to return to normal. The CRP also can be used to monitor the antibiotic treatment of an infection because of its rapid return to normal with resolution of the infection. The ESR may be elevated for weeks in a treated infection.

Leukocytosis is not especially helpful in diagnosing spinal infection. White blood cell counts may decrease in infants and debilitated patients. High white blood cell counts may indicate areas of infection other than the spine. Blood cultures are helpful if positive, which usually occurs in times of active sepsis with a febrile illness and may be adequate for the diagnosis and treatment of osteomyelitis, but this occurrence is rare.

IMAGING TECHNIQUES

The purpose of diagnostic techniques is confirmation of the clinical impression. In spinal infection, no single diagnostic technique is 100% effective as a confirmatory test. Culture of the organism from the infected tissue is the most definitive test, but results may be negative even under the most optimal conditions. Likewise, all imaging and laboratory studies may be inconclusive, depending on the time at which they are done relative to the onset of infection.

RADIOGRAPHY

Plain radiographs of the involved area are the most common initial study in patients with spinal infection. Radiographic findings, which appear 2 weeks to 3 months after the onset of the infection, include disc space narrowing, vertebral end plate irregularity or loss of the normal contour of the end plate, defects in the subchondral portion of the end plate, and

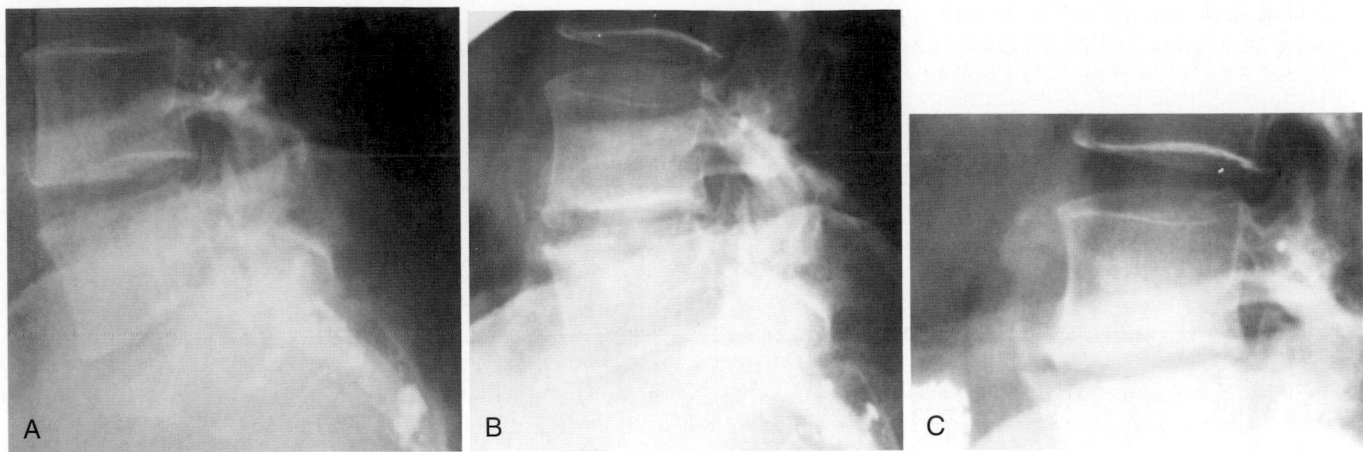

FIGURE 42-1 Radiographic appearance of spinal osteomyelitis. **A,** Minimal disc space narrowing, but normal end plate and subchondral region. **B,** Reduction of disc height associated with destruction of end plate and development of subchondral lytic defects. **C,** After successful treatment, note sclerotic vertebra and large osteophyte. (From Acker JD, Wood GW II, Moinuddin M, et al: Radiologic manifestations of spinal infection, State Art Rev Spine 3:403, 1989.)

hypertrophic (sclerotic) bone formation (Fig. 42-1). Occasionally, paravertebral soft-tissue masses may be noted with involvement of nearby areas of the spine. Late radiographic findings may include vertebral collapse, segmental kyphosis, and bony ankylosis. The sequence of events may range from 2 to 8 weeks for early findings to more than 2 years for later findings. The only definable abnormality on plain radiographs and CT scans related specifically to tuberculosis is fine calcification in the paravertebral soft-tissue space.

COMPUTED TOMOGRAPHY

CT adds another dimension to the plain radiographs. CT identifies paravertebral soft-tissue swelling and abscesses much more readily and can monitor changes in the size of the spinal canal. Some clinicians prefer CT to radiography for determining clinical progress. Findings with CT are similar to findings with plain radiographs, including lytic defects in the subchondral bone, destruction of the end plate with irregularity or multiple holes visible in the cross-sectional views, sclerosis near the lytic irregularities, hypodensity of the disc, flattening of the disc itself, disruption of the circumferential bone near the periphery of the disc, and soft-tissue density in the epidural and paraspinal regions. Postmyelogram CT more clearly defines compression of the neural elements by abscess or bone impingement and helps determine whether the infection extends to the neural structures themselves, but there is a risk of seeding the thecal space.

MAGNETIC RESONANCE IMAGING

High-quality MRI is an accurate and rapid method for identifying spinal infection. It identifies infected and normal tissues and probably best determines the full extent of the infection. MRI does not differentiate between pyogenic and nonpyogenic infections and cannot eliminate the need for diagnostic biopsy. To detect infection, T1- and T2-weighted views in the sagittal plane should be obtained. T1-weighted images have a decreased signal intensity in the vertebral bodies and disc spaces in patients with vertebral osteomyelitis. The margin between the disc and the adjacent vertebral body cannot be differentiated. In T2-weighted images, the signal intensity is increased in the vertebral disc and is markedly decreased in the vertebral body. Abscesses in the paravertebral soft tissue around the thecal sac can be readily identified as areas of increased uptake. Frequently, the delineation of infection in the paravertebral tissues with extension to the thecal tissues eliminates the need for additional myelography. MRI also is useful to identify primary spinal cord infections (myelitis) without epidural or bone involvement. The addition of gadolinium seems to enhance the delineation of epidural abscesses and to delineate further the extent of spinal infection.

Using serial MRI to follow the response to treatment of spine infections may not be clinically useful depending on what is being evaluated. Follow-up MRI has shown that bony findings of vertebral body enhancement, marrow edema, and compression fractures often appeared unchanged or worse in the setting of clinical improvement. Soft-tissue findings of paraspinal abscesses, epidural abscesses, and T2 disc space abnormalities tended to improve on follow-up MRI. Therefore, serial MRI should be used to monitor soft-tissue findings not bony findings. Furthermore, the clinical findings, such as decreased pain and improved neurologic function, seem to be better indicators than an improvement seen on MRI.

RADIONUCLIDE SCANNING

Radionuclide studies are relatively effective in identifying spinal infection. These techniques include technetium-99m (^{99m}Tc) bone scan, gallium-67 (^{67}Ga) scan, and indium-111-labeled leukocyte (^{111}In WBC) scan. The ^{99m}Tc bone scan has three basic phases: angiogram, blood pool images, and delayed static images. In infection, diffuse activity is seen on the blood pool images; the diffuse activity becomes focal on delayed views. This marked reactivity may persist for months. Bone scans are almost always positive in patients with infection, but they are not specifically diagnostic of infection. The ^{67}Ga scan is a good adjunct to bone scanning for the detection of osteomyelitis. A sensitivity of 90%, specificity of 100%, and accuracy of 94% in patients having combined ^{99m}Tc and ^{67}Ga scanning for infection have been reported. ^{67}Ga scans alone are not as accurate as the combination of bone scan and a ^{67}Ga scan for identifying infection. They also do not identify the type of organism involved. Because the ^{67}Ga scan changes rapidly with the resolution of the acute active infection, it may be useful to document clinical improvement.

The ^{111}In WBC scan is useful in detecting abscesses but does not differentiate between acute and chronic infections. False-negative ^{111}In WBC scans have been reported in chronic infections because the radionuclide accumulates with any inflammatory, noninfectious lesion. Likewise, neoplastic noninfectious inflammatory lesions may lead to similar false-positive results with all scanning techniques. One major advantage of ^{111}In WBC scanning is that it differentiates between noninfectious lesions, such as hematomas and seromas, which may appear as a mass or an abscess-like cavity on MRI or CT. Differentiation is important in the postoperative evaluation of potential infections.

DIAGNOSTIC BIOPSY

Biopsy of the suspected lesion is the best method of determining infection and identifying the causative agent so that appropriate antibiotics can be administered. Biopsy may be obtained percutaneously through a CT-guided needle procedure or by an open procedure. Biopsy, however, may not yield a pathogen. Administration of antibiotics before biopsy or the elapse of a long period between the onset of the disease and the biopsy may result in a negative biopsy.

Negative results from percutaneous biopsy should not preclude open biopsy if there is good clinical evidence of infection. Razak, Kamari, and Roohi reported only 22% positive results with percutaneous biopsy and 93% positive results with open biopsy. Marschall et al. likewise demonstrated that open biopsy had a higher microbiologic yield than needle biopsies.

DIFFERENTIAL DIAGNOSIS

The differential diagnosis of spinal osteomyelitis should include primary and metastatic malignancies; metabolic bone diseases with pathologic fractures; and infections in contiguous and related structures, including the psoas muscle, hip joint, abdominal cavity, and genitourinary system. Rheumatoid arthritis and ankylosing spondylitis and Charcot spinal arthropathy may also cause findings resembling osteomyelitis of the spine. Acquired immunodeficiency syndrome may be another underlying factor in these infections. Myelitis from bacterial infection also has similar findings and distinctive MRI findings.

NONOPERATIVE TREATMENT

Antibiotic treatment for vertebral osteomyelitis and discitis infections in adults is the primary therapy. Surgery is reserved for disease progression despite adequate empiric antimicrobial therapy, spinal instability with cord compression or impending cord compression, and drainage of epidural abscess. The antibiotic is chosen according to the positive stains, cultures, and sensitivities of the organism. Response to treatment is evaluated by observing clinical symptoms and serially following CRP and ESR.

The time for discontinuing antibiotic therapy also varies. Collert suggested that antibiotic therapy should be continued until the ESR returns to normal. Unfortunately the ESR can stay elevated for a prolonged period even in a treated infection. CRP values appear to decline more rapidly and may be a better gauge to base discontinuance of antibiotics, but currently this factor is still being studied. Intravenous antibiotics usually are continued for about 6 weeks and are followed by oral antibiotics as indicated by the CRP, ESR, and clinical response. A failure of improvement or continued persistence of symptoms should prompt a reevaluation of the therapy and possibly a repeat biopsy or even open biopsy for cultures or to remove sequestered and infected material.

With an adequate biopsy and a reliable patient who responds rapidly to antibiotics, hospitalization and bed rest usually are required only for the primary symptoms. Home-administered intravenous antibiotics allow the patient to complete treatment out of the hospital. A major risk with this technique is late pathologic fracture of the infected bone. In patients who are at risk for fracture or in pain, a brace is used. If ambulatory therapy is chosen, thorough education and close monitoring of the patient are mandatory.

PROGNOSIS

Even if an absolute diagnosis is not made, most spinal infections resolve symptomatically and radiographically within 9 to 24 months of onset. Recurrence of infection and periods of decreased immune response are always possible, as are delayed complications of kyphosis, paralysis, and myelopathy. These risks are greatest during the period when the infection is controlled but the bone is still soft, when the healing process has not advanced to the point where solid bone has formed around the infected tissue. Bracing is strongly recommended in these patients.

OPERATIVE TREATMENT

Surgical intervention is indicated when medical management has failed, when there is a neurologic deficit from either an abscess or mass causing instability or deformity, or when a diagnosis is not otherwise possible. The location of the infection dictates the surgical approach. Because vertebral osteomyelitis and discitis typically affect the anterior column, an approach that allows thorough debridement of the anterior column is necessary. In the cervical spine, an anterior approach allows this. The anterior body can be treated from an anterior or posterior approach in the thoracic or lumbar spine. Whether an anterior or posterior approach is used, the objective of surgery is to perform a thorough debridement with decompression of the neural elements and stabilization of the spine with correction of the deformity. Often this requires a corpectomy and the need for anterior stabilization with an interbody graft. The interbody graft can be a bone strut, mesh cage with allograft or autograft, or an expandable cage. Various studies have shown that all these interbody devices are acceptable. Often supplementation with posterior instrumentation is needed for added stability and to correct deformity.

SPECIFIC INFECTIONS

INFECTIONS IN CHILDREN

The syndrome of discitis in children is characterized by fever and an elevated CRP and ESR, followed by disc space narrowing on plain radiographs at 4 to 6 weeks from onset. The syndrome frequently is associated with difficulty in walking, malaise, irritability, and sudden inability to stand or walk comfortably. Most reports indicate that the cause is bacterial infection, although trauma also has been implicated. Most culture reports are positive for *S. aureus*. The average age at onset is 6 to 7 years. Symptoms usually are present for 4 weeks before hospitalization. Physical findings are limited. The child may refuse to walk or may cry when walking, and spinal flexion may be limited and so painful that the child holds himself or herself erect. Physical findings directly related to the spine are rare. Neurologic findings are uncommon but are ominous when present. In older children, abdominal pain may be a presenting symptom. Other, less frequent symptoms include hamstring tightness and spinal tenderness.

Diagnosing disc space infection (vertebral osteomyelitis) in children is difficult initially, and plain radiographs usually are negative. There may be a mild febrile reaction, but patients do not appear systemically ill. Laboratory investigation reveals only an elevated CRP and ESR in most patients. The best test to identify the infection probably is MRI or a combination of bone scanning and ^{67}Ga scanning. These scans should give the earliest indication of possible infection but are not totally diagnostic, and other possibilities, including inflammatory processes and tumors, may give false-positive results. Blood cultures may be helpful if obtained during the initial febrile period of the illness.

The treatment of discitis in children varies considerably. Some authors have suggested bed rest and immobilization, without antibiotics, whereas others have recommended organism-specific intravenous antibiotics and bed rest without immobilization until the child can walk and move around comfortably and then oral antibiotics for an additional period of time. Most patients are symptom free within several months. Spontaneous fusion occurs in about 25% of patients. Surgical procedures rarely are required, and persistent back pain rarely is a problem in children. Cast or brace immobilization has been recommended if pain or difficulty in walking persists; most frequently this is necessary in older children. Aggressive surgical treatment rarely is needed in children except in tuberculosis and other caseating diseases that have not responded well to antibiotics alone.

Special situations involving patients with immune suppression, suspected drug use, tumorous conditions, or poor response to conservative treatment require more vigorous evaluation by needle aspiration biopsy for culture and sensitivity. CT-controlled percutaneous biopsy, with the patient under a light general anesthesia, makes this a relatively safe procedure with high rates of positive culture. Definitive diagnosis and organism-specific antibiotic treatment constitute a more efficient method of dealing with these difficult situations.

In children younger than 6 years old, discitis may be viral in origin. Needle biopsy rarely is performed in these patients, and they may be the only group in whom careful monitoring without antibiotics is reasonable.

EPIDURAL SPACE INFECTION

Spinal epidural infections have a low reported incidence of 0.2 to 1.2 cases per 10,000 hospital admissions per year. The incidence of this infection is increased in immunosuppressed patients. Morbidity and mortality are high with epidural infections. The causes of infection are the same as those for osteomyelitis and discitis: direct extension from infected adjacent structure, hematogenous spread, and iatrogenic inoculation. Epidural abscess usually spans three to five vertebral segments. Longitudinal and circumferential extension of epidural infections is believed to be limited by the spinal canal anatomy. Using cryomicrotome sectioning, Hogan showed that epidural contents are discontinuous circumferentially and longitudinally. A spinal epidural abscess caused by direct extension from a vertebral osteomyelitis usually is on the ventral side of the canal anterior to the thecal sac.

The clinical findings are similar to those of osteomyelitis, but with several distinct differences: (1) a more rapid development of neurologic symptoms (days instead of weeks); (2) a more acute febrile illness; and (3) signs of meningeal irritation, including radicular pain with a positive straight-leg raising test and neck rigidity. The classic progression of the disease is generalized spinal ache, root pain, weakness, and finally paralysis, all occurring within 7 to 10 days. Confirmatory testing is similar to that for osteomyelitis. MRI is crucial to the determination of associated osteomyelitis. There is controversy over the etiology of neurologic impairment. Some authors believe that it is the result of a vascular insult, whereas others support mechanical compression.

Even before antibiotics the chance of complete recovery was reportedly better than 50% with early decompression (before the development of paralysis or within 36 hours of onset). Although progression of the process is slow enough to allow evaluation and preparation without endangering the patient, failure to provide prompt drainage can result in serious paralysis and possibly death. Compared with patients treated surgically, patients who have been treated with medical management have a higher failure rate with decreased motor function. A few authors have reported successful treatment without surgical drainage. For selected patients with an epidural abscess presenting with back pain alone or neurologic symptoms that have been stable for more than 72 hours this may be an option, but close clinical follow-up is necessary, and any deterioration of the patient's neurologic status or development of systemic sepsis requires urgent surgical decompression. Independent predictors of failure of nonoperative management of spinal epidural abscesses include age over 65 years, diabetes, methicillin-resistant *Staphylococcus aureus*, and neurologic compromise. Nonoperative medical management demands close observation and more active intervention if necessary. Medical management should be avoided in patients with cervical spinal epidural abscess. A recent study from Alton et al. reported a 75% failure rate and unacceptably poor motor score outcomes with medical management of cervical spinal epidural abscess when compared with surgical management. They recommended that all patients with cervical spinal epidural abscess have early decompression to optimize motor function.

The primary methods of treatment are surgical drainage and appropriate antibiotic therapy. The method of surgical treatment requires an accurate assessment of the location of the abscess and the presence of an associated osteomyelitis. Acute or chronic isolated dorsal (posterior), lateral, and some ventral (anterior) infections are best treated with total laminectomy for drainage, with closure over drains or secondary closure at a later date. Epidural infections associated with osteomyelitis are best exposed by anterior or posterolateral exposures that allow treatment of the osteomyelitis and the epidural infection. Laminectomy in patients with ventral (anterior) osteomyelitis results in late deformity and collapse, so posterior instrumentation should be used.

Other intraspinal infections include subdural abscess and spinal cord abscess. These infections are rare. Subdural abscesses progress at a slower pace than epidural abscesses and can be confused with tumors. Treatment requires durotomy without opening the arachnoid, thorough debridement, and dural closure if possible. Spinal cord abscesses cause pronounced incontinence and long tract signs. They frequently are confused with intramedullary tumors and transverse myelitis. In both of these conditions, the bone scan is normal, but the ^{67}Ga scan should be positive. MRI, preferably with gadolinium contrast, is extremely helpful in defining the extent of the abscess. Some spinal cord abscesses can be treated successfully with antibiotics alone.

MRI also may be useful in determining the outcome of spinal epidural abscesses. Tung et al. noted that weakness at follow-up was associated with 50% or more narrowing of the central canal, peripheral contrast enhancement, and abnormal spinal cord signal intensity. Incomplete recovery was associated with abscess size and the severity of canal narrowing.

POSTOPERATIVE INFECTIONS

Postoperative infections are usually pyogenic and occur shortly after an operation. Preventive measures should be taken to decrease the risk of infection (Table 42-1). Patients with instrumentation have been found to have significantly higher ESR and CRP values than patients without instrumentation, but these parameters normally decrease after surgery unless infection is present. Patients with postoperative infection usually have a renewed elevation of these parameters. Wound drainage was common and occurred at an average of 15 days after surgery; however, fever was uncommon. There usually is back pain and tenderness to palpation.

The Spine Patient Outcome Research Trial study of lumbar degenerative conditions showed the overall incidence of infection to be 2% after procedures for disc herniation, 2.5% after spinal stenosis surgery, and 4% after surgery for degenerative spondylolisthesis. Other studies have put the rate of infection after all spinal infections at 1.9% to 4.4%. Although this number is small, postoperative spinal infections are costly, and more important, can have a significant effect on a patient's clinical outcome.

The mode of transmission of postoperative infections usually is by direct inoculation of the surgical site with skin flora at the time of surgery. There are multiple patient-related and procedure-related risk factors believed to increase the incidence of postoperative infections. Patient-related risk factors include age over 65 years, obesity, chronic obstructive pulmonary disease, previous spinal surgery, hyperglycemia, diabetes, malnutrition, corticosteroid use, rheumatoid arthritis, coronary heart disease, and osteoporosis. Procedure-related risk factors associated with postoperative infection include duration of surgical procedure, number of people in the operating room, dural tear, blood loss, transfusion of packed red blood cells, retained wound drain, and instrumentation.

Use of topical intrawound vancomycin powder has been shown in early studies to decrease the risk of surgical site infections. A recent meta-analysis showed that vancomycin powder is protective against surgical site infections. Edin et al. reported no signs of tissue toxicity with vancomycin use and that it had little or no effect on osteoblasts at doses used in the surgical wound, which is usually 1 g.

TABLE 42-1

Recommendations for Minimizing Spinal Wound Infections

PREOPERATIVE RECOMMENDATIONS

- Whenever possible, identify and treat all infections remote to the surgical site before the elective procedure.
- Postpone elective operations on patients with remote site infections until the infection has resolved.
- Do not remove hair preoperatively unless it will interfere with the operation.
- If hair is removed, remove immediately before the operation, preferably with electric clippers.
- Adequately control serum blood glucose levels in all diabetic patients and avoid hyperglycemia perioperatively.
- Encourage tobacco cessation; at a minimum, instruct patients to abstain for at least 30 days before elective operation from smoking cigarettes, cigars, or pipes or from any other form of tobacco consumption (e.g., chewing/dipping).

OPERATING ROOM

- Prophylactic antibiotics should be given 30 minutes prior to the incision and redose after 3 to 4 hours or 1500 mL blood loss.
- Reduce traffic in and out of the operating room.
- Release soft-tissue retraction regularly.
- Irrigate regularly.
- Maintain strict aseptic techniques.
- Close and seal wounds.
- Maintain sterile dressings in the immediate postoperative period unless the wound is chemically sealed.

POSTOPERATIVE MANAGEMENT

- Concomitant infections (e.g., urinary tract infections, pneumonia) should be aggressively evaluated and treated.
- Sterile dressings should be maintained for 48 hours.
- Nutritional status of the patient should be carefully maintained, particularly during the postoperative period.

From Singh K, Heller JG: Postoperative spinal infections, Contemp Spine Surg 6:61, 2005.

Surgical treatment consists of initial drainage and debridement with primary closure done in layers over a drain. The patient is started on broad-spectrum intravenous antibiotics until cultures yield a pathogen. Once the organism is obtained with sensitivities the antibiotic may be changed. The patient stays on intravenous antibiotics for 6 weeks, and if there is improvement, intravenous antibiotics will be switched to oral antibiotics for roughly another 4 weeks. It is important to consult an infectious disease specialist for these patients. Repeat irrigation and debridement of the wound with cultures and layered closure over drains is done at 48-hour intervals until the wound is without necrotic tissue and cultures and Gram stain are negative. Instrumentation is to be assessed at the time of debridement. Well-fixed implants should be left in place. Numerous authors have shown that infections can be treated without removal of the instrumentation. Instrumentation is removed only when the fusion is solid or when fixation is lost. Bone graft pieces that are loose should be removed at the time of debridement. This is also our method of treatment of acute postoperative infections. Recalcitrant wounds may require negative pressure wound therapy, V-Y flaps, or free flaps when bone or implants are exposed. Recent literature has shown negative pressure wound therapy to be useful in treating postoperative spine infections. The technique involves packing a debrided wound with gauze or foam dressing. A drain is placed over the dressing, and then the wound is sealed with a drape. The end of the drain is attached to a vacuum to produce negative pressure. The dressing is changed sterilely every 2 to 3 days until wound can be closed.

BRUCELLOSIS

Brucellosis results in a noncaseating, acid-fast–negative granuloma caused by a gram-negative capnophilic coccobacillus. This infection occurs most frequently in individuals involved in animal husbandry and meat processing (workers in abattoirs). Pasteurization of milk and antibiotic treatment of animals have led to a significant decrease in the incidence of this disease. Symptoms include polyarthralgia, fever, malaise, night sweats, anorexia, and headache. Psoas abscesses are found in 12% of patients. Bone involvement, most frequently of the spine, occurs in 2% to 30% of patients. The lumbar spine is the most frequently involved spinal region.

Radiographic changes of steplike erosions of the margin of the vertebral body require 2 months or more to develop. Disc space thinning and vertebral segment ankylosis by bridging are similar to changes in other forms of osteomyelitis (Fig. 42-2). CT and MRI may show soft-tissue involvement. Moehring noted that ^{67}Ga scanning is not helpful in sacroiliac infections. MRI may be helpful in the early identification of the disease but has not been reported for this specific infection. The diagnosis usually is indicated by *Brucella* titers of 1:80 or greater; confirmatory cultures also should be done, if possible, using special techniques. Treatment usually consists of antibiotic therapy for 4 months and close monitoring of the *Brucella* titers. Persistence of a titer of 1:160 or greater after 4 months of treatment may indicate recurrence or resistance of the infection. Indications for surgical treatment are the same as for tubercular spinal infections. Because of the indolent nature of this disease, it can be mistaken for a degenerative process. Nas et al. recommended 6 months of antibiotic therapy (rifampicin and doxycycline) with surgery for spinal cord compression, instability, or radiculopathy.

FUNGAL INFECTIONS

Fungal infections generally are noncaseating, acid-fast–negative infections. They usually occur as opportunistic infections in immunocompromised patients. Difficulty in diagnosis often leads to delayed treatment. Symptoms usually develop slowly. Pain is less prominent as a physical symptom than in other forms of spinal osteomyelitis. Laboratory and radiographic findings are similar to those of pyogenic infections. Tubercular infection and tumors are the primary differential diagnoses. Direct culture by biopsy is the only method of absolute determination of the infecting organism.

Aspergillus and cryptococcal infections are of special note with regard to spinal infections. *Aspergillus* is an opportunistic infecting agent in most reported cases. One study noted spinal involvement in 63% and another study noted a predominant lumbar involvement and neurologic involvement in 30%. Pain, tenderness, and an elevated ESR and CRP are the most common symptoms, but white blood cell elevations are rare. The diagnosis requires biopsy. Most patients do not require further surgery.

Cryptococcal infection is a less opportunistic but more prevalent fungal infection. These organisms are found in

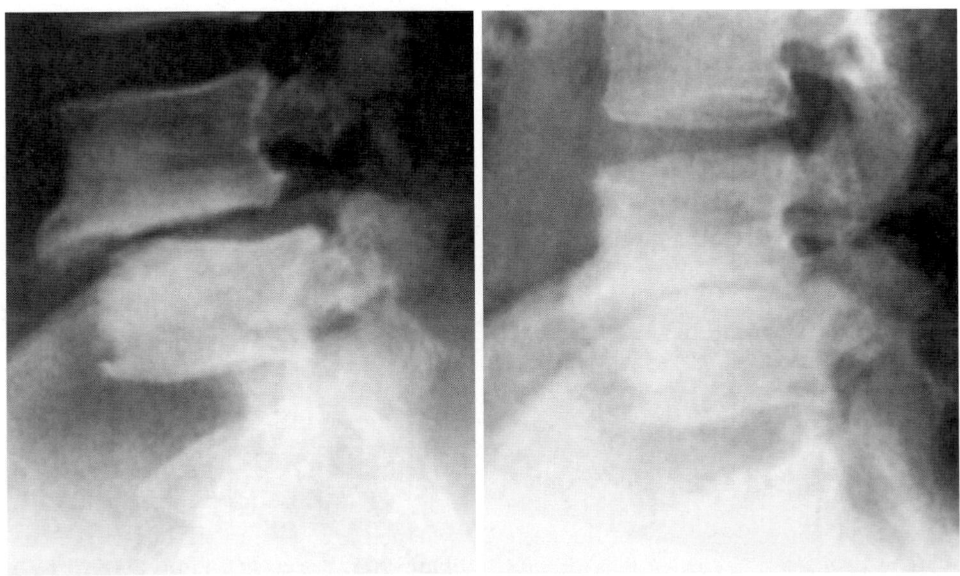

FIGURE 42-2 **Brucellosis of lumbar spine. Note vertebral sclerosis, spondylolisthesis, steplike irregularity in anterior vertebral body, and anterior osteophytes.** (From Lifeso RM, Harder E, McCorkell SJ: Spinal brucellosis, J Bone Joint Surg 67B:345, 1985.)

avian excreta and usually infect the human respiratory system. Spinal infection is rare and usually is associated with generalized cryptococcal dissemination. The primary findings are pain, weakness, and a mildly elevated ESR and CRP. Radiographs show lytic lesions that on biopsy reveal non–acid-fast, caseating granulomas without pus. The indications for radical surgery are the same as for tuberculosis.

TUBERCULOSIS

Tuberculosis was previously the primary cause of infectious spondylitis. Before the advent of effective chemotherapy, time and surgery for paralysis were the only treatment options. Laminectomy initially was performed for paralysis, but the results were disappointing until Ménard accidentally opened an abscess and the patient improved. Many patients treated in this manner died as a result of a secondary bacterial infection, and the practice was abandoned. Posterior spinal fusion, as described by Hibbs and Albee, was the preferred operation to prevent deformity and promote healing by internal immobilization. The first radical debridement and bone grafting procedure for abscess formation was reported in 1934. After the development of satisfactory chemotherapeutic agents, more aggressive surgery was attempted, including costotransversectomy with bone grafting and radical debridement with bone grafting as popularized by Hodgson. Tubercular bone and joint infections currently account for 2% to 3% of all reported cases of *M. tuberculosis*. Spinal tubercular infections account for one third to one half of the bone and joint infections. The thoracolumbar spine is the most commonly infected area. The incidence of infection seems to increase with age, but males and females are almost equally infected.

Pathologically, the infection is characterized by acid-fast–positive, caseating granulomas with or without pus. Tubercles composed of monocytes and epithelioid cells, forming minute masses with central caseation in the presence of Langerhans-type giant cells, are typical on microscopic examination. Abscesses expand, following the path of least resistance, and contain necrotic debris. Skin sinuses form, drain, and heal spontaneously. Bone reaction to the infection varies from intense reaction to no reaction. In the spine the infection spares the intervertebral discs and spreads beneath the anterior and posterior longitudinal ligaments. Epidural infection is more likely to result in permanent neurologic damage.

Slowly progressive constitutional symptoms are predominant in the early stages of the disease, including weakness, malaise, night sweats, fever, and weight loss. Pain is a late symptom associated with bone collapse and paralysis. Cervical involvement can cause hoarseness because of recurrent laryngeal nerve paralysis, dysphagia, and respiratory stridor (known as *Millar asthma*). These symptoms may result from anterior abscess formation in the neck. Sudden death has been reported with cervical disease after erosion into the great vessels. Neurologic signs usually occur late and may wax and wane. Motor function and rectal tone are good prognostic predictors.

Laboratory studies suggest chronic disease. Findings include anemia, hypoproteinemia, and mild elevation of ESR and CRP. Skin testing may be helpful but is not diagnostic. The test is contraindicated in patients with prior tuberculous infection because of the risk of skin slough from an intense reaction and is not useful in patients with suspected reactivation of the disease. Early radiographic findings include a subtle decrease in one or more disc spaces and localized osteopenia. Later findings include vertebral collapse, called "concertina collapse" by Seddon because of its resemblance to an accordion.

Definitive diagnosis depends on culture of the organism and requires biopsy of the lesion. Percutaneous techniques with radiographic or CT control usually are adequate. Percutaneous thoracoscopic or laparoscopic biopsy is another reported option. Open biopsy may be required if needle biopsy is dangerous or nonproductive or if other open procedures are required.

Delayed diagnosis and missed diagnosis are common. Differential diagnoses include pyogenic and fungal infections, secondary metastatic disease, primary tumors of bone (e.g., osteosarcoma, chondrosarcoma, myeloma, eosinophilic granuloma, and aneurysmal bone cyst), sarcoidosis, giant cell tumors of bone, and bone deformities such as Scheuermann disease.

TREATMENT OF TUBERCULAR SPINAL INFECTION

Definitive diagnosis by culture of a biopsy specimen is important because of the toxicity of the chemotherapeutic agents and the length of treatment required. If open biopsy is required, Hodgson et al. recommended definitive debridement, grafting, and arthrodesis at the same time. Their technique requires a more extensive excision of bone than that of Roaf et al., but their mortality was only 2.9%, and no deaths occurred in patients who had disease of limited extent or of short duration and who had no pulmonary involvement. No patient developed paraplegia after surgery. Hodgson et al. advised this method for all patients with early tuberculosis of the spine and proposed that it supplant conservative treatment in most patients. They operated on all patients, even patients in whom the disease was far advanced, and of the first 100 patients observed for 2 to 4 years, 93 had solid arthrodeses consisting of an uninterrupted bridge of mature bone and healing of the tuberculous focus. Yilmaz et al. concluded that anterior debridement, grafting, and anterior instrumentation was more effective than posterior instrumentation for stabilization and reduction of deformity.

Nonoperative and operative methods were extensively evaluated by the Medical Resource Council Working Party. Their reports indicated better results with regard to deformity, recurrence, development of paralysis, and resolution when radical surgery is performed with chemotherapeutic coverage. The resolution of paraplegia did not depend on surgical intervention. Long-term bed rest, with or without cast immobilization, was ineffective. If the facilities for radical surgery are unavailable, ambulatory chemotherapy is the treatment of choice. Their report identified the 6-month use of isoniazid with ethambutol or isoniazid with *p*-aminosalicylic acid to be inferior to isoniazid with rifampicin. They also stressed the use of adequate patient supervision for a successful result. Similar results have since been reported.

The indications for surgery in the absence of neurologic symptoms vary widely. Involvement of more than one vertebra significantly increases the risk of kyphosis and collapse. Open biopsy for diagnosis, debridement, and grafting with or without anterior instrumentation may offer the most direct approach in these patients. Resistance to chemotherapy and recurrence of the disease are other indications for radical surgical treatments as are severe kyphosis with active disease, signs and symptoms of cord compression, progressive impairment of pulmonary function, and progression of the kyphotic deformity. Primary contraindications to surgery are cardiac and respiratory failure.

Posterior fusion, with or without spinal instrumentation, is indicated after anterior decompression and grafting to prevent late collapse and stress fracture of the graft if more than two vertebrae are involved and if anterior instrumentation is not used. Posterior fusion alone rarely is indicated at this time. High incidences of failure and late progression of kyphotic deformity, with or without fatigue fracture of the fusion, have followed posterior fusion alone. Tricortical iliac crest is the preferred bone graft material for all levels, provided that it is long enough. If the ribs are strong, autogenous rib grafts can be used in the thoracic region, although frequent failure with the use of ribs as grafts has been reported. Fibular or humeral grafts may be required if the area of debridement is extensive and the available iliac crest graft is too short or if the ribs are not strong enough. The incidence of late stress fracture increases with the use of fibular or rib grafts (Table 42-2). External immobilization is mandatory whenever debridement and grafting are performed. Halo (vest, cast, or pelvic) immobilization for 3 months is used after cervical and cervicothoracic procedures. Removable or nonremovable thoracolumbar immobilization is used after thoracic and thoracolumbar procedures until the grafts have completely healed (9 to 12 months). Lumbosacropelvic immobilization is used after low lumbar procedures and should be from the hip to the knee of at least one leg for 6 to 8 weeks, followed by thoracolumbosacral immobilization until the graft has healed and the infection has resolved.

Cervical tuberculosis is a rare disease with a high complication rate. Hsu and Leong reported a 42.5% spinal cord compression rate in 40 patients. Children younger than 10 years old were more likely to develop abscesses, whereas older children were more likely to develop paraplegia. Drainage and chemotherapy were adequate for the younger children. For older patients, these researchers recommended radical anterior debridement and strut grafting followed by chemotherapy. Cervical laminectomy resulted in increased kyphosis, subluxation, and neurologic deficits. Posterior cervical fusion resulted in persistent pain, kyphosis, and neurologic deficits that required anterior debridement and strut grafting. Subluxation was treated with skull traction for reduction, followed by anterior decompression and strut grafting.

Lifeso recommended various treatments for three different stages of C1-2 tubercular infection. Stage 1 infections involve minimal bone and ligamentous destruction. Surgical treatment consists of transoral biopsy, decompression, and immobilization in an orthosis. Stage 2 infections involve ligamentous destruction, minimal bone loss, and anterior displacement of C1 on C2. The suggested treatment is transoral biopsy and decompression, followed by reduction with halo traction and later C1-2 posterior fusion. Stage 3 infections exhibit marked ligamentous and bone destruction with C1-2 displacement. The suggested treatment is transoral biopsy and decompression, followed by reduction with halo traction and later occiput to C3 posterior fusion.

The thoracic and lumbar spines are more commonly involved with tubercular infection. Rajasekaran and Shanmugasundaram compared the development of kyphosis with the degree of collapse at the time of presentation of tubercular disease and the institution of antibiotic treatment. They developed a formula to predict the degree of final gibbus deformity that was 90% accurate: $y = a + bx$ where y is the measurement of the final angle of gibbus deformity, x is the initial loss of vertebral body, and a and b are constants 5.5 and 30.5, respectively. Initial vertebral loss was determined by dividing the vertebra into tenths for each involved vertebra

TABLE 42-2

Analysis of Results in Relation to Type of Graft

TYPE OF GRAFT	NO.	NO. FOLLOW-UP	NONUNION OR INCOMPLETE FUSION	BODY FUSION	AVERAGE TIME TO FUSION (mo)	FINAL KYPHOSIS DECREASED	STATIC	INCREASED (AND AVERAGE)
Autologous rib	63	8	21	34 (62%)	24	1	30	24 (13 degrees)
Autologous ilium (series I)*	23	—	6	17 (74%)	14	1	21	1 (nil)
Autologous ilium (series II)*	18	—	1	17 (94.5%)	10	2	11	5 (7 degrees)
Homologous rib	1	—	—	1	24	—	1	—
Homologous tibia	7	—	2	5 (71%)	28	—	5	2
Heterologous	5	—	1	4 (80%)	18.5	—	3	2
Kiel bone†	4							
Heterologous Kiel bone† ilium	1							

From Kemp HBS, Jackson JW, Jeremiah JD, et al: Anterior fusion of the spine for infective lesions in adults, J Bone Joint Surg 55B:715, 1973.

*Autologous ilium: Series I denotes full-thickness ilium used as an inlay graft. Series II denotes full-thickness ilium crossing the coronal diameters of the affected vertebrae. The difference between the rate of fusion for autologous rib and autologous ilium was statistically significant ($p < 0.001$).

†Kiel bone = bovine bone.

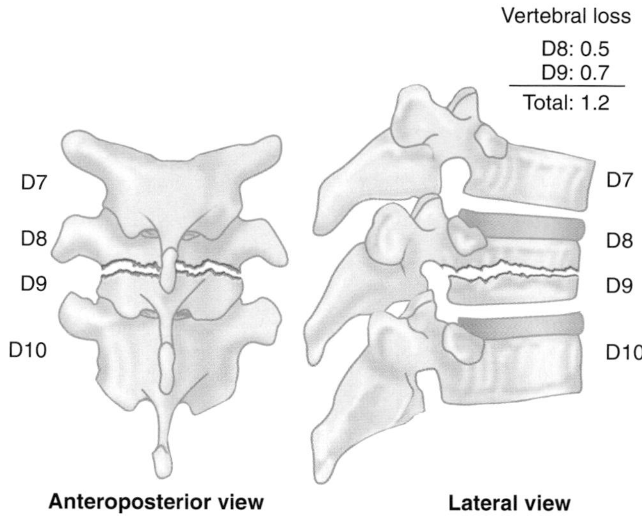

FIGURE 42-3 Line diagram showing method of assessment of loss of vertebral body.

(Fig. 42-3). According to the diagram the height loss of D8 is 0.5 and the height loss of D9 is 0.7, making the total vertebral height loss 1.2. Using the formula, the predicted degree of final kyphosis would be; 5.5 + 30.5 (1.2), which is 42.1 degrees. These researchers suggested that this formula can be used to identify patients most likely to develop significant kyphosis.

POTT PARAPLEGIA

The development of neurologic deficit is a strong indication for surgical treatment. Most patients with Pott paralysis recover. Paralysis caused by vascular embarrassment, penetration of the dura by the infection, and transection of the cord by a bony ridge portend a poorer prognosis. Paralysis persisting longer than 6 months was unlikely to improve.

Hodgson et al. (1964) described two basic groups: *group A, paraplegia with active disease,* which included subtypes 1 (external pressure on the cord) and 2 (penetration of the dura by infection) and *group B, paraplegia of healed disease,* which included subtypes 1 (transection of the cord by a bony ridge) and 2 (constriction of the cord by granulation and fibrous tissue). They recommended early surgery to prevent the development of dural invasion by the infection, which results in irreversible paralysis. A thorough preoperative examination, using MRI and CT of the involved segment, allows a complete evaluation of the extent of the disease and the development of a satisfactory approach for complete debridement and grafting. Late paralysis with inactive disease and significant kyphosis is much less responsive to treatment.

ATYPICAL TUBERCULAR INFECTIONS

Reports of atypical tubercular infections are limited to isolated case reports, usually in individuals who are elderly or immunocompromised by disease or medication. These atypical infections require much more aggressive surgical intervention because of the lack of antibiotic sensitivity and the risk of progression with standard tubercular therapy. The clinical manifestations and aggressive surgical treatment of atypical tubercular spinal infections and mycobacterial infections are similar.

ABSCESS DRAINAGE BY ANATOMIC LEVEL

Any abscess cavity around the spine and pelvis can be drained as summarized in the following techniques.

CERVICAL SPINE

If the cervical spine is involved, the abscess may be present retropharyngeally in the posterior triangle of the neck or supraclavicular area or the tuberculous detritus may gravitate downward under the prevertebral fascia to form a mediastinal abscess.

DRAINAGE OF A RETROPHARYNGEAL ABSCESS

Drainage of a retropharyngeal abscess through an incision in the posterior wall of the pharynx is warranted only in an emergency, as indicated by cyanosis and respiratory difficulty. Usually drainage should be through an extraoral approach (Fig. 42-4).

TECHNIQUE 42-1

- Make a 7.5-cm incision along the posterior border of the sternocleidomastoid muscle at the junction of its middle and upper thirds.
- Incise the superficial layer of cervical fascia and protect the spinal accessory nerve that pierces the sternocleidomastoid muscle and runs obliquely across the posterior triangle.
- Retract the sternocleidomastoid muscle medially, or divide it transversely.
- Using blunt dissection, expose the levator scapulae and splenius muscles, displace the internal jugular vein anteriorly, and palpate the abscess in front of the transverse processes and bodies of the vertebrae.
- Puncture the abscess wall with a hemostat, enlarge the opening, and gently but thoroughly evacuate the abscess.
- If the abscess is unusually large and symptoms are severe, do not close the wound; if the abscess is not large and symptoms are not severe, close the wound in layers.
- A tracheostomy set should be available in case the patient develops respiratory difficulty from edema of the larynx or in case the abscess ruptures into the pharynx.

DRAINAGE OF AN ABSCESS OF THE POSTERIOR TRIANGLE OF THE NECK

TECHNIQUE 42-2

- Incise the skin and superficial fascia obliquely for 6.3 cm along the posterior border of the sternocleidomastoid muscle.
- Retract this muscle medially, but carefully protect the superficial nerves and external jugular vein.

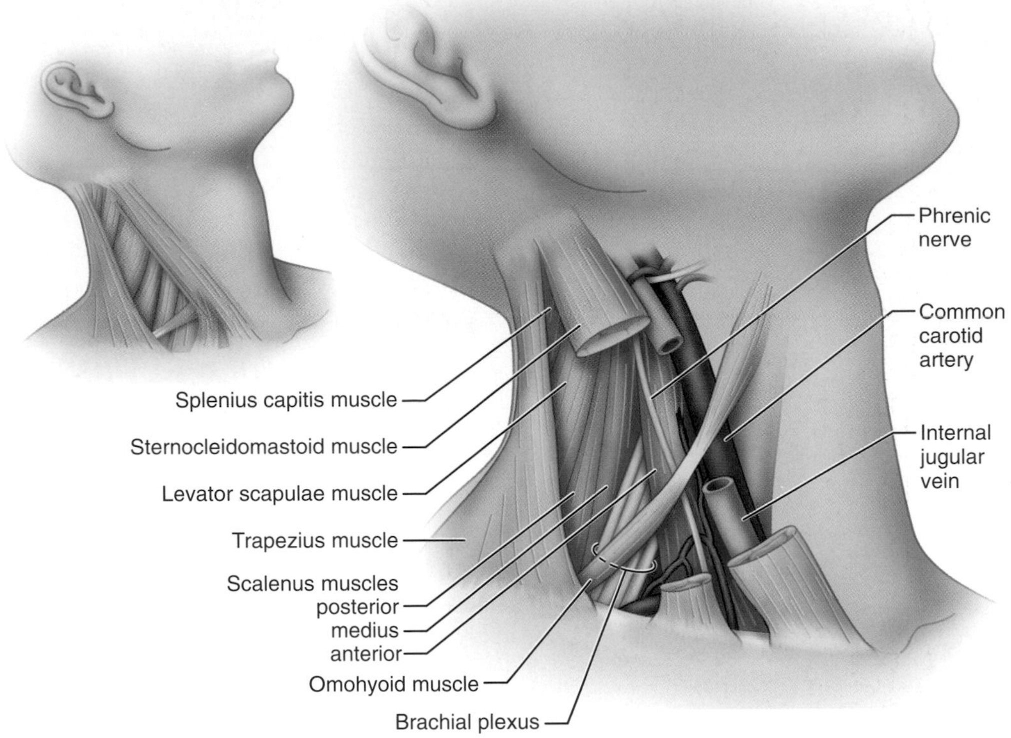

FIGURE 42-4 Drainage of tuberculous abscess of cervical spine. The *green line* indicates incision for extraoral approach. **SEE TECHNIQUE 42-1**.

- Identify the scaleni muscles without injuring the phrenic nerve.
- Locate and divide the line of cleavage between the scalenus anterior and longus colli muscles by blunt dissection obliquely inward to the abscess beneath the paravertebral fascia.
- Evacuate the cavity and close the wound.

ALTERNATIVE APPROACH FOR DRAINAGE OF A RETROPHARYNGEAL ABSCESS

Expose the anterior aspect of the cervical vertebrae as for standard anterior disc excision. This technique allows exposure from C2 to C7. A transverse incision is possible if only two or three vertebrae are involved. A longitudinal incision is made along the medial border of the sternocleidomastoid muscle if longer exposure is necessary.

TECHNIQUE 42-3

- Place the patient supine on the operating table with endotracheal anesthesia administered through a noncollapsible tube. Place the head turned to the right 10 to 20 degrees. The insertion of a small nasogastric tube may facilitate the positive identification of the esophagus.
- Place a small roll between the scapulas; the shoulders can be pulled downward with tape to allow easy radiography.
- Slightly extend the neck over a small roll placed beneath it. Place a head halter on the mandible and occiput and apply several pounds of traction.
- Prepare and drape the area from the mandible to the upper chest. It may be necessary to suture the initial drapes in place.
- Undermine the subcutaneous tissue above and below and divide the platysma muscle longitudinally in the direction of its fibers.
- Open the cervical fascia along the anteromedial border of the sternocleidomastoid muscle.
- Develop a plane between the sternocleidomastoid laterally and the omohyoid and sternohyoid medially.
- Palpate the carotid artery in this plane and gently retract it laterally with a finger.
- With combined blunt and sharp dissection, develop a relatively avascular plane between the carotid sheath laterally and the thyroid, trachea, and esophagus medially.
- Insert handheld retractors initially.
- Identify the esophagus by palpation of the nasogastric tube.
- Dissect free the filmy connective tissue on the posterolateral aspect of the esophagus along the entire exposed wound to prevent ballooning of the esophagus above and below the retractor.
- Expose the prevertebral fascia and open the abscess cavity.

- Insert a hypodermic needle into this material and obtain a lateral radiograph to confirm the proper level.
- Drain the wound in a standard fashion.
- Do not close the neck fascia, but let it fall together. The skin can be loosely closed or left open for delayed closure.

DORSAL SPINE

COSTOTRANSVERSECTOMY FOR DRAINAGE OF DORSAL SPINE ABSCESS

Most abscesses caused by disease of the dorsal spine can be evacuated by costotransversectomy (Fig. 42-5). This procedure, originally performed by Haidenhaim, was described by Ménard in 1894.

TECHNIQUE 42-4

- Make a midline incision over three spinous processes. Reflect the periosteum and soft tissues laterally from the spinous processes and laminae on the side containing the abscess.
- Expose fully the middle transverse process and resect it at its base.
- After reflecting the periosteum from the contiguous rib, resect its medial end by division 5 cm from the tip of the transverse process.
- Bevel the end of the rib; avoid puncturing the pleura.
- Open the abscess by blunt dissection close to the vertebral body. The opening should be large enough to permit thorough exploration of the cavity and removal of all debris. If resection of more than one rib is necessary, enlarge the initial incision accordingly.

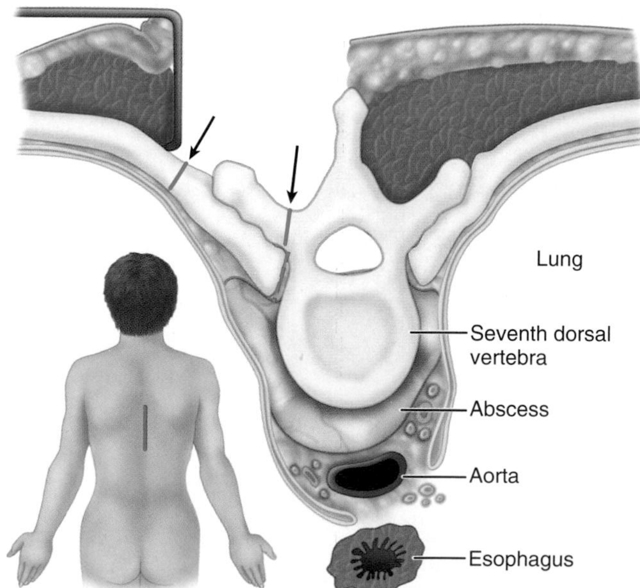

FIGURE 42-5 Costotransversectomy to drain tuberculous abscess of dorsal spine. **SEE TECHNIQUE 42-4.**

- After resecting the ribs, doubly ligate and divide the intervening neurovascular bundle.
- Close the wound in layers.

ALTERNATIVE COSTOTRANSVERSECTOMY FOR DRAINAGE OF DORSAL SPINE ABSCESS

TECHNIQUE 42-5

(SEDDON)

- Begin a semicircular skin incision in the midline about 10 cm proximal to the apex of the kyphos, curve it distally and laterally to a point 10 cm from the midline at this apex, and continue distally and medially to the midline at a point 10 cm distal to the apex (Fig. 42-6).
- If the infection is pyogenic without a kyphosis, a midline incision can be used.
- Elevate the skin flap and retract it medially.
- Cut the superficial muscles and turn them in whatever direction is appropriate for the particular level.
- Divide the erector spinae muscles transversely opposite the apex of the deformity.
- Using diathermy dissection, expose the medial 8.3 cm of not less than three ribs, the corresponding transverse processes, and the lateral third of the laminae (Fig. 42-7).
- Resect the rib that radiographs show to be level with the widest bulge of the abscess as follows.
- After dividing the costotransverse ligaments, remove the transverse process in one piece with large bone-cutting forceps.
- Using subperiosteal dissection, expose the rib, being careful not to perforate the pleura. If such a perforation occurs, place a small swab over it and try to close it as soon as the rib has been removed. The use of a Carlen tube allows deflation of the lung.
- Transect the rib at a point not less than 6.8 cm (in adults) lateral to the costotransverse joint.
- Use a curved gouge to free the medial end of the rib, pushing the gouge gently anteriorly and medially until it strikes the head of the rib or the vertebral column.

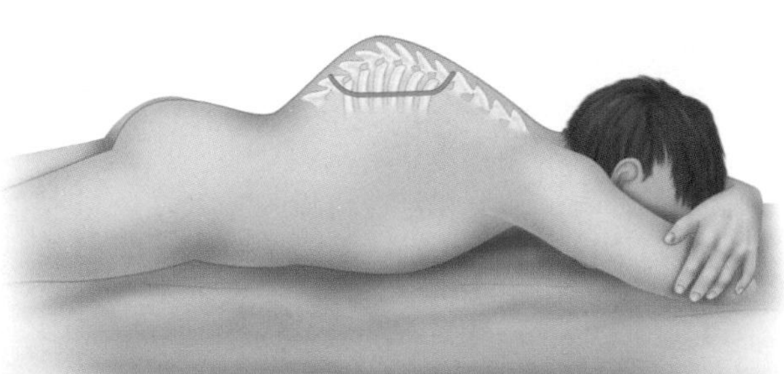

FIGURE 42-6 Incision for costotransversectomy or anterolateral decompression. **SEE TECHNIQUE 42-5.**

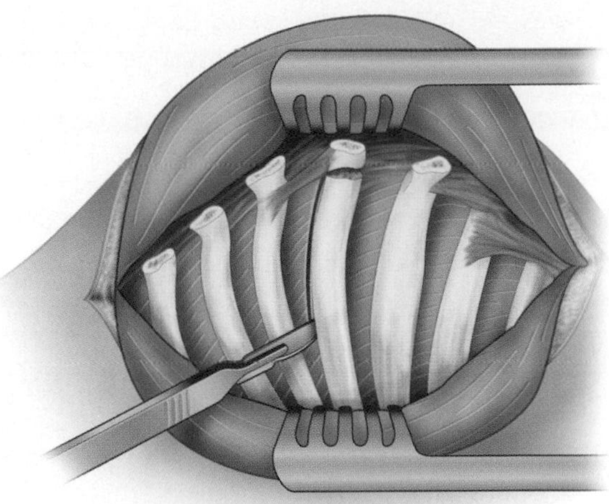

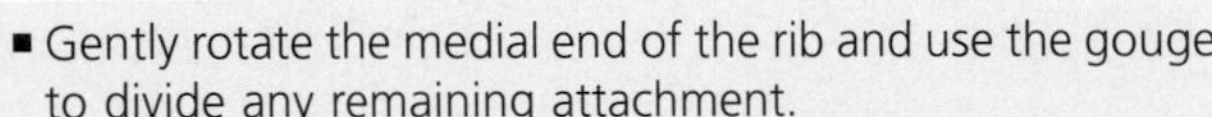

FIGURE 42-7 Exposure of ribs and resection of transverse processes. **SEE TECHNIQUE 42-5.**

- Gently rotate the medial end of the rib and use the gouge to divide any remaining attachment.
- If the operation is successful, pus pours out of the hole; remove it immediately with suction.
- Explore the abscess with a finger, reaching the vertebral bodies, opening small cavities, and dislodging necrotic material.
- If the abscess is unusually large, remove a second transverse process and rib for more exposure.
- Remove the tuberculous material from the abscess cavity and superficial tissues.
- After dusting the wound and the cavity with streptomycin powder, close the muscles and skin without a drain.

LUMBAR SPINE

DRAINAGE OF PARAVERTEBRAL ABSCESS

TECHNIQUE 42-6

- Make a 7.5- to 10-cm longitudinal incision 5 to 7.5 cm lateral to the midline parallel to the spinous processes.
- Divide the lumbodorsal fascia in line with the incision and pass a hemostat bluntly around the lateral and anterior borders of the erector spinae muscles to the transverse processes (Fig. 42-8).
- Usually the abscess is encountered immediately; if it is not, puncture the layer of lumbodorsal fascia that separates the quadratus lumborum muscle from the erector spinae group and force the hemostat along the anterior border of the transverse processes.
- After thorough evacuation of the abscess, close the incision in layers.

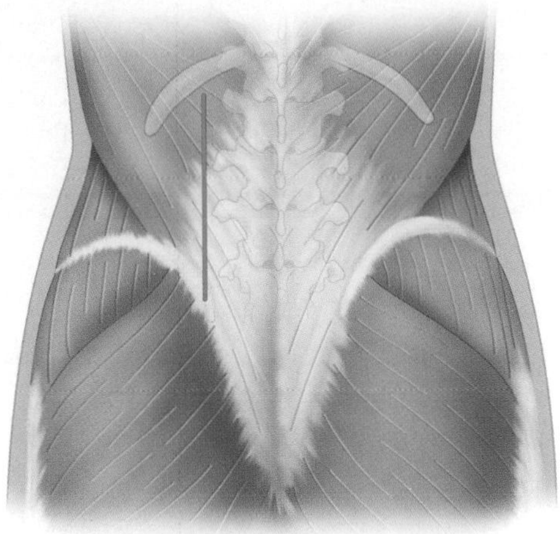

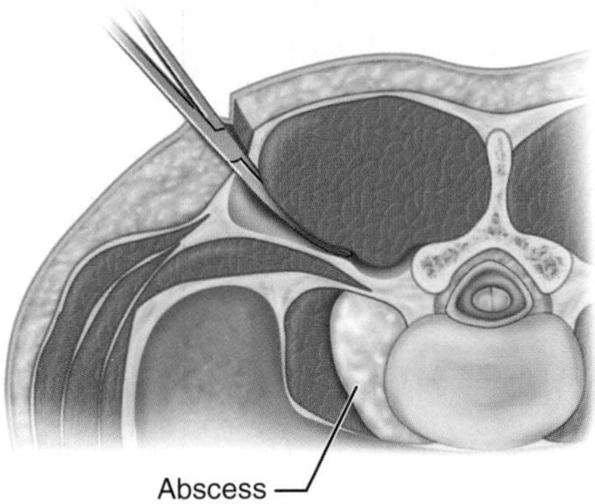

FIGURE 42-8 Drainage of paravertebral abscess. **SEE TECHNIQUE 42-6.**

PELVIS

PSOAS ABSCESS

Psoas abscesses are entirely extraperitoneal and follow the course of the iliopsoas muscle. Drainage can be done posteriorly through the Petit triangle, by a lateral incision along the crest of the ilium, or anteriorly under the Poupart ligament, depending on the size of the abscess and the area in which it appears. Occasionally, an abscess burrows beneath the Poupart ligament and is seen subcutaneously in the proximal third of the thigh in the adductor region (Fig. 42-9).

DRAINAGE THROUGH THE PETIT TRIANGLE

The sides of the Petit triangle are formed by the lateral margin of the latissimus dorsi muscle and the medial border of the obliquus externus abdominis muscle and its base by the crest of the ilium. The floor of the triangle is the obliquus internus abdominis muscle.

TECHNIQUE 42-7

- Make a 7.5-cm incision 2.5 cm proximal to and parallel with the posterior crest of the ilium, beginning lateral to the erector spinae group of muscles (Fig. 42-10).

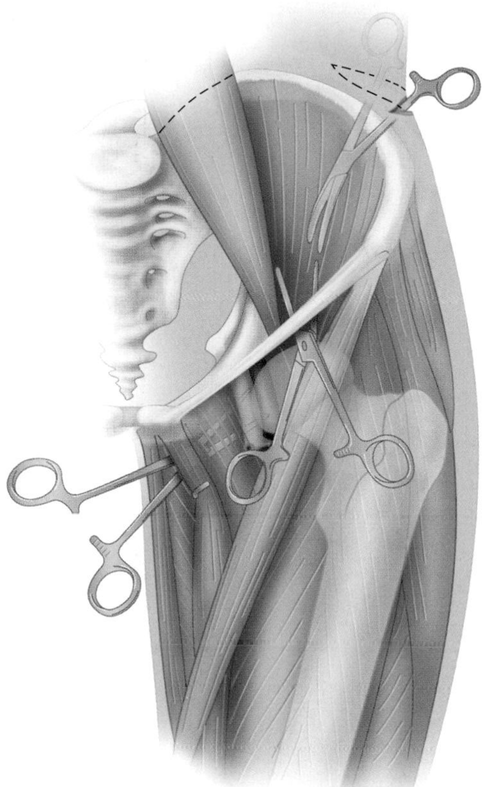

FIGURE 42-9 Drainage of psoas abscess. Hemostat in adductor region is pointed toward inferior edge of acetabulum; abscess usually is located nearer junction of femoral head and neck.

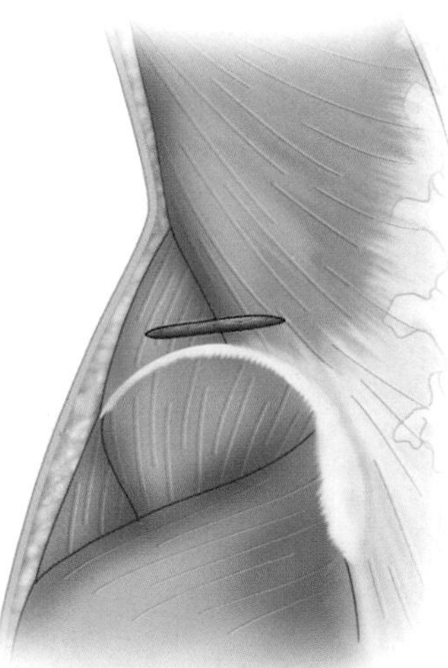

FIGURE 42-10 Drainage of pelvic abscess through Petit triangle. **SEE TECHNIQUE 42-7.**

- After exposure of the Petit triangle, bluntly dissect through the obliquus internus abdominis muscle directly into the abscess.
- After thorough evacuation of the abscess, close the incision in layers.

POSTOPERATIVE CARE. Because flexion contracture of the hip usually accompanies a psoas abscess, Buck traction should be used to correct the deformity and relax the spastic muscles until the hip is fully extended.

DRAINAGE BY LATERAL INCISION

TECHNIQUE 42-8

- Make a 10-cm incision along the middle third of the crest of the ilium and free the attachments of the internal and external obliquus abdominis muscles.
- With a hemostat, puncture the abscess, which can be palpated as a fluctuant extraperitoneal mass on the inner surface of the wing of the ilium.
- Avoid rupture of the peritoneum.

DRAINAGE BY ANTERIOR INCISION

TECHNIQUE 42-9

- Begin a longitudinal skin incision at the anterior superior spine and continue it distally for 5 to 7.5 cm on the anterior aspect of the thigh.
- Identify the sartorius muscle and carry the dissection deep to its medial border to the level of the anterior inferior spine. Protect the femoral nerve, which lies just medial to this area.
- Insert a long hemostat along the medial surface of the wing of the ilium under the Poupart ligament and puncture the abscess.
- Separate the blades of the hemostat to enlarge the opening and permit complete evacuation.
- Close the incision in layers.

Drainage by Ludloff Incision. When a psoas abscess points subcutaneously in the adductor region of the thigh, drainage is accomplished by a Ludloff incision, as described in Chapter 1.

Weinberg described a method of excising a psoas abscess when simpler treatment has failed or is likely to fail because of the size of the abscess, its chronicity, or involvement with mixed bacterial infection. He removed the abscess and any bony or cartilaginous sequestra lodged in the tract or in the diseased vertebrae.

COCCYGECTOMY FOR DRAINAGE OF A PELVIC ABSCESS

Lougheed and White noted that when tuberculosis involves the lower lumbar and lumbosacral areas, soft-tissue abscesses may gravitate into the pelvis, forming a large abscess anterior to the sacrum. These soft-tissue abscesses

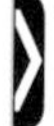

may point to the skin on the anterior surface of the thigh or above the iliac crest, but drainage at these sites alone is insufficient, resulting only in a chronically draining sinus despite antibacterial therapy. The pelvic abscess usually can be seen radiographically by retrograde injection of an opaque contrast medium. Lougheed and White devised a method of establishing dependent drainage posteriorly by coccygectomy. Their results in treatment of 10 patients by this method were uniformly good. The wound usually healed within 6 to 8 weeks, and the spinal lesions all became inactive.

TECHNIQUE 42-10

(LOUGHEED AND WHITE)

- Make a 15-cm elliptical incision over the coccyx, removing a strip of skin.
- After freeing the coccyx from soft tissues, disarticulate it from the sacrum.
- With careful hemostasis, carry the dissection upward, staying close to the sacrum until the resulting pyramidal tunnel communicates with the abscess cavity.
- After evacuating the purulent matter, insert an irrigating catheter to the top of the cavity and pack the wound with iodoform gauze.

POSTOPERATIVE CARE. For 2 to 3 weeks, the wound is irrigated through the catheter several times daily with a solution of streptomycin. The packing is changed at intervals until the wound has healed by granulation tissue from within.

OPERATIVE TECHNIQUES

RADICAL DEBRIDEMENT AND ARTHRODESIS

TECHNIQUE 42-11

(HODGSON ET AL.)

- Approach the upper cervical area (C1 and C2) through the transoral or transthyrohyoid approach. In either approach, perform a tracheostomy before operation. Have the anesthesia given through the tracheostomy opening, leaving the pharynx free of endotracheal tubing that would obstruct the view.
- For the transoral approach, place the head in hyperextension and pack the hypopharynx.
- Turn back the soft palate on itself and anchor it with stay sutures, exposing the nasopharynx.
- In the posterior pharyngeal wall, make a midline incision 5 cm long with its center one fingerbreadth inferior to the anterior tubercle of the atlas, which is palpable (Fig. 42-11A). Carry the incision down to bone.
- Strip the posterior pharyngeal wall subperiosteally as far laterally as the lateral margin of the lateral masses of the atlas and the axis.
- Retract the raised soft-tissue flaps with long stay sutures (Fig. 42-11B) and control any oozing of blood by packing. The anterior arch of the atlas, the body of the axis, and the atlantoaxial joints on either side now are exposed.
- For the transthyrohyoid approach, make a collar incision along the uppermost crease of the neck between the hyoid bone and the thyroid cartilage extending as far laterally as the carotid sheaths (Fig. 42-12A).
- Divide the sternohyoid and thyrohyoid muscles, exposing the thyrohyoid membrane. Detach this membrane as near to the hyoid bone as possible to avoid damaging the internal laryngeal nerve and the superior laryngeal vessels that pierce it from the side nearer to its inferior attachment (Fig. 42-12B).
- Enter the hypopharynx by cutting into the exposed mucous membrane from the side to avoid damaging the epiglottis.
- Expose the posterior pharyngeal wall by retracting the hyoid bone and the epiglottis; make a midline incision in it down to bone (Fig. 42-12C).
- Raise subperiosteally soft-tissue flaps on either side and retract them to expose the bodies of C2, C3, and C4 (Fig. 42-12D).
- As an alternative, approach the *upper cervical vertebrae* (anterior base of the skull and C1-4) through a transmaxillary approach (see Chapter 37).
- Approach the *lower cervical vertebrae* (C3-C7) through a collar incision or one along the anterior or posterior border of the sternocleidomastoid muscle (see Chapter 37). Incise the abscess longitudinally, exposing the spine.
- Approach the *lower cervical and upper thoracic vertebrae* (C7-T3) on the side with the larger abscess through a periscapular incision similar to that used for a first-stage thoracoplasty.
- Elevate the scapula with a mechanical retractor and resect the third rib.
- The pleura usually is opened, but if it is adherent, or if for other reasons it is necessary, make an extrapleural approach. Divide the superior intercostal artery at its origin, along with the accompanying vein.
- Approach the *midthoracic vertebrae* (T4-T11) usually from the left side.
- Select the rib that in the midaxillary line lies opposite the maximal convexity of the kyphos. It usually is two ribs superior to the center of the vertebral focus.
- Make an incision along this rib, resect it, and do a standard thoracotomy. The abscess usually is seen immediately, or there may be adhesions between it and the adjacent lung.
- Mobilize the lung and push it anteriorly.
- Make a longitudinal incision in the pleura close to the aorta in the groove between the aorta and the abscess.
- Displace the aorta anteriorly and medially, revealing the intercostal vessels; secure and divide these for the entire length of the abscess cavity.
- Divide also the elements of the splanchnic nerves.
- Displace the aorta anteriorly away from the spine and palpate the abscess across the anterior aspects of the vertebrae.
- Make a T-shaped incision through the abscess wall: The first incision is transverse and opposite the center of the

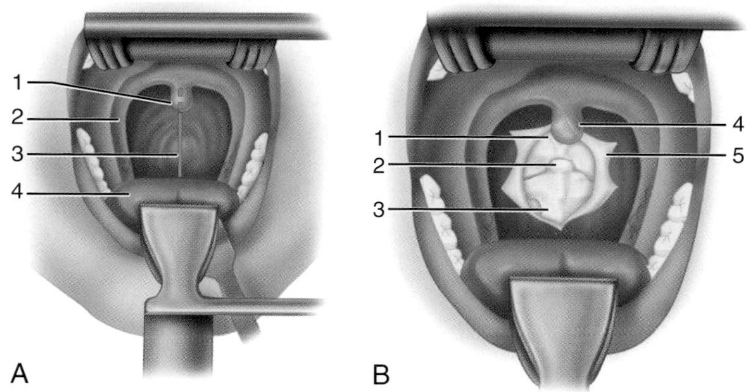

FIGURE 42-11 Transoral approach to upper cervical area. **A,** Incision in posterior pharyngeal wall. *1,* Uvula; *2,* soft palate; *3,* incision in posterior pharyngeal wall; *4,* tongue. **B,** Atlas and axis exposed. *1,* Atlas; *2,* odontoid process; *3,* axis; *4,* uvula; *5,* edge of posterior pharyngeal wall retracted. **SEE TECHNIQUE 42-11**.

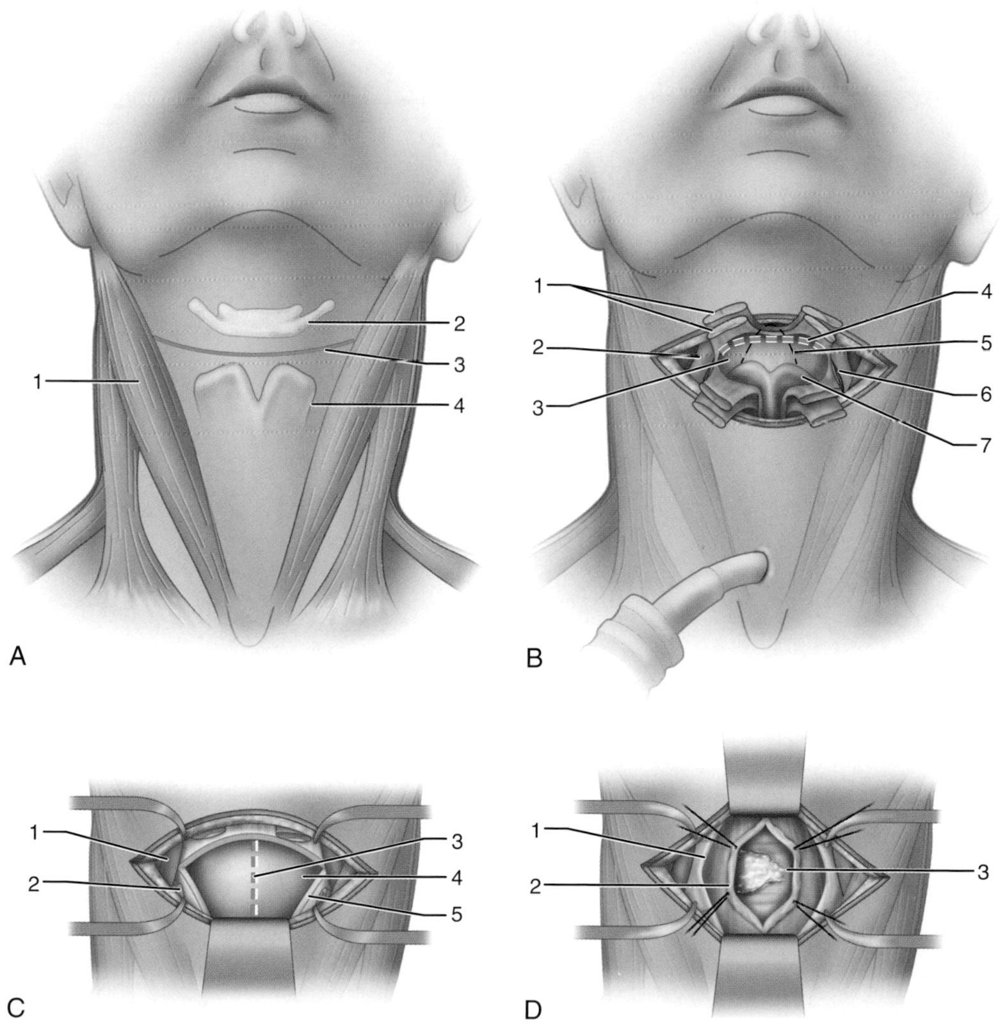

FIGURE 42-12 Transthyrohyoid approach to upper cervical area. **A,** Skin incision. *1,* Sternocleidomastoid muscle; *2,* hyoid bone; *3,* skin incision; *4,* thyroid cartilage. **B,** Incision in thyrohyoid membrane. *1,* Cut ends of sternohyoid and thyrohyoid muscles; *2,* omohyoid muscle; *3,* thyrohyoid membrane; *4,* incision in thyrohyoid membrane; *5,* epiglottis; *6,* internal laryngeal nerve and superior laryngeal artery; *7,* thyroid cartilage. **C,** Incision in posterior pharyngeal wall. *1,* Omohyoid muscle; *2,* cut ends of sternohyoid and thyrohyoid muscles; *3,* incision; *4,* posterior pharyngeal wall; *5,* cut edges of thyrohyoid membrane and hypopharyngeal mucosa. **D,** Vertebral bodies exposed. *1,* Cut edges of thyrohyoid membrane and hypopharyngeal mucosa; *2,* retracted edge of posterior pharyngeal wall; *3,* bodies of C2, C3, and C4 are exposed. **SEE TECHNIQUE 42-11**.

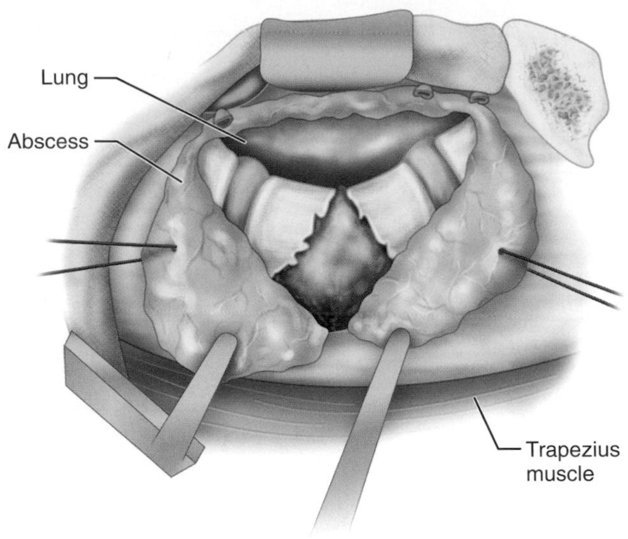

FIGURE 42-13 Abscess opened with T-shaped incision through its wall. **SEE TECHNIQUE 42-11.**

disease process, and the second is longitudinal and medial to the distally placed ligatures on the intercostal vessels.

- Raise the two triangular flaps, revealing the diseased area, including the inside of the abscess cavity (Fig. 42-13).
- Approach the *thoracolumbar area* (T12-L2) through an incision along the left 11th rib. Keep the dissection extrapleural and retroperitoneal and separate the diaphragm from the spine.
- Divide the psoas muscle transversely and turn it distally.
- Ligate the lumbar arteries and veins, as just described for the intercostals, and proceed with the approach as for the middorsal area.
- Expose the *lower lumbar vertebrae* (L3 and L4) through a renal approach, using a left 12th rib incision.
- The psoas muscle usually is divided transversely at a more distal level, often going through an ill-defined abscess between the muscle fibers. Avoid the trunks of the lumbar plexus posterior to the muscle.
- Expose the fifth lumbar and first sacral vertebrae through an extraperitoneal approach. Start the incision in the midline midway between the symphysis pubis and the umbilicus and carry it to the left in a lazy-S fashion to a point midway between the iliac crest and the lowest rib in the flank (Fig. 42-14A).
- Divide the skin, superficial fascia, and deep fascia in line with the incision. Divide the obliquus internus abdominis muscle in the same line but across its fibers. Divide also the transversus abdominis muscle and fascia in the same line.
- Expose and dissect the peritoneum from the lateral wall of the abdomen, the left psoas muscle, and the lower lumbar spine. If the bifurcation of the aorta is high, the easiest approach to the lumbosacral region is between the common iliac vessels. The only vessels encountered are the middle sacral artery and vein; cauterize and divide these (Fig. 42-14B).
- Retract or divide any fibers of the presacral plexus as necessary.
- If the bifurcation of the aorta is low, make the approach lateral to the aorta, the vena cava, and the common iliac vessels. Ligate and divide the iliolumbar and ascending lumbar veins to mobilize the left common iliac vein adequately (Fig. 42-14C and D). If necessary, ligate and divide the fifth lumbar artery and vein and, if a higher approach is required, the fourth lumbar artery and vein as well. Displace the large vessels to the right side and protect them with retractors.

EXCISION OF DISEASED TISSUE AND ANTERIOR ARTHRODESIS

- The technique of excision of the diseased tissue and of anterior arthrodesis is about the same at all levels of the spine.
- Remove debris, pus, and sequestrated bone or disc by suction or with a pituitary rongeur. If possible, pass the suction device anterior to or between diseased vertebrae into the abscess cavity on the opposite side and evacuate all material.
- Remove with an osteotome, rongeur, or chisel all diseased bone, soft and sclerotic, exposing the spinal canal for the whole length of the disease.
- Remove with a knife or rongeur the posterior common ligament and tuberculous granulation and fibrous tissue, exposing the dura.
- Excise the entire vertebral body affected by the disease because collections of pus or sequestrated bone or disc material often are found in the spinal canal posterior to apparently normal posterior parts of diseased bodies. If there is a definite indication, open the dura for inspection of the cord.
- Remove the disc at each end of the cavity, exposing normal bleeding bone (Fig. 42-15A).
- Partially correct the kyphosis by direct pressure posteriorly on the spine.
- After cutting a mortise in the vertebrae at each end, insert one or more strut grafts of the correct length, keeping the vertebrae sprung apart (Fig. 42-15B).
- For the dorsal area, fashion the grafts from the rib removed during thoracotomy (Fig. 42-16); bone bank grafts may be added. For the cervical area, obtain the grafts from the bone bank or from the iliac crest. For the lumbar area, take a massive graft from the iliac crest (Figs. 42-17 and 42-18).
- Put streptomycin and isoniazid into the cavity before closure. After thoracotomy, close the chest in the usual way and maintain suction drainage of the pleural space for 2 or 3 days.

POSTOPERATIVE CARE. The patient is placed in a plaster cast consisting of anterior and posterior shells and remains there until the spine is judged to have united clinically. The time of immobilization after surgery averages about 3 months. Mobilization is started gradually and is continued for 6 to 8 weeks; the patient is carefully watched for increasing kyphosis or other signs of disease activity.

Inferior vena cava
L5
L4
Ascending lumbar vein
Middle sacral vein
Iliolumbar vein
A
B
C
D

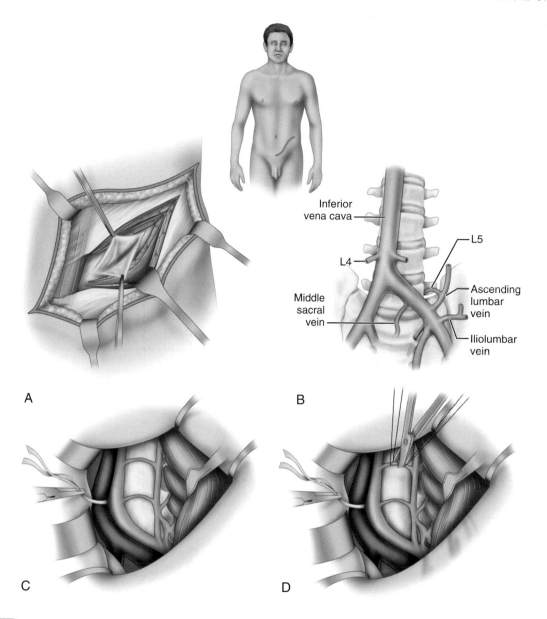

FIGURE 42-14 **A,** Extraperitoneal approach to fifth lumbar and first sacral vertebrae (see text). *Inset,* Skin incision. **B,** In high bifurcation of aorta, middle sacral artery and vein are cauterized and divided. In low bifurcation of aorta, iliolumbar and ascending lumbar veins are cauterized and divided. **C,** Exposed vertebrae are crossed by ascending lumbar vein. **D,** Ascending lumbar vein is ligated and divided. **SEE TECHNIQUE 42-11.**

DORSOLATERAL APPROACH

TECHNIQUE 42-12

(ROAF ET AL.)

- Expose the dorsal spine through a dorsolateral approach. Maintain careful hemostasis throughout.
- Select the side with the larger abscess shadow or, in the absence of an abscess, use the left side; make a curved incision. Begin posteriorly 3.8 cm from the midline and 7.5 cm proximal to the center of the lesion and curve distally and laterally to a point 12.5 cm from the midline at the center of the lesion; continue medially and distally, ending 3.8 cm from the midline and 7.5 cm distal to the center of the lesion (Fig. 42-19).
- Divide the superficial and deep fascia and the underlying muscles down to the ribs in the line of the incision. Retract the flap of the skin and muscle medially. Now locate the rib opposite the center of the focus and remove 7.5 to 10 cm of this rib and the one proximal and distal in the following manner.
- Free the ribs with a periosteal elevator and divide them with rib shears 7.5 to 10 cm from the tips of the transverse processes.
- Resect each at the tip of the transverse process.
- Divide under direct vision the ligaments and muscles attached to the rib heads and transverse processes and resect these bony parts.

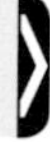

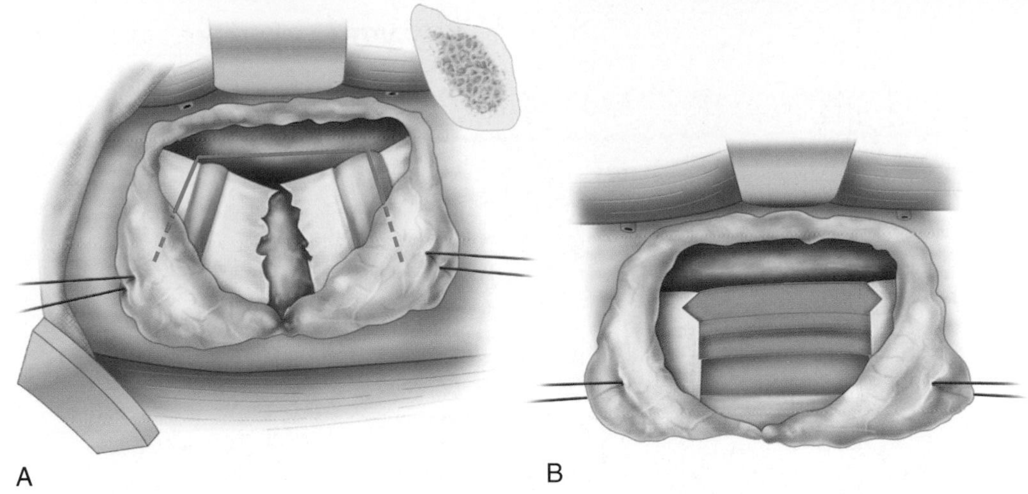

FIGURE 42-15 **A,** Excision of diseased bone. **B,** Grafts inserted, keeping vertebrae sprung apart. **SEE TECHNIQUE 42-11.**

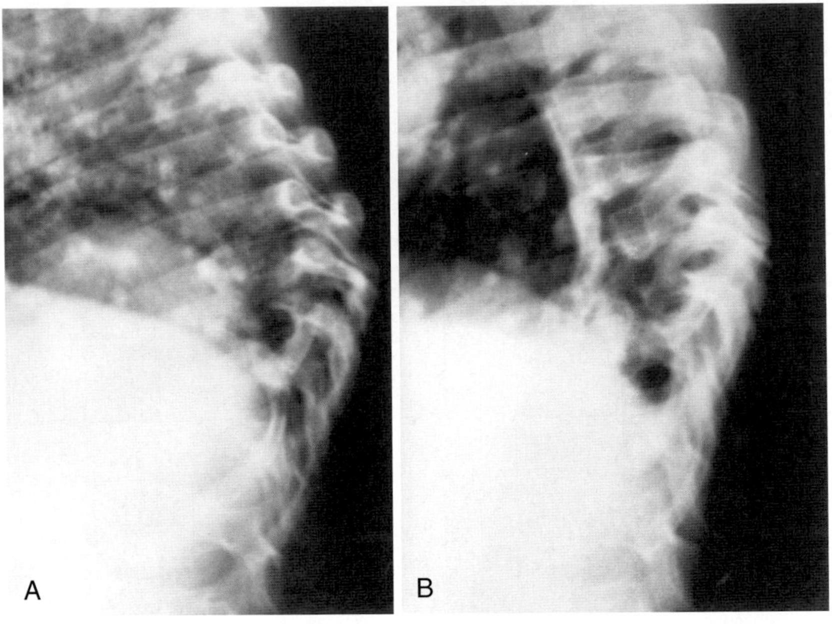

FIGURE 42-16 Tuberculosis of spine without paraplegia in 4-year-old girl. **A,** Destruction of vertebral bodies before surgery. **B,** Six months after thoracotomy approach, excision of diseased bone, and anterior fusion from T6 to T11 using resected ribs for grafts; 4.5 years later, pain and evidence of activity are absent. **SEE TECHNIQUE 42-11.**

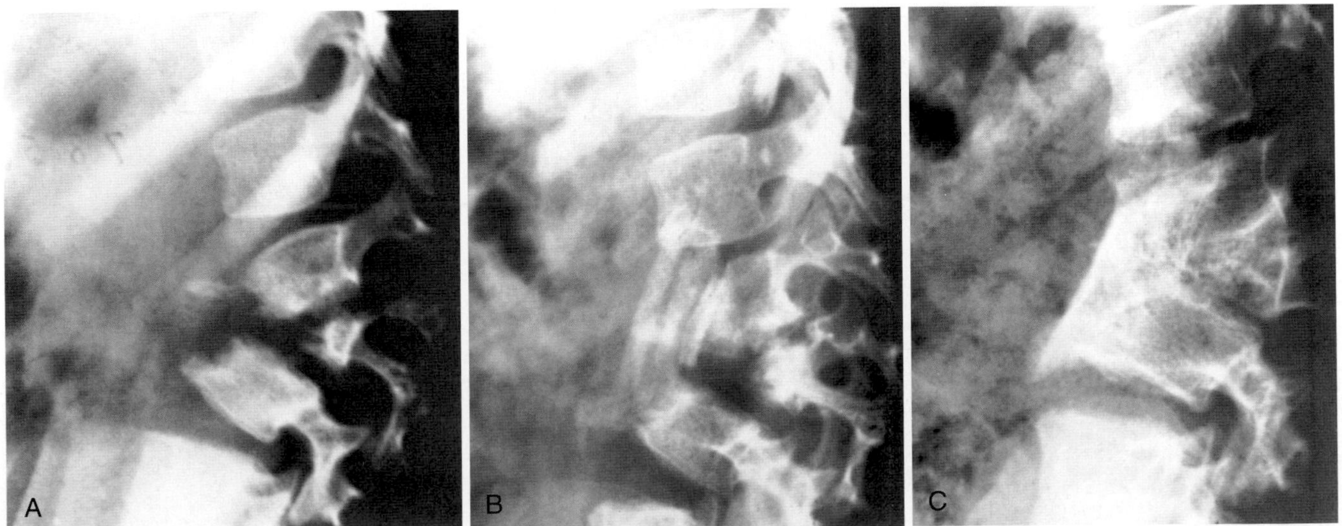

FIGURE 42-17 Tuberculosis of spine in 13-year-old girl. **A,** L2, L3, and L4 are destroyed, with resulting kyphosis. **B,** One month after excision of diseased bone and grafting of bone between L1 and L4 from resected 12th rib and from iliac crest. **C,** Three years after operation. Fusion is almost complete. (Courtesy Professor A.R. Hodgson.)**SEE TECHNIQUE 42-11.**

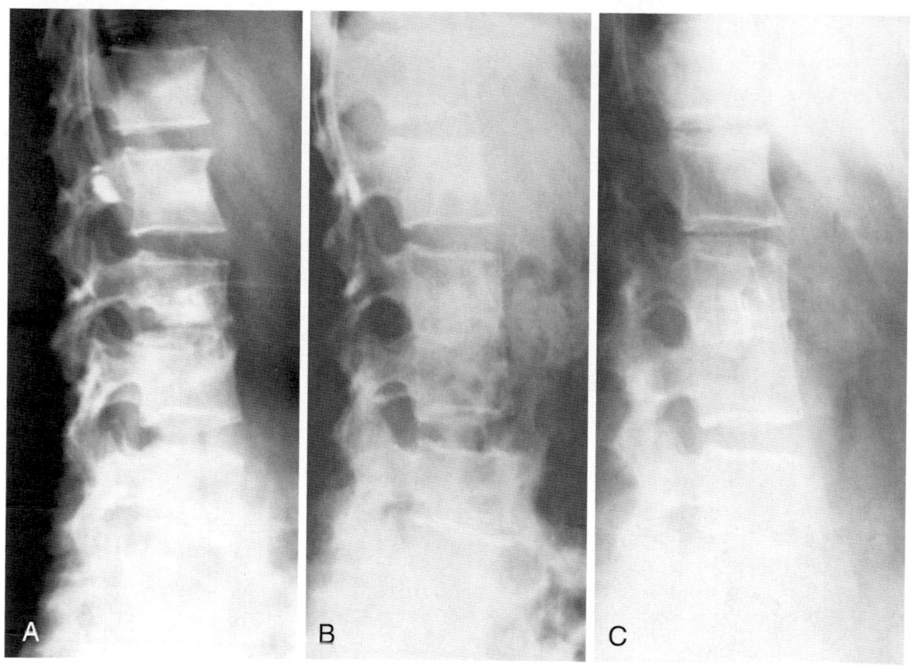

FIGURE 42-18 Tuberculosis of bodies of L2 and L3 without paraplegia in 23-year-old woman. **A,** Before surgery. **B,** Six months after debridement and anterior arthrodesis through left extraperitoneal approach; grafts were from ilium. **C,** Four years after surgery, fusion is complete. **SEE TECHNIQUE 42-11.**

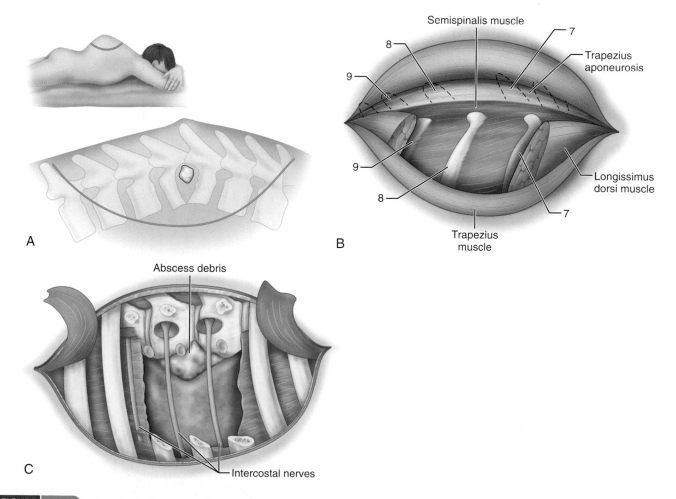

FIGURE 42-19 Dorsolateral approach to dorsal spine. **A,** Incision. **B,** Ribs and transverse processes exposed. **C,** Ribs and transverse processes resected, and abscess and vertebral bodies exposed. **SEE TECHNIQUE 42-12.**

- Identify two and preferably three intercostal nerves and trace them medially to the intervertebral foramina. These nerves, as they pass into the foramina, indicate the level of the cord in the spinal canal.
- Expose the intercostal vessels near the spinal column and cut them between clamps.
- Divide the intercostal muscles near the vertebral column.
- Separate the pleura from the spinal column by blunt dissection, exposing the lateral and anterolateral aspects of the vertebral bodies. Avoid perforating the pleura because it is often adherent and thickened; if a perforation occurs, suture it at once.
- Locate the center of the lesion by passing a finger into the wound anterior to the vertebral bodies. Remove all pus, granulation tissue, and necrotic matter.
- Occasionally, one or more vertebral bodies may be sequestrated and lying free in the abscess cavity. Usually two or three small bony sequestra and pieces of necrotic disc material are found. If the paravertebral shadow, thought to be an abscess, is found to be mainly fibrous tissue, it is more difficult to find the lesion. Under these circumstances, using radiographic control, explore the bone with a fine gouge, burr, and rongeur.
- After thorough debridement, decide whether bone grafts are advisable. The simplest method of grafting is to pack the cavity with bone chips.
- A more extensive procedure may be undertaken. With a chisel or gouge, roughen the lateral and anterolateral aspects of the diseased vertebral bodies and, if possible, of one healthy vertebra above and below and cut a groove in them, passing from healthy bone above to healthy bone below.
- Wedge a full-thickness rib graft into the groove and sink it deeply within the vertebral bodies.
- Place cancellous bone chips obtained from the remaining portion of the resected ribs in the groove and laterally along the roughened surface of the vertebral bodies.
- If the pleura has been accidentally opened, drain the pleural cavity with a chest tube inserted through a small stab incision in the eighth intercostal space in the midaxillary line and connected to an underwater seal for 48 hours after surgery.

COSTOTRANSVERSECTOMY

Costotransversectomy is discussed earlier in this chapter (see Techniques 42-4 and 42-5).

ANTEROLATERAL DECOMPRESSION (LATERAL RHACHOTOMY)

In 1933, Capener originated a procedure that he called *lateral rhachotomy,* which is now popularly known as *anterolateral decompression,* in which the spine is opened from its lateral side. This affords access to the front and side of the cord, permitting decompression by the removal of bony spurs, granulation tissue, and sequestra or the evacuation of abscesses. Because the procedure entails resection of one or more pedicles, it is contraindicated if the spine is unstable. The operation at best is difficult but is easiest when there is a sharp kyphos.

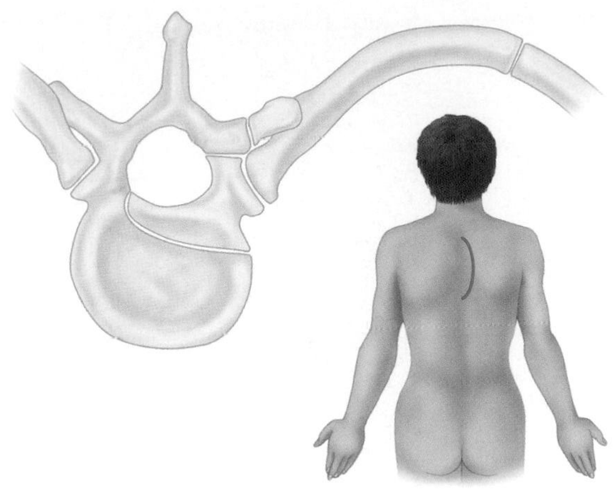

FIGURE 42-20 Capener anterolateral decompression for tuberculous abscess of dorsal spine. *Green areas,* Extent of bone resection. *Inset,* Skin incision. **SEE TECHNIQUE 42-13.**

TECHNIQUE 42-13

(CAPENER)

- If the disease is in the middorsal region, begin the incision in the midline at a point 10 cm proximal to the lesion, gently curve it laterally a distance of 7.5 cm, and return to the midline at a point 10 cm distal to the lesion (Fig. 42-20, inset). Reflect the skin and superficial and deep fasciae as a thick flap.
- Incise and retract laterally the origin of the trapezius muscle; divide the erector spinae muscles transversely over the rib leading to the affected intervertebral space, and retract them proximally and distally.
- After exposing the rib subperiosteally, resect it from its angle to the transverse process; if necessary, resect the rib proximal and distal in the same manner.
- Separate the intercostal nerve from its accompanying vessels and divide it using the proximal end as a guide to further dissection and later for traction on the cord.
- Carefully retract the pleura along with the intercostal vessels and remove the medial end of the rib and the transverse process and pedicle of the vertebra with a rongeur; a sphenoid punch and a motor-driven burr are helpful at this stage.
- The dura and the posterolateral aspect of the vertebral body are seen after anterior depression of the pleura and the intercostal vessels and traction on the intercostal nerve.
- Work from the more normal tissues in the vertebral canal toward the site of compression.
- Gently remove diseased bone with a curet; also remove all impinging and encroaching tissues so carefully that the dura is not even momentarily dented (Fig. 42-20).
- Thoroughly evacuate a paravertebral abscess if present.
- Close the wound in layers.

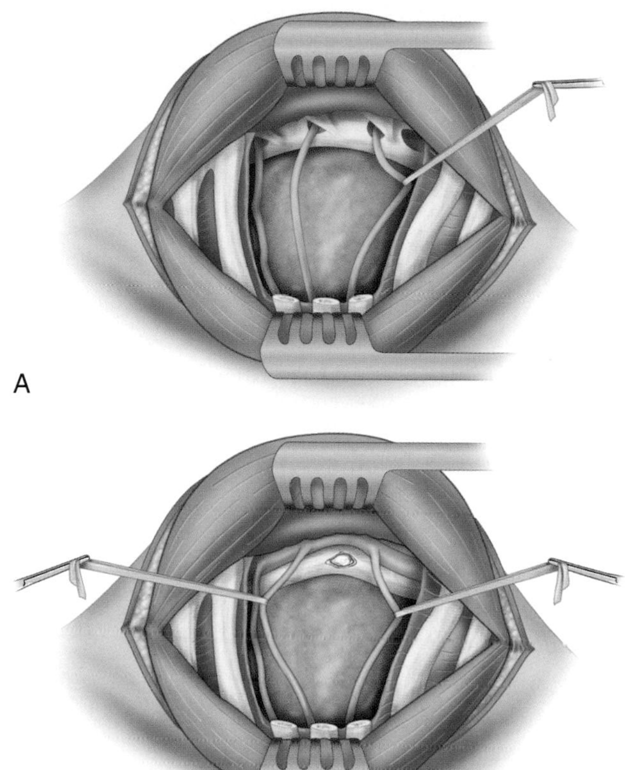

FIGURE 42-21 **A,** Intercostal nerves are isolated, and pedicles are exposed. **B,** Exposure of spinal cord after resection of three pedicles. Material anterior to cord can now be removed. Sequestrum is shown within abscess. **SEE TECHNIQUE 42-14.**

POSTOPERATIVE CARE. Anterior and posterior plaster shells, prepared before surgery, are applied; when the lesion is in the cervical or upper dorsal region, skeletal traction should be employed. Numerous authors recommend that three or more ribs be widely resected to provide better exposure.

ALTERNATIVE ANTEROLATERAL DECOMPRESSION (LATERAL RHACHOTOMY)

TECHNIQUE 42-14

(SEDDON)

- The approach and the method of rib resection are as described for costotransversectomy earlier (see Technique 42-5). Resect not less than three and not more than four ribs.
- Isolate the intercostal nerves and trace them medially to the intervertebral foramina; cut away the intervening intercostal muscles (Fig. 42-21A).
- Gently push the pleura anteriorly with the fingers and determine by palpation the position of the two or three pedicles to be resected.
- To increase exposure, cut away small parts of the overhanging neural arches. Remove as little bone as possible dorsal to the pedicles because anything in the least approaching hemilaminectomy is likely to be followed by a lateral subluxation of the spine.
- Resect the pedicles by nibbling away from their lateral surfaces with a rongeur (Fig. 42-21B). Use utmost care to avoid tearing the dura, which may be adherent to the inner surface of the pedicles. If a rent occurs, suture it as soon as possible.
- Remove the offending material, such as a caseous mass, granulation tissue, a necrotic disc, or a nest of sequestra. This may be accomplished easily, but the removal of a ridge of living bone is difficult.
- Do not retract the cord; leave it untouched and approach the bony ridge from the side or from beneath.
- Drill the ridge in several places with a slowly rotating hand drill and nibble away from the side and below with a small rongeur. The mass can be further broken up with an osteotome.
- The cord now rests on a shell of bone; gently push this bone anteriorly with a blunt instrument. Be sure to leave no offending ridges.
- Pass a probe along the anterior surface of the cord proximally and distally to locate any secondary cause of compression inside the spinal canal, such as an encapsulated caseous mass.
- Wash the wound with saline solution and dust it with streptomycin.
- Suture the muscles and skin without drainage.

POSTOPERATIVE CARE. Postoperative care is the same as for Technique 42-13.

TUMORS OF THE SPINE

BENIGN TUMORS

Of all primary benign bone tumors, 8% occur in the spine or sacrum. Benign lesions have a predilection for younger patients, usually occurring in the first three decades of life with 60% of benign lesions identified in the second and third decades (Box 42-1). Typically, benign lesions are in the posterior elements, anteriorly located lesions tend to be malignant (76%).

During operative treatment of tumors, certain fundamentals must be followed to maintain function and anatomy and to minimize the risk of recurrence or instability. These principles are most important in the region of the spinal cord. For cervical and thoracic lesions, the spinal cord must be preserved. Roots vary in importance depending on anatomic location and can be resected if long-term benefit is to be gained. Some paired vascular structures, including the vertebral arteries, also can be singly resected.

In the thoracic spine, laminectomy alone does not provide safe access to the anterior column. The risk of paralysis is significant, and alternative approaches must be used. For

BOX 42-1

Radiographic Diagnosis of Spine Tumors According to Age and Location

Diagnosis According to Age

10 to 30 Years Old
Aneurysmal bone cyst
Ewing sarcoma
Giant cell carcinoma
Histiocytosis X
Osteoblastoma
Osteoid osteoma
Osteochondroma
Osteosarcoma

30 to 50 Years Old
Chondrosarcoma
Chordoma
Hodgkin disease
Hemangioma

Older Than 50 Years
Metastatic
Myeloma

Diagnosis According to Location

Vertebral Body
Chordoma
Giant cell carcinoma
Hemangioma
Histiocytosis X
Metastatic disease
Multiple myeloma

Posterior Elements
Aneurysmal bone cyst
Osteoblastoma
Osteoid osteoma
Osteochondroma

Adjacent Vertebrae
Aneurysmal bone cyst
Chondrosarcoma
Chordoma

Multiple Vertebrae
Histiocytosis X
Metastatic
Myeloma

From Charbot JNC, Herkowitz HN: Spine tumors: patient evaluation, Semin Spine Surg 7:260, 1995.

patients who are unable to tolerate a thoracotomy, a costotransversectomy is a reasonable and safe approach to the anterior column. With aggressive lesions, the spinal canal may be contaminated. Nerve roots serve only the intercostal muscles, so sacrifice of some of the thoracic roots does not severely affect function, unless numerous roots are taken. As more thoracic roots are sacrificed, there is some effect on chest cage function and respiration because of interference with intercostal innervation.

Sacral tumors requiring wide excision are rare. Combined approaches often are necessary for wide excision and require complex reconstruction to stabilize the ilia to the distal lumbar spine. Resection of the sacrum and its associated nerve roots also affects continence. If both S1 nerve roots and a single S2 nerve root are preserved, 50% of patients retain continence. If only a single S3 root is taken, with S1 and S2 undisturbed, bowel and bladder function are retained. The nature of the tumor to be resected often dictates the anatomic level of resection.

STABILITY

Stability considerations after resection are different in adult and pediatric patients. In the cervical and thoracic regions, laminectomy creates instability in an immature spine, so arthrodesis should be done. The adult spine seems to tolerate laminectomy better, and some biomechanical considerations are useful when choosing instrumentation and fusion procedures. Instability created by anterior resection increases as more vertebral body is resected. As a rule of thumb, fusion should be done when any significant amount of vertebral body is resected. The exception to this is curettage; if adequate bone graft is placed after curettage, fusion usually is unnecessary. After anterior fusion, with or without instrumentation, immobilization with a TLSO generally is recommended. When incorporation of fusion bone is identified, usually 3 to 6 months postoperatively, the orthosis is discontinued.

Determination of instability after posterior spinal resections is not as straightforward as after anterior procedures. Important bony and ligamentous structures posteriorly contribute individually to overall stability in the intact spine. Soft-tissue restraints include the supraspinous, interspinous, and posterior longitudinal ligaments, the ligamentum flavum, and the facet capsules. The spinous processes, laminae, pars interarticularis, facet joints individually on the left and right, and posterior vertebral wall provide bony stability. Point systems have been created to assist in the determination of stability. Bridwell assigned 25% of posterior vertebral stability for each stabilizing structure, including the midline osteoligamentous complex (laminae, spinous processes, and intervening ligaments); the two facet joint complexes (left and right); and the posterior vertebral wall, disc, and annulus. Violation of two of the four complexes, or disruption of 50% of the stabilizing structures, is an indication for instrumentation and fusion. Bony involvement of tumors also contributes to impending pathologic fracture and instability. Considerations for impending instability or for determining stability after fracture include more than 50% collapse of the vertebral body, translation, segmental kyphosis of more than 20 degrees above normal, and involvement of anterior and posterior columns.

CLASSIFICATION

As with tumors in other locations, the Enneking classification is useful in determining treatment of spinal tumors (Fig. 42-22). Stage 1 tumors (e.g., osteoid osteoma, eosinophilic granuloma, osteochondroma, and hemangioma) are latent and typically require no treatment. If surgery is necessary, often intralesional excision is all that is required, with or without adjuvants such as liquid nitrogen, phenol, or PMMA. Stage 2 lesions are active, become symptomatic, and usually require only en bloc excision (i.e., removal of the tumor as a whole, as opposed to piecemeal). Intralesional excision often suffices for these tumors. Examples of stage 2 lesions include osteoid osteoma, osteoblastoma, eosinophilic granuloma,

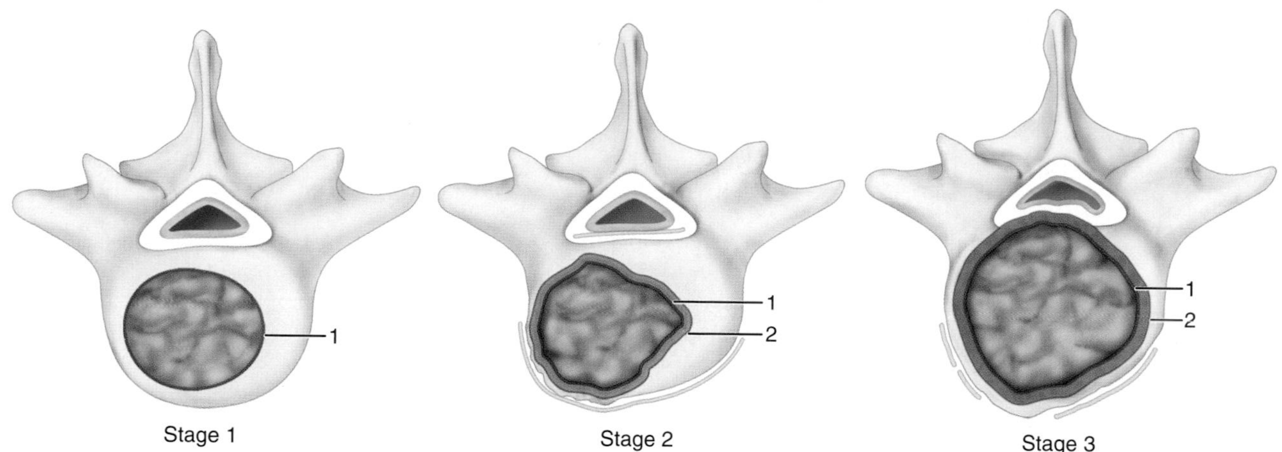

FIGURE 42-22 Enneking staging of benign spinal tumors. Capsule of tumor is indicated by *1,* and reactive pseudocapsule is indicated by *2.* Stage 3 aggressive benign tumors can expand through posterior vertebral wall and compress cord. Pseudocapsule is vascularized reactive tissue and can adhere to dura.

more aggressive hemangiomas, osteochondroma, and aneurysmal bone cysts. Aggressive lesions are characterized as stage 3. Despite being classified as benign tumors, lesions such as giant cell tumors and osteoblastomas are locally aggressive and have a tendency to recur. Wide excision is indicated for these lesions and consists of removal of the tumor with a cuff of normal tissue if possible. A marginal excision would result in a biopsy specimen that includes the reactive zone around the tumor. The exact type of excisional biopsy often is dictated by the anatomy of the spine and the location of the tumor.

POSTERIOR ELEMENT TUMORS

OSTEOID OSTEOMA

Osteoid osteoma is a lesion of bony origin that was first described by Jaffe in 1935. These lesions are most common in the spine (42%), affect men more often than women, and occur most often in the second decade. The lumbar spine is the most common location, the cervical next, and the thoracic last, and the lesion is almost invariably located in the posterior elements. A few cases of osteoid osteomas of vertebral bodies have been reported. This lesion is not locally aggressive and is defined by a size of less than 2 cm; larger lesions are classified as osteoblastomas.

Pain is the primary complaint in 83% of patients, is worse at night with awakening in nearly 30%, and is relieved by aspirin in 27%. Because of the location in the posterior elements, radiculopathy occurs in 28% of patients. A painful scoliosis may result, with the lesion usually present at the apex of the curve in the concavity. Although various curve types may result, the usual structural features of vertebral rotation normally present in idiopathic scoliosis are absent. The resultant scoliosis is rigid and rapidly progressive. Saifuddin et al., in a meta-analysis of spinal osteoid osteoma and osteoblastoma, determined that (1) 63% of patients had scoliosis, (2) scoliosis was significantly more common with osteoid osteomas than with osteoblastomas, (3) lesions were more common in the thoracic and lumbar regions than in the cervical region and more common in the lower cervical region than in the upper cervical region, and (4) lesions were more commonly located to one side of the midline. They concluded that these findings support the concept that in patients with spinal osteoid osteoma or osteoblastoma, scoliosis is secondary to asymmetric muscle spasm.

Diagnosis can be difficult because early radiographs may appear normal. Frequently, a sclerotic lesion of the pedicle is all that is apparent, and even this may be a subtle asymmetry. Later, the usual configuration of a central nidus with surrounding sclerosis may be found, but it is typical in appearance in only half of patients. Oblique radiographs can be helpful when the pedicle, facet, and pars interarticularis are studied. A radioisotopic bone scan is most helpful in accurate localization, and CT often shows the nidus.

Treatment should consist of surgical excision of the lesion if symptoms fail to improve or the scoliosis is progressive. Nidus excision can be confirmed by specimen CT. If the spine is considered unstable because of facet or pedicle removal, a single-level fusion is done simultaneously. Complete excision should result in improvement in the angular degree of the scoliosis, although resolution is less likely in patients 9 to 13.5 years old. Scoliosis persists in 20% to 30% of patients after successful resection. Curves that persist for more than 18 months after resection may require treatment. Brace management may be necessary in immature patients, and regular follow-up is advised. Surgery for spinal deformity usually is deferred until after treatment and resection of the osteoid osteoma and follows the same principles as for idiopathic scoliosis. Prompt relief of pain is the best postoperative indicator of successful removal of the tumor.

Other described treatment methods include high-frequency radiofrequency ablation. This involves CT-guided percutaneous insertion of a radiofrequency electrode. Although this technique has been used successfully in other parts of the body, the potential for neurologic damage around the spine makes it more challenging.

OSTEOBLASTOMA

Osteoblastoma accounts for 10% of all spinal tumors, and 32% appear in the spine. Similar to osteoid osteoma, osteoblastoma occurs most commonly in the second and third decades, with a male-to-female ratio of 2:1. These lesions almost always involve the pedicle or posterior elements or both, although contiguous levels may be affected. The predominant spinal region affected is the cervical region (40%), followed by the lumbar (23%), thoracic (21%), and sacral regions (17%). Osteoblastoma may be misdiagnosed as an osteosarcoma, Ewing sarcoma, lymphoma, or aneurysmal bone cyst, which all are high on the list of differential diagnoses. Differentiation from osteoid osteoma is based on size—these lesions exceed 2 cm.

Radiographic evaluation reveals a destructive, expansile lesion with a thin rim of cortical bone. Lytic features are predominant and occur in 50%, with purely blastic changes in 20%. Bone scanning always is positive and is helpful in identification. Although MRI is useful in identifying a soft-tissue mass, it may confuse the picture. A "flare" reaction may occur, suggesting extracompartmental extension and confusing the diagnosis of a benign lesion. As with other bony lesions, CT is best for definition of the extent of the tumor and for identification of the nidus.

Wide excision, if possible, is the treatment of choice. The tumor recurs 9 years after resection in 10% to 20% of patients with intralesional excision. The best indication of successful removal is relief of preoperative pain. Because of the possibility of recurrence and malignant transformation, however, long-term CT follow-up is mandatory. Operative treatment is necessary for recurrences because these lesions are not radiosensitive.

OSTEOCHONDROMA

Although rarely symptomatic, osteochondroma is the most common benign primary bone tumor. Half of patients with symptomatic tumors are younger than 20 years old, which is consistent with the growing cartilaginous cap. Males are affected three times more often than females, with most lesions protruding eccentrically from the neural arch. Because the spinal canal is occupied by spinal cord in the thoracic and cervical spine, lesions here are more frequently symptomatic. Ninety-one percent of osteochondromas occur in the cervical and upper thoracic spine, although the lumbar spine and sacrum also are affected. The lack of symptoms may result in underdiagnosis of lesions in the lumbar and sacral regions.

Radiographic evaluation often is diagnostic, with the lesions found most often in the posterior elements. Because of the radiolucent cartilaginous cap, however, MRI or myelography may be necessary to determine if impingement of the neural structures is present. These lesions are slow growing and require excision only if symptomatic. Malignant transformation occurs in less than 1% of tumors and is suspected when symptoms are rapid in onset with growth of a previously stable osteochondroma. A cartilaginous cap larger than 1 cm also is suspect. En bloc excision including all of the cartilaginous cap is done, with neurologic recovery the rule and recurrence the exception.

ANEURYSMAL BONE CYST

Aneurysmal bone cysts are relatively uncommon, accounting for only 1% to 2% of benign bone tumors. Although predominantly a posterior element lesion, an aneurysmal bone cyst may expand to include the pedicle and vertebral body. Of all aneurysmal bone cysts, 11% to 30% occur in the spine and are most frequent in patients younger than 20 years old. There does not seem to be a gender preference. Back pain is the predominant symptom in 95% of patients, although muscle spasms causing spinal rigidity or scoliosis also may be present. The differential diagnosis includes giant cell tumors, tuberculosis, fibrous dysplasia, eosinophilic granuloma, Ewing sarcoma, and osteoblastoma.

The characteristic radiographic finding with aneurysmal bone cysts is an expansile lesion with a reactive rim of cortical bone outlining the lesion as it expands from the cortex, although this may be absent in 30%. Another characteristic feature is that these lesions may affect contiguous levels. Arteriography may show a lesion with multiple septa and blood-filled spaces. MRI with gadolinium enhancement also shows the fluid levels within the septations.

Embolization may be successful, although some may require repeated embolizations. Low-dose irradiation has had limited success, with few side effects when dosages are less than 30 Gy. Radiation alone is successful, however, in only approximately 50%. Surgery has remained the standard of care for aneurysmal bone cysts. After embolization to decrease intraoperative blood loss, curettage and bone grafting are done. Despite intralesional margins, the recurrence is only 13%. Any instability created must be treated at the time of surgery and often requires a single-level fusion in skeletally immature patients.

VERTEBRAL BODY TUMORS

Typical benign lesions found in the vertebral bodies include hemangioma, eosinophilic granuloma, and giant cell tumors. Historically, lesions such as these were considered surgically inaccessible when in the vertebrae. The older literature recommended irradiation or chemotherapy. Although this still may be appropriate in special circumstances, such as in highly radiosensitive malignant tumors, angular deformity with potential paraplegia may result because of subsequent spinal instability. Benign tumors are best treated without irradiation to avoid secondary sarcomatous change. Optimal treatment of aggressive benign or solitary malignant tumors may be anterior resection of the tumor for cure or for tumor debulking.

HEMANGIOMA

Hemangioma is a common lesion, present in 10% to 12% of autopsy specimens. Most of these lesions are clinically silent and are detected only incidentally during evaluation for other problems. Occurrence may be single or multiple with contiguous levels affected, but the vertebral body is the most common location, especially in the lumbar and lower thoracic regions. The posterior elements are involved in 10% to 15% of patients; however, this is atypical and indicative of an aggressive lesion. Patients with symptomatic hemangiomas most commonly have pain (60%), neurologic compromise (30%), or symptomatic fracture (10%). Epidural cavernous hemangiomas are rare. Several case reports can be found in the recent literature.

Radiographs detect larger lesions, which have vertical striations and coarse, thick trabeculae, described as a "corduroy" vertebra. Expansion may be noted in aggressive hemangiomas, with erosion of the vertebral body. Axial CT shows a classic "polka dot" appearance. Bone scanning is not particularly helpful because lesions may be either hot or cold. MRI has become the standard for diagnosing these lesions. Typical hemangioma is identified by increased intensity on T1- and T2-weighted sequences and can be differentiated from Paget disease because pagetic bone has more cortical thickening and affects the entire vertebral body. Aggressive hemangiomas can involve the entire vertebral body, may be expansile, and may have a soft-tissue component, which is differentiated from typical hemangioma by hypointensity on T1-weighted images and hyperintensity on T2-weighted images.

Most hemangiomas do not require treatment, and other causes of pain must be excluded. For rare symptomatic lesions, radiation is successful in 50% to 80%. Embolization also is useful, especially in patients with progressive neurologic deficits, and may provide temporary relief of pain. Vertebroplasty has been used successfully for treatment of aggressive hemangiomas by stabilizing pathologic bone with an injection of bone cement into the vertebral body. Use of inflatable bone tamps has had similarly good short-term results. Direct intralesional injection of ethanol has been reported to be effective in obliterating symptomatic vertebral hemangiomas. CT angiography is required before injection to identify functional vascular spaces of the hemangioma and to direct needle placement. Less than 15 mL of ethanol should be used because pathologic fractures of the involved vertebrae have been reported in two patients who received 42 mL and 50 mL. For progressive neurologic deficit, radiation alone may be successful in arresting progression. With neurologic deficit and fracture, however, surgery is necessary to remove an aggressive hemangioma, and embolization should be done preoperatively to minimize bleeding intraoperatively.

EOSINOPHILIC GRANULOMA

Eosinophilic granuloma is most common in patients younger than 10 years old. It typically is a solitary lesion of bone, with 7% to 15% occurring in the spine, and has a predilection for the thoracic region. Symptoms usually include pain, muscular rigidity, and neurologic deficits; systemic symptoms may occur. The classic radiographic finding is vertebra plana seen as a complete collapse of the vertebral body on the lateral view. Bone scans are cold, and MRI often reveals a flare reaction on T2-weighted images, which can be mistaken for a malignant lesion. Differential diagnoses include Ewing sarcoma, aneurysmal bone cyst, infection, tuberculosis, leukemia, and neuroblastoma. Because radiographic findings are not pathognomonic, biopsy is necessary.

When the diagnosis is made, immobilization and observation alone often are sufficient treatment. These lesions typically regress spontaneously over time with some, although incomplete, restoration of vertebral deformity. Follow-up is important to detect instability. Operative intervention, including curettage and grafting, may speed healing. There presently is no role for radiation in the treatment of eosinophilic granuloma. Recurrence is unusual, and resolution of neurologic deficits usually occurs as the tumor regresses.

GIANT CELL TUMOR

Giant cell tumor is the most prevalent benign tumor of the sacrum, rarely affecting other spinal sites, and is second only to hemangioma as the most common benign spinal neoplasm. Giant cell tumors account for 4% to 5% of all primary bone tumors, occurring most often between the third and fifth decades. Females are affected twice as frequently as males, and 1% to 18% of giant cell tumors occur in the spine. Because of its lytic appearance, differential diagnoses include aneurysmal bone cysts, osteoblastoma, and metastasis.

Pain is the most common complaint and often has been present a long time before diagnosis. Neurologic deficits occur in 20% to 80% of patients with giant cell tumors of the spine. Radiographs show the lesions as lytic, septated, and expansile, often with cortical breakthrough and an associated soft-tissue mass. More than 50% of these lesions involve the vertebral body only. When present in the sacrum, the lesion is in the proximal aspect and eccentrically located.

Because of the aggressive nature of these lesions, en bloc resection with wide margins is necessary. Despite aggressive operative treatment, a 10% to 50% recurrence rate has been reported. Preoperative embolization is recommended, and embolization and radiation are reserved for lesions that cannot be resected or excised completely, or in which surgery would result in significant functional morbidity. Doses ranging from 3500 to 4500 cGy are safe and effective in controlling giant cell tumor. If intralesional excision is done, adjuvant cryotherapy should be considered. Metastases occur in 1% to 11% of patients, with a 10% incidence of sarcomatous change.

PRIMARY MALIGNANT TUMORS

Almost all patients with malignancies of the spine have pain. More than 95% seek medical care for pain, with radiculopathy occurring in about 20% of these patients.

CLASSIFICATION

The Enneking classification of malignant tumors also is useful for spinal tumors: stage I, low grade; stage II, high grade; and stage III, regional or distant metastases (Fig. 42-23). The site of the tumor is indicated by A, intracompartmental, or B, extracompartmental. This classification scheme is useful in determining if marginal or wide excision is best. Radical excision is impossible in the spine.

OSTEOSARCOMA

Primary osteosarcoma of the spine is rare, accounting for only 3% of all osteosarcomas, and frequently is fatal. Pain is the most common presenting complaint, but neurologic symptoms also are present in 70% of patients. These tumors are anterior column tumors, and 95% affect the vertebral body. Men and women are equally affected. Secondary osteosarcomas, which occur most commonly after irradiation or develop in patients with Paget disease, affect patients in their 60s. Soft-tissue extension, or extracompartmental disease, is the rule at the time of diagnosis, which is evident on MRI or at surgery.

Radiographs may show a lytic, blastic, or mixed picture affecting the vertebral body. Bone scanning is useful in identifying multicentric or metastatic disease, and axial CT scans are useful in delineating the bony anatomy. Intensive radiation therapy and chemotherapy are the primary treatments. Radical surgery has been suggested, including wide resection with adjuvant radiation therapy. The risk of local recurrence has been shown to be five times greater in patients with positive resection margins than in patients with tumor-free resection margins. Wide or marginal excision of the tumors improves survival; therefore, chemotherapy and at least marginal excision should be done if possible. Patients with metastases, large tumors, and sacral tumors have a poor prognosis. No association, however, has been found between

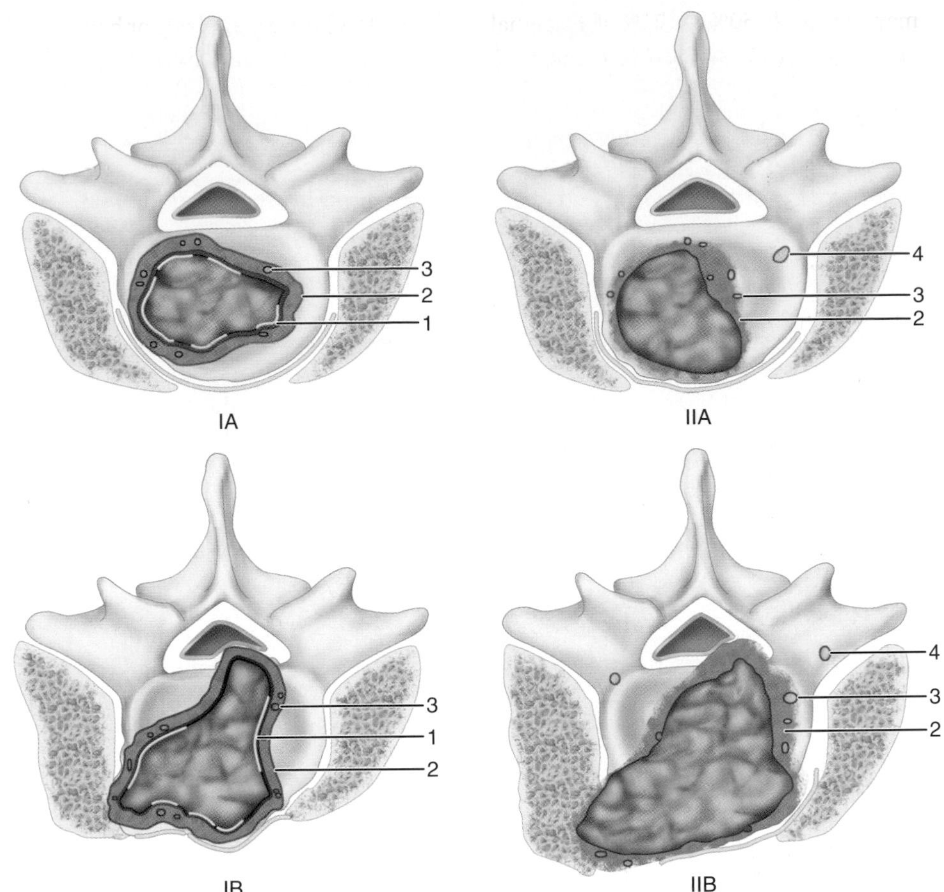

FIGURE 42-23 Enneking staging of malignant spinal tumors. Capsule of tumor is indicated by *1*, pseudocapsule is indicated by *2*, island of tumor within pseudocapsule (satellites) is indicated by 3 and at distance (skip metastases) is indicated by 4. Types IB and IIB tumors can compress cord if expanding posteriorly. Pseudocapsule is more or less infiltrated by neoplastic tissue, which can have direct contact with dural sac.

the affected spinal region and outcome. Total sacrectomy and reconstruction with PMMA, plate-and-screw devices, and custom-made prostheses have been reported to be successful in the treatment of sacral osteosarcoma.

EWING SARCOMA

Another anterior column primary bone tumor, Ewing sarcoma, is a permeative lesion that affects the spine only 3.5% to 8% of the time, with half of these tumors found in the sacrum. Neurologic deficits are present in many patients because of soft-tissue extension, and constitutional symptoms are common. Radiographic findings are confusing, with vertebra plana apparent in some patients, which may be confused with eosinophilic granuloma. Generally, these tumors are lytic, with a soft-tissue mass identified on MRI. Treatment is similar to that for appendicular Ewing sarcoma—chemotherapy and radiation. Surgical decompression is indicated only for tumors causing neurologic compromise and for potential instability to preserve neurologic function. Long-term survival is possible with this tumor; 5-year survival using chemotherapy and irradiation is 20% to 44%. The frequency of cerebral and skeletal metastasis is higher than in appendicular disease, where pulmonary metastasis is most prevalent.

CHORDOMA

Primarily a tumor of adults, chordoma is an uncommon tumor that affects the sacrum and coccyx. It originates embryologically from the notochord remnants and, as such, usually is a midline tumor. It is relatively slow growing but relentless in progression with high recurrence rates when a wide excision is not obtained. Symptoms usually are indolent with a palpable mass in the sacrum anteriorly on rectal examination. Men are affected twice as often as women, and the tumor affects an older population, with peak incidences during the fifth and seventh decades.

Radiographs reveal a lytic lesion in the midline of the sacrum with variable calcification. Bone scans often are negative because of the indolent biologic behavior of these tumors. MRI provides excellent delineation of the anterior soft-tissue extension that typically occurs with these tumors. Treatment involves a wide en bloc excision, which may be impossible in the proximal sacrum without sacrifice of the S2 nerve roots. Recurrence rates approach 28% with sacrectomy, and bowel and bladder continence are retained only if both the S2 roots and one of the S3 roots are preserved. If for any reason the tumor is incised during excision, recurrence may be 64%. As a result, great care is needed in resection of these tumors and radiation should be used for tumors with incisional margins.

Long-term survival may approach 50% to 75% if marginal resection or better is achieved.

MULTIPLE MYELOMA

Plasmacytoma is the single-lesion variety of multiple myeloma and is rare, accounting for only 3% of plasma cell dyscrasias. This diagnosis carries a 60% 5-year survival rate. Thereafter, gradual progression to multiple myeloma occurs, although extended survival has been reported. Multiple myeloma, in contrast, accounts for 1% of newly diagnosed malignancies and is uniformly fatal within 4 years of diagnosis in all patients when spinal disease is diagnosed. Men and women are equally affected during the sixth to eighth decades. These tumors result from unregulated proliferation of plasma cells, causing systemic manifestations. Diagnosis is confirmed by the presence of at least 10% abnormal plasma cells, lytic bone lesions, and monoclonal gammopathy diagnosed on serum protein electrophoresis or urine protein electrophoresis. Anemia and elevation of sedimentation rate also are characteristic on laboratory studies. Protein electrophoresis may be negative in 3% of patients with myeloma, which requires a low threshold for bone marrow aspiration in patients at risk. Treatment of plasmacytoma and multiple myeloma is irradiation, with operative intervention reserved for patients with neurologic deficits or progression despite maximal chemotherapy and irradiation.

METASTATIC TUMORS

Metastatic tumors are the most common malignant lesions found in bone, present 40 times more often than all other primary malignant bone tumors combined. Metastatic disease involves the spine in 50% to 85% of patients. The spine is the most common site of skeletal metastasis. Metastatic spread to the spine favors the thoracic region (70%), followed by the lumbar spine (20%), the cervical spine, and the sacrum. The vertebral body is the most common site of metastasis, followed by the pedicle and then the posterior elements. Ninety percent of tumors are extradural, 5% are intradural, and 1% are intramedullary. Breast, lung, and prostate are the most frequent tumors to metastasize to the spine, followed by thyroid, renal, and gastrointestinal cancer. Lymphoma is another tumor that commonly affects the spine and must be considered. Advances in chemotherapy, radiation therapy, and other cancer therapies have resulted in a significant improvement in survival for many of these types of cancer. With the improved survival, previously silent spinal metastases are becoming clinically apparent and significantly impair quality of life.

The chief complaint in most patients is pain, although 36% of spinal metastases do not cause symptoms. Pain usually is progressive and unremitting, and often no relief occurs even with rest or at night. A previous history of cancer, regardless of how remote, must prompt a search for metastatic disease in patients with progressive pain. Neurologic symptoms or signs may be present but are less frequent, occurring in 5% to 20% of patients with spinal metastases. For patients with thoracic metastasis, however, the rate of neurologic symptoms increases to 37%, probably because of the more sensitive spinal cord with less space available at this level compared with compression of the nerve roots in the lumbar spine. In patients who develop neurologic deterioration and paraparesis, only 25% to 35% regain lost motor function. Patients who are paraplegic or have complete bowel or bladder dysfunction are not likely to regain function regardless of treatment. Rapid onset of symptoms over less than 24 hours also indicates a poor prognosis for neurologic recovery, in contrast to a lesion with a slower onset of symptoms. With aggressive treatment, 60% of patients who retain the ability to walk before treatment of spinal metastasis maintain this function after treatment. In a study comparing radiation with surgery for patients with metastatic cord compression and neurologic symptoms, those who received surgery had greater benefits in terms of ambulation ability than those who had radiation. Imaging often is inconclusive and nondiagnostic in these patients. Plain radiographs of the spine are inconclusive in many with metastatic disease. The most sensitive study is bone scanning, which identifies most lesions larger than 2 mm, although false-negative studies occur in 5%. Multiple myeloma, breast, nasopharyngeal, lung, and renal tumors are the most likely neoplasms to appear falsely negative on bone scans. Use of CT is helpful in delineating soft-tissue extension from the bone or into the bone from extrinsic sources. Also, certain features of the CT scan are useful in determining whether a compression fracture is a result of osteoporosis or metastasis. Osteoporotic compression fractures reveal no evidence of cortical destruction, homogeneous involvement of the vertebral body, localized pathology, and the absence of a soft-tissue mass. MRI is more useful in evaluating soft-tissue masses, neural elements, and vertebral body lesions. Characteristic features of metastatic lesions are hypointensity on T1-weighted images, with enhancement on T2-weighted images and gadolinium-enhanced T1-weighted images. Myelography occasionally is necessary for tumors not well defined by other, less invasive, procedures but should be used cautiously because it can precipitate neurologic deterioration in 16% to 24% of patients, necessitating immediate decompression.

The standard methods of treatment for benign tumors, involving excision and grafting, usually are insufficient for the early mobilization of patients with symptomatic metastatic disease. An estimated 5% to 20% of patients with metastatic cancer develop spinal cord compression. Prostatic tumors are the most common cause of epidural impingement. Hypernephroma is the most common malignancy to cause neurologic impairment as the first sign of malignancy.

CLASSIFICATION

DeWald et al. suggested a classification of spinal metastases. Class I is destruction without collapse but with pain. This class is divided further into Ia, less than 50% vertebral body destruction; Ib, greater than 50% vertebral body destruction; and Ic, pedicle destruction. In this class, DeWald et al. considered surgery only for grades Ib and Ic. Class II is the addition of moderate deformity and collapse with immune competence. Patients in this class are considered a good risk for surgery. Class III patients are immunocompromised with moderate deformity and collapse. This class carries greater risk for surgery. Class IV includes patients with paralysis, collapse, and deformity with immune competence. This class is considered a relative surgical emergency. Class V adds immune incompetence to paralysis, collapse, and deformity. Patients in this class are not considered to be a good operative risk. Surgical reconstruction is recommended when more than 50% vertebral body destruction is identified or in the presence of involvement of one or both pedicles because of the risk of later fracture and deformity. This classification allows consideration of the tumor, potential instability, and patient physiology, which is a sensible approach to a difficult problem.

IRRADIATION

For most metastatic tumors, irradiation is sufficient for the palliation of symptoms of pain and neurologic deficit. Indications for irradiation include pain and mild, slowly progressive neurologic symptoms in the presence of a radiosensitive tumor; spinal canal compromise that results from soft-tissue compression and not bony retropulsion; and multifocal lesions compressing the spinal canal. Instability is a relative contraindication for irradiation because of the potential collapse and progression of deformity that could occur with tissue necrosis. Use of irradiation causes initial necrosis of tumor bone, which later is converted to lamellar bone and normal bone marrow. This process results in remineralization of the lesion at 2 months, formation of woven bone at 4 months, and reorganization into mature bone at 6 to 12 months. Initial necrosis after irradiation of large, potentially unstable lesions may result in acute instability and neurologic deterioration.

Successful treatment has been documented in 62% of patients with pain and in 52% of patients with neurologic impairment. Improvement in neurologic symptoms was noted in 25%. Surgery has failed to show a benefit in survival rates over irradiation; if symptoms can be controlled, radiation therapy seems to be the logical choice. Acute neurologic deterioration is an indication, however, for immediate surgical decompression.

OPERATIVE TREATMENT

Indications for surgical decompression include the requirement of tissue for diagnosis; treatment of an isolated lesion; treatment of a fracture causing instability, pain, or spinal canal compromise; radioresistant tumors, which usually include gastrointestinal and kidney metastases; recurrent tumor in a previously irradiated field; neurologic symptoms that are progressive despite adjuvant measures; and potential instability. Operative procedures often are extensive and involve significant blood loss; the patient must be in a physical state that allows for survival of the proposed procedure. Expected survival of more than 6 weeks is a relative indication for surgery in the presence of unremitting or progressive symptoms, although general physical condition also is important in operative decision-making. In patients with a reasonable long-term survival, bone grafting is recommended rather than PMMA because of the likely failure of such materials. Adjunctive radiation therapy must be planned carefully, however, to allow for incorporation of grafts when used. This is best accomplished by performing the irradiation preoperatively or delaying it until at least 3 weeks postoperatively if possible to improve fusion rates. Because of the hypercoagulable state of malignancy, especially in patients with paraplegia, the use of a preoperative inferior vena cava filter also should be considered.

Laminectomy has been shown to be of little value in the treatment of progressive paralysis caused by malignant spinal tumors in the anterior column. Successful results using this approach have been reported in only 30% to 40% of patients and are inferior to the results obtained with radiation alone. Radical laminectomy for tumor resection is of value, however, and should be considered when compression is caused by lesions in the posterior elements compressing the dura. Careful evaluation of diagnostic images is necessary for appropriate preoperative planning of the operative approach and subsequent procedures.

Because of the predominant vertebral body location of malignant tumors, anterior decompression is most often necessary to remove the pathologic process responsible for neurologic deterioration and pain. Other indications for anterior surgery include pathologic kyphosis with an intact posterior osteoligamentous complex. Improvement in pain is possible in 80% to 95% of patients, with restoration of neurologic function in 75%. Decompression often creates instability that requires reconstruction with instrumentation, allografts, and occasionally structural bone cement. Although circumferential instrumentation is definitely superior in stabilization, anterior instrumentation alone often suffices if the posterior osteoligamentous complex is intact and resection is less than a complete spondylectomy. Additional posterior decompression and stabilization in a combined approach often are necessary if the spinal canal is compressed anteriorly and posteriorly or if the posterior column is attenuated. If exposure of anterior and posterior columns is necessary, a two-stage approach combined under one anesthesia or a simultaneous approach can be used. High-grade instability, contiguous vertebral involvement, destruction of anterior and posterior columns, and need for en bloc resection are indications for these approaches. Solid fixation is possible with structural grafting anteriorly, and solid segmental instrumentation can be applied anteriorly and posteriorly if necessary to provide the most rigid surgical constructs.

For patients with anterior column involvement who are unable to tolerate a thoracotomy, or patients with circumferential spinal cord or neural constriction, a costotransversectomy is useful in the thoracic spine and a posterolateral approach is useful in the lumbar and cervical spines. Excision is intralesional, but decompression often is acceptable with the ability to restore stability using structural grafts or devices anteriorly with segmental instrumentation posteriorly. The morbidity of a thoracotomy is avoided, which is a necessity in some patients, especially patients with symptomatic metastasis from lung cancer. By excising the rib head, intercostal neurovascular bundle, and transverse process on the side of the lesion, the anterior and middle columns are accessible to about the midline using special curets. If the pedicle is uninvolved, this medial wall is preserved to avoid contamination of the spinal canal or damage to the spinal cord. Bilateral approaches occasionally are necessary for extensive posterior vertebral body involvement to allow access to both sides of the middle column. Care must be taken with soft-tissue extension to avoid inadvertent entry into the great vessels anteriorly. These procedures should be followed by instrumentation and fusion, and structural interbody grafting should be used if significant bony resection is done anteriorly to decrease tension stresses on the posterior implants.

There have been numerous reports on the efficacy of PMMA as an adjunct to internal fixation and bone grafting. Bone cement functions well in compression; however, results have been disappointing on the tension side of spinal reconstructions. Failure has been noted at a mean of 200 days after treatment, and its use has been recommended for patients with a short life expectancy or in salvage cases. Generally, if life expectancy is more than 3 to 6 months, bone graft incorporation is possible. Fear of neural injury from the use of PMMA has been a frequent concern. Wang et al. showed that although the temperature of the curing cement may reach 176° F to 194° F, the temperature measured beneath an intact lamina and under Gelfoam covering the dura at a laminar defect was significantly less (45° F). Later examination of the spinal cord in test animals did not show evidence of neural injury. Clinically, we have noted a decrease in amplitude of somatosensory evoked potentials during the curing phase that returns to normal within 20 to 30 minutes of insertion of PMMA. Injury from the use of the material near the spinal cord has not been reported. PMMA can be used to augment existing internal fixation devices; however, loosening is to be expected. If long-term survival is expected, provision for bone grafting and graft incorporation must be made.

Percutaneous vertebroplasty has been reported to be effective treatment for osteolytic spinal metastases and multiple myelomas. Cortet et al. reported decreased pain within 48 hours of vertebroplasty in 97% of patients with beneficial effects maintained in 89% at 3 months and 75% at 6 months. Although leakage of the cement outside the vertebral body occurred in 29, only two patients developed severe nerve root pain, owing to leakage into a neural foramen. Vertebroplasty should be done only in centers with experienced neurosurgeons or orthopaedic surgeons because of the possibility of severe complications.

ANTERIOR DECOMPRESSION FOR TUMOR OF THE SPINE

TECHNIQUE 42-15

- Approach the diseased spine using the standard anterior approach for that spinal segment from the side of the most prominent tumor mass, but choose an approach that allows for more radical or extensive exposure if necessary.
- Identify normal bone and disc cranially and caudally.
- Ligate segmental vessels first to allow discectomy, which is carried to the posterior longitudinal ligament. Ligation of the segmental vessel at the level of vertebral body involvement may be difficult because of encasement by soft-tissue extension.
- Decompression of the spinal canal or resection of tumor is possible if lesions are anteriorly situated. If decompression is necessary, create an access portal within the vertebral body anterior to the tumor and use curets to pull tumoral tissue anteriorly away from the spinal canal into the void. This allows decompression without forcing material against the already compressed dura.
- Piecemeal resection commonly is done for metastatic lesions; however, for en bloc resection, the tumor must not be violated. In these cases, osteotomize the pedicles after discectomy to allow en bloc resection. Be prepared for a cerebrospinal fluid leak because adherence of the tumor to the dura is possible.
- If any extension of tumor is present into the posterior elements, a staged posterior procedure for completion of vertebrectomy is done.
- When resection of tumor is complete, prepare for fixation. For patients with expected long-term survival of more than 1 to 2 years, place allograft or autograft for structural support. These grafts include allograft femur, humerus, fibula, and iliac crest. Autograft fibula and iliac crest are the only options unless a structural spacer, such as a mesh cage, is applied.
- Bone cement is a consideration in patients with a poor expected survival and allows for irradiation and immediate compressive strength when combined with anterior instrumentation. Cover the exposed dura or anterior longitudinal ligament or both with Gelfoam. Insert PMMA in a semiliquid or doughy state. Use of a reinforcement device is recommended; this may include Harrington or other hook-rod implants used as a distraction device, Steinmann pins, or a mesh titanium cage that engages the vertebral bodies and is totally covered with PMMA to provide a smooth external surface. Remove excess cement, which is especially important in the cervical spine where a large mass of cement can cause dysphagia. Avoid pushing the cement against the dura and spinal cord. As soon as the cement has been trimmed, begin continuous irrigation of the wound with normal saline. This theoretically keeps perineural temperatures at a minimum; although owing to cerebrospinal fluid convection, this may be unnecessary.
- Anterior instrumentation is added to provide maximal fixation. Numerous implants that are of low profile and provide at least four fixation points are available. For optimal fixation, place vertebral body screws in a bicortical fashion. If a later posterior instrumentation construct is planned, slight modification of screw placement is necessary to allow for placement of pedicle screws if these are to be used. Under these circumstances, identify the pedicle, and simply keep the vertebral body screws just inferior to these structures.
- When fixation is complete and compression of the interbody construct is maintained, test the construct for stability before closing. Remove and replace the cement and metal fixation if it is loose.
- Close the wound in the standard fashion.
- If corpectomy of more than a single level is done or if posterior column involvement is present, a combined approach with posterior instrumentation is preferred.

POSTOPERATIVE CARE. Rigid immobilization is preferable after these procedures, especially when the bone quality is in question because of osteoporosis or other metabolic causes. A TLSO is typically worn when getting out of bed and while up; however, it is unnecessary for the patient to wear this during sleep. When the graft incorporates over the next 3 to 6 months, the TLSO is discontinued. Radiation is deferred for 3 weeks if possible. Great attention is paid to nutrition during the perioperative period, and parenteral or enteral supplementation may be required.

COSTOTRANSVERSECTOMY FOR TUMOR OF SPINE

TECHNIQUE 42-16

- Using a standard posterior incision or a paramedian incision, expose the spinous processes and transverse processes bilaterally over the levels of anticipated instrumentation (see Chapter 37). When radiographic localization is complete, identify and expose the rib at the level and side of the pathologic process.
- To perform corpectomy, usually it is necessary to expose three ribs subperiosteally and disarticulate them at the costotransverse articulation and to excise the medial 8 to 10 cm of the ribs. Removal of the transverse processes aids in vertebral body exposure.
- When the ribs are removed, use peanut dissectors to elevate the pleura bluntly from the vertebral bodies.
- Create working portals between the intercostal neurovascular bundles for placement of retractors and instruments. During this step of the procedure, headlight illumination is mandatory to see into the retropleural space.
- Laminectomy or facetectomy can be done if necessary for posterior decompression. Ligation of the segmental vessels is possible, if necessary, under direct observation.
- Retention of the intercostal nerves is preferable; however, these can be sacrificed if they interfere with proper decompression. The tradeoff is chest wall anesthesia, intercostal paralysis, and potentially upper abdominal muscle paralysis below T7.
- Perform discectomy above and below the affected vertebral body in the standard fashion.
- Remove the tumor with curets and rongeurs to the level of the posterior longitudinal ligament or dura as necessary. Brisk bleeding as the tumor is curetted is to be expected but is minimized by preoperative embolization. Intermittent packing of the tumor also helps to control bleeding, with continuation of the procedure after bleeding subsides. When the tumor is excised, hemostasis usually occurs without much difficulty.
- For curative resections, it is difficult to obtain en bloc or wide margins using this approach. Osteotomes can be safely directed to parallel the posterior vertebral body wall; however, obtaining margins beyond the opposite lateral cortical wall of the vertebral body is impossible because of the risk of injury to the opposite segmental vessels. Nonetheless, the approach is useful in patients unable to tolerate thoracotomy when an anterior pathologic process is predominant and stabilization is necessary. Instrumentation is necessary for stabilization and can be used posteriorly at any time during the procedure, although we prefer to place implants before exposure of the spinal canal to minimize incidental dural tear while placing implants. Early placement of implants also can be helpful to distract the ligamentous structures and disc during the decompression. Pedicle fixation avoids the concerns of spinal canal compromise of hooks or wires and allows fixation of levels after laminectomy. Hook-rod or Luque-type constructs also are applicable, and the type used is determined by the surgeon's experience.
- Before closure, maintain positive-pressure ventilation momentarily while irrigation is allowed to cover the pleura. This is done to inspect the pleura for leaks that usually would necessitate placement of a chest tube.
- After bone grafting, standard closure is done over drains.

POSTEROLATERAL DECOMPRESSION FOR TUMOR OF THE SPINE

Posterolateral decompression is indicated for patients with tumors that involve the anterior, middle, and posterior columns simultaneously. This is done without the risks or the extensive exposure required for a simultaneous approach.

TECHNIQUE 42-17

- If a posterolateral approach is used, make a midline incision to expose the pathologic level.
- When identification of the correct level is confirmed, decompression can be done or posterior instrumentation can be placed. Regardless, because of the potential destabilization that occurs with laminectomy and pedicle resection, place posterior instrumentation before completion of the procedure.
- Begin decompression as the pedicle that leads into the tumor is sounded and use sequentially larger curets to remove bone through this access site.
- Hemilaminectomy is helpful to expose the medial border of the pedicle to avoid medial penetration, unless adequate decompression requires laminectomy, in which case this is done before the transpedicular decompression.
- Resect the lateral wall of the pedicle with a Leksell rongeur, which allows medialization of the curets.
- If the posterior vertebral body wall is retropulsed, resect the medial pedicle border as well.
- If compression is bilateral, a bilateral transpedicular approach is necessary.
- When the pedicle is resected, a reverse-angle curet or even a PLIF tamp can be placed ventral to the dura, against the tumor or retropulsed posterior vertebral wall so that it is tamped or pushed back into the vertebral body. Decancellation of the middle column often is necessary before this maneuver to create a space for the bone that is reduced.
- When the retropulsed material is pushed anteriorly, resect it with curets and pituitary rongeurs.
- Anterior column grafting depends on the procedure performed.
- Take care that morcellized graft is not retropulsed into the spinal canal after placement, creating the same problem the procedure was intended to correct.
- Perform appropriate bone grafting and instrumentation. If a large anterior vertebral body was resected, a structural device should be placed in addition to posterior segmental spinal instrumentation.

POSTOPERATIVE CARE. Patients are fitted for a TLSO, and immobilization is continued after the procedure for 3 to 6 months. Ambulation is started on the first postoperative day, unless neurologic deficit was preexistent, in which case bed-to-chair transfers are started. Anticoagulants are not used in spinal surgery patients because of the inherent risk of epidural hematoma, so lower extremity antiembolism stockings and compression foot devices are used until the patient is ambulatory. A vena cava filter should be considered for high-risk patients. Radiation is deferred, if possible, for at least 3 weeks when autogenous or allograft bone is used.

REFERENCES

INFECTIONS

BIOLOGY, DIAGNOSIS, AND TREATMENT OF SPINAL INFECTION

Bhavan KP, Marschall J, Olsen MA, et al: The epidemiology of hematogenous vertebral osteomyelitis: a cohort study in a tertiary care hospital, *BMC Infect Dis* 10:158, 2010.

Caroom C, Tullar JM, Benton G Jr, et al: Intrawound vancomycin powder reduces surgical site infections in posterior cervical fusion, *Spine* 38:1183, 2013.

Chaichana KL, Bydon M, Santiago-Dieppa DR, et al: Risk of infection following posterior instrumented lumbar fusion for degenerative spine disease in 817 consecutive cases, *J Neurosurg Spine* 20:45, 2014.

Edin ML, Miciau T, Lester GE, et al: Effect of cefazolin and vancomycin on osteoblasts in vitro, *Clin Orthop Relat Res* 333:245, 1996.

Ghobrial GM, Thakkar V, Andrews E, et al: Intraoperative vancomycin use in spinal surgery, *Spine* 39:550, 2014.

Khan MH, Smith PN, Rao N, Donaldson WF: Serum C-reactive protein levels correlate with clinical response in patients treated with antibiotics for wound infections after spinal surgery, *Spine J* 6:311, 2006.

Khan NR, Thompson CJ, DeCuypere M, et al: a meta-analysis of spinal surgical site infection and vancomycin powder, *J Neurosurg Spine* 21:974, 2014.

Koutsoumbelis S, Hughes AP, Girardi FP, et al: Risk factors for postoperative infection following posterior lumbar instrumented arthrodesis, *J Bone Joint Surg* 93A:1627, 2011.

Lim S, Edelstein AI, Patel AA, et al: Risk factors for postoperative infections following single-level lumbar fusion surgery, *Spine* 2014. [Epub ahead of print].

Nota SPFT, Braun Y, Ring D, Schwab JH: Incidence of surgical site infection after spine surgery: what is the impact of the definition of infection? *Clin Orthop Relat Res* 473:1612, 2015.

Pahys JM, Pahys JR, Cho SK, et al: Methods to decrease postoperative infections following posterior cervical spine surgery, *J Bone Joint Surg* 95A:549, 2013.

Ploumis A, Mehbod AA, Dressel TD, et al: Therapy of spinal wound infections using vacuum-assisted wound closure: risk factors leading to resistance to treatment, *J Spinal Disord Tech* 21:320, 2008.

Radcliff KE, Neusner AD, Millhouse PW, et al: What is new in the diagnosis and prevention of spine surgical site infections, *Spine J* 15:336, 2015.

Rao SB, Vasquez G, Harrop J, et al: Risk factors for surgical site infections following spinal fusion procedures: a case-control study, *Clin Infect Dis* 53:686, 2011.

Strom RG, Pacione D, Kalhorn SP, Frempong-Boadu AK: Decreased risk of wound infection after posterior cervical fusion with routine local application of vancomycin powder, *Spine* 38:991, 2013.

Thakkar V, Ghobrial GM, Maulucci CM, et al: Nasal MRSA colonization: impact on surgical site infection following spine surgery, *Clin Neurol Neurosurg* 125:94, 2014.

Theologis AA, Demirkiran G, Callahan M, et al: Local intrawound vancomycin powder decreases the risk of surgical site infections in complex adult deformity reconstruction, *Spine* 39:1875, 2014.

Weinstein JN, Lurie JD, Tosteson TD, et al: Surgical versus nonoperative treatment for lumbar disc herniation: four-year results for the spine patient outcomes research trial (SPORT), *Spine* 33:2789, 2008.

Weinstein JN, Lurie JD, Tosteson TD, et al: Surgical compared with nonoperative treatment for lumbar degenerative spondylolisthesis. Four-year results in the spine patient outcomes research trial (SPORT) randomized and observational cohorts, *J Bone Joint Surg* 91A:1295, 2009.

Weinstein JN, Tosteson TD, Lurie JD, et al: Surgical versus nonoperative treatment for lumbar spinal stenosis four-year results of the spine patient outcomes research trial, *Spine* 35:1329, 2010.

Xiong L, Pan Q, Jin G, et al: Topical intrawound application of vancomycin powder in addition to intravenous administration of antibiotics: a meta-analysis on the deep infection after spinal surgeries, *Orthop Traumatol Surg Res* 100:785, 2014.

PYOGENIC INFECTIONS

Canavese F, Gupta S, Krajbich JI, Emara KM: Vacuum-assisted closure for deep infection after spinal instrumentation for scoliosis, *J Bone Joint Surg* 90B:377, 2008.

Korovessis P, Repantis T, Hadjipavlou AG: Hematogenous pyogenic spinal infection: current perceptions, *Orthopedics* 35:885, 2012.

Kowalski TJ, Layton KF, Berbari EF, et al: Follow up MR imaging in patients with pyogenic spine infections: lack of correlation with clinical features, *AJNR Am J Neuroradiol* 28:693, 2007.

Lin CP, Ma HL, Wang ST, et al: Surgical results of long posterior fixation with short fusion in the treatment of pyogenic spondylodiscitis of the thoracic and lumbar spine: a retrospective study, *Spine* 37:E1572, 2012.

Marschall J, Bhavan KP, Olsen MS, et al: The impact of prebiopsy antibiotics on pathogen recovery in hematogenous vertebral osteomyelitis, *Clin Infect Dis* 52(7):867, 2011.

Mok JM, Guillaume TJ, Talu U, et al: Clinical outcome of deep wound infection after instrumented posterior spinal fusion: a matched cohort analysis, *Spine* 34:578, 2009.

Olsen MA, Nepple JJ, Riew KD, et al: Risk factors for surgical site infection following orthopaedic spinal operations, *J Bone Joint Surg* 90:62, 2008.

INFECTIONS IN CHILDREN

Fucs PM, Meves R, Yamada HH: Spinal infections in children: a review, *Int Orthop* 36:387, 2012.

Ho AK, Shrader MW, Falk MN, Segal LS: Diagnosis and initial management of musculoskeletal coccidioidmomycosis in children, *J Pediatr Orthop* 34:571, 2014.

Ryan SL, Sen A, Staggers K, et al: Texas Children's Hospital Spine Study Group: A standardized protocol to reduce pediatric spine surgery infection: a quality improvement initiative, *J Neurosurg Pediatr* 14:259, 2014.

Sandler AL, Thompson D, Goodrich JT, et al: Infections of the spinal subdural space in children: a series of 11 contemporary cases and review of all published reports. A multinational collaborative effort, *Childs Nerv Syst* 29:105, 2013.

Sponseller PD, Jain A, Shah SA, et al: Deep wound infections after spinal fusion in children with cerebral palsy: a prospective cohort study, *Spine* 38:2023, 2013.

EPIDURAL SPACE INFECTION

Alton TB, Patel AR, Bransford RJ, et al: Is there a difference in neurologic outcome in medical versus early operative management of cervical epidural abscesses? *Spine J* 15:10, 2015.

Kim SD, Melikian R, Ju KL, et al: Independent predictors of failure of nonoperative management of spinal epidural abscesses, *Spine J* 14:1673, 2014.

Patel AR, Alton TB, Bransford RJ, et al: Spinal epidural abscesses: risk factors, medical versus surgical management, a retrospective review of 128 cases, *Spine J* 14:326, 2014.

FUNGAL INFECTIONS

Iwata A, Ito M, Abumi K, et al: Fungal spinal infection treated with percutaneous posterolateral endoscopic surgery, *J Neurol Surg A Cent Eur Neurosurg* 75:170, 2014.

TUBERCULOSIS

Boachie-Adjei O, Papadopoulos EC, Pellisé F, et al: Late treatment of tuberculosis-associated kyphosis: literature review and experience from a SRS-GOP site, *Eur Spine J* 22(Suppl 4):641, 2013.

Chandra SP, Singh A, Goyal N, et al: Analysis of changing paradigms of management in 179 patients with spinal tuberculosis over a 12-year period and proposal of a new management algorithm, *World Neurosurg* 80:190, 2013.

Kaloostian PE, Gokaslan ZL: Current management of spinal tuberculosis: a multimodal approach, *World Neurosurg* 80:64, 2013.

Mohan K, Rawall S, Pawar UM, et al: Drug resistance patterns in 111 cases of drug-resistant tuberculosis spine, *Eur Spine J* 22(Suppl 4):647, 2013.

Pang X, Shen X, Wu P, et al: Thoracolumbar spinal tuberculosis with psoas abscesses treated by one-stage posterior transforaminal lumbar debridement, interbody fusion, posterior instrumentation, and postural drainage, *Arch Orthop Trauma Surg* 133:765, 2013.

Rajasekaran S, Khandelwal G: Drug therapy in spinal tuberculosis, *Eur Spine J* 22(Suppl 4):587, 2013.

Soares Do Brito J, Tirado A, Fernandes P: Surgical treatment of spinal tuberculosis complicated with extensive abscess, *Iowa Orthop J* 34:129, 2014.

TUMORS

Amendola L, Cappuccio M, De Iure F, et al: En bloc resections for primary spinal tumors in 20 years of experience: effectiveness and safety, *Spine J* 14:2608, 2014.

Buchowski JM, Sharan AD, Gokasaln ZL, Yamada J: *Modern techniques in the treatment of patients with metastatic spine disease*, Instructional Course Lecture #308, San Francisco, 2012, American Academy of Orthopaedic Surgeons, Annual meeting.

Gokaslan ZL, Yamada J, Buchowski JM, Sharan AD: *Modern techniques in the treatment of patients with metastatic spine disease*, Instructional Course Lecture #308, San Diego, CA, 2011, American Academy of Orthopaedic Surgeons, annual meeting.

Goldschlager T, Dea N, Boyd M, et al: Giant cell tumors of the spine: has denosumab changed the treatment paradigm? *J Neurosurg Spine* 22:526, 2015.

Hao DJ, Sun HH, He BR, et al: Accuracy of CT-guided biopsies in 158 patients with thoracic spinal lesions, *Acta Radiol* 52:1015, 2011.

Hillin TJ, Anchala P, Friedman MV, Jennings JW: Treatment of metastatic posterior vertebral body osseous tumors by using a targeted bipolar radiofrequency ablation device: technical note, *Radiology* 273:261, 2014.

Kim JM, Losina E, Bono CM, et al: Clinical outcome of metastatic spinal cord compression treated with surgical excision + radiation versus radiation therapy alone: a systematic review of literature, *Spine* 37:78, 2012.

Lange T, Stehling C, Fröhlich B, et al: Denosumab: a potential new and innovative treatment option for aneurysmal bone cysts, *Eur Spine J* 22:1417, 2013.

Liu JK, Laufer I, Bilsky MH: Update on management of vertebral column tumors, *CNS Oncol* 3:137, 2014.

Ma Y, Xu W, Yin H, et al: Therapeutic radiotherapy for giant cell tumor of the spine: a systematic review, *Eur Spine J* 2015. [Epub ahead of print].

Roper AE, Cahill KS, Hanna JW, et al: Primary vertebral tumors: a review of epidemiologic, histological, and imaging findings, Part I: benign tumors, *Neurosurgery* 69:1171, 2011.

Rose PS, Buchowski JM: Metastatic disease in the thoracic and lumbar spine: evaluation and management, *J Am Acad Orthop Surg* 19:37, 2011.

Sharan AD, Szulc A, Krystal J, et al: The integration of radiosurgery for the treatment of patients with metastatic spine diseases, *J Am Acad Orthop Surg* 22:447, 2014.

Tamburrelli FC, Proietti L, Scaramuzzo L, et al: Bisphosphonate therapy in multiple myeloma in preventing vertebral collapses: preliminary report, *Eur Spine J* 21(Suppl 1):S141, 2012.

White P, Kwon BK, Lindskog DM, et al: Metastatic disease of the spine, *J Am Acad Orthop Surg* 14:587, 2006.

Zadnik PL, Goodwin CR, Karami KJ, et al: Outcomes following surgical intervention for impending and gross instability caused by multiple myeloma in the spinal column, *J Neurosurg Spine* 22:301, 2015.

The complete list of references is available online at ***expertconsult.inkling.com****.*

CHAPTER 43

PEDIATRIC CERVICAL SPINE

William C. Warner Jr.

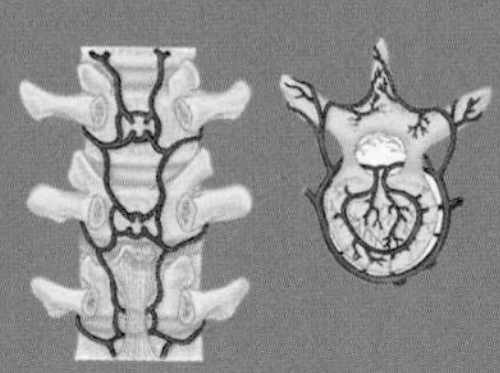

A variety of diseases and congenital anomalies may affect the pediatric cervical spine and increase the risk for neurologic compromise from instability or encroachment of the spinal cord. Multiple anomalies of the upper cervical spine are common within a single patient, so when a single anomaly is seen in a patient, others should be sought. An average of 3.4 cervical spine osseous anomalies per patient has been reported.

NORMAL EMBRYOLOGY AND GROWTH AND DEVELOPMENT

Most disorders of the spine are the result of aberrant growth and developmental processes. Knowledge of the normal embryology, growth, and development of the pediatric cervical spine is necessary to aid in the understanding of these conditions. In embryonic development of the spine, 42 to 44 pairs of somites (4 occipital, 8 cervical, 12 thoracic, 5 lumbar, 5 sacral, and 8 to 10 coccygeal) will form craniocaudally from the mesoderm on either side of the notochord. Each somite differentiates into either sclerotomes or dermomyotomes. Sclerotomes, precursors of the vertebral arch and body, collect at the embryonic midline, surrounding the neural tube and notochord, and proceed to separate into cranial and caudal portions. The cranial portion of each sclerotome then recombines with the caudal portion of the direct superior sclerotome, eventually forming vertebrae. In the cervical spine, eight pairs of embryonic somites create seven cervical vertebrae, with the cranial portion of the first cervical sclerotome contributing to the development of the occiput and the caudal portion of the eighth cervical sclerotome contributing to the formation of the T1 vertebrae.

The mechanism in the formation of the occiput-cervical junction is different and more complex. The first four spinal sclerotomes fuse to form the occiput and posterior foramen magnum. The cranial portion of the first cervical sclerotome remains as half a segment, eventually becoming part of the occipital condyle and tip of the odontoid (proatlas). The atlas is formed by cell contributions from the first cervical sclerotome and the fourth occipital sclerotome. However, unlike the other sclerotomes, the vertebral arch of the first sclerotome separates from the centrum to become the ring of C1 and fuses with the proatlas above and the centrum of C2, becoming the odontoid process and body of C2. Thus, the axis is created by cell contributions from the cranial half of the first cervical sclerotome (tip of the odontoid), the second cervical sclerotome, and the centrum, which becomes the body of the odontoid. The inferior portion of the axis body is formed from the second cervical sclerotome.

The *HOX* and *PAX* regulatory genes are believed to have a role in embryonic differentiation. *HOX* genes specify the vertebral morphology phenotype along the embryonic axis. The *PAX* genes are also integral in vertebral development and are thought to establish the intervertebral boundaries of the sclerotomes. Abnormalities of the *PAX1* sequence in humans are associated with Klippel-Feil syndrome.

At birth the atlas has three ossification centers, one for the body and one for each neural arch. Although the posterior arches usually fuse by 3 years of age, occasionally the posterior synchondrosis between the two fails to fuse, resulting in a bifid arch. The neurocentral synchondroses that connect the neural arches to the body close by 7 years of age.

The axis has four separate ossification centers: one for the dens, one for the body, and two for the neural arches. The neurocentral synchondroses connect the body to the adjacent lateral masses, and the dentocentral synchondrosis connects it to the dens. The dentocentral synchondrosis closes by 6 to 7 years of age; it may persist as a sclerotic line until 11 years. The neural arches of C2 fuse at 3 to 6 years of age. Occasionally, the tip of the odontoid is V shaped (dens bicornum), or a small separate summit ossification center may be present at the tip of the odontoid (ossiculum terminale).

Ossification of the third through seventh cervical vertebrae is similar: a single ossification center for the vertebral body and one for each neural arch. Between the ages of 2 and 3 years the neural arch fuses posteriorly, and by 3 to 6 years the neurocentral synchondroses between the neural arches and the vertebral body fuse. Until 7 to 8 years of age these vertebrae are normally wedge-shaped.

The clinical presentations of patients with pediatric cervical spine disorders are variable; however, most common presentations are deformity, pain, limited motion, or neurologic compromise.

ANOMALIES OF THE ODONTOID

Although congenital anomalies of the odontoid are rare, they can cause significant atlantoaxial instability. These anomalies usually are detected as incidental findings after trauma or when symptoms occur. Atlantoaxial instability can cause a compressive myelopathy, vertebral artery compression, or both.

Congenital anomalies of the odontoid can be divided into three groups: aplasia, hypoplasia, and os odontoideum (Fig. 43-1). Aplasia or agenesis is complete absence of the odontoid. Hypoplasia is partial development of the odontoid, and the bone varies from a small, peg-like projection to almost normal size. Odontoid hypoplasia and aplasia have been associated with spondyloepiphyseal dysplasia and mucopolysaccharidosis (Hunter, Hurler, Morquio, and Maroteaux-Lamy syndromes). In os odontoideum, the odontoid is an oval or round ossicle with a smooth, sclerotic border. It is separated from the axis by a transverse gap, leaving the apical segment without support (Fig. 43-1D). The ossicle is of variable size and usually is located in the position of the normal odontoid (orthotopic), although occasionally it appears near the occiput in the area of the foramen magnum (dystopic). Because this lesion is frequently asymptomatic and remains undiscovered until it is brought to the physician's attention by trauma or the onset of symptoms, the exact incidence of os odontoideum is unknown, but it is probably more common than appreciated. Odontoid anomalies have been reported to be more common in patients with Down syndrome, Klippel-Feil syndrome, Morquio syndrome, and spondyloepiphyseal dysplasia.

Knowledge of the embryology and vasculature of the odontoid is essential to understanding the etiologic theories of congenital anomalies of the odontoid. The odontoid is derived from mesenchyme of the first cervical vertebra. During development, it becomes separated from the atlas and fuses with the axis. A vestigial disc space between C1 and C2 forms a synchondrosis within the body of the axis. The apex, or tip, of the odontoid is derived from the most caudal occipital sclerotome, or proatlas. This separate ossification center, called *ossiculum terminale,* appears at age 3 and fuses by age 12. Anomalies of this terminal portion are rarely of clinical significance (Figs. 43-1C and 43-2).

The arterial blood supply to the odontoid is derived from the vertebral and carotid arteries (Fig. 43-3). The vertebral artery gives off an anterior ascending artery and a posterior ascending artery that begin at the level of C3 and ascend anterior and posterior to the odontoid, meeting superiorly to form an apical arcade. The most rostral portion of the extracranial internal carotid artery gives off "cleft perforators," which supply the superior portion of the odontoid. This peculiar arrangement of blood supply is necessary because of the

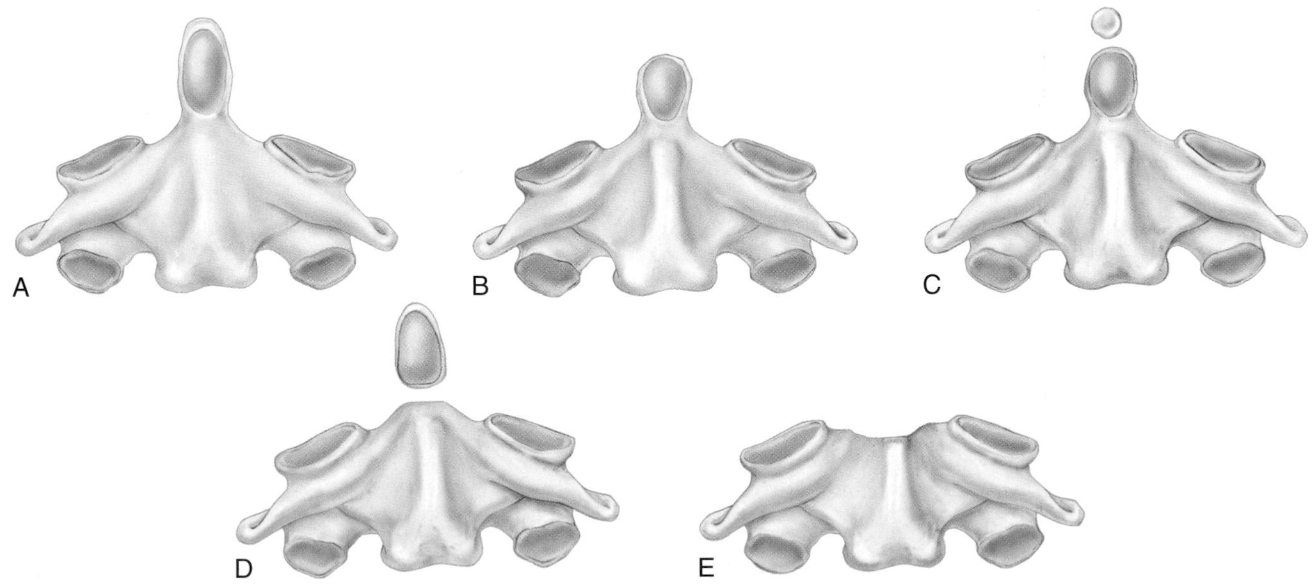

FIGURE 43-1 Types of odontoid anomalies. **A,** Normal odontoid. **B,** Hypoplastic odontoid. **C,** Ossiculum terminale. **D,** Os odontoideum. **E,** Aplasia of odontoid.

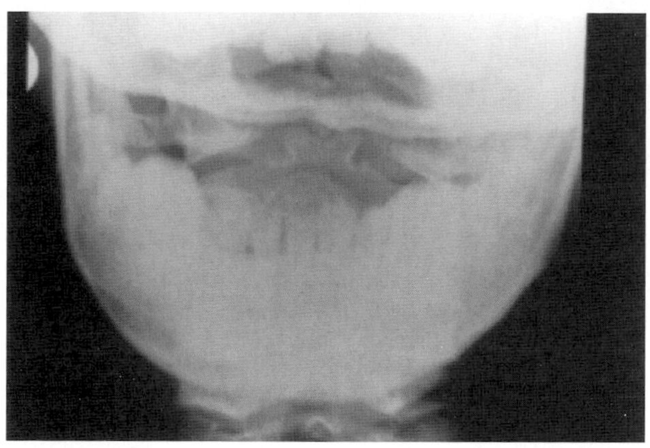

FIGURE 43-2 Anteroposterior open-mouth odontoid view showing V-shaped dens bicornis and ossiculum terminale.

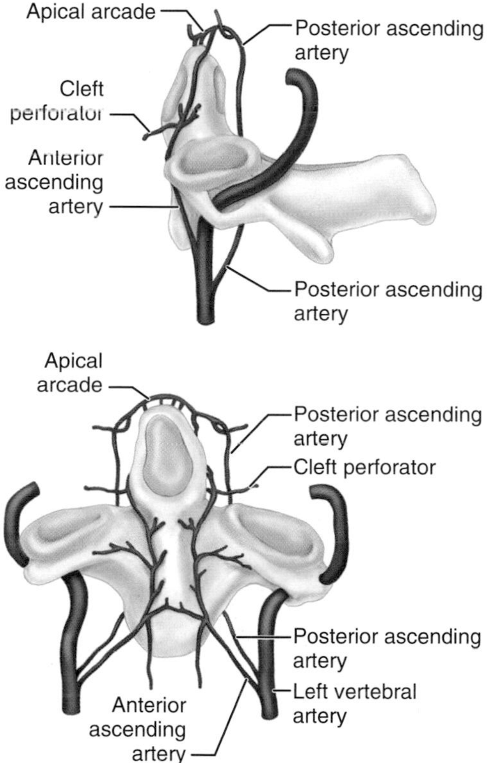

FIGURE 43-3 Blood supply to odontoid: posterior and anterior ascending arteries and apical arcade.

embryologic development and anatomic function of the odontoid. The synchondrosis prevents direct vascularization of the odontoid from C2, and vascularization from the blood supply of C1 cannot occur because of the synovial joint cavity surrounding the odontoid.

Congenital and acquired causes (posttraumatic) of odontoid anomalies have been suggested. Trauma has been reported in up to 50% of patients. Congenital causes include failure of fusion of the apex or ossiculum terminale and failure of fusion of the odontoid to the axis, neither of which explains all the findings in os odontoideum. The ossiculum terminale is usually too small to influence stability significantly, and the theory of failure of fusion of the odontoid to the axis does not explain the fact that the space between the ossicle and the axis is at the level of the articulating facets of C2, rather than below the level of the articulating facets where the synchondrosis occurs during development. A congenital etiology is supported by the increased incidence among patients with Down syndrome, Klippel-Feil malformation, multiple epiphyseal dysplasia, and other skeletal dysplasias compared with the general population. Os odontoideum can be acquired after infection or trauma or can result from osteonecrosis. Several authors have suggested that an unrecognized fracture at the base of the odontoid is the most common cause. A distraction force by the alar ligament pulls the tip of the fractured odontoid away from its base to produce a nonunion. Osteonecrosis after halo-pelvic traction has been reported.

DIAGNOSIS

The presentation of os odontoideum varies. Signs and symptoms can range from minor to frank compressive myelopathy or vertebral artery compression. Presenting symptoms may include neck pain, torticollis, or headache caused by local irritation of the atlantoaxial joint. Neurologic symptoms vary from transient episodes of paresis after trauma to complete myelopathy caused by cord compression. Symptoms may consist of weakness and loss of balance with upper motor neuron signs, although upper motor neuron signs may be completely absent. Proprioceptive and sphincter disturbances are common findings. Vertebral artery compression causes cervical and brainstem ischemia, resulting in seizures, syncope, vertigo, and visual disturbances. Lack of cranial nerve involvement helps differentiate os odontoideum from other occipitovertebral anomalies because the spinal cord impingement occurs below the foramen magnum.

RADIOGRAPHIC FINDINGS

Odontoid anomalies can be diagnosed on routine cervical spine radiographs that include an open-mouth odontoid view (Fig. 43-4). CT scans with reconstruction views and MRI are helpful in making the initial diagnosis of os odontoideum. Lateral flexion and extension radiographs can detect any instability. Odontoid aplasia appears as a slight depression between the superior articulating facets on the open-mouth odontoid view. Odontoid hypoplasia is seen as a short, bony remnant. With os odontoideum, a space is present between the body of the axis and a bony ossicle. The free ossicle of os odontoideum is usually half the size of a normal odontoid and is oval or round with smooth, sclerotic borders. The space differs from that of an acute fracture, in which the space is thin and irregular instead of wide and smooth. This space should not be confused with the neurocentral synchondrosis in children younger than 6 to 7 years of age.

The amount of instability can be documented by lateral flexion and extension plain films that allow measurement of the amount of anterior and posterior displacement of the atlas on the axis. In children, motion between the odontoid and the body of the axis must be shown before instability with os odontoideum can be diagnosed because the ossicle is fixed to the anterior arch of C1 and moves with it during flexion and extension. Measurement of the relation of C1 to the free

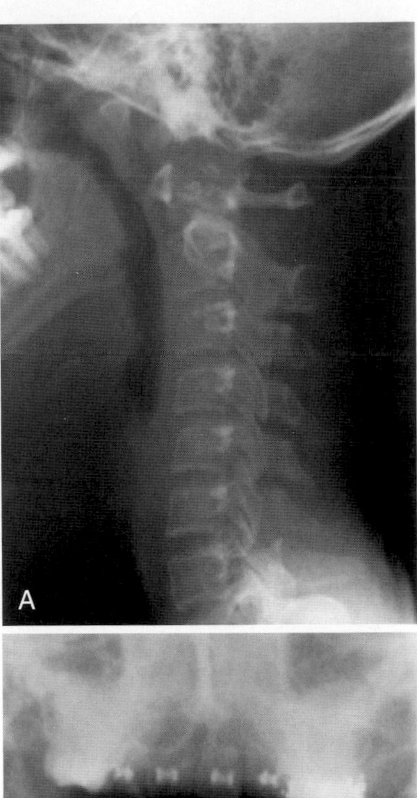

FIGURE 43-4 Lateral radiograph **(A)** and open-mouth odontoid radiograph **(B)** showing os odontoideum.

ossicle is of little value because this moves as one unit. A more significant measurement is made by projecting a line superiorly from the body of the axis to a line projected inferiorly from the posterior border of the anterior arch of the atlas. Measurements of more than 4 to 5 mm in children indicate significant instability.

The space available for the spinal cord also is a helpful measurement. This space is determined by measuring the distance from the posterior aspect of the odontoid or axis to the nearest posterior structure. Fielding reported that most symptomatic patients in his study had an average of 1 cm of movement. Cineradiography can also be helpful in determining motion around the C1-2 articulation.

Watanabe, Toyama, and Fujimura described two radiographic measurements that correlate with neurologic signs and symptoms. They found that if there is a sagittal plane rotation angle of more than 20 degrees or an instability index of more than 40%, a patient is likely to have neurologic signs and symptoms. The instability index is measured from lateral flexion and extension radiographs. Minimal and maximal distances are measured from the posterior border of the C2 body to the posterior arc of the atlas. The instability index is calculated by the following equation:

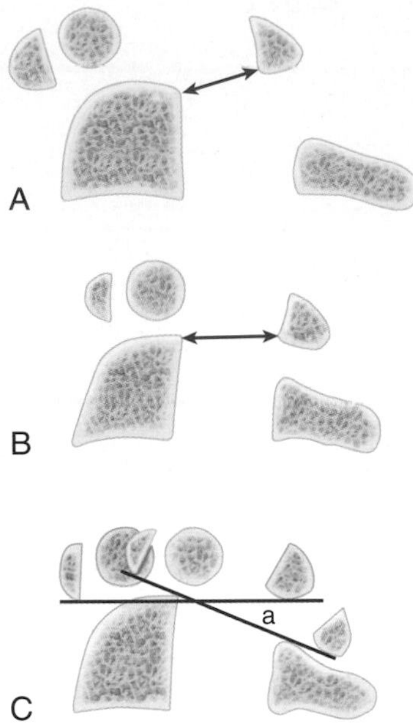

FIGURE 43-5 Radiographic parameters. Minimal **(A)** and maximal **(B)** distance from posterior border of body of C2 to posterior atlantal arch. **C,** Change of atlantoaxial angle between flexion and extension position. *a,* sagittal plane rotation.

$$\text{Instability index} = \text{maximum distance} - \text{minimum distance} + \text{maximum distance} \times 100(\%)$$

The sagittal plane rotation angle is measured by the change in the atlantoaxial angle between flexion and extension (Fig. 43-5). MRI can be useful in identifying reactive retrodental lesions that can occur with chronic instability. This reactive tissue is not seen on routine radiographs but can be responsible for a decrease in the space available for the spinal cord and compressive myelopathy. The prognosis of os odontoideum depends on the clinical presentation. The prognosis is good if only mechanical symptoms (torticollis or neck pain) or transient neurologic symptoms exist. It is poor if neurologic deficits slowly progress.

TREATMENT

The primary concern in congenital anomalies of the odontoid is that an already abnormal atlantoaxial joint can subluxate or dislocate with minor trauma and cause permanent neurologic damage or even death. Patients with local symptoms usually improve with conservative treatment, such as cervical traction or immobilization. The indications for operative stabilization are: (1) neurologic involvement (even if this is transient), (2) instability of more than 5 mm anteriorly or posteriorly, (3) progressive instability, and (4) persistent neck complaints associated with atlantoaxial instability and not relieved by conservative treatment (Box 43-1).

Prophylactic operative stabilization of odontoid instability less than 5 mm in asymptomatic patients is controversial. Because it may be difficult or impossible to restrict a child's activities, the safety of stability without restriction of activity must be weighed against the possible complications of surgery. The decision concerning prophylactic arthrodesis must be

BOX 43-1

Indications for Operative Stabilization of Os Odontoideum

- Neurologic involvement (even transient)
- Instability of greater than 5 mm posteriorly or anteriorly
- Progressive instability
- Persistent neck complaints

made after discussion with the patient and family concerning potential risks of operative and nonoperative treatment. Delayed neurologic injury has been reported in three patients who initially received conservative treatment. We, therefore, recommend prophylactic stabilization of os odontoideum.

In patients with neurologic deficits, skull traction should be used before surgery to achieve reduction, allow recovery of neurologic function, and decrease spinal cord irritation. Achieving and maintaining reduction are probably the most important aspects in the treatment of this anomaly.

Before C1-2 fusion, the integrity of the posterior arch of C1 must be documented. Incomplete development of the posterior ring of C1 is uncommon (3 cases in 1000) but is reported to occur with increased frequency in patients with os odontoideum.

POSTERIOR CERVICAL APPROACHES

ATLANTOAXIAL FUSION

Many variations of two basic techniques of atlantoaxial fusion exist (Box 43-2). The Gallie and the Brooks and Jenkins techniques have been the most frequently used for posterior atlantoaxial fusion (Figs. 43-6 to 43-8). The Gallie technique has the advantage of using only one wire passed beneath the lamina of C1, but tightening the wire can cause the unstable C1 vertebra to displace posteriorly and fuse in a dislocated position (see Fig. 43-6). The Brooks and Jenkins technique has the disadvantage of requiring sublaminar wires at C1 and C2 but gives greater resistance to rotational movement, lateral bending, and extension. The wire varies in size from 22 gauge to 18 gauge, depending on the age of the patient and the size of the spinal canal. Songer cables may also be used instead of wires for the Brooks and Jenkins fusion. In a very young child, wire fixation may be unnecessary; instead, the graft is placed along the decorticated fusion site, and a halo or Minerva cast is used for postoperative immobilization. With the use of fluoroscopy and image-guided systems, C1-2 transarticular screws can be used for stabilization in appropriately sized children.

BOX 43-2

Posterior Fusion Techniques

Atlantoaxial Fusion

Gallie

Advantage: One wire passed beneath lamina of C1

Disadvantage: Wire may cause unstable C1 vertebra to displace posteriorly and fuse in dislocated position

Brooks and Jenkins

Advantage: Greater resistance to rotational movement, lateral bending, and extension

Disadvantage: Requires sublaminar wires at C1 and C2

Harms and Melcher

Advantage: Individual placement of polyaxial screws simplifies technique and involves less risk to C1-C2 facet joint and vertebral artery.

Disadvantages: Possible irritation of the C2 ganglion from instrumentation. Technique is not possible in patients with aberrant course of the vertebral artery (20%).

Magerl and Seeman

Advantage: Significant improvement in fusion rates over traditional posterior wire stabilization and bone grafting techniques.

Disadvantage: Technically demanding and must be combined with Gallie or Brooks fusion for maximum stability.

Occipitocervical Fusion

Cone and Turner; Willard and Nicholson; Rogers

Required when other bony anomalies occur at occipitocervical junction

Wertheim and Bohlman

Wires passed through outer table of skull at occipital protuberance instead of through inner and outer tables near foramen magnum

Lessens risk of danger to superior sagittal and transverse sinuses (which are cephalad to occipital protuberance)

Koop, Winter, Lonstein

No internal fixation used

Autogenous corticocancellous iliac bone graft

Dormans et al.

Stable fixation is achieved by exact fit of autogenous iliac crest bone graft and fixation of the spinous process with button wire and fixation of the occiput with wires through burr holes.

Can be used in high-risk patients (Down syndrome) with increased stabilization and shorter immobilization time.

Contoured Rod, Screw, or Contoured Plate Fixation

Has the advantage of achieving immediate stability of the occipitocervical junction

POSTERIOR ATLANTOAXIAL FUSION

TECHNIQUE 43-1

(GALLIE)

- Carefully intubate the patient in the supine position while the patient is on a stretcher. Place the patient prone on the operating table with the head supported by traction, maintaining the head-thorax relationship at all times during turning. Obtain a lateral cervical spine radiograph to ensure proper alignment before surgery.
- Prepare and drape the skin in a sterile fashion and inject a solution of epinephrine (1 : 500,000) intradermally to aid hemostasis.

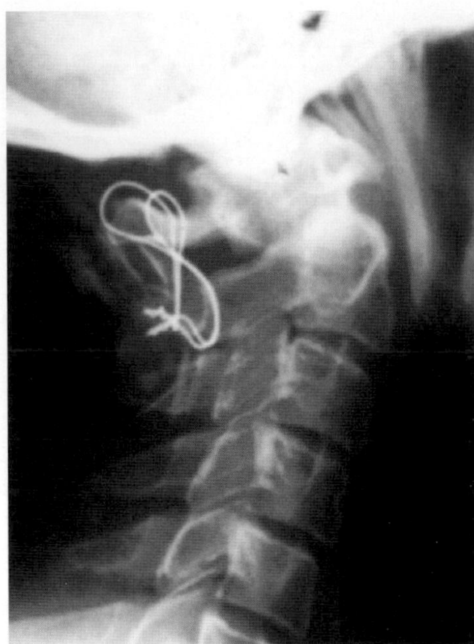

FIGURE 43-6 Posterior translation of atlas after C1-2 posterior Gallie fusion.

- Make a midline incision from the lower occiput to the level of the lower end of the fusion, extending it deeply within the relatively avascular midline structures, the intermuscular septum, or ligamentum nuchae. Do not expose any more than the area to be fused to decrease the chance of spontaneous extension of the fusion.
- By subperiosteal dissection, expose the posterior arch of the atlas and the laminae of C2.
- Remove the muscular and ligamentous attachments from C2 with a curet; dissect laterally along the atlas to prevent injury to the vertebral arteries and vertebral venous plexus that lie on the superior aspect of the ring of C1, less than 2 cm lateral to the midline.
- Expose the upper surface of C1 no farther laterally than 1.5 cm from the midline in adults and 1 cm in children. Decortication of C1 and C2 is generally unnecessary.
- From below, pass a wire loop of appropriate size upward under the arch of the atlas directly or with the aid of a nonabsorbable suture, which can be passed with an aneurysm needle.
- Pass the free ends of the wire through the loop, grasping the arch of C1 in the loop.
- Take a corticocancellous graft from the iliac crest and place it against the laminae of C2 and the arch of C1 beneath the wire.
- Pass one end of the wire through the spinous process of C2 and twist the wire on itself to secure the graft in place.
- Irrigate the wound and close it in layers with suction drainage tubes.

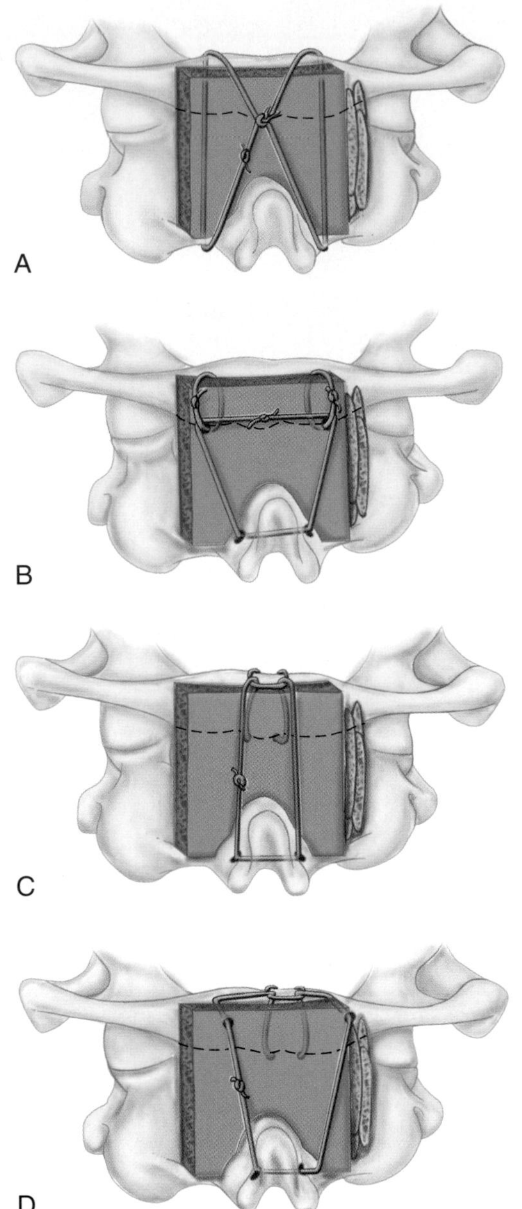

FIGURE 43-7 Fielding's modifications of wire techniques for holding graft in place. **A,** Wire passes under laminae of atlas and axis and is tied over graft. **B,** Wire passes through holes drilled in laminae of atlas and through spine of axis; holes are drilled through graft. **C,** Wire passes under laminae of atlas and through spine of axis and is tied over graft. This method is used most frequently. **D,** Wire passes under laminae of atlas and through spine of axis; holes are drilled through graft. **SEE TECHNIQUE 43-1.**

Fielding described several modifications of the Gallie fusion, as shown in Figure 43-7.

POSTOPERATIVE CARE. The patient is immobilized in a Minerva cast, halo cast or halo vest, or a cervicothoracic orthosis. Immobilization usually is continued for 12 weeks.

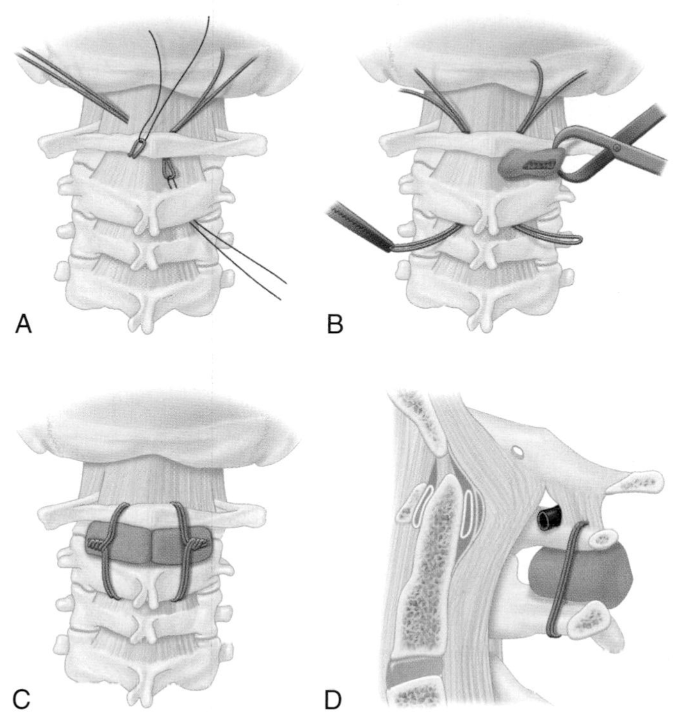

FIGURE 43-8 Brooks-Jenkins technique of atlantoaxial fusion. **A,** Insertion of wires under atlas and axis. **B,** Wires in place with graft being inserted. **C** and **D,** Bone grafts secured by wires (anteroposterior and lateral views). **SEE TECHNIQUE 43-2.**

POSTERIOR ATLANTOAXIAL FUSION USING LAMINAR WIRING

TECHNIQUE 43-2

(BROOKS AND JENKINS)

- Intubate and turn the patient onto the operating table as for the Gallie technique (Technique 43-1). Prepare and drape the operative site as described.
- Expose C1 and C2 through a midline incision.
- Using an aneurysm needle, pass a Mersilene suture from cephalad to caudad on each side of the midline under the arch of the atlas and then beneath the laminae of C2 (Fig. 43-8A). These sutures serve as guides to introduce two doubled 20-gauge wires. The size of the wire used varies depending on the size and age of the patient.
- Obtain two full-thickness bone grafts 1.25 to 3.5 cm from the iliac crest and bevel them so that the apex of the graft fits in the interval between the arch of the atlas and the lamina of the axis (Fig. 43-8B).
- Fashion notches in the upper and lower cortical surfaces to hold the circumferential wires and prevent them from slipping.
- Tighten the doubled wires over the graft and twist them on each side (Fig. 43-8C and D).
- Irrigate and close the wound in layers over suction drains.

POSTOPERATIVE CARE. The postoperative care is the same as that for the Gallie technique.

C1-2 TRANSARTICULAR SCREW FIXATION

Adult instrumentation and fusion techniques may be used in the pediatric cervical spine. The use of this instrumentation is dependent on the preoperative anatomy that would allow appropriate size screws to be placed safely. Adult instrumentation of the cervical spine usually can be used in adolescents and preteens. For smaller children, the use of these adult instrumentation techniques become more difficult but can be used safely in certain patients. Wang et al. reported good results in the management of pediatric atlantoaxial instability with C1-2 transarticular screw fixation and fusion, using a 3.5-mm screw in children 4 years old. Originally described for adult patients, it is technically demanding and requires fluoroscopic or stereotactic assistance for the proper placement of the transarticular screw (Fig. 43-9). Harms and Melcher reported posterior C1-C2 fusion using polyaxial screw and rod fixation in adults and children with good results. They cited the following advantages: individual placement of polyaxial screws in C1 and C2 allows direct manipulation of C1 and C2, simplifying reduction and fixation;

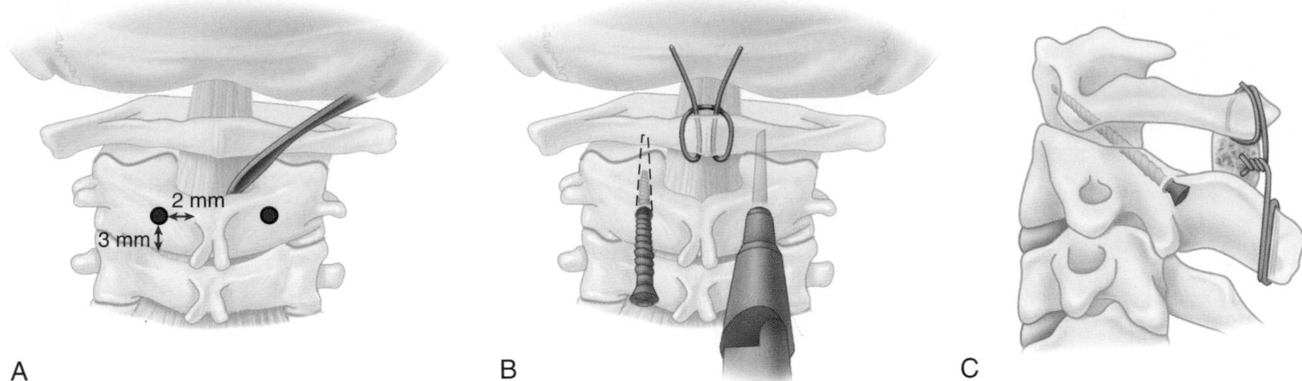

FIGURE 43-9 Magerl technique for atlantoaxial fusion.

superior and medial placement of the C2 screw carries less risk to the vertebral artery; the integrity of the posterior arch of C1 is not necessary for stable fixation (Fig. 43-10). Please refer to Chapter 41 for transarticular screw fixation technique in adults.

TRANSLAMINAR SCREW FIXATION OF C2

Translaminar screw fixation can be used as an alternative to polyaxial screw and rod fixation when the C2 isthmus or pedicle cannot be instrumented. Approximately 20% of patients have an abnormal path of the vertebral artery that will prevent placement of the C2 screw in Harms and Melcher's technique. Translaminar screw fixation may also be used in the lower cervical spine if needed.

TECHNIQUE 43-3

- Place the patient prone with the head in a neutral position in a Mayfield head holder.
- Expose the posterior arch of C1 and the spinous process, laminae, and medial and lateral masses of C2.
- Create a small cortical window at the junction of the C2 spinous process and the lamina on the left, close to the rostral margin of the C2 lamina (Fig. 43-11A).
- Using a hand drill, carefully drill along the length of the contralateral (right) lamina, with the drill visually aligned along the angle of the exposed contralateral laminar surface.
- Palpate the length of the drill hole with a small ball probe to verify that no cortical breakthrough into the spinal canal has occurred.
- Insert a 4-mm diameter polyaxial screw along the same trajectory. In the final position, the screw head is at the junction of the spinous process and lamina on the left, with the length of the screw within the right lamina.
- Create a small cortical window at the junction of the spinous process and lamina of C2 on the right, close to the caudal aspect of the lamina.

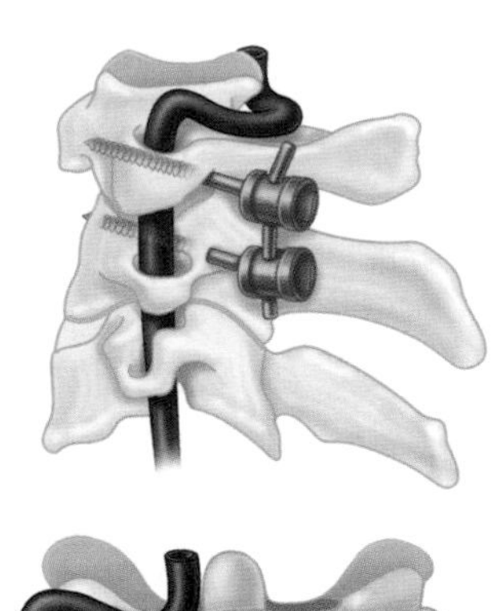

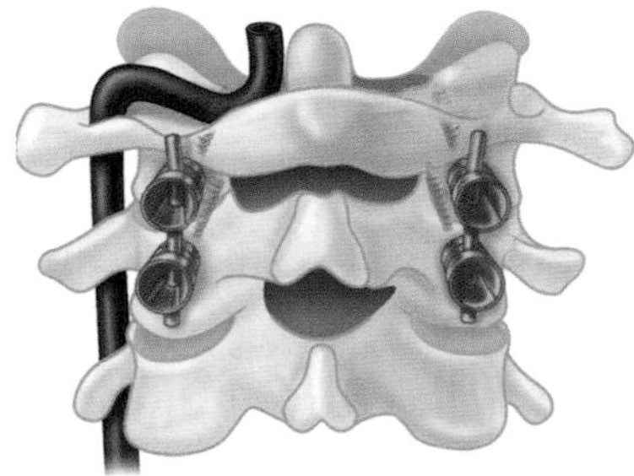

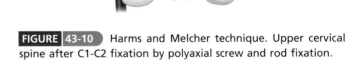

FIGURE 43-10 Harms and Melcher technique. Upper cervical spine after C1-C2 fixation by polyaxial screw and rod fixation.

- Using the same technique as above, insert a 4-mm diameter screw into the left lamina, with the screw head remaining on the right side of the spinous process.
- Place appropriate rods into the screw heads and attach to C1 screws or lateral mass screws below C2 (Fig. 43-11B).

POSTOPERATIVE CARE. The patient is immobilized in a cervical or cervicothoracic orthosis for 8 to 12 weeks.

OCCIPITOCERVICAL FUSION

When other bony anomalies occur at the occipitocervical junction, such as absence of the posterior arch of C1, the fusion can extend up to the occiput. The following technique for occipitocervical fusion includes features of techniques described by Cone and Turner, Rogers, Willard and Nicholson, and Robinson and Southwick.

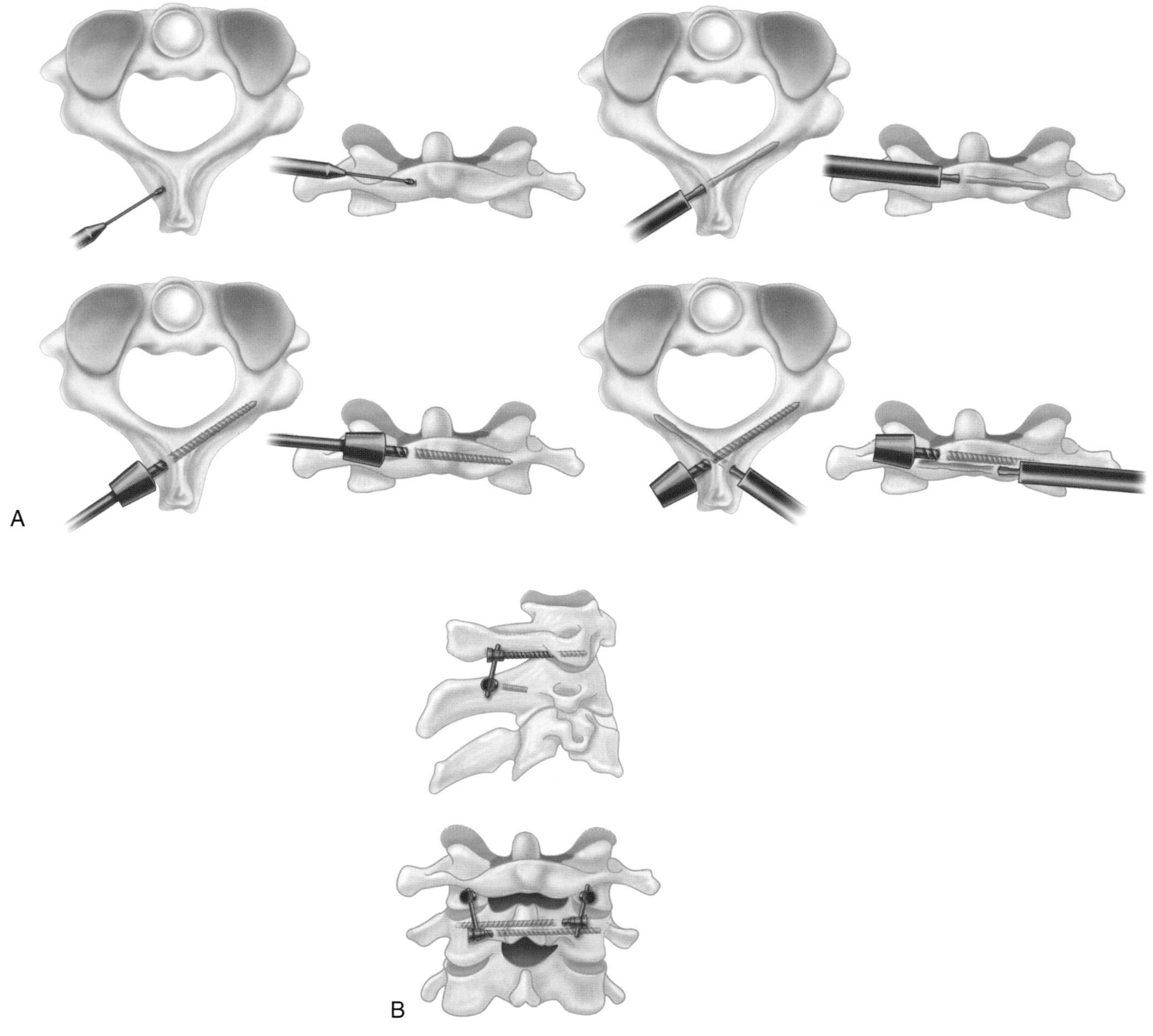

FIGURE 43-11 **A,** C2 translaminar screw placement. **B,** Lateral and anteroposterior views of completed C1-C2 fixation with C1 lateral mass screws connected to C2 laminar screws. **SEE TECHNIQUE 43-3.**

OCCIPITOCERVICAL FUSION

TECHNIQUE 43-4

- Approach the base of the occiput and the spinous processes of the upper cervical vertebrae through a longitudinal midline incision, extending it deeply within the relatively avascular intermuscular septum.
- Expose the entire field subperiosteally.
- Dissect the posterior occiput laterally to the level of the external occipital protuberance.
- Make two burr holes in the posterior occiput about 7 mm from the foramen magnum and 10 mm lateral to the midline (see Fig. 43-12).
- Separate the dura from the inner table of the skull by blunt dissection with a right-angle dissector.
- Pass short lengths of wire through the holes in the occiput and through the foramen magnum.
- Pass wires beneath the posterior arch of C1 on either side if the arch is intact.
- Drill holes in the outer table of the spinous processes of C2 and C3, completing them with a towel clip or Lewin clamp, and pass short lengths of wire through the holes.
- Obtain a corticocancellous graft from the iliac crest and make holes at appropriate intervals to accept the ends of the wires.
- Pass the wires through the holes in the graft and lay the graft against the occiput and the laminae of C2 and C3.

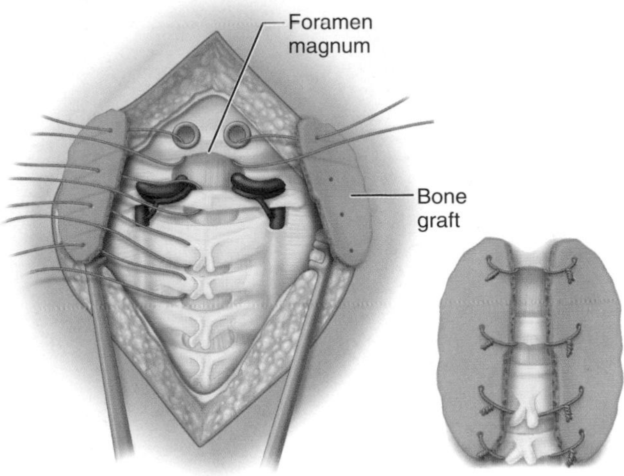

FIGURE 43-12 Robinson and Southwick method of occipitocervical fusion. **SEE TECHNIQUE 43-4.**

- Tighten the wires to hold the graft firmly in place (Fig. 43-12, *inset*).
- Lay thin strips of cancellous bone around the cortical grafts to aid in fusion.
- Inspect the graft and wires to ensure that they do not impinge on the dura or vertebral arteries. Irrigate and close the wound in layers over suction drains.

Robinson and Southwick pass individual wires beneath the laminae of C2 and C3 instead of through the spinous processes (Fig. 43-12).

POSTOPERATIVE CARE. Some form of external support is recommended. This support may vary from a Minerva cast or halo vest or halo cast to a cervicothoracic brace, depending on the degree of preoperative instability and the stability of fixation.

OCCIPITOCERVICAL FUSION PASSING WIRES THROUGH TABLE OF SKULL

Wertheim and Bohlman described a technique of occipitocervical fusion similar to that described by Grantham et al. in which wires are passed through the outer table of the skull at the occipital protuberance instead of through the inner and outer tables of the skull near the foramen magnum. Superior to the foramen magnum the occipital bone is very thin, but at the external occipital protuberance it is thick and allows passage of wires without passing through both tables. The transverse and superior sagittal sinuses are cephalad to the protuberance and are out of danger.

TECHNIQUE 43-5

(WERTHEIM AND BOHLMAN)

- Stabilize the spine preoperatively with cranial skeletal traction with the patient on a turning frame or cerebellar headrest.
- Place the patient prone and obtain a lateral radiograph to document proper alignment.
- Prepare the skin and inject the subcutaneous tissue with a solution of epinephrine (1 : 500,000).
- Make a midline incision extending from the external occipital protuberance to the spine of the third cervical vertebra.
- Sharply dissect the paraspinous muscles subperiosteally with a scalpel and a periosteal elevator to expose the occiput and cervical laminae, taking care to stay in the midline to avoid the paramedian venous plexus.
- At a point 2 cm above the rim of the foramen magnum, use a high-speed diamond burr to create a trough on either side of the protuberance, making a ridge in the center (Fig. 43-13A). With a towel clip, make a hole in this ridge through only the outer table of bone.
- Loop a 20-gauge wire through the hole and around the ridge and loop another 20-gauge wire around the arch of the atlas.
- Pass a third wire through a drill hole in the base of the spinous process of the axis and around this structure; three separate wires are used to secure the bone grafts on each side of the spine (Fig. 43-13B).
- Expose the posterior iliac crest and obtain a thick, slightly curved graft of corticocancellous bone of premeasured length and width.
- Divide this horizontally into two pieces and place three drill holes in each graft (Fig. 43-13C).
- Decorticate the occiput and anchor the grafts in place with the wires on both sides of the spine (Fig. 43-13D). Pack additional cancellous bone around and between the two grafts.
- Close the wound in layers over suction drains.

POSTOPERATIVE CARE. A rigid cervical orthosis or a halo cast is worn for 6 to 16 weeks, followed by a soft collar that is worn for an additional 6 weeks.

OCCIPITOCERVICAL FUSION WITHOUT INTERNAL FIXATION

Koop, Winter, and Lonstein described a technique of occipitocervical fusion without internal fixation for use in children. The spine is decorticated, and autogenous corticocancellous iliac bone is placed over the area to be fused. In children with vertebral arch defects, an occipital periosteal flap is reflected over the bone defect to provide an osteogenic tissue layer for the bone grafts. A halo cast is used for postoperative stability.

TECHNIQUE 43-6

(KOOP ET AL.)

- After the administration of endotracheal anesthesia, apply a halo frame with the child supine.
- Turn the child prone and secure the head with the neck in slight extension by securing the halo frame to a traction frame.

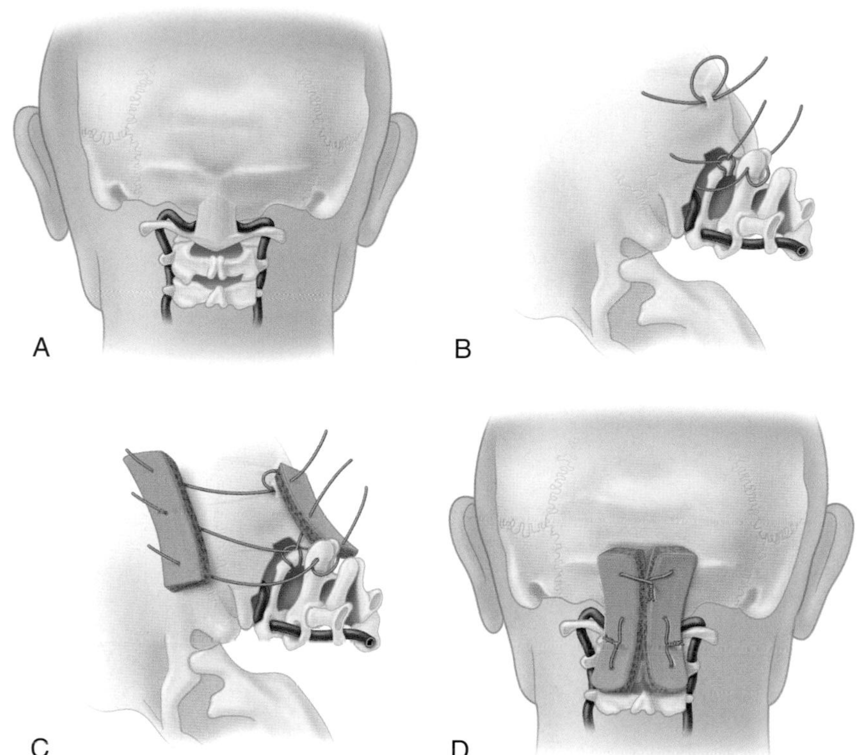

FIGURE 43-13 Wertheim and Bohlman method of occipitocervical fusion. **A,** Burr is used to create ridge in external occipital protuberance; hole is made in ridge. **B,** Wires are passed through outer table of occiput, under arch of atlas, and through spinous process of axis. **C,** Grafts are placed on wires. **D,** Wires are tightened to secure grafts in place. **SEE TECHNIQUE 43-5.**

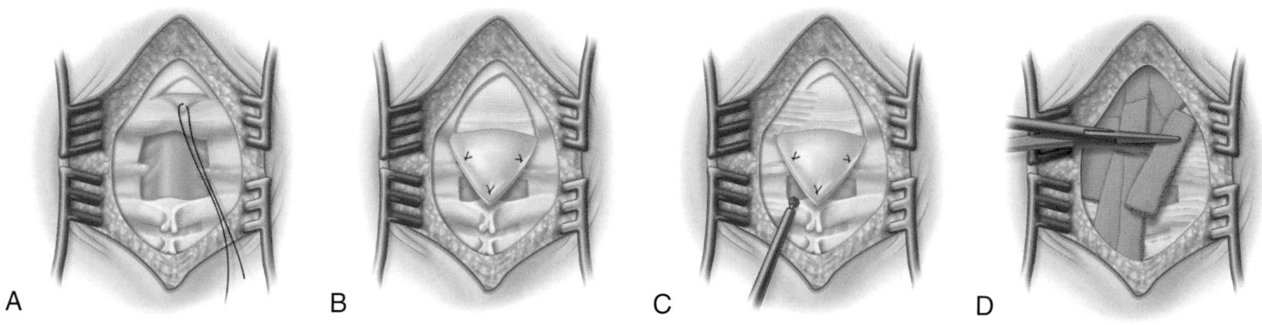

FIGURE 43-14 Koop, Winter, and Lonstein method of occipitocervical fusion used when posterior arch of C1 is absent. **A,** Exposure of occiput, atlas, and axis. **B,** Reflection of periosteal flap to cover defect in atlas. **C,** Decortication of exposed vertebral elements. **D,** Placement of autogenous cancellous iliac bone grafts. **SEE TECHNIQUE 43-6.**

- Make a midline incision. In patients with intact posterior elements, expose the vertebrae by sharp dissection.
- Decorticate the exposed vertebral elements and lay strips of autogenous cancellous iliac bone over the decorticated bone. Expose only the vertebrae to be included in the fusion. In patients with defects in the posterior elements, do not expose the dura, if possible.
- At the level of the occiput, dissect the nuchal tissue from the periosteum and retract it laterally (Fig. 43-14A).
- Elevate the occipital periosteum in a triangular-based flap attached near the margin of the foramen magnum.
- Reflect this flap caudally to cover the defects in the posterior vertebral elements and suture it in place (Fig. 43-14B).
- Decorticate the occiput and the remaining exposed vertebral elements with an air drill (Fig. 43-14C).
- Lay strips of autogenous cancellous bone in place over the entire area (Fig. 43-14D).
- Close the wound in layers over a suction drain.
- Turn the child supine and apply a halo cast.

POSTOPERATIVE CARE. The halo cast is worn until union is radiographically evident, usually at about 5 months. When union is documented by lateral flexion and extension radiographs, the halo cast is removed and a soft collar is worn for 1 month.

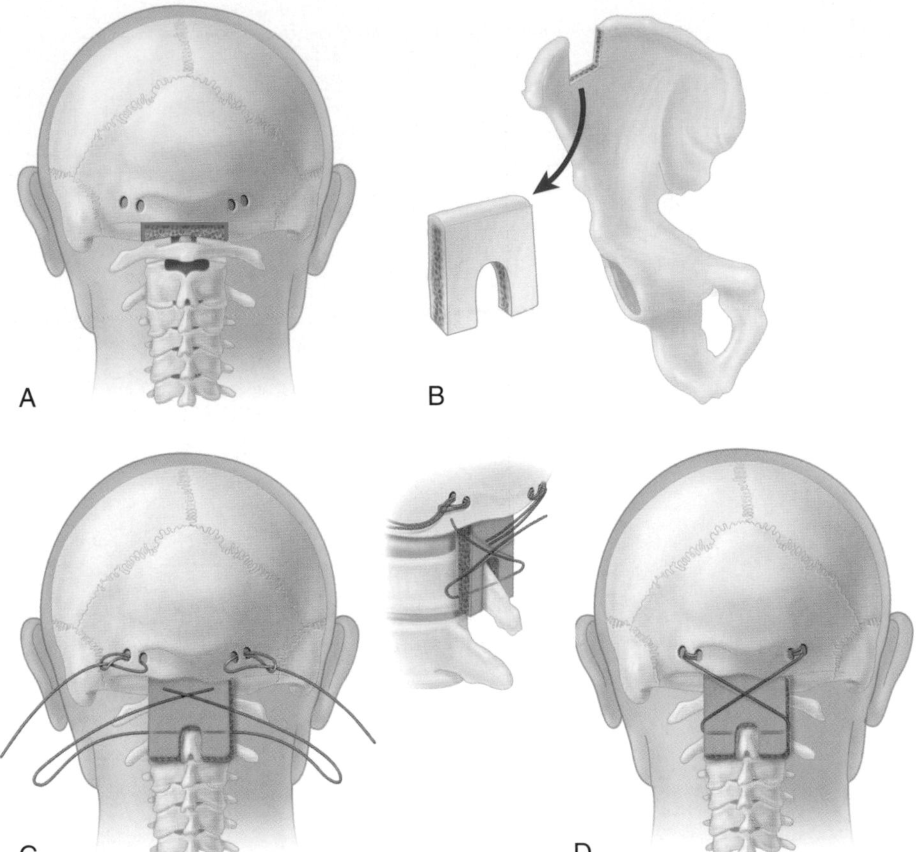

FIGURE 43-15 Occipitocervical fusion as described by Dormans et al. **A,** Placement of burr holes. **B,** Corticocancellous graft obtained from iliac crest. **C,** Looped 16- or 18-gauge wires passed through burr holes and looped on themselves. Graft positioned into occipital trough and around spinous process of cervical vertebra at caudal extent of fusion and locked into place by precise contouring of bone. **D,** Wires crossed, twisted, and cut. **SEE TECHNIQUE 43-7.**

OCCIPITOCERVICAL FUSION USING CROSSED WIRING

Dormans et al. described occipitocervical fusion using a different wiring technique in 16 children with an average age of 9.6 years (range 2.5 to 19.3 years). Fusion was achieved in 15 patients. Complications included pin track infection (four patients), pneumonia (one patient), additional level of fusion (one patient), and graft fracture and nonunion (one patient). The use of wire fixation, combined with inherent stability of the bone-graft construct, allowed for removal of the halo device relatively early (6 to 12 weeks).

TECHNIQUE 43-7

(DORMANS ET AL.)

- After halo ring application, place the patient prone and secure the halo frame to the operating table. Confirm alignment of the occiput and cervical spine with lateral radiographs.
- Expose the midline from the occiput to the second or third cervical vertebra. Limit the lateral dissection to avoid damaging the vertebral arteries.
- In patients who require decompression because of cervical stenosis or for removal of a tumor, remove the arch of the first or second cervical vertebra, or both, with or without removal of a portion of occipital bone to enlarge the foramen magnum.
- Use a high-speed drill to make four holes through both cortices of the occiput, aligning them transversely with two on each side of the midline and leaving a 1-cm osseous bridge between the two holes of each pair. The holes are placed caudad to the transverse sinuses (Fig. 43-15A).
- Fashion a trough into the base of the occiput to accept the cephalad end of the bone graft.
- Obtain a corticocancellous graft from the iliac crest and shape it into a rectangle, with a notch created in the inferior base to fit around the spinous process of the second or third cervical vertebra (Fig. 43-15B). The caudal extent of the intended fusion (the second or third cervical vertebra) is determined by the presence or absence of a previous laminectomy, congenital anomalies, or level of instability.
- Pass a looped 16- or 18-gauge Luque wire through the burr holes on each side and loop it onto itself.
- Pass Wisconsin button wires (Zimmer, Warsaw, IN) through the base of the spinous process of either the second or the third cervical vertebra (Fig. 43-15C). Pass the wire that is going into the left arm of the graft through the spinous process from right to left. Place the graft into the occipital trough superiorly and around the spinous process of the vertebra that is to be at the caudal level of the arthrodesis (the second or third cervical vertebra).
- Contour the graft precisely so that it fits securely into the occipital trough and around the inferior spinous process before the wires are tightened.
- Cross the wires, twist, and cut (Fig. 43-15D).

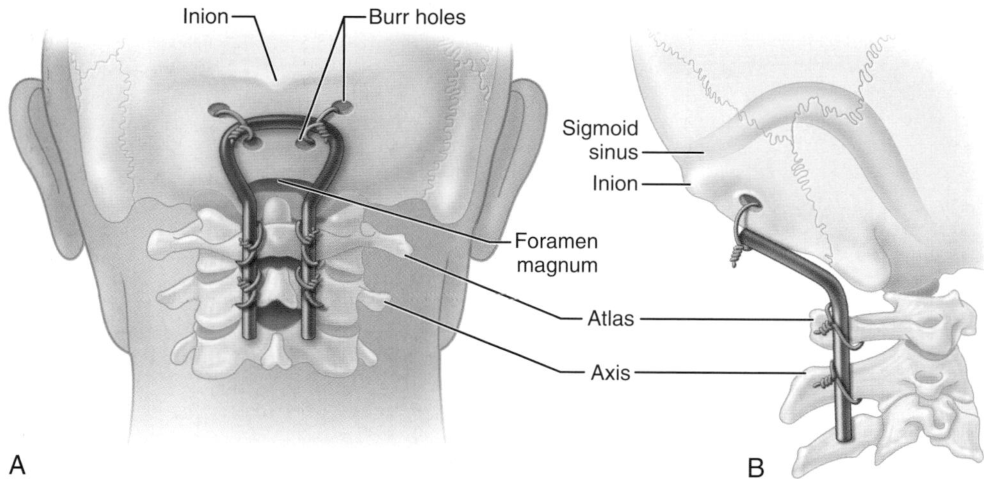

FIGURE 43-16 A and B, Occipitocervical fusion using contoured rod and segmental wire or cable fixation. **SEE TECHNIQUE 43-8.**

- Obtain a radiograph at this point to assess the position of the graft and wires and the alignment of the occiput and cephalad cervical vertebrae. Extension of the cervical spine can be controlled by positioning of the head with the halo frame, by adjustment of the size and shape of the graft, and, to a lesser extent, by appropriate tightening of the wires.
- For patients who have not had a decompression, pass the sublaminar wire caudal to the ring of the first cervical vertebra to secure additional fixation. In young children, this may be difficult or undesirable because of the small size of the ring of the first cervical vertebra or the failure of formation of the posterior arch of the first cervical vertebra.

POSTOPERATIVE CARE. A custom halo orthosis or halo cast is worn until a solid fusion is obtained; thereafter, a cervical collar is worn for 1 month.

OCCIPITOCERVICAL FUSION USING CONTOURED ROD AND SEGMENTAL ROD FIXATION

Occipitocervical fusion using a contoured rod and segmental wire or cable fixation, which has been described by several authors, has the advantage of achieving immediate stability of the occipitocervical junction. This stability allows the patient to move in a cervical collar after surgery, avoiding the need for halo cast immobilization. Smith et al. described occipitocervical arthrodesis using a contoured plate instead of a rod for fixation.

TECHNIQUE 43-8 *Figure 43-16*

- Approach the base of the occiput and the spinous processes of the upper cervical vertebrae through a longitudinal midline incision, extending it deeply within the relatively avascular intermuscular septum.
- Expose the entire field subperiosteally.
- Carry the dissection proximally above the inion and laterally to the level of the external occipital protuberance.
- Make a template of the intended shape of the stainless steel rod with the appropriate length of Luque wire.
- Make two burr holes on each side, about 2 cm lateral to the midline and 2.5 cm above the foramen magnum. Avoid the transverse and sigmoid sinus when making these burr holes. Leave at least 10 mm of intact cortical bone between the burr holes to ensure solid fixation.
- Pass Luque wires or Songer cables in an extradural plane through the two burr holes on each side of the midline. Pass the wires or cables sublaminar in the upper cervical spine.
- Bend the rod to match the template; this usually has a head-neck angle of about 135 degrees and slight cervical lordosis. A Bend Meister (Sofamor/Danek, Memphis) may be helpful in bending the rod.
- Secure the wires or cables to the rod.
- Decorticate the spine and occiput and perform autogenous cancellous bone grafting.

POSTOPERATIVE CARE. A Philadelphia collar or an occipitocervical orthosis is worn until the fusion is stable.

OCCIPITOCERVICAL FUSION USING A CONTOURED OCCIPITAL PLATE, SCREW, AND ROD FIXATION

This technique uses an adjustable-angle rod and a contoured occipital plate (VertexSelect, Medtronic, Memphis) for fixation.

TECHNIQUE 43-9 *Figure 43-17*

- Expose the spine posteriorly as described in Technique 43-8.
- Adjust the angle of each rod for the most preferable alignment; tighten the internal set screws to lock the angle.

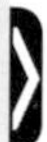

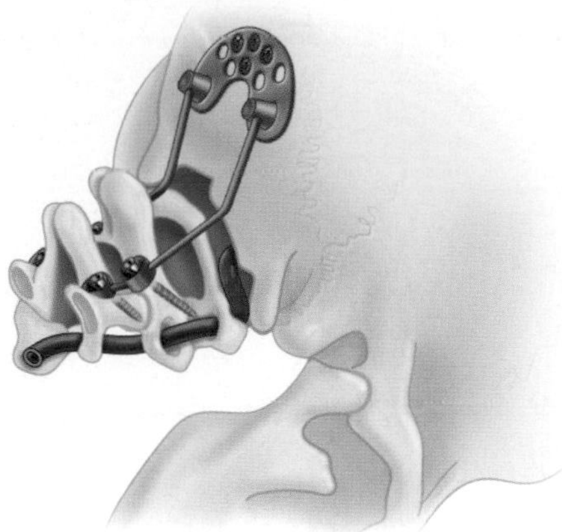

FIGURE 43-17 Occipitocervical fusion using contoured occipital plate, screw, and rod fixation (VertexSelect, Medtronic, Memphis). SEE TECHNIQUE 43-9.

Further bend the rods to best fit the patient's anatomy. Cut both ends of the rods to the required lengths.

- Position the rods in the previously placed cervical implants to determine the proper occipital plate size and make adjustments if necessary to align the rod.
- Position the occipital plate in the midline (occipital keel) between the external occipital protuberance and the posterior border of the foramen magnum. Contour the plate for an anatomic fit against the occiput. Avoid repeated bending of the plate because this may compromise its integrity. It may be necessary to contour the bone of the occiput.
- With an appropriate-size drill bit and guide that match the screw diameter, drill a hole in the occiput to the desired predetermined depth. Drilling must be done through the occipital plate to ensure proper drilling depth.
- Tap the hole, using a gauge to verify the depth. The occipital bone is very dense, and each hole should be completely tapped.
- Insert the appropriate size occipital screw and provisionally tighten it. Insert the rest of the screws as above and hand-tighten each.
- Place the rods into the implants and stabilize them by tightening the set screws. Perform final tightening of the occipital plate set screws and recheck all connections of the final construct before wound closure.

POSTOPERATIVE CARE. Immobilize the cervical spine in an orthosis for 8 to 12 weeks.

ANTERIOR CERVICAL APPROACHES

C1-2 subluxation or dislocation sometimes cannot be reduced with traction. If a patient has no neurologic deficits, a simple in situ posterior fusion can be done with little increase in risk. Posterior decompression by laminectomy has been associated with increased morbidity and mortality. Posterior decompression increases C1-2 instability unless accompanied by fusion from the occiput to C2 or C3. If posterior stabilization cannot be performed because of the clinical situation or anterior subluxation associated with cord compression is present, then an anterior approach should be considered. A subtotal maxillectomy, lateral retropharyngeal approach, or transoral approach can be used. The retropharyngeal approach usually is preferred because of the increased incidence of wound complications and infection associated with the transoral and maxillectomy approaches (Box 43-3).

BOX 43-3

Anterior Cervical Approaches

Transoral (Fang et al.)
High incidence of wound complications and infection

Transoral Mandible-Splitting and Tongue-Splitting (Hall, Denis, and Murray)
More extensive exposure of upper cervical spine

Subtotal Maxillectomy (Cocke et al.)
Extended maxillotomy and subtotal maxillectomy are used when exposure of base of skull is necessary and cannot be obtained by other approaches

Lateral Retropharyngeal (Whitesides and Kelly)
Extension of classic Henry approach to vertebral artery
Sternocleidomastoid muscle everted and retracted posteriorly
Dissection in plane posterior to carotid sheath
Potential for postoperative edema and airway obstruction

Modifications of Robinson and Southwick Approach (deAndrade and Macnab)
Anterior to sternocleidomastoid muscle
Dissection anterior to carotid sheath
Risk of injury to superior laryngeal nerve

McAfee et al.
Exposure from atlas to body of C3
No posterior dissection of carotid sheath
No entrance into oral cavity
Adequate for insertion of iliac or fibular strut grafts

TRANSORAL APPROACH

Fang and Ong achieved fusion by placing rectangular grafts into similarly shaped graft beds extending from the lateral mass of the atlas to the lateral mass and body of the axis. If only an anterior decompression is performed, it should be followed by a posterior fusion.

TECHNIQUE 43-10

(FANG AND ONG)

- Parenteral prophylactic antibiotics are given based on preoperative nasopharyngeal cultures. Endotracheal intubation is achieved using a noncollapsible tube and cuff. If extensive dissection is anticipated, a tracheostomy should be performed.

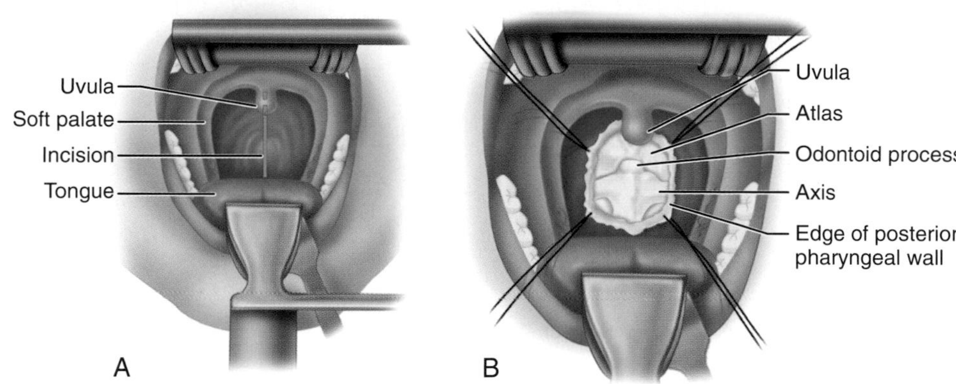

FIGURE 43-18 **A** and **B,** Transoral approach to upper cervical spine for exposure of anterior aspect of atlas and axis. **SEE TECHNIQUE 43-10.**

- Place the patient in the Trendelenburg position and insert a mouth gag to provide retraction. Identify the vertebral bodies by palpation.
- The ring of the first vertebra has a midline anterior tubercle, and the disc between the second and third vertebrae is prominent, providing another localizing landmark. Make a longitudinal incision in the midline of the posterior pharynx (Fig. 43-18A). The soft palate can be divided in the midline, making paresis after retraction less likely, or it can be folded back on itself.
- Continue the midline dissection down to bone and reflect the tissue laterally to the outer margin of the lateral masses of the axis (Fig. 43-18B). Beyond these margins are the vertebral arteries, and care should be taken not to harm them. The soft-tissue flap can be retracted using long stay sutures.
- After the procedure is complete, irrigate and close the wound loosely with interrupted absorbable sutures. Continue antibiotics for at least 3 days after surgery.

TRANSORAL MANDIBLE-SPLITTING AND TONGUE-SPLITTING APPROACH

Hall, Denis, and Murray described a mandible-splitting and tongue-splitting transoral approach to the cervical spine that gives more extensive exposure of the upper cervical spine than the approach of Fang and Ong.

TECHNIQUE 43-11

(HALL, DENIS, AND MURRAY)

- Apply a halo cast preoperatively and perform a tracheostomy through the fourth tracheal ring.
- With the patient under general anesthesia, prepare the operative field with povidone-iodine (Betadine), and drape it to exclude the halo cast and tracheostomy tube.
- Make an incision from the anterior gum margin through both surfaces of the lower lip and down over the middle of the mandible to the hyoid cartilage (Fig. 43-19A).
- Divide the tongue in the midline with electrocautery.
- Place traction sutures to allow better exposure of the midline raphe.
- Remove the lower incisor and make a step-cut with an oscillating saw in the mandible.
- Split the tongue longitudinally to the epiglottis through its central raphe (Fig. 43-19B).
- Fold the uvula on itself and suture it to the roof of the soft palate; retract the mandible and tongue down on each side to improve exposure.
- Open the mucosa over the posterior wall of the oral pharynx to expose the anterior cervical spine from the first cervical vertebra to the upper portion of the fifth cervical vertebra (Fig. 43-19C).
- Divide the anterior longitudinal ligament in the midline and reflect it laterally to allow enough exposure for removal of the anterior portion of the cervical spine and placement of bone grafts for fusion.
- Fix the posterior pharyngeal flap with 3-0 chromic suture.
- Thread a suction drain through the nose and insert it deep into the pharyngeal flap.
- Repair the tongue with 2-0 and 3-0 chromic sutures and fix the mandible with wires inserted through drill holes on each side of the osteotomy.
- Close the infralingual mucosa with 3-0 chromic sutures and close the subcutaneous tissue and skin.
- Preoperative and postoperative antibiotics are recommended.

POSTOPERATIVE CARE. A halo cast is worn until fusion is evident on radiographs. The halo cast is removed, and a soft collar is worn for 1 month.

SUBTOTAL MAXILLECTOMY

Cocke et al. described an extended maxillotomy with subtotal maxillectomy to be used when exposure of the base of the skull is needed and cannot be obtained by other approaches. This approach is technically demanding and requires a thorough knowledge of head and neck anatomy. A team of surgeons, including an otolaryngologist, a neurosurgeon, and an

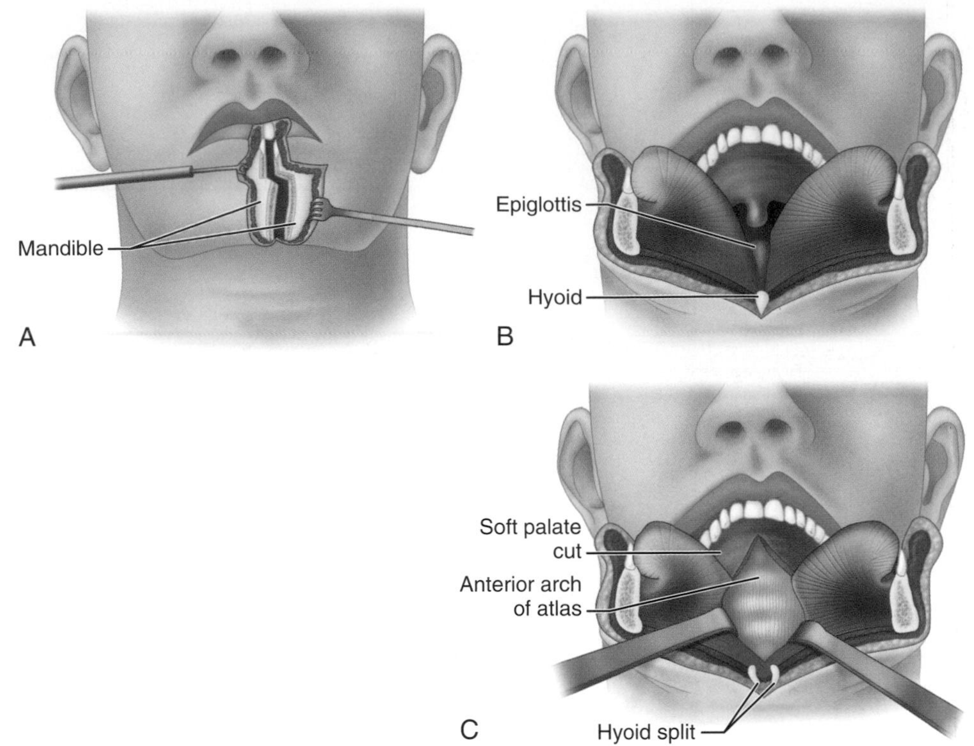

FIGURE 43-19 **A-C,** Mandible-splitting and tongue-splitting transoral approach. **SEE TECHNIQUE 43-11.**

orthopaedist, should perform this surgery. Please refer to older editions of *Campbell's Operative Orthopaedics* for the complete description.

Endoscopic approaches have also been described for anterior resection of the odontoid. The endoscopic approaches to the odontoid and anterior ring of C1 may be sublabial, transoral, or transcervical (Fig. 43-20).

LATERAL RETROPHARYNGEAL APPROACH

The lateral retropharyngeal approach described by Whitesides and Kelly is an extension of the classic approach of Henry to the vertebral artery. In this approach, the sternocleidomastoid muscle is everted and retracted posteriorly. The remainder of the dissection follows a plane posterior to the carotid sheath.

TECHNIQUE 43-12

(WHITESIDES AND KELLY)

- Make a longitudinal incision along the anterior margin of the sternocleidomastoid muscle. At the superior end of the muscle, carry the incision posteriorly across the base of the temporal bone.
- Divide the muscle at its mastoid origin.
- Partially divide the splenius capitis muscle at its insertion in the same area.
- At the superior pole of the incision is the external jugular vein, which crosses the anterior margin of the sternocleidomastoid; ligate and divide this vein. Branches of the auricular nerve also may be encountered and may require division.
- Evert the sternocleidomastoid muscle and identify the spinal accessory nerve as it approaches and passes into the muscle.
- Divide and ligate the vascular structures that accompany the nerve.
- Develop the approach posterior to the carotid sheath and anterior to the sternocleidomastoid muscle (Fig. 43-21A). The transverse processes of all the exposed cervical vertebrae are palpable in this interval.
- Using sharp and blunt dissection, develop the plane between the alar and prevertebral fascia along the anterior aspect of the transverse processes of the vertebral bodies. The dissection plane is anterior to the longus colli and capitis muscles and the overlying sympathetic trunk and superior cervical ganglion. (An alternative approach is to elevate the longus colli and capitis muscles from their bony insertion on the transverse processes and retract the muscles anteriorly, but this approach can disrupt the sympathetic rami communicantes and cause Horner syndrome.)
- When the vertebral level is identified, make a longitudinal incision to bone through the anterior longitudinal ligament.
- Dissect the ligament and soft tissues subperiosteally to expose the vertebral bodies.

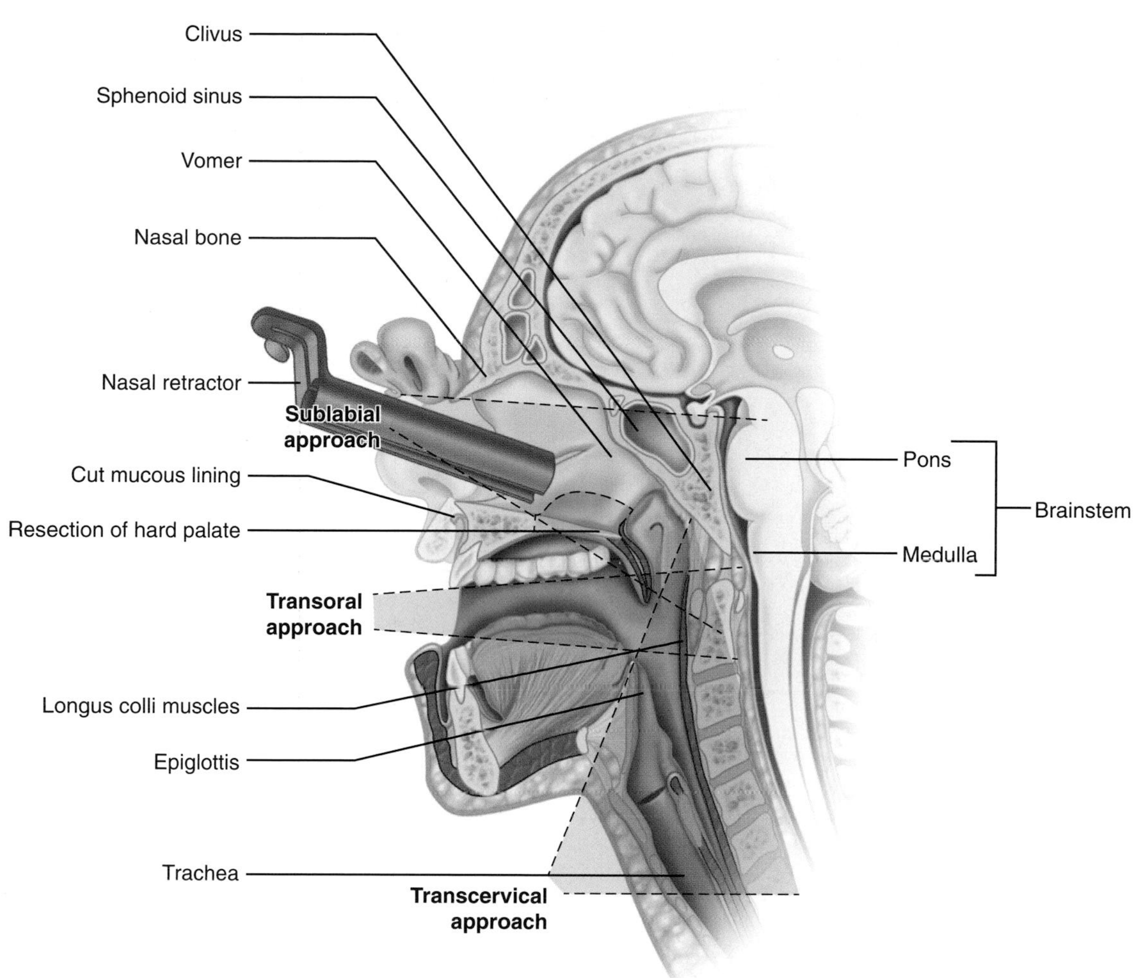

FIGURE 43-20 Endoscopic approaches to the cervical spine: relevant anatomy and operative angles for sublabial, transoral, and transcervical approaches to the cervical spine. (From Bettegowda C, Shajari M, Suk I, et al: Sublabial approach for the treatment of symptomatic basilar impression in a patient with Klippel-Feil syndrome, Neurosurgery 69[ONS Suppl 1]:ons77, 2011.)

- For fusion, place corticocancellous strips in a longitudinal trough made in the vertebral bodies.
- Irrigate and close the wound in layers over a suction drain in the retropharyngeal space.

POSTOPERATIVE CARE. Because of the potential for postoperative edema and airway obstruction, the patient should be monitored closely. Traction may be required for 1 to 2 days after surgery. When the traction is removed, the patient is immobilized in a cervicothoracic brace or halo vest or halo cast.

deAndrade and Macnab described an approach to the upper cervical spine that is an extension of the approach described by Robinson and Southwick and Bailey and Badgley. This approach is anterior to the sternocleidomastoid muscle (Fig. 43-21B), but the dissection is anterior to the carotid sheath rather than posterior. This approach carries an increased risk of injury to the superior laryngeal nerve.

ANTERIOR RETROPHARYNGEAL APPROACH

McAfee et al. used a superior extension of the anterior approach of Robinson and Smith to the cervical spine. This approach provides exposure from the atlas to the body of the third cervical vertebra without the need for posterior dissection of the carotid sheath or entrance into the oral cavity and gives adequate exposure for insertion of iliac or fibular strut grafts.

TECHNIQUE 43-13

(MCAFEE ET AL.)

- Place the patient supine on an operative wedge turning frame and perform a neurologic examination. Monitor the spinal cord during the operation using cortically recorded somatosensory-evoked potentials.

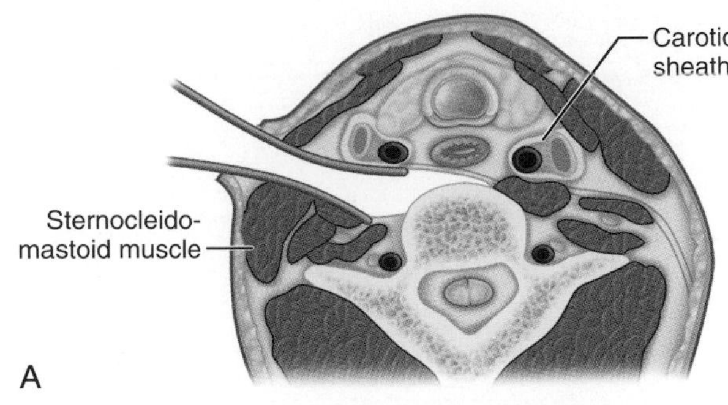

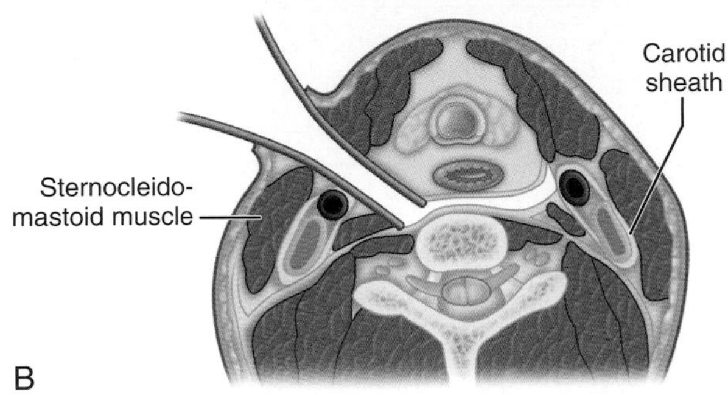

FIGURE 43-21 Lateral retropharyngeal approach to cervical spine. **A,** Whitesides and Kelly approach anterior to sternocleidomastoid muscle and posterior to carotid sheath. **B,** DeAndrade and Macnab approach anterior to sternocleidomastoid muscle and anteromedial to carotid sheath. **SEE TECHNIQUE 43-12.**

- Apply Gardner-Wells tongs with 4.5 kg of traction, if not already in place. Carefully extend the neck with the patient awake. Mark the maximal point of safe extension and do not exceed this at any time during the operative procedure.
- Perform fiberoptic nasotracheal intubation with the patient under local anesthesia. When the airway has been secured, place the patient under general anesthesia. Keep the patient's mouth free of all tubes to prevent any depression of the mandible inferiorly that may compromise the operative exposure.
- Make a modified transverse submandibular incision (the incision can be made on the right or left side depending on the surgeon's preference) (Fig. 43-22A). As long as the dissection does not extend caudad to the fifth cervical vertebra, this exposure is sufficiently superior to the right recurrent laryngeal nerve to prevent damage to this structure.
- Carry the incision through the platysma muscle and mobilize the skin and superficial fascia in the subplatysmal plane of the superficial fascia.
- Locate the marginal mandibular branch of the facial nerve with the aid of a nerve stimulator and by ligating and dissecting the retromandibular veins superiorly. Branches of the mandibular nerves usually cross the retromandibular vein superficially and superiorly. By ligating this vein as it joins the internal jugular vein and by keeping the dissection deep and inferior to the vein as the exposure is extended superiorly, the superficial branches of the facial nerve are protected.
- Free the anterior border of the sternocleidomastoid muscle by longitudinally transecting the superficial layer of deep cervical fascia.
- Locate the carotid sheath by palpation.
- Resect the submandibular salivary gland and suture its duct to prevent a salivary fistula. Identify the posterior belly of the digastric muscle and the stylohyoid muscle.
- Divide and tag the digastric tendon for later repair. Division of the digastric and stylohyoid muscles allows mobilization of the hyoid bone and the hypopharynx medially (Fig. 43-22B).
- Free the hypoglossal nerve from the base of the skull to the anterior border of the hypoglossal muscle and retract it superiorly throughout the remainder of the procedure (Fig. 43-22C).
- Continue the dissection between the carotid sheath laterally and the larynx and pharynx anteromedially.
- Beginning inferiorly and progressing superiorly, the following arteries and veins may need to be ligated for exposure: the superior thyroid artery and vein, the lingual artery and vein, and the facial artery and vein (Fig. 43-22C).
- Free the superior laryngeal nerve from its origin near the nodose ganglion to its entrance into the larynx (Fig. 43-22D).
- Transect the alar and prevertebral fascia longitudinally to expose the longus colli muscles (Fig. 43-22E).
- Ensure orientation to the midline by noting the attachment of the right and left longus colli muscles as they converge toward the anterior tubercle of the atlas. Detach the longus colli muscles from the anterior surface of the atlas and axis.
- Divide the anterior longitudinal ligament and expose the anterior surface of the atlas and axis. Do not carry the dissection too far laterally and damage the vertebral artery.
- McAfee et al. used a fibular or bicortical iliac strut graft contoured into the shape of a clothespin. The anterior body of C2 and the discs of C2 and C3 can be removed. Place the two prongs of the clothespin superiorly to straddle the anterior arch of the atlas. Tamp the inferior edge of the graft into the superior aspect of the body of C3, which is undercut to receive the graft. If the anterior aspect of the atlas must be removed, the superior aspect of the graft can be secured to the clivus.
- Begin closure by approximation of the digastric tendon.
- Place suction drains in the retropharyngeal space and the subcutaneous space.
- Suture the platysma and skin in the standard fashion.
- If the spine has been made unstable by the anterior decompression, perform a posterior cervical or occipitocervical fusion.
- If the hypopharynx has been inadvertently entered, have the anesthesiologist insert a nasogastric tube intraoperatively.
- Close the hole in two layers with absorbable sutures.

POSTOPERATIVE CARE. Parenteral antibiotics effective against anaerobic organisms should be added to the

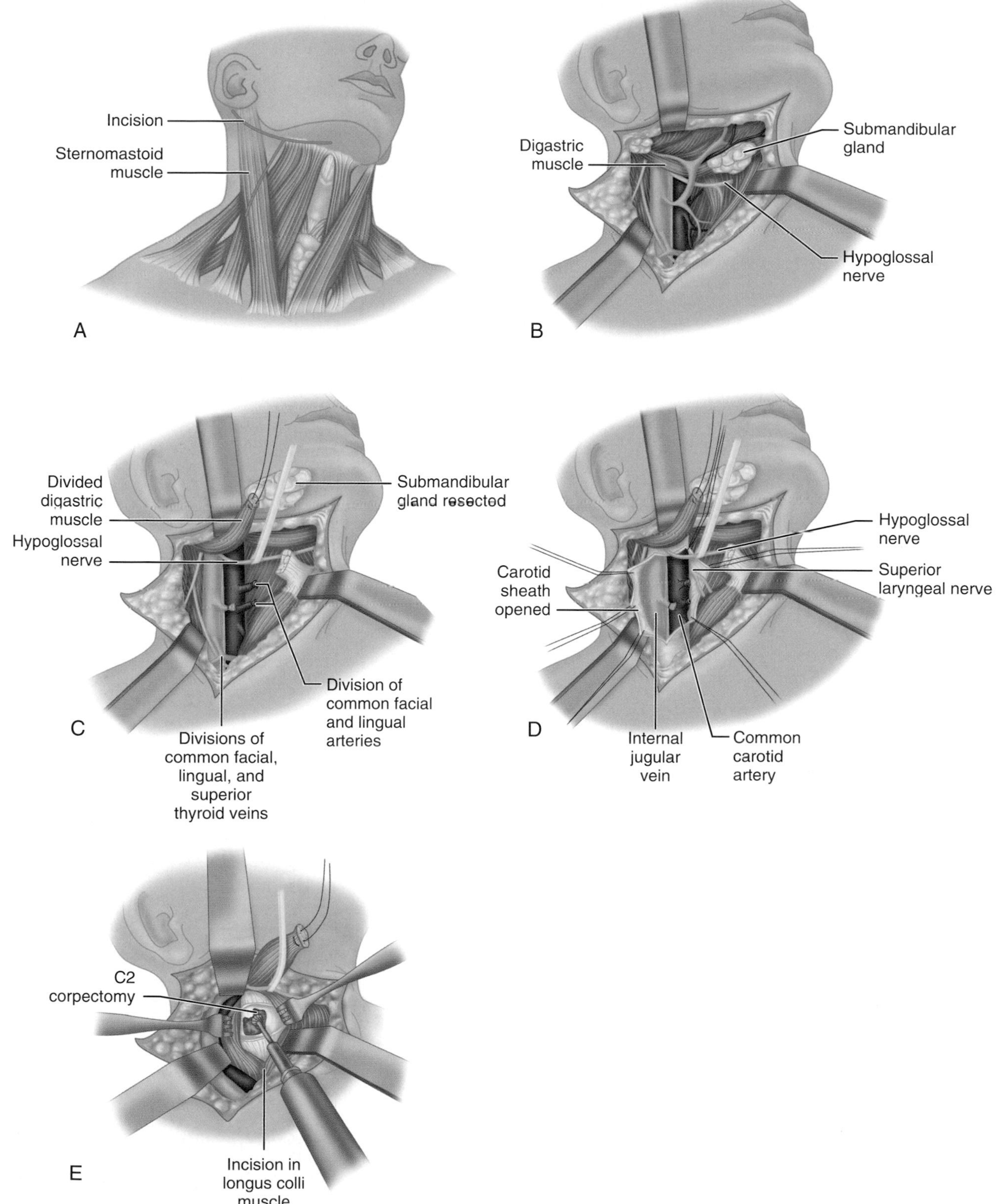

FIGURE 43-22 Anterior retropharyngeal approach to upper cervical spine described by McAfee et al. **A,** Submandibular incision. Lower limb of incision is used only if midcervical vertebrae must be exposed. **B** and **C,** Submandibular gland is resected, and digastric tendon is divided. Superior thyroid artery and vein also are divided. **D,** Hypoglossal nerve and superior laryngeal nerve are mobilized. Contents of carotid sheath are mobilized laterally, and hypopharynx is mobilized medially. **E,** Longus colli muscle is dissected laterally to expose anterior aspect of atlas and axis. **SEE TECHNIQUE 43-13.**

routine postoperative prophylactic antibiotics. The nasogastric tube is left in place for 7 to 10 days. Skull traction is maintained with the head elevated 30 degrees to reduce hypopharyngeal edema. Nasal intubation is maintained for 48 hours. If extubation is not possible in 48 to 72 hours, a tracheostomy can be performed. The Gardner-Wells tongs are removed 2 to 4 days after surgery, and a halo vest is applied and is worn for about 3 months. When the halo vest is removed, a cervical collar is worn for an additional month.

STERNAL-SPLITTING APPROACH

Mulpuri et al. described a sternal splitting approach to the cervicothoracic junction in children that is useful for complex spinal deformities around the cervicothoracic junction. The approach requires the assistance of a cardiothoracic surgeon.

TECHNIQUE 43-14

(MULPURI ET AL.)

- Make a standard extensile anterior cervical spine approach, incorporating an anterior sternal extension (Fig. 43-23A).
- Complete the neck dissection in a standard fashion.
- Make an incision along the medial border of the sternomastoid muscle, extending down to the sternal notch.
- Retract the sternomastoid muscle laterally with the neurovascular sheath, including the carotid artery, the jugular vein, and the vagus nerve. Division of the omohyoid, sternohyoid, and sternothyroid muscles facilitates extensile exposure.
- Extend the incision as a midline sternotomy approach.
- Use blunt digital dissection to mobilize the retrosternal soft tissues.
- Split the sternum using a sternal saw in a standard fashion.
- After opening the sternum, resect the thymus gland to provide exposure and mobilize and control the brachiocephalic trunk with a vessel loop.
- At this point, the anterior cervical spine and upper thoracic spine can be accessed contiguously (Fig. 43-23B).
- If necessary, the pericardium can be opened to increase mobility of the brachiocephalic trunk; however, the dissection of the brachiocephalic trunk can be done down to the pericardial reflection without opening the pericardium.
- Retract the trachea and esophagus slightly away from the midline with a right-angle retractor.
- Place a deep right-angle retractor under the innominate artery and pull it forward and downward as necessary to provide access to the lower cervical and upper thoracic spine (Fig. 43-23C).
- The distal extent of the exposure at this point depends on the patient's anatomy and deformity; in most patients, T4 can now be accessed and disc removal and instrumentation can be done safely. Aggressive distal exposure places the recurrent laryngeal nerve under traction and must be done carefully. Although left-sided anterior cervical approaches typically are preferred because of the distal course of the recurrent laryngeal nerve on that side, Mulpuri et al. used a right-sided approach with mobilization of the brachiocephalic trunk because medial displacement of the trunk exposes more segments of the thoracic spine on the right side (Fig. 43-23D).
- After completion of the orthopaedic procedure, obtain hemostasis and approximate the sternum with wires or sutures depending on the age of the child.
- Reattach the sternothyroid and omohyoid muscles.
- Close the neck incision in usual fashion. A small Silastic drain may be required under the sternothyroid muscle if hemostasis is a problem in the cervical portion of the approach.
- Place a mediastinal tube as in cardiac surgical procedures.

HALO VEST IMMOBILIZATION

The halo device, introduced by Perry and Nickel in 1959, provides immobilization for an unstable cervical spine and can be used for preoperative traction in certain situations. Successful use of the halo has been shown in infants and children with instabilities caused by injuries or by cervical malformations, although complications are more frequent in children than adults.

Most authors agree that the halo device provides the best immobilization of the cervical spine of all external immobilization methods, but reports have shown increased spinal motion (up to 70% of normal) and loss of reduction while in the halo. The halo vest has been well accepted by adult patients, and the vest can usually be easily fitted; in children, however, proper fit is rarely achieved with a prefabricated halo vest, and the use of a halo cast or custom-molded halo vest is a better choice.

Mubarak et al. recommended the following steps in the fabrication of a custom halo for a child: (1) the size and configuration of the head are obtained with the use of a flexible lead wire placed around the head; (2) the halo ring is fabricated by constructing a ring 2 cm larger in diameter than the wire model; (3) a plaster mold of the trunk is obtained for the manufacture of a custom bivalved polypropylene vest; and (4) linear measurements are made to ensure appropriate length of the superstructure. CT helps determine bone structure to plan pin sites to avoid suture lines or congenital malformations.

Skull thickness in children varies greatly up to age 6 years; it increases between ages 10 and 16 years, after which it is similar to that in adults. One study found that a 2-mm skull could be completely penetrated with a 160-lb load, which is below the recommended torque pressure for adult skulls.

Mubarak et al. described a technique for the application of a halo device in children younger than 2 years old. This multiple-pin technique differs from previously accepted recommendations in older children regarding pin number, pin placement, and torque. With multiple pins, significantly less torque can be used, allowing a greater range of pin placement sites in areas where the skull might otherwise be considered too thin. Perpendicular halo pin insertion has been recommended in an immature skull because this configuration results in increased load at the pin-bone interface and increases stability. Skull development is important to consider in halo device application in patients younger than 2 years old. Cranial suture interdigitation may be incomplete, and

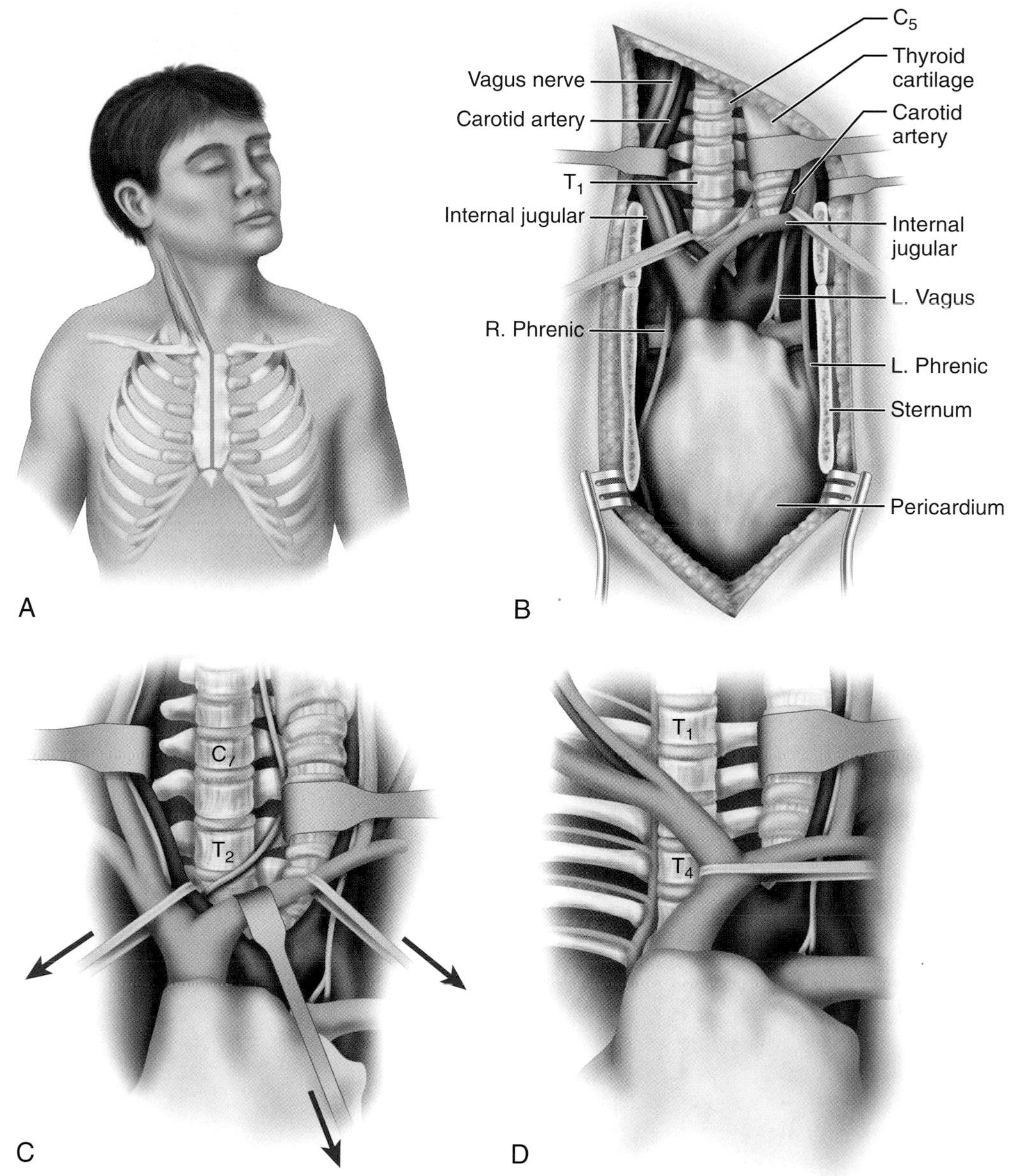

FIGURE 43-23 Mulpuri et al. sternal-split approach to cervicothoracic junction. **A,** Incision for right-sided approach. **B,** Sternum is opened, thymus gland is resected, and brachiocephalic trunk is mobilized to allow contiguous access to anterior cervical spine and upper thoracic spine. **C,** Retraction of trachea, esophagus, and innominate artery provides access to lower cervical spine and upper thoracic spine. **D,** Medial displacement of brachiocephalic trunk allows more distal access to thoracic spine. **SEE TECHNIQUE 43-14.**

fontanels may be open anteriorly in patients younger than 18 months old and posteriorly in patients younger than 6 months. Because of this, the halo device probably should not be used in children younger than 18 months old.

APPLICATION OF HALO DEVICE

Halo device applications for children in this age group require a custom-made halo ring and plastic jacket. Ten to 12 standard halo skull pins can be used. When constructed, the halo ring is applied with the patient under general anesthesia. In older children and adolescents, local anesthesia can be used.

TECHNIQUE 43-15

(MUBARAK ET AL.)

- Place the patient supine, with the head supported by an assistant or a cupped metal extension that cradles the head. If a metal extension is used, do not place the neck in flexion; a child's head is relatively large in proportion to the body.

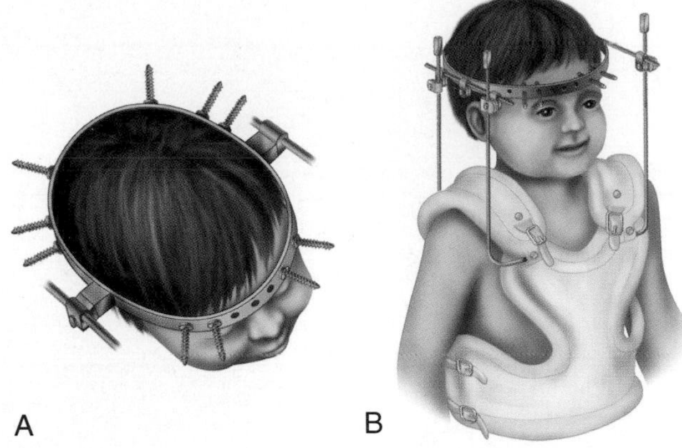

FIGURE 43-24 **A,** Ten pin placement sites for infant halo ring attachment using multiple-pin, low-torque technique. Usually, four pins are placed anteriorly, avoiding temporal area, and remaining six pins are placed in occipital area. **B,** Custom halo vest and light superstructure. **SEE TECHNIQUE 43-14.**

- Shave the immediate areas of pin insertion and prepare the skin with antiseptic solution.
- Infiltrate the skin and the periosteum in the selected areas with local anesthetic.
- Support the halo ring around the patient's head with the application device or the help of an assistant. Hold it below the area of greatest diameter of the skull, just above the eyebrows, and about 1 cm above the tips of the ears.
- Select the pin sites carefully so that the pins enter the skull as nearly perpendicular as possible. The best position for the anterior pins is in the anterolateral aspect of the skull, above the lateral two thirds of the orbit, and below the greatest circumference of the skull; this area is a relatively safe zone. Avoid the temporalis muscle because penetration of this muscle by the halo pin can be painful and may impede mandibular motion during mastication or talking; the bone in this area also is very thin, and pin loosening is likely.
- Place the posterior pins directly diagonal from the anterior pins, if possible, and inferior to the equator of the skull. Introduce the pins through the halo frame and tighten two diagonally opposed pins simultaneously.
- Ensure that the patient's eyes are closed while the pins are tightened to ensure that the forehead skin is not anchored in such a way as to prevent the eyelids from closing after application of the halo ring.
- In an infant or young child, insert 10 pins to finger tightness or 2 in-lb anterolaterally and posteriorly (Fig. 43-24A). If the skull thickness is of great concern, use finger tightness only to prevent penetrating the skull.
- In slightly older children, use 2 in-lb of torque (for halo device application in adults, see Chapter 41).
- In adolescents near skeletal maturity whose skull thickness is nearly that of an adult (as determined by CT), torque pressure can be increased to 6 to 8 in-lb.
- Secure the pins to the halo device with the appropriate lock nuts or set screws.
- Apply the polypropylene vest and superstructure after the halo ring and pins are in place (Fig. 43-24B).

POSTOPERATIVE CARE. The pins are cleansed daily at the skin interface with hydrogen peroxide or a small amount of povidone-iodine solution. The pins are retightened once at 48 hours after application.

COMPLICATIONS

Complications include pin loosening, infection, pin site bleeding, and dural puncture. If a pin becomes loose, it can be retightened as long as resistance is met. If no resistance is met, the pin should be removed and another pin inserted in an alternative site. If drainage develops around a pin, oral antibiotics and local skin care are begun. If the drainage does not respond to these measures or if cellulitis or an abscess develops, the pin should be removed and another pin should be inserted at an alternative site. If dural puncture occurs, the pin should be removed and another pin inserted at an alternative site; the patient should receive prophylactic antibiotic therapy. The dural tear usually heals in 4 or 5 days, at which time antibiotics can be discontinued.

BASILAR IMPRESSION

Basilar impression (basilar invagination) is a rare deformity in which there is an indention of the skull floor by the upper cervical spine. The tip of the odontoid is more cephalad than normal. The odontoid may protrude into the foramen magnum and encroach on the brainstem, causing neurologic symptoms because of the limited space available for the brainstem and spinal cord. Neurologic damage can be caused by direct pressure from the odontoid or from other constricting structures around the foramen magnum, circulatory compromise of the vertebral arteries, or impairment of cerebrospinal fluid flow. It is important that the orthopaedist be familiar with basilar impression and its presentation because this spinal deformity often goes unrecognized or is misdiagnosed as a posterior fossa tumor, bulbar palsy of polio, syringomyelia, amyotrophic lateral sclerosis, spinal cord tumor, or multiple sclerosis.

Basilar impression can be primary (congenital) or secondary (acquired). Primary basilar impression is a congenital structural abnormality of the craniocervical junction that often is associated with other vertebral defects (atlantooccipital fusion, Klippel-Feil syndrome, Arnold-Chiari malformation, syringomyelia, odontoid anomalies, hypoplasia of the atlas, and bifid posterior arch of the atlas); these associated conditions can cause the predominant symptoms. The incidence of primary basilar impression in the general population is 1%. Secondary basilar impression is an acquired deformity of the skull resulting from systemic disease that causes softening of the osseous structures at the base of the skull, such as Paget disease, osteomalacia, rickets, osteogenesis imperfecta, rheumatoid arthritis, neurofibromatosis, and ankylosing spondylitis. Secondary basilar impression occurs more commonly in types III and IV than in type I osteogenesis imperfecta.

Basilar impression causes neurologic symptoms because of crowding of the neural structures as they pass through the

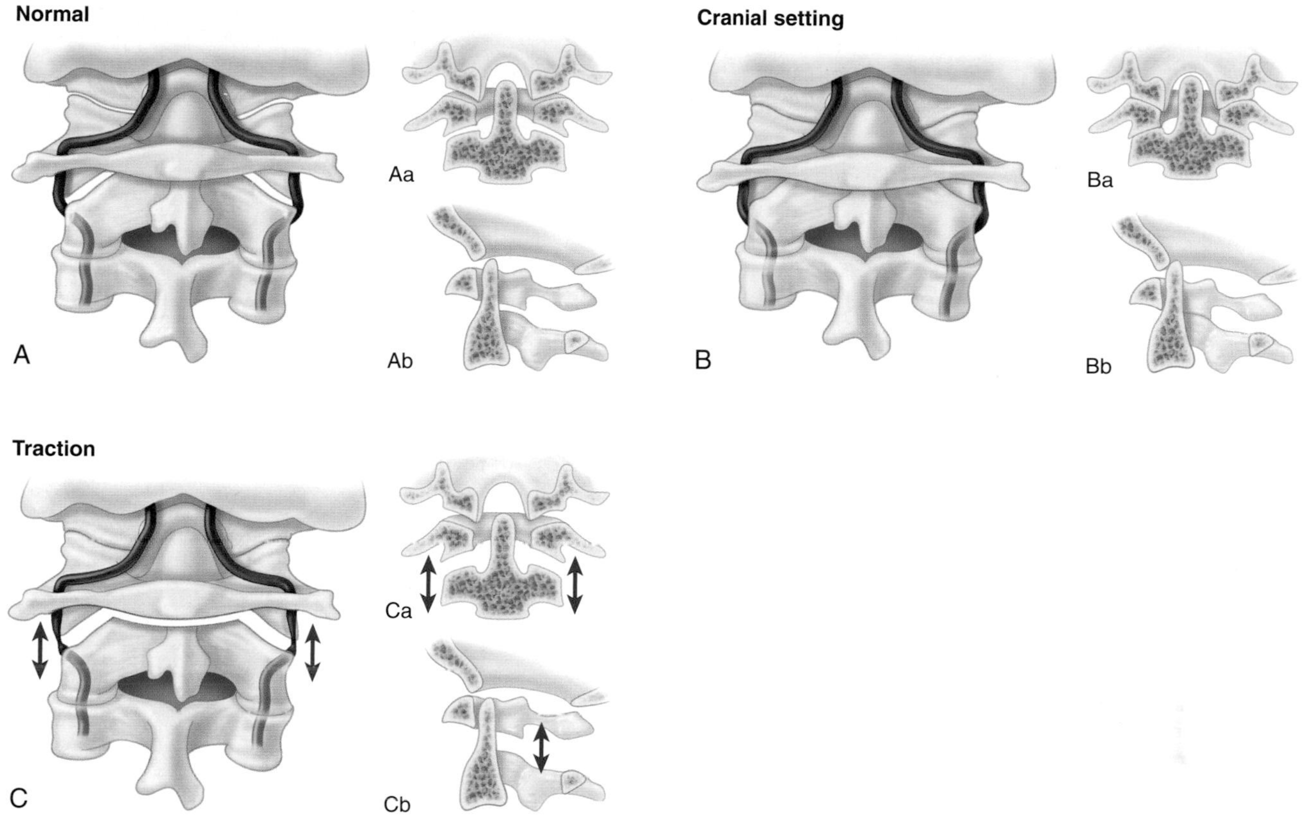

FIGURE 43-25 Schematic diagram showing cranial settling and possible vertebral artery injuries resulting from traction. **A,** Normal position of vertebral artery. *Aa* and *Ab,* Normal vertebral alignment. **B,** Position of vertebral artery after cranial settling. *Ba* and *Bb,* Vertebral alignment in cranial settling. **C,** Effect of traction on vertebral arteries. *Ca* and *Cb,* Effect of vertebral alignment.

foramen magnum. Clinical presentation varies, and patients with severe basilar impression may be totally asymptomatic. Symptoms usually appear during the second and third decades of life, probably because of increased ligamentous laxity and instability with age and decreased tolerance to compression of the spinal cord and vertebral arteries.

Most patients with basilar impression have short necks, asymmetry of the face or skull, and torticollis, but these findings are not specific for basilar impression and can be seen in patients with other congenital vertebral anomalies. Headache in the distribution of the greater occipital nerve is a frequent complaint. DeBarros et al. divided the signs and symptoms into two categories: those caused by pure basilar impression and those caused by the Arnold-Chiari malformation. They found that symptoms caused by pure basilar impression were primarily motor and sensory disturbances, such as weakness and paresthesia in the limbs, whereas patients with Arnold-Chiari malformation had symptoms of cerebellar and vestibular disturbances, such as ataxia, dizziness, and nystagmus. Involvement of the lower cranial nerves also occurs in basilar impression. The trigeminal, vagus, glossopharyngeal, and hypoglossal nerves may be compressed as they emerge from the medulla oblongata. DeBarros et al. also noted sexual disturbances, such as impotence and reduced libido in 27% of their patients.

Compression of the vertebral arteries as they pass through the foramen magnum is another source of symptoms. Bernini et al. found a significantly higher incidence of vertebral artery anomalies in patients with basilar impression and atlantooccipital fusion. Symptoms caused by vertebral artery insufficiency, such as dizziness, seizures, mental deterioration, and syncope, can occur alone or in combination with other symptoms of basilar impression. Children with occipitocervical anomalies may be more susceptible to vertebral artery injury and brainstem ischemia if skull traction is applied (Fig. 43-25).

RADIOGRAPHIC FINDINGS

Numerous measurements have been suggested for diagnosing basilar impression (Box 43-4), reflecting the difficulty of evaluating this area of the spine radiographically, and several methods of evaluation (plain radiography, CT, and MRI) may be needed to confirm the diagnosis. The most commonly used measurements are the lines of Chamberlain, McGregor, McRae, and Fischgold and Metzger. The Chamberlain, McGregor, and McRae lines are made on lateral radiographs of the skull (Fig. 43-26); the Fischgold and Metzger lines are made on an anteroposterior view (Fig. 43-27).

The Chamberlain line is drawn from the posterior edge of the hard palate to the posterior border of the foramen magnum. Symptomatic basilar impression can occur when the odontoid tip extends above this line. There are two disadvantages to the Chamberlain line: the posterior tip of the foramen magnum is difficult to define on the standard lateral

BOX 43-4

Measurements for Diagnosing Basilar Impression: Lateral Radiograph

Chamberlain Line

Extends from posterior edge of hard palate to posterior border of foramen magnum

Symptomatic basilar impression may occur if tip of odontoid is above this line

McGregor Line

Extends from upper surface of posterior edge of hard palate to most caudal point of occipital curve

Easier to identify on standard lateral view

Odontoid tip greater than 4.5 mm above this line considered an abnormal finding

Routine screening test; landmarks easily identified

McRae Line

Anteroposterior dimension of foramen magnum; line extends from anterior tip of foramen magnum to posterior tip

Patient usually asymptomatic if tip of odontoid is below this line

Helpful to determine clinical significance

Fischgold and Metzger (Digastric) Line

Extends between two digastric grooves (junction of medial aspect of mastoid process at base of skull)

Line normally passes 10.7 mm above odontoid tip and 11.6 mm above atlantooccipital joint

Confirms diagnosis

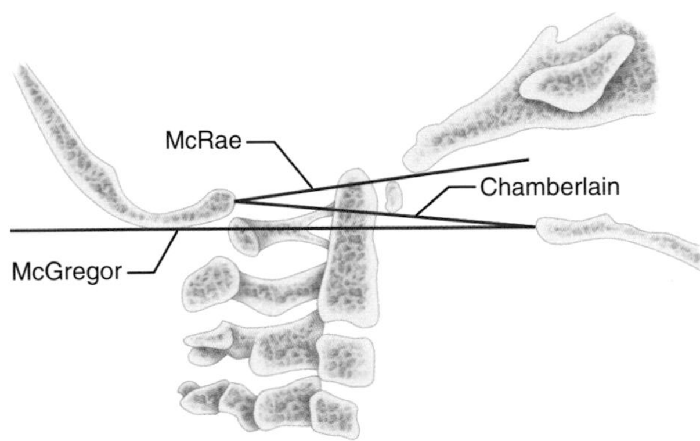

FIGURE 43-26 Base of skull and upper cervical spine showing location of McRae, McGregor, and Chamberlain lines.

view, and the posterior tip of the foramen magnum is often invaginated. McGregor modified the Chamberlain line by drawing a line from the upper surface of the posterior edge of the hard palate to the most caudal point of the occipital curve, which is much easier to identify on a standard lateral radiograph. The position of the tip of the odontoid is measured in relation to the McGregor line, and a distance of 4.5 mm above this line is considered the upper limit of normal. The McRae line determines the anteroposterior dimension of the foramen magnum and is formed by

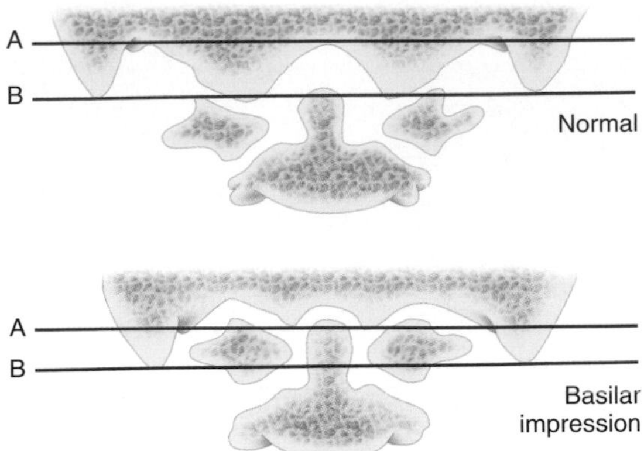

FIGURE 43-27 Fischgold and Metzger lines. Line was originally drawn from lower pole of mastoid process *B,* but because of variability in size of mastoid processes these researchers recommended drawing the line between digastric grooves *A.*

drawing a line from the anterior tip of the foramen magnum to the posterior tip. McRae observed that if the tip of the odontoid is below this line, then the patient usually is asymptomatic.

The lateral lines of McGregor and Chamberlain have been criticized because the anterior reference point (the hard palate) is not part of the skull, and measurements can be distorted by an abnormal facial configuration or a high-arched palate. To resolve these problems, Fischgold and Metzger described a method of assessing basilar impression that uses an anteroposterior tomogram or CT with anteroposterior reconstruction views (see Fig. 43-26). This assessment is based on a line drawn between the two digastric grooves (the junction of the medial aspect of the mastoid process at the base of the skull). Normally, the digastric line passes above the odontoid tip (10.7 mm) and the atlantooccipital joint (11.6 mm).

The Clark station, Redlund-Johnell criterion, and Ranawat criterion have been found useful to measure basilar impression in adults with rheumatoid arthritis. The Clark station is determined by dividing the odontoid process into three equal parts in the sagittal plane (Fig. 43-28). If the anterior ring of the atlas is level with the middle third (station II) or the caudal third (station III) of the odontoid process, basilar invagination is present. The Redlund-Johnell criterion is the distance between the McGregor line and the midpoint of the caudal margin of the second cervical vertebral body. Basilar invagination is present if the measurement is less than 34 mm in men and less than 29 mm in women. The Ranawat criterion is the distance between the center of the second cervical pedicle and the transverse axis of the atlas. Basilar invagination is present if this distance is less than 15 mm in men and less than 13 mm in women. The Redlund-Johnell and Ranawat criteria may not be applicable in small children.

The McGregor line is used as a routine screening test because the landmarks for this line can be defined easily on a standard lateral radiograph. If more information is needed, an MRI of the craniovertebral junction is used to confirm the

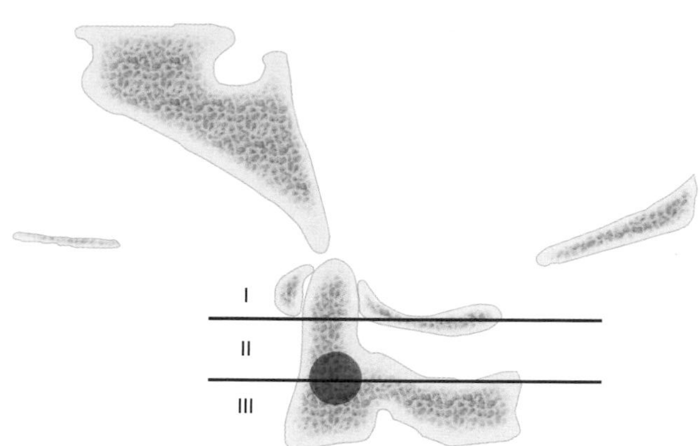

FIGURE 43-28 Clark stations of first cervical vertebra are determined by dividing odontoid process into three equal parts in sagittal plane. If anterior ring of atlas is level with middle third (station *II*) or caudal third (station *III*) of odontoid process, basilar impression is present.

diagnosis of basilar impression. CT and MRI are recommended; CT provides better osseous detail and MRI provides superior soft-tissue resolution. "Functional" MRI obtained with the cervical spine in flexion and then extension shows the dynamics of spinal cord compression caused by vertebral instability or anomaly.

TREATMENT

Conservative treatment of symptomatic patients with a collar or cervical orthosis has not been successful. Many patients with basilar impression have no neurologic symptoms, and some have minimal symptoms with no sign of progressive neurologic damage. These patients *can* be observed and examined periodically; surgery is indicated if the clinical picture becomes worse. The indications for surgery are based on the clinical symptoms and not on the degree of basilar impression. When a patient becomes symptomatic, progression of the disease and symptoms is likely.

If symptoms are caused by anterior impingement from the odontoid, stabilization in extension by an occipital C1-2 fusion is indicated. If symptoms and impingement persist, anterior excision of the odontoid can be done after posterior stabilization. Posterior impingement requires suboccipital craniectomy and laminectomy of C1 and possibly C2 to decompress the brainstem and spinal cord. The dura may need to be opened during this procedure to check for a tight posterior dural band that may be causing the symptoms instead of the bony abnormalities. Posterior fusion is recommended in addition to decompression if stability is in question.

ATLANTOOCCIPITAL FUSION

Atlantooccipital fusion (occipitalization) is a partial or complete congenital fusion between the atlas and the base of the occiput ranging from a complete bony fusion to a bony bridge or even a fibrous band uniting one small area of the atlas and occiput. Occipitalization is a failure of segmentation between the fourth occipital sclerotome and the first spinal sclerotome. This condition can lead to chronic atlantoaxial instability or basilar invagination and can produce a wide range of symptoms because of spinal cord impingement and vascular compromise of the vertebral arteries. The incidence of atlantooccipital fusion has been reported to be 1.4 to 2.5 per 1000 children, affecting males and females equally. Symptoms usually appear in the third and fourth decades of life. Atlantooccipital fusion frequently is associated with congenital fusion between C2 and C3 (reportedly in 70% of patients). Approximately half of patients with atlantooccipital fusion develop atlantoaxial instability. Kyphosis and scoliosis are also frequently associated with this deformity. Other associated congenital anomalies, such as anomalies of the jaw, incomplete cleft of the nasal cartilage, cleft palate, external ear deformities, cervical ribs, and urinary tract anomalies, occur in 20% of patients with atlantooccipital fusion.

Patients with atlantooccipital fusion commonly have low hairlines, torticollis, short necks, and restricted neck movement. Many patients complain of a dull, aching pain in the posterior occiput and the neck, with episodic neck stiffness, but symptoms vary depending on the area of spinal cord impingement. If the impingement is anterior, pyramidal tract signs and symptoms predominate; if the impingement is posterior, posterior column signs and symptoms predominate.

The shape and position of the odontoid are the keys to neurologic symptoms. When the odontoid lies above the foramen magnum, a relative or actual basilar impression is present. If the odontoid lies below the foramen magnum, the patient usually is asymptomatic. In this condition, the odontoid may be excessively long and angulated posteriorly, decreasing the anteroposterior diameter of the spinal canal. Autopsy findings have shown the brainstem indented by the abnormal odontoid. Anterior spinal cord compression with pyramidal tract irritation causes muscle weakness and wasting, ataxia, spasticity, pathologic reflexes (Babinski and Hoffman), and hyperreflexia. Posterior compression causes loss of deep pain, light touch, proprioception, and vibratory sensation. Nystagmus is a common finding. Cranial nerve involvement can cause diplopia, dysphagia, and auditory disturbances. Disturbances of the vertebral artery result in syncope, seizures, vertigo, and an unsteady gait.

Neurologic symptoms generally begin in the third and fourth decades of life, possibly because the older patient's spinal cord and vertebral arteries become less resistant to compression. Symptoms may be initiated by trauma or infection in the pharynx or nasopharynx.

RADIOGRAPHIC FINDINGS

Because this anomaly ranges from complete incorporation of the atlas into the occiput to a small fibrous band connecting part of the atlas to the occiput, routine radiographs usually are difficult to interpret, and CT or MRI may be needed to show the occipitocervical fusion (Fig. 43-29). Most commonly, the anterior arch of the atlas is assimilated into the occiput and displaced posteriorly relative to the occiput. About half of patients have a relative basilar impression caused by loss of height of the atlas. Posterior fusion usually is a small bony fringe or a fibrous band that frequently is not evident on a radiograph. This fringe is directed downward and into the spinal canal and can cause neurologic symptoms.

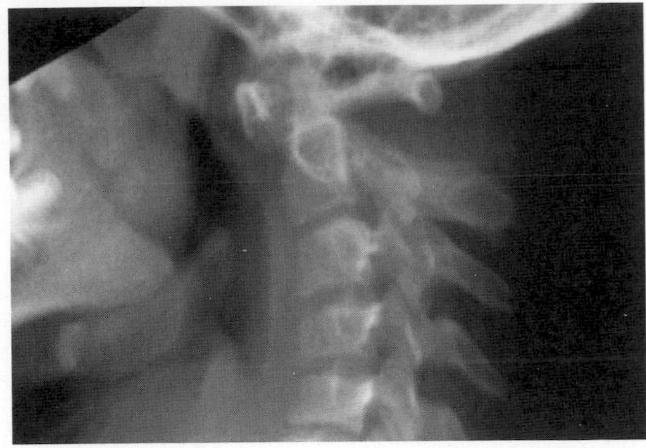

FIGURE 43-29 Lateral radiograph of patient with occipital cervical synostosis.

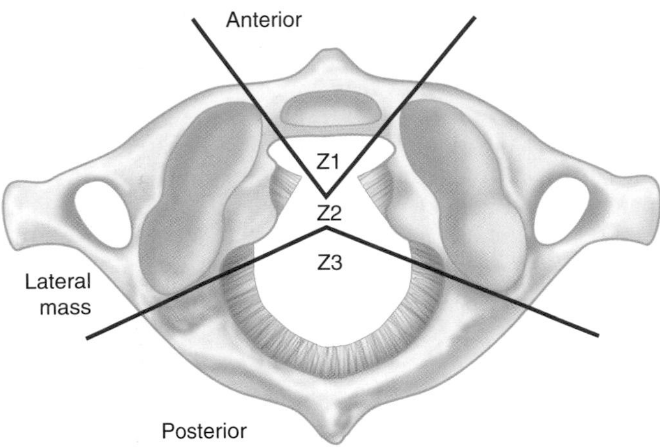

FIGURE 43-30 Morphologic classification of fusion of C1 to the occiput according to the anatomic site of occipitalization: *Z1*, a fused anterior arch; *Z2*, fused lateral masses; *Z3*, a fused posterior arch; and *Z4*, a combination of fused zones. (Redrawn from Gholve PA, Hosalkar HS, Ricchetti ET, et al: Occipitalization of the atlas in children. Morphologic classification, associations, and clinical relevance, J Bone Joint Surg Am 89:571, 2007.)

Gholve et al. classified fusion of C1 to the occiput into four zones. Zone 1 is a fused anterior arch, zone 2 a fusion of the lateral masses, zone 3 a fused posterior arch, and a combination of the zones (Fig. 43-30). In their 30 patients, zone 4 (a combination of zones) was the most common and patients with zone 2 fusion had the highest prevalence of spinal canal encroachment. Flexion and extension lateral cervical spine views should be part of the initial evaluation because of the frequency of atlantoaxial instability. McRae and Barnum measured the distance from the posterior aspect of the odontoid to the posterior arch of the atlas or the posterior lip of the foramen magnum, whichever was closer. When the distance was 19 mm or less, a neurologic deficit usually was present in their series. A sagittal diameter of 13 mm has been associated with neurologic symptoms. This measurement should be made on a flexion view because maximal narrowing of the canal usually occurs in flexion. Myelography or MRI can detect areas of encroachment on the spinal cord or medulla and is especially useful when a constricting fibrous band occurs posteriorly. Flexion and extension MRI often is needed to identify the pathology.

TREATMENT

Patients who have minor symptoms or become symptomatic after minor trauma or infection can be treated nonoperatively with immobilization in cervical orthosis. When neurologic symptoms occur, cervical spine fusion or decompression is indicated. Anterior symptoms usually are caused by a hypermobile odontoid; preliminary reduction of the odontoid with traction, followed by fusion from the occiput to C2, usually relieves the symptoms. If the odontoid is irreducible, the appropriateness of either in situ fusion without reduction or fusion with excision of the odontoid, with its associated risks and complications, must be determined. Posterior signs and symptoms usually are caused by bony compression or compression from a dural band. When this is documented by MRI or myelography, suboccipital craniectomy, excision of the posterior arch of the atlas, and removal of the dural band are indicated. This may need to be combined with a posterior fusion to prevent instability. Surgical results have been variable.

IDIOPATHIC ATLANTOOCCIPITAL INSTABILITY

Idiopathic atlantooccipital instability has been reported in five patients in one study. Neurologic signs included vertigo, syncope, and projectile vomiting, presumably caused by vertebral artery insufficiency from the mobility at the occipital-C1 junction. Posterior atlantooccipital fusion was successful in these patients.

KLIPPEL-FEIL SYNDROME

Klippel-Feil syndrome is a congenital fusion of the cervical vertebrae that may involve two segments, a congenital block vertebra, or the entire cervical spine. Congenital cervical fusion is a result of failure of normal segmentation of the cervical somites during the third to eighth week of life. The skeletal system may not be the only system affected during this time; cardiorespiratory, genitourinary, and auditory systems frequently are involved. In most patients, the exact cause is unknown. One proposed cause is a primary vascular disruption during embryonic development that results in fusion of the cervical vertebrae and other associated anomalies. Studies have suggested that this may be an inherited condition in some patients and have found autosomal dominant inheritance in those with C2-3 fusion. Evidence of a familial Klippel-Feil syndrome gene locus has been identified on the long arm of chromosome 8. Maternal alcoholism has also been suggested as a causative factor; a 50% incidence of cervical vertebral fusions has been found on radiographs of infants with fetal alcohol syndrome.

Occipitalization of the atlas, hemivertebrae, and basilar impression occur frequently in patients with Klippel-Feil syndrome, but their isolated occurrence is not considered part of this syndrome. The classic features of Klippel-Feil syndrome are a short neck, low posterior hairline, and limited range of neck motion. Patients may consult an orthopaedist because of neurologic problems, because of signs of instability of the cervical spine, or for cosmetic reasons. Because many patients are asymptomatic, the actual incidence of this condition is unknown, but estimates in the literature range from 1 in 42,400 births to 3 in 700. There is a slight male predominance (1.5:1). Feil classified the syndrome into three types: type I, block fusion of all cervical and upper thoracic vertebrae; type II, fusion of one or two pairs of cervical vertebrae; and type III, cervical fusion in combination with lower thoracic or lumbar fusion. Minimally involved patients with Klippel-Feil syndrome lead normal, active lives with no significant restrictions or symptoms. More severely involved patients have a good prognosis if genitourinary, cardiopulmonary, and auditory problems are treated early. Samartzis et al. developed the following radiographic classification: type I, a single congenitally fused cervical segment; type II multiple noncontiguous, congenitally fused segments; and type III multiple contiguous, congenitally fused cervical segments. Patients with type I have more long-term axial neck pain, and those with type II and III are more likely to have radiculopathy and myelopathy.

In patients with Klippel-Feil syndrome, neurologic compromise, ranging from radiculopathy to quadriplegia to death, can occur. The neurologic symptoms are caused by occipitocervical anomalies, instability, or degenerative joint and disc disease. Instability and degenerative joint disease are common when two fused areas are separated by a single open interspace. Patients with multiple short areas of fusion (three or more vertebrae) separated by more than one open interspace do not develop instability or degenerative joint disease as frequently, possibly because of a more equal distribution of stress in the cervical spine. Three patterns of cervical spine fusion with a potentially poor prognosis because of late instability or degenerative joint disease have been identified. Pattern 1 is fusion of C1-2 with occipitalization of the atlas. This pattern concentrates the motion of flexion and extension at the atlantoaxial joint; the odontoid becomes hypermobile and may dislocate posteriorly, narrowing the spinal canal and causing neurologic compromise. Pattern 2 is a long fusion with an abnormal occipitocervical junction, concentrating the forces of flexion, extension, and rotation through an abnormal odontoid or poorly developed C1 ring; with time, this abnormal articulation becomes unstable. This pattern should be differentiated from a long fusion with a normal C1-2 articulation and occipitocervical junction. Patients with pattern 2 fusions are not at high risk for instability and neurologic problems and have a normal life expectancy. Pattern 3 is a single open interspace between two fused segments with cervical spine motion concentrated at the single open interspace, which becomes hypermobile and causes instability and degenerative joint disease. On a lateral radiograph, the cervical spine with this pattern appears to hinge at an open segment.

ASSOCIATED CONDITIONS

Several congenital problems have been associated with congenital fusion of the cervical vertebrae, most commonly scoliosis, renal abnormalities, Sprengel deformity, deafness, synkinesis, and congenital heart defects (Box 43-5).

BOX 43-5

Conditions Commonly Associated With Klippel-Feil Syndrome

Scoliosis
Most frequent orthopaedic complication (60%)
Obtain radiographs of entire spine

Renal Abnormalities
Occur in approximately 30%
Usually asymptomatic
Obtain ultrasound or intravenous pyelogram

Cardiovascular Anomalies
Found in 4% to 14%
Ventricular septal defects most common

Deafness
Occurs in approximately 30%
Obtain audiometric testing

Synkinesis (Mirror Movements)
Occurs in approximately 20%
May restrict bimanual activities
Usually decreases with age

Respiratory Anomalies
Failure of lobe formation
Ectopic lungs
Restriction of lung function by shortened trunk, scoliosis, rib fusion, or deformed costovertebral joints

Sprengel Deformity
Occurs in approximately 20%
Unilateral or bilateral
Increases unsightly appearance
May affect shoulder motion

■ SCOLIOSIS

The most common orthopaedic anomaly is scoliosis. Studies have shown that 60% to 70% of patients with Klippel-Feil syndrome have scoliosis (curves > 15 degrees), kyphosis, or both. These patients may require treatment and should be followed closely until growth is complete. Two types of scoliosis have been identified. The first is congenital scoliosis caused by vertebral anomalies. The second occurs in a normal-appearing spine below an area of congenital scoliosis or cervical fusion; this type of curve tends to be progressive. Progression may be controlled with a brace. Surgery may be required to prevent progression in both types of scoliosis associated with Klippel-Feil syndrome. Radiographs of the entire spine should be obtained because a progressive curve may not be appreciated until significant deformity has occurred if attention is focused just on the congenital scoliosis or cervical fusion.

■ RENAL ANOMALIES

About one third of patients with Klippel-Feil syndrome have urogenital anomalies. Because the cervical vertebrae and genitourinary tract differentiate at the same time in the embryo, fetal maldevelopment between 4 and 8 weeks of development may produce genitourinary anomalies and Klippel-Feil syndrome. These renal anomalies usually are asymptomatic, and children with Klippel-Feil syndrome should be evaluated with an ultrasound, intravenous pyelogram, or MRI because the renal problems can be life threatening. The most common renal anomaly is unilateral absence of the kidney. Other anomalies include malrotation of kidneys, ectopic kidney, horseshoe kidney, and hydronephrosis from ureteral pelvic obstruction.

CARDIOVASCULAR ANOMALIES

The reported incidence of cardiovascular anomalies in children with Klippel-Feil syndrome ranges from 4.2% to 29%. Ventricular septal defects, alone or in combination, are the most common anomaly. Patients may have significant dyspnea and cyanosis. Other reported cardiovascular anomalies include mitral valve insufficiency, coarctation of the aorta, right-sided aorta, patent ductus arteriosus, pulmonic stenosis, dextrocardia, atrial septal defect, aplasia of the pericardium, patent foramen ovale, single atrium, single ventricle, and bicuspid pulmonic valve.

DEAFNESS

Approximately 30% of children with Klippel-Feil syndrome have some degree of hearing loss. McGaughran, Kuna, and Das reported that 80% of the 44 patients they studied had some type of audiologic abnormalities. Several reports document conduction defects with ankylosis of the ossicles, footplate fixation, or absence of the external auditory canal. Other reports suggest a sensorineural defect. There is no common anatomic lesion, and the hearing loss may be conductive, sensorineural, or mixed. All patients with Klippel-Feil syndrome should have audiometric testing. Early detection of hearing defects in a young child may improve speech and language development by permitting early initiation of speech and language training.

SYNKINESIS

Synkinesis (mirror movements) is involuntary paired movements of the hands and occasionally of the arms. One hand is unable to move without a similar reciprocal motion of the opposite hand. Synkinesis can be observed in normal children younger than 5 years old and is present in 20% of patients with Klippel-Feil syndrome. Synkinesis may be so severe as to restrict bimanual activities. The mirror movements become less obvious with increasing age and usually are not clinically obvious after the second decade of life.

In autopsy studies, incomplete decussation of the pyramidal tract in the upper cervical spinal cord has been observed, suggesting that an alternative extrapyramidal path is required to control motion in the upper extremity. Clinically normal patients with Klippel-Feil syndrome have been shown to have electrically detectable paired motion in the opposite extremity. These patients may be clumsier in two-handed activities. Occupational therapy can help the child disassociate the mirror movements and improve bimanual dexterity.

RESPIRATORY ANOMALIES

Pulmonary complications involving failure of lobe formation, ectopic lungs, or restrictive lung disease resulting from a shortened trunk, scoliosis, rib fusion, and deformed costovertebral joints have been reported.

SPRENGEL DEFORMITY

Sprengel deformity occurs in about 20% of patients with Klippel-Feil syndrome and can be unilateral or bilateral. Descent of the scapula coincides with the period of development of Klippel-Feil anomalies, and maldevelopment during this time (3 to 8 weeks of gestation) can cause both anomalies. Sprengel deformity increases the unsightly appearance of an already short neck and can affect the range of shoulder motion.

CERVICAL RIBS

Cervical ribs occur in 12% to 15% of patients with Klippel-Feil syndrome. When evaluating a patient with neurologic symptoms, the presence of a cervical rib and associated thoracic outlet syndrome should be investigated.

CLINICAL FINDINGS

The classic clinical presentation of Klippel-Feil syndrome is the triad of a low posterior hairline, a short neck, and limited neck motion (Fig. 43-31). This triad indicates almost complete cervical involvement and may be clinically evident at birth; however, fewer than half of patients with Klippel-Feil syndrome have all parts of the triad. Many patients with Klippel-Feil syndrome have a normal appearance, and the syndrome is diagnosed through incidental radiographs. Shortening of the neck and a low posterior hairline are not constant findings and may be overlooked; webbing of the neck (pterygium colli) is seen in severe involvement. The most constant clinical finding is limitation of neck motion. Rotation and lateral bending are affected more than flexion and extension. If fewer than three vertebrae are fused or if the lower cervical vertebrae are fused, motion is only slightly limited. Hensinger reported that some of his patients had almost full flexion and extension through only one open (unfused) interspace.

Symptoms usually are not caused by the fused cervical vertebrae but by open segments adjacent to areas of synostosis that become hypermobile in response to increased stress placed on the area. Symptoms can be caused by mechanical or neurologic problems. Mechanical problems are caused by stretching of the capsular and ligamentous structures near the hypermobile segment, resulting in early degenerative arthritis with pain localized to the neck. Neurologic problems result from direct irritation of or impingement on a nerve root or from compression of the spinal cord. Involvement of the nerve root alone causes radicular symptoms; spinal cord compression can cause spasticity, hyperreflexia, muscle weakness, and even complete paralysis.

RADIOGRAPHIC FINDINGS

Routine radiographs, cineradiograms, CT scans, and MR images may be useful in the evaluation of Klippel-Feil syndrome. Adequate radiographs can be difficult to obtain in severely involved children, but initial examination should include anteroposterior, odontoid, and lateral flexion and extension views of the cervical spine. Lateral flexion-extension views are the most important to identify atlantoaxial instability or instability near an open segment between two congenitally fused areas (Fig. 43-32). Spinal canal narrowing can occur from degenerative osteophytes or from congenital

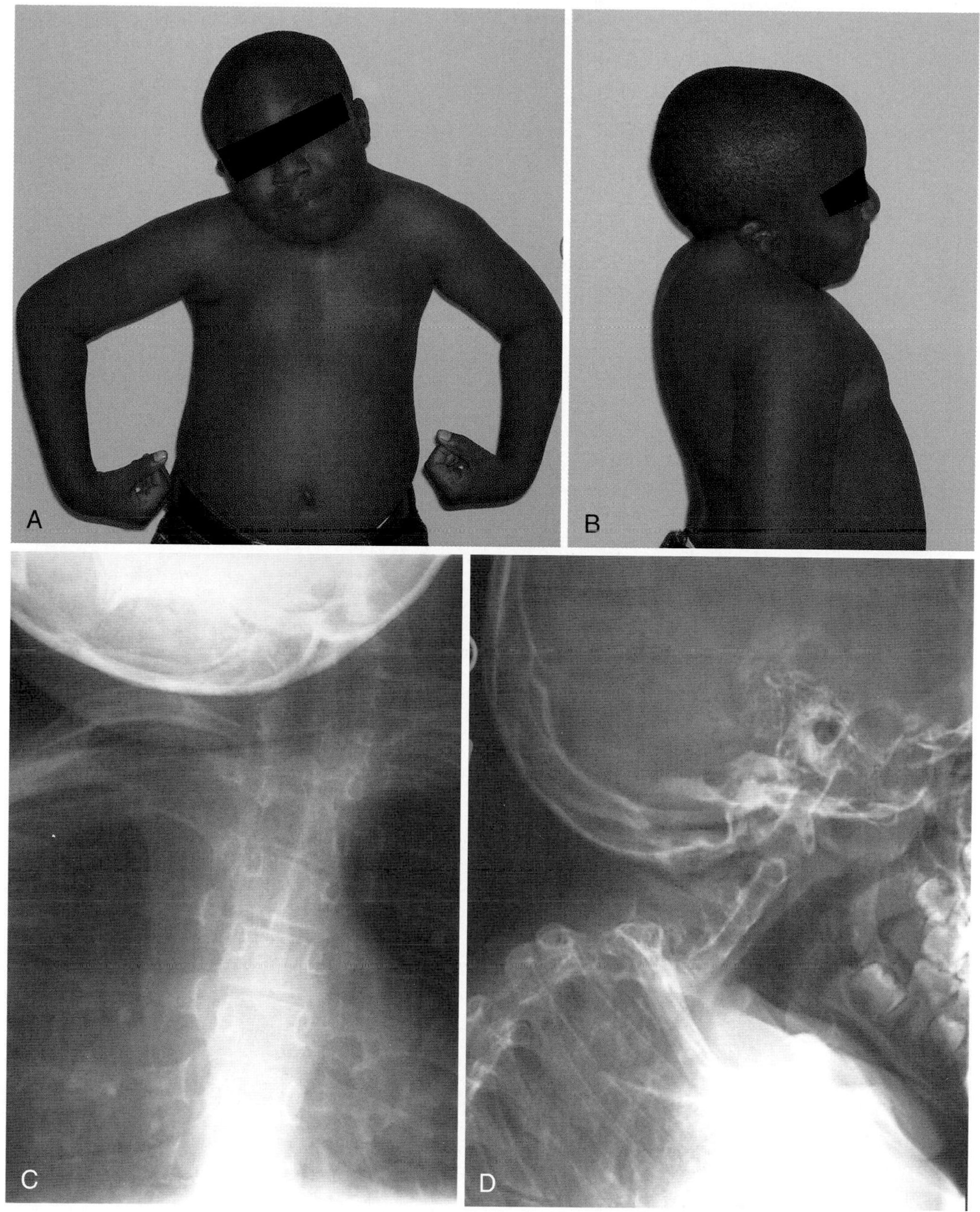

FIGURE 43-31 Clinical **(A** and **B)** and radiographic **(C** and **D)** features of Klippel-Feil syndrome in young boy.

spinal stenosis. If enlargement of the spinal canal is evident on radiographs, syringomyelia, hydromyelia, or Arnold-Chiari malformation should be suspected. In young patients with Klippel-Feil syndrome, serial lateral flexion-extension views should be obtained to evaluate instability at the atlantoaxial joint or at an open interspace between fused areas. Development of congenital or idiopathic scoliosis should be documented by radiographic examination of the entire spine. Cineradiography also may be helpful in determining the amount of vertebral instability. Besides vertebral fusion, flattening and widening of involved vertebral bodies and absent disc spaces are common findings. In young children, the spine may appear normal because of the lack of ossification. The posterior elements usually are the first to ossify and fuse, which aids in early diagnosis of Klippel-Feil syndrome. CT and MRI are helpful in diagnosing nerve root and spinal cord impingement by osteophyte formation. To evaluate instability and the risk of neurologic compromise, a flexion and extension MRI may be needed to give the soft-tissue definition necessary to show instability or spinal cord compromise.

TREATMENT

Mechanical symptoms caused by degenerative joint disease usually respond to traction, a cervical collar, and analgesics. Neurologic symptoms should be evaluated carefully

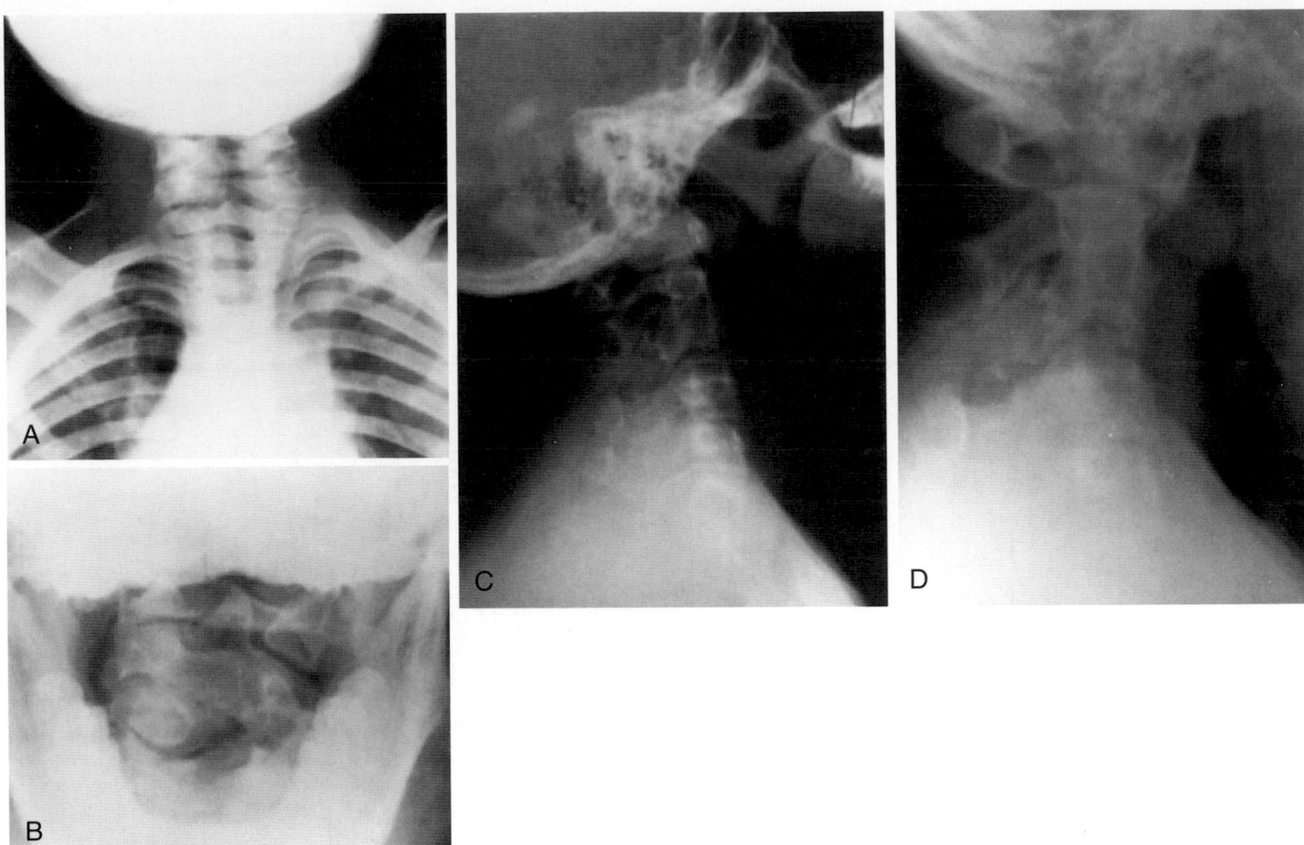

FIGURE 43-32 Radiographic features of Klippel-Feil syndrome in adolescent. **A,** Posteroanterior view shows congenital anomalies of cervical spine and left Sprengel deformity. **B,** Open-mouth odontoid view shows bony anomalies of cervical spine. **C,** Extension view shows odontoid in normal position. **D,** Flexion view shows increased atlantodens interval.

to locate the exact pathologic condition; surgical stabilization with or without decompression may be required. Prophylactic fusion of a hypermobile segment is controversial. The risk of neurologic compromise must be weighed against the further reduction in neck motion, and this decision must be made for each patient individually. Depending on the type of anatomic deformity and location of instability a posterior fusion, anterior fusion, or a combined anterior and posterior fusion may be needed. If anterior decompression and fusion are needed, this can be done with an anterior approach. Anterior decompression and interbody fusion can be performed with plate and screw fixation similar to adults if the anatomy allows for this (see Chapter 41). Cosmetic improvement after surgery has been limited, but surgical correction of Sprengel deformity can significantly improve appearance, and occasionally soft-tissue procedures such as Z-plasty and muscle resection improve cosmesis. Bonola described a method of rib resection to obtain an apparent increase in neck length and motion, but this is an extensive procedure with significant risk. Partial thoracoplasty is performed as a two-stage procedure: removal of the upper four ribs on one side and, after the patient has recovered from the first surgery, removal of the upper four ribs on the other side.

POSTERIOR FUSION OF C3-7

TECHNIQUE 43-16 *Figure 43-33*

- Administer general anesthesia with the patient in a supine position.
- Turn the patient prone on the operating table, maintaining traction and proper alignment of the head and neck. The head can be positioned in a headrest or maintained in skeletal traction.
- Obtain radiographs to confirm adequate alignment of the vertebrae and to localize the vertebrae to be exposed. There is a high incidence of extension of the fusion mass when extra vertebrae or spinous processes are exposed in the cervical spine.
- Make a midline incision over the chosen spinous processes and expose the spinous process and laminae subperiosteally to the facet joints.
- If the spinous process is large enough, make a hole in the base of the spinous process with a towel clip or Lewin clamp.

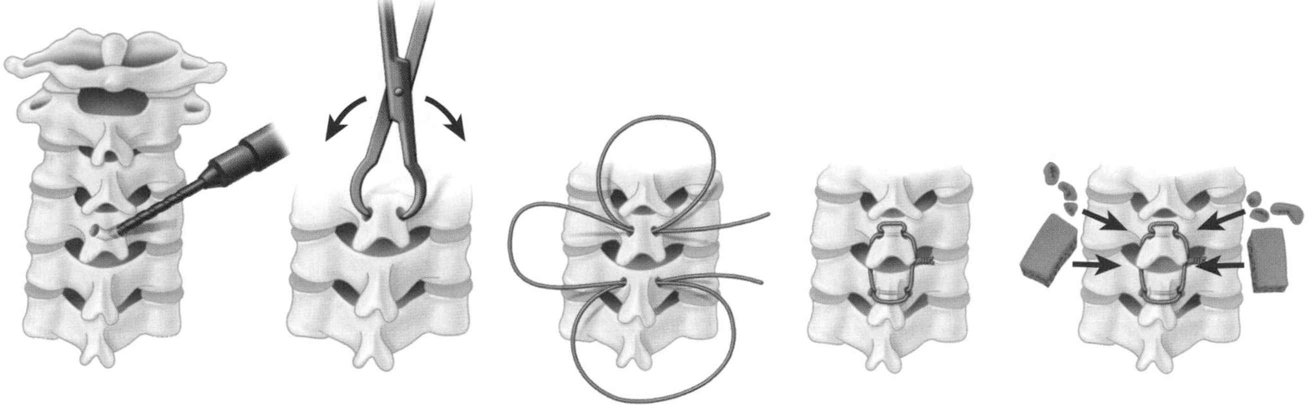

FIGURE 43-33 Modified Rogers wiring of cervical spine for posterior fusion. **SEE TECHNIQUE 43-16.**

- Pass an 18-gauge wire through this hole, loop it over the spinous process, and pass it through the hole again.
- Make a similar hole in the base of the spinous process of the inferior vertebra to be fused.
- Pass the wire through this hole, loop it under the inferior aspect of the spinous process, and pass it back through the same hole.
- Tighten the wire and place corticocancellous bone grafts along the exposed lamina and spinous processes.
- Close the wound in layers.
- If the spinous process is too small to pass wires, an in situ fusion can be performed and external immobilization can be used.

POSTOPERATIVE CARE. The patient should wear a rigid cervical orthosis until a solid fusion is documented radiographically.

POSTERIOR FUSION OF C3 TO C7 USING 16-GAUGE WIRE AND THREADED KIRSCHNER WIRES

TECHNIQUE 43-17

(HALL)

- Pass the threaded Kirschner wires through the bases of the spinous processes of the vertebrae to be fused, followed by a figure-of-eight wiring with a 16-gauge wire.
- After the 16-gauge wire has been tightened around the threaded Kirschner wires, pack strips of corticocancellous and cancellous bone over the posterior arches of the vertebrae to be fused (Fig. 43-34).
- Exposure and postoperative care are similar to those described for a Rogers posterior fusion and wiring.

Posterior instrumentation techniques (see Chapter 41) that are used in the adult spine (plate or rods and lateral mass screws) can be used in the pediatric cervical spine.

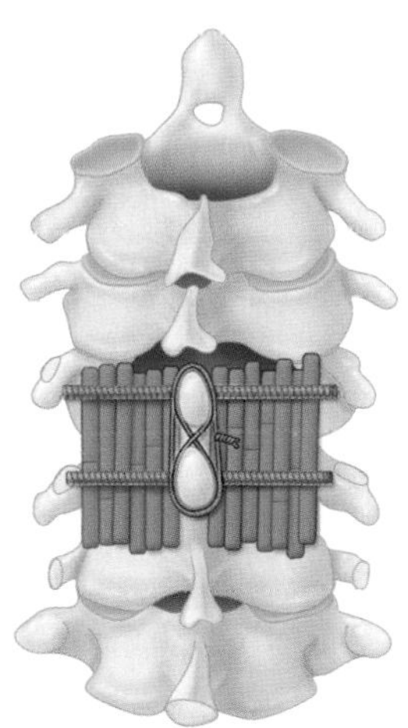

FIGURE 43-34 Hall technique of fixation for posterior arthrodesis of cervical spine. **SEE TECHNIQUE 43-17.**

Before the techniques are used, the size of the lateral masses must be evaluated to ensure there would be adequate room to place these screws.

POSTERIOR FUSION WITH LATERAL MASS SCREW FIXATION

Lateral mass screw fixation of the lower cervical spine can be used in older children or adolescents. The instrumentation should be matched to the size of the child. Techniques described differ primarily in the entry points and screw trajectories.

TECHNIQUE 43-18

(ROY-CAMILLE)

- Create an entry point for the screw 5 mm medial to the lateral edge and midway between the facet joint or at

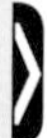

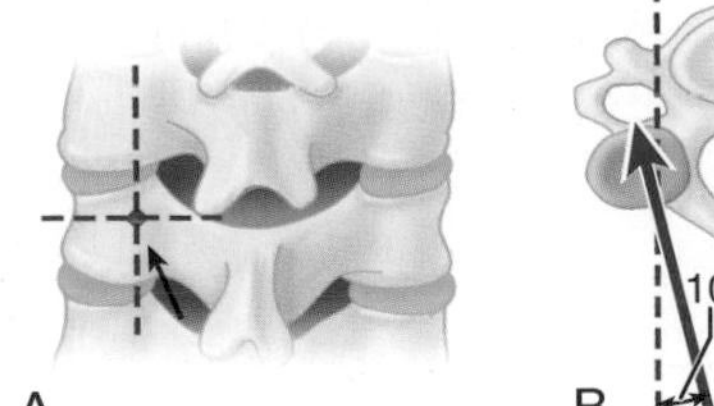

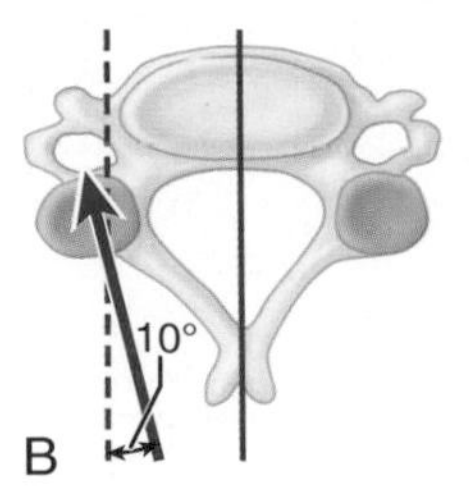

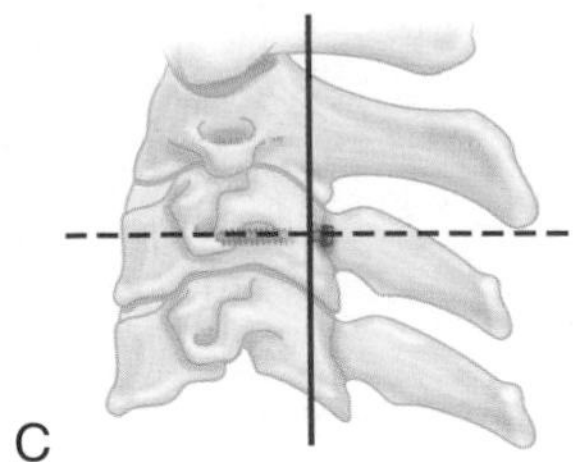

FIGURE 43-35 Roy-Camille technique of lateral mass screw insertion. **A,** Screw entry point. **B,** Drill directed perpendicular to posterior wall of vertebral body at 10-degree angle. **C,** Final screw position. **SEE TECHNIQUE 43-18.**

the center of the rectangular posterior face of the lateral mass (Fig. 43-35A).

- Direct the drill perpendicular to the posterior wall of the vertebral body with a 10-degree lateral angle (Fig. 43-35B). This trajectory takes the exit slightly lateral to the vertebral artery and below the existing nerve root. Use lateral fluoroscopic imaging to avoid penetration of the subadjacent facet.
- Set the depth guide to 10 to 12 mm to avoid penetration beyond the anterior cortex. For men the lateral mass depth from C3 to C6 ranges from 6 to 14 mm (average 8.7 mm) and in women 6 to 11 mm (average 7.9 mm). The depth can be increased if the local anatomy permits. If additional 20% of pullout strength with bicortical fixation is desired, place the screw to exit at the junction of the lateral mass and transverse process (Fig. 43-35C).

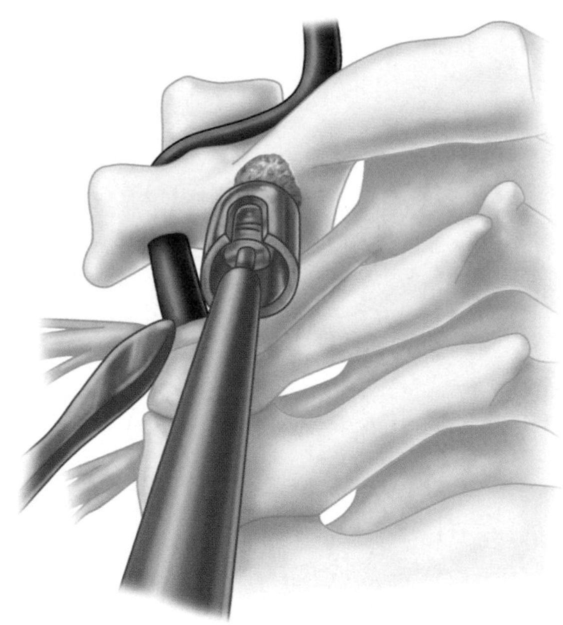

FIGURE 43-36 Posterior lateral mass screw and rod fixation. Drilling lateral mass for screw insertion. **SEE TECHNIQUE 43-19.**

POSTERIOR FUSION WITH LATERAL MASS SCREW AND ROD FIXATION

TECHNIQUE 43-19

- Select an entry portal 1 mm medial to the center of the lateral mass.
- Drill the lateral mass 25 to 35 degrees laterally and 15 degrees cephalad (parallel to the plane of the facet joint) for C3 to C6 (Fig. 43-36). The drilling should be 10 to 25 degrees medially and 25 degrees superiorly at C2 to avoid injuring the vertebral artery. Use a hand drill with a stop guide to prevent drilling of the opposite cortex. Tap the drill hole if necessary.
- Insert the proper length polyaxial screw into each lateral mass to be instrumented and check the position of the screws with posteroanterior and lateral C-arm images. Make adjustments as necessary.
- Insert the prebent rods into the screw head fixtures. Tighten the rods to the screws.

POSTOPERATIVE CARE. A cervical orthosis (cervical collar) is applied and worn for 6 to 8 weeks. Halo device immobilization may be considered if there is suboptimal fixation.

RIB RESECTION

TECHNIQUE 43-20

(BONOLA)

- Bonola described partial thoracoplasty with the use of local anesthesia, but general anesthesia can be used.
- Through a right paravertebral incision midway between the spinous processes and the medial margin of the scapula, divide the trapezius and rhomboid muscles to expose the posterior aspect of the first four ribs (Fig. 43-37A).
- Cut these ribs with a rib cutter a few centimeters from the costovertebral joint.
- Continue the dissection anteriorly along the ribs, dividing and removing the ribs as far anteriorly as the dissection allows (Fig. 43-37B).
- Close the wound in layers.

POSTOPERATIVE CARE. A cervical collar is fitted to help mold the resected area. The second stage of the procedure is performed on the opposite side after the patient has recovered from the initial surgery.

ATLANTOAXIAL ROTATORY SUBLUXATION

Atlantoaxial rotatory subluxation is a common cause of childhood torticollis, but the subluxation and torticollis usually are temporary. Rarely do they persist and become what is best described as atlantoaxial rotatory "fixation." Atlantoaxial rotatory subluxation occurs when normal motion between the atlas and axis becomes limited or fixed, and it can occur spontaneously, can be associated with minor trauma, or can follow an upper respiratory tract infection. The cause of this subluxation is not completely understood. Various causes that have been proposed include hyperemic decalcification of the arch of the atlas, causing inadequate attachment of the transverse ligaments; inflammation of the synovial fringes that act as an obstruction to reduction of subluxation; and disruption of one or both of the alar ligaments with an intact transverse ligament. A meniscus-like synovial fold in the C1-2 facet joints, which is primarily noted in children, caused subluxation in one study. Most authors now agree that the subluxation is related to increased laxity of ligaments and capsular structures caused by inflammation or trauma.

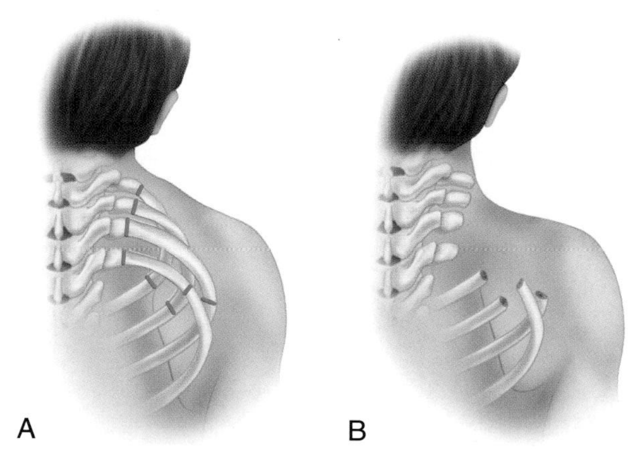

FIGURE 43-37 **A** and **B,** Bonola partial thoracoplasty for treatment of short neck in Klippel-Feil syndrome. **SEE TECHNIQUE 43-20.**

Fielding and Hawkins classified atlantoaxial rotatory subluxation into four types (Fig. 43-38): type I, simple rotatory displacement without anterior shift of C1; type II, rotatory displacement with an anterior shift of C1 on C2 of 5 mm or less; type III, rotatory displacement with an anterior shift of C1 on C2 greater than 5 mm; and type IV, rotatory displacement with a posterior shift. Type I displacement is the most common and occurs primarily in children. Type II is less common but has greater potential for neurologic damage. Types III and IV are rare but have high potential for neurologic damage.

Atlantoaxial rotatory subluxation usually occurs in children after an upper respiratory tract infection or minor or major trauma. The head is tilted to one side and rotated to the opposite side with the neck slightly flexed (the "cock robin" position). The sternocleidomastoid muscle on the long side is often in spasm in an attempt to correct this deformity. When the subluxation is acute, attempts to move the head cause pain. Patients are able to increase the deformity but cannot correct the deformity past the midline. With time, muscle spasms subside and the torticollis becomes less painful but the deformity persists. A careful neurologic examination should determine any neurologic compression or vertebral artery compromise.

RADIOGRAPHIC FINDINGS

Adequate radiographs of the cervical spine can be difficult to obtain in children with torticollis. Initial examination should include anteroposterior and odontoid views of the cervical spine. On the open-mouth odontoid view, the lateral mass that is rotated forward appears wider and closer to the midline and the opposite lateral mass appears narrower and farther away from the midline (Fig. 43-39). Apparent overlapping may obscure one of the facet joints of the atlas and axis. On the lateral view, the anteriorly rotated lateral mass appears wedge-shaped in front of the odontoid. The posterior arch of the atlas may appear to be assimilated into the occiput because

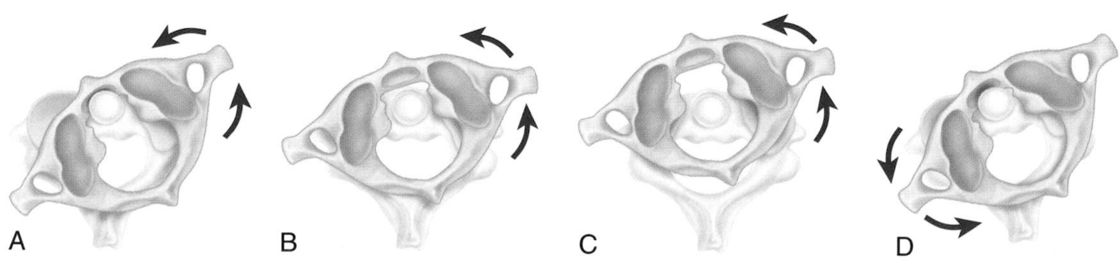

FIGURE 43-38 Fielding and Hawkins classification of rotatory displacement. **A,** Type I, simple rotatory displacement without anterior shift; odontoid acts as pivot. **B,** Type II, rotatory displacement with anterior displacement of 3 to 5 mm; lateral articular process acts as pivot. **C,** Type III, rotatory displacement with anterior displacement of more than 5 mm. **D,** Type IV, rotatory displacement with posterior displacement.

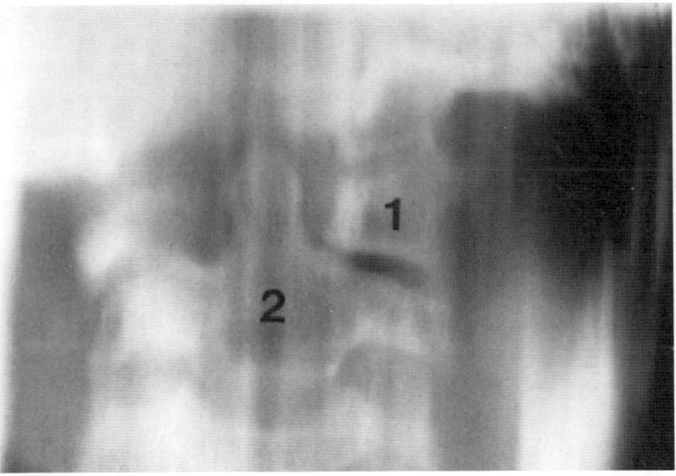

FIGURE 43-39 Atlantoaxial rotatory subluxation. Note lateral masses.

BOX 43-6

Treatment Plan for Rotatory Subluxation

Nonoperative Treatment

Present less than 1 week: immobilization in soft collar, analgesics, bed rest for 1 week; if no spontaneous reduction: hospitalization, halo traction

Present more than 1 week but less than 1 month: hospitalization, halo traction, cervical collar 4 to 6 weeks

Present more than 1 month: hospitalization, halo traction, cervical collar 4 to 6 weeks

Indications for Operative Treatment

Neurologic involvement

Anterior displacement

Failure to achieve and maintain correction of deformity that exists for longer than 3 months

Recurrence of deformity after an adequate trial of conservative management consisting of at least 6 weeks of immobilization

of the head tilt. A lateral radiograph of the skull may show the relative position of C1 and C2 more clearly than a lateral radiograph of the cervical spine. Lateral flexion and extension views should be obtained to document any atlantoaxial instability. Cineradiography confirms the diagnosis by showing the movement of atlas and axis as a single unit but is difficult to perform during the acute stage because movement of the neck is painful. Cineradiography is not routinely used because of the increased radiation exposure. CT with the head rotated as far to the left and right as possible during scanning to confirm the loss of normal rotation at the atlantoaxial joint confirms the diagnosis of rotatory subluxation. McGuire et al. classified the findings on dynamic CT scans (DCTS) into three stages: stage 0, torticollis but normal DCTS; stage 1, limitation of motion (<15 degrees difference between C1 and C2, but C1 crosses the midline of C2); and stage 2, fixed (C1 does not cross midline of C2). They found a significant trend between increasing intensity of treatment and stage of DCTS findings. The usefulness of DCTS, however, for the diagnosis of atlantoaxial rotatory subluxation has been questioned. MRI may be beneficial for evaluation of ligamentous pathology or spinal cord compression.

TREATMENT

The treatment plan should be based on the duration of the subluxation (Box 43-6). If rotatory subluxation has existed less than 1 week, immobilization in a soft collar, analgesics, and bed rest for 1 week are recommended. If reduction does not occur spontaneously, hospitalization and traction are indicated. If rotatory subluxation is present for longer than 1 week, but less than 1 month, hospitalization and cervical traction are indicated. Head-halter traction generally is used; but when torticollis persists longer than 1 month, halo traction may be required. Traction is maintained until the deformity corrects, then a cervical collar is worn for 4 to 6 weeks. Nonoperative treatment should be used only if no significant anterior displacement or instability is seen on radiographic evaluation.

Fielding listed the following as indications for operative treatment: (1) neurologic involvement, (2) anterior displacement, (3) failure to achieve and maintain correction if the deformity exists for longer than 3 months, and (4) recurrence of the deformity after an adequate trial of conservative management consisting of at least 6 weeks of immobilization. If operative treatment is indicated, a C1-2 posterior fusion is performed (Fig. 43-40). Fielding and Hawkins recommended preoperative traction for 2 to 3 weeks to correct the deformity as much as possible. Fusion is performed with the head in a neutral position. Halo immobilization is continued for 6 weeks after surgery to maintain correction while the fusion becomes solid. This can be accomplished with a halo cast or halo vest. Immobilization is continued until there is radiographic evidence of fusion.

CERVICAL INSTABILITY IN DOWN SYNDROME

In children with Down syndrome, generalized ligamentous laxity caused by the underlying collagen defect can result in atlantoaxial and atlantooccipital instability. Pizzutillo and Herman made a distinction between cervical instability and hypermobility in patients with Down syndrome. Instability implies pathologic intersegmental motion that jeopardizes neurologic integrity. Hypermobility refers to increased excursions that occur in the cervical spine of patients with Down syndrome compared with normal controls but do not result in loss of structural integrity of the anatomic restraints that protect neural tissues. Atlantoaxial instability, first described by Spitzer, Rabinowitch, and Wybar in 1961, occurs in 10% to 20% of children with Down syndrome. Instability can occur at more than one level and in more than one plane. Atlantooccipital instability also can occur in patients with Down syndrome; the incidence has been reported to be 60%. Despite these reports of atlantoaxial and atlantooccipital instability in patients with Down syndrome, the exact natural history related to this instability is unknown. In patients with Down syndrome, differentiating those with hypermobility and those with clinically significant instability may be difficult.

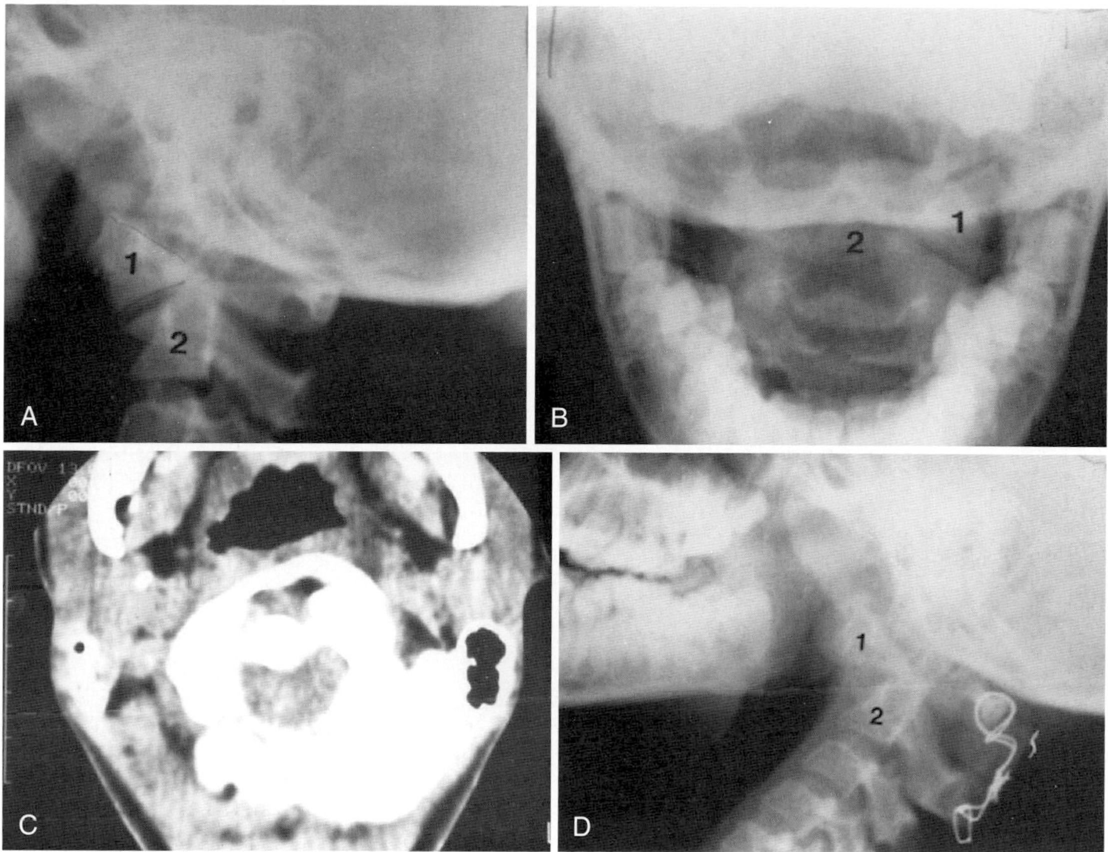

FIGURE 43-40 Atlantoaxial rotatory fixation. **A,** Lateral radiograph shows wedge-shaped mass anterior to odontoid. **B,** Open-mouth odontoid view. **C,** CT scan. **D,** After C1-2 in situ fusion.

The cervical spine in children with Down syndrome may be associated with congenital anomalies of the upper cervical spine, but whether the cervical anomalies are the cause or the result of ligamentous laxity is still controversial.

NEUROLOGIC FINDINGS

Neurologic symptoms are present in 1% to 2.6% of patients with cervical instability. Instability is usually discovered on routine screening examinations or on cervical radiographs obtained for other reasons. Progressive instability leading to neurologic symptoms is most common in boys older than 10.5 years of age. Involvement of the pyramidal tract usually results in gait abnormalities, hyperreflexia, and motor weakness. Other neurologic symptoms include neck pain, occipital headaches, and torticollis. Detailed neurologic examination is often difficult in patients with Down syndrome, and somatosensory evoked potentials may be beneficial in documenting neurologic involvement.

RADIOGRAPHIC FINDINGS

Radiographic examination should include anteroposterior, flexion and extension lateral, and odontoid views. CT scans in flexion and extension or cineradiography in flexion and extension also may be needed to evaluate the occipitoatlantal joint and the atlantoaxial joint for instability. MRI is useful in detecting any spinal cord signal changes in suspected instability and neurologic compromise in these patients in whom it is often difficult to obtain a detailed neurologic examination. Radiographic evidence of atlantooccipital instability is not as well defined as that for atlantoaxial instability, but the measurements described by Wackenheim (Fig. 43-41), Wiesel and Rothman (Fig. 43-42), Powers (Fig. 43-43), and Tredwell et al. are helpful. A Powers ratio of more than 1.0 is indicative

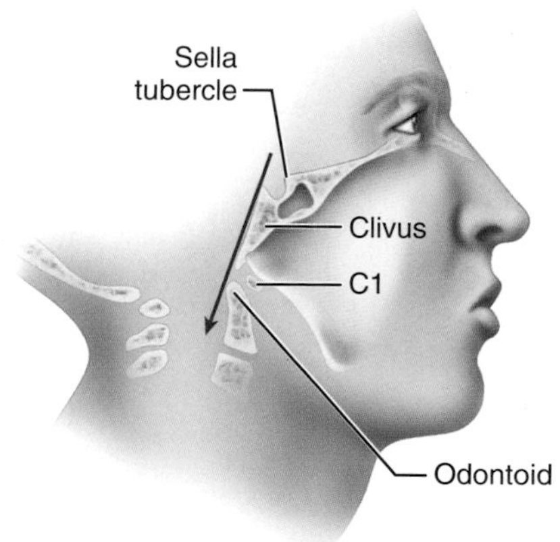

FIGURE 43-41 Drawing of Wackenheim clivus-canal line. This line is drawn along the clivus into the cervical spinal canal and should pass just posterior to the tip of the odontoid.

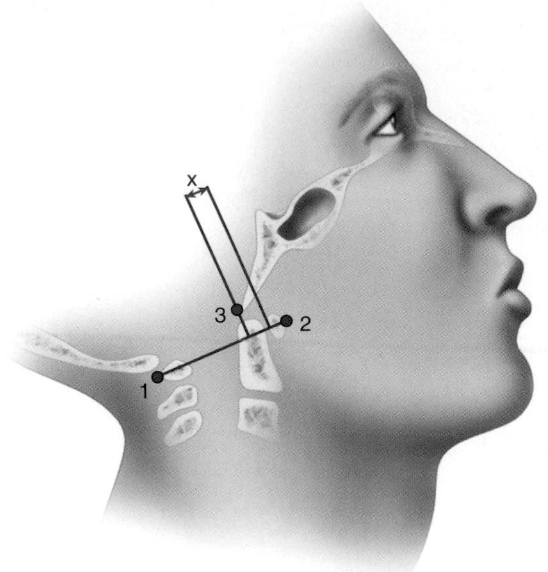

FIGURE 43-42 Method of measuring atlantooccipital instability according to Wiesel and Rothman. These lines are drawn on flexion and extension lateral radiographs, and translation should be no more than 1 mm. Atlantal line joins points *1* and *2*. Line drawn perpendicular to atlantal line at posterior margin of anterior arch of atlas. Point *3* is basion. Distance from point *3* to perpendicular line is measured in flexion and extension. Difference represents anteroposterior translation.

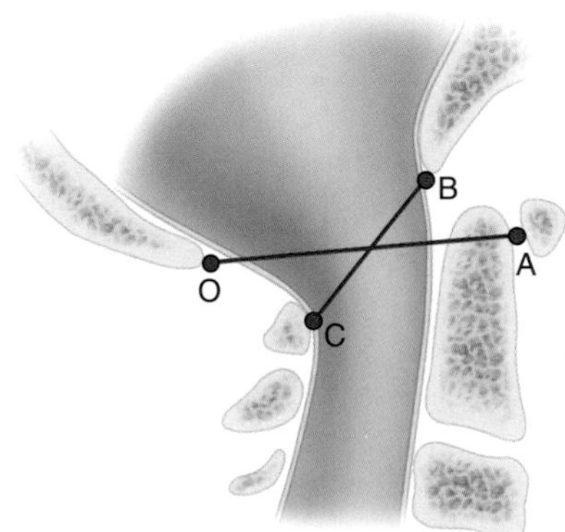

FIGURE 43-43 Powers ratio is determined by drawing a line from the basion *(B)* to the posterior arch of the atlas *(C)* and a second line from the opisthion *(O)* to the anterior arch of the atlas *(A)*. The length of line *BC* is divided by the length of line *OA*. A ratio greater than 1 is diagnostic of anterior atlantooccipital translation, and a ratio less than 0.55 is diagnostic of posterior translation.

of abnormal anterior translation of the occiput, and, according to Parfenchuck et al., a ratio of less than 0.55 indicates posterior translation. However, some studies have reported the poor reproducibility and reliability of these measurement techniques in children with Down syndrome, hindering the physician in providing well-supported treatment recommendations. CT scans in flexion and extension or cineradiography may be needed to give better detail and information about possible atlantooccipital instability.

An atlantodens interval (ADI) of 4.5 to 5 mm indicates instability in normal pediatric patients. Increased ADI in patients with Down syndrome has not been directly correlated with an increase in neurologic compromise. This suggests that radiographs of the cervical spine in Down syndrome must be evaluated by standards specific to that population and not by traditional standards for general pediatric patients because this may result in overdiagnosis of a pathologic process. Neurologic compromise occurs with a similar incidence in individuals with Down syndrome who have a normal ADI and those with an ADI from 4 to 10 mm. In Down syndrome, an ADI of less than 4.5 mm is normal; an ADI of 4.5 to 10 mm is considered hypermobile but not unstable unless neurologic findings are present; and an ADI of more than 10 mm is considered unstable, and the patient is at risk for neurologic compromise because of the decrease in the space available for the spinal cord.

TREATMENT

Hypermobility of the occipitoatlantal junction has been observed in more than 60% of patients with Down syndrome, but this usually is not associated with neurologic risk. If hypermobility of this joint is documented and the patient is neurologically normal, then restriction of high risk activities is recommended. If there is hypermobility and a neurologic deficit or an abnormal signal change in the spinal cord on MRI, then an occiput to C2 or 3 fusion is recommended.

When the ADI is less than 4.5 mm, no restriction of activities is necessary. In those who have an ADI of 4.5 to 10 mm with no neurologic symptoms, high-risk activities are limited. If there is a neurologic deficit or spinal cord changes on MRI, a C1-2 fusion is indicated. If the ADI is 10 mm or more, posterior fusion and instrumentation are recommended. Before fusion and instrumentation, the unstable C1-2 joint should be reduced by traction. If reduction cannot be obtained, an in situ fusion reduces the risk of neurologic compromise.

Complications are relatively common after cervical fusions in children with Down syndrome. Segal et al. reported frequent graft resorption after 10 posterior fusions and suggested as causes inadequate inflammatory response and collagen defects. Msall et al. reported the frequent development of instability above and below C1-2 fusion in patients with Down syndrome. Postoperative immobilization in a halo cast or halo vest should be continued for as long as possible because graft resorption 6 months after fusion has been reported. More stable fixation may decrease this complication.

C1-C2 transarticular screw fixation (see Figs. 43-9 and 43-10) or occiput to C2 instrumentation with plates or rods (Techniques 43-8 and 43-9) can be used successfully and give greater stability than wire fixation.

FAMILIAL CERVICAL DYSPLASIA

Saltzman et al. described a familial cervical dysplasia that affects the first cervical vertebra. Nine of 12 family members from three generations were affected by this inherited form of cervical vertebral dysplasia. The mode of transmission of this disorder is autosomal dominant, with apparently complete penetrance and variable expressivity. Most patients are asymptomatic, and clinical presentation varies from an incidental finding on radiographic examination to a passively correctable head tilt. Symptoms such as suboccipital headaches or decreased cervical motion may be present. CT scan and three-dimensional reconstructions best delineate the anatomic pathology. MRI is useful in identifying the potential for neurologic compromise and the need for surgical stabilization. If surgery is required for stabilization, an occiput-to-C2 fusion is usually needed.

CONGENITAL ANOMALIES OF THE ATLAS

Dubousset and Winter et al. described congenital hemiatlas or hypoplasia of the atlas that can cause marked torticollis if left untreated. Dubousset reported 17 patients with absence of the facet of C1 that led to severe, progressive, fixed torticollis. Initially, the deformity or torticollis was flexible, but with time it became fixed.

In most patients, the deformity is noted at birth as a lateral translation of the head on the trunk, with some degree of lateral tilt and rotation. The sternocleidomastoid muscle is not tight and there is often aplasia of the muscles in the nuchal concavity of the tilted side. Neurologic signs such as headaches, vertigo, or myelopathy occur in about 25% of patients. Plain radiographs are often difficult to interpret, and the diagnosis usually is made by CT. Other spinal cord anomalies may be detected by MRI, such as Arnold-Chiari malformations and stenosis of the foramen magnum. Angiography should be obtained preoperatively because vertebral arterial anomalies may occur on the aplastic side. This disorder has been classified into three types: type I is an isolated hemiatlas, type II is a partial or complete aplasia of one hemiatlas with other associated anomalies of the cervical spine, and type III is a partial or complete atlantooccipital fusion and symmetric or asymmetric hemiatlas aplasia, with or without anomalies of the odontoid and lower cervical spine. Initially the patient should be observed for progression of the deformity. Bracing will not stop progression of the deformity. Dubousset recommended using a halo cast to gradually correct the torticollis and obtain an acceptable position of the head and neck, followed by posterior fusion from occiput to C2. Seven of his 17 patients required surgical correction. Although the age at which the torticollis could be corrected was not specified, Dubousset obtained good results in patients 13 and 15 years of age.

LARSEN SYNDROME

Larsen syndrome is a rare disorder that may have vertebral anomalies such as spina bifida, hypoplastic vertebrae, cervical kyphosis, and anteroposterior dissociation. Patients with cervical kyphosis that may eventually lead to anteroposterior dissociation are difficult to treat. This is potentially the most serious manifestation of Larsen syndrome because of the risk of paralysis. The natural history of cervical kyphosis is variable. Both static and dynamic flexion and extension radiographs should be obtained to document the degree of deformity and any instability. Treatment is also variable and is based on the age of the patient, amount and flexibility of the kyphosis, and the presence of any neurologic deficits. Johnston et al. has advocated early posterior fusion in patients with Larsen syndrome and cervical kyphosis. He found gradual improvement of the cervical kyphosis from continued anterior vertebral body growth when a solid posterior fusion was obtained. In one patient, excessive lordosis occurred after posterior-only fusion. Sakaura et al. has recommended posterior spinal fusion for patients with mild and flexible cervical kyphosis and anterior decompression and circumferential arthrodesis for those with severe kyphotic deformity or in patients with neurologic deficits. The potential for dural ectasia should be considered in patients with Larsen syndrome. Jain et al. listed CT or MRI findings of enlargement of the dural sac, vertebral body scalloping, narrowing of the pedicles, and an enlarged spinal canal as highly indicative of dural ectasia.

POSTERIOR SPINAL FUSION FOR CERVICAL KYPHOSIS THROUGH A LATERAL APPROACH

TECHNIQUE 43-21

(SAKAURA ET AL.)

- Place the patient in the right decubitus position.
- Make an incision along the posterior margin of the sternocleidomastoid muscle (Fig. 43-44A) and bluntly dissect fascia of the posterior triangle of the neck to identify the levator scapulae muscle.
- Retract the carotid sheath and sternocleidomastoid muscle ventrally and the levator scapulae muscle dorsally to expose the scalene muscles.
- Identify the phrenic nerve and carefully dissect the insertions of the anterior scalene muscles from the anterior tubercles of the transverse processes from the C3 to C6 vertebrae. Also dissect the longus colli and capitis muscles from the anterior tubercles to identify the anterior aspect of the cervical spine.
- Identify the vertebral artery and C4 to C6 nerve roots lying posterior to the vertebral artery (Fig. 43-44A and B). Retract the vertebral artery anteriorly and resect the transverse process from C3 to C6 (Fig. 43-44C).
- Release and cut the tight cartilaginous tissue and anterior longitudinal ligaments attaching to the cervical vertebrae ventrally.
- Using a surgical microscope, expose the lateral aspect of the dura from C4 to C5 by removing the left lateral masses and pedicles of the C4 and C5 vertebrae with a rongeur and a diamond-headed airtome. This allows removal of the vertebral bodies of the C4 and C5 vertebrae including the discs between C3 and C4 and C5 and C6 with clear exposure of the nerve roots and dura.
- Remove the vertebral bodies and discs starting at the middle of the bodies and discs. Using a diamond burr, thin the dorsal cortices of the bodies to the width of the spinal canal.
- If the kyphosis cannot be manually corrected, then insert a thin spatula between the posterior longitudinal

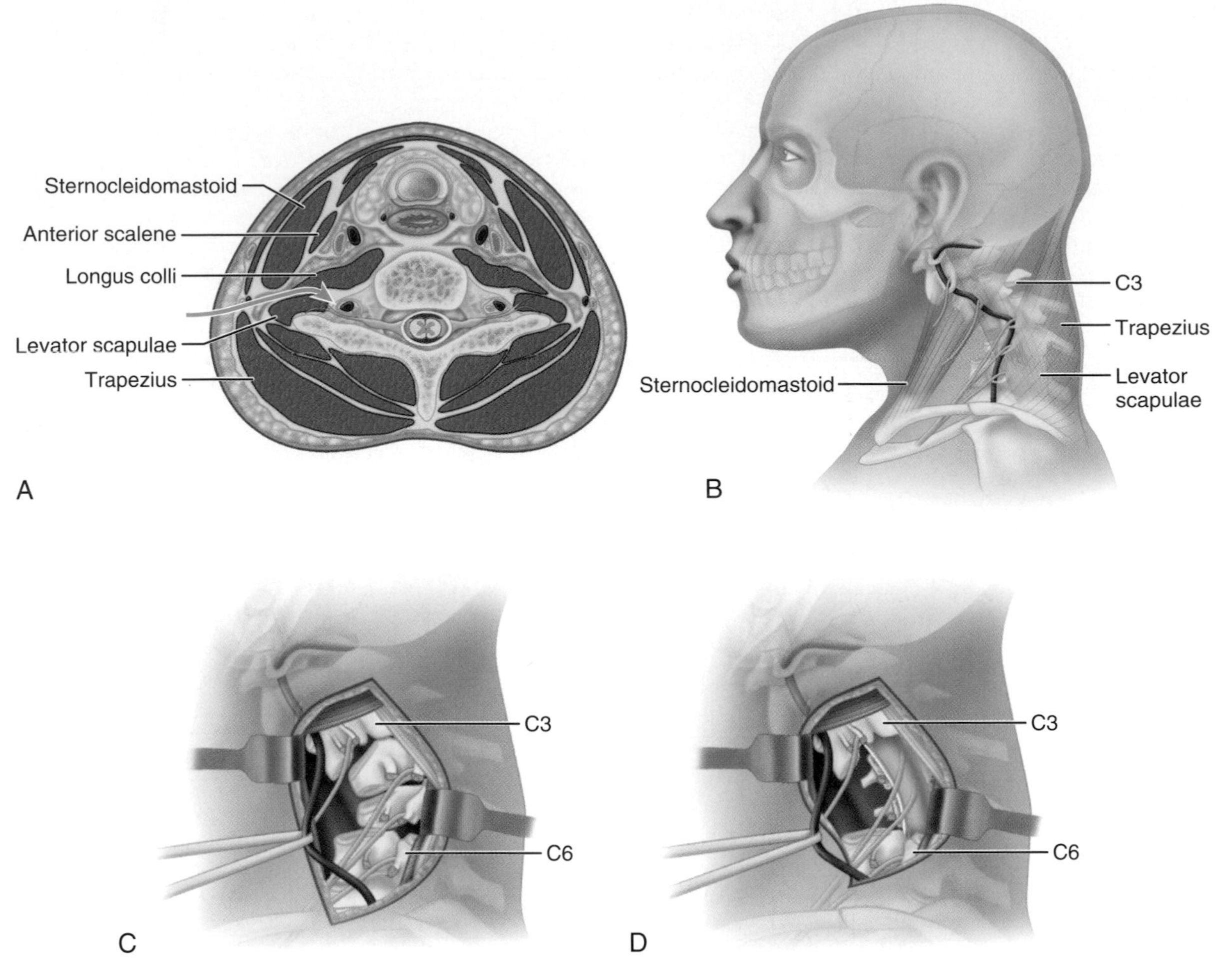

FIGURE 43-44 Sakaura et al. anterior decompression and arthrodesis through a lateral approach. **A,** Axial image of lateral approach to cervical spine. **B,** Vertebral artery and C4 to C6 nerve roots posterior to the vertebral artery. **C,** Vertebral artery anteriorly dislocated by resecting transverse processes from C3 to C6. **D,** Subtotal removal of C4 and C5 bodies and cutting of posterior longitudinal ligament. (**A** from Sakaura et al: Surgical treatment of cervical kyphosis in Larsen syndrome, Spine 32:E39, 2007.) **SEE TECHNIQUE 43-21.**

ligament and dura to avoid dural injury and cut the posterior longitudinal ligament at the middle of the exposed area (Fig. 43-44D). The vertebrae become slightly mobile, and the dura shifts ventrally. Under manual correction, insert an appropriate size strut from the tibia.

- Immobilize the patient in a halo device.

POSTOPERATIVE CARE. The patient is immobilized in a halo cast or vest or a cervicothoracic orthosis for 12 weeks.

INTERVERTEBRAL DISC CALCIFICATION

Intervertebral disc calcification is uncommon in children but does occur. This syndrome is characterized by an acute onset of cervical pain associated with torticollis and limited motion of the cervical spine. Although no definite cause has been identified, suggested causes include metabolic disease, local infection, and trauma. Most children with vertebral disc calcification are 5 months to 11 years old, and boys are more frequently affected than girls. Symptomatic disc calcification occurs most commonly in the lower cervical spine, usually at the C6-7 level, and approximately one third of patients have multiple levels involved. In children, calcification involves the nucleus pulposus, in contrast to the process in adults, which involves the annulus fibrosus (Fig. 43-45).

The most common symptoms of intervertebral disc calcification are neck pain, limitation of motion, and torticollis. Radicular pain or signs of nerve root compression are rare. Approximately 25% of patients have fever; 30% of patients have a history of trauma, and 15% have a history of upper respiratory tract infection. Pain usually begins suddenly and persists for 2 to 3 weeks; 75% of children are asymptomatic by 3 weeks, and 95% are asymptomatic within 6 months. Dai et al. found that the average time for symptoms to resolve was 34 days, and resolution of the calcifications was seen on radiographs by 15 months. Neurologic deficits, if present, improve in 90% of patients. Disc herniation is rare, but posterior herniations can cause spinal cord compression, and anterior herniations may result in dysphagia.

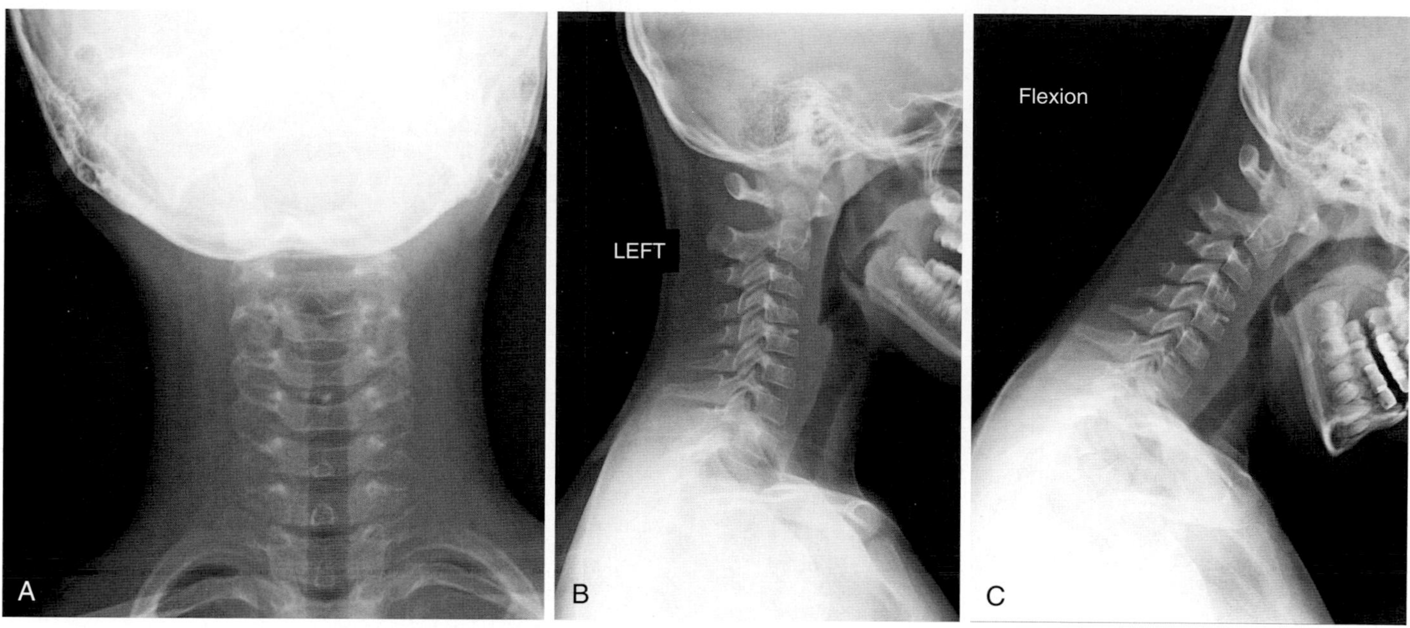

FIGURE 43-45 Intervertebral disc calcification in an 8-year-old boy.

Appropriate treatment consists of rest, cervical immobilization, and analgesics. Rarely, symptomatic nerve root or spinal cord impingement requires anterior discectomy and fusion. The long-term effects of intervertebral disc calcification are unknown, but permanent changes around the adjacent vertebral bodies that may be associated with early degenerative changes have been reported in young adults.

REFERENCES

EMBRYOLOGY AND GROWTH AND DEVELOPMENT

Gholve PA, Hosalkar HS, Ricchetti ET, et al: Occipitalization of the atlas in children: morphologic classification, associations, and clinical relevance, *J Bone Joint Surg* 89A:571, 2007.

Herring TA, editor: *Tachdjian's pediatric orthopaedics*, ed 4, Philadelphia, 2008, Elsevier.

Hosalkar HS, Sankar WN, Wills BPD, et al: Congenital osseous anomalies of the upper cervical spine, *J Bone Joint Surg* 90A:337, 2008.

Kaplan KM, Spivak JM, Bendo JA: Embryology of the spine and associated congenital abnormalities, *Spine J* 5:564, 2005.

McKay SD, Al-Omari A, Tomlinson LA, Dormans JP: Review of cervical spine anomalies in genetic syndromes, *Spine (Phila Pa 1976)* 37:E269, 2012.

SURGICAL APPROACHES

Mulpuri K, LeBlanc JG, Reilly CW, et al: Sternal split approach to the cervicothoracic junction in children, *Spine* 30:E305, 2005.

ANOMALIES OF THE ODONTOID

Arvin B, Fournier-Gosselin MP, Fehlings MG: Os odontoideum: etiology and surgical management, *Neurosurgery* 66:A22, 2010.

Kim IS, Hong JT, Jang WY, et al: Surgical treatment of os odontoideum, *J Clin Neurosci* 18:481, 2011.

Klimo P Jr, Coon V, Brockmeyer D: Incidental os odontoideum: current management strategies, *Neurosurg Focus* 31:E10, 2011.

Klimo P, Kan P, Rao G, et al: Os odontoideum: presentation, diagnosis, and treatment in a series of 78 patients, *J Neurosurg Spine* 9:332, 2008.

Leng LZ, Anand VK, Hartl R, Schwartz TH: Endonasal endoscopic resection of an os odontoideum to decompress the cervicomedullary junction: a minimal access surgical technique, *Spine* 34:E139, 2009.

Sankar WN, Wills BP, Dorman JP, Drummond DS: Os odontoideum revisited: the case for a multifactorial etiology, *Spine* 31:979, 2006.

Wada E, Matsuoka T, Kawai H: Os odontoideum as a consequence of a posttraumatic displaced ossiculum terminale. A case report, *J Bone Joint Surg Am* 91:1750, 2009.

Weng C, Tian W, Li ZY, et al: Surgical management of symptomatic os odontoideum with posterior screw fixation performed using the Magerl and Harms techniques with intraoperative 3-dimensional fluoroscopy-based navigation, *Spine (Phila Pa 1976)* 37:1839, 2012.

Zygourakis CC, Cahill KS, Proctor MR: Delayed development of os odontoideum after traumatic cervical injury: support for a vascular etiology, *J Neurosurg Pediatr* 7:201, 2011.

BASILAR IMPRESSION

Botelho RV, Neto EB, Patriota GC, et al: Basilar invagination: craniocervical instability treated with cervical traction and occipitocervical fixation. Case report, *J Neurosurg Spine* 7:444, 2007.

Dasenbrock HH, Clarke MJ, Bydon A, et al: Endoscopic image-guided transcervical odontoidectomy: outcomes of 15 patients, *Neurosurgery* 70:359, 2012.

Hedequist D, Bekelis K, Emans J, Proctor MR: Single stage reduction and stabilization of basilar invagination after failed prior fusion surgery in children with Down's syndrome, *Spine* 35:E128, 2010.

McGirt MJ, Attenello FJ, Sciobba DM, et al: Endoscopic transcervical odontoidectomy of pediatric basilar invagination and cranial settling. Report of 4 cases, *J Neurosurg Pediatr* 1:337, 2008.

Smith JS, Shaffrey CI, Abel MF, Menezes AH: Basilar invagination, *Neurosurgery* 66:39, 2010.

Wolinsky JP, Sciubba DM, Suk I, Gokaslan ZL: Endoscopic image-guided odontoidectomy for decompression of basilar invagination via a standard anterior cervical approach. Technical note, *J Neurosurg Spine* 6:184, 2007.

Yu Y, Hu F, Zhang X, et al: Endoscopic transnasal odontoidectomy combined with posterior reduction to treat basilar invagination: technical note, *J Neurosurg Spine* 19:637, 2013.

ATLANTOOCCIPITAL FUSION

Gholve PA, Hosalkar HS, Ricchetti ET, et al: Occipitalization of the atlas. Morphologic classification, association, and clinical relevance, *J Bone Joint Surg Am* 89:571, 2007.

Tubbs RS, Salter EG, Oakes WJ: The intracranial entrance of the atlantal segment of the vertebral artery in crania with occipitalization of the atlas, *J Neurosurg Spine* 4:319, 2006.

Wang S, Wang C, Liu Y, et al: Anomalous vertebral artery in craniovertebral junction with occipitalization of the atlas, *Spine* 34:2838, 2009.

KLIPPEL-FEIL SYNDROME

Auerbach JD, Kusuma SK, Hosalkar HS, et al: Spinal cord dimensions in children with Klippel-Feil syndrome: a controlled, blinded radiographic analysis with implications for neurologic outcomes, *Spine* 33:1366, 2008.

Bettegowda C, Sharjari M, Suk I, et al: Sublabial approach for the treatment of symptomatic basilar impression in a patient with Klippel-Feil syndrome, *Neurosurgery* 69(ONS Suppl 1):ons77, 2011.

Samartzis D, Herman J, Lubicky JP, Shen FH: Classification of congenitally fused cervical patterns in Klippel-Feil patients, *Spine* 31:E798, 2006.

Samartzis D, Herman J, Lubicky JP, Shen FH: Sprengel's deformity in Klippel-Feil syndrome, *Spine* 32:E512, 2007.

Samartzis D, Kalluri P, Herman J, et al: The extent of fusion within the congenital Klippel-Feil segment, *Spine* 33:1637, 2008.

Samartzis D, Kalluri P, Herman J, et al: 2008 Young Investigator Award: The role of congenitally fused cervical segments upon the space available for the cord and associated symptoms in Klippel-Feil patients, *Spine* 33:1442, 2008.

Samartzis D, Kalluri P, Herman J, et al: Cervical scoliosis in the Klippel-Feil patients, *Spine* 36:E1501, 2011.

Xue X, Shen J, Zhang J, et al: Klippel-Feil syndrome in congenital scoliosis, *Spine (Phila Pa 1976)* 39:E1343, 2014.

ATLANTOAXIAL ROTATORY SUBLUXATION

Been HD, Kerkhoffs GM, Maas M: Suspected atlantoaxial rotatory fixation-subluxation: the value of multidetector computed tomography scanning under general anesthesia, *Spine* 31:E163, 2007.

Beier AD, Vachhrajani S, Bayerl SH, et al: Rotatory subluxation: experience from the Hospital for Sick Children, *J Neurosurg Pediatr* 9:144, 2012.

Park SW, Cho KH, Shin YS, et al: Successful reduction for a pediatric chronic atlantoaxial rotatory fixation (Grisel syndrome) with long-term halter traction: case report, *Spine* 30:E444, 2005.

CERVICAL INSTABILITY IN DOWN SYNDROME

Bull MJ, Committee on Genetics: Health supervision for children with Down syndrome, *Pediatrics* 128:393, 2011.

Pizzutillo PD, Herman MJ: Cervical spine issues in Down syndrome, *J Pediatr Orthop* 25:253, 2005.

LARSEN SYNDROME

Jain VV, Anadio JM, Chang G, et al: Dural ectasia in a child with Larsen syndrome, *J Pediatr Orthop* 34:e44, 2014.

Katz DA, Hall JE, Emans JB: Cervical kyphosis associated with anteroposterior dissociation and quadriparesis in Larsen syndrome, *J Pediatr Orthop* 25:429, 2005.

Madera M, Crawford A, Mangano FT: Management of severe cervical kyphosis in a patient with Larsen syndrome: case report, *J Neurosurg Pediatr* 1:320, 2008.

Sakaura H, Matsuoka T, Iwasaki M, et al: Surgical treatment of cervical kyphosis in Larsen syndrome: report of 3 cases and review of the literature, *Spine* 3:E39, 2007.

INTERVERTEBRAL DISC CALCIFICATION

Bajard X, Renault F, Benharrats T, et al: Intervertebral disc calcification with neurological symptoms in children: report of conservative treatment in two cases, *Childs Nerv Syst* 26:973, 2010.

Beluffi G, Fiori P, Sileo C: Intervertebral disc calcifications in children, *Radiol Med* 114:331, 2009.

Chu J, Wang T, Pei S, Yin Z: Surgical treatment for idiopathic intervertebral disc calcification in a child: case report and review of the literature, *Childs Nerv Syst* 31:123, 2015.

Lernout C, Haas H, Rubio A, Griffet J: Pediatric intervertebral disk calcification in childhood: three case reports and review of the literature, *Childs Nerv Syst* 25:1019, 2009.

The complete list of references is available online at ***expertconsult.inkling.com.***

CHAPTER 44

SCOLIOSIS AND KYPHOSIS

William C. Warner Jr., Jeffery R. Sawyer

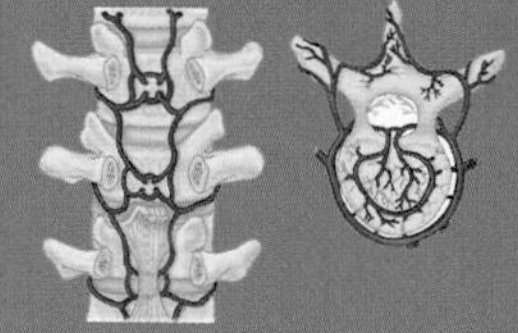

SCOLIOSIS

The word *scoliosis* is derived from the Greek word meaning "crooked." Scoliosis is defined as a lateral deviation of the normal vertical line of the spine. The lateral curvature of the spine also is associated with rotation of the vertebrae. This produces a three-dimensional deformity of the spine that occurs in the sagittal, frontal, and coronal planes.

The Scoliosis Research Society recommends that idiopathic scoliosis be classified according to the age of the patient when the diagnosis is made. Infantile scoliosis occurs from birth to 3 years of age; juvenile idiopathic scoliosis, between the ages of 4 and 10 years; and adolescent idiopathic scoliosis, between 10 years of age and skeletal maturity. This traditional chronologic definition of scoliosis is important because major differences exist between the subtypes (Table 44-1).

Scoliosis also can be classified based on the cause and associated conditions. Idiopathic scoliosis is the most common type, but the exact cause of this type of scoliosis is not known. Congenital scoliosis is caused by a failure in vertebral formation or segmentation of the involved vertebrae. Scoliosis also can be classified based on associated conditions, such as neuromuscular disorders (cerebral palsy, muscular dystrophy, or other neuromuscular disorders), associated syndromes, or generalized disease (neurofibromatosis, Marfan syndrome, bone dysplasia, tumors, or as a result of irradiation).

A distinction should be made between early-onset and late-onset scoliosis because the deformity may affect cardiopulmonary development. During childhood, not only do the lungs grow in size, but also the alveoli and arteries multiply and the pattern of vascularity changes. The alveoli in the pulmonary tree increase by about 10-fold between infancy and 4 years of age and are not completely developed until 8 years of age. Scoliotic deformity limits the space available for lung growth, and children who develop significant scoliosis before the age of 5 years generally have disabling dyspnea or cardiorespiratory failure. Currently, according to the classification as it relates to treatment, some infantile and early juvenile curves are being identified as early-onset scoliosis.

INFANTILE IDIOPATHIC SCOLIOSIS

Infantile idiopathic scoliosis is a structural, lateral curvature of the spine occurring in patients younger than age 3 years. James, who first used the term *infantile idiopathic scoliosis,* noted that these curves occurred before 3 years of age, were more frequent in boys than in girls, and were primarily thoracic and convex to the left.

Wynne-Davies noted plagiocephaly in 97 children in whom curves developed in the first 6 months of life; the flat side of the head was on the convex side of the curve. Other associated conditions that she found were intellectual impairment in 13%, inguinal hernias in 7.4% of boys with progressive scoliosis, developmental dislocation of the hip in 3.5%, and congenital heart disease in 2.5% of all patients. This led her to believe that the etiologic factors of infantile idiopathic scoliosis are multiple, with a genetic tendency that is either "triggered" or prevented by external factors.

Infantile idiopathic scoliosis is more common in Europe than in North America. In the early 1970s, infantile scoliosis was seen in 41% of patients with idiopathic scoliosis in Great Britain compared with less than 1% in the United States. This difference was believed to be from infant positioning (Fig. 44-1). Supine positioning was recommended in Europe, and prone positioning was recommended in the United States. Since the change to prone positioning, the incidence of

TABLE 44-1

Classification of Idiopathic Scoliosis by Age

PARAMETER	INFANTILE	JUVENILE	ADOLESCENT
Age at presentation	Birth to 3 yr	4 to 9 yr	10 to 20 yr
Male : female	1 : 1 to 2 : 1	<6 yr: 1 : 3 >6 yr: 1 : 6	1 : 6
Incidence	United States: 2% to 3% Great Britain: 30%	United States: 12% to 15% Great Britain: 12% to 15%	United States: 85% Great Britain: 55%
Curve types	Left thoracic L : R (2 : 1) Left thoracic/right lumbar	Right thoracic R : L (6 : 1)	Right thoracic R : L (8 : 1)
Associated findings	Mental deficiency, congenital hip dysplasia, plagiocephaly, congenital heart defects	None	None
Risk of cardiopulmonary compromise	High	Intermediate	Low
Risk of curve progression	<6 mo: low >1 yr: high	67%	23%
Rate of curve progression	Gradual progression: 2 to 3 degrees/yr Malignant progression: 10 degrees/yr	Progression at puberty: 6 degrees/yr Malignant progression: 10 degrees/yr	1 to 2 degrees/mo during puberty
Curve resolution	<1 yr: 90% >1 yr: 20%	20%	Rare
Curve magnitude and maturity	Gradual progression: 70 to 90 degrees Malignant progression: >90 degrees	Progression at puberty: 50 to 90 degrees Malignant progression: >90 degrees	Curves > 90 degrees are rare
Orthotic management	Effective at delaying and slowing rate of progression Ultimate progression: 100%	Decreases rate of progression until puberty (failure rate: 30% to 80%)	Effectively controls curves < 40 degrees (success rate: 75% to 80%)
Surgical treatment	Instrumentation without fusion <8 yr After 8 yr: ASF-PSF After 11 yr: PSF	Instrumentation without fusion <8 yr After 8 yr: ASF-PSF After 1 yr: PSF	PSF with instrumentation ASF if younger than 11 yr with open triradiate cartilage
Risk of crankshaft	High	High	Low

ASF, anterior spinal fusion; PSF, posterior spinal fusion.
Modified from Mardjetko SM: Infantile and juvenile scoliosis. In Bridwell KH, DeWald RL, editors: The textbook of spinal surgery, ed 2, Philadelphia, 1997, Lippincott-Raven.

infantile idiopathic scoliosis has declined in Great Britain from 41% to 4%.

Most curves in infantile idiopathic scoliosis are self-limiting and spontaneously resolve (70% to 90%); however, some curves may be progressive, usually increasing rapidly, are often difficult to manage, and may result in significant deformity and pulmonary impairment. Unfortunately, when a curve is mild, no absolute criteria are available for differentiating the two types and predicting progression. James et al. found that those with resolving scoliosis generally had a deformity that was noted before 1 year of age; most had smaller curves at presentation, and none had compensatory curves. Lloyd-Roberts and Pilcher found that curves associated with plagiocephaly or other molding abnormalities were more likely to be resolving, indicating an intrauterine positioning cause of this scoliosis. According to James, when compensatory or secondary curves develop or when the curve measures more than 37 degrees by the Cobb method when first seen, the scoliosis probably will be progressive.

Mehta developed a method to differentiate resolving from progressive curves in infantile idiopathic scoliosis based on measurement of the rib-vertebral angle (RVA). She evaluated the relationship of the convex rib head and vertebral body of the apical vertebra by drawing one line perpendicular to the apical vertebral endplate and another from the midneck to the midhead of the corresponding rib; the angle formed by the intersection of these lines is the RVA (Fig. 44-2). The RVA difference (RVAD) is the difference between the values of the RVAs on the concave and convex sides of the curve. Mehta reported that 83% of the curves resolved if the RVAD measured less than 20 degrees and that 84% of the curves progressed if the RVAD was greater than 20 degrees. She described a two-phase radiographic appearance based on the relationship of the apical ribs with the apical vertebra. In phase 1, the rib head on each side of the apical vertebra does not overlap the vertebral body. In phase 2, the rib head overlaps the convex side of the vertebral body. Phase 2 curves are progressive, and therefore the measurement of RVAD is

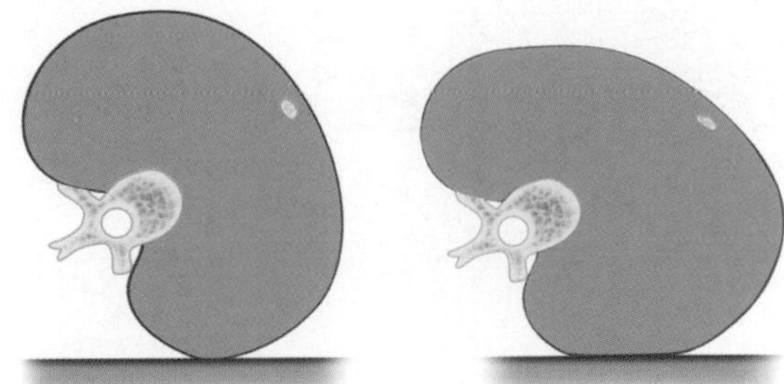

FIGURE 44-1 Diagram illustrates postural molding of thorax when infant is laid supine and partly turned toward the side.

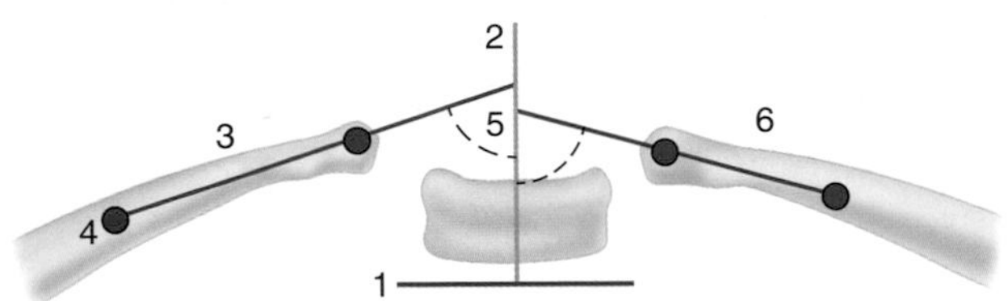

FIGURE 44-2 Construction of rib-vertebral angle (RVA) and rib-vertebral angle difference (RVAD). 1. Draw a line parallel to the bottom of the apical vertebra (apical vertebral endplate). 2. Draw a line perpendicular to the line drawn in Step 1. 3. Find the midpoint of the head of the rib. Find the midpoint of the neck of the rib. These landmarks are estimated and mental note is taken. 4. Draw a line from the midpoint of the head of the rib to the midpoint of the neck of the rib to the line from Step 2. 5. The resulting angle is the RVA for one side. 6. To calculate the RVAD, calculate the RVA for the other side. Use the lines created in Steps 1 and 2, and repeat Steps 3-5 for the other side. (From Corna J, Sanders JO, Luhmann SJ, et al: Reliability of radiographic measures for infantile idiopathic scoliosis, J Bone Joint Surg 94A:e86, 2012.)

unnecessary. These measurements are helpful in predicting curve progression, but the curves must be monitored closely to prevent severe progression with the resultant risk of restricted pulmonary disease. These measurements are helpful in predicting curve progression, but Corona et al. noted that these measurements should be used with care because of some variability of more than 10 degrees in 18% of paired observations. This highlights the necessity of closely monitoring curves both clinically and radiographically to prevent severe progression with the resultant risk of restricted pulmonary disease (Fig. 44-3).

An increased incidence of neural axis abnormalities (Chiari malformation, syrinx, low-lying conus, and brainstem tumor) has been noted on MRI in patients with infantile idiopathic scoliosis (21.7%). MRI evaluation is now recommended for infantile scoliosis for curves measuring more than 20 degrees. These patients usually require sedation for MRI. Pahys found a smaller percentage (13%) of patients with infantile scoliosis and intraspinal anomalies. Because of the need for sedation to obtain the MRI, close observation may be a reasonable alternative.

TREATMENT

Because of the favorable natural history in 70% to 90% of patients with infantile idiopathic scoliosis, active treatment often is not required. If the initial curve is less than 25 degrees

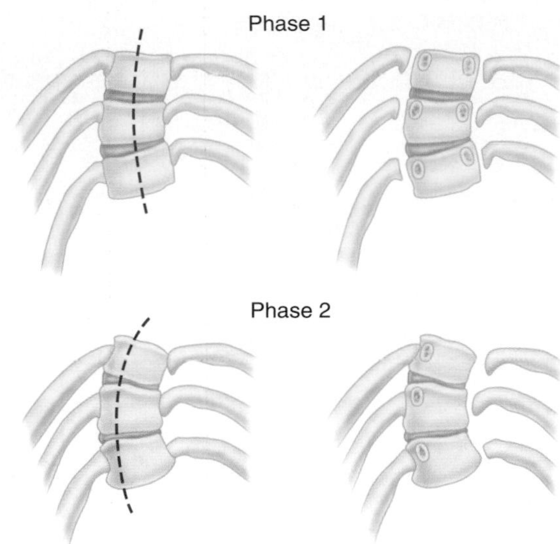

FIGURE 44-3 Two phases in progression of infantile scoliosis as seen on posteroanterior radiographs. Phase 1: rib head on convex side does not overlap vertebral body. Phase 2: rib head on convex side overlaps vertebral body. (Redrawn from Herring JA, editor: Tachdjian's pediatric orthopaedics, ed 4, Philadelphia, 2008, Elsevier, p 337.)

and the RVAD is less than 20 degrees, observation with radiographic follow-up every 6 months is recommended. Most resolving curves correct by 3 years of age (Fig. 44-4); however, follow-up should continue even after resolution because scoliosis may recur in adolescence.

CASTING

Treatment options for children with progressive infantile idiopathic scoliosis curves include serial casting, bracing, and later fusion; preoperative traction to correct the curve followed by fusion; and growing rod or vertical expandable prosthetic titanium rib (VEPTR) instrumentation without fusion (Synthes, West Chester, PA). Once the diagnosis of a progressive curve is made based on either a progressive Cobb angle or an RVAD of more than 20 degrees, rib phase 2, or a double curve, treatment is recommended. An orthotist can make a satisfactory thoracolumbosacral orthosis (TLSO) or cervicothoracolumbosacral orthosis (CTLSO) for curves that are not too large. Progression of many infantile curves can be prevented and significant improvement can be obtained with the use of a well-fitting orthosis during the early period of skeletal growth. In a very young child, serial casting with general anesthesia may be required until the child is large enough for a satisfactory orthosis. The interval between cast changes is determined by the rate of the child's growth, but a cast change usually is required every 2 to 3 months. Brace wear is continued full time until the curve stability has been maintained for at least 2 years. At that point, brace wear can be gradually reduced. McMaster reported control of the curves in 22 children with infantile scoliosis with an average brace time of more than 6 years.

Sanders et al. reported good results with early casting for progressive infantile idiopathic scoliosis using the technique of Cotrel and Morel (extension, derotation, flexion) cast correction. Best results were achieved if casting was started

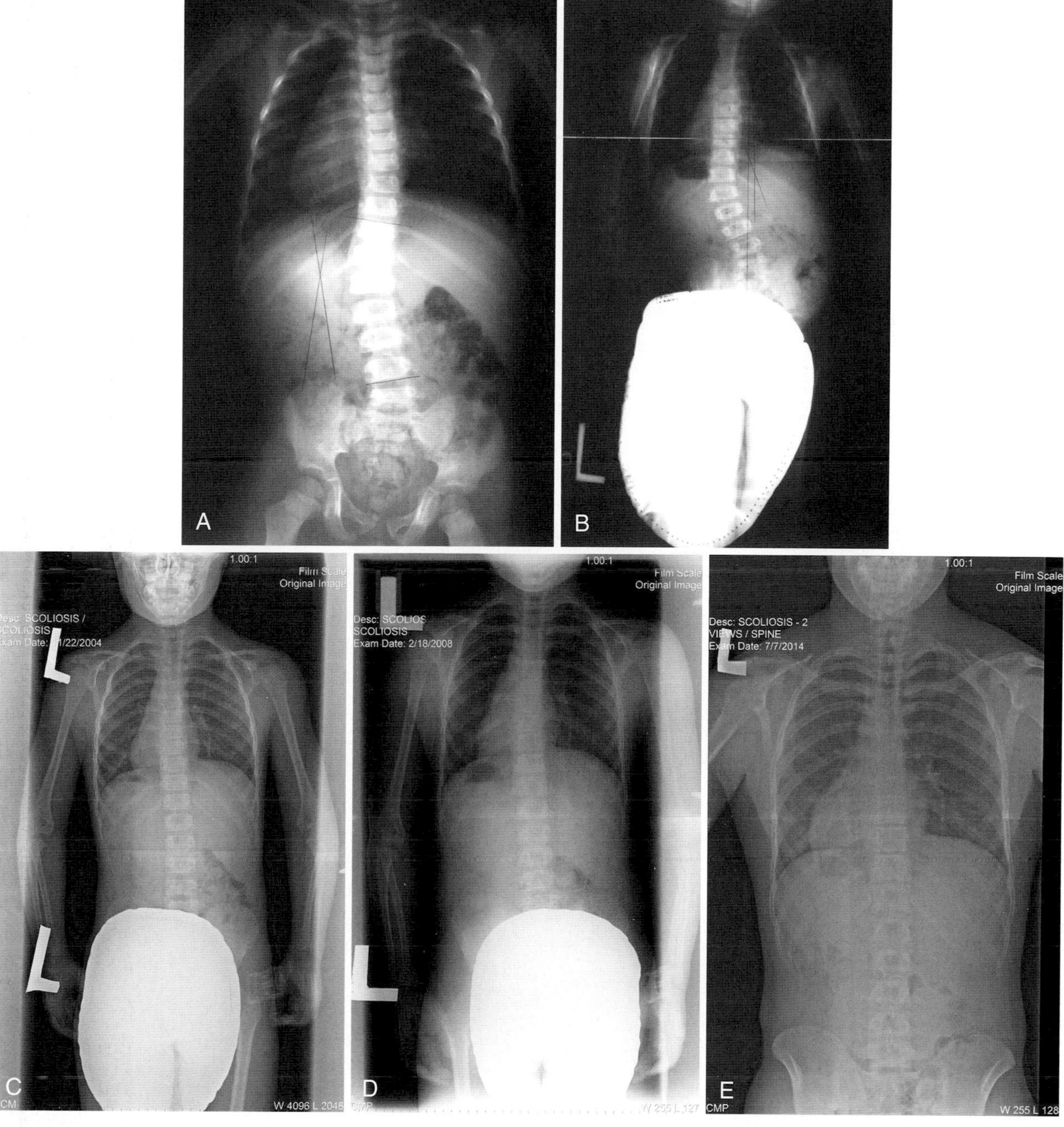

FIGURE 44-4 **A,** Infantile scoliosis in a 3-year-old child. **B,** At 4 years of age. **C,** At 6 years of age, curve has greatly improved and by 10 years of age **(D)** has resolved. **E,** At follow-up at age 16, there is no curve progression.

before 20 months of age and in curves less than 60 degrees. Cast correction in older patients with curves of more than 60 degrees frequently resulted in curve improvement (Fig. 44-5). Casts were changed every 2 to 4 months based on age and growth of the child. Once curves were corrected to less than 10 degrees, a custom-molded brace was used.

CASTING FOR IDIOPATHIC SCOLIOSIS

A proper casting table is crucial for this procedure. Although a standard Risser frame will suffice, it is quite large for small children. Sanders et al. have designed a table that leaves the head, arms, and legs supported but the body free for cast application.

TECHNIQUE 44-1

- Intubate the patient; thoracic pressure during cast molding can make ventilation temporarily difficult.
- Use a silver-impregnated shirt as the innermost layer. Head halter and pelvic traction also are used to assist in stabilizing the patient and in narrowing the body (Fig. 44-6A).
- A mirror slanted under the table is useful for viewing rib prominence, the posterior cast, and molds.
- Apply a thin layer of Webril with occasional felt on bony prominences.
- If there is a lumbar curve, flex the hips slightly to decrease lumbar lordosis and facilitate curve correction.

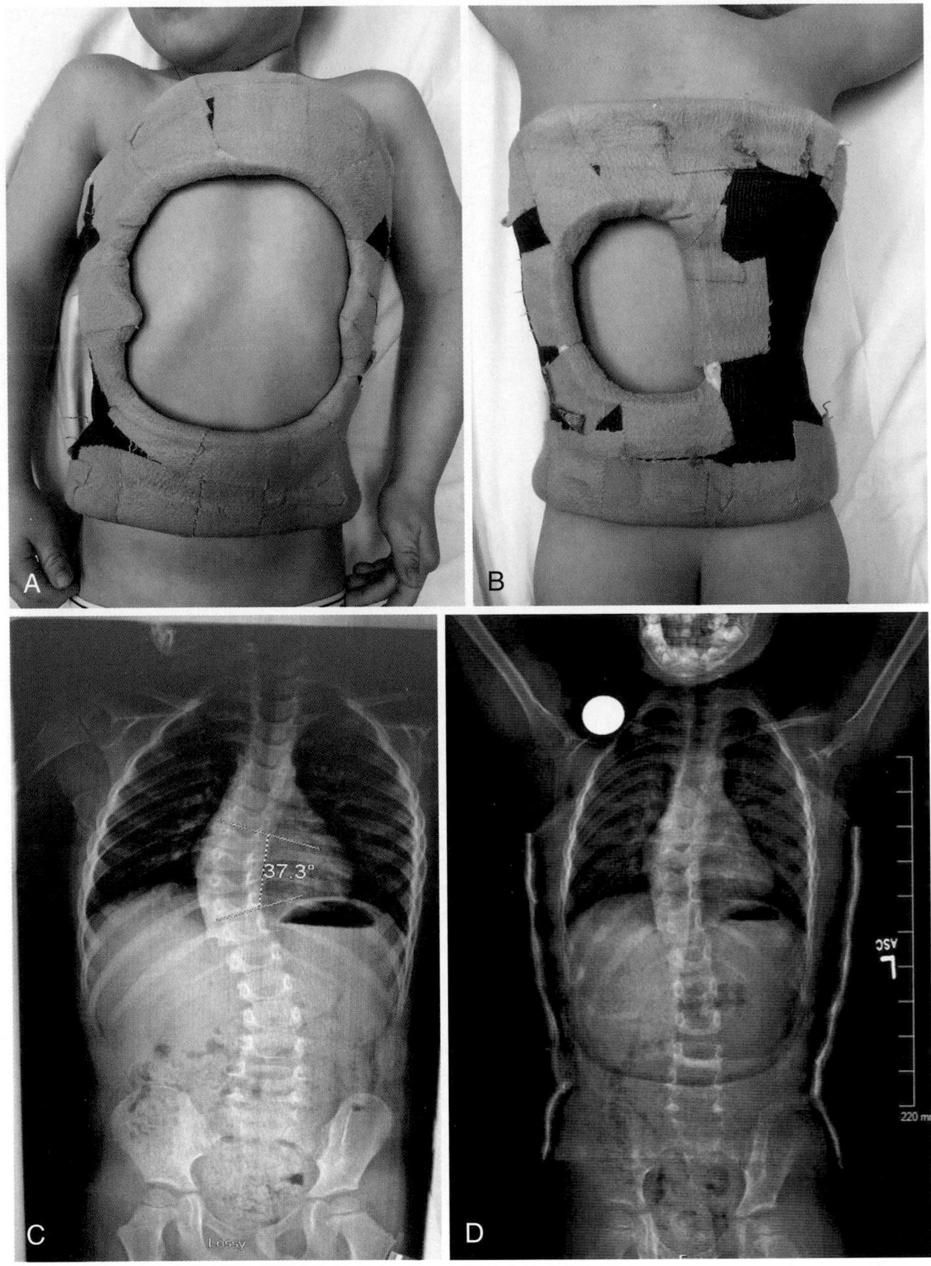

FIGURE 44-5 **A** and **B,** Mehta cast. **C,** Before cast wear. **D,** After 9 months of cast wear.

- Plaster is usually preferred over fiberglass because it is more moldable. The pelvic portion is the foundation of the cast and should be well molded.
- Apply pressure to the posteriorly rotated ribs with an attempt to anteriorly rotate these ribs to create a more normal chest configuration with counterrotation applied through the pelvic mold and upper torso. This is a derotation maneuver and should not push the ribs toward the spine in an attempt to correct the curve (Fig. 44-6B).
- If the apex is T9 or below, an underarm cast can be used, but the original technique used an over-the-shoulder cast.
- Create an anterior window to relieve the chest and abdomen while preventing the lower ribs from rotating. Create a posterior window on the concave side to allow the depressed concave ribs and spine to move posteriorly (Fig. 44-6C).

OPERATIVE TREATMENT

If a curve is severe or increases despite the use of an orthosis or casting, surgical stabilization is needed. Ideally, surgery should not only stop progression of the curve but also allow continued growth of the thorax and development of the pulmonary tree. Growing rods can be used to control curve progression and still allow for growth of the spine (see **Video 44-1**). This usually requires surgery every 6 months to

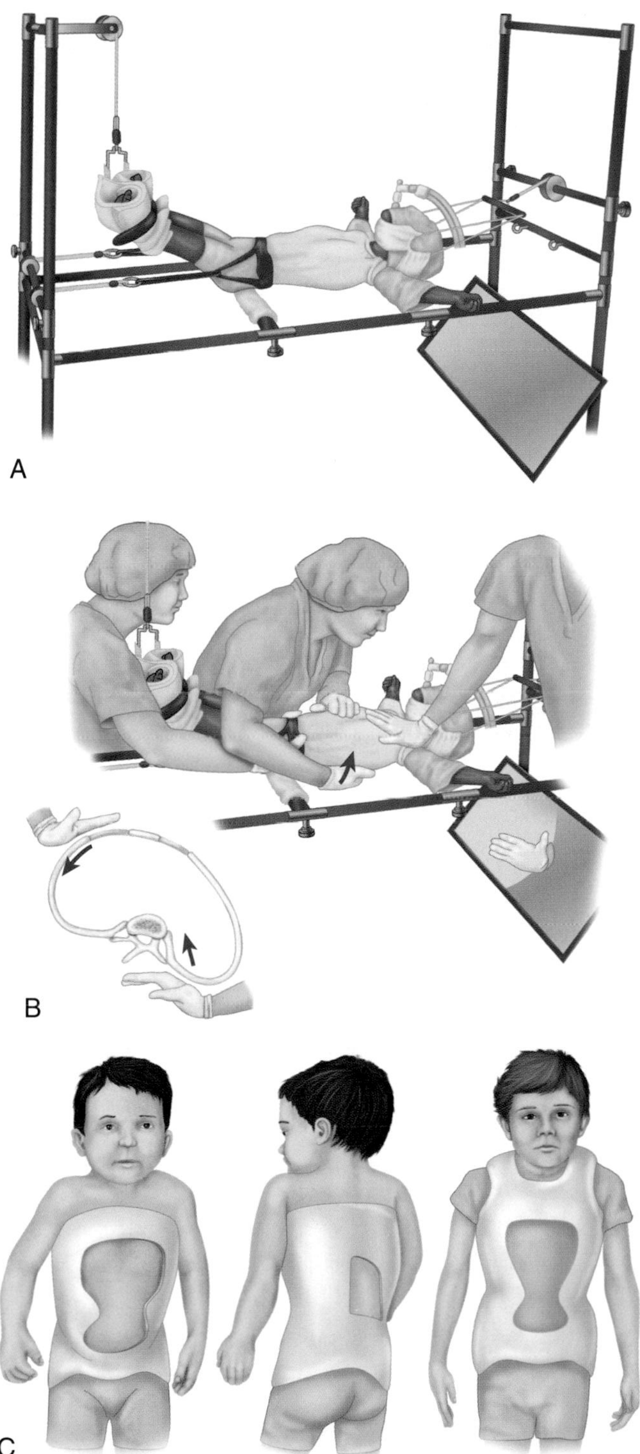

FIGURE 44-6 **A,** Position on table with traction applied to halter and pelvis. **B,** Example of correction maneuver for derotation of left thoracic curve. **C,** Underarm cast with windows. (Redrawn from Sanders JO, D'Astous J, Fitzgerald M, et al: Derotational casting for progressive infantile scoliosis, J Pediatr Orthop 29:581, 2009.) **SEE TECHNIQUE 44-1.**

lengthen the rods (see Technique 44-2 and **Video 44-2**). The use of magnetically controlled growing rods, such as the MAGEC Spinal Bracing and Distraction System (NuVasive, Aliso Viejo, CA), avoids a return to surgery every 6 months. VEPTR instrumentation has been reported as another alternative to correct the curve and allow for continued growth of the spine (see Technique 44-46). Schulz et al. reported this to be a safe and effective treatment of progressive curves in this patient population. When surgical fusion is necessary, a relatively short anterior and posterior arthrodesis should be considered, including only the structural or primary curve. Combined anterior and posterior arthrodesis is necessary to prevent the "crankshaft" phenomenon. The problem with this approach is that it leaves the child with a straight, shortened spine rather than a deformed spine of near-normal length. Karol reported that, despite early fusion surgery, revision surgery was required in 24% to 39% of patients. Restrictive pulmonary disease, defined as forced vital capacity less than 50% of normal, occurs in 43% to 64% of patients who have early fusion surgery. Thoracic growth after early surgery is an average of 50% of that seen in children with scoliosis who did not have early surgery. Because of the deleterious effect on the developing thoracic cage and lung function, fusionless instrumentation techniques are preferred.

JUVENILE IDIOPATHIC SCOLIOSIS

Juvenile idiopathic scoliosis appears between the ages of 4 and 10 years. Multiple patterns can occur, but the convexity of the thoracic curve usually is to the right. Juvenile idiopathic scoliosis accounts for 12% to 21% of idiopathic scoliosis cases. The female-to-male ratio is 1:1 in children between 3 and 6 years of age. This ratio increases with age, with the ratio of 4:1 from 6 to 10 years of age, and reaches a female-to-male ratio of 8:1 by the time the children are 10 years of age. The natural history of juvenile idiopathic scoliosis is usually slow to moderate progression until the pubertal growth spurt. Lonstein found that 67% of patients younger than age 10 years showed curve progression and that the risk of progression was 100% in patients younger than 10 years who had curves of more than 20 degrees. Robinson and McMaster reported curve progression in 95% of children with juvenile idiopathic scoliosis. Of those patients followed to maturity, 86% required spinal fusion. Most juvenile curves are convex right thoracic curve or double thoracic curve patterns and closely resemble those of adolescent idiopathic scoliosis. Few patients with juvenile idiopathic scoliosis have thoracolumbar or lumbar curves. Dobbs et al. modified the adolescent idiopathic scoliosis classification system of Lenke for juvenile idiopathic scoliosis (see Fig. 44-35). (There are the same six curve types, but instead of using side-bending radiographs to distinguish structural from nonstructural minor curves the authors used the deviation from the midline of the apex of the curve from the C7 plumb line for thoracic curves and the center sacral vertical line for thoracolumbar and lumbar curves. If the apex of the curve is completely off the line, a structural minor curve is present; if the apex is not off the line, a nonstructural minor curve is present.)

As in infantile idiopathic scoliosis, a high incidence of neural axis abnormalities has been found on MRI in children younger than 11 years with scoliosis (26.7%). Some may argue about the need for MRI in a routine preoperative workup, but most would agree that specific factors indicating a need for further MRI evaluation include pain, rapid progression, left thoracic deformity, neurologic abnormalities (alterations in the superficial abdominal reflex), and other neurologic findings, such as loss of bowel or bladder control. If operative intervention is planned, then preoperative MRI evaluation is recommended.

TREATMENT

Although it is likely to progress and often requires surgery, juvenile idiopathic scoliosis is treated according to guidelines similar to those for adolescent idiopathic scoliosis. For curves of less than 20 degrees, observation is indicated, with examination and standing posteroanterior radiographs every 4 to 6 months. Evidence of progression on the radiographs as indicated by a change of at least 5 to 7 degrees warrants brace treatment. If the curve is not progressing, observation is continued until skeletal maturity.

Although much of the earlier literature concerning orthotic treatment of juvenile idiopathic scoliosis had emphasized the Milwaukee brace, a TLSO is used for thoracic curves with the apex at T8 or below. Initially, the brace is worn full time (22 of 24 hours). If the curve improves after at least 1 year of full-time bracing, the hours per day of brace wear can be decreased gradually to a nighttime-only bracing program, which is much more tolerable, especially when the child reaches puberty. However, the patient is carefully observed for any sign of curve progression during this weaning process. If curve progression is noted, a full-time bracing program is resumed.

The success of nonoperative treatment is variable; 27% to 56% require spinal fusion for progressive curves. It often is not possible to predict which curves will increase from the curve pattern, the degree of curvature, or the patient's age at the time of diagnosis. Serial RVAD measurements have been useful to evaluate brace treatment; several guidelines can be formulated for evaluating brace treatment (Box 44-1).

Evidence of progression should be obtained before a brace is applied, unless the curve is greater than 30 degrees when the juvenile patient is first seen. Some curves, even in the range of 20 to 30 degrees, did not progress during a period of several months in one study; Mannherz et al. found progressive RVAD of more than 10 degrees over time to be associated with curve progression, and more frequent curve progression was noted in patients with less than 20 degrees of thoracic kyphosis. Double major curves tended to progress most often. Charles et al. reported that juvenile curves of more than 30 degrees had a 100% risk of progression to a surgical range, underscoring the importance of beginning treatment in curves of more than 30 degrees.

Kahanovitz, Levine, and Lardone found that patients who wore a Milwaukee brace part time (after school and at night) had good outcomes with curves of less than 35 degrees and RVADs of less than 20 degrees. Patients with curvatures of greater than 45 degrees at the onset of bracing and whose RVADs exceeded 20 degrees all eventually underwent spinal fusion. Patients with curvatures from 35 to 45 degrees at the onset of bracing had much less predictable prognoses. The part-time brace program consisted of wearing the brace after school and all night for approximately a year. The patients were then kept in the brace at night only for another 2.5 years. The brace was at that point worn every other night for an average of 1.2 years. Bracing generally was discontinued completely at an average of about 14 years of age. Individually, however, the numbers of hours spent wearing the brace depended on the amount of improvement and stability of the curvature. Part-time brace treatment may afford these children the social and psychological benefits not provided by a full-time brace program. Jarvis et al. reported the successful management (prevention of surgery) with part-time bracing in patients with juvenile idiopathic scoliosis. The Milwaukee brace may be preferred because it does not cause chest wall compression in these young patients. A total-contact TLSO often is prescribed, but rib cage distortion is possible because of the lengthy time the child must wear the brace. Robinson and McMaster found that the level of the most rotated vertebra at the apex of the primary curve was the most useful factor in determining the prognosis of patients with juvenile idiopathic scoliosis. Patients who had a curve apex at T8, T9, or T10 had an 80% chance of requiring spinal arthrodesis by 15 years of age. Khoshbin et al. reported that 50% of their patients progressed to surgery despite brace treatment. The operative rate was higher for patients with curves of more than 30 degrees at the start of brace treatment.

Even if the curve progresses, bracing may slow progression and delay surgery until the child is older, which may avoid a short trunk and lessen the possibility of a crankshaft phenomenon. If orthotic treatment fails, operative management of the curve should be considered. Important considerations in the operative treatment of patients with juvenile idiopathic scoliosis are the expected loss of spinal height and the limited chest wall growth and lung development after spinal fusion. Another important consideration is the crankshaft phenomenon. With a solid posterior fusion, continued anterior growth of the vertebral bodies causes the vertebral body and discs to bulge laterally toward the convexity and to pivot on the posterior fusion, causing loss of correction, increase in vertebral rotation, and recurrence of the rib hump. Dimeglio found that during the first 5 years of life the spine from T1 to S1 grows more than 2 cm a year. Between the ages of 5 and 10 years, it grows 0.9 cm per year, and then it grows 1.8 cm per year during puberty (Fig. 44-7). A solid spinal fusion stops the longitudinal growth in the posterior elements, but the vertebral bodies continue to grow anteriorly.

There is no full agreement about the exact parameters for which a child requires anterior and posterior fusions to prevent crankshaft deformity (Figs. 44-8 and 44-9). Shufflebarger and Clark recommended that patients with a Risser

BOX 44-1

Evaluation of Brace Treatment of Juvenile Idiopathic Scoliosis by the Rib–Vertebral Angle Difference (RVAD)

- If the RVAD values progress above 10 degrees during brace wear, progression can be expected.
- If the RVAD values decline as treatment continues, part-time brace wear should be adequate.
- Those patients with curves with RVAD values near or below 0 degrees at the time of diagnosis generally will require only a short period of full-time brace wear before part-time brace wear is begun.

sign of grade 0 or 1, a Tanner grade of less than 2, and a significant three-dimensional deformity have a preliminary anterior periapical fusion before posterior instrumentation and fusion. Sanders et al. noted that 10 of 43 patients with triradiate cartilage developed a crankshaft deformity after posterior-only fusion. An open triradiate physis in the pelvis indicates the need for supplementary anterior fusion. With superior correction and rotational control available with pedicle screw instrumentation, perhaps the need for anterior fusions could be lessened.

If the child is younger than 8 years, is small, and has a curve that cannot be controlled by nonoperative means, the ideal treatment is a growing rod system without fusion or growth modulation techniques. If the child is 9 or 10 years of age or large, growing rods or growth modulation may still be used but instrumentation and fusion may be appropriate. A

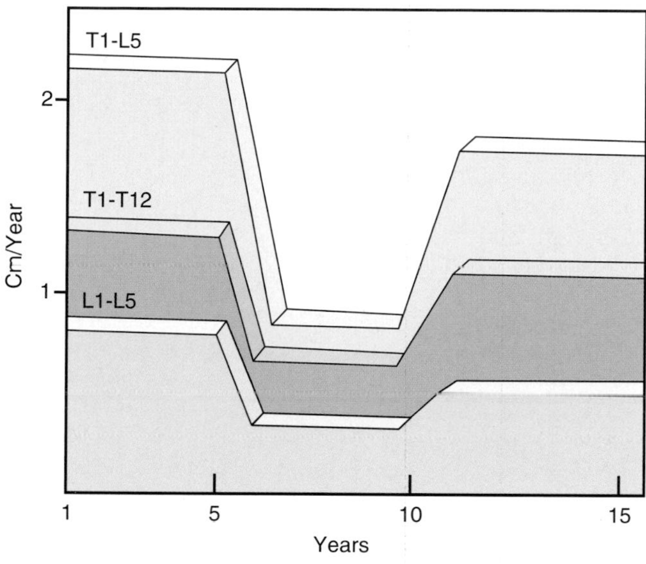

FIGURE 44-7 Growth velocity of T1-L5 segment, thoracic segment T1-12, and lumbar segment L1-L5. (From Dimeglio A: Growth of the spine before age 5 years, J Pediatr Orthop B 1:102, 1993.)

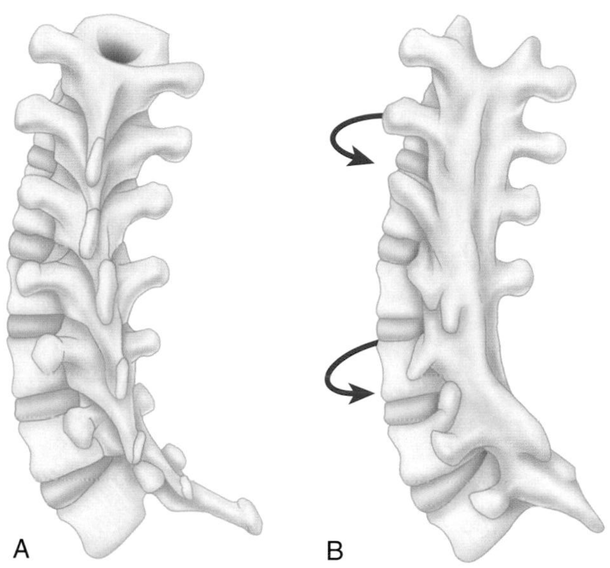

FIGURE 44-8 Crankshaft phenomenon. **A,** Spine with scoliosis. **B,** Despite solid posterior fusion, continued anterior growth causes increase in deformity.

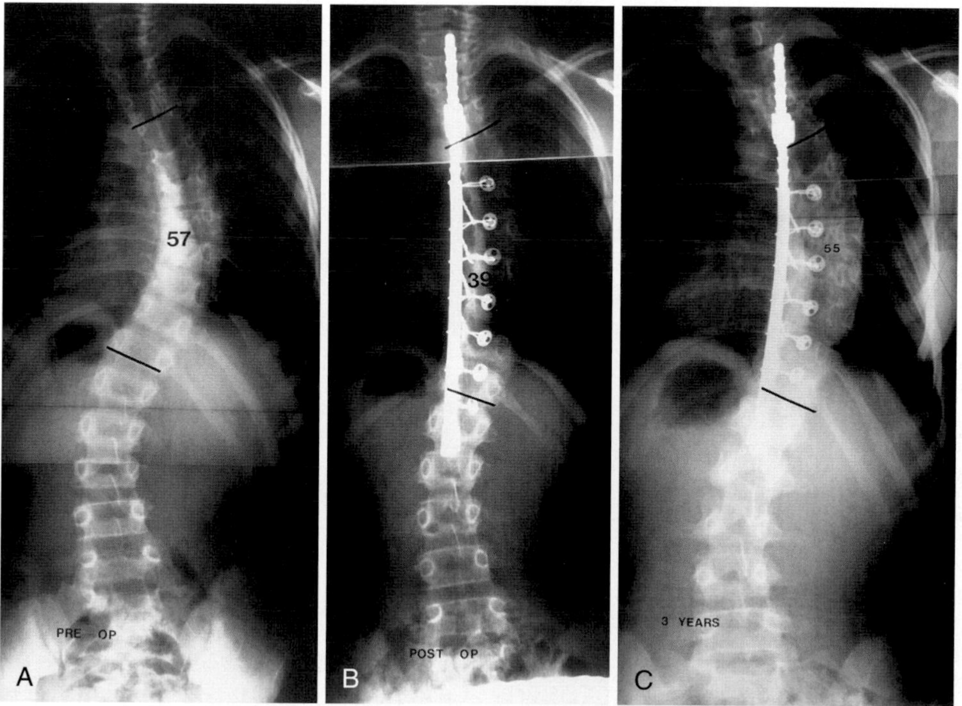

FIGURE 44-9 Fifty-seven-degree curve **(A)** was corrected to 39 degrees with posterior fusion and instrumentation **(B)**. **C,** Three years after surgery, deformity has recurred because of crankshaft phenomenon.

combined anterior and posterior spinal fusion to avoid the crankshaft phenomenon may be needed, but with the use of pedicle screws to allow better correction and derotation of the spine, an anterior fusion may not be necessary.

GROWING ROD INSTRUMENTATION

Growing rod instrumentation is a technique of posterior instrumentation that is sequentially lengthened to allow longitudinal growth while still attempting to control progressive spinal deformity.

Moe et al. described the use of a subcutaneous Harrington rod without fusion, followed by a full-time external orthosis, in certain flexible curves in growing children. The authors noted an average length gain in the instrumented area of 3.8 cm that ultimately required fusion. Complications, most frequently hook dislocation and rod breakage, occurred in 50% of patients. Currently, growing rod techniques include (1) a single growing rod, (2) dual growing rods, (3) VEPTR rods, (4) Luque trolley, and (5) Shilla technique. Magnetically controlled growing rods, such as the MAGEC rods (NuVasive, Aliso Viejo, CA), provide a noninvasive method for rod lengthening, avoiding the need for additional surgical procedures for lengthening.

The growing rod techniques should be considered in a cooperative patient with a stable family unit. This procedure usually is considered for patients younger than 10 years of age who have a curve of 60 degrees. Surgery is required every 6 months to lengthen the construct. A TLSO often is necessary for at least the first 6 months to protect the upper and lower levels of the instrumentation. Dual growing rods have been found to be effective in controlling severe spinal deformities and allowing spinal growth. With the use of dual rods, an apical fusion does not appear to be necessary during the course of treatment. We have had fewer instrumentation problems with the dual-rod technique than with previous single-rod techniques.

DUAL GROWING ROD INSTRUMENTATION WITHOUT FUSION

A multiple-hook segmental instrumentation system that is appropriate for the child's size is used. If the child weighs less than 30 lb, an infant spinal set may be necessary. If the infant set is used, the rod is quite flexible, and therefore some additional protection in the form of external immobilization is necessary until the system can be converted to a pediatric rod system of a larger diameter.

TECHNIQUE 44-2

- Place the patient prone on the operating table or frame; prepare and drape the back in the routine sterile fashion.
- Take care to select the stable vertebrae at both ends of the curve and make a single, long, straight incision into the subcutaneous tissue from the upper to the lower neutral vertebrae. Dede et al. described preservation of motion segments by using the "stable-to-be vertebra" on bending or traction films as the lowest instrumented vertebra. The stable-to-be vertebra is the vertebra that is transected by the center sacral line on traction or bending films (Fig. 44-10).
- Confirm appropriate levels with a radiograph.
- Carry the dissection down to the lamina and spinous process of the end vertebrae.
- Strip the periosteum from the concave and convex lamina out to the facet joint of the two vertebrae selected for hooks at each end of the curve.
- The upper and lower foundations for the growth rods can be done with either hooks or screws. If hooks are used to form the upper claw, insert a pedicle hook onto the lower of the two upper vertebrae and another superior transverse process hook on the upper of the two vertebrae on both the concave and convex sides.
- Form the lower claw by placing a supralaminar hook on the upper vertebra and the infralaminar hook on the lower vertebra. If it is anatomically feasible, pedicle screw fixation can be used in both the upper and lower foundations.
- Use two rods on the concave side and two rods on the convex side.
- Contour the rods to the natural contours of thoracic kyphosis and lordosis.
- Insert the rods under direct vision and use the appropriate set screws to hold the rods in the hooks or pedicle screws.
- Join the rods together with a low-profile growth rod connector (Fig. 44-11).
- Use bone chips to pack around the upper and lower foundation sites.
- Do not attempt subperiosteal dissection between the hook sites.

POSTOPERATIVE CARE. The child is placed in an orthosis for the first 6 months. At that time, the orthosis can be discontinued if the hook sites are solidly fused. The rods routinely are lengthened every 6 months. Lengthening is performed by exposing the connector and loosening the set screws. Distraction is applied, and the set screws are retightened. Lengthenings are stopped when no further distraction can be achieved. Sankar et al. found that with successive lengthenings, there is a law of diminishing returns: repeated lengthenings had decreased gains in length with each subsequent lengthening over time. When no further distraction can be achieved, the patient undergoes the final arthrodesis. The final arthrodesis usually necessitates removal of the rods, and in our experience, if the proximal and distal anchors are still solidly fixed and well fused, they are used as part of the final construct (Figs. 44-12 and 44-13).

Other growing rod constructs include the Luque trolley and the Shilla technique. The Luque trolley consists of sublaminar wires and rods without fusion. The Shilla technique consists of a nonlocking pedicle screw implant. The apex of the deformity is fixed and fused with pedicle screws while the ends of the construct are instrumented with screws that are not locked to the rod. This theoretically allows for apical control of the deformity and continued axial lengthening of the spine with growth.

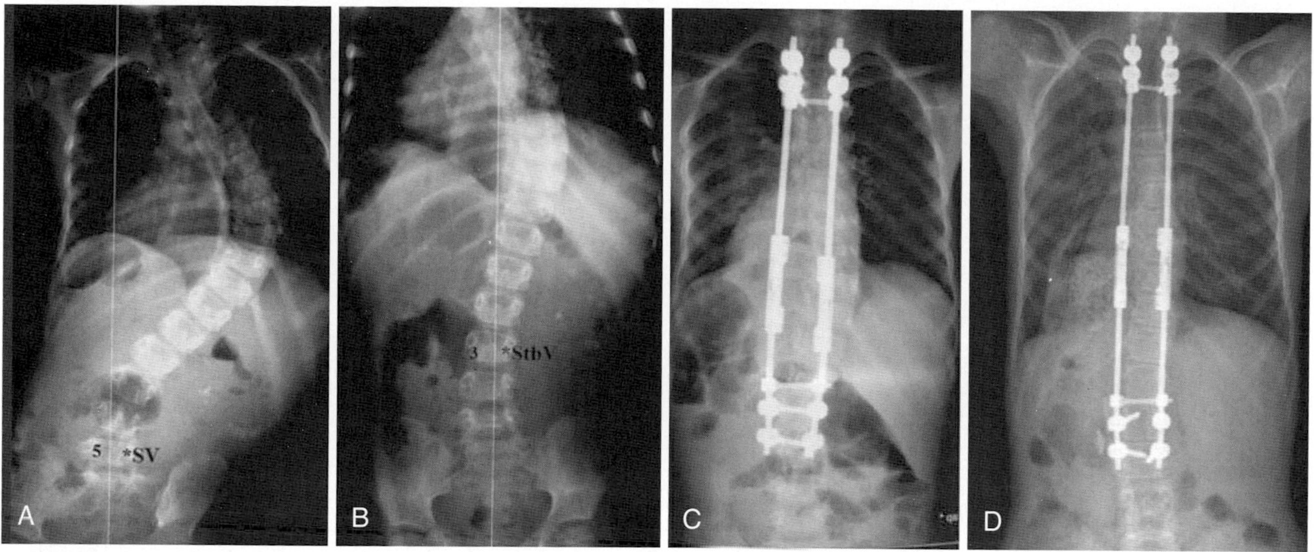

FIGURE 44-10 The "stable-to-be vertebra" (StbV) is the vertebra most closely bisected by the central sacral vertical (SV) line. **A,** In this patient, the stable-to-be vertebra is at L5. **B,** On the traction radiograph, it is at L3. **C,** The patient was treated with growing rod instrumentation extending to L3. **D,** At 6-year follow-up, correction is well maintained with no evidence of distal adding on. (From Dede O, Demirkiran G, Bekmez S, et al: Utilizing the "stable-to-be vertebra" saves motion segments in growing rods treatment of early-onset scoliosis, J Pediatr Orthop 36:336, 2016.)

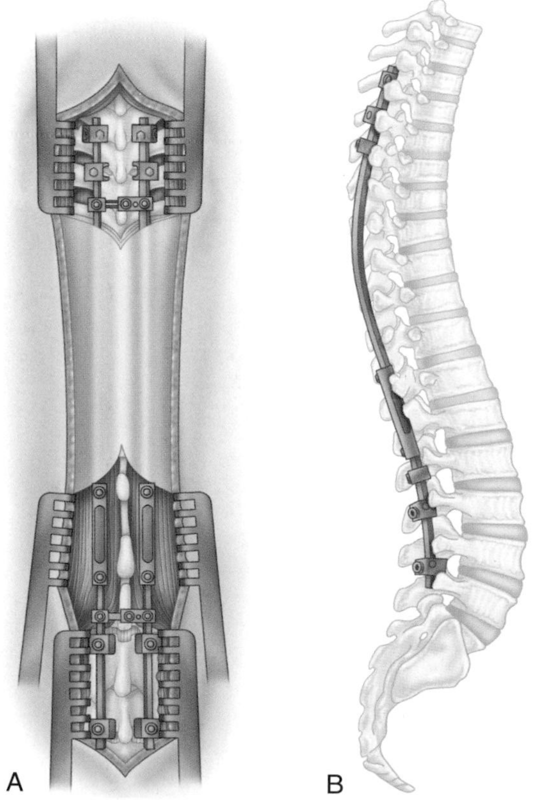

FIGURE 44-11 Technique of dual-rod instrumentation. **A,** Anteroposterior view. **B,** Lateral view showing construct contoured to maintain sagittal alignment. Extended tandem connectors are placed in thoracolumbar spine to minimize profile. **SEE TECHNIQUE 44-2.**

SHILLA GUIDED GROWTH SYSTEM

TECHNIQUE 44-3

(MCCARTHY ET AL.)

- Careful assessment of upright coronal and sagittal films, along with analysis of the flexibility of the curve by bending or traction films, is necessary to determine the location of the apical vertebral segments (Fig. 44-14). The apical three or four vertebral segments that are least corrected through flexibility testing are the apical levels for fusion and maximal correction.
- Place small needle markers in the spinous processes and obtain a radiograph to identify spinal levels.
- Make a single midline incision and perform subperiosteal dissection to only the apical levels.
- Incise the fascia 1 cm off the midline on both sides of the spinous processes from cephalad to caudad, merging with the subperiosteal dissection at the apex.
- Place bilateral fixed-head pedicle screws throughout the apical levels.
- Perform Ponte osteotomies (see Technique 44-24) between the apical segments if needed to enhance correction in all planes. Apical decortication is necessary for fusion of these levels.
- Place the growth guidance screws through the muscular layer with fluoroscopic visualization of bone. Use a cannulated polyaxial screw of sufficient diameter to fill the pedicle. A Jamshidi trocar system is helpful in placing the screw in the center of the pedicle.
- The location of the guidance screws depends on the curve; the screw should extend far enough into the lumbar spine to maintain the lordosis and coronal

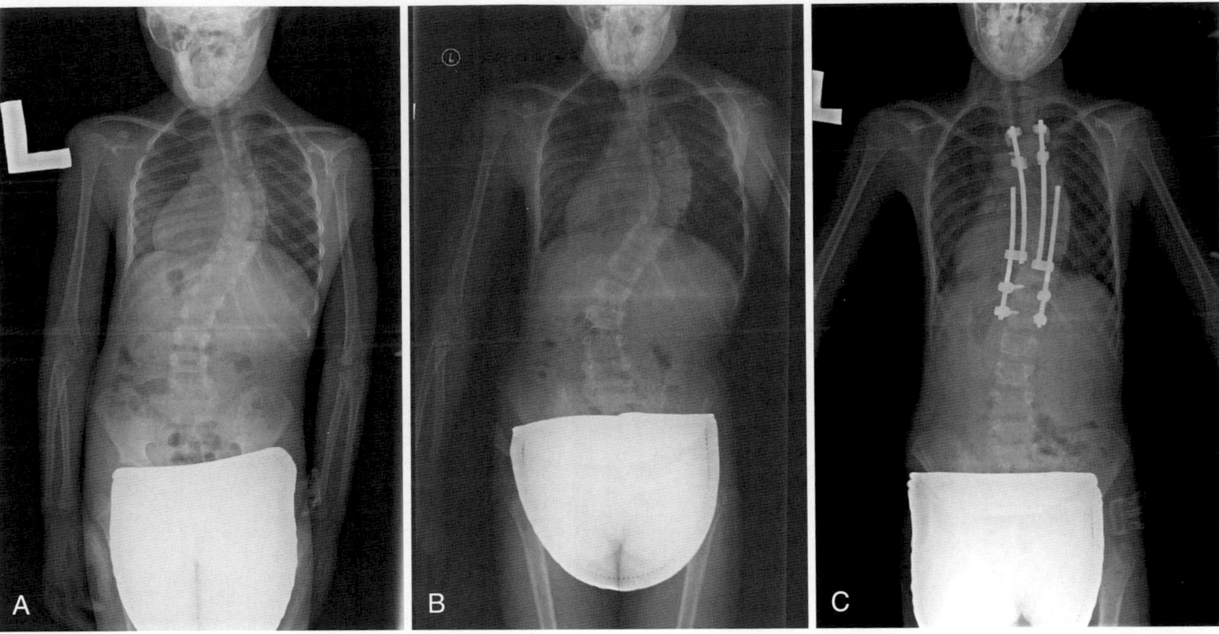

FIGURE 44-12 **A** and **B,** Anteroposterior and posteroanterior radiographs of child with infantile scoliosis treated with dual growing rods **(C).**

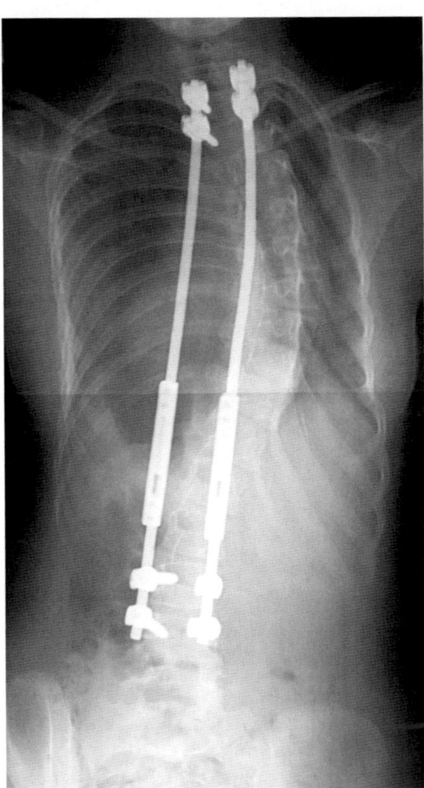

FIGURE 44-13 Growing rods. **SEE TECHNIQUE 44-2.**

correction. Avoid stopping the caudal instrumentation at the thoracolumbar junction because this may lead to prominence with flexion.

- Place the guidance screws at bilateral locations or staggered, making sure that they are separated by enough distance on the rod to allow for easy sliding.
- Because the guidance screws at the top of the construct are subjected to pull-out forces from kyphosis, place a sublaminar or transverse process cable or fiberwire (3 mm) one level above the upper screws to protect them.
- Choose a rod of the appropriate diameter for the size of the child, generally 4.5 mm, and contour it into normal sagittal curves, leaving the rod one vertebral level long at each length for growth.
- Before placement of the permanent rods, place a temporary (provisional) rod on the convex side and attach it loosely at the apex and one growing screw above and below the apex.
- Roll the provisional rod into a neutral position in the coronal and sagittal positions, translate it toward the concavity of the curve with coronal benders, and hold it there by tightening the apical plugs.
- Attach the permanent concave rod to the screws and remove the provisional rod.
- Derotate the apical levels with tube derotation devices or a vertebral column derotation device while holding the rods in place with vise grips to prevent rod rotation.
- The fixed-head screws lock the rods at the apical screws through the locking set screws that fix to the rods. The guidance screw caps capture the rods in the guidance screw head, leaving room for movement of the rod within the screw head.
- If needed to help maintain rod rotation, use a crosslink just below the apical fixation. If the child is younger than 5 years old, use a sliding type of crosslink to allow for growth in the canal diameter.
- Use the torque/countertorque device to snap off the caps at a preset torque pressure.
- Place bone graft at the apex only.
- Close the wound in routine fashion, using a small drain if necessary.

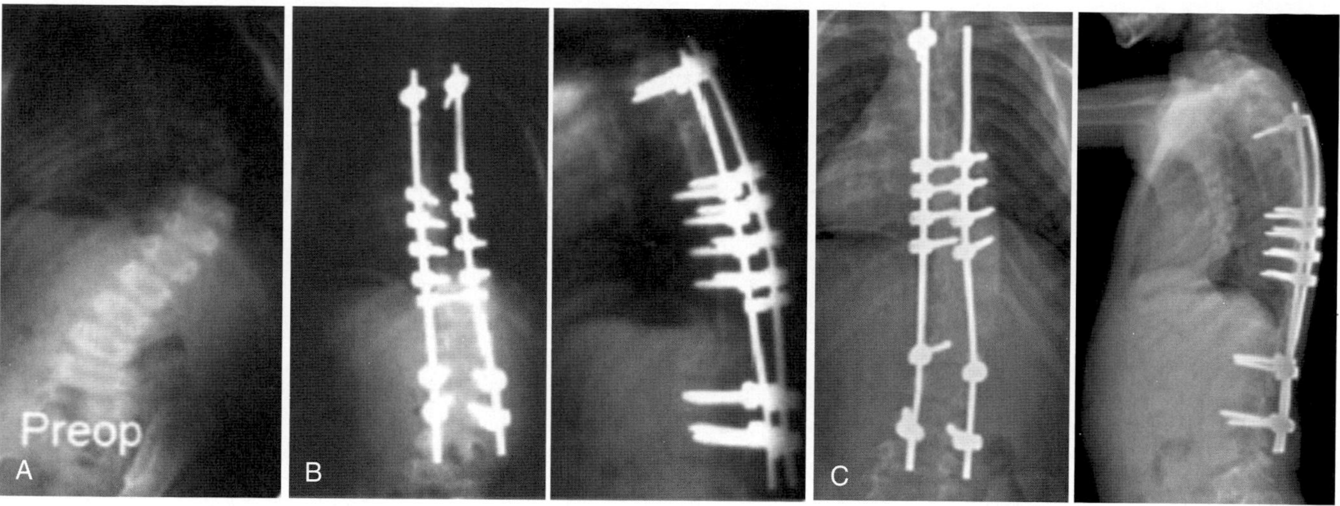

FIGURE 44-14 A, Preoperative standing radiograph of a 3-year-old child with infantile idiopathic scoliosis. B, Three-month postoperative radiographs after insertion of Shilla rods. C, Five-year postoperative radiographs. (From Medtronic: Shilla Growth Guidance System, Memphis, TN; 2012.) **SEE TECHNIQUE 44-3.**

POSTOPERATIVE CARE. The child is immobilized for 3 months. A bivalved form-fitting turtle-shell brace is used during daytime until the apical fusion is solid. A protective brace is not necessary after this period of immobilization unless excessively vigorous activities are expected.

Growing rods do have potential complications, and complications are common. Bess et al. found at least one complication in 58% of patients with early onset scoliosis who were treated with growing rods; submuscular placement of the rod resulted in fewer complications than subfascial placement. The most common complications are (1) rod breakage, (2) hook displacement or failure of proximal or distal fixation points, (3) infection, (4) skin breakdown over prominent rods, and (5) autofusion of the spine. Cahill et al. reported autofusion in 89% of children treated with growing rods. The average percentage of Cobb angle correction obtained at definitive fusion was 44%, and an average of seven osteotomies per patient was required at the time of definitive fusion because of autofusion. Flynn et al. also found that a deformity correction of less than 50% could be obtained when converting growing rods to a definitive instrumentation and fusion.

VEPTR instrumentation also can be used as a growing rod system (see Technique 44-46). The constructs can be rib-to-rib, rib-to-spine, or rib-to-pelvis. This has the advantage of minimal exposure of the spine and a theoretical decreased risk of spontaneous fusion of the spine. Another technique is to use a claw construct around ribs to act as the proximal attachment for dual growing rods. The advantage to using ribs as anchors instead of the spine is the preservation of motion between vertebrae, thereby preventing or delaying spontaneous fusion. The procedure is contraindicated in patients with kyphosis (upper thoracic kyphosis is poorly controlled with rib anchors) and patients who cannot tolerate repeated surgical procedures. This technique uses traditional spine implants with hooks that fit around the ribs. It is important to place the hook as close as possible to the transverse process to prevent the hook from sliding laterally (Fig. 44-15).

GROWING ROD ATTACHMENT USING RIB ANCHORS

TECHNIQUE 44-4

(SANKAR AND SKAGGS)

- Position the patient prone, taking care to pad all bony prominences. Neuromonitoring is essential when performing this procedure and should include both the upper and lower extremities.
- Make a midline skin incision or two separate incisions at the top and bottom of the construct, depending on the surgery.
- Dissect through the subcutaneous tissues and elevate a flap superficial to the paraspinal muscles laterally past the transverse processes. Confirm the location fluoroscopically.
- Alternatively, if the patient has multiple fused ribs and an open thoracostomy is planned, place the patient in the lateral decubitus position. Make a curvilinear J-shaped incision, starting halfway between the medial edge of the scapula and the posterior spinous process of T1-T2. Carry the incision distally and laterally across the 10th rib. Transect the muscle layers in line with the skin incision down to the level of the ribs and elevate an anterior flap to the costochondral junction. The paraspinal muscles are elevated from lateral to medial to the tips of the transverse process. In patients with multiple rib fusions and stiff chest walls, an opening wedge thoracostomy is indicated.
- For most patients, a thoracostomy usually is not necessary and has been shown to disrupt pulmonary function. The

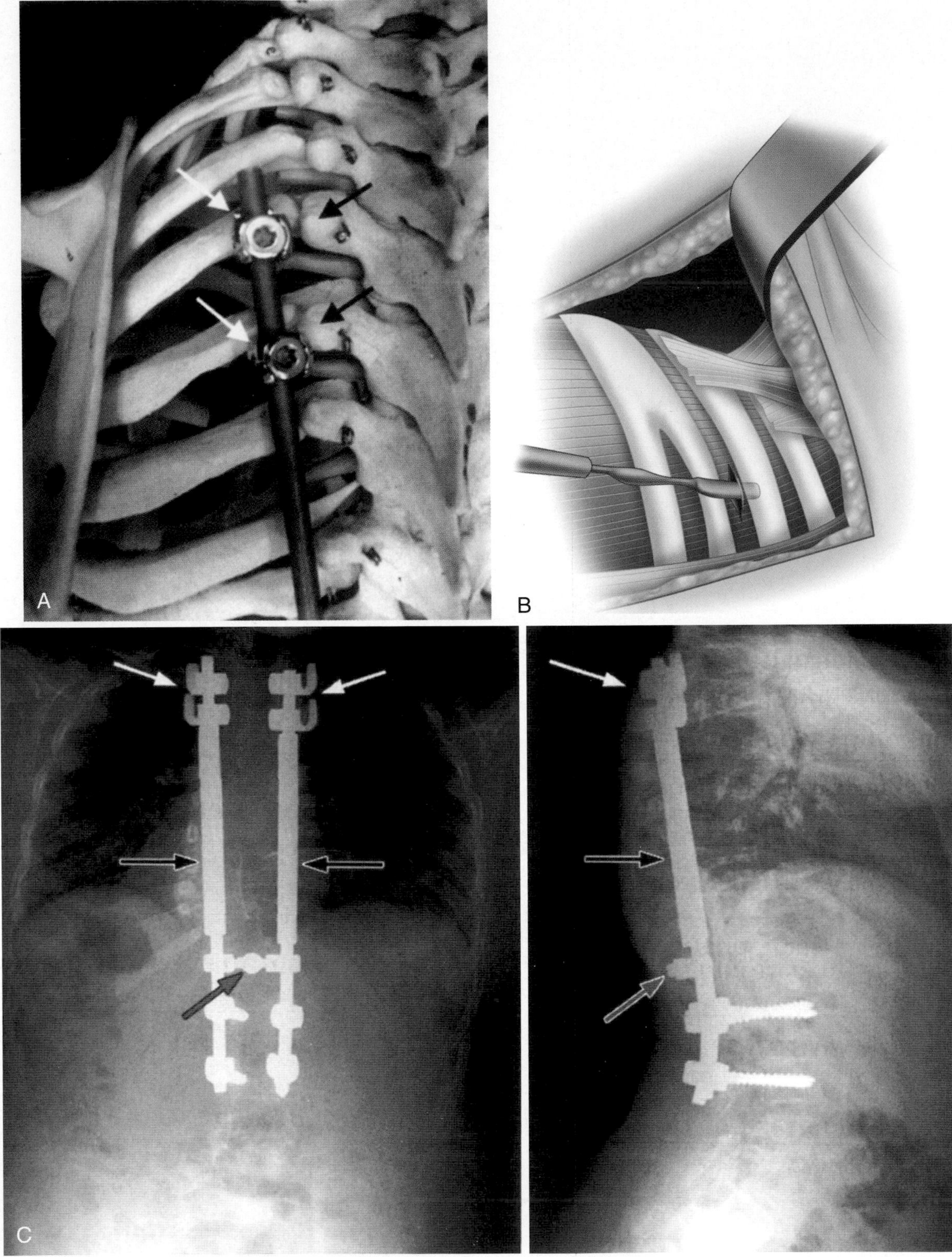

FIGURE 44-15 **A,** Model of thoracic chamber. Correct placement of rib anchors *(white arrows)* lateral to tips of transverse processes *(black arrows)*. **B,** Dissection of soft tissue anterior to rib. **C,** Postoperative posteroanterior and lateral radiographs after dual growing rods with proximal rib anchors *(white arrows)*. *Black arrows* indicate connectors and crosslink. (From Sankar WN, Skaggs DL: Rib anchors in distraction-based growing spine implants. In Wang JC, editor: Advanced reconstruction spine, Rosemont, IL, 2011, American Academy of Orthopaedic Surgeons.) **SEE TECHNIQUE 44-4.**

use of distraction-based rib implants is effective in opening up the rib spaces. Standard spine hooks can be used. Make a 5-mm transverse incision just distal to the neurovascular bundle using cautery (lateral to the transverse process). Make sure that the dissection on the top of the rib is immediately adjacent to the transverse process only (see Fig. 44-15A). If the soft tissues are dissected too far laterally, hooks tend to slide down. Use a Freer elevator to dissect the soft tissue anterior to the rib (see Fig. 44-15B). Preserve the periosteum around the rib to allow the rib to hypertrophy in response to stress.

- If a specialized device cradle is necessary, use a similar insertion technique, except stay subperiosteal with the rib dissection. Use a Freer elevator in both a superior and inferior direction around the rib to create a channel. Insert the rib cradle cap into the superior end of the channel and the rib cradle into the inferior end of the channel. Align the two devices and connect them with the cradle cap lock.
- Place a conventional upgoing spinal hook into the interval between the periosteum and pleura using a standard hook inserter or partial rod. Usually a second upgoing hook is placed around an adjacent rib to share the load. There is no need for a downgoing hook because distractive forces keep the rib in the hook.
- After proximal fixation, attention is turned to placement of the distal anchor. Through the same incision, subperiosteally dissect the lamina of the intended vertebrae. Either single-level fixation with a downgoing supralaminar hook or two-level fixation with pedicle screws can be used. If single-level fixation is used, preserve the interspinous ligament to avoid progressive kyphosis of the distal segment with distraction. If pedicle screws are used, place them at two adjacent levels because plowing of the implants could injure nerve roots.
- If two-level distal anchoring is chosen, use a narrow rongeur to destroy the facet joint and place cancellous crushed allograft into the joint. Decorticate the exposed bone and place bone graft before the rod to maximize bony contact.
- If one incision was used and if separate upper and lower rods were used, they can be connected with a longitudinal growing rod connector or side-to-side connector with the rods overlapping. It is prudent to use more than one connector. If two separate incisions were used for exposure, a soft-tissue tunnel should be made between the two anchor sites for passage of the rods. Sankar and Skaggs use a chest tube to facilitate passage of the rod.
- Although unilateral rods are less invasive, there are fewer anchor points to share the load, and balancing the curve can be problematic. Dual rods are more stable and less prone to loss of fixation and make balancing the spine easier. When dual rods are used, a crosslink should be included.
- If an opening wedge thoracostomy was performed, a second rib-to-rib device can be used laterally to assist in correction and to reduce the load on the medial rib-to-spine device. Place the superior cradle around the same ribs that have the medial hybrid device and place the inferior cradle on a stable rib no lower than the 10th rib.
- Before wound closure, fill the upper anchor site with warm saline and perform a Valsalva maneuver to look for a pleural leak. If bubbles are present, place a Hemovac (Zimmer, Inc., Warsaw, IN) or chest tube into the pleural space for a few days.
- Close the wound in layers using 1-0 braided absorbable suture for the musculocutaneous flap, a 2-0 suture for the dermis, and a running 3-0 monofilament absorbable suture for the final subcuticular layer.

POSTOPERATIVE CARE. Physical therapy is started on the first day after surgery. A TLSO should be used for 3 months if the arthrodesis was at a distal anchor site. Patients may return to sports at 3 months. Lengthenings are planned for every 6 months after the initial surgery (Fig. 44-15C).

GUIDED GROWTH AND PHYSEAL STAPLING

Growth modulation is an attempt to apply the principles of guided growth in the lower extremities with physeal stapling. Intervertebral stapling is used to produce a tethering effect on the convex side of the spine. This tether theoretically will allow for continued growth on the concave side of the spine deformity and gradual correction of the deformity with growth. Devices that have been used for this growth modulation are a flexible titanium clip, a nitinol staple, and an anterior spinal tether using anterior vertebral body screws and a polypropylene cord.

INTERVERTEBRAL STAPLING

Current indications for vertebral body stapling for scoliosis include age younger than 13 years in girls and 15 years in boys, skeletal maturity of Risser grade 0 or 1, with 1 year of growth remaining by wrist bone age, minimal rotation of both the thoracic and lumbar curves of 45 degrees and flexibility to less than 20 degrees, and a sagittal thoracic curve of 40 degrees or less. If the thoracic coronal curve is between 35 and 45 degrees and does not correct on bending films to less than 20 degrees, adding a posterior rib-to-spine hybrid construct may be considered. If the first erect radiograph does not measure 20 degrees or less after vertebral body stapling, Betz et al. recommended having the patient wear a corrective brace until the curve measures less than 20 degrees. Children younger than 8 years of age may not be ideal candidates for this surgery because of the possibility of overcorrection with growth.

TECHNIQUE 44-5

- Administer general anesthesia and place the patient in the lateral decubitus position with the convex side of the scoliosis facing upward.
- Fluoroscopic imaging should be used. Plan to staple all the vertebrae in the measured Cobb curve.
- For thoracic curves, a thoracoscopic-assisted approach is preferable.

- Create a portal in the posterior axillary line for insertion of the staples. Alternatively, two minithoracotomy incisions (< 5 cm) can be used, one centered at T4-5 and the other at T9-10. In most cases, the parietal pleura is not excised and the segmental vessels are preserved.
- Use a radiopaque trial instrument to determine the dimension of the staple (3 to 12 mm) and to create pilot holes. The smallest staple that spans the disc and growth plate is used.
- Insert a staple, which has been cooled in an ice water basin, into a pilot hole. Two single staples (two-prong) or one double staple (four-prong) are placed laterally, spanning each disc of the measured Cobb curve. Occasionally, at T4 and T5, the vertebrae are too small and can only accommodate a single two-prong staple.
- If there is significant hypokyphosis (kyphosis < 10 degrees) at the apex of the thoracic spine, place the staples more anteriorly to the midbody of the vertebra or place a third single staple along the anterolateral aspect of the vertebral body.
- Staples that cross the thoracolumbar junction require partial reflection of the diaphragm anteriorly off the spine to be applied in the proper position. The diaphragm then is repaired.
- For lumbar vertebrae, use a mini-open retroperitoneal approach.
- Ligate the segmental vessels of one or two levels to allow posterior retraction of the psoas. Place the staples in the posterior one third of the vertebral body to allow normal lordosis.
- In all cases, maximal correction is obtained on the operating room table first by positioning but also by pushing with the staple trial instrument (Fig. 44-16).

ANTERIOR VERTEBRAL TETHERING

Purported advantages of anterior vertebral tethering include that it allows the spine to grow and remain flexible, it is one-time surgery, and a later fusion can be done if needed. The indications for this technique have not been well established, but it is most likely beneficial for patients with enough growth remaining to substantially alter the shape of the spine and is most suited for primary thoracic curves with typical hypokyphotic apices (Fig. 44-17). Suggested contraindications include patients with no remaining growth, patients younger than 8 years of age, patients with curves of less than 40 degrees or more than 65 degrees, and patients with left-sided curves, pulmonary disease limiting single-lung ventilation, previous ipsilateral chest surgery, or poor bone quality.

TECHNIQUE 44-6

- With the use of single-lung ventilation and the patient in the lateral decubitus position, make a thoracoscopic approach.
- With fluoroscopy, mark the screw trajectories in the coronal plane, planning for three posterior axillary line 15-mm portals for screw placement. Use an 11-mm anterior axillary line portal for endoscopic placement.
- Open the pleura longitudinally 1 cm anterior to the rib heads.
- Coagulate and divide the segmental vessels and retract them anteriorly with sponges placed between the spine and the great vessels.
- Place bicortical transverse vertebral body screws through pronged washers using fluoroscopy to guide the screw trajectory.
- Introduce the tethering cord through a portal and capture it with a set screw into the proximal vertebral body screw. Adjust the portals to the appropriate interspace used to place the adjacent screws, and remove the long end of the tether from the chest through that portal, allowing a tensioning device to take slack out of the tether as the next set screw is tightened.
- Repeat this sequence for each screw, with more or less compression applied as indicated based on the deformity (generally more compression at the apex and less to none at the ends).
- Cut the tether distally and close the pleura over the device with the endoscopic suturing technique. Place a chest tube and reinflate the lungs.

POSTOPERATIVE CARE. The patient recovers in the hospital for 4 to 5 days. A thoracolumbosacral orthosis is recommended for 3 months after surgery. Noncontact activities can be resumed after 3 months.

INSTRUMENTATION WITH FUSION

If a child is older than 9 or 10 years or is unable to cooperate with the demands of growth rods, instrumentation and spinal fusion should be considered. A combined anterior and posterior procedure should be considered if the patient is deemed at risk for the crankshaft phenomenon (see Figs. 44-7 and 44-8). With the use of pedicle screws and the ability to get better correction of vertebral body rotation and the Cobb angle, an anterior fusion may not be needed in older juvenile patients undergoing a definitive instrumentation and fusion.

Preferably, if an anterior procedure is performed, the anterior release and fusion are done without sacrificing the segmental vessels. Anterior instrumentation is not used if posterior instrumentation is scheduled as a second procedure. Posteriorly, a multiple-hook or pedicle screw segmental system is used. Many of these systems have a variety of different size hooks, pedicle screws, and rods, depending on the size of the child. We have had good success, especially in younger children, with the use of freeze-dried crushed cancellous allograft bone, obtaining a successful fusion without the morbidity associated with an autologous posterior iliac crest graft. Karol et al., however, found that patients with proximal thoracic deformity who required fusion of more than four segments were at higher risk for the development of restrictive pulmonary disease. There was a significant correlation between poor pulmonary function and the proximal level of the thoracic fusion and the percentage of thoracic vertebrae fused.

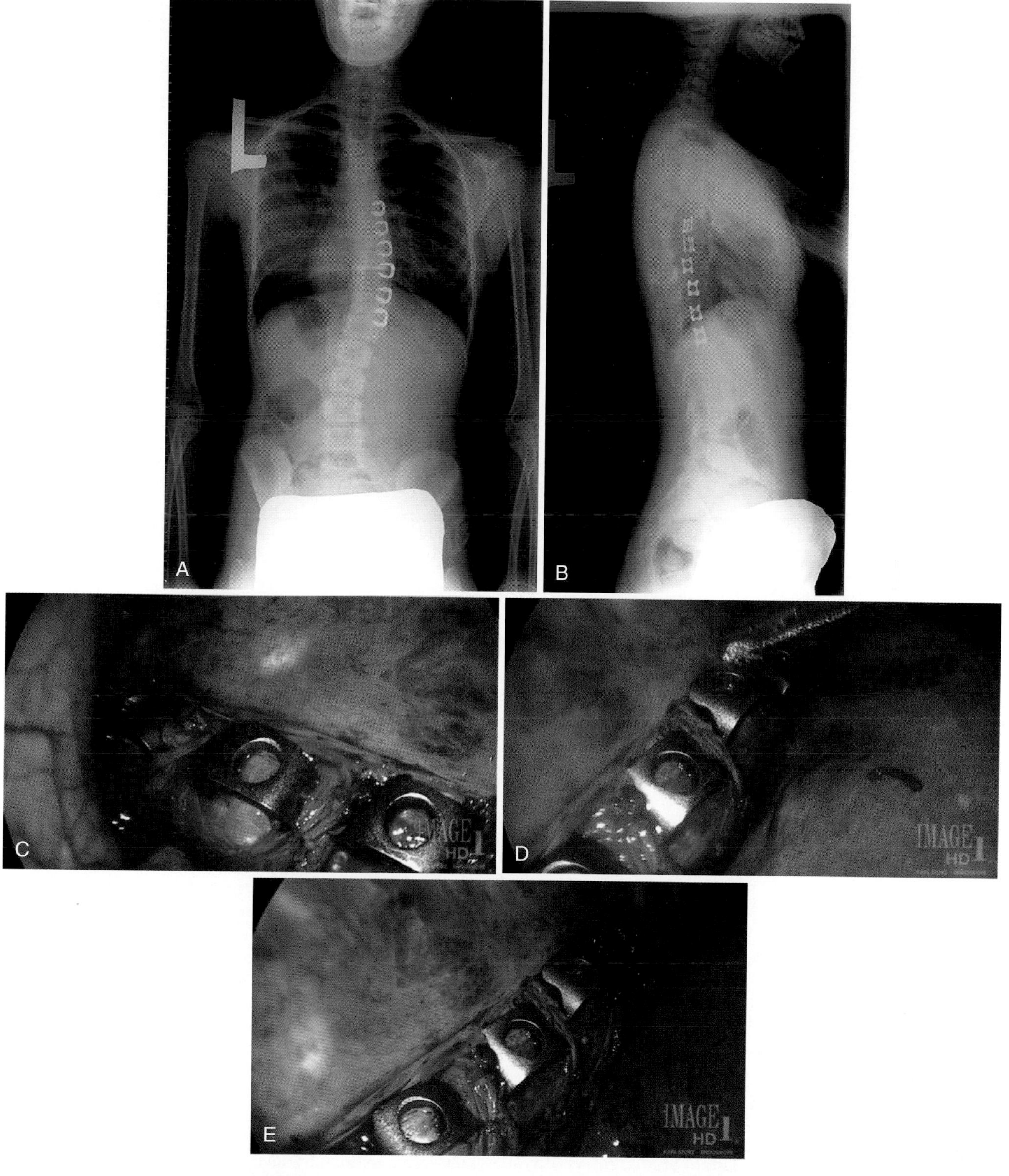

FIGURE 44-16 Guided growth and physeal stapling. **SEE TECHNIQUE 44-5.**

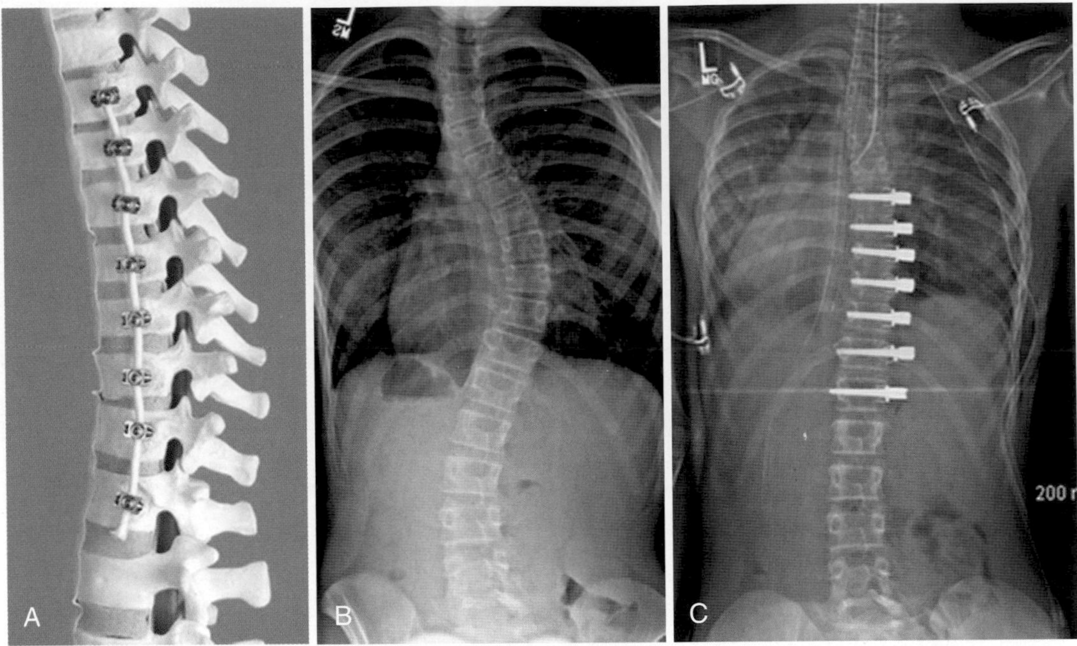

FIGURE 44-17 **A,** Anterior vertebral body tethering. **B,** Before tethering. **C,** After tethering. (From Shriners Hospital for Children Philadelphia Newsletter, June 18, 2014.) **SEE TECHNIQUE 44-6.**

ADOLESCENT IDIOPATHIC SCOLIOSIS

Adolescent idiopathic scoliosis is present when the spinal deformity is recognized after the child is 10 years of age but before skeletal maturity. This is the most common type of idiopathic scoliosis. The characteristics of adolescent idiopathic scoliosis include a three-dimensional deformity of the spine with lateral curvature plus rotation of the vertebral bodies. Most idiopathic curves are lordotic or hypokyphotic in the thoracic region, and this may represent an important factor in the etiology of idiopathic scoliosis.

ETIOLOGY

The exact cause of idiopathic scoliosis remains unknown. The consensus is that there is a hereditary predisposition and its actual cause is multifactorial. There are many proposed etiologic factors, but these can be divided into six general categories: (1) genetic factors, (2) neurologic disorders, (3) hormonal and metabolic dysfunctions, (4) skeletal growth, (5) biomechanical factors, and (6) environmental and lifestyle factors. The role of a genetic component in the cause of scoliosis is supported by several studies demonstrating an increased incidence of scoliosis in family members. Riseborough and Wynne-Davies found scoliosis in 11% of first-degree relatives of 207 patients with scoliosis. Genetic studies of families in which multiple members are affected have suggested several sites within the genome that appear to be linked to scoliosis. Currently genetic testing is being evaluated as a prognostic test for the risk of curve progression. Abnormalities in the central nervous system also have been thought to play a role in causing scoliosis. These neurologic factors can be divided into two major groups: neuroanatomic and neurophysiologic dysfunction. Studies have reported anatomic abnormalities in the midbrain, pons, and medulla and the vestibular system in scoliosis patients. Hindbrain abnormalities with cervicothoracic syrinx and low-lying cerebellar tonsils, with or without an abnormal cerebrospinal fluid dynamic, have been reported in patients with adolescent idiopathic scoliosis. Abnormalities of equilibrium and vestibular function have been noted as a possible cause. Differential growth between the right and left sides of the spine and a relative overgrowth of the anterior spinal column compared with the posterior column, resulting in a relative thoracic lordosis, have been postulated to cause scoliosis. Hormone abnormalities that have been proposed as causes are abnormalities in growth hormone, estrogen, melatonin, calmodulin, and leptin. Biomechanical causes are thought to be a result of asymmetric loading of the immature spine, which in turn causes asymmetric growth, resulting in a progressive deformity. Possible environmental or lifestyle factors include nutrition, diet, calcium and vitamin D intake, and exercise level. In summary, the exact cause of scoliosis remains unknown and may be multifactorial. Current research continues to try to better define these proposed causes.

NATURAL HISTORY

A knowledge of the natural history and prevalence of idiopathic scoliosis is essential to determine if treatment is necessary. Three important questions need to be answered:

What is the prevalence of idiopathic scoliosis in the general population?

What is the likelihood of curve progression necessitating treatment in a child with scoliosis?

What problems may occur in adult life if scoliosis is left untreated and the curve progresses?

Idiopathic scoliotic curves of more than 10 degrees are estimated to occur in 2% to 3% of children younger than 16 years of age. Larger curves of more than 30 degrees are estimated to occur in 0.15% to 0.3% of children. Weinstein

TABLE 44-2

Adolescent Idiopathic Scoliosis Prevalence

COBB ANGLE (DEGREES)	FEMALE:MALE	PREVALENCE (%)
>10	1.4-2:1	2-3
>20	5.4:1	0.3-0.5
>30	10:1	0.1-0.3
>40		<0.1

From Weinstein SL: Adolescent idiopathic scoliosis: prevalence and natural history. In Weinstein SL, editor: The pediatric spine: principles and practice, New York, 2001, Raven.

BOX 44-2

Factors Related to Progression of Adolescent Idiopathic Scoliosis

- Girls > boys
- Premenarchal
- Risser sign of 0
- Double curves > single curves
- Thoracic curves > lumbar curves
- More severe curves

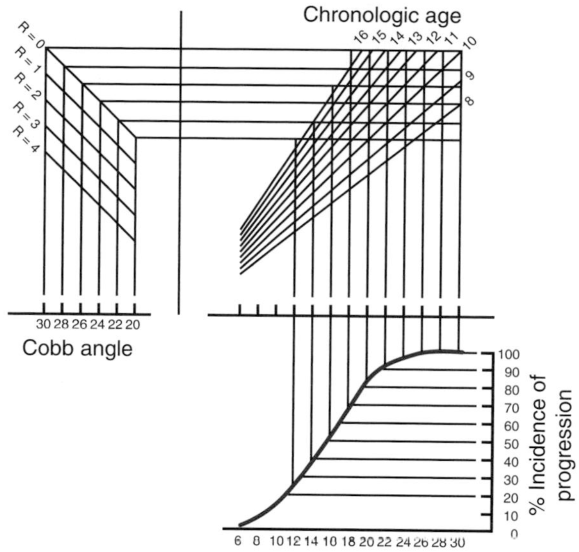

FIGURE 44-18 **Nomogram for prediction of progression of scoliotic curve.** (From Lonstein JE, Carlson JM: The prediction of curve progression in untreated idiopathic scoliosis during growth, J Bone Joint Surg 66A:1061, 1984.)

created a table of calculations that show decreasing prevalence with increasing curve magnitude (Table 44-2). The importance of these prevalence studies is that small degrees of scoliosis are common but larger curves occur much less frequently. Fewer than 10% of children with curves of 10 degrees or more require treatment.

Once scoliosis has been discovered in a child, the curve must be evaluated for the probability of progression. Most authors define progression as an increase of 5 degrees or more measured by the Cobb measurement over two or more visits. What is unknown is whether this progression will continue and what the final curve will be. Spontaneous improvement can occur in 3% of adolescents with idiopathic scoliosis, most of whom have curves of less than 11 degrees. Certain factors have been found to be related to curve progression (Box 44-2). Progression is more likely in girls than in boys. The time of curve progression in adolescent idiopathic scoliosis generally is during the rapid adolescent growth spurt before the onset of menses. This time of rapid growth has been called the peak height velocity (PHV), which is calculated from changes in a patient's height measurements over time and is reported to be about 8 cm per year for girls and 9.5 cm per year for boys. The incidence of progression decreases as the child gets older. The incidence of progression also has been found to be related to curve patterns. In general, double curves are more likely to progress than single curves and single thoracic curves tend to be more progressive than single lumbar curves. The incidence of progression also increases with the curve magnitude. Bunnell estimated that the risk of progression for a 20-degree curve is approximately 20% and the risk for a 50-degree curve is 90%. Lonstein and Carlson developed a nomogram to predict progression of a curve when a patient is first seen (Fig. 44-18). In a study of 89 female patients with scoliosis, a Risser sign of less than grade 2, major curve magnitude of more than 35 degrees, apical vertebral rotation of more than grade III, and spinal length increase of more than 20 mm in 1 year predicted curve progression. Sponseller et al. found that curve progression occurred after posterior spinal fusion with pedicle screws in 35% of patients with an open triradiate cartilage. In younger children with open triradiate cartilage and Risser grade 0, the Sponseller group advised against fusing "short of stable." Sanders et al. developed a simplified classification of skeletal maturity that has been shown to correlate highly with curve behavior (see Fig. 44-25).

The effect of progressive curves on adults with untreated scoliosis has been studied by several investigators. Five major considerations in the natural history of untreated adolescent idiopathic scoliosis in adults are (1) back pain, (2) pulmonary function, (3) psychosocial effects, (4) mortality, and (5) curve progression.

The incidence of back pain in the general population is between 60% and 80%, and the incidence in patients with idiopathic scoliosis is comparable. The incidence of frequent daily backache is slightly higher in patients with scoliosis (80% to 86%) than in patients without scoliosis. Patients with lumbar or thoracolumbar curves, especially those with translatory shifts at the lower end of the curves, have a slightly greater incidence of backache than patients with other curve patterns, but this is rarely disabling and is unrelated to the presence of osteoarthritic changes on radiographic examination. However, back pain has been found to be more severe than in adults without scoliosis.

In a 50-year follow-up study, the incidence of back pain in scoliosis patients was 77% compared with 37% in control subjects. Chronic back pain was reported by 61% of the scoliosis group and 35% of the control subjects. However, the ability of scoliosis patients to perform activities of daily living and work was similar to that of the control subjects. Studies have found that the most common symptom of patients with scoliosis is backache at the end of a strenuous day or after unusual activities that is relieved by rest. The location of pain was variable in these studies and generally unrelated to the location or magnitude of the curve.

In contrast, lumbar and thoracolumbar curves may arise in adult life and cause severe pain and discomfort. This degenerative type of scoliosis should not be confused with the natural history of untreated adolescent idiopathic scoliosis. Ultimately, it is important to determine whether the pain is related to scoliosis before treatment determinations are made.

A direct correlation has been noted between decreasing vital capacity and increasing curve severity. The respiratory impairment usually is restrictive lung disease and is seen only in thoracic scoliosis. There are reports that significant limitations of forced vital capacity do not occur until the curve approaches 100 to 120 degrees. Johnson et al. found significant respiratory impairment (pulmonary function < 65% predicted) in 19% of their preoperative patients with adolescent idiopathic scoliosis. The decrease in pulmonary function correlated with the severity of the main thoracic curve and sagittal plane hypokyphosis and was seen in patients with curves of 70 to 80 degrees.

Death in patients with adult idiopathic scoliosis also seems to be related to thoracic curves greater than 100 degrees, with resultant cor pulmonale. In a 40-year long-term study, the mortality rate was 15%, but only in one patient was cor pulmonale secondary to scoliosis the cause of death. In a subsequent 50-year follow-up, the number of deaths increased as expected but was no different from actuarially predicted rates for patients born in the same year. In yet another study, no patient with adolescent-onset idiopathic scoliosis died of respiratory failure. Most severe pulmonary effects of idiopathic scoliosis occur in curves that develop before the age of 5 years.

The psychologic effect of scoliosis has been studied by numerous authors. Unhappiness with the appearance often is correlated with the size of the rib prominence. Middle-aged patients tolerate the psychologic effects of scoliosis better than teenagers; however, many adult patients seeking treatment for untreated adolescent idiopathic scoliosis are most concerned with the cosmetic aspects of the disorder.

Curves may continue to progress throughout adult life. Weinstein et al. identified multiple factors that predict the likelihood of curve progression after maturity (Table 44-3). In general, curves in any area of less than 30 degrees at skeletal maturity did not tend to progress in adult life. Larger curves were more likely to progress throughout adult life, especially thoracic curves between 50 and 75 degrees. Lumbar curves also tend to progress in adulthood in curves less than 50 degrees if they are accompanied by a transitory shift between the lower vertebrae.

TABLE 44-3

Progression Factors in Curves More Than 30 Degrees at Skeletal Maturity

THORACIC	LUMBAR	THORACOLUMBAR
Cobb > 50 degrees	Cobb > 30 degrees	Cobb > 30 degrees
Apical vertical rotation > 30 degrees	Apical vertical rotation > 30 degrees	Apical vertical rotation > 30%
Mehta angle > 30 degrees	Curve direction Relation L5 to intercrest line Translatory shifts	Translatory shifts

From Weinstein SL: Natural history, Spine 24:2592, 1999.

PATIENT EVALUATION

The initial evaluation of the patient should include a thorough history, complete physical and neurologic examinations, and radiographs of the spine. After the general physical examination, the spine should be examined carefully and the characteristics of the deformity should be recorded.

Most patients with scoliosis present for evaluation because of their spine deformity. Back pain is present in about 32% of adolescents with idiopathic scoliosis (23% at presentation and 9% during treatment). Further workup may be needed if the patient's back pain is persistent, interferes with daily activities, occurs at night, or is associated with any abnormal neurologic findings. Menarchal status, parental height, and family history of scoliosis should be determined. Scoliosis occurs three times more frequently in children whose parents are affected and seven times more frequently if a sibling is affected. Also, if the parents or siblings have been treated for scoliosis, this may suggest a greater likelihood of curve progression in the patient. Surgical history is important in identifying scoliosis associated with congenital heart disease or with a prior thoracotomy.

On physical examination, the height of the patient should be measured. Serial measurement of height will detect when peak height velocity is occurring associated with an increase in progression of the curve. The height of the patient while standing and while sitting should be measured and recorded; these measurements are compared with later ones to determine changes in the patient's total height and whether any change is caused by growth of the lower extremities or by an increase or a decrease in the height of the trunk. On inspection of the spine, the examiner should look for any dimpling, hair patches, or skin abnormalities, such as hemangiomas or café au lait spots. Asymmetry of the shoulder, scapula, ribs, and waistline should be noted. Spinal balance can be determined by the alignment of the head over the pelvis. The head should be positioned directly above the gluteal crease. This can be assessed by dropping a plumb line from the base of the skull or from the spinous process of C7. The plumb line should not deviate from the center of the gluteal crease by more than 1 to 2 cm. In the sagittal plane, the spine is usually hypokyphotic. If hypokyphosis is absent clinically and radiographically, then a syrinx should be ruled out by MRI. The best clinical test for evaluating spinal curvature is the Adams forward bending test. As the patient bends forward at the waist until the spine is horizontal, the trunk is observed for rotation from behind (to asses midthoracic and lumbar rotation) and from the front (to assess upper thoracic rotation). The knees should be straight, the feet together, the arms dependent, and the palms in opposition. Because of vertebral rotation, this will produce a rib prominence in the thoracic region or a paraspinal fullness in the lumbar region. The patient should also be observed from the side to detect any

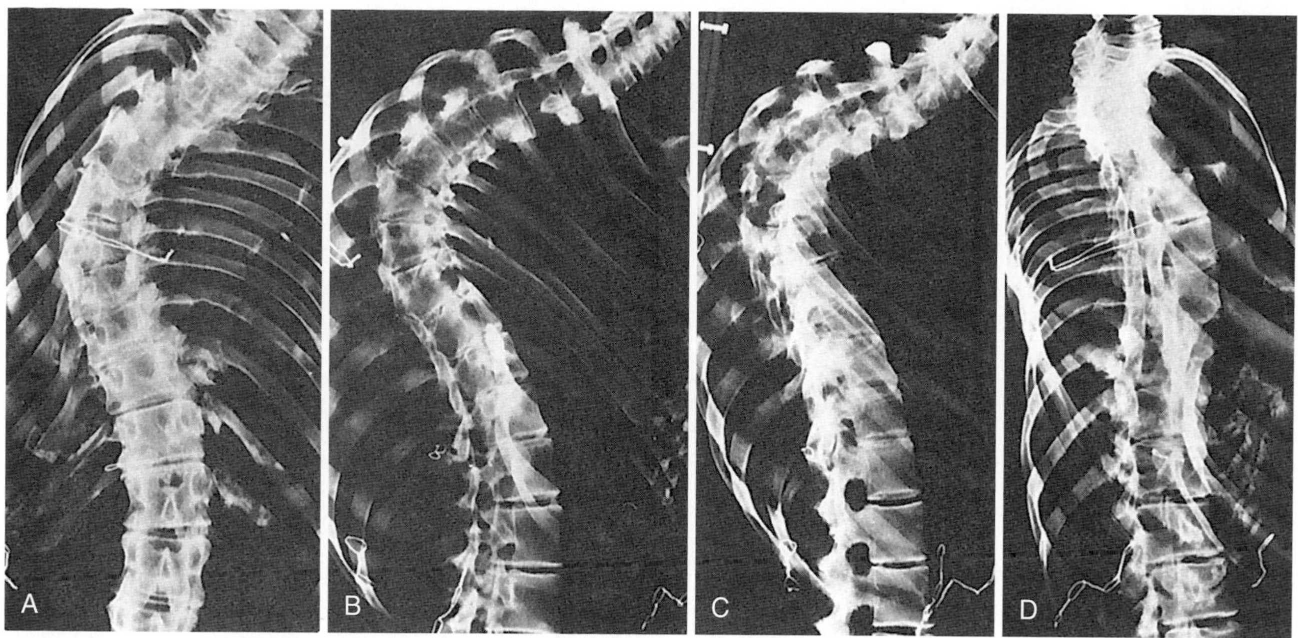

FIGURE 44-19 Radiographs at four points during rotational cycle of articulated scoliotic spine show changes in Cobb angle with rotation. On anteroposterior view, apparent Cobb angle of 87 degrees **(A)** and true Cobb angle of 128 degrees **(B)**. On lateral view, apparent kyphosis of 61 degrees **(C)** and true apical lordosis of 14 degrees **(D)**. (From Deacon P, Flood BM, Dickson RA: Idiopathic scoliosis in three dimensions: a radiographic and morphometric analysis, J Bone Joint Surg 66B:509, 1984.)

significant kyphosis. The scoliometer can be used in conjunction with the Adams forward bending test to evaluate truncal rotation. An angle of less than 7 degrees is considered within the limits of normal, and an angle of more than 7 degrees usually is associated with a curve of 15 to 20 degrees. Limb lengths should be measured because a discrepancy may cause a pelvic tilt and a compensatory scoliosis. A thorough neurologic examination should be done to determine if an intraspinal neoplasm or a neurologic disorder is the cause of scoliosis. Particular attention should be given to the abdominal reflexes because often they are the only neurologic abnormality found with some intraspinal disorders.

RADIOGRAPHIC EVALUATION

Posteroanterior and lateral radiographs of the spine, including the iliac crest distally and most of the cervical spine proximally, should be made with the patient standing. Inclusion of the iliac crest and the cervical spine generally requires 14 × 36-inch cassettes or digital equipment that allows accurate splicing of images. Patients should stand with their knees locked, with feet shoulder width apart, and looking straight ahead. The patient's shoulders are flexed forward, the elbows are fully flexed, and the fists should rest on the clavicles. The organs most at risk from radiation are the maturing breasts, and radiation is decreased by a factor of 5 to 11 by use of the posteroanterior view. Faster radiographic film and rare-earth screens also reduce the patient's exposure to radiation. New low-dose, digital slot-scanning techniques require approximately one eighth the radiation of standard radiographs.

Assessment of the flexibility of a scoliotic curve pattern is important when the patient is being evaluated for surgery or bracing. This can be assessed by right and left bending films, traction films, fulcrum bending films, or push-prone radiographs. Controversy remains regarding the best way to obtain bending films. If the lumbosacral junction is not well seen on the standing lateral radiograph, a spot lateral radiograph of the lumbosacral joint should be made to screen for spondylolisthesis.

Standard anteroposterior views of scoliosis curves can underestimate the magnitude of the curve. Also, true lateral views show a lordosis when the more standard lateral views give the erroneous impression of kyphosis (Fig. 44-19). Stagnara described a radiographic technique to eliminate this rotational component of the curve. In this technique, an oblique radiograph is made with the cassette parallel to the medial aspect of the rotational rib prominence and the x-ray beam positioned at right angles to the cassette (Fig. 44-20). A film made at 90 degrees to this provides the true lateral view, allowing a much more accurate measurement of the curve size and better evaluation of vertebral anatomy (Fig. 44-21).

Although no absolutely accurate method is available for determining skeletal maturity as an adolescent progresses through puberty, various radiographic parameters can be used to assess maturity. The most common method is assessment of bone age at the hand and wrist and development of the iliac apophysis (Risser sign), triradiate cartilage, olecranon apophysis ossification, and digital ossification.

The Risser sign is a measurement based on the ossification of the iliac apophysis, which is divided into four quadrants. The Risser sign proceeds from grade 0, no ossification, to grade 4, in which all four quadrants of the apophysis have ossification. Risser grade 5 is when the apophysis has fused completely to the ilium when the patient is skeletally mature. The Risser sign may not be as useful for predicting curve progression because grade 1 has been found to begin after the period of rapid adolescent growth or peak height velocity.

The peak height velocity (PHV) has been reported by several authors to be a better maturity indicator than the Risser sign, chronologic age, or menarchal age. PHV is calculated from serial height measurements and is expressed as centimeters of growth per year. Average values of PHV are 8 cm per year in girls and 9.5 cm per year in boys. Little et al., in a study of 120 girls with scoliosis, found that PHV reliably predicted cessation of growth (3.6 years after PHV in 90%) and likelihood of curve progression. Of 60 patients with curves of more than 30 degrees at PHV, 50 (83%) had curve progression to 45 degrees or more; of 28 with curves of 30 degrees or less at PHV, only one (4%) progressed to 45 degrees or more. Little et al. found similar results in boys with scoliosis and reported a 91% accuracy rate for predicting progression to 45 degrees or more. In both girls and boys, they found the PHV to be superior to the Risser sign, chronologic age, and menarchal age as a maturity indicator.

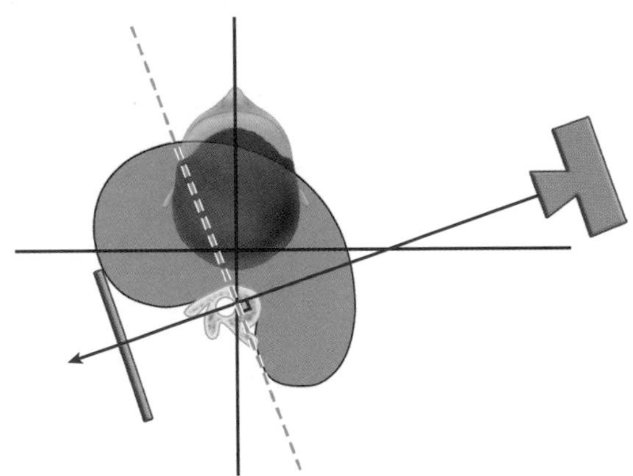

FIGURE 44-20 Diagram of Stagnara derotation view.

The triradiate cartilage begins to ossify in the early stages of puberty. In girls it is completely ossified after the period of PHV and before Risser grade 1 and menarche. In boys it is in the early stages of ossification when puberty begins. Sanders et al. evaluated the relationship of the PHV with the occurrence of the crankshaft phenomenon after posterior arthrodesis and instrumentation. They found that in patients with open triradiate cartilages, surgery done before or during the time of PHV was a strong predictor of the crankshaft phenomenon (Fig. 44-22).

Other methods for evaluating maturity and the risk of curve progression are based on hand and wrist or elbow radiographs. The Sauvegrain method determines skeletal age from anteroposterior and lateral radiographs of the left elbow. It is a 27-point system based on four anatomic structures about the elbow: lateral condyle, trochlea, olecranon apophysis, and the proximal radial epiphysis. Skeletal age is determined from this score. Charles et al. reported a method to assess maturity based on the olecranon apophysis. Five radiographic images demonstrated the typical characteristic of the olecranon during pubertal growth: two ossification nuclei, a half-moon image, a rectangular shape, the beginning of fusion, and complete fusion. This represented a simple but reliable method of skeletal age assessment and allowed for skeletal age to be determined in regular 6-month intervals from the age of 11 to 13 years in girls and from 13 to 15 years in boys. They found that this information complemented the

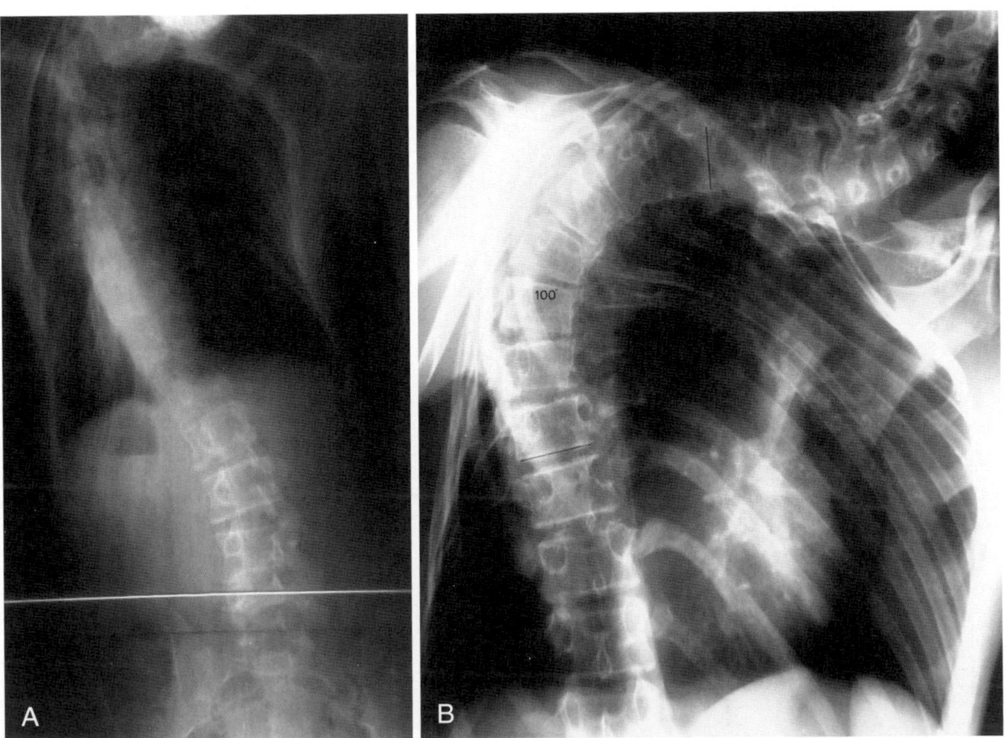

FIGURE 44-21 **A,** Standard posteroanterior radiograph of large scoliosis. **B,** Stagnara view showing better detail of curve, size, and vertebral anatomy.

Risser grade 0 and triradiate cartilage closure information (Figs. 44-23 and 44-24).

Both the Tanner-Whitehouse-III RUS score, based on the radiographic appearance of the epiphyses of the distal radius, ulna, and small bones of the hands, and the digital skeletal age maturity scoring system, based on the metacarpals and phalanges, highly correlate with peak height velocity and curve progression. However, these systems are cumbersome and not very practical to use in a busy clinical setting. Because of this, Sanders et al. reported a simplified classification based on the epiphyses of the phalanx, metacarpal, and distal radius. They were able to demonstrate that this method reliably predicted maturity and probability of progression to surgery (Fig. 44-25 and Table 44-4).

Davids et al. found a 10% incidence of central nervous system abnormalities in patients with presumed adolescent idiopathic scoliosis having subtle history, physical examination, or radiographic abnormalities (Fig. 44-26). The most valuable sign was absence of thoracic apical segment lordosis. Diab et al. and Richards et al. reported finding abnormalities on preoperative MRI in 9.9% and 6.8%, respectively, of patients with idiopathic scoliosis. Both studies found thoracic

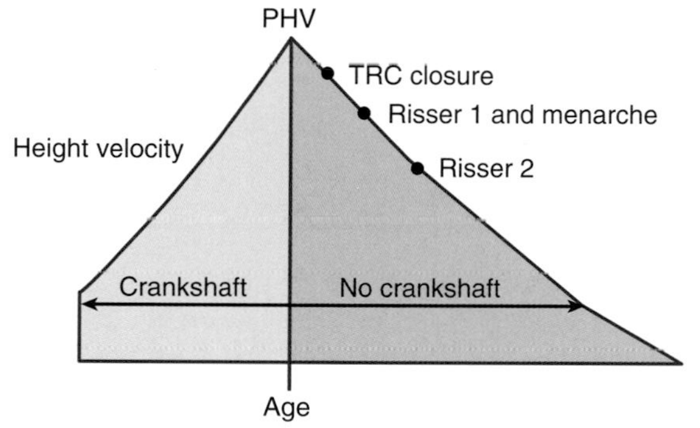

FIGURE 44-22 Height velocity. Triradiate cartilage (TRC) closure occurs after period of peak height velocity (PHV) and before Risser grade 1 and menarche. (Modified from Sanders JO, Little DG, Richards BS: Prediction of the crankshaft phenomenon by peak height velocity, Spine 22:1352, 1997.)

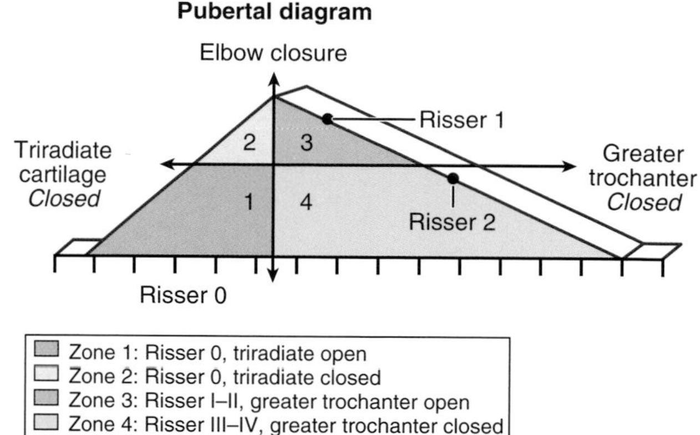

FIGURE 44-23 Pubertal diagram divided into four zones. Zone 1, ascending side, triradiate cartilage open, bone age between 11 and 13 years in girls and boys (Risser 0). Zone 2, ascending side, triradiate cartilage closed, bone age between 11 and 13 years in girls and between 13 and 15 years in boys (Risser 0). Zone 3, descending side, elbow closed but greater trochanter not fused, bone age between 13 and 16 years in girls and between 15 and 18 years in boys (Risser 1 to 2). Zone 4, descending side, elbow closed and greater trochanter fused, bone age between 13 and 16 years in girls and between 15 and 18 years in boys (Risser 3 to 4). (Redrawn from Dimeglio A, Canavese F, Charles P: Growth and adolescent idiopathic scoliosis: when and how much? J Pediatr Orthop 31:S28, 2011.)

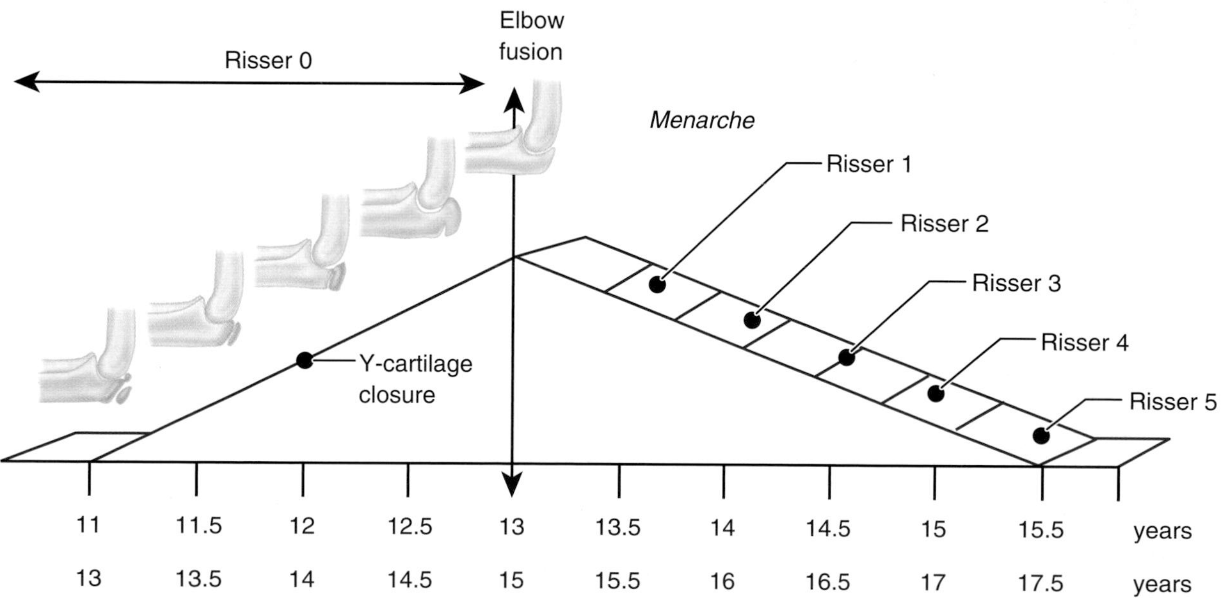

FIGURE 44-24 Simplified skeletal age assessment with the olecranon method during the accelerating pubertal growth phase of peak height velocity and Risser grade 0 from ages of 11 to 13 years in girls and from 13 to 15 years in boys, with a decelerating growth phase after elbow fusion. Y-cartilage closure = triradiate cartilage closure. (Redrawn from Charles YP, Dimeglio A, Canavese F, Dauers JP: Skeletal age assessment from the olecranon for idiopathic scoliosis at Risser grade 0, J Bone Joint Surg 89A:737, 2007.)

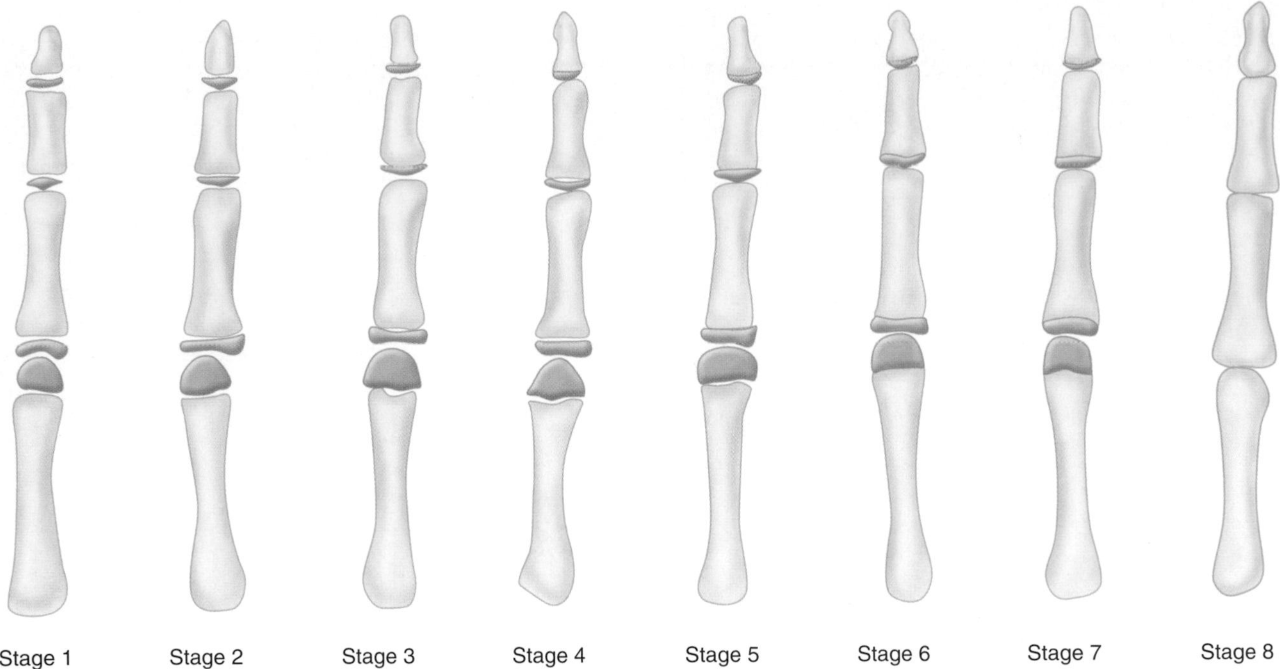

FIGURE 44-25 Sanders classification of skeletal maturity. Stage 1, juvenile slow; stage 2, preadolescent (Tanner 2); stage 3, adolescent rapid-early (Tanner 2 to 3, Risser 0); stage 4: adolescent rapid-late (Tanner 3, Risser 0); stage 5, adolescent steady-early (Risser 0); stage 6, adolescent steady-late (Risser > 0); stage 7, early mature; stage 8, mature stage (Risser 5). (From Crawford AH, et al: Clinical and radiographic evaluation of the scoliotic patient. In Newton PO, O'Brien MF, Shufflebarger HL, et al, editors: Idiopathic scoliosis: the Harms Study Group treatment guide, New York, 2010, Thieme, p 60.)

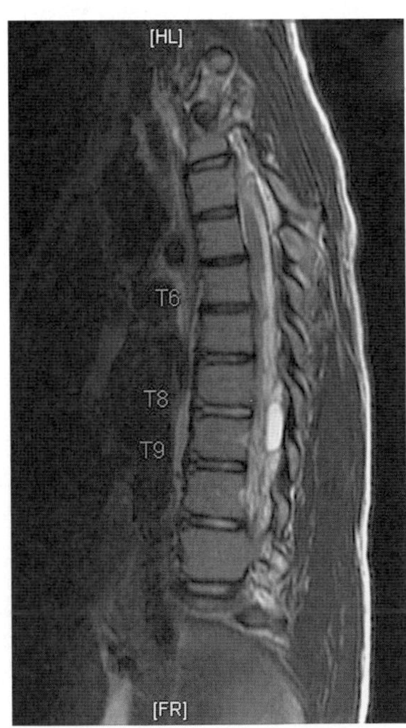

FIGURE 44-26 Preoperative MRI evaluation of what was presumed to be routine adolescent idiopathic scoliosis scheduled for surgical instrumentation and fusion. Total spine MR image reveals an epidural cyst at T8-9.

hyperkyphosis to be a risk factor for abnormal MRI findings. We obtain MRI of the total spine when any adolescent idiopathic scoliosis curve appears unusual or when there is a questionable history or physical findings, a rapidly progressive curve, or any large curve when the patient is first seen.

MEASUREMENT OF CURVES

The Cobb method of measurement recommended by the Terminology Committee of the Scoliosis Research Society (Fig. 44-27) consists of three steps: (1) locating the superior end vertebra, (2) locating the inferior end vertebra, and (3) drawing intersecting perpendicular lines from the superior surface of the superior end vertebra and from the inferior surface of the inferior end vertebra. The angle of deviation of these perpendicular lines from a straight line is the angle of the curve. If the endplates are obscured, the pedicles can be used instead. The end vertebra of the curve is the one that tilts the most into the concavity of the curve being measured. In general, on moving away from the apex of the curve, the next intervertebral space below the inferior end vertebra or above the superior end vertebra is wider on the concave side of the curve. Within the curve, the intervertebral spaces usually are wider on the convex side and narrower on the concave side. When significantly wedged, the vertebrae themselves, rather than the intervertebral disc spaces, may be wider on the convex side of the curve and narrower on the concave side. The reported interobserver and intraobserver variations in Cobb measurements average 5 to 7 degrees. These figures should be taken into account in determining whether a curve is truly progressing.

TABLE 44-4

Logistic Projection of the Probability of Lenke Type 1 and Type 3 Curves Progressing to Surgery Assuming a Threshold of More Than 50 Degrees*†

CURVE	STAGE 1	STAGE 2	STAGE 3	STAGE 4	STAGE 5	STAGE 6	STAGE 7,8
10°	2% (0% to 40%)	0% (0% to 15%)	0% (0% to 0%)	0% (0% to 0%)	0% (0% to 0%)	0% (0% to 0%)	0% (0% to 1%)
15°	23% (4% to 69%)	11% (1% to 58%)	0% (0% to 2%)	0% (0% to 0%)	0% (0% to 0%)	0% (0% to 0%)	0% (0% to 7%)
20°	84% (40% to 98%)	92% (56% to 99%)	0% (0% to 14%)	0% (0% to 1%)	0% (0% to 1%)	0% (0% to 1%)	0% (0% to 26%)
25°	99% (68% to 100%)	100% (92% to 100%)	29% (3% to 84%)	0% (0% to 5%)	0% (0% to 5%)	0% (0% to 2%)	0% (0% to 64%)
30°	100% (83% to 100%)	100% (98% to 100%)	100% (47% to 100%)	0% (0% to 27%)	0% (0% to 22%)	0% (0% to 11%)	0% (0% to 91%)
35°	100% (91% to 100%)	100% (100% to 100%)	100% (89% to 100%)	0% (0% to 79%)	0% (0% to 65%)	0% (0% to 41%)	0% (0% to 98%)
40°	100% (95% to 100%)	100% (100% to 100%)	100% (98% to 100%)	15% (0% to 99%)	0% (0% to 94%)	0% (0% to 83%)	0% (0% to 100%)
45°	100% (98% to 100%)	100% (100% to 100%)	100% (100% to 100%)	88% (2% to 100%)	1% (0% to 99%)	0% (0% to 98%)	0% (0% to 100%)

*Unshaded cells correspond with combinations of curve size and maturity stage for which surgery would be a plausible treatment if more than 50 degrees at maturity is accepted as the threshold for surgical treatment. Shaded cells correspond with combinations for which surgery would not be a plausible treatment.

†Cells with wide 95% confidence intervals (shown in parentheses) correspond with groups that had too few patients for accurate estimates (or groups that had no patients) and should be interpreted with caution.

Reproduced from Sanders JO, Khoury JG, Kishan S, et al: Predicting scoliosis progression from skeletal maturity: a simplified classification during adolescence, J Bone Joint Surg 90A:540, 2008.

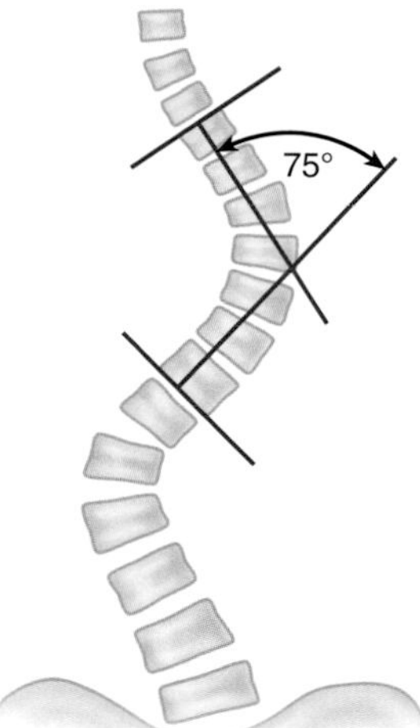

FIGURE 44-27 Diagram of Cobb method (see text).

VERTEBRAL ROTATION

The two most commonly used methods of determining vertebral rotation are those of Nash and Moe and of Perdriolle and Vidal. In the method of Nash and Moe, if the pedicles are equidistant from the sides of the vertebral bodies, no vertebral rotation is present (0 rotation). The grades progress to grade IV rotation, in which the pedicle is past the center of the vertebral body (Fig. 44-28). The Perdriolle torsion meter is a template that measures the amount of vertebral rotation on a spinal radiograph. The vertebra's pedicle-shadow offset and the edges of the vertebral body are marked and then measured with the torsion meter (Fig. 44-29). The advent of multiple-hook segmental and thoracic pedicle screw instrumentation systems has increased awareness of the rotational component of scoliosis and subsequently increased interest in postoperative measurement of rotation. Because both methods are subject to measurement errors, care must be taken in evaluating postoperative rotation information based on either the Nash and Moe or the Perdriolle and Vidal technique. Theoretically, a CT scan is much more accurate in evaluating vertebral rotation; CT usually is not used in routine scoliosis evaluation, however, due to increased radiation exposure. The Nash and Moe and the Perdriolle and Vidal techniques are subject to measurement error because of the three-dimensional torsion or dysplasia of the rotated segments, and postoperative measurements can be difficult or impossible because instrumentation may obscure the radiographic landmarks. Kuklo et al. evaluated the utility of alternative radiographic measures of vertebral rotation. They found that the rib hump as measured on the

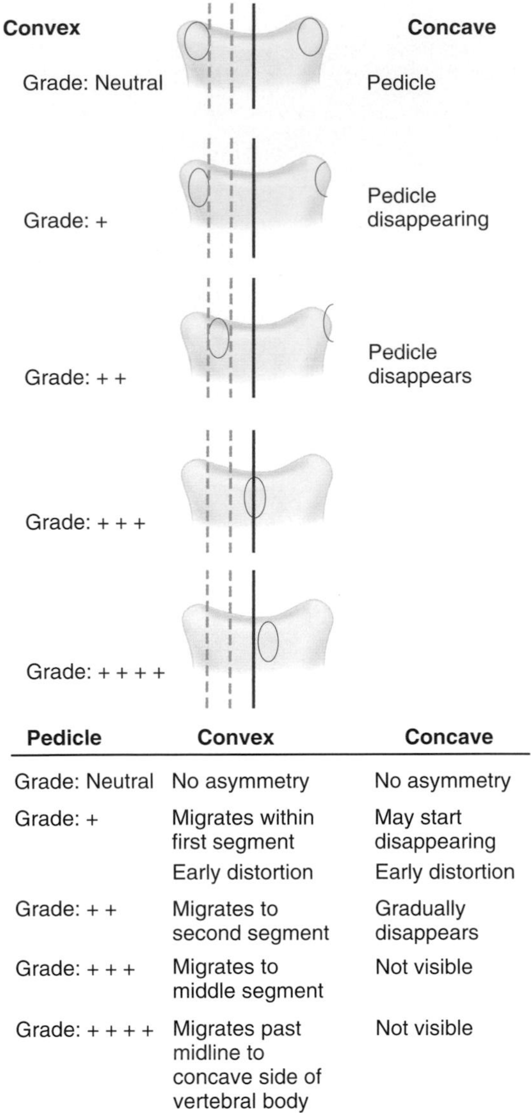

Pedicle	Convex	Concave
Grade: Neutral	No asymmetry	No asymmetry
Grade: +	Migrates within first segment Early distortion	May start disappearing Early distortion
Grade: + +	Migrates to second segment	Gradually disappears
Grade: + + +	Migrates to middle segment	Not visible
Grade: + + + +	Migrates past midline to concave side of vertebral body	Not visible

FIGURE 44-28 Pedicle method of determining vertebral rotation. Vertebral body is divided into six segments and grades 0 to 4+ are assigned, depending on location of pedicle within segments. Because pedicle on concave side disappears early in rotation, pedicle on convex side, easily visible through wide range of rotation, is used as standard.

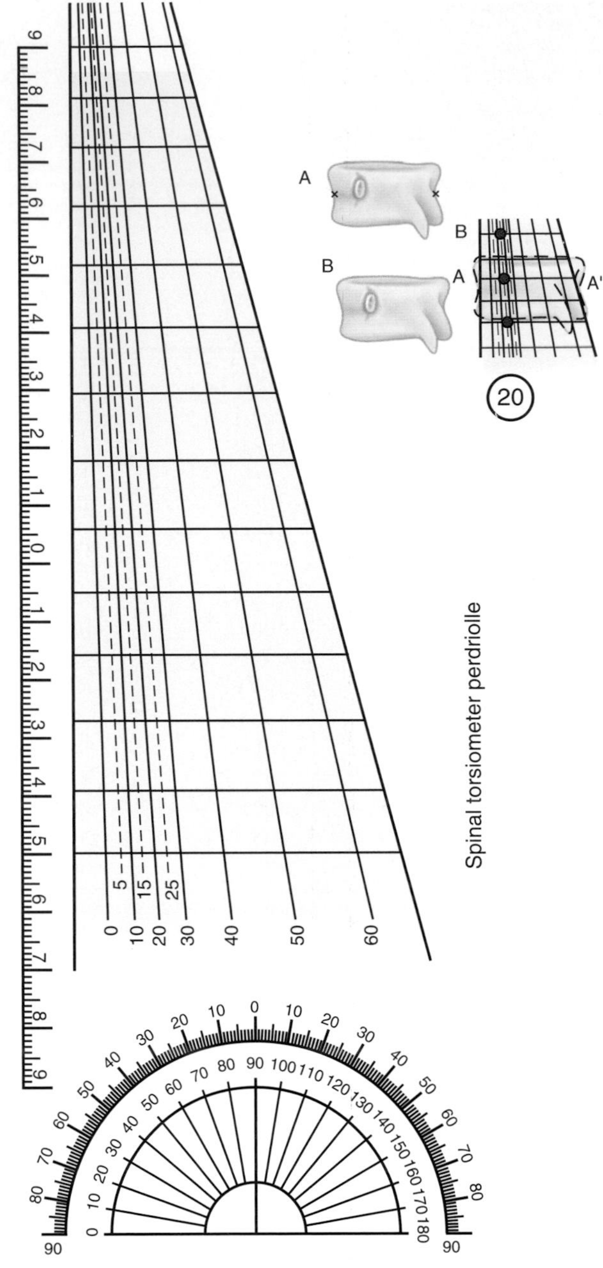

FIGURE 44-29 Perdriolle torsion meter for measuring vertebral rotation.

lateral radiograph (Fig. 44-30A) and the apical vertebral body-rib ratio (Fig. 44-30B) showed a strong correlation with vertebral rotation and can be used when CT is not feasible or when instrumentation obscures the landmarks necessary for rotation to be evaluated by the other techniques. New slot digital scanning imaging techniques (EOS Imaging, Paris, France) provide fast and accurate three-dimensional reconstructions of the spine that can better determine vertebral body rotation.

SAGITTAL BALANCE

The importance of normal sagittal alignment has become recognized in the management of patients with spinal deformity. Sagittal alignment can be considered on a segmental, regional, or global basis. Segmental analysis refers to the relationships between two vertebral bodies and the intervening disc. Regional sagittal balance includes that of the cervical, thoracic, or lumbar spines; the thoracolumbar junction often is considered separately. Global spinal alignment generally is considered to be an indication of overall sagittal balance.

Overall spinal sagittal balance is determined by a plumb line dropped from the dens. This plumb line usually falls anterior to the thoracic spine, posterior to the lumbar spine, and through the posterior superior corner of S1 (Fig. 44-31). On the standing long lateral films generally used in spinal deformity evaluation, the dens is not easily seen. The plumb line therefore usually is dropped from the middle of the C7 vertebral body. This plumb line is called the sagittal vertebral axis. A positive sagittal vertebral axis is considered present

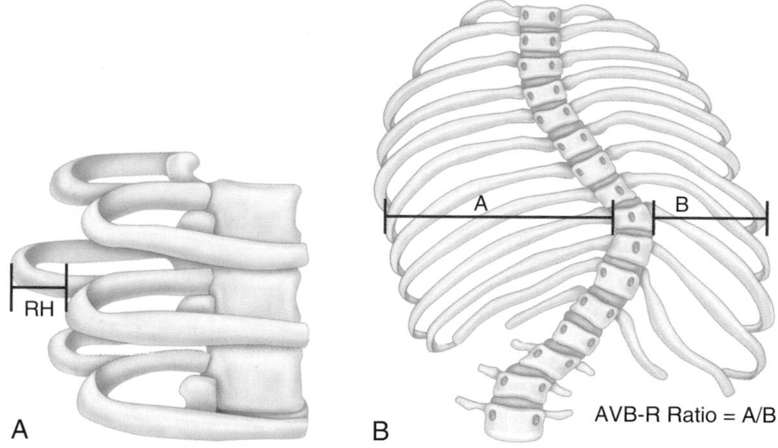

FIGURE 44-30 A, Diagram of measurement technique for assessing rib hump (RH) deformity. RH is linear distance between left and right posterior rib prominences at apex of rib deformity on lateral radiograph. B, Diagram of measurement technique for apical vertebral body/rib ratio (AVB-R). AVB-R is ratio of linear measurements from lateral borders of apical thoracic vertebrae to chest wall on anteroposterior radiographs. (Redrawn from Kuklo TR, Potter BK, Lenke WG: Vertebral rotation and thoracic torsion in adolescent idiopathic scoliosis: what is the best radiographic correlate? J Spinal Disord Tech 18:139, 2005.)

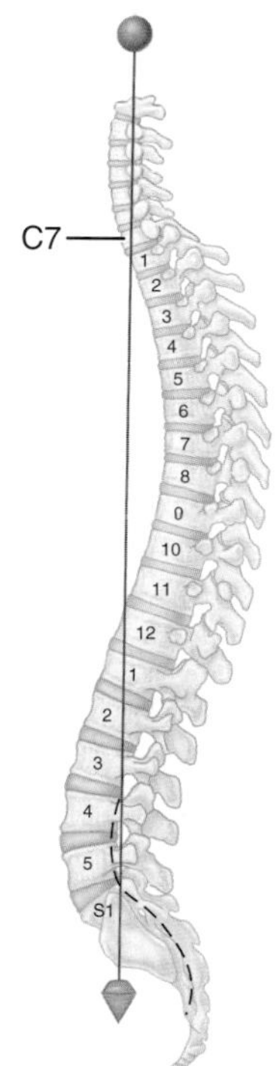

FIGURE 44-31 C7 sagittal plumb line is useful measurement of sagittal balance. Plumb line dropped from middle of C7 vertebral body falls close to posterosuperior corner of S1 vertebral body.

when the plumb line is anterior to the anterior aspect of S1. A negative sagittal vertebral axis occurs when this plumb line passes posterior to the anterior body of S1 (Fig. 44-32). The overall sagittal balance is probably a more important measurement than regional and segmental measurements. In general, for sagittal balance to be maintained, lumbar lordosis should measure 20 to 30 degrees more than the kyphosis. If overall sagittal balance is not considered, correction to the normal range of lordosis without similar correction of the kyphotic thoracic spine can lead to significant sagittal imbalance (Fig. 44-33).

In the thoracic spine, the normal sagittal curvature is kyphotic. The kyphosis begins at the first thoracic vertebra and reaches its maximal segmental kyphosis at T6 or T7. Ranges of thoracic kyphosis in normal patients, both adults and children, have been reported. Although the kyphosis begins at T1, this vertebra often cannot be seen on standing long-cassette lateral films. The T4 or T5 vertebra is more easily seen and measured. Gelb et al. found that the upper thoracic kyphosis from T1 to T5 in 100 adults averaged 14 ± 8 degrees. Adding this number to the kyphosis measured from T5 to T12 provides a reasonable estimate of overall regional kyphosis.

The normal regional lumbar sagittal alignment is lordotic. The normal apex of this lordosis is at the vertebral body of L3 or L4 or the disc space itself. The segments at L4-L5 and L5-S1 account for 60% of the overall lumbar lordosis. Wambboldt and Spencer reported that the lumbar discs account for −47 degrees of the lordosis; the vertebral bodies themselves account for only −12 degrees. This emphasizes the importance of preserving disc height during anterior procedures for the treatment of spinal deformities. Because 40% of the total lumbar lordosis is in the L5-S1 segment, it is important to measure to the top of the sacrum, although this can be difficult on standing lateral images. The lumbar lordosis is a dependent variable based on the amount of kyphosis. For sagittal balance to be maintained, lordosis generally is 20 to 30 degrees larger than thoracic kyphosis.

The orientation of the sacrum, the sacral slope, and the pelvic incidence are closely associated with the characteristics of lumbar lordosis and location of the apex of lumbar lordosis (Fig. 44-34). A sacral slope of less than 35 degrees and a low pelvic incidence are associated with a relatively flat, short lumbar lordosis. A sacral slope of more than 45 degrees and a high pelvic incidence are associated with a long, curved lumbar lordosis.

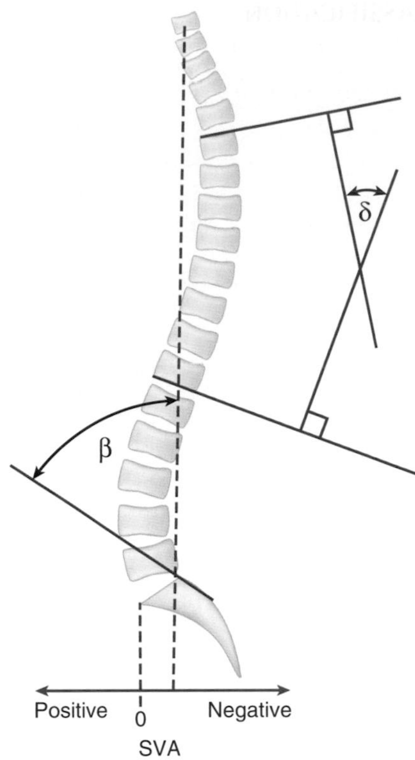

FIGURE 44-32 Method of measurement of various parameters of sagittal spinal alignment. Sagittal vertical axis (SVA) is horizontal distance from C7 plumb line to front corner of sacrum. Positive values indicate position anterior to sacrum; negative values are through or behind sacrum. β, Angle of sacral inclination, is angle subtended by tangent to posterior border of S1 and vertical axis. δ, Cobb angle between two vertebrae.

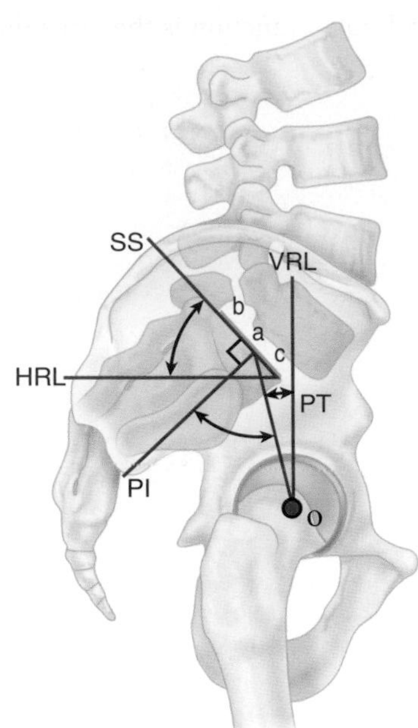

FIGURE 44-34 Sacral slope (SS) is angle subtended by horizontal reference line (HRL) and sacral endplate line (bc). SS shares common reference line (bc) with pelvic incidence (PI) and pelvic tilt (PT). PI is measured from static anatomic structures. PT and SS depend on angular position of sacrum/pelvis in relation to femoral heads, which changes with standing, sitting, and lying down. Relationship of PT and SS is affected by lumbosacropelvic flexion and extension. VRL, vertical reference line. (From Jackson R, Kanemura T, Kawakami N, Hales C: Lumbopelvic lordosis and pelvic balance on repeated standing lateral radiographs of adult volunteers and untreated patients with constant low back pain, Spine 25:575-586, 2000.)

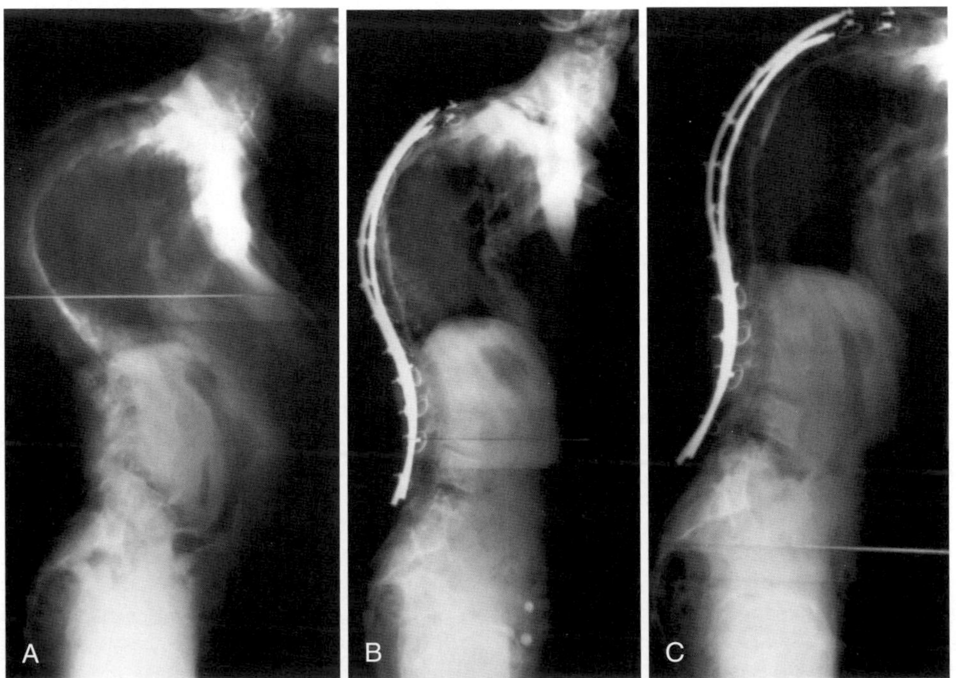

FIGURE 44-33 **A,** Preoperative standing lateral radiograph in patient with neuromuscular scoliosis. **B,** Standing lateral view 1 month later indicates imbalance between kyphosis and lordosis correction with signs of early increasing thoracic kyphosis. **C,** Further follow-up of same patient shows increasing falling off of thoracic kyphosis above instrumentation.

The thoracolumbar junction is the transition area from a relatively rigid kyphotic thoracic spine to a relatively mobile lordotic lumbar spine. Bernhardt and Bridwell showed that the thoracolumbar junction is nearly straight. This relationship must be maintained during reconstructive procedures to prevent a junctional kyphosis.

CURVE PATTERNS

PONSETI AND FRIEDMAN CLASSIFICATION

Idiopathic scoliosis curves were first classified by Ponseti and Friedman into five main patterns. A sixth curve pattern was described by Moe.

Single major lumbar curve. The lumbar curve has its apex between the L1-2 disc and L4. These curves produce an asymmetry of the waistline with prominence of the contralateral hip that parents often assume is caused by a short leg on the side of the curve.

Single major thoracolumbar curve. The thoracolumbar curve apex is at T12 or L1. This curve tends to produce more trunk imbalance than other curves. This decompensation from the midline often produces a severe cosmetic deformity.

Combined thoracic and lumbar curves (double major curves). Symmetric double major curves generally cause less visible deformities because the curves are nearly the same degree in size and the trunk usually is well balanced.

Single major thoracic curve. This curve pattern generally is a convex right pattern. Because of the thoracic location of the curve, rotation of the involved vertebrae may be obvious. The curve produces prominence of the ribs on the convex side, depression of the ribs on the concave side, and elevation of one shoulder, resulting in an unsightly deformity.

Single major high thoracic curve. There were only five patients with this curve pattern in the series of Ponseti and Friedman; although none of these curves became large, the deformity was unsightly because of the elevated shoulder and the deformed thorax. The apex of the curve usually was at T3, with the curve extending from C7 or T1 to T4 or T5.

Double major thoracic curve. This pattern was described by Moe and consists of a short upper thoracic curve, often extending from T1 to T5 or T6, with considerable rotation of the vertebrae and other structural changes in combination with the lower thoracic curve extending from T6 to T12 or L1. The upper curve usually is convex to the left, and the lower usually is convex to the right. Deformities in patients with this curve pattern usually are not as severe as in those with a single thoracic curve, but because of asymmetry of the neckline produced by the upper curve, this pattern is more deforming than combined thoracic and lumbar curves. In this curve pattern, the highly structural upper curve may be overlooked if the radiographs are not made on 14 × 36-inch cassettes and do not include the lower part of the cervical spine. If only the lower thoracic curve is corrected by fusion and instrumentation, the upper curve may not be flexible enough to allow correct posture and may lead to a cosmetically unacceptable result.

KING CLASSIFICATION

The classification system of King et al. is used to describe thoracic curves and aid in determining when the thoracic curve alone or both the thoracic and lumbar curves should be included in the instrumentation and fusion. Significant interobserver and intraobserver variability has been found in the use of this classification. Identification of curve types by the King classification begins with a careful physical examination. The location and magnitude of the thoracic rib hump and lumbar rotational prominence should be noted, as well as any elevation of the shoulder. Radiographic evaluation should include standing posteroanterior, lateral, and side-bending radiographs. The side-bending films are used to determine flexibility of the individual curves.

In a King type I curve, the lumbar curve is larger than the thoracic curve. On occasion, the thoracic and lumbar curves are nearly equal but the lumbar curve is less flexible on side bending. On clinical examination, the lumbar rotational prominence is larger than the rib hump.

Type II curves have created more confusion than any other curve pattern. As defined by King, type II thoracic scoliosis is a combined thoracic and lumbar curve pattern. On radiographs, the thoracic curve is larger than or equal to the lumbar curve. The lumbar curve must cross the center sacral line. On supine side-bending radiographs, the lumbar curve is more flexible than the thoracic curve. On clinical examination, the thoracic rib hump is larger than the lumbar rotational prominence.

A type III curve is a thoracic scoliosis with the lumbar curve not crossing the midline. The lumbar curve is very flexible on side-bending radiographs. On clinical examination, the thoracic rib hump is apparent and the lumbar prominence may be small or nonexistent.

A type IV curve is a single long thoracic curve, with L4 tilted into the curve and L5 balanced over the pelvis.

A type V curve is a double structural thoracic curve. On radiographs, the first thoracic vertebra is tilted into the concavity of the upper curve, which is structural on side-bending films. Clinical examination frequently finds an elevation of the left shoulder. On forward bending, there is an upper left thoracic rib hump and a lower right thoracic rib prominence.

LENKE CLASSIFICATION

Lenke et al. proposed a three-step classification system for adolescent idiopathic scoliosis that considers both frontal and sagittal plane deformity and is designed to guide surgical treatment decision making. Measurements are obtained from standard posteroanterior, lateral, and right and left bending radiographs. The three steps in this classification system are (1) identification of the primary curve, (2) assignment of the lumbar modifier, and (3) assignment of the thoracic sagittal modifier. The first step is to identify the primary curve. These curves should be divided by region: proximal thoracic, main thoracic, and thoracolumbar or lumbar. Curves are considered to be structural curves if they are more than 25 degrees on posteroanterior radiographs and do not bend to less than 25 degrees on side-bending radiographs. Based on these measurements the curve can be classified into six types (Fig. 44-35). The second step is to determine the lumbar spine modifier. This is determined by drawing a vertical line upward from the center of the sacrum

Curve type

Type	Proximal thoracic	Main thoracic	Thoracolumbar/ lumbar	Curve description
1	Nonstructural	Structural (major)	Nonstructural	Main thoracic (MT)
2	Structural	Structural (major)	Nonstructural	Double thoracic (DT)
3	Nonstructural	Structural (major)	Structural	Double major (DM)
4	Structural	Structural (major)	Structural	Triple major (TM)
5	Nonstructural	Nonstructural	Structural (major)	Thoracolumbar/lumbar (TL/L)
6	Nonstructural	Structural	Structural (major)	Thoracolumbar/lumbar—structural MT (Lumbar curve > thoracic by ≥ 10°)

Structural Criteria

Proximal thoracic:	Side-bending Cobb ≥ 25° T2-T5 kyphosis ≥ 120°
Main thoracic:	Side-bending Cobb ≥ 25°
Thoracolumbar/lumbar:	Side-bending Cobb ≥ 25° T10-L2 kyphosis ≥ +20°

Location of Apex
(SRS definition)

Curve	Apex
Thoracic	T2-T11-12 Disc
Thoracolumbar	T12-L1
Lumbar	L1-2 Disc-L4

Modifiers

Lumbar Spine Modifier	Center Sacral Vertical Line (CSVL) to Lumbar Apex	
A	CSVL between pedicles	A
B	CSVL touches apical body(ies)	B
C	CSVL completely medial	C

Thoracic Sagittal Profile T5-T12		
–	(Hypo)	< 10°
N	(Normal)	10°–40°
+	(Hyper)	> 40°

Curve type (1–6) + Lumbar spine modifier (A, B, or C) + Thoracic sagittal modifier (–, N, or +)
Classification (e.g., 1 B +): ____________

FIGURE 44-35 Curve types and criteria for structural curves and location of apex. (From Lenke LG, Betz RR, Harms J, et al: Adolescent idiopathic scoliosis: a new classification to determine extent of spinal arthrodesis, J Bone Joint Surg 83A:1169, 2001.)

(center sacral vertical line [CSVL]). The lumbar spine modifier is then determined by the relationship of the CSVL to the concave pedicle of the apical lumbar vertebra and can be assigned into A, B, or C. In type A, the CSVL is between the pedicles; in type B, it is between the medial pedicle wall and the lateral vertebra; and in type C, it is medial to the entire vertebra. The third step is to determine the thoracic sagittal modifier. The sagittal modifier is hypokyphotic (< 10 degrees), normal (10 to 40 degrees), or hyperkyphotic (> 40 degrees). Forty-two discrete curve classifications can be identified by this three-step process. Recommendations for fusion levels can be made based on these curve types. The recommendation is that the major and structural minor curves be included in the instrumentation and fusion and the nonstructural curves excluded. Overall, the classification is treatment directed. The purpose is to allow better organization of similar curve patterns and to provide comparisons of various treatment methods. This will then ultimately serve as a guide for optimal surgical treatment of each adolescent idiopathic scoliosis patient. This classification currently is the most popular and preferred classification for idiopathic scoliosis.

NONOPERATIVE TREATMENT

Various methods have been used to treat adolescent idiopathic scoliosis over the years, including physical therapy, manipulation, and electrical stimulation, but there is no scientific evidence supporting their effectiveness. The two most widely accepted nonoperative techniques for idiopathic scoliosis are observation and bracing.

OBSERVATION

Some degree of scoliosis is frequent in the general population, but few individuals have curves that require treatment. Unfortunately, no method is reliable for accurately predicting at the initial evaluation which curves will progress; thus, observation may be the primary treatment. A radiograph of the spine currently is the only definitive documentation of curve size and curve progression. Attempts have been made to monitor external contours with measurement of the rib hump, measurement of the trunk rotation angle with a "scoliometer," and use of contour devices such as moiré topography and ISIS scanning. These methods may be useful in certain small curves and for low-risk patients, but periodic evaluation of the spine with radiographs still is necessary.

In general, young patients with curves of less than 20 degrees can be examined every 6 to 9 months. Adolescents with larger degrees of curvature should be examined every 4 to 6 months. Skeletally mature patients with curves of less than 20 degrees generally do not require further evaluation. A curve of more than 20 degrees in a patient who has not reached skeletal maturity will need more frequent examination, usually every 4 to 6 months, with standing posteroanterior radiographs. If progression of the curve (an increase of 5 degrees during 6 months) beyond 25 degrees is noted, orthotic treatment may be considered. For curves of 30 to 40 degrees in a skeletally immature patient, orthotic treatment is recommended at the initial evaluation. Curves of 30 to 40 degrees in skeletally mature patients generally do not require treatment, but because studies indicate a potential for progression in adult life, these patients should be observed with yearly standing posteroanterior radiographs for 2 to 3 years after skeletal maturity and then every 5 years.

ORTHOTIC TREATMENT

The goal of brace treatment is to limit further progression of the scoliotic curve and avoid surgery. Correction may occur while in the brace, but the curve will generally settle to its pretreatment degree of curvature once the brace is discontinued. Brace correction of spinal curves is thought to occur through molding of the spine, trunk, and rib cage during growth, specifically through transverse loading of the spine through the use of corrective pads. The efficacy of brace treatment for patients with adolescent idiopathic scoliosis remains controversial. Numerous studies in the literature support the effectiveness of an orthosis in preventing curve progression and the need for surgical intervention. However, there are other studies that suggest bracing may not be effective. In one of the most recent bracing studies, Weinstein et al. showed successful treatment in 72% of braced patients compared with 48% success with observation. They concluded that bracing significantly decreased progression of high-risk curves to the threshold of surgery in patients with adolescent idiopathic scoliosis and that the benefit of bracing increased with longer hours of brace wear. The Scoliosis Research Society (SRS) Committee on Bracing and Nonoperative Management has recommended standardization of criteria for adolescent idiopathic scoliosis brace studies so that valid and reliable comparisons can be made. The optimal inclusion criteria consist of age 10 years or older when a brace is prescribed, Risser grades 0 to 2, primary curve angles of 25 to 40 degrees, no prior treatment, and, if female, either premenarchal or less than 1 year postmenarchal. Our indications for orthotic treatment of adolescent idiopathic scoliosis are similar to the SRS inclusion criteria. We recommend a brace for a flexible curve of 20 to 30 degrees in a growing child with documented progression of 5 degrees or more. Curves in the 30- to 40-degree range in growing children are treated at initial evaluation. Although surgery usually is indicated for curves in the 40- to 50-degree range in growing children, orthotic treatment may be considered for some curves, such as a cosmetically acceptable double major curve of 40 to 45 degrees. Orthotic treatment is not used in patients with curves of more than 50 degrees.

Underarm braces (Boston, Wilmington, and Miami) have replaced the Milwaukee brace in most centers. However, these low-profile braces are restricted to patients whose curve apex is at T7 or lower. The Charleston and Providence nighttime bending braces hold the patient in maximal side-bending correction and are worn only at night for 8 to 10 hours. These braces are best suited for single thoracolumbar or lumbar curves.

The orthoses were originally intended to be worn 23 hours a day, but concern about compliance has led to part-time bracing regimens. Most part-time bracing protocols call for approximately 16 hours or less of brace wear each day. A meta-analysis of the literature found a relationship between the duration of brace wear per day and prevention of curve progression, suggesting that the more time that is spent in a brace, the less likely it will be for the curve to progress. Katz et al. also found that the total number of hours of brace wear correlated with the lack of curve progression. This effect was most significant in patients who were at Risser grade 0 or 1 at the beginning of treatment and in patients with an open triradiate cartilage at the beginning of treatment. Curves did not progress in 82% of patients who wore the brace more than 12 hours per day compared with only 31% of those who wore the brace less than 7 hours per day. The number of hours of brace wear also was correlated inversely with the need for operative treatment.

The SpineCor brace (Biorthex Inc., Boucherville, Quebec, Canada) is an adjustable, flexible, dynamic brace with the cited advantages of simplicity of use, comfort, increased mobility, high patient compliance, and effectiveness. Outcomes of clinical studies indicate that prevention of curve progression is better with the brace than with no treatment, but comparative studies have shown it to be less effective than rigid orthoses in preventing curve progression. It appears to provide the greatest benefit for children between the juvenile and early adolescent stages, generally between the ages of 6 and 11 years, with Cobb angles of less than 30 degrees.

CASTING

UNDERARM CASTS

Before the development of posterior instrumentation, casting was used to obtain correction of curve prior to fusion. With newer instrumentation systems, postoperative casting seldom is used. If postoperative immobilization is needed, an orthotist often can make a TLSO that is comparable to a postoperative cast. Unlike a cast, a TLSO allows tightening or loosening as necessary and also trimming to relieve pressure areas. If an orthotist is not available,

however, a postoperative underarm cast can be used if postoperative immobilization is necessary.

TECHNIQUE 44-7

- Place the patient on a Risser table and apply a stockinette to extend from over the head to the knees.
- Position the removable crossbar at the level of the upper portion of the shoulders. Use felt to pad the canvas strap on which the patient is resting.
- Pass muslin straps around the waist over the stockinette and tie them at the level of the greater trochanter on the opposite side. Then pass the straps through the windlass at the end of the table and apply a slight amount of traction.
- Pad the iliac crest with felt.
- Use extrastrong, resin-reinforced plaster and extend the cast to the sternum anteriorly and the upper portion of the back posteriorly.
- Mold the cast well around the pelvis and iliac crest.
- As the cast dries, trim it at the level of the pubic symphysis anteriorly, extending proximally to about the level of the anterior superior iliac spine to allow 100 degrees of hip flexion. Posteriorly, trim low over the buttocks at the level of the greater trochanters. Then trim proximally to relieve pressure over the sacral prominence.
- Remove an abdominal window to free the upper portion of the abdomen, the lower costal margin, and the xiphoid process.

OPERATIVE TREATMENT

The accepted indications for surgical correction of spinal deformity are based on the natural history of the deformity and the potential consequences of the deformity for the patient in adult life. Natural history studies have been used to show the potential consequences of significant deformity and pain. Pulmonary complications usually result from unusual deformities and early-onset scoliosis. In children and adolescents, surgery is considered if the curve is likely to reach a magnitude that can be expected to become troublesome in adulthood. Although most authors recommend surgery when the curve reaches 50 degrees, other factors need to be considered. Smaller lumbar and thoracolumbar curves may cause significant trunk shift, coronal decompensation, and cosmetic deformity. Double 50-degree curves are not as cosmetically unacceptable as single curves, and if progression occurs in skeletally mature patients, it is likely to be gradual. In an immature patient, on the other hand, surgery may be considered for curves between 40 and 50 degrees, depending on the clinical appearance. Surgery is more likely to be required in a patient with a curve that progresses despite brace treatment. Patients with significant back pain should have further evaluation before surgery. Dickson et al. emphasized the importance of lordosis in treatment decision making. Thoracic lordosis has a detrimental effect on pulmonary function, and bracing worsens thoracic lordosis. Surgery is therefore more likely to be indicated for an adolescent with a progressive curve associated with significant thoracic lordosis. The general indications for operative treatment are summarized in Box 44-3.

BOX 44-3

Indications for Operative Treatment of Idiopathic Scoliosis

- Increasing curve in growing child
- Severe deformity (> 50 degrees) with asymmetry of trunk in adolescent
- Pain uncontrolled by nonoperative treatment
- Thoracic lordosis
- Significant cosmetic deformity

PREOPERATIVE PREPARATION

Once the decision to perform spinal fusion has been made, certain preliminary precautions should be taken and tests done to ensure that the patient is properly prepared for the operative procedure. Aspirin-containing products or nonsteroidal antiinflammatory agents should be discontinued before surgery because these medications may increase blood loss during surgery. Birth control pills should be discontinued 1 month before surgery because they have been shown to increase the possibility of thrombophlebitis in the postoperative period. Preoperative radiographic evaluation with posteroanterior, lateral, and side-bending films of the spinal levels to be fused is essential. Special imaging techniques, such as CT, MRI, and myelography, occasionally are needed to rule out conditions such as syringomyelia, diastematomyelia, and tethered cord.

Patients with adolescent idiopathic scoliosis should have preoperative pulmonary function studies if they have a history of poor exercise tolerance, a curve of more than 60 degrees associated with a history of reactive airway disease, or a curve of more than 80 degrees. Newton et al. looked at the magnitude of the thoracic curve, number of vertebrae involved in the thoracic curve, thoracic hypokyphosis, and coronal imbalance in patients and found that these were associated with an increased risk of moderate or severe pulmonary impairment, but there were some patients who had clinically relevant pulmonary impairment with much smaller curves. In fact, in some patients the pulmonary impairment was out of proportion to the severity of the scoliosis. Johnston et al. reported that 19% of their patients with adolescent scoliosis had less than 65% of predicted pulmonary function. Pulmonary function studies usually are indicated in patients with paralytic scoliosis or those with idiopathic or congenital scoliosis who have severe curves or significant kyphosis or lordosis. Nickel et al. advocated tracheostomy before surgery in any patient with paralytic scoliosis and a vital capacity of less than 30% of predicted normal. We have found that the indications for tracheostomy can be safely narrowed if the patient spends several days after surgery in an adequately staffed intensive care unit in which the patient can remain intubated, respiratory functions can be constantly supervised, and mechanical aids for respiration are readily available. If any doubt remains as to the patient's pulmonary status with these measures, however, a tracheostomy is better done at the time of surgery.

Preoperative autologous blood donations can be used in patients who qualify to decrease the risk of homologous blood transfusions. The risks of homologous blood transfusion include transmitted diseases, such as hepatitis, malaria,

TABLE 44-5

Quantity of Blood Taken at First Phlebotomy Based on Patient Body Weight

PATIENT WEIGHT (kg)	VOLUME OF BLOOD (mL)*
23.0-29.5	125-175
30.0-42.5	175-275
43.0-50.0	400-450
≥50.0	450-500

*If hematocrit level remained satisfactory, the quantity of blood to be withdrawn was increased within the range at subsequent phlebotomy.

Data from MacEwen GD, Bennett E, Guille JT: Autologous blood transfusions in children and young adults with low body weight undergoing spinal surgery, J Pediatr Orthop 10:750, 1990.

cytomegalovirus infection, and human immunodeficiency virus infection, as well as alloimmunization and graft-versus-host reactions. Most patients undergoing elective scoliosis surgery can avoid receiving homologous blood by using autologous blood transfusion. It is a safe method of blood replacement in children weighing less than 45.5 kg (100 lb). Patients are given oral iron supplements three times a day. Larger children are allowed to donate one unit of blood a week. The patient's hematocrit level is checked before each donation and must be at least 34%. If the level is low, the patient is asked to return the following week. For smaller patients, a lesser volume of blood should be obtained at each visit (Table 44-5). With improved collection and storage techniques, the blood can be stored in a liquid state for up to 45 days. Cryopreserved autologous blood also is an effective method for storing a sufficient volume of blood for scoliosis surgery; however, it requires expensive equipment that may not be universally available. Also, after the blood is thawed, the glycerol must be removed. Once the blood is thawed and washed, it must be used within 24 hours. Bess et al. found that in 51% of patients, a minimum of one unit of autologous blood donated preoperatively was wasted or the patients were transfused at a higher hematocrit (>30%). They suggested that a more precise autologous blood donation guideline is needed to limit unnecessary transfusion and wasted resources.

Roye et al. showed that erythropoietin is an effective means of increasing red cell mass and decreasing the need for homologous blood products. The difficulty with erythropoietin use is the cost, and we do not use it routinely.

INTRAOPERATIVE CONSIDERATIONS

Whether the surgery is done anteriorly or posteriorly, or both, certain intraoperative considerations are important. Because spinal surgery requires extensive dissection that may result in severe blood loss, a large-bore intravenous line is necessary. An arterial line is helpful for continuous monitoring of blood pressure. An indwelling urinary catheter is used to monitor urinary output. Electrocardiographic leads, blood pressure cuff, and esophageal stethoscope also are routine monitors. A pulse oximeter is a useful adjunct to the arterial line.

Spinal cord monitoring using both spinal somatosensory evoked potentials and motor evoked potentials has become the standard of care during scoliosis surgery. Cervical and cortical leads to the surgical area can record stimulation of the distal sensory nerves and can alert the surgeon to possible alteration of spinal cord transmission. Preoperative monitoring for a "baseline" is helpful for comparison during the operative procedure. When somatosensory evoked potentials are used, multiple recording sites must be used, including cortical, subcortical, and peripheral sites, and certain inhalation agents, such as halothane and isoflurane, should be avoided, as should diazepam and droperidol. The somatosensory evoked potential is a useful adjunct for monitoring spinal cord function, but it is not infallible, and false-positive and false-negative results have been reported. An important limitation of the somatosensory evoked potential is that it measures only the integrity of the sensory system.

The use of motor evoked potentials will monitor the spinal cord motor tracts. The combination of motor evoked potentials and somatosensory evoked potentials can significantly decrease the chance of unrecognized injury to the spinal cord. Transcranial electrical stimulation of the motor cortex generates an electrical impulse that descends the corticospinal tract and enters the peripheral muscle, where this electrical impulse can be recorded. This allows for monitoring of the ventral spinal cord, which is vulnerable to cord ischemia.

Triggered electromyographic monitoring is useful to detect a possible breach in the pedicle wall by a pedicle screw. A threshold of less than 6 mA should alert the surgeon to a possible breach.

If information is desired about individual nerve root functions, alternative neurophysiologic methods are necessary.

The first available spinal cord monitoring technique was the Stagnara wake-up test, described by Vauzelle, Stagnara, and Jouvinroux in 1973. In this test, the anesthesia is decreased or reversed after correction of the spinal deformity. The patient is brought to a conscious level and asked to move both lower extremities. Once voluntary movement is noted, anesthesia is returned to the appropriate level and the surgical procedure is completed. Engler et al. pointed out possible hazards in arousing a prone, intubated patient from anesthesia, and Brown and Nash stressed that this test documents only that spinal cord function has not suffered a major compromise at the time the test is done. It also does not allow continuous spinal cord monitoring. The ankle clonus test been reported as an alternative to the wake-up test. Clonus should be present for a brief period on emergence from anesthesia. The absence of clonus during this time is abnormal. The combination of the somatosensory and motor evoked potentials has made use of the wake-up test much less frequent.

Hypotensive anesthesia, in which mean arterial blood pressure is kept at 65 mm Hg, has been advocated as an effective way to decrease intraoperative blood loss. An arterial line is essential during this type of anesthesia. Care also must be taken in reducing blood pressure so that it does not lead to ischemia of the spinal cord. Hypotensive anesthesia should not be considered in patients with a heart condition or in patients with spinal cord compression in whom a decrease in arterial blood supply might restrict an already compromised spinal cord blood flow. Acute normovolemic hemodilution is a technique shown to reduce the need for allogenic blood transfusion. Removal of a volume of the patient's whole blood at the beginning of surgery is performed and replaced with colloid or crystalloid. The hematocrit is reduced to 28% during surgery, and the whole blood that was withdrawn is then transfused at the conclusion of surgery. This hemodilution technique requires an anesthesiologist skilled in its use.

The cell saver has been shown to save approximately 50% of the red cell mass, thereby reducing the need for intraoperative blood transfusions. The cell saver does add to the expense of the procedure, but if enough blood loss is anticipated, it is a reasonable option. Mann et al. reported a 40% red cell mass salvage in spinal surgery. The salvage rate was lower than in other procedures because spinal surgery does not allow pooling of lost blood. The surgical technique involves liberal use of sponges to tamponade vessels. The need for a narrow-diameter tip suction results in greater cell damage and thus a lower salvage. The cell saver is contraindicated in patients with malignant disease or infection. The surgeon should try to estimate preoperatively if enough blood will be salvaged to make the cell saver cost-effective.

Antifibrinolytics have been shown to reduce intraoperative blood loss. Verma et al. showed that both tranexamic acid and epsilon-aminocaproic acid reduced blood loss during surgery for adolescent idiopathic scoliosis but did not change the overall transfusion rate. Tranexamic acid was more effective in reducing total blood and postoperative drainage.

SURGICAL GOALS

The goals of surgery for spinal deformity are to correct or improve the deformity, to maintain sagittal balance, to preserve or improve pulmonary function, to minimize morbidity or pain, to maximize postoperative function, and to improve or at least not to harm the function of the lumbar spine. To accomplish these goals in patients with idiopathic scoliosis, surgical techniques may include anterior, posterior, or combined anterior and posterior procedures. The surgical indications, techniques, and procedures are divided into anterior and posterior sections.

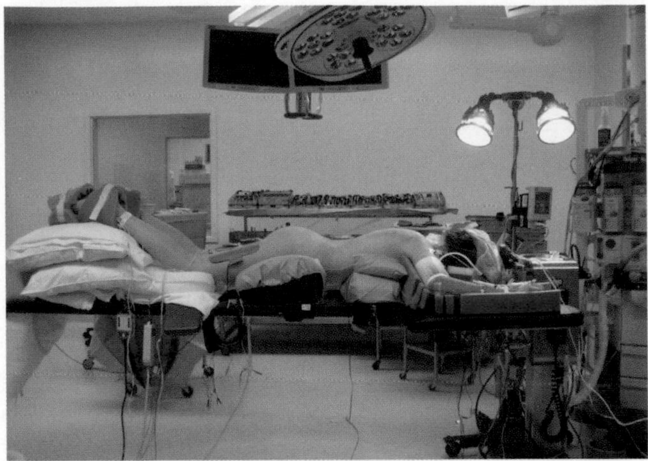

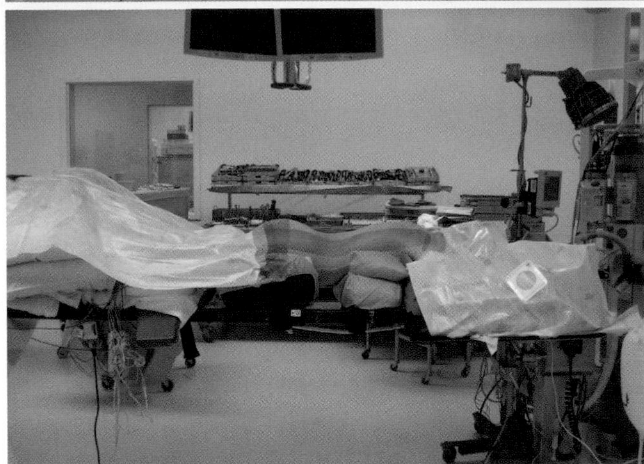

FIGURE 44-36 Patient positioning on Jackson table with hips in extension to maintain lumbar lordosis. **SEE TECHNIQUE 44-8.**

POSTERIOR SURGERIES FOR IDIOPATHIC SCOLIOSIS

POSTERIOR APPROACH

The posterior approach to the spinal column is the most commonly used. It is familiar to all orthopaedic surgeons and offers a safe and extensile approach that exposes the entire vertebral column.

TECHNIQUE 44-8

- Position the patient prone on a Jackson table (Mizuho OSI, Union City, CA) with the arms carefully supported and the elbows padded. The Jackson table eliminates intraabdominal pressure and helps reduce blood loss (Fig. 44-36).
- Do not abduct the shoulders more than 90 degrees to prevent pressure or stretch on the brachial plexus.
- The Jackson table maintains the hips in extension, which will maintain the lumbar lordosis, which is extremely important in obtaining proper sagittal alignment of the spine with instrumentation. The knees are well padded and slightly flexed to relieve some pressure from the hamstring muscles.
- Carefully pad the pressure points. The upper pads of the frame should rest on the chest and not in the axilla to avoid pressure on any nerves from the brachial plexus.
- When the patient is positioned on the frame with the hips flexed, lumbar lordosis is partially eliminated. If the fusion is to be extended into the lower lumbar spine, elevate the knees and thighs so that the patient lies with the hip joints extended to maintain normal lumbar lordosis.
- Scrub the patient's back with a surgical soap solution for 5 to 10 minutes and prepare the skin with an antiseptic solution. Drape the area of the operative site and use a plastic Steri-Drape (3M, St. Paul, MN) to seal off the skin.
- Make the skin incision in a straight line from one vertebra superior to the proposed fusion area to one vertebra inferior to it. A straight scar improves the postoperative appearance of the back (Fig. 44-37A). Make the initial incision through the dermal layer only. Infiltrate the intradermal and subcutaneous areas with an epinephrine solution (1 : 500,000).

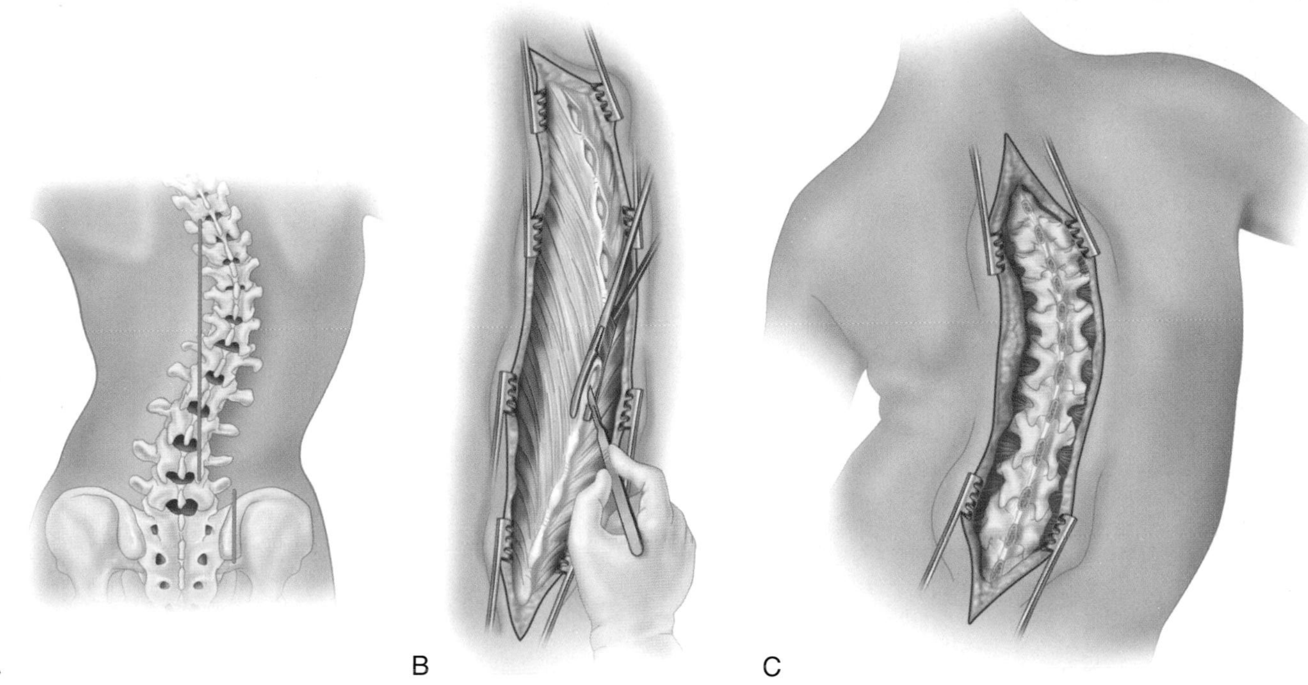

FIGURE 44-37 **A,** Skin incisions for posterior fusion and autogenous bone graft. **B,** Incisions over spinous processes and interspinous ligaments. **C,** Weitlaner retractors used to maintain tension and exposure of spine during dissection. **SEE TECHNIQUE 44-8.**

- Deepen the incision to the level of the spinous processes and use self-retaining Weitlaner retractors to retract the skin margins. Control bleeding with an electrocautery. Identify the interspinous ligament between the spinous processes; this often appears as a white line. As the incision is deepened, keep the Weitlaner retractors tight to help with exposure and to minimize bleeding. Now incise the cartilaginous cap overlying the spinous processes as close to the midline as possible (Fig. 44-37B). This midline may vary because of rotation of the spinous processes.
- With use of a Cobb elevator and electrocautery, expose the spinous processes subperiosteally after the cartilaginous caps have been moved to either side.
- After several of the spinous processes have been exposed, move the Weitlaner retractors to a deeper level and maintain tension for retraction and hemostasis.
- After exposure of all spinous processes, a localizing radiograph can be obtained. Alternatively, the T12 rib and the L1 transverse process can be used to localize the levels. Continue the subperiosteal exposure of the entire area to be fused, keeping the retractors tight at all times (Fig. 44-37C). It is easier to dissect from caudad to cephalad because of the oblique attachments of the short rotator muscles and ligaments of the spine.
- Extend the subperiosteal dissection first to the facet joints on one side and then the other side, deepening the retractors as necessary. Continue the dissection laterally to the ends of the transverse processes on both sides.
- Coagulate the branch of the segmental vessel just lateral to each facet.

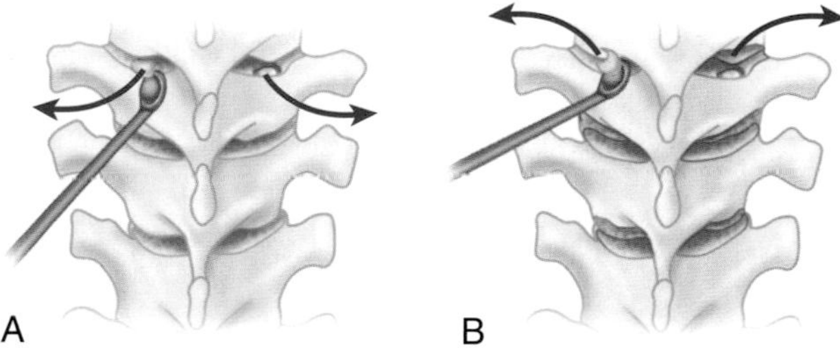

FIGURE 44-38 **A** and **B,** Cobb curets used to clean facets of ligament attachments. **SEE TECHNIQUE 44-8.**

- Place the self-retaining retractors deeper to hold the entire incision open and exposed.
- Sponges soaked in the 1 : 500,000 epinephrine solution can be used to maintain hemostasis.
- Use a curet and pituitary rongeur to completely clean the interspinous ligaments and the facets of all ligamentous attachments and capsule, proceeding from the midline laterally (Fig. 44-38) to decrease the possibility of the curet's slipping and penetrating the spinal canal.
- The entire spine is now exposed from one transverse process to another, all soft tissue has been removed, and the spine is ready for instrumentation and arthrodesis as indicated by the procedure chosen.

POSTERIOR FUSION

The long-term success of any operative procedure for scoliosis depends on a solid arthrodesis. The classic extraarticular

Hibbs technique has been replaced by intraarticular fusion techniques that include the facet joints. The success of spinal arthrodesis depends on surgical preparation of the fusion site, systemic and local factors, ability of the graft material to stimulate a healing process, and biomechanical features of the graft positioning. To obtain the best field for the fusion, soft-tissue trauma should be minimal. Avascular tissue should be removed from the graft bed. The surface of the bone and the facets should be decorticated to provide a large, maximally exposed surface area for vascular ingrowth and to allow delivery of more osteoprogenitor cells. The patient's condition should be improved as much as possible by nutrition and control of any medical problems. Smoking has been found to inhibit fusion significantly and should be discontinued before surgery. Autogenous bone graft from the iliac crest remains the "gold standard" for graft material, combining osteogenic, osteoconductive, and osteoinductive properties. Another excellent source of autogenous bone is rib obtained from a thoracoplasty. Allografts provide osteoconductive properties and have been shown to produce results equal to those of autogenous iliac crest graft in young patients. In certain conditions, such as paralytic scoliosis, in which large amounts of bone graft are needed and the iliac crests often are small or are used for instrumentation, allografts are used routinely. Several alternative graft materials include tricalcium phosphate, hydroxyapatite, and demineralized bone matrix. Bone morphogenetic protein can supply osteoinductive properties but has not been routinely used in multilevel fusions required in the treatment of scoliosis. In positioning the bone graft material, it should be remembered that bone graft generally does better under compression and is less effective with distraction. The farther the fusion is from the instantaneous axis of rotation, the better the fusion will prevent or minimize movement of that axis of rotation.

With improvements in surgical techniques and the inclusion of intraarticular fusion, together with meticulous dissection around the transverse processes, the pseudarthrosis rate has been decreased to 2% or less in adolescents with idiopathic scoliosis.

FACET FUSION

TECHNIQUE 44-9

(MOE)

- Expose the spine to the tips of the transverse processes as previously described (see Technique 44-8).
- Begin a cut over the cephalad articular processes at the base of the lamina and carry it along the transverse process almost to its tip. Bend this fragment laterally to lie between the transverse processes, leaving it hinged if possible.
- Thoroughly remove the cartilage from the superior articular process.
- Make another cut in the area of the superior articular facet with the Cobb gouge, beginning medially and working laterally to produce another hinged fragment.

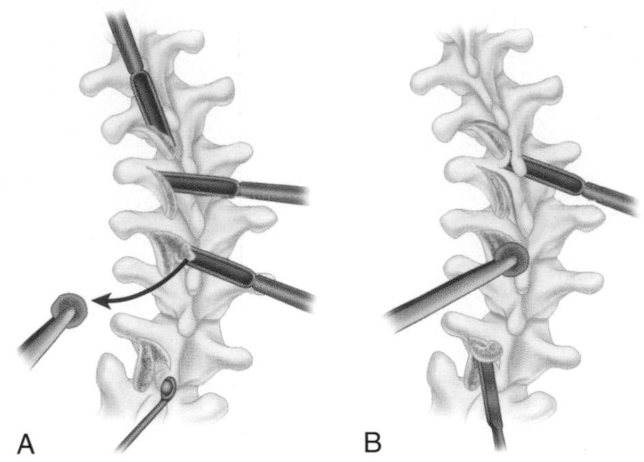

FIGURE 44-39 **A** and **B,** Moe technique of thoracic facet fusion. **SEE TECHNIQUE 44-9.**

- Place cancellous bone graft in the defect created (Fig. 44-39).
- In the lumbar spine, the facet joints are oriented in a more sagittal direction and a facet fusion is best accomplished by removal of the adjoining joint surface with a small osteotome or a needle-nose rongeur. This creates a defect that is packed with cancellous bone (Fig. 44-40).
- Decorticate the entire exposed spine with Cobb gouges from the midline, progressing laterally so that if the gouge were to slip it would be moving away from the spinal canal.
- Add cancellous bone graft. If the fusion is done for scoliosis and the amount of bone available is limited, concentrate the bone graft on the concave side of the curve because this bone will be subjected to compressive forces as opposed to tension forces on the convex side. The thoracolumbar and lumbar areas are the areas associated with the highest incidence of pseudarthrosis.

FACET FUSION

TECHNIQUE 44-10

(HALL)

- First, sharply cut the inferior facet with a gouge, remove this bone fragment to expose the superior facet cartilage, and remove this cartilage with a sharp curet.
- Create a trough by removing the outer cortex of the superior facet and add cancellous bone grafts (Fig. 44-41).
- Proceed with decortication as described in the Moe technique.
- At the completion of fusion, close the deep tissues with absorbable suture.
- Place a drain in the subcutaneous tissue or the deep layer, keeping the reservoir for this drain separate from the reservoir for the bone graft to allow monitoring of bleeding from the incision sites.

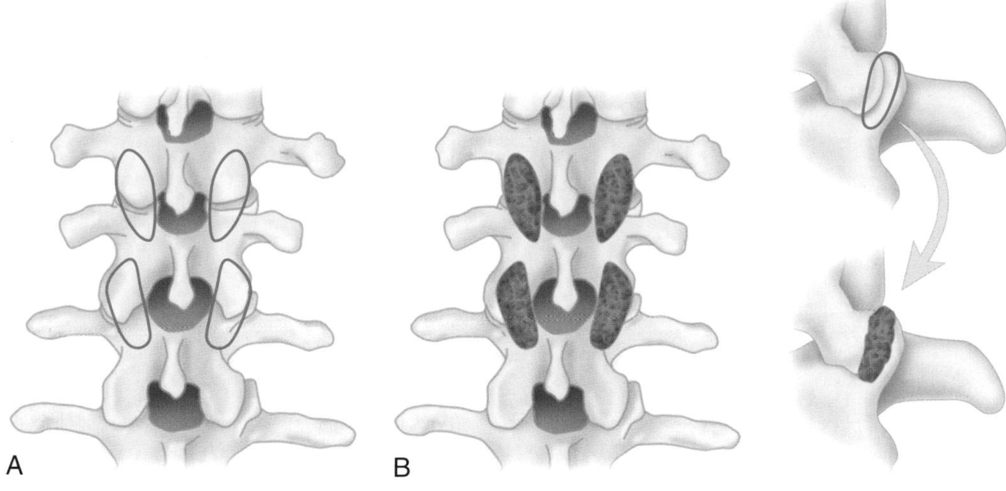

FIGURE 44-40 A and B, Moe technique of lumbar facet fusion. **SEE TECHNIQUE 44-9.**

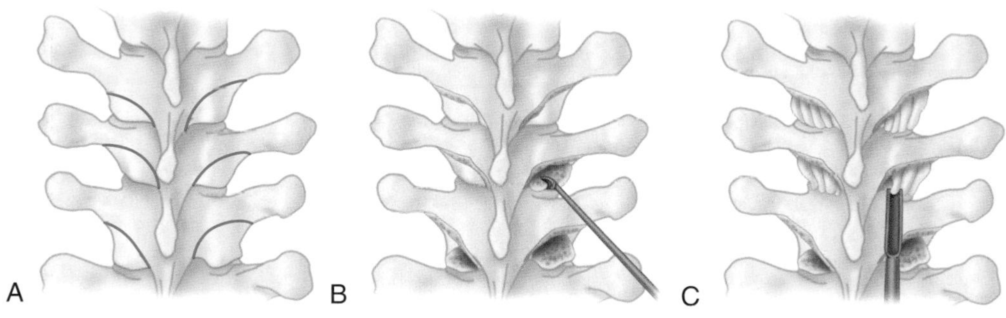

FIGURE 44-41 A-C, Hall technique of facet fusion. **SEE TECHNIQUE 44-10.**

- Approximate the subcutaneous tissues with 2-0 absorbable sutures and the skin edges with a running subcuticular absorbable stitch.
- Apply a bulky sterile dressing.

POSTOPERATIVE CARE. The patient is transferred to the bed from the operating table. Intravenous fluids are continued until the patient is able to tolerate oral intake and no longer requires any intravenous medication. Prophylactic preoperative, intraoperative, and postoperative intravenous antibiotics are given. Most patients have a Foley catheter inserted at the time of surgery; this is removed at 48 to 72 hours after surgery. Other postoperative treatment, such as casting, bracing, or ambulation, depends on the type of internal fixation, if any, used with the individual procedure.

BONE GRAFTING

Autogenous iliac crest bone graft has been considered the gold standard. The harvest of autogenous bone graft from the ilium can introduce the potential for intraoperative and postoperative morbidity associated with the procedure. Betz et al. described 91 patients with adolescent idiopathic scoliosis. Their results suggested that use of the rigid fixation provided by modern multisegmented hook or screw and rod systems combined with thorough decortication, facetectomy, and the inherent osteogenic potential of immature bone led to successful fusion rates without supplemental autogenous bone graft. Violas et al. found that local autograft bone produced fusion rates equal to those found with iliac crest autograft. The use of allograft does present the theoretical risk of disease transmission. Allograft also adds expense to the procedure, but this expense should be weighed against the decreased morbidity and decreased operative time. We have, likewise, found that the use of allograft definitely shortens operative time, postoperative pain, and blood loss. To date, we have not noted any increase in pseudarthrosis rates with use of allograft over previous cases done with autogenous iliac crest grafts.

AUTOGENOUS ILIAC CREST BONE GRAFT

TECHNIQUE 44-11

- Make an incision over the iliac crest to be used (Fig. 44-42A). If the original incision extends far enough distally into the lumbar spine, the iliac crest can be exposed through the same incision by subcutaneous dissection.

- Infiltrate the intradermal and subcutaneous areas with 1:500,000 epinephrine solution.
- Expose the cartilaginous apophysis overlying the posterior iliac crest and split it in the middle.
- With a Cobb elevator, expose the ilium subperiosteally.
- The superior gluteal artery emerges from the area of the sciatic notch (see Fig. 44-42A) and should be carefully avoided during the bone grafting procedure.
- If bicortical grafts are desired, expose the posterior crest of the ilium on the inner side and obtain two or three strips of bicortical graft with a large gouge. Otherwise, take cortical and cancellous strips from the outer table of the ilium (Fig. 44-42B).
- Place these bone grafts in a kidney basin and cover them with a sponge soaked in saline or blood.
- Control bleeding from the iliac crest with bone wax or Gelfoam.
- Approximate the cartilaginous cap of the posterior iliac crest with an absorbable stitch.
- Place a suction drain at the donor site and connect it to a separate reservoir to monitor postoperative bleeding here separately from the spinal fusion site.

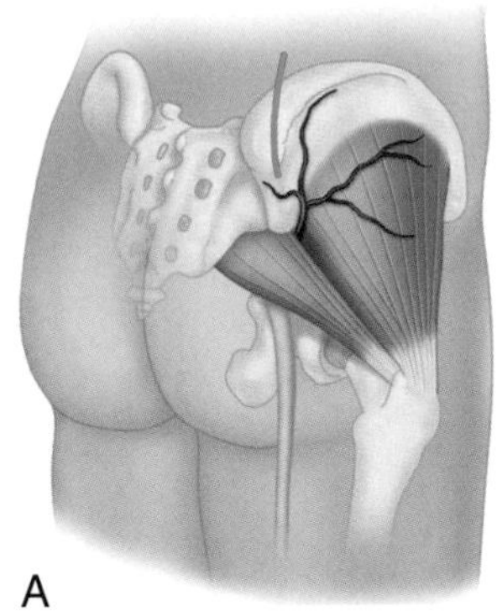

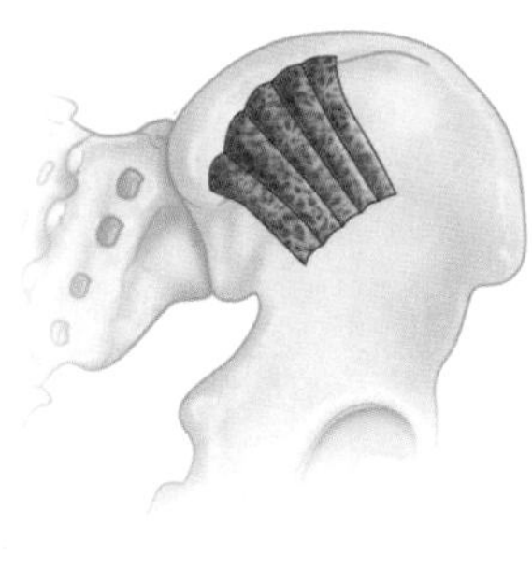

FIGURE 44-42 **A,** Superior gluteal artery as it emerges from area of sciatic notch. **B,** Cortical and cancellous strips removed from outer table of ilium for autogenous bone graft. **SEE TECHNIQUE 44-11.**

COMPLICATIONS OF BONE GRAFTING

The most common complication associated with bone graft harvesting from the posterior iliac crest is transient or permanent numbness over the skin of the buttock caused by injury of the superior cluneal nerves (Fig. 44-43A). The superior cluneal nerves supply sensation to a large area of the buttocks. They pierce the lumbodorsal fascia and cross the posterior iliac crest beginning 8 cm lateral to the posterior superior iliac spine. A limited incision, staying within 8 cm of the posterior superior iliac spine, which will avoid the superior cluneal nerves, is recommended.

The superior gluteal artery exits the pelvis, enters the gluteal region through the superiormost portion of the sciatic notch, and sends extensive branches to the gluteal muscles. Care should be taken when a retractor is inserted into the sciatic notch. Injury to the superior gluteal artery will cause massive hemorrhage, and the artery generally retracts proximally into the pelvis. Control of the bleeding frequently requires bone removal from the sciatic notch to obtain sufficient exposure. It may be necessary to pack the wound, turn the patient, and have a general surgeon locate and ligate the hypogastric artery. Ureteral injury also can occur in the sciatic notch from the sharp tip of a retractor.

Most of the stability of the sacroiliac joint is provided by the posterior ligamentous complex (Fig. 44-43B). Injury to the sacroiliac joint from removal of these ligaments can range from clinical symptoms of instability to dislocation.

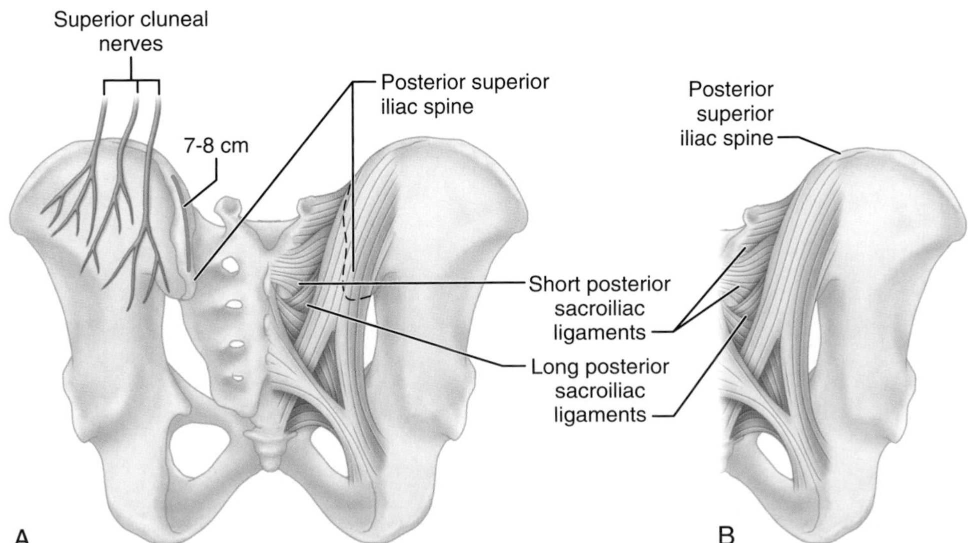

FIGURE 44-43 **A,** Superior cluneal nerve may be injured during harvest of bone graft from iliac crest. Limited incision *(green line)*, staying within 8 cm of posterior superior iliac spine, avoids nerve. **B,** Posterior ligament complex provides most of stability of sacroiliac joint.

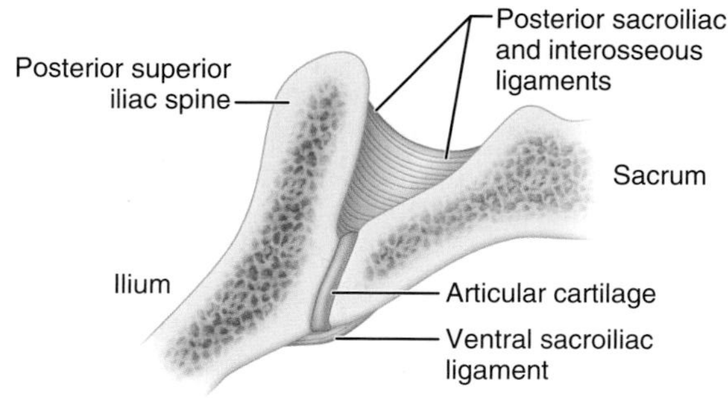

FIGURE 44-44 Full-thickness graft should not be obtained too close to sacroiliac joint to avoid damage to posterior ligamentous complex.

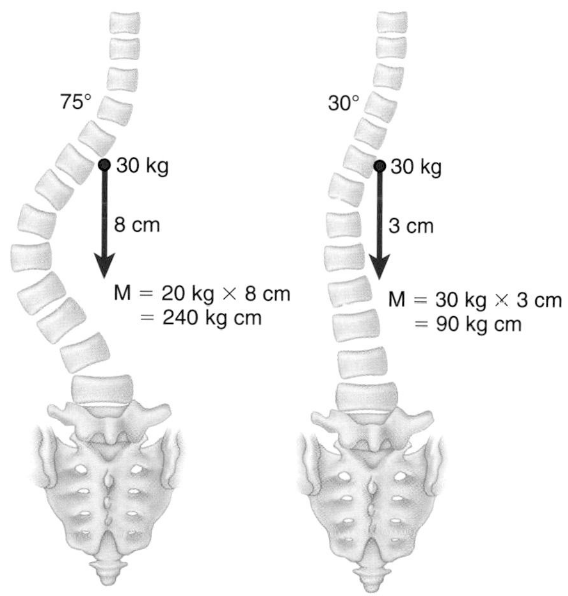

FIGURE 44-45 Comparative bending forces exerted at apexes of 75-degree curve and 30-degree curve.

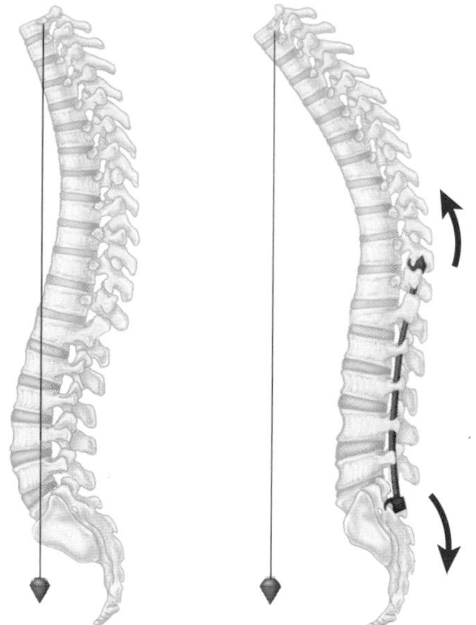

FIGURE 44-46 Effects of distraction rod in lumbar spine. If contouring for lordosis is inadequate, lumbar spine can be flattened by distracting force. Also note kyphotic deformity just superior to distraction rod.

Dislocation of the sacroiliac joint as a complication of full-thickness graft removal from the posterior ilium has been reported. If a full-thickness graft is obtained, it should not be obtained too close to the sacroiliac joint (Fig. 44-44).

POSTERIOR SPINAL INSTRUMENTATION

The goals of instrumentation in scoliosis surgery are to correct the deformity as much as possible and to stabilize the spine in the corrected position while the fusion mass becomes solid. The fusion mass in a well-corrected spine is subjected to much lower bending moments and tensile forces than is the fusion mass in an uncorrected spine (Fig. 44-45).

The ideal spinal instrumentation system is safe and reliable, with infrequent instrument failure and breakage. It should be strong enough to resist load from all directions without external support, be easy to use with little increase in operative time, and restore normal spinal contours in the coronal, sagittal, and transverse planes; it should not create new deformities as the instrumentation is applied. It also should be a cost-effective system. Numerous implants are available, although none meets all of the criteria for an ideal system. No one device is the best choice for every surgeon or every patient.

In 1962, Harrington introduced the first effective instrumentation system for scoliosis. For more than 30 years, use of the Harrington distraction rod, combined with a thorough posterior arthrodesis and immobilization in a cast or brace for 6 to 9 months, has been the standard surgical treatment of adolescent idiopathic scoliosis. The incidence of neurologic injury with this technique is less than 1%, and the pseudarthrosis rate is less than 10%. The major correcting force with the Harrington instrumentation is distraction.

Despite its success, the Harrington instrumentation system had several disadvantages. Correction with this system is achieved with distraction. As the curve is corrected with distraction, the efficiency of correction is decreased. The distraction forces are applied only at the ends of the construct where the hooks are seated. If the load exceeds the strengths of the lamina, fracture and loss of correction can result. With distraction, the spine is elongated and loss of sagittal contour occurs (Fig. 44-46). Finally, distraction does not deal with the rotational component of the idiopathic adolescent scoliotic curve. Posterior segmental instrumentation systems with multiple-hook, sublaminar wires, or pedicle screws have now largely replaced the Harrington system.

Posterior segmental spinal instrumentation systems provide multiple points of fixation to the spine and apply compression, distraction, and rotation forces through the same rod. These systems generally do not require any postoperative immobilization. They provide better coronal plane correction and better control in the sagittal plane. Hypokyphosis in the thoracic spine can be reduced and lumbar lordosis preserved when the instrumentation extends to the lower lumbar spine. With the use of pedicle screws there appears to be better transverse plane correction (vertebral rotation). These systems generally have implant failure and pseudarthrosis rates lower than those of Harrington instrumentation (see **Video 44-3**).

Three kinds of devices are available for fixation of posterior segmental instrumentation: wires or cables, hooks, and screws.

CORRECTION MANEUVERS

A variety of techniques and maneuvers can be used to achieve correction of spinal deformity. Distraction on the concave side of a thoracic curve will decrease scoliosis and thoracic kyphosis. Compression applied on the convex side of a lumbar curve will correct scoliosis and allow for restoration or maintenance of lumbar lordosis. Correction of a scoliotic curve also can be obtained by translating the apex of the curve into a more normal position. Translation can be achieved by a rod derotation maneuver. This classic derotation maneuver of Cotrel and Dubousset is accomplished by connecting the precontoured concave rod to each fixation site and then rotating the rod into the sagittal plane. This en bloc derotation maneuver results in a lateral translation of the apical vertebrae or an in situ relocation of the apex of the treated curve.

Pure translation is another method for correcting curves. This can be achieved with sublaminar wires or a reduction screw on the concave side. The rod is contoured into the desired amount of coronal and sagittal plane correction and placed into the proximal and distal fixation sites. The spine is then slowly and sequentially pulled to the precontoured rods using sublaminar wires or reduction screws.

In situ contouring is another correction technique. With the use of appropriate bending tools, in situ contouring in both the coronal and sagittal planes can improve spinal alignment in scoliosis. A cantilever technique can be used to reduce spinal deformity. With this technique the precontoured rod is inserted and fixed either proximally or distally and then sequentially reduced into each fixation site with a cantilever maneuver. This is usually followed by appropriate compression and distraction to finalize the correction. With the use of monoaxial and uniplanar pedicle screws, correction can be obtained by en bloc vertebral derotation over three or four apical vertebral segments or by direct segmental vertebral rotation in which the derotation maneuver is applied to individual vertebral segments.

SEGMENTAL INSTRUMENTATION: MULTIPLE HOOKS OR PEDICLE SCREWS

SURGICAL PLAN

Preoperative radiographs, including standing posteroanterior and lateral and bending films, should be evaluated and a surgical plan devised.

FUSION LEVELS AND HOOK SITE PLACEMENT

In determining fusion levels for multiple-hook segmental instrumentation, several basic principles must be considered.

Anteroposterior, lateral, and bending films are essential. Because standing bending films are not nearly as revealing, supine bending films are preferable. Traction, fulcrum, or push-prone bending films also may be needed in preoperative curve evaluation.

In the sagittal plane, all pathologic curves must be included. The goal of segmental instrumentation systems is to produce normal sagittal contours of the spine, if possible. The instrumentation should not be stopped in the middle of a pathologic sagittal curve, such as a thoracolumbar junctional kyphosis. The upper instrumentation should not stop at the apex of the kyphosis proximally. These levels are determined on standing lateral films.

In the transverse plane, the instrumentation should extend to a rotational neutral vertebra, if possible. This is determined on standing posteroanterior or bending films.

The instrumentation should be stopped at the level above disc space neutralization, as determined on bending films, as long as this level does not conflict with the sagittal and transverse plane requirements. In other words, the disc height should be equal on the right and left sides and should open on both the right and left sides with supine bending films. The rigid segment of the thoracic curve also is determined on coronal bending films and dictates the placement of intermediate hooks or pedicle screws.

The distal level should fall within the stable zone of Harrington (Fig. 44-47). The inferior vertebra ideally is bisected by the center sacral line, but this is necessary only on bending films, not on the upright standing posteroanterior film.

Once the proximal and distal levels of the fusion have been determined, if hooks are being used, hook placement patterns must be determined. To determine the appropriate hook patterns, the type of force that must be generated on the spine and what that force will do to the sagittal plane must be determined. The basic principles are as follows:

- Distraction forces (forces directed away from the apex of the curve) decrease lordosis or contribute to kyphosis.
- Compression forces (toward the apex of the curve) decrease kyphosis or create lordosis.
- To create kyphosis, the concave side must be approached first.

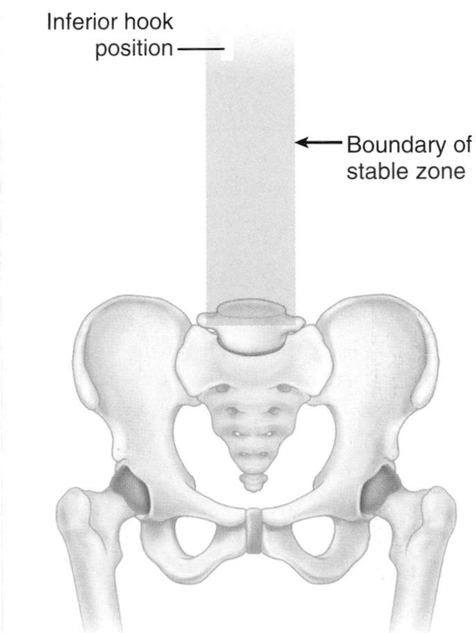

FIGURE 44-47 Stable zone for inferior vertebra as described by Harrington.

To create lordosis, the convex side must be approached first and the forces must be directed toward the apex of the curve.

At the thoracolumbar junction, distractive forces should not be applied, and in rod bending, the lordotic bend of the rod should be initiated at the T12-L1 interspace.

Some typical hook constructs and order of rod application are illustrated in Figures 44-48 to 44-53.

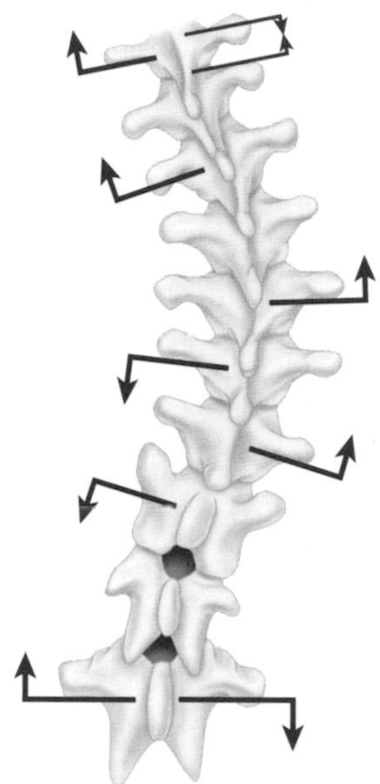

FIGURE 44-48 Typical hook site selection for Lenke 1A (King III).

Greater correction and derotation of the involved vertebrae can be obtained with the use of pedicle screw instrumentation, but this has led to problems with lumbar decompensation when a selective thoracic fusion is done. With greater correction being obtained in the primary structural curve, more attention needs to be focused on the proximal thoracic curve to avoid shoulder imbalance after surgery. Following Lenke's classification has been the best guide to aid in selection of appropriate fusion levels and avoidance of these complications. Trobisch et al., in a recent review, gave the following recommendations to aid in selecting fusion levels:

All Lenke structural curves should be included in the fusion and instrumentation. Also included are lumbar nonstructural curves of more than 45 degrees on standing posteroanterior radiographs or associated with clinically significant rotational deformity, or in the presence of wedging of apical vertebrae along the significant apical vertebral transition and rotation.

The upper instrumented vertebra should not end at a kyphotic disc.

T2 is selected as the upper instrumented vertebra when the left shoulder is elevated, T1 tilt is more than 5 degrees, and/or significant rotational prominences or trapezial fullness accompanies the proximal thoracic curve.

In lumbar modifier A curves, the lower instrumented vertebra is the vertebra touching the center sacral vertebral line; however, the spine is fused one or two levels farther distal when L4 is tilted in the direction of the thoracic curve.

In lumbar modifier B and C curves, the thoracolumbar stable vertebra is selected as the lower instrumented vertebra.

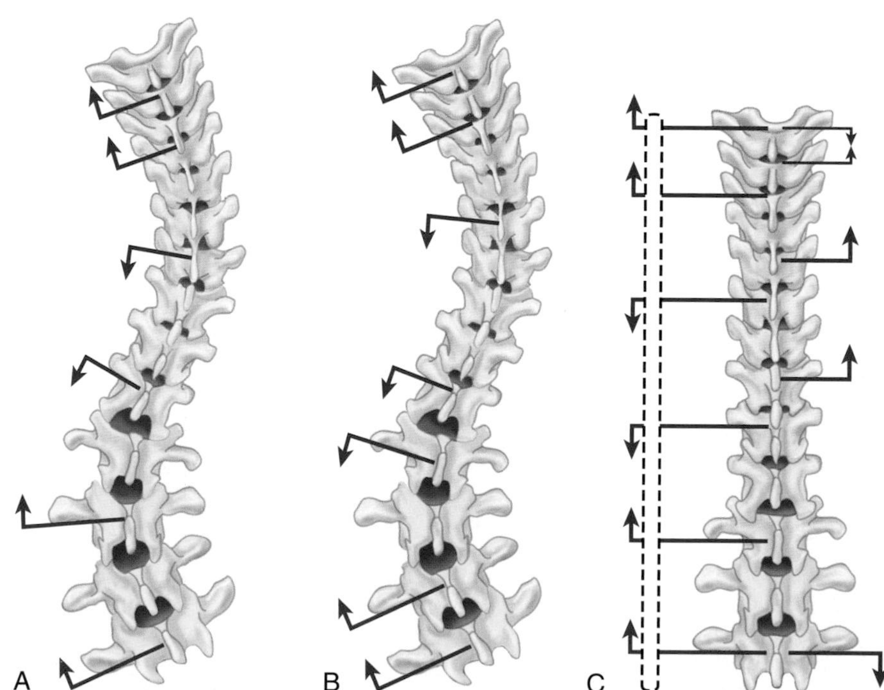

FIGURE 44-49 Instrumentation of Lenke 3 (double major) curve (see text). **A,** Hook placement for left rod. **B,** Two apical lumbar hooks can be used to apply compression at apex of lumbar curve. **C,** Hook placement for right rod after left rod rotation.

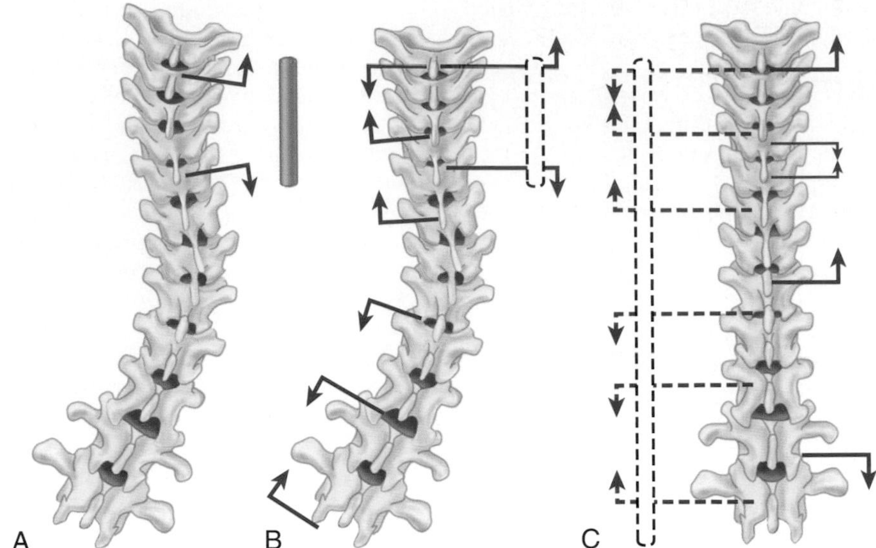

FIGURE 44-50 Instrumentation of Lenke 2 (King type V) double thoracic curve with temporary upper rod. **A,** Hook placement for insertion of short segment rod in concavity of high thoracic curve. **B,** Gentle distraction is applied, and rod is locked in place. **C,** Left rod is inserted to include both curves; compression is applied to convexity of upper curve, and distraction is applied to concavity of lower curve. Short rod is removed, and long rod is contoured with in situ benders.

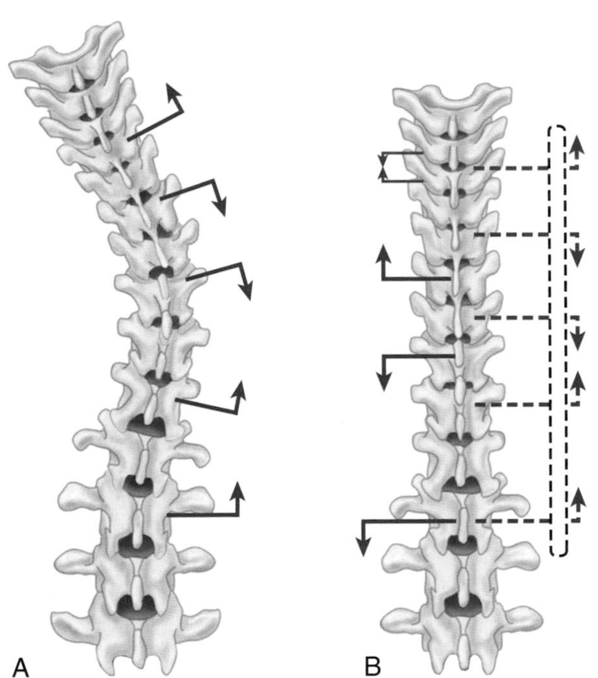

FIGURE 44-51 Instrumentation of Lenke 5 (thoracolumbar) curve by convex rod technique. **A,** Hook pattern for insertion of convex rod; hooks are compressed, and rod is rotated to obtain normal sagittal contour. **B,** Concave rod is inserted and seated with distraction, and crosslinks are applied.

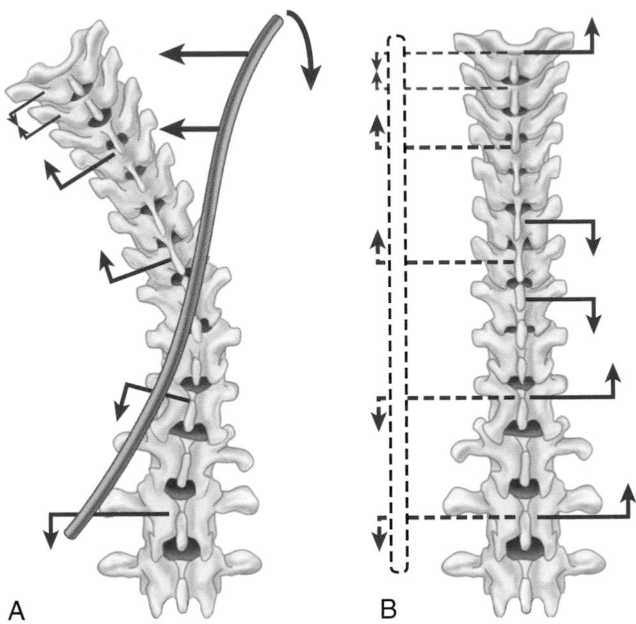

FIGURE 44-52 Instrumentation of Lenke 5 (thoracolumbar) curve with concave rod technique in which correction is produced by cantilever mechanism. **A,** Concave rod is inserted and rotated to convert lumbar scoliosis into lordosis as it is sequentially seated in each more-cephalad hook. **B,** Convex rod is inserted in hook pattern shown.

The lower instrumented vertebra in lumbar structural curves is influenced by curve flexibility (proposed by the lower instrumented vertebra translation) and rotation and correction on bending radiographs.

Even with these guidelines and using Lenke's classification, selection of fusion and instrumentation levels must be individualized for each patient.

HOOK SITE PREPARATION AND PLACEMENT

There are basically two types of hooks: pedicle and laminar. The pedicle hooks are designed for secure fixation in the thoracic spine by insertion into the facet with impingement on the thoracic pedicle. Pedicle hooks are used in an upgoing direction at T10 or higher. The laminar hooks can be used in the thoracic and lumbar spine. These can be placed around

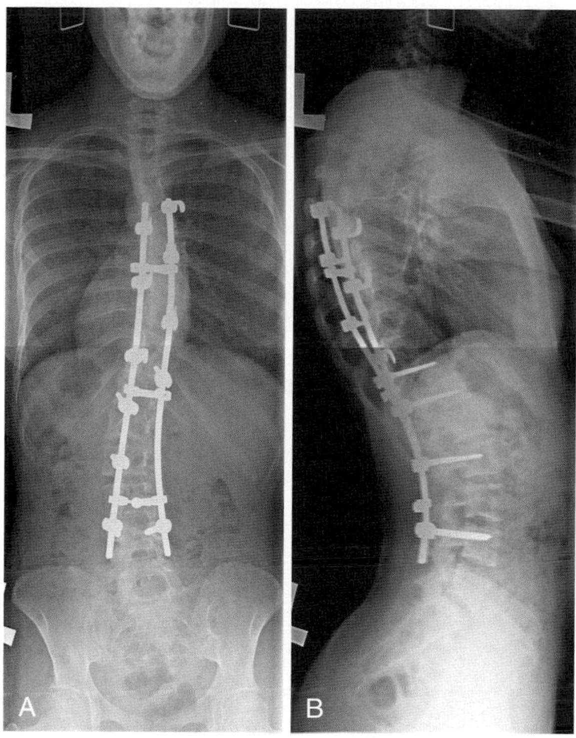

FIGURE 44-53 **A** and **B**, Hybrid fixation of Lenke 1A (King III) curve with pedicle screws at lower end of construct.

either the superior or inferior edge of the lamina or transverse process, according to the desired direction and point of application of forces.

PEDICLE HOOK IMPLANTATION

TECHNIQUE 44-12

- The pedicle hook is inserted in an upgoing direction from T1 to T10.
- The facet capsule is removed, and a portion of the inferior facet process is removed to facilitate insertion of the hook (Fig. 44-54A).
- After removal of the portion of the inferior facet process, use a curet to remove the hyaline cartilage from the facet joint.
- Introduce the pedicle finder into the facet joint and push gently against the pedicle (Fig. 44-54B). Take care in using this instrument that it is introduced into the intraarticular space and not into the bone of the inferior articular facet. It must find its way, sliding along the superior articular facet.
- Once the pedicle finder is in place, check the position by a laterally directed force applied to the finder. If the vertebra moves laterally when the pedicle finder is translated, the pedicle finder is in the correct place.
- Insert the pedicle hook with a hook inserter and holder if needed. Again, be certain that the horns of the bifid hook remain within the facet joint and do not hook into the remaining bone of the inferior facet (Fig. 44-55).

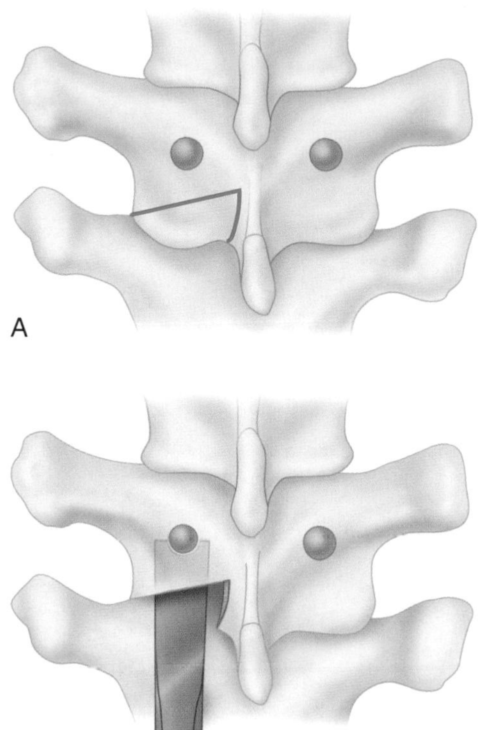

FIGURE 44-54 CD Horizon Legacy pedicle hook implantation. **A** and **B**, Hook site preparation and placement. **SEE TECHNIQUE 44-12.**

TRANSVERSE PROCESS HOOK IMPLANTATION

TECHNIQUE 44-13

- The transverse process hook is part of a pedicular-transverse claw system. In most scoliosis procedures, use this claw at the upper end of the convex side. The transverse process hook generally is a wide-blade lamina hook inserted in a downgoing manner around the superior portion of the transverse process.
- Prepare the area along the superior edge of the transverse process, using a transverse process elevator to separate the ligamentous attachment between the undersurface of the transverse process and the posterior arch of the rib medial to the rib transverse joint (Fig. 44-56).
- With use of a hook holder, insert the hook around the superior edge of the transverse process.

LAMINA HOOK IMPLANTATION

TECHNIQUE 44-14

- Place laminar hooks around either the superior or inferior edge of the lamina, according to the desired direction of

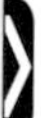

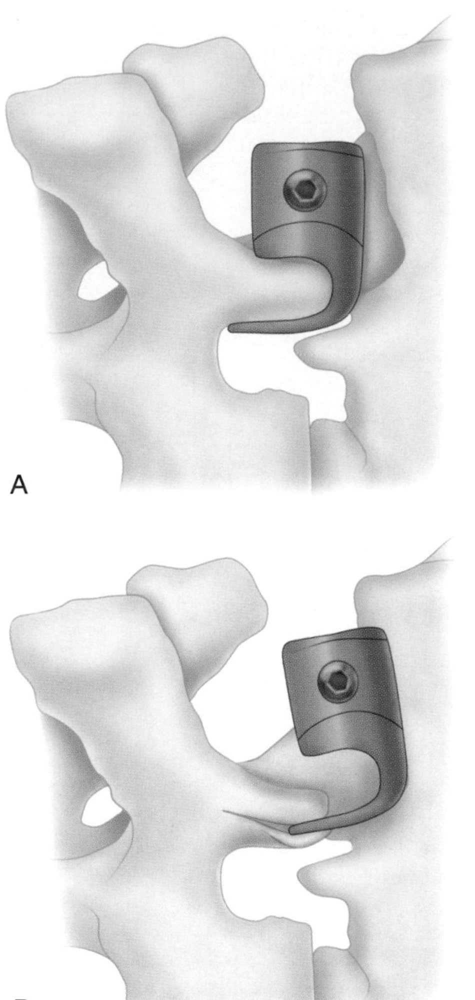

FIGURE 44-55 CD Horizon Legacy pedicle hook implantation. **A,** Correct placement of the hook. **B,** Incorrect placement of the hook. **SEE TECHNIQUE 44-12.**

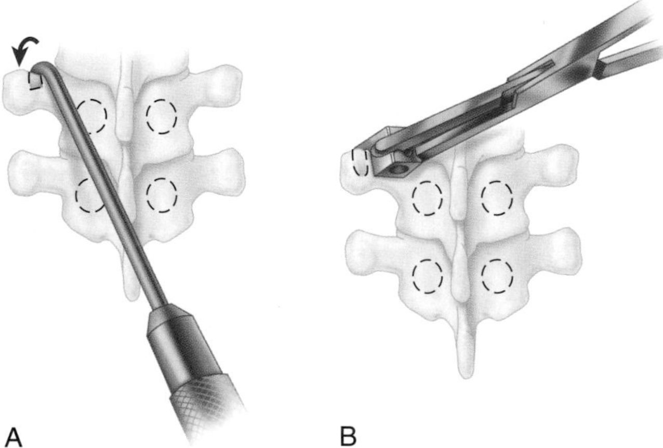

FIGURE 44-56 Area along superior edge of transverse process prepared using transverse process elevator. (Redrawn from Winter RB, Lonstein JW, Denis F, Smith MD, editors: Atlas of spine surgery, Philadelphia, 1995, WB Saunders, p. 263.) **SEE TECHNIQUE 44-13.**

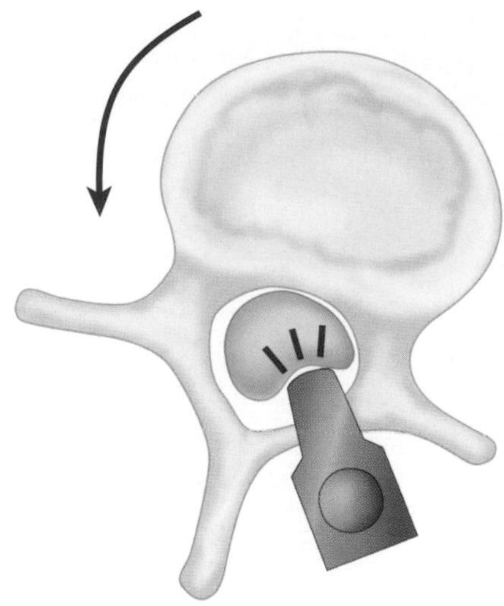

FIGURE 44-57 Lamina hook should be chosen carefully to match shape of lamina and to obtain closest possible fit to prevent hook impingement on spinal canal. **SEE TECHNIQUE 44-14.**

applied force. Carefully match the type of laminar hook to the shape of the lamina and obtain the closest possible fit to avoid the possibility of hook impingement on the spinal canal (Fig. 44-57).

- To insert the supralaminar hook, remove the ligamentum flavum with Kerrison rongeurs and curets (Fig. 44-58A). In the lumbar area, enough room generally exists between the vertebrae to allow implantation of the hook without removal of bone. In the thoracic area, however, the spinous process of the superior vertebra must be removed first.
- After the canal is open, obtain lateral extension of the area by excising the medial portion of the inferior articular facet of the superior vertebra. This will allow sufficient room for insertion of the thoracic laminar hook.
- When the infralaminar hook is inserted, partially remove the ligamentum flavum or separate it from the inferior surface of the lamina. If necessary, remove a piece of the inferior border of the lamina to allow proper seating of the hook on the lamina (Fig. 44-58B). Take care to preserve the lateral wall of the inferior facet to avoid lateral dislodgment of the hook.
- When the inferiormost laminar hook is inserted, preserve the interspinous ligament and facet capsule to prevent kyphosis distal to the rods.

PEDICLE FIXATION

Pedicle screw fixation from the posterior approach into the vertebral body has become an increasingly popular form of spinal fixation. Hamill et al. found that pedicle screws on the convex side of the lumbar spine improved coronal and sagittal correction, allowed the lower instrumented vertebra to be translated to the midline and brought to a horizontal position, and allowed improved restoration of segmental lordosis. A similar study found that the pedicle screws provided greater lumbar curve correction, better maintenance of correction,

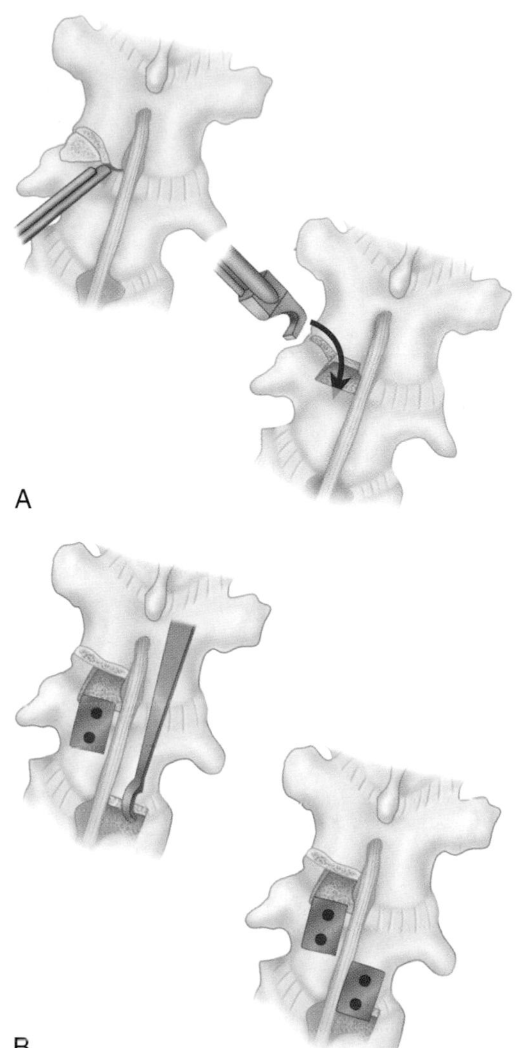

FIGURE 44-58 **A,** Supralaminar hook insertion. This insertion applies to lower two concave hooks in single thoracic curve instrumentation. Laminotomy is kept as small as possible to minimize risk of deep penetration into spinal canal during rod insertion. Tight fit is necessary, and thoracic laminar hook is used if laminar thickness is too small to allow lumbar laminar hook to be stable in anteroposterior plane. **B,** Infralaminar hook insertion. Lower convex hook in right thoracic curve is inserted in this manner. Ligamentum flavum is dissected off underside of lamina. Small inferior laminotomy provides horizontal purchase site for hook. Adjacent facet capsule should be spared because it is not included in fusion. **SEE TECHNIQUE 44-14.**

and greater correction of the uninstrumented spine below double major curves than laminar hooks. Neither study reported any complications associated with the placement of pedicle screws. Reported complication rates associated with the placement of pedicle screws have been low.

The use of thoracic pedicle screws in the treatment of adolescent idiopathic scoliosis has become more common (Fig. 44-59). In studies comparing hook fixation with thoracic pedicle screw fixation, thoracic posterior-only pedicle screw constructs were found to provide better correction than hook constructs. Correction obtained with hooks was 55%, and with segmental thoracic pedicle screws it was 72%. A 3% malposition rate for the thoracic pedicle screws based on plain radiographs was noted. No medial intracanal malpositions or neurologic complications were noted. The use of thoracic pedicle screw instrumentation often can eliminate the need for an anterior approach and may require a slightly shorter fusion length.

However, in a CT evaluation of 120 thoracic pedicle screws, 25% of the screws were found to have penetrated the pedicle cortex or the anterior cortex of the vertebral body. There were no neurologic complications. Anterior penetration of the vertebral body cortex by a pedicle screw in the thoracic spine has the most clinical relevance because of the proximity of the thoracic aorta (Fig. 44-60).

A thorough knowledge of the anatomy of the pedicles is necessary for the use of pedicle fixation. The pedicle connects the posterior elements to the vertebral body. Medial to the pedicle are the epidural space, nerve root, and dural sac. The exiting nerve root at the level of the pedicle is close to the medial and caudal cortex of the pedicle (Fig. 44-61). Close to the lateral and superior aspects of the pedicle cortex is the nerve root from the level above. At the L3 and L4 vertebral bodies, the common iliac artery and veins lie directly anterior to the pedicles (Fig. 44-62). In the sacral region, the great vessels and their branches lie laterally along the sacral ala. In the midline of the sacrum, a variable middle sacral artery can lie directly anterior to the S1 vertebral body. Anterior penetration of a vertebral body can occur without being apparent on the radiograph unless a "near-approach" view is obtained (Fig. 44-63).

In a study of the size of pedicles in mature and immature spines, the transverse pedicle width at the L5 and L4 levels reached 8 mm or more in children 6 to 8 years of age, but transverse width at L3 approaching 8 mm was not seen until 9 to 11 years of age (Fig. 44-64). The distance to the anterior cortex increased dramatically from the youngest age group until adulthood at all levels (Fig. 44-65). In patients with spinal deformities, the pedicles, especially the concave pedicles, often are deformed, and care must be taken in insertion of any pedicle fixation. Watanabe et al. studied thoracic pedicles in adolescents (14 to 16 years) with scoliosis to provide a classification that could be used for safe and accurate placement of pedicle screws. They found four pedicle types (Fig. 44-66): type A has a large cancellous channel in which the pedicle probe can be smoothly inserted without difficulty; type B has a small cancellous channel in which the probe fits snugly; type C is a cortical channel in which the probe must be tapped with a mallet to enter the body; and type D is an absent pedicle channel that requires a juxtapedicular screw position. Type A and B pedicles do not require special techniques for probe insertion, whereas type C and especially type D pedicles do require special methods. Pedicles located on the concave side of the curves were found to be significantly smaller than those on the convex side, regardless of whether they were cancellous or cortical. Of 1021 pedicles in which pedicle screws were placed, 61% were type A, 29.2% were type B, 6.8% were type C, and 3% were type D. CT validated the morphologic evaluation and description of the four pedicle types.

Various methods have been described for identifying the pedicle and placing the pedicle screw, but basic steps include (1) clearing the soft tissue, (2) exposing the cancellous bone

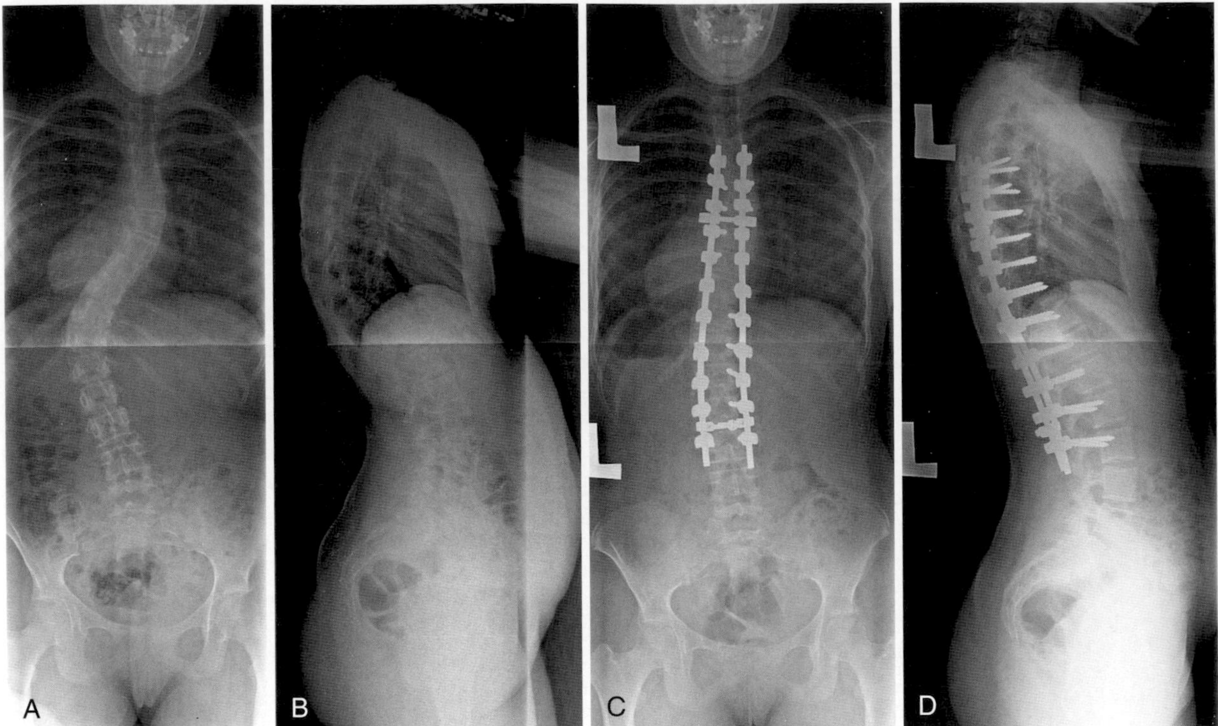

FIGURE 44-59 **A** and **B,** Preoperative posteroanterior and lateral radiographs of patient with idiopathic scoliosis treated with lumbar and thoracic pedicle screws. **C** and **D,** Postoperative posteroanterior and lateral radiographs of amount of correction and restoration of sagittal balance possible with this type of instrumentation.

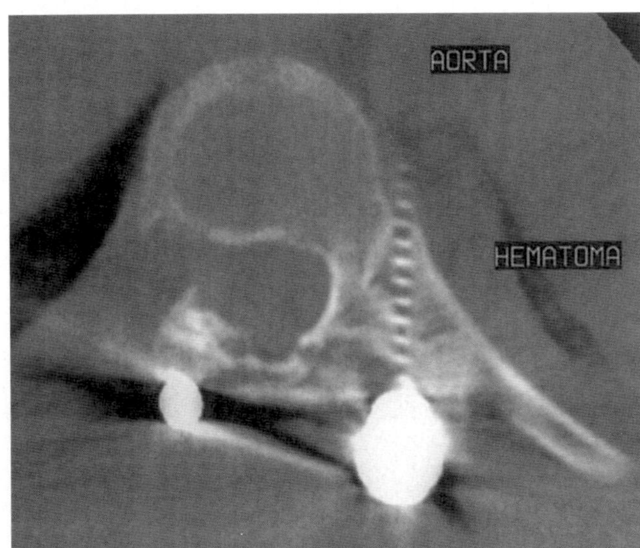

FIGURE 44-60 Complete lateral pedicle screw penetration at T10 on the concave side of King II scoliosis. Small hematoma probably was result of injury of segmental vessels. (From Liljenqvist UR, Halm HFH, Link TM: Pedicle screw instrumentation of the thoracic spine in idiopathic scoliosis, Spine 22:2239, 1997.)

of the pedicle canal by decortication at the intersection of the base of the facet and the middle of the transverse process, (3) probing the pedicle, (4) verifying the four walls of the pedicle canal by probing or obtaining radiographic confirmation, (5) tapping the pedicle, and (6) placing the screw.

In the lumbar spine, pedicle screws are commonly inserted with use of anatomic landmarks, and confirmatory radiographs are obtained. Because of the deformed pedicles associated with scoliosis, many surgeons use fluoroscopic guidance. Freehand pedicle screw placement in the thoracic spine may be safe in experienced hands. The technique significantly reduces exposure of both the surgeon and the patient to radiation. Because of the tight confines of the pedicle in the thoracic spine and the frequently altered normal anatomy, we still use fluoroscopy to identify the entry site into the thoracic pedicle and to confirm screw placement. Frameless stereotactic technology allows three-dimensional navigation and also can be used to guide and confirm pedicle screw placement.

INSERTION OF LUMBAR PEDICLE SCREWS

Zindrick described a "pedicle approach zone" (Fig. 44-67) that is decorticated before the pedicle is cannulated with either a probe or pedicle awl. Great care is taken to advance the instrument slowly and carefully. If resistance is encountered, the probe is repositioned. An intraoperative radiograph or C-arm image can be used to verify correct position. Instruments should pass relatively easily and should not be forced into the pedicle. In addition to radiographs or image intensification, laminotomy and medial pedicle wall exposure can be done to help confirm the intrapedicular passage of the instrument. Once satisfactory entry into the pedicle has been achieved and palpation from within the pedicle finds solid bone margins along the pedicle wall throughout 360 degrees, the screw can be inserted. If the screws are self-tapping, the screw itself is inserted. If the screws require tapping, the tap

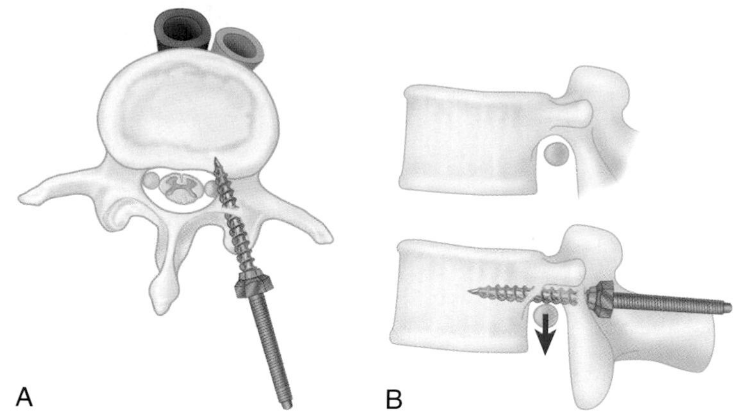

FIGURE 44-61 Errors in pedicle screw placement. **A,** Nerve root impingement by screw violating medial pedicle wall. **B,** Pedicle screw out inferiorly.

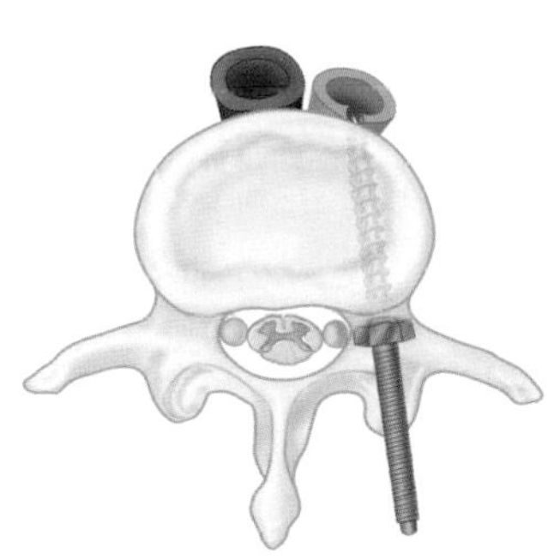

FIGURE 44-62 Vascular damage by insertion of screw beyond anterior cortex.

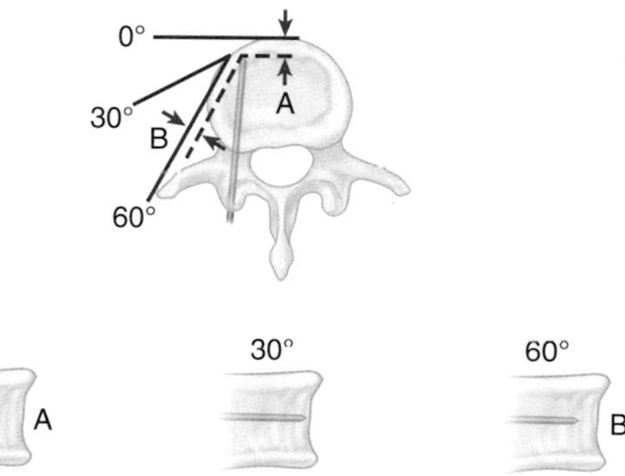

FIGURE 44-63 Near-approach radiographic view to decrease likelihood of anterior screw penetration. When drill (or screw or probe) tip is actually at anterior cortex, lateral view (0 degrees) misleadingly shows tip still to be some distance (A) away from cortex. When angle of view is too oblique (60 degrees), tip appears to be some distance (B) from cortex. Only when view is tangent to point of penetration (30 degrees in this illustration) does tip appear most nearly to approach actual breakthrough.

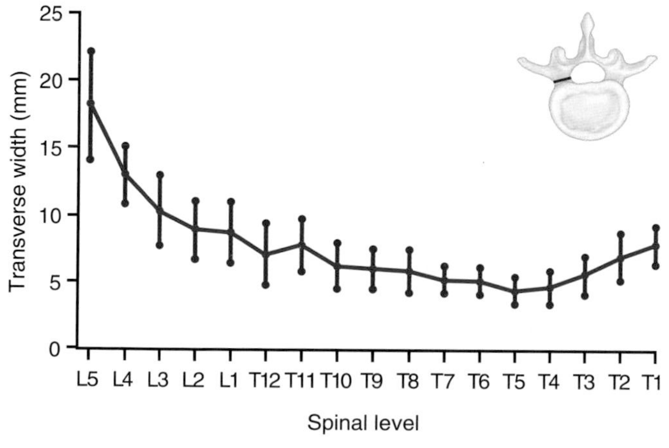

FIGURE 44-64 Transverse pedicle isthmus widths.

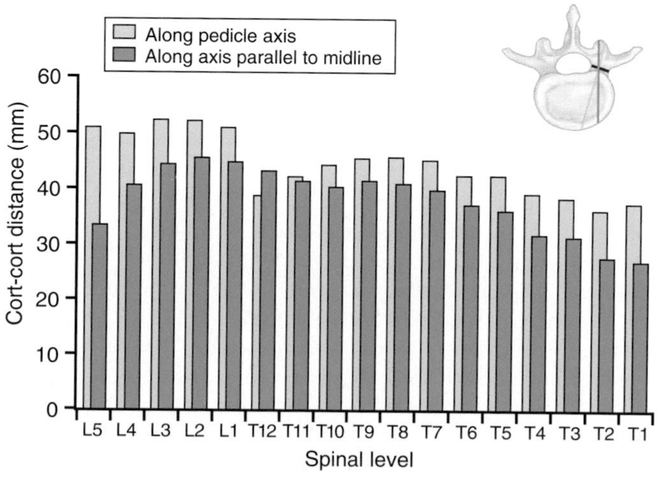

FIGURE 44-65 Distance to anterior cortex through pedicle angle axis versus through line parallel to midline axis of vertebra.

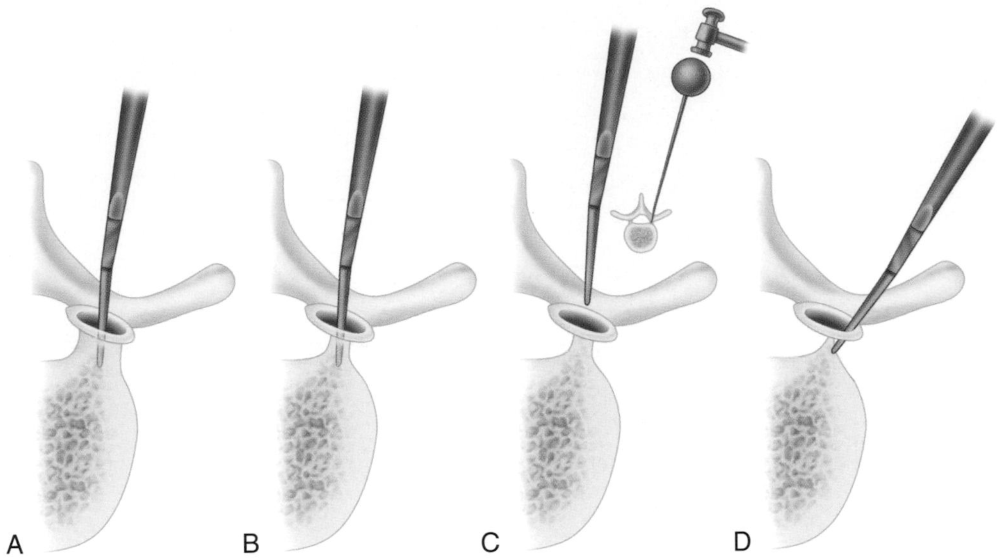

FIGURE 44-66 **Pedicle channel classification (see text).** (From Watanabe K, Lenke KG, Matsumoto M, et al: A novel pedicle channel classification describing osseous anatomy, Spine 35:1836, 2010.)

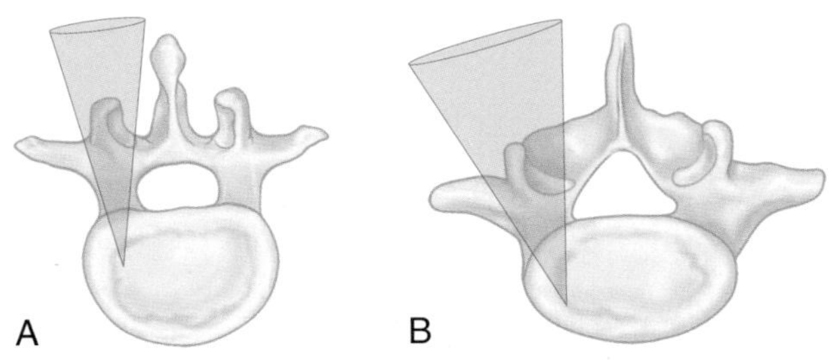

FIGURE 44-67 **A,** Funnel-shaped pedicle approach zone in upper lumbar region (L1). **B,** Funnel-shaped pedicle approach zone in lower lumbar region (L5). With increased pedicle size, pedicle approach zone funnel increases, especially in lower lumbar spine, allowing more latitude in pedicle screw insertion than in smaller upper lumbar and thoracic pedicles. (From Zindrick MR: Clinical pedicle anatomy, Spine: State of the Art Reviews 6:11, 1992.)

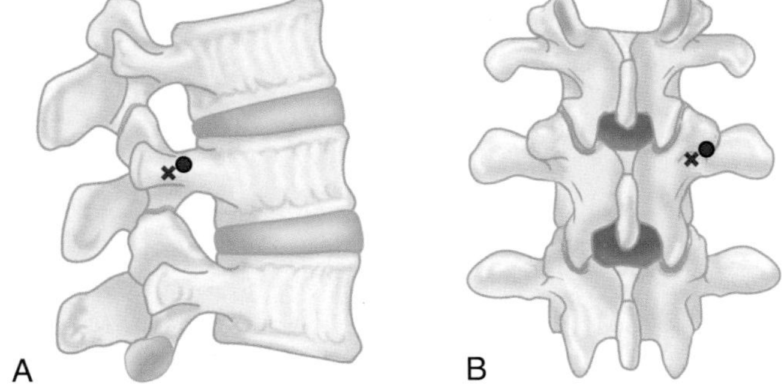

FIGURE 44-68 Entrance points for pedicle screw placement in lumbar spine as described by Roy-Camille (X) and Weinstein (•). **A,** Lateral view. **B,** Posterior view. Weinstein approach reduces interference with upper uninvolved lumbar motion segment.

is inserted first and then the screw. The common entry points in the lumbar spine are shown in Figure 44-68. The position of the pedicle in the sacrum is shown in Figure 44-69. In the lumbar spine, a medially directed screw allows the use of a longer screw and spares the facet joint, with less chance of injury to the common iliac vessels. Similarly, a medially directed sacral screw reduces the possibility of injury to anterior structures if the screw penetrates the anterior cortex.

When pedicle screws are used in the lumbar spine, screws usually are placed at every level on both the convex and concave sides. Each individual vertebra can be better derotated if it is instrumented on both sides (see deformity correction by direct vertebral rotation in Technique 44-15). In choosing the lowest instrumented vertebra, the standing posteroanterior films and the bending films must be considered. Bending films should be used in choosing the lowest instrumented lumbar vertebra. Instrumentation is stopped at the vertebra just above the first disc space that opens in the

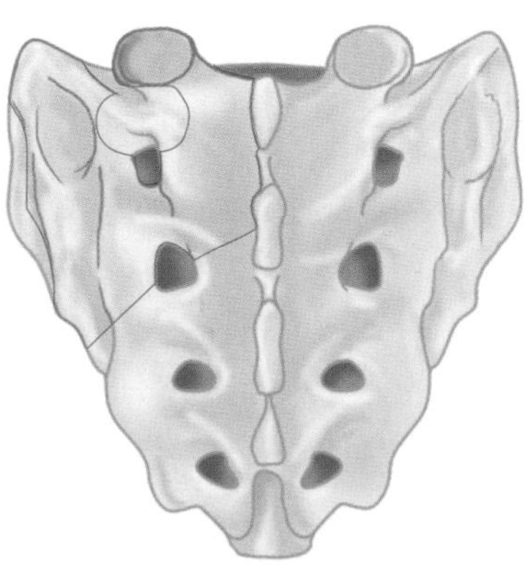

FIGURE 44-69 Coronal posterior view of contribution of sacrum and posterior element to pedicle approach zone.

BOX 44-4

Advantages and Disadvantages of Thoracic Pedicle Screws

Advantages

- When they are optimally placed, the screws are completely external to the spinal canal (supralaminar and infralaminar hooks, in contrast, are within the canal itself).
- Stronger fixation is possible than with hook implants.
- The screws are attached to all three columns, providing a rigid triangular crosslinked construct with a posterior-only implant.
- Facet joints, laminae, and transverse processes are free of implants; therefore, theoretically, there is more surface area for decortication.
- There is superior coronal correction and axial derotation.
- Most studies have shown slightly shorter fusion lengths than with hook constructs. With improved correction, there is a decreased need for anterior procedures and thoracoplasties.

Disadvantages

- The implants add significantly to the cost of the procedure.
- The potential complications in insertion of thoracic pedicle screws include injury to the spinal cord, nerve roots, pleural cavity, and aorta.
- Radiation exposure is significant to the surgeon and patient if routine fluoroscopy is used.

concavity of the lumbar curve on the bending film away from the concavity. Unless the curve is very flexible, the lower instrumented vertebra should at least touch the center sacral line on the standing posteroanterior radiograph.

INSERTION OF THORACIC PEDICLE SCREWS

The routine use of thoracic pedicle screws in adolescent idiopathic scoliosis has become more common. The advantages and disadvantages of thoracic screws are given in Box 44-4.

THORACIC PEDICLE SCREW INSERTION TECHNIQUES

TECHNIQUE 44-15

- Clean the facet joints of all capsular tissue. Perform a partial inferior articular process osteotomy to enhance fusion and to improve exposure of the entry site for the thoracic pedicle screws (Fig. 44-70A). Seeing the transverse processes, the lateral portion of the pars interarticularis, and the base of the superior articular process helps identify the starting points. In general, start the screw insertion from the neutrally rotated, most distal vertebra to be instrumented. Anatomic landmarks can be used as a guide for starting points and screw trajectory (Fig. 44-70B). Fixed-angle screws provide superior rotation in the thoracic spine and lumbar spine. Multiaxial screws can be used if needed.
- Perform a posterior cortical breach with a high-speed burr. A pedicle "blush" suggests entrance into the cancellous bone at the base of the pedicle, but this may not be seen in smaller pedicles because of the limited intrapedicular cancellous bone.
- Use a thoracic gearshift probe to find the cancellous soft spot indicating entrance into the pedicle.
- Point the tip first laterally to avoid perforation of the medial cortex (Fig. 44-70C).
- Advance the tip 20 to 25 mm (Fig. 44-70D).
- Remove the gearshift probe to reorient it so that the tip points medially and then place the probe carefully back into the base of the prior hole and advance it to the desired depth (Fig. 44-70E). The average depth is 30 to 40 mm in the lower thoracic region, 20 to 30 mm in the midthoracic region, and 20 to 25 mm in the proximal thoracic region in adolescents.
- Rotate the probe 180 degrees to ensure adequate room for the screw. Probing of the pedicle with the gearshift should proceed in a smooth and consistent manner with a snug feel. Any sudden advancement of the gearshift suggests penetration into soft tissue and pedicle wall or vertebral body violation.
- Once the gearshift probe is removed, view the track to make sure that only blood is coming out and not cerebrospinal fluid.
- With use of a flexible ball-tipped probe, advance the feeler probe to the base (floor) of the hole to confirm five distinct bony borders: the floor and four walls (medial, lateral, superior, and inferior) (Fig. 44-70F). Take special care in feeling the walls to the first 10 to 15 mm of the track.
- If a soft-tissue breach is palpated, redirect the screw. With the feeler probe at the base of the pedicle track, mark the length of the track with a hemostat and measure it (Fig. 44-70G).
- Undertap the pedicle track by 0.5 to 1 mm of the final screw diameter (Fig. 44-70H). After tapping, always palpate the tapped pedicle track again with the flexible feeler probe. This second palpation will allow identification of distinct bony ridges, confirming the intraosseous position of the track.
- Select the appropriate screw diameter and length by the preoperative radiographs, as well as by intraoperative measurement.
- Thread the screw onto either a fixed-angle or multiaxial screwdriver and slowly advance the screw down the pedicle to ensure proper tracking while allowing viscoelastic expansion (Fig. 44-70I). The smaller pedicle diameters are located at T6 and T7 and in the proximal thoracic concavity (e.g., T3 and T4).
- Confirm intraosseous screw placement.
- On the anteroposterior image intensification, make sure the screws are positioned correctly relative to each other. Screws should not go past the midline on the anteroposterior image. Use the lateral image primarily to gauge the length of the screws. No screw should extend past the anterior border of the vertebral body.
- Use electromyographic stimulation with real-time monitoring of the appropriate thoracic nerve root, recording

A

B

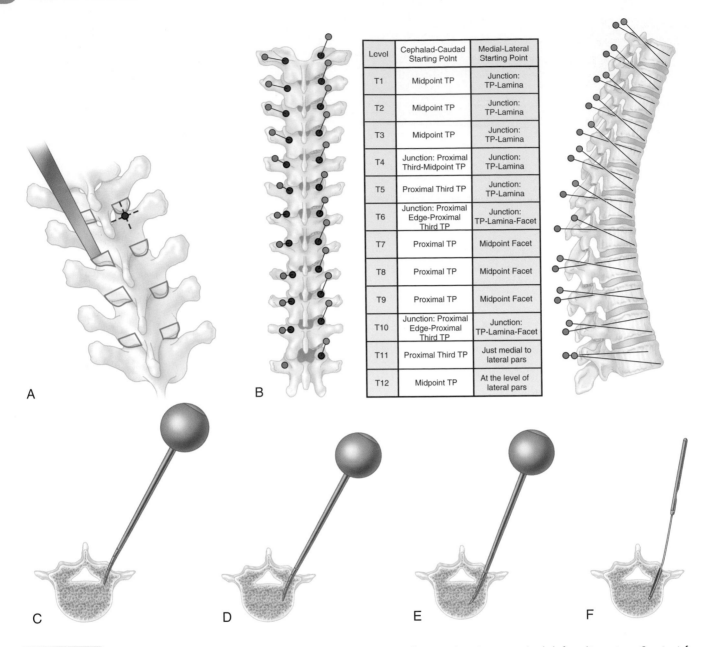

Level	Cephalad-Caudad Starting Point	Medial-Lateral Starting Point
T1	Midpoint TP	Junction: TP-Lamina
T2	Midpoint TP	Junction: TP-Lamina
T3	Midpoint TP	Junction: TP-Lamina
T4	Junction: Proximal Third-Midpoint TP	Junction: TP-Lamina
T5	Proximal Third TP	Junction: TP-Lamina
T6	Junction: Proximal Edge-Proximal Third TP	Junction: TP-Lamina-Facet
T7	Proximal TP	Midpoint Facet
T8	Proximal TP	Midpoint Facet
T9	Proximal TP	Midpoint Facet
T10	Junction: Proximal Edge-Proximal Third TP	Junction: TP-Lamina-Facet
T11	Proximal Third TP	Just medial to lateral pars
T12	Midpoint TP	At the level of lateral pars

C D E F

FIGURE 44-70 **A-T, Thoracic pedicle screw insertion techniques with use of CD Horizon Legacy spinal deformity system. See text for description.** (Redrawn from Lascombes P: CD Horizon Legacy Spinal System-deformity, surgical technique manual, Memphis, TN, 2005, Medtronic Sofamor Danek.) **SEE TECHNIQUE 44-15.**

from the rectus abdominis musculature. Below T12, the lumbar pedicle screws are tested by monitoring the appropriate lumbar nerve root. A triggered electromyographic threshold of less than 6 mA or a significant decrease from the average of all other screws may indicate a pedicle wall breach by the screw. If this is the case, remove the screw and palpate the pedicle wall before deciding whether to replace or to discard the screw.

SUBLAMINAR WIRES

Sublaminar wires generally are not used alone as anchors at the upper or lower instrumented vertebrae because they provide no axial stability. Sublaminar wires and cables are useful in and around the apex of curves to aid in the translation maneuver, in which the spine can be pulled to a precontoured rod, thus minimizing the need for derotational maneuvers. The more rigid the curve is, the more helpful these sublaminar wires or cables are (Fig. 44-71).

TECHNIQUE 44-16

- Expose the spine as described in Technique 44-8.
- With a needle-nose rongeur, gradually thin the ligamentum flavum until the midline cleavage plane is visible. In the thoracic spine, the spinous processes slant distally and must be removed before the ligamentum flavum can be

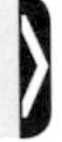

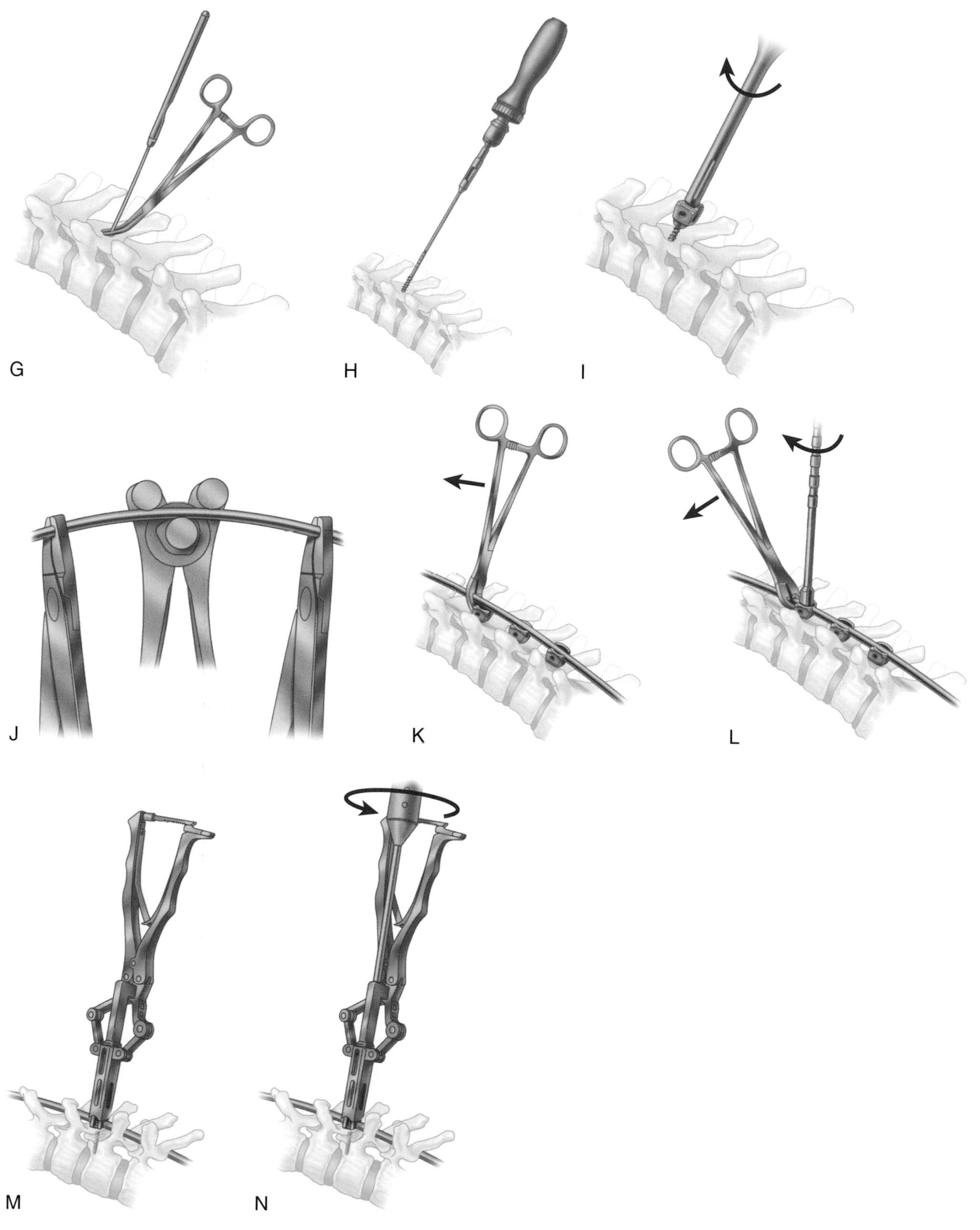

FIGURE 44-70, cont'd

Continued

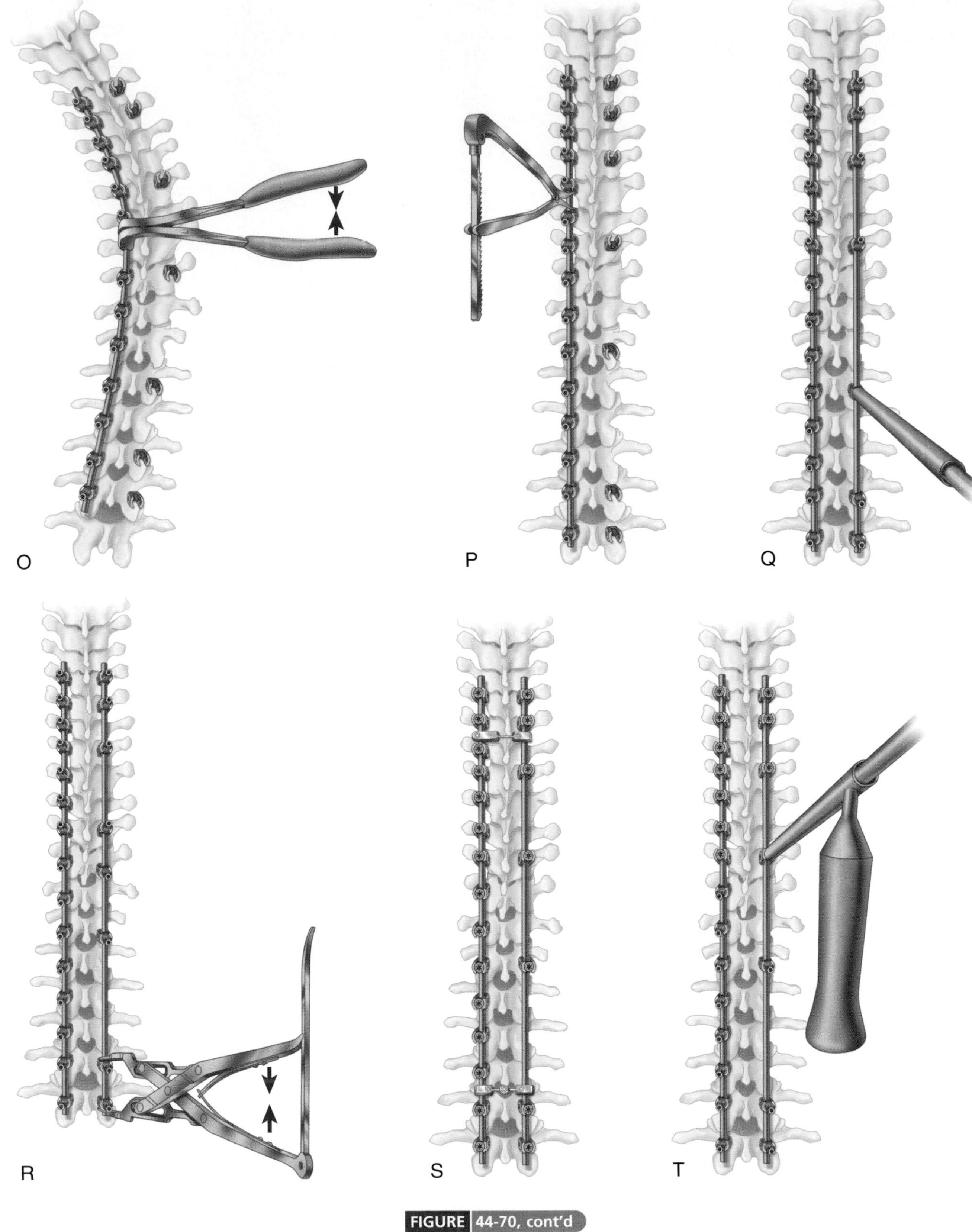

FIGURE 44-70, cont'd

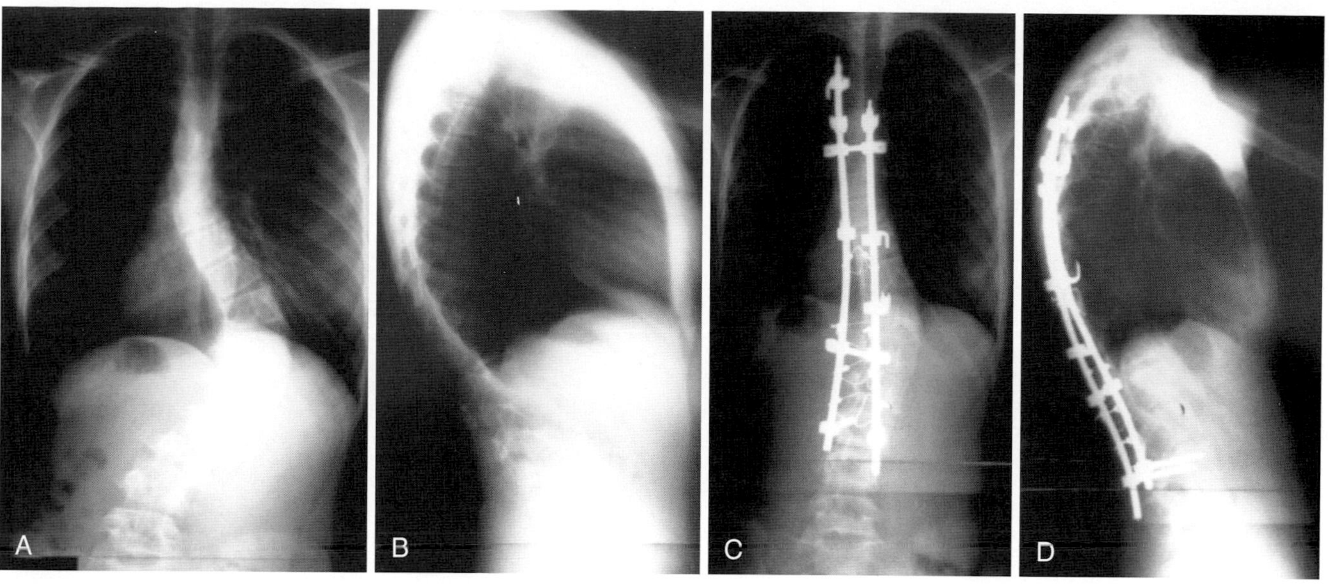

FIGURE 44-71 **A** and **B,** Preoperative anteroposterior and lateral standing scoliosis films. Thoracolumbar curve measures 77 degrees. **C** and **D,** Postoperative correction by hooks with sublaminar cables, correcting thoracolumbar curve to 22 degrees. **SEE TECHNIQUE 44-14.**

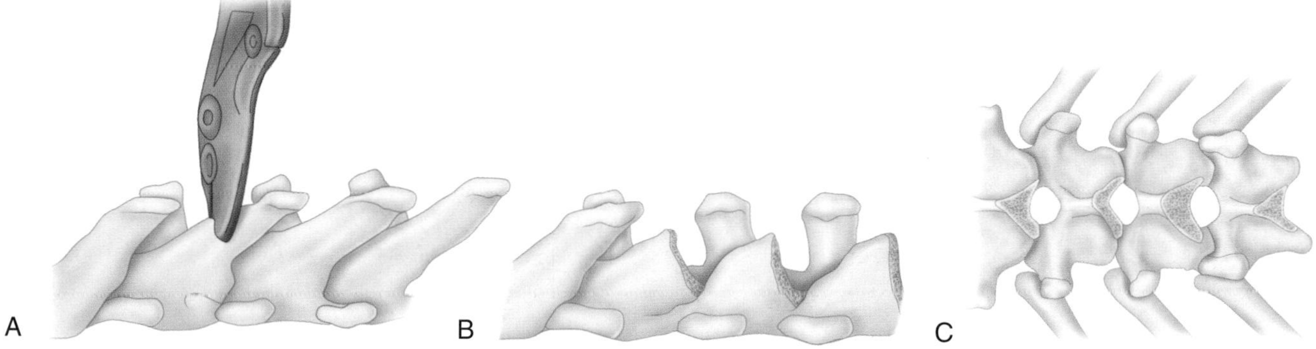

FIGURE 44-72 **A-C,** Removal of caudally slanting spinous processes to expose ligamentum flavum. **SEE TECHNIQUES 44-16 AND 44-17.**

adequately seen (Fig. 44-72). Once the midline cleavage is visible, carefully sweep a Penfield No. 4 dissector across the deep surface of the ligamentum flavum on the right and left sides (Fig. 44-73). Use a Kerrison punch to remove the remainder of the ligamentum flavum (Fig. 44-74). Take care during this step to avoid damaging the dura or epidural vessels.

- Johnston et al. showed that wire penetration into the neural canal during wire passage is substantial (up to 1 cm). Because the depth of penetration is less when a semicircular wire is used, shape the wire as shown in Figure 44-75. The largest diameter of the bend should be slightly larger than the lamina. Always pass the wire in the midline and not laterally and remove the spinous processes before wire passage. It is important that both the surgeon and the assistant be completely prepared for each step before passage of the wire and that they are careful about sudden movements and inadvertent touching or hitting of the wires that have already been passed.
- Passing of the wire is divided into four steps: (1) introduction, (2) advancement, (3) roll-through, and (4)

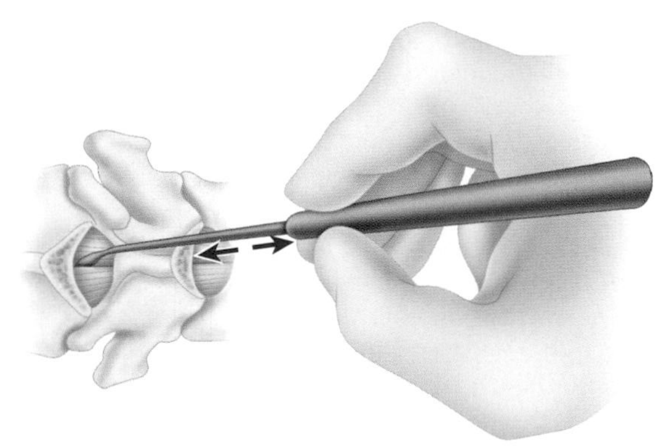

FIGURE 44-73 Penfield No. 4 dissector for freeing deep surfaces of ligamentum flavum. **SEE TECHNIQUES 44-16 AND 44-17.**

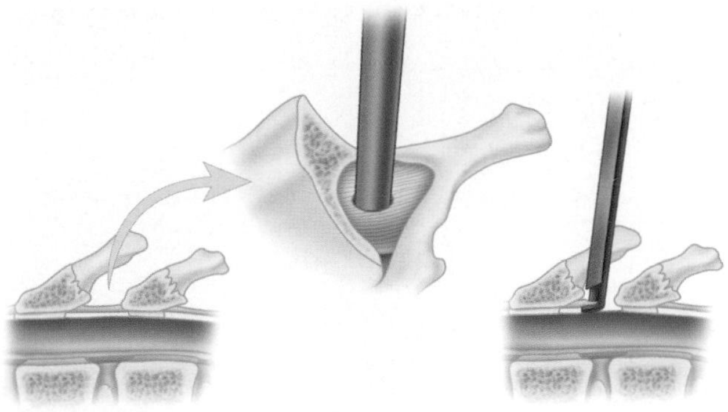

FIGURE 44-74 Kerrison punch for removal of remainder of ligamentum flavum. **SEE TECHNIQUES 44-16 AND 44-17.**

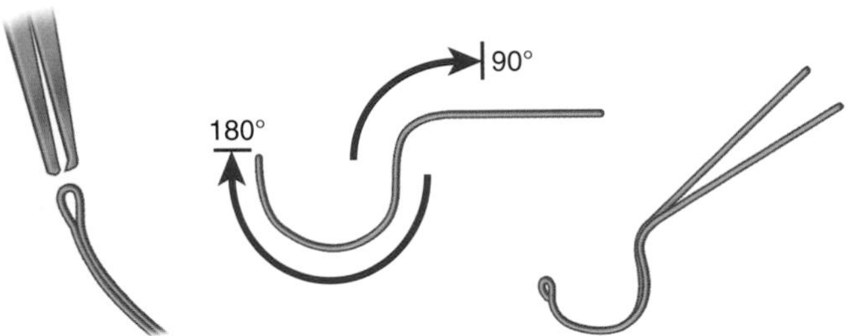

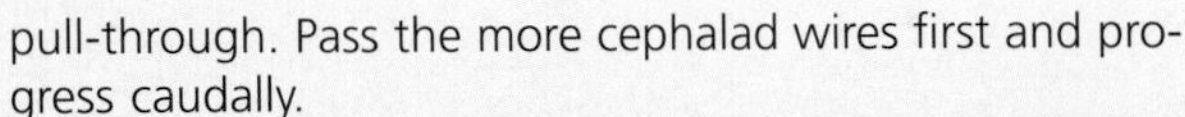

FIGURE 44-75 Shape of double wire before it passes under lamina. **SEE TECHNIQUES 44-16 AND 44-17.**

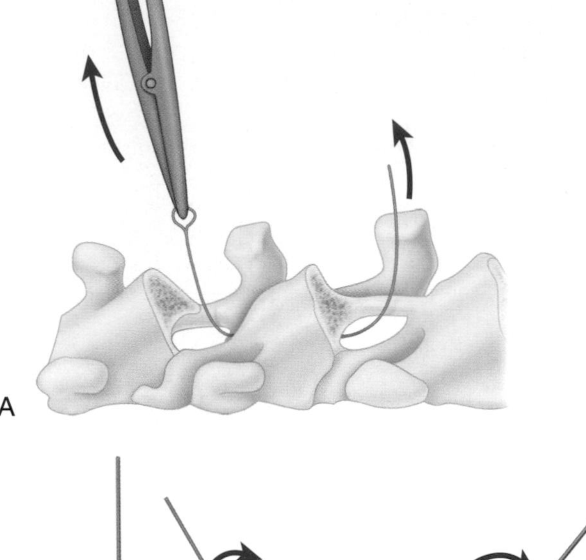

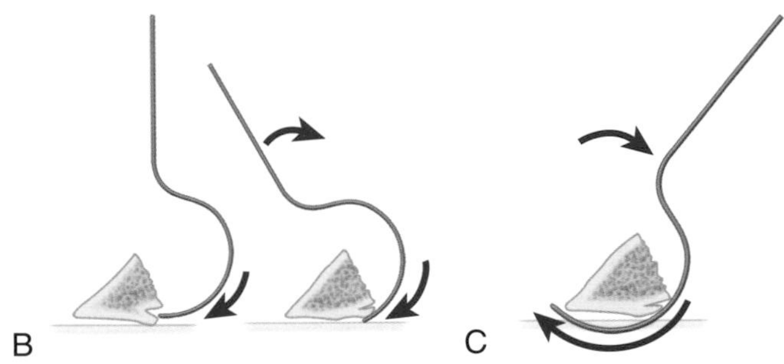

FIGURE 44-76 **A-C,** Passage of segmental wire beneath lamina. **SEE TECHNIQUES 44-16 AND 44-17.**

pull-through. Pass the more cephalad wires first and progress caudally.

- Gently place the tip of the wire into the neural canal at the inferior edge of the lamina in the midline. Hold the long end of the doubled wire in one hand and advance the tip with the other. Rest the hand that is advancing the tip firmly on the patient's back. Lift the tails of the wire slightly, pulling them to keep the wire snugly against the undersurface of the lamina (Fig. 44-76A).
- Once the wire has been introduced, advance it 5 to 6 mm. Beginning roll-through too soon will cause the tip of the wire to strike the inferior portion of the vertebral arch, and the wire can be pushed more deeply into the neural canal (Fig. 44-76B).
- After advancement, roll the tip of the wire so that it emerges on the upper end of the lamina (Fig. 44-76C). As the tip of the wire emerges, use a nerve hook to pull the end farther up from the lamina to allow enough room for a needle holder, wire holder, or Kocher clamp to be placed into the loop of the wire by the assistant. Take the clamp from the assistant and pull the wire with the clamp until it is positioned beneath the lamina, with half its length protruding above and half below the lamina. As the clamp is pulled, gently feed the wire superiorly from the long end. This must be a coordinated maneuver and must be done by the surgeon.
- Once the wire has been pulled through, cut off the tip of the wire and place one length of the wire on the right side and the other length on the left side of the lamina.
- As an alternative, leave double wires on one side and pass another wire so that double wires are present on both sides.
- Crimp each wire into the surface of the lamina to prevent any wire from being pushed accidentally into the neural canal (Fig. 44-77).
- As more wires are passed, it becomes more likely that the other wires will be accidentally hit. Even though the wires are crimped over the lamina, hitting them can be dangerous, and care must be taken to avoid these previously placed wires. Crimp the superior wire toward the midline and crimp the inferior wire laterally.

SUBLAMINAR CABLES

Songer et al. recommended the use of sublaminar cables instead of monofilament stainless steel wire because wire breakage and migration have been serious complications of sublaminar wiring. They also suggested that cable flexibility prevents repeated contusions to the spinal cord that can occur during insertion of the rod and tightening of the wire.

TECHNIQUE 44-17

- Remove the spinous processes and ligamentum flavum (see Figs. 44-72 to 44-74).

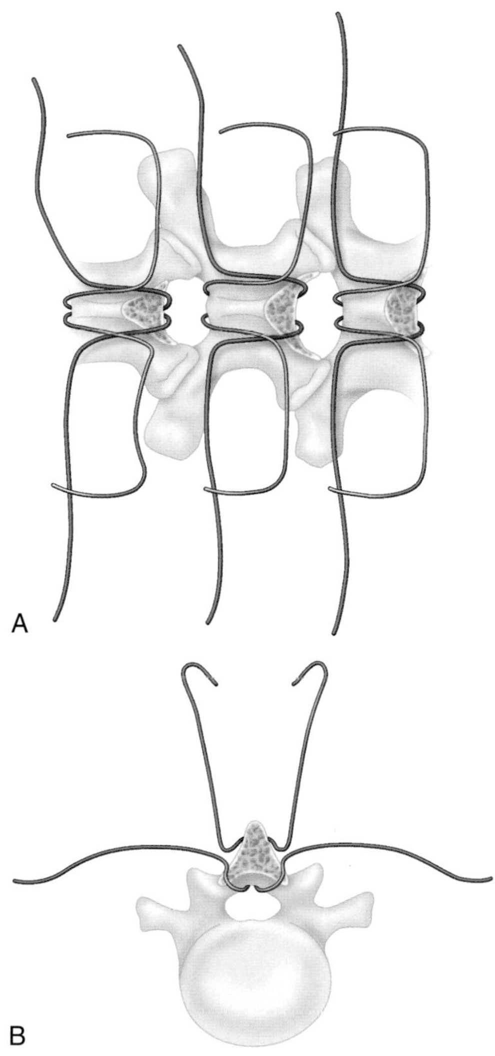

FIGURE 44-77 **A** and **B,** After division, wire is crimped on laminar surface of each side of spinous process. **SEE TECHNIQUE 44-16.**

- Contour the monofilament cable leader into a C shape and pass it beneath the lamina. Grasp the leader and pull it through, leaving equal amounts of cable above and below the lamina (Fig. 44-78A). Cut the tip of the leader and separate the two cables. Pass one arm of the cable through the inferior loop to "lasso" the lamina (Fig. 44-78B).
- After the cables have been passed, contour the rods as indicated. Place the rods through the noose of the cable and use the cable to lasso the rod into position (Fig. 44-78C). The cables currently have an integral crimp. Pass a provisional crimp over the cable.
- Prepare the cable tensioner by depressing the release lever and sliding the release button, which allows the tension to fully retract (Fig. 44-79A).
- Insert the cable through the tensioner. The cable leader must be straight and short. Once the cable has been threaded through the tensioner, lift the cam lever to lock the cable. Depress the tension arm repeatedly until the desired tension is obtained. After appropriate tension is obtained, lock the provisional crimp into place (Fig. 44-79B). The tension on any other cables can be adjusted and retightened by use of the provisional crimp and tensioner.
- After all cables have been tightened, compress the integral crimp (Fig. 44-79C).

INSTRUMENTATION SEQUENCE IN TYPICAL LENKE 1A CURVE

The following is a typical instrumentation sequence for a Lenke 1A (King III) curve with use of the CD Horizon Legacy spinal deformity system. Multiple other systems are available to accomplish the same result. Readers are referred to the technique manual for further details of the system that best fits their practice.

TECHNIQUE 44-18

- Once the hook sites are prepared, remove the laminar hooks. They are not stable before rod insertion and can be jarred loose during decortication.
- At this point in the surgery, perform facetectomy (Fig. 44-80A).
- Curet the intervening cartilage to expose subchondral bone. Decortication of the laminae, spinous processes, and transverse processes along with bone graft placement will be done at completion of instrumentation.
- After facetectomy, place the laminar hooks back in their original positions.
- At this point, cut the correction rod that will be placed on the concave side to the appropriate length, which generally is 2 to 3 cm longer than the overall hook-to-hook length.
- Bend the rod to achieve correct sagittal plane contour. This is accomplished with small, incremental steps by use of the French bender (Fig. 44-80B). The CD Horizon Legacy rod has an etched line to maintain the same plane orientation of the rod and to prevent a spiral-type bend. If the scoliosis is flexible, bend the rod to achieve the planned postoperative sagittal contours. If the curve is stiff, contour the rod to fit easily within the hooks; this rigid scoliosis will be corrected mainly with derotation and in situ bending.
- Place the contoured rod into the implants. This can be started from either the superior or inferior hook. Place the set screws into the first hooks where the rod seats perfectly. After the rod is inserted into the first one or two hooks, it then becomes necessary to use one of several methods to facilitate rod reduction and fully seat the rod into the saddle of the implants.
- The "forceps rocker" method is effective for seating the rod into the implant when there is only a slight height difference between the rod and the implant saddle. To use the rocker, grasp the sides of the implant with a rocker cam above the rod and the forceps tips facing the same direction as the hook blade (Fig. 44-80C). Lever the

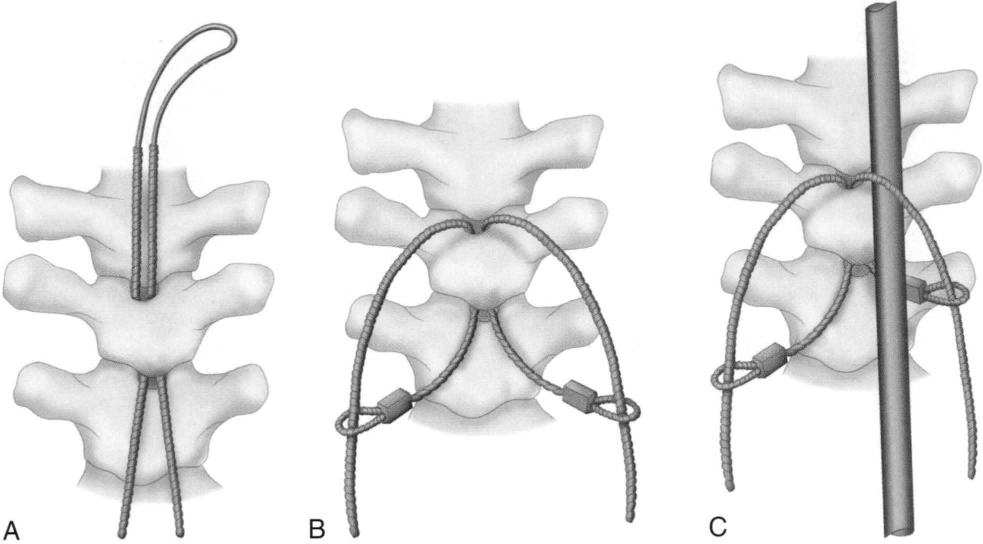

FIGURE 44-78 Sublaminar cable technique. **A,** C-shaped cable leader is passed through lamina. **B,** Cable ends are passed through inferior loops to lasso lamina. **C,** Rod in place beneath cable. **SEE TECHNIQUE 44-17.**

rocker backward over the rod to seat the rod into the saddle of the implant. The set screw is then inserted into the hook (Fig. 44-80D).

- In situations in which the difference between the hook and rod is such that the rocker cannot be used, use the Beale rod reducer. This reducer is placed over the implant with the ratchet portion parallel to the rod.
- Slowly close the reducer by squeezing the handles together, allowing the attached sleeve to slide down and seat the rod into the saddle of the implant (Fig. 44-80E).
- Place a set screw through the set screw tube of the reducer, using the provisional driver (Fig. 44-80F).
- Once the contoured rod and all of the set screws have been placed, perform the rod rotation maneuver. This is done slowly, and it is essential to watch all of the hooks because the hooks can sometimes be dislodged during this rotational maneuver. The hooks in the center of the construct are those most likely to back out during rod rotation. Using two rod grippers (Fig. 44-81A), rotate the rod to translate the apex of the curve toward the midline. If the hooks begin to dislodge, place one of the rod grippers next to the hook and reseat the hook by use of a distractor. Once the rod rotation is complete, tighten the set screws.
- In situ benders are then used for correction and final adjustment of the rod in the sagittal plane. Bend the rod in small, incremental steps by use of the two bender tips positioned near each other on the rod (Fig. 44-81B).
- Once the contouring has been completed, perform distraction or compression to seat the hooks in their final positions. It is recommended to use a rod gripper as a stop for distraction maneuvers rather than any portion of the implant (Fig. 44-82A). Compression maneuvers generally are carried out on two hooks (Fig. 44-82B). Take care that these instruments are placed against the implant body and not against the set screw.
- After these maneuvers are complete, tighten the set screws further. Place the convex stabilizing rod, measure the length, and cut the rod to length. With use of the French bender, contour the rod according to the curvature of the spine in the residual position of alignment from the correction rod. Place the contoured rod into the hooks and provisionally secure the rods with set screws (Fig. 44-82C).
- Once the rod is secured to the implants, apply distraction and compression.
- Measure the length and apply appropriate side crosslinks. Transverse crosslinks are necessary to provide rotational stability to the construct. Ideally, the crosslinks should be placed close to the ends of the construct. Tighten the set screws.
- Place the countertorque instrument over the implant and rod (Fig. 44-82D). Place the break-off driver through the cannulated countertorque. The self-retaining break-off driver provides leverage for breaking the set screw heads. Tighten the handle clockwise and shear off the set screw head (Fig. 44-82E).
- In this system, the broken-off part of the set screw is captured in the cannulated portion of the driver.
- After final tightening, the sheared-off portions of the set screws accumulated in the driver are removed with an obturator (Fig. 44-82F). These are then counted and compared against the number of implants.
- Perform decortication with either a power burr or Cobb gouge.
- Apply bone graft.
- Close the wound in the routine manner.

POSTOPERATIVE CARE. Postoperatively, most patients have a temporary ileus. For this reason, food and liquids

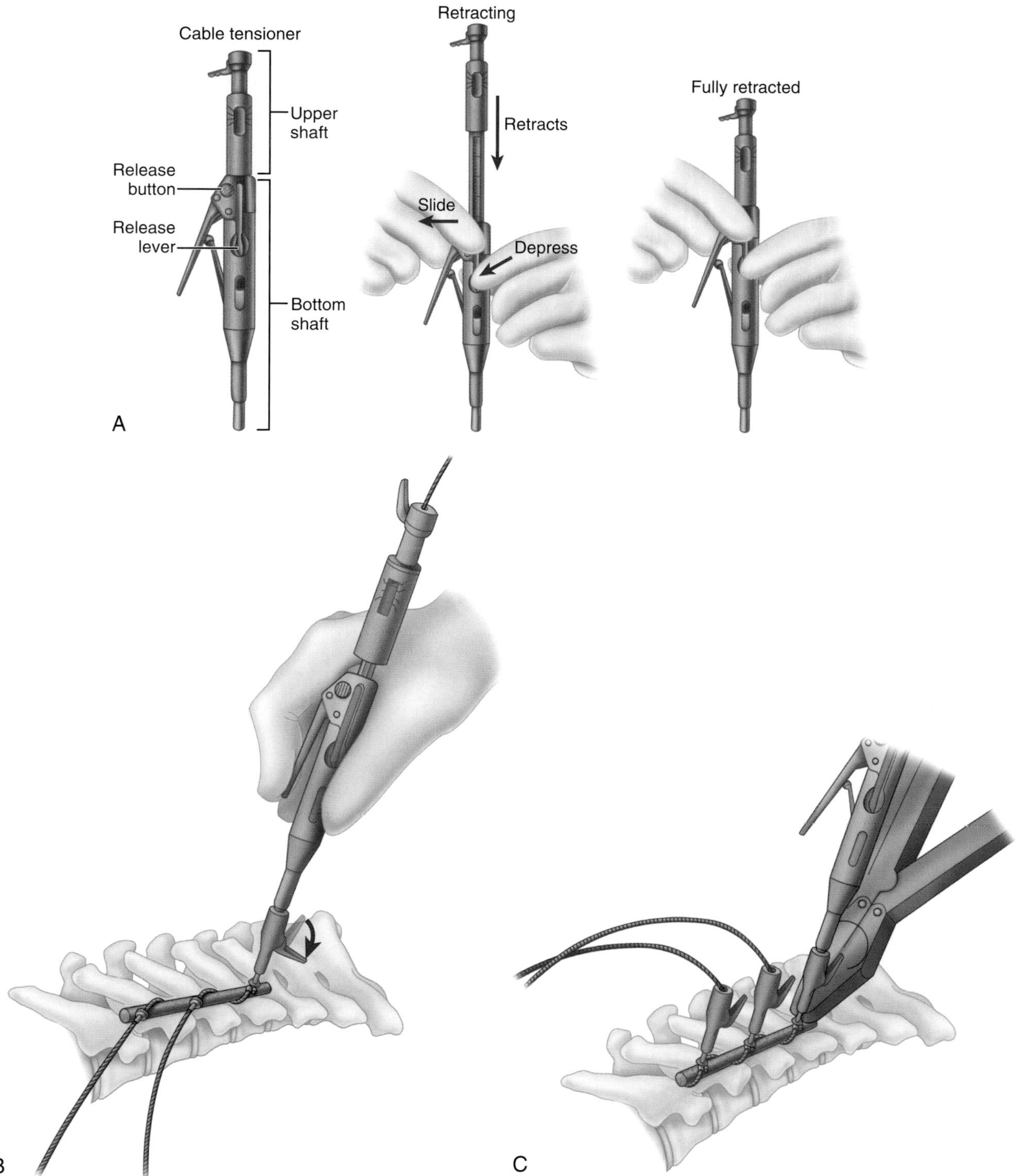

FIGURE 44-79 **A,** Tensioner device. **B,** After appropriate tension is applied, provisional crimp is locked into place. **C,** After all cables have been tightened, top hats are crimped. (Redrawn from Cable tensioner instruction sheet, Danek Cable Instruments, Memphis, TN, Sofamor Danek.) **SEE TECHNIQUE 44-17.**

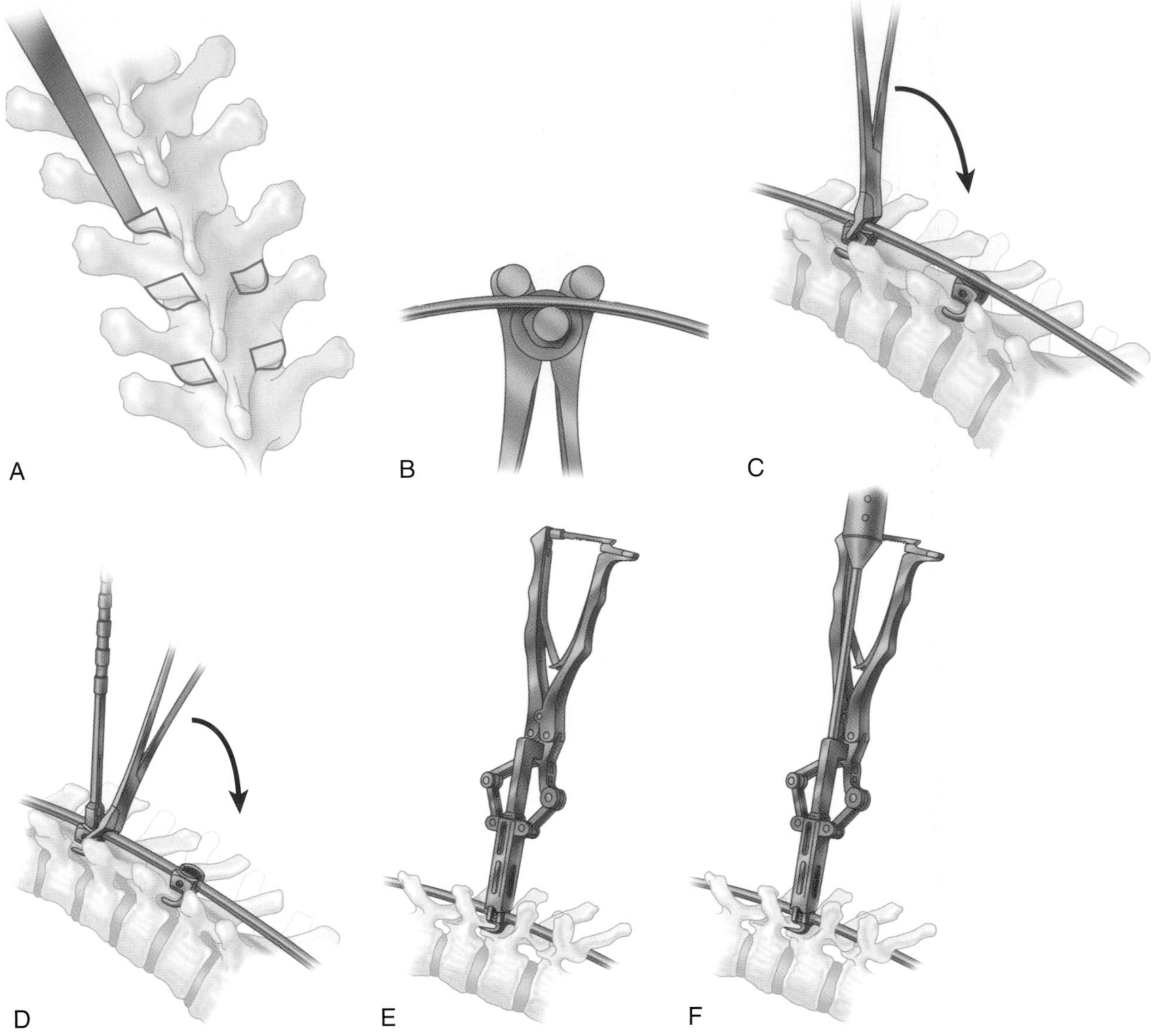

A B C D E F

FIGURE 44-80 **A-F,** Instrumentation sequence for Lenke 1A (King III) curve with CD Horizon Legacy spinal deformity system (see text). Decortication, rod contouring, and reduction. (Redrawn from Lascombes P: CD Horizon Legacy Spinal System-deformity, surgical technique manual, Memphis, TN, 2005, Medtronic Sofamor Danek.) **SEE TECHNIQUE 44-18.**

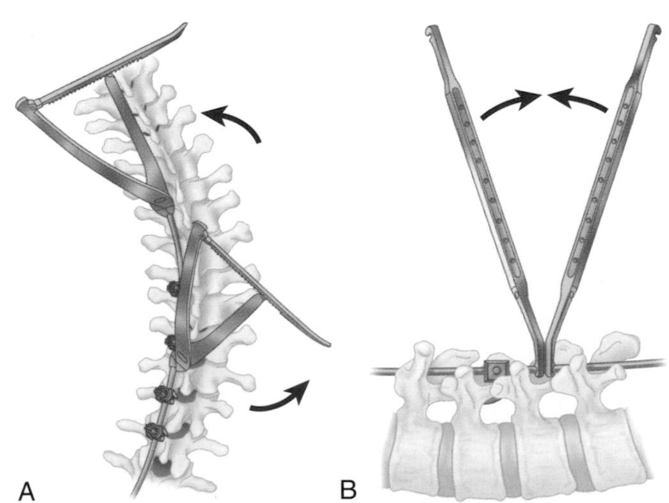

FIGURE 44-81 **A** and **B,** Deformity correction by CD Horizon Legacy spinal deformity system. See text for description. (Redrawn from Lascombes P: CD Horizon Legacy Spinal System-deformity, surgical technique manual, Memphis, TN, 2005, Medtronic Sofamor Danek.) **SEE TECHNIQUE 44-18.**

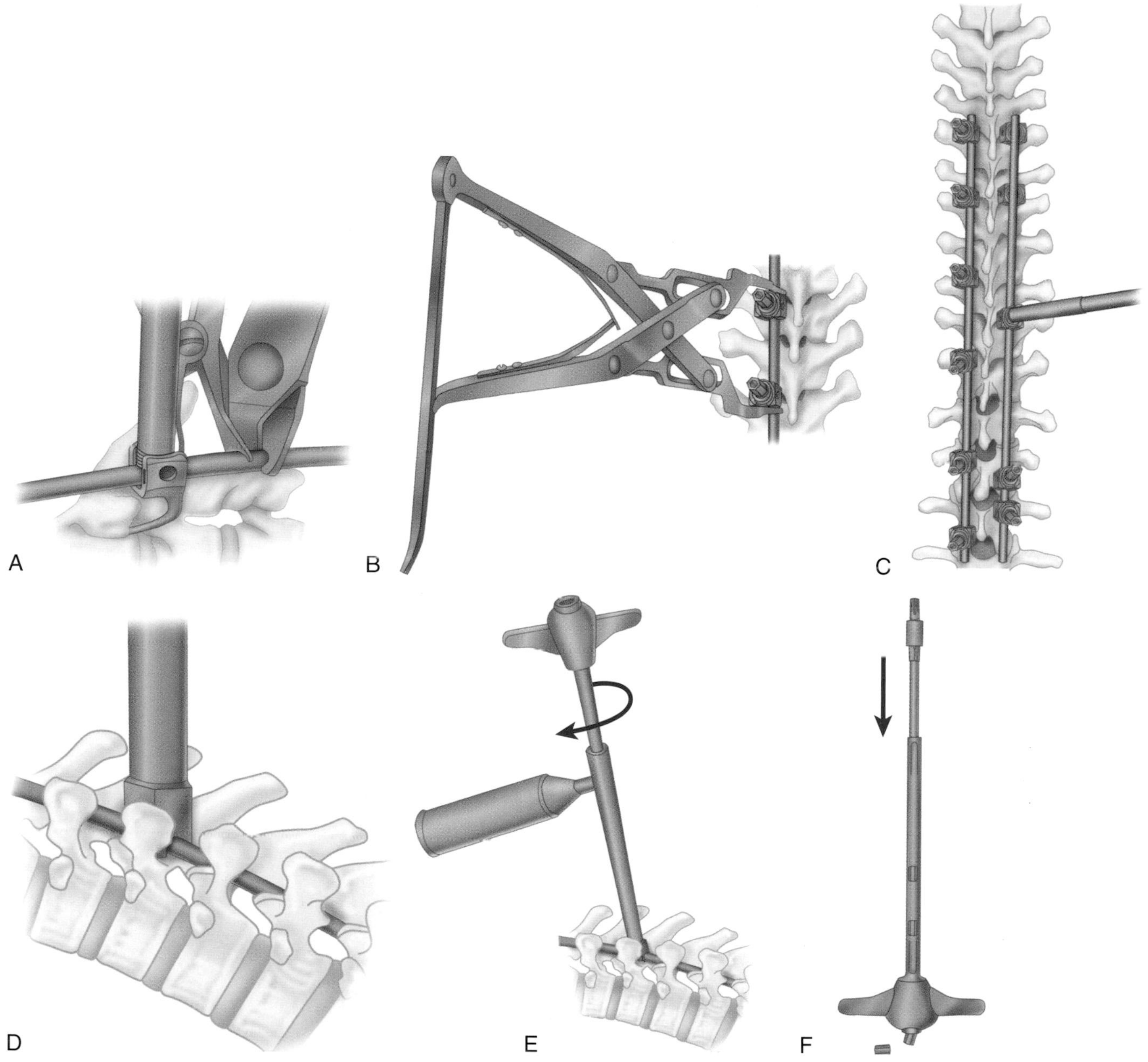

FIGURE 44-82 **A-F,** **Rod compression and distraction, stabilization, and final tightening for CD Horizon Legacy spinal deformity system (see text). Decortication, rod contouring, and reduction.** (Redrawn from Lascombes P: CD Horizon Legacy Spinal System-deformity, surgical technique manual, Memphis, TN, 2005, Medtronic Sofamor Danek.) **SEE TECHNIQUE 44-18.**

are advanced slowly. Frequently, they have atelectasis and a low-grade fever, and intravenous antibiotics may be continued for 24 hours. The suction drain is removed at 24 to 48 hours, depending on the amount of drainage. The patient is mobilized from bed to chair as quickly as pain allows. The instrumentation usually is stable enough that no external support or brace is needed. Patients are discharged from the hospital as soon as they tolerate food and liquids, their temperature decreases, and they are independent with household-type activities.

DEFORMITY CORRECTION BY USE OF TRANSLATIONAL TECHNIQUES WITH MULTIPLE THORACIC PEDICLE SCREWS

TECHNIQUE 44-19

- Once the correct screw placement has been verified by image and by triggered electromyography, contour a trial rod in the sagittal and coronal planes.

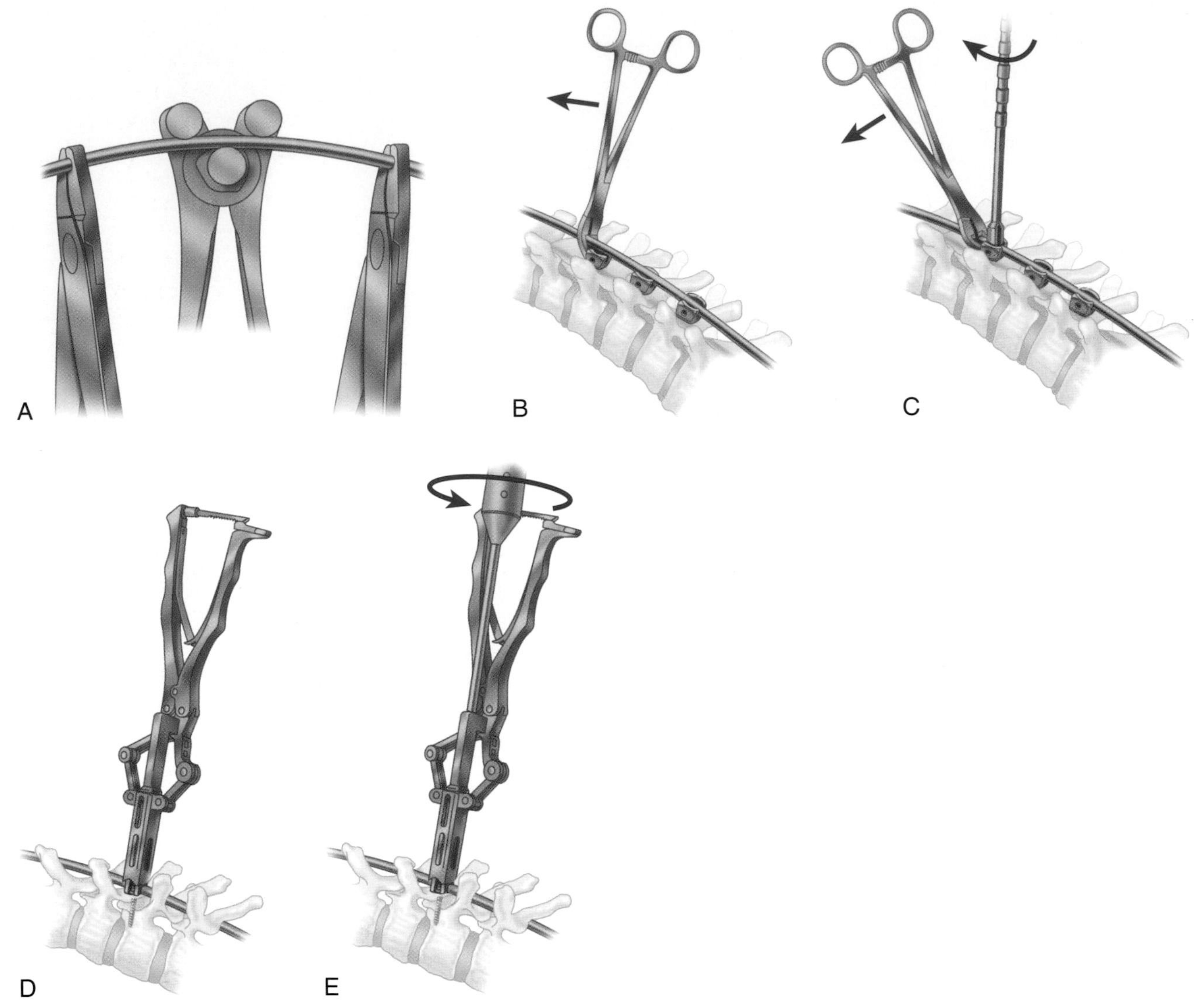

FIGURE 44-83 **A-K,** Thoracic screw insertion techniques with use of CD Horizon Legacy spinal deformity system. See text for description. (Redrawn from Lascombes P: CD Horizon Legacy Spinal System-deformity, surgical technique manual, Memphis, TN, 2005, Medtronic Sofamor Danek.) **SEE TECHNIQUE 44-19.**

- Hold the rod with rod grippers to prevent it from rotating during contouring (Fig. 44-83A). For hypokyphotic deformities, which are the most common, place the rod on the concavity first.
- Place the contoured rod into the screws. There are several instruments that can be used to fully seat the rod into the saddle of the implant. A forceps rocker is effective for seating the rod into the implant when there is only a slight height difference between the rod and the implant saddle. To use the rocker, grasp the sides of the implant with a rocker cam above the rod (Fig. 44-83B). Lever backward over the rod. The levering action allows the rod to be fully seated in the saddle of the implant.
- Introduce a set screw plug into the screw (Fig. 44-83C).
- If the rod rests over the implant but is too far superior for the rocker, use a rod reducer.
- Place the reducer over the implant with the ratchet portion parallel to the rod (Fig. 44-83D).
- Slowly close the reducer, allowing the attached sleeve to slide down and seat the rod into the implant saddle.
- Place a set screw through the plug tube and provisionally tighten it (Fig. 44-83E). The set screws are tightened on each end of the rod but kept loose in the center.
- Slowly straighten the concave rod with the left and right coronal benders. Each straightening of the concave rod is performed over a pedicle screw. Only small corrections are made each time, and several passes are generally required to allow viscoelastic relaxation (Fig. 44-83F).
- Once correction is obtained, perform desired compression or distraction (Fig. 44-83G). Distraction can sometimes be useful in correcting any residual endplate tilt either proximally or distally.

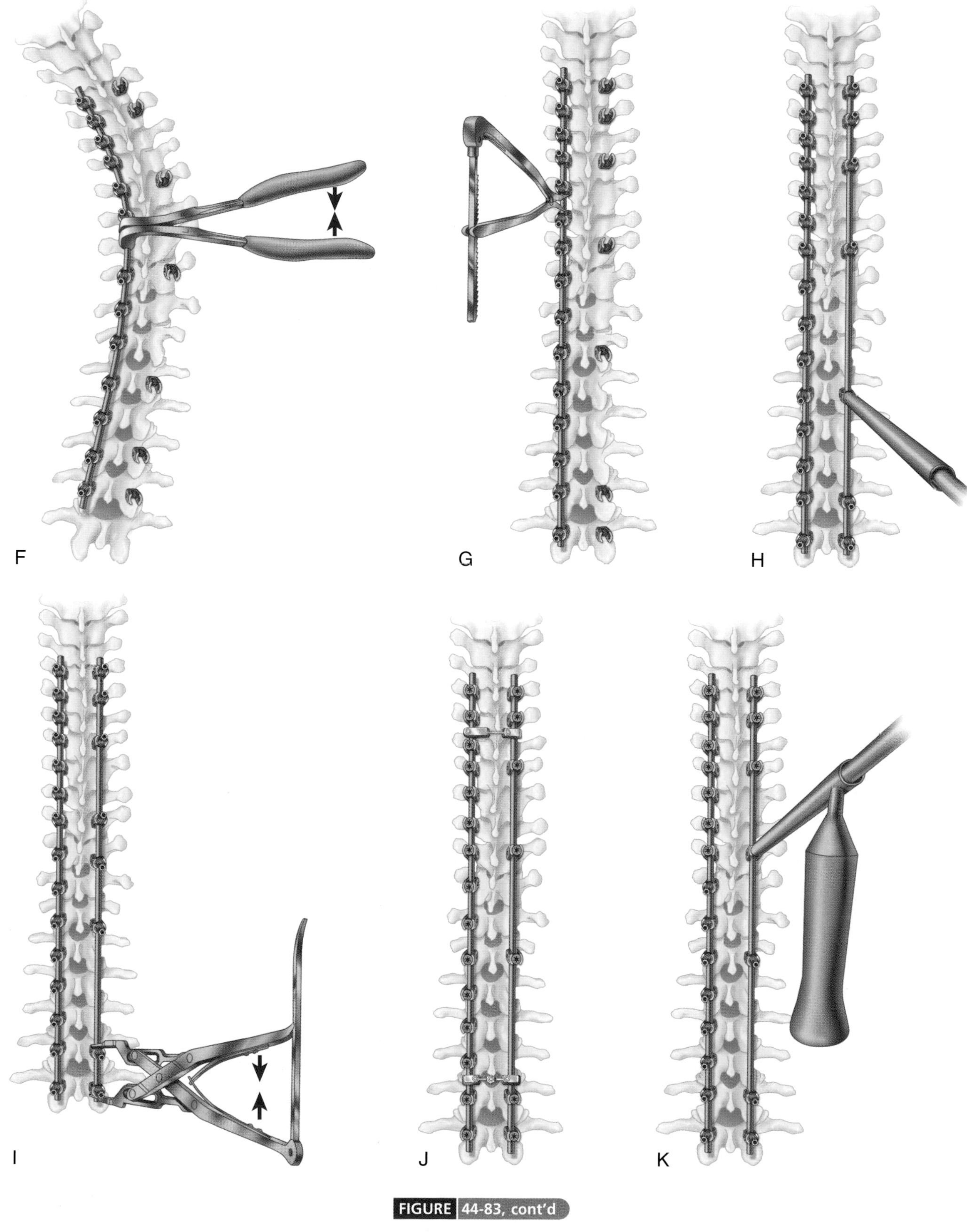

FIGURE 44-83, cont'd

- Contour a second rod and place it in the convex screw heads (Fig. 44-83H).
- Place compressive forces on segments on the convex side to horizontalize the lowest instrumented vertebra and mildly compress the convexity of the deformity (Fig. 44-83I).
- In situ bending in the sagittal plane may be needed to re-create sagittal balance.
- Apply appropriate-sized crosslinks (Fig. 44-83J).
- In this particular instrumentation system, a countertorque and a self-retaining break-off driver are used. Shear the heads of the set screws off and lock the rod into place (Fig. 44-83K).
- Decorticate the posterior elements with a bur and place a bone graft.

DEFORMITY CORRECTION BY DIRECT VERTEBRAL ROTATION

TECHNIQUE 44-20

- In this technique, we routinely use bilateral pedicle screws at every level to be fused in the thoracic spine. The direct vertebral rotation is opposite to that of the vertebral rotation in the thoracic curve; apical and juxtaapical vertebrae are rotated clockwise in the transverse plane.
- Insert screw derotators onto the pedicle screws of the juxtaapical vertebrae on both the concave and convex sides and derotate the vertebrae as much as possible.
- Remove the screw derotators on the concave side and contour the rod to fit into the pedicle screws on the concave side while holding the vertebrae derotated.
- Rotate the rod as the convex screws are held in a derotated position (Fig. 44-84). During the rod derotation, rotate the convex screws in the opposite direction (clockwise) of the rod derotation maneuver.
- After completion of the derotation, lock the rod into position by tightening the set screws fully.
- If the curve is rigid, we have found that often little rod derotation is possible. In these cases, while holding the convex screws in the derotated position, use the coronal rod bender to correct the deformity in the coronal plane. Again, this is done in incremental steps, each one around a pedicle screw.
- Once the coronal correction is obtained, temporarily tighten the set screws.
- Place the concave rod derotator over the appropriate pedicle screw and a convex rod derotator on the pedicle screw on the other side of the same vertebra.
- Loosen the concave set screw and derotate the vertebra farther in a clockwise manner and tighten the screw. In this manner, individual derotation of each vertebra can be performed.
- After this, apply the stabilizing rod in the screws on the convex side and attach the set screws.
- Apply appropriate crosslinks. Shear the set screws off, decorticate the posterior element, and apply bone graft.

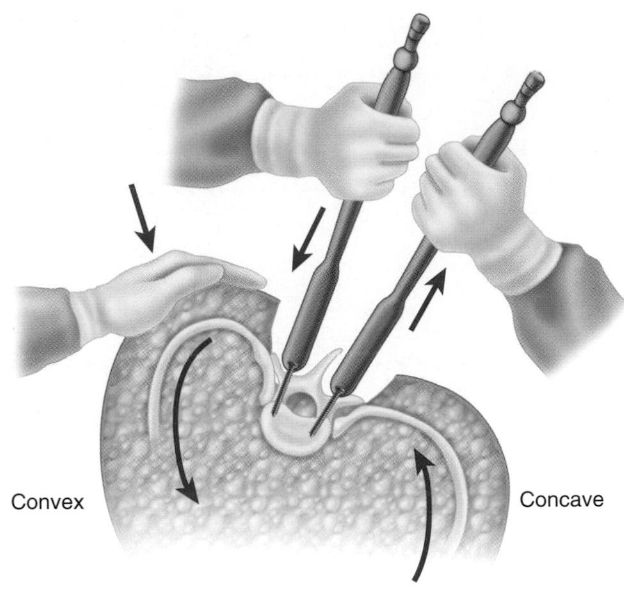

FIGURE 44-84 **Direct vertebral rotation.** (Redrawn from Newton PO, O'Brien MF, Sufflebarger HL, et al, editors: Idiopathic scoliosis: the Harms Study Group treatment guide, New York, 2010, Thieme.) **SEE TECHNIQUE 44-20.**

COMPLICATIONS AND PITFALLS IN SEGMENTAL INSTRUMENTATION SYSTEMS

In addition to the complications inherent in any spinal arthrodesis, segmental instrumentation systems have several potential pitfalls. These generally can be divided into strategic mistakes and technical mistakes.

One of the more common strategic mistakes is stopping the instrumentation at the middle of a sagittal or frontal pathologic curve. If the instrumentation is stopped at the level of a thoracolumbar kyphosis, a postoperative distal junctional kyphosis often occurs (Fig. 44-85). This mistake is prevented by closely following the principles of instrumentation site selection and avoiding ending instrumentation at a level of thoracolumbar kyphosis on a standing lateral radiograph.

Kim et al. defined proximal junctional kyphosis as a Cobb angle of more than 10 degrees and of 10 degrees greater than the preoperative measurement when measured from the lower end point of the uppermost instrumented vertebra and the upper endplate of two supraadjacent vertebrae. They found an incidence of 26% at 7.3 years after surgery. The proximal junctional kyphosis did not progress after 2 years.

Another common strategic mistake is failure to recognize the significance of the upper thoracic curve preoperatively. If the upper thoracic curve does not correct on supine bending films to the predicted correction of the lower thoracic curve, elevation of the left shoulder and an unsightly deformity will occur (Fig. 44-86). This mistake is prevented by carefully evaluating the clinical appearance of the shoulders and the bending films, as well as the standing radiographs, with special attention to this upper curve. Useful measurements from standing radiographs are the T1 tilt angle, the clavicle angle, and the radiographic shoulder height. The T1 tilt angle is measured by the intersection of a line drawn along the T1 cephalad endplate and a line parallel to the horizontal

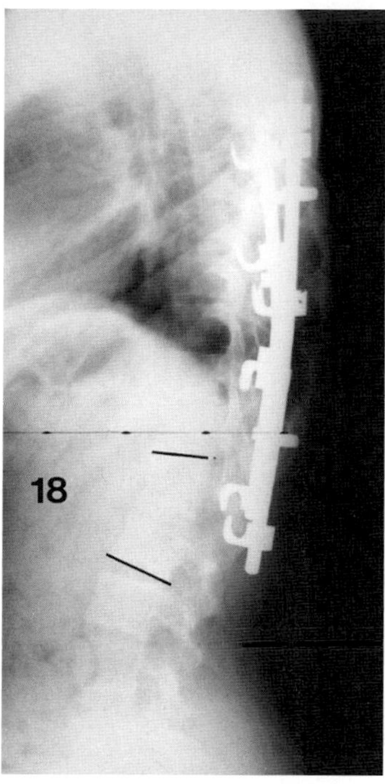

FIGURE 44-85 Postoperative junctional kyphosis in King type II thoracic curve; instrumentation stopped at level of thoracolumbar kyphosis.

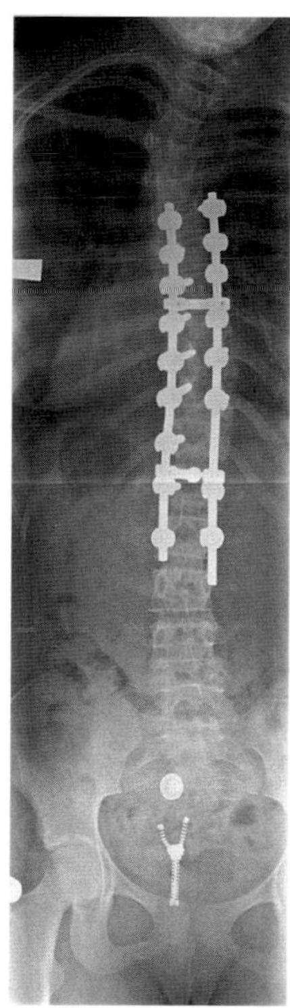

FIGURE 44-86 Elevation of shoulder caused by undercorrection of upper thoracic curve.

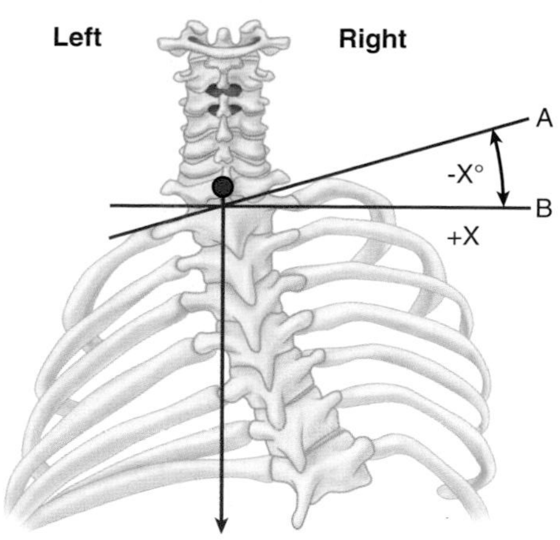

FIGURE 44-87 When right edge of vertebral body is up, tilt angle is defined as negative. When left edge of vertebral body is up, tilt angle is defined as positive. (Redrawn from O'Brien MF, Kuklo TR, Blanke KM, Lenke LG, editors: Spinal deformity study group radiographic measurement manual, Memphis, TN, 2004, Medtronic Sofamor Danek, p. 55.)

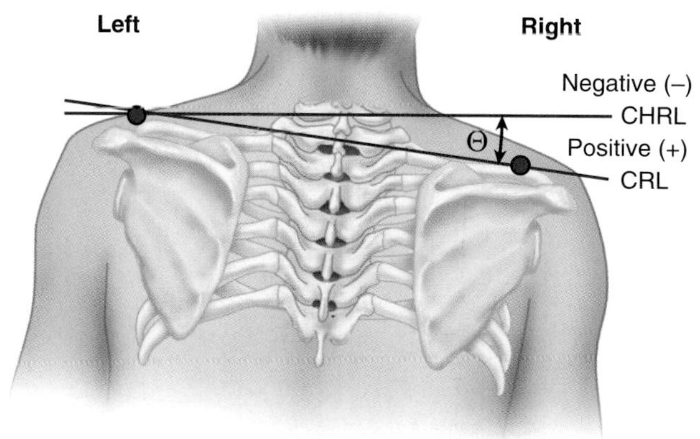

FIGURE 44-88 Clavicular angle. CHRL, Clavicle horizontal reference line; CRL, clavicle reference line. (Redrawn from O'Brien MF, Kuklo TR, Blanke KM, Lenke LG, editors: Spinal deformity study group radiographic measurement manual, Memphis, TN, 2004, Medtronic Sofamor Danek, p. 56.)

reference line (Fig. 44-87). The clavicular angle is measured by the intersection of a line touching the two highest points of the clavicle and a line parallel to the horizontal reference line (Fig. 44-88). The radiographic shoulder height is determined by the difference in the soft-tissue shadow directly superior to each acromioclavicular joint on a standing posteroanterior radiograph (Fig. 44-89). A proximal curve should be considered structural if (1) the curve size is more than 30 degrees and remains more than 20 degrees on side-bending radiographs; (2) the Nash-Moe apical rotation is above grade 1; (3) there is more than 1 cm of apical translation from the C7 plumb line; (4) there is a positive T1 tilt; and (5) clinical elevation of either shoulder (frequently the left) is noted, depending on the curve type. The other problem frequently described in the coronal plane is decompensation with selective fusion of the thoracic curve (Fig. 44-90). When using pedicle screws for distal fixation, we have found that this problem can be minimized by careful evaluation of the lumbar curve according to the Lenke criteria and also by the clinical appearance of the lumbar curve. If the curve is

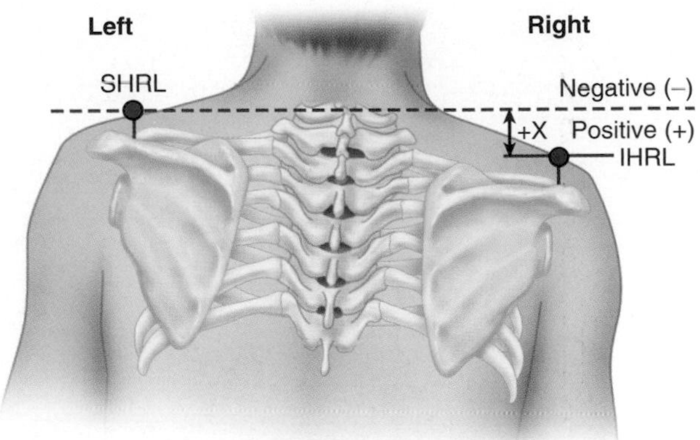

FIGURE 44-89 Radiographic shoulder height. IHRL, Inferior horizontal reference line; SHRL, superior horizontal reference line. (Redrawn from O'Brien MF, Kuklo TR, Blanke KM, Lenke LG, editors: Spinal deformity study group radiographic measurement manual, Memphis, TN, 2004, Medtronic Sofamor Danek, p. 57.)

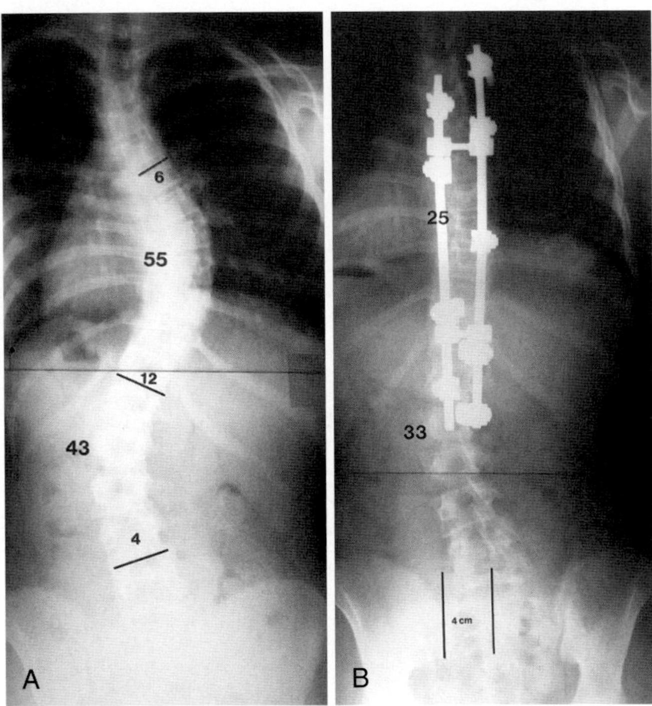

FIGURE 44-90 **A,** King type II curve. **B,** Decompensated lumbar curve after fusion of thoracic curve only.

severely rotated clinically, it probably will need to be incorporated in the fusion. If a selective thoracic fusion is performed, the lower instrumented vertebra should at least touch the center sacral line on the standing posteroanterior preoperative radiograph. A well-balanced correction of the spine after a selective thoracic fusion is more likely if the preoperative ratio of the thoracic to lumbar curve magnitude is greater than 1:2, the apical vertebral rotation ratio of the thoracic to lumbar curve is greater than 1:0, and the apical vertebral translation of the thoracic to the lumbar curve is 1:2.

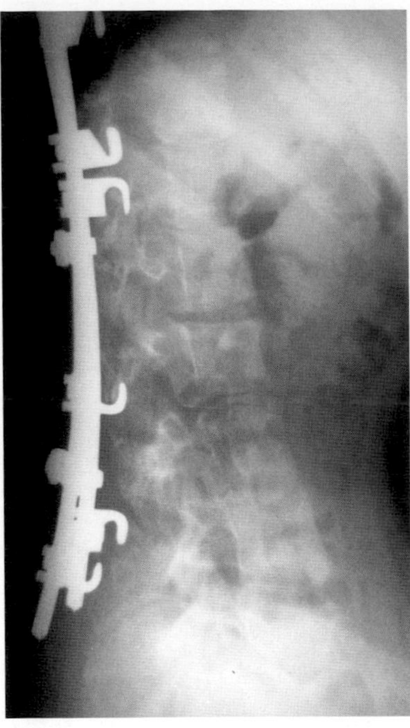

FIGURE 44-91 Cut-out of lower hooks caused by improper contouring of rods.

When a multiple-hook segmental instrumentation system is used, several potential technical problems should be avoided during the surgical procedure. During insertion of the pedicle hooks, the hooks should not be inserted too horizontally or else the inferior facet of the superior vertebra may be fractured; if the hooks are inserted too vertically, the superior facet of the inferior vertebra may be fractured. The pedicle hook should be carefully inserted into the intraarticular space, and care should be taken to be certain that the pedicle is incorporated into the bifid area of the hook. During insertion of the laminar hooks, the most frequent problem is insufficient insertion of the hook under the lamina. If this hook is not well seated, when the rod is applied and rotated and a posterior-directed force is applied, the hook often pulls out and the lamina breaks. The lower laminar edge runs in a backward and downward direction; therefore, when infralaminar hooks are inserted in the lumbar spine, the hooks must be inserted in the same direction. Often, shaving down of the lamina is required to allow the hook to be well seated.

The goal of the surgery is to restore normal sagittal contours. In contouring the rod, excessive bending of the rod should be avoided, if possible. If a large lumbar curve is present and the rod is contoured in the coronal plane to correspond exactly to the lumbar curve, as the rod is rotated, an excessive posterior force is applied to the lower hooks, and these hooks can then cut out posteriorly (Fig. 44-91). If, however, the distance between the rod and hook is too large, the lamina can break as the rod is being inserted into the hook. In this case, it may be necessary to contour the rod further.

As the rod rotation maneuver is done, the intermediate hooks of the thoracic spine tend to unload and can pull out with rotation. These hooks generally have to be reseated at least once during the rod rotation maneuver. Also, when a lordotic rod bend with a reverse hook pattern is applied at the thoracolumbar junction, the infralaminar hook at the distal end often needs to be reset with rod rotation. As the rod is rotated, the upper end vertebra hook tends to medially rotate into the canal and may cause neurologic injury, such as a Brown-Séquard syndrome. This hook should be watched carefully during the rotation maneuver.

The lower intermediate hook on the concave side can be forced accidentally into the spinal canal during rod insertion. The spinal cord generally is shifted toward the concave side of the scoliosis curve, and therefore extreme caution should be exercised when the rod is inserted. When the rod is rotated, however, the lower intermediate hook is pulled backward and away from the spinal cord. The lower intermediate hook is therefore of more concern during rod insertion, whereas the upper end vertebral hook is of more concern during rod rotation.

When the convex rod is applied, a downward force is applied to the apical vertebra. Therefore this hook should be a pedicle hook and not a laminar hook. In general, the upper end vertebra in scoliosis should be instrumented on both sides with at least one pedicle–transverse process claw. Because compression is applied to the convex rod, the pedicle–transverse process claw generally is used on the convex side. The hook that most frequently dislodges is the inferior, convex, cranially directed hook. An additional caudally directed hook at the level above can give a two-level claw configuration to this hook and decrease the possibility of hook cutout.

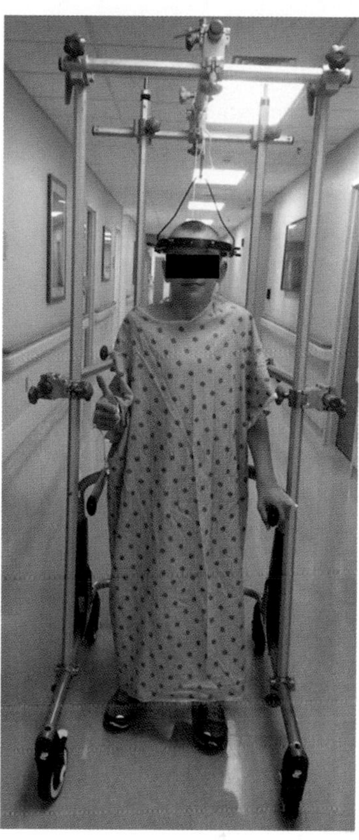

FIGURE 44-92 Child in halo-gravity traction. SEE TECHNIQUE 44-21.

RIGID CURVES

HALO-GRAVITY TRACTION

Rigid curves of the spine in adolescents have historically been treated with halo traction as an adjunct to surgery. However, it is not always indicated, especially if the deformity includes the cervical spine or distal spine with hip flexion contractures, kyphosis, or stenosis (Fig. 44-92). It also is associated with complications and requires prolonged hospital stays.

TECHNIQUE 44-21

(SPONSELLER AND TAKENAGA)

- Sedation and local anesthesia should be used for this procedure.
- Place the halo just below the equator of the skull, above the eyebrows and pinnae of the ears.
- Six to eight pins are used in children younger than 6 years of age and tightened to 4 in-lb of torque. In older children or adults (if there is normal bone density), the pins are tightened to 8 in-lb. Place the anterior pins lateral to the midportion of the eyebrows to avoid the supraorbital nerves. Place the posterior pins diametrically opposite the anterior pins. Retighten the pins after 24 to 48 hours. If there is loosening after this, the pin should be relocated.
- Begin traction immediately with 5 lb of weight for young children and 10 lb for children close to maturity.
- Gradually increase the traction weight by 2 to 3 lb/day as tolerated, with the goal being a weight of 33% to 50% of the patient's body weight. Incline the bed downward caudally.
- Inspect the patient's skin regularly because pressure sores from bony prominences are common, especially in patients who have trouble turning themselves.
- Continue traction throughout the day. Patients should be upright in a halo wheelchair or walker for part of the day. The goal is to suspend the patient's trunk as much as possible. Traction also may be applied when the patient is standing in a specially designed walker. Decrease the traction weight when the patient is sleeping, especially when the weight is near its maximum.
- Check the patient's neurologic status in the upper and lower extremities three times daily, as well as cranial nerve function.
- The duration of preoperative halo-gravity traction may range from 2 to 12 weeks depending on the severity of the curve, its response to traction, and the overall condition of the patient.
- Obtain radiographs approximately every week to assess the improvement obtained.
- Longer periods of traction may help to optimize nutrition and minimize pulmonary problems in those with borderline pulmonary or nutritional reserve.

TEMPORARY DISTRACTION ROD

The use of temporary internal distraction rods in advance of the corrective surgical procedure has been described as an alternative to halo traction for severe rigid curves. Improved curve correction and restoration of sagittal and coronal contours have been cited as advantages to this technique. Placement of one or two temporary rods, soft-tissue releases, and osteotomies are performed usually 1 week before the permanent final implants are placed and fusion performed. The time between procedures can be longer than 1 week if necessary.

Before surgery, standard anteroposterior and lateral plain radiographs of the spine should be obtained with the patient standing or sitting, depending on the neurologic status. Traction films are helpful in predicting the amount of correction that can be obtained with a temporary rod. In addition, MRI and CT of the cervical, thoracic, and lumbar spine should be obtained to evaluate the precise spinal anatomy. Preoperative antibiotics should be administered.

TECHNIQUE 44-22

(BUCHOWSKI ET AL.)

- Place the patient prone on a Jackson table or alternatively on a flat radiolucent table. Place longitudinal chest rolls. The goal when positioning the patient on the table is to obtain as much correction of body alignment as possible to lessen the force required to achieve intraoperative correction. Gardner-Wells tongs can be helpful to obtain temporary intraoperative traction. The tongs can be released once instrumentation is placed and the spine is distracted.
- Neuromonitoring is absolutely necessary during distraction of the spine.
- Make a skin incision in the standard fashion. Through a midline incision, carry subperiosteal dissection along the laminae down to the osseous cephalad anchor points.
- Place two infralaminar or pedicle hooks in a standard fashion in the laminae that are not intended to be the final cephalad fixation points. Alternatively, the ribs may be used as temporary cephalad anchor points. This requires subperiosteal dissection along the lamina and then laterally over the transverse processes until the medial aspects of the ribs are palpated. To avoid entering the chest, dissect the ribs subperiosteally along their anterior surfaces (before closure, check to make sure the chest has not been entered). Place standard laminar hooks on the rib in an upgoing fashion.
- For placement of the caudal anchors, use standard lumbar pedicle screws, placing two screws (or more, depending on bone quality) at adjacent vertebrae. Alternatively, sublaminar hooks can be used. The vertebrae cephalad to the end vertebrae of the final construct should be chosen because some loosening of the temporary anchor points is expected to occur with distraction.
- If the pelvis is used for anchoring points, expose the iliac spine. Place an iliac screw in the posterior superior iliac crest close to (but not entering) the sciatic notch. It should be placed parallel and at least 2 cm lateral to where the permanent iliac screw will be placed. Alternatively, an S-shaped hook may be used, and this may be easier to connect to the distraction rod with a side-to-side connector.
- Although there are several possibilities for placement of internal distraction rod constructs, the simplest is to attach one distraction rod to the cephalad anchor points and a second rod to the caudal anchor points. Connect the two rods using a side-to-side connector with overlap of the rods. In some patients with extreme deformity, it may be necessary to attach two short rods (one attached cephalad and one caudal) to a third distraction rod using multiaxial crosslink connectors.
- Apply distraction across these two rods serially by loosening and tightening the side-to-side connector. Careful attention should be given to spinal cord function during the distraction process. If a depression in spinal cord signal is noticed, the amount of correction should be decreased and a wake-up test performed.
- Once the temporary rod or rods have been placed, expose the rest of the spine subperiosteally. Perform releases and osteotomies as necessary to allow additional correction of the spine. Although technically more difficult, additional anchor points can be placed after releases and osteotomies if necessary.
- Small amounts of distraction should be performed throughout the procedure to allow maximal correction with minimal stress. With time, soft-tissue release, facetectomies, and osteotomies, additional correction can be obtained with the goal at the end of surgery to have correction greater than that shown on the supine traction film with 50% or more correction in the Cobb angle. Bone graft is not used at this time but can be stored for the final procedure.
- Irrigate the wound thoroughly. Buchkowski et al. recommend jet lavage and antibiotic-detergent solution to decrease the risk of infection.
- Closure is difficult because substantial soft-tissue lengthening occurs with distraction and the rods usually are lateral to the transverse processes. If necessary, raise thick local flaps including the paraspinal muscles to make closure possible. Use closed suction drains in the space created during the closure.

STAGE II DEFINITIVE SURGERY

- Reexpose the spine. Leaving the temporary rod(s) in place if feasible, create the anchor points for the final construct. There should be a substantial increase in the ability to correct the spine at this point, and it may be possible to gain additional distraction.
- Remove the temporary instrumentation and insert the final implants.
- Perform repeat pulsed irrigation and drainage and close the wound.

POSTOPERATIVE CARE. Between the first and second stages, parenteral nutrition is recommended until the patient can optimize oral intake. Sitting, standing, and walking are encouraged to avoid pulmonary complications. Casting or bracing is not required.

ANTERIOR RELEASE

Complete anterior release of the thoracic or lumbar spine, or both, allows improved mobilization of a curve and correction of deformity. Additional posterior release with instrumentation may be necessary in more severe or rigid deformity.

TECHNIQUE 44-23

(LETKO ET AL.)

- In the thoracic spine, resect the convex rib heads and attempt to rupture the concave costovertebral joints.
- In both the thoracic and lumbar spine, remove the disc and posterior annulus. Release the posterior longitudinal ligament.
- Resect the convex inferior endplate with or without resection of the convex superior endplate to allow mobilization and correction in the coronal plane. By shortening the anterior column, hypokyphosis in the thoracic sagittal profile can be corrected to normal.
- Anterior structural support of the lumbar spine and thoracolumbar junction is recommended to prevent kyphosis.
- After complete anterior release, anterior instrumentation can be performed if the curve is not too rigid or large.

OSTEOTOMY IN COMPLEX SPINAL DEFORMITY

Spinal osteotomy should be considered for patients with large, stiff curves for whom instrumentation alone cannot correct the deformity or restore balance. The classic indication for this procedure was a long rounded kyphosis as in Scheuermann kyphosis; however, it is a versatile procedure that can be performed safely to aid in the gradual correction of rigid scoliotic curves. If soft-tissue releases are insufficient in obtaining correction, proceeding to osteotomy is the next step. The Ponte, Smith-Petersen osteotomy is performed for scoliosis greater than 70 to 75 degrees that does not bend down to less than 40 degrees or for kyphosis that corrects to greater than 40 to 50 degrees in hyperextension. Each millimeter of resection equals 1 degree of correction, with a possible correction of 5 to 10 degrees per level. Multiple levels can be resected to obtain more correction. A collapsed or immobile disc may be a contraindication to this technique. The choice of osteotomy depends on the apex of the deformity.

TECHNIQUE 44-24

Figure 44-93

(PONTE, SMITH-PETERSEN OSTEOTOMY)

- Place the patient prone on an open-frame radiolucent table that allows the abdomen to hang free and places the lumbar spine in lordosis.
- After exposing the spine as described in Technique 44-6, perform complete facetectomies for complete exposure.
- Develop the screw tracks for subsequent pedicle screw placement (without placing the screws) to help guide the osteotomy.
- Remove the lamina, ligamentum flavum, and superior and inferior articular processes bilaterally, and resect the spinous process of the vertebra just cephalad to the osteotomy site.
- Create a wedge-shaped osteotomy 7 to 10 mm in width and carry it laterally to the intervertebral notch with small Kerrison rongeurs. The point should be oriented distally. Both limbs of the wedge should be symmetric unless some coronal plane correction is desired. Take care to avoid the pedicles above and below the osteotomy and the nerve roots. If there is significant rotational deformity, open the osteotomy to a larger degree on the convex side.
- When closing the osteotomy site, widening the osteotomy by removing more superior facet may prevent impingement of the superior nerve root.
- At this point, instrumentation can be added as indicated to achieve necessary correction.

POSTERIOR THORACIC VERTEBRAL COLUMN RESECTION

Vertebral column resection is indicated for patients with complex, rigid, spinal deformities that cannot be corrected by less aggressive osteotomies. Circumferential access is provided to the vertebral column and neural elements for decompression and stabilization. This procedure is quite challenging and entails resection of one or more entire vertebral segments, including the posterior elements, vertebral body, and adjacent discs. Patients with cardiopulmonary comorbidities may not be suitable candidates.

TECHNIQUE 44-25

(POWERS ET AL.)

- Position the patient on a Jackson table with adjustable pads. Intraoperative halo-gravity traction can be used. Neuromonitoring is necessary for this procedure.
- Subperiosteally expose the spine out to the tips of the transverse process (Fig. 44-94A).
- Place pedicle screws using a freehand technique at the preplanned levels of fusion, a minimum of three levels above and three below the vertebral column resection (Fig. 44-94C). The spine is considered unstable from the time resection begins until final correction is achieved. A minimum of six points of fixation, both cephalad and caudal to the resection, is recommended. Multiaxial reduction screws can be placed at the apical concave regions of severe scoliosis or at the proximal or distal regions of severe kyphoscoliosis or kyphosis. In the lumbar spine, they should be placed in the concavity of the lumbar region.
- Expose 4 to 5 cm of the medial ribs corresponding with the level of resection. Remove the ribs by cutting each laterally and then disarticulating the costovertebral joints,

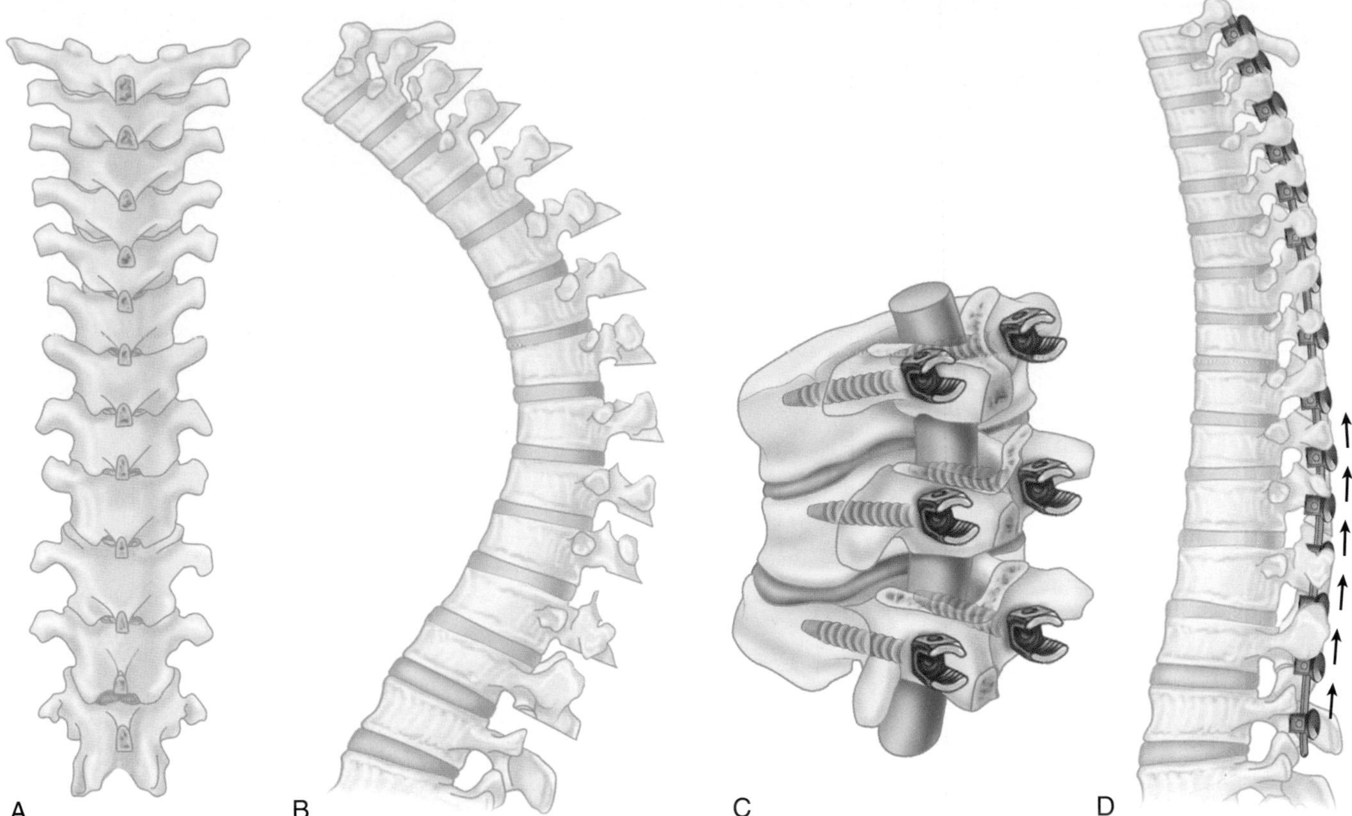

FIGURE 44-93 Ponte osteotomies for correction of kyphosis. **A** and **B,** Wedge-shaped osteotomies. **C** and **D,** Placement of rod for correction. (Redrawn from Geck MJ, Macagno A, Ponte A, Shufflebarger HL: Posterior only treatment of Scheuermann's kyphosis using segmental posterior shortening and pedicle screw instrumentation, J Spinal Disord Tech 20:586, 2007.) **SEE TECHNIQUE 44-24.**

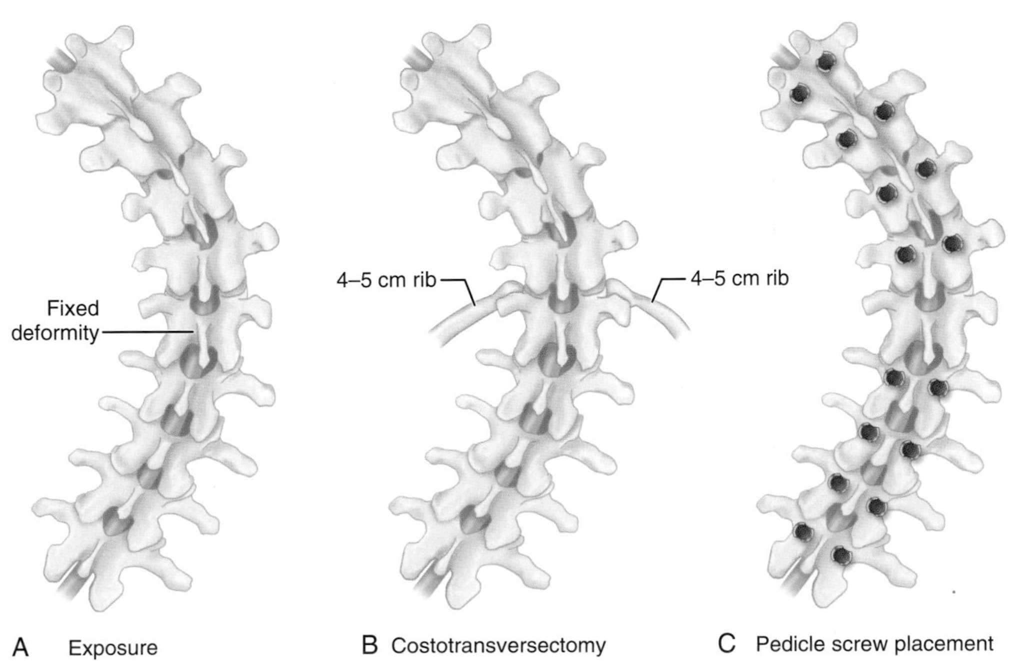

FIGURE 44-94 **A,** Posterior thoracic vertebral column resection. Spine exposed to tips of transverse processes. **B,** Medial 4 to 5 cm of ribs attached to vertebra excised to base of vertebral body. **C,** Pedicle screws placed segmentally, periadjacent to planned vertebrectomy site. (Redrawn from Powers AK, et al: Posterior thoracic vertebral column resection. In Wang JC: Advanced reconstruction: spine, Rosemont, IL, 2011, American Academy of Orthopaedic Surgeons, p. 265.) **SEE TECHNIQUE 44-25.**

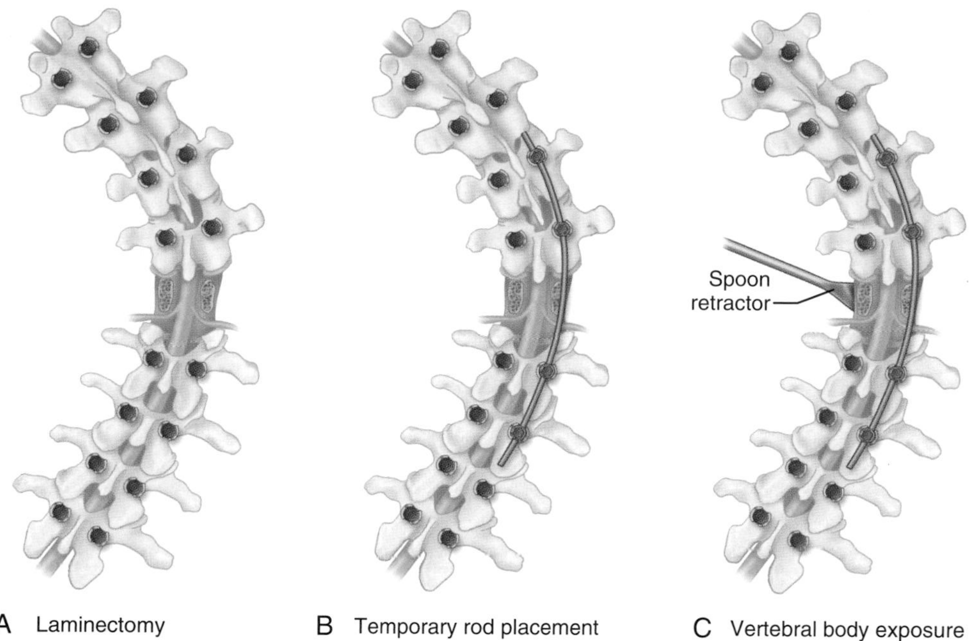

FIGURE 44-95 **A,** Complete laminectomy performed from inferior pedicles of level above to superior pedicles of level below planned resection. **B,** Temporary rod placed either unilaterally or bilaterally, depending on amount of instability anticipated. **C,** Vertebral body exposed superperiosteally or subperiosteally laterally and then anteriorly. Spoon retractor placed anterior to body. (Redrawn from Powers AK, et al: Posterior thoracic vertebral column resection. In Wang JC, editor: Advanced reconstruction: spine, Rosemont, IL, 2011, American Academy of Orthopaedic Surgeons, p. 265.) **SEE TECHNIQUE 44-25.**

or resect the transverse process at the level of the resection bilaterally to weaken the attachment of the rib head. The removal of the ribs and transverse process allows access to the lateral pedicle wall and vertebral body and can be used as a graft to fill the laminectomy defect later.

- After bilateral costotransversectomy, dissect the vertebral body wall anteriorly until the anterior vertebral body is exposed. Protect the thoracic sympathetic chain, anterior and posterior vessels, and pleura with a retractor.
- Perform bilateral laminectomies and facetectomies at the levels to be resected and complete the posterior decompression by removing the lamina cephalad to the pedicles above the resection and caudal to the pedicles below the resection (Fig. 44-95A). Posterior column exposure should be 5 to 6 cm to allow access to the spinal cord and to prevent dural buckling or impingement. Ligate the corresponding nerve roots medial and dorsal to the root ganglion.
- Once the osteotomies are complete, insert a temporary stabilizing rod and fix with two or three pedicle screws above and below the vertebral column resection (Fig. 44-95B and C). Depending on the deformity, one or two rods can be used to prevent subluxation of the spine.
- Identify the pedicles to be resected and enter through their lateral wall to gain access to the vertebral body. Complete the corpectomy by curetting the cancellous bone out of the vertebral body. Save this bone for later bone grafting. Most of the vertebral body removed should be from the convexity of the deformity. Powers prefers to perform resection from the concave side before the convex side removal to minimize bleeding and to remove some tension from the concave side before proceeding. Except for the anterior shell, remove the entire vertebral body. Keep a thin rim of bone intact on the anterior longitudinal ligament for fusion. Thin the anterior bone if it is thick and cortical.
- Perform discectomies above and below the resected body to expose the adjacent vertebral body endplates; however, avoid violating these because this can lead to interbody cage subsidence (Fig. 44-96).
- For removal of the posterior wall, inspect the dura and free it of any attachments, such as the anterior epidural venous plexus, the posterior longitudinal ligament, or osteophytes. Control epidural bleeding, which can be significant, with bipolar electrocautery. Once the dura is freed, the thin posterior vertebral body can be tamped away from the spinal cord into the corpectomy defect (Fig. 44-97A). Inspect the dura after posterior vertebral body removal and remove any points of attachment or compression.
- Once the resection is complete, closure of the defect and deformity correction are performed. In this procedure, the spinal column is always shortened, not lengthened, with compression. Obtain correction with pedicle screws or using a construct-to-construct closure method performed by placing a construct rod above and one below to distribute forces of correction over several pedicle screw levels. Compression should proceed slowly because subluxation or dural impingement may occur (Fig. 44-97B).
- In any deformity with a degree of kyphosis, Powers et al. recommend using an anterior structural cage to prevent overshortening and to help provide extra kyphosis correction.

- Once the vertebral column resection has been completed, place a permanent contralateral rod and remove the temporary rod. Then place a second permanent rod on the ipsilateral side and perform appropriate correction compression or distraction maneuvers as necessary.
- Confirm alignment by intraoperative radiographs (Fig. 44-98) and perform a final circumferential dural inspection.
- Place split-thickness rib autograft over the laminectomy defect and secure it to the rods using sutures or a crosslink.

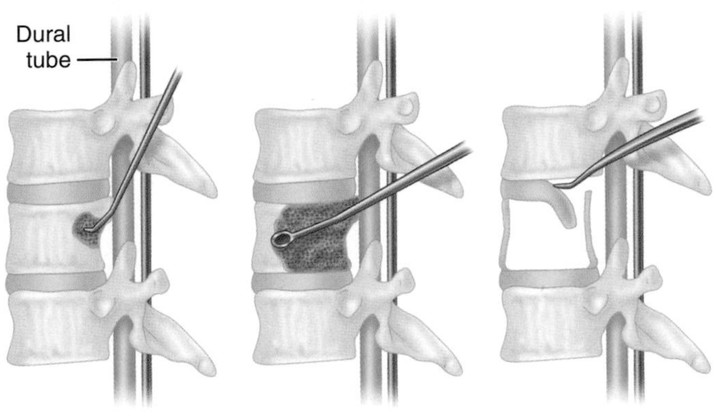

FIGURE 44-96 **Vertebral body corpectomy and discectomy.** (Redrawn from Powers AK, et al: Posterior thoracic vertebral column resection. In Wang JC editor: Advanced reconstruction: spine, Rosemont, IL, 2011, American Academy of Orthopaedic Surgeons, p. 265.) **SEE TECHNIQUE 44-25.**

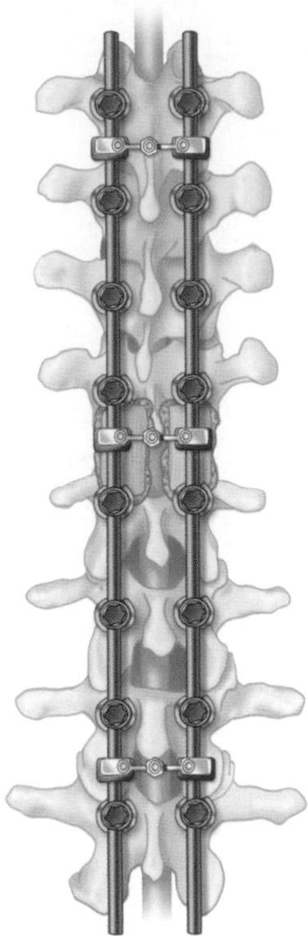

FIGURE 44-98 **Permanent rods with rib bridge graft.** (Redrawn from Powers AK, et al: Posterior thoracic vertebral column resection. In Wang JC, editor: Advanced reconstruction: spine, Rosemont, IL, 2011, American Academy of Orthopaedic Surgeons, p. 265.) **SEE TECHNIQUE 44-25.**

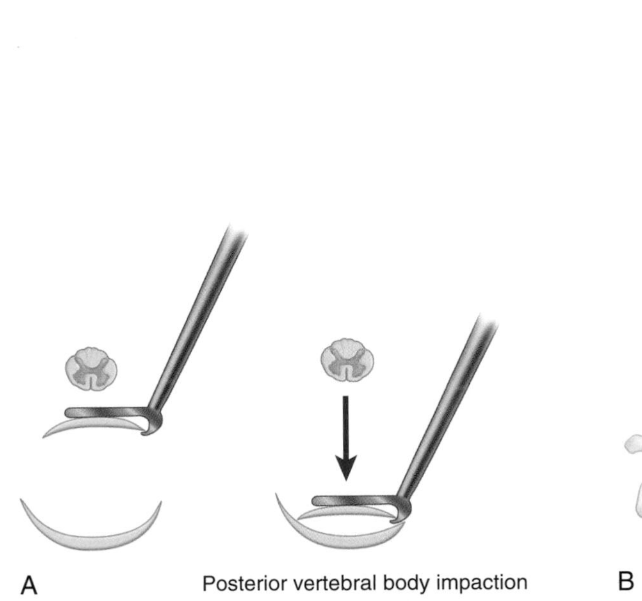

FIGURE 44-97 **A,** Impaction of posterior wall of vertebral body into defect created. **B,** Correction of deformity using compression. (Redrawn from Powers AK, et al: Posterior thoracic vertebral column resection. In Wang JC, editor: Advanced reconstruction: spine, Rosemont, IL, 2011, American Academy of Orthopaedic Surgeons, p. 265.) **SEE TECHNIQUE 44-25.**

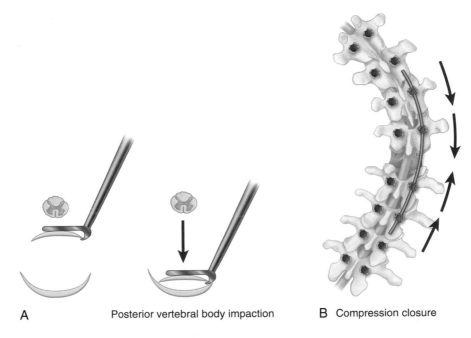

- Irrigate the wound with saline. Decorticate the posterior spine and facet joints with a high-speed burr and place copious amounts of bone graft.
- Place subfascial and suprafascial Hemovac drains through separate stab incisions and close the wound in layers with interrupted absorbable sutures.

POSTOPERATIVE CARE. The suction drain is removed once the drainage is less than 50 mL per 8-hour shift or at 48 hours postoperatively. Most patients will develop a postoperative ileus. Food or liquids are begun slowly and advanced as tolerated. Most patients also develop a postoperative atelectasis and temperature elevation. This is managed with routine "pulmonary toilet" and incentive spirometer. Intravenous antibiotics are administered for 24 hours. If the patient is old enough, a patient-controlled pain medication pump is used. Postoperative continuous epidural analgesia using local anesthetic agents or opioids, or both, can be used in appropriate situations. The patient is gradually gotten out of bed as allowed by pain tolerance. A postoperative brace or no immobilization may be used depending on the stability of the instrumentation construct. When the temperature has subsided and the patient is relatively independently ambulatory and tolerating food and liquid intake, the patient is discharged. At the 6-month checkup, if the fusion appears solid, most limitations are lifted. We generally advise against contact sports after this type of spinal surgery.

COMPLICATIONS OF POSTERIOR SCOLIOSIS SURGERY

EARLY COMPLICATIONS

NEUROLOGIC INJURY

The most feared and unpredictable complication in scoliosis surgery remains neurologic injury. For patients undergoing spinal fusion for adolescent idiopathic scoliosis, the incidence of neurologic injury is relatively low, between 0.32% and 0.69%. It may be caused by inadvertent entry of the instrumentation into the spinal canal. Newer and more complex instrumentation systems require the surgeon to be aware of potential problems with instrumentation (see Box 44-4). Other possible causes of neurologic injury during surgery are unrecognized spinal cord tethers or other spinal anomalies and ischemic damage as the spine is lengthened during the correction procedure. Management of an intraoperative neurologic deficit begins with a series of corrective actions. The first step is to bring the patient's mean arterial pressure above 90 mm Hg combined with administration of an increased concentration of inspired oxygen. The patient's wound also should be irrigated with warm saline in an effort to increase perfusion. If the neurologic injury is associated with curve correction, the spine should be allowed to return to its precorrection state and consideration given to removal of the implants. The use of corticosteroids is controversial and is determined on a case-by-case basis. (Spinal cord monitoring and the wake-up test are discussed in the section on intraoperative considerations for operative treatment of adolescent idiopathic scoliosis.)

INFECTION

Moe et al. reported two types of wound infections after scoliosis surgery. The first is obvious because a high fever develops, usually within 2 to 5 days after surgery, and the wound almost always appears infected. In the second type, the temperature is elevated only slightly or moderately and the wound appears relatively normal. Diagnosis of this latter type of wound sepsis may be difficult. Patients often have postoperative temperature elevation of up to 102°F, which should decline gradually during the first 4 postoperative days. Any spike of temperature above 102°F should strongly suggest a deep wound infection, especially if the patient's general condition does not steadily improve. The appearance of the wound can be deceiving, with no significant erythema or tenderness. Prompt aspiration of the wound in several sites is recommended. Culture specimens should be submitted, but results should not be awaited, and reoperation should be planned immediately.

The most common organism associated with postoperative infection is *Staphylococcus aureus.* When the wound infection is diagnosed, the wound is opened widely and thorough irrigation and debridement are done. The implants and most of the bone graft usually are left in, and the wound is closed over drains, although Ho et al. found nearly a 50% rate of persistent infection, despite multiple incisions and debridements if the implants were retained. Appropriate antibiotics are administered for 3 to 6 weeks, depending on the severity of the infection. If the wound infection is discovered late, it may be necessary to debride the wound, to irrigate copiously, and to pack the wound open or use a vacuum-assisted closure (VAC) sponge. The patient is brought back to the operating room in 3 to 5 days, and the wound is closed over suction tubes. In severe infections or gram-negative infections, such as those caused by *Pseudomonas* or *Escherichia coli,* it may be necessary to leave the wound packed open or use a VAC sponge for prolonged periods and allow it to granulate in from the bottom. This also is occasionally necessary if the infection recurs a few days after the wound is closed over suction drains.

With the use of prophylactic preoperative, intraoperative, and postoperative antibiotics, the incidence of postoperative wound infections in surgery for idiopathic scoliosis is less than 1%.

ILEUS

Ileus is a common complication after both anterior and posterior spinal fusion. Oral feedings are resumed slowly after surgery. Intravenous fluids are continued until a full diet is tolerated. Malnutrition is uncommon in teenagers with idiopathic scoliosis, but patients requiring a two-stage corrective procedure may become malnourished as a result of the limited oral calorie intake associated with closely spaced surgical procedures. Combined anterior and posterior procedures also are more likely to be done in patients with neuromuscular disorders, and parenteral hyperalimentation should be considered for these patients.

ATELECTASIS

Atelectasis is a common cause of fever after scoliosis surgery. Frequent turning of the patient and deep breathing and coughing usually control or prevent serious atelectasis. Inhalation therapy with intermittent positive-pressure breathing may be beneficial in cooperative patients, but inflation of the stomach during this type of treatment must be avoided. Incentive spirometry now is commonly used instead. The atelectasis and the fever secondary to the atelectasis generally resolve rapidly once the patient is mobilized.

PNEUMOTHORAX

At the time of subperiosteal posterior spine exposure, the pleura may be entered inadvertently between the transverse processes on the concave side of the scoliosis. If a thoracoplasty is done at the same time, a pneumothorax is more likely to occur. Observation of the pneumothorax is probably appropriate if it is less than 20%, but chest tube insertion is needed for larger pneumothoraces.

DURAL TEAR

If a dural tear occurs during removal of the ligamentum flavum or insertion of a hook or wire, repair should be attempted. The laminotomy often must be enlarged to allow access to the ends of the dural tear. If repair is not done, drainage of the cerebrospinal fluid through the wound can cause problems postoperatively.

WRONG LEVELS

Care should be taken in the operating room to correctly identify the vertebral levels. If the fusion extends to the sacrum, it can be used as a landmark and the vertebrae accurately counted. For other curves, we routinely obtain an intraoperative radiograph with use of a marker on the vertebra to be identified. Alternatively, the level can be confirmed by palpation of the T12 rib and the L1 transverse process.

URINARY COMPLICATIONS

The syndrome of inappropriate antidiuretic hormone secretion develops in the immediate postoperative period in a high percentage of patients undergoing spinal fusion. This causes a decline in urinary output and is maximal on the evening after surgery. If the serum osmolality is diminished and the urine osmolality is elevated, this syndrome should be considered and fluid overload should be avoided. The urinary output gradually increases in the next 2 to 3 days after surgery.

VISION LOSS

Postoperative loss of vision has an incidence of 0.02% to 0.2%. In a review of a nationwide database including over 40,000 patients under the age of 18 who had surgery for idiopathic scoliosis, De la Garza-Ramos et al. found that vision loss was reported in 0.16%. Prone positioning, particularly in the Trendelenburg position, has been noted to increase intraocular pressure. This is thought to be a risk factor for postoperative loss of vision as the result of decreased perfusion of the optic nerve. Other suggested risk factors include a younger age, a history of deficiency anemia, and long-segment fusions. The loss of vision manifests itself during the first 2 postoperative days. Most deficits are permanent.

LATE COMPLICATIONS

PSEUDARTHROSIS

In adolescents with idiopathic scoliosis, the pseudarthrosis rate is approximately 1%; the rate is higher in patients with neuromuscular scoliosis. The most common areas of pseudarthrosis are at the thoracolumbar junction and at the distally fused segment. With more rigid and stronger implants, the pseudarthrosis may not be apparent for years. In a review of cases of nonunion with segmental instrumentation, the average time to presentation of nonunion was 3.5 years. In 23% of patients with nonunion, implant failure was detected 5 to 10 years postoperatively. The diagnosis of pseudarthrosis usually is made by oblique radiographs, a broken implant, tomograms, CT, or bone scanning. After successful posterior fusion, the disc height anteriorly should diminish as the vertebral body continues to grow at the expense of the disc space. A large disc space anteriorly may indicate a posterior pseudarthrosis. Often, however, the pseudarthrosis cannot be confirmed even with the most sophisticated radiographic evaluation and can be detected only by surgical exploration.

If a pseudarthrosis does not cause pain or loss of correction, surgery may not be necessary. Asymptomatic pseudarthrosis is more common in the distally fused segments. A pseudarthrosis at the thoracolumbar junction is more likely to cause loss of correction and pain.

At surgical exploration, the cortex is smooth and firm over the mature and intact areas of the fusion mass and the soft tissues strip away easily. Conversely, at a pseudarthrosis, the soft tissues usually are adherent and continuous into the defect; however, a narrow pseudarthrosis may be difficult to locate, especially if motion is slight. In this instance, decortication of the fusion mass in suspicious areas is indicated and a search always should be made for several pseudarthroses. An extremely difficult type of pseudarthrosis to determine is a solid fusion mass posteriorly that is not well adherent to the underlying spine and lamina. Once the pseudarthrosis has been identified, it is cleared of fibrous tissue, and the curve is reinstrumented by the application of compression over the pseudarthrosis. If this is not done, kyphotic deformity may worsen because of incompetent spinal extensor muscles from the previous surgical exposure. The pseudarthroses are treated as ordinary joints to be fused: their edges are freshened and decorticated, and autogenous bone graft is applied in addition to the instrumentation.

LOSS OF LUMBAR LORDOSIS

If distraction is applied across the lumbar spine, normal physiologic lumbar lordosis may be diminished or eliminated, causing the patient to stand with a forward tilt that results in upper back pain, lower back pain, and even pain in the hips (Fig. 44-99). Care also must be taken in positioning the patient on the spinal frame and ensuring that the hips are not flexed (see Technique 44-8). Positioning of patients on a Jackson frame equipped with two chest pads, two anterior pelvic pads, and two proximal thigh pads has been shown to maintain the preoperative lumbar lordosis when measured from T12 to S1 and from L1 to L5. Patients with pedicle screw placement to L3 or L4 have been found to have statistically greater increase in instrumented lumbar lordosis after the completion of the instrumentation process than patients with only hook placement from T12 to L2. The best treatment for the loss of lumbar lordosis is prevention, which includes careful patient positioning, avoidance of distraction in the lumbar spine, and use of newer segmental instrumentation systems.

CRANKSHAFT PHENOMENON

If posterior fusion alone is done in patients with a significant amount of anterior growth remaining, a crankshaft

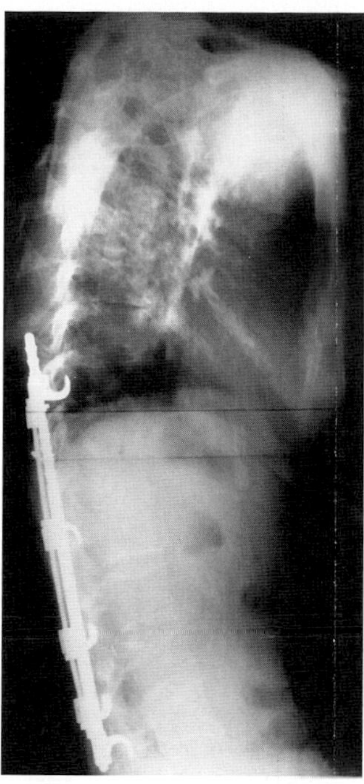

FIGURE 44-99 Loss of lumbar lordosis (lumbar "flat back").

phenomenon usually occurs (see section on treatment of juvenile idiopathic scoliosis). This is prevented by combining anterior and posterior fusions in younger children. More recent reports in the literature indicate that the use of posterior segmental pedicle screw instrumentation may obviate the need for combined fusions. Tao et al. reported that none of 46 patients with interval or continuous pedicle screw instrumentation had experienced crankshaft phenomenon at 3-year follow-up.

SUPERIOR MESENTERIC ARTERY SYNDROME

Rarely, superior mesenteric artery syndrome may cause small bowel obstruction after spinal fusion. The transverse portion of the duodenum crosses the midline anterior to the spine and the aorta and posterior to the superior mesenteric artery. As the space between these structures decreases, obstruction of the duodenum can occur. The patient develops nausea and bilious vomiting. An upper gastrointestinal series often is required for the diagnosis to be made. The average onset of superior mesenteric artery syndrome has been reported to be 5 to 7 days after surgery. Initial treatment should consist of nasogastric drainage and intravenous fluid replacement, alimentation through feeding tubes, or intravenous hyperalimentation. This often allows swelling in the duodenum to subside. If nonoperative treatment fails, general surgical procedures, such as release of the ligament of Treitz or duodenojejunostomy, may be necessary.

TRUNK DECOMPENSATION

Problems with trunk decompensation have been noted with the newer segmental instrumentation systems in the treatment of King type II curves. As noted earlier, decompensation can be prevented and a well-balanced correction obtained if the preoperative ratio of the thoracic to lumbar curve magnitude is greater than 1:2, the apical vertebral rotation ratio of the thoracic to the lumbar curve is greater than 1:0, and the apical vertebral translation of the thoracic to lumbar curve is greater than 1:2. If decompensation occurs and is mild with minimal trunk imbalance, treatment may not be needed. The patient can be observed periodically for lumbar curve progression. For more severe decompensation, an orthosis can be used for treatment of the lumbar curve. If bracing is unsuccessful, it may be necessary to extend the fusion to the distal stable vertebra of the lumbar curve.

As noted in an earlier section on Complications and Pitfalls in Segmental Instrumentation Systems, a proximal curve should be considered structural if (1) the curve size is more than 30 degrees and remains more than 20 degrees on side-bending radiographs; (2) the Nash-Moe apical rotation is above grade 1; (3) there is more than 1 cm of apical translation from the C7 plumb line; (4) there is a positive T1 tilt; and (5) clinical elevation of the left shoulder is noted.

LATE INFECTION

Delayed deep wound infections requiring removal of instrumentation because of pain, swelling, and spontaneous drainage have been reported. Causes have been attributed to an inflammatory response to micromotion and corrosion of the components and intraoperative seeding of low-virulence skin organisms. Treatment may include removal of instrumentation and primary wound closure, with parenteral, followed by oral, antibiotics.

POSTERIOR THORACOPLASTY

Of all the deformities caused by idiopathic scoliosis, the posterior rib prominence is generally the patient's main concern. With thoracic pedicle instrumentation and derotation techniques, we now rarely find it necessary to perform a thoracoplasty. Chen et al. found that posterior instrumentation in combination with thoracoplasty led to a significant decrease in pulmonary function at 3 months. Eventually, the function returned to normal at 1 year postoperatively. In our experience, the addition of a thoracoplasty also significantly increases the postoperative pain and not infrequently requires the insertion of a chest tube or at least pleural aspiration. If necessary for cosmetic reasons, resection of the convex ribs can improve the postoperative cosmetic result of this surgery.

THORACOPLASTY

TECHNIQUE 44-26

(BETZ)

- Position the patient as for a standard posterior spinal fusion for idiopathic scoliosis (see Technique 44-8). Prepare and drape the patient in a standard fashion. For adequate exposure of the rib prominence, place the lateral drapes at the posterolateral axillary line or wider.
- Make a routine midline incision (see Technique 44-8).
- Perform the thoracoplasty through this midline posterior incision by retracting the fascia and working under it and the latissimus dorsi, or, alternatively, make a separate parallel vertical incision centered over the rib hump as described by Steel. If the single, midline posterior incision

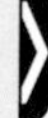

is used, extend the skin incision distally to approximately L2 or L3 for a right thoracic curve to adequately retract the thoracolumbar fascia from the midline.

- Stopping the skin incision at T12 does not provide adequate lateral exposure. Likewise, proximally, carry the skin incision approximately ½ to 1 inch farther. Despite the slight increase in length, this incision is much more cosmetically appealing than the two-incision technique. The advantage of the two-incision technique is easier access to the lateral rib. With newer instrumentation techniques, better translation of the apex of the curve to the midline is possible and less of the rib needs to be resected laterally than is necessary with Harrington rod techniques.
- After the skin incision is made, outline the spinous processes and incise the thoracolumbar fascia off the spinous process.
- In the L2-3 region, be careful to identify the very thin layer of thoracolumbar fascia. By sharp and blunt dissection, elevate this fascia off the paravertebral muscle fascia, working laterally and proximally at the same time to develop a plane. Sequentially incise the thoracolumbar fascia off the spinous processes, proceeding proximally.
- Once the fascia has been retracted laterally, palpate the ribs starting at the apex of the deformity. Symmetric resection is done working distally and proximally one rib at a time.
- Mark the apical rib with an electrocautery.
- Make a midline incision into the paraspinal muscles medially and outline the ribs for the periosteal cut.
- Use an elevator to pull the periosteum off the surface of the rib to the lateral edge. The elevator should be pulled and not pushed to prevent penetration of the pleura. Usually between four and six ribs are outlined.
- Once the periosteum has been stripped to the side of the rib, use the elevator to strip the periosteum and muscle around the inferior edge of the rib.
- With a Cobb elevator, strip the periosteum from the anterior aspect of the rib in a medial to lateral direction. This is the time the pleura is most likely to be entered.
- Once the anterior aspect of the rib has been stripped with a Cobb elevator, pass a Doyen retractor circumferentially and medial to lateral on the exposed rib. Identify the most medial attachment of the rib to the transverse process and pass a rib cutter around the rib and push it as far medially as possible.
- Hold the rib with a towel clip or Kocher clamp to prevent it from plunging through the pleura when it is cut. Cut the rib medially, keeping the cut as parallel to the floor as possible, and then make the lateral cut. For a standard rib resection in a patient with a 55-degree right thoracic curve, 2 cm of rib should be cut initially.
- Take care not to resect too much rib because more rib can be removed if necessary.
- If the thoracoplasty is done before instrumentation of the spine, the apex of the curve will translate to the midline when the curve is corrected, leaving a much larger gap than is apparent at the time of the original rib resection.
- Apply bone wax to the ends of the rib and pack Gelfoam into the periosteal bed.
- Cut additional ribs in an identical fashion, but going proximally and distally from the apex, progressively removing less rib.
- Once the resection has been completed, lift the edges of the wound and pour saline into the wound. Have the anesthesiologist perform a Valsalva maneuver to look for a leak in the pleura.
- Place a suction drain over the resected rib bed.
- Close the thoracolumbar fascia with a running absorbable suture, starting at the distal aspect of the wound.
- Cut the removed segments of rib into small pieces for use as autogenous bone graft in the spinal arthrodesis.
- Alternatively, the thoracoplasty procedure can be done after spinal instrumentation. This allows better evaluation of the rib hump after the instrumentation but also can lead to increased blood loss if this procedure is done after the major dissection of the spine in the midline.

POSTOPERATIVE CARE. After skin closure and dressing application, a protective plaster shell is applied over the rib resection area. This shell is essential to help prevent a postoperative flail chest and to minimize motion of the cut ribs on top of the pleura and the possibility of pleural effusion. The shell is made of plaster with foam underneath to protect the skin. The mold is made while the patient is prone on the operating table to prevent a plaster burn, but the shell is not applied until the patient is in the recovery room. A chest radiograph is obtained in the recovery room to rule out a pneumothorax, and then the shell is applied and wrapped with 6-inch elastic wraps. Alternatively, the posterior shell of a TLSO that was made preoperatively can be used. The patient's back is examined 2 days after surgery. If there is no evidence of a flail chest and the rib resection gap measures less than the width of the palm of the hand, no prolonged postoperative immobilization is needed. If there is a larger gap or a flail chest, a postoperative rib protector, such as the posterolateral half of a TLSO, is fitted. This rib protector is worn for 3 months. Alternatively, a full TLSO brace can be used for the first 3 months after surgery to protect the chest cage while the ribs regenerate.

COMPLICATIONS AND PITFALLS

During rib resection, a hole may be made in the parietal pleura. No attempt should be made to repair the pleura. The hole in the rib bed should be gently packed with Gelfoam, and the intercostal muscles should be closed with a running suture from the most medial to the lateral aspect. As the last sutures are tightened, the anesthesiologist expands the patient's lung, expressing as much air from the pleural cavity as possible before the final sutures are tied. The purpose of closing the hole is to prevent blood from seeping into the pleural cavity. An expanding pneumothorax should not occur because only the parietal pleura is violated and not the visceral pleura. Suction drains are used routinely. Less than 50% of patients with pleural holes require chest tubes. Daily semierect and lateral decubitus radiographs are made for 3 days. A thoracentesis is done if fluid accumulation persists and the patient is symptomatic. If a second thoracentesis becomes necessary, a chest tube is considered.

On occasion, even without a pleural hole, a pleural effusion may develop. The use of a protective shell postoperatively minimizes this complication. For expanding, symptomatic effusions, a thoracentesis is done; a chest tube is inserted if it occurs a second time.

Resection of too much rib will cause rib concavity. This complication is preventable, and it is better to resect too little rib than too much. Six ribs should be the maximum taken, and never more than 8 cm in length.

The most common error leading to residual rib prominence is not resecting enough ribs and not resecting the ribs medially enough. This risk must be weighed against the risk of causing a rib concavity. If a long rib deformity requires resection of more than six ribs, the risk of causing a rib concavity is high. In this situation, it is better to do a second procedure later than to risk a rib concavity.

CONCAVE RIB OSTEOTOMIES

The concept of concave rib osteotomies was introduced by Flinchum in 1963. Kostuik, Tolo, Goldstein, and Mann et al. reported the use of concave osteotomies and their possible value as a release procedure. Halsall et al., in cadaver studies, tested flexibility before and after sectioning of the ribs on the tension side. They found an average increase in deflection of 53%. Flexibility increased most when five or six ribs were resected. The addition of concave rib osteotomies to instrumentation and fusion procedures increases the risk of pulmonary morbidity. Goldstein reported five pleural effusions and three pneumothoraces in 17 patients who had resection of 5 to 6 cm of concave ribs. Mann et al. decreased the incidence of complications by performing rib osteotomies rather than rib resections. They reported two pleural effusions and one pneumothorax in 10 patients. Although concave osteotomies can increase the flexibility of right curves, with pedicle screw fixation and correction we have rarely needed to include this as part of our procedure. If concave rib osteotomies are done, a prophylactic chest tube should be inserted.

OSTEOTOMY OF THE RIBS

TECHNIQUE 44-27

(MANN ET AL.)

- Approach the concave ribs through the midline incision used for the instrumentation and spinal fusion.
- Retract the paraspinous muscles lateral to the tips of the concave transverse processes. When needed, use electrocautery to incise overlying tissue along the rib axis.
- Incise the periosteum along the rib axis for 1.5 cm lateral to the transverse process and use small elevators to expose the rib periosteally.
- Protect the pleura with the elevators and use a rib cutter to section the rib approximately 1 cm lateral to the transverse process (Fig. 44-100A).
- Lift the lateral rib segment with a Kocher clamp and allow it to posteriorly overlap the medial segment (Fig. 44-100B).
- Rongeur any jagged ends and place a small piece of thrombin-soaked Gelfoam between the rib and pleura for protection and hemostasis.
- Make four to six osteotomies over the apical concave vertebrae.
- Approximate the paraspinous muscles with an absorbable suture.
- Complete the instrumentation and fusion and insert a chest tube.

ANTERIOR INSTRUMENTATION FOR IDIOPATHIC SCOLIOSIS

Anterior instrumentation and fusion for idiopathic scoliosis is a well-accepted procedure for certain thoracolumbar and lumbar curves. A Lenke type 4 curve pattern in which the thoracolumbar or lumbar curve is the structural component and the main thoracic or proximal thoracic curves are nonstructural is the ideal situation for this type of procedure. Anterior instrumentation can provide derotation and correction of the curve in the coronal plane. On occasion, the deformity can be corrected by fusing fewer motion segments than if the same curve were approached posteriorly, although with pedicle screw instrumentation of the lumbar spine, this often is not the case. The thoracolumbar or lumbar curve should be flexible. The thoracic curve should be nonstructural and reducible to 25 degrees or less on the bending films. The incomplete curve between the lumbar or thoracolumbar curve and sacrum must be carefully evaluated because it also must be flexible enough to correct on bending films (Fig. 44-101). The child must be old enough for the vertebrae to be large enough to allow screw fixation. Caution is advised in using these systems in children younger than 9 years. In general, the lowest instrumented vertebra is the lower end vertebra of the Cobb measurement. The proximal level usually is the neutral vertebra. The fusion should not extend into the compensatory thoracic curve above. On the convex bending film, the disc below the lowest instrumented vertebra should open up on both sides. This indicates that the lower vertebra selected can be made horizontal with the anterior approach. If there is a discrepancy in the levels indicated on the bending films and the standing posteroanterior film with the Cobb measurement, the method that indicates the longest segment of instrumentation and fusion should be selected.

The anterior approach for thoracolumbar and lumbar curves has several potential disadvantages: chylothorax; injury to the ureter, spleen, or great vessels; retroperitoneal fibrosis; and prominent instrumentation that must be carefully isolated from the great vessels. Without careful attention to detail, a kyphosing effect can occur even with solid-rod and dual-rod anterior instrumentation systems. The attachment to the spine is through relatively cancellous vertebral bodies, and proximal screw dislodgement also is a risk. Many orthopaedic surgeons require the assistance of a thoracic or general surgeon with anterior approaches.

Shufflebarger et al. recommended a posterior rather than anterior approach and pedicle screw fixation for lumbar and thoracolumbar scoliosis with posterior shortening. After a wide posterior release (Fig. 44-102), the spine is instrumented with pedicle screws and a 5-mm rod. With this technique, the same levels are fused as would be fused with anterior instrumentation. The morbidity of the anterior approach is avoided,

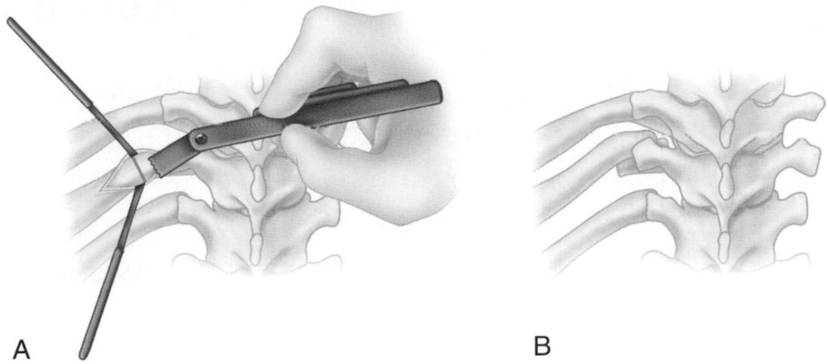

FIGURE 44-100 Rib osteotomy. **A,** Rib is exposed subperiosteally 1 cm lateral to transverse process. Osteotomy is completed with microsagittal saw. **B,** Overlap of lateral rib segment. **SEE TECHNIQUE 44-27.**

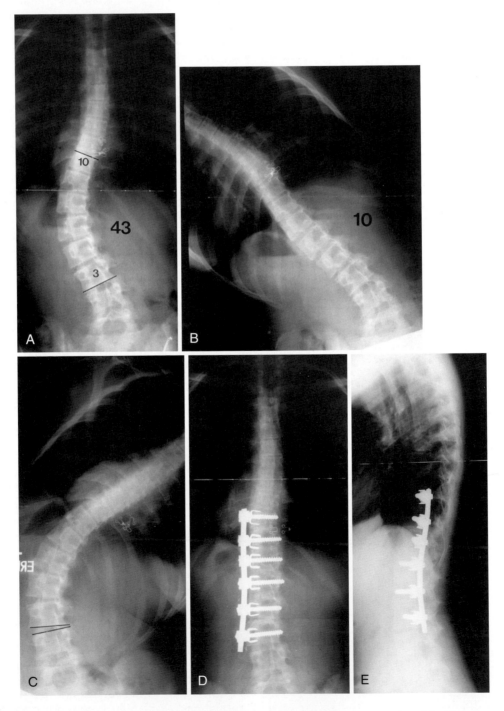

FIGURE 44-101 **A,** Flexible 43-degree thoracic curve. **B,** Correction on bending film. **C,** Correction of fractional curve on bending film. **D** and **E,** After anterior fusion with Texas Scottish Rite Hospital (TSRH) instrumentation.

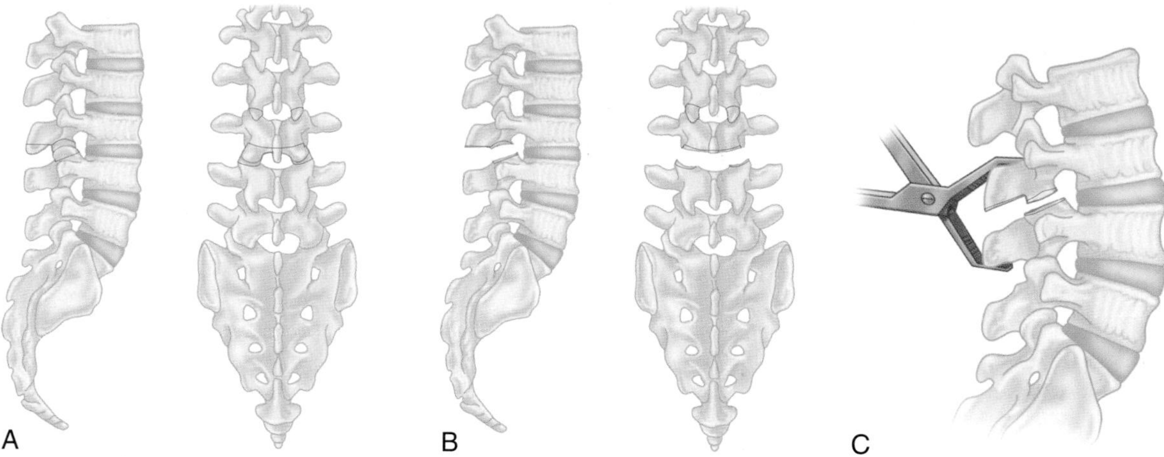

FIGURE 44-102 Posterior approach and pedicle screw fixation. **A,** Areas in *blue* indicate bony resection to be accomplished for posterior shortening procedure. Interspinous ligament and ligamentum flavum must be removed, including intracanal portion of capsular ligament of facet joint. **B,** Facet joints and all posterior ligamentous structures have been excised. **C,** Ability to produce lordosis after posterior shortening is shown. (Redrawn from Shufflebarger HL, Geck MJ, Clark CE: The posterior approach for lumbar and thoracolumbar adolescent idiopathic scoliosis: posterior shortening and pedicle screws, Spine 29:269, 2004.)

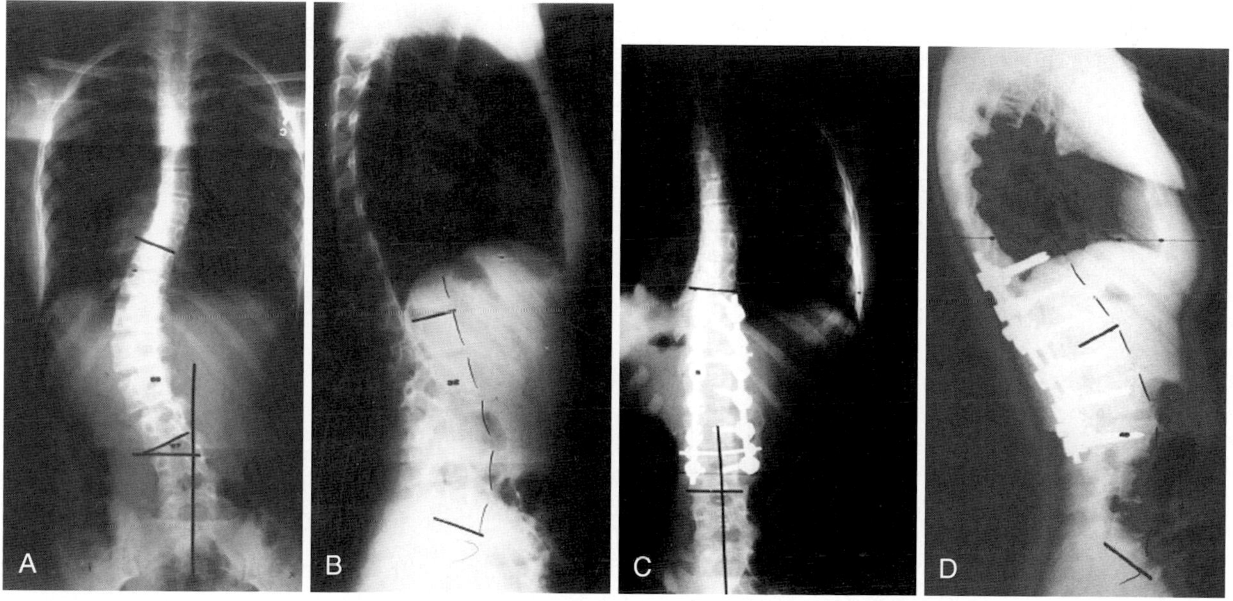

FIGURE 44-103 **A** and **B,** Anteroposterior and lateral preoperative radiographs show significant thoracolumbar curve of 55 degrees from T10-L3, with shift of C7 plumb line off center sacral line with 27 degrees angulated and significantly translated distal end vertebra. Trunk shift is present. Sagittal lumbar lordosis is only 32 degrees. **C** and **D,** Postoperative standing views show centralization and leveling of lowest instrumented vertebra, end of Cobb measurement. Lumbar lordosis is normalized to 45 degrees. (From Shufflebarger HL, Geck MJ, Clark CE: The posterior approach for lumbar and thoracolumbar adolescent idiopathic scoliosis: posterior shortening and pedicle screws, Spine 29:269, 2004.)

and the patient is managed with a posterior approach familiar to all spine surgeons. They reported excellent correction of the coronal and sagittal deformities (Fig. 44-103).

Anterior instrumentation and fusion also can be used in the treatment of thoracic curves. Betz et al. formed a study group to prospectively evaluate anterior spinal instrumentation and fusion with a threaded rod anterior system and to compare it with posterior spinal fusion with various multiple-segmented hook-rod systems in patients with adolescent idiopathic thoracic scoliosis. Initially, there was an unacceptably high rod breakage rate, but this was reduced by a stronger, solid-rod system. Advantages of the anterior thoracic approach are a more complete three-dimensional correction of the deformity because of thorough disc and annular excision, curve correction by convex compression that shortens the spinal column and avoids distraction of neural elements, fusion of end vertebra to end vertebra often resulting in a shorter fusion construct than would be

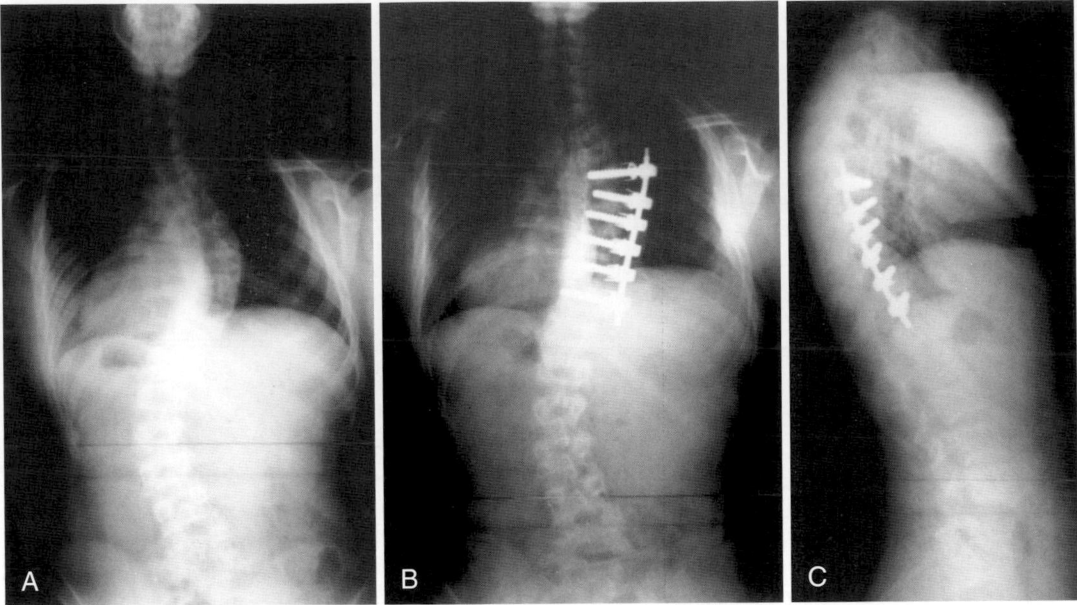

FIGURE 44-104 **A,** Standing posteroanterior radiograph of patient with idiopathic scoliosis. With posterior approach, this patient would require fusion well down into the lumbar spine. **B** and **C,** Postoperative posteroanterior and lateral radiographs after anterior instrumentation. Although some loss of fixation of proximal screw is noted, patient achieved satisfactory correction and well-balanced spine in both coronal and sagittal planes by instrumentation of only thoracic spine deformity.

required posteriorly (Fig. 44-104), possible reduction of the number of upper and midlumbar fusion levels, avoidance of a crankshaft phenomenon in skeletally immature patients, decreased frequency of decompensation in primary thoracic curves with compensatory lumbar curves, kyphosis or lordosis of the vertebral segment to improve the sagittal profile after disc excision, and avoidance of problems with prominent posterior instrumentation that occurs in thin patients even with the newer low-profile instruments. Potential disadvantages of this approach include chest cage disruption, with its effects on pulmonary function, the need for the assistance of a thoracic surgeon, an increased risk of progressive kyphosis because of posterior spinal growth in skeletally immature patients (Risser grade 0), and smaller vertebrae and less secure fixation, especially of the proximal screw (see Fig. 44-104). The aorta can be very close to the screw tips if bicortical fixation is achieved (Fig. 44-105). Potter et al. compared curve correction by posterior spinal fusion and thoracic pedicle screws with anterior spinal fusion by single-rod instrumentation in Lenke type 1 curves. They found that posterior spinal fusion by thoracic pedicle screw instrumentation provided superior instrumented correction of the main thoracic curves and spontaneous correction of the thoracolumbar and lumbar curves. They also found that the posterior approach showed improved correction of thoracic torsion and rotation. Our experience is similar in that we rarely see the need for anterior instrumentation of thoracic curves.

If the curve to be instrumented is a thoracolumbar curve, a thoracoabdominal approach is required. If the curve is purely lumbar, a lumbar extraperitoneal approach can be used.

THORACOABDOMINAL APPROACH

TECHNIQUE 44-28

- Place the patient in the lateral decubitus position with the convex side of the curve elevated.
- Make a curvilinear incision along the rib that is one level higher than the most proximal level to be instrumented. This generally is the ninth rib in most thoracolumbar curves. Make the incision along the rib and extend it distally along the anterolateral abdominal wall just lateral to the rectus abdominis muscle.
- Expose and excise the rib.
- Enter the chest and retract the lung.
- Identify the diaphragm as a separate structure; it tends to closely approximate the wall of the thoracic cage. The diaphragm can be removed in two ways. We prefer to remove it from the chest cavity and then continue with retroperitoneal dissection distally. Alternatively, the retroperitoneum can be entered below the diaphragm, and then the diaphragm can be divided. To remove the diaphragm from the chest cavity, enter the chest cavity transpleurally through the bed of the rib. Then use electrocautery to divide the diaphragm close to the chest wall. Leave a small tag of diaphragm for reattachment.
- Once the diaphragm has been reflected, expose the retroperitoneal space.
- Dissect the peritoneal cavity from underneath the internal oblique muscle and the abdominal musculature.

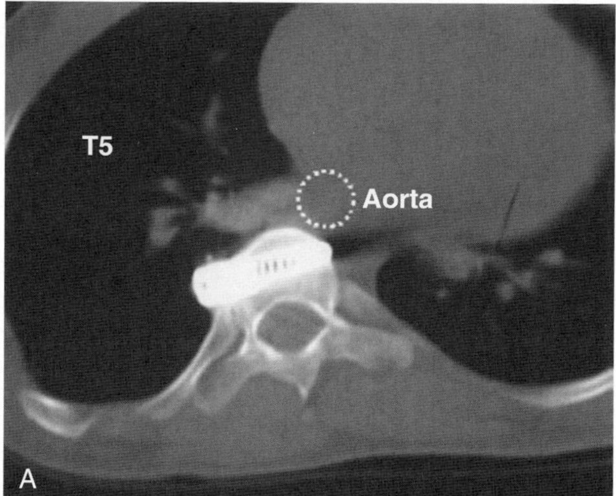

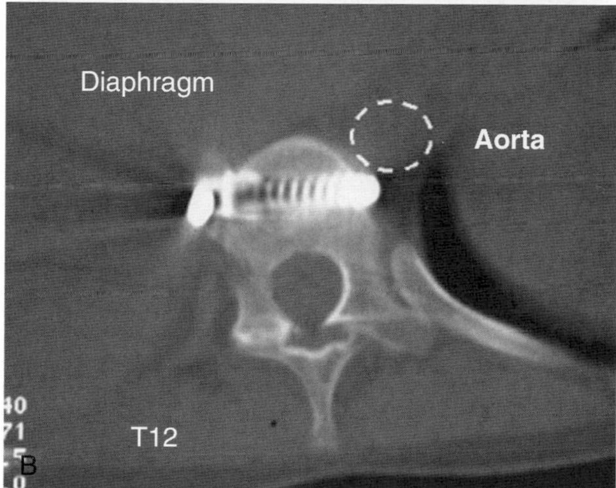

FIGURE 44-105 **A,** CT image at T5 showing good screw position. **B,** With descending aorta at 2-o'clock position, 26% of distal screw was thought to be adjacent to aorta at 2 mm or less. (From Kuklo TR, Lehman RA Jr, Lenke LG: Structures at risk following anterior instrumented spinal fusion for thoracic adolescent idiopathic scoliosis, J Spinal Disord Tech 18:S58, 2005.)

- Split the internal oblique and the transverse abdominal muscles in line with the skin incisions and extend the exposure distally as far as necessary.
- Identify the vertebral bodies and carefully dissect the psoas muscle laterally off the vertebral disc spaces. The psoas origin usually is at about L1.
- Divide the prevertebral fascia in the direction of the spine.
- Identify the segmental arteries over the waist of each vertebral body and isolate and ligate them in the midline.
- Expose the bone extraperiosteally.
- The exposure from T10 to L2 or L3 with this approach is simple; but more distally the iliac vessels overlie the L4 and L5 vertebrae, and exposure in this area requires more meticulous dissection and displacement of these vessels.

LUMBAR EXTRAPERITONEAL APPROACH

TECHNIQUE 44-29

- Place the patient in the lateral decubitus position with the convex side up.
- Make a midflank incision from the midline anteriorly to the midline posteriorly (Fig. 44-106A).
- Divide the abdominal oblique muscles in line with the incision (Fig. 44-106B and C).
- As the dissection leads laterally, identify the latissimus dorsi muscle as it adds another layer: the transversalis fascia and the peritoneum. The transversalis fascia and the peritoneum diverge posteriorly as the transversalis fascia lines the trunk wall, and the peritoneum turns anteriorly to encase the viscera. Posterior dissection in this plane allows access to the spine without entering the abdominal cavity.
- Repair any inadvertent entry into the peritoneum immediately because it may not be identifiable later.
- Reflect all the fat-containing areolar tissue back to the transverse fascia and the lumbar fascia, reflecting the ureter along with the peritoneum (Fig. 44-106D).
- Locate the major vessels in the midline, divide the lumbar fascia, and carefully retract the great vessels.
- Divide the segmental arteries and veins as they cross the waist of the vertebra in the midline and ligate them to control hemorrhage.
- The skin incision must be placed carefully to ensure that the most cephalad vertebra to be instrumented can be easily seen.

DISC EXCISION

TECHNIQUE 44-30

- Once the anterior portion of the spine has been exposed, the discs can be felt as soft, rounded, protuberant areas of the spine compared with the concave surface of the vertebral body.
- Divide the annulus sharply with a long-handled scalpel (Fig. 44-107) and remove it.
- Remove the nucleus pulposus with rongeurs and curets. It is not necessary to remove the anterior or posterior longitudinal ligaments.
- Once the disc excision has been completed, remove the cartilaginous endplates with use of either ring curets or an osteotome. The posterior aspects of the cartilaginous endplates often are more easily removed with angled curets.
- Obtain hemostasis with Gelfoam soaked in thrombin unless a cell saver is in use.
- Significant correction of the curve usually occurs during the discectomies, and it becomes more flexible and more easily correctable.

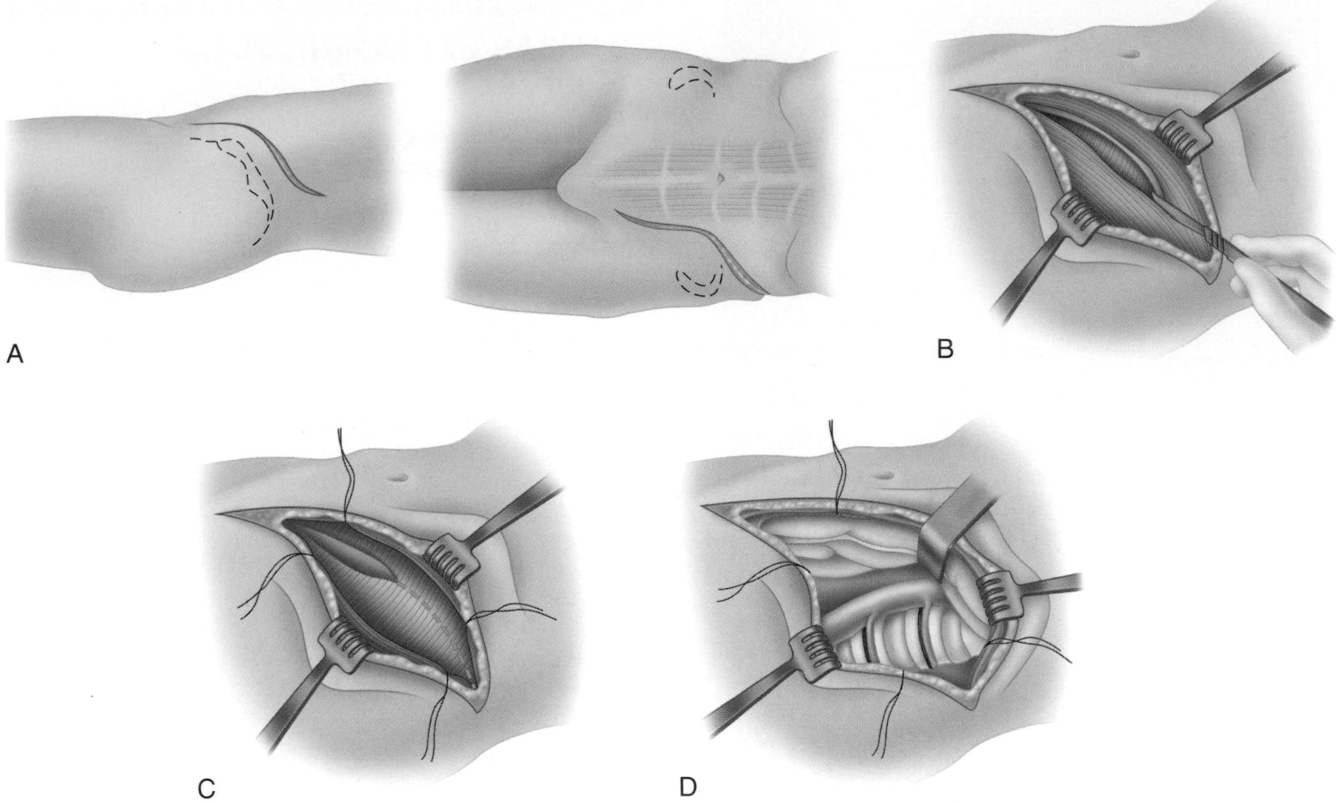

FIGURE 44-106 **A,** Skin incision for extraperitoneal approach to lumbar and lumbosacral spine. **B,** Incision of fibers of external oblique muscle. **C,** Incision into fibers of internal oblique muscle. **D,** Exposure of spine before ligation of segmental vessels. **SEE TECHNIQUE 44-29.**

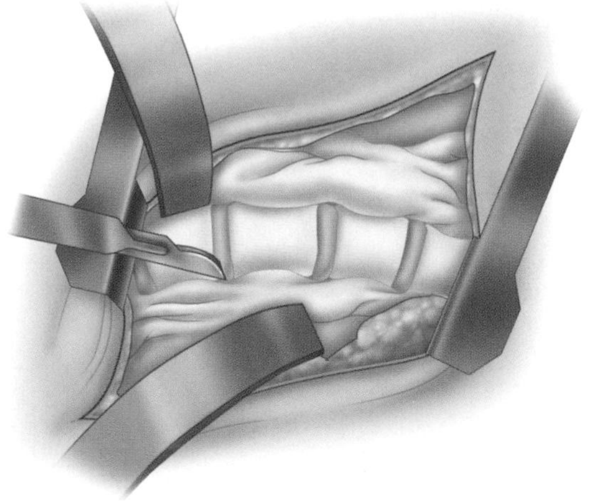

FIGURE 44-107 Disc excision. Annulus is divided with long-handled scalpel and removed. **SEE TECHNIQUE 44-30.**

ANTERIOR INSTRUMENTATION OF A THORACOLUMBAR CURVE WITH DUAL-ROD INSTRUMENTATION

TECHNIQUE 44-31

- After exposure of the spine and removal of the discs, staples and screws are inserted into each vertebral body, beginning proximally and working distally.
- Place an appropriate-sized staple on the lateral aspect of the vertebral body, being sure to be posterior enough to allow placement of the anterior screw. Various staple lengths are available to accommodate different-sized patients. Normally, in the lower thoracic spine, the staple is placed just anterior to the rib head.
- Impact the staple into the vertebral body (Fig. 44-108A and B). Make a pilot hole with an awl in the vertebral body, which eliminates the need to tap the screws (Fig. 44-108C).
- In the posterior hole, insert a screw of appropriate diameter and length angled approximately 10 degrees posterior to anterior, perpendicular to the base of the staple. Leave the screw slightly elevated off the staple surface until the

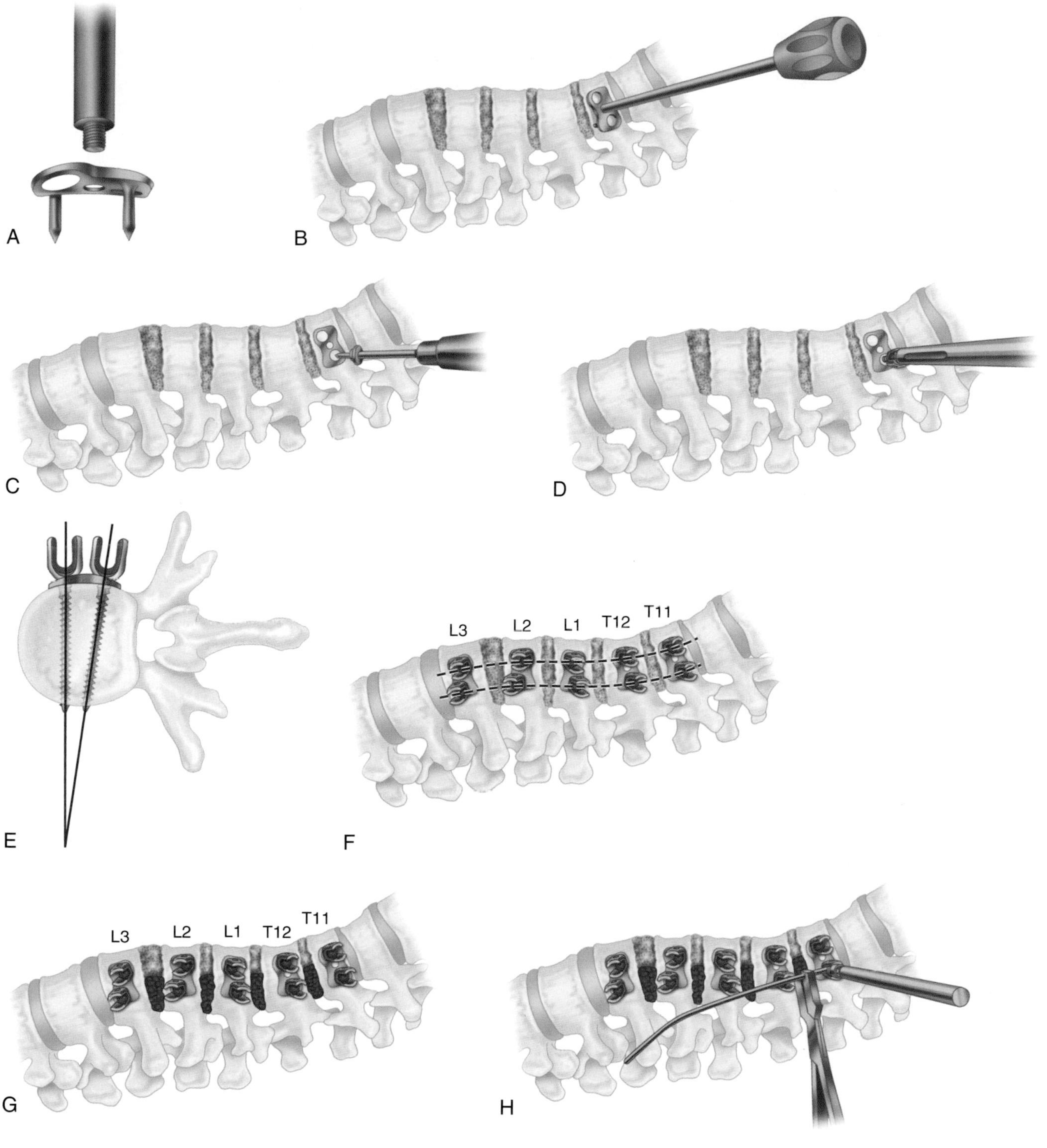

FIGURE 44-108 **A-Q, Anterior instrumentation of thoracolumbar curve with CD Horizon Legacy dual-rod instrumentation. See text for description.** (Redrawn from Lenke LG: CD Horizon Legacy Spinal System anterior dual-rod surgical technique manual, Memphis, TN, 2002, Medtronic Sofamor Danek.) **SEE TECHNIQUE 44-31.**

Continued

anterior screw is fully seated to prevent tilting of the staple (Fig. 44-108D).

- Place the anterior screws in a neutral but slightly anterior to posterior angular position. Once again, the goal is to place the screw perpendicular to the base of the staple (Fig. 44-108E). Bicortical purchase is required at the ends of the construct and is suggested in the intermediate levels as well. Figure 44-108F shows the staples and screws inserted from T11 to L3 before rod insertion.
- Decorticate the endplates before graft placement.
- Place intervertebral structural grafts beginning in the most caudal disc and working in a proximal direction.

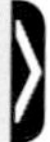

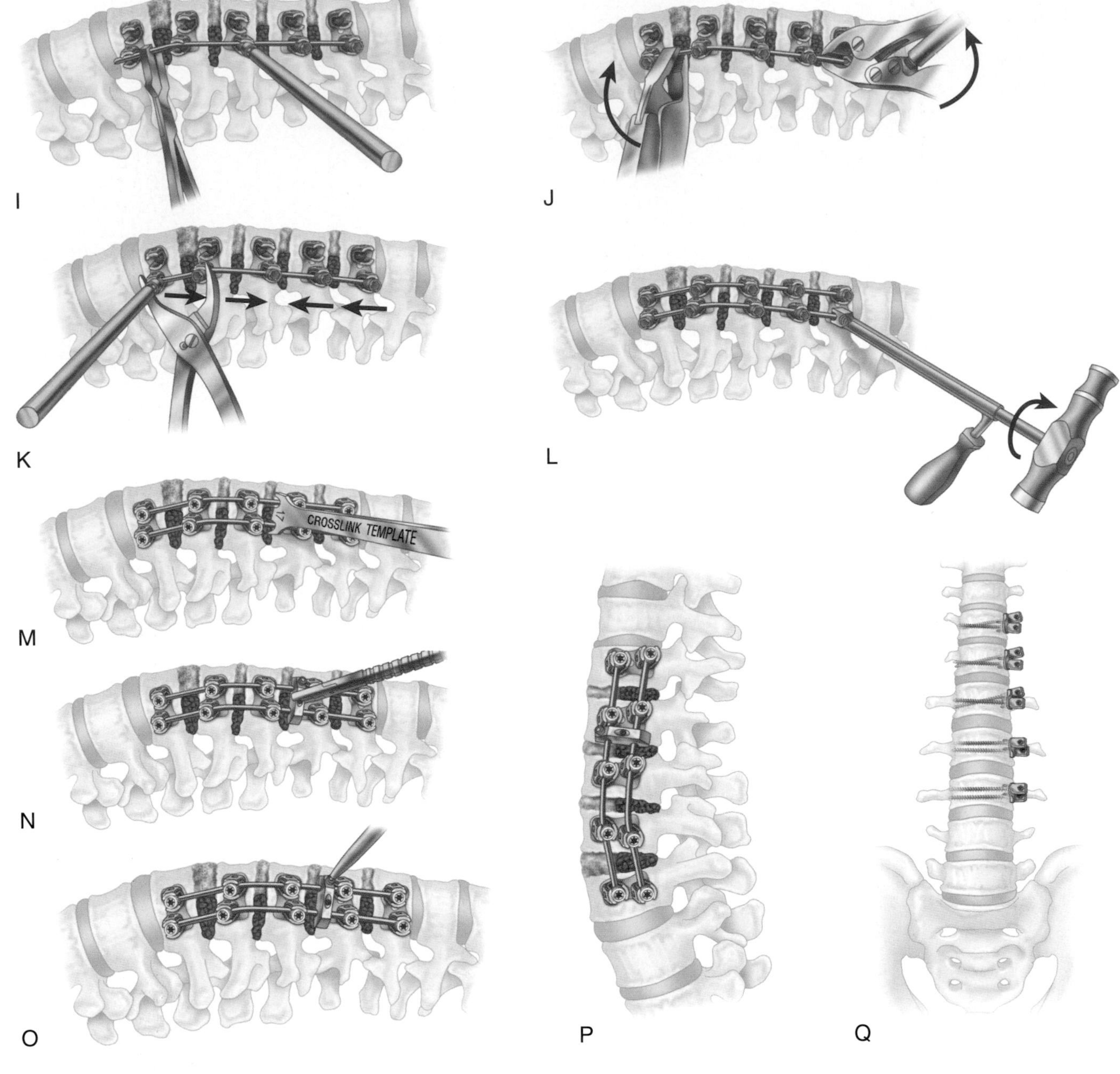

FIGURE 44-108, cont'd

Structural grafts are placed in the anterior aspect of the disc to facilitate lordosis (Fig. 44-108G). Posteriorly, autogenous morselized rib graft is placed against the decorticated endplates.

- Perform appropriate biplanar bending of the posterior rod.
- Engage the posterior rod proximally and cantilever it into the distal screws. Capture the rod at each level with set screws (Fig. 44-108H). The orientation of the posterior rod is shown in Figure 44-104I prior to the rod rotation maneuver.
- Place the rod grippers onto the rod and rotate it 90 degrees from posterior to anterior. This will facilitate both scoliosis correction and the production of sagittal lordosis (Fig. 44-108J).
- Perform intervertebral compression across the posterior screws after locking the apical screw and compressing from the apex to both ends (Fig. 44-108K).
- Place the anterior rod sequentially into the screws and seat and lock it with mild compression forces. This is just a stabilizing rod, and no further correction is attempted. Correction in the coronal and sagittal planes can be determined on intraoperative anteroposterior radiographs.
- Once the final position is confirmed, break off the set screws with the counterforce device (Fig. 44-108L).

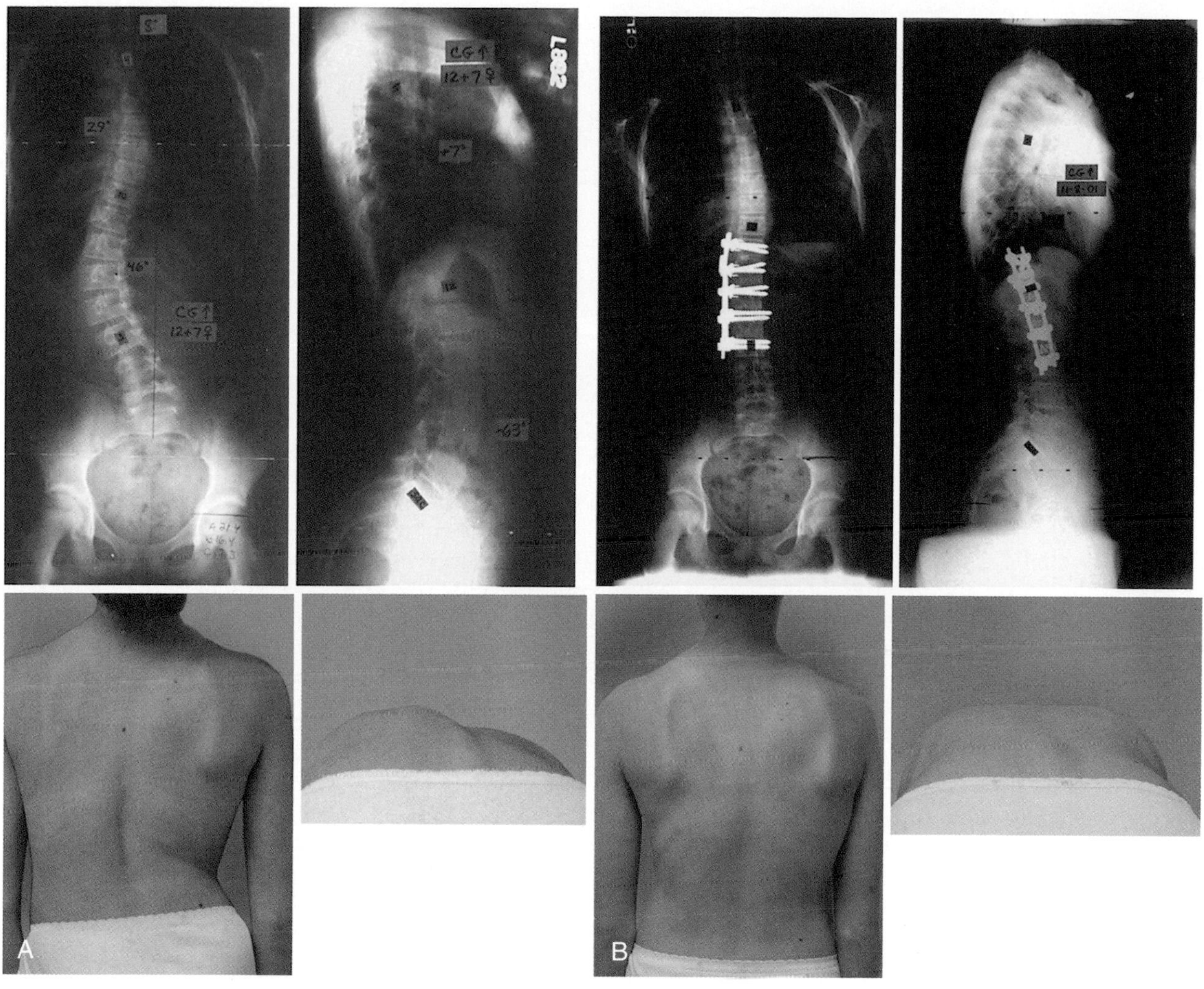

FIGURE 44-109 **A,** Preoperative clinical and radiographic views of 12-year-old, skeletally immature patient. **B,** Clinical and radiographic views after anterior spinal fusion and instrumentation from T11-L3. (From Lenke LG: CD Horizon Legacy Spinal System anterior dual-rod surgical technique manual, Memphis, TN, 2002, Medtronic Sofamor Danek.) **SEE TECHNIQUE 44-31.**

- Place one or two crosslink plates to create a rectangular construct, which increases rigidity of the system. Use the crosslink plate measuring tools to determine the required implant size (Fig. 44-108M) and then grasp the appropriate-sized crosslink and place it on the rods (Fig. 44-108N and O).
- The lower profile of this anterior instrumentation (Fig. 44-108P and Q) allows the closure of the pleura distally to the junction of the pleura and the diaphragm.
- Complete the closure procedure. Close the diaphragm, deep abdominal layers, chest wall (after chest tube placement), muscle layers, subcutaneous tissues, and skin.

POSTOPERATIVE CARE. The patient is allowed up on the first postoperative day. The chest tube usually is left in place for 48 to 72 hours. It is removed when the drainage decreases to less than 50 mL for two consecutive 8-hour periods. A TLSO can be used for immobilization, but if the screws have good purchase, no postoperative immobilization is used. A Foley catheter is necessary to monitor urine output because urinary retention is common. An ileus is to be expected after anterior surgery and usually lasts 2 to 3 days. Temperature elevation consistent with atelectasis is common and usually responds to pulmonary therapy and ambulation as soon as the patient is capable (Fig. 44-109).

COMPLICATIONS AND PITFALLS OF ANTERIOR INSTRUMENTATION

Pitfalls and complications may be related to poor patient selection, poor level selection, or instrument technical difficulties. A common technical problem is failure of the most proximal screw (see Fig. 44-104), which can be prevented by watching this screw carefully during the derotation maneuver.

At any sign of screw loosening, the correction maneuver should be stopped. Another technical problem is encountered if the screw heads are not aligned properly and one screw head is offset from the others. If one screw is off just slightly, rod placement can be difficult. Variable-angle screws or polyaxial screws allow some adjustment to account for this offset.

A number of studies have emphasized the potential complications associated with an anterior approach to the spine, including respiratory insufficiency requiring ventilatory support, pneumonia, atelectasis, pneumothorax, pleural effusion, urinary tract infection, prolonged ileus, hemothorax, splenic injury, retroperitoneal fibrosis, and partial sympathectomy.

Neurologic injury can occur during discectomy or screw insertion. The screws should be placed parallel to the vertebral endplates. When the segmental vessels are ligated, the anastomosis at the intervertebral foramina should be avoided to minimize the chance of injury to the vascular supply of the spinal cord. A scoliotic deformity is approached from the convex side of the curve, and because the great vessels are inevitably on the concave side of the curve, the risk of injury to them is low. To increase purchase of the screws, however, the opposite cortex of the vertebra should be engaged by the screw, and care must be taken to be certain that the screw is not too prominent on the concave side.

ANTERIOR THORACOPLASTY

The advantages of anterior thoracoplasty are the same as for posterior thoracoplasty. For the patient, reduction of the rib deformity is among the most important aspects of operative correction and fusion. The bone graft obtained from a thoracoplasty may obviate the need for an iliac bone graft that contributes to the postoperative morbidity.

ANTERIOR THORACOPLASTY

TECHNIQUE 44-32

(SHUFFLEBARGER)

- After thoracotomy, reflect the parietal pleura over the chest wall, exposing the ribs.
- From within the thoracotomy, divide the periosteum in line with the rib.
- Use an elevator to complete circumferential subperiosteal dissection of the rib in the posterior axillary line.
- Divide the rib with an end-cutting instrument. Then grasp the rib and bring it into the chest.
- Perform circumferential dissection of the periosteum and intercostal muscles to the costotransverse articulation.
- Disarticulate the rib head from the costotransverse and costocorporeal articulation.
- Remove the posterior portion of the remaining ribs in a similar manner to complete the thoracoplasty. This thoracoplasty not only improves the appearance and provides bone graft but also significantly softens the chest wall to facilitate exposure in patients with rigid deformities.

VIDEO-ASSISTED THORACOSCOPY

Video-assisted thoracoscopic surgery in the treatment of pediatric spinal deformity can be used for anterior release. Endoscopic anterior instrumentation also can be used for correction of thoracic scoliosis. At this time, our preference for the instrumentation of thoracic curves is a posterior approach with segmental instrumentation by hooks or cables or thoracic pedicle screws. Advantages of thoracoscopic surgery over open thoracotomy, in addition to better illumination and magnification at the site of surgery, include less injury to the latissimus muscle and chest wall with less long-term pain, decreased blood loss, better cosmesis, shorter recovery time, improved postoperative pulmonary function, and potentially shorter hospital stays. The primary disadvantages of thoracoscopy are related to a steep learning curve and the technical demands of the procedure.

Specialized equipment is required for these procedures. A general, pediatric, or thoracic surgeon familiar with thoracoscopy and open thoracotomies should be available to assist in the initial stages of the procedure and should remain scrubbed for the entire case. The anesthesiologist should be skilled in the use of double-lumen tubes with one-lung ventilation.

Indications for video-assisted thoracoscopic surgery include neuromuscular scoliosis in patients with compromised pulmonary function requiring anterior release, rigid curves requiring anterior release and posterior fusion, and skeletal immaturity in patients in whom anterior surgery is needed to prevent the crankshaft phenomenon. Relative indications include rigid thoracic idiopathic curves that do not correct on bending and rigid kyphotic deformities. With the more rigid posterior instrumentation systems currently available, anterior release in most idiopathic spinal deformities is not needed. Crawford extended his indications to include all procedures to the thoracic spine previously approached by thoracotomy.

Contraindications to the procedure include the inability to tolerate single-lung ventilation, severe or acute respiratory insufficiency, high airway pressures with positive-pressure ventilation, emphysema, and previous thoracotomy.

The equipment required for spinal thoracoscopic surgery is similar to that for general thoracoscopy. The basic equipment includes telescopes, light sources, cameras, monitors, and appropriate instrumentation. The most commonly used telescope is a 30-degree angled, 10-mm scope. In some pediatric cases, a smaller telescope may be needed, but it does not provide the same magnitude of illumination and resolution as the 10-mm scope. Telescopes with a lens-washing and site irrigation system are useful in defogging and cleaning the end of the scope. Other equipment includes flexible portals and long-handled manual instruments, such as curets, pituitary rongeurs, fan retractors, suction irrigation systems, endoscopic clip appliers, and periosteal elevators.

VIDEO-ASSISTED THORACOSCOPIC DISCECTOMY

Some surgeons prefer to work facing the patient with the patient in a lateral decubitus position (Fig. 44-110A), whereas others prefer to work from behind the patient, therefore working away from the spinal cord (Fig. 44-110B).

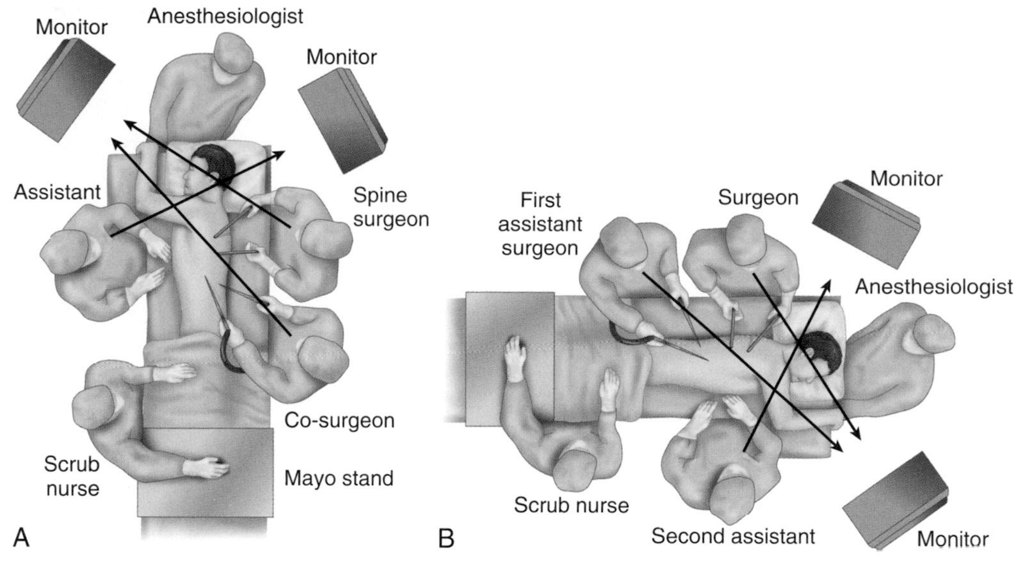

FIGURE 44-110 **A,** Conventional setup for video-assisted thoracoscopic spinal surgery. **B,** Setup with surgeon working away from spine. **SEE TECHNIQUE 44-33.**

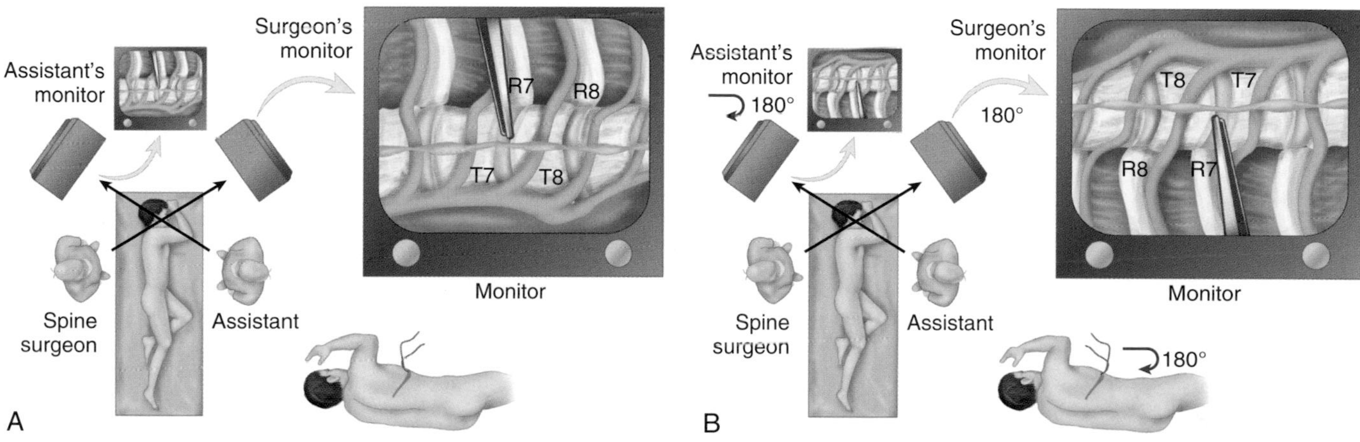

FIGURE 44-111 **A,** Thoracoscopic traditional technique. **B,** Thoracoscopic inversion technique. **SEE TECHNIQUE 44-33.**

Two monitors are positioned so that they can be seen from each side of the table. Because the traditional setup for most endoscopic procedures requires members of the surgical team to be on opposite sides of the patient, and because working opposite the camera image can lead to disorientation, Horton described turning the assistant's monitor upside down. The monitor on the posterior aspect of the patient is inverted, and once the visualization port for the camera is established, the scope is inserted into the camera and rotated 180 degrees on the scope mount so that the camera is upside down. The assistant holding the inverted camera views the inverted monitor, which projects a normal monitor image as would be seen in an open thoracotomy (Fig. 44-111A and B).

TECHNIQUE 44-33

(CRAWFORD)

- After general anesthesia is obtained by either a double-lumen endotracheal tube or a bronchial blocker for single-lung ventilation, turn the patient into the lateral decubitus position. Prepare and drape the operative field as the anesthesiologist deflates the lung. About 20 minutes is required for complete resorption atelectasis to be obtained.
- Place the upper arm on a stand with the shoulder slightly abducted and flexed more than 90 degrees to allow placement of portals higher into the axilla. Use an axillary roll to take pressure off the axillary structures.
- Identify the scapular borders, 12th rib, and iliac crest, and outline them with a marker.
- Place the first portal at or around the T6 or T7 interspace in the posterior axillary line (Fig. 44-112A).
- Make a skin incision with a scalpel and then continue with electrocautery through the intercostal muscle to enter the chest cavity. To avoid damage to the intercostal vessels and nerves, make the incision over the top of the rib. Insert a finger to be sure the lung is deflated and that it is away from the chest wall so it will not be injured when the trocar is inserted.

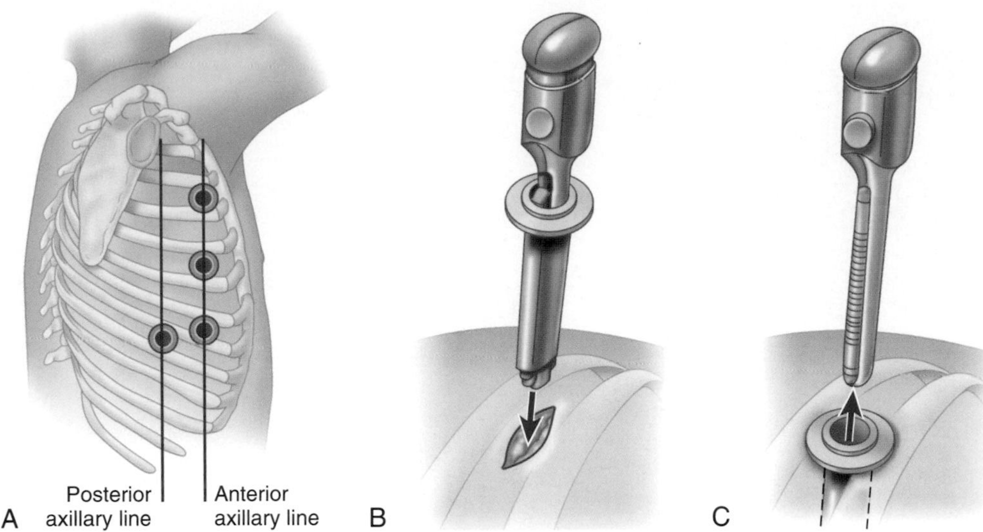

FIGURE 44-112 **A,** First portal for anterior thoracoscopic release of spine created along posterior axillary line between T6 and T8 intercostal spaces. Subsequent portals are created along anterior axillary line. **B,** Technique of portal insertion. Fifteen- to 20-mm incision is made parallel to superior surface of rib. Flexible portal is inserted with trocar. **C,** Trocar is removed, leaving flexible portal in place. **SEE TECHNIQUE 44-33.**

- Insert flexible portals through the intercostal spaces with a trocar (Fig. 44-112B and C).
- Insert a 30-degree angled, 10-mm rigid thoracoscope. Prevent fogging of the endoscope by prewarming it with warm irrigation solution and wiping the lens with a sterile fog-reduction solution. Wipe the endoscope lens intermittently with this solution to optimize visibility. Some endoscopes have incorporated irrigating and windshield-like cleaning mechanisms to further simplify the procedure.
- Evaluate the intrathoracic space to determine anatomy, as well as possible sites for other portals. The superior thoracic spine usually can be seen without retraction of the lung once the lung is completely deflated; however, some retraction usually is necessary below T9-10 because the diaphragm blocks the view.
- Once the spinal anatomy has been identified, continue to identify levels. The first rib usually cannot be seen, and the first visually identifiable rib is the second rib. Count the ribs sequentially to identify the levels to be released. Insert a long, blunt-tipped needle into the disc space and obtain a radiograph to confirm the levels intraoperatively.
- Select other portal sites after viewing from within. View the trocars with the endoscope as they are inserted. Take care on inserting the inferior portal to avoid perforation of the diaphragm. Use a fan retractor to retract the diaphragm, but take care not to lacerate the lung.
- Divide the parietal pleura with an endoscopic cautery hook.
- Place the hook in the parietal pleura in the region of the disc, midway between the head of the rib and the anterior spine.
- Pull the pleura up and cauterize in successive movements proximally and distally, avoiding the segmental vessels.
- Identify the intervertebral discs as elevations on the spinal column and the vertebral bodies as depressions.
- For a simple anterior release, do not ligate the segmental vessels because of the risk of tearing. Bleeding can be difficult to control endoscopically. Crawford recommended coagulation of any vessels that appear to be at risk for bleeding.
- Once the pleura has been completely resected, proceed directly to excision of the annulus at the level of the intervertebral discs to be removed. The rib heads provide excellent landmarks for localization. The rib head articulates with the base of the pedicle and the vertebral body just caudad to or at the level of the disc space; for example, the T9 rib head leads to the T8-9 disc space (Fig. 44-113).
- Make a transverse cut with cautery across the vertebral body, parallel to the disc, cephalad and caudad to it.
- Elevate the periosteum toward the vertebral endplate to isolate the disc
- Make a transverse cut across the annulus fibrosus, continuing down to the level of the nucleus pulposus.
- Use rongeurs, curets, and periosteal elevators as necessary to ensure complete removal of the disc materials and endplates.
- Control bleeding of the subchondral bone by packing the disc space with Surgicel (Johnson & Johnson, Somerville, NJ).
- Stress the spinal column segment with moderate force after each release to see if mobility has been accomplished.
- After the discectomies have been done, harvest of rib graft can be done through the portal sites if needed (Fig. 44-114).
- The pleura can be closed or left open.
- Place a chest tube through the most posterior inferior portal. Use the endoscope to observe the chest tube as it is placed along the vertebral column. Connect the chest tube to a water seal.
- Once the anesthesiologist has inflated the lung to determine whether an air leak exists, close the portals in routine fashion.

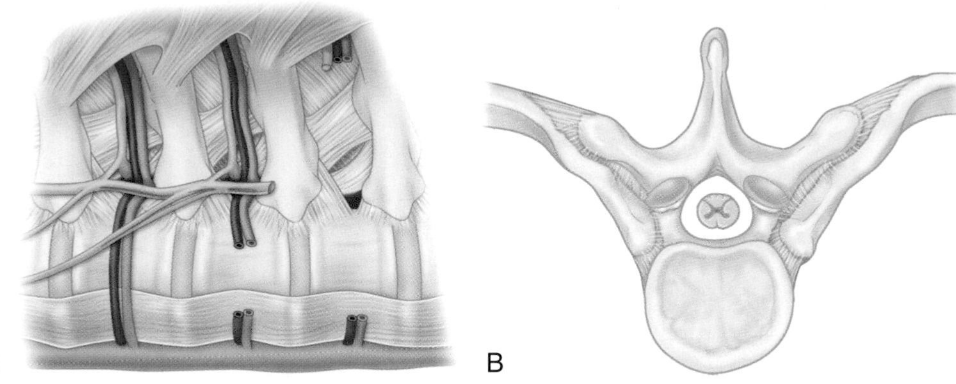

FIGURE 44-113 **A,** Thoracic vertebral anatomy. Ribs attach to vertebrae by costotransverse and costovertebral ligaments. Head of ribs articulate with base of pedicle and vertebral body just below disc or at disc space. Segmental vessels cross over middle of concave surface of vertebral bodies. **B,** Cross section of thoracic vertebra showing relationship of rib and pedicle to spinal cord. **SEE TECHNIQUE 44-33.**

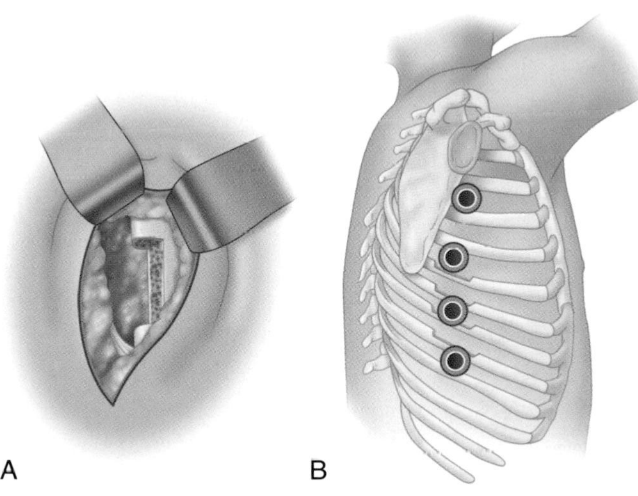

FIGURE 44-114 **A** and **B,** Three or four rib sections removed and morselized until enough bone graft has been obtained. **SEE TECHNIQUE 44-33.**

PITFALLS AND COMPLICATIONS

Bleeding can be difficult to control with endoscopic surgery. A radiopaque sponge with a heavy suture attached and loaded on a sponge stick should be available at all times to apply pressure. The suture allows later retrieval of the sponge. After application of direct pressure, electrocautery should be used for hemostasis. If necessary, endoscopic clip appliers or another hemostatic agent should be used. Instrumentation for open thoracotomy should be set up on a sterile back table to avoid delays or confusion if an immediate thoracotomy is needed to control bleeding.

Lung tissue can be damaged during the procedure. If an air leak occurs, it can be repaired with an endoscopic stapler. A dural tear can be recognized by leakage of clear cerebrospinal fluid from the disc space. Hemostatic agents can sometimes seal small cerebrospinal fluid leaks. If a dural tear continues to leak cerebrospinal fluid, a thoracotomy and vertebrectomy with dural repair may be required.

Cloudy fluid in the intervertebral disc space after irrigation and suctioning may indicate a lymphatic injury, which can be closed with an endoscopic clip applier. The thoracic duct is especially vulnerable to injury at the level of the diaphragm. If a chylothorax is discovered after closure, it is treated with a low-fat diet.

The sympathetic nerve chain on the operative side often is transected. This causes little or no morbidity; however, the surgeon needs to inform the patient and family members of the possibility of temperature and skin color changes below the level of the surgery.

Postoperative pulmonary problems often involve the downside lung, in which mucous plugs can form. The anesthesiologist should suction both lungs before extubation.

ENDOSCOPIC ANTERIOR INSTRUMENTATION OF IDIOPATHIC SCOLIOSIS

As experience with video-assisted thoracoscopy has increased, techniques have been developed for anterior instrumentation of the thoracic spine through a thoracoscopic approach. The goal is to allow thoracoscopic anterior discectomy, fusion, and instrumentation comparable to that for open thoracotomy.

CD HORIZON ECLIPSE SPINAL INSTRUMENTATION

TECHNIQUE 44-34

(PICETTI)

- Obtain appropriate preoperative radiographs and determine the fusion levels by Cobb angles.
- After general anesthesia is obtained by a double-lumen intubation technique (children weighing less than 45 kg may require selective intubation of the ventilated lung) and one-lung ventilation has been achieved, place the

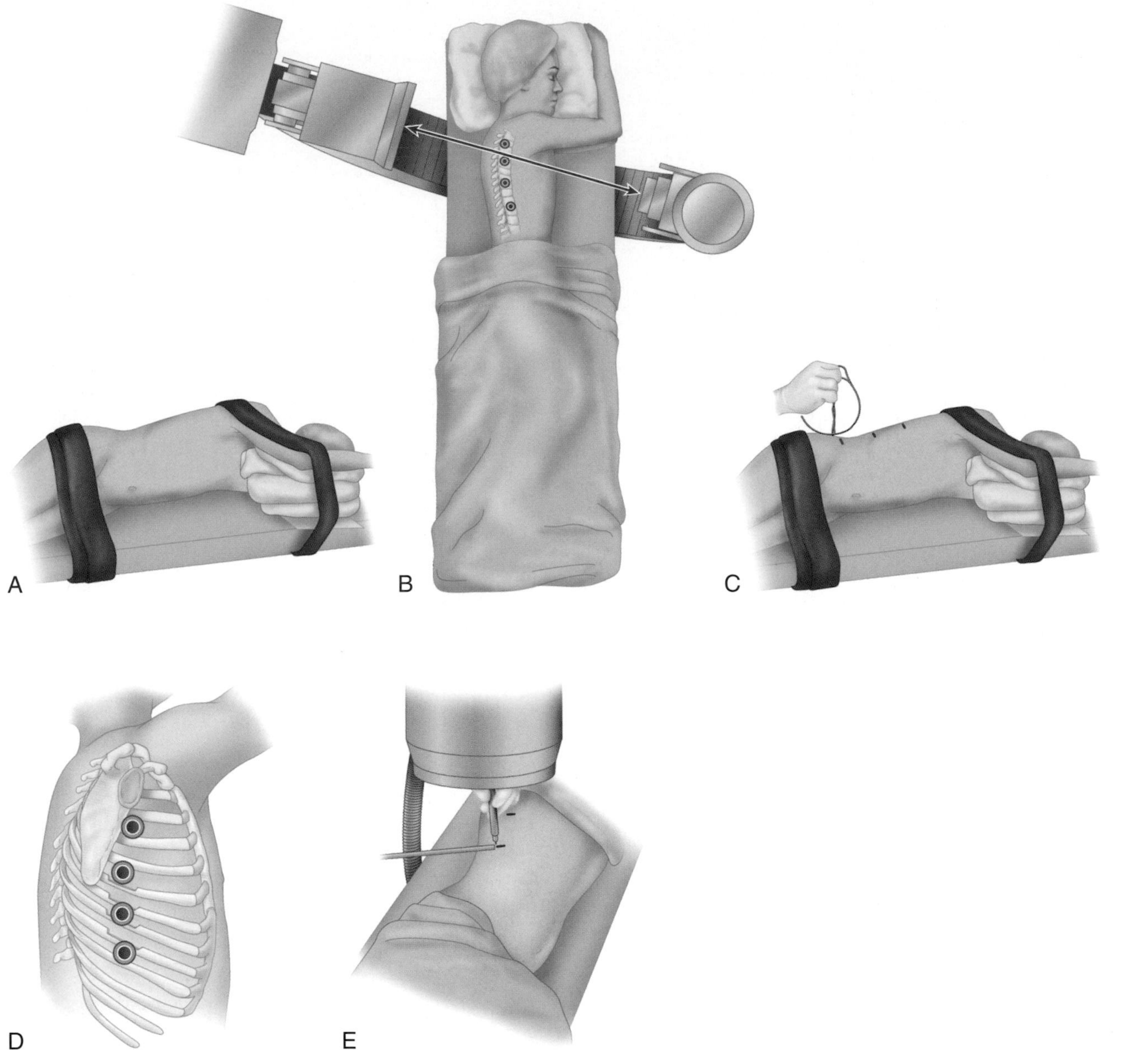

FIGURE 44-115 **A,** Patient positioning. **B,** C-arm in posteroanterior plane used to determine proper incision placement. **C,** Marker positioned posterior to patient and aligned with every other vertebral body. **D,** Three to five incisions are made, depending on number of levels to be instrumented. **E,** Cross mark is then placed on previous line. This is location of center of portals. (Redrawn from Picetti GD III: CD Horizon Eclipse Spinal System surgical technique manual, Memphis, TN, 1999, Sofamor Danek.) **SEE TECHNIQUE 44-34.**

patient into the direct lateral decubitus position, with the arms at 90/90 and the concave side of the curve down. It is imperative to have the lung completely collapsed in this procedure. If the patient's oxygen saturation drops on placement into the lateral decubitus position, have the anesthesiologist readjust the tube.

- Tape the patient's hips and the shoulders to the operating table (Fig. 44-115A). Have a general or thoracic surgeon assist in the first part of the procedure if necessary.
- With the use of C-arm intensification, identify the vertebral levels and portal sites. A straight metallic object is used as a marker to identify the vertebral levels and portal sites. The superior and inferior access incisions are the most critical because the vertebrae at these levels are at the greatest angle in relation to the apex of the curve.
- View the planes with a C-arm in the posteroanterior plane and make sure the endplates are parallel and well defined. Rotate the C-arm until it is parallel to the vertebral body endplates, not perpendicular to the table (Fig. 44-115B).
- Position the marker posterior to the patient and align with every other vertebral body (Fig. 44-115C).
- Obtain a C-arm image at each level.
- Once the marker is centered and parallel to the endplates, make a line on the patient at each portal site in line with

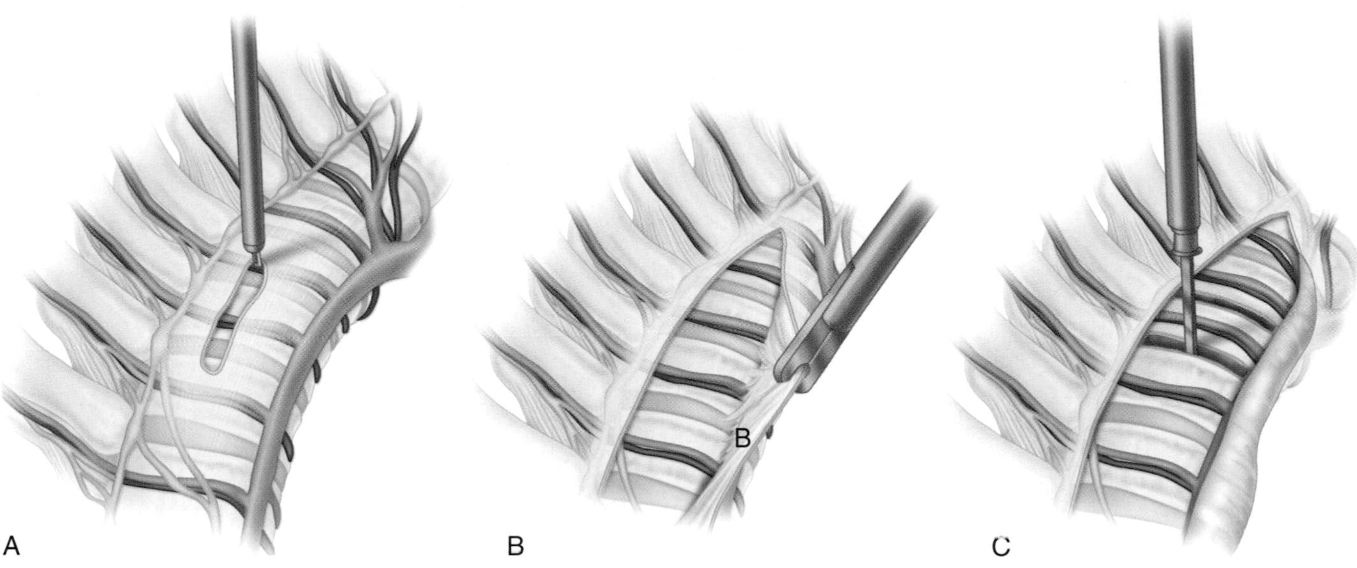

FIGURE 44-116 **A,** Incision of pleura along entire length without injury to segmental vessels. **B,** Pleura is dissected off vertebral bodies and discs, anteriorly off anterior longitudinal ligament and posteriorly off rib heads by peanut or endoscopic grasper. **C,** Kirschner wire is placed into disc space, and C-arm images are used to confirm level. Electrocautery is used to incise disc annulus. (Redrawn from Picetti GD III: CD Horizon Eclipse Spinal System surgical technique manual, Memphis, TN, 1999, Sofamor Danek.) **SEE TECHNIQUE 44-34.**

the marker. Marks should be two interspaces apart to allow placement of portals above and below the rib at each level and to provide access to two levels through a single skin incision. Use three to five incisions, depending on the number of levels to be instrumented (Fig. 44-115D).

- Once marks are made at all portal sites, rotate the C-arm to the lateral position. Place the marker end on each line and adjust the marker position until the C-arm image shows the end of the marker at the level of the rib head on the vertebrae. Place a cross mark on the previous line (Fig. 44-115E). This is the location of the center of the portals and will show the degree of rotation of the spine.
- The spine surgeon's position at the patient's back allows all of the instruments to be directed away from the spinal cord.

EXPOSURE AND DISCECTOMY

- Prepare and drape the patient, including the axilla and scapula.
- Check positioning to confirm that the patient has remained in the direct lateral decubitus position. This orientation provides a reference to gauge the anteroposterior and lateral direction of the guidewires and the screws.
- Make a modified thoracotomy incision at the central mark. The incision can be smaller because it is used only for the central discectomies, screw placement, and viewing. The other discectomies and screw placements are done through the access portals because they provide better alignment to the end disc spaces and vertebral bodies.
- After the lung has been deflated completely, make the initial portal in the sixth or seventh interspace by use of the alignment marks made previously. Make sure that the portal is in line with the spine and positioned according to the amount of spinal rotation. Insertion of the first portal at this level will avoid injury to the diaphragm, which normally is more caudal.
- Once the portal is made, use a finger to confirm that the lung is deflated and make sure there are no adhesions.
- Place 10.5- to 12-mm access portals under direct observation at the predetermined positions. Count the ribs to ensure that the correct levels are identified on the basis of preoperative plans.
- Incise the pleura longitudinally along the entire length of the spine to be instrumented.
- Place a Bovie hook on the pleura over a disc and make an opening. Insert the hook under the pleura and elevate it and incise along the entire length (Fig. 44-116A). Use suction to evacuate the smoke from the chest cavity.
- Dissect the pleura off the vertebral bodies and discs. Continue pleural dissection anteriorly off the anterior longitudinal ligament and posteriorly off the rib heads by use of a peanut or endoscopic grasper (Fig. 44-116B).
- Place a Kirschner wire into the disc space and confirm the level with C-arm intensification.
- With electrocautery, incise the disc annulus (Fig. 44-116C).
- Remove the disc in standard fashion with use of various endoscopic curets and pituitary, Cobb, and Kerrison rongeurs. If necessary, use endoscopic shavers and rasps to assist in discectomy.
- Once the disc is completely removed, thin the anterior longitudinal ligament from within the disc space with a pituitary rongeur. Thin the ligament to a flexible remnant that is no longer structural but will contain the bone graft.
- Remove the disc and annulus posteriorly back to at least the rib head. Use a Kerrison rongeur to remove the

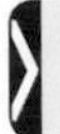

annulus posterior to the rib heads. Leave the rib head intact at this point because it will be used to guide screw placement.

- Once the disc has been evacuated, remove the endplate completely and inspect the disc space directly with the scope. Pack the disc space with Surgicel to control endplate bleeding.

GRAFT HARVEST

- Use an Army-Navy retractor to stabilize the rib.
- With a rib cutter, make two vertical cuts through the superior aspect of the rib and perpendicular to the rib extending halfway across it. Use an osteotome to connect the two cuts while the retractor supports the rib.
- Remove and morselize the rib section.
- Remove three or four other rib sections in a similar fashion until enough bone graft has been obtained (see Fig. 44-114).
- If a rib is removed through an access incision, retract the portal anteriorly as far as possible. Dissect the rib subperiosteally and carry posterior dissection as far as the portal can be retracted. This technique yields an adequate amount of graft and preserves the integrity of the rib, thus protecting the intercostal nerve and decreasing postoperative pain.
- If the patient has a large chest wall deformity, perform thoracoplasties and use rib sections for grafting.
- Do not remove the rib heads at this time because they function as landmarks for screw placement.

SCREW PLACEMENT

- Position the C-arm at the most superior vertebral body to be instrumented. It is imperative to have the C-arm parallel to the spine to give an accurate image.
- The vessels are located in the depression or middle of the vertebral body and serve as an anatomic guide for screw placement.
- Grasp the segmental vessels and coagulate at the mid–vertebral body level with the electrocautery (Fig. 44-117A). Hemoclip and cut larger segmental vessels if necessary.
- Check positioning again to ensure that the patient is still in the direct lateral decubitus position.
- Place the Kirschner guidewire onto the vertebral body just anterior to the rib head (Fig. 44-117B). Check this position with the C-arm to verify that the wire will be parallel to the endplates and in the center of the body (Fig. 44-117C and D).
- Check the inclination of the guide in the lateral plane by examining the chest wall and the rotation. The guide should be in a slight posterior to anterior inclination, directing the wire away from the canal. If there is any doubt or concern about the anterior inclination, obtain a lateral C-arm image to verify position.
- Once the correct alignment of the guide has been attained, insert the Kirschner wire into the cannula of the Kirschner guide that is positioned centrally on the vertebral body.
- Drill the guidewire to the opposite cortex, ensuring that it is parallel to the vertebral body.
- Confirm the position with the C-arm as the wire is inserted. Take care not to drill the wire through the opposite cortex because this can injure the segmental vessels and the lung on the opposite side.
- The most superior mark on the guidewire represents a length of 50 mm, and the etched lines are at 5-mm increments. The length of the Kirschner wire in the vertebral body can be determined by these marks. Start at the 50-mm mark and subtract 5 mm for each additional mark that is showing (Fig. 44-117E). For example, if there are four marks, in addition to the 50-mm mark, the length of the Kirschner wire would be 30 mm.
- Remove the guide and place the tap over the Kirschner wire onto the vertebral body. To maximize fixation strength, use the largest-diameter tap that will fit in the vertebral bodies, based on the preoperative radiographs. Grasp the distal end of the wire with a clamp (Fig. 44-117F) and hold it as the tap is inserted so that the wire will not advance. This is important to avoid a pneumothorax in the opposite chest cavity. Tap only the near cortex (Fig. 44-117G). Use the C-arm to monitor tap depth and Kirschner wire position.
- Place the appropriate-sized screw, based on the Kirschner wire measurement and tap diameter, over the wire with the Eclipse screwdriver and advance it (Fig. 44-117H). To ensure bicortical fixation, select a screw that is 5 mm longer than the width of the vertebral body as measured with the Kirschner wire. Grasp the wire again to avoid advancement while the screw is inserted.
- Remove the wire when the screw is approximately halfway across the vertebral body.
- Check the screw direction with the C-arm as it is advanced and seated against the vertebral body. The screw should penetrate the opposite cortex for bicortical fixation.
- Instrument all Cobb levels.
- Use each rib head as a reference for subsequent screw placement to help ensure that the screws are in line and will produce proper spinal rotation when the rod is inserted. With the screws properly aligned, the screw heads form an arc that can be verified with a lateral image (Fig. 44-117I).
- Adjust the side walls of the screws (saddles) to be in line for insertion of the rod (Fig. 44-117J). If a screw is sunk more than a few millimeters deeper than the rest of the screws, reduction of the rod into the screw head may be difficult. The C-arm image can confirm depth of screw placement as the screws are inserted.
- Once all the screws have been placed, remove the Surgicel and use the graft funnel and plunger to deliver the graft into the disc spaces (Figs. 44-117K and L). Fill each disc space all the way across to the opposite side.

ROD MEASUREMENT AND PLACEMENT

- Determine the rod length with the rod length gauge. Place the fixed ball at the end of the measuring device into the saddle of the inferior screw. Then guide the ball at the end of the cable through all of the screws with a pituitary rongeur to the most superior screw and insert it into the saddle (Fig. 44-118A). Pull the wire tight and take a reading from the scale. The scale is in centimeters.
- Cut the 4.5-mm-diameter rod to length and insert it into the chest cavity through the thoracotomy. The rod has slight flexibility, so do not bend it before insertion.

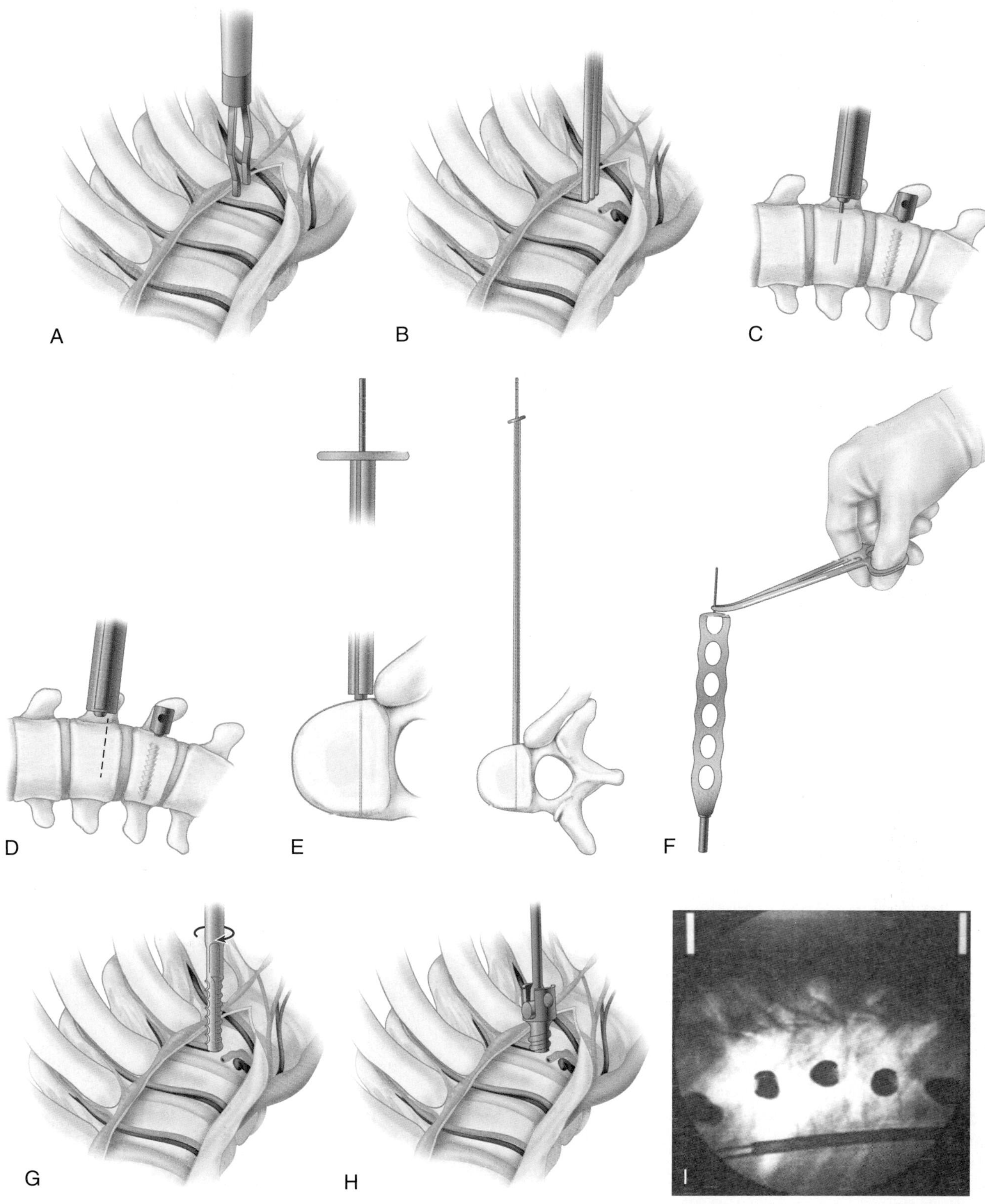

FIGURE 44-117 **A,** Segmental vessels are grasped and ligated at midvertebral body level with electrocautery. **B,** Kirschner guidewire is placed onto vertebral body just anterior to rib head. **C** and **D,** Position is checked with C-arm to verify that wire will be parallel to endplates in center of body. **E,** Most superior mark on guidewire represents length of 50 mm, and etched lines are at 5-mm increments. Length of Kirschner wire is determined by these marks. **F,** Distal end of Kirschner wire grasped with clamp and held as tap is inserted. **G,** Only near cortex is tapped. **H,** Appropriate-sized screw is placed over Kirschner wire with Eclipse screwdriver and advanced. **I,** Alignment of screw heads verified by lateral image.

Continued

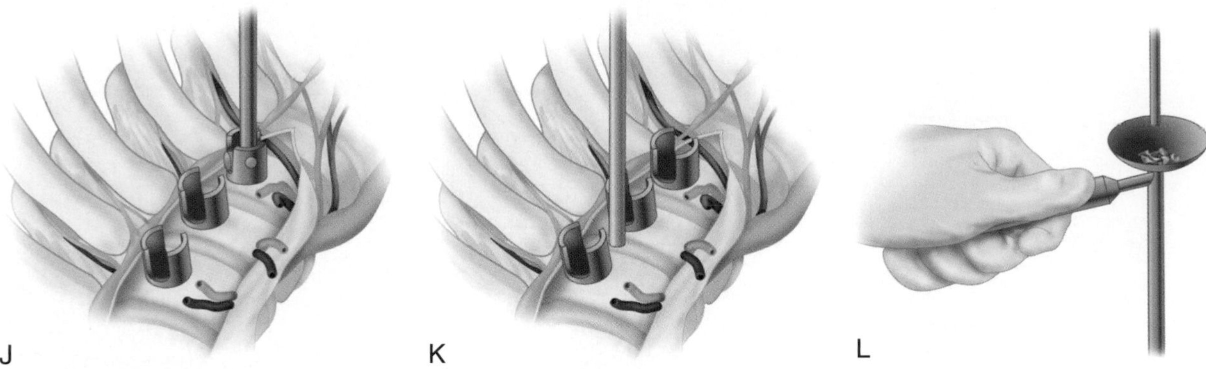

FIGURE 44-117, cont'd **J,** Side walls of screws adjusted to be in line for receipt of rod. **K** and **L,** Graft delivered to disc space by graft funnel and plunger. Disc space should be filled totally across to opposite side. (Redrawn from Picetti GD III: CD Horizon Eclipse Spinal System surgical technique manual, Memphis, TN, 1999, Sofamor Danek.) **SEE TECHNIQUE 44-34.**

- Apply anterior compression to obtain kyphosis in the thoracic spine.
- Do not cut the rod longer than measured because the total distance between the screws will be reduced with compression.
- Manipulate the rod into the inferior screw with the rod holder (Fig. 44-118B). The end of the rod should be flush with the saddle of the screw to prevent the rod from protruding and irritating or puncturing the diaphragm.
- Once the rod is in place, remove the portal and place the plug introduction guide over the screw to guide the plug and to hold the rod in position (Fig. 44-118C).
- Place the obturator in the tube to assist in the insertion through the incision if necessary.
- Load a plug onto the plug-capturing T25 driver (Fig. 44-118D). Insert the plug with the flat side and the laser etching up.
- Once the plug is placed on the driver, turn the sleeve clockwise to engage the plug with the sleeve.
- Place the plug through the plug introduction guide and insert it into the screw. Do not place the plug without using the introduction guide and the plug inserter.
- To ensure proper threading, turn the sleeve once counterclockwise before advancing the plug.
- Once the plug has been correctly started, hold the locking sleeve to prevent any further rotation. This will disengage the plug from the inserter as the plug is placed into the screw (Fig. 44-118E).
- Remove the driver and introduction guide and torque the screw with the torque-limiting wrench. This is the only plug that is tightened completely at this time.
- Sequentially insert the rod into the remaining screws with use of the rod pusher (Fig. 44-118F). Place the rod pusher on the rod several screws above the screw into which the rod is being placed.
- Apply the plugs through the plug introduction guide as described. To allow compression, do not fully tighten the plugs at this time.
- Once the rod has been seated and all the plugs are inserted into the screws, apply compression between the screws.

COMPRESSION: RACK AND PINION

- Insert the compressor through the thoracotomy incision. Once it is in the thoracic cavity, manipulate it by holding the ball-shaped attachment with the compressor holder. The rack and pinion compressor fits over two screw heads on the rod; turning the compressor driver clockwise compresses the two screws (Fig. 44-119A). Start compression at the inferior end of the construct with the most inferior screw's plug fully tightened.
- Once satisfactory compression has been obtained on a level, tighten the superior plug with the plug driver through the plug introduction guide.
- Apply compression sequentially superiorly until all levels have been compressed, then torque each plug to 75 in-lb with the torque-limiting wrench. The construct is complete at this point (Figs. 44-119B and C).

COMPRESSION: CABLE COMPRESSOR

- Insert each end of the cable through one of the distal holes on the side of the guide (not the larger central hole). The actuator should be in the position closest to the compressor body.
- Form a 3-inch loop at the end of the guide (Fig. 44-120A), with the two cable ends passing through the actuator body.
- Engage the lever arm by use of one of the plug drivers through the cam mechanism (Fig. 44-120B).
- Place the end of the compressor through the distal portal. With the portal removed, place a plug introduction guide through the adjacent incision, through the loop, and over the next screw to be compressed.
- Place the foot of the compressor over the rod and against the inferior side of the end screw (Fig. 44-120C).
- Fully tighten the plug in the end screw. Squeeze the handle of the compressor several times to compress.
- Once satisfactory compression has been obtained at a level, tighten the superior plug with the plug driver through the plug introduction guide.
- To disengage the compressor, tilt it toward the superior screw until the foot disengages from the inferior screw.

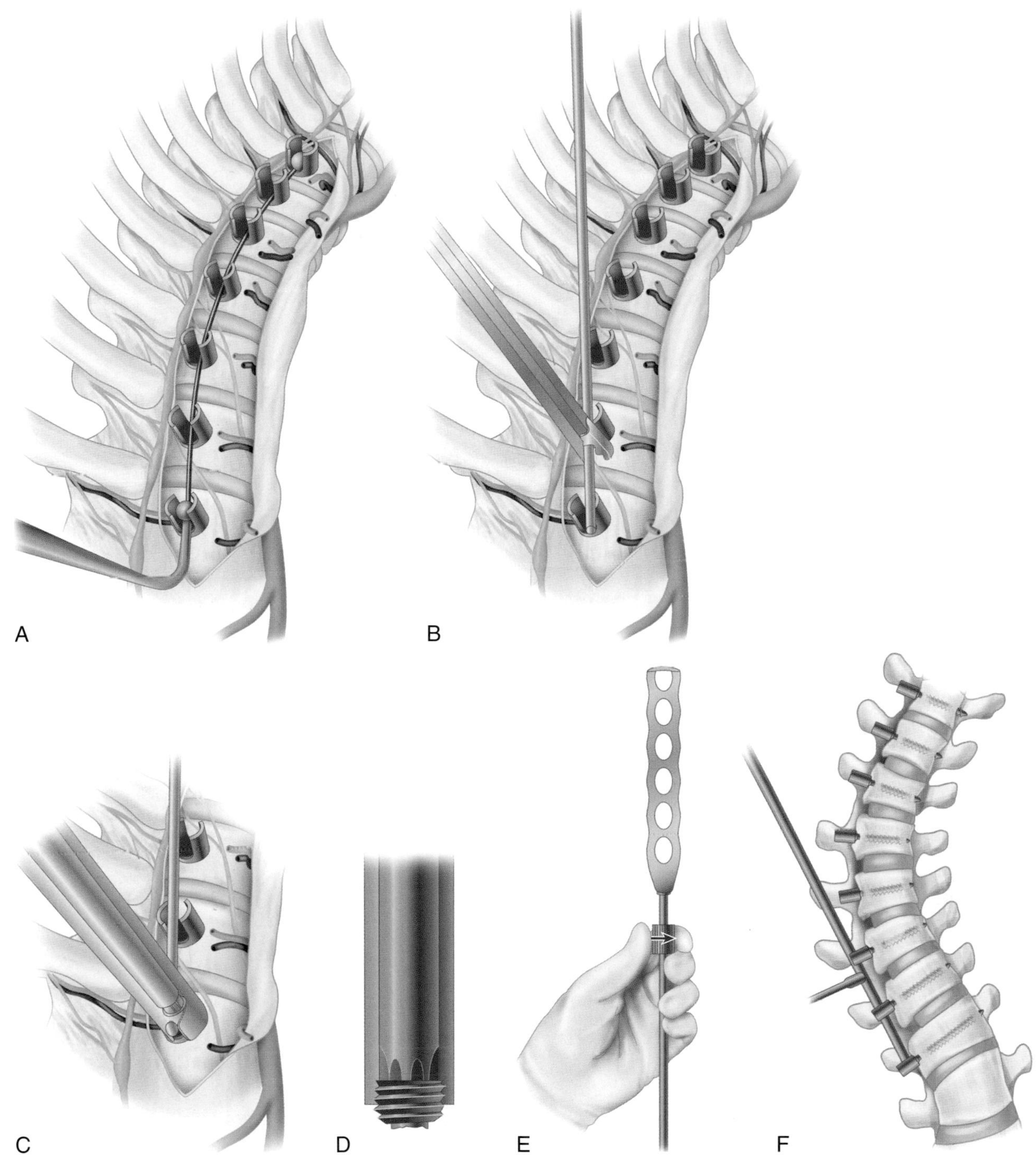

FIGURE 44-118 **A,** Ball at end of cable is guided through all screws with pituitary rongeur to superiormost screw and inserted into saddle. **B,** Rod manipulated into inferior screw with rod holder. **C,** Plug introduction guide placed over screw to guide plug and to hold rod in position. **D,** Plug loaded onto plug-capturing T25 driver. **E,** Holding locking sleeve to prevent further rotation disengages plug from inserter as plug is inserted into screw. **F,** Rod reduced into remaining screws with use of rod pushers. (Redrawn from Picetti GD III: CD Horizon Eclipse Spinal System surgical technique manual, Memphis, TN, 1999, Sofamor Danek.) **SEE TECHNIQUE 44-34.**

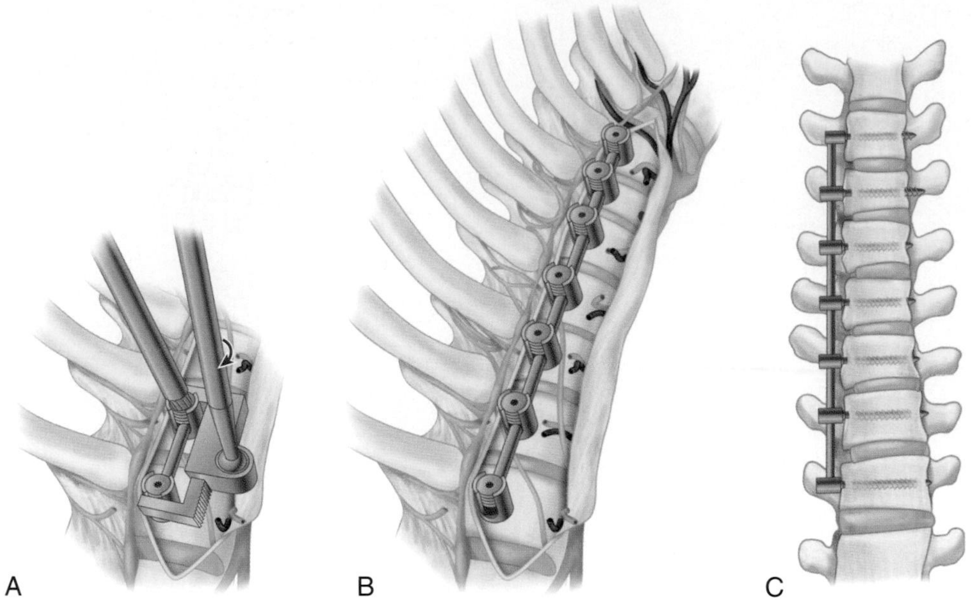

FIGURE 44-119 **A,** Rack-and-pinion compressor fits over two screw heads on rod. **B** and **C,** Completed construct. (Redrawn from Picetti GD III: CD Horizon Eclipse Spinal System surgical technique manual, Memphis, TN, 1999, Sofamor Danek.) **SEE TECHNIQUE 44-34.**

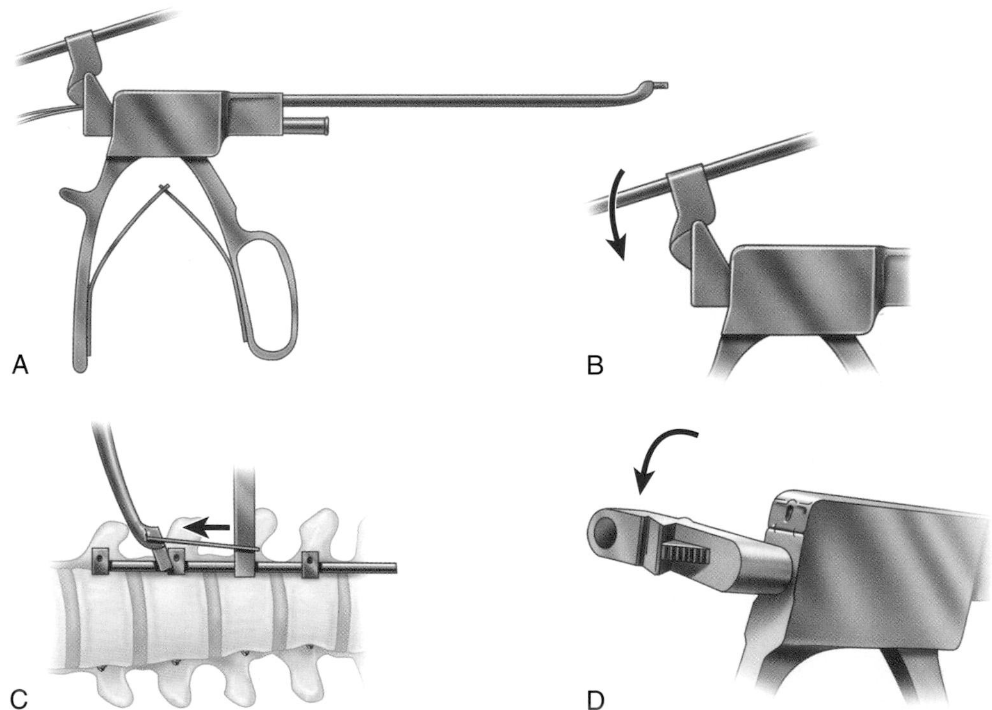

FIGURE 44-120 **A-D,** Cable compression. See text for description. (Redrawn from Picetti GD III: CD Horizon Eclipse Spinal System surgical technique manual, Memphis, TN, 1999, Sofamor Danek.) **SEE TECHNIQUE 44-34.**

- Turn the actuator mechanism 90 degrees to disengage the ratchet (Fig. 44-120D).
- With the cable loop still around the plug introduction guide that is on the superior screw, pull the compressor until the actuator is next to the compressor body.
- Repeat the steps described on subsequent screws. Apply compression sequentially until all levels have been compressed and then torque each plug to 75 in-lb with the torque-limiting wrench. The construct is complete at this point.
- Place a 20-French chest tube through the inferior portal and close the incisions. Obtain anteroposterior and lateral radiographs before the patient is transferred to the recovery room.

POSTOPERATIVE CARE. The chest tube is left in until drainage is less than 100 mL every 8 hours. Patients can be ambulatory after the first postoperative day, and they can be discharged from the hospital the day after the chest tube is removed. A brace should be worn for 3 months.

NEUROMUSCULAR SCOLIOSIS

The specific causes of neuromuscular scoliosis are unknown, but several contributing factors are well known. Loss of muscle strength or voluntary muscle control and loss of sensory abilities, such as proprioception, in the flexible and rapidly growing spinal column of a juvenile patient are believed to be factors in development of these curves. As the spine collapses, increased pressure on the concave side of the curve results in decreased growth of that side of the vertebral body and wedging of the vertebral body itself. The vertebrae also can be structurally compromised by malnutrition or disuse osteopenia.

The Scoliosis Research Society has established a classification for neuromuscular scoliosis (Box 44-5).

Neuromuscular curves develop at a younger age than do idiopathic curves, and a larger percentage of neuromuscular curves are progressive. Unlike idiopathic curves, even small neuromuscular curves may continue to progress beyond skeletal maturity. Many neuromuscular curves are long, C-shaped curves that include the sacrum, and pelvic obliquity is common. Patients with neuromuscular scoliosis also may have pelvic obliquity from other sources, such as hip joint and other lower extremity contractures, all of which can affect the lumbar spine. The progressing neurologic or muscular disease also can interfere with trunk stability. These patients generally are less tolerant of orthotic management than are patients with idiopathic scoliosis, and brace treatment often is ineffective in preventing curve progression. Spinal surgery in this group is associated with increased bleeding and less satisfactory bone stock; longer fusions, often to the pelvis, are needed.

Many neuromuscular spinal deformities require operative intervention. The goal of treatment is to maintain a spine balanced in the coronal and sagittal planes over a level pelvis. The basic treatment methods are similar to those for idiopathic scoliosis: observation, orthotic treatment, and surgery.

BOX 44-5

Scoliosis Research Society Classification of Neuromuscular Spinal Deformity

- Primary neuropathies
- Upper motor neuron neuropathies
  - Cerebral palsy
  - Spinocerebellar degeneration
    - Friedreich ataxia
    - Roussy-Levy disease
    - Spinocerebellar ataxia
  - Syringomyelia
  - Spinal cord tumor
  - Spinal cord trauma
- Lower motor neuron pathologies
  - Poliomyelitis
  - Other viral myelitides
  - Traumatic
  - Charcot-Marie-Tooth disease
  - Spinal muscular atrophy
    - Werdnig-Hoffmann disease (SMA type 1)
    - Kugelberg-Welander disease (SMA type 2)
  - Dysautonomia
    - Riley-Day syndrome
  - Combined upper and lower pathologies
    - Amyotrophic lateral sclerosis
    - Myelomeningocele
    - Tethered cord
- Primary myopathies
  - Muscular dystrophy
    - Duchenne muscular dystrophy
    - Limb-girdle dystrophy
    - Facioscapulohumeral dystrophy
  - Arthrogryposis
  - Congenital hypotonia
  - Myotonia dystrophica

NONOPERATIVE TREATMENT

OBSERVATION

Not all neuromuscular spinal deformities require immediate treatment. Small curves of less than 20 to 25 degrees can be observed carefully for progression before treatment is begun. Similarly, large curves in severely mentally retarded patients in whom the curve is not causing any functional disability or hindering nursing care can be observed. If progression of a small curve is noted, orthotic management may be considered if the patient can tolerate this form of treatment. If the functional ability of severely impaired patients is compromised by increasing curvature, treatment may be instituted.

ORTHOTIC TREATMENT

Progressive neuromuscular scoliosis in very young patients can be treated with an orthosis. The scoliosis often continues to progress despite orthotic treatment, but the rate of progression can be slowed, and further spinal growth can occur before definitive spinal fusion. The brace also can provide flaccid patients with trunk support, allowing the use of the upper extremities.

A custom-molded, total-contact TLSO usually is required for these children because their trunk contours do not accommodate standard braces. Most patients with neuromuscular scoliosis lack voluntary muscle control, normal righting reflexes, and the ability to cooperate with an active brace program; therefore, passive-type orthotics have been more successful in our experience in managing these neuromuscular curves. Patients with severe involvement and no head control frequently require custom-fabricated seating devices combined with orthoses or head-control devices.

A more malleable type of spinal brace, the soft Boston orthosis, is fabricated from a soft material that is well tolerated by patients, yet it is strong enough to provide good trunk support. The major complaint with the use of this brace has been heat retention.

Because of problems with brace treatment of neuromuscular patients, growing rods and rib-based techniques have been successfully used to control progressive neuromuscular curves. Several authors have reported improvement in the Cobb angle and pelvis with these techniques, but a deep wound infection rate of 30% also has been reported.

OPERATIVE TREATMENT

The goal of fusion in patients with neuromuscular scoliosis is to produce solid arthrodesis of the spine, balanced in both the coronal and sagittal planes and over a level pelvis. In doing so, the surgery should maximize function and improve the quality of life. To achieve this goal, a much longer fusion is necessary than usually is indicated for idiopathic scoliosis. Because of a tendency for cephalad progression of the deformity when fusion ends at or below the fourth thoracic vertebra, fusion should extend to T4 or above. The decision on the distal extent of the fusion generally is whether to fuse to the sacrum or to attempt to stop short of it. On occasion, the fusion can exclude the sacrum if the patient is an ambulator who requires lumbosacral motion, has no significant pelvic obliquity, and has a horizontal L5 vertebral body. Many of these patients, unfortunately, are nonambulators with a fixed spinopelvic obliquity. If the spinopelvic obliquity is fixed on bending or traction films (> 10 to 15 degrees of L4 or L5 tilt relative to the interiliac crest line), the caudal extent of the fusion usually is the sacrum or the pelvis. Maintaining physiologic lordosis in the lumbar spine is important in insensate patients who require fusion to the pelvis. This permits body weight to be distributed more equally beneath the ischial tuberosities and the posterior region of the thigh, reducing the risk of pressure sores over the coccyx and ischium. Bone-bank allograft usually is used to obtain a fusion.

PREOPERATIVE CONSIDERATIONS

Patients with neuromuscular scoliosis must have complete medical evaluations, including cardiac, pulmonary, and nutritional status. Many conditions, such as Duchenne muscular dystrophy and Friedreich ataxia, are associated with cardiac involvement. Most patients with neuromuscular scoliosis have diminished pulmonary function, and careful preoperative evaluation is essential. Nickel et al. found that patients with vital capacities of less than 30% of predicted normal required respiratory support postoperatively, and those with a similar decrease of vital capacity and without a voluntary cough reflex required tracheostomy. Some surgeons prefer to use a nasotracheal tube for postoperative respiratory assistance as long as necessary. Preoperatively, the patient should have pulmonary function studies if the patient is able to cooperate, and the vital capacity and forced expiratory volume in the first second are evaluated. This information is considered along with the patient's ability to cough and with measurement of arterial blood gas levels. Postoperative pulmonary management is then formulated in close consultation with a pulmonary specialist before surgery.

Patients with neuromuscular scoliosis often have suboptimal nutrition because of gastrointestinal problems, such as a hiatal hernia or gastroesophageal reflux. Surgery intensifies the preexisting state by raising the patient's metabolic requirements. The lack of coordination of the muscles around the mouth and pharynx often causes difficulties in swallowing. Appropriate nutritional therapy, including preoperative hyperalimentation, may help improve wound healing and decrease the possibility of postoperative infection. Surgical procedures such as a gastrostomy and a Nissen fundoplication can be helpful in improving nutrition and decreasing the possibility of problems with gastroesophageal reflux. Procedures to control oral secretions also can be beneficial, especially in patients with cerebral palsy.

Seizure disorders are common in patients with neuromuscular scoliosis, and preoperative anticonvulsant levels should be optimized within a therapeutic range. Osteopenia may be present because of the anticonvulsant medications. The preoperative use of valproic acid has also been shown to be associated with increased blood loss and need for blood transfusions.

Ambulatory status should be evaluated carefully before surgery. Often a patient with marginal ambulation capabilities and progressive scoliosis may not walk again after spinal surgery. The patient and the parents must understand this before surgery.

Techniques to minimize blood loss intraoperatively should be available, including electrocautery, hypotensive anesthesia, hemodilution techniques, and a cell saver. Use of antifibrinolytics has been shown to decrease intraoperative blood loss during posterior spinal fusion and instrumentation in neuromuscular scoliosis surgery. Dhawale et al. reported that tranexamic acid was more effective than epsilon-aminocaproic acid in decreasing blood loss in neuromuscular patients. Because of chronic anemia and poor nutrition, most patients with neuromuscular scoliosis are not suitable candidates for preoperative autodonation of blood.

Most patients with neuromuscular disease have insufficient autogenous bone; allograft bone usually is used to obtain a fusion and is an acceptable alternative.

As in other types of scoliosis surgery, the fusion levels and instrumentation must be determined preoperatively. The source of pelvic obliquity must be determined (Fig. 44-121). Ko et al. reported that more than half of cerebral palsy patients had more than 10 degrees of asymmetry in the transaxial plane between right and left sides of the pelvis. There was greater asymmetry in patients with windswept hips. Combined anterior and posterior arthrodeses may be required for severe pelvic obliquity. Other indications for a combined anterior and posterior approach include necessity for an anterior release for further correction of severe kyphosis, severe and rigid scoliosis that cannot be corrected by bending or traction to less than 60 degrees, and deficient posterior elements, such as those in patients with myelomeningocele. With the use of pedicle screws the need for anterior surgery has decreased. Most neuromuscular deformities can be treated with segmental

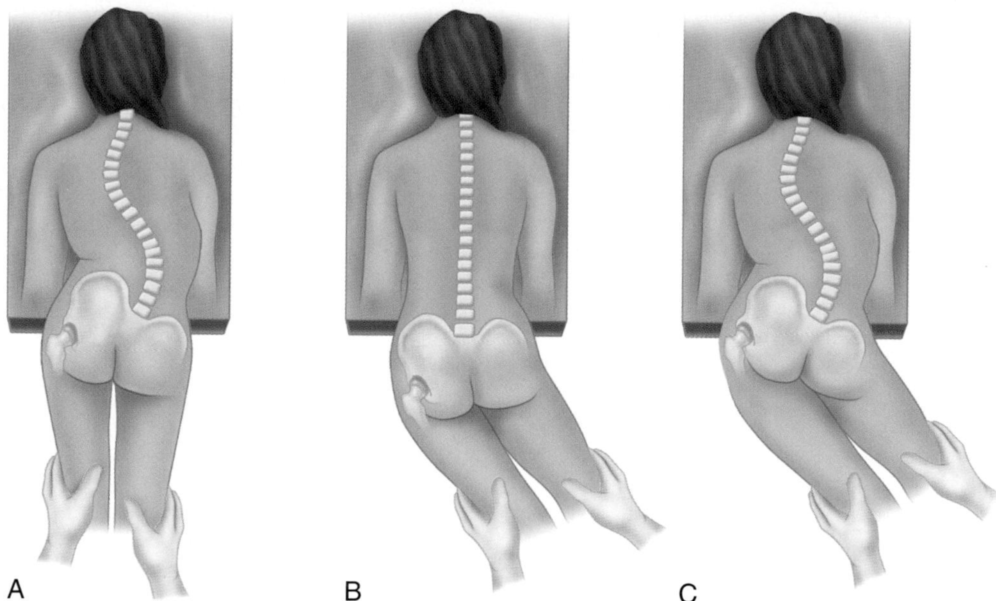

FIGURE 44-121 A, Pelvic obliquity. B, If pelvic obliquity is eliminated by abduction or adduction of hips, pelvic-femoral muscle contracture is cause. C, If obliquity persists despite abduction or adduction of hips, fixed spinal-pelvic deformity exists. (From Shook JE, Lubicky JP: Paralytic scoliosis. In Bridwell KH, DeWald RL, editors: The textbook of spinal surgery, ed 2, Philadelphia, 1997, Lippincott-Raven.)

instrumentation using pedicle screw fixation and supplemented with sublaminar cables as needed.

Finally, the patient's family should be clearly informed of the potential benefits and risks of any surgical procedure. The surgery is directed toward functional goals, such as sitting balance, pain relief, and improvement in fatigability, rather than toward any cosmetic improvement. These functional goals must be weighed against the potential risks of the procedure and must be documented in the patient's medical record.

OPERATIVE CONSIDERATIONS

The potential for intraoperative complications in patients with neuromuscular scoliosis is great. Death can result from anesthesia problems, although more frequently it occurs from postoperative pulmonary deterioration. Relative hypothermia can easily occur in a lengthy spinal operation in which a large area of tissue is exposed and can cause myocardial depression and arrhythmias. Spinal surgery is associated with greater blood loss in patients with neuromuscular disease than in patients with idiopathic scoliosis. The anesthesiologist should be aware of both of these potential problems and should be prepared for them with an arterial line, a central venous pressure line, temperature probes, and careful management of urine output. Because the curves generally are larger, more rigid, and more difficult to instrument, neurologic complications can occur during surgery. Many patients with neuromuscular scoliosis are unable to cooperate with an intraoperative wake-up test. Spinal cord monitoring can be a valuable technique in these patients. Schwartz et al. evaluated the safety of using transcranial motor-evoked potentials in neuromuscular patients. There were no episodes of seizures in any neuromuscular patients, including those with a history of epilepsy.

The surgical technique must include meticulous debridement of the soft tissue off the posterior elements of the spine. Ablation of the facet joints and a massive amount of bone graft are necessary. The bone frequently is osteopenic, and appropriate stable segmental instrumentation should be used. Anterior release and fusion can be considered in patients with large curves with a fixed spinal pelvic obliquity or in patients with posterior element deficiencies. Anterior instrumentation in neuromuscular curves may be used if needed, but it is rarely used. A 29% failure rate has been reported with pelvic fixation in neuromuscular patients. Myung et al. recommended placing bilateral pedicle screws at L5 and S1, in addition to two iliac screws, to decrease the failure rate of pelvic fixation in neuromuscular patients.

POSTOPERATIVE CONSIDERATIONS

Pulmonary problems are the most likely complications in the immediate postoperative period, and the assistance of a pulmonary specialist is invaluable. Ventilatory support may be necessary, and such techniques as suctioning, spirometers, and intermittent positive-pressure breathing may be appropriate. Possibly the best measure to prevent postoperative pulmonary problems is a spinal construct strong enough to allow early mobilization.

Fluid balance must be monitored carefully. After spinal surgery, especially in patients with neuromuscular scoliosis, antidiuretic hormone levels may be increased, leading to oliguria. If fluids are increased to overcome the oliguria, fluid overload may occur. This is especially disastrous in patients with impaired renal function, pulmonary compromise, and cardiac difficulties.

The necessity for postoperative orthotic support must be determined for each patient. If a complication, such as extremely osteopenic bone, compromises spinal fixation, or if less than ideal instrumentation is used, the use of postoperative external support may be wise. If the patient is so large, spastic, or dyskinetic that the spinal instrumentation may be excessively stressed, a postoperative orthosis may be considered.

Infection is a frequent problem in patients with neuromuscular scoliosis, probably because of the metabolically compromised host and the lengthy spinal fusions necessary. Patients with myelomeningocele and cerebral palsy have the highest infection rates. A major source of postoperative infection is the urinary tract. Any organisms found in the urine should be aggressively treated for 48 hours before surgery and for 3 months after surgery. Spinal infection is treated in the same manner as in patients with idiopathic scoliosis (see section on complications of posterior scoliosis surgery).

Pseudarthrosis with subsequent instrumentation failure is a potential late problem. If the pseudarthrosis causes pain or loss of correction, repair probably will be necessary, but asymptomatic pseudarthrosis without curve progression or pain can be observed.

LUQUE ROD INSTRUMENTATION WITH SUBLAMINAR WIRING

Eduardo Luque is credited with popularizing the use of long L-shaped rods and sublaminar wires in the surgical treatment of spinal deformity. The rods can be contoured, and the spine is corrected as the wires are tightened.

Wilber et al. noted neurologic changes in 17% of their patients with idiopathic scoliosis, but since surgeons have become more proficient with the technique, the incidence of neurologic injury has been much lower. The neurologic complications from sublaminar wires are of three types: cord injury, root injury, and dural tears. Root injuries are the most common and lead to hyperesthesia, but these generally resolve within 2 weeks. Delayed paraplegia and neurologic deficits have been reported in patients months after sublaminar wiring techniques. In a canine model, epidural and intramedullary hemorrhage, reactive epidural fibrosis, dural thinning and perforation, indentation of the dorsal surface of the spinal cord, cellular destruction within the spinal cord, and uncontrolled displacement of the sharp ends of the wires into the dural sac during wire extraction, were reported. Although sublaminar wires or cables have potential risks, we have found that for neuromuscular curves, the advantages of this type of segmental instrumentation far outweigh the potential risks.

The original Luque rods were L-shaped rods that were contoured to appropriate sagittal contours. Appropriately sized alloy rods are contoured to the appropriate sagittal contours and are connected proximally and distally with crosslinks. Originally, stainless-steel wires in diameters of 16- and 18-gauge were used. We now usually use sublaminar cables as opposed to the wire (see Technique 44-17).

LUQUE ROD INSTRUMENTATION AND SUBLAMINAR WIRES WITHOUT PELVIC FIXATION

TECHNIQUE 44-35

- The spine is exposed posteriorly as described in Technique 44-8.
- Wires or cables are passed as described in Technique 44-17.
- Two rods are used for most scoliosis corrections, with the first rod applied either to the convex or concave side of the curve. Lumbar scoliosis generally is more easily corrected by the concave rod technique. and because most neuromuscular curves include the lumbar spine and pelvis, the concave rod technique is most frequently used.
- Bend the appropriate amount of lordosis and kyphosis into the rods with the rod benders.
- Place the initial rod with its short limb passing transversely across the lamina of the lowermost vertebra to undergo instrumentation on the concave side.
- Pass it through the hole at the base of the spinous process if possible.
- Tighten the inferior double wire or cable on the concave side to supply firm fixation at the distal level. Now tighten the wires or cables to the lamina of the vertebra above the curve.
- Loosely attach the convex rod proximally after the short end has been placed loosely under the long limb of the concave rod. Once the concave rod has been completely tightened, it often is difficult to pass this short limb under the long limb of the concave rod.
- Reduce the spine to the rod by manual correction and a wire or cable tightener. An assistant can apply appropriate manual correction by pressure on the trunk as the wires or cables are tightened beneath the apex of the curvature (Fig. 44-122).
- As each wire or cable is tightened, more correction is obtained, and the twisting maneuver must be repeated two or three times on each wire to ensure a tight fit.
- Securely fasten the convex rod, tightening wires or cables from cephalad to caudad.
- Once in position, both rods usually can be brought into firm contact with the lamina by squeezing them together with the rod approximator. As this is done, the concave wires or cables will again loosen and must be tightened.
- Trim the wires to about ½ inch in length and bend them toward the midline.
- With the internal fixation device in place, very little bone is exposed for decortication and facet excision. We prefer to excise the facets if at all possible.
- A large volume of bone graft is necessary, and cancellous bone is harvested from the posterior iliac crest. Because the instrumentation often includes the iliac crest (see Technique 44-37), allograft bone usually is necessary. Place the graft lateral to the rods on both sides of the spine and out to the tips of the transverse processes. If possible, place bone graft between the wires, along the laminae.

SACROPELVIC FIXATION

Many patients with neuromuscular problems require instrumentation and fusion to the sacrum. O'Brien described three fixation zones for sacropelvic fixation (Fig. 44-123). Examples of zone I fixation include S1 sacral screws and a McCarthy S-rod. Zone II fixation includes S2 screws and the Jackson intrasacral rod technique (see later section on combined

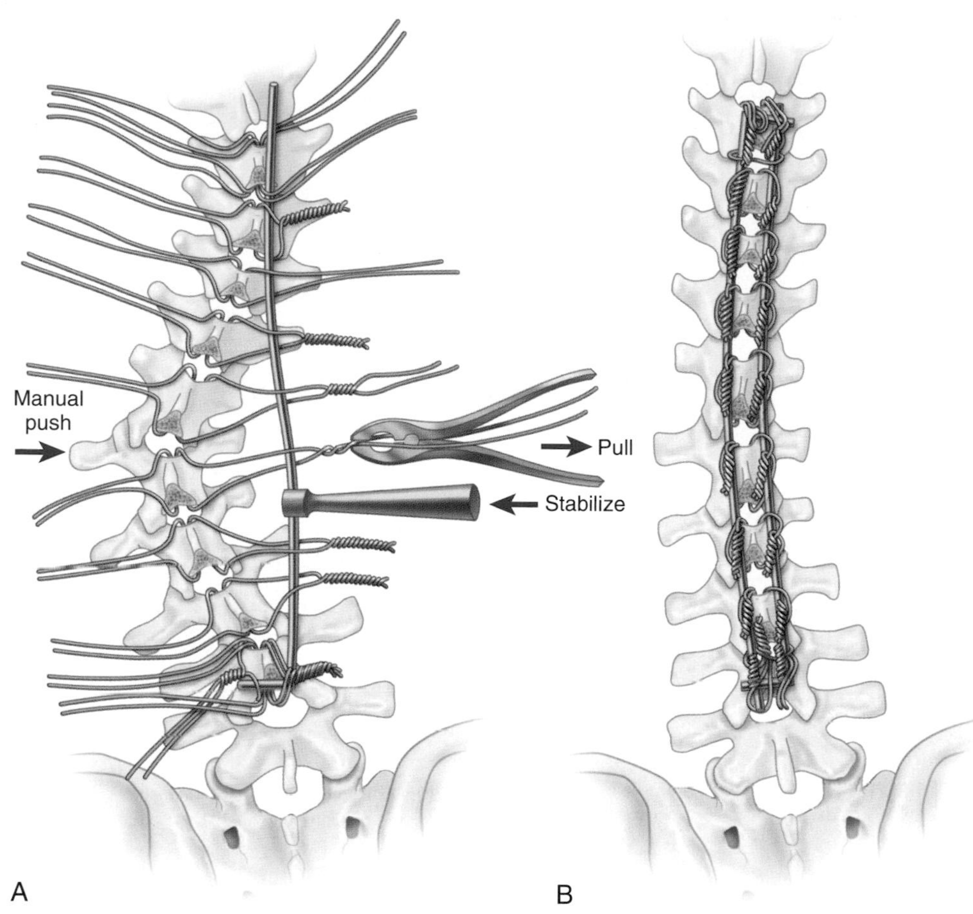

FIGURE 44-122 **A and B, Concave rod technique for correction of lumbar scoliosis.** (From Segmental spinal fixation and correction using Richards' L-rod instrumentation, Memphis, TN, Smith & Nephew Richards.) **SEE TECHNIQUE 44-35.**

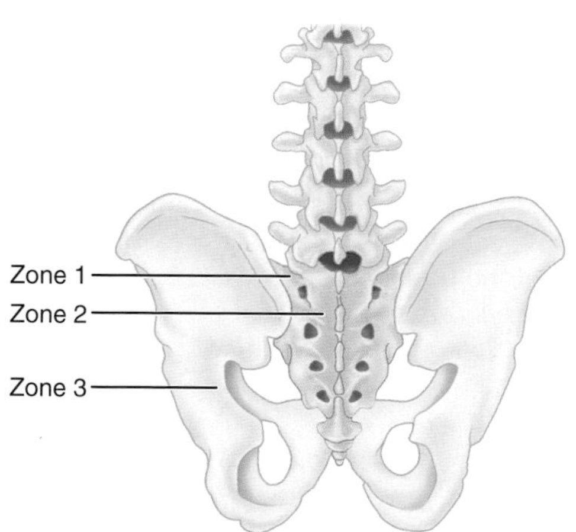

FIGURE 44-123 Sacropelvic fixation zones.

anterior and posterior fusion for scoliosis in patients with myelomeningocele). Zone III fixation includes the Galveston L-rod technique and sacroiliac screws.

If fixation to the pelvis is necessary, McCarthy has described an S-rod technique (Fig. 44-124). These two rods are crosslinked at the lumbosacral junction (Fig. 44-125) and then fixed with a combination of hooks, pedicle screws, and sublaminar wires or cables bilaterally throughout the lumbar and thoracic spine. The rods generally are crosslinked below the upper fixation to provide further stability against migration or rotation of the rods. We have found that if hooks or screws are not used at the upper end, wires alone provide no support against axial loading.

The advantages of the S-rod are that firm fixation is provided around the sacral ala without crossing the sacroiliac joint and that harvesting of bone graft from the ilium is not a problem because the ilium is not violated as it is when the Galveston technique is used. Prebent S-rods are available; complex bends cannot be done effectively at the time of surgery. The rods can be further contoured with a rod bender at the time of surgery to accommodate the size of the sacrum and to provide the appropriate sagittal plane correction.

SACROPELVIC FIXATION

TECHNIQUE 44-36

(MCCARTHY)

- Expose the spine posteriorly as described in Technique 44-8.
- Perform careful dissection of the sacral ala, using a curet to clean the superior edge. Use finger dissection ventrally.

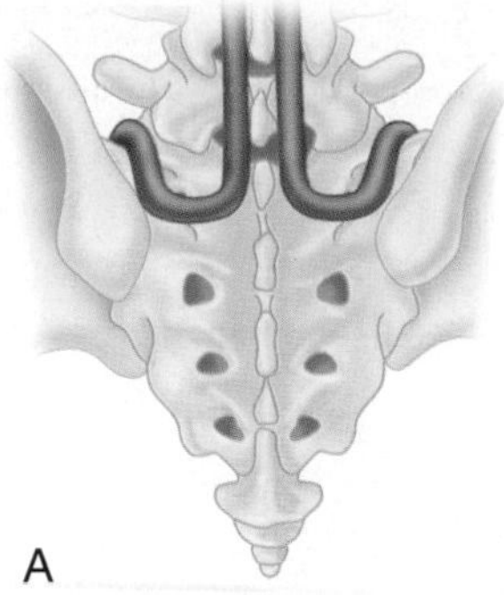

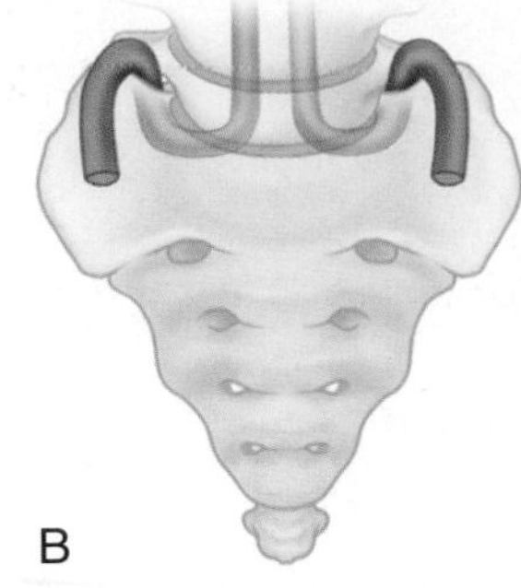

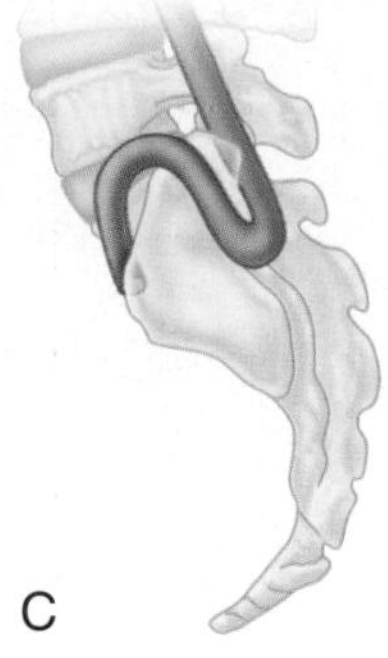

FIGURE 44-124 **A-C,** S-rods are manufactured as a pair to fit over the right and left sacral alae for fixation to the sacrum without crossing the sacroiliac joint. They are available in $\frac{3}{16}$-inch and $\frac{1}{4}$-inch rods.

- The rods come in different sizes and contours. In most instances, a 5.5-mm rod provides satisfactory fit to the sacral ala.
- Contour the rods to appropriate sagittal contours.
- Place the S-rod over the sacral ala from posterior to anterior in a position adjacent to the anterior border of the sacroiliac joint. It lies posterior to the L5 nerve root and roughly parallel to it.
- Seat the S-portion of the rod firmly against the sacral ala by distraction between an L4-level hook or pedicle screw. The rods then can be used as a firm fixation point for translation or correction of scoliotic deformities or by placing the right and left rods simultaneously and cross-linking them, applying a strong cantilever corrective force for correction of pelvic obliquity. Crosslinking the two S-rods provides stability and eliminates the increased time and difficulty of insertion of rods into the ilium.
- Elevate the medial aspect of the iliac apophysis and rotate it over the top of the S-rod on the sacral ala.
- Provide bone graft to encase the S-rod into the sacrum.

GALVESTON SACROPELVIC FIXATION

Another popular method for achieving sacropelvic fixation is the Galveston technique described by Allen and Ferguson in which the pelvis is stabilized by driving a segment of the L-rod into each ilium (Fig. 44-126). The rod is inserted into the posterior iliac crest and rests between the cortices above the sciatic notch. This fixation provides immediate firm stability and is biomechanically a stable construct. There are potential disadvantages, however, because the rod crosses the sacroiliac joint. It is postulated that motion in the sacroiliac joint is responsible for a "halo" that is often seen around the end of the Galveston rod in the iliac wing. Whether this radiographic phenomenon actually results in clinical problems is unknown. In a biomechanical comparison of 10 lumbosacral fixation techniques, McCord et al. found that the most secure fixation of the lumbosacral joint was obtained by extending the fixation anterior to the projected lateral image of the middle column as in the Galveston technique.

TECHNIQUE 44-37

(ALLEN AND FERGUSON)

- Expose both iliac crests from the midline incision at the level of the posterior superior iliac spine. Expose the iliac crest to the sciatic notch. The area just proximal to the sciatic notch provides the most satisfactory fixation.
- Use a large, smooth Steinmann pin corresponding to the size of the rod diameter or a pedicle awl to create a tunnel for the rod. The insertion site is just posterior to the sacroiliac joint at the level of the posterior inferior iliac spine, distal to the posterior superior iliac spine, along the transverse bar of the ilium. The area for insertion often is difficult to identify, and the rod may be inserted too superiorly.
- Carefully identify the area for insertion and use a rongeur to carefully remove soft tissue and bone to expose the inner and outer tables of the ilium.
- Drill the Steinmann pin to a depth of 6 to 9 cm.
- Asher et al. described use of a pedicle awl for pin insertion. This allows tactile perception to determine whether the awl is perforating the cortex of the ilium.
- Use a rongeur to remove enough cartilage and cortical bone to create a 1 × 1-cm entry site into the inferior portion of the posterior superior iliac spine. This exposes the intramedullary space.
- Introduce a blunt-tipped pedicle awl into the intracortical space and advance it by gentle oscillating pressure on the handle of the awl.
- Direct the awl to 2 cm above the sciatic notch and advance it to the appropriate depth of the rod in the ilium (Fig. 44-127).
- Now use a flexible ball-tipped pedicle probe to ensure that the hole made by the blunt-tipped probe is completely intracortical. Place the smooth Steinmann pin into the iliac hole.

ROD CONTOURING (ASHER)

- Preparation of the rod is made easier by the use of a variable-radius bender set. To prepare the rod for iliac (Galveston) placement, four measurements are needed: (1) the length of the intrailiac portion of the rod (Fig. 44-128A), (2) the transverse plane angle of the iliac

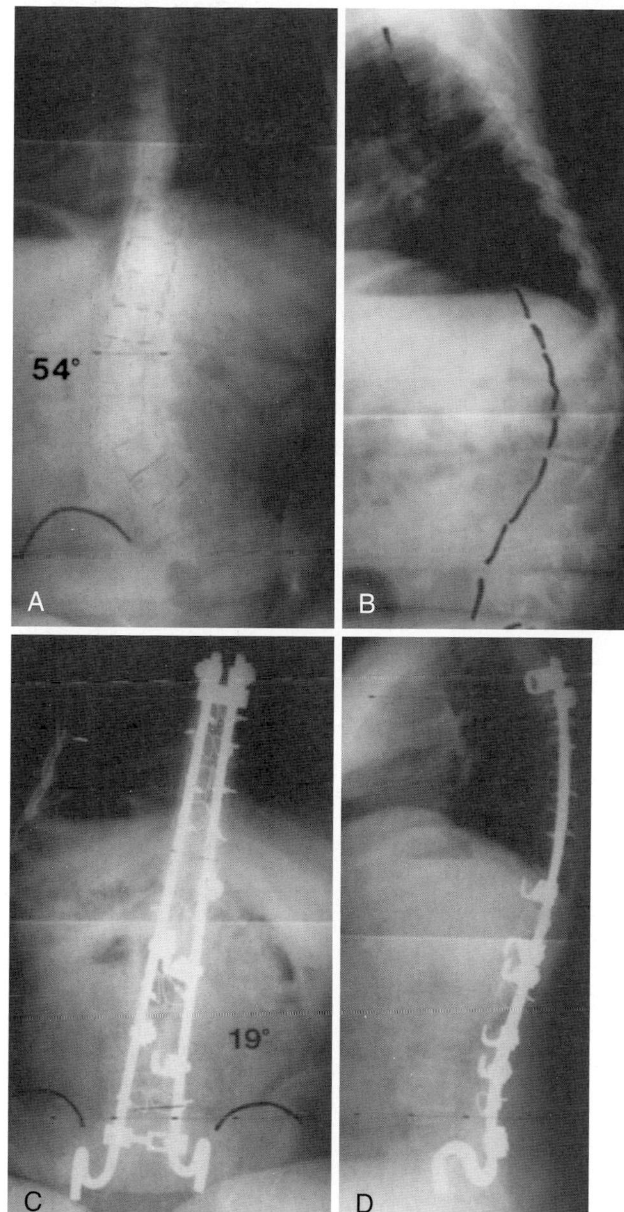

FIGURE 44-125 Nine-year-old girl with spinal muscular atrophy and curve of 54 degrees and pelvic obliquity measuring 15 degrees. She was treated with combination of S-rods, TSRH hooks, and Songer cables. Her postoperative curve measured 19 degrees with pelvic obliquity of 0 degrees. **A** and **B,** Preoperative anteroposterior and lateral views. **C** and **D,** Postoperative anteroposterior and lateral views. (From McCarthy RE, Saer EH: The treatment of flaccid neuromuscular scoliosis. In Bridwell KH, DeWald RL, editors: The textbook of spinal surgery, ed 2, Philadelphia, 1997, Lippincott-Raven.)

fixation site to the midsagittal plane (Fig. 44-128B), (3) the medial-lateral distance from the iliac entry site to the intended line of longitudinal passage of the rod along the spine (Fig. 44-128C), and (4) the length of the rod needed from the sacrum to the most cephalad instrumentation site.

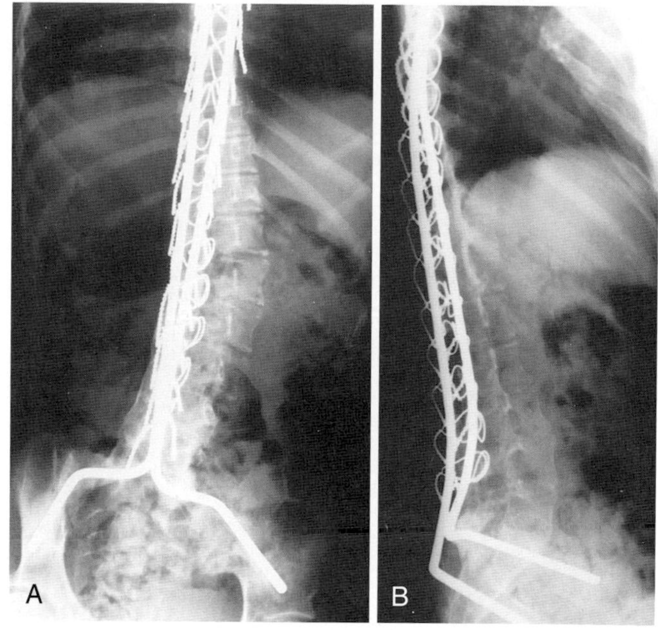

FIGURE 44-126 **A** and **B,** Stabilization of pelvis with Galveston technique. Segment of rod is driven into each ilium. **SEE TECHNIQUE 44-37.**

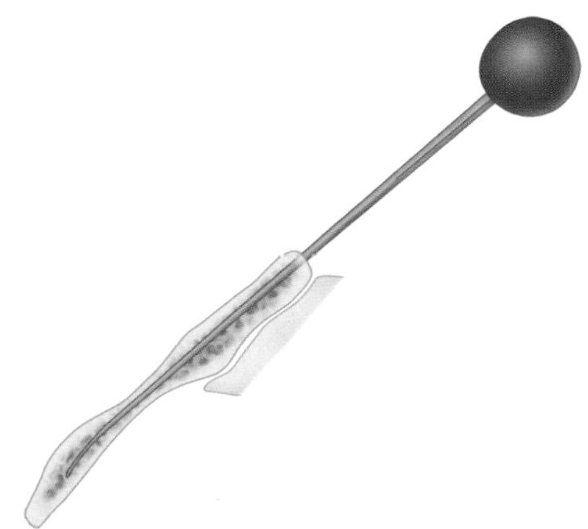

FIGURE 44-127 Intracortical passage of pedicle probe in ilium. **SEE TECHNIQUE 44-37.**

- Lay suture along the spine line from the sacrum to the facet above the last instrumented vertebra; its length plus 1 cm is the usual length for this portion of the rod.
- Add the first and third measurements; a right-angle bend is placed at this distance from one end (Fig. 44-128D); this is the iliosacral portion of the rod.
- The medial-lateral distance (measurement 3) minus approximately 3 mm to allow for the bend is from the middle of the right-angle bend. Mark this at the iliosacral portion of the rod.
- After the right-left orientation is verified, place an angle identical to that of the iliac fixation site to the midsagittal plane at this second mark (Fig. 44-128E). This separates the iliosacral portion of the rod into the iliac and sacral portions.

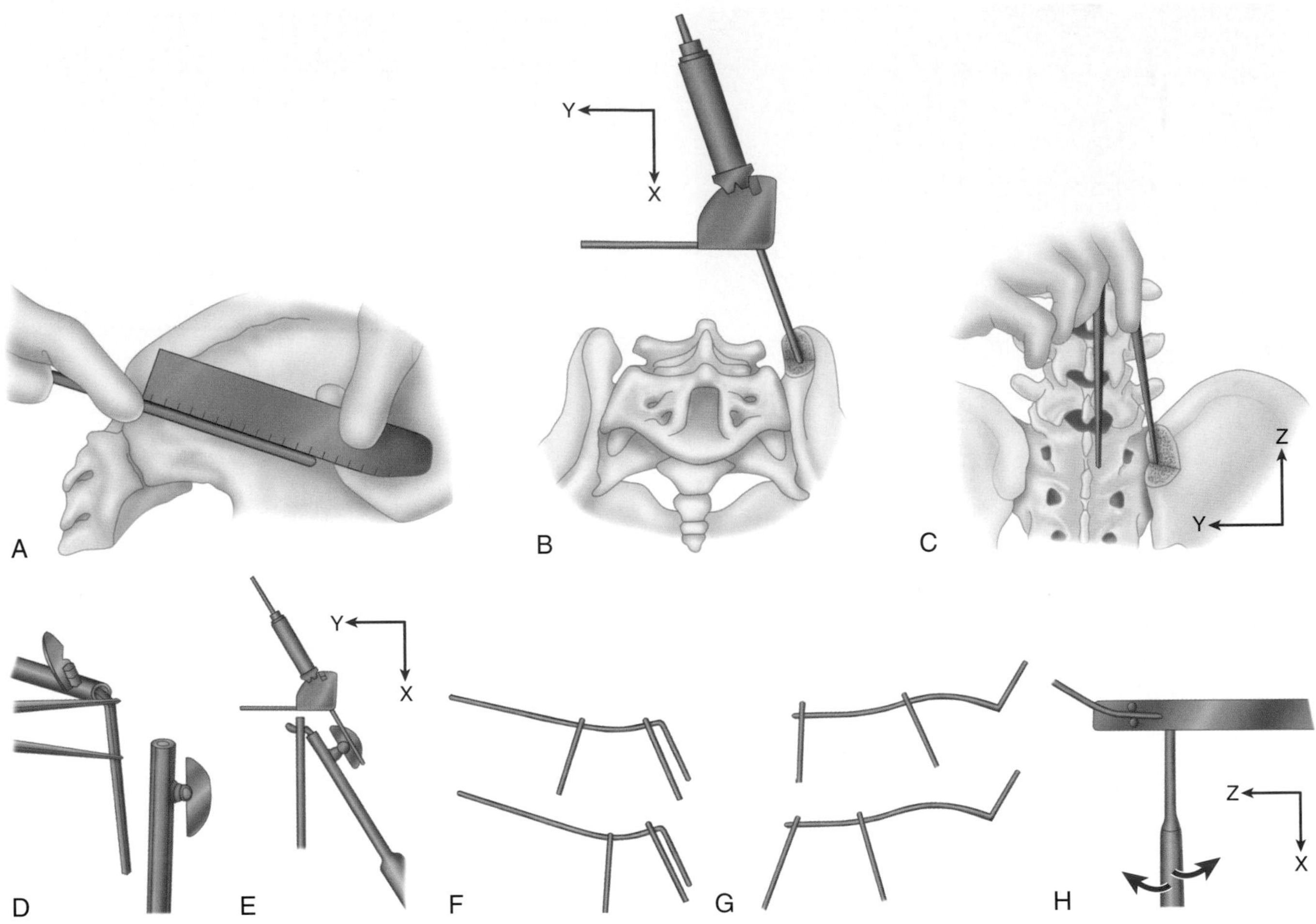

FIGURE 44-128 Technique of Asher. **A,** Length of intrailiac portion of rod. **B,** Transverse angle of iliac fixation site in midsagittal plane. **C,** Coronal plane distance from iliac entry site to intended line of longitudinal passage along spine. **D,** Right-angle bend. **E,** Iliosacral axial plane bend. **F,** Placement of long- and short-radius lordosis. **G,** Placement of long and short thoracic kyphosis. **H,** Sagittal plane iliac angle adjustment. (Redrawn from Boachie-Adjei O, Asher MA: Isola instrumentation for scoliosis. In McCarthy R, editor: Spinal instrumentation techniques, vol 2, Rosemont, IL, 1998, Scoliosis Research Society.) **SEE TECHNIQUE 44-37.**

- Add sagittal plane bends, beginning at L5-S1, thus leaving a straight portion over the sacrum. Because lordosis is not uniform but is greater in the lower lumbar spine, two contours are necessary. The contour for the entire lumbar spine is a long radius, whereas that for the lower lumbar spine is shorter (Fig. 44-128F).
- Add thoracic kyphosis, again by use of the flat benders (Fig. 44-128G).
- Attempt a trial placement to check whether the sagittal plane bend of the sacroiliac bend is correct. This can be determined by measuring the distance from the rod to the spine at the cephalad and caudal levels of the rod.
- Make final sagittal plane iliac angle adjustments with flat bender posts and a tube bender (Fig. 44-128H).
- The Galveston technique can be combined with a multiple-hook or pedicle screw segmental system with crosslinks if desired (Fig. 44-129A and B).

UNIT ROD INSTRUMENTATION WITH PELVIC FIXATION

When two unlinked L-rods are used, the rods may translate with respect to one another and compromise control of pelvic obliquity. In addition, twisting within the laminar wires can result in rotation of one rod relative to another. The $\frac{1}{4}$-inch rods generally used in neuromuscular patients are difficult to bend so that they can conform to the complex three-dimensional curves of the spine. In response to these problems, Bell et al. developed the unit rod. The unit rod is a single continuous $\frac{1}{4}$-inch stainless-steel rod with a U bend at the top and "bullet-ended" pelvic legs for implantation into the pelvis (Fig. 44-130). The three-dimensional preshaped kyphosis, lordosis, and pelvic legs were devised from a database of patients without spinal deformity. Eight lengths of rod are available, increasing in

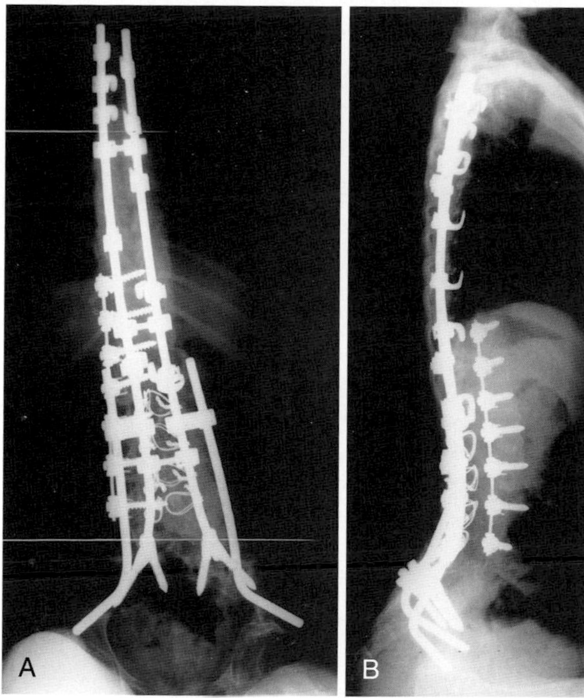

FIGURE 44-129 A and B, Instrumentation with multiple-hook segmental fixation and domino-type crosslinks. **SEE TECHNIQUE 44-37.**

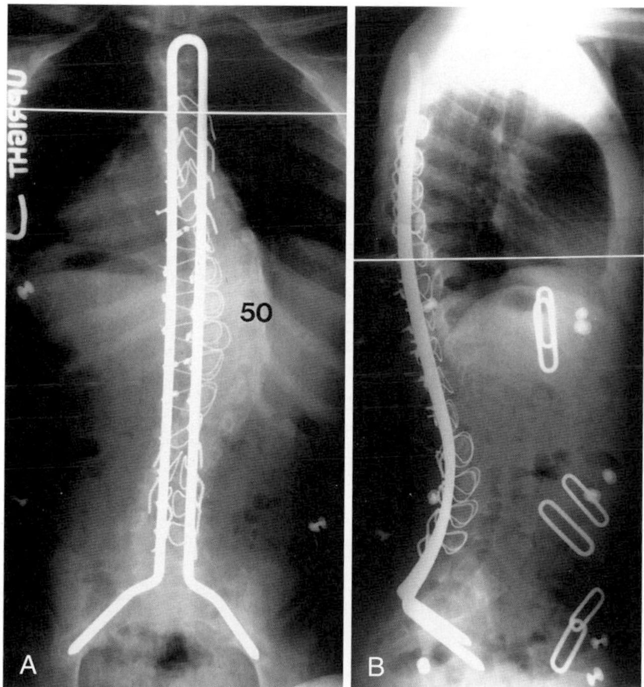

FIGURE 44-130 A and B, Unit rod for neuromuscular scoliosis developed by Bell, Moseley, and Koreska. Single, continuous ¼-inch stainless steel rod has U-shaped bend at top and bullet-shaped ends for insertion into pelvis. **SEE TECHNIQUE 44-38.**

20-cm increments from 310 to 450 cm. Right and left iliac guides facilitate drilling into the posterior ilia and subsequent introduction of the pelvic legs. The length of the iliac legs decreases proportionally as the rod shortens. The unit rod attempts to normalize body alignment in both the sagittal and coronal planes by establishing normal lordosis and kyphosis and correcting pelvic obliquity. We have not found the unit rod satisfactory for extremely rigid curves unless an anterior release or wedge osteotomies are done to reduce the spinal stiffness. If, however, the curves seem relatively flexible on bending films or physical examination, correcting to less than 40 degrees, we have had excellent results with the use of the unit rod.

TECHNIQUE 44-38

- Expose the spine as described in Technique 44-6. Expose both iliac crests to the posterior superior iliac spine and down to the sciatic notch.
- Mark a ¼-inch drill with a marking pen at 15 mm longer than the sciatic notch if the child weighs more than 45 kg and at 10 mm if the child weighs less than 45 kg.
- Place the appropriate right or left drill guide into the sciatic notch. Keep the lateral handle of the drill guide parallel to the pelvis (Fig. 44-131A) and the axial handle of the drill guide parallel to the body axis (Fig. 44-131B).
- Start the drill hole as far inferiorly on the posterior superior iliac crest as possible (Fig. 44-131C).
- Drill a hole in the ilium to the marked depth and check the hole with a wire to make certain the cortex has not been penetrated.
- Use a similar technique on the opposite iliac crest.
- Pass the sublaminar wires.
- Measure the length of the rod by placing the rod upside down, with the corner of the rod at the drilled hole on the elevated side of the pelvis. If kyphosis is severe, choose one length shorter because the kyphotic spine shortens as it corrects. If pelvic obliquity is severe, test the length from both the high and low sides and choose an intermediate length. If the rod is placed and turns out to be too long, it may be necessary to cut off the superior end; the upper end then can be connected with a crosslink.
- Cross the legs of the appropriate-length rod and insert them first into the hole on the low side of the pelvic obliquity (Fig. 44-132A). Cross the rod so that the leg going into the low side is underneath the other leg.
- Insert approximately one half to three fourths of the leg length into the hole. Then insert the next leg by holding it with a rod holder and guiding it into the correct direction of the hole.
- Use the impactor and drive the rod leg in by alternately impacting each leg (Fig. 44-132B). Be certain that each rod leg is impacted in the exact direction of the hole or the cortex may be penetrated.
- Once the rod is firmly seated, use the proximal end of the rod as a "rudder" to bring the distal end of the rod to the spine (Fig. 44-132C).
- Do not push the rod down completely into the wound in one move because this may pull the legs out of the pelvis or fracture the ilium. Instead, push the rod to line it up

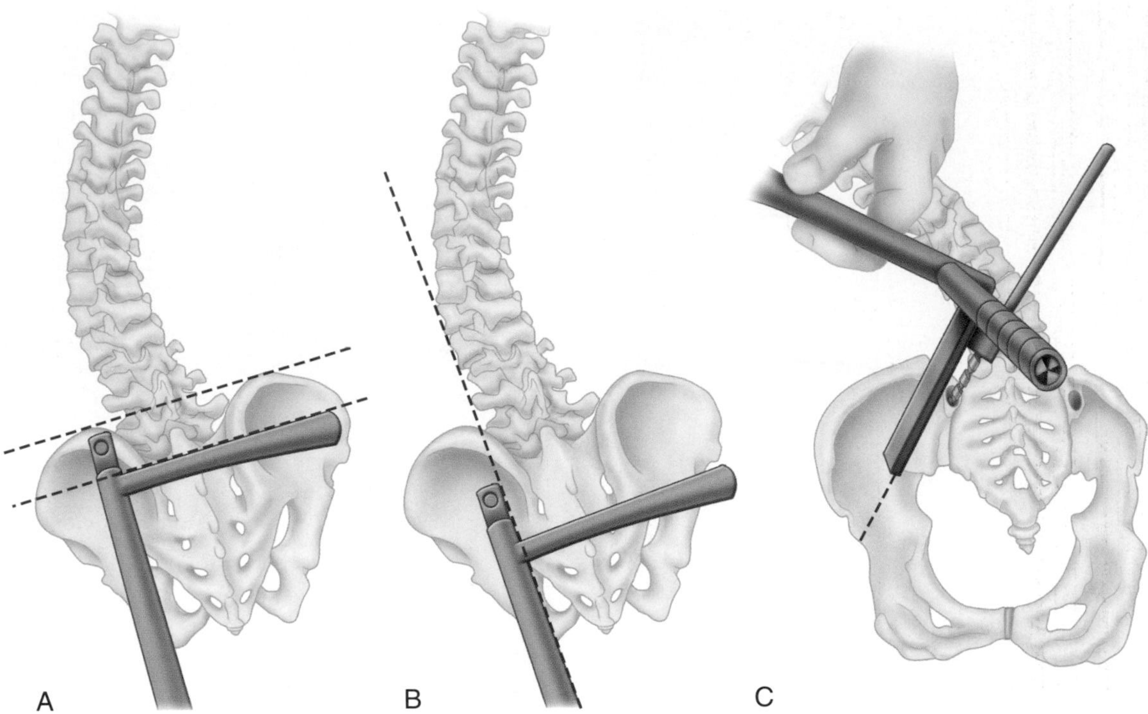

FIGURE 44-131 **Unit rod instrumentation. A, Lateral handle of drill guide is kept parallel to pelvis. B, Axial handle is kept parallel to body axis. C, Drill hole started inferiorly on posterior superior iliac crest.** (**C** redrawn from Miller F, Dabney KW: Unit rod procedure for neuromuscular scoliosis. In McCarthy R, editor: Spinal instrumentation techniques, vol 2, Rosemont, IL, 1998, Scoliosis Research Society.) **SEE TECHNIQUE 44-38.**

with the L5 lamina only and tie these wires down with a jet wire twister.

- Now push the rod to the L4 vertebra, twist the wires, and cut them off.
- Tighten the wires from caudad to cephalad one level at a time. Do not relax the push on the rod between the levels of the major curve or too much load may be applied to the end vertebra. Do not use the wires themselves to pull the rod down to the lamina or the wires will cut through the lamina.
- After all the wires have been tightened, go back and verify that all previously tightened wires are well seated.
- Cut the wires at 10- to 15-mm lengths.
- Bend all wires into the midline of the rod and direct them caudally (Fig. 44-132D).
- Apply bone graft. Bank bone usually is needed because the iliac crest is used for pelvic fixation.

ILIAC FIXATION WITH ILIAC SCREWS

Iliac screws provide secure and rigid pelvic fixation, which has the advantage of not having prefixed angles for pelvic fixation.

TECHNIQUE 44-39

- After the spine is exposed, dissect laterally underneath the spinal fascia to reach the medial aspect of the iliac wing at its very distal aspect.
- Identify the posterior superior iliac spine. The starting point for screw placement is 1 cm inferior to the posterior superior iliac spine and 1 cm proximal to the distal edge of the posterior superior iliac spine (Fig. 44-133A). If required, expose the lateral aspect of the iliac wing to help with the trajectory of the pathway down the iliac bone (Fig. 44-133B).
- With a 4-mm burr, create a medial cortical defect at the appropriate starting point.
- By use of an iliac probe or pedicle probe with the tip facing medially and the trajectory 45 degrees caudal and lateral, tunnel down between the cortices of the ilium (Fig. 44-133C). It is more likely to exit laterally than medially. That is the reason for the probe to face medially. The ideal placement of the screw will be just cephalad to the superior gluteal notch, which is the thickest part of the ilium.
- Once the tunnel has been formed with the probe, use a flexible ball-tip sounding probe to palpate the intraosseous borders of the ilium to confirm intraosseous placement of the screw. Tap the tunnel if necessary.
- Various angles are available on the screw heads to allow easier placement of the connector rods. Screw trials are used to determine which type of screw best fits the patient's anatomy. Select an appropriate-sized screw.
- Insert the screw with the screwdriver. If angled screw heads are used, each angle screw has its own screwdriver. Once the screw is placed snuggly into the ilium, it is important that the top of the screw head rest below the

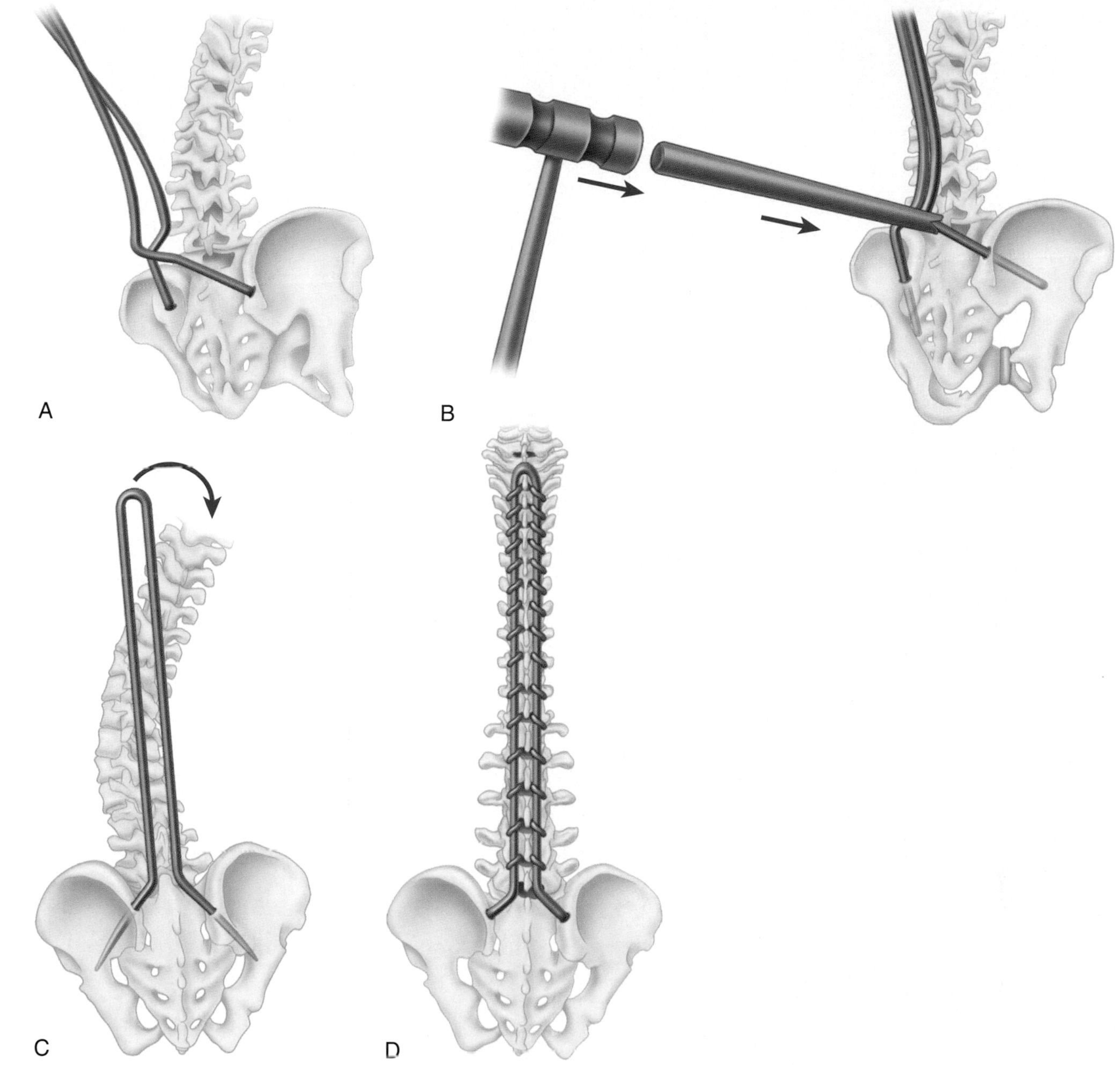

FIGURE 44-132 Unit rod instrumentation, *continued.* **A,** One leg of rod is placed into low side of pelvic obliquity first. **B,** Impactor is used to drive rod legs into pelvis. **C,** Once rod is firmly seated, proximal end can be used as rudder to bring distal end to spine. **D,** Wires are bent into midline of rod and directed caudally. **SEE TECHNIQUE 44-38.**

top of the posterior superior iliac spine (Fig. 44-133D). This ensures that the screw will not be prominent postoperatively.

- Position the screw head facing directly medial to allow the lateral connector to engage and thus keep the rod vertical in its orientation.
- Determine the length of the lateral connector after placing and aligning the more cephalad spinal instrumentation; the goal is a vertical rod with only sagittal plane and minimal coronal plane bending.
- Once the offset is determined, cut the lateral connector to length and insert it into the screw head and provisionally tighten the screw.
- Insert the rod into the lateral connector and cantilever it down into the cephalad spinal instrumentation (Fig. 44-133E).
- Place the set screw for the lateral connector and provisionally tighten it.
- When all implants are securely in place, perform final tightening and break off the set screw head (Fig. 44-133F).

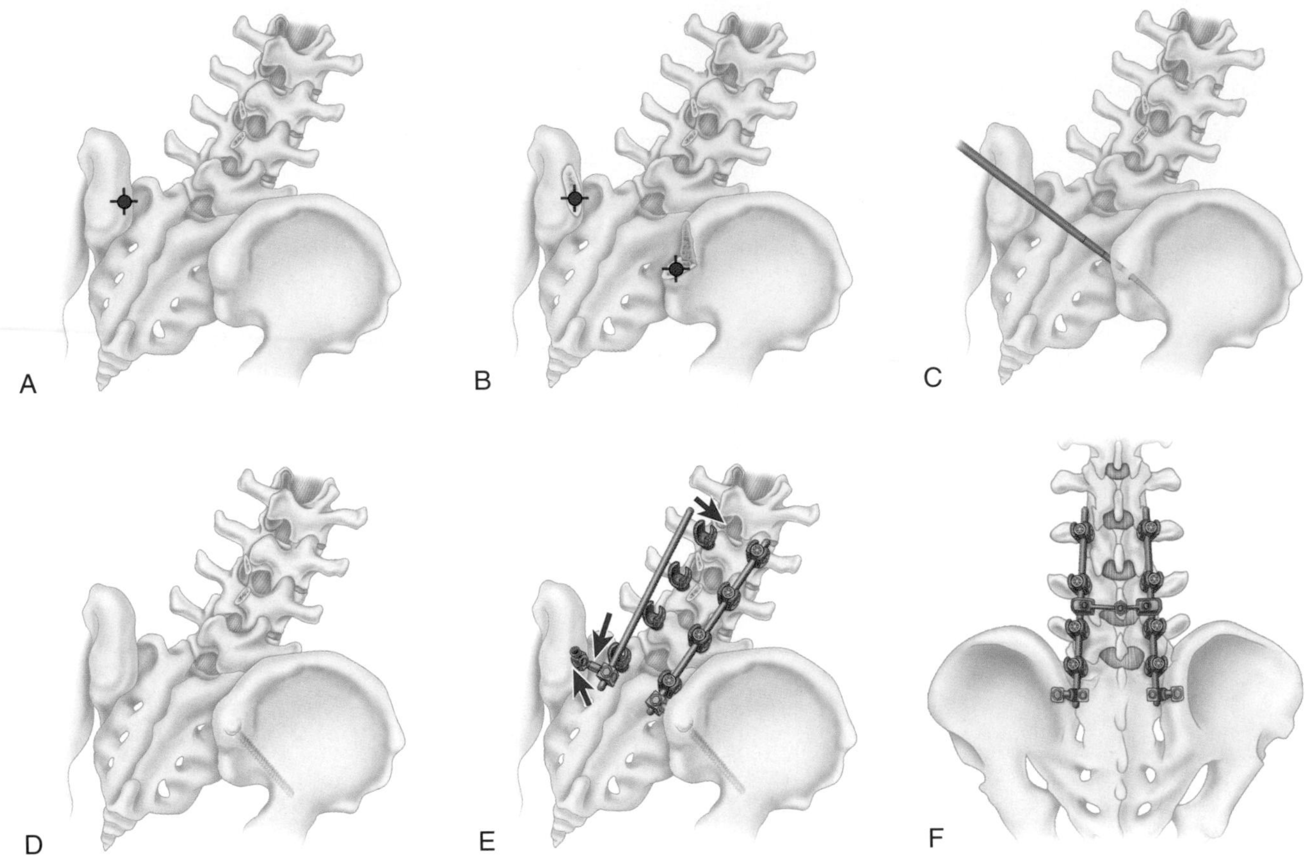

FIGURE 44-133 **A-F, Iliac fixation with CD Horizon Legacy spinal system. See text for description.** (Redrawn from Lenke LG, King AG: CD Horizon Legacy iliac fixation spinal system technical guide, Memphis, TN, 2004, Medtronic Sofamor Danek.) **SEE TECHNIQUE 44-39.**

POSTOPERATIVE CARE. Postoperative immobilization is not recommended after L-rod or unit-rod instrumentation. However, because neuromuscular curves frequently are associated with osteoporosis, spasticity, inability of the patient to cooperate, and severe curves, postoperative immobilization in a TLSO for 3 to 6 months may be needed if there is any question about stability of the instrumentation construct.

S2 ILIAC LUMBOPELVIC SCREW PLACEMENT

The screws in this technique do not require a separate skin or fascial incision, and average lengths of 70 to 100 mm are attainable. Additionally, this fixation does not interfere with aggressive iliac crest harvest. However, O'Brien et al. reported articular cartilage violation in 60% and noted that biomechanical strength of the S2 iliac screw technique has not been evaluated. The advantages of this technique are reduced implant prominence and placement of the iliac screw in line with other spinal anchors, thus avoiding acute bends in the rod to obtain pelvic fixation. Myung et al. recommended this technique to allow for six points of fixation distal to L4 with pelvic instrumentation.

ILIAC AND LUMBOSACRAL FIXATION WITH SACRAL-ALAR-ILIAC SCREWS

TECHNIQUE 44-40

- Place the patient prone on a radiolucent table, ensuring that the pelvis is as neutral as possible with minimal rotation.
- Extend a midline skin incision to expose the dorsal foramina of the sacrum, specifically the S1 and S2 foramina. Additional lateral dissection to the iliac crest is not needed.
- Stand on the contralateral side of the patient to identify the starting point. Find the midpoint between the S1 and S2 dorsal foramina and the lateral border of the foramen; the starting point is where these two lines intersect (Fig. 44-134A). This starting point should be in line with the S1 pedicle screw.
- Be aware that the entry point may vary with the local anatomy of the patient. If the pelvis is asymmetric in the transverse plane, as is common in patients with genetic or neuromuscular disorders, the starting point may need to vary in the mediolateral plane.

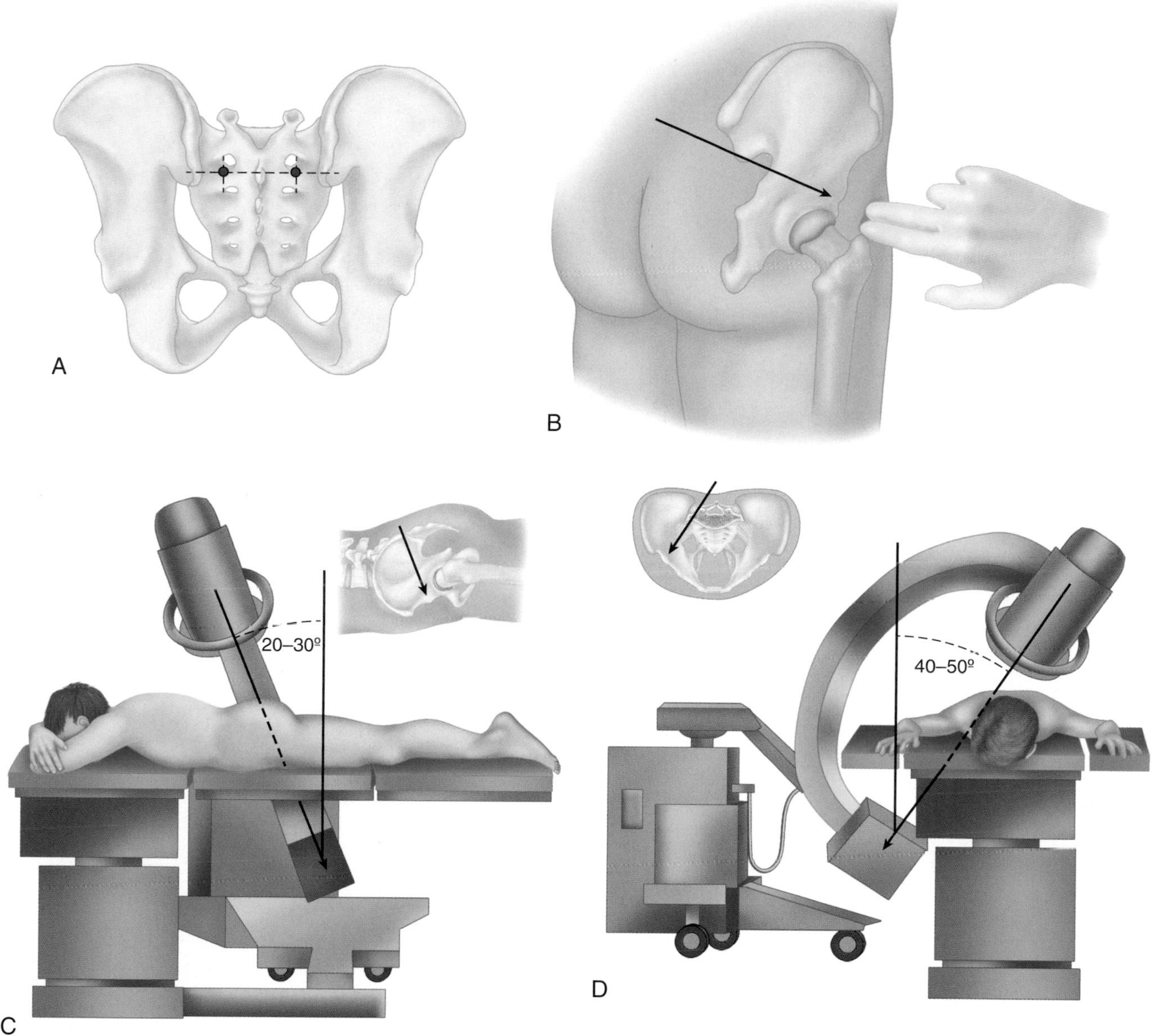

FIGURE 44-134 Iliac and lumbosacral fixation with sacral-alar-iliac screws. **A,** Starting point for screw insertion. **B,** Screw trajectory. **C** and **D,** Fluoroscopic confirmation of appropriate trajectory.

Continued

- Determine the proper trajectory of the sacral-alar-iliac fixation. Aim for the anterior inferior iliac spine, which can be found by palpating the top of the greater trochanter (Fig. 44-134B). The trajectory should pass immediately above the sciatic notch.
- To use fluoroscopy to identify the appropriate trajectory, orient the C-arm in the intended trajectory and position it above the starting point. Then angle the C-arm 20 to 30 degrees caudal (Fig. 44-134C) and 40 to 50 degrees to the vertical plane (Fig. 44-134D), aiming for the anterior inferior iliac spine. With this trajectory, the iliac teardrop should be visible on the anteroposterior fluoroscopic image (Figs. 44-134E).
- Use an awl and probe or pelvic 2.5-mm drill bit to verify the correct trajectory. The path of the probe or drill should be within 20 mm of the greater sciatic notch and aiming toward the anterior inferior iliac spine (Fig. 44-134F). This trajectory may vary with pelvic obliquity and lumbar lordosis.
- If using a drill, feel for the bony end point after each advancement of the drill. Once the drill crosses the sacroiliac joint, use a 3.2-mm drill bit to avoid breaking the smaller bit in the ilium. Alternatively, an awl can be used in a dysplastic pelvis.
- Obtain a teardrop fluoroscopic image to ensure that the anterior-posterior trajectory is within the thickest part of the ilium, without a cortical breach.
- Use a ball-tipped probe to palpate the course of the screw and confirm the bony end point. Note the appropriate screw length as shown on the ball-tipped probe or on the tap.

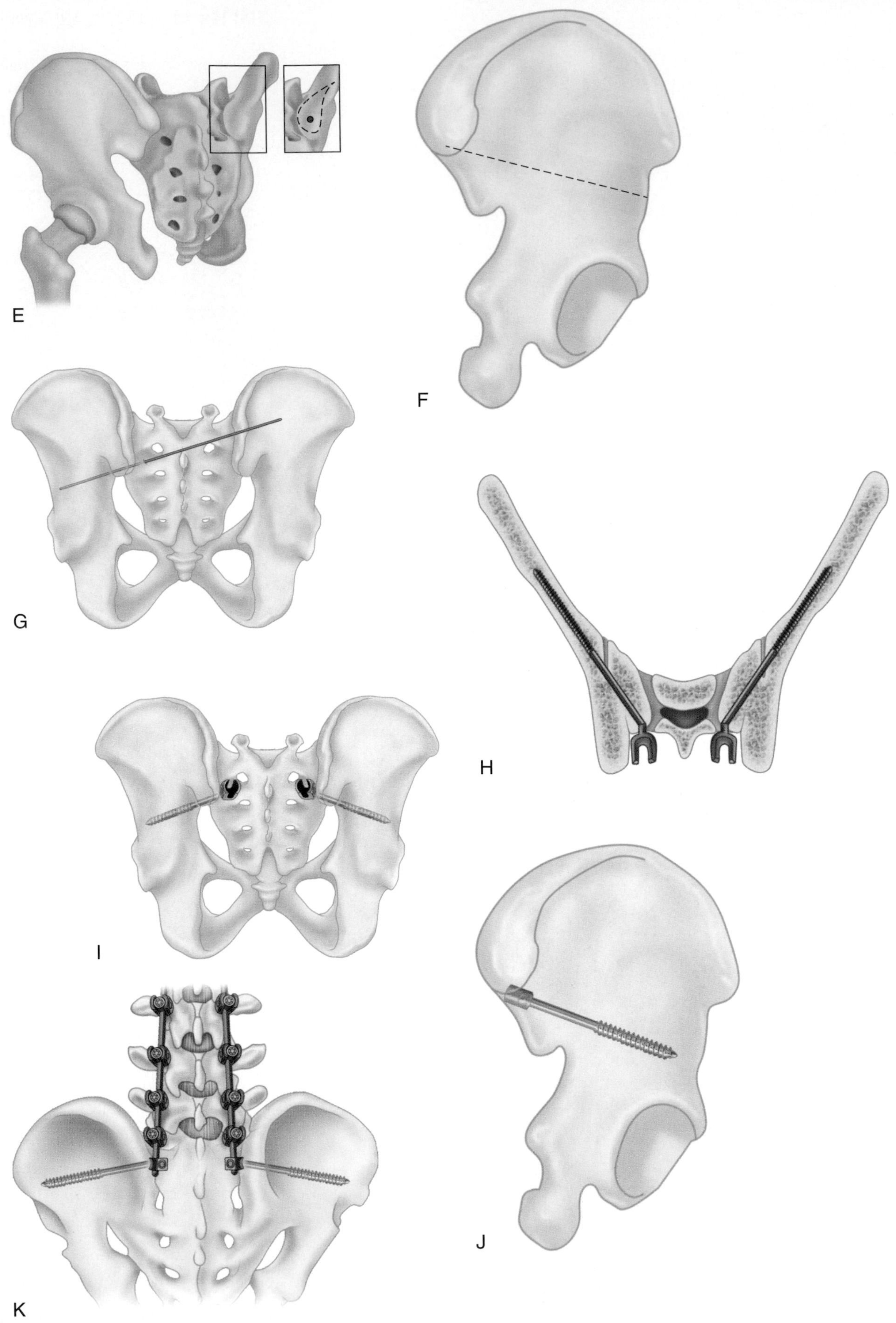

FIGURE 44-134, cont'd **E,** With proper trajectory, iliac teardrop should be visible on anteroposterior image. **F,** Path of probe or drill within 20 mm of the greater sciatic notch and aimed toward the anterior inferior iliac spine. **G,** Guidewire placed through drilled hole. **H-J,** Fluoroscopic teardrop view to confirm screw placement. **K,** Final position of rods. (Courtesy DePuy Synthes Companies of Johnson & & Johnson.) **SEE TECHNIQUE 44-40.**

- Place a guidewire through the probed or drilled hole to preserve the trajectory (Fig. 44-134G) and confirm its position with fluoroscopy.
- Tap the hole using the same-size pedicle tap as the intended screw diameter. Make sure that the guidewire does not advance during advancement of the tap.
- Insert the screw, aiming for the anterior inferior iliac spine with the trajectory within 20 mm above the greater sciatic notch. Before the screw is fully seated, remove the guidewire to prevent bending or breakage.
- Using the teardrop fluoroscopy view, confirm screw placement (Figs. 44-134H to J).
- Choose a rod length that will span the full length of the construct. Sagittally contour the rod before implanting it.
- Check to ensure that the sacral-alar-iliac screws are in line with the S1 screws and proximal screws in the construct. Rods can be inserted from caudal to cranial (most commonly) or from cranial to caudal in the case of severe proximal deformity.
- Insert the set screw to capture the rod. Tighten the rod to fix the rod to the distal screw and continue in a cephalad direction, capturing the rod with the rest of the screws in the construct (Fig. 44-134K), and tighten the set screws.

CEREBRAL PALSY

The prevalence of spinal deformities in patients with cerebral palsy varies according to the degree of neuromuscular involvement. Less than 10% of ambulatory patients with spastic hemiplegia have scoliosis; however, of those, 21% have scoliosis greater than 10 degrees and 6% have scoliosis greater than 30 degrees. Madigan and Wallace found scoliosis in 65% of patients with spastic quadriplegia who required total care. Most authors agree that the severity of the curve is directly proportional to the degree of neurologic impairment. Scoliosis in patients with cerebral palsy can continue to progress into the third decade. The greatest progression has been noted in patients who are unable to walk and have thoracolumbar or lumbar curves (average progression 0.8 degree per year in curves less than 50 degrees and 1.4 degrees per year in curves more than 50 degrees).

Scoliosis in patients with cerebral palsy is best managed by early recognition and control of the curve before the deformity becomes severe. Unlike idiopathic scoliosis, scoliosis caused by cerebral palsy can be painful. If the scoliosis is left untreated, function may be lost. If the patient is ambulatory, the trunk may become so distorted that standing erect becomes impossible. Sitting may become more difficult with increasing pelvic obliquity. If supplemental support by the hands is needed to sit, the patient will lose the ability to perform activities that require use of the upper extremity.

Bonnett et al. listed the following seven goals of scoliosis treatment in patients with cerebral palsy:

Improvement in assisted sitting to make positioning and transfer easier for nursing attendants and family

Relief of pain in the hips and back

Increased independence because of a decreased need for assistance, both for the positioning required to relieve pain and to prevent pressure areas and for feeding

Improvement in upper extremity function and table-top activities by eliminating the need to use the upper extremities for trunk support

Reduction of the equipment needed, making possible the use of other equipment

Placement of the patient in a different facility, one in which less care is provided

Improved eating ability made possible by a change in position

Each patient must be evaluated individually to determine the potential for achieving these rehabilitation goals.

CLASSIFICATION

Lonstein and Akbarnia classified cerebral palsy curves into two groups (Fig. 44-135). Group I curves—double curves with both thoracic and lumbar components—occurred in 40% of their patients. These curves, which are similar to curves of idiopathic scoliosis, occurred more commonly in patients with only intellectual impairment who were ambulatory and lived at home. Group II curves were present in 58% of patients. These curves were more severe lumbar or thoracolumbar curves that extended into the sacrum, with marked pelvic obliquity. Patients with these curves usually were nonambulatory with spastic quadriplegia, generally were not cared for at home, and were more likely to have the classic form of cerebral palsy rather than intellectual impairment alone.

NONOPERATIVE TREATMENT

If the curve is small, careful observation is indicated. If the curve progresses or is more than 30 degrees in a growing child who is an independent ambulator or sitter, treatment should be instituted. If a child is skeletally mature, bracing is not likely to be effective and surgery is indicated if the curve is 50 degrees or more. If neurologic involvement is extreme in a patient who is severely impaired and the curve is not causing any significant functional problems or pain, observation is appropriate.

Most nonambulatory patients with cerebral palsy do not have head or neck control during the first years of life. Custom seating may be effective in providing these patients with a straight spine and a level pelvis. Custom seating also can effectively accommodate severe spinal deformities and allow an upright posture in severely involved individuals.

If the curve is progressive, an orthotic device may be helpful as a temporizing device but will not provide permanent control of the curve. Orthoses generally are used for curve control during growth in a child who is ambulatory or who has independent sitting ability. The orthosis often provides enough trunk support to free the upper extremities for functional use. The orthosis of choice is a passive, total-contact TLSO with either a one-piece front-opening or a two-piece bivalved design or the soft Boston orthosis.

OPERATIVE TREATMENT

The operative treatment of scoliosis in cerebral palsy is complex. Determining which type of surgery is needed, and even whether any surgical procedure is warranted, is difficult. Before the introduction of newer techniques and instrumentation, the operative treatment of these patients was likely to fail, but the ability to treat these individuals has improved greatly.

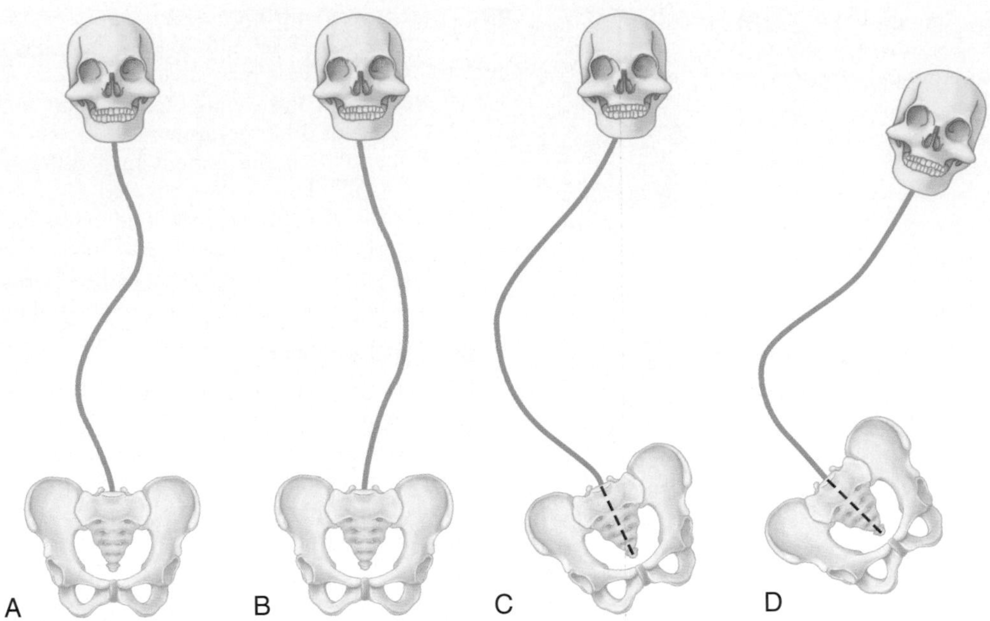

FIGURE 44-135 **A** and **B**, Group I double curves with thoracic and lumbar component and little pelvic obliquity. **C** and **D**, Group II large lumbar or thoracolumbar curves with marked pelvic obliquity.

The indications for surgical stabilization depend on the degree of mental involvement and the functional state of the individual with cerebral palsy. Determining which functional abilities would be helped by surgery is not always easy. Certainly, in ambulatory children and in those of near-normal intelligence, operative indications are similar to those for idiopathic scoliosis (curves of 40 to 45 degrees or more during adolescence; curves of more than 50 to 60 degrees in young, skeletally mature adults; and progressive curves that do not respond to nonoperative treatment). The decision concerning treatment of a child with total body involvement, seizure disorder, no head or trunk control, and major nutritional problems is difficult. If a practical, functional gain is not likely, the risks of surgery may not be acceptable.

The surgical techniques available for scoliosis in patients with cerebral palsy have improved significantly. A pseudarthrosis rate of 20% has been reported in patients with posterior spinal fusion and Harrington instrumentation. Combined anterior and posterior procedures with anterior and posterior instrumentation result in adequate correction with a low incidence of pseudarthrosis. The introduction of Luque rods and segmental instrumentation also has greatly improved the results of surgery for scoliosis in cerebral palsy patients. In a comparison study of a two-stage technique (anterior spinal instrumentation and fusion using the Zielke apparatus followed by posterior Luque procedures to the pelvis) with a single-stage posterior technique using Luque rods, the pseudarthrosis rate was 40% in the single-stage procedure and only 9.5% in the combined procedure. Allen and Ferguson questioned the need for anterior instrumentation because anterior instrumentation actually decreases the overall correction. They recommended an anterior release and fusion followed by a second-stage Luque procedure to the pelvis. With posterior segmental instrumentation systems, the technique of anterior release and fusion without instrumentation followed by posterior instrumentation also has produced satisfactory results. In patients with cerebral palsy and scoliosis, segmental instrumentation has the advantage of allowing distraction and compression along the rods in addition to bending and rotational forces. The principles remain the same in that a large, stiff curve before surgery may need an anterior release, discectomy, and anterior bone grafting. Posterior instrumentation to the pelvis is completed at a second stage. The use of double sacral screws or iliosacral screws for fixation to the pelvis has been recommended. With pedicle screw instrumentation and posterior-only surgery, results are reported to be similar to those of anterior and posterior surgery. There probably is no one ideal technique for managing these complex curves. In general, we use pedicle screws, and pelvic fixation is preferred when possible. The rods can be crosslinked to increase stability. Our preference at this time for pelvic fixation is the iliac screw technique or S2 iliac screw technique (see Techniques 44-35 and 44-36). If the pelvis is too small to accept screw fixation, we use the McCarthy S-rod technique (see Technique 44-32) with crosslinking for pelvic fixation.

The type of surgery also depends on the type of scoliosis. According to Lonstein and Akbarnia, patients with group I curves usually require only a posterior fusion, with fusion to the sacrum rarely needed (Fig. 44-136). A combined anterior and posterior approach to group I curves is needed only when there is a significant lumbar component, in which case an anterior release and fusion and posterior instrumentation add correction and reduce the rate of pseudarthrosis. Group II curves usually require a long fusion to the sacrum because the sacrum is part of the curve and pelvic obliquity is present. Traction radiographs should be obtained. If a level pelvis and balanced spine can be obtained, a one-stage posterior approach is indicated. However, if the traction radiograph shows significant residual pelvic obliquity, or if the torso is not balanced over the pelvis, a two-stage approach is indicated. In general, the larger the lumbar curve, the more severe

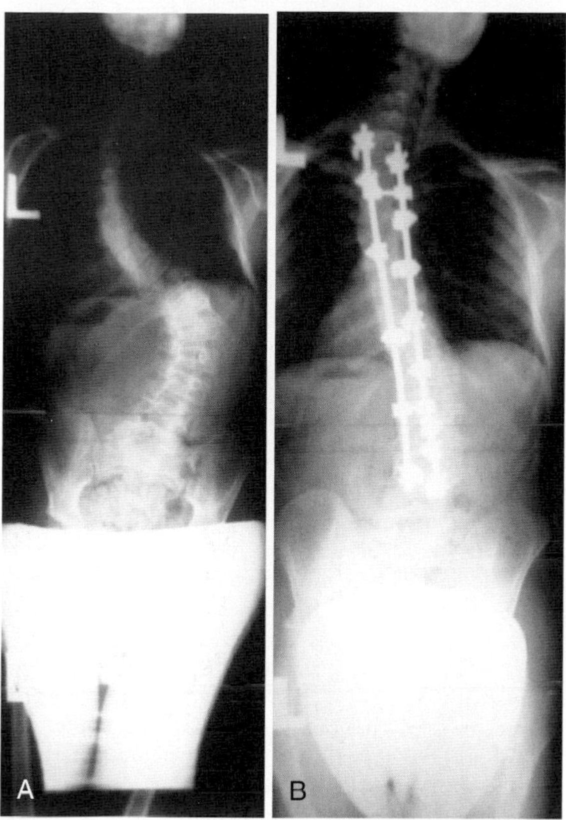

FIGURE 44-136 **A,** Preoperative standing radiograph of patient with cerebral palsy and significant group I scoliosis. **B,** Postoperative appearance 4 years after posterior instrumentation not including the sacrum.

the pelvic obliquity; and the more rigid the curve, the more likely a two-stage procedure will be needed, although with current segmental instrumentation with pedicle screws, anterior and posterior procedures are not needed as often.

Radiographic evaluation of patients with contractures around the hips can lead to erroneous conclusions. The radiograph often is made with the patient supine and the hips extended. If one hip has an adduction contracture and the opposite hip has an abduction contracture, it may appear that pelvic obliquity is present. An appropriate radiographic evaluation should include a supine view obtained with the hips in a relaxed position, whatever the contractures dictate. This allows the spine and pelvis to assume a neutral alignment without the influence of hip contractures. Kyphosis can be caused by tight hamstrings and should be evaluated carefully because if the hamstrings are not released, increased stress will be placed on the instrumentation.

Several technical points should be considered in instrumentation of patients with cerebral palsy. The most proximal level of the fusion should be above T4 to prevent "falling off" of the kyphosis above the instrumentation. Only small portions of the ligamentum flavum on either side of the superior interspinous space to be instrumented should be removed. If possible, the supraspinous and interspinous ligaments at the superior level should be preserved to prevent an increase in kyphosis above instrumentation. Pedicle hooks or screws are used for fixation at the most proximal level to add axial load support to the system.

Immobilization after the spinal fusion depends on the activity level of the child and the security of the internal fixation. If a child can tolerate external support without any detrimental effect on function, it can be used no matter how secure the internal fixation. If, however, external support would significantly hinder the patient's functional ability and the internal fixation is secure, it should not be used. If the bone is obviously osteopenic or instrumentation is less than ideal, postoperative external support may be necessary.

COMPLICATIONS

Improved techniques of instrumentation and preoperative and postoperative management have decreased complications, but a much higher complication rate should be expected after surgery for this type of scoliosis than after that for idiopathic curves. Complications in patients with cerebral palsy have been reported in up to 81%, including infection in 15% to 19%. Patients with cerebral palsy are believed to be at an increased risk for infection. Deep infections can be treated by irrigation and debridement, administration of systemic antibiotics, and delayed primary closure or closure over a suction drain.

Pulmonary complications often develop in these patients because they cannot cooperate in deep breathing and coughing exercises, and appropriate prophylactic pulmonary measures are needed.

If the upper limit of the fusion is not selected carefully (above T4), kyphosis cephalad to the upper limit of the fusion can occur. Pseudarthrosis is less frequent with newer instrumentation systems, but it still occurs and often results in implant failure. Other possible complications are those inherent in any spinal operation, such as urinary tract infection, ileus, and blood loss.

Although the complications can be significant in these patients, the functional improvement or prevention of deterioration of function may be worth the effort and the risks of surgery. Complications should be expected and planned for; prompt treatment will lessen their severity.

FRIEDREICH ATAXIA

Friedreich ataxia is a recessively inherited condition characterized by spinocerebellar degeneration. The genetic cause has been found to be a flaw within the frataxin gene on chromosome 9q13. The clinical onset takes place between the ages of 6 and 20 years. Primary symptoms include progressive ataxic gait, dysarthria, decreased proprioception or vibratory sense, muscle weakness, and lack of deep tendon reflexes. Secondary symptoms include pes cavus, scoliosis, and cardiomyopathy. Affected children frequently are wheelchair bound in the first or second decade of life. The cardiomyopathy often leads to death in the third or fourth decade of life.

Labelle et al. evaluated 56 patients with a diagnosis of Friedreich ataxia and found that all 56 patients had scoliosis. The most common pattern was double structural thoracic and lumbar curves (57%). The typical neuromuscular thoracolumbar curve with pelvic obliquity was found in only 14%. Milbrandt et al. reported that 63% of their patients developed scoliosis. Because no significant correlation could be established between overall muscle weakness and curve progression, as would be expected in neuromuscular scoliosis, Cady and Bobechko postulated that the pathogenesis of scoliosis in patients with Friedreich ataxia may be a disturbance of equilibrium and postural reflexes rather than muscle weakness. Not all curves in patients with Friedreich ataxia are progressive (49% are progressive); the onset of the disease at an early age and the presence of scoliosis before puberty have been found to be major factors in progression. Scoliosis appearing in the late teens or early 20s is less likely to be progressive.

Most authors have not found bracing to be useful for progressive curves in patients with Friedreich ataxia. The orthosis fails to control the curve, and by the time scoliosis develops, the patients often have a significant degree of ataxia and the restriction of a spinal orthosis makes ambulation more difficult. Curves of less than 40 degrees should be observed, curves of more than 60 degrees should be treated operatively, and curves of between 40 and 60 degrees should be observed or treated operatively, depending on the age of the patient, the onset of the disease, and such characteristics of the scoliosis as the patient's age when it is recognized and evidence of progression of the curve. If the curve is observed too long, cardiomyopathy may have progressed to the point that surgery is risky, if not impossible; early surgical treatment is therefore recommended for progressive curves.

Cardiology evaluation is mandatory before any surgery is considered in these patients. Patients with Friedreich ataxia frequently are unable to walk with postoperative immobilization. Prolonged bed rest postoperatively must be kept to a minimum, or weakness can increase rapidly. For these reasons, the ideal instrumentation for these patients is segmental spinal instrumentation with multiple fixation devices, such as hooks, sublaminar cables, or pedicle screws, that do not require external support postoperatively. In general, these patients require a long fusion with attention to sagittal contours to prevent later problems with thoracic kyphosis. Milbrandt recommended segmental instrumentation and fusion from T2 to the sacrum. The pelvis usually is not included in these fusions unless pelvic obliquity is significant. Spinal cord monitoring usually is not effective in these patients, and plans for a wake-up test should be made preoperatively to evaluate the neurologic status after instrumentation and correction.

CHARCOT-MARIE-TOOTH DISEASE

Classic Charcot-Marie-Tooth disease is a demyelinating neuropathy. The condition is dominantly inherited, with considerable variation in severity. The reported incidence of spinal deformity in Charcot-Marie-Tooth disease varies from 10% to 26%. Some authors have found brace treatment to be well tolerated, whereas others have had little success, with curve progression reported in 71% and with 33% requiring instrumentation and fusion. The sagittal plane deformity accompanying this scoliosis most frequently is kyphosis, and fusion to the pelvis generally is not necessary unless pelvic obliquity exists. Intraoperative monitoring rarely is possible in patients with Charcot-Marie-Tooth disease; therefore, preoperative plans for intraoperative assessment of possible neurologic compromise with a wake-up test should be considered.

SYRINGOMYELIA

Syringomyelia is a cystic, fluid-filled cavitation within the spinal cord. Scoliosis may be the first manifestation of a syringomyelia. Syringomyelia can exist with or without Chiari I malformations. The proposed cause of syringomyelia associated with Chiari I malformation is disturbed or obstructed cerebrospinal fluid flow. Syringomyelia without associated Chiari I malformation is described as a noncommunicating syrinx. Scoliosis has been reported in 63% to 73% of children with syringomyelia. Physical findings that may indicate syringomyelia include neurologic deficits and pain associated with the scoliosis, intrinsic muscle wasting of the hands, cavus deformity, asymmetric muscle bulk, occipital and upper cervical headaches, and loss of superficial abdominal reflexes. Radiographic features suggestive of syringomyelia include Charcot changes in joints and a left thoracic curvature. Patients with syringomyelia and scoliosis have been found to have thoracic kyphosis (> 40 degrees) instead of thoracic hypokyphosis seen with idiopathic scoliosis. Cervical lordosis also is increased in this patient population. If the diagnosis of syringomyelia is suspected, MRI should be done (Fig. 44-137). In obtaining the MRI study, care must be taken to include the craniocervical junction to rule out the presence of an Arnold-Chiari malformation.

The association of syringomyelia with scoliosis may have a significant influence on treatment. Paraplegia and rupture of a large cyst in the cord resulting in death have been reported in patients with syringomyelia who had instrumentation and fusion. Because of the possibility of these complications, surgery for scoliosis in patients with syringomyelia should be approached cautiously. The rate of progression of the neurologic deficit and the prognosis of the curve should be considered carefully before any extensive surgery is considered. Drainage of the cyst, followed by observation to determine if the subsequent curve stabilizes, has been recommended as initial treatment. In one study, improvement was noted in three of 15 patients, and progression did not occur in any patient. Another study showed that drainage of the syrinx delayed but did not prevent curve progression in immature patients; however, drainage of the syrinx did allow use of distraction-type instrumentation without complications. At our institution, the pediatric neurosurgeons believe that the syrinx usually is associated with Chiari I malformations. Their preferred management is decompression of the posterior fossa. If the curve continues to progress after posterior fossa decompression, surgery may be indicated. If instrumentation is necessary in these patients, distraction should be avoided if at all possible. This can be accomplished by either anterior instrumentation or posterior thoracic pedicle instrumentation with a direct vertebral rotation technique. Direct communication with the neurosurgeon always is indicated preoperatively in these patients to minimize the possibility of spinal cord injury.

SPINAL CORD INJURY

Several series in the literature have reported an incidence of spinal deformity in 99% of children with spinal cord injuries before the adolescent growth spurt. Spinal deformity is much more common and the rate of curve progression much greater in preadolescents than in older patients.

Increasing curvature with pelvic obliquity in a child with a spinal cord injury can lead to a loss of sitting balance that requires the use of the upper extremities for trunk support rather than for functional tasks. Pressure sores may occur on the downside of the ischium, and hip subluxation can occur on the high side of the pelvic obliquity.

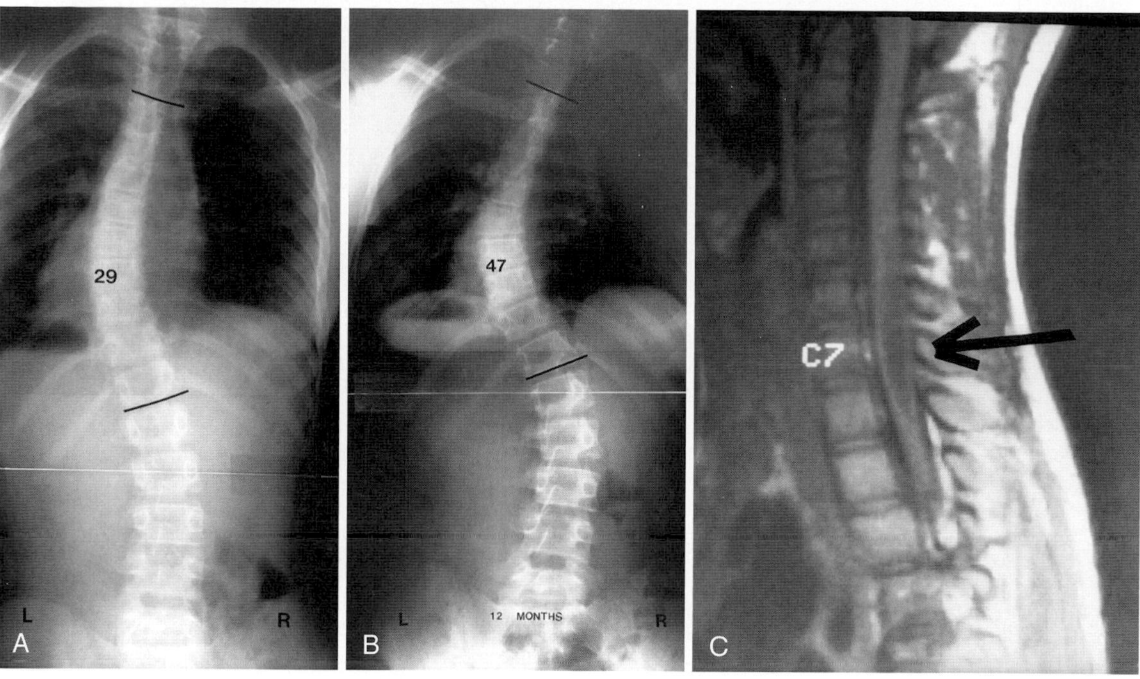

FIGURE 44-137 Progressive curve in patient with syringomyelia. **A**, Initial curve. **B**, One year later. **C**, MRI shows syrinx at C7 *(arrow)*.

ORTHOTIC TREATMENT

Although some authors believe that alteration of the natural progression of scoliosis in these patients is impossible with devices such as braces and corsets, other authors indicated that orthotic treatment does have a place in the management of scoliosis in preadolescent patients with spinal cord injuries. Orthotic treatment is difficult because of potential skin problems, but effective slowing of progression has been noted. The use of an orthosis may delay the need for surgery in preadolescent patients until longitudinal growth of the spine is more complete. Orthotic treatment requires close cooperation among the physician, the family, and the patient. A custom-fitted, well-padded, plastic total-contact TLSO generally is used. Close attention must be paid to any evidence of pressure changes on the skin. The brace can be removed at night and used only during sitting.

OPERATIVE TREATMENT

Most preadolescent children with spinal cord injuries ultimately require surgical stabilization of their scoliosis (50% to 60%). If the curve progresses despite orthotic treatment, operative intervention is indicated. If the curve is more than 60 degrees when the child is first seen, surgery should be considered. Curves treated with an orthosis are considered for surgery if they progress beyond 40 degrees, and curves between 40 and 60 degrees are considered individually.

The prevalence of pseudarthrosis in these patients reported in the literature ranges from 27% to 53%. Dearolf et al. found pseudarthrosis in 26% of their patients, and they attributed the lower figure to the use of segmental fixation in recent years. Segmental instrumentation allows more rigid fixation, and postoperative immobilization can be avoided (Fig. 44-138). Complete urinary tract evaluation should be done before surgery because urinary tract infections are common in patients with spinal cord injuries. The urine should be cultured 2 weeks before surgery. If the culture is positive, the patient is treated with antibiotics for 10 days and then the culture is repeated. If the organism is sensitive to a medication delivered orally, surgery is done when the culture is negative and the antibiotic is continued through surgery. If the organism is sensitive only to intravenous antibiotics, surgery is delayed until the cultures are negative for 10 days after discontinuation of the antibiotics. Postoperatively, oral antibiotic prophylaxis should be continued for 3 months. Rapidly progressive curves in patients with spinal cord injury should be evaluated with MRI for the possibility of a posttraumatic syrinx.

If possible, surgery should be delayed until the patient weighs more than 100 lb. This allows the use of larger rods and more stable fixation. With the increased use of thoracic pedicle screws and lumbar pedicle screws, anterior release is becoming less necessary. It still should be considered, however, in a patient who has a large, rigid curve. For patients younger than 10 years with progressive curves of more than 50 degrees, a dilemma still exists. Luque instrumentation or subcutaneous Harrington rods without fusion failed in all four patients treated in this manner by Dearolf et al. If the child is very young, a dual growing rod technique will provide more stable fixation and fewer failures than the subcutaneous Harrington rod technique. If a definitive fusion is required in a young child at risk for future crankshaft problems, a first-stage anterior release and fusion should be considered, followed by posterior segmental spinal instrumentation and fusion. With the better correction in the coronal, sagittal, and axial planes provided by posterior pedicle screw instrumentation, anterior fusion may not be necessary in young children.

Dearolf et al. reported pseudarthroses in three of 10 preadolescent patients and in one mature patient who had fusion to the sacrum. They believed that if there was little residual pelvic obliquity, fusion to L4 or L5 would be

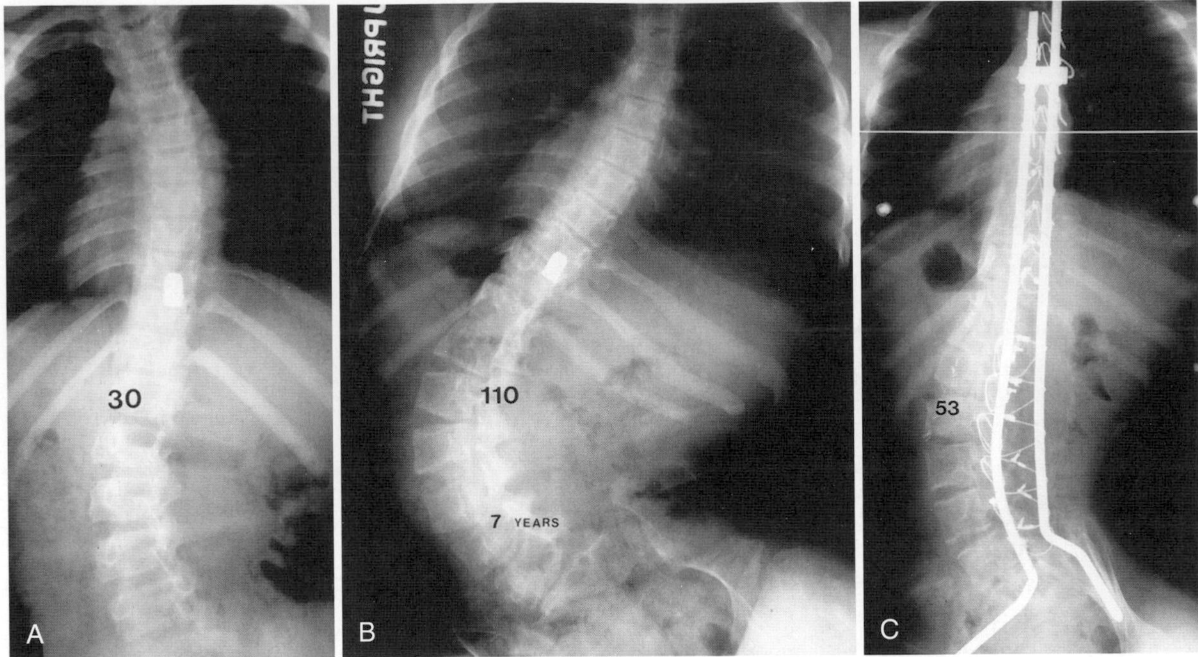

FIGURE 44-138 Progressive paralytic scoliosis after gunshot wound. **A,** Initial curve of 30 degrees. **B,** Seven years later, curve is 110 degrees. **C,** After fusion and segmental instrumentation, correction to 53 degrees.

sufficient. If, on the other hand, the pelvis was significantly involved in the curve, fusion probably should include the sacrum with pelvic instrumentation. For patients who are ambulators and in whom adequate correction can be obtained without involving the pelvis, an effort should be made to end the instrumentation above the pelvis. In carefully selected patients, Shook and Lubicky used short anterior spinal fusion with instrumentation alone. They reported that this provided excellent curve correction over a short segment and allowed a number of open disc spaces below the fused segment (Fig. 44-139).

If laminectomy was used to treat the initial spinal cord injury, an increased incidence of kyphosis can be expected. A kyphosis that is rigid and cannot be corrected to less than 50 degrees on hyperextension views may need to be treated with a first-stage anterior release and spinal fusion, followed by a long posterior fusion with segmental instrumentation.

POLIOMYELITIS

Because the Salk and Sabin vaccines have made poliomyelitis in children rare in the United States, most recent experience in treating postpolio spinal deformities is in adult patients. The basic principles of treatment, however, are no different from those of treatment of spinal deformities resulting from other neuromuscular diseases. Bonnett et al. outlined the indications for correction and posterior spine fusion in patients with poliomyelitis (Box 44-6).

As in any other neuromuscular curve, the length of fusion is much greater in patients with poliomyelitis than in those with idiopathic scoliosis. Segmental instrumentation is recommended. In evaluation of the distal extent of the fusion in a patient with poliomyelitis, it must be determined whether the pelvic obliquity is caused by the spinal curvature itself or by other factors, such as iliotibial band contractures.

BOX 44-6

Indications for Correction and Posterior Spine Fusion in Patients With Poliomyelitis

- Collapsing spinal deformity because of marked paralysis
- Progressive spinal deformity that does not respond to nonoperative treatment
- Reduction of cardiorespiratory function associated with progressive restrictive lung disease
- Decreasing independence in functional activities because of spinal instability that necessitates use of the upper extremities for trunk support rather than for tabletop activities
- Back pain and loss of sitting balance associated with pelvic obliquity, which frequently causes ischial pain and pressure necrosis on the downside of the gluteal region

SPINAL MUSCULAR ATROPHY

Spinal muscular atrophy is an autosomal recessive condition in which the anterior horn cells of the spinal cord, and occasionally the bulbar nuclei, atrophy. Daher et al. proposed that this disorder is caused by one episode of neural destruction at different times in childhood. Children affected earlier in life have more severe involvement than do those affected later. Spinal muscular atrophy can be classified into three types based on the severity of disease and the age of the patient at the time of clinical onset. Type I, or acute infantile Werdnig-Hoffmann disease, is the most severe form and is usually diagnosed within the first 6 months of life. The course of the disease is progressive, with most of these children dying within the first 2 to 3 years of life. Children with type 2 spinal muscular atrophy (chronic or intermediate form) manage to

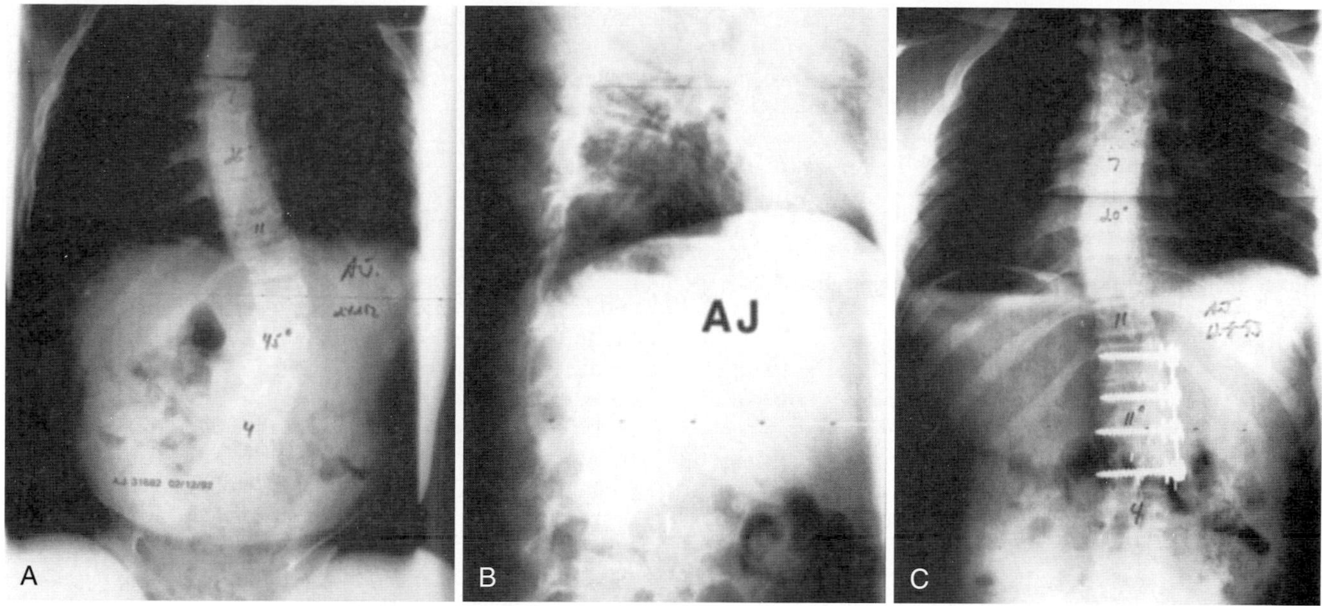

FIGURE 44-139 Fourteen-year-old boy who was paraplegic as result of gunshot wound to spine. **A** and **B**, Anteroposterior and lateral sitting thoracolumbar spine views showing 45-degree right lumbar curve with minimal pelvic obliquity. Lateral view shows thoracolumbar junction to be fairly straight. Because patient wanted to continue walking with braces, preservation of as many mobile segments below fusion was thought advantageous. Because of behavior of lumbar curve on side bending, it was thought that anterior fusion alone with instrumentation would provide correction of scoliosis and maintain sagittal contour. **C**, Anteroposterior sitting thoracolumbar spine view postoperatively shows excellent correction of scoliosis and preservation of sagittal contour. Anterior procedure was done with subperiosteal stripping of spine, and fusion healed rapidly within a few months. (From Shook JE, Lubicky JP: Paralytic scoliosis. In Bridwell KH, DeWald RL, editors: The textbook of spinal surgery, ed 2, Philadelphia, 1997, Lippincott-Raven.)

achieve normal motor milestones until 6 to 8 months of age. They often are very weak but can usually sit without support. Patients will usually survive into the third or fourth decade. Type III, or Kugelberg-Welander disease, usually is seen after 2 years of age. It is more slowly progressive, and most patients are able to ambulate independently.

On clinical examination, children with spinal muscular atrophy have severe weakness of the trunk and limb muscles. Fasciculations of the tongue and tremors of the extremities are frequent. Reflexes are diminished. Most patients have normal intelligence, and the heart is unaffected by the disease process. Motor and sensory nerve conduction velocities are normal, but electromyography demonstrates denervation with fibrillation potentials. The cause of death usually is pulmonary insufficiency. Ninety percent of these patients have scoliosis, and it is the most severe problem in those who survive childhood. Once patients with spinal muscular atrophy are wheelchair bound, their scoliosis develops rapidly. Aprin et al. noted that scoliosis usually is diagnosed between 6 and 8 years of age, and the more severe the disease, the more likely the curve is to be progressive. The scoliosis is a typical neuromuscular spinal deformity with a long C-shaped curve pattern. Thoracolumbar curves are seen in 80% of patients, and thoracic curves are noted in only 20% of patients.

ORTHOTIC TREATMENT

Bracing has been reported to slow progression of the curve and allows sitting for longer periods. However, patients treated in braces have been found to be less functional because of decreased flexibility of the spine and therefore tend to be noncompliant. When the scoliosis in a skeletally immature patient reaches 20 degrees in the sitting position, orthotic treatment should be considered, usually with a total-contact TLSO. This is used only during sitting to minimize progression of the curve and to provide an extremely weak child with a stable sitting support. Severe chest wall deformities can occur from bracing, and developing chest wall deformities are a contraindication to brace treatment. Although bracing may not eliminate the need for surgical stabilization, it may delay surgery until the child is closer to the end of growth. Surgery at a young age would require anterior and posterior approaches to prevent the crankshaft phenomenon, and the anterior fusion adds considerably to the risk of the procedure in these patients. The anterior approach almost invariably involves "taking down" the diaphragm, which is the main respiratory muscle in patients with spinal muscular atrophy. Thoracoscopic anterior release and fusion (see Technique 44-28) may be a satisfactory alternative in these patients at great risk of crankshaft development. Chandran et al. described the use of a growing rod construct as an effective option in the treatment of scoliosis in patients with spinal muscular atrophy. This is the preferred option until a definitive posterior fusion can be done.

OPERATIVE TREATMENT

Surgical treatment of the spinal deformity is posterior spinal fusion with posterior segmental instrumentation and adequate bone grafting. Because fusion to the sacrum is needed for many of these patients, fixation to the pelvis can be obtained by the Galveston or iliac screw technique (see Techniques

44-33 and 44-35). Augmentation of the fusion with bone-bank allograft bone usually is necessary. If the vertebrae are extremely osteoporotic, external support, such as a bivalved body jacket, can be used. For a severe fixed lumbar curve with pelvic obliquity, anterior release and fusion may be needed in addition to posterior instrumentation. It should be understood, however, that anterior surgery in patients with severe pulmonary compromise carries a great risk, and this risk must be evaluated carefully before surgery. With posterior pedicle screw instrumentation, which provides better correction in the coronal, sagittal, and axial planes, anterior fusion usually is not necessary. Preoperative traction can offer an excellent method to improve the flexibility of the spine and also improves pulmonary function before posterior fusion and instrumentation.

Complications should be expected in this group of patients (45%). Pseudarthrosis, atelectasis, pneumonitis, and death have been reported. Brown et al. reduced their complication rate from 35% to 15% with the use of Luque segmental instrumentation and the elimination of postoperative immobilization.

Frequent pulmonary complications in patients with spinal muscular atrophy require respiratory support for a longer than normal period after surgery and rapid mobilization when possible. Patients with spinal muscular atrophy may be especially sensitive to medications that depress the respiratory centers, and the use of these drugs in the postoperative period should be minimal. Lonstein and Renshaw found that patients with forced vital capacity of less than 20% of that predicted are at great risk for postoperative death. A vigorous preoperative and postoperative physical therapy program is mandatory.

The patient and the family should be warned of the possibility of some loss of function after spinal instrumentation and fusion. A flexible spine allows a weak trunk to collapse forward to increase the reach of the upper extremity. Also, flexibility of the spine and extremities allows the center of gravity to be placed where weak muscles have the best mechanical advantage. Spinal fusion creates a longer lever arm that weak hip muscles are unable to control. Gross motor activities, such as transfers, rolling, bathing, dressing, and toileting, have been noted to decline after spinal fusion. This loss of function, however, must be weighed against the predicted functional loss and pulmonary compromise from severe, untreated spinal deformity. During the long, progressive course of this disease, the advantages of a stable trunk far outweigh the disadvantages.

FAMILIAL DYSAUTONOMIA

Familial dysautonomia (Riley-Day syndrome), first described in 1949, is a rare autosomal recessive disorder found mostly in Jewish children of Eastern European extraction. Its clinical features include absence of overflow tears and sweating, vasomotor instability that often leads to hyperthermia, and relative indifference to pain. Other frequent findings include episodic hypertension, postural hypotension, transient blotching of the skin, hyperhidrosis, episodic vomiting, disordered swallowing, dysarthria, and motor incoordination. Death is caused most often by pulmonary disease. Scoliosis is the major orthopaedic problem in patients with this disease. The scoliosis may be progressive and may be large enough to contribute to early death because of kyphoscoliotic cardiopulmonary decompensation. Kyphosis also is a frequent sagittal plane deformity in these patients. If surgery for the scoliosis is considered, however, features of the syndrome such as vasomotor and thermal instability can cause troublesome and sometimes fatal operative or postoperative complications. Brace treatment, although beneficial in some patients, often is complicated by the tendency for pressure ulcers to develop.

Posterior spinal fusion with instrumentation was required in 13 of 51 patients in the Israeli series of Kaplan et al. All children undergoing surgery had severe pulmonary problems. Intraoperative and postoperative respiratory and dysautonomic complications were frequent. Because of osteopenic bone, only minor improvement of the spinal deformity was possible, and a small loss of correction was common; however, those surviving noted a marked decrease in the frequency of pneumonia and, for some reason, an improvement in the degree of ataxia. Albanese and Bobechko reported surgical stabilization of kyphoscoliosis in seven patients. Intraoperative complications included transient hypertension, failure of the lamina because of osteopenia, and an endotracheal tube that was plugged by thick secretions after the lung was collapsed for an anterior approach. All patients had at least one complication, although there were no intraoperative or immediate postoperative deaths.

One technical problem in instrumenting these curves is the frequent occurrence of severe kyphosis combined with weak bone. Anterior procedures should be approached with caution because of the frequency of respiratory problems. Despite the significant dangers and high complication rates in patients with familial dysautonomia, surgery can be done successfully with proper precautions and can improve the quality of life.

ARTHROGRYPOSIS MULTIPLEX CONGENITA

Arthrogryposis multiplex congenita is a syndrome of persistent joint contractures that are present at birth. A myopathic subtype is characterized by muscle changes similar to those found in progressive muscular dystrophy. In the neuropathic subtype, anterior horn cells are reduced or absent in the cervical, thoracic, and lumbosacral segments of the spinal cord. In the third subtype, joint fibrosis and contractures alone are the main problems.

Scoliosis is common in patients with arthrogryposis multiplex congenita (20% to 66%). A single thoracolumbar curve is the predominant curve pattern. The scoliosis usually is detected at birth or within the first few years of life. Brace treatment rarely is successful and should be used only with small, flexible curves (< 30 degrees) in patients who were ambulators. In patients who are nonambulatory or have a curve of more than 30 degrees, the brace is ineffective in controlling the curve. Rib-based distraction using the vertical expandable prosthetic titanium rib (VEPTR) has been reported to be effective in controlling scoliosis and kyphosis and maintaining thoracic growth in patients with arthrogryposis.

The onset of pelvic obliquity is a serious problem. If treatment of the pelvic obliquity by release of the contractures in the hip area does not halt progression of the curve, spinal fusion to the sacrum may be necessary. The onset of thoracic lordosis also requires prompt treatment. Because of the severity and rigidity of the curves, postoperative complications are frequent. The connective tissue is tough, and the bones are osteoporotic. An average blood loss of 2000 mL has been reported, and Herron et al. obtained a maximal correction of only about 25% with Harrington instrumentation and posterior fusion. Combined anterior and posterior spinal arthrodesis has been recommended in these patients because it is more effective in terms of curve correction and in the least loss of correction at follow-up. If patients have less than 90 degrees of passive flexion of the hip, caution should be exercised in extending spinal arthrodesis to the pelvis because this is likely to make sitting difficult. If a significant pelvic obliquity is present that does not correct to acceptable levels on preoperative bending films, a first-stage anterior release and fusion are indicated. This is then followed by posterior instrumentation and fusion to the pelvis.

DUCHENNE MUSCULAR DYSTROPHY

Duchenne muscular dystrophy is an inherited X-linked recessive condition caused by a frameshift mutation in the dystrophin gene at the Xp21.2 locus of the X chromosome. The clinical course is one of progressive weakness, loss of the ability to walk at 10 to 14 years of age, and eventual wheelchair dependence. Death from pulmonary or cardiac compromise usually occurs in the second or third decade of life. Scoliosis develops in most patients with Duchenne muscular dystrophy, although the use of corticosteroids may decrease the development of spinal deformity in these patients. Before steroids were used in Duchenne patients, scoliosis developed in more than 90%; since steroid use began, the rate has fallen to only 10% to 20% (Fig. 44-140). A review of the Nationwide Inpatient Sample from 2001 to 2012 demonstrated a significant decrease in the rate of scoliosis surgery in patients with Duchenne muscular dystrophy. Lebel et al. reported that only 20% of their patients receiving steroids went on to undergo spinal fusion, but 90% of patients not receiving steroids had spinal fusions.

Spinal deformity usually occurs after the patient becomes confined to a wheelchair, although very early scoliosis has been detected in some ambulatory patients. The curves are predominantly long thoracolumbar curves with pelvic obliquity, the collapse of which is caused by absence of muscles and not by asymmetric muscle activity or contracture. Once a curve develops, it generally is progressive and cannot be controlled by braces or wheelchair seating systems. In patients with Duchenne muscular dystrophy, pulmonary function deteriorates approximately 4% each year after the age of 12 years. If orthotic treatment is continued while pulmonary function deteriorates significantly, surgical stabilization may become impossible. When the forced vital capacity decreases to less than 35%, surgery probably is not advisable because of the potential pulmonary problems postoperatively. Patients with Duchenne muscular dystrophy have reduced cardiac function that may alter the anesthetic management. Hypotensive anesthesia to minimize blood loss may not be possible. Increased intraoperative blood loss is commonly seen in patients with Duchenne muscular dystrophy. This may be due to having to dissect through dystrophic and fibrotic muscle, loss of vasoconstriction of blood vessels from the absence of dystrophin, and altered platelet function.

Lonstein and Renshaw's indications for spinal fusion in patients with Duchenne muscular dystrophy are curves of more than 30 degrees, forced vital capacity of more than 30% of normal, and prognosis of at least 2 years of life remaining. Because the scoliosis invariably increases, many authors recommended spinal fusion at the onset of the deformity in patients who use a wheelchair full time even when the curves are as small as 20 degrees or less. In decision making, the patient's pulmonary function probably is more important than the size of the curve. The vital capacity should be 40% to 50% of normal. If the curve is allowed to progress beyond 30 to 40 degrees, the forced vital capacity can be less than 40% of predicted normal. Most patients with Duchenne muscular dystrophy generally have a forced vital capacity of 50% to 70% of normal when they begin to use a wheelchair full time. Surgery is recommended during the first few years of full-time wheelchair use, when the patient almost always

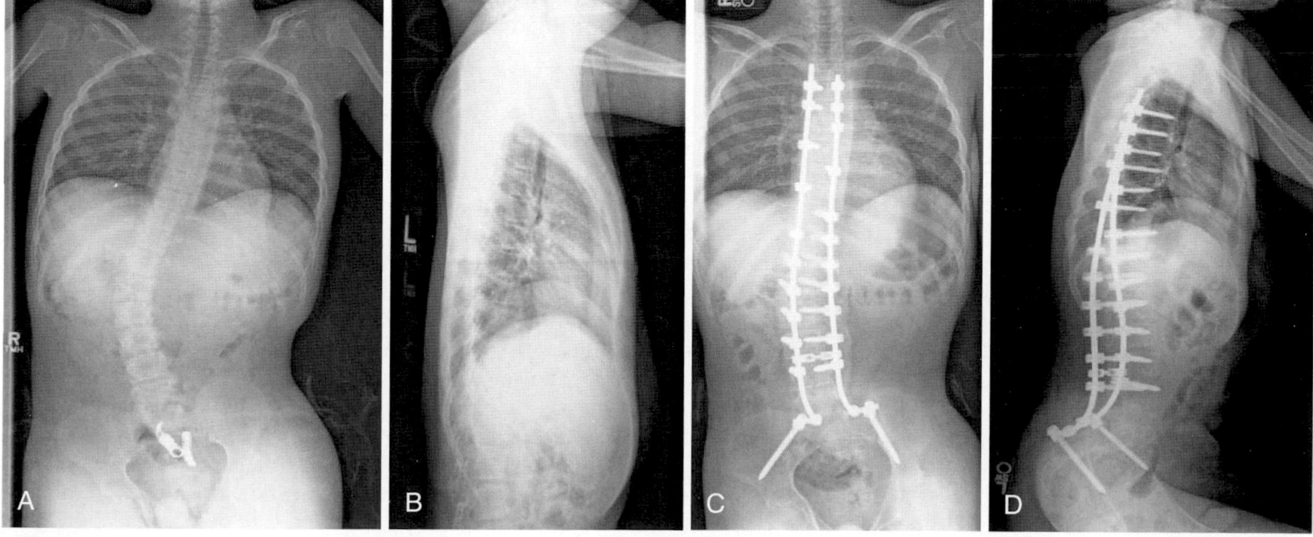

FIGURE 44-140 **A** and **B**, Progressive scoliosis in patient with Duchenne muscular dystrophy. **C** and **D**, After fusion with Luque rod instrumentation.

has a small, flexible curve and little or no pelvic obliquity but still has a forced vital capacity of 40% or more. Suk et al. found that surgery in patients who had Duchenne muscular dystrophy with scoliosis improved function and decreased the deterioration of forced vital capacity compared with patients treated conservatively; however, the muscle power and forced vital capacity continued to decrease in both groups.

Treatment of scoliosis in patients with Duchenne muscular dystrophy consists of segmental instrumentation with sublaminar wires or cables, hooks, or pedicle screws and fusion from T2 to the pelvis. In patients with smaller curves and no fixed pelvic obliquity, the fusion and instrumentation can end at L5. If fixed pelvic obliquity is more than 15 degrees, fusion to the pelvis with iliac screw or S-rod pelvic fixation is indicated. Correction of pelvic obliquity is reported to be more certain with instrumentation and fusion to the sacrum in larger curves (average, 61 degrees), and better maintenance of correction of pelvic obliquity has been reported in patients who had fusions that extended to the pelvis than in patients in whom the distal extent of fusion was in the lumbar spine. The fusion should extend to the high upper thoracic spine (T2), to prevent proximal or junctional kyphosis. The sagittal contours of the spine, especially lumbar lordosis, should be maintained for sitting balance and pressure distribution. Bone-bank allograft is needed because a massive amount of bone graft will be necessary to obtain a solid fusion. Because of the pulmonary compromise in these patients, rapid postoperative mobilization is important. When segmental spinal instrumentation is used, postoperative bracing usually is not necessary.

Lonstein and Renshaw listed the following benefits of spinal fusion in patients with Duchenne muscular dystrophy: preserves sitting balance, prevents back pain, improves spinal decompensation, frees the arms of the necessity of trunk support, improves body image, and possibly slows the deterioration of pulmonary function. However, the rate of decline of forced vital capacity is not changed by preventing scoliosis with spinal fusion. The use of corticosteroids in patients with Duchenne muscular dystrophy has been shown to prolong the time that patients are able to walk. The use of corticosteroids also appears to have a positive effect on the prevention of spinal deformity.

VARIANTS OF MUSCULAR DYSTROPHY OTHER THAN DUCHENNE TYPE

Spinal curvature in association with non–Duchenne muscular dystrophy is uncommon. The occurrence of scoliosis in patients with non–Duchenne muscular dystrophy depends on the specific type of dystrophic disease, and the prognosis is related to the severity of the primary problem. For instance, Siegel found that childhood dystrophia myotonica is not associated with spinal curvature. Facioscapulohumeral dystrophy is more rapidly progressive when the onset occurs in childhood. Frequently, it also is asymmetric in distribution, and structural scoliosis can occur. None of the 11 patients described by Daher et al. had pelvic obliquity. Thoracic lordosis was present in 36% of their patients, all of whom developed poor vital capacity and shortness of breath. The use of an orthosis during the juvenile years controlled the curve until the pubertal growth spurt, when progression occurred. The brace should not be used, however, when a thoracic lordosis exists. Spinal fusion is effective in maintaining correction and preventing curve progression in these patients.

CONGENITAL SCOLIOSIS

Congenital scoliosis is a lateral curvature of the spine caused by the presence of vertebral anomalies that result in an imbalance of the longitudinal growth of the spine. The prevalence rate of congenital scoliosis is thought to be approximately 1 in 1000 live births. The critical time in the development of the spine embryologically is the fifth to sixth week—the time of segmentation processes—and congenital anomalies of the spine develop during the first 6 weeks of intrauterine life. Some type of anomaly must be visible on the radiographs of the spine before a diagnosis of congenital scoliosis can be made. Because congenital scoliosis often is rigid and correction can be difficult, it is important to detect these curves early and to institute appropriate treatment while the curve is small rather than to attempt salvage-type procedures that are necessary when the deformity is severe.

A specific cause for congenital scoliosis has not been identified. Environmental factors, genetics, vitamin deficiency, chemicals, and drugs have all been implicated in the development of vertebral abnormalities. Currently, researchers hypothesize that environmental factors affect the delivery of genetic instructions during the critical stages of development of the spine, resulting in vertebral anomalies. A family of genes referred to as the homeobox, or HOX, genes have been shown to direct and regulate the processes of embryonic differentiation and segmentation of the axial skeleton. Loder et al. suggested that environmental factors, such as low oxygen tension, may modulate the expression of the sonic hedgehog or homeobox genes that are involved in normal vertebral segmentation. Research suggests that maternal exposure to toxins, such as carbon monoxide, may cause congenital scoliosis. Associations with maternal diabetes and ingestion of antiepileptic drugs during pregnancy also have been postulated as possible causes. However, most congenital scoliosis cases are believed to be caused by nongenetic, fetal environmental factors, but usually these factors cannot be determined by a history.

CLASSIFICATION

Classification of congenital scoliosis is based on the abnormal embryologic development of the spine and the type of vertebral anomaly. Then it is further classified by the site at which the anomaly occurs. The classification proposed by MacEwen et al. and later modified by Winter, Moe, and Eilers is the one most uniformly accepted (Box 44-7; Figs. 44-141 and 44-142). The vertebral anomalies may be caused by a failure of formation or a failure of segmentation, or by a combination of these two factors, resulting in a mixed deformity. The congenital curve also should be classified according to the area of the spine involved because this is indicative of the prognosis of the specific deformity. The areas generally distinguished are the cervicothoracic spine, thoracic spine, thoracolumbar spine, lumbar spine, and lumbosacral spine. The purpose of this classification is to distinguish curves with a poor prognosis that may require early intervention from curves that have a more benign natural history that may be observed. Kawakami et al. recommended a three-dimensional

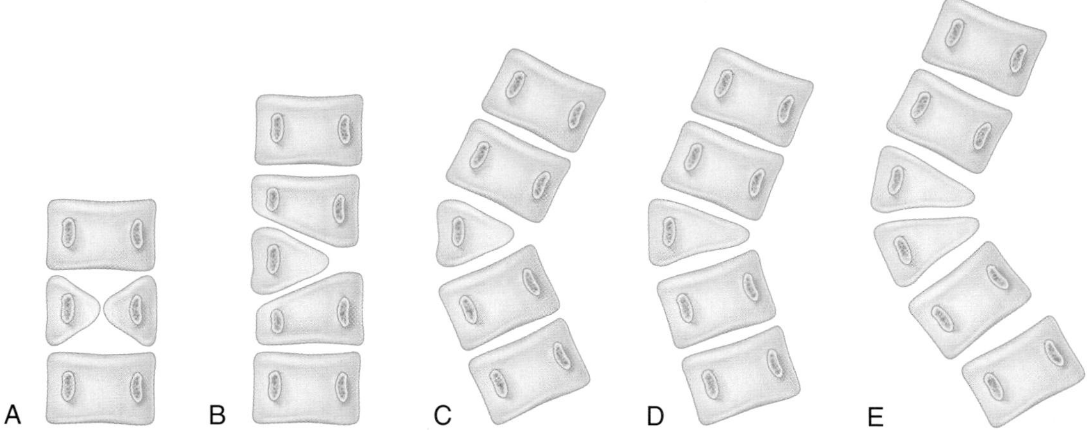

FIGURE 44-141 Defects of formation. **A**, Anterior central defect. **B**, Incarcerated hemivertebra. **C**, Free hemivertebra. **D**, Wedge vertebra. **E**, Multiple hemivertebrae.

BOX 44-7

Classification of Congenital Scoliosis

- Failure of formation (see Fig. 44-136)
  Partial failure of formation (wedge vertebra)
  Complete failure of formation (hemivertebra)
- Failure of segmentation
  Unilateral failure of segmentation (unilateral unsegmented bar; see Fig. 44-148)
  Bilateral failure of segmentation (block vertebra; see Fig. 44-142)
- Miscellaneous

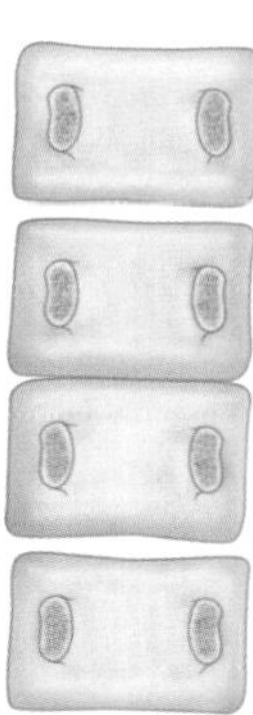

FIGURE 44-142 Block vertebra.

classification based on three-dimensional CT images. They found that congenital spinal deformity could be classified into four types: type I, solitary simple; type 2, multiple simple; type 3, complex; and type 4, segmentation failure (Table 44-6).

PATIENT EVALUATION

In addition to the routine spinal evaluation, some specific physical findings should be sought in patients with congenital scoliosis. The skin of the back should be carefully examined for signs such as hair patches, lipomas, dimples, and scars, which may indicate an underlying anomalous vertebra. The neurologic evaluation should be thorough. Evidence of neurologic involvement, such as clubfoot, calf atrophy, absent reflexes, and atrophy of one lower extremity compared with the other, should be noted carefully. Many children with congenital scoliosis have other anomalies.

Neural axis abnormalities are present in up to 35% of patients. Congenital heart disease has been reported to be present in up to 25% of patients with congenital scoliosis. Patients who are undergoing surgery for congenital scoliosis should have a screening echocardiogram and evaluation by a cardiologist. Genitourinary anomalies have been reported in 20% to 40% of patients with congenital scoliosis. A renal ultrasound remains the standard for urologic screening in these patients, but also may be evaluated on MRI if this is being obtained for other reasons. MacEwen, Winter, and

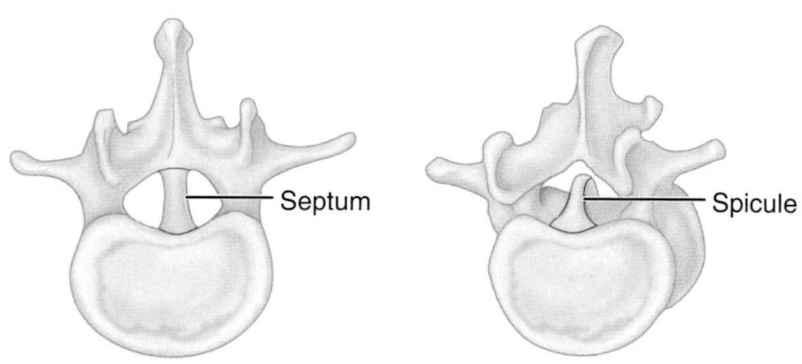

FIGURE 44-143 Diastematomyelia spicule invaginates dura and divides spinal cord, either partially or completely.

Hardy emphasized the importance of a complete evaluation of the genitourinary system: 18% of their patients had urologic anomalies, including 2.5% who had obstructive disease that could be life-threatening. Other musculoskeletal anomalies also occur frequently in association with congenital spine anomalies (Figs. 44-143 and 44-144).

A high-quality series of routine radiographs is essential to evaluate the deformity. The congenital curve should be classified as a failure of segmentation or a failure of formation, and the radiographs should be examined carefully for any evidence of widening of the pedicles or midline bony defects that may indicate an underlying cord anomaly.

TABLE 44-6

Algorithm for Evaluating Congenital Spinal Deformities

Step 1	Count the number of vertebral anomalies	Solitary or multiple
Step 2	Detect the abnormal formation	(+), (–), or (±)
Step 3	Determine the site of abnormal formation	Anterior or posterior, or both
Step 4	Determine the type of abnormal formation	Anterior: hemivertebra, anterior wedge, lateral wedge, butterfly Posterior: bilamina (wedged), incomplete bilamina, hemilamina Spina bifida
Step 5	Detect the mismatched formation	(+) or (–)
Step 6	Detect the abnormal formation	(+), (–), or (±)
Step 7	Determine the type of segmentation	Anterior: fully segmented, semisegmented, nonsegmented Posterior: fully segmented, semisegmented, nonsegmented
Step 8	Determine the site of abnormal segmentation	Anterior, unilateral, or posterior, or all
Step 9	Detect the discordant segmentation	(+) or (–)

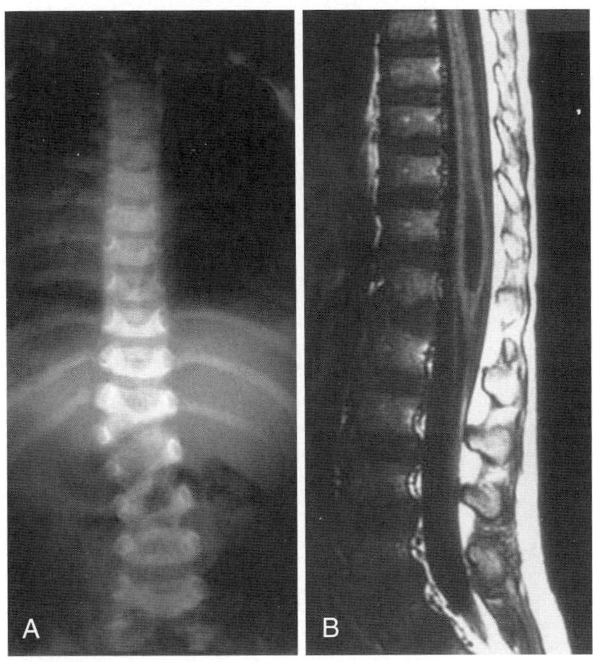

FIGURE 44-144 **A,** Congenital scoliosis with hemivertebrae. **B,** MRI shows occult syrinx extending from C4 to the conus. (From Prahinski JR, Polly DW Jr, McHale K, Ellenbogen RG: Occult intraspinal anomalies in congenital scoliosis, J Pediatr Orthop 20:59, 2000.)

Probably more important than classification of the curve is an analysis of the growth potential of the curve to better determine the possibility of curve progression. All congenital curves should be carefully measured with the Cobb technique, including compensatory or secondary curves in seemingly normal parts of the spine. Measurements should include each end of the anomalous area, as well as each end of the entire curve generally considered for treatment. CT and MRI have allowed us to better study the spinal anatomy and to screen for spinal dysraphism (see Fig. 44-144). There is a high risk of congenital intraspinal anomalies in patients with congenital scoliosis and a lack of cutaneous manifestations in a significant number of patients. MRI during infancy may help delineate the anatomic deformity, which may not be visible on plain radiographs, and also better delineates the physis. MRI is helpful in evaluating patients whose curves are not too large, but the scans are difficult to interpret in patients with major scoliosis. Winter et al. found the incidence of spinal dysraphism to be 10%. The prevalence rate of spinal dysraphism on MRI examination approaches 43% in patients with congenital spinal deformities.

NATURAL HISTORY

Progression of congenital scoliosis is dependent on the type and location of the vertebral anomaly. Curve progression occurs more rapidly during the first 5 years of life and during the adolescent growth spurt. These two periods represent the most rapid stages of spinal growth. Analysis of the growth status is the most important factor in predicting the possibility of progression of these congenital deformities. Dubousset et al. emphasized the importance of considering growth of the spinal canal in three dimensions (Fig. 44-145). Analysis of the potential growth on both sides of the curve will help with the prognosis. For example, if normal convex growth is expected and deficient concave growth is likely, major deformity will occur (Fig. 44-146); however, if growth is deficient on both the convex and concave sides, progressive lateral deformity may not occur. If both sides are deficient in growth potential over many levels, shortening of the trunk may occur without lateral curvature.

The deformity produced by a failure of formation is much more difficult to predict than that caused by failure of segmentation. A hemivertebra produces scoliosis through an enlarging wedge on the affected side of the spine, whereas a unilateral unsegmented bar retards growth on the affected side. The growth imbalance in patients with hemivertebrae is not as severe as in those with unilateral unsegmented bars. A hemivertebra can exist tucked into the spine between adjacent normal vertebrae without causing a corresponding deformity. Winter called this an "incarcerated hemivertebra." When the hemivertebra is separated from either of the adjacent vertebrae by a disc, it is a segmented hemivertebra with two functioning physes on either side and is likely to cause a

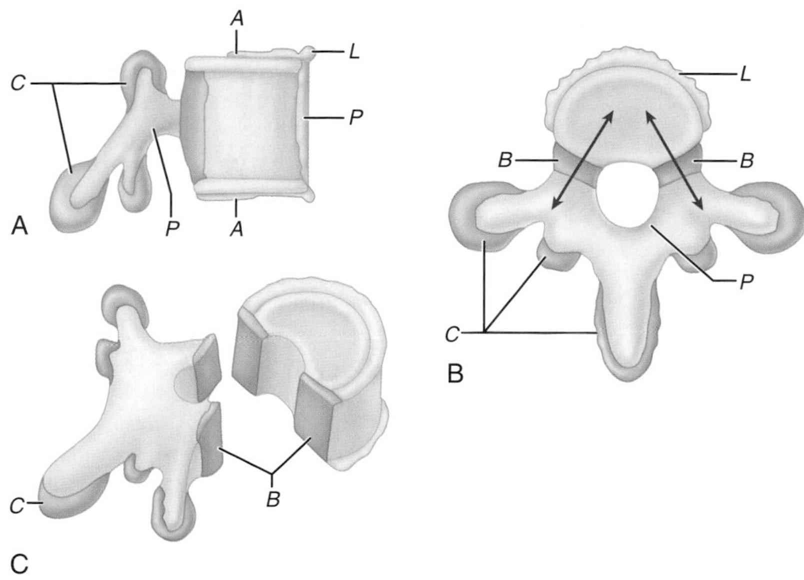

FIGURE 44-145 Vertebral growth. **A,** Body endplates (superior and inferior; labeled as *A*). **B,** Neurocentral cartilage (bipolar) fusion at age 7 or 8 years (labeled as *B*). **C,** Posterior elements cartilage (labeled as *C*). L, Ring apophysis (begins at age 7 to 9 years, closed at age 14 to 24 years); P, periosteum. (Redrawn from Dubousset J, Katti E, Seringe R: Epiphysiodesis of the spine in young children for congenital spinal deformations, J Pediatr Orthop B 1:123, 1993.)

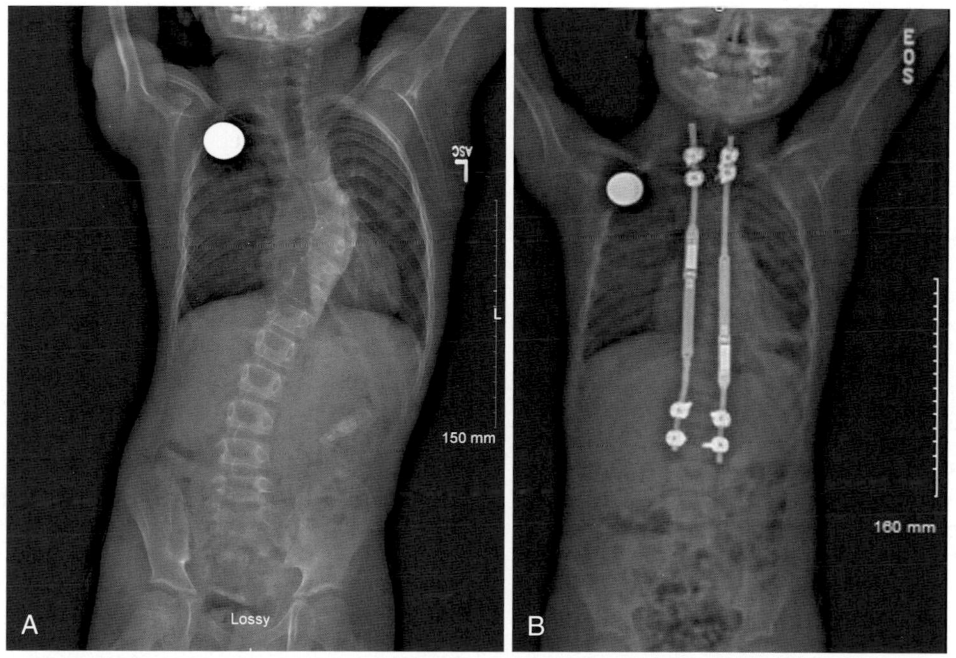

FIGURE 44-146 **A,** Eight-year-old boy with congenital scoliosis. Deficient concave growth has resulted in a major deformity. **B,** After insertion of MAGEC growing rods.

slowly progressive curve (Fig. 44-147). If the hemivertebra has only one adjacent disc and is fused to an adjacent vertebra, this is called a semisegmented hemivertebra, and if there are no adjacent discs associated with a hemivertebra, this is termed a nonsegmented hemivertebra and it has little growth potential.

Several excellent studies have outlined the natural history of congenital scoliosis and have found that the rate of deterioration and the ultimate severity of the curve depend on both the type of anomaly and the site at which it occurs. The most progressive of all anomalies is a concave, unilateral unsegmented bar with a convex hemivertebra (Fig. 44-148). The mean rate of curve progression is 6 to 7 degrees per year before 10 years of age. The majority of curves will exceed 50 degrees by 2 years of age. Second in severity is a unilateral unsegmented bar. A mean of three vertebrae usually are affected. The mean rate of curve progression is 5 degrees per year, with the curve exceeding 50 degrees by 10 years of age and 70 degrees by skeletal maturity. Next in severity of risk of progression is a double convex hemivertebra. These curves usually progress at 3 to 4 degrees per year, with most exceeding 50 degrees by 10 years of age and exceeding 70 degrees by skeletal maturity. A fully segmented hemivertebra will progress relatively slowly, at 1 or 2 degrees per year. For each type of anomaly, the rate of deterioration usually is less severe if the abnormality is in the upper thoracic region, more severe in the thoracic region, and most severe in the thoracolumbar region (Fig. 44-149). The rate of deterioration of the curve is not constant, but if the curve is present before the patient is 10 years of age, it usually increases, especially during the adolescent growth spurt. The least severe scoliosis is caused by a block vertebra.

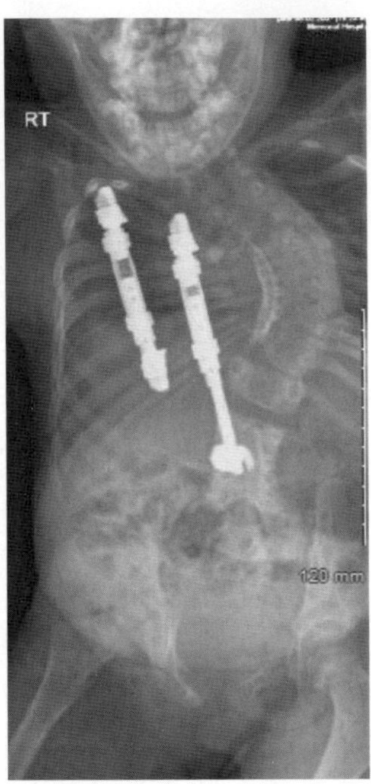

FIGURE 44-147 Progression of deformity in a 5-year-old girl with arthrogryposis and a large unsegmented bar treated with rib-based distraction (VEPTR).

NONOPERATIVE TREATMENT

Nonoperative treatment is of limited value in patients with congenital scoliosis. Nonprogressive curves require regular observation during periods of rapid growth (0 to 5 years of age and 10 to 15 years of age) with quality radiographs twice a year. Observation also is helpful in patients with multiple anomalies in whom the prognosis is difficult to determine.

Bracing sometimes can be used to control secondary curves when the primary congenital curve is being treated

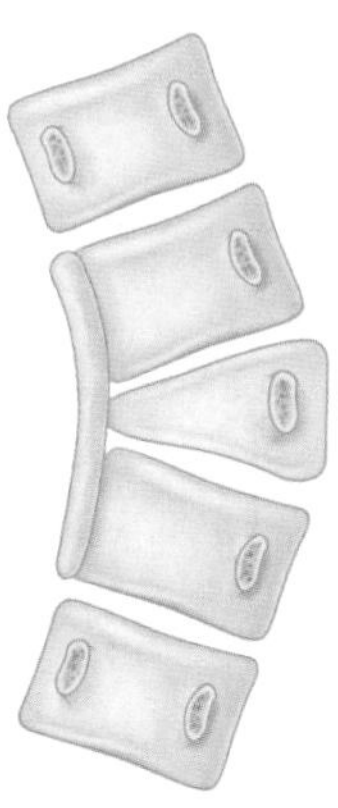

FIGURE 44-148 Unilateral and unsegmented bar with contralateral hemivertebra.

No treatment required / May require spinal fusion / Requires spinal fusion / * Too few or no curves

Site of curvature	Block vertebra	Wedged vertebra	Hemivertebrae: Single	Hemivertebrae: Double	Unilateral unsegmented bar	Unilateral unsegmented bar and contralateral hemivertebrae
Upper thoracic	< 1° – 1°	* – 2°	1° – 2°	2° – 2.5°	2° – 4°	5° – 6°
Lower thoracic	< 1° – 1°	1° – 2°	2° – 2.5°	2° – 3°	5° – 6.5°	6° – 7°
Thoracolumbar	< 1° – 1°	1.5° – 2°	2° – 3.5°	5° – *	6° – 9°	> 10° – *
Lumbar	< 1° – *	< 1° – *	< 1° – 1°	*	> 5° – *	*
Lumbosacral	*	*	< 1° – 1.5°	*	*	*

FIGURE 44-149 Median yearly rate of deterioration without treatment for each type of single congenital scoliosis in each region of spine. Numbers on left in each column refer to patients seen before 10 years of age; numbers on right refer to patients seen at age 10 years or older.

BOX 44-8

Treatment of Congenital Scoliosis

- Prevention of future deformity
  In situ fusion
- Correction of deformity—gradual
  Hemiepiphysiodesis and hemiarthrodesis
  Growing rod nonfusion
  Vertical expandable prosthetic titanium rib (VEPTR)
- Correction of deformity—acute
  Instrumentation and fusion
  Hemivertebra excision
  Osteotomy

BOX 44-9

Common Errors in Instrumentation in Patients With Congenital Scoliosis

- Use of rods in small children in whom the bone structure is not strong enough to add any stability
- Excessive distraction leading to paralysis
- Failure to preoperatively evaluate for a tethered cord or other intraspinal abnormalities
- Failure to do a wake-up test after rod insertion
- Failure to perform adequate fusion because of reliance on internal stability
- Failure to supplement the instrumentation with adequate external immobilization

nonoperatively. Also, bracing may prevent progression of a secondary curve that is causing balance problems. If orthotic treatment is elected, careful measurement and comparison of spine radiographs at 6-month intervals must be made. Because of the slow progression of some curves, it is important to compare current radiographs with all previous films, including the original films, to detect curve progression.

OPERATIVE TREATMENT

Because 75% of congenital curves are progressive, surgery remains the fundamental treatment. Congenital spinal deformity can be treated by procedures that prevent further deformity or procedures that correct the present deformity. If treatment is aimed at correcting the present deformity, the curve can be corrected gradually or immediately. The surgical methods available for treatment of congenital scoliosis are outlined in Box 44-8.

POSTERIOR FUSION WITHOUT INSTRUMENTATION

In situ fusion allows for stabilization of a curve that has shown documented progression or is predicted to progress. It is ideally done early for small curves to prevent the curve from becoming unacceptably large. A controversy with in situ fusion is whether a combined anterior and posterior fusion is required. Posterior fusion alone can control curve progression, but if there is significant anterior growth in the involved vertebra, progression of the deformity may occur in some young children owing to the crankshaft phenomenon. If anterior fusion is needed, then this may be performed either through an anterior open technique, thoracoscopically, or with a posterior approach through the pedicles. In situ fusion for unilateral unsegmented bars usually only includes the involved vertebra. One level cephalad and one level caudad to the involved vertebrae are included in the fusion.

The basic posterior spinal fusion technique is described in Technique 44-6. Correction is achieved postoperatively by a corrective cast or brace. Smaller-sized implants that are appropriate for the patient's size may be used for stabilization of in situ fusion and lessen the time needed in a cast or brace.

POSTERIOR FUSION WITH INSTRUMENTATION

The advantages of instrumentation in congenital scoliosis are that slightly more correction can be obtained, the rate of pseudarthrosis can be reduced somewhat, and the need for a postoperative cast or brace is less. These advantages must be weighed against the risks of paralysis and infection. Congenital scoliosis is the condition in which paraplegia occurs most often after Harrington instrumentation. The risk of neurologic injury can be lowered but not eliminated with careful preoperative evaluation by myelography or MRI, by intraoperative spinal cord monitoring with somatosensory evoked potentials and motor-evoked potentials, and by the routine use of the wake-up test. Instrumentation does not alter the length of the fusion or the necessity for facet fusion, decortications, or abundant bone graft (Box 44-9). Instrumentation usually should be reserved for larger curves in older children in whom obtaining and maintaining correction of the curves would be difficult in a plaster cast alone. The curves should be flexible, and no intraspinal abnormalities should be present. Ideally, kyphosis should not be significant. The goal of this surgery is modest correction and curve control. In addition to spinal cord monitoring with somatosensory evoked potentials and motor-evoked potentials, a wake-up test also is needed in these patients. The instrumentation is used to increase the fusion rate and as a stabilizing strut, rather than to obtain significant correction.

COMBINED ANTERIOR AND POSTERIOR FUSIONS

The main indications for anterior and posterior fusions instead of isolated posterior fusion are to treat sagittal plane problems, to increase the flexibility of the scoliosis by discectomy, to eliminate the anterior physis to prevent bending or torsion of the fusion mass with further growth (crankshaft phenomenon), and to treat curves with a significant potential for progression. The anterior procedure consists of removal of the disc, cartilage endplates, and bony endplates. Bone graft in the form of bone chips is placed into the disc space for fusion. No anterior instrumentation is used. The spine is exposed on the convex side, but the approach is dictated by the level of the curve. The anterior fusion can be done through an open anterior approach or thoracoscopically. After the anterior fusion, a posterior procedure is done. Instrumentation may or may not be used, depending on such factors as the severity of the curve. The postoperative management is the same as after posterior fusion with or without instrumentation. Dubousset et al. recommended anterior and posterior fusions in young patients who are fused at the lumbar level before Risser grade 0 and who have significant residual deformity of 30 degrees and 10 degrees of rotation. For thoracic curves, the amount of crankshaft effect that can be tolerated is weighed against the risks of the thoracotomy necessary to perform the anterior epiphysiodesis.

TRANSPEDICULAR CONVEX ANTERIOR HEMIEPIPHYSIODESIS AND POSTERIOR ARTHRODESIS

King et al. described a technique of transpedicular convex anterior hemiepiphysiodesis combined with posterior arthrodesis for treatment of progressive congenital scoliosis. In effect, a combined anterior and posterior fusion can be done through a single posterior approach. These authors reported arrest of curve progression in all nine of their patients after this procedure. The average age of patients at surgery was 9 years. Their technique is based on the work of Michel and Krueger, who described a transpedicular approach to the vertebral body, and Heinig, who described the "eggshell" procedure, so called because the vertebral body is hollowed out until it is eggshell thin before it is collapsed. King et al. found the pedicle dimensions to be adequate for this technique even in infants; however, they recommended preoperative CT through the center of each pedicle to be included in the epiphysiodesis.

TECHNIQUE 44-41

(KING)

- Position the patient prone on a radiolucent operating table, with a frame or chest rolls. After preparation and draping, obtain a radiograph over a skin marker to identify the appropriate level for the incision.
- Make a single midline posterior incision and retract the paraspinous muscles on both sides of the curve as far as the tips of the costotransverse processes in the thoracic spine and lateral to the facet joints in the lumbar spine.
- Remove the cortical bone in the area of the pedicle to be mined caudad to the facet joint and at the base of the costotransverse process in the thoracic spine.
- Use the curet to remove the cancellous bone. The medullary cavity of the pedicle can now be seen. The cortex medially indicates the boundary of the spinal canal, and caudally and cranially it indicates the margins of the intervertebral neural foramina. Use progressively larger curets until only the cortical rim of the pedicle remains (Fig. 44-150A). The pedicle margins then expand into the vertebral body.
- Remove cancellous bone, creating a hole in the lateral half of the vertebral body, and use curved curets to remove cancellous bone from the vertebral body in the cephalad and caudal directions until the endplate bone, the physis, and the intervertebral disc are encountered. Brisk bleeding may occur, and the surgeon should be prepared for it.
- For a single hemivertebra, mine the pedicle of the hemivertebra itself, along with that of the adjacent vertebrae in the cephalad and caudal directions (Fig. 44-150B). Communication with each pedicle hole across the physis and disc space is readily achieved (Fig. 44-150C).
- Pack autogenous bone from the iliac crest down the pedicles and across the vertebral endplates and discs.
- Posteriorly, excise the convex and concave facet joints and pack with cancellous bone. Carry out decortication bilaterally.
- Use autologous iliac crest bone graft or allograft bone graft.
- If internal fixation is needed, a wire, compression device, or pedicle screw device can be used.

POSTOPERATIVE CARE. The patient is placed in a TLSO for 4 to 6 months. After that, no further immobilization is used.

COMBINED ANTERIOR AND POSTERIOR CONVEX HEMIEPIPHYSIODESIS (GROWTH ARREST)

Gradual correction of congenital scoliosis may be obtained through the use of a convex hemiepiphysiodesis. This technique is used for curves that are the result of failure of formation. There is no role for this technique in failures of segmentation. Correction of deformity relies on the future growth of the spine on the concave side. In deformities caused by failure of segmentation, there is really no growth potential on the concave side. This technique is best for treating a single hemivertebra that has not resulted in a large curve at the time of surgery. This technique is appropriate in children younger than 5 years who meet certain criteria: a documented progressive curve, a curve of less than 50 degrees, a curve of six segments or fewer, concave growth potential, and no pathologic congenital kyphosis or lordosis. Even if the concave side ceases to grow, the anterior and posterior fusions obtain a good result as far as stabilizing the curve. Epiphysiodesis of the entire curve, not merely the apical segment, should be done. Rigid spinal immobilization is used until the fusions are solid, usually at least 6 months after surgery.

Preoperative planning is important. Each vertebra should be considered a cube divided into four quadrants, with each quadrant growing symmetrically around the spinal canal (Fig. 44-151). When growth is unbalanced, the zones that must be fused to reestablish balanced growth are determined preoperatively. King et al. noted a true epiphysiodesis effect after transpedicular convex anterior hemiepiphysiodesis (see Technique 44-41) in four of their nine patients, all four of whom had a single hemivertebra. On the basis of these results, they recommended transpedicular hemiepiphysiodesis with posterior hemiarthrodesis in selected patients with a single hemivertebra. Demirkiran et al. reported that a convex growth arrest could be obtained with a posterior fusion and pedicle screw instrumentation at each involved level, with results similar to those of an anteroposterior convex hemiepiphysiodesis.

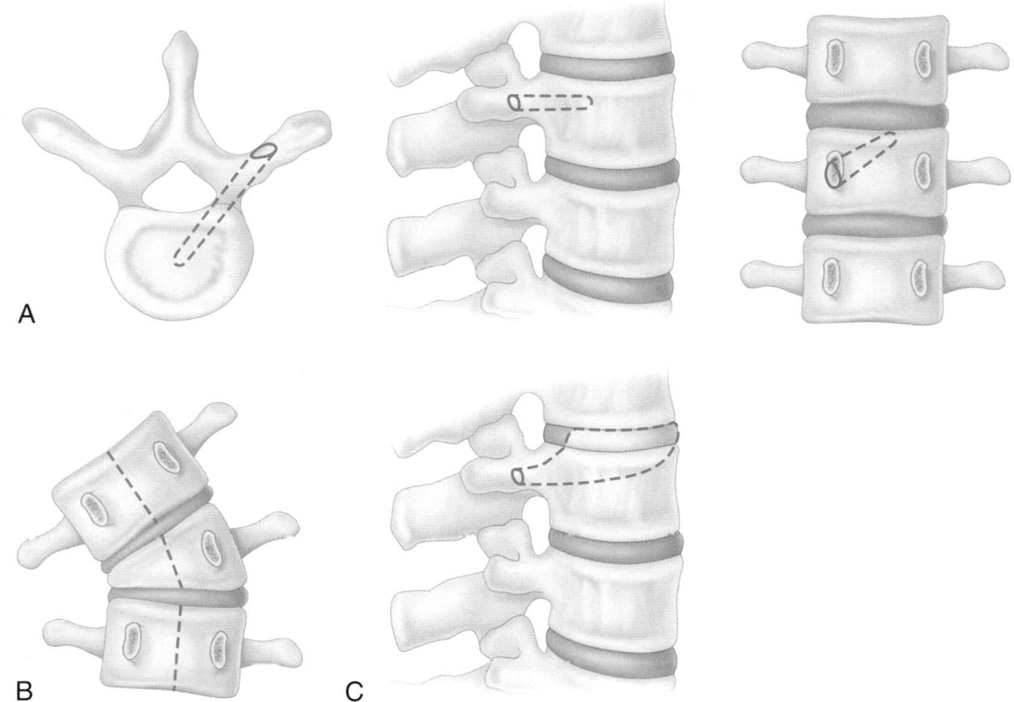

FIGURE 44-150 **A,** How pedicles are curetted. **B,** Anterior view of bone removed during "eggshell" procedure. **C,** Bone is almost completely hollowed out, and endplates and discs have been removed. **SEE TECHNIQUE 44-41.**

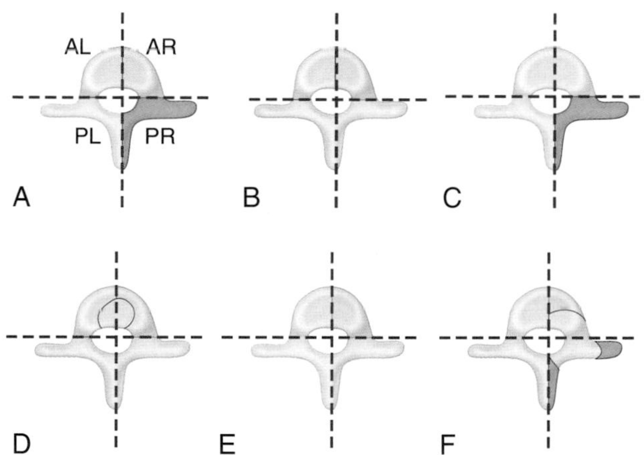

FIGURE 44-151 **A,** Vertebral growth on horizontal plane, four segments: AL, anterior left; AR, anterior right; PL, posterior left; and PR, posterior right. **B,** Congenital posterior bar involving PL and PR; level of epiphysiodesis must be AL and AR. **C,** Anterior defect involving AL and AR; epiphysiodesis must involve PL and PR. **D,** Anterior excess of growth potential involving both AR and AL; epiphysiodesis must involve both AR and AL above and below. **E,** Congenital posterolateral bar involving PL only; epiphysiodesis must involve only AR. **F,** Excess (hemivertebra) growth involving only AR and part of PR; hemiepiphysiodesis must involve AR and PR. (Modified from Dubousset J, Katti E, Seringe R: Epiphysiodesis of spine in young children for congenital spinal deformation, J Pediatr Orthop B 1:23, 1992.)

CONVEX ANTERIOR AND POSTERIOR HEMIEPIPHYSIODESES AND FUSION

TECHNIQUE 44-42

(WINTER)

- Place the patient in a straight lateral position with the convexity of the curve upward. Prepare and drape the back and side in the same field. The anterior approach technique varies according to the level to be fused (see Techniques 44-28 and 44-29). The posterior approach is a standard subperiosteal exposure (see Technique 44-8) but is always only on the convex side of the curve.
- Once the curve has been exposed, insert needles or other markers both anteriorly and posteriorly so that both are visible on one cross-table radiograph. Failure to place the fusion precisely in the proper area can lead to a poor result.
- Once the proper area has been identified, incise the periosteum of the anterior vertebral bodies and peel it forward to the lateral edge of the anterior longitudinal ligament and backward to the base of the pedicle (Fig. 44-152A).
- Incise the annulus of the disc at its superior and inferior margins and remove the superficial portion of the nucleus pulposus.

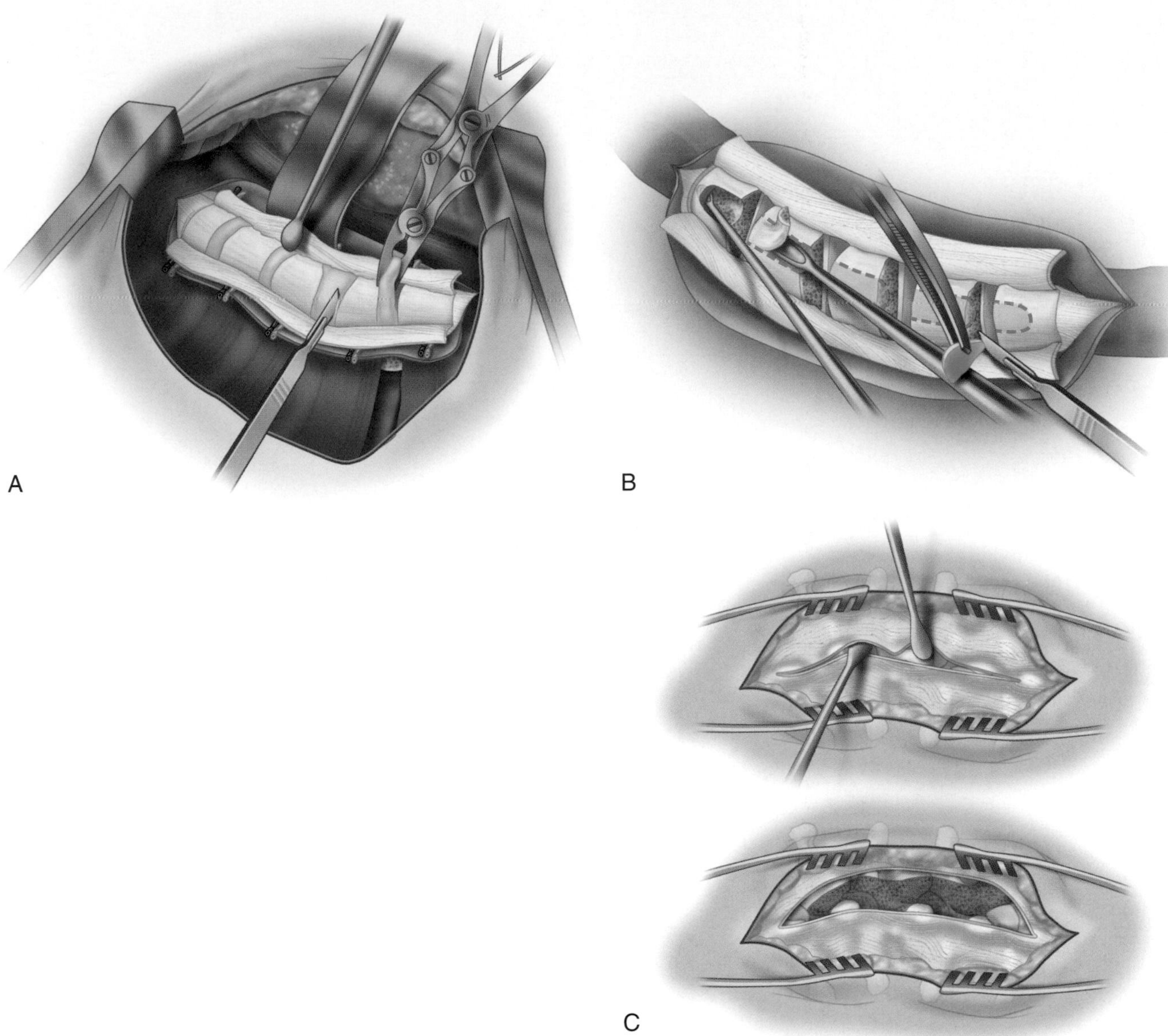

FIGURE 44-152 Combined anterior and posterior convex hemiepiphysiodesis. **A,** Periosteum of anterior vertebral bodies incised and peeled forward and backward. **B,** Trough created in lateral side of vertebral bodies. Autogenous rib graft placed in trough. **C,** Area to be fused exposed through standard, unilateral, subperiosteal exposure. Area is decorticated, and bone graft is applied. **SEE TECHNIQUE 44-42.**

- Carefully remove the cartilaginous endplates, which are thick in children, taking at least one third of the physes but never more than half.
- Once the cartilaginous endplates have been removed, remove the cortical bony endplate with a curet.
- Make a trough in the lateral side of the vertebral bodies (Fig. 44-152B) and lay the autogenous rib graft in the trough. Use cancellous bone to augment the autogenous rib graft. If autogenous rib is not available, use iliac or bone-bank bone.
- The posterior procedure consists of a standard, unilateral, subperiosteal exposure of the area to be fused (Fig. 44-152C).
- Excise the facet joints, remove any facet cartilage, decorticate the entire area, and apply a bone graft.
- Apply a corrective Risser cast while the child is still under anesthesia to avoid having to use a second anesthetic.

POSTOPERATIVE CARE. Casting is continued for 6 months, and the cast is changed as frequently as necessary. Follow-up must be continued until the end of growth. Results may appear excellent for years but can deteriorate during the adolescent growth spurt.

Growing rods and VEPTR instrumentations that have been used to treat early-onset scoliosis also have been used

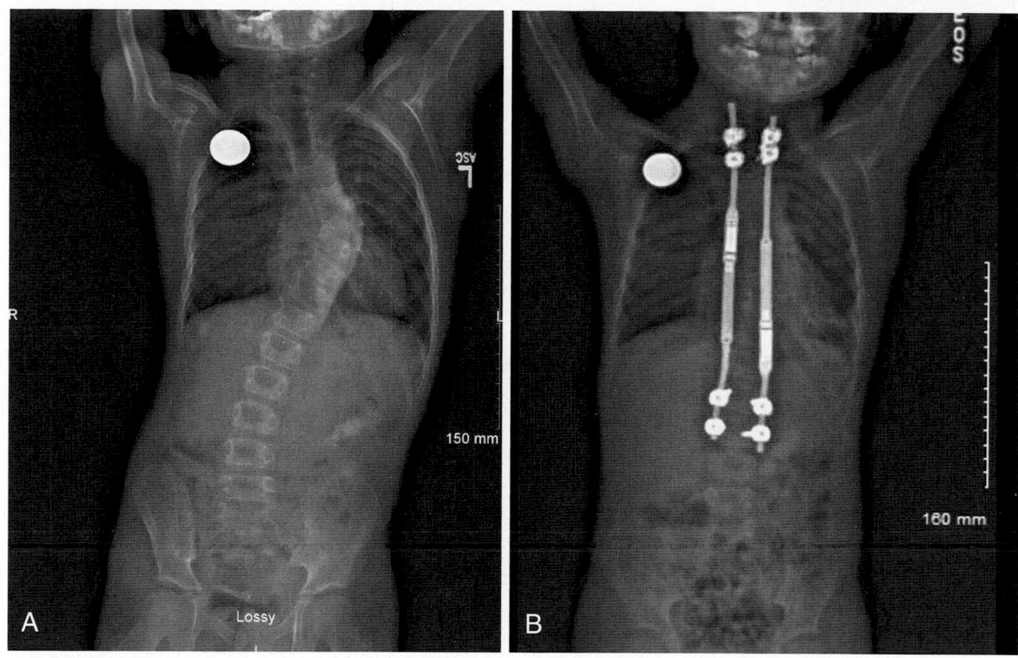

FIGURE 44-153 **A,** Eight-year-old boy with congenital scoliosis. **B,** After correction and insertion of MAGEC growing rods. **SEE TECHNIQUE 44-42.**

for gradual correction and stabilization of progressive congenital curves. Several authors have reported good results with these techniques, with acceptable complication rates. The growing rod technique is suggested for patients with primary vertebral anomalies (Fig. 44-153); patients with rib fusion or associated thoracic insufficiency syndrome with congenital scoliosis usually are treated with a VEPTR.

HEMIVERTEBRA EXCISION

Hemivertebra excision can produce immediate correction of a congenital spine deformity. This technique will remove the cause of and prevent further worsening of the deformity. Hemivertebra excision usually is reserved for patients with pelvic obliquity or with fixed, lateral translation of the thorax that cannot be corrected by other means. At the lumbosacral area, excision of the hemivertebra can improve trunk imbalance. The L3, L4, or lumbosacral level, below the level of the conus medullaris, is the safest level at which to excise a hemivertebra. Hemivertebra excision in the thoracic area has more risk because this area of the spinal canal is the narrowest and has the least blood supply, but with spinal cord monitoring (somatosensory evoked potentials and motor-evoked potentials) the excision can still be performed.

The curves best managed by hemivertebra excision are angular curves in which the hemivertebra is the apex. This technique has been reported mostly in lumbosacral hemivertebrae that produce lateral spinal decompensation in patients for whom curve-stabilizing techniques cannot achieve adequate alignment. Hemivertebra resection can be done at any age, but the optimal indication of hemivertebra resection is a patient younger than 5 years with a thoracolumbar, lumbar, or lumbosacral hemivertebra that is associated with truncal imbalance or a progressive curve. Chang et al. recommended early resection before structural changes occur above and below the hemivertebra. They also found that if resection was done before 6 years of age, the patients had significantly better deformity correction and did not have any negative effects on the growth of the vertebral body or spinal canal compared with patients treated after 6 years of age. Yaszay et al. found that while hemivertebra resection had a higher complication rate than either hemiepiphysiodesis/in situ fusion or instrumented fusion without resection, posterior hemivertebra resection in younger patients resulted in a better percentage of correction than the other two techniques.

Hemivertebra excision should be considered a convex osteotomy at the apex of the curve. The entire curve front and back must be fused. Neurologic risk is inherent in hemivertebra excision because the spinal canal is entered both anteriorly and posteriorly. Winter described two patients with lumbar root problems after hemivertebra excision.

Leatherman and Dickson recommended a two-stage procedure in which the vertebral body is removed through an anterior exposure; then, in a second stage, the posterior elements are removed and fusion is done. Other authors have reported acceptable results with one-stage anterior and posterior hemivertebra resection. If there is significant associated kyphosis, the hemivertebra can be excised from a posterior-only technique as described by Ruf and Harms or through a costotransversectomy as described by Smith. In general, postoperative cast or brace immobilization is prescribed for 6 months. The use of instrumentation with downsized implants will give adequate fixation and may permit a brace to be worn rather than a cast, but the bone stock must be adequate to accept the instrumentation or a postoperative cast will be needed.

Heinig described a decancellation procedure done with curets through the pedicle. Lubicky recommended both internal fixation and external immobilization with this technique. He found that the amount of immediate correction from this technique was unpredictable, but it did generally

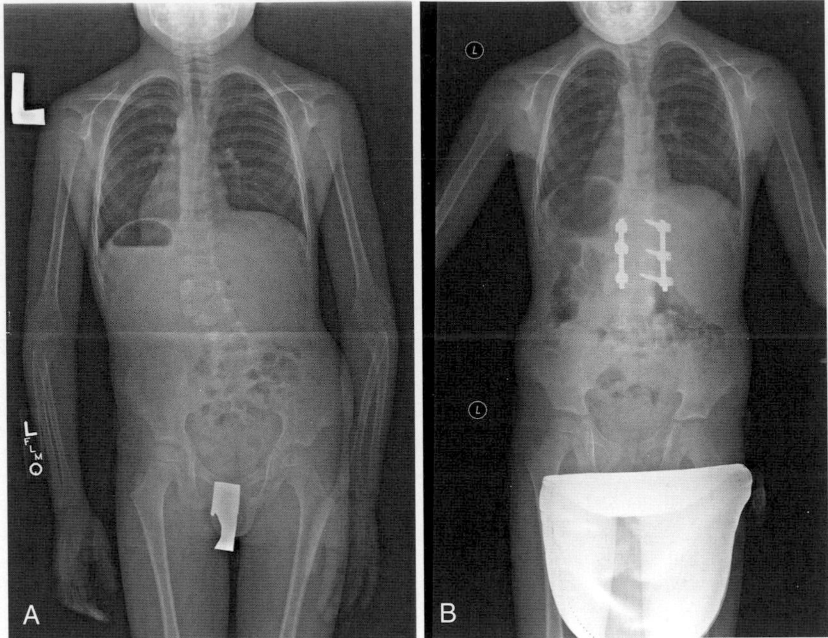

FIGURE 44-154 **A,** Congenital scoliosis in a 7-year-old boy. **B,** After hemivertebra excision and fusion with short-segment rods and pedicle screws.

lead to a hemiepiphysiodesis when it was combined with a convex posterior fusion at the same level. He recommended that the technique be done with C-arm control (Figs. 44-154 and 44-155). Heinig and Lubicky advised leaving the hemilamina in place until the vertebral body resection is complete to protect the neural tube while the curet is used. This technique can be useful if the hemivertebra is located posteriorly next to the spinal canal, where seeing the hemivertebra from anteriorly can be difficult.

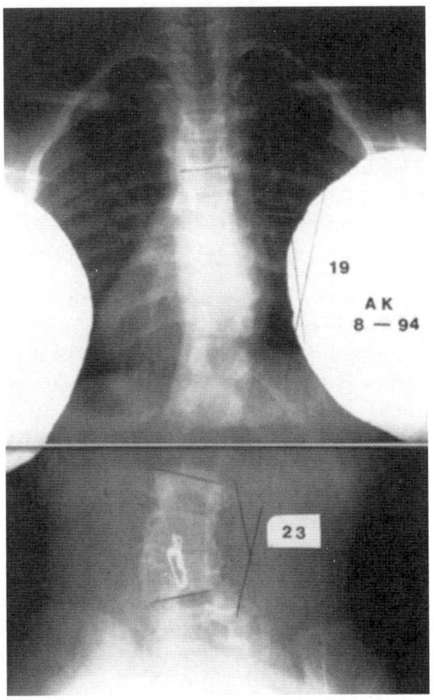

FIGURE 44-155 **Posteroanterior standing view of spine in 8½-year-old girl shows nicely balanced spine and solid hemiepiphysiodesis on left in lumbar spine 7 years after procedure similar to eggshell technique.** (From Lubicky JP: Congenital scoliosis. In Bridwell KH, DeWald RL, editors: The textbook of spinal surgery, ed 2, Philadelphia, 1997, Lippincott-Raven.)

HEMIVERTEBRA EXCISION: ANTEROPOSTERIOR APPROACH

TECHNIQUE 44-43

(HEDEQUIST AND EMANS)

- Place the patient in the lateral decubitus position for simultaneous anteroposterior approach. The anterior approach is on the convex side and should be marked before surgery (Fig. 44-156A).
- For the anterior procedure, approach the spine through a standard transthoracic, transthoracic-retroperitoneal, or retroperitoneal approach, depending on the location of the hemivertebra. The only exposure needed is of the hemivertebra and the discs above and below it.
- For the posterior approach, make a standard posterior midline incision and carry the dissection out to the tips of the transverse process, taking care when dissecting over the areas of laminar deficiency.
- After the dissection is complete, obtain a spot radiograph or fluoroscopic view to confirm the appropriate level.

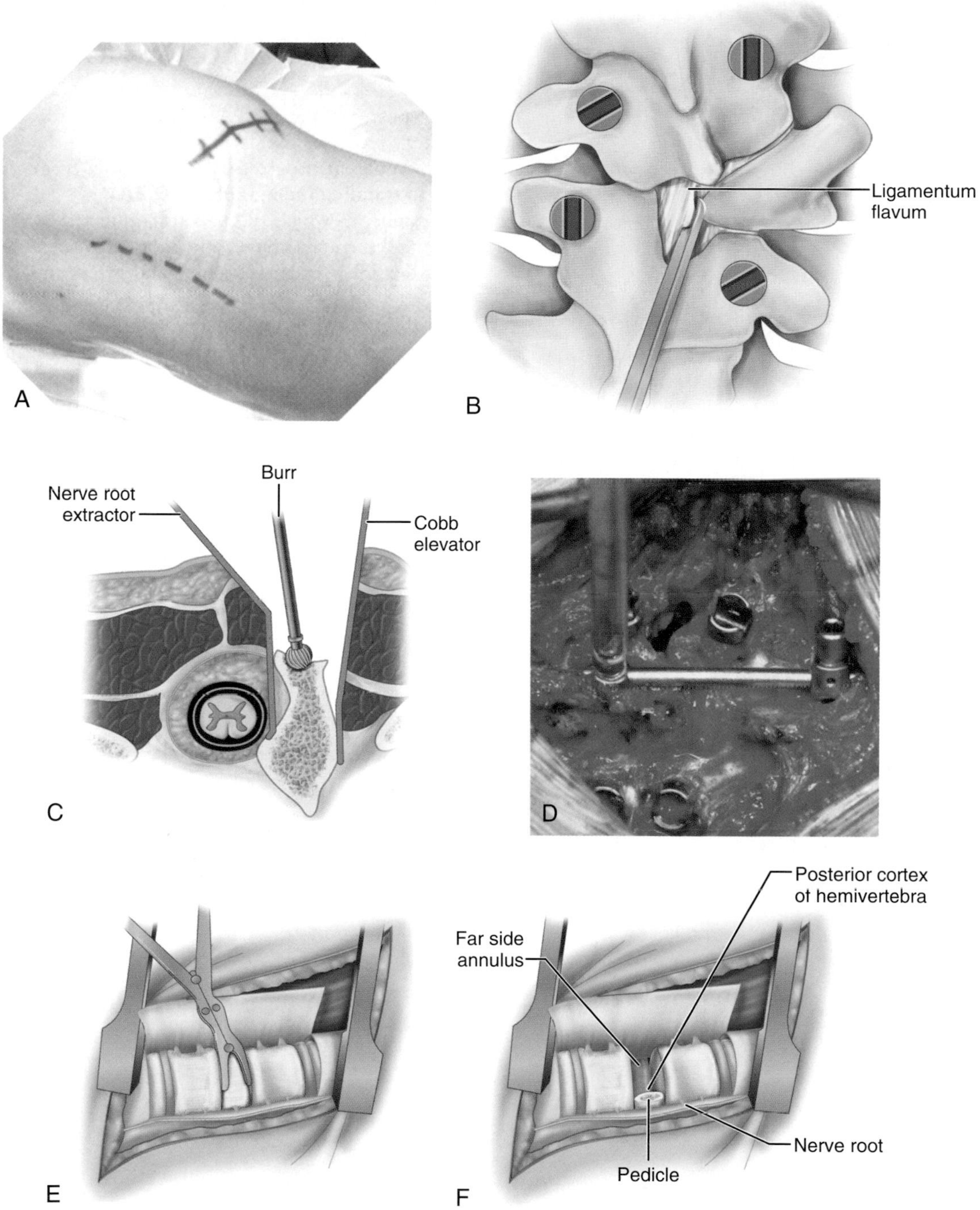

Ligamentum flavum

Nerve root extractor

Burr

Cobb elevator

Posterior cortex of hemivertebra

Far side annulus

Nerve root

Pedicle

FIGURE 44-156 Hemivertebra excision. **A,** Patient positioning for anteroposterior excision. **B** and **C,** Resection of posterior hemilamina with Kerrison rongeur. **D,** Compression of laminar hooks with closure of excision site. **E,** Anterior resection. **F,** Resection carried back to pedicle. (From Hedequist DJ, Emans JB: Hemivertebra excision. In Wiesel SW, editor: Operative techniques in orthopaedic surgery, Philadelphia, 2011, Wolters Kluwer/Lippincott Williams & Wilkins, p. 1466.) **SEE TECHNIQUE 44-43.**

HEMIVERTEBRA EXCISION

- Begin the excision by dissecting over the edge of the transverse process and down the lateral wall of the body with a Cobb elevator and a curve-tipped device. Place a curved retractor. If the hemivertebra is in the thoracic region, resect the rib head first to obtain access.
- Resect the cartilaginous surfaces of the concave facet to encourage fusion.
- With a Kerrison rongeur, begin resection in the midline with the ligamentum flavum followed by resection of the hemilamina (Fig. 44-156B). Extend the resection over to the facet, protecting the nerve roots above and below the

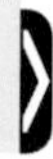

hemivertebra. Resect the transverse process and cortical bone over the pedicle until cancellous bone of the pedicle and cortical outlines of its walls are seen. Once again, take care to avoid nerve roots. Gelfoam and cottonoids can be used to protect the dura during resection.

- Develop the subperiosteal plane down the lateral wall of the pedicle and body with the use of a Cobb elevator to facilitate retraction and protection. The dural contents can be protected with a nerve root retractor. Blood loss can be controlled by bipolar sealing of the epidural vessels. Use a diamond-tipped burr to continue resection to the pedicle and into the hemivertebral body to protect against unwanted injury to the soft tissues. Work stepwise within the walls of the pedicle and confines of the body to make removal of the cortical shells easier (Fig. 44-156C). Resect the walls of the pedicle and the remaining walls of the hemivertebral body. Generally, the dorsal cortex of the vertebral body is removed last. The resection is wedge shaped and includes the discs above and below, as well as the concave area of the disc.
- While protecting the dura and its contents, remove the disc material with a pituitary rongeur and curet. Do not remove the disc material above or below or correction will be limited. Proceed with wedge closure and deformity correction.

CLOSURE OF WEDGE RESECTION

- Place resected vertebral cancellous bone and allograft chips into the wedge resection site anteriorly.
- Closure of the wedge resection is achieved with the use of laminar hooks and external three-point pressure on the body.
- Place a downgoing supralaminar hook at the superior level and an upgoing infralaminar hook on the inferior level.
- To close the resection site, insert the rod, using compression to obtain correction. Using the rod avoids having to place large compression forces across the pedicle screws and allows the screws to maintain correction without plowing of the screws into the immature bone. The compression should be slow and controlled. Observe the dura to make sure it does not get caught in the closure of the posterior elements (Fig. 44-156D). If insufficient correction is obtained, resect further along the edges of the laminae.
- Place two additional rods on either side of the spine connected to the corresponding screws. Apply a crosslink if possible.
- Decorticate the spine and place vertebral corticocancellous allograft.

ANTEROPOSTERIOR EXCISION

- If anteroposterior excision is performed, place the posterior implant anchors before resection. Once complete exposure has been performed, place the posterior screws.
- Create a full-thickness subperiosteal flap over the hemivertebra after localization is confirmed (Fig. 44-156E).
- Starting at the inferior endplate of the adjacent superior body and the superior endplate of the adjacent inferior body, create longitudinal full-thickness cuts in the periosteum, working anteriorly to the contralateral side. Then move posteriorly until the hemivertebral pedicle is seen.
- Resect the discs above and below the hemivertebra all the way posterior to the posterior longitudinal ligament.
- Resect the hemivertebral body back to the posterior cortical wall of the body with rongeurs and a diamond-tipped burr. The posterior wall can be resected off the posterior longitudinal ligament starting at the level of the disc resections. The part of the pedicle that can be seen can be resected.
- For posterior resection, start with the hemilamina and proceed to the pedicle (Fig. 44-156F). With both incisions open and fields exposed, the pedicle can be resected though both incisions.
- Once the hemivertebra has been resected, wedge closure and correction of the deformity can proceed as described earlier.

POSTOPERATIVE CARE. Postoperative care is similar to that for other spinal correction procedures. If fixation is adequate, patients can be placed in a custom-molded TLSO for 3 months. In children younger than 2 years or if fixation is not adequate, a Risser type cast is recommended for 2 months followed by brace wear for 6 months. It may be necessary to remove the implants after a year if prominence is a problem.

HEMIVERTEBRA EXCISION: LATERAL-POSTERIOR APPROACH

Li et al. described a lateral-posterior approach for hemivertebra resection that gave a safe and stable resection through a single incision (Fig. 44-157).

TECHNIQUE 44-44

(LI ET AL.)

- After administration of general anesthesia, place the patient in a lateral decubitus position, with the convex

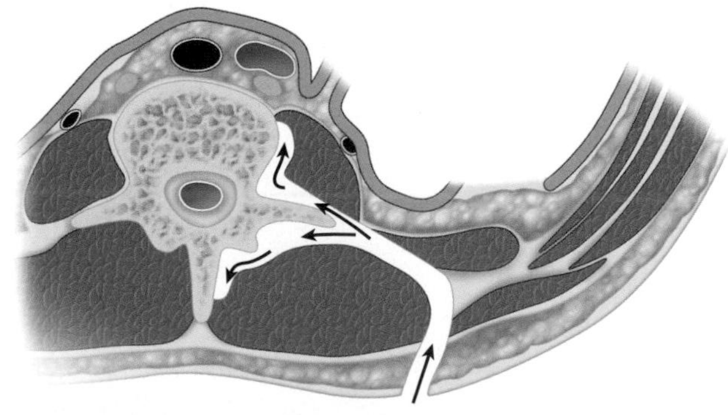

FIGURE 44-157 **Lateral-posterior approach for hemivertebra resection.** (Redrawn from Li X, Luo Z, Li X, et al: Hemivertebra resection for the treatment of congenital lumbar spinal scoliosis with lateral-posterior approach, Spine 33:2001, 2008.) **SEE TECHNIQUE 44-44.**

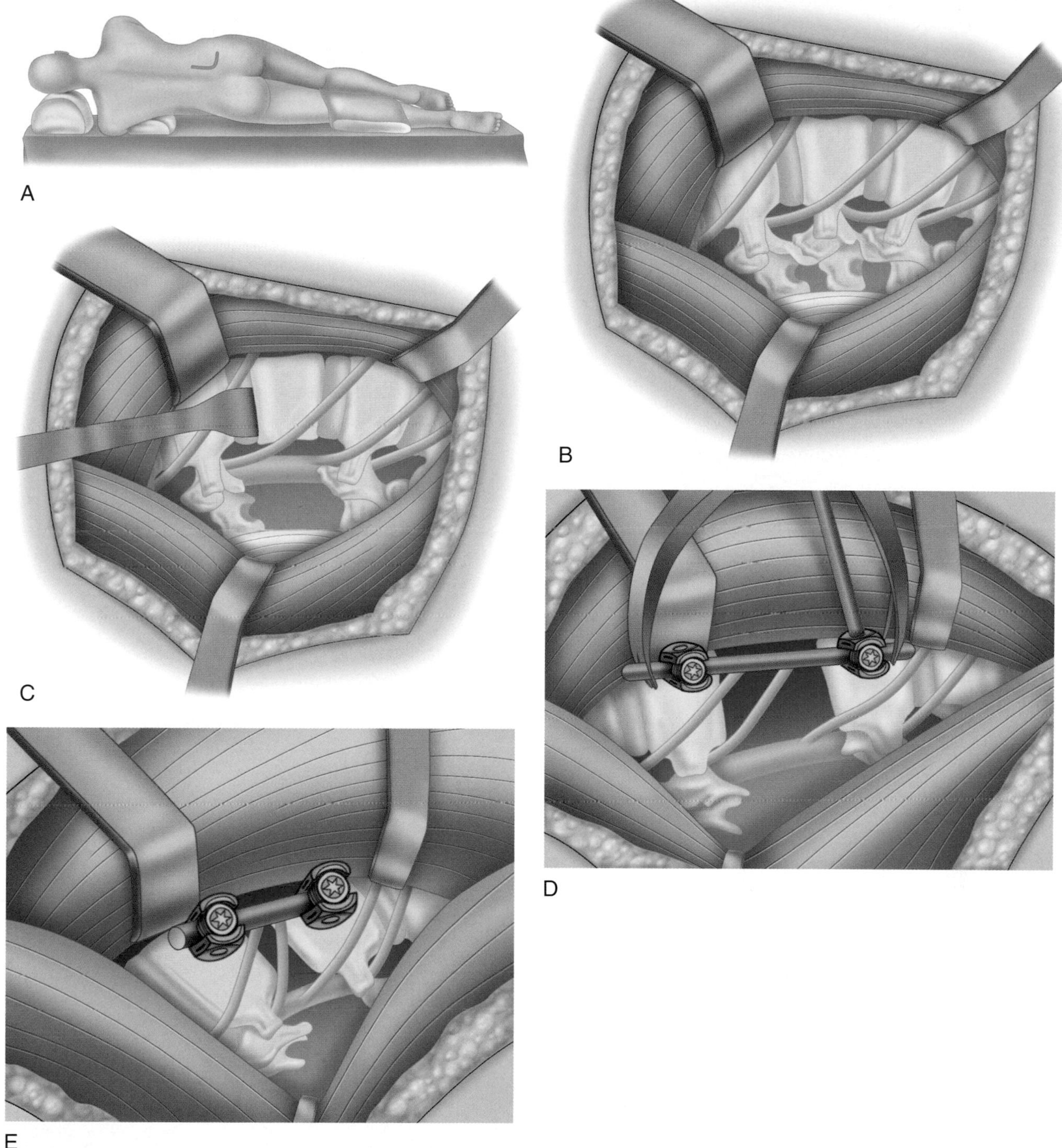

FIGURE 44-158 Hemivertebra excision through lateral-posterior approach. **A,** Patient positioning. **B,** Exposure of hemivertebra. **C,** Resection of hemivertebra. **D,** Compression and stabilization. **E,** Fusion. (Redrawn from Li X, Luo Z, Li X, et al: Hemivertebra resection for the treatment of congenital lumbar spinal scoliosis with lateral-posterior approach, Spine 33:2001, 2008.) **SEE TECHNIQUE 44-44.**

side of the curve up. Prepare and drape the flank in routine fashion.

- Use an L-shaped lateral-posterior approach to expose the hemivertebra (Fig. 44-158A). Make a straight longitudinal incision about 3.5 cm lateral to the spinous process from one segment cephalad to one segment caudad to the hemivertebra, and then turn to the lateral.
- Carry the dissection down to the lumbodorsal fascia and retract the skin and subcutaneous tissue on either side.
- Make a fascial incision and pull the sacrospinal muscle medially.
- Expose the lumbar transverse processes, facet joints, lamina, and spinous process subperiosteally.

- After pulling the psoas major laterally, proceed with dissection directly anteriorly on the pedicle to the vertebral body.
- After segmental vessels have been ligated, the hemivertebra and the appendage, which have been identified radiographically, are exposed (Fig. 44-158B).
- Remove the lamina of the hemivertebra with its attached transverse process, facet joint, and the remaining portion of the pedicle and spinous process.
- Completely excise the disc material on both sides of the hemivertebra.
- Remove the vertebral physes.
- Remove the hemivertebra, starting dissection from the convex aspect to the concave aspect. If the dura has been exposed, place a Gelfoam sponge over it.
- Cut the removed hemivertebral body into morsels and carefully lay it as a graft in the gap that was created by the resection.
- Carry out compression and stabilization on the convex side with short-segmental instrumentation (Cotrel-Dubousset Horizon, Medtronic Sofamor Danek, Memphis, TN), including vertebrae cephalad and caudad to the hemivertebra to correct the scoliosis deformity (Fig. 44-158D).
- Decorticate the facets and the laminae cephalad and caudad to the hemivertebra on the convex side of the curve.
- Cut any bone that is removed during the laminectomy into morsels and place it as graft material through the area extending from one vertebra cephalad to one vertebra caudad to the hemivertebra (Fig. 44-158E).
- Control bleeding with thrombin-soaked Gelfoam and place thrombin-soaked Gelfoam over the dural sac. Close the wound in a routine manner.
- Obtain radiographs to confirm curve correction.

POSTOPERATIVE CARE. A rigid brace is worn full time or part time for an average of 4 months, depending on when the fusion appears solid on radiographs (Fig. 44-159).

TRANSPEDICULAR EGGSHELL OSTEOTOMIES WITH FRAMELESS STEREOTACTIC GUIDANCE

Mikles et al. described a technique for transpedicular eggshell osteotomies for congenital scoliosis with frameless stereotactic guidance. This technique is recommended in older patients who have congenital scoliosis with multiplanar spinal abnormalities. The guidance system was used to locate the pedicles intraoperatively for accurate screw placement. They thought that screw placement was difficult because of the abnormal anatomy, and they found the use of the guidance system to be helpful in obtaining screw placement proximally and distally and, therefore, a rigid instrumentation construct.

TECHNIQUE 44-45

(MIKLES ET AL.)

- Obtain an operative CT scan with 1-mm cuts from one level above to one level below the spinal deformity, with use of the appropriate protocol for the frameless stereotactic guidance system. Three-dimensional reconstructions are assimilated. With newer fluoroscopic image guidance systems, CT may not be necessary.
- Determine the level of the osteotomy before surgery. This usually corresponds with an eggshell osteotomy of the hemivertebra but is individualized for each patient.
- Monitor spinal cord and cauda equina function by somatosensory evoked potentials.
- Position the patient prone on a Jackson spinal table. Carefully pad bony prominences.
- Make a midline posterior incision and subperiosteally dissect to the deformity.
- Confirm the location and identification of the vertebral elements by plain radiographs.
- Place an appropriate reference arc on the upper thoracic spinous processes.

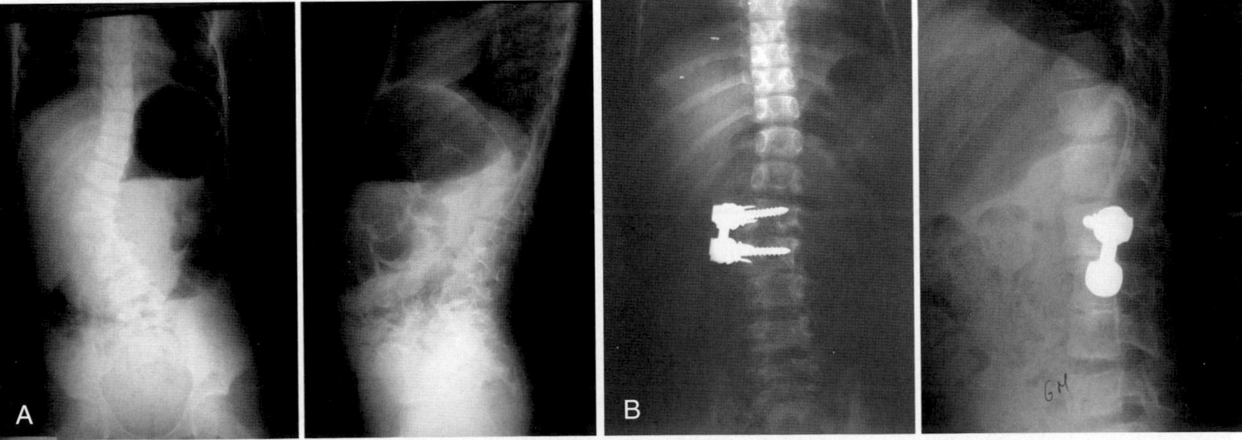

FIGURE 44-159 **A,** Preoperative radiographs of 9-year-old girl with congenital scoliosis due to L2 hemivertebra. **B,** Six months after hemivertebra resection and scoliosis correction. (From Li X, Luo Z, Li X, et al: Hemivertebra resection for the treatment of congenital lumbar spinal scoliosis with lateral-posterior approach, Spine 33:2001, 2008.) **SEE TECHNIQUE 44-44.**

- Register numerous skeletal sites by paired-point and surface-matching techniques. Registration points are determined for only two levels above and below the osteotomy site.
- By use of the guidance system, locate the pedicles with the digitized probe, a digitized drill guide, or a digitized pedicle tap.
- Probe the pedicle with a pedicle probe to the appropriate depth and angle. Insert a digitized ball-tipped probe into the pedicle hole to check the length of the hole and to verify the intrapedicular position.
- Place the screws approximately two levels above and below the chosen osteotomy site.
- After screw placement, identify the transverse processes at the osteotomy level bilaterally; identify the foramina above and below the pedicle and check with fluoroscopy.
- Trim the midline region down carefully with a burr until a thin layer of lamina is left.
- Perform a central laminectomy at the chosen level, including any overhanging lamina from the levels above or below.
- Start the posterior decancellation osteotomy on the side of the most accurately detailed anatomy. Identify the pedicle circumferentially and remove it with its transverse process while visual protection of the nerve root is maintained.
- Identify the pedicle opposite the proposed osteotomy and perform a similar exposure.
- After pedicle removal, expose the vertebral body and inferior floor of the spinal canal.
- Elevate the dura off the posterior wall of the vertebral body and begin the decancellation of the body through the pedicle remnants. Use angled curets to remove the cancellous bone from the vertebral body. Remove the disc spaces if necessary. Push the floor of the canal into the created space with reverse curets and subsequently remove it. Complete vertebrectomy is attempted but not always achieved. This allows the best correction of the curve.
- After completion of the osteotomy, apply gentle pressure to the posterior spine with extension of the hips to close the osteotomy site. Spinal cord monitoring is followed carefully during this time. The dura and nerve roots are continuously viewed to prevent entrapment. Titanium instrumentation is used. Some additional coronal correction is obtained with compression and distraction of the osteotomy site. Additional lordosis can be obtained with in situ contouring.
- Place two crosslinks and local autogenous bone graft, which was harvested from the vertebral body, laterally along the decorticated transverse processes of the instrumented segment.
- Close the deep fascial layer and place a suction drain subcutaneously.
- Perform a Stagnara wake-up test in the operating room.

POSTOPERATIVE CARE. The patient is fitted with a well-molded TLSO, which is worn for 12 weeks, starting on the second postoperative day.

THORACIC INSUFFICIENCY SYNDROME

Growing rod techniques can be used to treat congenital deformities involving long sections of the spine or deformities with large compensatory curves in normally segmented regions above and below a congenital deformity. Thoracic insufficiency syndrome may be associated with congenital scoliosis and fused ribs. When this occurs, it is best managed during growth by expansion thoracostomy and insertion of expandable VEPTR devices.

Campbell defined thoracic insufficiency syndrome as the inability of the thorax to support normal respiration or lung growth. This condition occurs in patients with hypoplastic thorax syndromes, such as Jeune and Jarcho-Levin syndromes, progressive infantile scoliosis with reductive distortion of the thoracic volume from spinal rotation, and congenital scoliosis associated with fused ribs on the concave side of the curve. In a hypoplastic thorax associated with congenital scoliosis, "extrinsic" restrictive lung disease can be caused by volume restriction of the underlying growing lungs and motion restriction of the ribs with reduction of the secondary breathing mechanism, as well as altered diaphragmatic mechanics. Thoracic and, therefore, lung volume increases to 30% of adult size by the age of 5 and to 50% of adult size by the age of 10.

Lung growth is limited to the anatomic boundaries of the thorax, so any spine or rib cage malformation that reduces the thoracic volume early in life may adversely affect the size of the lungs at skeletal maturity (Fig. 44-160). Maximizing thoracic height and volume is especially important in very young patients because lung growth between birth and the age of 8 years is related to increases in alveolar number and size and because growth of the lung between 8 years and maturity is primarily a result of increases in alveolar size.

Patients with early onset scoliosis have been shown to have a higher mortality rate from respiratory failure than those with adolescent idiopathic scoliosis. A review of the literature found that young patients treated with thoracic fusions had a high rate of revision surgery (24% to 39%) and restrictive lung disease (43% to 64%), with those patients having upper thoracic fusions being at the highest risk. Long thoracic fusions by limiting thoracic and lung growth in young patients should be avoided to prevent the development of iatrogenic thoracic insufficiency.

Because of the inability of traditional spinal correction techniques to increase the dimensions of the thorax, Campbell developed a technique to directly treat chest wall deformity with indirect correction of the congenital scoliosis. This procedure treats the total global deformity of the thorax, allowing the spine to grow undisturbed by surgical intervention, with increased height of the thoracic spine and the thorax.

Gruca described a technique of operative compression of the ribs to obtain correction of idiopathic scoliosis on the convex side of the curve; however, concerns exist about this limiting thoracic and therefore lung growth. Campbell developed rib distraction instrumentation techniques for treatment of primary hemithorax constriction in severe spinal deformity in young children. He postulated that indirect correction of scoliosis could be obtained by surgical expansion of the chest through rib distraction on the concave side of the curve. He compared this technique with an opening wedge osteotomy of a malunion of a long bone. In this technique, the thoracic

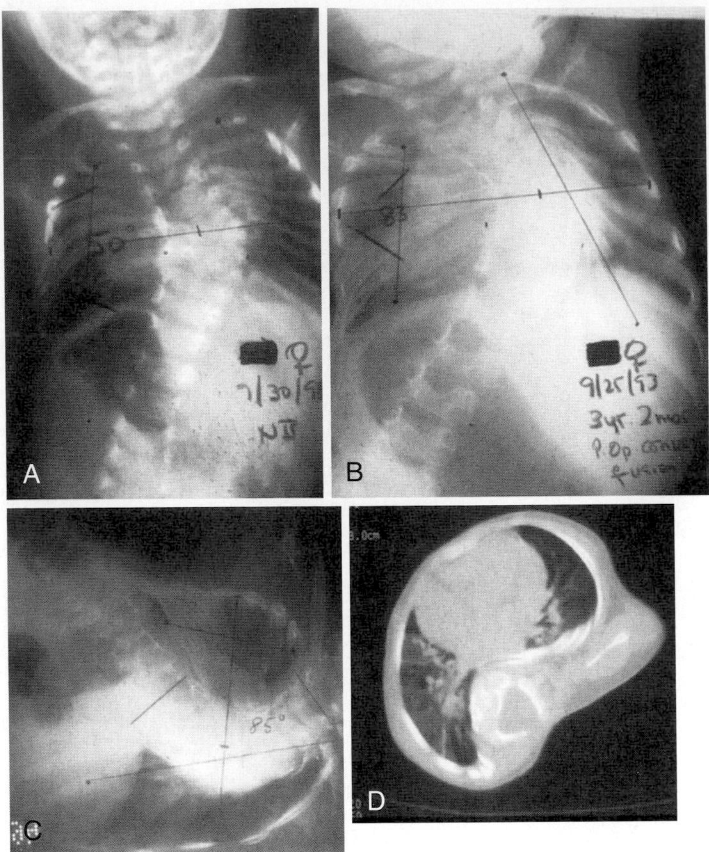

FIGURE 44-160 **A,** Birth radiograph of girl with 50-degree congenital scoliosis due to multiple vertebral anomalies. **B,** Curve had increased to 83 degrees by age 3 years. She underwent anterior convex spinal fusion and developed respiratory insufficiency 6 months after surgery, requiring supplemental nasal oxygen. **C,** "False" lateral decubitus view, better showing changes in dimensions of thorax in addition to spinal curvature. **D,** CT scan shows extreme hypoplasia of chest and underlying lungs. (From Campbell RM: Congenital scoliosis due to multiple vertebral anomalies associated with thoracic insufficiency syndrome, Spine: State of the Art Reviews 14:210, 2000.)

deformity is corrected by an "opening wedge thoracostomy" in the center of the deformity of the concave constricted hemithorax. Once the constricted hemithorax is lengthened, the thorax is equilibrated, with indirect correction of the scoliosis. Correction is maintained with an expandable titanium rib prosthesis. A substantial correction of the hemithorax deformity, an average curve correction of approximately 20 degrees, and the continued growth of the spine were noted as well. Elongation of unilateral unsegmented bars over time in patients treated with chest wall distraction techniques also has been noted (Fig. 44-161). The advantages of this technique are that it directly treats the anatomic causes of thoracic insufficiency syndrome and does not interfere with any subsequent spinal procedures that may be needed later in life.

Campbell treated 34 patients who had progressive congenital scoliosis associated with fused ribs of the concave hemithorax with expansion thoracoplasty and a titanium rib prosthesis. He recommended consideration of spinal growth-sparing techniques, such as growth rods and expansion thoracoplasty, for patients with multiple levels of malformation in the thoracic spine (jumbled spine) with associated areas of either rib deletion or fusion (jumbled thorax). Patients treated with rib-based distraction have been shown to have improvement in their coronal and sagittal spine deformities, pulmonary status, hemoglobin levels, and nutritional status. Although Cobb angle correction with this technique is well described, it has been shown to correlate poorly with pulmonary function and so the exact method(s) of physiologic improvement remain unknown.

Since the initial reports, rib-based distraction has now been used in the treatment of thoracic insufficiency and scoliosis in other conditions such as neuromuscular scoliosis and myelomeningocele. Because this is a posterior-based distraction technique, there is a potential for the development of increased kyphosis, especially in patients with increased preoperative kyphosis. Increased kyphosis may also play a role in proximal rib anchor failure. Longer constructs from the pelvis to ribs have been used to prevent excessive kyphosis; however, these should be avoided in ambulatory patients because of the increased incidence of postoperative crouch gait caused by changes in the lumbosacral mechanics. Intraoperative neuromonitoring is recommended for all initial insertions and in lengthening in which patients have neurologic changes at the time of their initial insertion. The role of its use in routine lengthenings in neurologically normal patients remains controversial. A large multicenter study found a rate of eight neurologic injuries in 1736 consecutive procedures (0.5%) of which five were at the time of initial implantation (1/5%). When used, it should include monitoring of the upper extremities because the upper extremity was

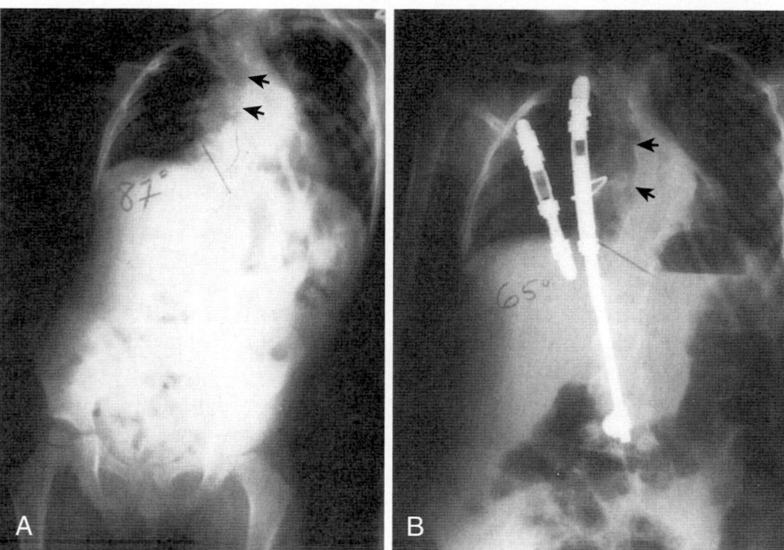

FIGURE 44-161 **A,** Multiple congenital anomalies of thoracic spine, including hemivertebra on convex side of curve and long unilateral unsegmented bar on concave side *(arrows),* in 2½-year-old girl with 87-degree scoliosis. **B,** At 6-year follow-up, curve is corrected to 65 degrees. Length of large central, unilateral segmented bar from T5 to T11 on concave side of curve *(arrows)* compared preoperatively and postoperatively suggests growth on concave side of curve. (From Campbell RM: Congenital scoliosis due to multiple vertebral anomalies associated with thoracic insufficiency syndrome, Spine: State of the Art Reviews 14:210, 2000.)

involved in six of eight cases, which may have been related to brachial plexus injury.

EXPANSION THORACOPLASTY

The vertical expandable prosthetic titanium rib (VEPTR) device comes in two forms. The device with a radius of 220 mm is most commonly used in the treatment of fused ribs and scoliosis. The titanium alloy permits the use of MRI postoperatively. There are three anchors available: rib, spine, and pelvis. The rib anchor consists of two C-shaped clamps that, when locked, form a loose encirclement around the rib to avoid vascular compromise of the underlying rib. Lateral stability is provided by the surrounding soft tissues. The spine anchor consists of a low-profile closed laminar hook. The pelvic anchor consists of an S-shaped modified McCarthy hook that is placed over the iliac crest. The central portion of the device consists of two sliding rib sleeves. The superior sleeve is attached to the cranial anchor, which is usually a rib, and the inferior sleeve is attached to the caudal anchor, which can be a rib, the spine, or the pelvis. The device is locked inferiorly by a peg-type lock through one of two holes, 5 mm apart in the distal rib sleeve, into partial-thickness holes in the inferior rib cradle post. This provides variable expandability for the device in increments of 5 mm. It is important to insert the device with the sleeves completely overlapped to maximize the excursion of the construct before revision is necessary (Fig. 44-162).

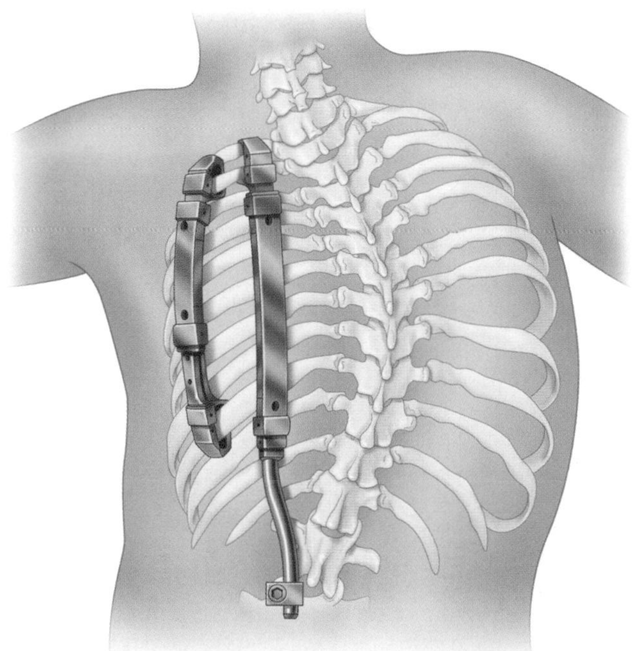

FIGURE 44-162 Expandable prosthetic rib device. (Redrawn from Campbell RM, personal communication.) **SEE TECHNIQUE 44-46.**

TECHNIQUE 44-46

(CAMPBELL)

- Place the patient in a lateral decubitus position with the concave side of the hemithorax upward. A small padded bolster can be placed at the apex of the curve to help with correction.
- Intraoperative spinal monitoring of both upper and lower extremities is used. Begin prophylactic intravenous antibiotics.
- Make a thoracotomy incision around the tip of the scapula and carry it anteriorly. Often in patients with fused ribs, the scapula is both hypoplastic and elevated

proximally. In these patients, the skin incision may need to be brought more distal as it courses around the scapula.

- If a hybrid device is to be used, make a second incision 1 cm lateral to the midline over the proximal lumbar spine (Fig. 44-163A).
- Through the thoracotomy incision, elevate the muscle flaps and proximally identify the middle scalene muscle. Place devices on the second rib posterior to the scalene muscle. Anterior to the middle scalene muscle device, attachment is not done proximally because of the risk of impingement on the neurovascular bundle (Fig. 44-163B).
- Once exposure has been completed, identify the central rib fusion mass by the absence of intercostal muscles. This is the center of the apex of thoracic deformity where the concave hemithorax is most tightly constricted by rib fusion and is best seen on preoperative bending radiographs.
- Before the opening wedge thoracostomy is performed, prepare the rib prosthesis cradle sites proximally and distally. Make 1-cm incisions by use of an electrocautery in the intercostal muscles under the second rib, with a second 5-mm incision above it in the muscle.
- Use an elevator to carefully strip off only the anterior portion of the rib periosteum without violating the pleura (Fig. 44-163C).
- Insert a second elevator into the proximal intercostal muscle incision to encircle the rib.
- Prepare the inferior rib cradle site in the same fashion.
- Insert the rib cradle cap into the proximal intercostal muscle incision sideways and then turn it distally to encircle the rib, similar to insertion of a spinal laminar hook.
- Pass the superior rib cradle into the inferior intercostal muscle incision (Fig. 44-163D), mate it with the cradle cap, and lock it into place with pliers (Fig. 44-163E).
- The sites for the cradles should be just lateral to the transverse processes of the spine. The superior cradle site should be at the top of the area of the constricted hemithorax. If that site does not allow enough distance between the cradle sites for a device of sufficient length to have reasonable expansion capability, the site can be moved superiorly. In very flexible spines, however, care must be taken not to induce a large compensatory curve in the spine above the primary hemithorax constriction by placing the rib cradle too far superiorly. The inferior cradle site should be in a stable base of the area of the constricted hemithorax, below the line of the opening wedge thoracostomy, and usually encircling two fused ribs.
- Select the inferior rib cradle site by picking a rib of attachment that is clinically stable, as horizontal as possible, and at the inferior edge of the thoracic constriction. Avoid unstable rib attachments distally (vestigial rib) because of the high loads placed on the device in the expansion of a fused chest wall.
- Insert the superior cradle before the opening wedge thoracostomy is made. The inferior cradle is not placed at this point because the size of the device required to hold acute hemithorax correction is not known until the hemithorax is lengthened by the opening wedge thoracostomy.
- The deformity of the concave hemithorax is corrected by an opening wedge thoracostomy (Fig. 44-163F). This corrects the "angulated thorax," similar to the use of an opening wedge osteotomy to correct malunion of a long bone.
- Place the thoracostomy in the apex of the thoracic constriction where it can best correct the concave hemithorax, lengthen the constricted segment, and flare out the superior ribs laterally to increase thoracic volume. In most patients, this line of correction passes not through the apex of the scoliosis but above it.
- To confirm the correct position, place metal markers on the chest wall and verify the location with C-arm radiographs and then compare with the preoperative plan.
- The line of cleavage for the primary opening wedge thoracostomy may be through a mass of fused ribs, an area of fibrous adhesions between two ribs, or vestigial intercostal muscle. If the chosen interval is osseous, use a rongeur and Kerrison punches to make the thoracostomy. Be careful not to reflect periosteum from the rib incision site, which will devascularize the rib. Strip away the underlying periosteum with a No. 4 Penfield elevator. The line of the thoracostomy extends from the sternum, along the contours of the ribs, to the transverse processes of the spine posteriorly.
- Reflect the paraspinous muscles from lateral to medial. Take care not to expose the spine to minimize the risk of inadvertent fusion.
- Once exposure is completed, gently spread the thoracostomy interval apart with two vein retractors to allow a lamina spreader to be inserted between the ribs in the midaxillary line of the thorax. Then complete the opening wedge thoracostomy by gradually widening the lamina spreader about 5 mm every 3 minutes (Fig. 44-163G) until the thoracic interval is widened to approximately 1 cm.
- If the ribs are easily distracted and there is at least 0.5 cm of soft tissue between the ribs as they articulate with the spine medially, no further resection is necessary.
- If rib distraction is difficult, additional rib fusion mass probably requires resection medially. If further resection is needed, cut a 1-cm-wide channel medially at the posterior apex of the opening wedge thoracostomy, resecting the remaining fused rib anterior to the transverse process and following it down to the vertebral body for complete removal.
- Expose the bone to be removed a few millimeters at a time by subperiosteal dissection with a Freer elevator.
- Use a rongeur to remove the exposed bone. Take care to resect only visible bone, avoiding the spinal canal posteriorly and the esophagus and great vessels anteriorly. Preserve anomalous segmental vessels.
- Disarticulate the last 5 mm of fused rib from the spine with an angled curet, avoiding the neuroforamen, until the cartilage articular disc is visible.
- Secure hemostasis with bipolar cautery.
- Place bone wax over any raw bone surfaces.
- If the maximal thoracostomy interval distraction is 2 cm or less, the underlying pleura generally stretches and remains intact. If distraction is more than 2 cm, the pleura may begin to tear. Small tears in the pleura require no

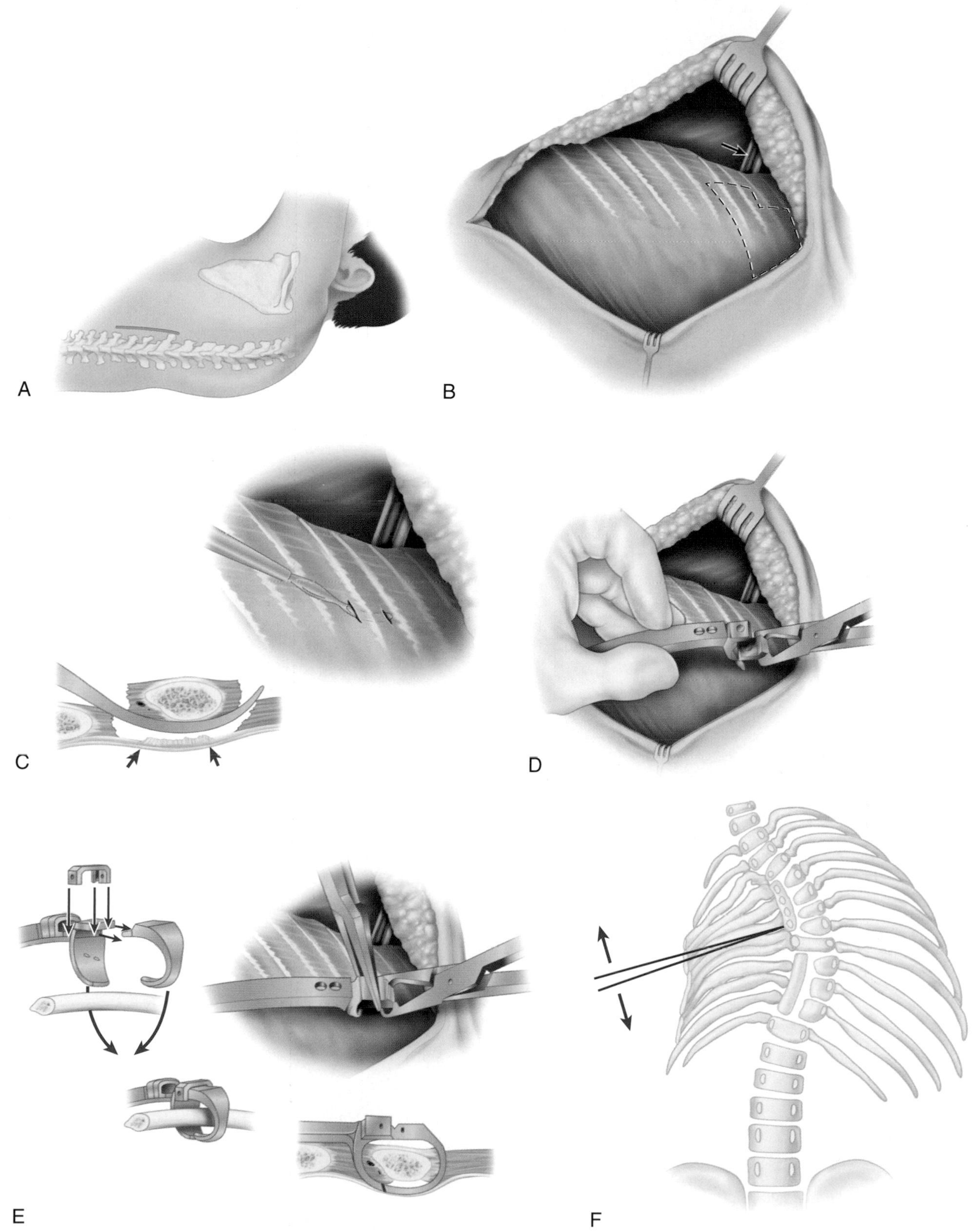

FIGURE 44-163 **A-J,** Campbell technique of expansion thoracoplasty. See text for description. (Redrawn from Campbell RM, personal communication, 2000.) **SEE TECHNIQUE 44-46.**

Continued

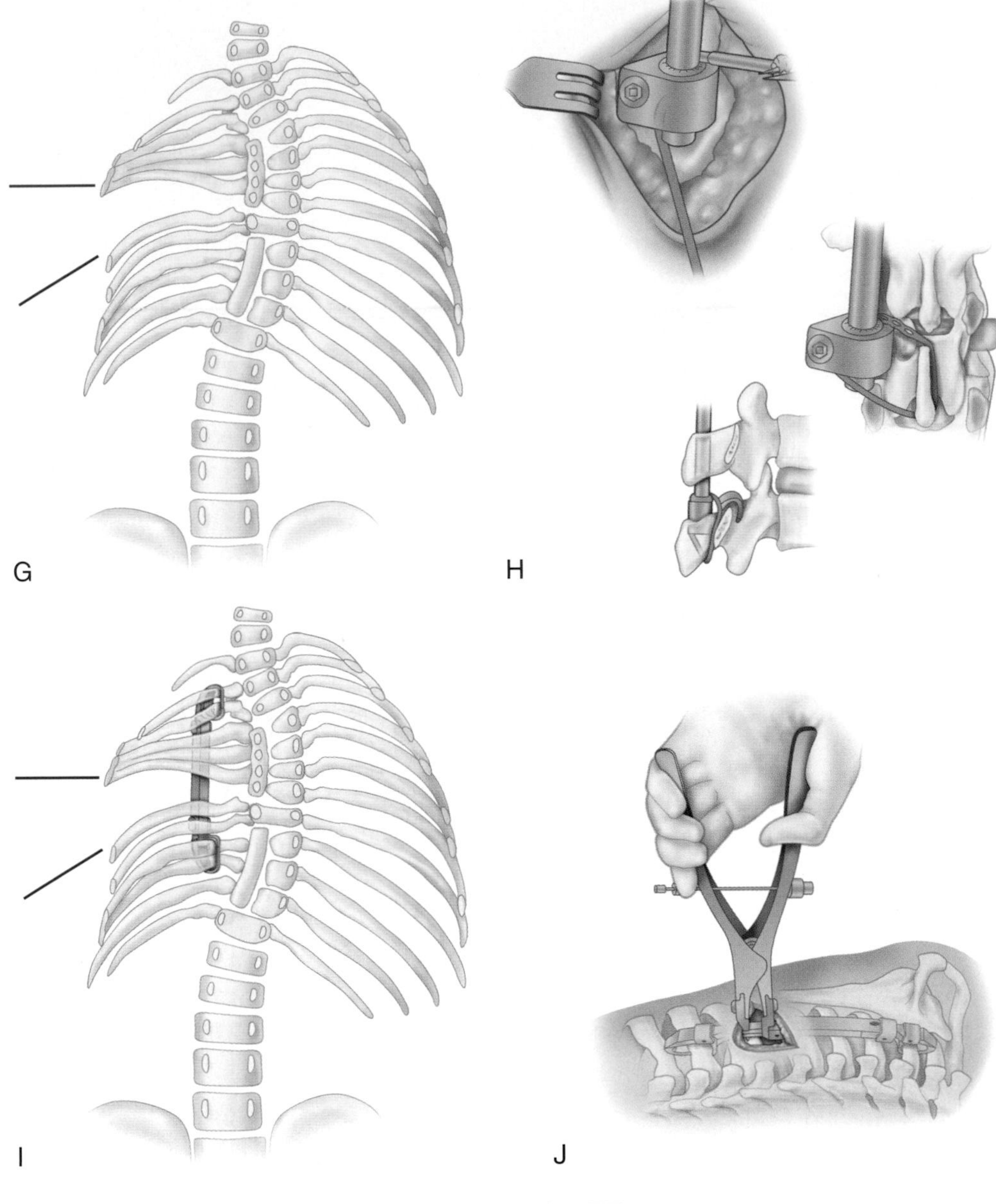

FIGURE 44-163, cont'd

treatment, but substantial defects are treated with a Gore-Tex sheet (WL Gore and Assoc., Newark, DE) sutured to the edges of the intact pleura. Avoid attaching it to rib, muscle, or periosteum because it will become a tether. A Gore-Tex sheet of 0.6-mm thickness is used for small defects, and a 2-mm sheet is used for larger defects. The Gore-Tex sheet usually is placed after the device has been implanted to allow accurate sizing of the sheet needed for maximal thoracic volume. The surface of the sheet is brought outward to maximize volume.

- After the chest is expanded by the lamina spreader, measure the distance between the superior and inferior cradle sites to determine the size of the device needed. The inferior rib cradle and the rib sleeve should be of compatible sizes. An inferior rib cradle that is substantially shorter than the rib sleeve will reduce the device's ability for later expansion and require more frequent change-outs.
- Assess the orientation of the device and cradle after acute thoracostomy expansion so that they conform best to the corrected anatomy.
- After the device is sized and the orientation for the inferior cradle is chosen, relax the lamina spreader to ease access to the cradle sites.
- Insert the cradle cap inferiorly, implant the inferior cradle, and lock the components together with a cradle lock.
- If a hybrid device is used to span down to the lumbar spine, place this in a supralaminar position by resecting the intraspinous ligament and ligamentum flavum using a Kerrison rongeur.

- Place a bone graft on the lamina down to the hook to further stabilize a construct with a one-level fusion. Alternatively, a two-level claw construct can be used to increase stability, especially in older patients.
- If the superior cradle has not been previously inserted, implant it now.
- Reinsert the lamina spreader between medial ribs at the apex of the opening wedge thoracostomy. Reexpand the interval, expanding the thorax by bringing the device components out to length.
- Assemble the device by threading the rib sleeve over the inferior cradle and levering the rib sleeve in line with the superior rib cradle by the device wrenches. The acute correction obtained by the opening wedge thoracostomy is now stabilized by the rib device (Fig. 44-163H).
- For primary thoracic scoliosis in children younger than 18 months, only a single thoracic device is placed posteriorly, adjacent to the transverse processes of the spine. If a patient is older than 18 months and has adequate lumbar canal size and laminae, more support of the thoracostomy can be provided by a hybrid device and a second thoracic prosthesis added posterolaterally.
- Place the thoracic prosthesis in the posterior axillary line to further expand the constricted hemithorax, with proximal attachment just posterior to the middle scalene muscle with at least 0.5 cm between the superior rib cradles.
- Once assembled, tension both devices by expanding them 0.5 cm to fit snugly without excessive distraction pressure and then place two distraction locks on the rib sleeve.
- If the chest wall defect created by the opening wedge thoracostomy is larger than 2 cm, potential chest wall instability will need to be considered. A chest wall defect up to 3 cm wide is well tolerated proximally because of the splinting effect of the scapula posteriorly and the pectoralis muscle anteriorly. A distal chest wall defect of more than 2 cm and a proximal defect of more than 3 cm may need augmentation to provide chest wall stability by centralization of surgically created "pseudoribs" in the defect, addition of more devices, or implantation of a Gore-Tex sheet (2 mm thick) over the defect.
- In the first technique, called transport centralization, separate a single rib or pseudorib of two or three fused ribs away from the superior border of the opening wedge thoracostomy and rotate it downward, like a "bucket handle," to lie centrally in the chest wall defect. The goal of this technique is to divide the chest wall defect into a series of smaller defects, none larger than 2 cm. If the defect is too large for a single rib, separate another rib or pseudorib from the inferior border of the open wedge thoracostomy and bring it into the defect, dividing the larger defect into three smaller ones. Take care to preserve all soft-tissue attachments to avoid devascularization of the rib.
- The second method of augmentation is to add additional devices if transport centralization is not feasible or bone stock is inadequate. This method is practical only in larger patients with adequate soft tissue for device coverage, and usually three devices are the maximum that can be used safely.
- Finally, a 2-mm Gore-Tex sheet can be used to supplement either of the other two methods. When the scoliosis extends from the thorax into the lumbar spine, use a lumbar hybrid rod extension. This lumbar extension can be used only in patients with adequate lumbar spinal canal size for hook placement, and generally the patient should be at least 18 months of age. Preoperatively assess the width of the canal by CT. The usual site of distal insertion is at either L1 or L2; but if the scoliosis extends well distally into the lumbar spine, L3 can be used. Avoid more distal insertion sites on the spine if possible.
- Spinal dysraphism of the proximal lumbar spine may require that the laminar hook be placed in the distal lumbar spine or that a modified McCarthy hook for the pelvis be coupled to the hybrid lumbar extension.
- Through a separate skin incision over the lumbar spine, insert the hybrid distraction device and pass it percutaneously from proximal to distal through the paraspinal muscles. Because of the kyphosis of the thorax, if the device is passed in a proximal direction, it may inadvertently penetrate the chest. Size the device similar to the all-thoracic technique and complete the opening wedge thoracostomy.
- Implant the superior cradle with an empty rib sleeve sized to extend to the inferior border of the thorax at the 12th rib.
- Size a hybrid rod lumbar extension to match the rib sleeve and select for implantation.
- Insert the inferior hook sublaminar. Size a hybrid rod lumbar extension to match the rib sleeve.
- With a lamina spreader in place to maintain the correction obtained with the opening wedge thoracostomy, use in situ benders to bend the hybrid rod into a slight kyphosis proximally and slight valgus and lordosis distally to best fit the lamina hook. The length of the rod should allow it to extend 1 cm distal to the hook.
- With a Kelly clamp, create a tunnel from the proximal incision through the paraspinal muscles, moving proximally to distally, with a finger in the lumbar incision to palpate the tip of the clamp as it exits the muscle. Use the Kelly clamp to grasp a small chest tube and pull it into the proximal incision.
- Attach the hybrid device to the tube and, by use of the tube, thread it proximally to engage the rib cradle and then into the hook.
- Distract the rib and tighten the hook.
- Place bone graft over the laminae.
- A large amount of correction may push the anterior portion of the proximal fused ribs proximally into the brachial plexus. To check for acute thoracic outlet syndrome, bring the scapula back into position while the anesthesiologist monitors pulses and ulnar nerve function is monitored by somatosensory potentials. If both are normal, close the muscle flaps with absorbable suture and close the skin in standard fashion with absorbable subcutaneous sutures.
- If either the pulse or ulnar nerve function is abnormal, retract the scapula and subperiosteally resect 2 cm of the proximal two ribs that are anterior under the brachial plexus.

- Bring the scapula back into position and check somatosensory potentials again. If they are normal, close the incision.

POSTOPERATIVE CARE. The patient is placed in the intensive care unit until extubation, which will depend on the severity of the preoperative pulmonary compromise. In general, we leave our uncomplicated thoracostomy patients intubated overnight and wean respiratory support as tolerated. No bracing is used postoperatively to avoid constriction of chest wall growth. At intervals of approximately 6 months after the initial implantation, the device is expanded in an outpatient procedure. Prophylactic intravenous antibiotics are administered, and the distal end of the device is exposed with an incision through the thoracostomy incision if possible. Once the underlying muscle is exposed, it is split along its fibers or cut vertically either on the medial or lateral side of the device to form a thick muscle flap. Incisions directly over the device(s) should be avoided owing to the potential for skin breakdown and implant infection. The distraction lock over the device is removed, and distractor pliers are inserted to lengthen the device (Fig. 44-163I and J). The prosthesis is lengthened slowly, approximately 2 mm every 3 minutes, to avoid fracture. Once maximal reactive pressure is reached, the device is locked in place with a new distraction lock. Lengthening usually is a minimum of 0.5 cm and up to 1.5 cm. Once the device has exhausted its expandability, a change-out operative procedure is done through small proximal and distal transverse incisions. The sleeves are removed and replaced with larger components (implants). Devices that extend well under the scapula may be difficult to exchange and often require opening of a large portion of the old thoracotomy incision to change the components.

KYPHOSIS

In the sagittal plane, the normal spine has four balanced curves: the cervical spine is lordotic; the thoracic spine is kyphotic (20 to 50 degrees), with the curve extending from T2 or T3 to T12; the lumbar region is lordotic (31 to 79 degrees); and the sacral curve is kyphotic. On standing, the thoracic kyphosis and lumbar lordosis are balanced. Normal sagittal balance is defined as a plumb line dropped from C7 and intersecting the posterosuperior corner of the S1 vertebra (Fig. 44-164). Positive sagittal balance occurs when the plumb line falls in front of the sacrum, and negative sagittal balance occurs when the plumb line falls behind the sacrum.

In the upright position, the spine is subjected to the forces of gravity, and several structures maintain its stability: the disc complex (nucleus pulposus and annulus), the ligaments (anterior longitudinal ligament, posterior longitudinal ligament, ligament flavum, apophyseal joint ligaments, and intraspinous ligament), and the muscles (the long spinal muscles, short intrinsic spinal muscles, and abdominal muscles). Kyphosis of 50 degrees or more in the thoracic spine usually is considered abnormal. Kyphotic deformity may occur if the anterior spinal column is unable to withstand

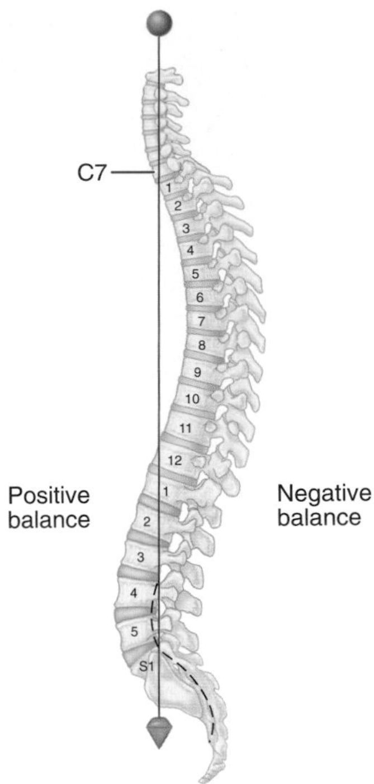

FIGURE 44-164 Plumb line is dropped from middle of C7 vertebral body to posterosuperior corner of S1 vertebral body. (Redrawn from Bernhardt M: Normal spinal anatomy: normal sagittal plane alignment. In Bridwell KH, DeWald RL, editors: The textbook of spinal surgery, ed 2, Philadelphia, 1997, Lippincott-Raven.)

compression, causing shortening of the anterior column. Disruption of the posterior column and inability to resist tension can lead to relative lengthening of the posterior column and kyphosis (Fig. 44-165).

SCHEUERMANN DISEASE

Scheuermann originally described a rigid juvenile kyphosis in 1920. Scheuermann disease is a structural kyphosis of the thoracic or thoracolumbar spine that occurs in 0.4% to 8.3% of the general population. It occurs slightly more often in males. The age at onset usually is during the prepubertal growth spurt, between 10 and 12 years of age.

CLASSIFICATION

Scheuermann disease is divided into two distinct groups: a typical form and an atypical form. These two types are determined by the location and natural history of the kyphosis, including symptoms occurring during adolescence and after growth is completed. Typical Scheuermann disease usually involves the thoracic spine. This classic form of Scheuermann kyphosis has three or more consecutive vertebrae, each wedged 5 degrees or more, producing a structural kyphosis. In contrast, atypical Scheuermann disease usually is located in the thoracolumbar junction or the lumbar spine. It is characterized by vertebral endplate changes, disc space narrowing, and anterior Schmorl nodes but does not necessarily have three consecutively wedged vertebrae of 5 degrees. Thoracic Scheuermann disease is the most common form.

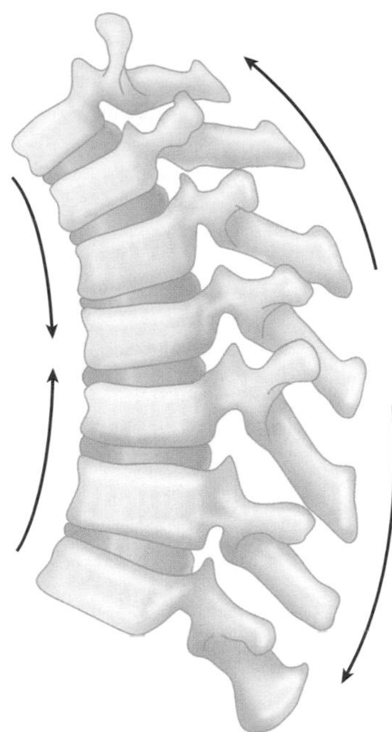

FIGURE 44-165 Forces that contribute to kyphotic deformity of thoracic spine. Anterior vertebral bodies are in compression, and posterior vertebral elements are in tension.

ETIOLOGY

The cause of Scheuermann disease is probably multifactorial. Scheuermann thought that the kyphosis resulted from osteonecrosis of the ring apophysis of the vertebral body. However, the ring apophysis lies outside the true cartilaginous physis and contributes nothing to the longitudinal growth of the body; therefore, a disturbance in the ring apophysis should not affect growth of the vertebra or cause vertebral wedging. In 1930, Schmorl suggested that the vertebral wedging is caused by herniation of disc material into the vertebral body; these herniations now are known as Schmorl nodes. Schmorl theorized that as the disc material is extruded into the vertebral body the height of the intervertebral disc is diminished, which causes increased pressure anteriorly and disturbances of enchondral growth of the vertebral body and subsequent wedging. However, Schmorl nodes are relatively common and frequently occur in patients with no evidence of Scheuermann disease. Ferguson implicated the persistence of anterior vascular grooves in the vertebral bodies during preadolescence and adolescence. He suggested that these vascular defects create a point of structural weakness in the vertebral body, which leads to wedging and kyphosis.

Bradford and Moe and Lopez et al. found that osteoporosis may be responsible for the development of Scheuermann disease. However, a study of bone density in a group of trauma patients and teenagers with Scheuermann disease, as well as a cadaver study, found no evidence of osteoporosis in the vertebrae.

Mechanical factors are a likely cause of Scheuermann disease. Lambrinudi and others suggested that the upright posture and the tightness of the anterior longitudinal ligament of the spine contribute to the deformity. Scheuermann kyphosis is more common in patients who do heavy lifting or manual labor. The fact that some correction of the kyphosis can be obtained by bracing that relieves pressure on the anterior vertebral regions also indicates that mechanical factors are important. The kyphosis probably increases pressure on the vertebral endplates anteriorly, causing uneven growth of the vertebral bodies as a response to the law of Wolff.

A biochemical abnormality of the collagen and matrix of the vertebral endplate cartilage also has been suggested as an important factor in the cause. Abnormal collagen fibers and a decrease in the ratio between collagen and proteoglycan have been found in the matrix of the endplate cartilage in patients with Scheuermann disease.

Several authors have found support for a genetic basis for Scheuermann disease. A high familial predilection has been noted in several studies. The disease may be inherited in an autosomal dominant fashion. Additional support for a genetic basis is provided by Carr et al. in a report of Scheuermann disease occurring in identical twins. In summary, many causes have been suggested but none has been proved. Further research is required to better investigate the ultimate causes of Scheuermann disease.

CLINICAL FINDINGS

Scheuermann disease usually appears around the adolescent growth spurt. The presenting complaint is either pain in the middle or lower back or concern about posture. Frequently, the parents believe that the kyphosis is postural, so diagnosis and treatment are delayed. Pain usually is located in the area of the deformity or in the lower back, is made worse by activity, and typically improves with the cessation of growth. If pain is present in the lumbar area and the deformity is in the thoracic region, the possibility of spondylolysis should be considered.

Physical examination shows an angular thoracic or thoracolumbar kyphosis with compensatory hyperlordosis of the lumbar spine. The kyphosis is sharply angular and does not correct with the prone extension test (Fig. 44-166). The lumbar lordosis below the kyphosis usually is flexible and corrects with forward bending. Tight hamstrings and pectoral muscles are common. On forward bending, a small structural scoliosis may be present in as many as 30% of patients.

Physical findings in patients with atypical (lumbar) Scheuermann disease may differ from those in patients with thoracic deformity. These patients usually have low back pain, but, unlike patients with the more common form of Scheuermann disease, they do not have as noticeable a deformity. Pain with spinal movement is the primary symptom. The condition is especially common in males involved in competitive athletics and in farm laborers, suggesting that it represents an injury to the vertebral physes from repeated trauma rather than true Scheuermann disease.

Abnormal neurologic findings have been reported in 9% to 15% of patients with Scheuermann kyphosis; such findings emphasize the importance of a detailed neurologic examination. Spinal cord compression from kyphosis, thoracic disc herniation, epidural cysts, and epidural lipomatosis have been reported. If lower extremity weakness, hyperreflexia, sensory changes, or other neurologic findings are detected, MRI of the kyphotic area should be done.

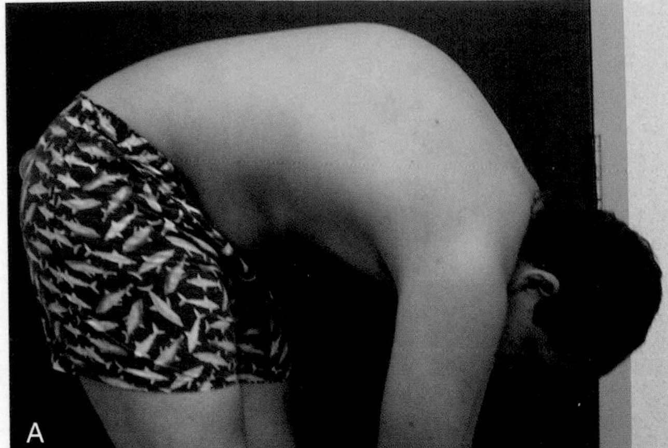

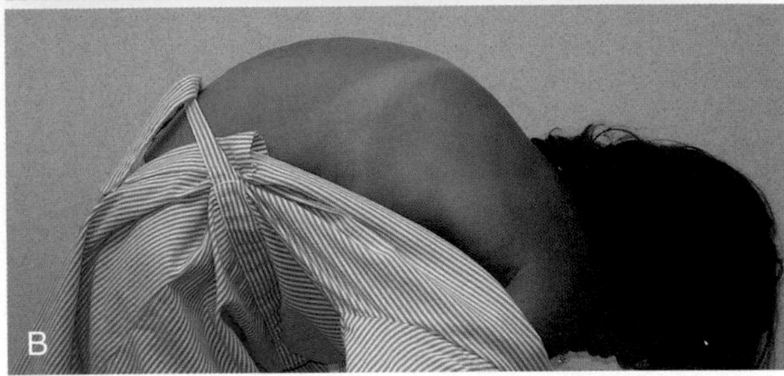

FIGURE 44-166 **A,** Scheuermann kyphosis. **B,** Postural kyphosis. (From Warner WC: Kyphosis. In Morrissy RT, Weinstein SL, editors: Lovell and Winters pediatric orthopaedics, ed 6, Philadelphia, 2006, Lippincott Williams & Wilkins, p. 797.)

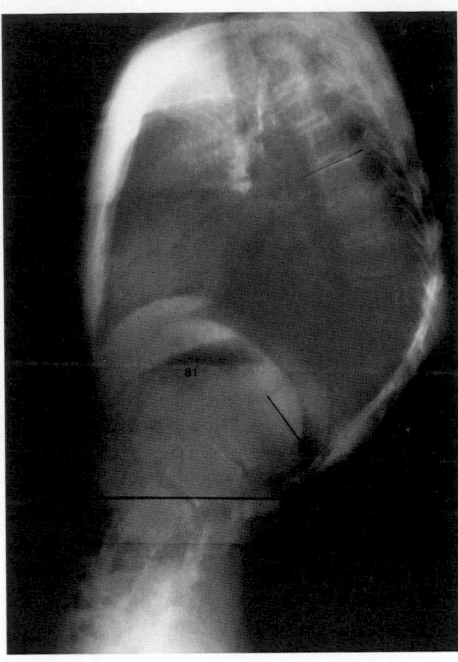

FIGURE 44-167 Scheuermann kyphosis. Kyphotic deformity of 81 degrees and Schmorl nodes.

RADIOGRAPHIC FINDINGS

Standing anteroposterior and lateral radiographs of the spine should be obtained. The amount of kyphosis is determined by the Cobb method on a lateral radiograph of the spine. The cranial and most caudal tilted vertebrae in the kyphotic deformity are selected. A line is drawn along the superior endplate of the cranial vertebra and the inferior endplate of the most caudal vertebra. Lines are drawn perpendicular to the line along the endplates, and the angle they form is the degree of kyphosis. The criteria for the diagnosis of typical Scheuermann disease are more than 5 degrees of wedging of at least three adjacent vertebrae at the apex of the kyphosis and vertebral endplate irregularities with a thoracic kyphosis of more than 50 degrees (Fig. 44-167). Bradford suggested that three wedged vertebrae are not necessary for the diagnosis but rather an abnormal, rigid kyphosis is indicative of Scheuermann disease. Flexibility and the structural nature of the deformity are determined by taking a lateral posteroanterior radiograph with the patient lying over a bolster placed at the apex of the deformity to hyperextend the spine. On a lateral radiograph, most patients will be in negative sagittal balance measured by dropping a plumb line from the center of the C7 vertebral body and measuring the distance from this line to the posterosuperior corner of the S1 vertebra. Scoliosis is evident on posteroanterior radiographs in approximately a third of patients. A lateral radiograph should be made with the patient in the hyperextended position over a bolster to determine the structural nature of the deformity.

Atypical Scheuermann disease of the lumbar spine is characterized by irregularity of the vertebral endplates, the presence of Schmorl nodes, and narrowing of the intervertebral discs, without wedging of the vertebral bodies or kyphosis. Late degenerative changes such as disc space narrowing and Schmorl nodes occur as in Scheuermann disease of the thoracic spine.

NATURAL HISTORY

In most cases, Scheuermann disease results in minimal deformity and few symptoms. The kyphotic deformity can progress rapidly during the adolescent growth spurt. Back pain and fatigue are common complaints during adolescence but usually disappear with skeletal maturity. Factors that contribute to the risk of continued progression of kyphosis include the number of years of growth remaining and the number of wedged vertebrae. Neurologic injury occasionally has been reported in adolescents because of herniation of a thoracic disc, an epidural cyst, or the severe kyphotic deformity alone with subsequent compression of the cord.

The true natural history of untreated Scheuermann disease in adulthood is not well established. Travaglini and Conte found that the kyphosis increased during adulthood in 80% of their patients, although few developed severe deformity. During middle age, degenerative spondylosis is common, but radiographic findings do not always correlate with the presence or absence of back pain. If the kyphosis is less than 60 degrees, these changes usually do not occur in adulthood.

Patients with Scheuermann kyphosis were found in one study to have more intense back pain, jobs that tend to have lower requirements for activity, loss of extension of the trunk, and different localization of pain. However, the level of education, number of days absent from work because of back pain, pain that interfered with activities of daily living, self-esteem,

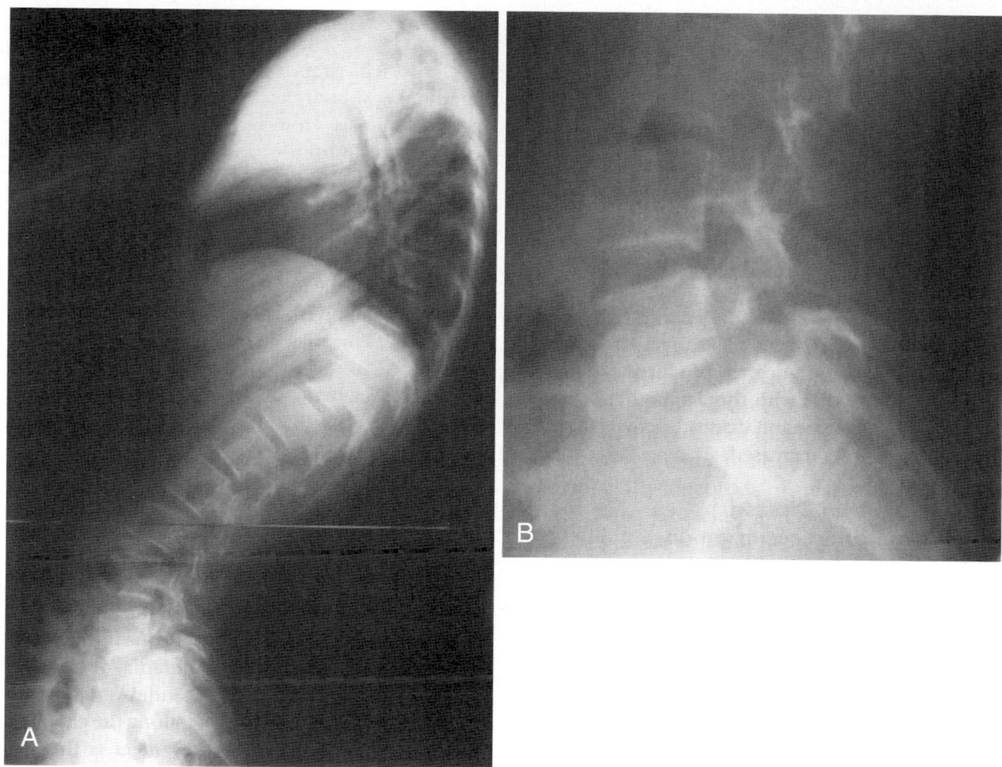

FIGURE 44-168 **A** and **B,** Lateral radiographs show spondylolisthesis with kyphosis. (From Warner WC: Kyphosis. In Morrissy RT, Weinstein SL, editors: Lovell and Winter's pediatric orthopaedics, ed 6, Philadelphia, 2006, Lippincott Williams & Wilkins.)

social limitations, use of medication for back pain, or level of recreational activities were not significantly different from those without Scheuermann disease. Most patients reported little preoccupation with their physical appearances. Normal or above-normal averages of pulmonary function were found in patients in whom the kyphosis was less than 100 degrees. Patients who have Scheuermann kyphosis may have some functional limitation, but it does not significantly affect their lives. Patients who have not had surgery for the kyphosis adapt reasonably well to their condition.

Lumbar Scheuermann disease, which usually is associated with strenuous physical activity, generally becomes asymptomatic within several months after restriction of activities. It has not been shown to have any long-term sequelae in adult life, as long as those affected avoid strenuous jobs.

ASSOCIATED CONDITIONS

Mild-to-moderate scoliosis is present in about one third of patients with Scheuermann disease, but the curves tend to be small (10 to 20 degrees). Scoliosis associated with Scheuermann disease usually has a benign natural history. Deacon et al. divided scoliotic curves in patients with Scheuermann disease into two types on the basis of the location of the curve and the rotation of the vertebrae into or away from the concavity of the scoliotic curve. In the first type of curve, the apices of the scoliosis and kyphosis are the same and the curve is rotated toward the convexity. The rotation of the scoliotic curve is opposite to that normally seen in idiopathic scoliosis. They suggested that the difference in direction of rotation is caused by scoliosis occurring in a kyphotic spine, instead of the hypokyphotic or lordotic spine that is common in idiopathic scoliosis. In the second type of curve, the apex of the scoliosis is above or below the apex of the kyphosis and the scoliotic curve is rotated into the concavity of the scoliosis, more like idiopathic scoliosis. This type of scoliosis seen with Scheuermann kyphosis is the more common, and it rarely progresses or requires treatment.

Lumbar spondylolysis is frequently found in patients with Scheuermann kyphosis (Fig. 44-168). The suggested reason for the increased incidence of spondylolysis (50% to 54%) is that increased stress is placed on the pars interarticularis because of the associated compensatory hyperlordosis of the lumbar spine. This increased stress causes a fatigue fracture at the pars interarticularis, resulting in spondylolysis. Other conditions reported in patients with Scheuermann disease include endocrine abnormalities, hypovitaminosis, inflammatory disorders, and dural cysts.

DIFFERENTIAL DIAGNOSIS

The most common entity to be differentiated from Scheuermann disease is postural round-back deformity. This deformity characteristically produces a slight increase in thoracic kyphosis, which is mobile clinically and is easily correctable on the prone extension test. Radiographs show normal vertebral body contours without vertebral wedging. The kyphosis is more gradual than the angular kyphosis commonly seen in Scheuermann disease. A normal radiograph, however, may not rule out Scheuermann disease because radiographic changes may not be apparent until a child is 10 to 12 years of age.

If pain is a presenting symptom, infectious spondylitis must be considered. This usually can be excluded, however, by clinical and laboratory studies and by MRI, CT, or bone scan of the spine. On occasion, traumatic injuries can confuse the differential diagnosis, but usually the wedging caused by a compression fracture involves only a single vertebra rather than the three or more vertebrae involved in true Scheuermann kyphosis. Osteochondrodystrophies, such as Morquio and Hurler syndromes, as well as tumors and congenital deformities, especially congenital kyphosis, also must be considered. In young men, ankylosing spondylitis must be ruled out, and this may require an HLA-B27 blood test.

TREATMENT

The indications for treatment of patients with Scheuermann kyphosis can be grouped into five general categories: pain, progression of deformity, neurologic compromise, cardiopulmonary compromise, and cosmesis. Treatment options include observation, conservative methods, and surgery.

NONOPERATIVE TREATMENT

OBSERVATION

Adolescents with mildly increased kyphosis of less than 50 degrees without evidence of progression can be evaluated with repeated standing lateral radiographs every 4 to 6 months. When growth is complete, further follow-up is not needed. Exercises alone have not been shown to provide any correction of the deformity in patients with Scheuermann disease. An exercise program, however, can help maintain flexibility, correct lumbar lordosis, and strengthen the extensor muscles of the spine and may improve any postural component of the deformity. Stretching exercises should be prescribed for patients with associated tightness of the hamstring or pectoralis muscles. Patients with lumbar Scheuermann disease and back pain should avoid heavy lifting and should be prescribed an exercise program for the lower back.

ORTHOTIC TREATMENT

The Milwaukee brace has been recommended for the treatment of Scheuermann disease. This brace acts as a dynamic three-point orthosis that promotes extension of the thoracic spine. Low-profile braces, without a chin ring and with anterior shoulder pads, can be used for curves with an apex at the level of T9 or lower. Indications for brace treatment are at least 1 year of growth remaining in the spine, some flexibility of curve (40% to 50%), and kyphosis of more than 50 degrees. The brace is worn full time for the first 12 to 18 months. If the curve has stabilized and no progression is noted, then a part-time brace program can be used until skeletal maturity. An improvement in lumbar lordosis of 35% and in thoracic kyphosis of 49% has been reported in teenagers with Scheuermann kyphosis treated in this manner. Overall, at long-term follow-up, some loss of correction had occurred, but 69% of patients had improvement from the initial kyphosis. Others have reported less correction (30% initially), but the final kyphosis correction averaged only 10%.

Although the Milwaukee brace has been shown to effectively prevent kyphosis progression and offers some modest permanent correction, full-time brace wear often is resisted by adolescents. Gutowski and Renshaw found that the Boston lumbar kyphosis orthosis was satisfactory for correction of curves of less than 70 degrees and had better compliance. They recommended the Boston lumbar orthosis as an acceptable alternative to the Milwaukee brace in patients with flexible kyphotic curves of less than 70 degrees and in whom compliance may be a problem. The rationale for the Boston lumbar orthosis is that reduction of the lumbar lordosis will cause the patient to dynamically straighten the thoracic kyphosis to maintain an upright posture. This presupposes a flexible kyphosis, a normal neurovestibular axis, and the absence of hip flexion contractures.

Lowe used a modified underarm TLSO with padded anterior, infraclavicular outriggers for patients with thoracolumbar-pattern Scheuermann disease (apex T9 and below) and found that it was as effective as the Milwaukee brace and was cosmetically more acceptable to patients.

Hyperextension casting has been used with excellent results in Europe, but this method is associated with frequent problems with the skin, restrictions of physical activity, and the need for frequent cast changes.

OPERATIVE TREATMENT

The indications for surgery in patients with Scheuermann kyphosis are a progressive kyphosis of more than 75 degrees and significant kyphosis associated with pain that is not alleviated by conservative treatment methods. The biomechanical principles of correction of kyphosis include lengthening the anterior column (anterior release), providing anterior support (interbody fusion), and shortening and stabilizing the posterior column (compression instrumentation and arthrodesis). Surgical correction can be achieved by a posterior approach, an anterior approach, or a combined anterior and posterior approach. The combined anterior and posterior approach has been the most frequently recommended, but with the development of pedicle screw fixation and posterior spinal osteotomy techniques, such as the Ponte procedure, posterior-only surgery has become the preferred approach. A posterior procedure without osteotomy can be considered if the kyphosis is flexible and can be corrected to, and maintained at, less than 50 degrees while a posterior fusion occurs (Fig. 44-169). Historically, the use of Harrington compression rods was common, but these have been replaced by segmental hook and pedicle screw instrumentation.

Anterior instrumentation was described by Kostuik and consisted of anterior interbody fusion and anterior instrumentation with a Harrington distraction system augmented by postoperative bracing. Although Kostuik reported good results with this technique, the anterior-only instrumentation approach for treatment of Scheuermann kyphosis is not widely used.

When a combined anterior and posterior procedure is used for Scheuermann disease, the anterior release and fusion are done first. The anterior release can be done through an open anterior procedure or by thoracoscopy. Herrera-Soto et al. showed good sagittal correction, with no loss of correction or junctional kyphosis, with a thoracoscopic technique. Interbody cages have been used in an effort to improve sagittal correction; however, Arun et al. found no difference in outcomes between patients with anterior fusion using interbody cages and those with anterior fusion using autogenous rib grafting. The posterior fusion and instrumentation can be done on the same day as the anterior release and fusion or as a staged procedure. Segmental instrumentation systems using multiple hooks or pedicle screws are used for the posterior spinal fusion.

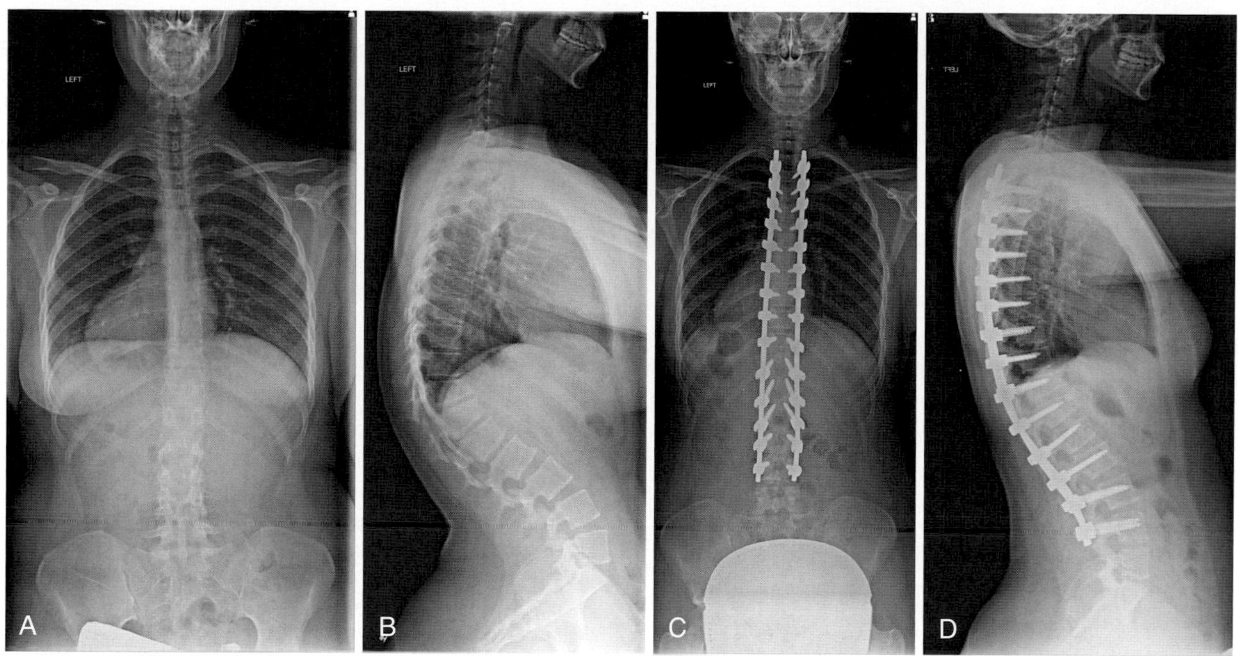

FIGURE 44-169 A and B, Scheuermann kyphosis. C and D, After correction and posterior fusion.

Other instrumentation techniques have been used for correction of Scheuermann kyphosis. Sturm, Dobson, and Armstrong reported good results with posterior fusion alone by use of large, threaded Harrington compression rods rather than small ones. Coscia et al. reported an average 23-degree improvement with a combined anterior and posterior approach with Luque sublaminar wires and rods used posteriorly for internal fixation. However, junctional kyphosis above the instrumented area developed in 13 of their 19 patients, probably because the interspinous ligament and ligamentum flavum must be removed to allow wire passage. The Luque rods can translate the kyphosis posteriorly, but they cannot shorten the posterior column, which is an important aspect in treating kyphotic deformity.

The use of posterior spinal osteotomies such as the Ponte osteotomy allows for relative shortening of the posterior column and greater correction of the kyphosis. Several studies have shown similar sagittal correction with combined anterior and posterior procedures and posterior-only procedures with Ponte osteotomies. Posterior fusion and instrumentation should include the proximal vertebra in the measured kyphotic deformity and the first lordotic disc distally. If the fusion and instrumentation end in the kyphotic deformity, a junctional kyphosis at the end of the instrumentation may occur. Cho et al. reported the occurrence of distal junctional kyphosis despite inclusion of the first lordotic disc. They recommended inclusion of the lumbar vertebral body bisected by a vertical line drawn from the posterosuperior corner of the sacrum to prevent distal junctional kyphosis.

Junctional decompensation has been reported to occur in as many as 30% of patients. Overcorrection of the deformity should be avoided to prevent junctional kyphosis. No more than 50% of the preoperative kyphosis should be corrected, and the final kyphosis should not be less than 40 degrees. Lowe found that patients with Scheuermann disease tend to be in negative sagittal balance and become further negatively balanced after surgery, which may predispose them to develop a junctional kyphosis. Lonner et al. found that the pelvic incidence may be related to the amount of proximal junctional kyphosis and that distal junctional kyphosis was related to fusion that ended cranial to the neutral sagittal vertebra. Denis et al. suggested that the incidence of proximal junctional kyphosis can be minimized by the appropriate selection of the upper end vertebra and avoiding disruption of the junctional ligamentum flavum. They also recommended incorporation of the first lordotic disc into the fusion construct.

ANTERIOR RELEASE AND FUSION

TECHNIQUE 44-47

- The levels of the anterior release are those with the most wedging and the least flexibility on hyperextension lateral views. This region generally includes seven or eight interspaces centered on the apex of the kyphosis.
- Select the appropriate anterior approach for the levels to be fused. If there is no associated scoliosis, make the approach through the left side. If there is a concomitant scoliosis, approach the spine on the convexity of the scoliosis.
- Release the anterior longitudinal ligament and excise the entire disc and cartilaginous endplate, leaving only the posterior portion of the annulus and the posterior longitudinal ligament.
- Curet the bony endplates but do not remove them completely.
- Use a laminar spreader to loosen or to mobilize each joint.

- Pack each disc space temporarily with Gelfoam or Surgicel to minimize blood loss.
- Perform an interbody fusion with use of the morselized rib graft.
- Anterior instrumentation can be used to aid in correction of the deformity and stabilization until a solid fusion occurs.

POSTERIOR MULTIPLE HOOK AND SCREW SEGMENTAL INSTRUMENTATION

With multiple hook and screw segmental instrumentation systems, several techniques are available for reduction of kyphosis. The cantilever method (Fig. 44-170) consists of inserting the precontoured rod into the pedicle–transverse process claws or thoracic pedicle screws above the apex of the kyphosis. With the apex of the deformity as a fulcrum, the distal end of the rod is pushed into the lower hood or pedicle screws at the caudal end of the deformity by a cantilever maneuver. The disadvantage of this method is that the correction is a three-point cantilever maneuver and the correction is therefore somewhat abrupt and forces are concentrated at the ends of the construct. Reduction pedicle screws and instruments can be used to make this reduction maneuver more gradual. Another method for correction is an apical compression technique using multisegmental hooks or pedicle screw constructs on either side of the apex. A combination of the cantilever and compression techniques also can be used. These two techniques often are combined with a posterior column shortening procedure, allowing gradual correction of the kyphosis. Rigid posterior instrumentation systems can be combined with posterior column shortening (Ponte osteotomies) to correct the kyphosis without the need for anterior release and fusion.

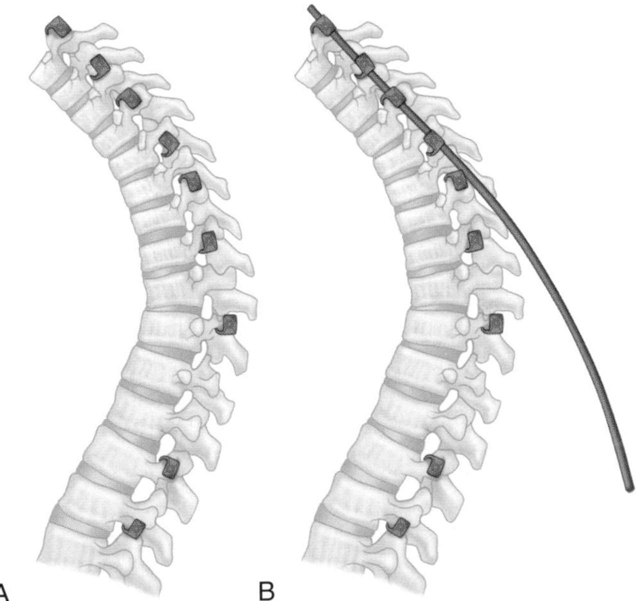

FIGURE 44-170 Reduction of kyphosis, standard method. **A,** Insertion of hooks. Note three sets of pedicle-transverse claws above apex of kyphosis. **B,** Rod passed through hooks of proximal segment and distal end of rod pushed to lower spine with rod pusher. Note that lower tip bend in rod facilitates hook insertion under distal lamina. **SEE TECHNIQUE 44-48.**

TECHNIQUE 44-48

(CRANDALL)

- Place the patient prone on a Jackson frame. The spine is approached posteriorly. The instrumentation frequently extends proximally to T2 to T3.
- Determine the apex of the kyphosis on preoperative radiographs.
- Use at least two sets of pedicular-transverse process claws or thoracic pedicle screws above the apex if the curve is flexible. In very large patients with rigid curves, extra fixation sites may be needed. A third set of fixation points may be used. Below the apex, reduction pedicle screws are used. At least three sets of screws are recommended.
- Debride the facet joints at each level to allow posterior column compression and to provide a bony surface for fusion.
- Perform osteotomies if necessary.
- Bend both rods above the kyphosis to approximate the normal spinal contour. Proper rod contouring is important. Leave the distal rods uncontoured.
- Insert the upper end of both rods into the proximal points. If hooks are being used, compress each claw construct to ensure that each hook claw remains seated. Tighten the threaded plugs to hold the upper hooks or pedicle screws securely in the rod.
- After all the rods are in the proximal fixation points, place a crosslink plate on the rods. Attach the distal ends of both rods into the reduction screws (Fig. 44-171A).
- Begin the incremental reduction process with all reduction screws to pull the spine up to the rod (Fig. 44-171B).
- Cut the distal ends of the rods to the appropriate length (Fig. 44-171C).
- As the intermediate points of fixation come in contact with the rod, lock them to the rod and compress them to the proximal points of fixation. Gradual, repeated tightening, a few turns at a time with "two-finger" force on the driver, will bring the spine up in a safe and controlled fashion (Fig. 44-172). The spine is directly translated to the rod from any direction, achieving simultaneous correction in both the coronal and sagittal plane. Importantly, this correction should not proceed too quickly. A gradual reduction allows the spine to stretch the soft-tissue structures contracted in the kyphosis and allows the least amount of stress on the construct and spinal cord.
- After full kyphosis correction, fully compress the posterior column and lock it into position. Place a crosslink plate distally and proximally (Figs. 44-173 and 44-174).
- During tightening of the reduction crimps (every 3 to 5 minutes), harvest bone graft and decorticate the spine and facets.

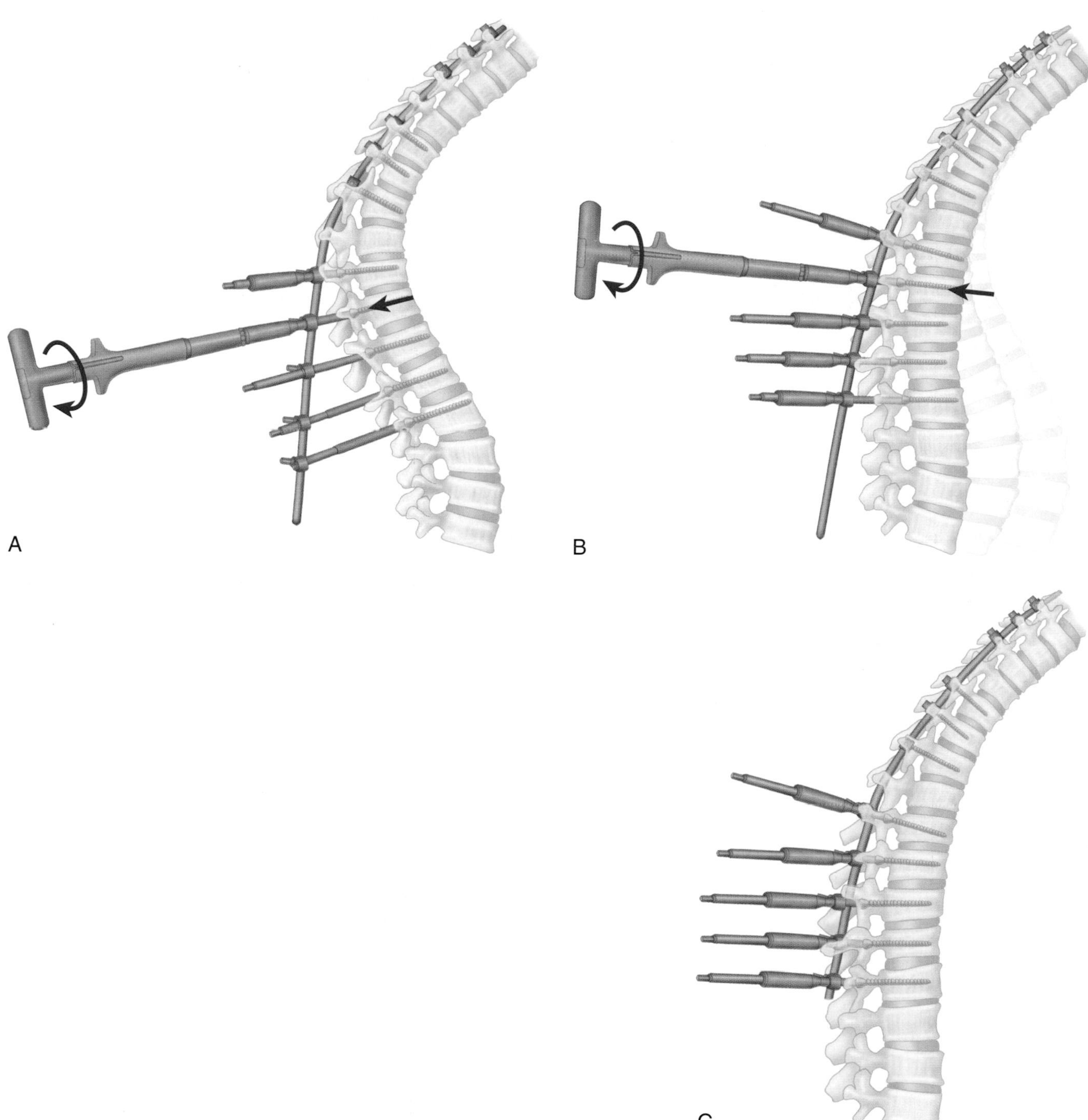

FIGURE 44-171 Posterior multiple-hook and screw segmental instrumentation. **A,** Reduction crimps are attached. **B,** Incremental reduction. **C,** Distal end of rod cut to appropriate length. **SEE TECHNIQUE 44-48.**

- At the completion of the instrumentation, add abundant autogenous bone graft.

POSTOPERATIVE CARE. Unless the bone quality is poor and fixation is tenuous, postoperative bracing is not required. If there is any concern about fixation, an extension orthosis, such as a Jewett brace, can be used until the fusion begins to consolidate, usually in 3 to 6 months. Ambulation is started as soon as possible. All patients start isometric and isotonic back exercise programs when the fusion appears solid. In adolescents, the fusion generally is solid in approximately 6 months. The patient generally is allowed to sit up on the second or third day postoperatively.

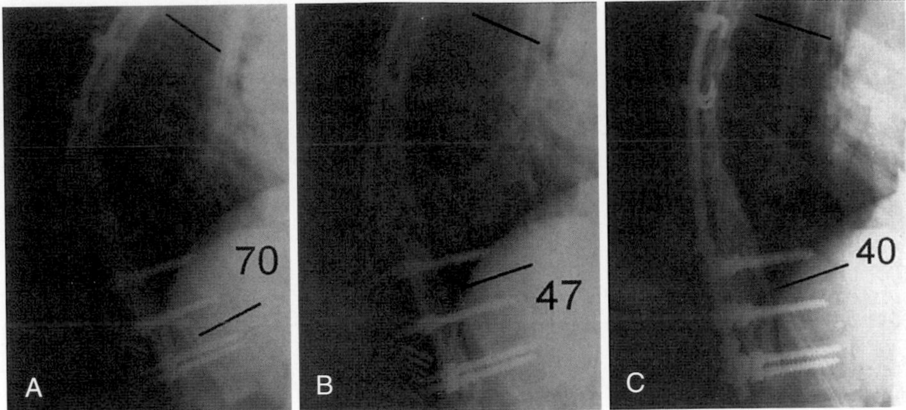

FIGURE 44-172 **A,** Beginning of correction, 70 degrees of kyphosis. **B,** Midpoint of correction, 47 degrees of kyphosis. **C,** Final construct, 40 degrees of kyphosis. **SEE TECHNIQUE 44-48.**

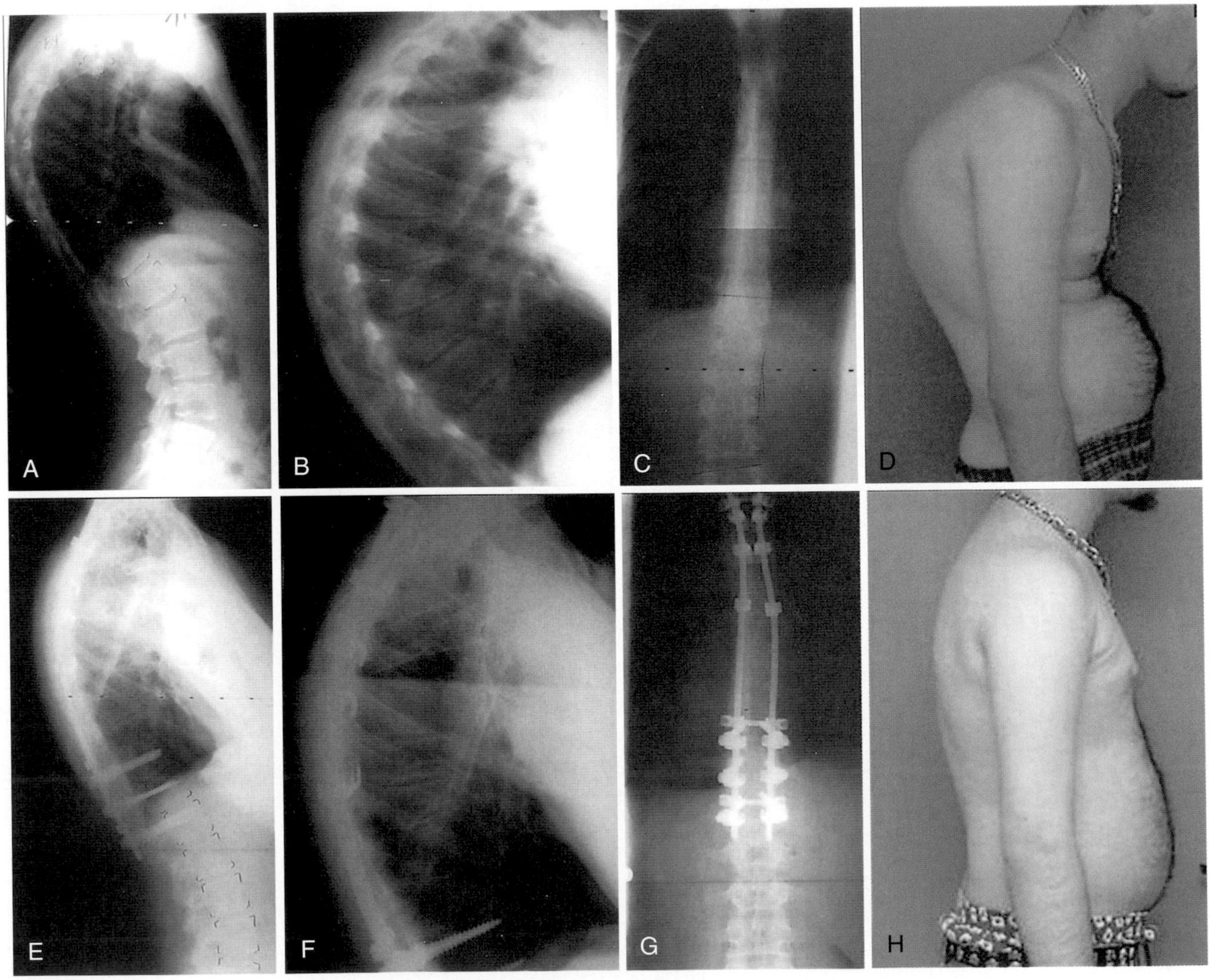

FIGURE 44-173 **A-C,** Preoperative radiographs of patient with Scheuermann kyphosis. **D,** Preoperative clinical photograph. **E-G,** Postoperative radiographs. **H,** Postoperative photograph. **SEE TECHNIQUE 44-48.**

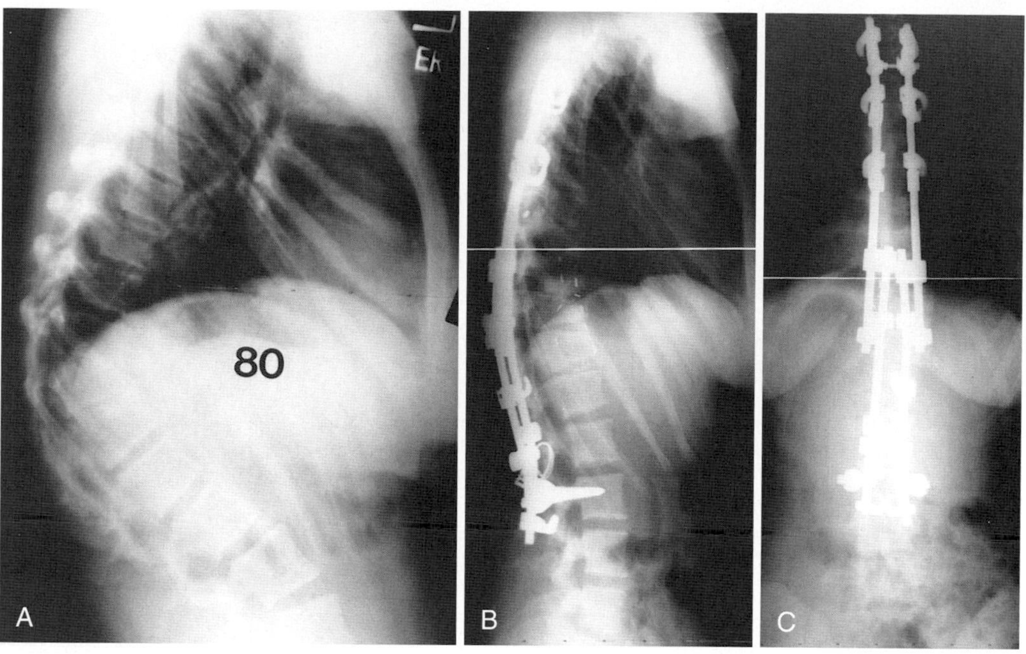

FIGURE 44-174 A, Kyphosis of 80 degrees. B and C, After posterior fusion and instrumentation with four rods connected by domino crosslinks. **SEE TECHNIQUE 44-48.**

POSTERIOR COLUMN SHORTENING PROCEDURE FOR SCHEUERMANN KYPHOSIS

Ponte, Gebbia, and Eliseo described a posterior column shortening technique for the correction of Scheuermann kyphosis. The potential advantages of this technique include that it is a single-stage posterior procedure; the posterior spine is shortened rather than the anterior spine lengthened, thereby increasing safety; a gradual correction is obtained; there are no complications from a thoracotomy or thoracoscopy; and there is no surgical interference with anterior blood supply to the spinal cord.

TECHNIQUE 44-49

(PONTE)

- A posterior midline approach is performed.
- Expose the spine subperiosteally to include one vertebra above and one vertebra below the fusion levels. The proximal extent of the fusion may need to include T1 to minimize the risk of cranial junctional kyphosis. The caudal limit must always be included and is determined by the first lordotic disc (open anteriorly) on lateral standing films.
- Resect the spinous processes and perform wide facetectomies and partial laminectomies of both the inferior and superior laminar borders at every intersegmental level of the fusion area. Ideally, gaps of 4 to 6 mm should be obtained (Fig. 44-175A). A generous resection of the facet joints as far as the pedicles is an essential step of this technique.
- Remove the ligamentum flavum entirely at all levels. The gaps extend uniformly over the entire width of the posterior spine (Fig. 44-175B to D).
- Insert the rods into the supralaminar hooks. If closed hooks are used, preload the hooks onto the rod and insert it as a unit. Pass the rod through the hooks just proximal to the apex. If open hooks are used, use appropriate set screws to hold the rod in the hooks or screws above the apex of the kyphosis.
- Leave the apical vertebra uninstrumented (Fig. 44-175D to I).
- Apply minimal compression force to keep the hooks in place. Any corrective tightening at this point would narrow the gaps and make placement of the hooks for the second rod difficult.
- Repeat the same sequence for the second rod. Apply compressive forces, beginning with the two opposing hooks facing the apex and then continuing sequentially to the cranial and caudal ends (see Fig. 44-175G).
- Repeat these maneuvers alternately on both sides and several times, always beginning at the apex. As compression proceeds, the rods will gradually straighten out and the intersegmental gaps will close. Creating small notches for the hook blades will prevent their interference with the closure of the gaps.
- Obtain an intraoperative radiograph to assess the magnitude of the correction. Fine-tuning is performed as needed to obtain a harmonious distribution of intersegmental correction.
- Secure two transverse connectors if they are needed for additional stability.
- Perform decortication and add morselized bone graft.

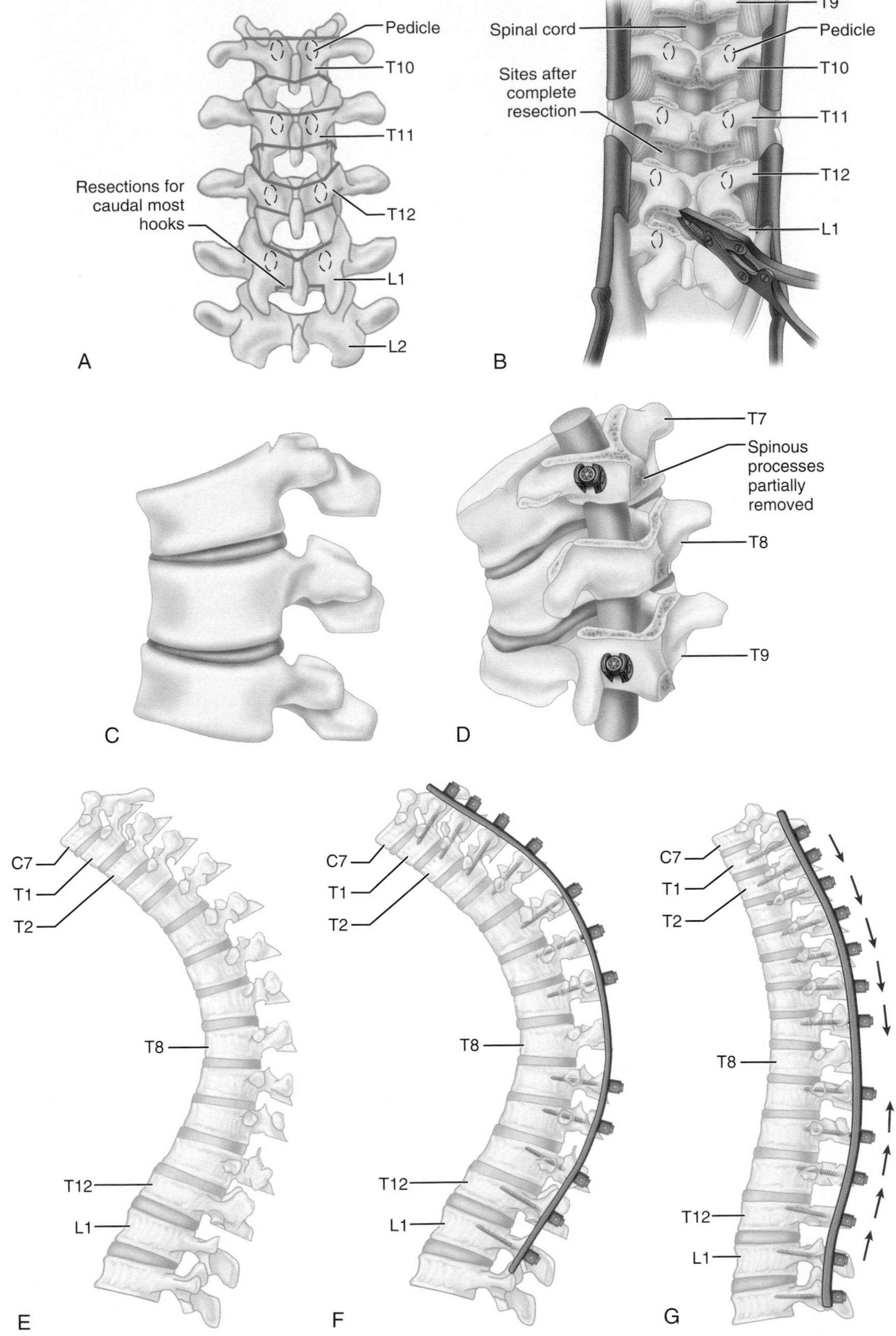

FIGURE 44-175 Posterior column shortening for Scheuermann kyphosis. **A,** Broad posterior resection *(shaded parts)* at every intersegmental level of entire area of fusion and instrumentation. **B,** Posterior view showing levels of completed resections. **C,** Lateral view showing gaps from osteotomies. Correction is achieved by closing gaps. **D,** Oblique view showing three apical vertebrae after completion of bone resections. Apical vertebra is left uninstrumented. **E** to **G,** Schematic representation of reduction of kyphosis.

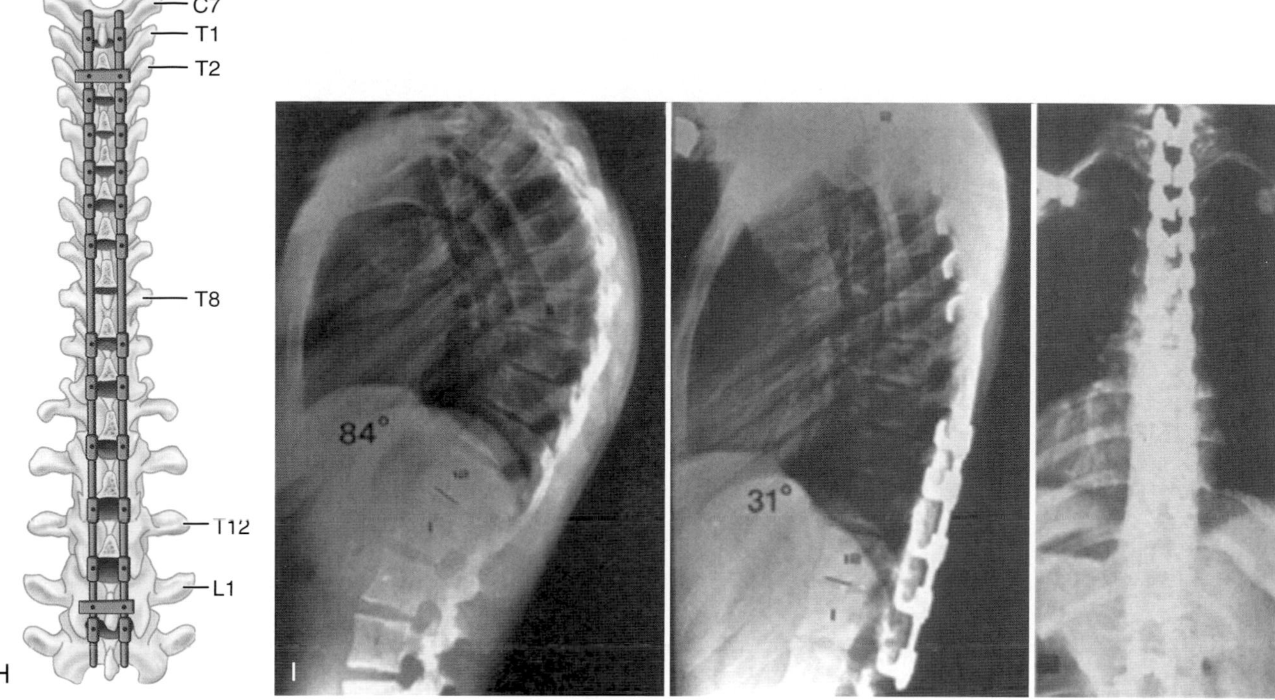

FIGURE 44-175, cont'd H, Posterior view showing hook pattern of construct and two transverse connectors. I, Severe thoracic kyphosis in 42-year-old woman preoperatively *(left)* and at 31 months postoperatively *(middle);* standing anteroposterior radiograph shows the fully segmental construct from T1 to L1 *(right).* (Redrawn from Ponte A: Posterior column shortening for Scheuermann's kyphosis. An innovative one-stage technique. In Haher TR, Merola AA, editors: Surgical techniques for the spine, New York, 2003, Thieme.) **SEE TECHNIQUE 44-49.**

- The same principle, with Ponte osteotomies, can be used with different instrumentation, including pedicle screws. Pedicle screws provide secure fixation without the problem of multiple hooks within the spinal canal and without the problem of the hooks potentially blocking the closure of the osteotomies. Gradual reduction-type pedicle screws can be used distally to allow a more gradual correction of the kyphosis.

POSTOPERATIVE CARE. The patient is allowed to sit out of bed on the first postoperative day. There is no need for external support, such as bracing. Physical activities, such as sports or lifting of more than 5 or 10 lb, are restricted for 3 to 6 months. Radiographic assessment of the fusion at 6 months is performed, and if the fusion appears solid, gradual return to full activities is then allowed. Patients with an osteopenic spine or who are overweight or noncompliant may require a brace until the fusion is solid.

COMPLICATIONS

Complications are more frequent after the operative treatment of Scheuermann kyphosis than adolescent idiopathic scoliosis; in the case of major complications, Loner et al. reported that they were four times more likely in Scheuermann kyphosis. Proximal junctional kyphosis has been reported to be present in as many as 30% and distal junctional kyphosis in 12% of surgically treated patients. To decrease the risk of junctional kyphosis, Denis et al. suggested that the fusion should include all vertebrae involved in the kyphosis, disruption of the ligamentous complex at the ends of the fusion should be avoided, and the fusion should extend distally to include the vertebra below the first lordotic disc. Distal and proximal implant failure is caused by the increased stresses placed on the instrumentation.

CONGENITAL KYPHOSIS

Congenital kyphosis is an uncommon deformity, but neurologic deficits resulting from this deformity are frequent. Congenital kyphosis occurs because of abnormal development of the vertebrae consisting of a failure of formation or failure of segmentation of the developing segments. The spine may be either stable or unstable, or it may become unstable with growth. Spinal deformity in congenital kyphosis usually will progress with growth, and the amount of progression is directly proportional to the number of vertebrae involved, the type of involvement, and the amount of remaining normal growth in the affected vertebrae. Winter et al. described 130 patients with congenital kyphosis of three types. Type I is congenital failure of vertebral body formation. Type II is failure of vertebral body segmentation (Fig. 44-176). Type III is a combination of both of these conditions. McMaster and Singh further subdivided type I congenital kyphosis into posterolateral quadrant vertebrae, posterior hemivertebrae, butterfly (sagittal cleft) vertebrae, and anterior or anterolateral wedged vertebrae (Fig. 44-177). This classification is important in predicting the natural history of these congenital

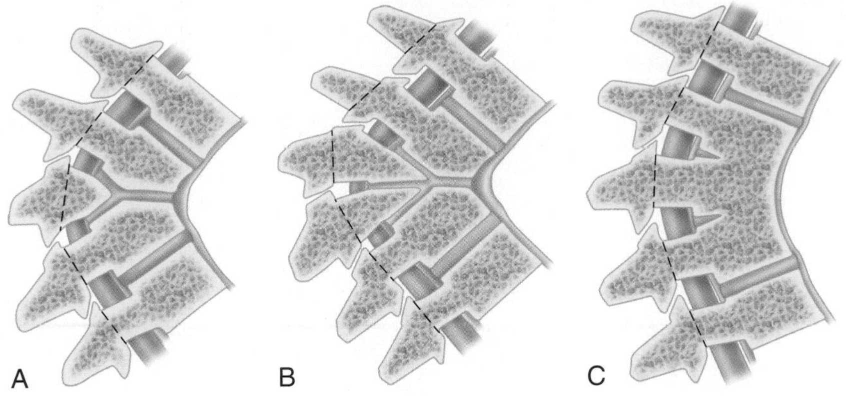

FIGURE 44-176 Classification of congenital kyphosis. **A** and **B,** Type I. **C,** Type II. (Type III is not shown.)

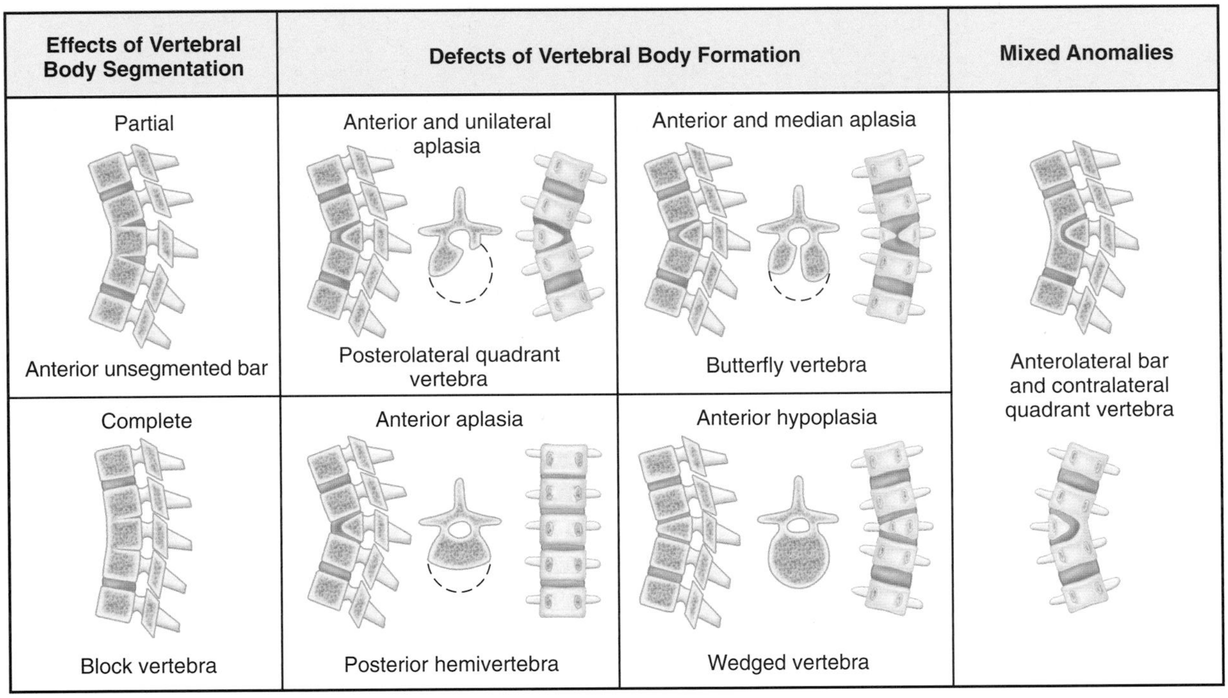

Effects of Vertebral Body Segmentation	Defects of Vertebral Body Formation		Mixed Anomalies
Partial Anterior unsegmented bar	Anterior and unilateral aplasia Posterolateral quadrant vertebra	Anterior and median aplasia Butterfly vertebra	Anterolateral bar and contralateral quadrant vertebra
Complete Block vertebra	Anterior aplasia Posterior hemivertebra	Anterior hypoplasia Wedged vertebra	

FIGURE 44-177 **Different types of vertebral anomalies that produce congenital kyphosis or kyphoscoliosis.** (From McMaster MJ, Singh H: Natural history of congenital kyphosis in kyphoscoliosis: a study of 112 patients, J Bone Joint Surg 81A:1367, 1999.)

kyphotic deformities. Dubousset and Zeller et al. added a rotatory dislocation of the spine, and Shapiro and Herring further divided type III displacement into type A (sagittal plane only) and type B (rotatory, transverse, and sagittal planes). Any classification can be further subdivided into deformities with or without neurologic compromise.

The natural history of congenital kyphosis is well known and based on the type of kyphosis. Type I deformities are more common than type II deformities and occur more commonly in the thoracic spine and at the thoracolumbar junction. They are extremely rare in the cervical spine. In the series of McMaster and Singh, progression was most rapid in type III kyphosis, followed by type I. Kyphosis caused by two adjacent type I vertebral anomalies progressed more rapidly and produced a more severe deformity than did a single anomaly. Approximately 25% of patients with type I deformities had neurologic deficits, and deformities in the upper thoracic spine were more likely to be associated with neurologic problems. No patient in whom the apex of the kyphosis was at or caudad to the 12th thoracic vertebra had neurologic abnormalities. However, type I kyphosis progressed relentlessly during growth and usually accelerated during the adolescent growth spurt before stabilizing at skeletal maturity. An anterior failure of vertebral body formation produces a sharply angular kyphosis that is much more deforming and potentially dangerous neurologically than a curve with a similar Cobb measurement, owing to an anterior failure of segmentation that affects several adjacent vertebrae and produces a smooth, less obvious deformity.

Type II deformities (failure of segmentation) are less common. An absence of physes and discs anteriorly in one or more vertebrae results in the development of an anterior unsegmented bar. The amount of kyphosis produced is proportional to the discrepancy between the amounts of growth in the anterior and posterior portions of the defective vertebral segments. Mayfield et al. reported that these deformities progress at an average rate of 5 degrees a year and are not as severe as type I deformities. Paraplegia usually is not reported in patients with type II kyphosis; however, low back pain and cosmetic deformities are significant and early treatment is warranted.

CLINICAL AND RADIOGRAPHIC EVALUATION

The diagnosis of a congenital spine problem usually is made by a pediatrician before the patient is seen by an orthopaedist. The deformity may be detected before birth on a prenatal ultrasound examination or noted as a clinical deformity in a neonate. If the deformity is mild, congenital kyphosis can be overlooked until a rapid growth spurt makes the condition more obvious. Some mild deformities are found by chance on radiographs that are obtained for other reasons. Clinical deformities seen in the neonate tend to have a worse prognosis than those discovered as an incidental finding on plain radiographs.

Physical examination usually reveals a kyphotic deformity at the thoracolumbar junction or in the lower thoracic spine. A detailed neurologic examination should be done to look for any subtle signs of neurologic compromise. Associated musculoskeletal and nonmusculoskeletal anomalies should be sought on physical examination. High-quality, detailed anteroposterior and lateral radiographs provide the most information in the evaluation of congenital kyphosis (Fig. 44-178). Failure of segmentation and the true extent of failure of formation may be difficult to detect on early films because of incomplete ossification. Flexion and extension lateral radiographs are helpful in determining the rigidity of the kyphosis and possible instability of the spine. CT with three-dimensional reconstructions can identify the amount of vertebral body involvement and can determine whether more kyphosis or scoliosis might be expected (Fig. 44-179). CT can only identify the nature of the bony deformity and the size of the cartilage anlage; it does not show the amount of growth potential in the cartilage anlage and therefore only estimates the possible progression. An MRI study should be obtained in most patients because of the significant incidence of intraspinal abnormalities. In addition, the location of the spinal cord and any areas of spinal cord compression caused by the kyphosis can be seen on MRI. The cartilage anlage will be well defined by MRI in patients with failure of formation (Fig. 44-180).

Genitourinary abnormalities, cardiac abnormalities, Klippel-Feil syndrome, and intraspinal abnormalities are frequent in these patients. Cardiac evaluation and renal ultrasonography should be done. Myelograms have been used for documenting spinal cord compression but generally have been replaced by MRI. If myelography is used, Winter et al. emphasized that the patient should be placed supine for the myelographic evaluation so that the contrast medium pools at the apex of the kyphosis. If scoliosis is present, the patient must be turned to a semilateral position to place the convexity of the kyphoscoliosis in a dependent position.

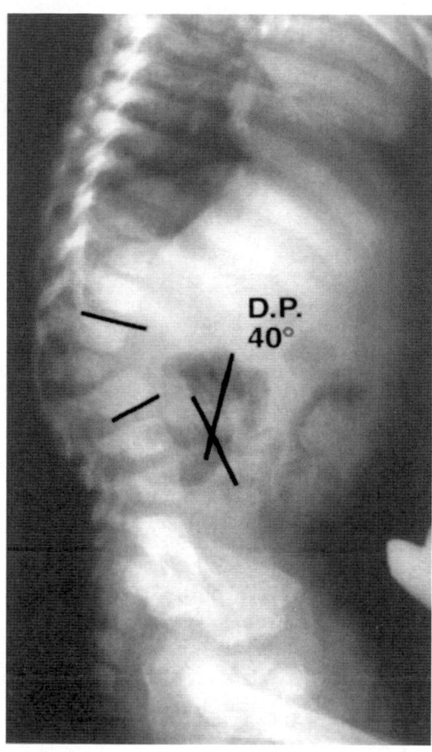

FIGURE 44-178 Two-year-old child with type I congenital kyphosis measuring 40 degrees. Radiograph shows failure of formation of anterior portion of first lumbar vertebra. (From Warner WC: Kyphosis. In Morrissy RT, Weinstein SL, editors: Lovell and Winter's pediatric orthopaedics, ed 6, Philadelphia, 2006, Lippincott Williams & Wilkins.)

OPERATIVE TREATMENT

The natural history of this condition usually is one of continued progression and an increased risk of neurologic compromise. Therefore surgery is the preferred method of treatment. If the diagnosis is uncertain or the deformity is mild, close observation may be an option. Unless compensatory curves are being treated above or below the congenital kyphosis, bracing has no role in the treatment of congenital kyphosis because it neither corrects the deformity nor stops the progression of kyphosis.

Surgery is recommended for congenital kyphosis. The type of surgery depends on the type and size of the deformity, the age of the patient, and the presence of neurologic deficits. Procedures include posterior fusion, anterior fusion, combined anterior and posterior fusion, anterior osteotomy with posterior fusion, posterior column shortening and fusion, and vertebral body resection. Fusion can be done with or without instrumentation.

TREATMENT OF TYPE I DEFORMITY

The treatment of type I deformity depends on the stage of the disease. For type I deformity, the best treatment is early posterior fusion. In a patient younger than 5 years old with a deformity of less than 50 or 55 degrees, posterior fusion

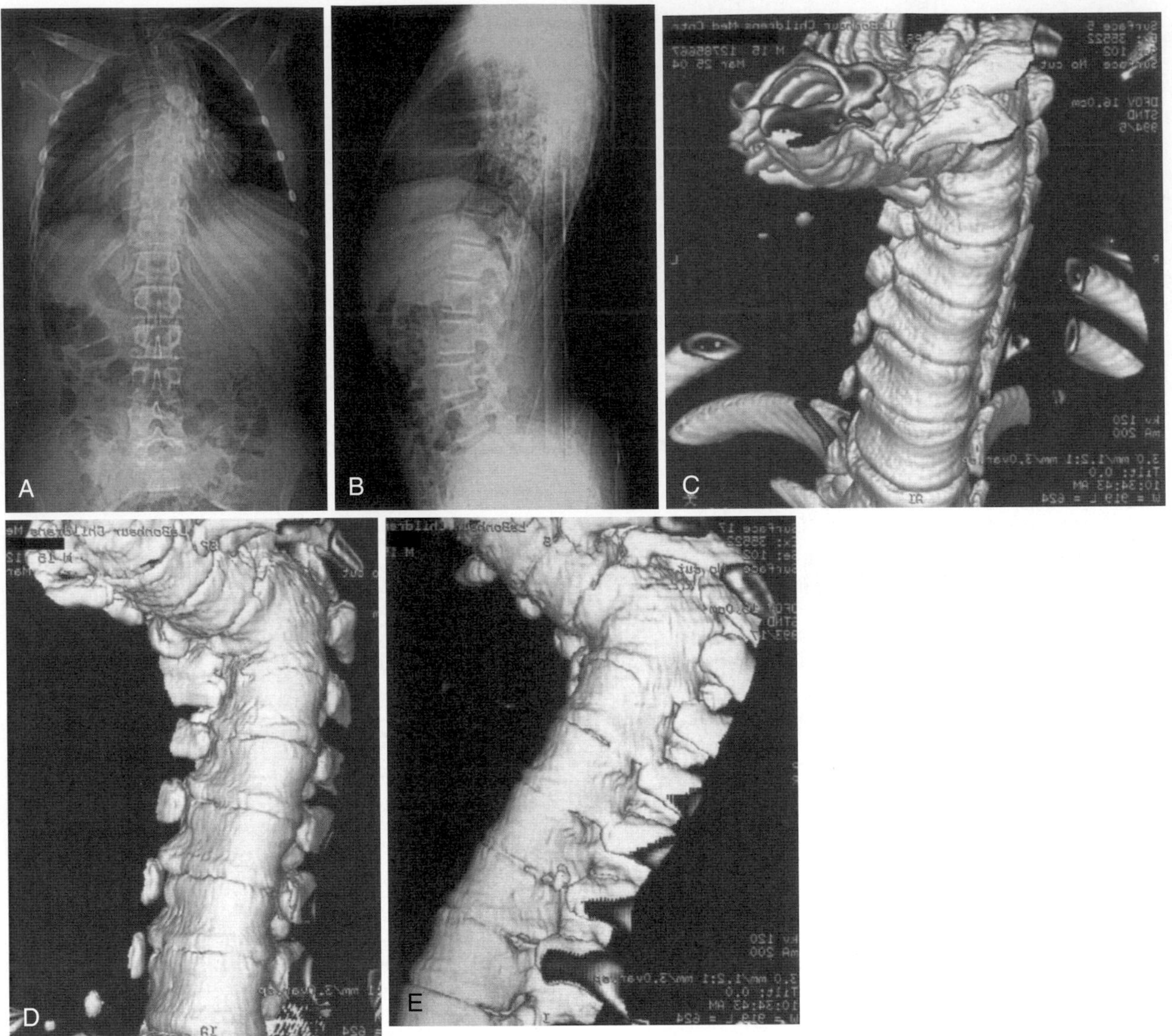

FIGURE 44-179 Congenital kyphosis. **A** and **B,** Anteroposterior and lateral radiographs. Note inadequate detail of kyphosis on lateral radiograph of spine. **C-E,** CT three-dimensional reconstruction views that clearly show bony anatomy of congenital kyphosis. (From Warner WC: Kyphosis. In Morrissy RT, Weinstein SL, editors: Lovell and Winter's pediatric orthopaedics, ed 6, Philadelphia, 2006, Lippincott Williams & Wilkins.)

alone, extending from one level above the kyphotic deformity to one level below, is recommended. This allows for some improvement because growth continues anteriorly from the anterior endplates of the vertebrae one level above and below the kyphotic vertebrae that are included in the posterior fusion. Although McMaster and Singh reported 15 degrees of correction in most patients treated with this technique, Kim et al. reported that correction of kyphosis occurred with growth only in patients younger than 3 years of age with type II and type III deformities. In curves of more than 60 degrees, anterior and posterior spinal fusions at least one level above and one level below the kyphosis are indicated. This halts the progression of the kyphotic deformity, but because the anterior physes are ablated, there is no possibility of correction with growth.

Posterior fusion alone may be successful if the kyphosis is less than 50 to 55 degrees in older patients with type I kyphotic deformity. If the deformity is more than 55 degrees, anterior and posterior fusion produces more reliable results. Anterior fusion alone will not correct the deformity, and anterior strut grafting with temporary distraction and posterior fusion, with or without posterior compression instrumentation, is necessary for deformity correction (Fig. 44-181). Posterior instrumentation may allow for some correction of the kyphosis but should be regarded more as an internal stabilizer than as a correction device. Although instrumentation has been reported to decrease the occurrence of pseudarthrosis, it should be used with caution in rigid, angular curves because of the high incidence of neurologic complications. If anterior strut grafting is done, the strut graft should be placed anteriorly under compression. If the goal of surgery is to stop the progression of deformity without correction, an anterior interbody fusion with a posterior fusion can be done. Simultaneous anterior and posterior approaches through a

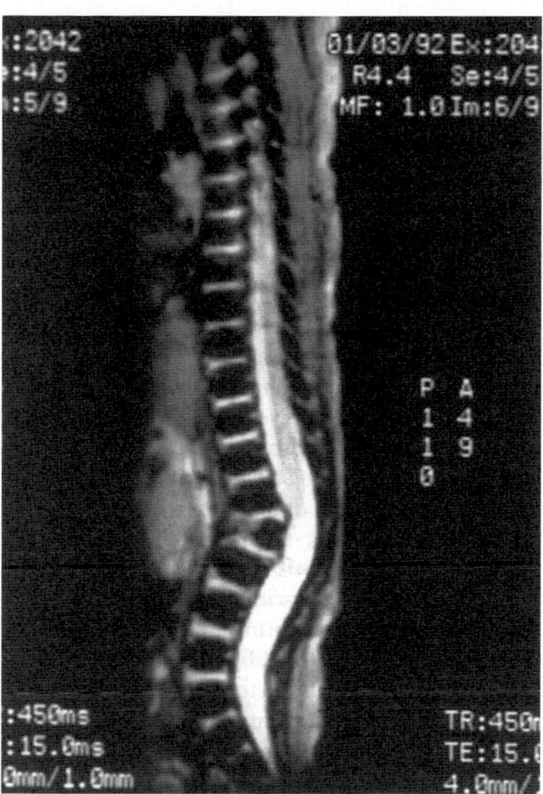

FIGURE 44-180 MRI of type I congenital kyphosis. Failure of formation of anterior vertebral body is shown, but growth potential of involved vertebra cannot be determined. Note pressure on dural sac. (From Warner WC: Kyphosis. In Morrissy RT, Weinstein SL, editors: Lovell and Winter's pediatric orthopaedics, ed 6, Philadelphia, 2006, Lippincott Williams & Wilkins.)

costotransversectomy that allows resection of the posterior hemivertebra and correction of the kyphosis with posterior compression instrumentation have been described. After removal of the hemivertebra, correction can be obtained safely and the thecal sac observed during correction. Use of skeletal traction (halo-pelvic, halo-femoral, or halo-gravity) to correct the deformity is tempting but is not recommended because there is a risk of paraplegia (Fig. 44-182). Traction pulls the spinal cord against the apex of the rigid kyphosis, which can lead to neurologic compromise in a patient with a rigid gibbus deformity.

Late treatment of a severe congenital kyphotic deformity that is accompanied by spinal cord compression is difficult; laminectomy has no role in the treatment of this condition. If there is an associated scoliosis, the anterior approach for decompression may need to be on the concavity of the scoliosis to allow the spinal cord to move both forward and into the midline after decompression. After adequate decompression, the involved vertebrae are fused with an anterior strut graft. Posterior fusion, with or without posterior stabilizing instrumentation, is then performed. Postoperative support using a cast, brace, or halo cast may be required. Posterior vertebral column resection or decompression and subtraction osteotomy, followed by stabilizing instrumentation, also can be used. Chang et al. described circumferential decompression and cantilever bending correction with posterior instrumentation.

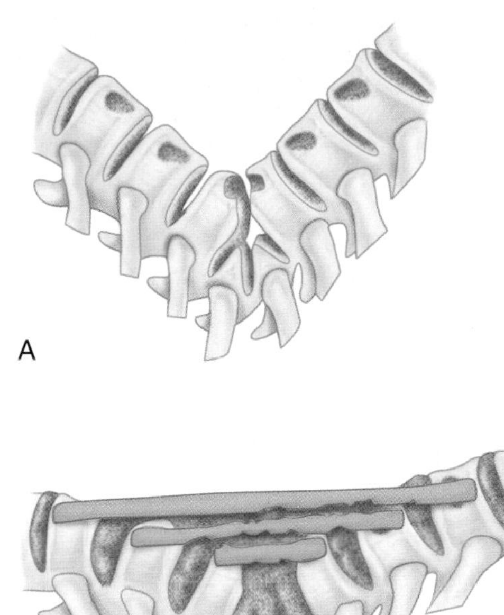

FIGURE 44-181 **A,** Preparation of tunnels for strut grafts. **B,** Insertion of strut grafts into prepared tunnels with cancellous bone graft in disc spaces.

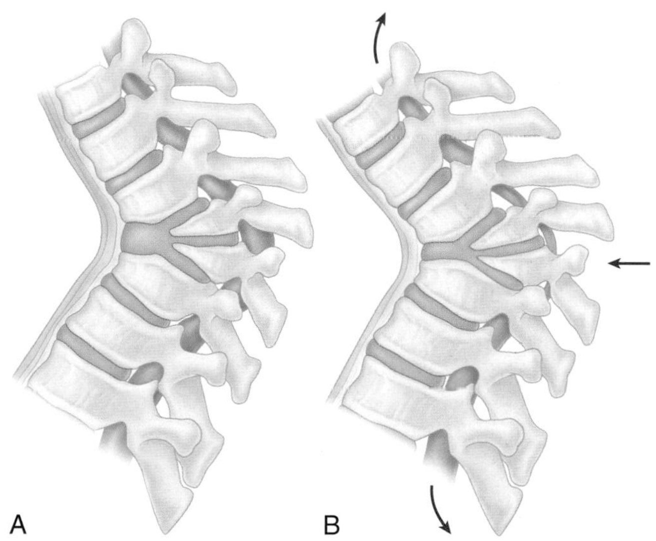

FIGURE 44-182 Effect of traction on rigid congenital kyphosis. **A,** Apical area does not change with traction, but adjacent spine is lengthened. **B,** As spine lengthens, so does spinal cord, producing increased tension in cord and aggravating existing neurologic deficits.

TREATMENT OF TYPE II DEFORMITY

If a type II kyphosis is mild (<50 degrees) and detected early, posterior fusion using compression instrumentation can be done. All the involved vertebrae plus one vertebra above and one vertebra below the congenital kyphosis should be included in the posterior fusion.

Because the kyphosis is rounded and affects several segments in type II deformity, instead of being sharply angular as in type I, compression instrumentation can be safely used. If the deformity is severe and detected late, correction can be obtained only with anterior osteotomies and fusion, followed by posterior fusion and compression instrumentation.

ANTERIOR OSTEOTOMY AND FUSION

TECHNIQUE 44-50

(WINTER ET AL.)

- Expose the spine through an appropriate anterior approach (see Chapter 37).
- Ligate the segmental vessels and expose the spine by subperiosteal stripping (Fig. 44-183A). The anterior longitudinal ligament usually is thickened and must be divided at one or more levels. Make sure that a circumferential exposure is made all the way to the opposite foramen before beginning the osteotomy.
- Divide the bony bar with a sharp osteotome or high-speed burr. Start the division anteriorly and work posteriorly until the remaining disc material is entered.
- Once the remaining disc material is seen, use a laminar spreader and excise the disc material back to the level of the posterior longitudinal ligament (Fig. 44-183B). If the bony bar is complete, make the osteotomy all the way through the posterior cortex at the level of the foramina. Take care in the area of the posterior longitudinal ligament because the ligament may be absent.
- Once the osteotomies have been completed, insert strut grafts, slotting them into bodies above and below the area of the kyphos. Hollow out the cancellous bone of each body with a curet. With rib, fibula, or iliac crest grafts of sufficient length, insert the upper end of the graft into the slot first. As manual pressure is applied posteriorly against the kyphos, use an impactor to tap the lower end of the graft into place. Place additional grafts in the disc space defects and close the pleura over them if possible. More than one strut graft may be necessary, depending on the severity of the curve. The grafts should be placed as far anterior to the axis of the flexion deformity as possible.
- Winter et al. found that failures of anterior fusion in their patients generally were associated with strut grafts that were too short or placed too close to the apex of the kyphosis or with inadequate removal of the intervertebral discs in the fusion area.

ANTERIOR CORD DECOMPRESSION AND FUSION

TECHNIQUE 44-51

(WINTER AND LONSTEIN)

- Expose the spine through an appropriate anterior approach.
- Identify the apical vertebra and the site of compression and remove the intervertebral disc completely on each side of the vertebral body or bodies.
- Remove the vertebral body laterally at the apex of the kyphosis with curets, rongeurs, or high-speed burrs.
- Remove the cancellous bone back to the posterior cortex of the vertebral body from pedicle to pedicle, removing a wedge-shaped area of bone (Fig. 44-184A).
- Beginning on the side away from the surgeon, use angled curets to remove the posterior cortical shell. Removal of the bone farthest away first prevents the spinal cord from falling into the defect and blocking vision on the far side (Fig. 44-184B).
- Next, remove the closest bony shell, working toward the apex. Control epidural bleeding with thrombin-soaked Gelfoam.
- Once the cord has been decompressed, perform an anterior strut graft fusion (Fig. 44-184C).
- Close and drain the incision in the routine manner.
- At a second stage, a posterior fusion with or without instrumentation is done.

ANTERIOR VASCULAR RIB BONE GRAFTING

Bradford et al. noted frequent fracture of strut grafts when the grafts were not in contact with the vertebral bodies and simply spanned an open area between vertebrae. A rib or fibular graft may take up to 2 years for replacement, and it is weakest approximately 6 months after surgery. To prevent graft fracture, Bradford developed a technique of vascular pedicle bone graft for the treatment of severe kyphosis when the strut must be placed more than 4 cm from the spine. He credited Rose et al. with first describing the technique in 1975.

TECHNIQUE 44-52

(BRADFORD)

- Plan the thoracotomy to remove enough rib to bridge the kyphosis. For a severe kyphotic deformity from T6 to T12, a vascularized fifth rib would be used to strut the deformity.
- Make a skin incision as in the routine transthoracic exposure. Take care to identify the appropriate rib and avoid the use of electrocautery over the rib periosteum.
- Divide the intercostal muscles sharply off the cranial portion of the rib. This rib dissection is always extraperiosteal. Divide the rib distally to provide enough length to span the area of deformity.
- At the level of the distal rib osteotomy, ligate the intercostal vessels and sharply cut the intercostal nerve and allow it to retract. The intercostal muscles attached to the caudal portion of the rib should remain attached to provide protection for the intercostal vessels that will perfuse the rib.
- At the level for the proximal rib osteotomy, mobilize the periosteum away from the rib.

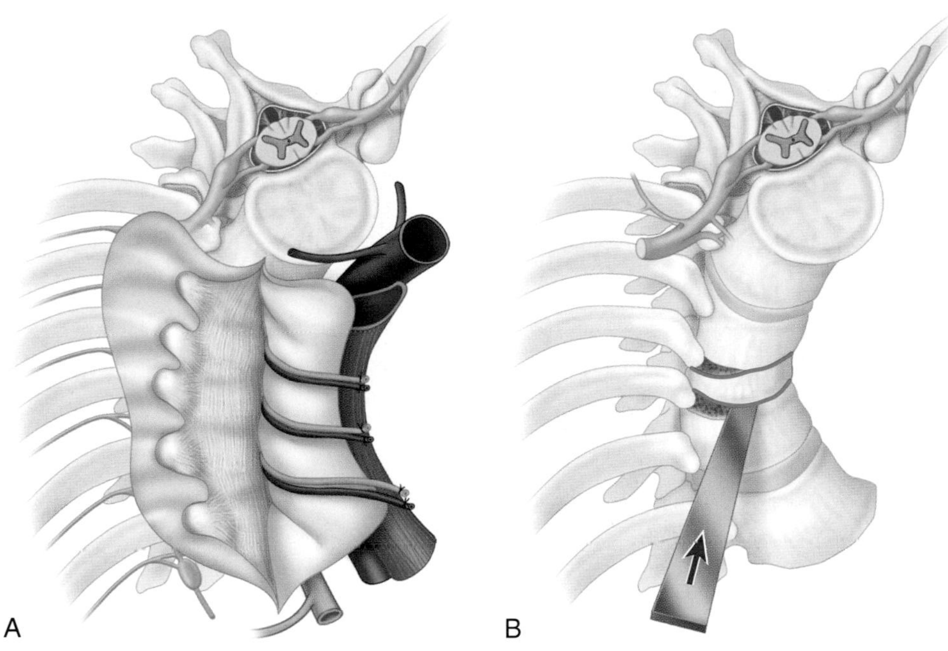

FIGURE 44-183 **A,** Anterolateral exposure of spine in preparation for anterior osteotomy. **B,** Completion of osteotomy with osteotome. **SEE TECHNIQUE 44-50.**

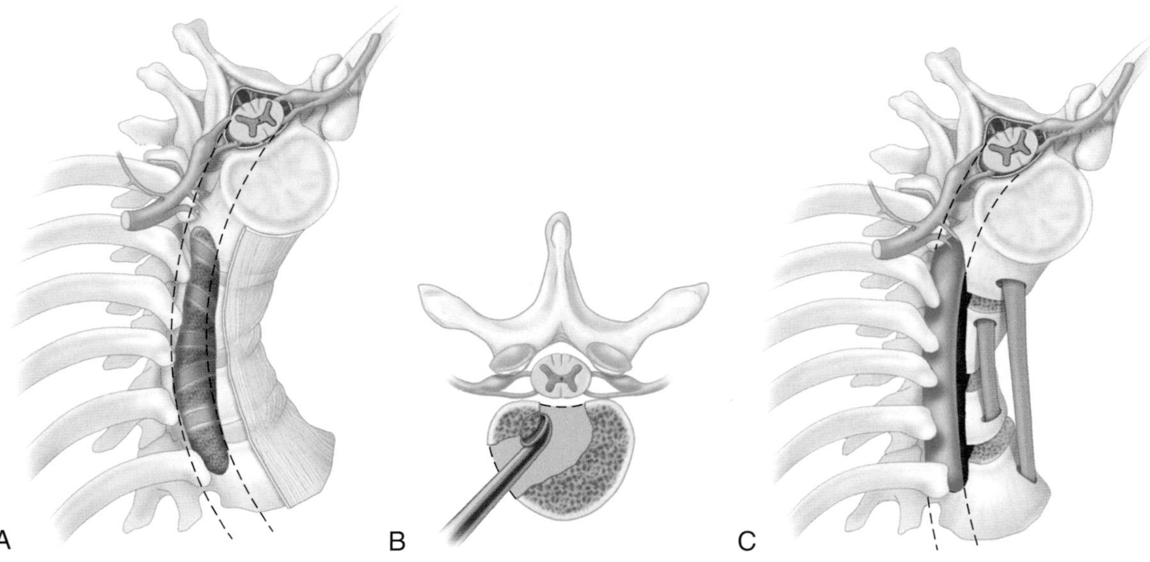

FIGURE 44-184 **A,** Anterolateral exposure of spine and partial removal of apex of kyphosis. **B,** Posterior cortex is removed, allowing decompression of spinal cord. **C,** Cord is decompressed and strut grafts are in place. **SEE TECHNIQUE 44-51.**

- Once the osteotomy is completed, the rib is connected only to the caudal intercostal muscle and its intercostal vascular pedicle. Carefully divide the intercostal vessels below the rib in the direction of the costovertebral joint, retaining the muscle around the intercostal pedicle. Do not dissect out the intercostal artery and vein.
- If the rib and muscle are poorly perfused, dissect the vascular pedicle away from the intercostal vessels (Fig. 44-185).
- Mobilize the rib with its intact intercostal musculature and artery and vein complex (Fig. 44-186A).
- Carefully peel back the periosteum on the rib graft for 2 or 3 mm on each end to provide bone-to-bone contact

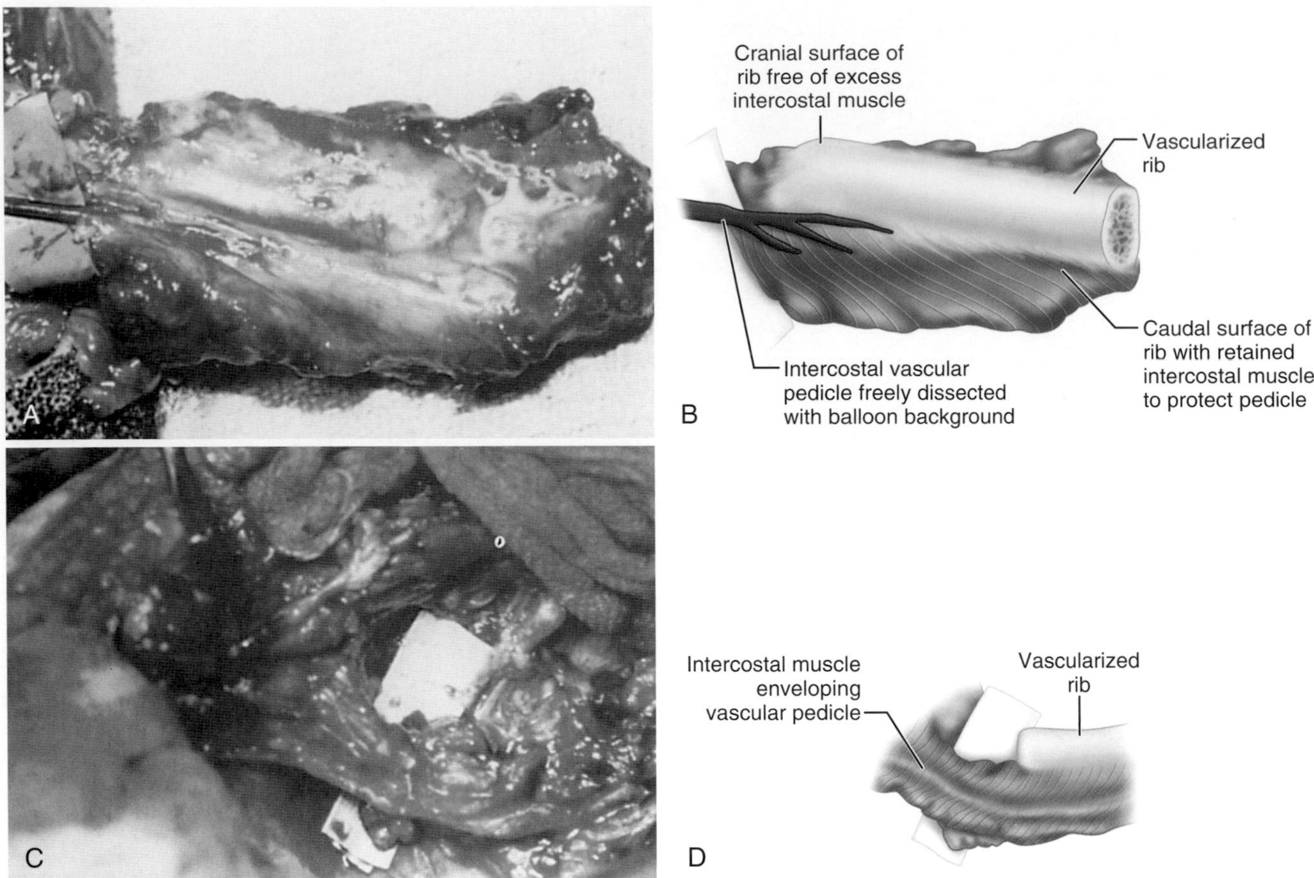

FIGURE 44-185 **A and B,** Background balloon placed behind intercostal vascular pedicle. Ordinarily, it is not necessary to dissect out vascular pedicle. **C and D,** Retaining portion of intercostal muscle with vessel as shown here reduces likelihood of pedicle injury during harvest. (From Shaffer JW, Bradford DS: The use of and techniques for vascularized rib pedicle grafts. In Bridwell KH, DeWald RL, editors: The textbook of spinal surgery, ed 2, Philadelphia, 1997, Lippincott-Raven.) **SEE TECHNIQUE 44-52.**

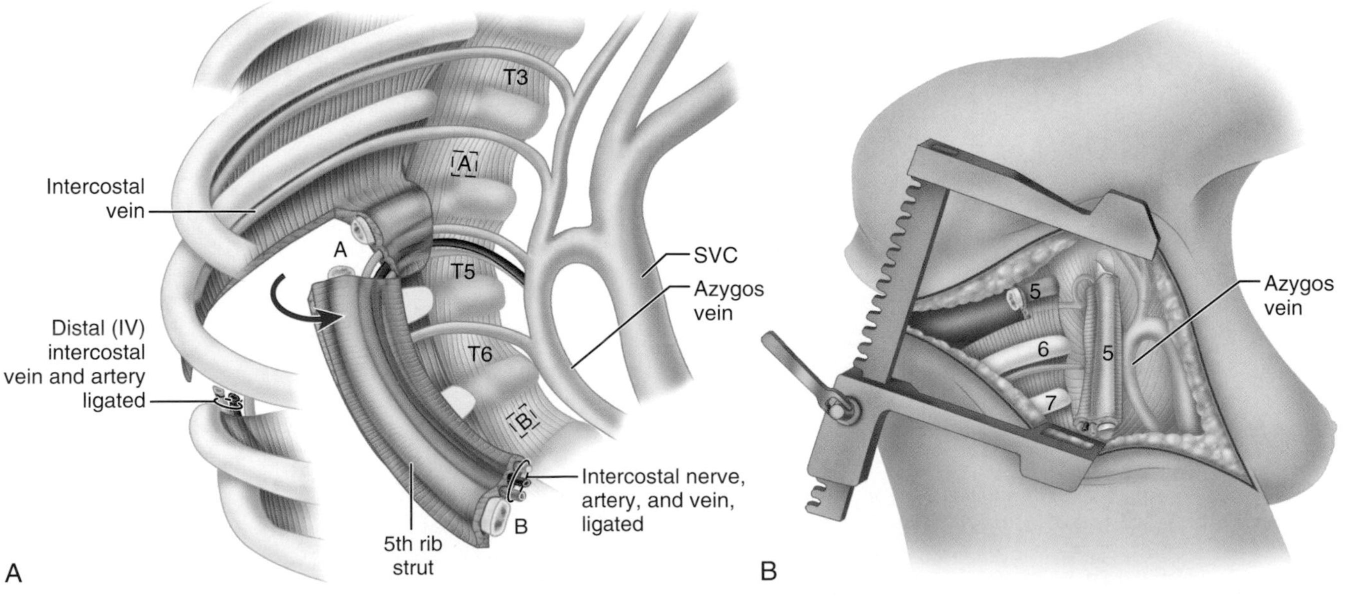

FIGURE 44-186 Thoracotomy. **A,** Wide margin of intercostal muscle left attached to rib to ensure intact blood supply. **B,** Rib graft rotated 90 degrees on its axis and keyed into vertebral bodies over length of kyphosis to be fused. **SEE TECHNIQUE 44-52.**

without soft-tissue intervention when the graft is rotated into position.
- Identify the vertebral bodies proximally and distally to be included in the fusion.
- Make a hole in the anterior aspect of the vertebral body above and below to accept the ends of the rib graft.
- Trim the rib so that the ends will match the length of the spine to be fused.
- Rotate the rib on its axis approximately 90 degrees and wedge it into the vertebrae above and below (Fig. 44-186B).
- Close the chest in a routine fashion over chest tubes.
- Immobilization of the spine after vascular grafting is the same as after nonvascular graft procedures.

CIRCUMFERENTIAL DECOMPRESSION AND CANTILEVER BENDING

TECHNIQUE 44-53

(CHANG ET AL.)
- With the patient prone and somatosensory evoked potential monitoring initiated, make a straight posterior midline incision.
- After subperiosteal dissection, expose three to five vertebrae (depending on the bone quality) above and below the apex to the tips of the transverse process.
- Insert pedicle screws segmentally except at the levels of circumferential decompression, where at least three segments of fixation are made at either end of the decompression.
- Carry dissection out laterally, exposing the ribs corresponding to the levels of circumferential neurologic decompression as determined by preoperative radiographic analysis (most often at the apex of the kyphotic deformity).
- Remove the transverse process and the corresponding ribs on both sides of the neurologic decompression to expose the lateral wall of the pedicle.
- Deepen the subperiosteal dissection, following the lateral wall of the vertebral body, until a comfortable working space for neurologic decompression is evident beneath the compromised cord.
- Take care to avoid damaging segmental vessels during the exposure. Injured segmental vessels should be clamped, ligated, and cut under spinal cord monitoring to ensure that there are no changes in somatosensory evoked potentials.
- Carry out total laminectomy and facetectomy at the apex to expose the compromised neural tissue. In thoracic vertebrae, cut the nerve roots to facilitate thorough neurologic decompression; in the lumbar vertebrae, keep the nerve roots intact.
- Remove the pedicle to expose the lateral portion of the compromised dural tube.
- Connect pedicle screws on both sides by two rods contoured to the shape of the deformity to facilitate rigid fixation.
- Because of the marked angular change in segments around the apex, the rods can be situated nearly on the same coronal plane as the compromised cord by adjusting the protruding height of the screw heads at the levels immediately cephalad and caudad to the apex (the level of circumferential neurologic decompression) and properly precontouring the rods (Fig. 44-187A).
- Create a tunnel beneath the compromised cord by penetrating a blunt-end cage trial from one side of the apical vertebral body to the other. Enlarge the tunnel and use rongeurs, curets, and pituitary forceps to remove the portion of the apical vertebral body above the tunnel and adjacent to the anterior compromised dural tube (including the posterior vertebral wall).
- After completion of this neurologic decompression, check to ensure that the canal is clear of any residual compression at the resection margins. Use a curet to remove cancellous bone within the portion of the apical vertebral body; deepen the tunnel to the depth of the anterior vertebral cortex. Weaken the cortex at several points by penetration with a blunt-end cage trial to facilitate its fracture while applying cantilever bending for correction.
- Connect one pair of in situ benders to each contoured rod at the levels immediately cephalad and caudad to the apex (Fig. 44-187B). Fix the position of the benders by using wire to tie the free ends at the desired location (Fig. 44-187C).
- Fracture the apical vertebral body anterior to the cord and open it with the correction hinge in the compromised cord.
- Slowly increase the bending force. If resistance is felt, stop the correction and fix.
- After correction, perform a wake-up test.
- Measure the height of the anterior interbody gap. Fill a titanium mesh with bone chips and insert it into the anterior gap, and place an autogenous iliac bone graft around the titanium mesh. Insert the mesh cage from the lateral side to fit on the cephalad and caudal bone base.
- Confirm proper cage position by direct observation and fluoroscopy. Make sure there is ample space between the cage and the cord before releasing the benders and locking the cage in place (Fig. 44-187D).
- Connect two transverse links to the rods at the cephalad and caudad levels to the level of neurologic decompression.
- Perform posterior fusion at all instrumented levels.
- Close the wound in the usual fashion over suction drains.

POSTOPERATIVE CARE. Patients are fitted with a custom-made, plastic thoracolumbosacral orthosis and are allowed out of bed 72 hours after surgery. The orthosis is worn for 6 months.

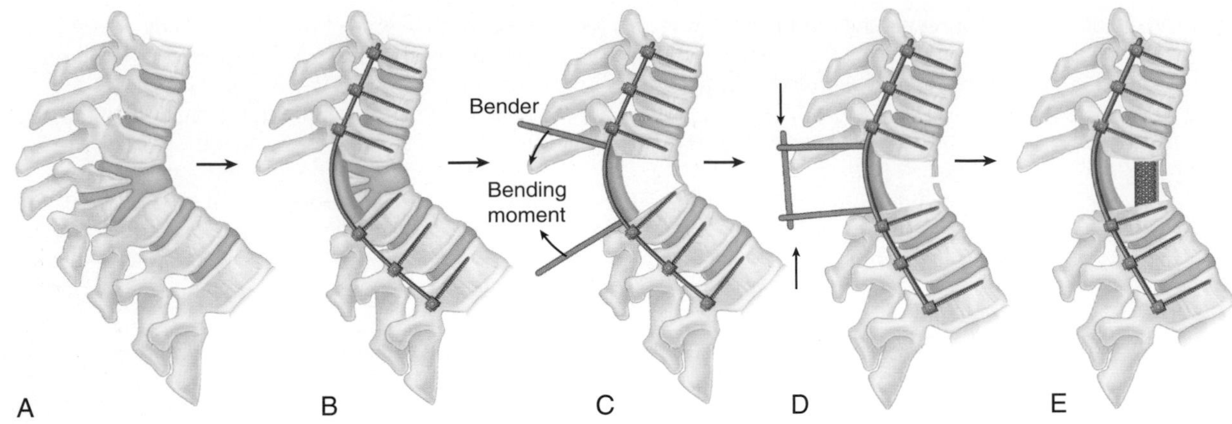

FIGURE 44-187 Hinge technique for correction of severe, rigid kyphotic deformity. **A,** Severe angular kyphosis. **B,** Laminectomy, pediculectomy, and rods placed on same plane as the cord. **C,** Complete circumferential decompression and placement of rod benders. **D,** Cantilever bending to correct kyphosis. **E,** Insertion of mesh cage to provide anterior support.. (Redrawn from Chang KW, Cheng CW, Chen HC, Chen TC: Correction hinge in the compromised cord for severe and rigid angular kyphosis with neurologic deficits, Spine 34:1040, 2009.) **SEE TECHNIQUE 44-53.**

POSTERIOR HEMIVERTEBRA RESECTION WITH TRANSPEDICULAR INSTRUMENTATION

TECHNIQUE 44-54

(RUF AND HARMS)

- Carefully expose the posterior elements of the spine at the affected levels, including the lamina, transverse processes, and facet joints, and, in the thoracic spine, the surplus rib head on the convex side.
- Mark the entry points for the pedicle screws with a fine needle and check their position with image intensification in an anteroposterior view. In the lumbar region, the entry point is the base of the transverse process at the lateral border of the superior articular facet. In the thoracic region, the entry point is at the superior margin of the transverse process, slightly lateral to the lower lateral edge of the articular facet. On image intensification, the tips of the cannulas should project onto the oval of the pedicles, ideally slightly lateral to the center.
- Open the bone at the entry point with a sharp awl or small burr, and advance a 2-mm drill through the pedicle into the vertebral body. Mark the drill holes with Kirschner wires and check their correct position with fluoroscopy. After tapping, insert the screws.
- Remove the posterior elements of the hemivertebra, including the lamina, facet joints, transverse process, and posterior part of the pedicle. Identify the spinal cord and the nerve roots above and below the pedicle of the hemivertebra. In the thoracic spine, resect the rib head and the proximal part of the surplus rib at the convex side also.
- After resection of the transverse process and the rib head, expose the lateral-anterior part of the hemivertebra by blunt dissection; this exposure is retroperitoneal in the lumbar spine and extrapleural in the thoracic spine.
- Remove the remnants of the pedicle and expose the posterior aspect of the vertebral body of the hemivertebra; this is made easier by the fact that the hemivertebra lies far laterally on the convex side, whereas the spinal cord usually is shifted to the concave side.
- Cut the discs adjacent to the hemivertebra and mobilize and remove the body of the hemivertebra, using a blunt spatula to protect the anterior structures.
- Completely remove the remaining disc material of the upper and lower disc spaces and debride the endplates down to bleeding bone. Make sure that disc removal reaches the contralateral side.
- Complete the instrumentation and apply compression on the convex side until the gap left after resection is closed completely. If a void remains, fill it with cancellous bone.
- When kyphosis is present, anterior column support can be added to create a fulcrum to achieve lordosis. The neural structures must be controlled and protected at all times during the resection and during the corrective maneuver.
- If there is a single hemivertebra without bars, rib synostosis, or other major structural changes of the neighboring vertebrae, only the two vertebrae adjacent to the resected hemivertebra are fused. If major structural changes are present in the adjacent vertebrae or there is a more severe kyphotic deformity, one or two additional segments may be included in the fusion.
- For contralateral bar formation and rib synostosis, the synostosed rib heads on the concave side are removed and the bar is cut. The fusion is extended with segmental instrumentation over the whole length of the bar formation to the adjacent vertebrae.

POSTOPERATIVE CARE. Postoperative management is as described for Technique 44-53.

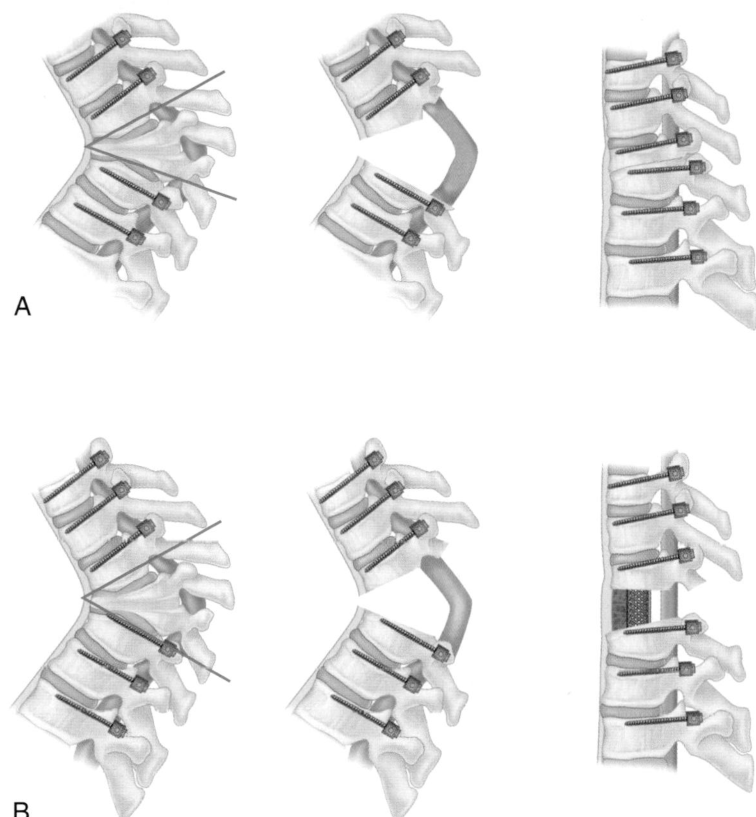

FIGURE 44-188 Pedicle subtraction osteotomy and posterior vertebral column resection for congenital kyphosis. **A,** Pedicle subtraction osteotomy. **B,** Posterior vertebral column resection. (Redrawn from Zeng Y, Chen Z, Qi Q, et al: The posterior surgical correction of congenital kyphosis and kyphoscoliosis: 23 cases with minimum 2 years follow-up, Eur Spine J 22:372, 2013.) **SEE TECHNIQUE 44-54.**

Zeng et al. described pedicle subtraction osteotomy and posterior vertebral column resection (Fig. 44-188) in 23 patients with kyphosis or kyphoscoliosis. Overall, satisfactory correction was obtained in 91%, with comparable complications.

COMPLICATIONS OF OPERATIVE TREATMENT

Some of the more frequent complications of treatment of congenital kyphosis are pseudarthrosis, progression of kyphosis, and paralysis. Pseudarthrosis and progression of the kyphotic deformity can be minimized by performing anterior and posterior fusions for deformities of more than 50 degrees. The posterior fusion should extend from one level above to one level below the involved vertebra.

Paralysis is perhaps the most feared complication of spinal surgery. The risk of this complication can be lessened by not attempting to maximally correct the deformity with instrumentation. Instrumentation should be used more for stabilization of rigid deformities rather than correction. Halo traction in rigid congenital kyphotic deformities has been associated with an increased risk of neurologic compromise. Another long-term problem, occurring in approximately 38% of patients with kyphosis, is low back pain caused by increased lumbar lordosis that is needed to compensate for the kyphotic deformity.

PROGRESSIVE ANTERIOR VERTEBRAL FUSION

Progressive anterior vertebral fusion is an uncommon cause of kyphosis in children that may be confused with type II congenital kyphosis if it is discovered late. However, it is distinguishable from type II congenital kyphosis in that the disc spaces and vertebral bodies are normal at birth and later become anteriorly fused. Knutsson first described progressive anterior vertebral fusion in 1949, and fewer than 100 cases have since been reported. The cause is unknown, and it is probably a distinct clinical condition; however, it may possibly represent a delayed type II congenital kyphosis.

Certain forms of type II congenital kyphosis (failure of segmentation) can be inherited with failure of segmentation and delayed fusion of the anterior vertebral elements, which are not visible on radiographs until 8 or 10 years of age. Familial occurrence has been reported by several authors. Associated anomalies, including hearing defects, tibial agenesis, foot deformities, Klippel-Feil syndrome, Ito syndrome, pulmonary artery stenosis, and hemisacralization of L5, also have been reported.

Neurologic deficits usually do not occur in patients with progressive anterior vertebral fusion, but spinal cord compression resulting from an acutely angled kyphosis has been reported.

Van Buskirk et al. described five stages of progressive anterior vertebral fusion: stage 1, disc space narrowing that occurs to a greater extent anteriorly than posteriorly; stage 2, increased sclerosis of the vertebral endplates of the anterior and middle columns; stage 3, fragmentation of the anterior vertebral endplates; stage 4, fusion of the anterior and sometimes the middle columns; and stage 5, development of a kyphotic deformity.

Kyphosis that occurs in the last stage of progressive anterior vertebral fusion is the result of the anterior disc space fusing while the posterior disc space remains open. Growth continues in the posterior disc space and the posterior column. Patients with thoracic progressive anterior vertebral fusion have a better prognosis than those with lumbar involvement. This is probably because of the normal kyphotic posture of the thoracic spine. Nonoperative treatment is recommended for most thoracic progressive anterior vertebral fusion deformities. If it occurs in the lumbar spine, a posterior spinal fusion is indicated for stage 1 through stage 3 deformity. For stages 4 and 5, the kyphotic deformity has already occurred in a normal lordotic lumbar spine and posterior fusion will only stop progression of the deformity. An anterior osteotomy with posterior fusion and instrumentation is necessary to obtain normal sagittal alignment.

INFANTILE LUMBAR HYPOPLASIA

Thoracolumbar kyphosis secondary to lumbar hypoplasia was reported by Campos et al. in seven normal infants in whom the thoracolumbar kyphosis resolved spontaneously with growth. It began improving with walking age and corrected to normal by 6 years of age. The average initial kyphosis was 34 degrees. The patients had a clinically apparent kyphotic deformity during the first year of life, and on radiographs they had a relatively sharply angled kyphosis, with the apex at the affected vertebra (Fig. 44-189A). The affected vertebra was wedge shaped with an anterosuperior indentation, giving it the appearance of a beak (Fig. 44-189B and C). Only one vertebra was involved in all seven infants, either L1 or L2. Campos et al. recommended an initial period of observation to get a better assessment of the deformity as ossification progresses and to avoid overtreatment of lumbar hypoplasia that will improve with growth.

SPONDYLOLYSIS AND SPONDYLOLISTHESIS

Herbiniaux, a Belgian obstetrician, noted a bone prominence in front of the sacrum that caused problems in delivery. He generally is credited with having first described spondylolisthesis. The term *spondylolisthesis* was used by Kilian in 1854 and is derived from the Greek *spondylos,* meaning "vertebra," and *olisthenein,* meaning "to slip." Spondylolisthesis is defined as anterior or posterior slipping of one segment of the spine on the next lower segment. Spondylolysis is a unilateral or bilateral defect of the pars interarticularis.

CLASSIFICATION

Wiltse, Newman, and Macnab's classification of spondylolisthesis is illustrated in Figure 44-190 and Box 44-10. Marchetti and Bartolozzi suggested that the classification of Wiltse et al. is based on a mixture of etiologic and topographic criteria, that it is difficult to predict progression or response to surgery with this classification, and that it also is difficult to identify the type of spondylolisthesis precisely. They therefore attempted to further classify spondylolisthesis by dividing the condition into developmental and acquired forms (Box 44-11). Their classification removes the isthmic or lysis part of spondylolisthesis from the primary role in causation and emphasizes the developmental and dysplastic aspects. In analyzing the spondylolisthesis, the surgeon must first decide if the condition is developmental or acquired. If it is developmental, the degree of dysplasia must be determined as high (severe) or low (mild) by evaluation of the quality of the posterior bony hook (Fig. 44-191). The degree of lordosis and the position of the gravity line also are important; the farther anterior the gravity line is, the more likely the spondylolisthesis is to increase. The competency of the disc at the level of the spondylolisthesis also is important; MRI may be required to determine this. Indications of an unstable situation include a significant localized kyphosis (high slip angle) of the slip. Bony changes, such as a trapezoid-shaped L5 vertebral body and a dome-shaped sacrum, also are indicative of instability and significant dysplasia. The implications of the classification system are that the more dysplastic and unstable the situation is, the more aggressive the surgical procedure should be to solve the problem.

Herman and Pizzutillo proposed a new classification for spondylolysis and spondylolisthesis in children and adolescents that uses pertinent elements of the Wiltse et al. and the Marchetti and Bartolozzi classifications. This four-part classification was based on clinical presentation and morphology of the spinal abnormality. Type I is a dysplastic spondylolysis and spondylolisthesis similar to the Wiltse et al. dysplastic category. Type II is referred to as developmental spondylolysis and spondylolisthesis. This type usually is an incidental finding. Type III refers to traumatic spondylolysis and spondylolisthesis and is subdivided into acute and chronic types. The chronic type is further subdivided into (1) stress reaction, (2) stress fracture, and (3) spondylolytic defect or nonunion of pars. Type IV is pathologic spondylolysis and spondylolisthesis (Box 44-12).

Hollenberg et al. described an MRI classification system for spondylolysis: grade 0, normal; grade 1, bone edema and intact cortices compatible with stress reaction; grade 2, incomplete fracture; grade 3, complete active fracture with accompanying bone edema; and grade 4, complete fracture without accompanying bone marrow edema.

Developmental spondylolisthesis and the acquired stress fracture type of spondylosis are the focus of this section. Acquired degenerative spondylolisthesis is discussed in Chapter 40.

ETIOLOGY AND NATURAL HISTORY

The prevalence of spondylolisthesis in the general population is 5% to 8%. The male-to-female ratio for this condition is 2:1. Developmental spondylolisthesis with lysis is considered to be the result of a fatigue fracture caused by repetitive mechanical stresses on the lower lumbar spine in children

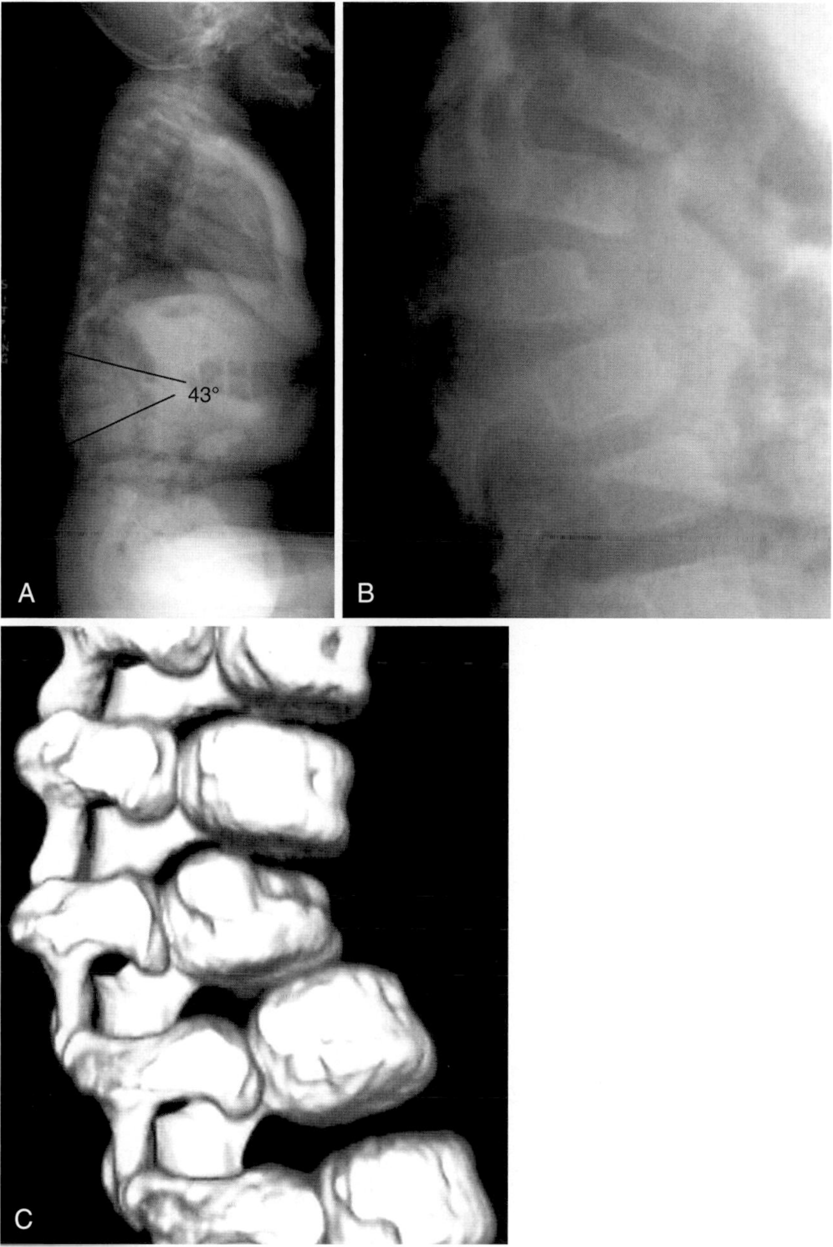

FIGURE 44-189 **A** and **B**, L2 hypoplasia in patient with spontaneous resolution. Note beaked vertebra at L2. **C**, Three-dimensional CT showing beaked L2 vertebra. (From Campos MA, Fernandes P, Dolan LA, Weinstein SL: Infantile thoracolumbar kyphosis secondary to lumbar hypoplasia, J Bone Joint Surg 90A:1726, 2008.)

with a genetic predisposition for the defect. During flexion and extension, the load on the posterior bony arch increases considerably from L1 to L5, with the highest mechanical stress concentrated at the pars interarticularis of L5. The defect has not been noted at birth or in chronically bedridden patients. Wiltse et al. postulated that lumbar lordosis is accentuated by the normal flexion contractures of the hip in childhood and that this posture places the weight-bearing forces on the pars interarticularis. Letts et al. suggested that shear stresses are greater on the pars interarticularis when the lumbar spine is extended. Cyron and Hutton found that the pars interarticularis is thinner and the vertebral disc is less resistant to shear in children and adolescents than in adults. It also is more common in certain types of sporting activities with repetitive hyperextension and rotational loads applied to the lumbar spine. Adequate separation between the adjacent articular facets allows the posterior elements to overlap one another during hyperextension. As reported by Ward et al., a lack of sufficient interfacetal distance in the cranial to caudal direction is likely to pinch the L5 lamina between the inferior facets of L4 and the superior facets of S1 during repetitive hyperextension of the lumbar spine, leading to the development of a spondylolytic defect. The prevalence of spondylolysis and spondylolisthesis increases in children and adolescents who are active in sports that involve repetitive hyperextension of the lumbar spine, such as gymnastics, weight lifting,

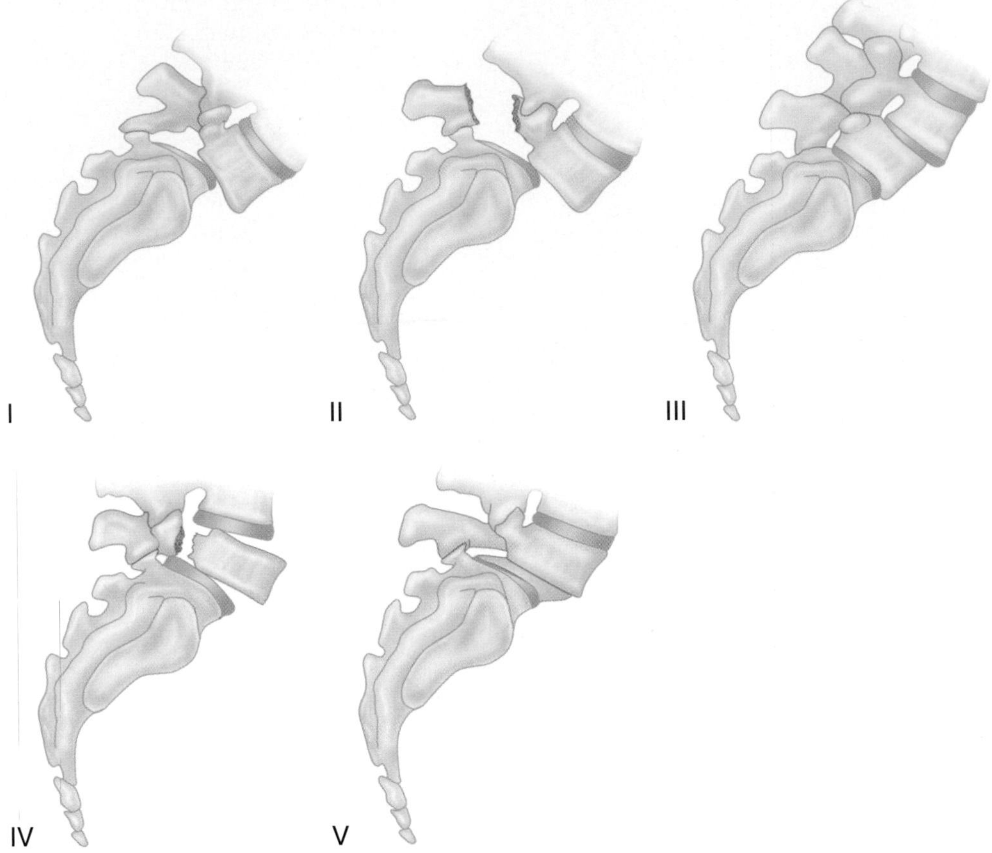

FIGURE 44-190 Five types of spondylolisthesis: type I, dysplastic; type II, isthmic; type III, degenerative; type IV, traumatic; type V, pathologic. (Redrawn from Hensinger RN: Spondylolysis and spondylolisthesis in children, Instr Course Lect 32:132, 1983.)

BOX 44-10

Classification of Spondylolisthesis (Wiltse et al.)

- Type I, dysplastic—Congenital abnormalities of the upper sacral facets or inferior facets of the fifth lumbar vertebra that allow slipping of L5 on S1. No pars interarticularis defect is present in this type.
- Type II, isthmic—Defect in the pars interarticularis that allows forward slipping of L5 on S1. Three types of isthmic spondylolistheses are recognized:
  - Lytic—a stress fracture of the pars interarticularis
  - An elongated but intact pars interarticularis
  - An acute fracture of the pars interarticularis
- Type III, degenerative—This lesion results from intersegmental instability of a long duration with subsequent remodeling of the articular processes at the level of involvement.
- Type IV, traumatic—This type results from fractures in the area of the bony hook other than the pars interarticularis, such as the pedicle, lamina, or facet.
- Type V, pathologic—This type results from generalized or localized bone disease and structural weakness of the bone, such as osteogenesis imperfecta.

BOX 44-11

Classification of Spondylolisthesis (Marchetti and Bartolozzi)

Developmental

- High dysplastic
  - With lysis
  - With elongation
- Low dysplastic
  - With lysis
  - With elongation

Acquired

- Traumatic
  - Acute fracture
  - Stress fracture
- Postsurgery
  - Direct surgery
  - Indirect surgery
- Pathologic
  - Local pathology
  - Systemic pathology
- Degenerative
  - Primary
  - Secondary

From DeWald RL: Spondylolisthesis. In Bridwell KH, DeWald RL, editors: The textbook of spinal surgery, ed 3, Philadelphia, 2011, Lippincott Williams & Wilkins.

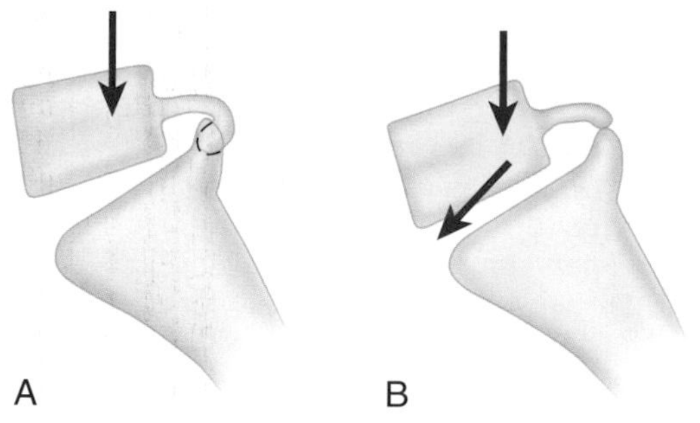

FIGURE 44-191 **A,** Pedicle, pars interarticularis, inferior facets of L5, and sacral facets all form bony hook that prevents L5 vertebra from sliding forward along slope of sacral endplate. **B,** Difference between normal bony hook and dysplastic bony hook that is incapable of providing resistance to forward slippage of the L5 vertebra under weight-bearing stresses in upright spine.

BOX 44-12

Classification of Spondylolisthesis and Spondylolysis (Herman and Pizzutillo)

- Type I—Dysplastic
- Type II—Developmental
- Type III—Traumatic
  - Acute
  - Chronic
    - Stress reaction
    - Stress fracture
    - Spondylolytic defect
    - Nonunion of pars
- Type IV—Pathologic

From Herman MJ, Pizzutillo PD: Spondylolysis and spondylolisthesis in the child and adolescent, Clin Orthop Relat Res 434:46, 2005.

swimming, wrestling, and rowing. The incidence can vary from 11% to 30% but has been reported to be as high as 47% in elite athletes who participate in high-risk sports such as diving and gymnastics. These observations indicate that the condition is acquired rather than congenital. However, as many as 50% of Eskimos are reported to have spondylolisthesis, whereas only 6% to 7% of white males and 1.1% of adult black women have the condition, indicating a definite genetic predisposition.

Beutler et al. followed up on a prospective study started in the early 1950s by Dr. Daniel Baker to determine the incidence and natural history of spondylolysis and spondylolisthesis. From 1955 to 1957, radiographs were taken of all first-grade children in a northern Pennsylvania town, a study population of 500 children. A lytic defect of the pars interarticularis was found in 4.4%. By adulthood, lumbar lytic lesions had developed in additional subjects, bringing the total incidence to 6%. Four decades later, all subjects with a pars defect were observed. Subjects with unilateral defects never experienced slippage during the course of the study. Progression of spondylolisthesis slowed with each decade. There was no association of slip progression and low back pain. There was no statistically significant difference between the SF-36 scores of the study population and those of the general population of the same age. Their findings indicated a benign course for the first 50 years of life. Only a small percentage of subjects developed symptomatic slippage progression in long-term follow-up studies. Their findings confirm that there is no justification for advising children and adolescents with spondylolysis and low-grade spondylolisthesis not to participate in competitive sports.

Progression of spondylolisthesis is uncommon if it is less than 30%. If increased slipping occurs, it usually occurs between the ages of 9 and 15 years and seldom after the age of 20 years. Harris and Weinstein, in a long-term follow-up of untreated patients with grade III and grade IV spondylolistheses, found that 36% of patients were asymptomatic, 55% had mild symptoms, and only one patient had significant symptoms. All patients led active lives, and all had required only minor adjustments in their lifestyles. None of the patients was dissatisfied with his or her appearance, and none stated that it had interfered with social or business relationships. In a similar group of patients treated with in situ posterior interlaminar arthrodeses, 57% were asymptomatic and 38% had mild symptoms.

CLINICAL FINDINGS

Patients with spondylolysis and spondylolisthesis usually present with symptoms of mechanical low back pain that is aggravated by high activity levels or competitive sports. Pain is diminished with activity restriction and rest. Often no symptoms will be present and the patient seeks medical evaluation because of a postural deformity or gait abnormality. Pain most often occurs during the adolescent growth spurt and is predominantly backache, with only occasional leg pain. Symptoms are aggravated by high activity levels or competitive sports and are diminished by activity restriction and rest. The back pain probably results from instability of the affected segment, and the leg pain usually is related to irritation of the L5 nerve root.

Back pain on lumbar hyperextension is a common clinical finding. Pain can be reproduced by performing the one-leg hyperextension test or "stork test." This usually reproduces pain on the affected side. Buttock pain radiating into the posterior thighs is common during walking or standing. A neurologic deficit affecting the L5 or S1 nerve root is present in 15% of patients. With a significant slip, a step-off at the lumbosacral junction is palpable, motion of the lumbar spine is restricted, and hamstring tightness is evident on straight-leg raising. Tightness of the hamstrings is present in 80% of symptomatic patients. As the vertebral body is displaced anteriorly, the patient assumes a lordotic posture above the level of the slip to compensate for the displacement. The sacrum becomes more vertical, and the buttocks appear heart shaped because of the sacral prominence. With more severe slips, the trunk becomes shortened and often leads to complete absence of the waistline. These children walk with a peculiar gait, described as a "pelvic waddle" by Newman, because of the hamstring tightness and the lumbosacral kyphosis. Children, unlike adults, seldom have objective signs of nerve root compression, such as motor weakness, reflex change, or sensory deficit. Tight hamstrings often are the only positive physical finding.

Scoliosis is relatively common in younger patients with spondylolisthesis and is of three types: (1) sciatic, (2)

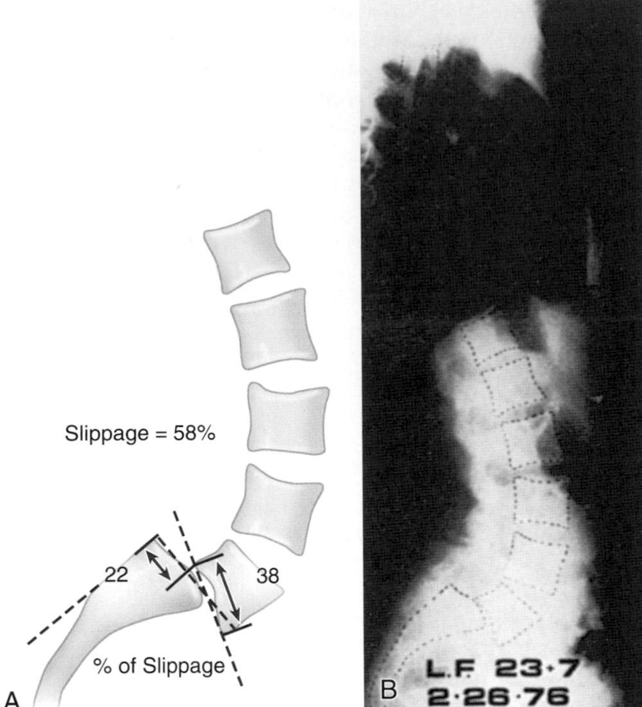

FIGURE 44-192 **A** and **B**, Percentage of slipping calculated by measurement of distance from line parallel to posterior portion of first sacral vertebral body to line parallel to posterior portion of body of L5; anteroposterior dimension of L5 inferiorly is used to calculate percentage of slipping.

olisthetic, or (3) idiopathic. Sciatic scoliosis is a lumbar curve caused by muscle spasm. Usually, this is not a structural curve, and it resolves with recumbency or relief of symptoms. Olisthetic scoliosis is a torsional lumbar curve with rotation that blends with the spondylolytic defect and results from asymmetric slipping of the vertebra. These lumbar curves generally resolve after treatment of the spondylolisthesis. Severe curves, however, may become structural, and treatment is more complicated. Fusion of the lumbosacral area has been found to have no corrective effect on thoracic or thoracolumbar curves. When idiopathic scoliosis and spondylolisthesis occur together, they should be treated as separate problems.

RADIOGRAPHIC FINDINGS

The key to diagnosis of spondylolysis and spondylolisthesis lies in routine radiographs. The initial evaluation should include anteroposterior views, standing lateral views, and a Ferguson coronal view. The Ferguson coronal view is obtained by angling the x-ray beam parallel to the L5-S1 disc. With this view, the profiles of the L5 pedicles, transverse processes, and sacral ala are more easily seen. The lateral view should be taken with the patient standing because a 26% increase in slipping has been noted on standing films compared with recumbent films. In spondylolysis without slippage, the pars interarticularis defect often is difficult to see. Oblique views of the lumbar spine can put the pars area in relief apart from the underlying bony elements, making viewing of the defect easier. A recent study has called into question whether routine oblique radiographs are useful and needed in the evaluation of a patient with spondylolysis or spondylolisthesis. A bone scan may be indicated in children in whom an acquired pars defect is believed to be present but cannot be confirmed by plain films. The bone scan may detect the stress reaction stage before the fracture occurs. Isotope imaging with single-photon emission computed tomography (SPECT) is considered an extremely sensitive technique for early diagnosis of acute spondylolysis. Unfortunately, SPECT is nonspecific, detects only 17% of chronic lesions, and cannot distinguish between stress reactions and complete fractures.

Computed tomography (CT) has long been considered the gold standard for detecting pars interarticularis fractures. Limitations of CT, however, include low accuracy in distinguishing between a recent active fracture or a stress reaction and a chronic nonunion. Another drawback is the increased radiation exposure associated with CT scanning.

MRI can identify stress reactions and fractures in the pars; however, it is technique dependent, and T2-weighted fat-suppressed images in the oblique and sagittal planes are needed to evaluate bone marrow edema in acute lesions. MRI is useful for evaluation of disc pathology and any nerve root compression. Disadvantages are cost, availability, and need for an experienced radiologist in reading the image. Hollenberg et al. described an MRI classification system for spondylolysis: grade 0, normal; grade 1, bone edema and intact cortices compatible with a stress reaction; grade 2, incomplete fracture; grade 3, complete active fracture with accompanying bone edema; and grade 4, complete fracture without accompanying bone marrow edema.

The most commonly used radiographic grading system for spondylolisthesis is that of Meyerding. In this system, the slip grade is calculated by determining the ratio between the anteroposterior diameter of the top of the first sacral vertebra and the distance the L5 vertebra has slipped anteriorly (Fig. 44-192). Grade I spondylolisthesis is displacement of 25% or less; grade II, between 25% and 50%; grade III, between 50% and 75%; and grade IV, more than 75%. A grade V spondylolisthesis represents the position of L5 completely below the top of the sacrum. This also is termed *spondyloptosis*.

Bourassa-Moreau et al. emphasized the importance of standardizing the measurement techniques for determining slip severity in spondylolisthesis. They used two measurement techniques: technique 1 used a line drawn from the posteroinferior corner of the L5 vertebra that is perpendicular to the S1 vertebral endplate, and technique 2 used a line tangential to the posterior wall of the L5 vertebra that intersects the S1 vertebral endplate (Fig. 44-193). They found a significant difference between the two measurement techniques, highlighting the need to standardize and specify the measurement techniques used to plan and assess any intervention in spondylolisthesis (Fig. 44-194).

DeWald recommended a modification of the Newman system to better define the amount of anterior roll of L5 (Fig. 44-195). The dome and the anterior surface of the sacrum are divided into 10 equal parts. The scoring is based on the position of the posterior inferior corner of the body of the fifth lumbar vertebra with respect to the dome of the sacrum. The second number indicates the position of the anterior inferior corner of the body of the L5 vertebra with respect to the anterior surface of the first sacral segment.

The angular relationships are the best predictors of instability or progression of the spondylolisthesis deformity. These relationships are expressed as the slip angle, which is formed by the intersection of a line drawn parallel to the inferior or superior aspect of the L5 vertebra and a line drawn perpendicular to the posterior aspect of the body of the S1 vertebra (Fig. 44-196). The normal slip angle in a patient without spondylolisthesis should be lordotic. With a high-grade spondylolisthesis, the angle is commonly kyphotic. The degree of kyphosis may become large, representing a severe form of segmental kyphosis at L5-S1. Boxall et al. found an association between a high slip angle (> 55 degrees) and progression of the deformity, even after a solid posterior arthrodesis.

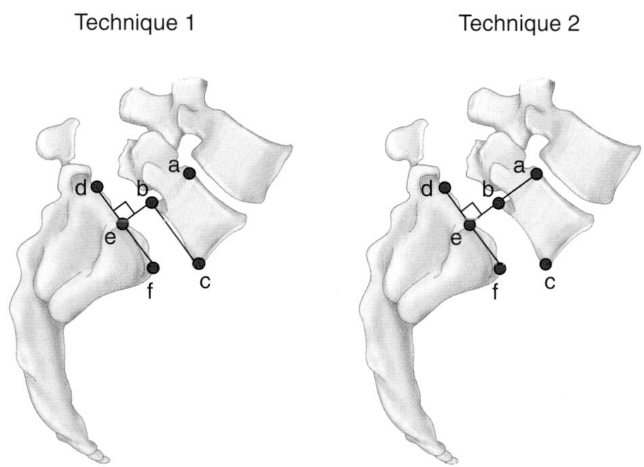

FIGURE 44-193 Two techniques for spondylolisthesis measurement. Technique 1 uses the b-f line perpendicular to the S1 endplate (line e-d); technique 2 uses a tangent to the L5 posterior wall, line a-b. These lines indicate the position of L5 on S1 in point f. (Redrawn from Bourassa-Moreau E, Mac-Thiong JM, LaBelle H: Redefining the technique for the radiologic measurement of slip in spondylolisthesis, Spine 35:1401, 2010.)

Restoration of spinopelvic balance is important in the treatment of spondylolisthesis. Hresko et al. described two patterns of deformity in patients with a high-grade spondylolisthesis, based on the alignment of the sacrum and pelvis. The first group was classified as balanced, and the sacral slope and pelvic tilt were similar to those of patients without spondylolisthesis in this balanced group. The second group was classified as unbalanced and had marked retroversion of the sacropelvic complex. The balanced group is characterized by a high sacral slope and low pelvic tilt. The unbalanced group has a vertical sacrum, a low sacral slope, and a high pelvic tilt (Fig. 44-197).

TREATMENT OF ACQUIRED SPONDYLOLYSIS

Treatment of acquired spondylolysis from a stress fracture in children and adolescents depends on whether the spondylolysis is acute or chronic. Micheli, Jackson et al., and Rabushka et al. described children and adolescents in whom acute

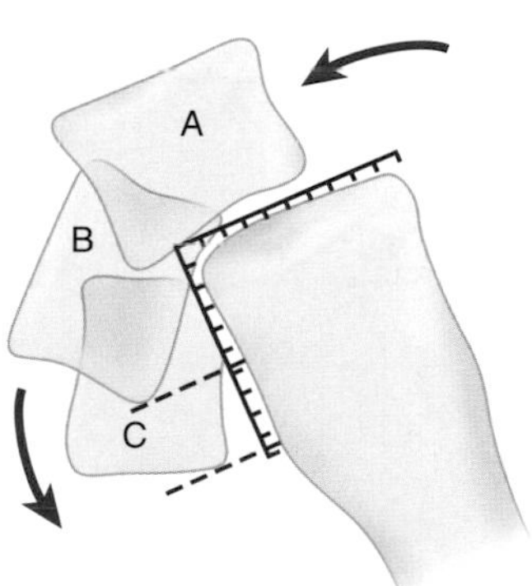

FIGURE 44-195 Modified Newman spondylolisthesis grading system. Degree of slip is measured by two numbers, one along sacral endplate and second along anterior portion of sacrum: A = 3 + 0; B = 8 + 6; and C = 10 + 10.

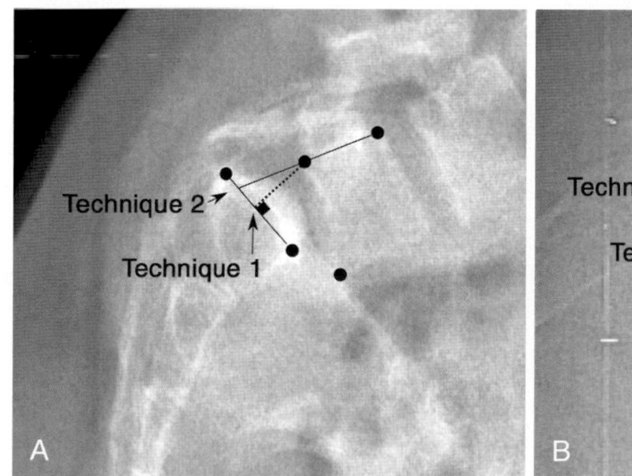

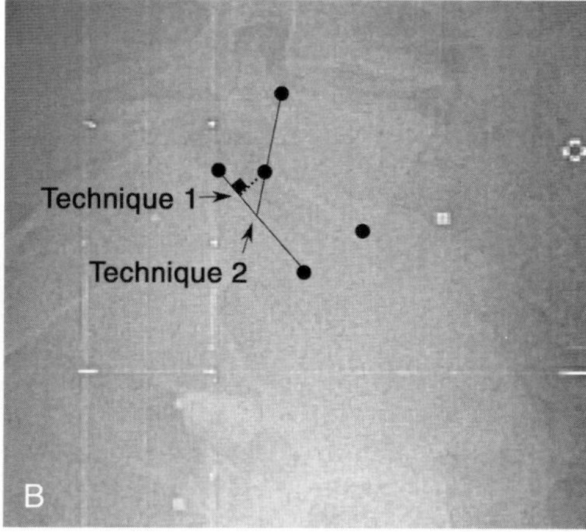

FIGURE 44-194 Two clinical cases illustrating how the differences between technique 2 and technique 1 (see Fig. 44-193) vary with respect to the orientation of L5 over S1. **A,** In a kyphotic alignment (high LSA), technique 2 underestimates the value obtained. **B,** In a lordotic alignment (low LSA), technique 2 overestimates the technique 1 value. These cases illustrate a negative correlation between LSA and technique 2 difference. LSA, lumbosacral angle. (From Bourassa-Moreau E, Mac-Thiong JM, LaBelle H: Redefining the technique for the radiologic measurement of slip in spondylolisthesis, Spine 35:1401, 2010.)

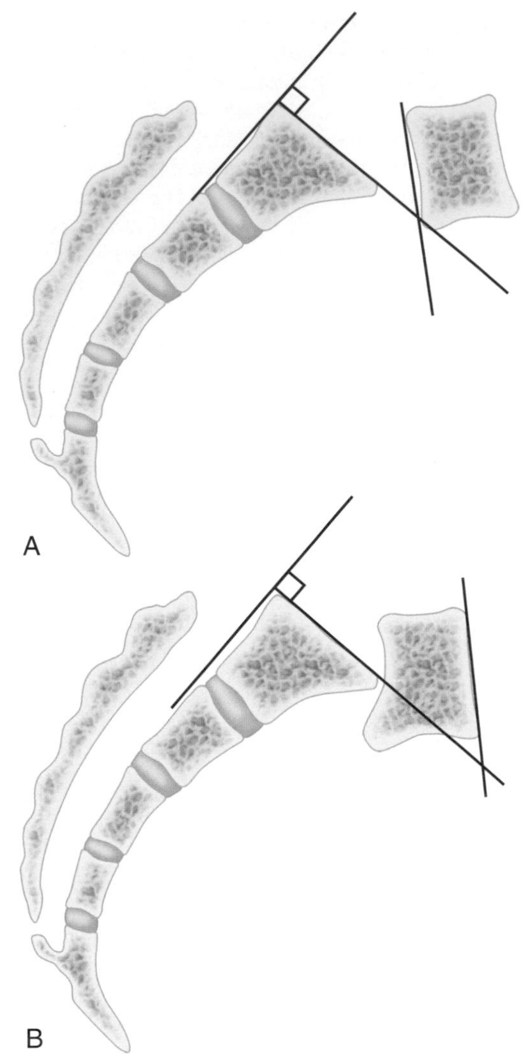

FIGURE 44-196 Schematic representation of slip angle or kyphotic malalignment of lumbosacral junction present in high-grade isthmic dysplastic spondylolisthesis. **A,** Standard method of measurement. **B,** Method used when inferior L5 endplate is irregularly shaped.

spondylolytic defects healed with cast or brace immobilization. Typically, these children have an acute onset of symptoms and the episode of injury is clearly documented. Often they are participating in a sport, such as gymnastics, that causes repetitive hyperextension of the spine. A SPECT scan or MRI can be helpful in determining whether the process is acute or chronic. If the SPECT scan detects an abnormality or MRI shows edema in the pedicle, a CT scan of the suspected area can be obtained to distinguish between a stress reaction and an acute stress fracture. CT scanning is the most helpful radiographic technique for determining the presence or absence of healing.

Nonoperative treatment will return most adolescents to normal activities. The spectrum of nonoperative treatment recommendations ranges from rest and restriction of activities to bracing and a structured rehabilitation program. Treatment begins with rest and restriction of activities; however, El Rassi et al. found that there was only a 42% compliance rate with restriction of activities; this finding highlights the need for participation by the patient, parents, and coaches in the treatment plan. Brace treatment has been controversial because of the inability of a standard TLSO to completely immobilize the lumbosacral junction. A brace will give some global restriction of motion of the lumbar spine but is probably most effective in forcing restriction of activities. Electrical stimulation has been used with varied results in attempts to heal an acute pars fracture.

A structured rehabilitation program is essential to return the patient to sports. This program has four phases: (1) acute, (2) subacute, (3) pre-sport, and (4) sport-conditioning. The acute phase focuses on relief of pain and inflammation and rehabilitation of the lumbopelvic stabilizers. The subacute phase emphasizes core strengthening and restoration of trunk range of motion. Nonimpact cardio activities can be begun during this stage. The therapist initiates sports-simulated movements to increase the patient's strength and endurance during the pre-sport phase. In the final sports-conditioning phase, sport-specific drills and impact cardio training are begun with the goal of returning the patient to his or her desired sport. The nonoperative treatment and structured rehabilitation program usually requires 12 weeks to complete. Patients with a stress reaction may progress faster, but some patients may require 4 to 5 months of rehabilitation before they are ready to return to sports.

Children and adolescents in whom the spondylolysis is of long duration are treated with routine nonoperative measures. Activities are restricted, and back, abdominal, and core-strengthening exercises are prescribed. If the symptoms are more severe, a brief period of bed rest or brace immobilization may be required. Once the pain has improved and the hamstring tightness has lessened, the child is allowed progressive activities. Yearly examinations with standing spot lateral radiographs of the lumbosacral spine are advised to rule out the development of spondylolisthesis. If the patient remains asymptomatic, limitation of activities or contact sports is not necessary. Most children with spondylolysis have excellent relief of symptoms or only minimal discomfort at long-term follow-up. If a child does not respond to conservative measures, other causes of back pain, such as infection, tumor, osteoid osteoma, and herniated disc, should be ruled out. Special attention should be paid to children whose symptoms do not respond to bed rest or who have objective neurologic findings. A very small percentage of children with spondylolysis who do not respond to conservative measures and in whom the other possible causes of back pain have been eliminated may require operative treatment.

REPAIR OF SPONDYLOLYTIC DEFECT

The primary indication for operative treatment of spondylolysis is failure of a 6-month conservative treatment program. The principles of pseudarthrosis repair are the same as for any long bone: debridement, grafting of the site with autogenous bone graft, and compression across the fracture. The type of surgery is based on the location of the spondylolysis and any associated disc pathology or associated vertebral dysplasia.

The surgical treatment of spondylolysis can be either an intervertebral fusion or a repair of the pars defect. When the lesion is at L5, direct repair of the pars defect and an L5 to S1 fusion will give similar results. If there is associated disc pathology at L5 or S1 or any associated dysplasia, fusion is

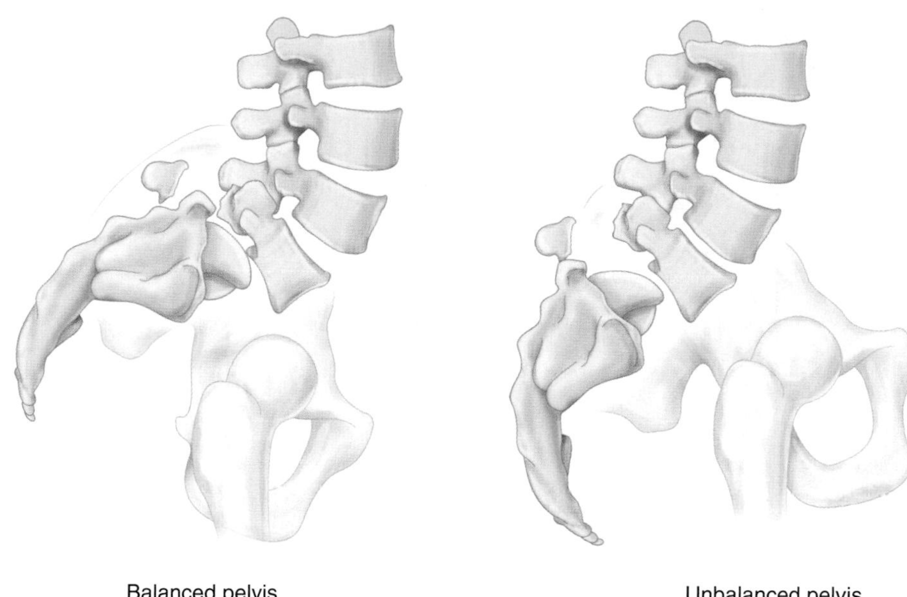

FIGURE 44-197 **Sagittal view of spinopelvic alignment in high-grade spondylolisthesis.** (From Hresko MT, LaBelle H, Roussouly P, Berthonnaud E: Classification of high-grade spondylolistheses based on pelvic version and spine balance, Spine 32:2208, 2007.)

the preferred treatment. When the pars lesion is at L4 or L3, direct repair is recommended. Four repair techniques have been described: (1) Scott wiring, (2) Buck screw, (3) pedicle screw and hook, and (4) V-rod or U-rod technique. With all techniques, the rate of return to sports is reported to be 80% to 90%. The Scott technique places wires around the transverse process on each side and through the spinous process to compress the pars defect. This is the least rigid of all the fixation methods, but it nonetheless has a healing rate of nearly 80%. Direct intralaminar screw fixation of a pars defect, described by Buck in 1970 with good outcomes in 93%, offers a minimally invasive and motion-preserving technique. The use of pedicle screws and infralaminar hoods attached to a short rod allows compression of the pars defect along the rod to stabilize the defect. This is the most rigid construct. A similar technique uses a U-shaped rod placed inferior to the spinous process for stabilization and compression of the pars defect. Sairyo et al. described restoration of disc stresses to normal at the cranial and caudal levels of the pars defect after direct intralaminar screw fixation using the Buck technique. Several other studies also have shown a superior biomechanical advantage of the Buck technique relative to other common fixation techniques; however, according to a biomechanical study of the four different techniques, all of which restored normal intervertebral rotation, the Scott and Buck constructs were found to be less stable than the screw-hook or U-rod constructs. Mihara et al. found that the Buck screw technique restored more normal motion at the involved level and adjacent level.

Kakiuchi reported successful union of pars defects with the use of a pedicle screw, laminar hook, and rod system. A pedicle screw is placed in the pedicle above the pars defect. The pars defect is bone grafted. A rod is placed in the pedicle screw and then into the caudal laminar hook, and compression is applied. This gives a more stable construct than that afforded by wire techniques. A second surgery for removal of prominent implants after healing may be necessary.

SPONDYLOLYSIS REPAIR

TECHNIQUE 44-55

(KAKIUCHI)

- Place the patient prone on a Hall frame.
- Expose the involved vertebra, including the defect of the pars interarticularis, through a midline posterior incision. Remove the fibrous tissue in and behind the defect with a Cobb elevator, rongeur, or curet. To maintain the length of the pars interarticularis, do not remove the sclerotic bone on both sides of the defect.
- Clean the lateral aspect of the inferior half of the superior articular process and the medial third of the posterior aspect of the transverse process of soft tissue without interfering with the capsule of the facet.
- Decorticate the posterior aspect of the pars interarticularis and adjoining portion of the lamina with use of a small chisel (Fig. 44-198A). Do not decorticate the lateral and inferior aspects of the superior articular process to maintain the strength of the osseous structures for pedicle screw placement.
- If nerve root decompression is indicated, remove the bone spurs over the nerve root with an osteotome (Fig. 44-198B). Bury free fat tissue in the defect created above the nerve root to prevent bone graft from falling onto the nerve root.
- To achieve a wider area for bone grafting, the starting point for the insertion of the pedicle screw is near the

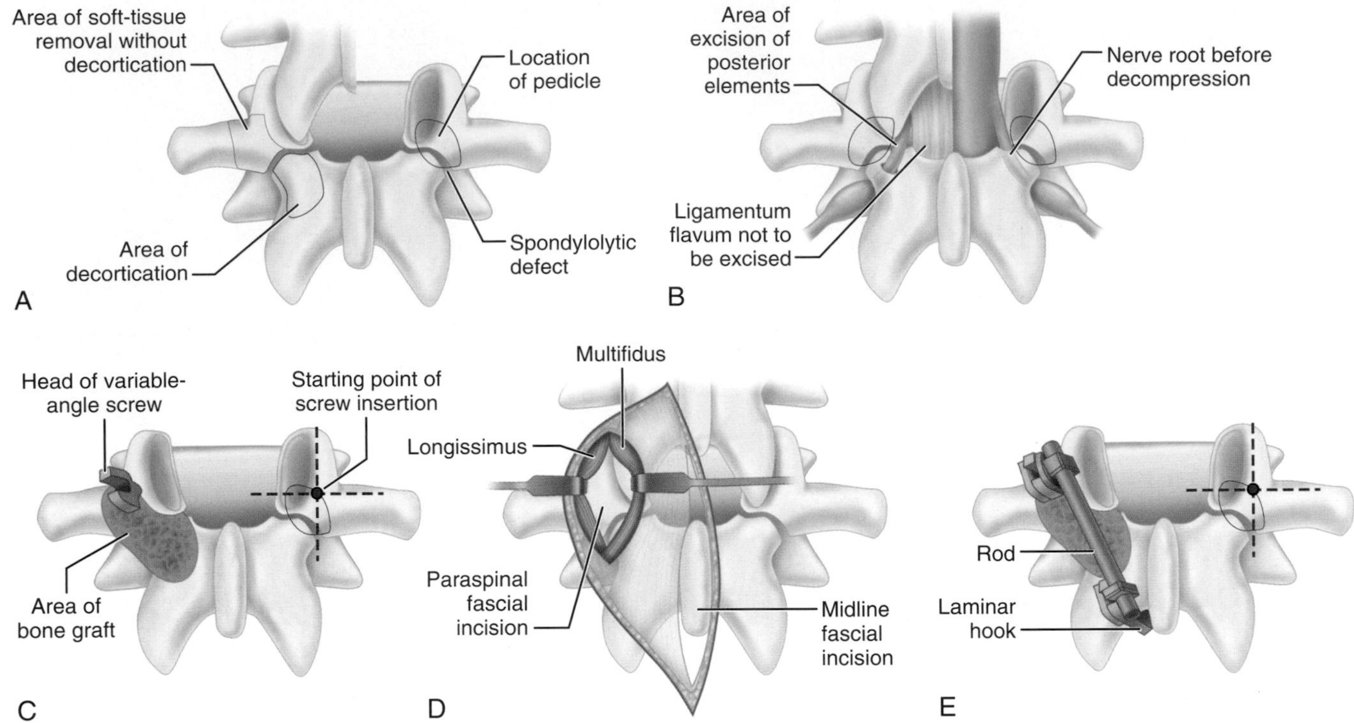

FIGURE 44-198 **A,** Recipient bed prepared for autogenous cancellous bone graft. **B,** Posterior elements overlying affected nerve root are excised. **C,** Variable-angle pedicle screw and bone graft inserted. **D,** A paraspinal approach may be used when the multifidus muscle is too tight for pedicle screw insertion through the midline. **E,** Rod attached to head of screw with variable-angle eyebolt. Laminar hook attached to rod. (From Kakiuci M: Repair of the defect in spondylolysis, J Bone Joint Surg 79A:818, 1997.) **SEE TECHNIQUE 44-55.**

intersection of a vertical line through the center axis of the pedicle and a horizontal line at the superior border of the pedicle (Fig. 44-198C).

- Direct the screw slightly caudally so that it enters the vertebral body at the center axis of the pedicle.
- After insertion of the pedicle screw, take strips of cancellous bone from the posterior aspect of the ilium through the same incision in the skin.
- Pack the cancellous bone as an onlay graft from the medial third of the transverse process to the decorticated portion of the lamina to form a sheet of bone about 1 cm thick (see Fig. 44-198C).
- If the multifidus muscle is too tight for pedicle screw insertion through this midline approach (which is more common at L5 than more cephalad levels), the starting point for insertion of the pedicle screw on the superior articular process should be exposed through the paraspinal approach over the pedicle through the same midline incision in the skin and additional small fascial incisions made 2 to 3 cm lateral to the midline (Fig. 44-198D). Insert a finger through the natural cleavage plane between the multifidus and longissimus muscles to the insertion point over the pedicle.
- Cut the rod to the appropriate length and attach it to the head of the variable-angle screw. Insert a laminar hook to the inferior edge of the lamina and attach it to the rod (Fig. 44-198E).
- To reduce the size of the defect of the pars interarticularis, apply a mild compression force between the hook and the head of the screw with the hook compressor before tightening the locknut in the eyebolt.
- Repeat the procedure on the contralateral side.

POSTOPERATIVE CARE. Usually patients are allowed to stand and walk on the second or third postoperative day. A hard lumbosacral corset is worn for 2 months, but its use should be determined on an individual basis. Patients are allowed unrestricted activity after 6 months.

MODIFIED SCOTT REPAIR TECHNIQUE

van Dam reported success in 16 patients with a modification of the Scott repair technique. In 26 direct pars repairs, union was achieved in 22.

TECHNIQUE 44-56

(VAN DAM)

- Approach the lumbar spine posteriorly.
- Identify and debride the area of the pars pseudarthrosis.

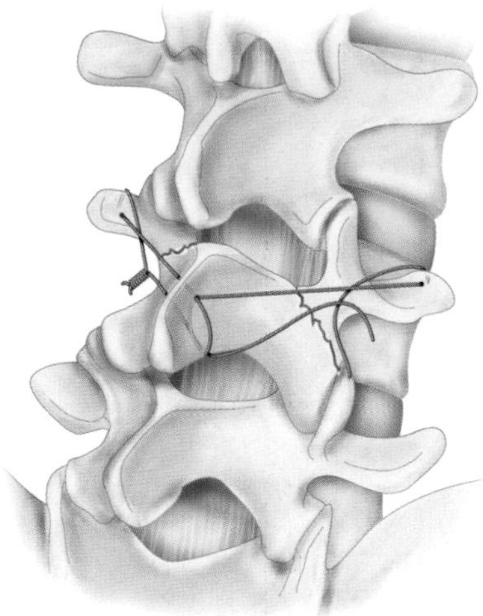

FIGURE 44-199 Scott wiring technique. (Redrawn from Rechtine G II: Spondylolysis repair. In Vaccaro A, Albert TJ, editors: Spine surgery tricks of the trade, New York, 2003, Thieme.) **SEE TECHNIQUE 44-56.**

- Place a 6.5-mm cancellous screw approximately two thirds of the way into the ipsilateral pedicle.
- Loop an 18-gauge wire around the screw head and pass the wire through a hole at the base of the spinous process.
- Pass the ends of the wire through a metal button and tighten the wire loop around the screw head.
- Twist the wire ends tightly against the metal button and cut the excess wire away.
- Place autogenous cancellous bone in and around the debrided pars defect.
- Fully seat the screw to accomplish final tightening of the wire (Fig. 44-199).
- Taddonio described the use of pedicle screws attached to Cotrel-Dubousset rods and offset laminar hooks to accomplish the same mechanical stability as in the Buck technique and Bradford technique. Roca et al. described the use of a titanium variable-angle pedicular-laminar hook-screw especially designed for direct spondylolysis repair.

POSTOPERATIVE CARE. The patient should use a lumbosacral orthosis for a minimum of 3 months and up to 6 months after surgery. Healing of the pars is ascertained by follow-up CT scan.

INTRALAMINAR SCREW FIXATION OF PARS DEFECT (BUCK SCREW TECHNIQUE)

TECHNIQUE 44-57

PEDICLE SCREW FIXATION

- With the patient prone in a position to minimize lordosis, use fluoroscopy to localize the level of the defect.

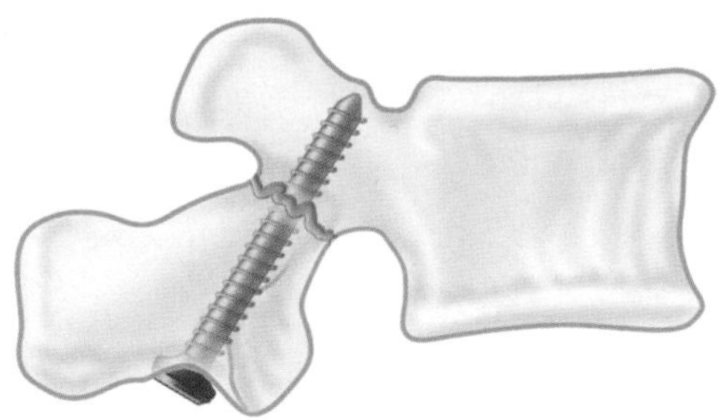

FIGURE 44-200 Technique of Buck screw fixation of pars defect. **SEE TECHNIQUE 44-57.**

- Make a midline incision approximately 5 cm long lateral to the corresponding spinous process to expose the lamina and the defect.
- Use a curet to clean the defect.
- Under fluoroscopy, and alternating between anteroposterior and lateral views, make a percutaneous stab wound with a 4.5-mm cannulated screw guidewire.
- Drill the wire through the caudal laminar surface, bisecting the pedicle to the superior cortex of the pedicle and traversing the pars defect (Fig. 44-200).
- Use a 3.2-mm cannulated drill to drill over the guidewire.
- Remove the wire and use a ball-tipped probe to feel the cortices.
- Measure and tap the screw length.
- If the lamina is large enough, overdrill it distally.
- Insert a solid (rather than cannulated) 4.5-mm screw of the appropriate size, with compression as needed.
- Through the same incision, harvest a posterior iliac crest bone graft and place the cancellous graft in the defect. Overlay a corticocancellous strip from the lamina to the transverse process.

SPONDYLOLYSIS REPAIR WITH U-ROD OR V-ROD

TECHNIQUE 44-58

(SUMITA ET AL.)

- With the patient prone, make a midline incision and elevate the paraspinal musculature laterally to expose the lamina, pars, and base of the transverse process. Take care not to injure the capsule of the facet joint.
- Expose the defect in the pars and use a curet to remove the fibrocartilage.
- Use a burr to decorticate the defect and the corresponding lamina and transverse process.
- Using anatomic landmarks and fluoroscopy, determine the starting point for the pedicle screw.
- Create the starting hole with a burr and use a pedicle finder to enter the pedicle.

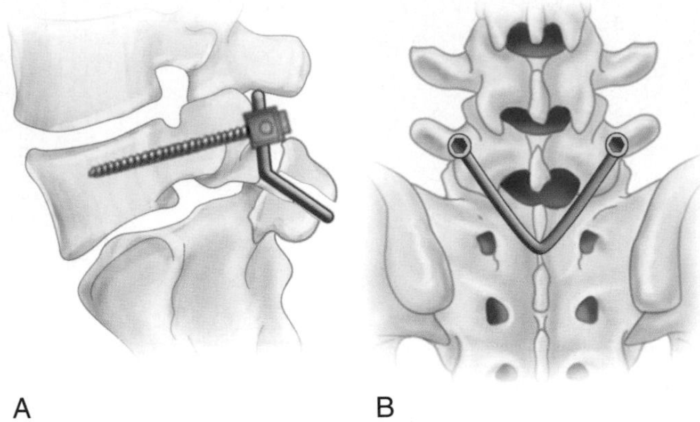

FIGURE 44-201 Sagittal **(A)** and axial **(B)** position of the pedicle screw instrumentation for V-rod fixation. **SEE TECHNIQUE 44-58.**

- Assess the walls and floor with a ball-tipped probe and tap the hole for a 5-mm pedicle screw.
- Harvest bone graft from the iliac crest, place it in the defect, and impact it before insertion of the screw.
- After the screws are placed, contour a rod into a U shape or V shape (Fig. 44-201) and place it just caudal to the interspinous ligament of the affected level; attach the rod to each pedicle screw, and tighten the screws to compress the defect.
- Confirm correct placement of the screw and rod with fluoroscopic imaging.

POSTOPERATIVE CARE. Intravenous antibiotics are administered until the wound is dry. The patient is mobilized without a brace.

POSTEROLATERAL FUSION

Posterolateral fusion is the conventional operative treatment of symptomatic spondylolysis at L5 unresponsive to conservative treatment. Pedicle instrumentation and fusion often are done to avoid the necessity of postoperative bracing. If no internal fixation is used, the patient is immobilized in a TLSO. A pantaloon cast or a TLSO with a thigh extension also may be used for greater immobilization. Fusion rates of approximately 90% have been reported with similar percentages of relief of symptoms after fusion of L5 to the sacrum. Extension of the fusion to L4 is not necessary. The Gill procedure or a wide laminectomy in a child is not necessary.

TREATMENT OF DEVELOPMENTAL SPONDYLOLISTHESIS

NONOPERATIVE TREATMENT

Surgery is not always necessary for spondylolisthesis. Restriction of the patient's activities, muscle rehabilitation (spinal, abdominal, and trunk), and other nonoperative measures, including the intermittent use of a rigid back brace, often are sufficient if the symptoms are minimal and the slippage is mild. If symptoms improve, progressive increases in activity are permitted. Activity restrictions are unnecessary for patients with mild degrees of spondylolisthesis. For symptom-free patients with slips of more than 25% but less than 50%, contact sports and activities that carry a high probability of back injury should be avoided. Standing spot lateral radiographs of the lumbosacral junction are made every 6 to 12 months until the completion of growth. This is especially important in female patients and in patients who have high-risk characteristics for progression of the slip.

OPERATIVE TREATMENT

Indications for surgery include persistent symptoms despite conservative treatment for 6 months to 1 year, persistent tight hamstrings, abnormal gait, and pelvic-trunk deformity. Development of a neurologic deficit is an indication for operative intervention, as is progression of the slip, which is indicative of a severe dysplasia. Early surgery may prevent more difficult or risky surgeries at a later time. If a patient is asymptomatic and has a slip of more than 50%, severe dysplasia (high dysplastic spondylolisthesis) is likely and surgery is indicated.

A posterolateral fusion between L5 and the sacrum is recommended for slips of less than 50% in children and adolescents whose symptoms persist despite conservative treatment. This degree of slippage is a mild dysplasia (low dysplastic type), usually without a significant slip angle. In our experience, these children do well with a posterolateral fusion in situ. We have not seen the need for any attempts at reduction of these patients unless there is significant lumbosacral kyphosis. We generally instrument these patients with pedicle screw fixation to avoid the need of postoperative immobilization. Extremely tight hamstrings, decreased Achilles tendon reflexes, and even footdrop may improve after a solid arthrodesis. Laminectomy as an isolated technique in a growing child is contraindicated because further slipping will occur. Hensinger et al. and Boxall et al. expressed doubt as to whether decompression with removal of the posterior element of L5 should ever be done in children with slips of less than 50%, no matter which signs and symptoms of neurologic compromise are present. Obtaining a true anteroposterior (Ferguson) view of the lumbosacral junction is important in evaluating the success of arthrodesis. This view provides a true coronal profile of the L5-sacral ala region. For L5-S1 fusion with pedicle screws, see Technique 44-56.

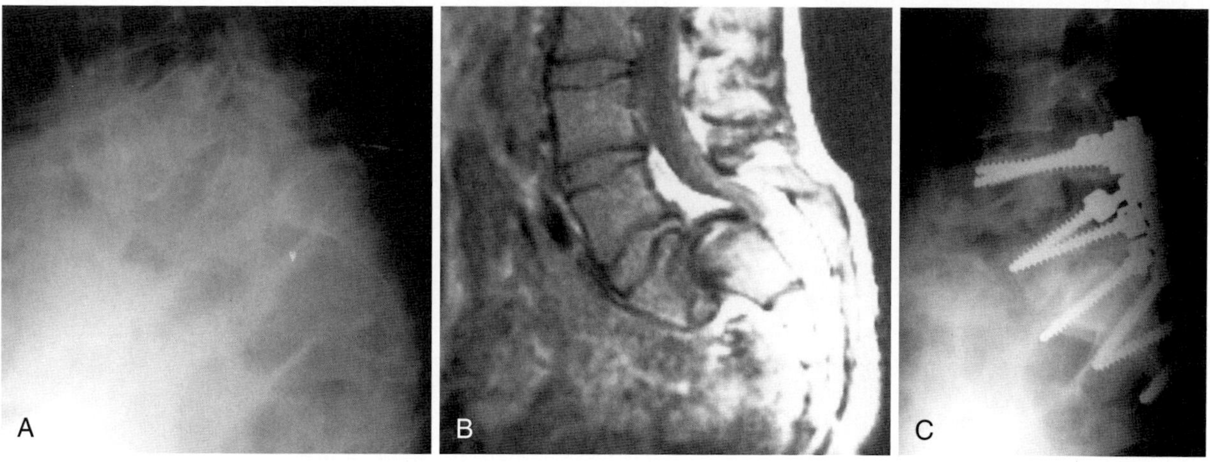

FIGURE 44-202 A, Severe spondylolisthesis. B, MR image shows slip. C, After anterior and posterior reduction and fusion with posterior instrumentation.

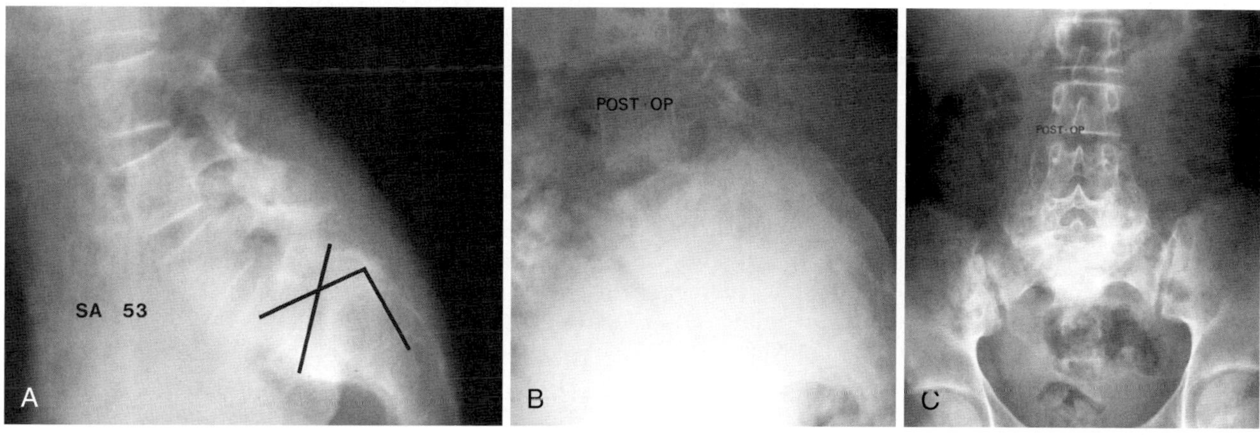

FIGURE 44-203 A, Severe spondylolisthesis. B and C, After in situ fusion.

TREATMENT OF SEVERE (HIGH DYSPLASTIC) SPONDYLOLISTHESIS

Operative treatment of high dysplastic spondylolisthesis is more controversial. Most authors agree that slippage of more than 50% requires fusion. The operative options, however, are many: posterior in situ fusion, adding instrumentation to a posterior in situ fusion; posterior decompression, partial reduction, instrumentation, and fusion; posterior decompression, complete reduction, instrumentation, and posterior fusion; posterior fusion with postoperative cast reduction; posterior instrumentation and fusion combined with posterior lumbar interbody fusion; anterior release; intradiscal graft or structural cage combined with posterior instrumentation and fusion; and reduction and circumferential fusion with or without instrumentation. For patients with a grade V spondyloptosis, Gaines and Nichols described an L5 spondylectomy with fusion of L4 to the sacrum.

Lenke et al. found that 21% of 56 in situ bilateral transverse process fusions for spondylolisthesis were definitely not fused, but despite this low fusion rate, overall clinical improvement was noted in more than 80% of patients. Other authors recommended combined anterior fusion and reduction with posterior spinal instrumentation for high dysplastic slips because of problems with the healing of a posterior arthrodesis alone. In addition to improving the appearance, the reduction of spondylolisthesis with instrumentation improves the chance of fusion, but these procedures have many risks and potential complications (Fig. 44-202). Johnson and Kirwan and Wiltse et al. reported excellent results in patients with slips of more than 50% treated with bilateral lateral fusions. Freeman and Donati found similar results after in situ fusion in patients observed for an average of 12 years (Fig. 44-203). Poussa et al. compared the results of in situ fusion of spondylolisthesis of more than 50% with results of reduction by a transpedicular system and found no differences between the groups in functional improvement or pain relief. In situ fusion gave a satisfactory cosmetic appearance; reduction procedures were associated with increased operative time, complications, and reoperations. Also, long-term findings showed that the in situ fusion group performed better in almost all clinical parameters measured. Other reports have recorded an increased rate of nonunion with bending of the fusion mass and delayed neurologic complications when posterolateral fusion in situ has been performed in high-grade slips.

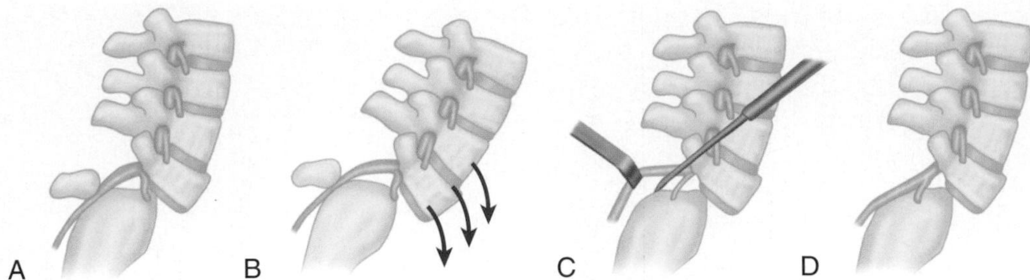

FIGURE 44-204 **A,** Severe spondylolisthesis. **B,** Increase that may occur intraoperatively. **C,** Operative decompression of cauda equina with sacroplasty. **D,** Appearance of sacrum after excision of posterior superior aspect.

Instrumentation with pedicle screws has been used in an attempt to prevent further deterioration of the spondylolisthesis with in situ fusion. The goal of surgical treatment in patients with a high-grade spondylolisthesis is to restore the global sagittal balance of the spinopelvic complex. The degree of reduction of the translatory displacement in high-grade slips is less important than improving the lumbosacral kyphosis and restoring sagittal imbalance. In severe cases, the fusion may need to be extended to L4. The potential advantages of reduction of high-grade spondylolisthesis include reduction of the slip angle (lumbosacral kyphosis), which improves the sagittal lumbosacral orientation and places the fusion mass in more compression, and improves the global sagittal balance and the cosmetic appearance. Direct neural decompression also is allowed with this procedure. Disadvantages are that more extensive surgery is required, an additional anterior procedure often is needed, and there is an increased risk for neurologic injury. The theoretical advantages of complete reduction of spondylolisthesis should be weighed against the natural history studies of Murray et al. in untreated spondylolisthesis, with satisfactory clinical results with fusion in situ.

Cauda equina injuries may occur after in situ fusions. In severe spondylolisthesis, the sacral roots are stretched over the back of the body of S1 and are sensitive to any movement of L5 on S1. It has been postulated that muscle relaxation after general anesthesia and the surgical dissection may lead to additional slippage that further stretches these sacral roots. Patients most at risk have an initial slip angle of more than 45 degrees. Thorough neurologic evaluation before and after in situ arthrodesis is recommended in all patients with grade III or grade IV spondylolisthesis. Examination should include clinical assessment of perineal sensation, function of the bladder, and rectal tone. If a patient has a detectable neurologic deficit preoperatively, decompression of the cauda equina at the time of the arthrodesis with removal of the posterior superior lip of the sacrum (Fig. 44-204) can be done. Because this decompression causes additional instability, segmental instrumentation with pedicle screws is required. Alternatively, decompression of the cauda equina can be combined with reduction of the forward slip with posterior pedicle segmental instrumentation. If injury to the cauda equina is evident after an otherwise uneventful in situ arthrodesis, prompt decompression with removal of the posterior aspect of S1 is recommended. In situ pedicle segmental instrumentation should be considered to further stabilize the area.

There are no definite guidelines regarding the appropriate surgical treatment of children and adolescents with high dysplastic spondylolisthesis. Intuitively, it seems that the more dysplastic and unstable the spine is, the more justifiable is some type of reduction and instrumentation. Boachie-Adjei et al. proposed a technique of partial reduction of the lumbosacral kyphosis, decompression of the nerve roots, posterolateral fusion, and pedicle screw transvertebral fixation of the lumbosacral junction. This technique has the advantage of providing three-column fixation by the lumbosacral transfixation, yet it is performed through a single posterior approach. It also allows interbody grafting to be done if necessary without a formal anterior procedure. Lenke and Bridwell also found that this approach provided the best fusion rates and clinical outcomes with acceptable complication rates.

POSTEROLATERAL FUSION AND PEDICLE SCREW FIXATION

TECHNIQUE 44-59

(LENKE AND BRIDWELL)

- Place the patient prone on a radiolucent table. Initially, the patient can be positioned with the knees and hips flexed to facilitate decompression.
- Approach the spine through a standard posterior midline lumbosacral incision.
- Perform a Gill laminectomy and bilateral L5 and S1 nerve root decompressions. It is extremely important to decompress the L5 nerve roots widely past the tips of the L5 transverse processes.
- Place pedicle screws at L5 and S1. For additional sacropelvic fixation points, use bilateral distal iliac wing screws. In high-grade slips, instrumentation to L4 may be needed.
- Apply mild distraction to the L5-S1 segment and perform a sacroplasty to shorten the sacrum and decrease the stretch of the L5 nerve roots.
- At this point, if the hips and knees are flexed, extend them to flex the pelvis to meet the L5 segment.
- Attempt to access the L5-S1 disc space from the posterior approach. If this can be done, remove the disc and use morselized bone graft or place structural cages in the L5 disc.

- Contour the rod and place it into the distal fixation segment; flex the sacrum with the rod to meet the L5 segment.
- Place the graft anterior just before locking the instrumentation into place.
- Review the intraoperative anteroposterior and lateral radiographs.
- Perform a formal wake-up test to assess bilateral foot and ankle movement.
- Place iliac crest bone graft harvested proximal to the iliac screw site over the decorticated transverse process and sacral ala bilaterally (Fig. 44-205).
- If an adequate anterior spinal fusion could not be performed posteriorly, the patient is brought back 5 to 7 days later for an anterior procedure.
- Depending on the degree of reduction obtained, a formal discectomy with structural grafts or metallic cages is used with the anterior iliac crest graft for fusion.
- If the slip angle and translation correction have not been enough to allow access to the L5 disc anteriorly, ream over a Kirschner wire that is placed from the midportion of the L5 through the L5-S1 disc and into the proximal sacrum and insert the fibular allograft.

POSTOPERATIVE CARE. Depending on the security of the fixation obtained, a single pantaloon brace or TLSO may be needed. The brace can be discontinued when it appears that the fusion is solid enough to safely do so, usually at 3 to 4 months postoperatively.

INSTRUMENTED REDUCTION

In high dysplastic spondylolisthesis, reduction and fusion with internal fixation and a sagittally aligned spine can eliminate the complication of progression of the deformity that can occur after in situ fusion. Lumbar root pain or deficit may require decompression of the L5 symptomatic roots and internal fixation. Internal fixation makes it possible to decompress these roots fully without fear of residual instability or progressive slipping (Fig. 44-206). Sacral radiculopathy caused by stretching of the sacral roots over the posterosuperior corner of the sacrum theoretically can be relieved by restoring the lumbar spine to its proper position over the sacrum. This relieves the anterior pressure from the sacral roots, shortens their course, and relaxes the cauda equina. Correction of the slip angle (kyphosis) greatly reduces the bending moment and tensile stress that works against the posterior lumbosacral graft. When normal biomechanics are restored by correction of the deformity, it may be possible to fuse fewer lumbosacral segments. Theoretically, restoring body posture and mechanics to normal may lessen future problems in the proximal areas of the spine. Physical appearance is a concern of adolescents with high-grade spondylolisthesis, and this can be improved with reduction of the deformity.

These theoretical advantages, however, should be weighed carefully against the potential risks of the surgery. These procedures are technically demanding and carry with them a significant risk of nerve root injury. As techniques are evolving, these risks are decreasing but are undeniably still present. Numerous techniques to obtain complete reduction of high-grade dysplastic spondylolisthesis have been described. The following technique is just one of those described.

TECHNIQUE 44-60

(CRANDALL)

- After general anesthesia is obtained, place the patient prone on a radiolucent table.
- Use a routine midline approach to the lumbosacral spine.
- Perform a full L5 laminectomy, inferior facetectomy, and nerve root decompression. A discectomy at L5-S1 will also make L5 more mobile for reduction.
- Prepare and tap the pedicles at L5-S1 and insert long post screws bilaterally at L5.
- Screws also should be placed bilaterally at S1.
- For high-grade spondylolisthesis, a distal point of fixation is needed to form a strong and stable base from which L5 can be pulled into position. Options include iliac screws (Fig. 44-207A) and S2 alar screws (Fig. 44-207B and C).
- Aim the S2 multiaxial screws laterally into the beak of the sacral ala.
- After all screws are placed, select a rod of the appropriate length and diameter, along with the corresponding three-dimensional connectors, and preassemble the construct.
- Place screw extenders on the post of the S1 screws to ease insertion.
- Slide the preassembled construct down the screw extenders at S1 and the threaded post of the long post screw at L5 and into the multiaxial screw heads at S2.
- Repeat the same process on the contralateral side of the spine.
- Once the connectors are in place, temporarily secure them at S1 with a lock screw. When the construct is in place, each rod creates a "diving board" over L5 (Fig. 44-207D).
- Place a low-profile crosslink plate between the S1 and S2 levels of the construct. If iliac screws are used, this is not necessary.
- Place the provisional reduction crimps on both the long post three-dimensional screws at L5 (Fig. 44-207E). Place the crimp driver on the threaded posts of the screws. Advance the driver down the threaded post to the provisional reduction crimp. Sequentially tighten the driver by rotating clockwise and pushing down on the reduction crimps (Fig. 44-207F). By use of the provisional reduction crimps, the spine is brought into its correct anatomic position in a gradual and highly controlled way (Fig. 44-207G and H).
- If the L5 connector "bottoms out" onto the screw head before full reduction is achieved (Fig. 44-207I), there are two options for getting the last few millimeters of correction.
- Contour the rod with more lordosis at L5 to increase the reduction distance for L5 to be pulled back (Fig. 44-207J), or place the connector at S1 at the very top of the post, which creates more reduction distance (Fig. 44-207K).
- Once the spondylolisthesis is fully corrected, compress L5 to S1 with the compressor to make the alignment as

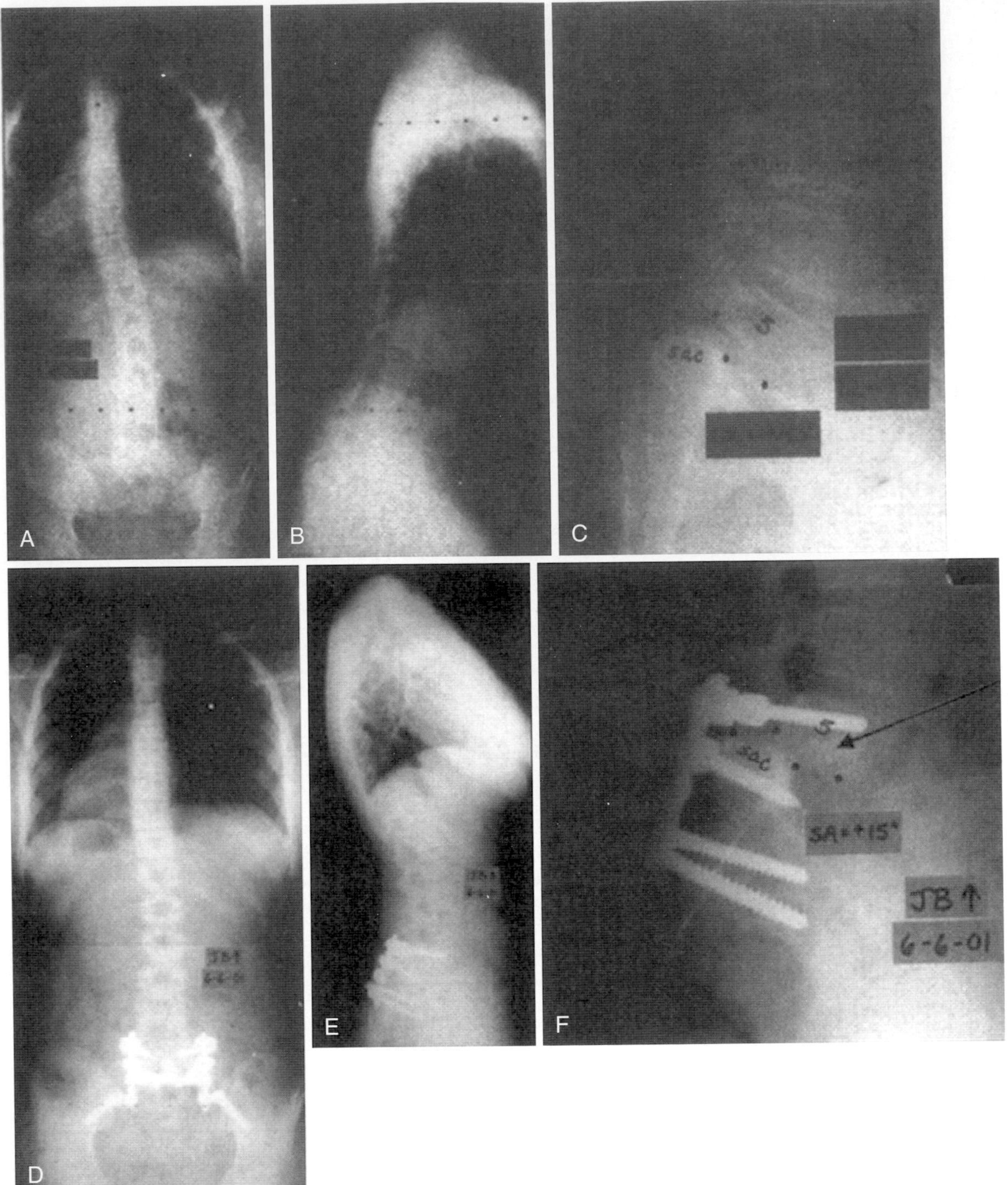

FIGURE 44-205 Radiographs of 12-year-old girl with high-grade IV isthmic dysplastic spondylolisthesis. Patient has small amount of sciatic scoliosis on coronal view **(A and B).** Sacrum is vertical on sagittal radiograph **(C),** and she is positioned with her trunk anterior to her pelvis, showing anterior sagittal imbalance. Patient had posterior decompression, partial reduction, sacral dome osteotomy, and posterolateral fusion with instrumentation from L5 to sacrum. One week later, she had anterior fibular dowel graft placement from L5 to sacrum. Radiographs **D** to **F** show improved position of L5 on sacrum and excellent alignment in overall coronal **(D)** and sagittal **(E)** radiographs. **F,** *Arrow* points to anterior edge of fibular graft. (From Lenke LG, Bridwell KH: Evaluation and surgical treatment of high-grade isthmic dysplastic spondylolisthesis, Instr Course Lect 52:525, 2003.) **SEE TECHNIQUE 44-59.**

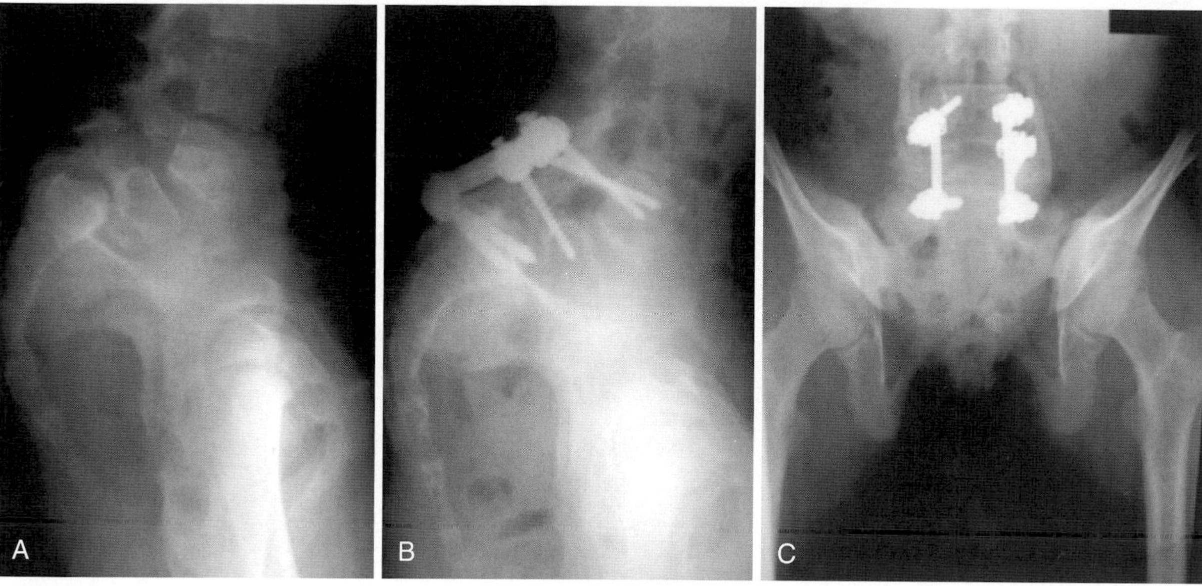

FIGURE 44-206 **A,** Standing lateral radiograph of high dysplastic spondylolisthesis, L5 on S1, in 12-year-old patient who had significant leg pain. It was thought that decompression of L5 nerve roots was important part of surgical procedure. **B** and **C,** Postoperative lateral and Ferguson views of lumbosacral junction after decompression of L5 nerve roots with limited reduction and internal fixation L4 to S1. Postoperatively, patient's back and leg symptoms were completely relieved.

stable as possible. The correction is more likely to be maintained if bone or a small cage is placed into the disc space through a posterior lumbar interbody fusion or transforaminal lumbar interbody fusion before L5 is compressed to S1.

- Place lock screws in the three-dimensional connectors at L5 and S1 (Fig. 44-207L) and tighten all four lock screws. As the tightening occurs, the break-off portion of the set screw will shear off and remain in the sleeve of the driver.
- Use a "cutter" to cut the long post flush with the assembly (Fig. 44-207M and N).

PARTIAL REDUCTION AND INTERBODY FUSION

Satisfactory results have been reported with partial reduction and posterior interbody fusion for the management of high-grade spondylolisthesis in pediatric and adult patients. Partial reduction can be augmented with an anterior fusion using morselized bone graft or a structural cage in the L5 disc. Placement of a transsacral fibular graft or direct placement of sacral screws across the L5 disc into the L5 vertebral body also can be used to augment a partial reduction and fusion, as described by Smith et al.

TECHNIQUE 44-61

(SMITH ET AL.)

- Place the patient prone on a four-poster frame. Neuromonitoring is strongly recommended for this technique, including an intraoperative wake-up test in adult patients.
- Perform standard subperiosteal dissection of the posterior elements from L2 to the sacrum. Perform decompression and sacral laminectomies of S1 and S2.
- Place a temporary distracting rod from the inferior aspect of the lamina of L2 to the sacral ala, allowing distraction with concomitant extension moment applied by extension of the thighs. If distraction prevents reduction of the slip angle, the primary reduction maneuver is extension of the hip joints.
- If the sacral dome is thought to cause significant anterior impingement of the dural sac, perform partial sacral dome resection to decompress the neural elements further.
- Sweep the dural sac toward the midline in the vicinity of the S1-S2 disc.
- While protecting the neural elements under fluoroscopic control, advance a guidewire through the body of S1, across the L5-S1 disc space, and up to the anterior cortex of L5.
- Overream the guidewire under fluoroscopic guidance, beginning at 6 mm and increasing by 2 mm increments, usually up to 12 mm.
- Measure a single fibular allograft. Cut it and impact it into position. Remove the temporary distraction rod.
- To augment the transsacral fibula, place pedicle screw fixation in L4 and transsacral pedicle screws capturing L5. Direct the sacral screws along the same sagittal trajectory as the fibula to capture L5 with subsequent placement of rods connecting the pedicle screws.
- Perform a posterolateral fusion from L4 to the sacral ala after harvest of iliac crest bone graft.

POSTOPERATIVE CARE. Postoperative care is the same as that after the one-stage decompression and posterolateral interbody fusion.

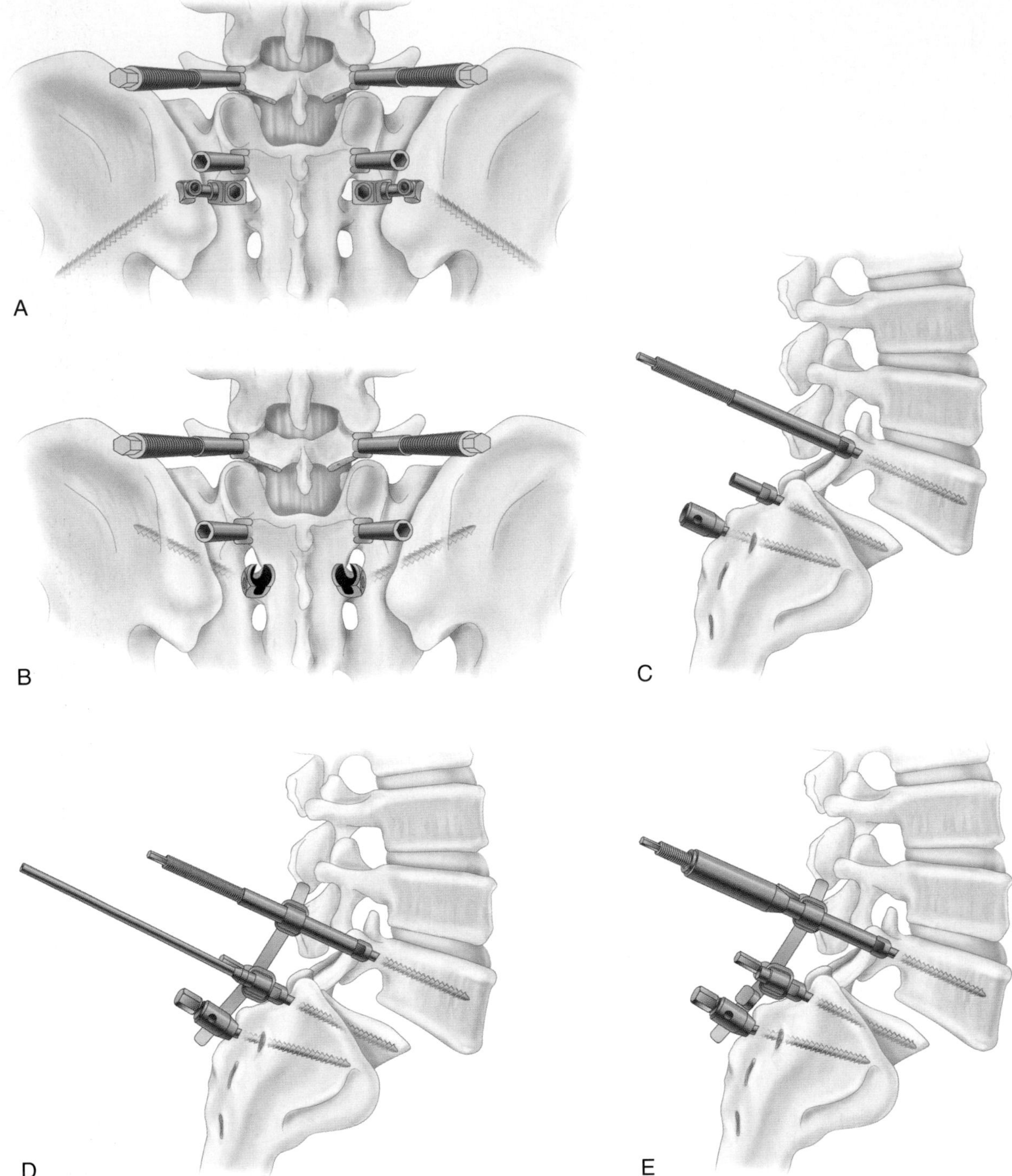

FIGURE 44-207 **A-N,** Reduction and fusion in high dysplastic spondylolisthesis with internal fixation. See text for description. (Redrawn from Crandall D: TSRH-3D Plus MPA spinal instrumentation-deformity and degenerative, surgical technique manual, Memphis, TN, 2005, Medtronic Sofamor Danek.) **SEE TECHNIQUE 44-60.**

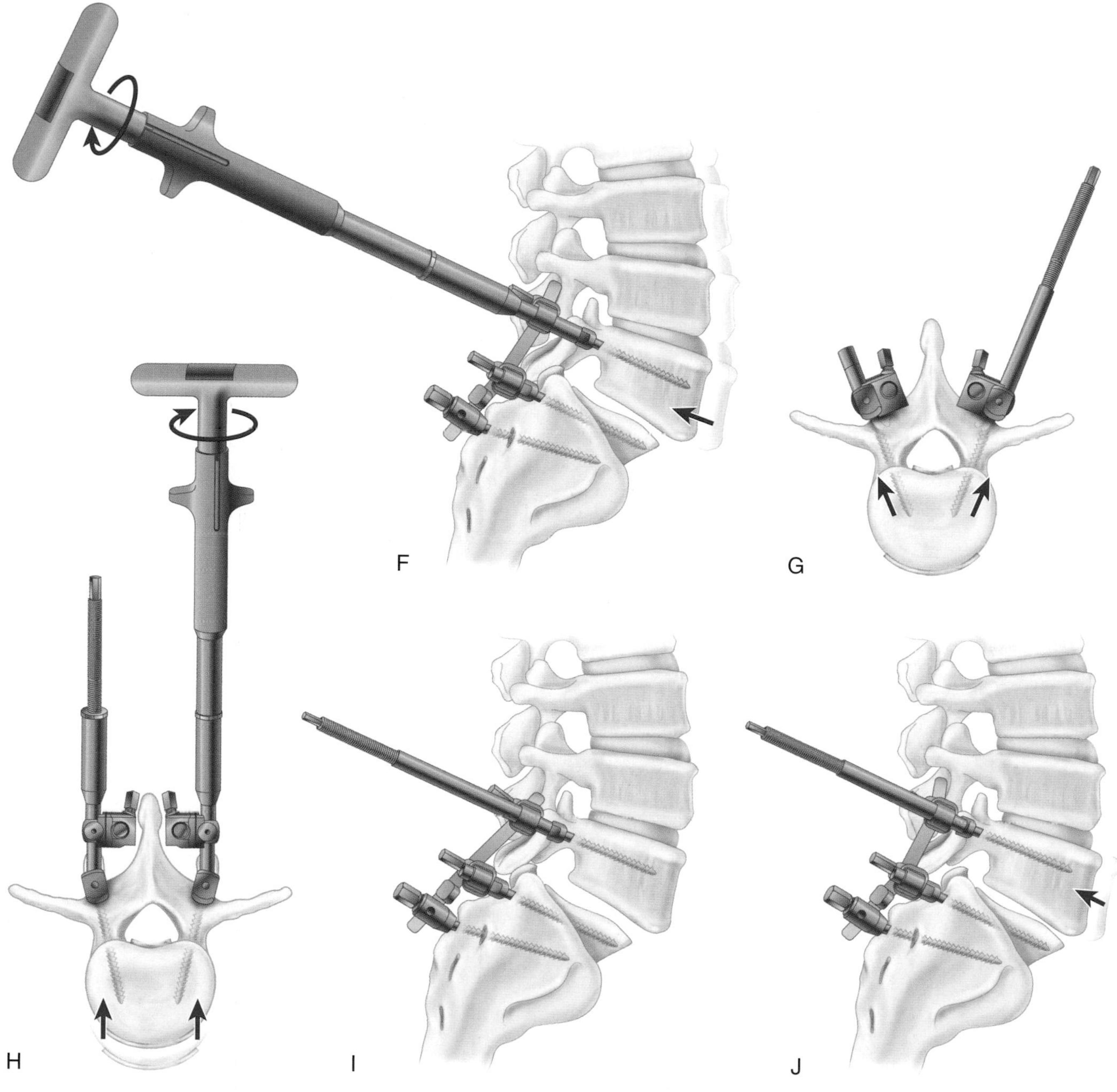

FIGURE 44-207, cont'd

Continued

ONE-STAGE DECOMPRESSION AND POSTEROLATERAL INTERBODY FUSION

TECHNIQUE 44-62

(BOHLMAN AND COOK)

- Place the patient prone, with the right leg draped free as the graft donor site.
- Approach the spine through a standard midline incision from the third lumbar level to the second sacral level. Subperiosteally strip muscle to the tip of the transverse process and sacral ala on each side.
- Remove the posterior elements of the fifth lumbar and first sacral vertebrae (and fourth lumbar vertebra if necessary).
- Perform a wide foraminotomy to decompress the fifth lumbar and first sacral nerve roots.
- Gently free the dura from the posterosuperior prominence of the first sacral vertebral body with a Penfield elevator. Osteotomize the sacral prominence with a curved osteotome to create a ventral trough for the dura and to eliminate all pressure on the dura (Fig. 44-208A).

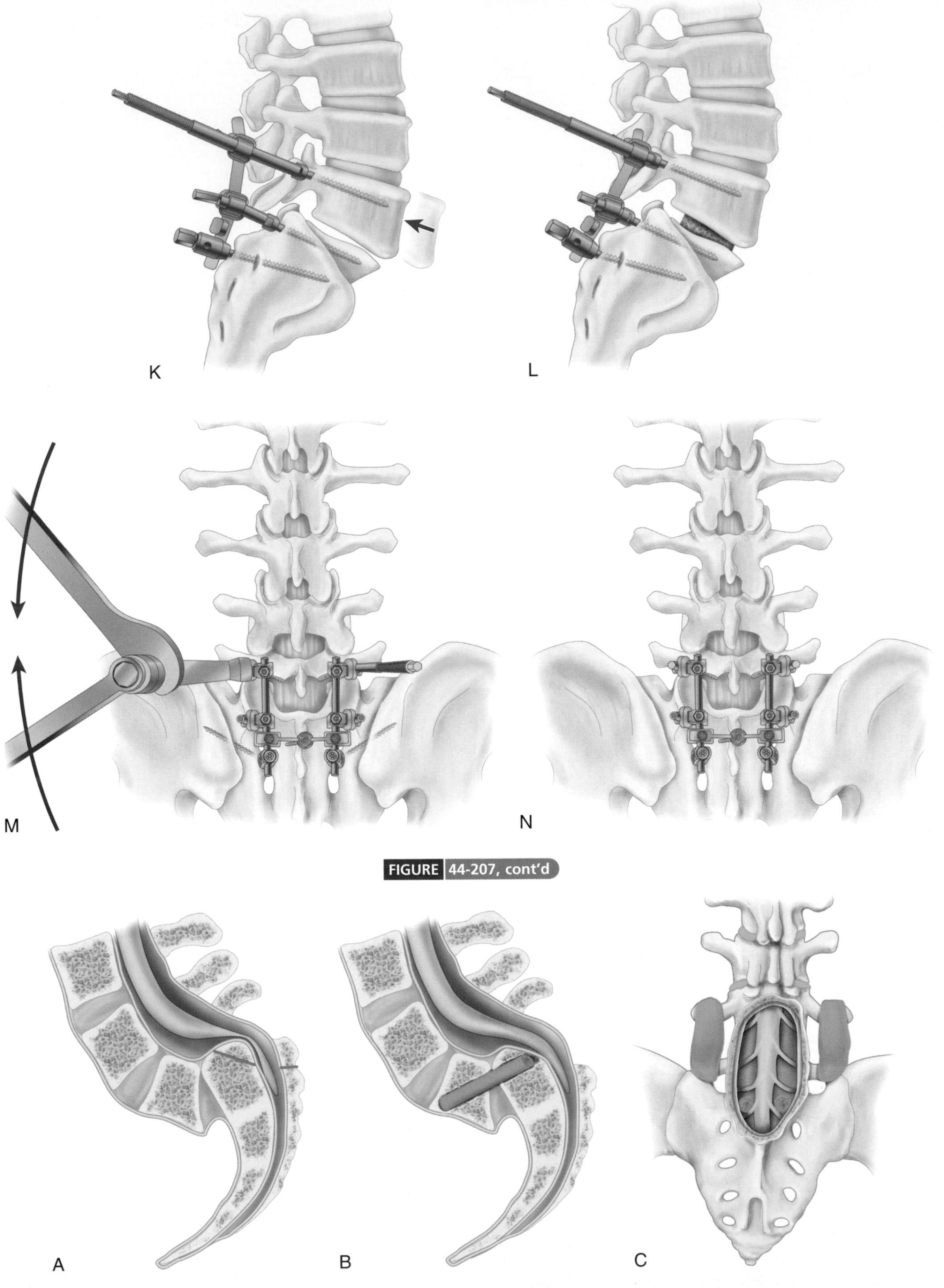

FIGURE 44-208 **A,** Amount of first sacral vertebral body resected to decompress dura *(blue line).* **B,** Insertion of interbody fibular graft and posterior decompression. **C,** After posterior decompression and fusion. *Colored area* represents posterolateral fusions. Ends of two fibular grafts are shown just above first sacral nerve roots. (From Bohlman HH, Cook SS: One-stage decompression and posterolateral and interbody fusion for lumbosacral spondyloptosis through a posterior approach, J Bone Joint Surg 64A:415, 1982.) **SEE TECHNIQUE 44-62.**

- Introduce a guide pin between the fifth lumbar and first sacral nerve roots on each side. Each pin is approximately 1 cm lateral to the midline and is directed through the first sacral vertebral body anteriorly. Confirm the proper position of each guidewire with radiographs.
- Drill a ⅜-inch epiphyseodesis bit over each guide pin to the appropriate depth, being careful not to violate the anterior cortex of the fifth lumbar vertebra (≈ 5 cm).
- Obtain a fibular graft from the right leg and divide it longitudinally. Insert one half of the graft into each hole and countersink it 2 mm so as not to impinge on the dura (Fig. 44-208B).
- Perform a standard bilateral, posterolateral transverse process fusion from the third or fourth lumbar vertebra to the sacral ala using iliac crest grafts (Fig. 44-208B and C).
- Close the wound over a drain.

POSTOPERATIVE CARE. The patient is kept at bed rest for 7 to 10 days and then is mobilized in a lumbosacral orthosis. The drain is removed in 48 hours.

UNINSTRUMENTED CIRCUMFERENTIAL IN SITU FUSION

Circumferential in situ fusion has been used for the treatment of high-grade spondylolisthesis in children with better long-term results reported than after posterolateral or anterior fusion alone. The Scoliosis Research Society recommends that if reduction is performed, circumferential fusion with instrumentation should be done at the time of reduction.

TECHNIQUE 44-63

(HELENIUS ET AL.)

- Place the patient prone on a four-poster Relton frame.
- Make a posterior midline skin incision and develop the space bilaterally through the erector spinae muscles, 3 cm from the midline. Identify the L5 transverse process, the L5-S1 facet joint, and the sacral ala.
- Expose the posterior iliac wing through the same incision and obtain corticocancellous bone graft material.
- Open the L5-S1 facet joint with an osteotome and decorticate and curet the L5 transverse process and sacral ala. Place autogenous graft over the decorticated bone and impact it into the L5-S1 facet joint space.
- Close the fasciae on both sides as well as the subcutaneous tissues and skin with running absorbable suture.
- Place the patient supine, with both hips extended and the lower extremities spread apart. Place a small bolster under the lumbar spine to obtain lumbar lordosis. A Trendelenburg position of the table helps to keep the abdominal contents cephalad to the operating area.
- Make a longitudinal midline incision from just caudal to the umbilicus to just cephalad to the symphysis pubis.
- Open the fascia over the rectus abdominis muscle and develop the internervous plane between the abdominal muscles.
- After opening the peritoneum, extend the approach cephalad by cutting through the linea alba and packing the abdominal contents superiorly. Take care not to enter the dome of the bladder caudally.
- Open the posterior peritoneum (Fig. 44-209A) and assess the anatomy of the iliac vessels. Usually, the presacral intervertebral disc can be approached between the great vessels. Protect the left iliac vein across the L5 vertebral body and caudal to the aortic bifurcation.
- With a forceps, use blunt dissection to expose the L5-S1 disc.
- Identify the anterior longitudinal ligament and ligate the middle sacral artery. To help retract the iliac vessels, two Steinmann pins can be inserted on either side of the L5 vertebral body. Try to preserve all the parasympathetic nerve fibers in this area by approaching the disc space in the midline.
- Open the anterior longitudinal ligament horizontally, just cephalad to the L5-S1 disc space (Fig. 44-209B). The lower anterior lip of the L5 vertebra can be resected along the anterior longitudinal ligament to better expose the disc space.
- Carefully remove all intervertebral disc material up to the posterior longitudinal ligament, as well as the ring apophysis on both sides. Prepare the endplates with curettage.
- Obtain two to three tricortical wedge-shaped bone grafts (15 mm anterior and 10 mm posterior dimension) from either anterior iliac wing. The length of this graft is approximately 20 mm but may vary some. The grafts must fit into the disc space as prepared (Fig. 44-209C). A moderate increase in disc height and proper patient positioning reduce the spondylolisthesis and lumbosacral kyphosis. Using three structural autogenous grafts provides the best stability.
- In slips of nearly 100%, it may be necessary to increase the area for anterior spinal fusion. In these cases, an osteotomy of the sacrum may be necessary. Continue the release of the anterior ligament inferiorly, producing an osteoperiosteal flap over the S1 vertebral body. Apply corticocancellous bone grafts beneath this flap to increase the area for anterior intervertebral fusion.
- Reattach the anterior longitudinal ligament with absorbable sutures through osseous channels in the L5 vertebra.
- Close the posterior peritoneal and laparotomy incision (Fig. 44-209D).

POSTOPERATIVE CARE. A postoperative custom-molded TLSO is worn, and the patient is allowed to mobilize 2 to 3 days after surgery. Bending, lifting, and sports are restricted for 3 to 6 months or until a solid fusion is obtained.

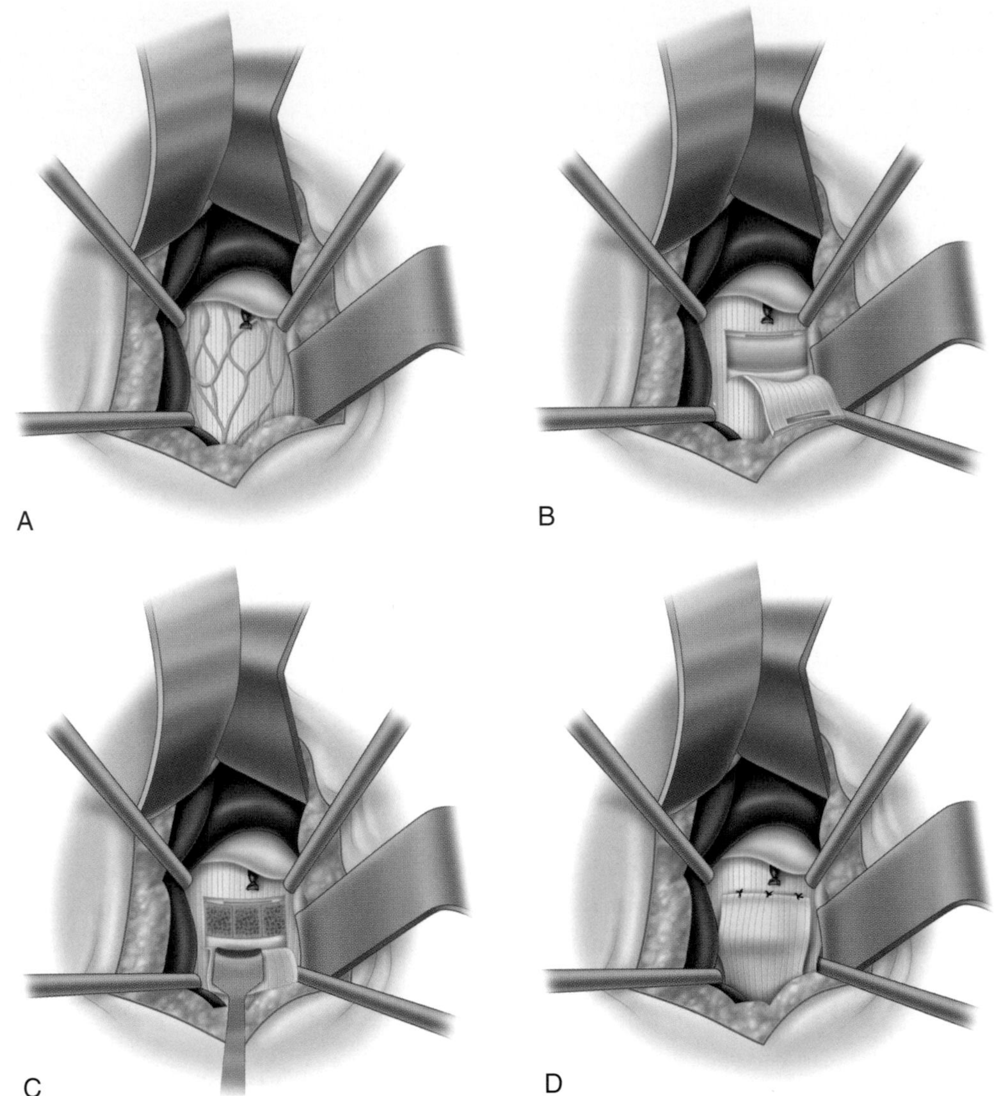

FIGURE 44-209 **A,** Posterior peritoneum opened and middle sacral artery ligated. **B,** Anterior longitudinal ligament opened, and small piece of bone removed from lower lip of L5. **C,** After discectomy, structural autogenous grafts placed. **D,** Anterior longitudinal ligament reattached through osseous channels and posterior peritoneal and laparotomy incisions are subsequently closed. (From Helenius I, Remes V, Poussa M: Uninstrumented in situ fusion for high-grade childhood and adolescent isthmic spondylolisthesis: long-term outcome, J Bone Joint Surg 90A:145, 2008.) **SEE TECHNIQUE 44-63.**

TREATMENT OF SPONDYLOPTOSIS

L5 VERTEBRECTOMY

Spondyloptosis exists when the entire body of L5 on a lateral standing radiograph is totally below the top of S1. Gaines popularized a two-stage L5 vertebrectomy procedure for this difficult problem (Fig. 44-210). The objective is to restore sagittal plane balance to avoid nerve root damage from cauda equina and nerve root stretching during reduction. This is a challenging procedure and should be done only by surgeons experienced in the surgical treatment of patients with high-grade isthmic dysplastic spondylolisthesis.

TECHNIQUE 44-64

(GAINES)

- This technique is performed in two stages, during either a single anesthetic or two separate anesthetic procedures.
- In the first stage, perform an L5 vertebrectomy and totally remove the L4-L5 and L5-S1 discs through a transverse abdominal incision (Fig. 44-211A).
- Excise the L5 body back to the base of the pedicles and control epidural bleeding with Gelfoam.
- Do not attempt reduction of the deformity at this time.
- Remove the caudal cartilage endplate of L4 after the L5 vertebrectomy is completed.

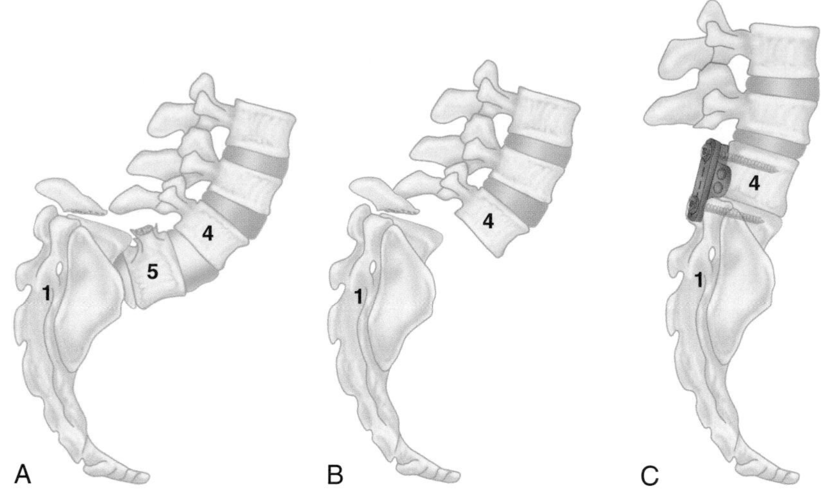

FIGURE 44-210 **A-C,** Diagram of two-stage L5 vertebrectomy for spondyloptosis. **SEE TECHNIQUE 44-64.**

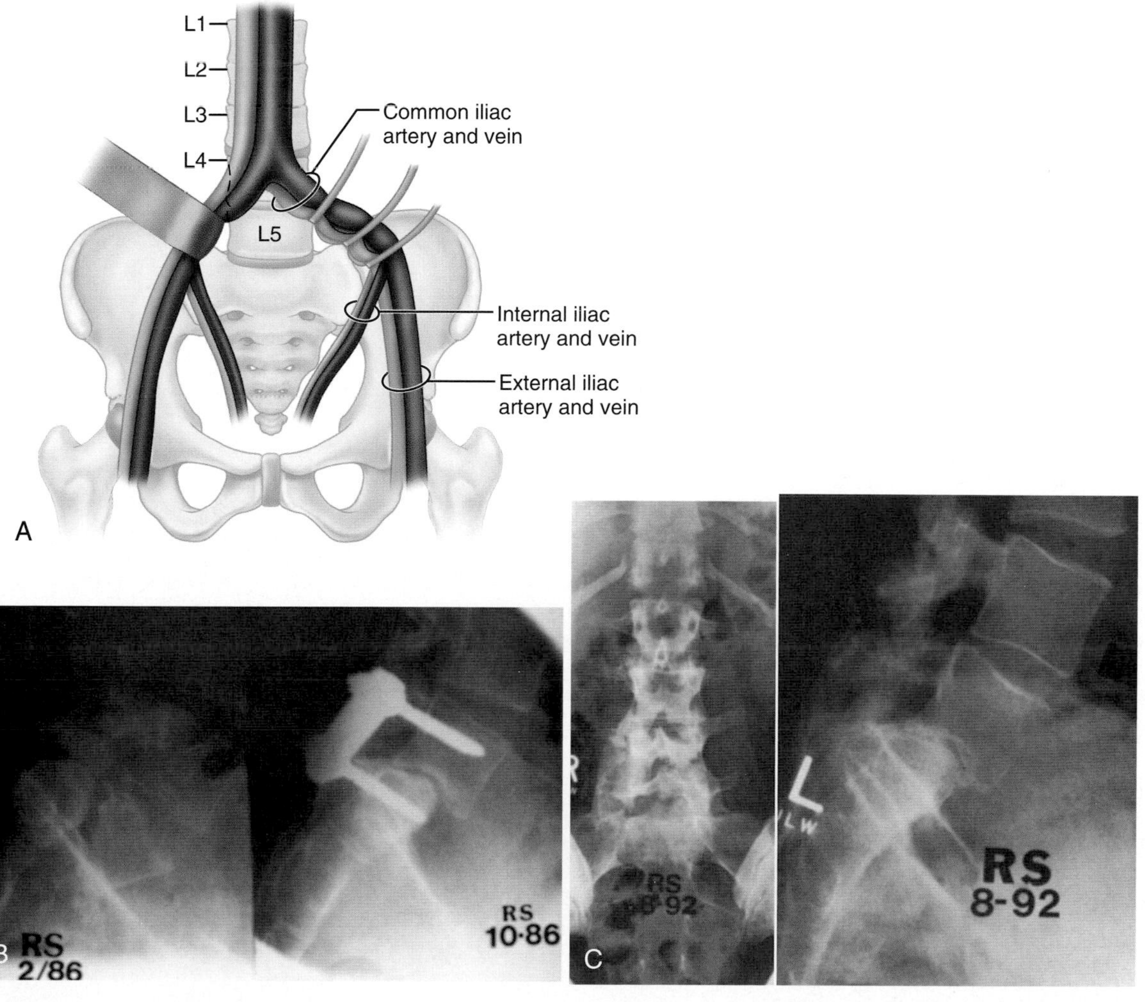

FIGURE 44-211 **A,** Anterior approach for resection of L4-L5 disc, vertebral body of L5, and L5-S1 disc is made through incision extending transversely across both rectus abdominis muscles. Great vessels are mobilized laterally after being carefully identified, and structures to be resected are seen between bifurcation of vena cava and aorta. **B,** Preoperative and postoperative lateral radiograph. **C,** Radiographs of same patient 7 years later. Solid intertransverse fusion and interbody fusion are shown. Reconstructed L4-S1 intervertebral foramen is wide open on lateral radiograph. (**A** redrawn from and **B** and **C** from Gaines RW Jr: The L5 vertebrectomy approach for the treatment of spondyloptosis. In Bridwell KH, DeWald RL, editors: The textbook of spinal surgery, ed 2, Philadelphia, 1997, Lippincott-Raven.) **SEE TECHNIQUE 44-64.**

- For the second stage, place the patient prone.
- Through a posterior approach, remove the L5 pedicles, facets, and laminar arch bilaterally.
- Place the pedicle screws into L4 and S1.
- Clean the upper surface of the sacrum of the cartilage endplate, but preserve the cortical endplate for docking with the inferior endplate of L4. Bone from the vertebrectomy is left between the L4 and S1 screws posterolaterally (Fig. 44-211B and C). L4 must touch S1 directly after the reduction, and the L5 and S1 nerve roots must both be free. Direct exposure of the L5 nerve roots and dural tube is the most important way to avoid serious iatrogenic injury to the cauda equina.

KYPHOSCOLIOSIS

MYELOMENINGOCELE

Treatment of patients with myelomeningocele spinal deformities is the most challenging in spine surgery. It requires a team effort, with cooperation of consultants in several subspecialties. These children often have multiple system dysfunctions that influence the treatment of their spinal deformity.

INCIDENCE AND NATURAL HISTORY

Scoliosis and kyphosis with secondary adaptive changes are common in patients with myelomeningocele. Spinal deformity may be the result of developmental deformities that are acquired and related to the level of paralysis or congenital deformities that are the result of vertebral malformation. Developmental and congenital forms of spinal deformity may exist concurrently in patients with myelomeningocele. These deformities often are progressive and can lead to significant disabilities. The incidence of scoliosis increases with increasing age and neurologic level. Trivedi et al. found the prevalence of scoliosis to be 93%, 72%, 43%, and less than 1%, respectively, in patients with thoracic, upper lumbar, lower lumbar, and sacral motor levels. Congenital scoliosis in myelomeningocele is associated with structural disorganization of the vertebrae with asymmetric growth and includes all of the congenital anomalies associated with scoliosis: hemivertebrae, unilateral unsegmented bars, and various combinations of the two. Congenital scoliosis occurs in 15% to 20% of patients with myelomeningocele, and most curves in myelomeningocele patients are paralytic. In these patients, the spine is straight at birth and gradually develops a progressive curvature because of the neuromuscular problems. These generally are long, C-shaped curves with the apex in the thoracolumbar or lumbar spine (Fig. 44-212). These paralytic curves often extend into the lumbosacral junction and often are associated with pelvic obliquity. In these children, spinal curvatures often develop at a younger age than in children with idiopathic scoliosis, beginning at 3 to 4 years of age, and can become severe before the patient is 10 years old. Future trunk growth and final trunk height are considerations in treatment, although Lindseth noted that children with myelomeningocele have slow growth because of growth hormone deficiency and mature earlier than usual, often by 9 to 10 years in girls and 11 to 12 years in boys.

CLINICAL EVALUATION

Thorough evaluation is critical for determining the appropriate management of patients with myelomeningocele and spinal deformity. The following areas are closely investigated: presence of hydrocephalus, any operative procedures for shunting, bowel and bladder function, frequency of urinary tract infections, use of an indwelling catheter or intermittent catheterization, possible latex allergies, current medications, mental status, method of ambulation, level of the defect, any noticeable progression of the curve, and any lower extremity contractures. The spine is examined to determine the type and flexibility of the deformity and to detect any evidence of pressure sores or lack of sitting balance. In patients with progressive paralytic scoliosis, hydromyelia, disturbed ventricular shunts, syringomyelia, tethered cord, or compression

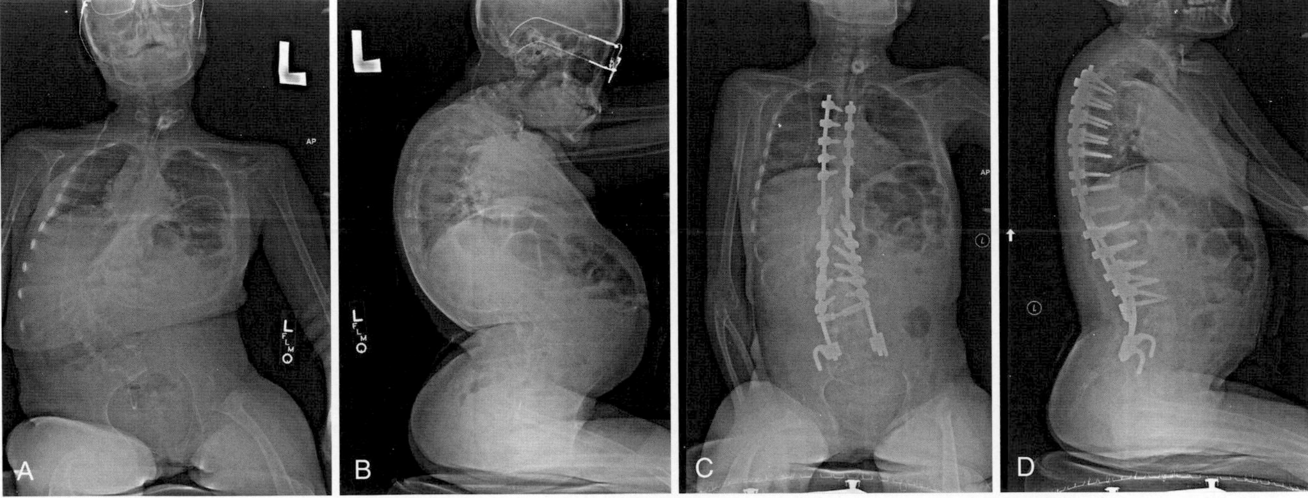

FIGURE 44-212 **A** and **B**, Congenital scoliosis in a patient with myelomeningocele; note C-shaped curve. **C** and **D**, After posterior fusion and instrumentation.

from an Arnold-Chiari syndrome may contribute to the progression of scoliosis. Most patients with myelomeningocele have radiographic tethering of the spinal cord at the site of the sac closure, but the mere presence of radiographic tethering does not necessarily imply traction on the cord. Other clinical signs and symptoms of cord tethering should be observed, including back pain, new or increased spasticity, changes in muscle strength, difficulty with gait, changes in bowel or bladder function, and the appearance of lower extremity deformities.

Careful evaluation of any pelvic obliquity is necessary. Because patients with myelomeningocele are prone to development of contractures around the hips, careful physical examination of the hip adductors, extensors, and flexors is important in evaluating the cause of pelvic obliquity. Lubicky noted a difficult but unusual problem in some patients with myelomeningocele and extension contractures of the hips. In these patients, flexion through the thoracolumbar spine was needed for them to sit upright. Spinal fusion would make sitting impossible and would place significant mechanical stresses on the instrumentation (Fig. 44-213). Physiologic hip flexion should be restored in these patients before spinal instrumentation and fusion are undertaken.

RADIOGRAPHIC FINDINGS

Radiographs should be taken with the patient upright and supine. If the patient can ambulate, standing films should be made. If the patient is nonambulatory, sitting films should be made. The upright films allow better evaluation of the actual deformity of the spine and will demonstrate the contribution of the paralytic component to the spine deformity. Supine films show better detail of various associated spinal deformities. The flexibility of the curves is determined with traction or bending films.

Radiographic evaluation of the pelvic obliquity should include a supine view obtained with the hips in the "relaxed" position. In this view, the hips are flexed and abducted or adducted as dictated by the contractures. Alternatively, radiographs can be made with the patient prone and the hips off the edge of the radiographic table and placed in abduction or adduction (see Fig. 44-121).

Various specialized radiographs are helpful. Myelography and MRI are useful for evaluating such conditions as hydromyelia, tethered cord (Fig. 44-214), diastematomyelia, and Arnold-Chiari malformation. CT with reconstruction views will give better bone detail for associated congenital spine anomalies. Renal ultrasound or intravenous pyelography should be done at regular intervals, according to the urologist's recommendation.

SCOLIOSIS AND LORDOSIS IN MYELOMENINGOCELE

ORTHOTIC TREATMENT

Although the natural history of paralytic curves in patients with myelomeningocele is not changed by orthotic treatment, bracing may be useful to delay spinal fusion until adequate spinal growth has occurred. Bracing may accomplish this in paralytic curves but does not affect congenital curves. The brace also can improve sitting balance and free the hands for other activities. Custom-fitted braces are used but require close and frequent observation by the parents. The skin must be examined frequently for pressure areas; any sign of pressure requires immediate brace adjustment. Bracing usually is not instituted until the curve is beginning to cause clinical problems, and generally it is worn only when the patient is upright. If the curve fails to respond to bracing or if bracing becomes impossible because of pressure sores or noncompliance, surgery is indicated. The patient and the parents need to understand that the brace is not the definitive treatment of these curves.

Flynn et al. reported that VEPTR is a reasonable treatment option for spinal deformity in immature, nonambulatory myelomeningocele patients for correcting spinal deformity, allowing spinal growth, and maintaining adequate respiratory function until definitive fusion is needed.

OPERATIVE TREATMENT

Several authors have indicated that surgery on the myelomeningocele spine is accompanied by potentially serious complications. Although the operative procedures varied considerably in these reports, some observations could be made. Because of densely scarred and adherent soft tissue, spinal exposure often is lengthy and hemorrhagic. The deformity often is rigid, and correction may be limited. The quality of the bone often provides poor fixation for instrumentation systems, and the inadequacy of the posterior bone mass provides a poor bed for bone grafting. The lack of normal posterior vertebral elements makes instrumentation and achieving a solid fusion difficult. The abnormal placement of the paraspinal muscles results in the lack of usual soft-tissue coverage of the spine and instrumentation systems. Newer techniques of surgery and instrumentation, bank bone, and prophylactic antibiotics have lessened but not eliminated these problems. The parents must be aware of these potential problems before surgery and must accept these as inherent in the operative treatment.

Emans et al. called attention to the problem of latex allergy in patients with myelomeningocele. Repeated exposures to latex during daily catheterization and multiple operations most likely accounts for sensitization of these patients to natural latex. The allergy is to the residual plant proteins in natural latex products and is an immunoglobulin E–mediated, immediate type of hypersensitivity. Anaphylaxis may occur intraoperatively and easily can be confused with other intraoperative emergencies. Patients with myelomeningocele should be closely questioned about any preoperative reactions to latex. Latex allergy testing can now be performed. We routinely treat all patients with myelomeningocele as if they have a latex allergy.

Congenital abnormalities that cause scoliosis in patients with myelomeningocele are treated in the same manner as in other patients with congenital scoliosis with early operative intervention. Paralytic scoliosis is more common than congenital scoliosis, and lordoscoliosis is the most common type. The combined anterior and posterior fusion method provides the best chance to achieve a durable fusion. Stella et al. also reported that the best correction was obtained in patients who had instrumented anterior and posterior fusions. High pseudarthrosis rates have been reported in patients with myelomeningocele and are related to the surgical approach, type, and presence of instrumentation or the use of a posterior-only approach. The reported pseudarthrosis rates are 0% to 50% for anterior fusion, 26% to 76% for isolated posterior fusion, and 5% to 23% for combined anterior and

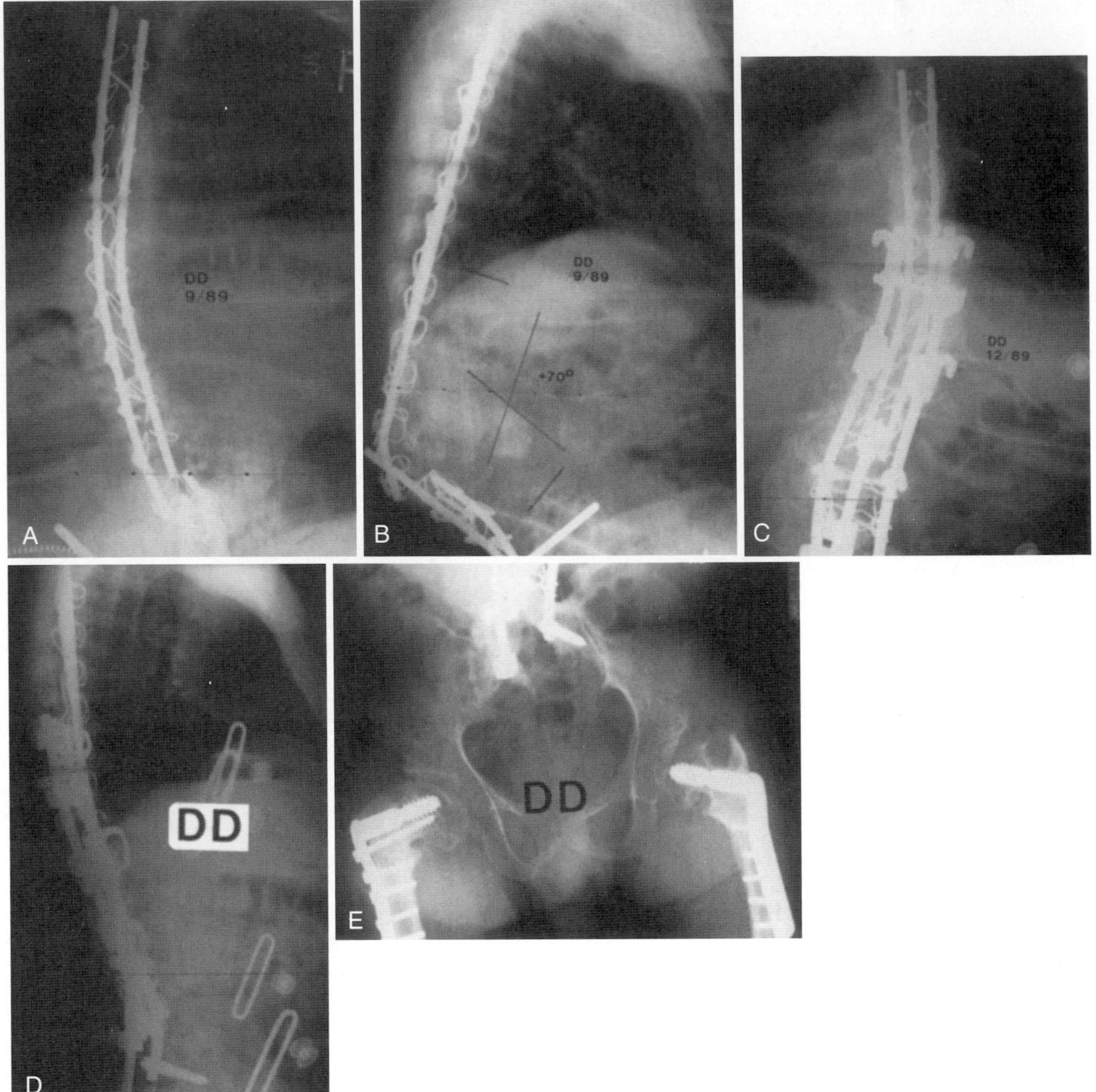

FIGURE 44-213 Thoracic-level myelomeningocele in 16-year-old boy who had progressive scoliosis and underwent anterior interbody fusion and posterior Luque instrumentation. Unfortunately, he had extremely poor hip flexion. Three years later, he had increasing deformity. Anteroposterior **(A)** and lateral **(B)** radiographs at time of presentation show broken rods and severe kyphotic deformity. Pseudarthrosis provided flexion for sitting because hips could not. Anteroposterior **(C)** and lateral **(D)** radiographs after revision of pseudarthrosis anteriorly and posteriorly. After these procedures and during same hospitalization, patient underwent femoral shortening osteotomies, which allowed him to sit properly and prevented stress on instrumentation **(E)**. (From Lubicky JP: Spinal deformity in myelomeningocele. In Bridwell KH, DeWald RL, editors: The textbook of spinal surgery, ed 2, Philadelphia, 1997, Lippincott-Raven.)

posterior fusions. Infection rates have approached 43% and are highest when surgery is performed with concurrent urinary tract infections. Preoperative urinary cultures are mandatory, as is treatment with antibiotics preoperatively and postoperatively. Prophylactic antibiotic use has reduced the infection rate to 8%.

Selection of Fusion Levels. The levels of fusion depend on the age of the child, location of the curve, level of paralysis, ambulatory status, and presence or absence of pelvic obliquity. Spinal fusion generally should extend from neutral vertebra to neutral vertebra, with the end vertebra of the scoliotic curve located within the stable zone. Paralytic curves often tend to be fused too short, especially proximally. In deciding whether to stop the fusion short or long, the longer fusion usually is safer. In the past, instrumentation was extended to the pelvis because deficient posterior elements of the lumbar spine made adequate fixation impossible. With pedicle screw fixation, fusion and instrumentation sometimes can be stopped short of the pelvis. Mazur et al. and Müller et al. showed that spinal fusion to the pelvis in ambulatory patients

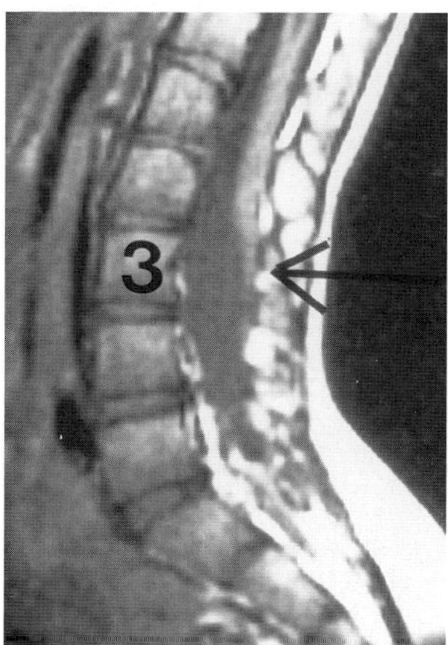

FIGURE 44-214 MRI shows tethered cord at L3 in patient with kyphoscoliosis.

diminished their ambulatory status. They therefore recommended fusion short of the pelvis, if possible, in ambulatory patients. Ending the fusion above the pelvis eliminates the stresses on the instrumentation and fusion areas at the lumbosacral junction and allows some motion for adjustment of lordosis in those who have mild hip flexion contractures. In nonambulatory patients, unless the lumbar curve can be corrected to less than 20 degrees and the pelvic obliquity to less than 15 degrees, the scoliosis will continue to progress if the lumbosacral junction is not fused.

Attention to the sagittal contour is extremely important. Even in a nonambulatory patient, maintenance of lumbar lordosis is important. If the lumbar lordosis is flattened, the pelvis rotates and much of the sitting weight is placed directly on the ischial tuberosities; this can result in the development of pressure sores.

Anterior-Only Fusion. Sponseller et al. recommended anterior fusion and instrumentation alone in selected patients with myelomeningocele and paralytic scoliosis. Their indications for this procedure include thoracolumbar curves of less than 75 degrees, compensatory proximal curves of less than 40 degrees, no significant kyphosis in the primary curve, and no evidence of syrinx. Fourteen patients were treated with this technique. A rod and vertebral body screw construct was used most frequently anteriorly. A decrease in quadriceps strength was noted immediately after surgery in two patients, and it was hypothesized that the amount of correction achieved with the anterior instrumentation systems was so great that traction was placed on the cord. Intraoperative monitoring of quadriceps function may be needed in these patients.

POSTERIOR INSTRUMENTATION AND FUSION

Posterior instrumentation and fusion alone has been reserved for flexible curves with most of the posterior elements intact so that adequate fixation can be obtained with pedicle screws. However, the curve must be flexible and correction must allow almost normal coronal and sagittal balance. Posterior-only instrumentation and fusion has been associated with the highest pseudarthrosis rates.

TECHNIQUE 44-65

- Place the patient prone on a radiolucent frame.
- Prepare and drape the back in a sterile manner.
- Make a midline incision from the area of the superior vertebra to be instrumented down to the sacrum.
- In the area of the normal spine, carry out subperiosteal dissection. An inverted-Y incision has been described to prevent exposure of the sac in the midline, but we have had difficulty with skin necrosis with use of this technique and have had better results with a midline incision that follows the scarred area of the skin posteriorly and careful dissection around the sac in the midline area.
- Make the skin incision carefully because the dural sac is just beneath the skin. If a dural leak is noted, repair it immediately.
- Carry the dissection laterally over the convex and concave facet areas and down to the ala of the sacrum (Fig. 44-215A) to expose the area of normal spine to be fused and the bony elements in the region of the abnormal sac area.
- Hooks, pedicle screws, or sublaminar wires can be used to instrument the normal vertebra above the sac area.
- In the area of the defect, attempt to achieve segmental fixation. Pass a wire around a pedicle and twist it on itself to secure fixation (Fig. 44-215B). Pass wires on both the concave and the convex sides of the curve. Because these pedicles often are osteoporotic, take care in tightening the wires so that they do not "cut through."
- On the concave side of the curve, distraction can help correct pelvic obliquity.
- If the iliac wing is large enough to accept the Galveston fixation, make a Galveston bend in short rods and insert the short rods in the iliac crests. Alternatively, an iliac screw with connectors can be used.
- Connect two longer rods to the spine with the segmental wires and connect the long rods to the Galveston-type rods with domino-type crosslinks (see Technique 44-37).
- Alternatively, if the iliac wings are too small, use the McCarthy technique (see Technique 44-36). Take care to preserve normal lumbar lordosis and secure the rods in place by tightening the segmental wires.
- Apply copious bone-bank allograft to any areas of bony structures posteriorly.
- It is important to link the two rods with a crosslink system.

COMBINED ANTERIOR AND POSTERIOR FUSION

The most commonly required procedure for progressive scoliosis in patients with myelomeningocele combines anterior and posterior fusions with posterior instrumentation. Posterior instrumentation consists of a standard rod with hooks, pedicle screws, sublaminar wires, or cables, or a combination of these in the areas of normal posterior

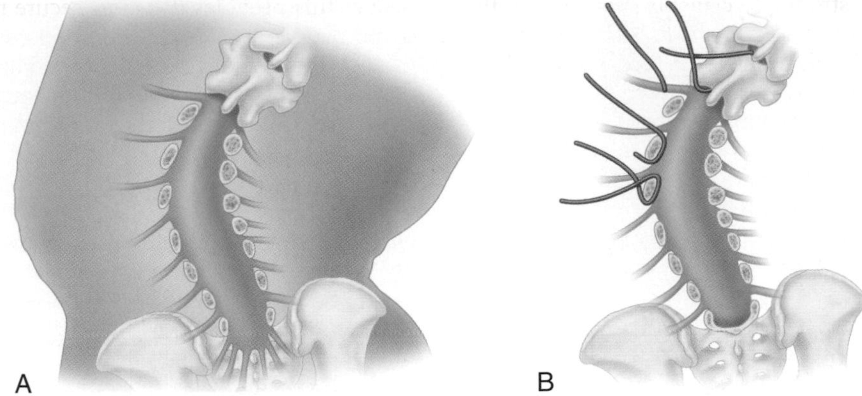

FIGURE 44-215 Correction of scoliosis in myelomeningocele. **A,** Spinal exposure; dural sac is not dissected. **B,** Sublaminar wires placed in normal spine; in area of spina bifida, wires encircle pedicle for segmental fixation. **SEE TECHNIQUE 44-65.**

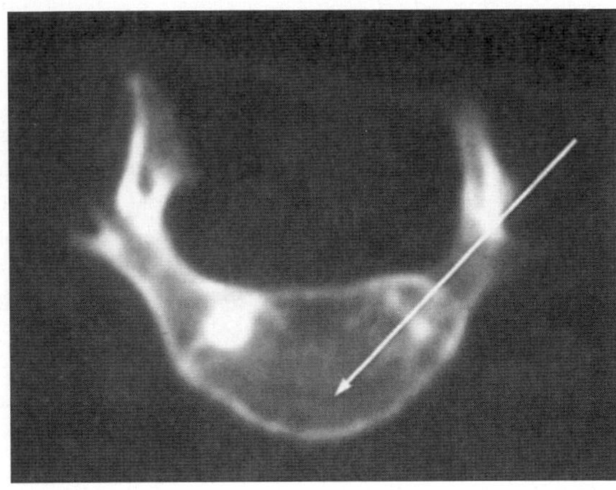

FIGURE 44-216 CT scan shows abnormal pedicle orientation in dysraphic vertebra. (From Rodgers WB, Frim DM, Emans JB: Surgery of the spine in myelodysplasia: an overview, Clin Orthop Relat Res 338:19, 1997.)

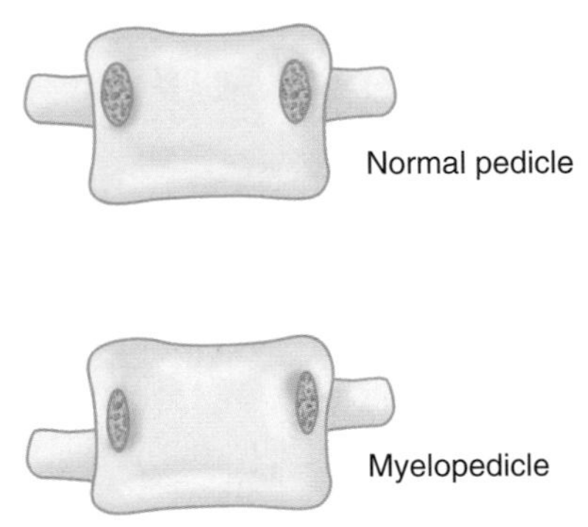

FIGURE 44-217 Diagram shows alteration in anatomic relationship of pedicle-transverse process.

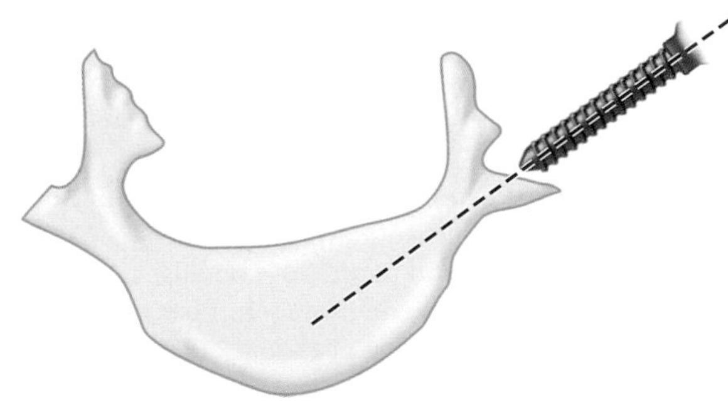

FIGURE 44-218 Pedicle screw insertion.

elements. The hooks and pedicle screws allow distraction or compressive forces to be applied, and the wires or cables allow a translational force to be applied. The wires or cables also have the advantage of distributing the corrective forces over multiple vertebral levels and providing secure fixation of all instrumented levels.

The absence of posterior elements in the dysraphic portion of the spine makes fixation more of a problem, so various instrumentation systems need to be available (Fig. 44-216). Rodgers et al. noted that pedicle screws greatly improved fixation and correction of the dysraphic portion of the spine. In widely dysraphic vertebrae, the orientation and landmarks of the pedicle are altered (Fig. 44-217), and direct viewing of the pedicle is necessary to insert pedicle screws in these areas. The pedicle is exposed either by resection of a sufficient amount of facet or by dissection along the medial wall of the spinal canal and retraction of the meningocele sac to identify the medial wall of the pedicle. During probing of the pedicle, remaining within the cortices of the pedicle is imperative. The pedicle screws do not necessarily need to penetrate the anterior vertebral cortex. In the dysraphic spine, the pedicle screws often have to be inserted at an angle from lateral to medial (Fig. 44-218). This requires special attention to rod contouring to attach the rod to the screw because of the lateral position of the screw head. The small vertebral bodies and osteopenic bone often make the purchase of pedicle screws questionable.

Two other techniques for fixation of the dysraphic spine can be used. Drummond spinous process button wires can be passed through laminar remnants (Fig. 44-219), or segmental wires can be looped around each pedicle. When Drummond button wires are used, the dysraphic laminae are exposed and dissection is done between the sac and the adjacent laminae while the sac is carefully retracted medially. A hole is placed through the strongest available portion of the laminar remnant, and the wire is passed from medial to lateral, leaving the button on the inner surface of the lamina. Segmental wires can be looped around each pedicle by passing from one foramen around the pedicle and other posterior remnants medial to the pedicle and then back through the next foramen and back to the original wire. The passage of these wires usually is blind. The wires then attach to the rod. The wire also can be looped around a pedicle bone screw if it is difficult to contour the rod to easily fit in the screw (see Fig. 44-215A and B).

Instrumentation to the pelvis frequently is necessary to correct associated pelvic obliquity in nonambulatory children. Fixation to the pelvis and sacrum is especially difficult in children with myelomeningocele because the bone often is osteoporotic and the pelvis is small, making secure instrumentation difficult. The stresses placed on distal fixation in scoliosis tend to displace sacral or sacropelvic instrumentation laterally. If there is associated kyphosis, these forces tend to displace sacral or pelvic instrumentation dorsally.

Several techniques have been described for extending fixation to the pelvis, including Galveston, Dunn-McCarthy, Jackson, Fackler, sacral bar, and pedicle screws. Our preferred technique for pelvic fixation in patients with paralytic scoliosis is the Galveston technique (see Technique 44-37). We believe this provides the most secure pelvic fixation for scoliotic curves. However, many patients with myelomeningocele have hypoplastic iliac crests, and in these patients, L-rods are fixed to the sacrum with the technique described by McCarthy (see Technique 44-36). This technique does not restrict lateral displacement as well as the Galveston intrapelvic fixation does, but crosslinking of the two rods may help decrease lateral displacement. Once the two rods are crosslinked, pelvic obliquity can be corrected by cantilevering the crosslinked rods. The Jackson intrasacral rod technique consists of inserting the rods through the lateral sacral mass and into the sacrum. The rod then penetrates the anterolateral cortex and usually is attached to a sacral screw, providing fixation in flexion and extension. The anatomy of the sacrum in patients with myelomeningocele makes this technique quite difficult. Widmann et al. described a technique using a sacral bar connected to standard Cotrel-Dubousset–like rods in 10 patients and found it to be effective (Fig. 44-220). Pelvic fixation by sacral pedicle screws is not reliable in these small osteopenic patients.

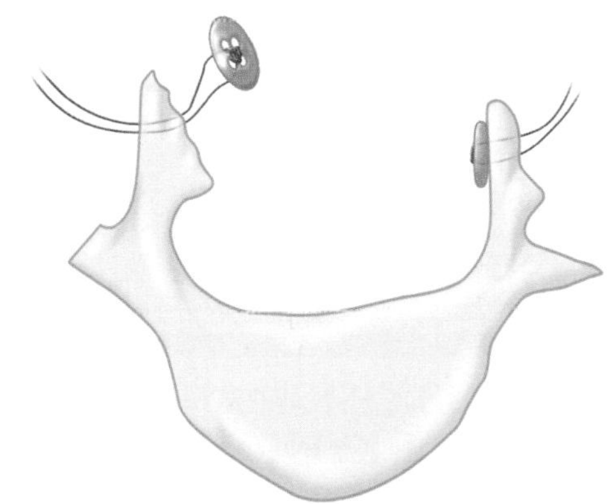

FIGURE 44-219 Diagram of Wisconsin button wire fixation of dysraphic vertebra.

In patients who are treated with combined anterior and posterior fusion, the necessity for anterior instrumentation is controversial. One study found no statistical differences in fusion rate, curve correction, or change in pelvic obliquity with anterior and posterior instrumentation and fusion compared with anterior arthrodesis with only posterior instrumentation and fusion. However, other studies have reported better correction and a decrease in the rate of implant failure and postoperative loss of correction with instrumented anterior and posterior fusions. If anterior instrumentation is used, care must be taken to not cause a kyphotic deformity in the instrumented spine.

KYPHOSIS IN MYELOMENINGOCELE

INCIDENCE AND NATURAL HISTORY

Kyphosis in patients with myelomeningocele may be either developmental or congenital. Developmental kyphosis is not present at birth and progresses slowly. It is a paralytic kyphosis that is aggravated by the lack of posterior stability. Congenital kyphosis, which is a much more difficult problem, usually measures 80 degrees or more at birth. The level of the lesion usually is T12 with total paraplegia. The kyphosis is rigid and progresses rapidly during infancy. Children with severe

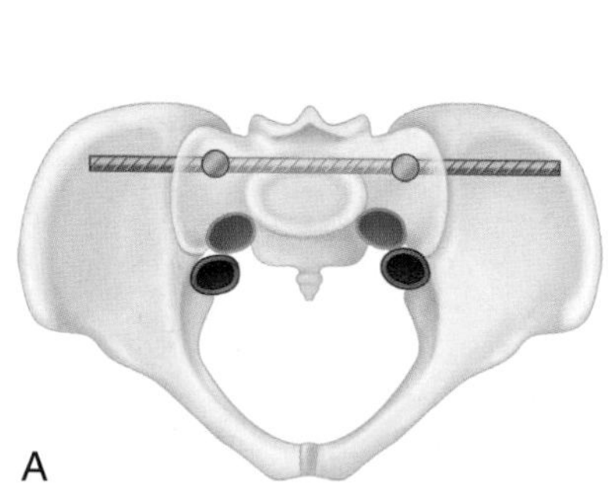

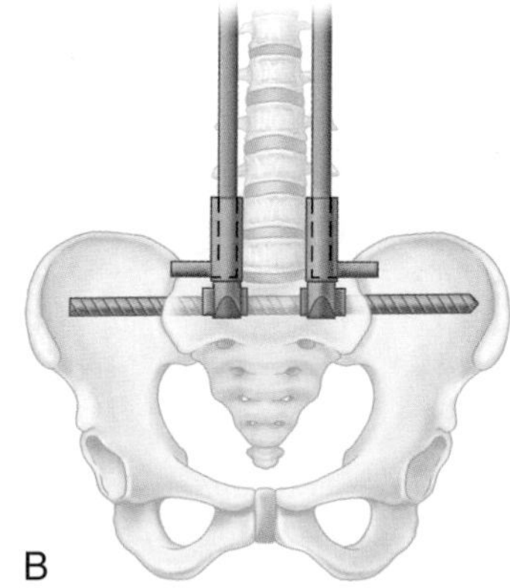

FIGURE 44-220 **A,** Correct passage of sacral bar through body of sacrum, posterior to great vessels and anterior to spinal canal. **B,** Connection between sacral bar and vertical rods.

kyphosis are unable to wear braces and often have difficulty sitting in wheelchairs because the center of gravity is displaced forward. An ulceration may develop over the prominent kyphosis and make skin coverage difficult. Progression of the kyphosis may lead to respiratory difficulty because of incompetence of the inspiratory muscles, crowding of the abdominal contents, and upward pressure on the diaphragm. Increased flexion of the trunk can interfere with urinary drainage and also may cause problems if urinary diversion or ileostomy becomes necessary.

Hoppenfeld described the anatomy of this condition and noted that the pedicles are widely spread and the rudimentary laminae actually are everted. The anterior longitudinal ligament is short and thick. The paraspinal muscles are present but are displaced far anterolaterally (Fig. 44-221); thus, all muscles act anterior to the axis of rotation, which tends to worsen the kyphosis.

OPERATIVE TREATMENT

Apical vertebral ostectomy, as proposed by Sharrard, makes closure of the skin easier in neonates but provides only short-term improvement, and the kyphotic deformity invariably recurs. Crawford et al. reported kyphectomies performed at the time of dural sac closure in the neonate. They found this to be a safe procedure with excellent initial correction.

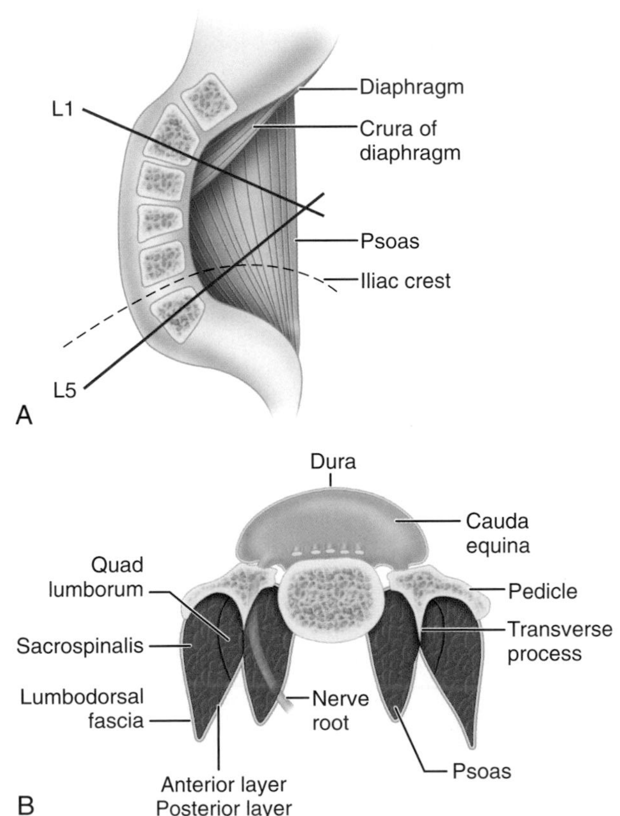

FIGURE 44-221 **A,** Sagittal diagram showing deforming effect of psoas muscle on kyphosis. **B,** Transverse section of lumbar spine and attached muscles in region of kyphosis. Pedicles and laminae of vertebrae are splayed laterally; erector spinae muscles enclosed in thoracolumbar fascia lie lateral to vertebral bodies and act as flexors.

Eventual recurrence is expected despite the procedure. The recurrence, however, is a longer, more rounded deformity that is technically less demanding to correct. Lindseth and Selzer reported vertebral excision for kyphosis in children with myelomeningocele. Their most consistent results were obtained with partial resection of the apical vertebra and the proximal lordotic curve, which was done in 12 patients. If only the apical vertebra and other vertebrae on either side were excised, correction of the kyphotic prominence was lost. Others have found that the Warner and Fackler type of sacral anchoring (see Fig. 44-223) provides a rigid construct, good correction, and low-profile instrumentation. That has also been our experience and is our preferred method of sacral anchoring in kyphectomies. Other techniques using a Dunn-McCarthy technique, intrasacral fixation, and pedicle screws also have been described. The optimal instrumentation and distal fixation technique is yet to be determined.

Although all severe congenital kyphoses in patients with myelomeningocele progress, not all patients require surgery. Kyphectomy is indicated to improve sitting balance or when skin problems occur over the apex. The trend is to delay surgery until the patient is 7 or 8 years of age, if possible. The surgery should be done before skeletal maturity, however. Delaying the surgery allows more secure internal fixation with less postoperative loss of correction.

Sarwark reported a subtraction osteotomy of multiple vertebrae at the apex, which creates lordosing osteotomies at each level. The vertebral body is entered and subtracted via the pedicles with a curet, distal to proximal. A closing osteotomy is done posteriorly to obtain correction. The spine is instrumented from the midthoracic level to the sacrum. The reported advantages include less blood loss, decreased morbidity, no need for cordotomy, and continued growth because the endplates are not violated.

VERTEBRAL EXCISION AND REDUCTION OF KYPHOSIS

TECHNIQUE 44-66

(LINDSETH AND SELZER)

- Use a midline posterior incision (Fig. 44-222A), which can be varied somewhat, depending on local skin conditions.
- Expose subperiosteally the more normal vertebrae superiorly and the area of the abnormality, continuing the exposure past the lateral bony ridges.
- At this point, remove the sac.
- Dissect inside the lamina until the foramina are exposed on each side of the spine.
- Expose, divide, and coagulate the nerve, artery, and vein within each foramen, exposing the sac distally where it is scarred down and thin.
- At its distal level, cross-clamp the sac with Kelly clamps and divide it between the clamps (Fig. 44-222B).
- Close the scarred ends with a running stitch. Dissect the sac proximally.
- As this proximal dissection is done, large venous channels connecting the sac to the posterior vertebral body will be

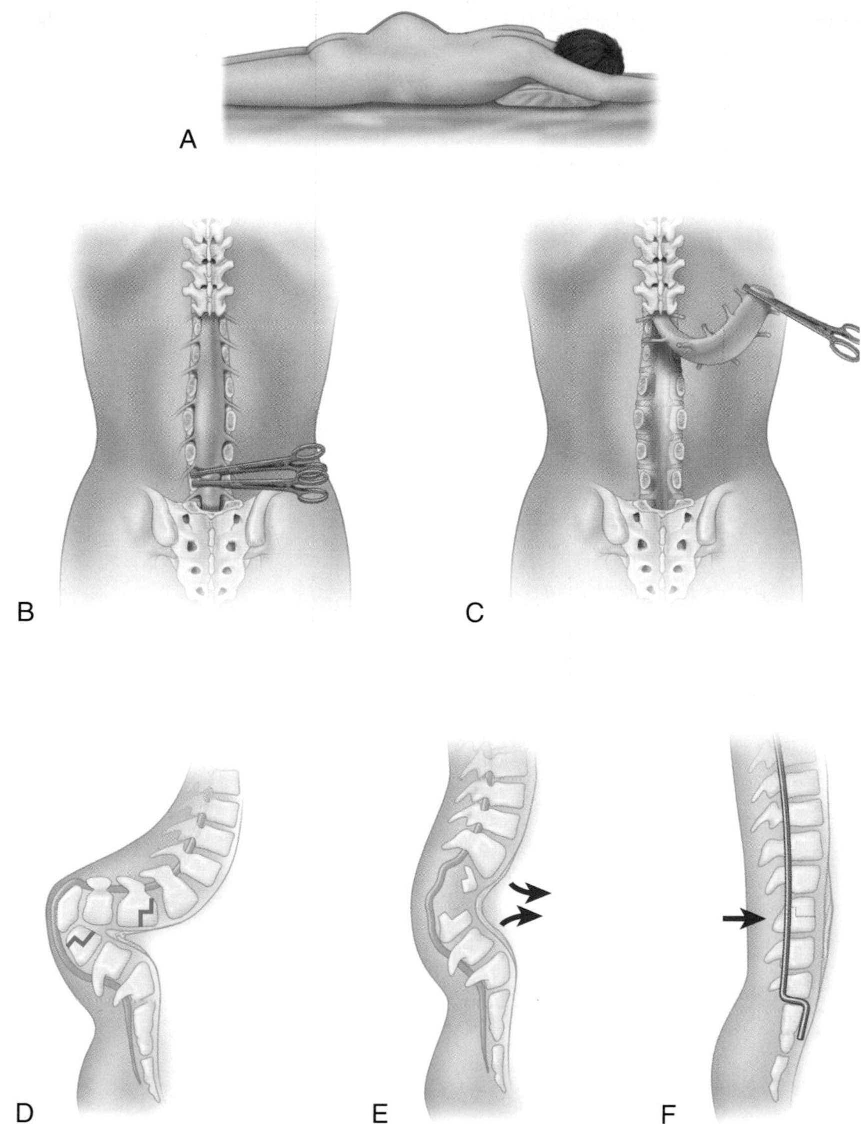

FIGURE 44-222 Technique of vertebral excision (Lindseth and Selzer). **A,** Patient positioning. **B,** Exposure of area of kyphosis and dural sac. **C,** Sac is divided distally and dissected proximally. **D,** Vertebrae between apex of lordosis and apex of kyphosis are removed. **E,** Kyphosis is reduced. **F,** Reduction is maintained with stable internal fixation (in this instance, with Luque rods and segmental wires). **SEE TECHNIQUE 44-66.**

encountered; control the bleeding from the bone with bone wax and from the soft tissue with electrocautery.

- Dissect the sac up to the level of the dura that appears more normal (Fig. 44-222C).
- The sac can be transected at this point. If this is done, close the dura with a purse-string suture. Do not suture the cord itself shut, but leave it open so that the spinal fluid can escape from the central canal of the cord into the arachnoid space.
- If the sac is not removed, it can be used at the completion of the procedure to further cover the area of the resected vertebra.
- Once the sac has been reflected proximally, continue dissection around the vertebral bodies, exposing only the area to be removed. If the entire kyphotic area of the spine is exposed subperiosteally, osteonecrosis of these vertebral bodies may occur.
- Remove the vertebrae between the apex of the lordosis and the apex of the kyphosis (Fig. 44-222D). Remove the vertebra at the apex of the kyphosis first by removing the intervertebral disc with a Cobb elevator and curets. Take care to leave the anterior longitudinal ligament intact to act as a stabilizing hinge.
- Once this vertebra has been removed, temporarily correct the spine to determine how many cephalad vertebrae should be removed. Remove enough vertebrae to correct the kyphosis as much as possible but not so many that approximation is impossible (Fig. 44-222E).
- Morselization of these vertebral bodies provides additional bone graft.

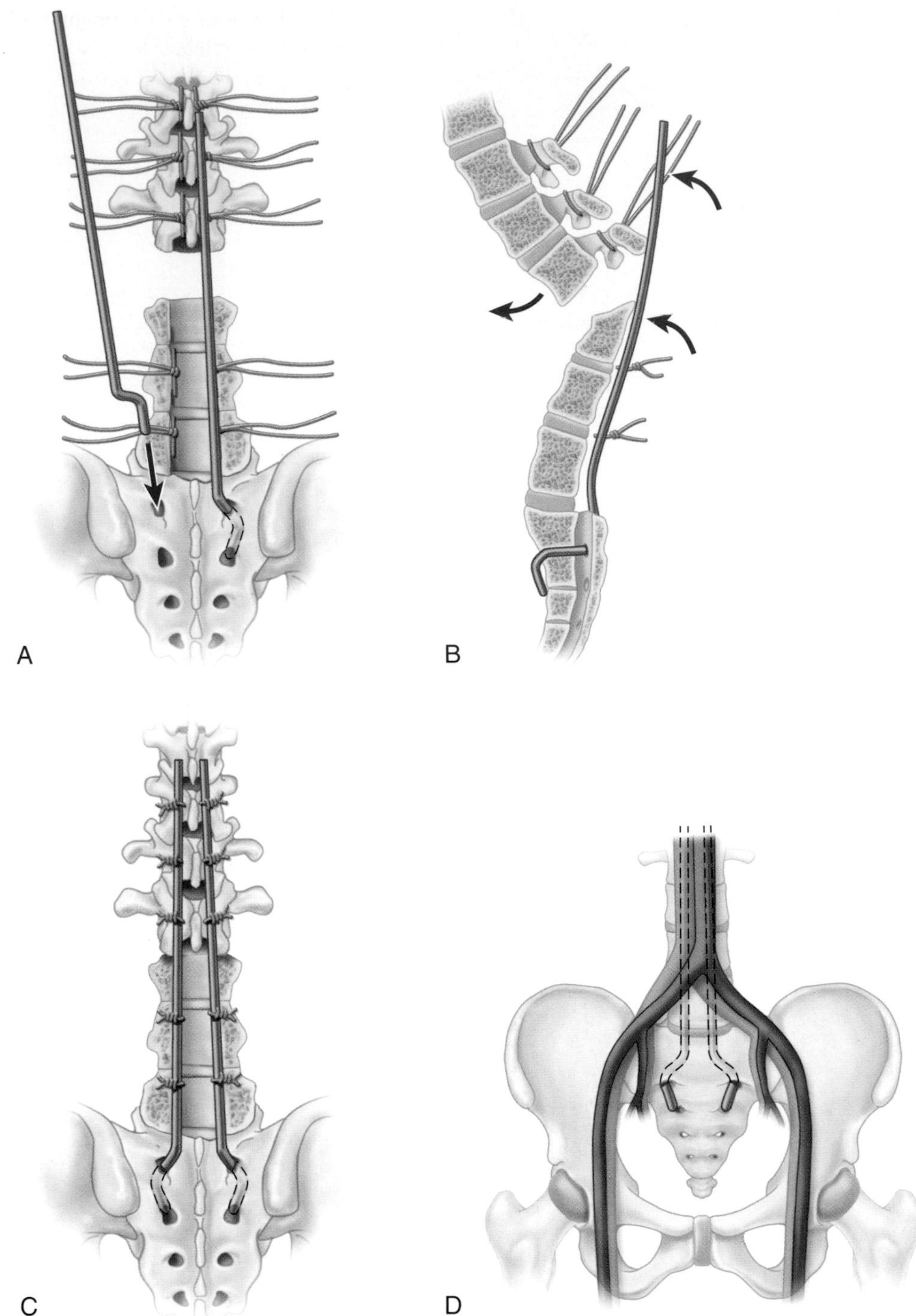

FIGURE 44-223 **A-D, Anterior fixation of kyphotic deformity in patients with myelomeningocele.** (From Warner WC Jr, Fackler CD: Comparison of two instrumentation techniques in treatment of lumbar kyphosis in myelodysplasia, J Pediatr Orthop 13:704, 1993.) **SEE TECHNIQUE 44-66.**

- Many techniques have been described for fixation of the kyphotic deformity, but L-rod instrumentation to the pelvis with segmental wires is our preferred method (Fig. 44-222F). The distal end of the rod can be contoured. We prefer to use a prebent, right-angled rod and pass the bend through the S1 foramen rather than around the ala of the sacrum. This is the method of Warner and Fackler (Fig. 44-223).
- Move the distal segment to the proximal segment and tighten the segmental wires.

POSTOPERATIVE CARE. If fixation is secure, the patient may be mobilized in a wheelchair as tolerated. Some patients in whom the bone is too osteoporotic and the stability of internal fixation is in doubt may be kept at bed rest or may require postoperative custom bracing. The fusion usually is solid in 6 to 9 months.

The postoperative care of these patients requires close observation by all subspecialty consultants involved. Postoperative infections, urinary tract problems, skin problems, and pseudarthrosis are frequent. The improved function, however, and the prevention of progression of the kyphosis make surgery worth the risks.

Paralytic kyphosis is treated with more standard techniques. When surgery becomes necessary, anterior fusion over the area of the apex and all levels of deficient posterior elements is done. This is followed by posterior fusion and instrumentation.

SACRAL AGENESIS

Sacral agenesis is a rare lesion that often is associated with maternal diabetes mellitus. Renshaw postulated that the condition is teratogenically induced or is a spontaneous genetic mutation that predisposes to or causes failure of embryonic induction of the caudal notochord sheath and ventral spinal cord. The dorsal ganglia and the dorsal (sensory) portion of the spinal cord continue to develop. The vertebrae and motor nerves are not subsequently induced, and the sacral agenesis results. Sensation remains intact because the dorsal ganglia and the dorsal portion of the spinal cord have been derived from the neural crest tissue. This disturbance in the normal sequence of development explains the observation that the lowest vertebral body with pedicles corresponds closely to the motor level, whereas the sensory level is distal to the motor level.

Renshaw proposed the following classification: type I, either total or partial unilateral sacral agenesis (Fig. 44-224A); type II, partial sacral agenesis with partial but bilaterally symmetric defects and a stable articulation between the ilia and a normal or hypoplastic S1 vertebra (Fig. 44-224B); type III, variable lumbar and total sacral agenesis with the ilia articulating with the sides of the lowest vertebra present (Fig. 44-224C); and type IV, variable lumbar and total sacral agenesis with the caudal endplate of the lowest vertebra resting above either fused ilia or an iliac amphiarthrosis (Fig. 44-224D). Type II defects are most common, and type I are least common. Types I and II usually have a stable vertebral-pelvic articulation, whereas types III and IV produce instability and possibly a progressive kyphosis.

The clinical appearance of a child with sacral agenesis ranges from one of severe deformities of the pelvis and lower extremities to no deformity or weakness whatsoever. Those with partial sacral or coccygeal agenesis may have no symptoms. Those with lumbar or complete sacral agenesis may be severely deformed, with multiple musculoskeletal abnormalities, including foot deformities, knee flexion contractures with popliteal webbing, hip flexion contractures, dislocated hips, spinal-pelvic instability, and scoliosis. The posture of the lower extremities has been compared with a "sitting Buddha" (Fig. 44-225). Anomalies of the viscera, especially in the

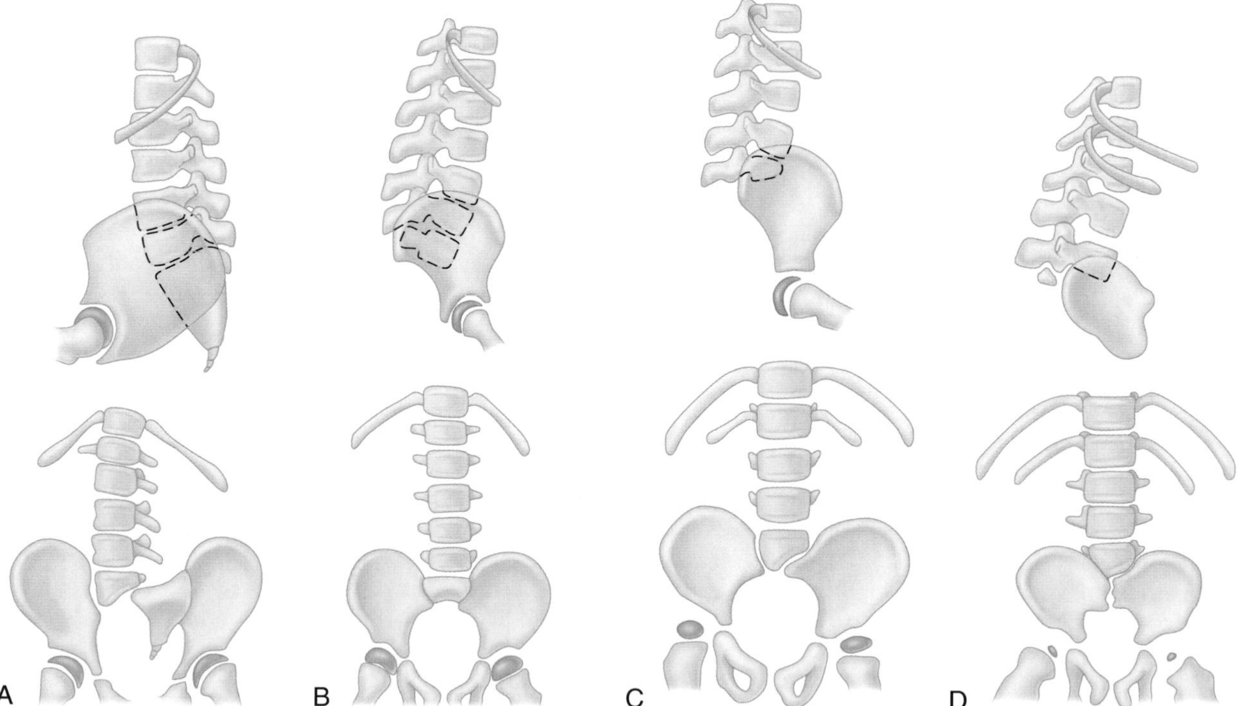

FIGURE 44-224 Types of sacral agenesis. **A,** Type I, total or partial unilateral sacral agenesis. **B,** Type II, partial sacral agenesis with partial, bilateral symmetric defects in stable articulation between ilia and normal or hypoplastic S1 vertebra. **C,** Type III, variable lumbar and total sacral agenesis; ilia articulate with lowest vertebra. **D,** Type IV, variable lumbar and total sacral agenesis; caudal endplate of lowest vertebra rests above fused ilia or iliac amphiarthrosis.

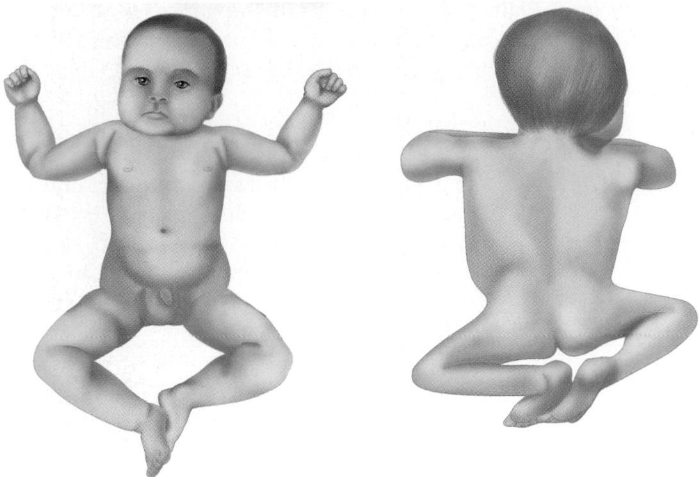

FIGURE 44-225 Severe knee flexion contractures with popliteal wedging and hip flexion deformities or contractures in children with lumbosacral agenesis result in the "sitting Buddha" position.

genitourinary system and the rectal area, are common. Inspection of the back reveals a bone prominence representing the last vertebral segment, often with gross motion between this vertebral prominence and the pelvis. Flexion and extension may occur at the junction of the spine and pelvis rather than at the hips.

Neurologic examination usually reveals intact motor power down to the level of the lowest vertebral body that has pedicles. Sensation, however, is present down to more caudal levels. Even patients with the most severe involvement may have sensation to the knees and spotty hypesthesia distally. Bladder and bowel control often is impaired.

■ TREATMENT

Phillips et al. reviewed the orthopaedic management of lumbosacral agenesis and concluded that patients with partial absence of the sacrum only (types I and II) have an excellent chance of becoming community ambulators. Management of more severe deformities (types III and IV) is more controversial.

Scoliosis is the most common spinal anomaly associated with sacral agenesis. No correlation has been found between the type of defect and the likelihood of scoliosis. Scoliosis may be associated with congenital anomalies, such as hemivertebra, or with no obvious spinal abnormality above the level of the vertebral agenesis. Progressive scoliosis or kyphosis requires operative stabilization as for similar scoliosis without sacral agenesis.

The treatment of spinal-pelvic instability is more controversial. Perry et al. noted that the key to rehabilitation of a patient with an unstable spinal-pelvic junction is establishment of a stable vertebral-pelvic complex around which lower extremity contractures can be stretched or operatively released. Renshaw also emphasized that patients with type III or type IV defects must be observed closely for signs of progressive kyphosis. If progressive deformity is noted, he recommended lumbopelvic arthrodesis as early as is consistent with successful fusion. In his series, fusion was done in patients 4 years of age or older. Ferland et al. reported successful spinopelvic fusion using vascularized rib grafts, with good outcomes in their patients. Phillips et al., however, found that spinal-pelvic instability was not a problem in 18 of the 20 surviving patients at long-term follow-up. Others noted an actual decrease in the ability to sit after stabilization of the lumbopelvic area. Proper care of patients with sacral agenesis is best provided by a treatment team, including an orthopaedic surgeon, urologist, neurosurgeon, pediatrician, physical therapist, and orthotist-prosthetist.

BOX 44-13

Clinical Criteria for Diagnosis of Neurofibromatosis

For the diagnosis of neurofibromatosis to be made, two of the following features are necessary:

- A minimum of six café au lait spots larger than 1.5 cm in diameter in a postpubertal patient and larger than 5 mm in diameter in prepubertal patients
- Two or more neurofibromas of any type or one plexiform neurofibroma
- Freckling in the inguinal or axillary regions
- Optic glioma
- Two or more iris Lisch nodules by slit-lamp examination
- A distinctive osseous lesion
- A first-degree relative with a definitive diagnosis of neurofibromatosis

UNUSUAL CAUSES OF SCOLIOSIS

NEUROFIBROMATOSIS

Neurofibromatosis is a hereditary hamartomatous disorder of neural crest derivation. These hamartomatous tissues may appear in any organ system of the body. The most widely described clinical forms of neurofibromatosis are the peripheral (NF1) and central (NF2) types.

The classic neurofibromatosis (NF1) described by von Recklinghausen is an autosomal dominant disorder that affects approximately 1 in 4000 people. Patients with NF1 develop Schwann cell tumors and pigmentation abnormalities. Orthopaedic problems are frequent in patients with this type of neurofibromatosis, with spinal deformity being the most common.

Central neurofibromatosis (NF2) also is an autosomal dominant disorder; however, it is much less common. It is characterized by bilateral acoustic neuromas. NF2 usually does not have any bone involvement or orthopaedic manifestations.

The diagnosis of NF1 is based on clinical criteria (Box 44-13). Scoliosis is the most common osseous defect associated with neurofibromatosis. Studies have reported spinal disorders in 10% to 60% of patients with neurofibromatosis.

The spinal deformities of neurofibromatosis are of two basic forms: nondystrophic and dystrophic. Nondystrophic deformities mimic idiopathic scoliosis and behave accordingly; the neurofibromatosis seems to have little influence on the curve or its treatment. Functional scoliosis also may develop and is caused by a leg-length discrepancy resulting

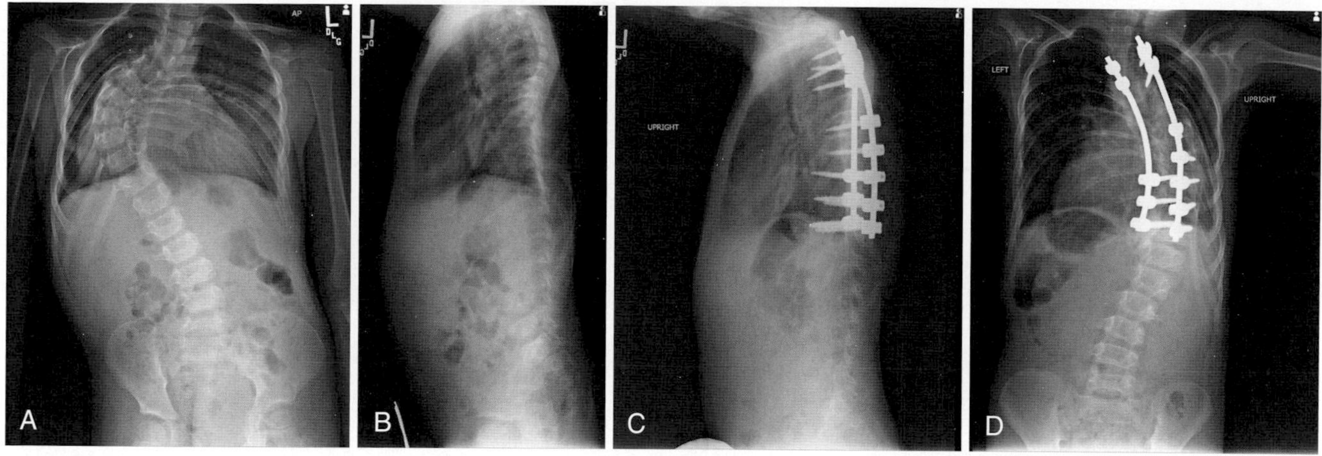

FIGURE 44-226 **A** and **B**, Dystrophic scoliosis. **C** and **D**, After posterior thoracic fusion and instrumentation.

from lower extremity hypertrophy or dysplasia of the long bones. Dystrophic scoliosis characteristically is a short-segment, sharply angulated curve with severe wedging of the vertebral bodies, severe rotation of the vertebrae, scalloping of the vertebral bodies, spindling of the transverse processes, foraminal enlargement, and rotation of the ribs 90 degrees in the anteroposterior direction that makes them appear abnormally thin. Rib penetration into the spinal canal has even been reported. Curves with significant sagittal plane deformity are common in dystrophic scoliosis. Dystrophic curves usually progress without treatment in patients with neurofibromatosis. Lykissas et al. found that the presence of three or more dystrophic features was highly predictive of curve progression and the need for operative stabilization (Fig. 44-226). Neurofibromatosis kyphoscoliosis is characterized by acute angulation in the sagittal plane and striking deformity of the vertebral bodies near the apex. Paraplegia has been reported in patients with this type of kyphoscoliosis. Severe thoracic lordoscoliosis also has been described in patients with neurofibromatosis.

MANAGEMENT OF NONDYSTROPHIC CURVES

Nondystrophic curves have the same prognosis and evolution as do idiopathic curves, except for a higher risk of pseudarthrosis after operative fusion. Dystrophic vertebral body changes may develop over time in nondystrophic curves. A spinal deformity that develops before 7 years of age should be observed closely for potential evolving dystrophic features (modulation). If the curve then acquires either three penciled ribs or a combination of three dystrophic features, clinical progression is almost a certainty. The general guidelines for treating nondystrophic curves are the same as for idiopathic curves other than watching closely for any modulation. Curves of less than 20 to 25 degrees are observed; if no dystrophic changes occur, a brace is prescribed when the deformity progresses to 30 degrees. If the deformity exceeds 40 to 45 degrees, a posterior spinal fusion with segmental instrumentation will produce results similar to those obtained in patients with idiopathic scoliosis. Also common in these patients are spinal canal neurofibromas, which may grow and cause pressure-induced dysplasia of the canal. CT myelography or MRI should be done before surgery to rule out the presence of any intraspinal canal neurofibroma.

MANAGEMENT OF DYSTROPHIC SCOLIOSIS

Brace treatment is probably not indicated for the typical dystrophic curve of neurofibromatosis. Appropriate operative treatment is determined by the presence or absence of a kyphotic deformity and by the presence or absence of neurologic deficits.

Before operative treatment of dystrophic curves in patients with neurofibromatosis, the presence of an intraspinal lesion, such as pseudomeningocele, dural ectasia, or intraspinal neurofibroma (dumbbell tumor), should be ruled out. Impingement of these lesions against the spinal cord has been reported to cause paraplegia after instrumentation of these curves. MRI or complete high-volume CT myelography in the prone, lateral, and supine positions should be done before operative treatment. Although myelography is adequate to evaluate the presence of intraspinal tumors or dural ectasia, MRI is better to evaluate displacement of the cord, subarachnoid extent of neurofibroma, or anterior abnormalities; however, MRI may be inadequate for the severe kyphoscoliotic deformity associated with dystrophic kyphoscoliosis, and high-volume computed myelography often is necessary. In a study by Ramachandran et al., 37% of patients in both the nondystrophic and dystrophic groups were found to have intraspinal and paraspinal neurofibromas. Significantly more tumors were identified adjacent to the convexity of the curve in the dystrophic group. Routine neural axis MRI evaluation in patients with NF1 and spinal deformity should be performed, particularly if surgical intervention is planned.

SCOLIOSIS WITHOUT KYPHOSIS

Patients with dystrophic scoliosis without kyphosis should be observed at 6-month intervals if the curve is less than 20 degrees. As soon as the progression of the curve is noted, a posterior spinal fusion should be done. If this fusion is done before the curve becomes too large, anterior fusion will not be necessary (Fig. 44-227). Traditionally, combined anterior and posterior fusion is recommended unless there are contraindications to the anterior approach (e.g., patients with anterior neurofibromas, excessive venous channels, poor medical condition, or thrombocytopenia caused by splenic obstruction by a fibroma or peculiar anatomic configurations). However, more recent studies have suggested that posterior fusion alone can stabilize curves less than 90

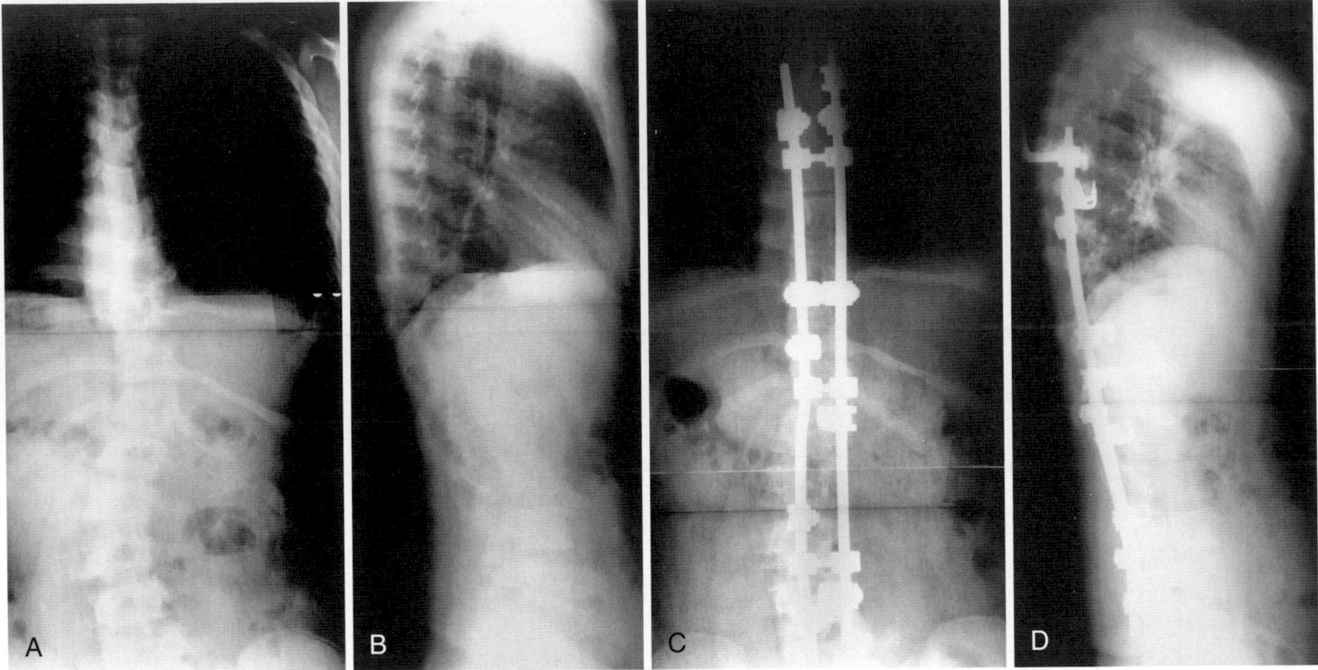

FIGURE 44-227 A and B, Dystrophic scoliosis. C and D, After posterior fusion and instrumentation.

degrees. Curves with kyphosis or with the apex below T8 should be considered for combined anterior and posterior fusion to decrease the rate of pseudarthrosis and curve progression. Segmental hook or screw instrumentation systems provide correction and permit ambulation with or without postoperative bracing. Sublaminar wires can be used to augment the instrumentation, particularly at the proximal end of the construction and across the apex of the curve. If instrumentation is tenuous, bracing should be used. The fusion mass must be followed carefully. If there is any question as to the status of the fusion mass, the surgical area is explored 1 year after surgery and additional autogenous bone grafting is done. Similarly, if progression of more than 10 degrees occurs, the fusion mass is explored and reinforced.

KYPHOSCOLIOSIS

Patients with dystrophic scoliosis and angular kyphosis have been shown to respond poorly to posterior fusion alone. Good results are obtained by combined anterior and posterior fusion. Reasons for fusion failure may include too little bone and too limited an area for fusion; therefore, Winter et al. recommended that the entire structural area of the deformity be fused anteriorly, with complete disc excision and strong strut grafts, preferably from the fibula, as well as rib and iliac crest grafts. Ideally, all anterior grafts should be in contact throughout with other grafts or with the spine. Grafts surrounded by soft tissue tend to be resorbed in the midportion. Early diagnosis and treatment by combined anterior and posterior fusion with internal fixation, if possible, is recommended. If anterior fusion is necessary for kyphoscoliotic deformities, vascularized rib graft augmentation as described by Bradford (Fig. 44-228) may be considered.

However, some authors have questioned the necessity of an anterior approach in all dystrophic kyphoscoliotic curves. For smaller dystrophic scoliosis with kyphosis of less than 40 degrees, posterior spinal instrumentation with arthrodesis is considered as soon as possible. The fusion mass should be explored at 1 year after surgery or sooner if progression of more than 10 degrees occurs.

KYPHOSCOLIOSIS WITH SPINAL CORD COMPRESSION

Spinal cord or cauda equina compression caused by spinal angulation, rib penetration, or tumor has been described. Cord compression caused by an intraspinal lesion must be distinguished from kyphotic angular cord compression by MRI or high-volume CT myelography in the prone, lateral, and supine positions. Patients with severe scoliosis without significant kyphosis and with evidence of paraplegia should be assumed to have an intraspinal lesion until proved otherwise. If cord compression is caused by kyphoscoliotic deformity, laminectomy is absolutely contraindicated. Removal of the posterior elements adds to the kyphosis and also removes valuable bone surface for a posterior fusion. If spinal cord compression is minor and no intraspinal tumor is present, halo-gravity traction can be used. The patient's neurologic status must be monitored carefully even if the kyphosis is mobile. As the alignment of the spinal canal improves and the compression is eliminated, anterior and posterior fusions can be done without direct observation of the cord. However, significant cord compression in patients with severe structural kyphoscoliosis requires anterior cord decompression. Anterior strut graft fusion must be done with this decompression, and posterior fusion is done as a second stage. If a tumor causes spinal cord compression anteriorly, anterior excision, spinal cord decompression, and fusion are indicated. If the lesion is posterior, a hemilaminectomy with tumor excision may be necessary. Instrumentation and fusion should be done at the time of decompression to prevent a rapidly increasing kyphotic deformity and neurologic injury.

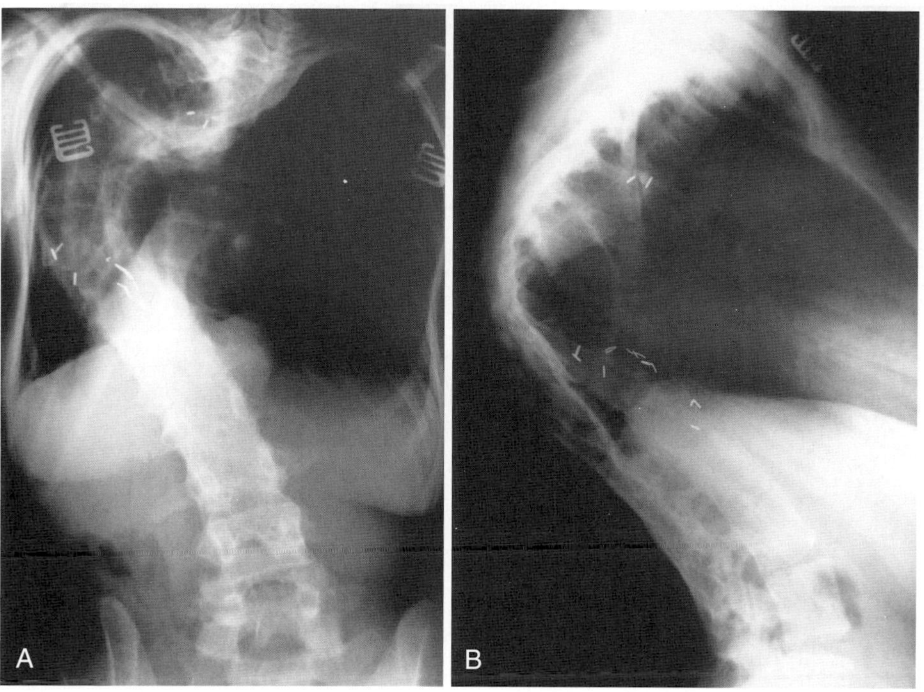

FIGURE 44-228 **A** and **B,** After anterior fusion with vascularized rib graft in patient with dystrophic kyphoscoliosis.

POSTOPERATIVE MANAGEMENT

Patients with nondystrophic curves are managed the same as those with idiopathic curves. If, however, the instrumentation is tenuous, casting or bracing is used. However, patients with dystrophic scoliosis should be considered for immobilization in a cast or brace until fusion is evident on anteroposterior, lateral, and oblique radiographs. Exploration of the fusion mass at 6 to 12 months after surgery may be necessary in dystrophic curves, and prolonged immobilization often is needed. Even after the fusion is solid, the patient should be observed annually to be certain that no erosion of the fusion mass is occurring.

COMPLICATIONS OF SURGERY

In addition to the complications inherent in any major spinal surgery, several complications are related to the neurofibromatosis. Plexiform venous anomalies can be present in the soft tissues surrounding the spine and can impede the operative approach to the vertebral bodies, leading to excessive bleeding. The increased vascularity of the neurofibromatous tissue itself also may increase blood loss. The angular deformity of the neurofibromatosis may cause significant mechanical problems with anterior strut grafting. The apical bodies may have subluxed into bayonet apposition or be so rotated that they no longer are in alignment with the rest of the spine. This malalignment does not allow the anterior strut grafts to be placed in the concavity of the kyphosis and makes them mechanically less effective in preventing its progression. Adequate anterior fusion may be difficult to obtain and should be performed on the concave side, with multiple strut grafts. Convex discectomies may further destabilize the spine, and placement of struts from the convex approach is technically difficult. Pheochromocytoma, a tumor arising from chromaffin cells, can be associated with neurofibromatosis and can create an anesthetic challenge. Patients with neurofibromatosis have a general tendency for decreased bone mineral density and osteopenia, possibly increasing the challenge of obtaining stable implant fixation to the spine.

Many patients with neurofibromatosis and scoliosis have cervical spine abnormalities (Fig. 44-229). Deformities of the cervical spine that cause cord compression and paraplegia have been reported in patients with neurofibromatosis. Cervical lesions associated with scoliosis or kyphoscoliosis have been classified into two groups: abnormalities of bone structure and abnormalities of vertebral alignment. Cervical anomalies are most common in patients with short kyphotic curves or thoracic or lumbar curves that measure more than 65 degrees. These patients are more likely to require anesthesia, traction, and operative stabilization of the spine. Routine radiographic evaluation of the cervical spine is recommended in all patients with neurofibromatosis before anesthesia for any reason and before traction for treatment of the scoliosis. High-grade spondylolisthesis of the lower lumbar spine also has been reported in association with neurofibromatosis. The entire spinal column must be carefully assessed for cervical and lumbosacral abnormalities.

Postoperative paralysis caused by contusion of the spinal cord by the periosteal elevator during exposure has been reported in two patients with unsuspected areas of laminar erosion because of dural ectasia. A total-spine MRI study or a complete high-volume myelography series in the prone, lateral, and supine positions would have alerted the surgeon to this before surgery. The most dangerous situation for neurologically intact patients with neurofibromatosis is instrumentation and distraction of the spine in the presence of unrecognized intraspinal lesions.

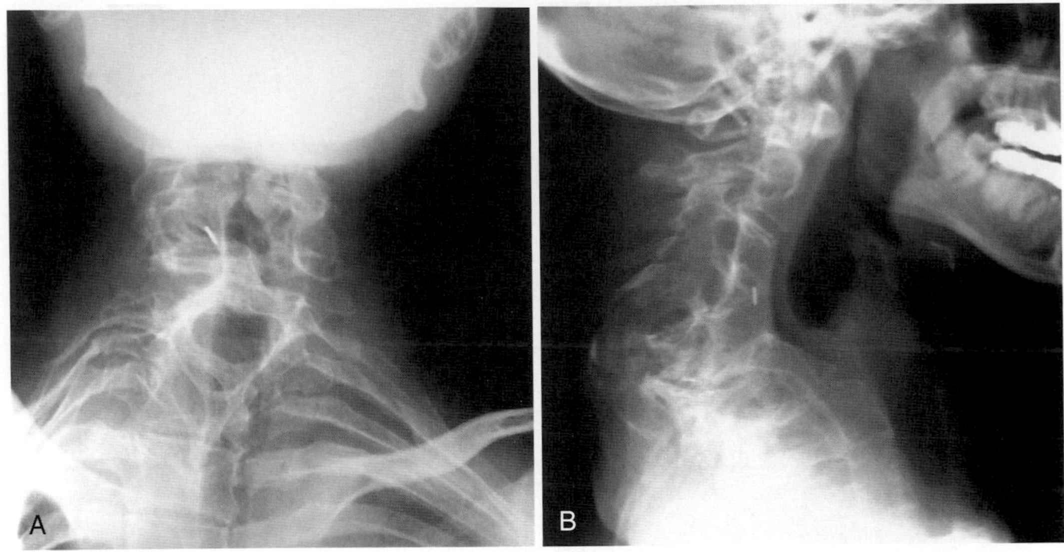

FIGURE 44-229 A and B, Cervical spine deformity in patient with neurofibromatosis.

MARFAN SYNDROME

Marfan syndrome is a disorder of connective tissue inherited as an autosomal dominant trait. It occurs in 1 to 2 per 10,000 persons and affects males and females equally. Sporadic occurrences reportedly account for 25% of patients. In most cases, a mutation in the fibrillin-1 *(FBN1)* gene has been implicated, resulting in abnormalities in a protein essential to proper formatting of elastic fibers found in connective tissue.

DIAGNOSIS

Genetic testing for *FNB1* mutations lacks sensitivity and specificity and is not efficient in all cases; therefore, the diagnosis of Marfan syndrome relies on physical findings, which have traditionally been divided into two categories: major and minor signs. Major signs include ectopia lentis, aortic dilation, severe kyphoscoliosis, and pectus deformity. Minor signs include myopia, tall stature, mitral valve prolapse, ligamentous laxity, and arachnodactyly. Newer diagnostic criteria place greater weight on cardiovascular manifestations; therefore, in the absence of a family history, the presence of both aortic root aneurysm and ectopia lentis is sufficient for the unequivocal diagnosis of Marfan syndrome. Screening tests for the Marfan phenotype in the orthopaedic examination include the thumb sign (the thumb extends well beyond the ulnar border of the hand when it is overlapped by the fingers), the wrist sign (the thumb overlaps the fifth finger as the patient grasps the opposite wrist), and the knee sign (the patient has the ability to touch the toes on the floor when sitting with the knees crossed). The diagnosis of Marfan syndrome frequently is delayed because cardiovascular involvement is a major diagnostic criterion and may not be evident until adolescence or adulthood. Scoliosis is reported to occur in 40% to 60% of patients with Marfan syndrome. These curves develop in patients with multiple major signs (definite diagnosis of Marfan), as well as those with only minor signs (Marfan phenotype). Marfan curves of less than 40 degrees in adults tend not to progress, whereas curves of more than 40 degrees progress (an average of 2.8 degrees a year in a study by Sponseller et al.); the curve patterns of scoliosis in Marfan syndrome are similar to those in idiopathic scoliosis. Double major curves are more frequent, and the scoliosis progresses more frequently in the infantile age group. Disabling back pain is more frequently a presenting complaint in patients with scoliosis associated with Marfan syndrome than in patients with idiopathic scoliosis. Sagittal plane deformities are common (Fig. 44-230). A thoracolumbar kyphosis can be found in patients with Marfan syndrome (Fig. 44-231). Characteristic vertebral anomalies also are found in these patients, including narrow pedicles, wide transverse processes, and vertebral scalloping. Spondylolisthesis associated with Marfan syndrome also has been reported in one study. Cervical spine abnormalities also are common in patients with Marfan syndrome, but clinical problems from these abnormalities are rare. Basilar impression and focal cervical kyphosis are the most commonly reported cervical spine abnormalities. The focal cervical kyphosis usually is associated with a lordotic thoracic spine.

NONOPERATIVE TREATMENT

OBSERVATION

For young patients with small curves of less than 25 degrees, observation every 3 to 4 months is indicated. The family should be made aware, however, that many of these curves progress.

ORTHOTIC TREATMENT

Brace treatment is less successful in patients with Marfan syndrome than in those with idiopathic scoliosis. Sponseller et al. reported successful brace treatment in 4 of 22 patients. Chest wall deformity, with narrowing of the inferior portion of the thoracic cage, also has been noted with the use of an underarm TLSO. Bracing should be considered for patients with flexible progressive curves between 25 and 40 degrees who do not have associated thoracic lordosis or lumbar kyphosis. Bracing is not indicated for large, rigid curves or curves associated with thoracic lordosis.

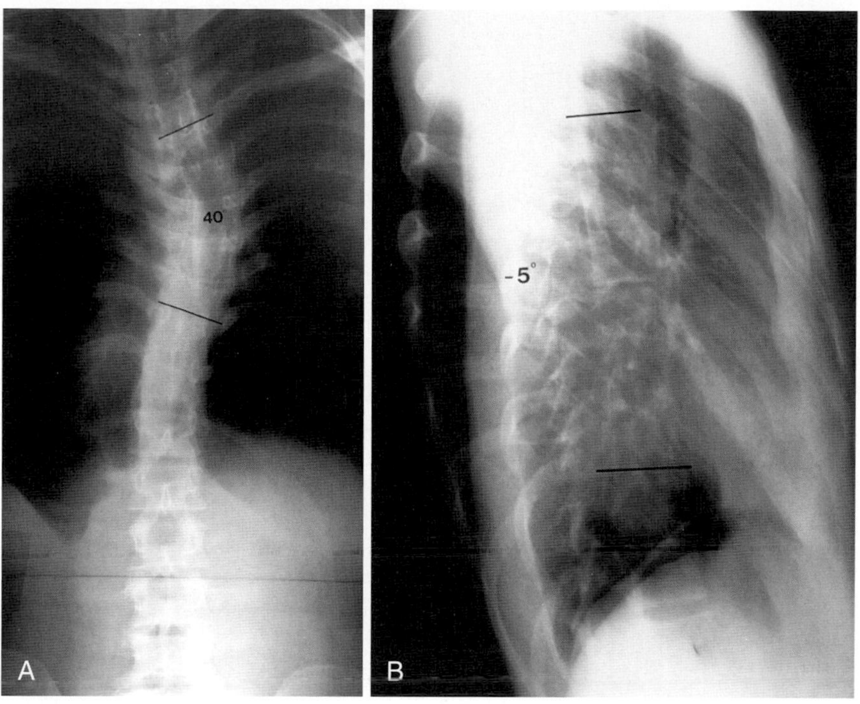

FIGURE 44-230 A and B, Thoracic lordosis in patient with Marfan syndrome.

OPERATIVE TREATMENT

If progression occurs despite bracing or if the curve exceeds 40 degrees, spinal fusion is recommended. If nonoperative treatment is continued too long, cardiovascular involvement may progress to the point of making surgery dangerous, if not impossible. Before operative intervention is considered, a complete cardiovascular evaluation is mandatory. Aortic dilation can develop in these patients at any time from childhood to late adolescence or adulthood. Echocardiography is recommended because its sensitivity for aortic root dilation greatly exceeds that of auscultation. Any evidence of aortic dilation should be treated medically or operatively before treatment of the spinal deformity.

Scoliosis in patients with Marfan syndrome can be corrected similar to the way it is corrected in idiopathic scoliosis, and solid fusion and maintenance of correction can be anticipated; however, Jones et al. and Gjolaj et al. found that the number of surgical complications was higher in patients with Marfan syndrome. Complications included increased blood loss, pseudarthroses (10%), dural tears (8%), infection (10%), and failure of fixation (21%). The development of scoliosis or kyphosis at the upper or lower fusion levels (adding on) can occur after surgery. Jones et al. found this complication to occur in the coronal plane in 8% of their patients and in the sagittal plane in 21%.

Large bone grafts, secure segmental internal fixation, and careful postoperative observation for pseudarthrosis are required in these patients. In general, the technique of instrumentation and selection of hook or screw levels are the same as for idiopathic scoliosis, but selection of the lowest instrumented vertebrae is ideally the neutral and stable vertebra in both the coronal and sagittal planes. Jones et al. recommended that any curve of more than 30 degrees should be included in the arthrodesis. As with all scoliotic deformity correction, care must be taken in determining the distal extent of the fusion to avoid junctional kyphosis.

Thoracic lordosis is relatively common in patients with Marfan syndrome and spinal deformity, and sagittal plane balance must be obtained in addition to improvement of the coronal plane deformity. Segmental instrumentation systems using hooks and pedicle screws or all pedicle screws are effective in correcting this problem. Surgical treatment should provide a more normal anteroposterior diameter of the chest, because this frequently is narrow.

Growing rod constructs have been used with success for patients with Marfan syndrome with early-onset scoliosis for which definitive spinal fusion is not possible because of skeletal immaturity. Dual rod constructs are recommended. Because these children will require multiple lengthening procedures, careful monitoring of the cardiovascular manifestations of Marfan syndrome is essential. Not all adolescents with Marfan syndrome and kyphosis require surgery, but those who do often require anterior fusion and posterior instrumentation and fusion. Typically, kyphosis in Marfan syndrome has a low thoracic or thoracolumbar apex and involvement of the lumbar spine.

Severe spondylolisthesis associated with Marfan syndrome has been reported. It has been postulated that the spondylolisthesis may be more likely to progress because of poor musculoligamentous tissues. Successful treatment of grade IV spondylolisthesis with in situ fusion has been reported.

VERTEBRAL COLUMN TUMORS

Because of their variable presentation, tumors of the vertebral column often present diagnostic problems. A team composed of a surgeon, a diagnostic radiologist, a pathologist, and often a medical oncologist and radiotherapist is necessary for

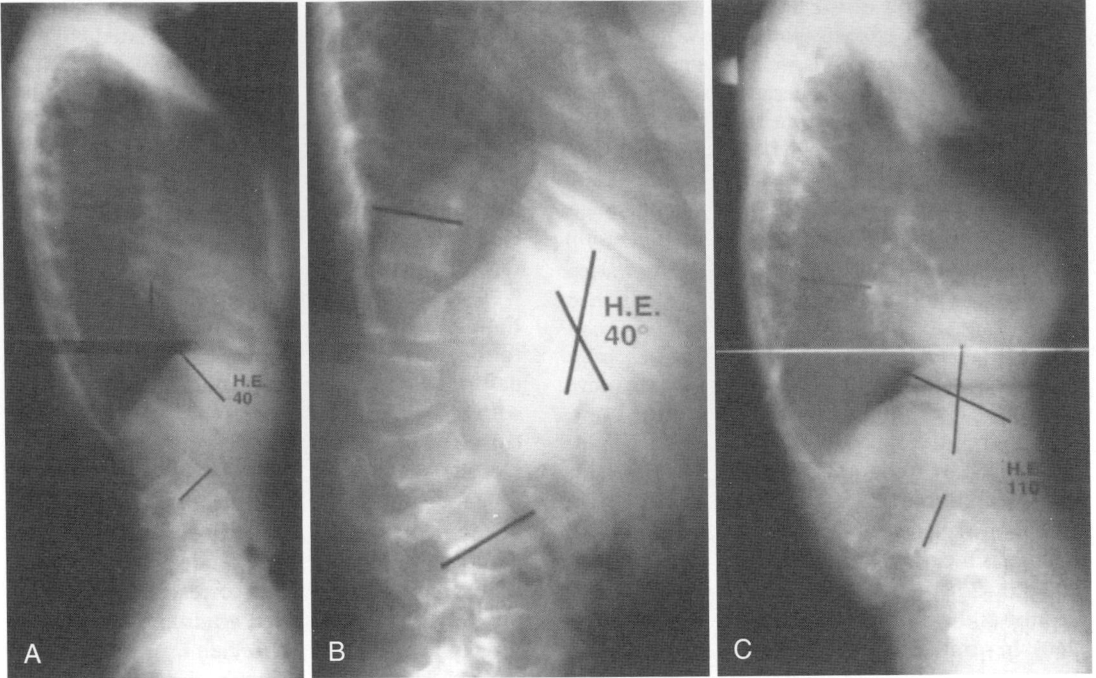

FIGURE 44-231 **A** and **B**, Lateral radiographs of 17-year-old child with Marfan syndrome and 40-degree progressive thoracolumbar kyphosis. **C**, Lateral radiograph of same patient 3 years later shows that thoracolumbar kyphosis has progressed to 110 degrees. (From Warner WC: Kyphosis. In Morrissy RT, Weinstein SL, editors: Lovell and Winter's pediatric orthopaedics, ed 6, Philadelphia, 2006, Lippincott Williams & Wilkins.)

treatment of the spectrum of tumors that involve the spine. The discussion in this section is on the most common primary tumors of the vertebral column in children.

CLINICAL FINDINGS

A complete history is the first step in the evaluation of any patient with a tumor. The initial complaint of patients with tumors involving the spine generally is pain. The exact type and distribution of pain vary with the anatomic location of the pathologic process. In general, pain caused by a neoplasm is not relieved by rest and often is worse at night. On occasion, constitutional symptoms such as anorexia, weight loss, and fever may be present. The age and sex of the patient may be important in the differential diagnosis.

Physical examination should include a general evaluation in addition to careful examination of the spine. The tumor may produce local tenderness, muscle spasm, scoliosis, and limited spine motion. Painful scoliosis can be the result of a spinal tumor. In such cases, the tumor is usually located at the concavity of the curve. Spine deformity also may be secondary to vertebral collapse or muscular spasms caused by pain. More than 50% of patients with malignant tumors of the spine present with neurologic symptoms. A careful neurologic examination is essential.

Laboratory studies should include a complete blood cell count, urinalysis, and sedimentation rate, as well as determination of serum calcium, phosphorus, and alkaline phosphatase concentrations. Alkaline phosphatase may be elevated two to three times normal in patients with osteosarcoma. Lactate dehydrogenase is a reliable indicator of the tumor burden in patients with Ewing sarcoma. An elevated white blood cell count with thrombocytopenia is characteristic of leukemia. Further laboratory studies may be indicated based on the clinical course.

RADIOGRAPHIC EVALUATION AND TREATMENT

Radiographs of the spine should be made in at least two planes at 90-degree angles. The radiographs should be evaluated for the presence of scoliosis, kyphosis, loss of lumbar lordosis, destruction of pedicles, congenital vertebral anomalies, lytic lesions, altered size of neural foramina, abnormal calcifications, and soft-tissue masses. If a scoliotic curve is present, the curve usually shows significant coronal decompensation. There is an absence of the usual compensatory balancing curve above or below the curve containing the lesion. The scoliosis lacks the usual structural characteristics associated with idiopathic scoliosis, such as vertebral rotation and wedging. Curves with these characteristics should raise the index of suspicion for an underlying cause of the scoliosis.

Bone scanning is helpful in certain tumors of the spine, especially osteoid osteoma. CT has greatly improved evaluation of the extent of the lesion and the presence of any spinal canal compromise; sagittal and coronal reformatted images are necessary to define the exact anatomic location and extent of the lesion. MRI is useful in evaluating the extent of soft-tissue involvement of the tumor and for determining the level and extent of neurologic compromise in patients with a neurologic deficit.

Arteriography may be indicated to evaluate the extent of the tumor and to localize major feeder vessels.

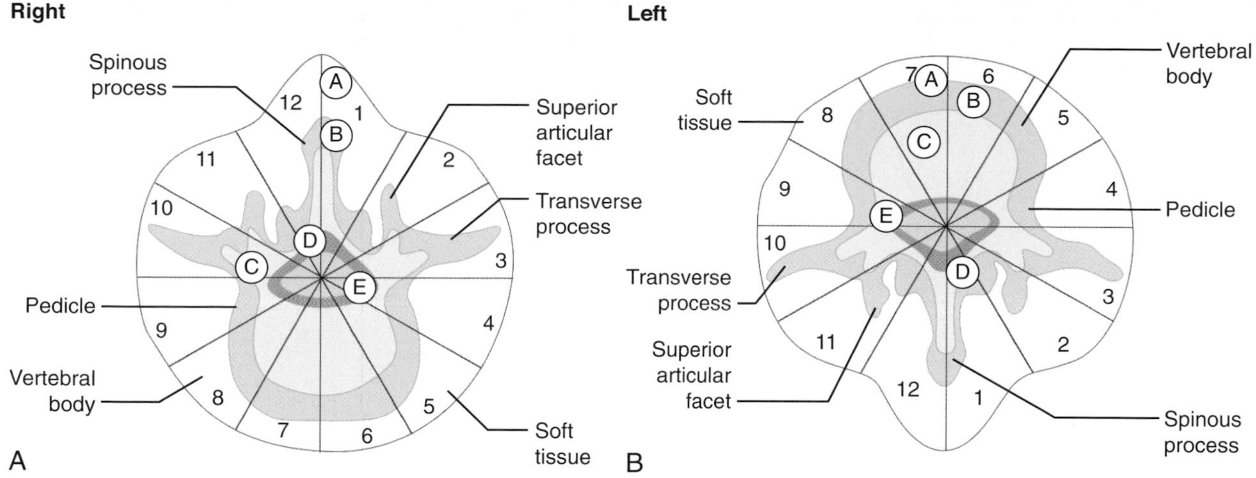

FIGURE 44-232 **A,** Weinstein-Boriani-Biagini tumor classification system. The vertebra is divided into 12 radiating zones that are numbered clockwise, beginning at one half of the spinous process. The concentric layers are lettered sequentially from extraosseous soft tissues to the intradural space. **B,** The Spine Oncology Study Group modified the classification by numbering the radial zones in a counterclockwise fashion, beginning at the left half of the spinous process to allow for a more anatomic orientation of the diagram for ease of use. **Circled letters:** *A,* extraosseous soft tissues; *B,* intraosseous (superficial); *C,* intraosseous (deep); *D,* extraosseous (extradural); *E,* extraosseous (intradural). (**A** redrawn from Boriani S, Weinstein JN, Biagini R: Primary bone tumors of the spine: terminology and surgical staging, Spine 22:1036, 1997. **B** redrawn from Chan P, Boriani S, Fourney DR, et al: An assessment of the reliability of the Enneking and Weinstein-Boriani-Biagini classifications for staging of primary spinal tumors by the Spine Oncology Study Group, Spine 34:384, 2009.)

Surgical staging classification systems specific to spine tumors have been designed to guide treatment and aid in defining the prognosis. The surgical staging systems proposed by Boriani et al. and Tomita et al. were devised to aid in surgical planning and are used to delineate the margins of the tumor. The Weinstein-Boriani-Biagini (WBB) classification is an alphanumeric system that can be used to evaluate the extent of a lesion in the axial plane by dividing the vertebrae into 12 radial zones and five concentric layers with a designation for the presence of metastasis (Fig. 44-232). The Spine Oncology Study Group modified this system by orienting the diagram to correspond to the orientation of the vertebrae on axial tomograms. The tumor is reported according to the spinal level or levels affected in the cephalocaudal dimension. The method of surgical excision is based on the zone or zones that the tumor occupies. Tomita et al. classified tumors based on their anatomic location in the axial and sagittal planes using a numeric system that reflects the most common progression of tumor growth (Figs. 44-233 and 44-234); this classification is used to guide surgical management.

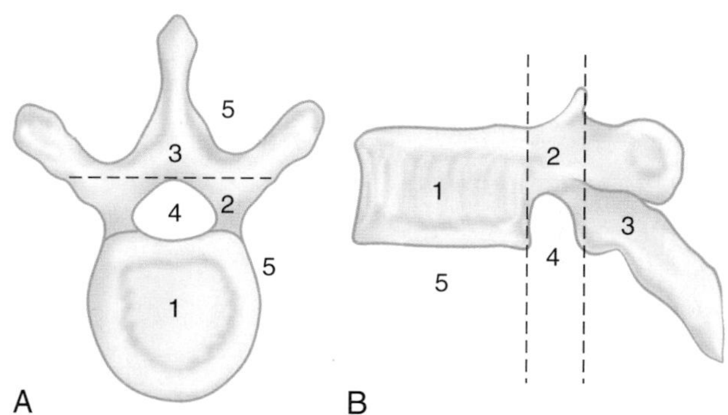

FIGURE 44-233 Axial **(A)** and lateral **(B)** illustrations of the Tomita anatomic classification of primary spinal malignant tumors. Lesions are classified by their location on the vertebra using a numeric scheme that reflects the most common progression of tumor growth: 1, vertebral body; 2, pedicle; 3, lamina and transverse and spinous processes; 4, spinal canal and epidural space; and 5, paravertebral space. (Redrawn from Tomita K, Kawahara N, Baba H, et al: Total en bloc spondylectomy: a new surgical technique for primary malignant vertebral tumors, Spine 22:324, 1997.)

■ BIOPSY

Certain tumors, such as osteochondroma and osteoid osteoma, generally can be diagnosed by their clinical presentation and radiographic appearance. Other benign tumors, such as osteoblastoma, aneurysmal bone cyst, and giant cell tumors, often are difficult to diagnose preoperatively. Biopsy is the ultimate diagnostic technique for evaluating neoplasms. The biopsy may be incisional (removal of a small portion of the tumor) or excisional (removal of the entire tumor).

Percutaneous CT-guided needle biopsy is an excellent diagnostic tool. Ghelman et al. obtained histologic diagnoses in 85% of 76 biopsy specimens, and Kattapuram, Khurana, and Rosenthal obtained accurate diagnoses in 92%. Metastatic diseases were most often diagnosed accurately (95%), and benign primary tumors were diagnosed least often (82%). Fine-needle cytologic aspirates are satisfactory for diagnosis of metastatic disease and most infections, but large-core biopsy specimens are preferable for primary bone tumors.

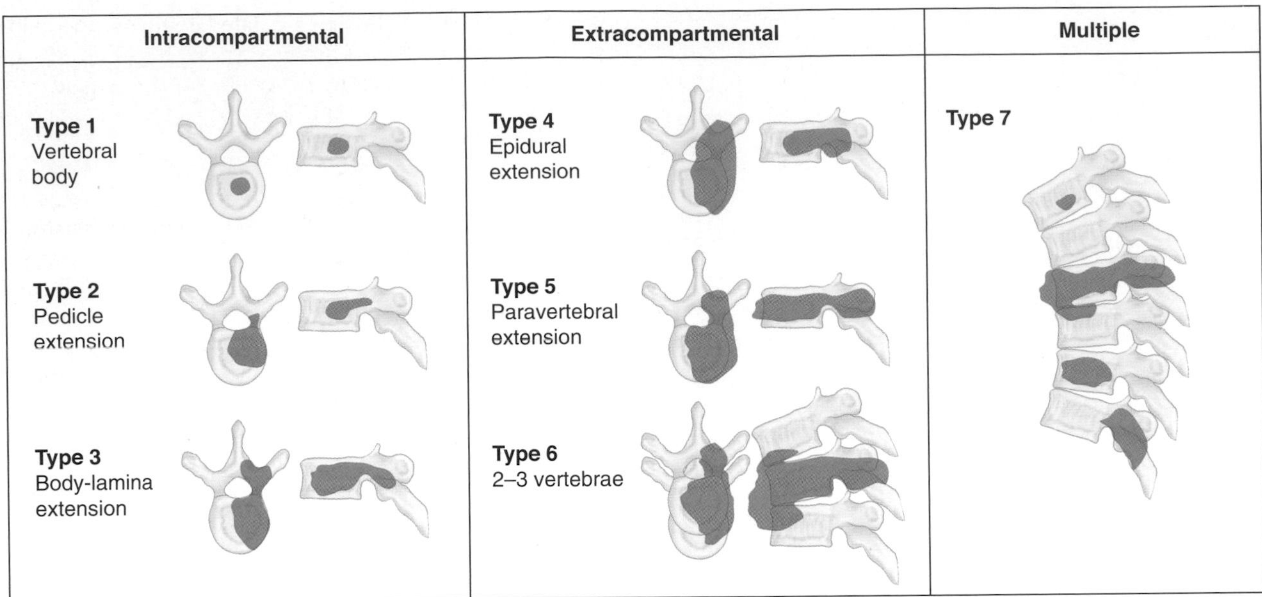

FIGURE 44-234 **Tomita surgical classification of spinal tumors. Tumor types are categorized based on the number of vertebral areas affected.** (Redrawn from Tomita K, Kewahara N, Baba H, et al: Total en bloc spondylectomy: a new surgical technique for primary malignant vertebral tumors, Spine 22:324, 1997.)

OPEN BIOPSY OF THORACIC VERTEBRA

If the needle biopsy is not diagnostic, an open biopsy or transpedicular biopsy will yield more tissue. Care must be taken that the open biopsy does not interfere with the definitive surgery if total resection is anticipated.

TECHNIQUE 44-67

(MICHELE AND KRUEGER)

- With the patient prone, make an incision over the side of the spinous process of the involved vertebra.
- Retract the muscles and expose the transverse process.
- Perform an osteotomy at the base of the transverse process at its junction with the lamina (Fig. 44-235A).
- By depressing or retracting the transverse process, expose the isthmus of the vertebra, revealing the cancellous nature of its bone structure. Radiographic verification of the level is important.
- Insert a $\frac{3}{16}$-inch trephine with $\frac{1}{4}$-inch markings through the fenestra and guide it downward with slight pressure so that a mere twisting action leads the trephine into the pedicle and finally into the body (Fig. 44-235B). Remove the trephine repeatedly and in each instance check that the contents consist of cancellous bone, which indicates that the trephine is in the medullary substance of the pedicle and has created a channel from the posterior elements directly into the vertebral body.
- Remove the pathologic tissue with a small blunt curet.
- Alternatively, after the osteotomy of the base of the transverse process, expose the vertebral body by retracting the transverse process and depressing the adjacent rib to expose the junction of the pedicle and the body.
- Use the trephine to penetrate this junction at an angle of 45 degrees toward the midline and remove the material with a curet (Fig. 44-235C).

BENIGN TUMORS OF THE VERTEBRAL COLUMN

The most common benign tumors of the vertebral column in children are osteoid osteoma, osteoblastoma, aneurysmal bone cyst, eosinophilic granuloma, and hemangioma.

OSTEOID OSTEOMA

Osteoid osteoma is a benign growth that consists of a discrete osteoid nidus and reactive sclerotic bone thickening around the nidus. No malignant change of these tumors has ever been documented. The lesion occurs more frequently in males than in females. Spinal lesions occur predominantly in the posterior elements of the spine, especially the lamina and the pedicles. Osteoid osteoma of the vertebral body has been reported but is rare. The lumbar spine is the most frequently involved area.

Typically, patients with spinal osteoid osteoma have pain that is worse at night and relieved by aspirin. The pain increases with activity and often is localized to the site of the lesion. Radicular symptoms are especially common with lesions of the lumbar spine. Lesions in the cervical spine can produce radicular-type symptoms in the shoulders and arms, but the results of the neurologic examination usually are normal.

Physical examination reveals muscle spasm in the involved area of the spine. The patient's gait may be abnormal because of pain, and localized tenderness over the tumor may be moderate to severe.

Osteoid osteoma is the most common cause of painful scoliosis in adolescents, especially if the vertebral column

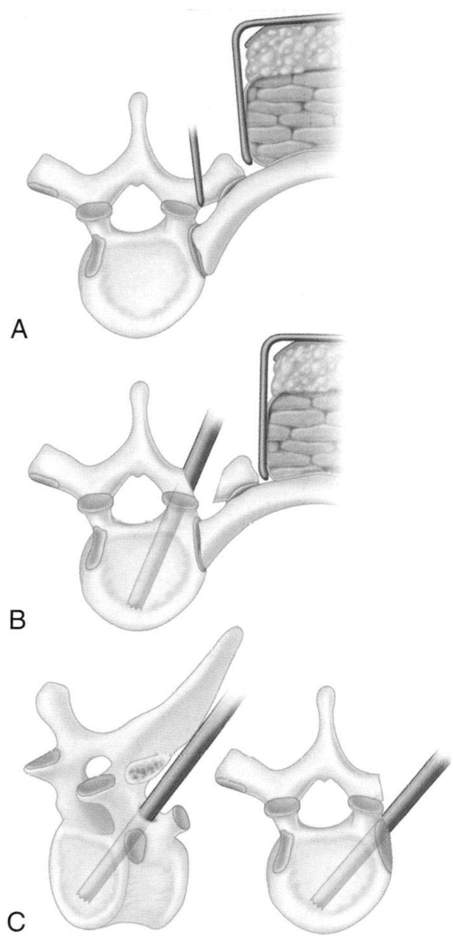

FIGURE 44-235 **A,** Transverse osteotomy at base of thoracic transverse process. **B,** Trephine through fenestra of isthmus, into pedicle and body. **C,** Trephine inserted into body at junction of pedicle. **SEE TECHNIQUE 44-67.**

is involved. The scoliosis associated with osteoid osteoma usually is described as a C-shaped curve, but only 23% to 33% of patients have this classic curve pattern. The osteoid osteoma usually is located on the concave side of the curve and in the area of the apical vertebra.

When the osteoid osteoma is visible on plain radiographs, its appearance is diagnostic—a central radiolucency with a surrounding sclerotic bony reaction; however, the lesion often is not visible on plain films. Technetium bone scanning should be considered in any adolescent with painful scoliosis (Fig. 44-236A). False-negative bone scans have not been reported in patients with osteoid osteoma of the spine. CT with very narrow cuts will precisely define the location of the tumor and the extent of the osseous involvement (Fig. 44-236B).

Patients with spinal tumors and scoliosis reach a critical point after which the continuation of a painful stimulus results in structural changes in the spine. Pettine and Klassen found that 15 months is the critical duration of symptoms if antalgic scoliosis is to undergo spontaneous correction after excision of the tumor. Although the natural course of many osteoid osteomas is spontaneous remission, spinal lesions in children or adolescents should be removed when they are diagnosed to prevent the development of structural scoliosis. The operative treatment of an osteoid osteoma is complete removal; recurrence is likely after incomplete removal. If pain and deformity persist after removal of the lesion, incomplete removal or perhaps a multifocal lesion should be suspected. Exact localization of the tumor is imperative. Rinsky et al. reported the intraoperative localization of the lesion by radionuclide imaging and the use of a gamma camera, but the camera is bulky, and it is often difficult to pinpoint the location of the nidus of the osteoid osteoma in this manner. The best way to determine the exact location of the nidus preoperatively is with high-resolution CT. Technetium can be injected 2 to 3 hours before surgery, and the specimen can be sent for in vitro radionuclide evaluation. If the specimen can be excised en bloc, a CT scan of the specimen may show the nidus.

Excision of these lesions usually does not require spinal fusion, but if removal of a significant portion of the facet

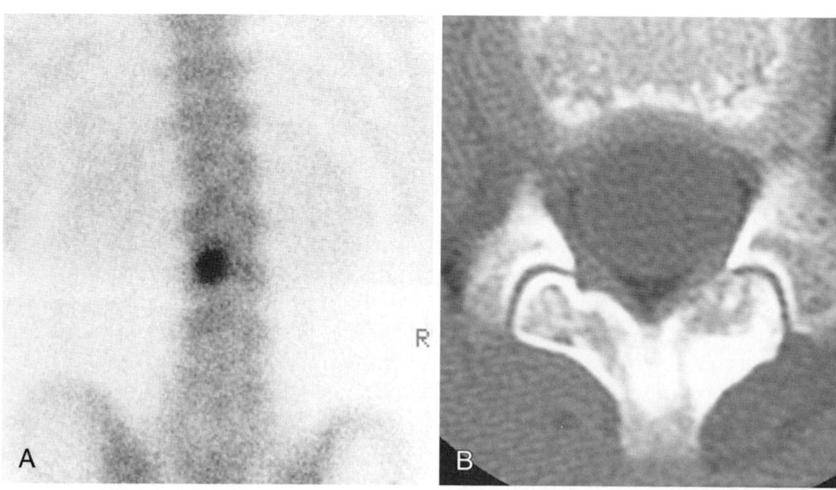

FIGURE 44-236 Bone scan **(A)** and CT scan **(B)** of patient with spinal osteoid osteoma.

joints and pedicles makes the spine unstable, spinal fusion can be done at the time of tumor removal. Surgical navigation systems such as the O-arm can be used intraoperatively to evaluate the adequacy of resection. This is the preferred method if it is available in the treating institution.

OSTEOBLASTOMA

Most authors believe that osteoid osteoma and osteoblastoma are variant manifestations of a benign osteoblastic process, resulting in an osteoid nidus surrounded by sclerotic bone. The lesions are histologically similar. The primary difference is the tendency of the osteoblastoma to form a less sclerotic but more expansile mass. Lesions larger than 1.5 cm in diameter are defined as osteoblastomas and those less than 1.5 cm as osteoid osteomas.

Benign osteoblastoma is an uncommon primary bone tumor that accounts for less than 1% of all bone tumors. Of these reported tumors, however, 40% have been located in the spine and more than one half were associated with scoliosis. The presenting symptom for most patients is pain; however, often the nonspecificity of symptoms may contribute to a delay in diagnosis. In one study, pain was present for an average of 16 months before the diagnosis was made, and scoliosis was present in 50% of patients with osteoblastomas involving the thoracic or lumbar spine. The osteoblastomas were always located in the concavity of the curve, near its apex.

In contrast to osteoid osteoma, plain radiographs often are sufficient to confirm the diagnosis of osteoblastoma. CT scans and bone scans (Fig. 44-237), however, can be helpful for a cross-sectional evaluation and localization of the tumor before operative excision. Osteoblastoma of the spine involves predominantly the posterior elements (66%) or the posterior elements and vertebral bodies (31%). A neoplasm involving only a vertebral body is unlikely to be an osteoblastoma. Spinal osteoblastomas are typically expansile with a scalloped or lobulated contour, well-defined margins, and frequently a sclerotic rim.

The treatment of osteoblastoma of the spine is complete operative excision. Recurrences after incomplete curettage are not rare, and malignant change has been reported after incomplete curettage; complete excision is therefore advised whenever possible. Because of the possibility of late sarcomatous changes, irradiation of this lesion is not recommended. The scoliosis associated with vertebral column osteoblastoma usually is reversible after excision if the diagnosis is made early and treatment is undertaken at that time. Akbarnia and Rooholamini found that the scoliosis improved in three patients who had symptoms for 9 months or less before excision of the tumor; the scoliosis did not improve in two patients whose symptoms had been present for longer periods.

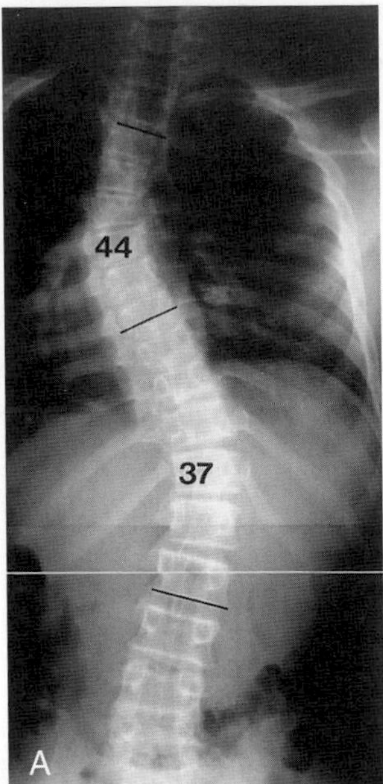

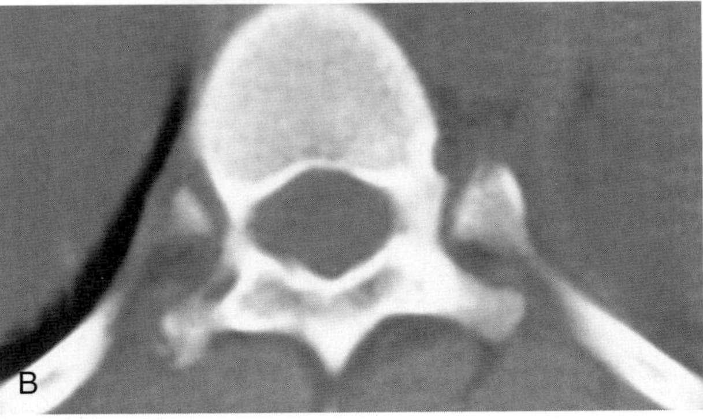

FIGURE 44-237 Radiograph **(A)** and CT scan **(B)** of patient with osteoblastoma on right side of spine that caused left thoracic curve.

ANEURYSMAL BONE CYSTS

An aneurysmal bone cyst is a nonneoplastic, vasocystic tumor originating on either a previously normal bone or a preexisting lesion. It is most common in children and young adults, and vertebral involvement is common. Its radiographic appearance is characteristic—an expansile lesion confined by a thin rim of reactive bone. The lesion can occur in the vertebral body but is more commonly seen in the posterior elements of the spine. An aneurysmal bone cyst is the only benign tumor that can cross the disc and involve more than one spinal level. Pain is the most common symptom, and radicular symptoms may be caused by cord compression.

Treatment is operative excision whenever possible. The tumors can be quite vascular, and if operative resection is contemplated, preoperative embolization should be considered. Embolization should be done in addition to the operative excision, and vessels supplying important segments of the spinal cord or brain should not be embolized. The indications for embolization are benign vascular tumors in central locations. In one study, three of the four tumors that were embolized were aneurysmal bone cysts. Contraindications include avascular tumors and tumors supplied by vessels that also supply important segments of the spinal cord because embolization of these vessels may infarct the spinal cord. Dick et al. suggested that malignant tumors that are to be treated with radiation should not be embolized, because effective radiation requires high oxygenation of the cells. Good clinical results have been reported after arterial embolization; however, the major disadvantage is the need for repeated procedures and repeated CT scans and angiography. Radiation therapy should be used only in those lesions that cannot be operatively excised.

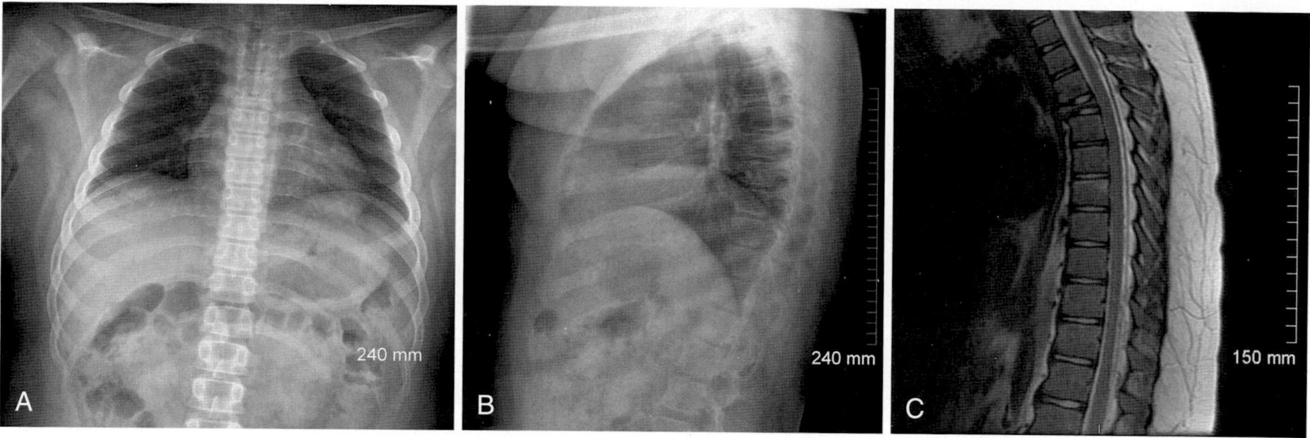

FIGURE 44-238 Eosinophilic granuloma in a 10-year-old child resulting in vertebra plana at T4. **A** and **B**, Radiographic appearance. **C**, Appearance on sagittal MRI.

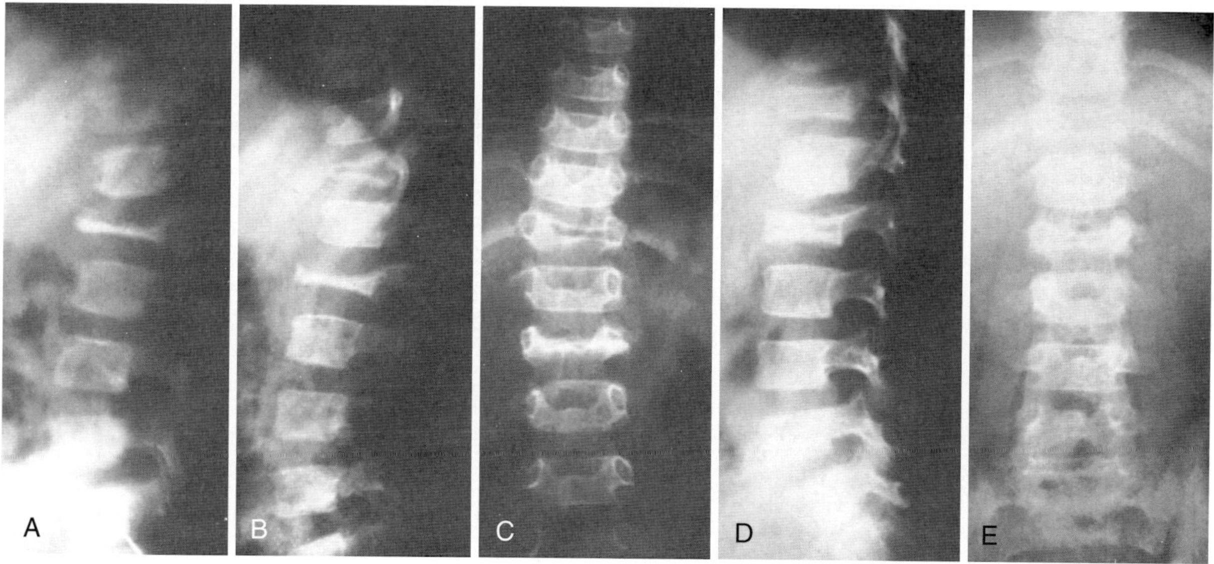

FIGURE 44-239 **A**, Eosinophilic granuloma of spine in 3½-year-old patient. **B**, Sudden collapse of T12 3 weeks later, in addition to vertebra plana at L2. **C**, Collapse of T12 and L2. **D** and **E**, Considerable reconstitution of the vertebral height of T12 and L2 16 months later. (From Seiman LP: Eosinophilic granuloma of the spine, J Pediatr Orthop 1:371, 1981.)

Many patients with aneurysmal bone cysts of the vertebral column have neurologic symptoms (30%), including complete or incomplete paraplegia or root signs or symptoms. When these neurologic symptoms occur, complete excision of the aneurysmal bone cyst with decompression of the spinal canal is indicated. The approach, whether anterior, posterior, or combined anterior and posterior, is dictated by the location of the lesion.

EOSINOPHILIC GRANULOMA

Eosinophilic granuloma in childhood usually is a solitary lesion. The cause of this lesion, which may not represent a true neoplasm, is unknown. Approximately 10% involve the spine. Eosinophilic granuloma may produce varying degrees of vertebral collapse, including the classic picture of a vertebra plana (Fig. 44-238). Considerable collapse of the vertebral body may occur without neurologic compromise, and significant reconstitution in height may occur after treatment (Fig. 44-239). Bone scan may show increased uptake. A lytic radiographic image without vertebra plana with normal bone scan uptake probably is a benign lesion, but biopsy must still be done. The differential diagnoses include aneurysmal bone cyst, acute leukemia, metastatic neuroblastoma, Ewing sarcoma, or multifocal osteomyelitis. MRI can be helpful in distinguishing eosinophilic granuloma from a malignant neoplasm. Eosinophilic granuloma will most often not have a prominent soft-tissue mass associated with the vertebral collapse. A malignant tumor, such as Ewing sarcoma, often has extensive soft-tissue involvement (Fig. 44-240). The treatment of vertebra plana generally focuses on relief of symptoms. The usual result is spontaneous healing. Spinal deformity may be minimized by the use of an appropriate orthosis. Other reported treatment alternatives include curettage and bone grafting, radiotherapy, and interlesional instillation of corticosteroids, but they rarely are needed.

HEMANGIOMA

Hemangioma is the most common benign vascular tumor of bone. Most hemangiomas involve the vertebral bodies or skull, and involvement of other bones is rare. Vertebral involvement usually is an incidental finding and requires surgery only when neurologic function is compromised (Fig. 44-241C). Hemangioma has been reported in as many as 12% of spines studied by autopsy. The lesion usually produces a characteristic, vertical, striated appearance (see Fig. 44-241A and B). Laredo et al. divided vertebral hemangiomas into three subcategories. The most common is the asymptomatic vertebral hemangioma; the second is a compressive vertebral hemangioma that compresses the cord or cauda equina; and the third is the rare vertebral hemangioma that causes clinical symptoms (symptomatic vertebral hemangioma). Six radiographic criteria were noted that were indicative of vertebral hemangioma leading to compressive problems: thoracic location (from T3 to T9), entire vertebral body involvement, neural arch (particularly pedicles) involvement, irregular honeycomb appearance, expanded and poorly defined cortex, and swelling of the soft tissue. It was suggested in patients with vertebral hemangioma and back pain of uncertain origin that the presence of three or more of these signs may indicate a potentially symptomatic vertebral hemangioma. Laredo et al. also compared MRI findings in asymptomatic and symptomatic vertebral hemangiomas. They found that vertebral hemangiomas with low-signal intensity on T1-weighted images had a significant vascular component, which might have been a major contributing factor to the patient's symptoms. Most vertebral hemangiomas contained predominant fat attenuation values on CT and showed high-signal intensity on T1-weighted imaging, indicating a predominantly fatty content. These researchers emphasized, however, as has been our experience, that most vertebral hemangiomas are not symptomatic and are an incidental finding. If neurologic dysfunction and anterior collapse occur, operative excision of the lesion, perhaps with adjuvant embolization as described by Dick et al., is recommended.

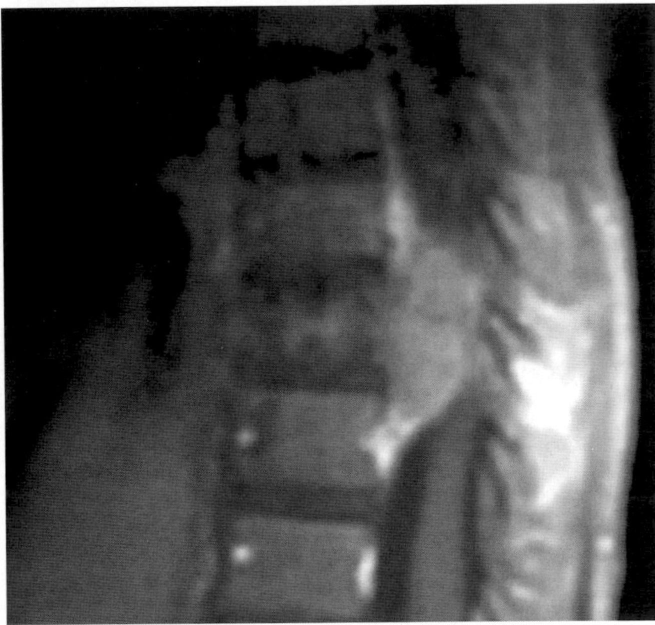

FIGURE 44-240 Sagittal T1-weighted MRI of spine in 8-year-old boy with epidural Ewing sarcoma. Note extensive soft-tissue mass that is characteristic of malignant neoplasms in spine. (From Garg S, Dormans JP: Tumors and tumor-like conditions of the spine in children, J Am Acad Orthop Surg 13:372, 2005.)

PRIMARY MALIGNANT TUMORS OF THE VERTEBRAL COLUMN

Primary malignant tumors of the vertebral column are uncommon. In children, the most common are Ewing sarcoma and osteogenic sarcoma.

EWING SARCOMA

Ewing sarcoma is a relatively rare, primary malignant tumor of bone. The tumor occurs most frequently in males in the second decade of life. All bones, including the spine, may be affected. The tumor most commonly begins in the pelvis or long bones and rapidly metastasizes to other skeletal sites, including the spine, especially the vertebral bodies and pedicles.

The currently recommended treatment of Ewing sarcoma is radiotherapy and adjuvant chemotherapy. On occasion, surgery may be necessary to stabilize the spine because of compression of the neural elements and bony instability. If decompression of the neural elements is necessary, stabilization usually is needed at the same time.

OSTEOGENIC SARCOMA

Osteogenic sarcoma is the most common primary malignant bone tumor, excluding multiple myeloma, but less than 2%

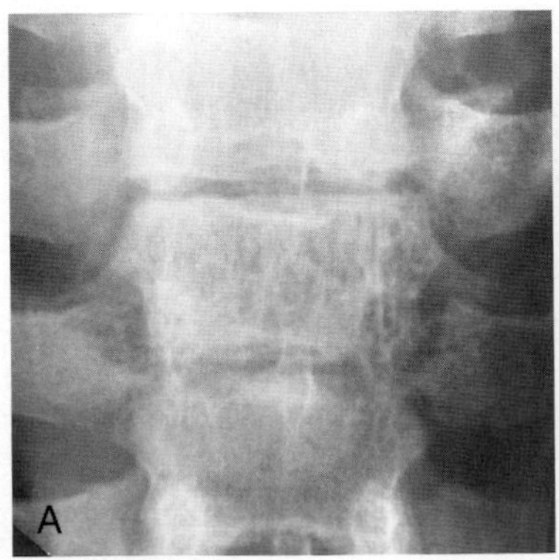

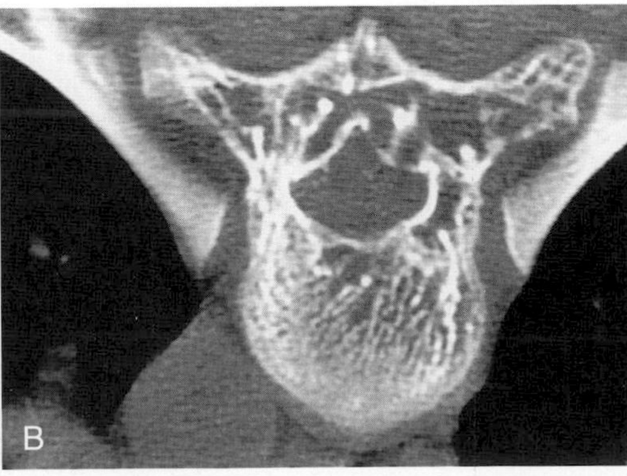

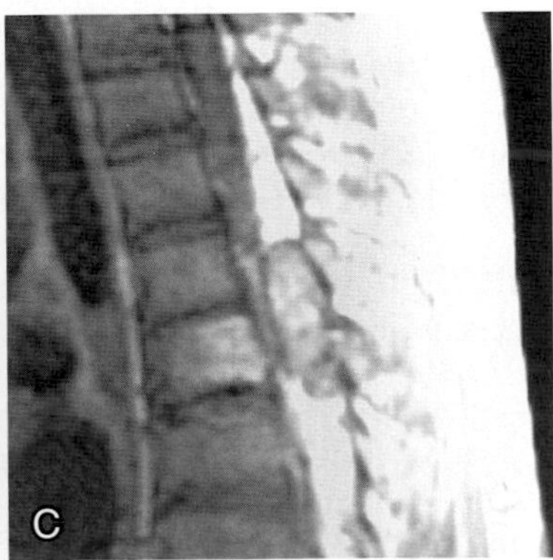

FIGURE 44-241 Radiograph **(A)**, CT scan **(B)**, and MRI **(C)** of patient with spinal hemangioma with canal compromise.

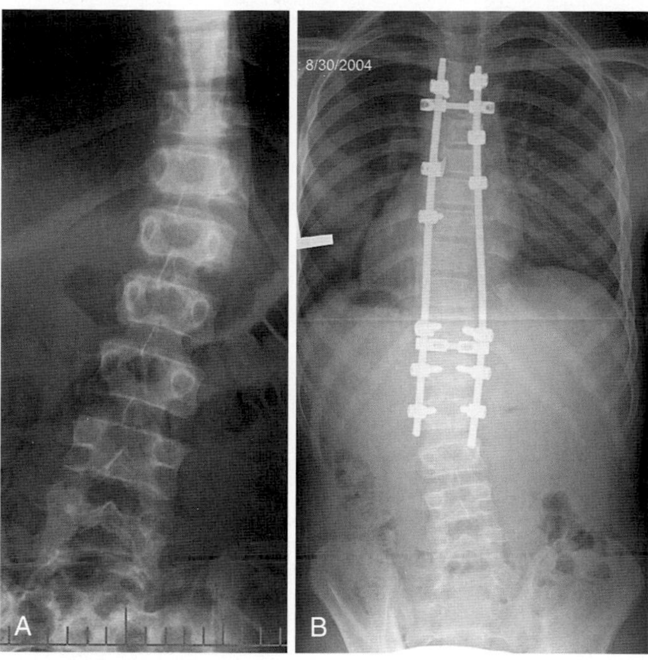

FIGURE 44-242 **A,** Osteogenic sarcoma in an 14-year-old child. **B,** After tumor resection and stabilization.

originate in the spine. It is a malignant tumor of bone in which tumor cells form neoplastic osteoid or bone, or both. Classic osteogenic sarcoma is more common in boys 10 to 15 years of age. This is a rapidly progressive malignant neoplasm, and multiple metastatic lesions to the vertebral column are more common than primary involvement (Fig. 44-242). The role of surgery for vertebral involvement is based on whether the spinal lesion is solitary, primary, or metastatic. If decompression of the spinal cord becomes necessary, or if structural integrity of the vertebral column is compromised, stabilizing procedures usually are required. If aggressive operative debridement is required, the neural structures limit the margin of the resection, making it impossible to achieve as wide a margin of resection as in the extremities.

POSTIRRADIATION SPINAL DEFORMITY

Perthes in 1903 first described inhibition of osseous development by irradiation. Later studies indicated that the physis is particularly sensitive to radiation. A physis exposed to 600 rad or more showed some growth retardation, and complete inhibition of growth was produced by doses of more than 1200 rad. The longitudinal growth of a vertebral body takes place by means of true physeal cartilage, similar to the longitudinal growth of the metaphysis of the long bones. The three most common solid tumors of childhood for which radiation therapy is part of the treatment regimen and in which the vertebral column is included in the radiation fields are neuroblastoma, Wilms tumor, and medulloblastoma.

■ INCIDENCE

Mayfield et al. studied spinal deformity in children treated for neuroblastoma, and Riseborough et al. studied spinal deformity in children treated for Wilms' tumor. Several principles can be summarized from these studies. A direct relationship seems to exist between the amount of radiation and the severity of the spinal deformity. In general, a dose of less than 2000 rad is not associated with significant deformity, a dose between 2000 and 3000 rad is associated with mild scoliosis, and a dose of more than 3000 rad is associated with more severe scoliosis. Irradiation in younger children, especially those 2 years of age or younger, produces the most serious disturbance in vertebral growth. Radiation treatment in children older than 4 years is less frequently associated with spinal deformity. Asymmetric irradiation is associated with significant spinal deformity. Engel and Arkin et al. produced experimental scoliosis by asymmetric irradiation, either internal or external. Progression usually occurs during the adolescent growth spurt. Scoliosis is the most frequent deformity, and the direction of the curve usually is concave toward the side of the irradiation. Kyphosis may occur in association with the scoliosis, or kyphosis alone may be present, most frequently at the thoracolumbar junction. Children who require a laminectomy because of epidural spread of tumor are especially prone to the development of moderate-to-severe spinal deformity. Similarly, those children whose disease causes paraplegia also are prone to rapid progression of the deformity. Without these two complicating features, most radiation-induced scoliotic deformities remain small and do not require treatment. Because progression of these curves generally occurs during the adolescent growth spurt, any child undergoing radiation therapy to the spine should have orthopaedic consultation and regular follow-up until skeletal maturity.

■ RADIOGRAPHIC FINDINGS

Neuhauser et al. described the radiographic changes in previously irradiated spines, and Riseborough et al. divided the radiographic findings into four groups. The earliest noted changes were alterations in the vertebral bodies within the irradiated section of the spine, which are expressions of irradiation impairment of physeal enchondral growth at the vertebral endplates. The most obvious features of these lesions were growth arrest lines that subsequently led to the bone-in-bone picture (28%) (Fig. 44-243). Endplate irregularity with an altered trabecular pattern and decreased vertebral body height were seen most frequently (83% of patients). Contour abnormalities, causing anterior narrowing and beaking of the vertebral bodies, such as those seen in Morquio disease (Fig. 44-244), were present in 20% of patients. Asymmetric or symmetric failure of vertebral body development was apparent on the anteroposterior radiographs of all 81 patients studied. The second group of radiographic changes included alterations in spinal alignment. Scoliosis was present in 70% of patients and kyphosis in 25%. The third group of radiographic findings included skeletal alterations in bones other than the vertebral column, the most common of which were iliac wing hypoplasia (68%) and osteochondroma (6%). The fourth group consisted of patients with no evidence of deformity of the axial skeleton (27%).

■ TREATMENT

Most studies indicate that the curves usually remain slight until the adolescent growth spurt, when progression can be severe and rapid. Orthoses for treatment of postirradiation spinal deformity may or may not (50%) improve or stop progression of the deformity, especially if severe changes in the architecture of the vertebrae and excessive soft-tissue

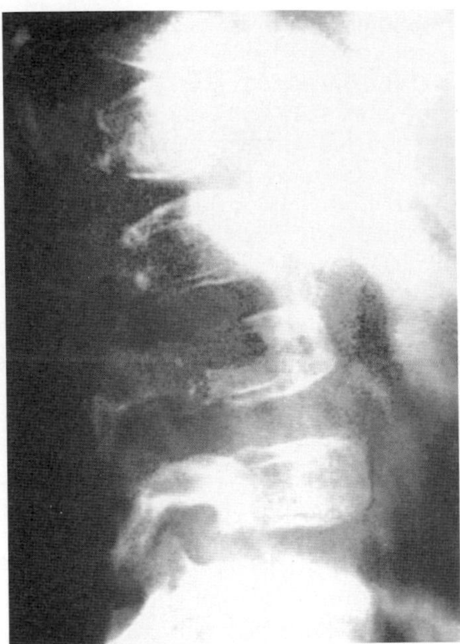

FIGURE 44-243 "Bone-in-bone" appearance of irradiated spine, equivalent of growth arrest line in long bone. (From Katzman H, Waugh T, Berdon W: Skeletal changes following irradiation of childhood tumors, J Bone Joint Surg 51A:825, 1969.)

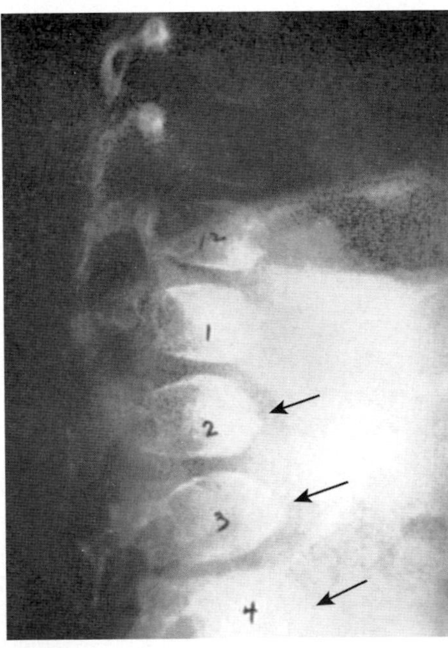

FIGURE 44-244 Contour abnormalities of vertebral bodies after radiotherapy for Wilms tumor in 8-month-old patient. (From Katzman H, Waugh T, Berdon W: Skeletal changes following irradiation of childhood tumors, J Bone Joint Surg 51A:825, 1969.)

scarring are present. The indications for operative treatment are a scoliosis of more than 40 degrees and a thoracolumbar kyphosis of more than 50 degrees. Patients with progression despite brace treatment also are considered candidates for operative intervention. Riseborough et al. outlined the difficulties in obtaining adequate correction and fusion of these curves, which frequently are rigid. Extensive soft-tissue scarring may further complicate the surgery. Many patients requiring operative treatment have a kyphoscoliotic deformity, and many also have had previous laminectomies, which will inhibit solid fusion. Healing can be prolonged, and pseudarthrosis is common.

Combined anterior and posterior fusions with an anterior strut graft or anterior interbody fusion and posterior instrumentation should be considered for patients with kyphotic deformities of more than 40 degrees. Because of the unpredictable nature of the irradiated anterior bone stock, anterior instrumentation may not be possible. Segmental hook or screw instrumentation systems, with their ability to apply both compression and distraction, are ideal for posterior instrumentation in these patients. If irradiation was for a tumorous process, consideration should be given to titanium implants, which would allow better follow-up MRI, if necessary. The fusion area is selected by the same criteria as for idiopathic curves (see earlier section on fusion levels and hook site placement). A large quantity of bone from the nonirradiated iliac crest should be used. Ogilvie suggested exploration of the fusion 6 months after surgery for repeated bone grafting of any developing pseudarthrosis. Because of problems with bone stock, postoperative immobilization in a TLSO often is indicated until complete fusion is obtained.

COMPLICATIONS AND PITFALLS

Pseudarthrosis, infection, and neurologic injury are more frequent after spinal fusion for radiation-induced deformity than for other spinal deformities. The increase in pseudarthrosis is attributed to poor bone quality, decreased bone vascularity, kyphotic deformity, and absence of posterior bone elements after laminectomy. Poor vascularity and skin quality have been associated with an increased infection rate. Severe scarring sometimes is present in the retroperitoneal space, making the anterior exposure more difficult. Because viscera can be damaged by radiation, bowel obstruction, perforation, and fistula formation may occur after spinal fusion. This can be difficult to differentiate from postoperative cast syndrome. Paraplegia also has been reported in two patients who had radiation treatment for neuroblastoma and surgical correction. It is believed that they had a subclinical form of radiation myelopathy and that spinal correction compromised what little vascular supply there was to the cord. The surgeon should be aware of this possibility and avoid overcorrection of these kyphotic deformities.

OSTEOCHONDRODYSTROPHY

DIASTROPHIC DWARFISM

Diastrophic dwarfism is inherited as an autosomal recessive disease. The diagnosis usually can be made at birth on the basis of clinical features and, for families at risk, before birth by ultrasound examination and molecular genetic testing. Clinical and radiographic findings are short limbs, short stature, multiple joint contractures, and early degeneration of joints. Spinal deformities, including cervical kyphosis, scoliosis, and exaggerated lumbar lordosis, often are seen. Remes et al. found scoliosis in 88% of patients with diastrophic dwarfism. They subdivided the scoliotic curves into three subtypes: early progressive, idiopathic-like, and mild nonprogressive. The early progressive type resembled the progressive form of infantile idiopathic scoliosis, with early onset, rapid progression, and severe outcome. Patients with the idiopathic-like scoliosis had features similar to patients with adolescent idiopathic scoliosis.

The indications for treatment of scoliosis in diastrophic dwarfism have not been fully established. Patients with diastrophic dwarfism already have many abnormalities in their appearance. The benefits of surgical treatment should therefore be evaluated critically. Brace treatment has been found to be useful only for small curves in these patients. If the curve cannot be braced successfully, the spinal deformity can progress to a severe scoliosis causing imbalance of the trunk. This can lead to difficulties in gait and a reduction in the already short standing height. The most important factors to be considered are the rate of progression and the time at onset: the earlier the time at onset, the more rapid and severe the progression and curve type. The early progressive type of scoliosis virtually always develops into a severe deformity unless surgery is performed. In very young children, growth rod–type instrumentation can be considered. However, because growth is limited, repeated surgeries to lengthen the rods are done at 15- to 18-month intervals instead of the usual 6-month interval. If a significantly progressive curve is noted in a very young child not appropriate for growing rods, combined anterior and posterior fusion should be considered. If a growth rod can be successfully used, by the age of 10 years, most of the spinal growth in a diastrophic dysplastic patient is complete and definitive fusion is then done.

Cervical kyphosis occurs commonly, and although it usually resolves with age, it can cause quadriplegia. Radiographic evaluation of the cervical spine is mandatory in these patients. If the cervical kyphosis worsens, surgical treatment is necessary. If the kyphosis is mild, posterior fusion alone, combined with a halo brace, should be considered. In an older child with a more severe kyphosis, combined anterior and posterior fusion should be considered. If the kyphosis is causing neurologic problems, decompression anteriorly at the apex of the kyphosis is needed along with anterior and posterior fusion.

SPONDYLOEPIPHYSEAL DYSPLASIA

Orthopaedic aspects of spondyloepiphyseal dysplasia are discussed in Chapter 32.

The spinal problems most commonly associated with this condition are scoliosis, kyphoscoliosis, and odontoid hypoplasia with atlantoaxial instability (Fig. 44-245). If the scoliosis and kyphoscoliosis are progressive, orthotic treatment sometimes is useful for delaying the fusion until the patient is older. Bethem et al. found that the Milwaukee brace was more successful in managing the kyphotic deformity than the scoliotic deformity. Kopits found a 30% to 40% incidence of atlantoaxial instability in patients with spondyloepiphyseal dysplasia. In children with this condition who are not walking by 2 to 3 years of age, the most likely explanation is spinal cord compression at the upper cervical region. Flexion-extension lateral cervical spine radiographs should be obtained. If ossification delay in vertebral bodies makes accurate determination of movement at this level impossible, a flexion-extension lateral MRI study is indicated. Once the instability is diagnosed, the treatment is surgical fusion.

If the scoliotic curve continues to progress despite bracing, surgical fusion is considered. Unlike in achondroplasia, spinal stenosis generally is not present in patients with spondyloepiphyseal dysplasia.

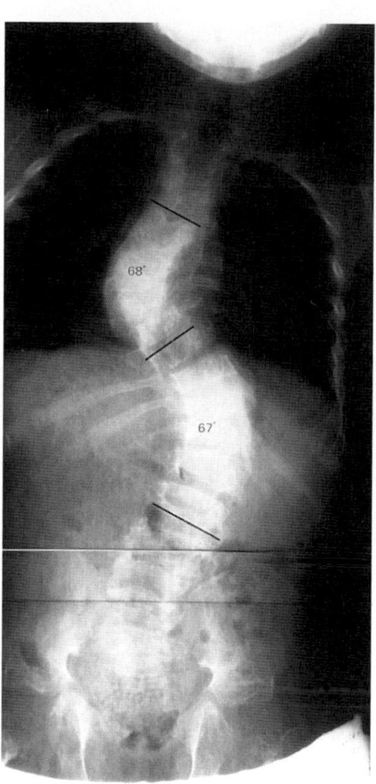

FIGURE 44-245 Spinal deformity in patient with spondyloepiphyseal dysplasia.

OSTEOGENESIS IMPERFECTA

Patients with osteogenesis imperfecta have abnormal collagen production that results in defective bone and connective tissue. Other orthopaedic aspects of osteogenesis imperfecta are described in Chapter 32.

The reported incidence of spinal deformity in patients with osteogenesis imperfecta ranges from 40% to 90%. Hanscom et al. developed a classification system based on the degree of bone involvement and the likelihood of development of a spinal deformity. Patients with type A disease have mild bony abnormalities with normal vertebral contours. Patients with type B disease have bowed long bones and wide cortices with biconcave vertebral bodies and a normal pelvic contour. Patients with type C disease have thin, bowed long bones and protrusio acetabuli, which develop around the age of 10 years. Patients with type D disease have deformities similar to type C, with the addition of cystic changes around the knee by the age of 5 years. Patients with type E disease are totally dependent functionally. Scoliosis occurred in 46% of their patients with type A disease and in all patients with types C and D. Benson et al., in a review of 100 patients with osteogenesis imperfecta, also concluded that the severity of the disease correlates with the risk of development and the severity of the scoliosis. Anissipour et al. reviewed 157 patients with osteogenesis imperfecta and scoliosis. Using the modified Sillence classification, they were able to follow patients having mild (type I), intermediate (type IV), and severe (type III) disease. There were high rates of scoliosis progression in types II and IV osteogenesis imperfecta, with a benign course in type I patients. Bisphosphonate therapy initiated before the patient reached the age of 6 years modulated the curve progression in type III patients.

The natural history of scoliosis in patients with osteogenesis imperfecta is continued progression. Scoliosis present at a young age almost always is progressive, and progression may continue into adulthood. Severe and disabling spinal deformities have been found in many adults with osteogenesis imperfecta.

ANESTHESIA PROBLEMS

There are several areas of concern in the administration of anesthesia for a patient with osteogenesis imperfecta. The primary concern is the risk of fractures. Extreme care must be taken in handling these patients, including positioning on the operating table with adequate padding and care in transfer. Care also should be taken in establishment of the intravenous line or application of a blood pressure cuff because both can result in fracture. Intubation and airway control also can be problematic because these patients have large heads and short necks, as well as tongues that often are disproportionately large. Extension of the head to facilitate intubation could cause a cervical spine fracture or a mandibular fracture. Because many patients with osteogenesis imperfecta have thoracic deformities, poor respiratory function should be expected.

A tendency for hyperthermia to develop in patients with osteogenesis imperfecta also has been noted. This does not appear to be a malignant type, however, and it may be related to elevated thyroid hormone levels, which are found in at least half of the patients with osteogenesis imperfecta. Hyperthermia can be induced by various anesthetic agents, as well as by atropine, and atropine should be avoided in these patients. If hyperthermia occurs, it is controlled with cooling, supplemental oxygen, sodium bicarbonate, cardiovascular stimulants, and dantrolene sodium. Libman suggested preoperative treatment with dantrolene sodium to perhaps prevent hyperthermia. He also recommended minimizing fasciculations associated with succinylcholine chloride. If possible, other agents should be used. If succinylcholine chloride is necessary, the fasciculations may be minimized by prior administration of a nondepolarizing muscle relaxant.

ORTHOTIC TREATMENT

Most authors agree that bracing does not control progressive scoliosis in patients with severe osteogenesis imperfecta. Brace treatment has been found to be ineffective in stopping progression of scoliosis in patients with osteogenesis imperfecta even if the curves are small, although Hanscom et al. suggested that orthotic treatment under carefully controlled circumstances may be a reasonable alternative to operative intervention in patients with type A or type B osteogenesis imperfecta. It is doubtful whether any effective forces from an orthosis can be transmitted to the spine of a patient with preexisting deformity of the chest wall, fragile ribs, and deformed vertebral bodies.

OPERATIVE TREATMENT

Spinal fusion is recommended for curves of more than 50 degrees in patients with osteogenesis imperfecta, regardless of the age of the patient, provided there are no medical contraindications (Fig. 44-246). The decision to fuse the spine should depend on the extent of the curvature and the presence of progression rather than on the age of the patient. In a series by Yong-Hing and MacEwen, one third of patients had some complications; five of 60 patients developed pseudarthroses, nine lost more than 2.5 L of blood, and 14 had problems related to instrumentation. In the absence of a pseudarthrosis or kyphosis, late bending of the fused spine did not occur. Fusion is recommended for prevention of progression of the spinal deformity and cardiopulmonary problems in patients with types B, C, and E osteogenesis imperfecta.

Segmental hook or screw instrumentation systems can be considered in patients with type A osteogenesis imperfecta. Patients with the milder form of the disease can be treated in the same manner as patients with idiopathic scoliosis, although significant correction of the curve should not be attempted. Bone graft should be obtained from the iliac crest, but often the amount of bone available is inadequate and allograft is required for a supplement. If the patient is small, pediatric instrumentation may be needed. The rod must be bent carefully to conform to the contours of the spine in both the coronal and sagittal planes to prevent excessive pull-out forces on the hooks. Methyl methacrylate has been used to supplement hook placement in these patients.

In patients with more severe disease (type C or type D), the use of L-rods with segmental wires (Fig. 44-247) has been recommended. Great care in tightening these wires should be taken to prevent a wire from pulling through the lamina posteriorly. An alternative is to use Mersilene tapes. Anterior procedures should not be necessary if spinal deformities are stabilized before they become too severe.

Because of poor bone quality, immobilization in a two-piece TLSO often is necessary for 6 to 9 months after surgery until the fusion is solid.

UNUSUAL CAUSES OF KYPHOSIS

POSTLAMINECTOMY SPINAL DEFORMITY

Laminectomies most often are done in children for the diagnosis and treatment of spinal cord tumors, although they also may be needed in other conditions, such as neurofibromatosis and syringomyelia. Several authors reported the frequency of spinal deformities after laminectomy in children. The incidence of spinal deformity ranged from 33% to 100%.

Kyphosis is the most common deformity that occurs after multiple-level laminectomies (Fig. 44-248). Spinal deformity after laminectomy has been found to be more frequent in children younger than 15 years; also noted was the higher the level of the laminectomy, the greater the likelihood of spinal deformity or instability. All cervical or cervicothoracic laminectomies were followed by deformity in two studies. Lonstein et al. described two basic types of kyphosis, depending on the status of the facet joints posteriorly: sharp and angular or long and gradually rounding.

Scoliosis also may occur after laminectomy and generally is in the area of the laminectomy and associated with the kyphotic deformity. Scoliosis may occur at levels below the laminectomy, but this is usually caused by the paralysis from the cord tumor or its treatment rather than by the laminectomy.

The causes of instability of the spine after multiple laminectomies include skeletal and ligamentous deficiencies,

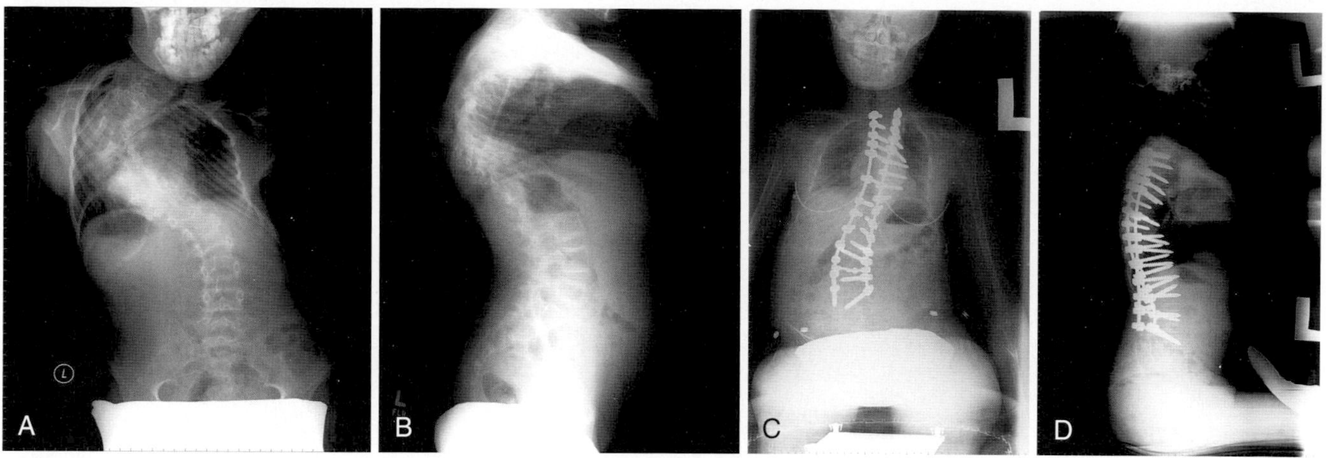

FIGURE 44-246 **A** and **B,** Spinal deformity in patient with osteogenesis imperfecta. **C** and **D,** Postoperative radiographs after posterior fusion and instrumentation.

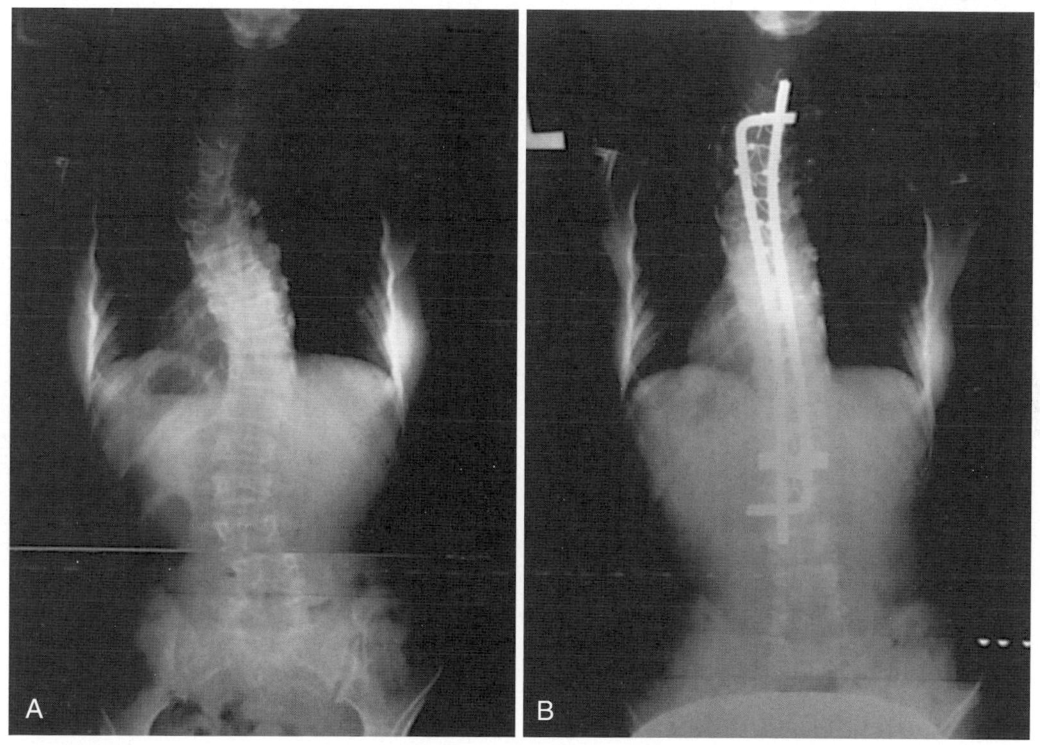

FIGURE 44-247 **A,** Preoperative posteroanterior radiographs of patient with osteogenesis imperfecta with progressing curvature. **B,** Postoperative radiographs after instrumentation with sublaminar cables and Luque rods.

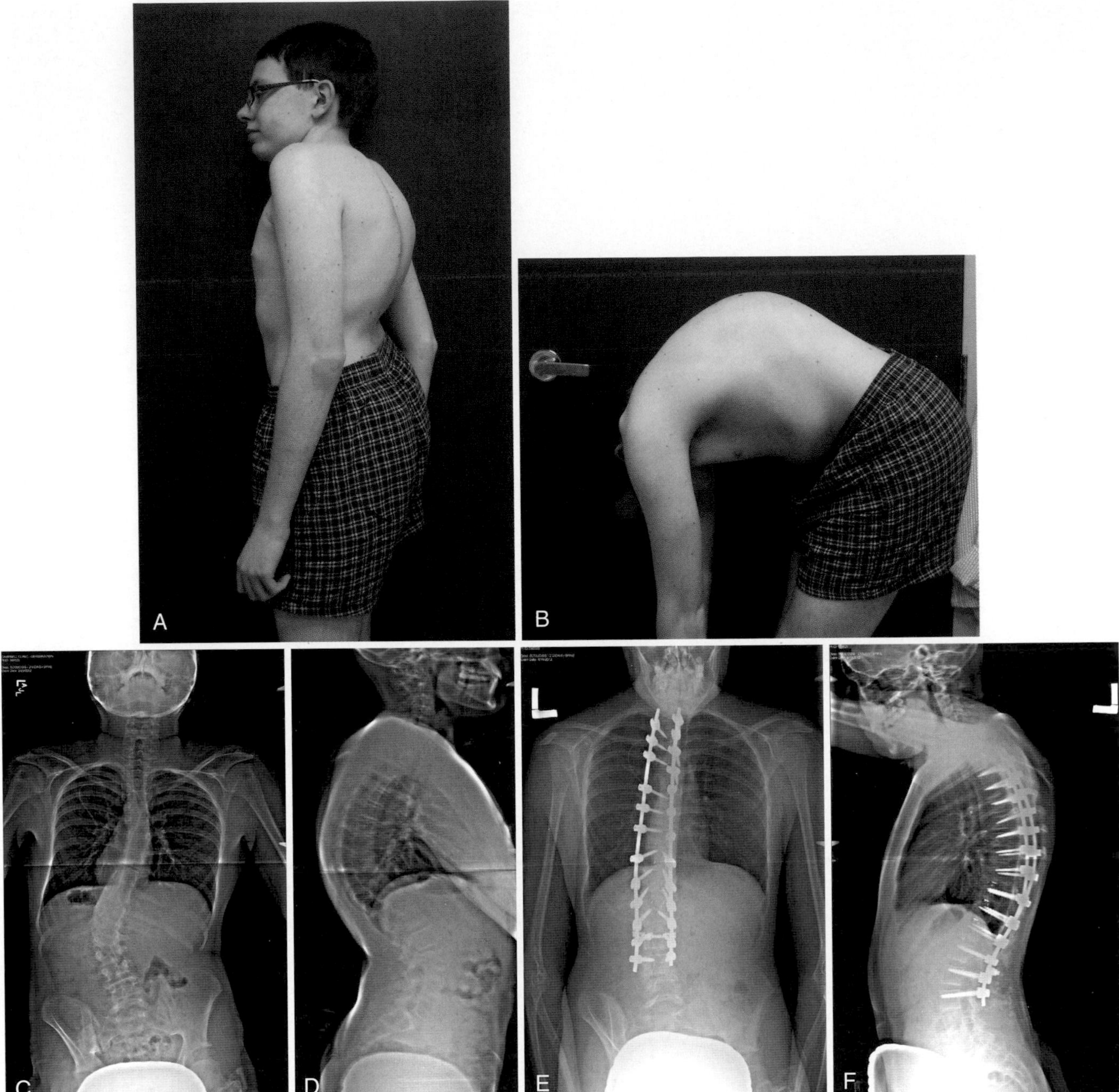

FIGURE 44-248 Postlaminectomy kyphosis. **A** and **B**, Clinical appearance. **C** and **D**, Radiographic appearance. **E** and **F**, After posterior fusion with pedicle screw instrumentation.

neuromuscular imbalance, progressive osseous deformity, and radiation therapy. Increased wedging or excessive motion has been noted in children rather than subluxation as occurs in adults, possibly because, after laminectomy, pressure is increased on the cartilaginous endplates of the vertebral bodies anteriorly and, with time, cartilage growth is decreased and vertebral wedging occurs (Fig. 44-249). Panjabi et al. showed that the loss of posterior stability caused by removal of interspinous ligaments, spinous processes, and laminae allows the normal flexion forces to produce a kyphosis. Lonstein et al. emphasized the importance of the facet joints posteriorly in these deformities. They showed that when the facet joints are completely removed at one level, gross instability results, with maximal angulation at that level causing a sharp, angular kyphos, enlargement of the intervertebral foramen, and opening of the disc space posteriorly (Fig. 44-250). If complete removal is on one side only, the angular kyphosis is accompanied by a sharp scoliosis with the apex at the same level. If all the facets are preserved, a gradual rounding kyphos results in the area of the laminectomy. Many authors have reported extremely high incidences of spinal deformity in children younger than 10 years with complete

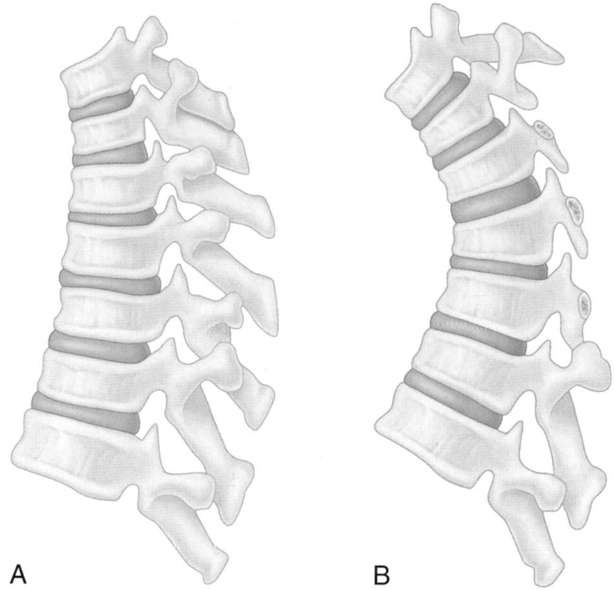

FIGURE 44-249 Drawings of thoracic spine before and after repeated laminectomy show effects on growth of vertebral bodies. **A,** Before laminectomy, anterior vertebral bodies are rectangular in configuration. **B,** Spine that has had multiple laminectomies will have increased compression anteriorly because of loss of posterior supporting structures. This compression results in less growth in anterior portion of vertebral body than in posterior portion. In time, this will result in wedging of vertebral bodies, causing kyphotic deformity.

paralysis. Children with extensive laminectomies and paralysis as a result of spinal cord tumors or their treatment are likely to have increasing spinal deformities. Radiation therapy, used to treat many spinal tumors, has been associated with injury to the vertebral physis and subsequent spinal deformity (see Postirradiation Spinal Deformity, earlier). The cause of postlaminectomy spinal deformity is therefore multifactorial.

TREATMENT

The treatment of postlaminectomy kyphosis is difficult, and, if at all possible, it is best to prevent the deformity from occurring. When laminectomy is necessary, the facet joints should be preserved whenever possible. Localized fusion at the time of facetectomy or laminectomy may help prevent progression of the deformity, but because of the loss of bone mass posteriorly, localized fusion may not produce a large enough fusion mass to prevent kyphosis. The surgical technique of laminoplasty to expose the spinal cord may lessen the chance of progressive deformity. This approach involves suturing the laminae back into place after removal or removing just one side of the laminae and allowing them to hinge open like a book to expose the spinal cord and then suturing that side of the lamina back in place. This procedure may provide a fibrous tether connecting the laminae to the spine, and Mimatsu has shown a decreased incidence of postlaminectomy kyphosis when it has been used. After surgery in which the laminae have been removed, the child should be examined regularly by an orthopaedic surgeon. If a spinal deformity is detected, brace treatment can be considered. The patient's long-term prognosis, however, should be considered before definitive treatment plans are made. If the prognosis for survival is poor, spinal fusion may not be appropriate. With modern treatment protocols and improved survival rates for tumors, fusion usually is indicated for progressive deformity.

Most authors recommend combined anterior and posterior fusions for this condition because of the small amount of bone surface posteriorly after a wide laminectomy. Also, many of these deformities have a kyphotic component and anterior spinal fusion is more successful biomechanically than posterior fusion. Anteriorly, the fusion mass is under compression rather than distraction forces. Of 45 patients treated for postlaminectomy scoliosis, Lonstein reported pseudarthroses in 33% with posterior fusion alone, in 22% with anterior fusion alone, and in 9.5% with combined anterior and posterior fusion. At the first stage, anterior fusion is done by removal of all of the disc material, taking special care to remove the entire disc back to the posterior longitudinal ligament to prevent growth in the posterior aspect of the vertebral endplate with increasing kyphotic deformity. Strut grafting, with the rib graft obtained during the approach, or a fibular graft can be used to provide correction in addition to the fusion. Additional bone obtained locally from the vertebral bodies or ilium or remaining rib should be packed into the open disc spaces. Posterior fusion and instrumentation are done either immediately or a week after the anterior fusion. Because of the absence of the posterior elements, instrumentation of the involved spine is desirable but not always possible. Pedicle screw fixation has been helpful in allowing the use of posterior instrumentation for postlaminectomy kyphosis and scoliosis. This procedure provides secure fixation while the spinal fusion is maturing. The use of titanium rod instrumentation has been recommended at the time of laminectomy. The instrumentation provides stability postoperatively, and the titanium rods allow postoperative MRI to evaluate spinal cord tumors. Often, the extent of the deformity and the absence of the posterior elements make instrumentation impossible, and a halo cast or vest may be necessary in these patients after surgery.

SKELETAL DYSPLASIAS

ACHONDROPLASIA

Achondroplasia, the most common of the bony dysplasias, is caused by a mutation of fibroblast growth factor receptor 3. The most frequent spinal deformity associated with this condition is thoracolumbar kyphosis that is present at birth (Fig. 44-251). The frequency of kyphosis in achondroplasia is 87% from age 1 to 2 years, 39% from age 2 to 5 years, and 11% from age 5 to 10 years. As muscle tone develops and walking begins, the kyphotic deformity usually resolves, although persistent kyphosis has been reported and can become severe in some patients. This kyphosis is poorly tolerated by the patient with achondroplasia because of the decreased size of the spinal canal related to a marked decrease in the interpedicular distance in the lower lumbar region and to shortened pedicles, which cause a reduction in the anteroposterior dimensions of the spinal canal.

It is important to be aware of the possibility of persistent or progressive thoracolumbar kyphosis in these patients.

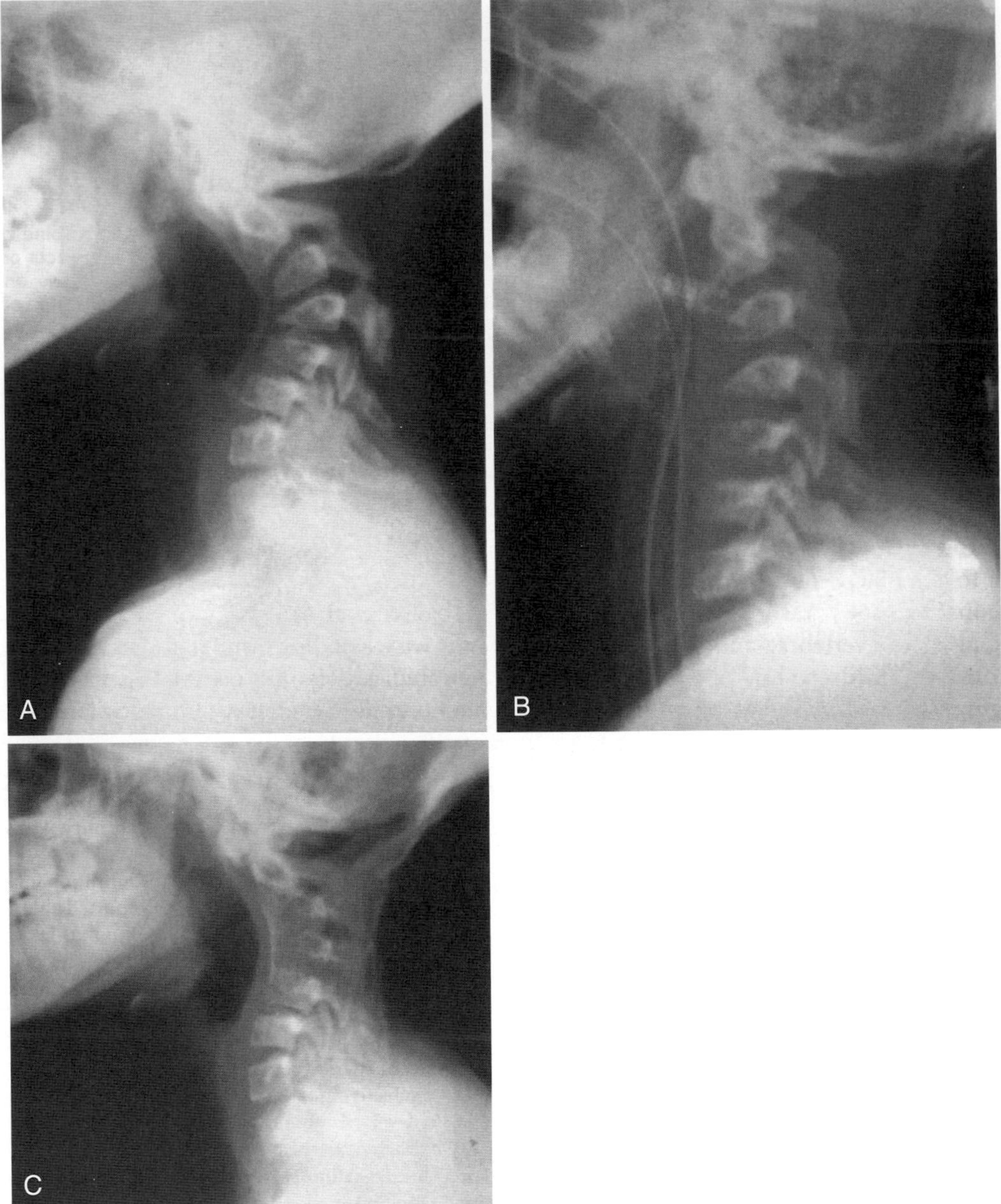

FIGURE 44-250 Radiographs of 13-year-old girl treated for low-grade astrocytoma. She had resection of the tumor, a portion of occiput, and laminae of C1-C4, followed by radiotherapy at a dose of 5400 cGy. **A,** Progressive cervical kyphosis developed. Note wedging of anterior vertebral body. **B,** Radiograph in halo traction shows partial reduction of kyphosis. **C,** Postoperative radiograph after anterior and posterior fusion. (From Warner WC: Kyphosis. In Morrissy RT, Weinstein SL, editors: Lovell and Winter's pediatric orthopaedics, ed 6, Philadelphia, 2006, Lippincott Williams & Wilkins.)

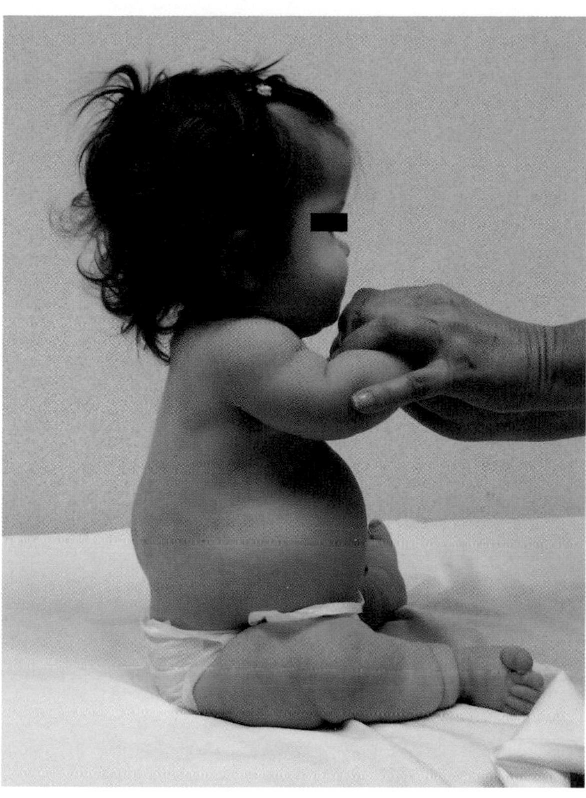

FIGURE 44-251 Kyphosis in infant with achondroplasia.

Early bracing to prevent progression and correction of any associated hip flexion contractures to prevent hyperlordosis below the kyphosis are recommended. Pauli et al. showed the efficacy of early prohibition of unsupported sitting and bracing in a series of 66 infants with achondroplasia. The parents were advised to prevent unsupported sitting and to keep young children from sitting up more than 60 degrees even with support. If the kyphosis developed and became greater than 30 degrees (as measured on prone lateral radiographs), TLSO bracing was begun and continued until the child was walking independently and there was evidence of improvement in vertebral body wedging and kyphosis. With this form of early intervention, they reported no recurrences of progressive kyphosis.

If the kyphosis progresses despite conservative treatment, operative stabilization is indicated. The indications for surgery include a documented progression of a kyphotic deformity, kyphosis of more than 50 degrees, and neurologic deficits relating to the spinal deformity. Unless the kyphosis is rapidly progressive or there are neurologic deficits, surgery is delayed until 4 years of age. Neurologic deficits can occur as a direct result of the kyphotic deformity and also as a result of the lumbar stenosis. Neurologic deficits in infants with achondroplasia may indicate narrowing of the foramen magnum and basilar impression. Evaluation of neurologic deficits therefore should include appropriate imaging studies of the foramen magnum and the occipitocervical junction. A thorough physical examination and diagnostic study, including a CT scan or MRI, may be necessary to determine the source of neurologic deficits.

Most patients with progressive thoracolumbar kyphosis require combined anterior and posterior fusion. The traditional approach has been to avoid posterior instrumentation because of the small canal. Ain and Browne recommended an anterior approach when the pedicle was too small to accommodate screw instrumentation. Corpectomy to relieve anterior impingement was needed when hyperextension over a bolster failed to correct the kyphosis to less than 50 degrees. Patients in whom no instrumentation was used posteriorly had repeated posterior bone grafting 4 months after the original procedure. If pedicle screw instrumentation was used, the pedicle screws were placed under fluoroscopic guidance. In patients with achondroplasia, the pedicles are directed cranially at all levels, and the average pedicle length is nearly 10 mm shorter than in individuals without achondroplasia. In Ain and Browne's patients, all kyphotic segments were included in the fusion. If a concomitant decompression was done, the fusion was ended at least one level cephalad to the most superior level of laminectomy to avoid development of junctional kyphosis (Fig. 44-252). They found that pedicle instrumentation of the pediatric achondroplastic spine did not cause intraoperative neurologic monitoring difficulties or lead to postoperative neurologic deficits. Posterior column shortening with pedicle screws and posterior instrumentation also has been used to successfully treat neurologic deficits secondary to thoracolumbar kyphosis.

Symptomatic spinal stenosis usually does not occur until the third or fourth decade of life, but it may develop before adolescence. The reported incidence of symptomatic spinal stenosis ranges from 37% to 89%. The interpedicular distance typically decreases from L1 to L5 and the pedicle diameter increases in the same direction, resulting in a 40% reduction in size of the sagittal and coronal diameter of the spinal canal. Approximately one fourth of all patients with achondroplasia will require surgery for spinal stenosis. Surgical indications are progressive symptoms, urinary retention, severe claudication (symptoms after walking less than two city blocks), and neurologic symptoms at rest. Surgical management of spinal stenosis is a decompressive laminectomy. Laminectomy alone is not always sufficient for decompression, and the nerve root recesses on both sides should be explored because lateral stenosis usually is present. Because of the high risk of developing a postlaminectomy kyphosis, concurrent posterior instrumentation and fusion are recommended.

MUCOPOLYSACCHARIDOSES

Of the many types of mucopolysaccharidoses, Morquio, Hurler, and Maroteaux-Lamy syndromes are the types most commonly associated with structural changes of the spine. The spinal deformity commonly seen in children with these conditions is kyphosis, usually in the thoracolumbar junction (Figs. 44-253 and 44-254). The vertebral bodies of these patients are deficient anteriorly and are flattened, beaked, or notched. The intervertebral discs are thick and bulging, often larger than the bodies. Thus in time, the thoracolumbar spine collapses into kyphosis. The kyphosis is flexible in childhood but with progression becomes increasingly rigid. Treatment of the condition depends on the degree of the deformity, as well as the child's prognosis. Hurler syndrome usually is rapidly progressive, and affected children usually die before the age of 10 years (Fig. 44-255).

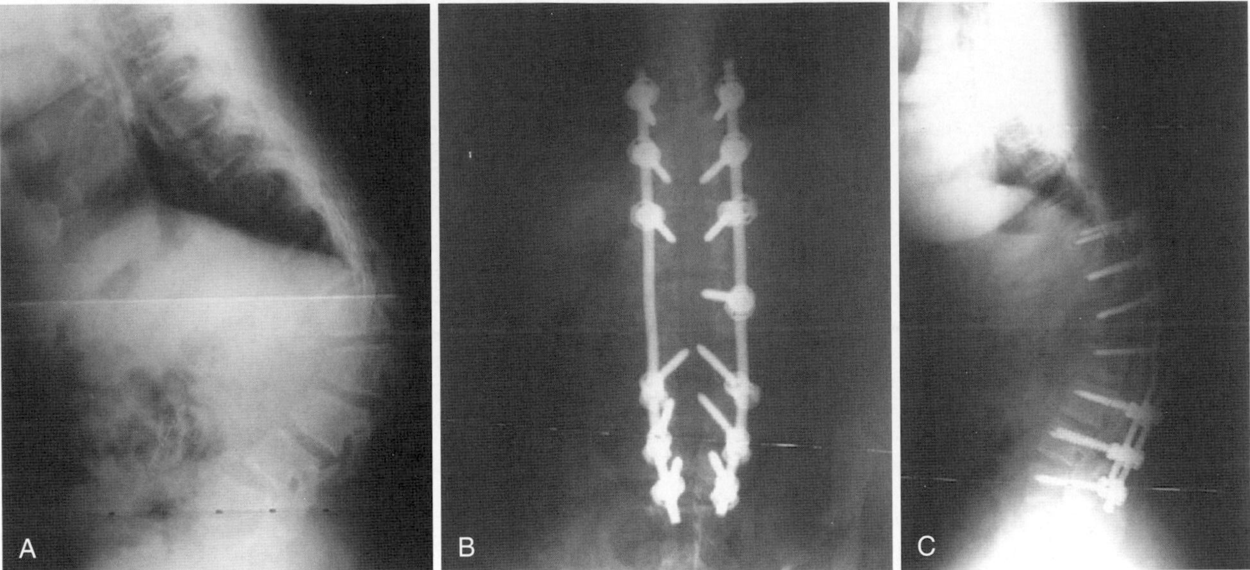

FIGURE 44-252 Spinal arthrodesis with instrumentation in pediatric achondroplasia. **A,** Preoperative lateral radiograph. **B,** Postoperative anteroposterior radiograph. **C,** Postoperative lateral radiograph. (From Ain MC, Browne JA: Spinal arthrodesis with instrumentation for thoracolumbar kyphosis in pediatric achondroplasia, Spine 29:2075, 2004.)

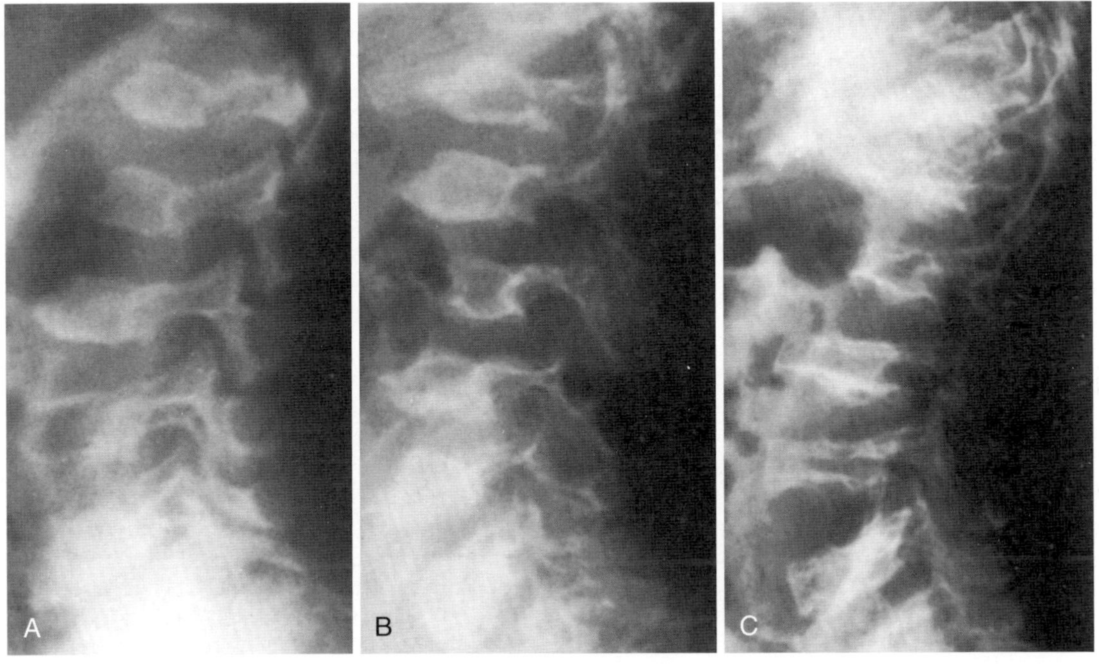

FIGURE 44-253 Spinal deformity in Morquio syndrome. **A,** Hook-shaped bodies in young child. **B,** Further anterior ossification in older child. **C,** Flattened, rectangular vertebral bodies in adult. (From Langer LO, Carey LS: The radiographic features of the KS mucopolysaccharidosis of Morquio, Am J Roentgenol 97:1, 1966.)

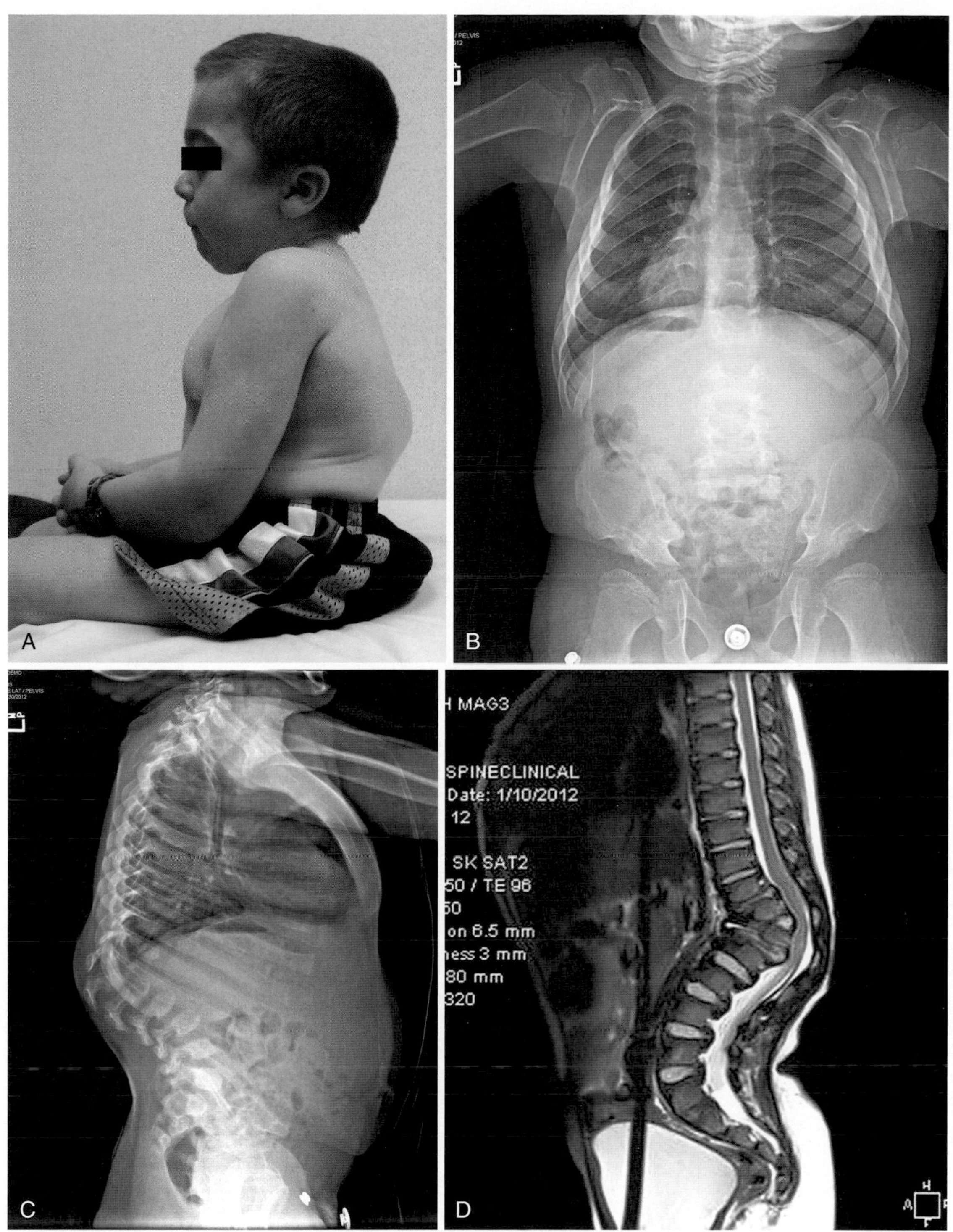

FIGURE 44-254 Kyphotic deformity in patient with mucopolysaccharidosis. **A,** Clinical appearance. **B** and **C,** Radiographic appearance. **D,** MRI.

Morquio syndrome is the most common of the mucopolysaccharidoses. Children with this condition may well live into adult life and have normal mentality. Many authors, including Blaw and Langer, Kopits, Langer, and Lipson, have emphasized the frequent occurrence of atlantoaxial instability in patients with Morquio syndrome. The most common presenting symptom is reduced exercise tolerance, followed by progressive upper motor neuron deficits. Blaw and Langer stated that neurologic problems in the first 2 decades of life usually are related to odontoid abnormalities or atlantoaxial instability; later, symptoms primarily are caused by the kyphosis or gibbus. Posterior fusion of C1 to C2 is the recommended treatment of atlantoaxial instability as soon as any signs of a myelopathy are identified. Blaw and Langer recommended that the developing gibbus during childhood be treated with an appropriate spinal orthosis to prevent neurologic deficits. Dalvie et al. described the use of anterior discectomy and anterior instrumentation to correct the thoracolumbar gibbus in these patients. The advantages of this technique are the opportunity for anterior decompression by excision of the bulging disc before correction of the kyphosis; the number of levels included in the fusion is less than required posteriorly; the posterior elements in these children are not strong enough to hold instrumentation, and, furthermore, associated canal stenosis, because of soft-tissue deposition, makes intracanal instrumentation unsafe; the interbody fusion obtained is of excellent quality; and anterior surgery can be performed, dissecting fewer muscle planes. The primary difficulty with this technique is technical in nature. The vertebral bodies are very small, and great care must be taken to ensure central placement of the screws. If the correction maneuver places excess stress on the implants, they may cut through the bone. The corrective maneuver must therefore include an external corrective force. Good correction of the kyphosis was obtained and maintained throughout the follow-up period (Fig. 44-256).

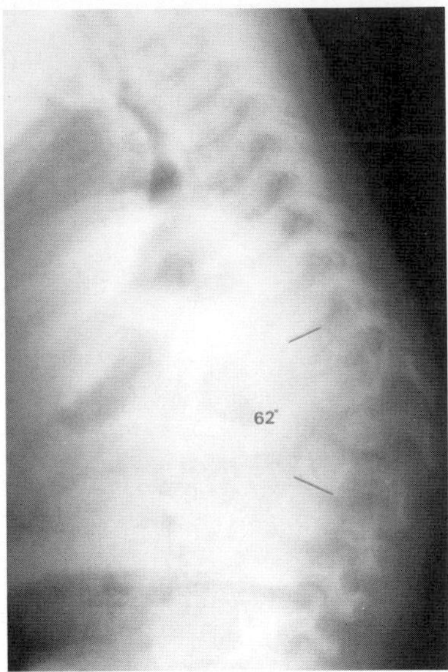

FIGURE 44-255 Kyphosis at thoracolumbar junction in patient with Hurler syndrome.

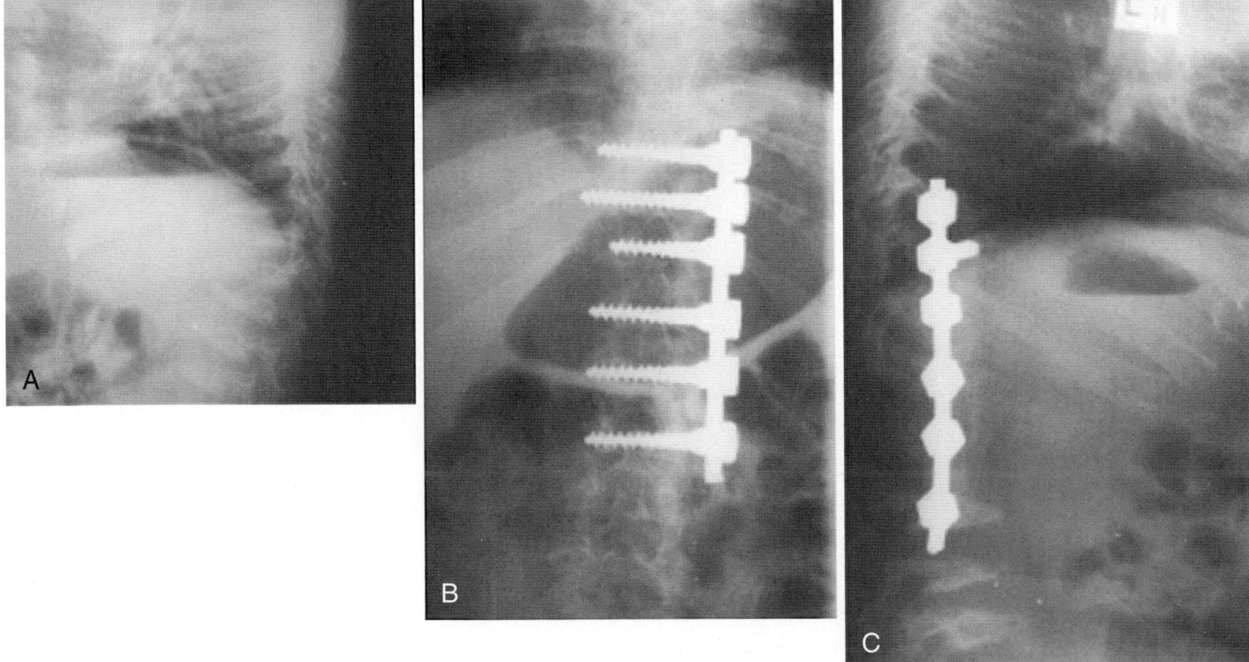

FIGURE 44-256 Anterior fusion for thoracolumbar kyphosis in mucopolysaccharidosis. **A,** Preoperative radiograph. **B,** Anteroposterior radiograph showing instrumentation in place. **C,** Radiograph at 3 years shows correction of gibbus with instrumentation and solid bony fusion. (From Dalvie SS, Noordeen MH, Vellodi A: Anterior instrumented fusion for thoracolumbar kyphosis in mucopolysaccharidosis, Spine 26:E539, 2001.)

REFERENCES

INFANTILE AND JUVENILE IDIOPATHIC SCOLIOSIS

Akbarnia BA: Management themes in early onset scoliosis, *J Bone Joint Surg* 89A:42, 2007.

Bess S, Akbarnia BA, Thompson GH, et al: Complications of growing-rod treatment for early-onset scoliosis: analysis of one hundred and forty patients, *J Bone Joint Surg* 92A:2533, 2010.

Cahill PJ, Marvil S, Cuddihy L, et al: Autofusion in the immature spine treated with growing rods, *Spine* 35:E1199, 2010.

Charles YP, Daures JP, de Rosa V, Dimeglio A: Progression risk of idiopathic juvenile scoliosis during pubertal growth, *Spine* 31:1933, 2006.

Corona J, Sanders JO, Luhmann SJ, et al: Reliability of radiographic measures for infantile idiopathic scoliosis, *J Bone Joint Surg* 94A:e86, 2012.

Crawford CH 3rd, Lenke LG: Growth modulation by means of anterior tethering resulting in progressive correction of juvenile idiopathic scoliosis: a case report, *J Bone Joint Surg* 92A:202, 2010.

Dede O, Demirkiran G, Bekmez S, et al: Utilizing the "stable-to-be vertebra" saves motion segments in growing rods treatment for early-onset scoliosis, *J Pediatr Orthop* 36:336, 2016.

Dobbs MB, Lenke LG, Szymanski DA, et al: Prevalence of neural axis abnormalities in patients with infantile idiopathic scoliosis, *J Bone Joint Surg* 84A:2230, 2002.

Flynn JM, Tomlinson LA, Pawelek J, et al: Growing-rod graduates: lessons learned from ninety-nine patients who completed lengthening, *J Bone Joint Surg* 95A:1745, 2013.

Jain V, Lykissas M, Trobisch P, et al: Surgical aspects of spinal growth modulation in scoliosis correction, *Instr Course Lect* 63:335, 2014.

Jarvis J, Garbedian S, Swamy G: Juvenile idiopathic scoliosis: the effectiveness of part-time bracing, *Spine* 33:1074, 2008.

Kager AN, Marks M, Bastrom T, et al: Morbidity of iliac crest bone graft harvesting in adolescent deformity surgery, *J Pediatr Orthop* 26:132, 2006.

Karol LA, Johnston C, Mladenov K, et al: Pulmonary function following early thoracic fusion in non-neuromuscular scoliosis, *J Bone Joint Surg* 90A:1272, 2008.

Khoshbin A, Caspi L, Law PW, et al: Outcomes of bracing in juvenile idiopathic scoliosis until skeletal maturity or surgery, *Spine* 40:50, 2015.

Lavelle WF, Samdani AF, Cahill PJ, Betz RR: Clinical outcomes of nitinol staples for preventing curve progression in idiopathic scoliosis, *J Pediatr Orthop* 31:S107, 2011.

Lenke LG, Dobbs MB: Management of juvenile idiopathic scoliosis, *J Bone Joint Surg* 89A:55, 2007.

McCarthy RE, Luhmann S, Lenke L, McCullough FL: The Shilla growth guidance technique for early-onset spinal deformities at 2-year follow-up: a preliminary report, *J Pediatr Orthop* 34:1, 2014.

McCarthy RE, McCullough FL: Shilla growth guidance for early-onset scoliosis: results after a minimum of five years of follow-up, *J Bone Joint Surg* 97A:1578, 2015.

Pahys JM, Samdani AF, Betz RR: Intraspinal anomalies in infantile idiopathic scoliosis: prevalence and role of magnetic resonance imaging, *Spine* 34:E434, 2009.

Redding G, Song K, Inscore S, et al: Lung function asymmetry in children with congenital and infantile scoliosis, *Spine J* 8:639, 2008.

Samdani AF, Ames RJ, Kimball JS, et al: Anterior vertebral body tethering for idiopathic scoliosis: two-year results, *Spine* 39:1688, 2014.

Sanders JO, D'Astous J, Fitzgerald M, et al: Derotational casting for progressive infantile scoliosis, *J Pediatr Orthop* 29:581, 2009.

Sankar WN, Skaggs DL, Yazici M, et al: Lengthening of dual growing rods and the law of diminishing returns, *Spine* 36:806, 2011.

Sarlak AY, Atmaca H, Buluc L, et al: Juvenile idiopathic scoliosis treated with posterior arthrodesis and segmental pedicle screw instrumentation before the age of 9 years: a 5-year follow-up, *Scoliosis* 4:1, 2009.

Schulz JF, Smith J, Cahill PJ, et al: The role of the vertical expandable titanium rib in the treatment of infantile idiopathic scoliosis: early results from a single institution, *J Pediatr Orthop* 30:659, 2010.

Sucato DJ: Management of severe spinal deformity: scoliosis and kyphosis, *Spine* 35:2186, 2010.

Thompson GH, Akbarnia BA, Campbell RM Jr: Growing rod techniques in early-onset scoliosis, *J Pediatr Orthop* 27:354, 2007.

Thompson GH, Lenke LG, Akbarnia BA, et al: Early onset scoliosis: future directions, *J Bone Joint Surg* 89A:163, 2007.

Yang JS, McElroy MJ, Akbarnia BA, et al: Growing rods for spinal deformity: characterizing consensus and variation in current use, *J Pediatr Orthop* 30:264, 2010.

NATURAL HISTORY OF ADOLESCENT IDIOPATHIC SCOLIOSIS

Buchowsky JM, Skaggs DL, Sponseller PD: Temporary internal distraction as an aid to correction of severe scoliosis: surgical technique, *J Bone Joint Surg* 89A(Suppl 2):297, 2007.

Coillard C, Circo AB, Rivard CH: A prospective randomized controlled trial of the natural history of idiopathic scoliosis versus treatment with the SpineCor brace: Sosort Award 2011 winner, *Eur J Phys Rehabil Med* 50: 479, 2014.

Horacek O, Mazanec R, Morris CE, Kobesova A: Spinal deformities in hereditary motor and sensory neuropathy: a retrospective qualitative, quantitative, genotypical, and familial analysis of 175 patients, *Spine* 32:2502, 2007.

Kruse LM, Buchan JG, Gurnett CA, Dobbs MB: Polygenic threshold model with sex dimorphism in adolescent idiopathic scoliosis: the Carter effect, *J Bone Joint Surg* 94A:1485, 2012.

Ogilvie JW: Update on prognostic genetic testing in adolescent idiopathic scoliosis (AIS), *J Pediatr Orthop* 31(1 Suppl):S46, 2011.

Sanders JO, Khoury JG, Kishan S, et al: Predicting scoliosis progression from skeletal maturity: a simplified classification during adolescence, *J Bone Joint Surg* 90A:540, 2008.

Sitoula P, Verma K, Holmes L Jr, et al: Prediction of curve progression in idiopathic scoliosis: validation of the Sanders Skeletal Maturity Staging System, *Spine* 40:1006, 2015.

Verma K, Errico T, Diefenbach C, et al: The relative efficacy of antifibrinolytics in adolescent idiopathic scoliosis: a prospective randomized trial, *J Bone Joint Surg* 96A:e80, 2014.

Walick KS, Kragh JE Jr, Ward JA, Crawford JJ: Changes in intraocular pressure due to surgical positioning: studying potential risk for postoperative vision loss, *Spine* 32:2591, 2007.

Wang WJ, Yeung HY, Chu WC, et al: Top theories for the etiopathogenesis of adolescent idiopathic scoliosis, *J Pediatr Orthop* 31(1 Suppl):S14, 2011.

PATIENT EVALUATION IN ADOLESCENT IDIOPATHIC SCOLIOSIS

Charles YP, Diméglio A, Canavese F, Daures JP: Skeletal age assessment from the olecranon for idiopathic scoliosis at Risser grade 0, *J Bone Joint Surg* 89A:2737, 2007.

Chen ZQ, Wang CF, Bai YS, et al: Using precisely controlled bidirectional orthopedic forces to assess flexibility in adolescent idiopathic scoliosis: comparisons between push-traction film supine side bending suspension, and fulcrum bending films, *Spine* 36:1679, 2011.

Escalada F, Marco E, Duate E, et al: Assessment of angle velocity in girls with adolescent idiopathic scoliosis, *Scoliosis* 4:20, 2009.

Gille O, Champain N, Benchikh-El-Fegoun A, et al: Reliability of 3D reconstruction of the spine of mild scoliotic patients, *Spine* 32:568, 2007.

Hans SD, Sanders JO, Cooperman DR: Using the Sauvegrain method to predict peak height velocity in boys and girls, *J Pediatr Orthop* 28:836, 2008.

Herring JA, editor: *Tachdjian's pediatric orthopaedics*, ed 4, Philadelphia, 2008, Elsevier Saunders.

Ilharreborde B, Steffen JS, Nectoux E, et al: Angle measurement reproducibility using EOS three-dimensional reconstructions in adolescent idiopathic scoliosis treated by posterior instrumentation, *Spine* 36:E1306, 2011.

Johnston CE, Richards BS, Sucato DJ, et al: Correlation of preoperative deformity magnitude and pulmonary function test in adolescent idiopathic scoliosis, *Spine* 36:1096, 2011.

Luk KD, Cheung WY, Wong Y, et al: The predictive value of the fulcrum bending radiographs in spontaneous apical vertebral derotation in adolescent idiopathic scoliosis, *Spine* 37:E922, 2012.

Nault ML, Parent S, Phan P, et al: A modified Risser grading system predicts the curve acceleration phase of female adolescent idiopathic scoliosis, *J Bone Joint Surg* 92A:1073, 2010.

Sanders JO, Khoury JG, Kishan S, et al: Predicting scoliosis progression from skeletal maturity: a simplified classification during adolescence, *J Bone Joint Surg* 90A:540, 2008.

Takahashi S, Passuti N, Delecrin J: Interpretation and utility of traction radiography in scoliosis surgery: analysis of patients treated with Cotrel-Dubousset instrumentation, *Spine* 22:2542, 1997.

NONOPERATIVE MANAGEMENT OF IDIOPATHIC SCOLIOSIS

Gammon SR, Mehlman CT, Chan W, et al: A comparison of thoracolumbar orthoses and SpineCor treatment of adolescent idiopathic scoliosis patients using the Scoliosis Research Society standardized criteria, *J Pediatr Orthop* 30:531, 2010.

Guo J, Lam TP, Wong MS, et al: A prospective randomized controlled study on the treatment outcome of SpineCor brace versus rigid brace for adolescent idiopathic scoliosis with follow-up according to the SRS standardized criteria, *Eur Spine J* 23:2650, 2014.

Gutman G, Benoit M, Joncas J, et al: The effectiveness of the SpineCor brace for the conservative treatment of adolescent idiopathic scoliosis: comparison with the Boston brace, *Spine J* 16:626, 2016.

Harfouch BF, Weinstein SL: Intraoperative push-prone test: a useful technique to determine the lowest instrumented vertebra in adolescent idiopathic scoliosis, *J Spinal Disord Tech* 27:237, 2014.

Katz DE, Herring JA, Browne RH, et al: Brace wear control of curve progression in adolescent idiopathic scoliosis, *J Bone Joint Surg* 92A:1343, 2010.

Ohrt-Nissen S, Hallager DW, Gehrchen M, Dahl B: Flexibility predicts curve progression in Providence nighttime bracing of patients with adolescent idiopathic scoliosis, *Spine (Phil Pa 1976)* 2016. [Epub ahead of print].

Pellios S, Kenanidis E, Potoupnis M, et al: Curve progression 25 years after bracing for adolescent idiopathic scoliosis: long term comparative results between two matched groups of 18 versus 23 hours daily bracing, *Scoliosis Spinal Disord* 11:3, 2016.

Sanders JO, D'Astous J, Fitzgerald M, et al: Derotational casting for progressive infantile scoliosis, *J Pediatr Orthop* 29:581, 2009.

Sponseller PD: Bracing for adolescent idiopathic scoliosis in practice today, *J Pediatr Orthop* 31(1 Suppl):S53, 2011.

Sponseller PD, Takenaga R: The use of traction in treating large scoliotic curves in idiopathic scoliosis. In Newton PO, O'Brien MF, Shufflebarger HL, et al, editors: *Idiopathic scoliosis: the Harms Study Group treatment guide*, New York, 2010, Thieme.

Weinstein SL, Dolan LA, Wright JG, Dobbs MB: Effects of bracing in adolescents with idiopathic scoliosis, *N Engl J Med* 369:1512, 2013.

OPERATIVE TREATMENT OF IDIOPATHIC SCOLIOSIS

Bess RS, Lenke LG, Bridwell KH, et al: Wasting of preoperatively donated autologous blood in the surgical treatment of adolescent idiopathic scoliosis, *Spine* 31:2375, 2006.

Betz RR, D'Andrea L: Proteus™ shape memory alloy staple surgical technique. In *Medtronic technique manual*, Memphis, TN, 2006, Medtronic Sofamor Danek.

Betz RR, Ranade A, Samdani AF, et al: Vertebral body stapling: a fusionless treatment option for a growing child with moderate idiopathic scoliosis, *Spine* 35:169, 2010.

Bollini G, Docquier PL, Viehweger E, et al: Lumbar hemivertebra resection, *J Bone Joint Surg* 88A:1043, 2006.

Cahill PJ, Marvil SC, Cuddihy L, et al: Autofusion of the skeletally immature spine treated with growing rod instrumentation, *Spine* 35: E1199, 2010.

Caubet JF, Emans JB, Smith VT, et al: Increased hemoglobin levels in patients with early onset scoliosis: prevalence and effect of a treatment with vertical expandable prosthetic titanium rib (VEPTR), *Spine* 34:2534, 2009.

Coe JD, Warden KE, Herzig MA, McAfee PC: Influence of bone mineral density on the fixation of thoracolumbar implants: a comparative study of transpedicular screws, laminar hooks, and spinous process wires, *Spine* 21:1759, 2007.

de Mendonca RG, Sawyer JR, Kelly DM: Complications after surgical treatment of adolescent idiopathic scoliosis, *Orthop Clin North Am* 47:395, 2016.

Devlin VJ, Schwartz DM: Intraoperative neurophysiologic monitoring during spinal surgery, *J Am Acad Orthop Surg* 15:549, 2007.

Diab MG, Franzone JM, Vitale MG: The role of posterior spinal osteotomies in pediatric spinal deformity surgery: indications and operative treatment, *J Pediatr Orthop* 31:S88, 2011.

Diab M, Landman Z, Lubicky J, et al: Use and outcome of MRI in the surgical treatment of adolescent idiopathic scoliosis, *Spine* 36:667, 2011.

Diab M, Smith AR, Kuklo TR, Spinal Deformity Study Group: neural complications in the surgical treatment of adolescent idiopathic scoliosis, *Spine* 32:2759, 2007.

Ho C, Skaggs DL, Weiss JM, Tolo VT: Management of infection after instrumented posterior spine fusion in pediatric scoliosis, *Spine* 32:2739, 2007.

Jain V, Kykissas M, Trobisch P, et al: Surgical aspects of spinal growth modulation in scoliosis correction, *Instr Course Lect* 63:335, 2014.

Karol LA: Early definitive spinal fusion in young children: what we have learned, *Clin Orthop Relat Res* 469:1323, 2011.

Karol LA, Johnston C, Mladenov K, et al: Pulmonary function following early thoracic fusion in non-neuromuscular scoliosis, *J Bone Joint Surg* 90A:1272, 2008.

Kim YJ, Bridwell KH, Lenke LG, et al: Pseudarthrosis in adult spinal deformity following multisegmental instrumentation and arthrodesis, *J Bone Joint Surg* 88A:721, 2006.

Letko L, Jensen RG, Harms J: The treatment of rigid idiopathic scoliosis: releases, osteotomies, and apical vertebral column resection. In Newton PO, O'Brien MF, Shufflebarger HL, et al, editors: *Idiopathic scoliosis: the Harms Study Group treatment guide*, New York, 2010, Thieme.

McCarthy KP, Chafetz RS, Mulcahey MJ, et al: Clinical efficacy of the vertebral wedge osteotomy for the fusionless treatment of paralytic scoliosis, *Spine* 35:403, 2010.

McCarthy RE, Sucato D, Turner JL, et al: Shilla growing rods in a caprine animal model: a pilot study, *Clin Orthop Relat Res* 468:705, 2010.

Newton PO, Upasani VV: Surgical treatment of the right thoracic curve pattern. In Newton PO, O'Brien MF, Shufflebarger HL, et al, editors: *Idiopathic scoliosis: the Harms Study Group treatment guide*, New York, 2010, Thieme.

Powers AK, O'Shaughnessy BA, Lemke LG: Posterior thoracic vertebral column resection. In Wang JC, editor: *Advanced reconstruction: spine*, Rosemont, IL, 2011, American Academy of Orthopaedic Surgeons, p 265.

Sankar WN, Skaggs DL: Rib anchors in distraction-based growing spine implants. In Wang JC, editor: *Advanced reconstruction: spine*, Rosemont, IL, 2011, American Academy of Orthopaedic Surgeons.

Sariak AY, Atmaca H, Buluc L, et al: Juvenile idiopathic scoliosis treated with posterior arthrodesis and segmental pedicle screw instrumentation before the age of 9 years: a 5-year follow-up study, *Scoliosis* 4:1, 2009.

Schulz JF, Smith J, Cahill P, et al: The role of the vertical expandable titanium rib in the treatment of infantile idiopathic scoliosis: early results from a single institution, *J Pediatr Orthop* 30:659, 2010.

Skaggs DL, Choi PD, Rice C, et al: Efficacy of intraoperative neurologic monitoring in surgery involving a vertical expandable prosthetic titanium rib for early-onset spinal deformity, *J Bone Joint Surg* 91A:1657, 2009.

Skaggs DL, Sankar WN, Albrekston J, et al: Weight gain following vertical expandable prosthetic titanium ribs surgery in children with thoracic insufficiency syndrome, *Spine* 34:2530, 2009.

Smith JT: Bilateral rib-to-pelvis technique for managing early-onset scoliosis, *Clin Orthop Relat Res* 469:1349, 2011.

Sponseller PD, Jain A, Newton PO, et al: Posterior spinal fusion with pedicle screws in patients with idiopathic scoliosis and open triradiate cartilage: does deformity progression occur? *J Pediatr Orthop* 2015. [Epub ahead of print].

Sui WY, Ye F, Yang JL: Efficacy of tranexamic acid in reducing allogeneic blood products in adolescent idiopathic scoliosis surgery, *BMC Musculoskelet Disord* 17:187, 2016.

Tao F, Zhao Y, Wu Y, et al: The effect of differing spinal fusion instrumentation on the occurrence of postoperative crankshaft phenomenon in adolescent idiopathic scoliosis, *J Spinal Disord Tech* 23:e75, 2010.

Thompson GH, Akbarnia BA, Campbell RM Jr: Growing rod techniques in early-onset scoliosis, *J Pediatr Orthop* 27:354, 2007.

Trobisch PD, Ducoffe AR, Lonner BS, Errico TJ: Choosing fusion levels in adolescent idiopathic scoliosis, *J Am Acad Orthop Surg* 21:519, 2013.

White KK, Song KM, Frost N, Daines BK: VEPTR™ growing rods for early-onset neuromuscular scoliosis: feasible and effective, *Clin Orthop Relat Res* 469:1335, 2011.

NEUROMUSCULAR SCOLIOSIS (GENERAL)

Brooks JT, Sponseller PD: What's new in the management of neuromuscular scoliosis, *J Pediatr Orthop* 2015. [Epub ahead of print].

Funk S, Lovejoy S, Mencio G, Martus J: Rigid instrumentation for neuromuscular scoliosis improves deformity correction without increasing complications, *Spine* 41:46, 2016.

Myung KS, Lee C, Skaggs DL: Early pelvic fixation failure in neuromuscular scoliosis, *J Pediatr Orthop* 35:258, 2015.

Schwartz DM, Sestokas AK, Dormans JP, et al: Transcranial electric motor evoked potential monitoring during spine surgery: is it safe? *Spine* 36:1046, 2011.

Sponseller PD, Zimmerman RM, Ko PS, et al: Low-profile pelvic fixation with the sacral alar iliac technique in the pediatric population improves results at two-year minimum follow-up, *Spine* 35:1887, 2010.

White KK, Song KM, Frost N, Daines BK: VEPTR growing rods for early-onset neuromuscular scoliosis: feasible and effective, *Clin Orthop Relat Res* 469:1335, 2011.

CEREBRAL PALSY

Auerbach JD, Spiegel DA, Zgonis MH, et al: The correction of pelvic obliquity in patients with cerebral palsy and neuromuscular scoliosis: is there a benefit of anterior release prior to posterior spinal arthrodesis? *Spine* 34:E766, 2009.

Beckmann K, Lange T, Gosheger G, et al: Surgical correction of scoliosis in patients with severe cerebral palsy, *Eur Spine J* 25:506, 2016.

Dhawale AA, Shah SA, Sponseller PD, et al: Are antifibrinolytics helpful in decreasing blood loss and transfusions during spinal fusion surgey in children with cerebral palsy scoliosis? *Spine* 37:E549, 2012.

Ko PS, Jameson PG 2nd, Chang TL, Sponseller PD: Transverse-plane pelvic asymmetry in patients with cerebral palsy and scoliosis, *J Pediatr Orthop* 31:277, 2011.

McElroy MJ, Sponseller PD, Dattilo JR, et al: Growing rods for the treatment of scoliosis in children with cerebral palsy: a critical assessment, *Spine* 37:E1504, 2012.

Modi HN, Hong JY, Mehta SS, et al: Surgical correction and fusion using posterior-only pedicle screw construct for neuropathic scoliosis in patients with cerebral palsy: a three-year follow-up study, *Spine* 34:1167, 2009.

INHERITABLE NEUROLOGIC DISORDERS

Abdulian MH, Liu RW, Son-Hing JP, et al: Double rib penetration of the spinal canal in a patients with neurofibromatosis, *J Pediatr Orthop* 31:6, 2011.

Feldman DS, Jordan C, Fonesca L: Orthopaedic manifestation of neurofibromatosis type I, *J Am Acad Orthop Surg* 18:346, 2010.

Karol LA, Elerson E: Scoliosis in patients with Charcot-Marie-Tooth disease, *J Bone Joint Surg* 89A:1504, 2007.

Lykissas MG, Schorry EK, Crawford AH, et al: Does the presence of dystrophic features in patients with type 1 neurofibromatosis and spine deformities increase the risk of surgery? *Spine* 38:1595, 2013.

McElroy MJ, Shaner AC, Crawford TO, et al: Growing rods for scoliosis in spinal muscular atrophy: structural effects, complications, and hospital stays, *Spine* 36:1305, 2011.

Milbrandt TA, Kunes JR, Karol LA: Friedreich's ataxia and scoliosis: the experience at two institutions, *J Pediatr Orthop* 28:234, 2008.

Miller F: Spinal deformity secondary to impaired neurologic control, *J Bone Joint Surg* 89A:143, 2007.

Tsirikos AL, Smith G: Scoliosis in patients with Friedreich's ataxia, *J Bone Joint Surg* 94B:684, 2012.

SYRINGOMYELIA

Akhtar OH, Rowe DE: Syringomyelia-associated scoliosis with and without the Chiari I malformation, *J Am Acad Orthop Surg* 16:407, 2008.

Godzik J, Holekamp TF, Limbrick DD, et al: Risks and outcomes of spinal deformity surgery in Chiari malformation, type 1, with syringomyelia versus adolescent idiopathic scoliosis, *Spine J* 15:2002, 2015.

Sha S, Qiu Y, Sun W, et al: Does surgical correction of right thoracic scoliosis in syringomyelia produce outcomes similar to those in adolescent idiopathic scoliosis? *J Bone Joint Surg* 98A:295, 2016.

Strahle J, Smith BW, Martinez M, et al: The association between Chiari malformation type I, spinal syrinx, and scoliosis, *J Neurosurg Pediatr* 15:607, 2015.

Zebala LP, Bridwell KH, Baldus C, et al: Minimum 5-year radiographic results of long scoliosis fusion in juvenile spinal muscular atrophy patients: major curve progression after instrumented fusion, *J Pediatr Orthop* 31:480, 2011.

Zhang ZX, Feng DX, Li P, et al: Surgical treatment of scoliosis associated with syringomyelia with no or minor neurologic symptoms, *Eur Spine J* 24:1555, 2015.

ARTHROGRYPOSIS MULTIPLEX CONGENITA

Astur N, Flynn JM, Flynn JM, et al: The efficacy of rib-based distraction with VEPTR in the treatment of early-onset scoliosis in patients with arthrogryposis, *J Pediatr Orthop* 34:8, 2014.

Campbell RM Jr: Spine deformities in rare congenital syndromes: clinical issues, *Spine* 34:1815, 2009.

Greggo T, Martikos K, Pipitone E, et al: Surgical treatment of scoliosis in a rare disease: arthrogryposis, *Scoliosis* 5:24, 2010.

DUCHENNE MUSCULAR DYSTROPHY

Cheuk DK, Wong V, Wraige E, et al: Surgery for scoliosis in Duchenne muscular dystrophy, *Cochrane Database Syst Rev* (10):CD005375, 2015.

Chua K, Tan CY, Chen Z, et al: Long-term follow-up of pulmonary function and scoliosis in patients with Duchenne's muscular dystrophy and spinal muscular atrophy, *J Pediatr Orthop* 36:63, 2016.

Karol LA: Scoliosis in patients with Duchenne muscular atrophy, *J Bone Joint Surg* 89A:155, 2007.

Lebel DE, Corston JA, McAdam LC, et al: Glucocorticoid treatment for the prevention of scoliosis in children with Duchenne muscular dystrophy: long-term follow-up, *J Bone Joint Surg* 95A:1057, 2013.

Raudenbush BL, Thirukumaran CP, Li Y, et al: Impact of a comparative study on the management of scoliosis in Duchenne muscular dystrophy: are corticosteroids decreasing the rate of scoliosis surgery in the United States? *Spine* 2016. [Epub ahead of print].

Scannell BP, Yaszay B, Bartley CE, et al: Surgical correction of scoliosis in patients with Duchenne muscular dystrophy: 30-year experience, *J Pediatr Orthop* 2016. [Epub ahead of print].

Sucato DJ: Spine deformity in spinal muscular atrophy, *J Bone Joint Surg* 89A:148, 2007.

Suk KS, Lee BH, Lee HM, et al: Functional outcomes in Duchenne muscular dystrophy scoliosis: comparison of the differences between surgical and nonsurgical treatment, *J Bone Joint Surg* 96A:409, 2014.

CONGENITAL SCOLIOSIS

Bowen RE, Scaduto AA, Banuelos S: Does early thoracic fusion exacerbate preexisting restrictive lung disease in congenital scoliosis patients? *J Pediatr Orthop* 28:506, 2008.

Chang DG, Kim JH, Ha KY, et al: Posterior hemivertebra resection and short segment fusion with pedicle screw fixation for congenital scoliosis in children younger than 10 years: greater than 7-year follow-up, *Spine* 40:484, 2015.

Chang DG, Suk SI, Kim JH, et al: Surgical outcomes by the age at the time of surgery in the treatment of congenital scoliosis in children under age 10 years, *Spine J* 15:1783, 2015.

Flynn JM, Emans JB, Smith JT, et al: VEPTR to treat nonsyndromic congenital scoliosis: a multicenter, mid-term follow-up study, *J Pediatr Orthop* 33:679, 2013.

Hedden D: Management themes in congenital scoliosis, *J Bone Joint Surg* 89A:72, 2007.

Hedequist D, Emans J: Congenital scoliosis: a review and update, *J Pediatr Orthop* 27:107, 2007.

Hensinger RN: Congenital scoliosis: etiology and associations, *Spine* 34:1745, 2009.

Imrie MN: A "simple" option in the surgical treatment of congenital scoliosis, *Spine J* 11:119, 2011.

Jalanko T, Rintala R, Puisto V, Helenius I: Hemivertebra resection for congenital scoliosis in young children, *Spine* 36:41, 2011.

Kawakami N, Tsuji T, Imagama S, et al: Classification of congenital scoliosis and kyphosis: a new approach to the three-dimensional classification for progressive vertebral anomalies requiring operative treatment, *Spine* 34: 1756, 2009.

Li X, Luo Z, Li X, et al: Hemivertebra resection for the treatment of congenital lumbarspinal scoliosis with lateral-posterior approach, *Spine* 33:2001, 2008.

Li XF, Liu ZD, Hu GY, et al: Posterior unilateral pedicle subtraction osteotomy of hemivertebra for correction of the adolescent congenital spinal deformity, *Spine J* 11:111, 2011.

Louis ML, Gennari JM, Loundou AD, et al: Congenital scoliosis: a frontal plane evaluation of 251 operated patients 14 years old or older at follow-up, *Orthop Traumatol Surg Res* 96:741, 2010.

Marks DS, Qaimkhani SA: The natural history of congenital scoliosis and kyphosis, *Spine* 34:1751, 2009.

McMaster MJ, McMaster ME: Prognosis for congenital scoliosis due to a unilateral failure of vertebral segmentation, *J Bone Joint Surg* 95A:972, 2013.

Mik G, Drummond DS, Hosalkar HS, et al: Diminished spinal cord size associated with congenital scoliosis of the thoracic spine, *J Bone Joint Surg* 91A:1698, 2009.

Murphy RF, Moisan A, Kelly DM, et al: Use of vertical expandable prosthetic titanium rib (VEPTR) in the treatment of congenital scoliosis without fused ribs, *J Pediatr Orthop* 36:329, 2016.

Shen J, Wang Z, Liu J, et al: Abnormalities associated with congenital scoliosis: a retrospective study of 226 Chinese surgical cases, *Spine* 38:814, 2013.

Vitale MG, Matsumoto H, Bye MR, et al: A retrospective cohort study of pulmonary function, radiographic measures, and quality of life in children with congenital scoliosis: an evaluation of patient outcomes after early spinal fusion, *Spine* 33:1242, 2008.

Wang S, Zhang J, Qiu G, et al: Dual growing rods technique for congential scoliosis: more than 2 years outcomes: preliminary results of a single center, *Spine* 37:E1639, 2012.

Yaszay B, O'Brien M, Shufflebarger HL, et al: Efficacy of hemivertebra resection for congenital scoliosis: a multicenter retrospective comparison of three surgical techniques, *Spine* 36:2052, 2011.

Yazici M, Emans J: Fusionless instrumentation systems for congenital scoliosis: expandable spinal rods and vertical expandable prosthetic titanium rib in the management of congenital spine deformities in the growing child, *Spine* 34:1800, 2009.

SCHEUERMANN DISEASE

Abul-Kasim K, Schlenzka D, Selariu E, Ohlin A: Spinal epidural lipomatosis: a common imaging feature in Scheuermann disease, *J Spinal Disord Tech* 25:356, 2012.

Arun R, Mehdian SMH, Freeman BJC, et al: Do anterior interbody cages have a potential value in comparison to autogenous rib graft in the surgical management of Scheuermann's kyphosis? *Spine J* 6:413, 2006.

Cho W, Lenke LG, Bridwell KH, et al: The prevalence of abnormal preoperative neurological examination in Scheuermann kyphosis: correlation with X-ray, magnetic resonance imaging, and surgical outcome, *Spine* 39:1771, 2014.

Coe JD, Smith JS, Berven S, et al: Complications of spinal fusion for Scheuermann kyphosis: a report of the Scoliosis Research Society Morbidity and Mortality Committee, *Spine* 35:99, 2009.

Damborg F, Engell V, Andersen M, et al: Prevalence, concordance, and heritability of Scheuermann kyphosis based on a study of twins, *J Bone Joint Surg* 88A:2133, 2006.

Denis F, Sun EC, Winter RB: Incidence and risk factors for proximal and distal junctional kyphosis following surgical treatment for Scheuermann kyphosis, *Spine* 34:E729, 2009.

Fotiadis E, Kenanidis E, Samoladas E, et al: Scheuermann's disease: focus on weight and height role, *Eur Spine J* 17:673, 2008.

Geck MJ, Macagno A, Ponte A, Shufflebarger HL: The Ponte procedure: posterior only treatment of Scheuermann's kyphosis using segmental posterior shortening and pedicle screw instrumentation, *J Spinal Disord Tech* 20:586, 2007.

Jansen RC, van Rhijn LW, van Ooij A: Predictable correction of the unfused lumbar lordosis after thoracic correction and fusion in Scheuermann kyphosis, *Spine* 31:1227, 2006.

Koptan WMT, El Miligui YH, El Sebaie HB: All pedicle screw instrumentation for Scheuermann's kyphosis correction: is it worth it? *Spine J* 9:296, 2009.

Lee SS, Lenke LG, Kuklo TR, et al: Comparison of Scheuermann kyphosis correction by posterior-only thoracic pedicle screw fixation versus combined anterior/posterior fusion, *Spine* 31:2316, 2006.

Lonner BS, Newton P, Betz R, et al: Operative management of Scheuermann's kyphosis in 78 patients: radiographic outcomes, complications, and technique, *Spine* 32:2644, 2007.

Lonner BS, Toombs CS, Guss M, et al: Complications in operative Scheuermann kyphosis: do the pitfalls differ from operative adolescent idiopathic scoliosis? *Spine* 40:305, 2015.

Lowe TG, Line BG: Evidence based medicine: analysis of Scheuermann kyphosis, *Spine* 32:S115, 2007.

Makurthou AA, Oei L, El Saddy S, et al: Scheuermann disease: evaluation of radiological criteria and population prevalence, *Spine* 38:1690, 2013.

Tsirikos AI, Jain AK: Scheuermann's kyphosis: current controversies, *J Bone Joint Surg* 93B:857, 2011.

Wood KB, Melikian R, Villamil F: Adult Scheuermann kyphosis: evaluation, management, and new developments, *J Am Acad Orthop Surg* 20:113, 2012.

Zeng Y, Chen Z, Qi Q, et al: The posterior surgical correction of congenital kyphosis and kyphoscoliosis: 23 cases with minimum 2 years follow-up, *Eur Spine J* 22:372, 2013.

CONGENITAL KYPHOSIS

Alyvaz M, Olgun ZD, Demirkiran HG, et al: Posterior all-pedicle screw instrumentation combined with multiple chevron and concave rib osteotomies in the treatment of adolescent congenital kyphoscoliosis, *Spine J* 14:11, 2014.

Atici Y, Sököcü S, Uzümcügil O, et al: The results of closing wedge osteotomy with posterior instrumented fusion for the surgical treatment of congenital kyphosis, *Eur Spine J* 22:1368, 2013.

Campos MA, Fernandes P, Dolan L, Weinstein SL: Infantile thoracolumbar kyphosis secondary to lumbar hypoplasia, *J Bone Joint Surg* 90A:1726, 2008.

Cheh G, Lenke LG, Padberg AM, et al: Loss of spinal cord monitoring signals in children during thoracic kyphosis correction with spinal osteotomy, *Spine* 33:1093, 2008.

Demirkiran G, Dede O, Karadeniz E, et al: Anterior and posterior vertebral column resection versus posterior-only technique: a comparison of clinical outcomes and complications in congenital kyphoscoliosis, *Clin Spine Surg* 2016. [Epub ahead of print].

Giglio CA, Volpon JB: Development and evaluation of thoracic kyphosis and lumbar lordosis during growth, *J Child Orthop* 1:187, 2007.

Hamzaoglu A, Ozturk C, Tezer M, et al: Simultaneous surgical treatment in congenital scoliosis and/or kyphosis associated with intraspinal abnormalities, *Spine* 32:2880, 2007.

Hansen-Algenstaedt N, Gessler R, Goepfert M, Knight R: Percutaneous three column osteotomy for kyphotic deformity correction in congenital kyphosis, *Eur Spine J* 22:2139, 2013.

Helgeson MD, Shah SA, Newton PO, et al: Evaluation of proximal junctional kyphosis in adolescent idiopathic scoliosis following pedicle screw, hook, or hybrid instrumentation, *Spine* 35:177, 2010.

McMaster MJ: Congenital kyphosis. In Bridwell KH, DeWald RL, editors: *The textbook of spinal surgery*, ed 3, Philadelphia, 2011, Wolters Kluwer/Lippincott-Raven.

McMaster MJ, Glasby MA, Singh H, Cunningham S: Lung function in congenital kyphosis and kyphoscoliosis, *J Spinal Disord Tech* 20:203, 2007.

Noordeen MHH, Garrido E, Tucker SK, Elsebaie HB: The surgical treatment of congenital kyphosis, *Spine* 34:1808, 2009.

Reinker K, Simmons JW, Patil V, Stinson Z: Can VEPTR® control progression of early-onset kyphoscoliosis? A cohort study of VEPTR® patients with severe kyphoscoliosis, *Clin Orthop Relat Res* 469:1342, 2011.

Spiro AS, Rupprecht M, Stenger P, et al: Surgical treatment of severe congenital thoracolumbar kyphosis through a single posterior approach, *Bone Joint J* 95:1527, 2013.

Tsirikos AI, McMaster MJ: Infantile developmental thoracolumbar kyphosis with segmental subluxation of the spine, *J Bone Joint Surg* 92B:40, 2010.

Winter RB, Lonstein JE, Denis F: Sagittal spinal alignment: the true measurement, norms, and description of correction for thoracic kyphosis, *J Spinal Disord Tech* 22:311, 2009.

Zeller RD, Dubousset J: Progressive rotational dislocation in kyphoscoliotic deformities: presentation and treatment, *Spine* 25:1092, 2000.

Zeng Y, Chen Z, Qi Q, et al: The posterior surgical correction of congenital kyphosis and kyphoscoliosis: 23 cases with minimum 2 years follow-up, *Eur Spine J* 22:372, 2013.

PROGRESSIVE ANTERIOR VERTEBRAL FUSION

Bollini G, Guillaume JM, Launay F, et al: Progressive anterior vertebral bars: a study of 16 cases, *Spine* 36:E423, 2011.

SPONDYLOLYSIS AND SPONDYLOLISTHESIS

Altaf F, Osei NA, Garrido E, et al: Repair of spondylolysis using compression with a modular link and screws, *J Bone Joint Surg* 93B:73, 2011.

Beck NA, Miller R, Baldwin K, et al: Do oblique views add value in the diagnosis of spondylolysis in adolescents? *J Bone Joint Surg* 95A:e65, 2013.

Bhatia NN, Chow G, Timon SJ, Watts HG: Diagnostic modalities for the evaluation of pediatric back pain: a prospective study, *J Pediatr Orthop* 28:230, 2008.

Bourassa-Moreau E, Mac-Thiong JM, Joncas J, et al: Quality of life of patients with high-grade spondylolisthesis: minimum 2-year follow-up after surgical and nonsurgical treatments, *Spine J* 13:770, 2013.

Cavalier R, Herman MJ, Cheung EV, Pizzutillo PD: Spondylolysis and spondylolisthesis in children and adolescents, part I. Diagnosis, natural history, and nonsurgical management, *J Am Acad Orthop Surg* 14:417, 2006.

Cheung EV, Herman MJ, Cavalier R, Pizzutillo PD: Spondylolysis and spondylolisthesis in children and adolescents, part II. Surgical management, *J Am Acad Orthop Surg* 14:488, 2006.

Cohen E, Stuecker RD: Magnetic resonance imaging in diagnosis and follow-up of impending spondylolysis in children and adolescents: early treatment may prevent pars defects, *J Pediatr Orthop B* 14:63, 2005.

El Rassi G, Takemitsu M, Glutting J, Shah SA: Effect of sports modification on clinical outcome in children and adolescent athletes with symptomatic lumbar spondylolysis, *Am J Phys Med Rehabil* 92:1070, 2013.

Fadell MF, Gralla J, Bercha I, et al: CT outperforms radiographs at a comparable radiation dose in the assessment for spondylolysis, *Pediatr Radiol* 45:1026, 2015.

Fan J, Yu GR, Liu F, et al: A biomechanical study on the direct repair of spondylolysis by different techniques of fixation, *Orthop Surg* 2:46, 2010.

Helenius I, Remes V, Lamberg T, et al: Long-term health-related quality of life after surgery for adolescent idiopathic scoliosis and spondylolisthesis, *J Bone Joint Surg* 90A:1231, 2008.

Helenius I, Remes V, Poussa M: Uninstrumented in situ fusion for high-grade childhood and adolescent isthmic spondylolisthesis: long-term outcome: surgical technique, *J Bone Joint Surg* 90A:145, 2008.

Hresko MT, Hirschfeld R, Buerk AA, Zurakowski D: The effect of reduction and instrumentation of the spondylolisthesis on spinopelvic sagittal alignment, *J Pediatr Orthop* 29:157, 2009.

Hresko MT, Labelle H, Roussouly P, Berthonnaud E: Classification of high-grade spondylolistheses based on pelvic version and spine balance: possible rationale for reduction, *Spine* 32:2208, 2007.

Klein G, Mehlman CT, McCarty M: Nonoperative treatment of spondylolysis and grade I spondylolisthesis in children and young adults: a meta-analysis of observational studies, *J Pediatr Orthop* 29:146, 2009.

Lamberg T, Remes V, Helenius I, et al: Uninstrumented in situ fusion for high-grade childhood and adolescent isthmic spondylolisthesis: long-term outcome, *J Bone Joint Surg* 89A:512, 2007.

Leone A, Cianfoni A, Cerase A, et al: Lumbar spondylolysis: a review, *Skeletal Radiol* 40:683, 2011.

Mac-Thiong JM, Duong L, Parent S, et al: Reliability of the SDSG classification of lumbosacral spondylolisthesis, *Spine* 37:E95, 2012.

Mac-Thiong JM, Labelle H: A proposal for a surgical classification of pediatric lumbosacral spondylolisthesis based on current literature, *Eur Spine J* 15:1425, 2006.

Mac-Thiong JM, Wang Z, de Guide JA, Labelle H: Postural model of sagittal spino-pelvic alignment and its relevance for lumbosacral developmental spondylolisthesis, *Spine* 33:2316, 2008.

McCarty ME, Mehlman CT, Tamai J, et al: Spondylolisthesis: intraobserver and interobserver reliability with regard to the measurement of slip percentage, *J Pediatr Orthop* 29:755, 2009.

Menga EN, Jain A, Kebaish KM, et al: Anatomic parameters: direct intralaminar screw repair of spondylolysis, *Spine* 39:E153, 2014.

Menga EN, Kebaish KM, Jain A, et al: Clinical results and functional outcomes after direct intralaminar screw repair of spondylolysis, *Spine* 39:104, 2014.

Nitta A, Sakai T, Goda Y, et al: Prevalence of symptomatic lumbar spondylolysis in pediatric patients, *Orthopedics* 39:e434, 2016.

Poussa M, Remes V, Lambert T, et al: Treatment of severe spondylolisthesis in adolescence with reduction or fusion in situ: long-term clinical, radiologic, and functional outcome, *Spine* 31:583, 2006.

Rush JK, Astur N, Scott S, et al: Use of magnetic resonance imaging in the evaluation of spondylolysis, *J Pediatr Orthop* 35:271, 2015.

Sairyo K, Goel VK, Faizan A, et al: Buck's direct repair of lumbar spondylolysis restores disc stresses at the involved and adjacent levels, *Clin Biomech (Bristol, Avon)* 21:1020, 2006.

Sairyo K, Katoh S, Takata Y, et al: MRI signal changes of the pedicle as an indicator for early diagnosis of spondylolysis in children and adolescents: a clinical and biomechanical study, *Spine* 31:206, 2006.

Sakai T, Goda Y, Tezuka F, et al: Characteristics of lumbar spondylolysis in elementary school age children, *Eur Spine J* 25:602, 2016.

Sakai T, Sairyo K, Mima S, Yasui N: Significance of magnetic resonance imaging signal change in the pedicle in the management of pediatric lumbar spondylolysis, *Spine* 35:E641, 2010.

Snyder LA, Shufflebarger H, O'Brien MF, et al: Spondylolysis outcomes in adolescents after direct screw repair of the pars interarticularis, *J Neurosurg Spine* 21:329, 2014.

Sumita T, Sairyo K, Shibuya I, et al: V-rod technique for direct repair surgery of pediatric lumbar spondylolysis combined with posterior apophyseal ring fracture, *Asian Spine J* 7:115, 2013.

Tanguay F, Labelle H, Wang Z, et al: Clinical significance of lumbosacral kyphosis in adolescent spondylolisthesis, *Spine* 37:304, 2012.

Tsirikos AI, Garrido EG: Spondylolysis and spondylolisthesis in children and adolescents, *J Bone Joint Surg* 92B:751, 2010.

Tsirikos AI, Sud A, McGurk SM: Radiographic and functional outcome of posterolateral lumbosacral fusion for low grade isthmic spondylolisthesis in children and adolescents, *Bone Joint J* 98:88, 2016.

Wang Z, Parent S, Mac-Thiong JM, et al: Influence of sacral morphology in developmental spondylolisthesis, *Spine* 33:2185, 2008.

Warner WC: Kyphosis. In Morrissy RT, Weinstein SL, editors: *Lovell and Winter's pediatric orthopaedics*, ed 6, Philadelphia, 2006, Lippincott Williams & Wilkins.

KYPHOSCOLIOSIS IN MYELOMENINGOCELE

Akbar M, Bremer R, Thomsen M, et al: Kyphectomy in children with myelodysplasia: results 1994-2004, *Spine* 31:1007, 2006.

Altiok H, Finlayson C, Hassani S, Sturm P: Kyphectomy in children with myelomeningocele, *Clin Orthop Relat Res* 469:1272, 2011.

Ferland CE, Sardar ZM, Abuljabbar F, et al: Bilateral vascularized rib grafts to promote spino-pelvic fixation in patients with sacral agenesis and spino-pelvic dissociation: a new surgical technique, *Spine J* 15:2583, 2015.

Flynn JM, Ramirez N, Emans JB, et al: Is the vertebral expandable prosthetic titanium rib a surgical alternative in patients with spina bifida? *Clin Orthop Relat Res* 469:1291, 2011.

Guille JT, Sarwark JF, Sherk HH, Kumar SJ: Congenital and developmental deformities of the spine in children with myelomeningocele, *J Am Acad Orthop Surg* 14:294, 2006.

Ko AL, Song K, Ellenbogen RG, Avellino AM: Retrospective review of multilevel spinal fusion combined with spinal cord transection for treatment of kyphoscoliosis in pediatric myelomeningocele patients, *Spine* 32:2493, 2007.

Kocaoglu B, Erol B, Akgülle H, et al: Combination of Luque instrumentation with polyaxial screws in the treatment of myelomeningocele kyphosis, *J Spinal Disord Tech* 21:199, 2008.

Samagh SP, Cheng I, Elzik M, et al: Kyphectomy in the treatment of patients with myelomeningocele, *Spine J* 11:e5, 2011.

Smith JT, Novais E: Treatment of the gibbus deformity associated with myelomeningocele in the young child with the use of the vertical expandable prosthetic titanium rib (VEPTR): a case report, *J Bone Joint Surg* 92A:2211, 2010.

MARFAN SYNDROME

Gjolaj JP, Sponseller PD, Shah SA, et al: Spinal deformity correction in Marfan syndrome versus adolescent idiopathic scoliosis: learning from the differences, *Spine* 37:1558, 2012.

Qiao J, Xu L, Liu Z, et al: Surgical treatment of scoliosis in Marfan syndrome: outcomes and complications, *Eur Spine J* 2016. [Epub ahead of print].

Shirley ED, Sponseller PD: Marfan syndrome, *J Am Acad Orthop Surg* 17:572, 2009.

Sponseller PD, Bhimani M, Solacoff D, Dormans JP: Results of brace treatment of scoliosis in Marfan syndrome, *Spine* 25:2350, 2000.

Sponseller PD, Erkula G, Skolasky RL, et al: Improving clinical recognition of Marfan syndrome, *J Bone Joint Surg* 92A:1868, 2010.

Sponseller PD, Thompson GH, Akbarnia BA, et al: Growing rods for infantile scoliosis in Marfan syndrome, *Spine* 34:1711, 2009.

Zenner J, Hitzl W, Meier O, et al: Surgical outcomes of scoliosis surgery in Marfan syndrome, *J Spinal Disord Tech* 27:48, 2014.

VERTEBRAL COLUMN TUMORS

Boriani S, Weinstein JN, Biagini R: Primary bone tumors of the spine: terminology and surgical staging, *Spine* 22:1036, 1997.

Chan P, Boriani S, Fourney DR, et al: An assessment of the reliability of the Enneking and Weinstein-Boriani-Biagini classifications for staging of primary spinal tumors by the Spine Oncology Study Group, *Spine* 34:384, 2009.

Chunguang Z, Limin L, Rigao C, et al: Surgical treatment of kyphosis in children in healed stages of spinal tuberculosis, *J Pediatr Orthop* 30:271, 2010.

Kalra KP, Dhar SB, Shetty G, Dhariwal Q: Pedicle subtraction osteotomy for rigid posttuberculous kyphosis, *J Bone Joint Surg* 88B:925, 2006.

Kelly SP, Ashford RJ, Rao AS, Dickson RA: Primary bone tumours of the spine: a 42-year survey from the Leeds Regional Bone Tumour Registry, *Eur Spine J* 16:405, 2007.

Kim HJ, McLawhorn AS, Goldstein MJ, Boland PJ: Malignant osseous tumors of the pediatric spine, *J Am Acad Orthop Surg* 20:646, 2012.

Maheshwari AV, Cheng EY: Ewing sarcoma family of tumors, *J Am Acad Orthop Surg* 18:94, 2010.

Moon MS, Kim SS, Lee BJ, et al: Surgical management of severe rigid tuberculous kyphosis of the lumbar spine, *Int Orthop* 35:75, 2011.

Rajasekaran S, Vijay K, Shetty AP: Single-stage closing-opening wedge osteotomy of spine to correct severe post-tubercular kyphotic deformities of the spine: a 3-year follow-up of 17 patients, *Eur Spine J* 19:583, 2010.

Sinigaglia R, Gigante C, Bisinella G, et al: Musculoskeletal manifestations in pediatric acute leukemia, *J Pediatr Orthop* 28:20, 2008.

Zhang HQ, Wang YX, Guo CF, et al: *One-stage posterior approach and combined interbody and posterior fusion for thoracolumbar spinal tuberculosis with kyphosis in children*. Available at orthosupersite.com.

OSTEOCHONDRODYSTROPHY

Anissipour AK, Hammerberg KW, Caudill A, et al: Behavior of scoliosis during growth in children with osteogenesis imperfecta, *J Bone Joint Surg* 96A:237, 2014.

Borkhuu B, Nagaraju DK, Holems L, Mackenzie WG: Factors related to progression of thoracolumbar kyphosis in children with achondroplasia: a retrospective cohort study of forty-eight children treated in a comprehensive orthopaedic center, *Spine* 34:1699, 2009.

Kopits SE: Thoracolumbar kyphosis and lumbosacral hyperlordosis in achondroplastic children, *Basic Life Sci* 48:241, 1988.

Qi X, Matsumoto M, Ishii K, et al: Posterior osteotomy and instrumentation for thoracolumbar kyphosis in patients with achondroplasia, *Spine* 17:E606, 2006.

Shirley ED, Ain MC: Achondroplasia: manifestations and treatment, *J Am Acad Orthop Surg* 17:231, 2009.

Yilmaz G, Hwang S, Oto M, et al: Surgical treatment of scoliosis in osteogenesis imperfecta with cement-augmented pedicle screw instrumentation, *J Spinal Disord Tech* 27:174, 2014.

POSTLAMINECTOMY SPINAL DEFORMITY

Ain MC, Shirley ED, Pirouzmanesh A, et al: Postlaminectomy kyphosis in the skeletally immature achondroplast, *Spine* 31:197, 2006.

Simon SL, Auerbach JD, Garg S, et al: Efficacy of spinal instrumentation and fusion in the prevention of postlaminectomy spinal deformity in children with intramedullary spinal cord tumors, *J Pediatr Orthop* 28:244, 2008.

The complete list of references is available online at ***expertconsult.inkling.com****.*

INDEX

Page numbers followed by "*f*" indicate figures, "*t*" indicate tables, and "*b*" indicate boxes.

A

D

E

F

G

H

I

J

K

L

M

N

O

Q

R

S

T

U

V

W

X

Y

Z